CARDIOLOGY
AN ILLUSTRATED TEXT/REFERENCE

CARDIOLOGY
AN ILLUSTRATED TEXT/REFERENCE
VOLUME 2

CARDIOVASCULAR DISEASE

EDITORS

KANU CHATTERJEE, MB, FRCP
*Professor of Medicine
University of California,
San Francisco
Associate Chief of Cardiology
Moffitt/Long Hospital
San Francisco, California*

JOEL KARLINER, MD
*Professor of Medicine
University of California,
San Francisco
Chief of Cardiology
Ft. Miley Veterans
Administration Hospital
San Francisco, California*

ELLIOT RAPAPORT, MD
*Professor of Medicine
University of California,
San Francisco
Chief of Cardiology
San Francisco General Hospital
San Francisco, California*

MELVIN D. CHEITLIN, MD
*Professor of Medicine
University of California,
San Francisco
Associate Chief of Cardiology
San Francisco General Hospital
San Francisco, California*

WILLIAM W. PARMLEY, MD
*Professor of Medicine
University of California,
San Francisco
Chief of Cardiology
Moffitt/Long Hospital
San Francisco, California*

MELVIN SCHEINMAN, MD
*Professor of Medicine
University of California,
San Francisco
Chief of Electrophysiology
Moffitt/Long Hospital
San Francisco, California*

FOREWORD BY
RICHARD GORLIN, MD
*Mt. Sinai Medical Center
New York, New York*

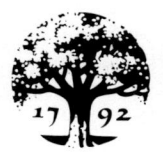

J.B. LIPPINCOTT COMPANY
Philadelphia

GOWER MEDICAL PUBLISHING
New York ▪ London

LIBRARY OF CONGRESS CATALOGING-IN-PUBLICATION DATA
Cardiology: an illustrated text/reference / editors, Kanu Chatterjee,
  William W. Parmley; foreword by Richard Gorlin.
    p.   cm.
    Includes bibliographical references.
    Includes index.
    Contents: v. 1. Physiology, pharmacology & diagnosis—v.
  2. Cardiovascular disease.
    ISBN 0-397-44611-X
    1. Cardiology.   2. Cardiovascular system—Diseases.
  I. Chatterjee, Kanu.   II. Parmley, William W. (William Watts), 1936-

  [DNLM: 1. Heart Diseases.   WG 200 C26553]
RC667.C383   1991
616. 1'2—dc20
DNLM/DLC   91-6641
for Library of Congress   CIP

BRITISH LIBRARY CATALOGING IN PUBLICATION DATA
Cardiology.
  Rev. ed.
  1. Stet.
  I. Chatterjee, Kanu, 1934–   II. Parmley, William W. *1936*
  –
  616.12

  ISBN 0-397-44611-X

DRUG DOSAGE The authors and publisher have exerted every effort to ensure that drug selection and dosage set forth in this text are in accordance with current recommendations and practice at the time of publication. However, in view of ongoing research, changes in government regulations, and the constant flow of information relating to drug therapy and drug reactions, the reader is urged to check the package insert for each drug for any change in indications and dosage and for added warnings and precautions. This is particularly important when the recommended agent is a new or infrequently used drug.

© **COPYRIGHT 1991 BY GOWER MEDICAL PUBLISHING,** 101 Fifth Avenue, New York, NY 10003. All rights reserved. No part of this publication may be reproduced, stored in a retrieval system, or transmitted in any form or by any means electronic, mechanical, photocopying, recording, or otherwise without prior written permission of the publisher.

DISTRIBUTED IN USA AND CANADA BY:
J.B. Lippincott Company
East Washington Square
Philadelphia, PA 19105 USA

DISTRIBUTED ELSEWHERE (EXCEPT JAPAN) BY:
Wolters Kluwer Ltd.
Middlesex House
34-42 Cleveland Street
London W1P 5FB UK

DISTRIBUTED IN JAPAN BY:
Nankodo Co., Ltd.
42-6, Hongo 3-Chome
Bunkyo-Ku
Tokyo 113 Japan

EDITORS:
William B. Millard
Leah Kennedy

ART DIRECTOR:
Jill Feltham

DESIGNER:
Kathryn Greenslade

ILLUSTRATION DIRECTOR:
Laura Pardi Duprey

ILLUSTRATORS:
Susan Tilberry (schematics)
Patricia Gast
Vantage Art, Inc. (charts)

COMPOSITOR:
Tapsco, Inc.

10 9 8 7 6 5 4 3 2 1

**PRINTED IN SINGAPORE
BY IMAGO PRODUCTIONS (FE) PTE, LTD.**

CONTENTS

VOLUME 1
PHYSIOLOGY, PHARMACOLOGY, DIAGNOSIS

Section 1
NORMAL AND ABNORMAL CARDIOVASCULAR PHYSIOLOGY
Section Editor: William W. Parmley

CHAPTER 1 *Cardiac Anatomy* 1.2
Melvin D. Cheitlin Walter E. Finkbeiner

2 *Physiology of Cardiac Muscle Contraction* 1.19
William W. Parmley Joan Wikman-Coffelt

3 *Cardiovascular Adrenergic and Muscarinic Cholinergic Receptors* 1.41
Patricia L. Wisler Frank J. Green August M. Watanabe

4 *Myocardial Hypertrophy, Failure, and Ischemia* 1.68
William W. Parmley Joan Wikman-Coffelt

5 *Ventricular Function* 1.85
William W. Parmley

6 *Physiology of the Coronary Circulation* 1.101
Francis J. Klocke Avery K. Ellis

7 *The Circulation in the Limbs: Normal Function and Effects of Disease* 1.114
John T. Shepherd Paul M. Vanhoutte

8 *Physiology and Pathophysiology of Exercise* 1.129
C. Gunnar Blomqvist

9 *Pulmonary Edema* 1.144
Max Harry Weil Eric C. Rackow Carter E. Mecher

10 *Principles in the Management of Congestive Heart Failure* 1.154
William W. Parmley

11 *Orthostatic Hypotension* 1.163
C. Gunnar Blomqvist

Section 2
CARDIOVASCULAR PHARMACOLOGY
Section Editor: William W. Parmley

12 *Basic Principles of Clinical Pharmacology* 2.2
Raymond L. Woosley Dan M. Roden

13 *Diuretics* 2.19
Arnold M. Chonko Jared J. Grantham

14 *Digitalis, Catecholamines, and Other Positive Inotropic Agents* 2.34
Kanu Chatterjee

15 *Nitrates* 2.75
Jonathan Abrams

16 *The Alpha- and Beta-Adrenergic Blocking Drugs*   2.91
   William H. Frishman   Shlomo Charlap

17 *Calcium Channel Blockers in Therapeutics*   2.105
   Bramah N. Singh   Martin A. Josephson   Koonlawee N. Nademanee

18 *Vasodilator Drugs in the Treatment of Heart Failure*   2.123
   William W. Parmley

19 *Hypolipidemic Agents*   2.137
   Mary J. Malloy   John P. Kane

20 *Antithrombotic Therapy in Cardiac Disease*   2.143
   John H. Ip   Valentin Fuster   James H. Chesebro   Lina Badimon

21 *Cardiovascular Drug Interactions*   2.172
   Neal L. Benowitz

Section 3
BEDSIDE EVALUATION OF THE PATIENT
Section Editor: Kanu Chatterjee

22 *The History*   3.2
   Kanu Chatterjee

23 *Bedside Evaluation of the Heart: The Physical Examination*   3.11
   Kanu Chatterjee

24 *Examination of the Lungs*   3.54
   Thomas Killip

25 *Bedside Diagnosis of Congenital Heart Disease*   3.58
   Alvin J. Chin   William F. Friedman

Section 4
NONINVASIVE TESTS
Section Editor: Kanu Chatterjee

26 *The Chest X-Ray Film and the Diagnosis of Heart Disease*   4.2
   Melvin D. Cheitlin

27 *Electrocardiogram*   4.14
   Borys Surawicz

28 *Echocardiography and Doppler in Clinical Cardiology*   4.33
   Nelson B. Schiller   Ronald B. Himelman

29 *The Scintigraphic Evaluation of the Cardiovascular System*   4.107
   Elias H. Botvinick   Michael Dae   William O'Connell   Douglas Ortendahl   Robert Hattner

30 *New Cardiac Imaging Modalities*   4.163
   Charles B. Higgins

31 *Exercise Stress Testing: Principles and Clinical Application*   4.183
   Myrvin H. Ellestad   Robert J. Stuart

32 *Exercise Evaluation of Cardiorespiratory Function*   4.202
   Karl T. Weber   Joseph S. Janicki

33 *Noninvasive Evaluation of Peripheral Vascular Disease*   4.213
   D. E. Strandness, Jr.

Section 5
INVASIVE TESTS
Section Editor: Kanu Chatterjee

34 *Cardiac Catheterization* 5.2
 Blase A. Carabello

35 *Coronary Arteriography Including Quantitative Estimation of Coronary Artery Stenosis* 5.20
 George T. Kondos Jeffrey G. Shanes Bruce H. Brundage

36 *Cardiac Digital Angiography* 5.43
 Neal Eigler James S. Forrester

37 *Assessment of Ventricular Diastolic Function* 5.55
 Derek G. Gibson

38 *Cardiac Biopsy* 5.67
 Margaret E. Billingham Henry D. Tazelaar

39 *Bedside Hemodynamic Monitoring* 5.80
 Kanu Chatterjee

Section 6
ELECTROPHYSIOLOGY
Section Editor: Melvin M. Scheinman

40 *Mechanisms of Cardiac Arrhythmias* 6.2
 Richard J. Kovacs John C. Bailey Douglas P. Zipes

41 *Pharmacodynamics of Antiarrhythmic Drugs* 6.14
 Peter Danilo, Jr. Michael R. Rosen

42 *Use of Antiarrhythmic Drugs: General Principles* 6.31
 Kelley P. Anderson Roger A. Freedman Jay W. Mason

43 *Clinical Use of Newer Antiarrhythmic Drugs* 6.44
 Samuel Levy

44 *Invasive Cardiac Electrophysiology Studies: An Introduction* 6.54
 Masood Akhtar

45 *Measurements and Clinical Application of Monophasic Action Potentials* 6.68
 Michael R. Franz

46 *Ambulatory Holter Electrocardiography: Technology, Clinical Applications, and Limitations* 6.87
 Joel Morganroth Harold L. Kennedy

47 *The Sick Sinus Syndrome and Evaluation of the Patient with Sinus Node Disorders* 6.100
 J. Anthony Gomes

48 *Bundle Branch Block and Atrioventricular Conduction Disorders* 6.111
 Robert W. Peters Melvin M. Scheinman

49 *Supraventricular Tachycardia* 6.128
 John M. Herre Melvin M. Scheinman

50 *Ventricular Arrhythmias* 6.142
 John M. Miller Mark E. Josephson

51 *Right Ventricular Tachycardias*   6.156
     Guy Fontaine   Robert Frank   Fabrice Fontaliran   Gilles Lascault   Joelice Tonet

52 *Devices for the Management of Rhythm Disorders: Pacemakers and Defibrillators*   6.170
     Jerry C. Griffin

53 *Surgical Treatment of Cardiac Arrhythmias*   6.185
     T. Bruce Ferguson, Jr.   James L. Cox

54 *Catheter Ablation for Cardiac Arrhythmias*   6.215
     Melvin M. Scheinman

55 *Syncope*   6.224
     Fred Morady

56 *Evaluation and Treatment of Patients with Aborted Sudden Death*   6.237
     David J. Wilber   Hasan Garan   Jeremy N. Ruskin

57 *Cardiopulmonary Resuscitation*   6.249
     James T. Niemann   J. Michael Criley

58 *Congenital and Acquired Long QT Syndromes*   6.258
     Anil K. Bhandari   Phuc Tito Nguyen   Melvin M. Scheinman

VOLUME 2
CARDIOVASCULAR DISEASE

Section 7
CORONARY HEART DISEASE
Section Editor: Joel S. Karliner

59 *Epidemiology, Established Major Risk Factors, and the Primary Prevention of Coronary Heart Disease*   7.2
     Jeremiah Stamler

60 *Lipid Abnormalities: Mechanisms, Clinical Classifications, and Management*   7.36
     Robert W. Mahley   Thomas P. Bersot

61 *Evaluation of the Patient with Signs and Symptoms of Ischemic Heart Disease*   7.48
     Louis J. Dell'Italia   Robert A. O'Rourke

62 *Stable Anginal Pectoris*   7.62
     Joel S. Karliner

63 *Acute and Chronic Ischemic Heart Disease: Unstable Angina*   7.75
     Carl J. Pepine

64 *Silent Ischemia*   7.91
     William W. Parmley

65 *Variant Angina*   7.100
     John Speer Schroeder

66 *Acute Myocardial Infarction: Pathophysiology*   7.112
     Wilbur Y. W. Lew   Martin M. LeWinter

67 *Measurement of Myocardial Infarction Size*   7.134
   L. Maximilian Buja   James T. Willerson
68 *Management of Uncomplicated Acute Myocardial Infarction*   7.142
   Gabriel Gregoratos
69 *Reperfusion in Acute Myocardial Infarction*   7.163
   David W. Muller   Eric J. Topol
70 *Complications of Acute Myocardial Infarction*   7.179
   Prediman K. Shah   H. J. C. Swan
71 *Cardiac Rehabilitation*   7.204
   Victor F. Froelicher
72 *Management of the Postmyocardial Infarction Patient*   7.217
   Nora Goldschlager
73 *Transluminal Coronary Angioplasty and Newer Catheter-Based Interventions*   7.237
   Paul G. Yock
74 *Coronary Artery Bypass Surgery*   7.249
   Joel S. Karliner
75 *The Role of Cardiac Surgery in the Management of Acute Myocardial Infarction*   7.262
   Jack M. Matloff   Richard J. Gray

Section 8
HYPERTENSION
Section Editor: William W. Parmley

76 *Pathophysiology of Essential Hypertension*   8.2
   Gordon H. Williams   Norman K. Hollenberg
77 *Evaluation and Management of the Patient with Essential Hypertension*   8.16
   Edward D. Frohlich
78 *Evaluation of Secondary Forms of Hypertension*   8.28
   Michael D. Cressman   Ray W. Gifford, Jr.
79 *Effects of Antihypertensive Treatment on Left Ventricular Hypertrophy and Coronary Blood Flow*   8.44
   Pierre Wicker   Fetnat M. Fouad   Robert C. Tarazi[†]
80 *Hypertension in the Elderly*   8.53
   Robert C. Tarazi[†]

[†]Deceased.

Section 9
VALVULAR HEART DISEASE
Section Editor: Elliot Rapaport

81 *The Use of Afterload-Reducing Agents in Acute Valvular Regurgitation*   9.2
   Jack Kron   J. David Bristow
82 *Chronic Valvular Insufficiency*   9.11
   Hans P. Krayenbuehl   Otto M. Hess
83 *Mitral Valve Prolapse Syndrome*   9.30
   Pravin M. Shah

84 *Valvular Heart Disease: Prosthetic Valve Replacement* 9.40
   L. Henry Edmunds, Jr.   V. Paul Addonizio, Jr.   Nicholas A. Tepe

85 *Catheter Balloon Valvuloplasty* 9.54
   James P. Srebro   Thomas A. Ports

86 *Infective Endocarditis* 9.73
   Gabriel Gregoratos

87 *Tricuspid Valve Disease* 9.91
   Gordon A. Ewy

88 *Aortic Stenosis* 9.106
   Robert C. Schlant

89 *Mitral Stenosis* 9.116
   Elliot Rapaport

Section 10
MYOCARDIAL, PERICARDIAL, AND ENDOCARDIAL DISEASES
Section Editor: Melvin D. Cheitlin

90 *Dilated Cardiomyopathy* 10.2
   Ralph Shabetai

91 *Hypertrophic Cardiomyopathy* 10.18
   E. Douglas Wigle

92 *Diseases of the Pericardium* 10.38
   David H. Spodick

93 *Noninfective Endocardial Disease* 10.65
   Edwin L. Alderman

94 *Pulmonary Heart Disease Including Pulmonary Embolism* 10.70
   John A. Paraskos

95 *Myocarditis* 10.84
   George Cherian   M. Thomas Abraham

96 *Rheumatic Fever* 10.98
   M. Thomas Abraham   George Cherian

97 *Restrictive and Obliterative Cardiomyopathy* 10.107
   Walter H. Abelmann

Section 11
CONGENITAL HEART DISEASE IN THE ADULT
Section Editor: Elliot Rapaport

98 *The Adult with Surgically Corrected Heart Disease: The Unnatural History* 11.2
   Melvin D. Cheitlin

99 *Coronary Arterial Anomalies* 11.14
   Melvin D. Cheitlin

100 *Cyanotic Congenital Heart Disease* 11.27
   Mary Allen Engle

101 *Interatrial Septal Defect in the Adult* 11.43
   Melvin D. Cheitlin   Elliot Rapaport

102 *Ductus Arteriosus and Ventricular Septal Defect in the Adult*   11.51
  Warren G. Guntheroth

103 *Congenital Valvular and Other Isolated Obstructive Lesions in the Adult*   11.61
  Mary J.H. Morriss   Dan G. McNamara

104 *Pulmonary Vascular Disease in Adults with Congenital Heart Disease*   11.77
  Joseph S. Alpert   James E. Dalen

105 *Echocardiography in Congenital Heart Disease*   11.88
  Kyung J. Chung   David J. Sahn

Section 12
OTHER DISORDERS OF THE CARDIOVASCULAR SYSTEM
Section Editor: Melvin D. Cheitlin

106 *Alcohol and the Heart*   12.2
  Timothy J. Regan

107 *Cardiovascular Injury as the Internist Sees It*   12.13
  Melvin D. Cheitlin

108 *Diseases of the Aorta and Peripheral Arteries*   12.27
  John A. Spittell, Jr.   Peter C. Spittell

109 *Cardiac Neoplasms*   12.45
  Emilio R. Giuliani   Jeffrey M. Piehler

Section 13
SECONDARY DISORDERS OF THE HEART
Section Editor: Melvin D. Cheitlin

110 *Collagen Diseases and the Heart*   13.2
  Jonathan L. Halperin

111 *Pregnancy in the Cardiac Patient*   13.19
  John H. McAnulty   James Metcalfe   Kent Ueland

112 *The Elderly Patient with Cardiovascular Disease*   13.28
  Nanette Kass Wenger

113 *Assessment and Management of the Cardiac Patient Before, During, and After Noncardiac Surgery*   13.41
  Lee Goldman

114 *Respiratory and Hemodynamic Management After Cardiac Surgery*   13.52
  Michael A. Matthay   Kanu Chatterjee

115 *The Relationship of Emotions and Cardiopathology*   13.67
  Robert S. Eliot   Hugo M. Morales-Ballejo

116 *Cardiac Complications of Substance Abuse*   13.74
  Michael L. Callaham   Kanu Chatterjee

117 *Endocrine Diseases and the Cardiovascular System*   13.82
  Leon Resnekov

118 *Cardiac and Cardiopulmonary Transplantation*   13.92
  Mark E. Thompson   J. Stephen Dummer   Bartley P. Griffith

SECTION 7

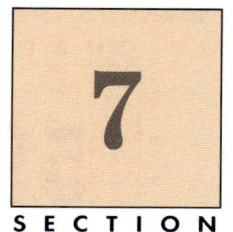

Section Editor
Joel S. Karliner, MD

Coronary Heart Disease

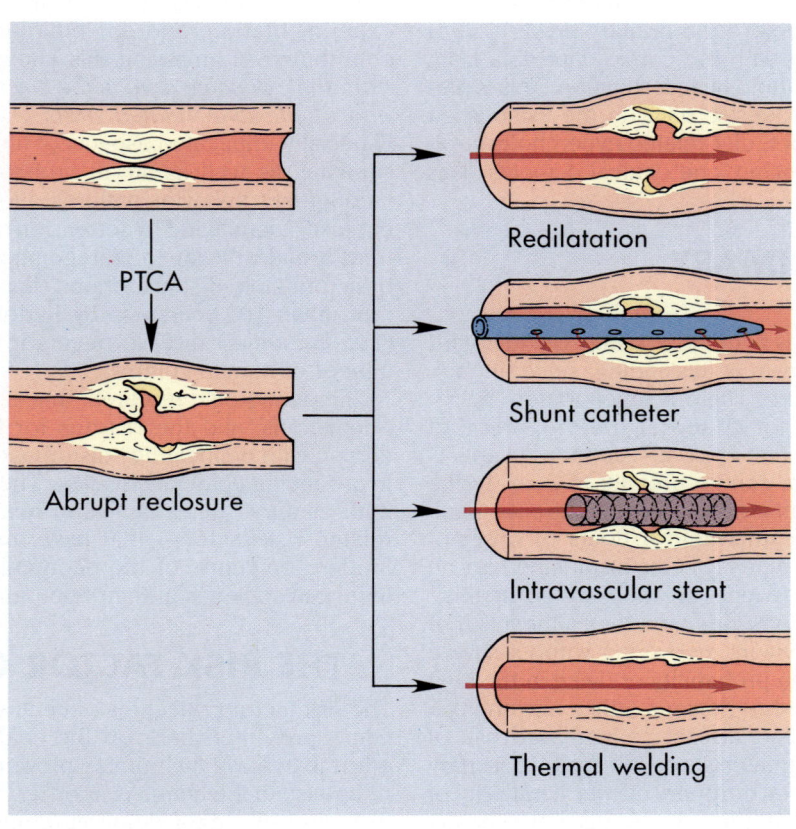

EPIDEMIOLOGY, ESTABLISHED MAJOR RISK FACTORS, AND THE PRIMARY PREVENTION OF CORONARY HEART DISEASE

Jeremiah Stamler

The findings of epidemiologic research constitute one of the key foundations for the mounting effort to achieve the primary prevention of coronary heart disease (CHD), along with the concordant data from animal–experimental, clinical, and pathologic investigation. This is particularly the case in regard to the extensive data on the established major risk factors for CHD—"rich" diet, diet-related hypercholesterolemia and hypertension, cigarette smoking, and clinical diabetes. This chapter reviews these matters.

ESSENTIALITY OF PRIMARY PREVENTION

It is an old aphorism that "prevention is better than cure." But in regard to coronary heart disease, this aphorism is misleading, since, in fact, once CHD is manifest, there is no cure. There is amelioration, palliation, care—but not cure. Moreover, for all too high a proportion of people developing clinical CHD, the first episode—sudden death—is the last, manifest before medical care can be brought to bear. In the prime of life, more than a quarter of first major coronary events manifest as sudden death (defined as death within 3 hours of onset of symptoms, with many of these deaths actually being instantaneous); an additional almost 20% of first major events are nonsudden deaths.[1] Thus, all told (counting sudden plus nonsudden deaths), almost half of first events terminate fatally. For survivors recovering without severe impairment of ventricular function, the probability of dying in the next 5 years is increased fivefold compared to persons of like age and sex who are free of clinical coronary heart disease.[2,3] Increased risk of mortality is due overwhelmingly to greater susceptibility to coronary death. With both first and recurrent fatal coronary events, a majority of the deaths (about 70%) are so rapid that they occur outside the hospital.[4] These findings, originally gathered in the 1960s, are the pattern of the 1980s as well. In American communities with comprehensive modern emergency services able to save any sizable numbers of lives acutely, the additional fact has clearly emerged that persons saved by resuscitation are at very high risk of dying in subsequent years.

These basic facts about the natural history of CHD lead to only one conclusion: major progress against its epidemic onslaught requires primary prevention, that is, prevention of first events, starting from early childhood on. Despite the importance of all therapeutic aspects for those already clinically ill with CHD, such as emergency care, acute care (coronary care unit and post-coronary care unit), long-term care (secondary prevention), and rehabilitation, the strategic key to controlling this epidemic is primary prevention.

SCIENTIFIC FOUNDATIONS OF THE PRIMARY PREVENTION EFFORT

The scientific foundations of the effort to prevent coronary heart disease are the extensive data sets on its etiology and pathogenesis accumulated by over 100 years of research, with major advances in the decades since World War II. As indicated above, all methods available to biomedical research—clinical and pathologic investigation, animal experimentation, and epidemiologic research—have synergistically contributed in amassing this knowledge. *The central generalization from the extensive data is the key role of multiple aspects of life-style and of life-style–related traits as major risk factors causing CHD.* Especially implicated aspects of life-style are "rich" diet and cigarette smoking, as well as, in all probability, sedentary habit and possibly incongruent behavior patterns; life-style–related traits include hypercholesterolemia and hypertension, as well as clinical diabetes mellitus. In its broadest form, the foregoing generalization is a reaffirmation of a basic principle first elaborated (based on studies of infectious disease) more than 100 years ago by Rudolf Virchow, that is, whenever mass (*i.e.*, epidemic) disease occurs it is a consequence of ". . . disturbances of human culture."[5]

Epidemiologic research, that is, research on patterns of disease in populations, and the reasons for these patterns, is particularly concerned with delineating "disturbances in human culture" and their role in producing epidemic disease. Thus, the focus of this chapter is on the 20th century "disturbances of human culture"—the major life-style–related risk factors—that have made premature CHD the principal modern epidemic of the economically developed countries (*i.e.*, of industrial societies in their economic maturity).

THE RISK FACTOR CONCEPT

The risk factor concept is of central importance in regard to the inferences presented here on the epidemiologic findings underlying the effort to achieve the primary prevention of CHD. Therefore, a summary of its essential features is in order. The risk factor concept is based on the extensive data demonstrating that for most diseases afflicting humans, the relationship between exposure to causative environmental factors and occurrence of clinical illness is probabilistic. That is, the relationship is not one-to-one, exposure → disease, but rather exposure → varying probabilities of disease (subclinical, clinical), depending on extent of exposure (dose) and multiple modifying factors in the environment and in the host. (A corollary is that almost all human diseases are due to multiple factors, even though for some there is a primary and essential cause without which the disease will not develop, *e.g.*, a bacterium.) A risk factor then is in its broadest sense a trait associated with increased risk of developing disease. This broad definition, while pragmatically useful, especially in the early stages of active research on the etiology of a disease of obscure or unknown causation, begs a vital question: Is an observed association an etiologically significant one? Much epidemiologic research is concerned with seeking answers to this question in regard to exposures putatively implicated in disease causation.

Epidemiology, like astronomy, evolutionary biology, and geology, is primarily a descriptive, not an experimental, science. Therefore, in assessing the etiologic significance of associations observed in populations, epidemiology uses a set of guidelines as aids in making judgments. Based on these judgments, more refined and precise inferences are drawn concerning risk factors than the broad elementary one described above. That is, etiologic conclusions are drawn as to whether available knowledge warrants classifying a trait associated with a disease as an established risk factor, that is, a cause of the disease at a very high level of probability; a probable or possible risk factor, in terms of etiology; a hypothetical risk factor; or a spurious risk factor.

CRITERIA FOR ASSESSING THE ETIOLOGIC SIGNIFICANCE OF EPIDEMIOLOGIC ASSOCIATIONS

Seven criteria are generally used as guidelines in the assessment of the etiologic significance of epidemiologic associations:

1. *Strength* of the association, as expressed by the relative risk, that is, the ratio of the disease incidence rate for people exposed to the trait (*e.g.*, cigarette smoking) compared to those not exposed.
2. *Graded nature* of the association, that is, does relative risk rise with exposure to higher doses of the trait (*e.g.*, 10 vs. 20 vs. 30 cigarettes per day, serum cholesterol of 200 vs. 220 vs. 240 vs. 260).
3. *Time sequence* of the association, that is, are data available from prospective studies demonstrating that the trait precedes the disease, so that the possibility can be ruled out that the disease caused the trait.
4. *Consistency* of the association, that is, its repeated demonstration in several different populations under varying circumstances.
5. *Independence* of the association, that is, its persistence as a significant relationship with simultaneous consideration of other traits known or suspected to be involved in the etiology of the disease.
6. *Predictive capacity* of the association, that is, ability based on findings in one or more populations to predict disease incidence rates in other independent populations and strata of these populations.
7. *Coherence* (plausibility) of the association, in two senses: first, that the findings of epidemiologic research are coherent with those from other biomedical investigative modalities (animal experimentation, clinical and pathologic research), and second, that there are one or more plausible pathogenetic pathways whereby the trait functions as an etiologic agent, and data are available indicating the operation of the pathway or pathways.

Based on these guidelines, expert groups have over the last quarter century, both in the United States and internationally, designated several traits as *established risk factors* for CHD.

ESTABLISHED MAJOR RISK FACTORS FOR CORONARY HEART DISEASE

Traits are designated *established major risk factors* when three criteria are met: (1) they are assessed to be implicated in CHD causation; (2) they are common (*i.e.*, widely prevalent) in the population; and (3) they are amenable to prevention and control. To make the distinction clear, it is established that in western industrialized countries CHD risk rises with age, and at any age until late in life it is greater for men than women—several-fold greater in young adulthood and middle age. These strong, consistent relations are independent of the associations of other traits with CHD. Hence, both age and male sex are established CHD risk factors of importance. But they are not designated *major* risk factors, since they are not amenable to intervention for CHD prevention. (Possibly in the decades ahead, with advances in genetic manipulation, the aging process will become subject to influence, and this intervention will be added to CHD prevention.)

"Rich" diet, diet-dependent hypercholesterolemia and hypertension, cigarette smoking, and diabetes (especially the much more common non-insulin-dependent diabetes) are established major risk factors for CHD. Their prevention and control are therefore of decisive importance for the primary prevention of CHD. Hence they are the central focus of this chapter.

☐ THE EPIDEMIOLOGIC FINDINGS
"RICH" DIET AND CORONARY HEART DISEASE RISK: AN OVERVIEW
DEFINITION OF "RICH" DIET

"Rich" diet is defined as a habitual pattern of eating foods high in cholesterol (>450 mg/day) and saturated fat (>15% of calories); it is also usually high in total fat (>35% of calories), in refined and processed sugars (>15% of calories), in total calories (for level of energy expenditure), and in sodium (>4 g/day). It is a diet with a high proportion of calories from lipid-rich animal products (meats, eggs, dairy products) and from separated (visible) fats, a sizable proportion of which are of animal origin and from hydrogenated vegetable oils (at least until recently in the United States).[6-8] For many people it is also a diet high in alcohol (>4 drinks/day, >50 g alcohol or about 350 calories/day from alcohol). For all these reasons, it is a diet of high caloric density, high in empty calories (from highly caloric products containing few or no essential nutrients), often suboptimal in ratios of essential nutrients to calories.

EMERGENCE OF "RICH" DIET AS A MASS PHENOMENON

The availability of this type of "rich" diet for most of the population of the United States and several other western industrialized countries is a recent development in human nutrition largely unique to the 20th century. It is a byproduct of industrial society in its maturity, with consequent high-yield agriculture and animal husbandry and high per capita incomes making relatively expensive foodstuffs of animal origin generally available. As such, it is a marked departure from the situation that prevailed for most people for millenia, from the beginning of agriculture to the late 19th or early 20th century (*i.e.*, subsistence overwhelmingly on grains, starchy tubers, and legumes). Bread is no longer the staff of life for the relatively affluent populations in the western industrialized countries (a minority of the human race). In these countries, for the first time in recorded history, most people have daily access in sizable quantity to lipid-rich animal products (meats, dairy products, eggs). Moreover, in the United States over the last several decades a high proportion of the meat (particularly beef) has been coming from feedlots and not off the range, with the great majority of the grain produced for domestic food consumption going to fodder. The result is highly fattened livestock and fat-laden marbleized beef and pork. Animal products plus refined and processed sugars have progressively replaced grains and potatoes in the national mix of foodstuffs, resulting in a continuous increase, until recent years, in availability of dietary lipid high in saturated fats and cholesterol.[6,7] Even with the favorable trends in American eating patterns over the last decades, foodstuffs high in total fat, saturated fat, cholesterol, and refined and processed sugars continue to be widely used (Table 59.1).[8]

THE MULTIPLE EFFECTS OF "RICH" DIET ON CORONARY HEART DISEASE RISK

"Rich" diet increases CHD risk in several ways. High intakes of cholesterol and saturated fat, plus caloric imbalance with resultant obesity, account for the high prevalence rates of hypercholesterolemia–hyperbetalipoproteinemia in the population. Both the composition of "rich" diets and the associated overweight (aided and abetted by sedentary living habits) also contribute to high prevalence rates of hypertension, with high intakes of sodium and alcohol playing important roles. Marked overweight is a key risk factor for the common form of diabetes, non-insulin-dependent diabetes (NIDD). As already noted, hypercholesterolemia, hypertension, and diabetes are established major risk factors for CHD. Further, in addition to its aforementioned consequences, marked obesity adds independently to CHD risk, at least for young adults and persons under age 50. Data are also available indicating that diets high in saturated fats and cholesterol may enhance tendencies to thrombogenesis. Finally, "rich" diet, especially high dietary lipid, most particularly high dietary cholesterol, relates significantly to CHD risk independent of (*i.e.*, over and above) its key role in producing high prevalence rates of the foregoing risk factors.

SERUM CHOLESTEROL–LIPOPROTEINS AND CORONARY HEART DISEASE RISK

As noted above, both dietary lipid composition and calorie balance influence levels of serum total cholesterol (TC). These factors largely account for the marked differences in *mean* TC among different *populations*. They also largely account for population differences in mean levels of the atherogenic fractions of serum TC (*e.g.*, serum low density lipoprotein cholesterol [LDL-C]). However, diet is not the only factor influencing an individual's serum cholesterol and its atherogenic subfractions. Individuals differ in their metabolic responses to diet, at least in part due to genetic influences, through pathways that in the main are not yet clearly elucidated. Therefore, although there is habitual ingestion of more or less similar diets by people within a population, they differ widely in their serum TC and LDL-C levels (*e.g.*, standard deviations of the group TC mean in the order of 40 mg/dl or more for middle-aged Americans). Even when people are fed identically, under controlled experimental conditions, interindividual variation remains sizable (*e.g.*, for TC in the order of 30 mg–35 mg/dl with usual American diets). This phenomenon makes it possible to rank people by serum TC, LDL-C, and so on, over a wide range, and to relate these

TABLE 59.1 MAJOR CONTRIBUTORS OF SATURATED FAT, CHOLESTEROL, TOTAL FAT, AND CALORIES IN THE UNITED STATES DIET

Food Group*	Saturated Fat %	Cum%	Cholesterol %	Cum%	Total Fat %	Cum%	Calories %	Cum%
Hamburgers, cheeseburgers, meat loaf	9.3	9.3	7.3		7.0		4.4	
Whole milk, whole milk beverages	9.1	18.4	5.4		6.0		4.7	
Cheeses, excluding cottage cheese	7.3	25.7	3.0		4.5		2.4	
Beef steaks, roasts	7.3	33.0	8.7		5.4		4.1	
Hot dogs, ham, lunch meats	7.0	40.0	4.3	28.7	6.4	29.3	3.2	18.8
Doughnuts, cookies, cake	4.8	44.9	3.6		6.0		5.7	
Eggs	4.5	49.4	35.9		4.6		2.5	
Pork, including chops, roast	4.0	53.4	3.6		4.0		2.3	
Butter	3.7	57.0	1.7		2.4		0.9	
White bread, rolls, crackers	3.2	60.3	0.7	74.2	4.9	51.2	9.6	39.8
Ice cream, frozen desserts	3.1	63.4	1.7		2.0		1.7	
Margarine	2.6	65.9			4.5		1.6	
2% Milk	2.5	68.4	0.8		1.4		1.7	
Mayonnaise, salad dressings	2.4	70.8	0.6		4.3		1.7	
French fries, fried potatoes	1.9	72.7		77.3	2.7	66.1	2.5	49.0
Salty snacks	1.5	74.2	0.2		2.0		1.4	
Bacon	1.4	75.6	0.5		1.4		0.6	
Nondairy coffee creamers	1.3	76.9			0.5			
Sausage	1.3	78.2	0.6		1.3		0.6	
Chili	1.2	79.5	0.5	79.1	1.0	72.3	0.8	52.4
Gravy, other meat sauces	1.2	80.6			1.1		0.5	
Candy (chocolate)	1.1	81.8			1.0		0.8	
Pies, excluding pumpkin	1.1	82.9	0.8		1.5		1.3	
Chicken, turkey, excluding fried	1.1	84.0	2.5		1.2		1.1	
Fried fish	1.0	85.0	0.6	83.0	1.2	78.3	0.9	57.0
Peanuts, peanut butter	1.0	86.0			1.9		0.9	
Spaghetti with tomato sauce	1.0	87.0	1.5		1.3		1.6	
Salad and cooking oils	0.8	87.8			2.6		0.9	
Pinto, navy, other dried beans	0.8	88.6	0.2		0.7		1.2	
Beef stew, pot pie	0.8	89.4	0.8	85.5	0.6	85.4	0.5	62.1
Alcoholic beverages							5.6	
Regular soft drinks							3.6	
Sugar							1.5	
Potatoes, excluding fried	0.7		0.6		0.9		1.5	
Orange juice		90.1		86.1		86.3	1.4	75.7
Meat and poultry products		33.3		28.8		29.4		17.6
Dairy products, including butter		25.7		12.6		16.3		11.4
Eggs		4.5		35.9		4.6		2.5
Baked goods		9.1		5.1		12.4		16.6
Visible fats, excluding butter		5.8		0.6		11.4		20.8

* The 35 items are the main ones from an overall list of 50 which supply most of the specified nutrient.

(Data from Block G, Dresser CM, Hartman AM, Carroll MD: Nutrient sources in the American diet: Quantitative data from the NHANES II Survey. II. Macronutrients and fats. Am J Epidemiol 122:27–40, 1985) variables to risk of future CHD. (Since the epidemiologic data on TC are the most comprehensive, TC is the focus of attention here. Given that LDL-C is the main component of serum TC, making up a majority of TC in most persons, the findings set down here in regard to TC as a CHD risk factor apply as well to LDL-C.)

In contrast to some other variables (see below), it is possible with a single determination of serum cholesterol to characterize and classify a person accurately and validly, since the ratio of intraindividual variance to interindividual variance for serum TC is about 1:3 (*i.e.*, people differ much more from each other than from themselves in regard to this variable).[9] (Blood pressure shares this characteristic.)

Highly *consistent* data on the relationship of serum cholesterol to risk of CHD are available in great quantity, from studies of over 50 population cohorts in the United States and many other countries.[10] For all the American cohorts, serum cholesterol at baseline was significantly related to subsequent risk of clinical CHD in univariate analyses, and in multivariate analyses as well (done in most studies). In the two population studies reporting analyses of postmortem data, entry serum cholesterol of individuals was also related to severity of coronary atherosclerosis at autopsy.[11,12] A significant positive relationship between baseline serum TC and incidence of clinical CHD was also recorded for most of the cohorts from other countries.

Overall, the findings of the large number of prospective epidemiologic studies across the world are impressive in regard to their consistency, including consistency of results among the many studies in both the United States and abroad. The positive findings, demonstrating a strong independent relationship of serum cholesterol to CHD incidence for individuals within a population, are of a scope rare in medical research on chronic noninfectious disease.

As to the quantitative aspects of this significant relationship, Tables 59.2 and 59.3 display recently acquired data from far and away the largest prospective study done to date, involving 356,222 men screened in 18 United States cities in the recruitment effort for the Multiple Risk Factor Intervention Trial (MRFIT).[3,13] These men were age 35 to 57 and free of a history of hospitalization for myocardial infarction at entry. As these data forcefully demonstrate, the relationship between serum cholesterol and CHD risk is a *strong* one, that is, a more than fourfold higher risk for men in the highest decile of serum cholesterol (levels ≥264 mg/dl) compared to men in the lowest decile (≤167 mg/dl). Further, in regard to other criteria for assessing the etiologic significance of epidemiologic associations, it is a *graded* relationship. Over the range from about 180 mg/dl on up, the higher the serum cholesterol, the greater the risk. The relationship is a *continuous* one, with about 80% of the population at progressively increased risk. Since these are prospective data (mean follow-up of 6 years), the trait clearly preceded the disease event (*i.e.*, the important criterion of appropriate *temporal* sequence is met). With this unprecedentedly large sample size, numbers were adequate to assess the relationship for five specific age groups (35–39, 40–44, 45–49, 50–54, 55–57), and for normotensive nonsmokers, normotensive smokers, hypertensive nonsmokers, hypertensive smokers, all normotensives, all hypertensives, all nonsmokers, and all smokers.[13] The results were the same in each of these analyses: 6-year CHD death rate, age-specific or age-adjusted, was progressively higher for quintiles 2, 3, 4, and 5 of the baseline serum cholesterol distribution, consistently in a strong and graded fashion. The relationship prevailed irrespective of age, blood pressure, or smoking status at entry (*i.e.*, it was *independent* of these other traits, which were also significantly related to CHD risk). Other similar analyses on this large cohort show that serum cholesterol related to CHD risk for men with and without a clinical diagnosis of diabetes requiring drug treatment.[3] Multiple logistic regression analyses confirmed that serum cholesterol was significantly related to risk of death within 6 years from CHD, all cardiovascular diseases, and all causes with control for age, cigarette use, blood pressure, and diabetes, for both white and black men in this large MRFIT cohort. These analyses further showed that for CHD death, a difference in serum cholesterol of 20 mg/dl was associated with a 17% difference in risk of CHD death, that is, a difference in serum cholesterol of about 10% (cohort baseline mean level: 214.6 mg/dl) was associated with a difference in CHD risk of almost 20%, an estimate in quantitative agreement with others.[14–16]

These findings from within-population prospective epidemiologic studies, with the unit of analysis an individual person, are consistent with those of cross-population investigations, with the unit an entire cohort. The Seven Countries Study is the most comprehensive research undertaking of this latter type.[17,18] This long-term prospective study of 16 population samples in seven countries (Finland, Greece, Italy, Japan, The Netherlands, United States, and Yugoslavia) included 12,763 men age 40 to 59 at the start of the study. Follow-up data at 5,

TABLE 59.2 DECILES OF SERUM CHOLESTEROL AND AGE-ADJUSTED 6-YEAR CORONARY HEART DISEASE MORTALITY FOR 356,222 MEN AGE 35 TO 57 FREE OF A HISTORY OF HOSPITALIZATION FOR MYOCARDIAL INFARCTION (MRFIT PRIMARY SCREENEES)

Serum Cholesterol Decile	mg/dl	Mean Serum Cholesterol (mg/dl)	Coronary Heart Disease Mortality Number of Deaths	Rate per 1,000	Relative Risk
1	<168	153.2	95	3.16	1.00
2	168–181	175.0	101	3.32	1.05
3	182–192	187.1	139	4.15	1.31
4	193–202	197.6	149	4.21	1.33
5	203–212	207.5	203	5.43	1.72
6	213–220	216.1	192	5.81	1.84
7	221–231	225.9	261	6.94	2.20
8	232–244	237.7	272	7.35	2.33
9	245–263	253.4	352	9.10	2.88
10	≥264	289.5	494	13.05	4.13

(Data from Stamler J, Wentworth D, Neaton JD, for the MRFIT Cooperative Research Group: Is the relationship between serum cholesterol and risk of death from coronary heart disease continuous and graded? Findings on the 356,222 primary screenees of the Multiple Risk Factor Intervention Trial [MRFIT]. JAMA 256:2823–2828, 1986)

10, and 15 years demonstrated a significant relationship between baseline median serum cholesterol of the 16 samples and CHD risk.

As shown below, when the findings for serum cholesterol and other major risk factors (blood pressure, cigarette use) from one or a set of prospective studies are applied to entirely different populations, it is possible accurately to predict CHD risk; that is, the criterion of *predictive* power is met.

Finally, the criterion that the relationship be a *coherent* one is also met, in two senses. First, the epidemiologic data are consistent with the pathologic, clinical, and animal–experimental data on the relationship of serum cholesterol level to risk of atherosclerotic coronary heart disease. For example, there are the pathologic findings and correlations of the International Atherosclerosis Project (see below).[19] There are the observations on this association of the first generation of clinical cardiologists, a crucial early contribution.[20-22] In the last 15 years, many reports of angiographic studies have been published, showing significant relationships between serum cholesterol–lipoprotein levels and severity of coronary atherosclerosis.[10,23,24] Further, there is the vast fund of confirmatory evidence from thousands of animal experiments over the last 75 years, in virtually all species employed in the laboratory, avian and mammalian, herbivorous, carnivorous, and omnivorous, including the extensive recent work with nonhuman primates. These studies clearly show that sustained hypercholesterolemia (usually induced by increased intake of cholesterol and fat) leads to atherosclerosis. The animal work has included feeding only small amounts of cholesterol to rabbits, chickens, and monkeys at levels present in usual human diets in western industrialized countries. Although little or no hypercholesterolemia supervened, atherosclerotic lesions developed nonetheless. In recent monkey studies with dietary cholesterol at only 43 mg or 129 mg/1,000 calories, serum total cholesterol remained in the normal range, but LDL-cholesterol rose, HDL-cholesterol fell, and atherosclerotic intimal changes developed.[25] Feeding a usual American diet to monkeys induced hypercholesterolemia and atherosclerosis, whereas a ration of human foods with a lipid composition akin to southern European fare resulted in little rise in serum cholesterol and little atherosclerosis.[26] Atherosclerotic lesions of every degree of severity and their complications (*e.g.*, peripheral gangrene, fatal myocardial infarction) have been produced by dietary cholesterol-fat in animals, including nonhuman primates. After discontinuation of the atherogenic diet, hypercholesterolemia quickly clears and lesions gradually regress. After induction of coronary atherosclerosis in monkeys by feeding them a high cholesterol diet, lesions regressed when a diet was fed to maintain a serum cholesterol level of about 200 mg/dl, but not when the level was about 300 mg/dl.[27] Animal experiments in several species have also shown that hypertension *per se* is not atherogenic, but it significantly accelerates and intensifies atherogenesis when the lipid nutritional–metabolic prerequisites, including altered serum cholesterol–lipoprotein levels, are present.

All these findings lend coherence to the conclusion that such lipid nutritional–metabolic changes are a primary etiologic factor in the mass occurrence of premature severe atherosclerosis and its disease consequences in human populations, and that such habits and traits as cigarette smoking and hypertension are secondary (adjuvant) causes

TABLE 59.3 QUINTILES OF SERUM CHOLESTEROL, DIASTOLIC BLOOD PRESSURE, SMOKING STATUS, AND 6-YEAR AGE-ADJUSTED CORONARY HEART DISEASE DEATH RATE PER 1,000 IN 356,222 MEN AGE 35 TO 57 AT BASELINE AND FREE OF A HISTORY OF HOSPITALIZATION FOR MYOCARDIAL INFARCTION (MRFIT PRIMARY SCREENEES)

Serum Cholesterol Quintile (mg/dl)	Diastolic Pressure < 90 mm Hg			Diastolic Pressure ≥ 90 mm Hg					
	No. of Deaths	No. of Men	Rate per 1,000	No. of Deaths	No. of Men	Rate per 1,000	No. of Deaths	No. of Men	Rate per 1,000
Nonsmokers							**All Nonsmokers**		
1 <182	47	35,741	1.6	36	9,612	3.7	83	45,353	2.1
2 182–202	82	34,553	2.5	51	11,599	4.0	133	46,152	2.9
3 203–220	87	31,939	2.7	80	12,839	5.6	167	44,778	3.5
4 221–244	126	30,431	3.8	94	14,500	5.6	220	44,931	4.4
5 ≥245	188	26,996	6.4	200	16,930	10.7	388	43,926	8.0
All	530	159,660	3.3	461	65,480	6.4	991	225,140	4.3
Smokers							**All Smokers**		
1 <182	82	20,017	5.2	31	5,002	6.3	113	25,019	5.4
2 182–202	95	19,675	5.5	60	5,977	10.0	155	25,652	6.7
3 203–220	128	18,812	7.3	100	6,397	15.5	228	25,209	9.5
4 221–244	186	19,119	10.2	127	7,533	16.6	313	26,652	12.1
5 ≥245	250	18,907	13.3	208	9,643	21.4	458	28,550	16.0
All	741	96,530	8.4	526	34,552	15.1	1,267	131,082	10.3
All							**All**		
1 <182	129	55,758	2.8	67	14,614	4.6	196	70,372	3.2
2 182–202	177	54,228	3.5	111	17,576	6.0	288	71,804	4.2
3 203–220	215	50,751	4.3	180	19,236	8.8	395	69,987	5.6
4 221–244	312	49,550	6.2	221	22,033	9.2	533	71,583	7.1
5 ≥245	438	45,903	9.1	408	26,573	14.4	846	72,476	11.1
All	1,271	256,190	5.2	987	100,032	9.3	2,258	356,222	6.3

(Data from Stamler J, Wentworth D, Neaton JD, for the MRFIT Cooperative Research Group: Is the relationship between serum cholesterol and risk of death from coronary heart disease continuous and graded? Findings on the 356,222 primary screenees of the Multiple Risk Factor Intervention Trial [MRFIT]. JAMA 256:2823–2828, 1986) contributing importantly once habitual diet high in cholesterol and saturated fat leads to high prevalence of hypercholesterolemia with its attendant imbalance in lipoprotein levels.

The criterion of coherence is also met in its second sense, that is, reasonable mechanisms of pathogenesis have been identified whereby the factor of concern leads to the disease, in this instance elevated serum cholesterol and its role in producing atherosclerotic CHD. Here animal–experimental research, given its unique capabilities, has made major contributions, particularly in recent years. Fundamental data are available tracing the results of a diet high in cholesterol and saturated fat, from the intestine into the lymph, the bloodstream, the hepatic and fat cells, and into the arterial wall. These encompass the effects of hypercholesterolemia and its attendant changes in serum lipoproteins (qualitative and quantitative) on the cells of the arterial wall, for example, endothelial injury, cholesterol (especially cholesterol ester) accumulation, proliferation of smooth muscle and other cells, cell death, enhanced thrombogenesis, and other components of the pathologic process.

To return to the findings from prospective epidemiologic studies, the age-specific data show that while relative risk (*e.g.*, the *ratio* of CHD death rates for quintile 5 compared to quintile 1) tends to decrease with age, absolute excess risk (*e.g.*, the *difference* in risk between quintile 5 and quintile 1) has the opposite pattern, that is, it tends to increase with age, reflecting the absolute rise in CHD rate with age. Thus, absolute excess risk of CHD in six years was almost three times higher for men age 55 to 57 in quintile 5 of the serum cholesterol distribution compared to corresponding men age 35 to 39.[13] This increase with age in absolute excess risk attributable to hypercholesterolemia—a central concern for clinicians working with patients and public health professionals dealing with populations—indicates the potential benefit throughout middle age of safe measures for preventing and controlling hypercholesterolemia.

The data from the MRFIT and other cohorts also demonstrate that for any quintile of serum cholesterol above optimal (*i.e.*, above about 180 mg/dl) excess CHD risk is a function not only of age, but also of status in regard to other established major risk factors. Thus, for men in quintile 5 of the serum cholesterol distribution, age-adjusted absolute excess risk is progressively greater for nonsmoking hypertensives, smoking normotensives, and smoking hypertensives, compared to nonsmoking normotensives (Table 59.3).[13] Correspondingly, hypercholesterolemic people with diabetes are at much greater excess risk than hypercholesterolemic people without diabetes (see below).

The data in Tables 59.2 and 59.3 make possible detailed estimates of the absolute excess risks attributable to hypercholesterolemia for the several strata of the population, that is, the number and proportion of coronary deaths attributable to hypercholesterolemia of varying degrees.[13] Thus, of the 356,222 middle-aged men in the MRFIT cohort, men in serum cholesterol quintiles 2, 3, 4, and 5—compared to men in quintile 1—experienced 66, 167, 290, and 592 excess CHD deaths, respectively (*i.e.*, a total of 1,115 excess CHD deaths in quintiles 2–5). Of this total of excess CHD deaths, 6% were in quintile 2, 15% in quintile 3, 26% in quintile 4, and 53% in quintile 5. Thus, almost half the excess CHD deaths (47%) were in quintiles 2 to 4, with serum cholesterol in the range 182 mg to 244 mg/dl. These data illuminate the population-wide nature of the problem of serum cholesterol levels above optimal and the limitations of a preventive strategy focused exclusively on the highest risk people, for example, those in quintile 5 or decile 10 of the serum cholesterol distribution, or the 2.5% with levels two standard deviations above the population mean, or those with monogenetic abnormalities (*e.g.*, familial hyperbetalipoproteinemia, occurring in heterozygote form about once in every 500 live births).

For the MRFIT cohort, with a total of 2,258 CHD deaths in six years, the estimate from the foregoing data is that altogether 49% (1,115/2,258), almost one half, of the CHD deaths were excess deaths attributable to serum cholesterol levels ≥182 mg/dl.[13] With control for age, diastolic pressure, cigarette use, and diabetes, the estimate of population attributable risk from the multiple logistic regression analysis was similar: 46% of all CHD deaths in this cohort were excess deaths attributable to serum cholesterol levels ≥180 mg/dl. These data afford insights into the possibilities for preventing CHD by shifting downward the population serum cholesterol distribution through improved eating habits from early childhood on.

Data on two sizable cohorts of men recovered from myocardial infarction (2,789 placebo-treated men in the Coronary Drug Project and 5,440 men among the total of 361,662 MRFIT screenees) further demonstrate that serum cholesterol is significantly and independently related to prognosis post-myocardial infarction.[2,28] The slope of relative risk tends to be less steep than for men without prior myocardial infarction, but given the much greater absolute risk of death post–myocardial infarction, absolute excess risk is as high or higher.

BLOOD PRESSURE AND CORONARY HEART DISEASE RISK

Most of the prospective epidemiologic studies performed to date have also presented data on the relationship in their cohorts of blood pressure to CHD risk.[10] As with serum total cholesterol, the data on both systolic blood pressure (SBP) and diastolic blood pressure (DBP) and CHD risk meet the seven criteria set down above for judging the etiologic significance of an observed epidemiologic association. Also, as with elevated serum cholesterol, blood pressure levels above optimal are common in the adult population and are amenable to prevention and control by nonpharmacologic means, especially dietary means (*e.g.*, prevention and control of obesity, high sodium intake, and heavy alcohol ingestion).[3,29] For people with definite clinical high blood pressure (HBP) by current clinical criteria (*e.g.*, mean of multiple DBP readings ≥90 mm Hg), control can be accomplished by pharmacologic, along with nonpharmacologic, means.[30] All these facts warrant designating blood pressure above optimal as an established major CHD risk factor, as already noted.

As with serum cholesterol, the ratio of intraindividual to interindividual variances for both SBP and DBP are well below 1.0 (*i.e.*, people differ from each other a good deal more than they vary over time within themselves). Therefore, a single determination of blood pressure, particularly when carefully done in a standardized way, generally suffices for epidemiologic purposes to classify and rank people by SBP and DBP within a population, and to distinguish one person from another with high-level validity.

As with serum cholesterol, the large size of the MRFIT screenee cohort and the standardized data collection procedure make possible assessments of the relationship of blood pressure to CHD risk in a detailed fashion and with a degree of precision hitherto unprecedented. The data permit a clear definition not only of the risks of hypertension, as currently defined in clinical practice, but also—more broadly—of the total blood pressure problem in the middle-aged population.

DIASTOLIC BLOOD PRESSURE

In the MRFIT study, optimal DBP was a level <75 mm Hg. Of the total cohort age 35 to 37 at entry, only 18% had mean DBP levels in this optimal low normal range. Another 15%, with DBP 75 to 79 mm Hg, had an apparent increase in risk of 9%. For those with levels in the ranges 80 to 84 mm Hg and 85 to 89 mm Hg (22% and 16%, respectively, of the total cohort), appropriately designated nowadays as persons with *high normal DBP*, 6-year risks of fatal CHD were increased by 19% and 56%, respectively. For successive strata, with DBPs in the hypertensive ranges, risk rose progressively. For those with so-called mild hypertension (mean DBP in the 90–94 mm Hg, 95–99 mm Hg, and 100–104 mm Hg range) relative risks were 1.69, 2.23, and 2.60, respectively, with 2.00 overall for this 90 to 104 mm Hg stratum. With a 100% increase in risk, the term "mild" hypertension hardly seems sound for this stratum. These men with entry DBP 90 to 104 mm Hg made up 25% of the total cohort and 87% of those with high blood pressure (HBP), that is, with mean DBP 90 mm Hg or greater.

Those with DBP levels definitely above optimal (*i.e.*, those with baseline mean DBP ≥80 mm Hg) made up two thirds (66.7%) of the total cohort (Table 59.4).[31] This is a measure of the scope—of the population-wide nature—of the blood pressure problem among middle-aged American men.[29] It is by no means limited to the large numbers of men (28% of the MRFIT cohort) with DBP ≥90 mm Hg.

Estimates of numbers of excess CHD deaths attributable to DBP levels above optimal shed further light on the nature of the blood pressure problem (see Table 59.4).[31] The 58,324 men with DBP 85 to 89 mm Hg made up the stratum contributing the most excess CHD deaths, 157 deaths compared to 154 for the 90 to 94 mm Hg stratum, 153 for the 95 to 99 mm Hg stratum, and 113 for the 100 to 104 mm Hg stratum. Given their relatively small numbers, the strata with more severe hypertension accounted for relatively few excess deaths, despite their high relative risk. The 87,133 men with so-called mild hypertension, DBP 90 to 104 mm Hg, accounted for a majority (51.6%) of all excess CHD deaths attributable to DBP ≥80 mm Hg, and 72% of all excess CHD deaths attributable to DBP ≥90 mm Hg. Clearly this most common hypertensive stratum is of central importance in terms of strategy for the prevention and control of HBP and of CHD due to HBP. Of considerable relevance also is the high-normal group, those with mean DBP 80 to 89 mm Hg, who accounted for 28% of all excess CHD deaths, more than the 20% of excess CHD deaths attributable to DBP ≥105 mm Hg.

In regard to the issues of strategy concerning the total blood pressure problem, these data demonstrate that as urgent and important is the need to identify and treat people with more severe hypertension (*i.e.*, mean DBP ≥115 mm Hg), this cannot be the main and central concern, from an overall medical care and public health strategy point of view. Rather, the essence of the problem is first and foremost in regard to the 90 to 104 mm Hg stratum, and also the 80 to 89 mm Hg stratum, and the prevention and control of these degrees of DBP elevation. Correspondingly, given that fully two thirds of middle-aged men have DBP levels above optimal, a critical need is to address—in the whole population, from early childhood on—the aspects of life-style accounting for this population-wide problem. The aims must include not only early recognition, evaluation, and optimal comprehensive long-term care for those who already have HBP—the high-risk arm of the strategic effort; it must also embrace sustained efforts to prevent HBP from ever developing, that is, primary prevention, shifting the entire distribution of blood pressure downward—the population-wide arm of the strategic effort. Both are required to bring the epidemic of premature CHD under control.

The MRFIT data permit an estimate of the overall proportion of CHD deaths attributable to DBP ≥80 mm Hg: altogether almost one third (32%) of the CHD deaths in six years were excess deaths due to DBP ≥80 mm Hg (Table 59.4).[31]

SYSTOLIC BLOOD PRESSURE

The findings for SBP were similar to those for DBP, with an even greater (eight-fold) spread of relative risk of 6-year CHD death (Table 59.5).[31] Similar data were also recorded for the end points for all cardiovascular and all causes mortality. As with DBP, only a small minority of the cohort of middle-aged men had an optimal SBP.

Progressive increase in risk of 6-year CHD death was clearly manifest for all strata from SBP 125 to 129 mm Hg on, and relative risk was high for all strata from 130 to 134 mm Hg (relative risk 1.76) on. Although SBP 130 to 139 mm Hg is still widely regarded as within the normal range for middle-aged men, almost one quarter (24.3%) of all excess CHD deaths attributable to SBP above optimal stemmed from this stratum. The 140 to 149 mm Hg stratum accounted for almost another quarter (23.9%) of all excess CHD deaths; the 150 to 159 mm Hg stratum, for almost another fifth (19.5%). Both strata are still often designated "borderline" hypertension. Together, these three large strata, making up 42% of the cohort, accounted for over two thirds (67.7%) of all excess CHD deaths attributable to SBP levels above optimal. As with DBP, more severe elevations of SBP (*e.g.*, SBP 160 mm Hg and greater), while associated with markedly higher relative risks (3.82–8.05), generated a minority of all excess CHD deaths, given the relatively small numbers of men with these levels. Thus, again the blood pressure problem is demonstrated to be one affecting broad strata of middle-aged men in the population, and not just a small minority with frankly hypertensive SBP by usual clinical criteria.[29]

Based on these SBP data, 42% of all CHD deaths in six years in this cohort were attributable to SBP levels above optimal; 38% were attributable to SBP levels of 130 mm Hg or greater (Table 59.5).[31] Again, these are estimates of the potential for CHD prevention through control of blood pressure levels above optimal.

EFFECT OF SYSTOLIC BLOOD PRESSURE ON CORONARY HEART DISEASE RISK OF PERSONS WITH ELEVATED DIASTOLIC BLOOD PRESSURE

As shown above, both SBP and DBP—considered separately as risk factors—relate in a similar fashion to CHD risk. With the unprecedentedly large numbers in the MRFIT screenee sample, assessed at baseline

TABLE 59.4 BASELINE DIASTOLIC BLOOD PRESSURE AND 6-YEAR AGE-ADJUSTED CORONARY HEART DISEASE MORTALITY IN 356,222 MEN AGE 35 TO 57 AND FREE OF MYOCARDIAL INFARCTION AT BASELINE (MRFIT PRIMARY SCREENEES)

Baseline Diastolic Blood Pressure (mm Hg)	No. of Men	No. of CHD Deaths	Age-Adjusted CHD Death Rate per 1,000	Relative Risk	Estimated Number of Excess CHD Deaths
<75	64,309	276	4.8	1.00	0
75–79	54,334	260	5.1	1.06	16.3
80–84	79,223	445	5.7	1.19	71.3
85–89	58,324	445	7.5	1.56	157.4
90–94	46,601	394	8.1	1.69	153.8
95–99	25,838	291	10.7	2.23	152.5
100–104	14,694	197	12.5	2.60	113.2
105–109	6,491	113	16.4	3.42	75.3
110–114	3,718	63	15.3	3.19	39.1
≥115	2,690	73	23.6	4.92	50.6
All	356,222	2,557	7.2		829.5

in standardized fashion, it became possible to assess the additional question: for persons with elevated DBP by usual clinical criteria, does level of SBP independently relate to CHD risk? Numbers were adequate to explore this matter for 5 mm Hg strata of DBP over the ranges 90 to 94 mm Hg, 95 to 99 mm Hg, 100 to 104 mm Hg, and 105 to 109 mm Hg. For each stratum of DBP, age-adjusted 6-year rate of CHD death was progressively and markedly higher with higher levels of SBP. For example, for the DBP stratum 90 to 94 mm Hg, the 6-year rate was lowest with SBP 120 to 129 mm Hg, 63% higher with SBP 130 to 139 mm Hg, 84% higher with SBP 140 to 149 mm Hg, 155% higher with SBP 150 to 159 mm Hg, and 318% higher with SBP ≥160 mm Hg. These new data demonstrate clearly that for persons with HBP defined based on DBP criteria, including less severe HBP, the level of SBP has a significant, important, independent positive relationship to CHD risk.

These massive data sets on the United States experience in the 1970s and 1980s are further forceful confirmation that hypertension is one of the established major CHD risk factors. Voluminous consistent data to this effect have been amassed over many years by all the key research methodologies. In addition to the findings from the many prospective population studies, underscored in exquisite detail by the cited MRFIT results, meaningful confirmatory evidence relevant to the mechanisms involved is available from autopsy and from animal-experimental studies. Thus, in the International Atherosclerosis Project, persons with hypertension had consistently more coronary and aortic atherosclerosis at autopsy than persons without hypertension for all age, sex, race, or geographic location groups.[19] A further important finding was that for decedents from the nonindustrialized countries, with habitual diets relatively low in saturated fat and cholesterol and with correspondingly low serum cholesterol levels, atherosclerosis in persons with hypertension only rarely reached a level of severity great enough to lead to clinical CHD. This is in keeping with the evidence from animal experimentation with rabbits, chickens, dogs, and nonhuman primates: in the absence of an atherogenic diet (*i.e.*, a diet supplemented with cholesterol-fat, with consequent alteration in serum lipids-lipoproteins), hypertension by itself induces little or no atherosclerosis. On the other hand, when the nutritional-metabolic prerequisites for atherogenesis prevail, high blood pressure significantly accelerates and aggravates lesion development.[20-22]

Prospective epidemiologic data from cross-population studies, with an entire cohort the unit of study, have also yielded findings coherent with those from the within-population investigations, focused on individuals. In the Seven Countries Study, for example, 10-year CHD incidence and mortality rates of the 16 population groups were significantly and independently related to both the entry group mean blood pressure and serum cholesterol level (Fig. 59.1).[17] The Seven Countries Study data also demonstrate (*e.g.*, with the findings for the two Japanese cohorts) that for samples with habitual diets low in saturated fat and cholesterol, with resultant low mean serum cholesterol levels, incidence of CHD was comparatively low despite a sizable prevalence of hypertension. These interpopulation findings reinforce the evidence from other studies on the additive impact of the established major risk factors and on the pivotal role of diet, especially dietary lipid and diet-lipid-related serum cholesterol.

The available data indicate that the optimal situation in regard to blood pressure is to reach adulthood with consistent readings of systolic less than 120 mm Hg and diastolic less than 80 mm Hg, and to remain at those levels over the next decades—an experience registered by only a small minority of persons in modern society even in the absence of obesity.[22] Clearly the problem of nonoptimal blood pressure readings is a common one, including its important component of frankly hypertensive levels (*i.e.*, average diastolic values ≥90 mm Hg).

ISOLATED SYSTOLIC HYPERTENSION

The findings on the MRFIT screenees show that for middle-aged persons, as well as for the elderly, isolated systolic hypertension (*i.e.*, an elevated SBP with a DBP under 90 mm Hg) is associated with in-

TABLE 59.5 BASELINE SYSTOLIC BLOOD PRESSURE AND 6-YEAR AGE-ADJUSTED CHD MORTALITY IN 356,222 MEN AGE 35 TO 57 AND FREE OF MYOCARDIAL INFARCTION AT BASELINE (MRFIT PRIMARY SCREENEES)

Baseline Systolic Blood Pressure (mm Hg)	No. of Men	No. of CHD Deaths	Age-Adjusted CHD Death Rate per 1,000	Relative Risk	Estimated Number of Excess CHD Deaths
<110	21,378	73	3.9 ⎫ 3.8	1.00	0
110–114	28,458	93	3.7 ⎭		
115–119	37,611	157	4.5	1.18	26.3
120–124	52,621	191	4.0	1.05	10.5
125–129	46,195	213	4.9	1.29	50.9
130–134	45,793	303	6.7	1.76	132.8
135–139	33,502	246	7.2	1.89	113.9
140–144	27,252	251	8.7	2.29	133.5
145–149	17,132	193	10.2	2.68	109.6
150–154	13,404	190	11.9	3.13	108.6
155–159	8,067	142	14.9	3.92	89.5
160–164	5,953	100	14.5	3.82	63.7
165–169	3,354	65	15.0	3.95	37.6
170–174	2,528	56	16.4	4.32	31.9
175–179	1,485	48	30.6	8.05	39.8
≥180	3,190	107	24.9	6.55	67.3
All	347,923*	2,428	7.0		1,015.9

* Of the total cohort of 356,222 men, systolic blood pressure determinations were reported for these 347,923. (Data from Stamler J, Wentworth D, Neaton JD, for the MRFIT Cooperative Research Group: Is the relationship between serum cholesterol and risk of death from coronary heart disease continuous and graded? Findings on the 356,222 primary screenees of the Multiple Risk Factor Intervention Trial [MRFIT]. JAMA 256:2823–2828, 1986)

creased CHD risk.[32,33] Again, the large size of the MRFIT primary screenee cohort made possible a detailed high-precision estimate. For example, for 78,177 men with mean DBP 80 to 84 mm Hg at baseline, the 6-year age-adjusted CHD mortality rate was progressively higher when SBP was ≥130 mm Hg, by 19%, 98%, 74%, and 181%, respectively, for those with SBP 130 to 139 mm Hg, 140 to 149 mm Hg, 150 to 159 mm Hg, and ≥160 mm Hg, respectively, compared to those with SBP 110 to 119 mm Hg. Findings were similar for the end-points all cardiovascular disease and all causes mortality.[33] These data support the judgment that with a mean SBP ≥140 mm Hg and a mean DBP <90 mm Hg, a middle-aged or elderly person is appropriately designated as having isolated systolic hypertension (ISH), with consequent increased CHD risk.

CIGARETTE SMOKING AND CORONARY HEART DISEASE RISK

Data from many prospective studies in the United States and many other countries demonstrate that cigarette smoking is significantly and independently related to CHD risk (nonfatal plus fatal heart attack, CHD death, sudden CHD death) for both middle-aged and elderly men and women.[1,3,10,22,34–38] This is particularly the case in populations consuming "rich" diets, with consequent high prevalence rates of hypercholesterolemia and hypertension. In the United States, investigations on cigarette smoking include four studies of very large sample sizes—one of 294,000 veterans; two by the American Cancer Society involving about 188,000 and 800,000 persons, respectively;[10,38] and the ongoing study of MRFIT primary screenees (Table 59.3).[3,13] Other large studies in other countries encompass a Canadian sample of 78,000 veterans, and British samples of 41,000 physicians and 20,000 Whitehall civil servants.[10,38] Most of these long-term investigations were undertaken in the late 1940s, 1950s, and 1960s. The new data from the large cohort of MRFIT primary screenees, giving experience in the 1970s and 1980s, underscore the great increase in CHD risk due to cigarette use, including both "moderate" (1–15 cigarettes/day) and heavy smoking. Overall, age-adjusted 6-year risk of CHD death was 2.3 times higher for cigarette smokers compared to nonsmokers. Of the 2,258 CHD deaths in the entire cohort of 356,222 men, 697 (31%) were excess deaths attributable to the smoking habit. In agreement with these findings, data from long-term prospective studies show that users of filter-tip cigarettes have as high a CHD risk as users of non-filter cigarettes.[10,38,39] Cigarette smoking and use of oral contraceptive pills have a marked joint impact on risk of premature CHD for women, with an increase in risk of ten times or more. Excess risk with continued cigarette use is also great for persons with clinical CHD including those post–myocardial infarction. Evidence also is accumulating on the risks associated with passive smoking.

Cross-population studies have yielded data consistent with the foregoing findings. Thus, in analyses for 18 economically developed countries, statistically significant correlations were found between the average number of cigarettes smoked per person per year in the years 1954 to 1965 and CHD mortality in the early 1970s for the age group 35 to 74. Average total tobacco consumption (kg/person/year) was also significantly related to CHD mortality. This was true for both men and women.[40] The trends (slopes) in cigarette use in recent years in these countries were significantly related to the trends (slopes) of mortality from premature CHD.

Concordant with these findings, autopsy studies have shown severe atherosclerosis of major arteries to be more frequent among cigarette smokers than among nonsmokers. The relationship is a graded one, that is, the more cigarettes smoked per day, the more frequently was severe atherosclerosis manifest. In decedents from the Framingham and the Hawaiian populations, this relationship prevailed with control for hypercholesterolemia and hypertension, as well as age. Postmortem analyses have also found smokers frequently to have sclerosis of small arteries and arterioles in the heart muscle. Several recent angiographic studies have also presented data on the relationship of cigarette smoking to severity of coronary arteriosclerosis.[10,38]

In addition to increased risk of CHD, cigarette smokers are significantly more prone than nonsmokers to sickness, disability, and death from other atherosclerotic diseases (peripheral vascular disease, atherothrombotic cerebral infarction, and nonluetic aortic aneurysm) and from hypertensive cardiovascular disease as well.

Unquestionably, the mass adoption of the cigarette habit by tens of millions of people in the United States and in other western industrialized countries in the 20th century is one of the most important causes of the epidemic of premature coronary heart disease.

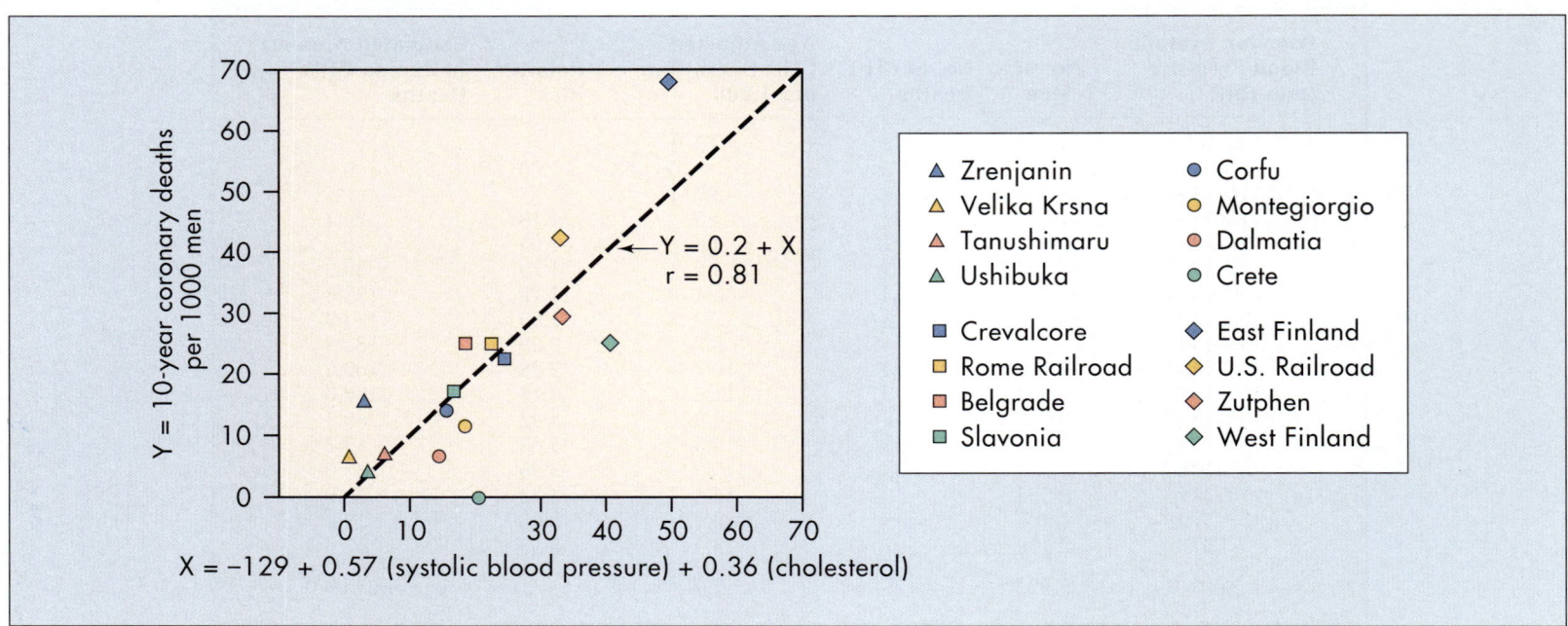

FIGURE 59.1 Cohort systolic blood pressure and serum cholesterol concentration medians at entry versus 10-year age-standardized death rate from coronary heart disease of men originally age 40 to 59 in seven countries, without cardiovascular disease at entry, Seven Countries Study. The multiple regression solution indicates agreement with the observed coronary death rate of $r = 0.81$, and the slope, $b = 1.00$, has $SE = 0.19$. (Modified from Keys A (ed): Seven Countries—A Multivariate Analysis of Death and Coronary Heart Disease. Cambridge, Harvard University Press, 1980)

CLINICAL DIABETES AND CORONARY HEART DISEASE RISK

Clinical diabetes mellitus has repeatedly been implicated as a contributor to accelerated and aggravated atherosclerotic disease, coronary, peripheral, and cerebral, at least for populations in western industrialized countries. Recent data from United States prospective epidemiologic studies in progress in the 1970s and 1980s lend strong further support to this conclusion. Thus, the 9-year follow-up findings of the Chicago Heart Association Detection Project in Industry show much higher CHD mortality rates for persons with diabetes at baseline, compared to those free of this diagnosis (Table 59.6).[41] This was the outcome for both men and women. It prevailed after adjustment for age and the other established major risk factors. For men, the 9-year adjusted CHD death rate for diabetics was 4.8 times higher than for nondiabetics, with an absolute excess mortality rate for the diabetics of 86 per 1,000. For women, the relative risk of the diabetics compared to the nondiabetics was higher still, 5.8. However, given the much lower CHD death rate for women compared to men, absolute excess risk of diabetic women (23 per 1,000) was considerably less than for diabetic men. The CHD death rate for diabetic women was somewhat higher than for nondiabetic men (28 vs 23 per 1,000), but not nearly as high as for diabetic men (109 per 1,000). Thus, these data, while clearly showing increased risk of premature CHD for diabetic women, do not support the oft-heard statement that diabetes abolishes the sex differential in susceptibility to CHD; a more sound characterization is that diabetes decreases the sex differential in CHD risk. The data from the Chicago study also demonstrate that at least under conditions prevailing in the United States, diabetes is significantly related to CHD risk of men and women independent of other established major risk factors. Results of multivariate analyses with use of the Cox regression model also support this conclusion.[41]

Among the 361,662 MRFIT screenees, 5,625 (1.6%) gave a history at baseline of drug treatment for diabetes, 5,245 without and 380 with a concomitant history of myocardial infarction. For the 5,245 diabetic men free of myocardial infarction, 6-year age-adjusted CHD death rate was 3.2 times higher than for the 350,977 nondiabetic men without a myocardial infarction history.[3] The findings were similar for the endpoints all cardiovascular deaths and mortality from all causes. Correspondingly, for the 380 diabetic men with a history of myocardial infarction, age-adjusted risk of death from CHD was greater than for the 5,060 nondiabetic men with a history of myocardial infarction.

When the 5,245 diabetic and 350,977 nondiabetic MRFIT screenees free of myocardial infarction at baseline were stratified by serum cholesterol quintiles and 6-year age-adjusted CHD death rates were computed, two findings were apparent: first, for both diabetics and nondiabetics, serum cholesterol was signifcantly related to CHD risk. Second, for each of the five serum cholesterol strata, CHD mortality was considerably higher (by 2.8 to 5.5 times) for diabetics than for nondiabetics.[3] The findings were similar with stratification of diabetics and nondiabetics by quintiles of blood pressure and by cigarette smoking status at baseline. That is, for diabetics, as for nondiabetics, CHD risk is related to serum cholesterol, blood pressure, and cigarette use; in addition, diabetes is related to CHD risk over and above the impact of these three other established major risk factors.

These conclusions are reinforced when all four traits—diabetic status, serum cholesterol, blood pressure, and cigarette use—are considered together (Table 59.7).[3] With the large size of the MRFIT screenee sample, the four traits could be dichotomized, with enough men in each of the 16 strata to permit assessment of 6-year age-adjusted CHD death rate with reasonable precision. The first fact of note is that the stratum with serum cholesterol <220 mg/dl, DBP <90 mm Hg, and no cigarette use at baseline made up only a small minority of all diabetics and of all nondiabetics—25% and 28%, respectively. (As data sets presented above clearly demonstrate, neither the <220 mg/dl nor the <90 mm Hg cut points for serum cholesterol and DBP, respectively, define people at optimal risk. Had use been made of the cut points defining the lowest quintile of risk, <182 mg/dl and <76 mm Hg, respectively, the proportion of both diabetic and nondiabetic men at relatively low CHD risk would have been even smaller.) As Table

TABLE 59.6 NINE-YEAR CORONARY HEART DISEASE MORTALITY RATES AND ABSOLUTE EXCESS RISK PER 1,000, CRUDE, AGE-ADJUSTED,* MULTIPLE RISK FACTOR-ADJUSTED,* BY BASELINE DIABETES† DIAGNOSIS AND BY SEX IN 19,250 WHITE MEN AND WOMEN AGED 35 TO 64 AT BASELINE

Group	N	No. of CHD Deaths	CHD Mortality Rate (per 1,000)		
			Crude	Age-Adjusted	Multiple Risk Factor‡-Adjusted
All men	11,220	286	25.5	26.7	25.9
Diabetic men	377	44	116.7	111.5	109.5
Nondiabetic men	10,843	242	22.3	23.7	23.0
		Absolute excess risk in men	94.4	87.8	86.5
All women	8030	47	5.9	4.2	5.3
Diabetic women	170	6	35.3	30.8	28.0
Nondiabetic women	7,860	41	5.2	3.6	4.8
		Absolute excess risk in women	30.1	27.2	23.2

* Adjustment is based on the linear model.

† Diabetes previously diagnosed by physician.

‡ Age, serum cholesterol, systolic blood pressure, number of cigarettes smoked per day, electrocardiographic abnormalities, education.

(Data from Pan W-H, Cedres LB, Liu K et al: Relationship of clinical diabetes and asymptomatic hyperglycemia to risk of coronary heart disease mortality in men and women. Am J Epidemiol 123:504–556, 1986)

59.7 shows, 44% of the diabetic and 42% of the nondiabetic men had at least one of the three other major risk factors, based on the cut points used; 31% and 30%, respectively, had any two or all three traits.

For both diabetic and nondiabetic men, 6-year age-adjusted CHD death rates were progressively higher with any one only, any two only, or all three of the other major risk factors (Table 59.7).[3] Highest relative risk was 2.8 for the diabetic men and 8.9 for the nondiabetic men. For each of the eight strata defined on the basis of dichotomized criteria for serum cholesterol, DBP, and cigarette use, CHD mortality was much higher for diabetics than for nondiabetics. Hence, absolute excess risk attributable to hypercholesterolemia, hypertension, or cigarette use was generally greater for diabetics than for nondiabetics, even though relative risk was less (Table 59.7).

Multiple logistic regression analyses for the entire cohort of 356,222 men free of myocardial infarction at baseline confirmed the significant independent relationship of all four of these traits to risk of death from CHD, all cardiovascular diseases, and all causes.[3] Similar analyses for the 5,245 diabetic and 350,977 nondiabetic men also confirmed that for both sets of men serum cholesterol, DBP, and cigarette smoking were independently related to 6-year risk of CHD death.

The extensive autopsy analyses of the International Atherosclerosis Project yielded data generally confirming the role of diabetes as a coronary risk factor.[19] In contrast to its findings for Americans and Norwegians, for decedents from nonindustrialized countries, with diets relatively low in saturated fat and cholesterol, and consequently with lower population mean serum cholesterol levels, the degree of coronary atherosclerosis attained with diabetes was only rarely severe enough to lead to clinical coronary heart disease. This finding is consistent with other reports from countries with similar socioeconomic and nutritional circumstances.

At present, findings with regard to the relationship of asymptomatic hyperglycemia to atherosclerotic disease are inconsistent and contradictory.[41,42] Further research is needed to elucidate the reasons for the anomalous results and resolve present uncertainties.

Most adults with clinical diabetes mellitus have the non-insulin-dependent maturity-onset form of the disease. Marked obesity is the one trait clearly established as the major factor contributing strongly to the likelihood of its occurrence.[43]

COMBINATIONS OF ESTABLISHED MAJOR RISK FACTORS AND CORONARY HEART DISEASE RISK

Earlier in this chapter, data were presented on the relationship of each of the individual established major risk factors to occurrence of CHD. These included analyses in which impact of one of these factors was considered while controlling for the others (*e.g.*, impact of serum cholesterol over quintiles of its distribution for normotensive nonsmokers, normotensive smokers, hypertensive nonsmokers, and hypertensive smokers (see Table 59.3)[13] or impact of diabetes for eight groups identified based on status in regard to serum cholesterol, DBP, and cigarette use[3]). With the large sample size of the MRFIT primary screenee cohort, these relationships could be examined with precision by this classical straightforward epidemiologic method of multiple cross-classification. These analyses also demonstrate with a high degree of accuracy the influence on CHD risk of *combinations* of these established major risk factors. Thus, as shown in Table 59.3, the range of risk across the 20 strata was more than 13-fold: a 6-year age-adjusted CHD death rate of 21.4 per 1,000 for cigarette smoking hypertensive men with baseline serum cholesterol ≥245 mg/dl, compared to a rate of only 1.6 per 1,000 for nonsmoking normotensive men with serum cholesterol <182 mg/dl. Only 10% of the entire cohort were in this lowest risk subgroup; 90% were at higher risk.

The problem of increased risk is population-wide; it is not confined to a minority (see also below). Increase in risk was substantial for all 19 of the other groups, for example, a relative risk of 1.56 for the group of non-smoking normotensive men in the second quintile of the serum cholesterol distribution (182 mg–202 mg/dl). For each higher quintile of serum cholesterol, risk of CHD death was higher, and risk rose progressively for men with one or the other or both of the other two traits. For example, for men in serum cholesterol quintile 4, with moderate hypercholesterolemia, levels of "only" 221 mg to 244 mg/dl, the following increases in relative risk of 6-year CHD death were recorded, depending on their status in regard to high blood pressure (HBP) and cigarette use: DBP < 90 mm Hg, nonsmoker—"only" a 2.4 times increase in risk (3.8/1.6); DBP ≥ 90 mm Hg, nonsmoker—a 3.5 times increase; DBP < 90 mm Hg, smoker—a 6.4 times increase; DBP ≥ 90 mm Hg, smoker—a 10.4 times increase (see Table 59.3).[13] Absolute excess risk, that is, the difference in risk for a given group compared to the group at lowest risk, also increased progressively and steeply with various combinations of these three traits (*e.g.*, for the aforementioned strata, from 2.2 [3.8 minus 1.6], to 4.0, to 8.6, to 15.0 per 1,000 in the six years from average age of about 45 to 51 years). The three major risk factors act synergistically to increase risk.

Results were similar when four factors—diabetes, serum cholesterol, blood pressure, and smoking—were considered simultaneously (see Table 59.7).[3] In this analysis, each of the four traits was dichotomized, with 220 mg/dl the cut point for serum cholesterol, rather than 182 mg/dl as in the previous analysis. Nevertheless, only about a quarter of the men were in the lowest stratum of risk—nondiabetic, nonsmoker, serum cholesterol <220 mg/dl, DBP <90 mm Hg. Their

TABLE 59.7 BASELINE MAJOR RISK FACTORS AND 6-YEAR AGE-ADJUSTED CORONARY HEART DISEASE MORTALITY IN 5,245 DIABETIC AND 350,977 NONDIABETIC MEN AGE 35 TO 57 AND FREE OF MYOCARDIAL INFARCTION AT BASELINE (MRFIT PRIMARY SCREENEES)

Serum Cholesterol	Cigarette Use	Diastolic Blood Pressure	% of Cohort		Mortality per 1,000		Relative Risk		Absolute Excess Risk per 1,000	
			Diabetic	*Nondiabetic*	*Diabetic*	*Nondiabetic*	*Diabetic*	*Nondiabetic*	*Diabetic*	*Nondiabetic*
<220	No	<90	24.6	28.3	13.4	2.1	1.00	1.00	0.0	0.0
<220	No	≥90	13.5	9.3	16.3	4.1	1.22	1.95	2.9	2.0
<220	Yes	<90	15.7	16.1	18.7	5.7	1.40	2.71	5.3	3.6
≥220	No	<90	14.7	16.6	24.9	4.7	1.86	2.24	11.5	2.6
<220	Yes	≥90	6.4	4.7	24.8	10.6	1.85	5.05	11.4	8.5
≥220	No	≥90	10.8	9.0	17.1	8.1	1.28	3.86	3.7	6.0
≥220	Yes	<90	9.0	11.0	24.5	11.5	1.83	5.48	11.1	9.4
≥220	Yes	≥90	5.3	4.9	37.6	18.8	2.81	8.95	24.2	16.7

age-adjusted 6-year CHD death rate was 2.1 per 1,000. At the other extreme, CHD mortality rate for diabetic cigarette smoking men with hypercholesterolemia and HBP was 37.6 per 1,000, 18 times higher.

In another analysis of the experience of this MRFIT cohort (free of a history of previous myocardial infarction), a group at optimal low risk was identified based on the following five criteria: in the lowest quintile of serum cholesterol (<182 mg/dl) and DBP (<76 mm Hg), SBP <120 mm Hg, nonsmoker, nondiabetic. Of the 356,222 men age 35 to 57 at baseline, only 7,948 (only 2.2%) met these criteria.[3] This is the most forceful documentation to date of the fact that, given prevailing American life-styles in the middle of the 20th century, virtually the entire population was at varying levels of excess CHD risk by the time it attained middle age. The 7,948 men in the MRFIT cohort with optimal status for the five risk factors at baseline experienced only six CHD deaths during the 6-year follow-up period, an age-adjusted CHD mortality rate of only 0.8 per 1,000. This was a rate about one fiftieth (2.1%) that of the group with all four risk factors, as defined above. If all 356,222 men had had a 6-year CHD death rate of only 0.8 per 1,000, there would have been 285 CHD deaths instead of the 2,258 recorded. Thus, 1,973 CHD deaths (87% of all the CHD deaths) were excess deaths attributable to various combinations of the established major risk factors prevalent among most middle-aged American men. This statistic, 87% excess CHD deaths, is a measure of the potential for controlling the epidemic of premature CHD in the United States by improving life-styles to reduce the high prevalence rates of the major life-style–related risk factors.

Data on long-term follow-up of Harvard and University of Pennsylvania college entrants show that at least from the teens on, status with regard to blood pressure and cigarette use (and overweight as well) all relate strongly, in additive fashion, to risk of CHD in middle age.[44] (Serum cholesterol was not measured for these youngsters decades ago.) These data demonstrate the need—underscored by recent autopsy data on children[45,46]—for attention to population life-styles from early childhood on (*i.e.*, to primary formation of healthful living habits) to prevent the major risk factors from developing in the first place.[47,48]

As indicated above, the data emerging from the in-depth analyses made possible by the size of the MRFIT screenee cohort reinforce the soundness, relevance, and urgency of the population-wide strategy for the primary prevention of CHD. With a scope and precision not previously attainable, based on data from the 1970s and 1980s, they confirm conclusions reached on the basis of data from earlier prospective epidemiologic studies begun in the late 1940s, 1950s, and 1960s (*e.g.*, those of the national cooperative Pooling Project). The Pooling Project life-table analyses add a further dimension concerning the combined impact of three of the major risk factors, because they give data on long-term cumulative risk from age 40 through age 64, that is, a 25-year span of middle age (Table 59.8).[49,50] In these data, the full scope of the modern CHD epidemic is laid bare: for the entire cohort, the overall risk of a first major coronary event (nonfatal myocardial infarction or CHD death) before age 65 was almost one in four (221 per 1,000). For the 20% of men in the lowest quintile of risk, based on joint assessment of the three established major risk factors, the probability of a first major coronary event was about 1 in 17 (58 per 1,000). For American men in the 1950s and 1960s, this was a relatively low risk, but hardly a miniscule risk absolutely. Moreover, it was a good deal higher than that in all Japanese and Chinese men over this age span, reflecting first and foremost contrasting patterns of diet and serum cholesterol. Whereas men in the Pooling Project in the lowest quintile of risk had a mean serum cholesterol of 206 mg/dl, representative groups of middle-aged men in Japan and China have repeatedly shown overall mean levels no greater than 180 mg/dl and as low as 158 mg/dl.[17,42,51] Thus, as the data for the lowest risk group in the MRFIT screenee cohort also show, the status of men in quintile 1 of the Pooling Project may be viewed as a first, but by no means an optimal and final, goal for American men. This is further evidenced from the rates of hypercholesterolemia, hypertension, and cigarette smoking prevalent even in this quintile.[49,50]

As to the men of the United States Pooling Project in the highest 20% of risk (quintile 5) based on their high levels of the three major risk factors, their risk of a first major coronary event by age 65 was well over 1 in 3 (396 per 1,000), almost seven times greater than that in the lowest quintile (see Table 59.8).[49,50]

Excess risk was widely spread throughout the cohort, twice as great for the second quintile as for the first, three times greater for the third quintile, and four times greater for the fourth quintile (Table 59.8).[49,50] More than half (51%) the total excess risk was in quintiles 2, 3, and 4; the remaining 49%, in quintile 5. These findings, along with the MRFIT and multiple other data sets on the ubiquity of excess risk in the United States population, document the essentiality of a two-pronged strategy for the prevention and control of epidemic premature CHD, that is, the need for population-wide improvements in life-styles to shift the distributions of the major risk factors downward for the whole population plus special pinpointed efforts for the higher risk strata. Actual achieve-

TABLE 59.8 THREE MAJOR RISK FACTORS AND RISK OF A FIRST MAJOR CORONARY EVENT BETWEEN AGES 40 TO 64 IN 8,162 WHITE MEN, POOL 5, POOLING PROJECT, FINAL REPORT

Quintile of Level	Number of Events	Risk of an Event per 1,000	Relative Risk	Absolute Excess Risk per 1,000	Per Cent of All Excess
I	23	57.9	1.00		
II	66	118.3	2.04	60.4	8.7%
III	107	168.0	2.90	110.1	15.9%
IV	167	241.1	4.16	183.2	26.5%
V	271	395.7	6.83	337.8	48.9%
All	634	221.0			

$$\frac{\text{QII–V Excess Events, 4,000 Men}}{\text{All Events, 5,000 Men}} = \frac{691.5}{981.0} = 70.5\% \text{ of all events are excess events, attributable to the three major risk factors.}$$

(Data from Pooling Project Research Group: Relationship of blood pressure, serum cholesterol, smoking habit, relative weight and ECG abnormalities to incidence of major coronary events: Final report of the Pooling Project. J Chronic Dis 31:210–306, 1978)

ments by the United States population in the last decade or two are summarized below. Because people with clinically manifest CHD are at especially high risk of acute events and death, and because their prognosis is significantly and sizably influenced by their status in regard to the major risk factors, they must be included among the higher risk strata deserving special attention as part of this two-pronged strategy.

The data in Table 59.8 also permit an estimate of the proportion of all first major coronary events that were excess events, attributable to the presence of hypercholesterolemia, hypertension, or cigarette smoking, or a combination of these, to a degree greater than that in quintile 1. The excess risk of an event before age 65, over and above the risk for quintile 1 (57.9 per 1,000 men), was 60.4, 110.1, 183.2, and 337.8 per 1,000 men for quintiles 2, 3, 4, and 5, respectively, with an average excess risk for these four quintiles of 172.9 per 1,000 men. These excess risks summate to 691.5 excess events per 4,000 men in quintiles 2 to 5. Total or absolute risk per 5,000 men in quintiles 1 to 5 is the sum of the age-adjusted rates per 1,000 persons, that is, 981.0 per 5,000 men (57.9 + 118.3 + 168.0 + 241.1 + 395.7, Table 59.8).[49,50] Therefore, the proportion of all events that were excess events is 691.5 of 981.0 (*i.e.*, 70.5%).

This calculation is also an estimate of the potential that existed for prevention of premature CHD among middle-aged American men in the 1950s and 1960s. With shifts downward in the distributions of the established major risk factors (*e.g.*, as a first goal) to levels for the whole middle-aged population like those prevailing for the lowest quintile of risk, it may be projected that about 70% of all first major coronary events before age 65 could have been prevented. Over the last two decades, the distributions of the three major risk factors have indeed been moving downward, with sizable declines in mean levels of serum cholesterol and in prevalence rates of hypercholesterolemia, hypertension, and cigarette smoking for the adult population (see below). Concomitantly, death rates from premature CHD have decreased steadily and substantially from the mid or late 1960s to the early 1980s, by about 40% overall (see below). These data support the central thesis of this chapter, that the contemporary mass onslaught of CHD, like earlier forms of epidemic disease, is preventable.

THE PRIMARY AND ESSENTIAL ROLE OF "RICH" DIET, PARTICULARLY DIETARY LIPID, IN THE CAUSATION OF EPIDEMIC PREMATURE CORONARY HEART DISEASE

Extensive data on the role of "rich" diet are now available from epidemiologic investigations of both the interpopulation and intrapopulation type. In the former, also called cross-population or ecologic studies, the units under investigation are whole groups, and the data used in the analyses are for whole groups, for example, the mean intake of dietary lipids for the populations of several countries and their relationship to CHD death rates of these populations. In such a study, and many like it, data on the individuals making up the groups are not even available to the investigators. In contrast, the focus of intrapopulation studies is on the individual members of a population—traits of individuals and how they relate to disease risk.

The interpopulation or ecologic studies take advantage of opportunities to evaluate the effects of markedly different life-styles of different populations, for example, the contrasting levels of mean per capita dietary lipid intake in different populations. This is their strength. Inability to characterize individuals and their risk is their main limitation, plus constraints in dealing with possible confounding variables.

Interpopulation research on diet and CHD has used three types of data: (1) data generally available on countries and their subunits, from official sources (*e.g.*, government departments, the United Nations and its related bodies, including the Food and Agriculture Organization [FAO], and the World Health Organization [WHO]; (2) autopsy data, gathered from the records of routine autopsies or systematically collected in special investigations; and (3) data on samples of living populations undergoing systematic investigation. The many interpopulation studies over the decades, particularly since World War II, have yielded highly consistent findings on the relationship of "rich" diet, especially high intake of cholesterol and saturated fat, to CHD risk.

INTERPOPULATION EPIDEMIOLOGIC RESEARCH

ANALYSES OF DATA FROM OFFICIAL SOURCES. At least 12 multinational analyses have been reported based on data from FAO and WHO.[10,40,52] All of them consistently show statistically significant univariate associations between dietary constituents and mortality from CHD. These encompass significant positive associations between dietary saturated fat, cholesterol, animal fat, total fat, total protein, animal protein, animal foodstuffs (meats, dairy products, eggs), refined and processed sugars, total calories and CHD mortality rates in middle age. Significant negative correlations with CHD mortality were shown for vegetable protein, vegetable fat, vegetable foodstuffs (grains, legumes, vegetables, and fruits), total carbohydrate, and, in one study, wine.

Univariate analyses using these official data on mean per capita intake of macronutrients and major food groups yield high-order significant positive associations between many of these variables and CHD death rates. In the evaluation of these data and their possible etiologic import it is relevant that most of these nutritional variables are themselves highly intercorrelated, reflecting the fact that "richness" of national diets is a function of per capita national income. When variables are highly intercorrelated (*e.g.*, a simple correlation coefficient ≥ 0.5), they cannot be entered simultaneously into multiple regression and partial correlation analyses due to the likelihood of spurious results. Moreover, even with as many as 20 or 30 countries in the analyses, this is a relatively small number, limiting the number of independent variables that can simultaneously be considered in multivariate analyses. Given these problems, analyses have been done of two variables at a time, with use of the techniques of bivariate cross-classification and analysis of variance, rather than bivariate regression and partial correlation. As shown in Table 59.9, such analyses indicate that the dietary lipid components—cholesterol, saturated fat, and polyunsaturated fat, considered together by means of the equations of Keys and co-workers and Hegsted and co-workers—relate to CHD mortality independently of several other nutrients–foodstuffs.[52] This was not the case for either refined and processed sugars or per capita estimated intake of fiber from vegetable products.

Evaluation of the etiologic import of these statistically significant associations requires their assessment in relation to the totality of the data, that is, along with multiple other data sets collected by different methods (epidemiologic, pathologic, clinical, animal–experimental), and use of the above-cited guidelines to weigh causative implications —strength of the associations, their graded relationship, temporal relationship, consistency, independence, predictive capacity, and coherence.

International data from official sources have also been used to assess whether there is a relationship between the time-trend of dietary factors and the time-trend of CHD mortality. Significant associations were found between the slopes of dietary cholesterol intake and the slopes of CHD death rate, and between the slopes of animal product intake and the slopes of CHD death rate.[40,52,53]

Concordant findings have also come from similar analyses of these kinds of data, to evaluate trends over time within individual countries. One of the most seminal of such studies was by Malmros, shortly after World War II, on pre-war and wartime death rates due to atherosclerotic disease for several European countries.[20,54] The data indicate that wartime dietary restriction, including marked curtailment of egg, dairy product, and total fat intake, was associated with a definite decrease in deaths due to atherosclerosis. Other investigators presented similar findings from Finland and Russia.[20] The monograph by Keys and associates, *The Biology of Human Starvation*, reviewed additional data from Germany, France, and Belgium.[55]

Official data have also been used to assess effects of migration, for example, CHD death rates in Italy and Japan have been compared with those for Italian–Americans and Japanese–Americans.[21] The latter groups tend to have CHD death rates similar to those of their fellow Americans and considerably higher than age-matched and sex-matched Italians and Japanese. This is in accordance with the inference that life-styles, including dietary habits, acquired in the adopted country play the key role in influencing CHD risk, and not population genetics.

AUTOPSY STUDIES. As long ago as the 1920s, the German pathologist Aschoff commented that autopsy findings indicated regression of atherosclerosis in central Europe during the post-World War I years of famine, "when a shortage of eggs, milk and butter was an outstanding characteristic of the diet."[56] Beitzke reported a like finding in autopsy material during those years of fat-poor nourishment in Germany.[57] Similar data and inferences emerged from European research centers studying the effects of famine during and right after World War II.[55,58]

In the early 1950s, an analysis was done of 10,000 postmortem records in Kyushu, Japan, and the findings were compared with those reported from Minnesota (Fig. 59.2).[59,60] Myocardial infarction (MI) was found in only 75 cases in the Japanese material; severe coronary atherosclerosis was also rare, about one-tenth that of persons of the

TABLE 59.9 DIETARY LIPID SCORE, REFINED AND PROCESSED SUGAR (1954–1965) AND CORONARY HEART DISEASE MORTALITY RATES (1969–1973), MEN AND WOMEN AGE 35 TO 74, 20-COUNTRY STUDY

	Bivariate Classification of 20 Countries				
Variable	Lipid Score* ≤45.5 Sugar <14.1% Calories	Lipid Score >45.5 Sugar <14.1% Calories	Lipid Score ≤45.5 Sugar ≥14.1% Calories	Lipid Score >45.5 Sugar ≥14.1% Calories	All
Men					
No. of countries	7†	3‡	3§	7‖	20
Lipid score	34.6 ± 12.0	51.6 ± 3.4	35.0 ± 6.5	54.5 ± 7.2	44.2 ± 12.8
Sugar (% calories)	11.1 ± 2.6	12.8 ± 1.4	15.6 ± 1.1	16.0 ± 1.2	13.7 ± 2.8
CHD death rate (per 100,000/year)	346.3	659.9	472.1	705.9	538.1
Analysis of variance: lipid score, $P = 0.002$; sugar, $P = 0.264$; interaction, $P = 0.599$					
Women					
No. of countries	7*	3†	3‡	7§	20
Lipid score	34.6 ± 12.0	51.6 ± 3.4	35.0 ± 6.5	54.5 ± 7.2	44.2 ± 12.8
Sugar (% calories)	11.1 ± 2.6	12.8 ± 1.4	15.6 ± 1.1	16.0 ± 1.2	13.7 ± 2.8
CHD death rate (per 100,000/year)	146.8	239.9	185.6	275.7	211.7
Analysis of variance: lipid score, $P = 0.021$; sugar, $P = 0.313$; interaction, $P = 0.967$					

* Lipid score was calculated by Keys equation, $1.35(2S-P) + 1.5Z$, where S is the percent of calories from saturated fatty acids, P is the percent of polyunsaturated fatty acids, and Z is the square root of dietary cholesterol in mg per 1000 calories.

† Austria, France, German Fed. Rep., Israel, Italy, Japan, Switzerland

‡ Belgium, Finland, Ireland

§ Netherlands, Norway, Venezuela

‖ Australia, Canada, Denmark, New Zealand, Sweden, United Kingdom, United States

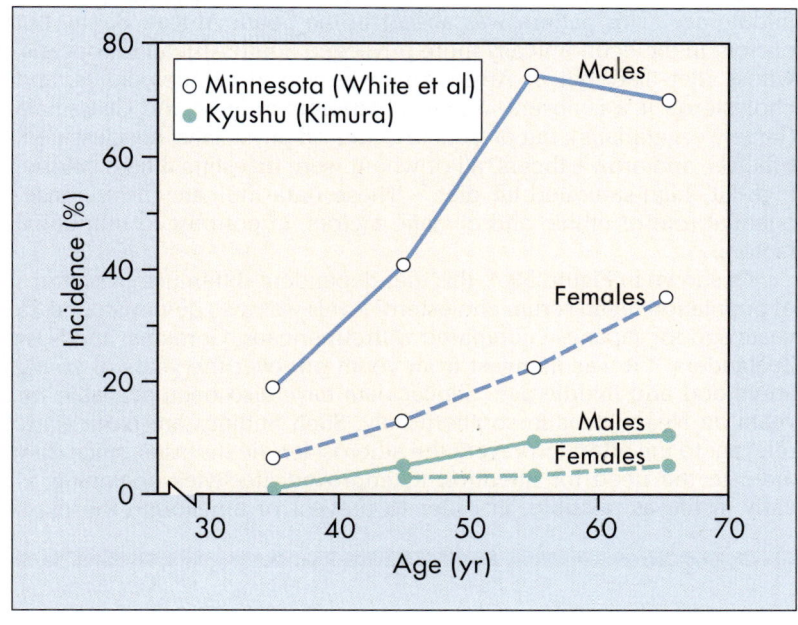

FIGURE 59.2 High-grade coronary sclerosis in consecutive autopsies, by age and sex, United States versus Japan. (Data from Kimura N: Analysis of 10,000 postmortem examinations in Japan. In Keys A, White PD (eds): World Trends in Cardiology: I. Cardiovascular Epidemiology, p 22. New York, Hoeber-Harper, 1956; and White NK, Edwards JE, Dry TJ: The relationship of the degree of coronary atherosclerosis with age, in men. Circulation 1:645–654, 1950)

same age in the United States. These findings corresponded with the marked differences in diet and in age-specific death rates from CHD in the two countries.

Throughout the post–World War II era, Japan has continued to be distinctive among the highly industrialized countries for its comparatively low CHD mortality rates. Japan is also unusual among these countries in regard to low per capita intake of total fat, saturated fat, cholesterol, and calories.[10,17,21,22,40,52]

Other reports in the 1950s noted the rarity of MI and severe coronary atherosclerosis at autopsy among the peoples of Africa, Asia, and Latin America.[21,22]

The International Atherosclerosis Project (IAP) has been the most systematic and comprehensive study of this type.[19] It quantified the degree of atherosclerosis of the aorta and coronary arteries at autopsy in over 31,000 persons age 10 to 69 who died between 1960 and 1965 in 15 cities and countries throughout the world, two of them highly industrialized populations (New Orleans and Oslo) with relatively high annual per capita income and the remaining 13 largely nonindustrialized low-income populations of Latin America, Africa, and the Far East. Marked differences among populations were recorded in the extent of severe atherosclerosis (aortic and coronary), and strong correlations were noted between percentage of calories from total fat in the habitual diets of the populations and population mean serum cholesterol levels, between dietary fat and occurrence of advanced atherosclerotic lesions, and between population mean serum cholesterol and occurrence of advanced atherosclerotic lesions.[19] Data on saturated fat and dietary cholesterol were not reported; egg intake, a major source of dietary cholesterol, was reported as generally paralleling total fat and protein intake, but the data were too fragmentary for reliable ranking. Level of animal protein consumption was also significantly related to severity of atherosclerosis. The authors commented, ". . . it was not considered etiologically important because of the strong supporting evidence for a primary role of fat, rather than protein, in determining . . . severity of atherosclerosis, and incidence of CHD."[19] Other dietary variables, including sugar consumption, were not significantly related to severity of atherosclerosis.

The IAP also noted that findings indicative of hypertension and diabetes were also related to severity of atherosclerosis, conspicuously and consistently for the decedents of the industrialized countries, and less clearly and regularly for those from the nonindustrialized nations.[19] These findings are in accord with two basic conclusions about atherosclerotic disease: first, its multifactorial etiology and pathogenesis; second, the central and essential role of "rich" diet in establishing the metabolic prerequisites for mass occurrence of severe atherosclerosis. Thus, authors reporting Far Eastern experience had earlier observed that with the predominantly vegetarian diets there (*i.e.*, diets high in complex carbohydrates and low in cholesterol, saturated fat, and total fat), mild maturity-onset diabetes was not associated with a tendency to severe atherosclerotic disease, in contrast to the situation in the West.[61] Recently, others have arrived at the same conclusion.[62] Data from Africa and Japan, as well as animal–experimental evidence, have also pointed to a similar inference concerning the role of "rich" diet as a precondition for hypertension-induced aggravation of atherogenesis.

The foregoing anatomical studies of the IAP involved gross, not microscopic, grading of lesions. They distinguished grossly between fatty streaks, regarded as early-stage atherosclerotic lesions, and advanced raised atherosclerotic lesions (including fibrous plaques and lesions complicated by ulceration, thrombosis, hemorrhage, or calcification), regarded as developing from fatty streaks.[19] The IAP investigators also did histologic studies of randomly selected coronary artery and aortic fatty streaks of males age 10 to 39 years from seven location–race groups exhibiting a wide range of extent of advanced lesions in later decades. Microscopically assessed amounts of intimal lipid and cellular infiltration of coronary fatty streaks were significantly correlated, and both of these were significantly related to fibrous plaques.

Populations with higher fat intakes and serum cholesterol levels tended to have more coronary fatty streaks in youth and young adulthood (as seen grossly), more lipid and cellular infiltration in these fatty streaks (as seen microscopically), and more advanced lesions in middle age.[19,63] These data give added meaning to the significant associations shown by the IAP among dietary lipid, serum cholesterol, and gross grading for advanced atherosclerosis (aortic and coronary).

STUDIES OF LIVING POPULATION SAMPLES. Among the many investigations comparing living population samples in different countries, the Seven Countries Study is the most comprehensive.[1,17,18] This prospective study of 16 population samples in seven countries—Finland, Greece, Italy, Japan, Netherlands, United States, and Yugoslavia—included 12,763 men originally age 40 to 59. It has yielded key data on the interrelationships among habitual diet, serum cholesterol, and CHD. Analyses of the diets on random samples of the populations showed that amount and type of lipid habitually eaten, especially saturated fat (and inevitably cholesterol), varied markedly among the population samples. While saturated fat intake was low for the Japanese villagers and several of the southern European groups, it was high for the men in Finland, the Netherlands, and the United States, 17% to 22% of calories (total fat 35%–40%). Polyunsaturated fat intake was never high (3%–5% of calories). Baseline saturated fat intakes and 5-year and 10-year CHD rates for these population samples were highly and significantly correlated, as were saturated fat intake and serum cholesterol, and serum cholesterol and CHD rates (Figs. 59.1 and 59.3).[1,17]

Most of the other components of the chemically analyzed diets—total calories, monounsaturated fat, polyunsaturated fat, and total protein—were not significantly related to serum cholesterol levels or CHD rates. Total fat intakes and CHD rates were correlated, but the correlation with saturated fat was much more significant. Dietary cholesterol was not evaluated. Sucrose intakes, significantly correlated with saturated fat intakes ($r = 0.84$), were significantly correlated with CHD rates in univariate analyses, but not after controlling for saturated fat intake; saturated fat intakes remained significantly related to CHD rates after controlling for sucrose intakes.[1,17]

Many other international comparisons have yielded data in accordance with those of the Seven Countries Study. These have included reports on the markedly different findings in the nonindustrialized and industrialized sectors of the world. Consistently, groups of clinically normal people in the economically less developed nations, ingesting predominantly vegetarian diets low in cholesterol, lipids, and calories, had mean plasma cholesterol–lipid–betalipoprotein levels significantly lower than groups of clinically normal persons in the United States. Moreover, they exhibited a different pattern of change in plasma cholesterol level with age. Thus, for Americans, plasma cholesterol levels tended to rise sizably with each decade of life, from youth well into middle age. This pattern was absent in the South African Bantu, but present in the economically more privileged South African Europeans, whose diet, like that of Americans, was rich in calories, lipids, and cholesterol. It was absent in manual laborers in India and Guatemala (largely vegetarians), but present in better-off physicians, businessmen, officials, and army officers, all of whom were ingesting a high-calorie, high-fat, high-saturated-fat diet.[21] These data indicate the inconsequential role of ethnic and climatic factors, in contrast to nutritional factors.

As shown in Figure 59.4, this diet-dependent difference in patterns of population mean serum cholesterol levels was also demonstrated 25 years ago for Japanese compared with Americans, Germans, and New Zealanders.[64] It was manifest from youth on, over the years of young adulthood and middle age. Similar data have also been available for years on Neapolitans in southern Italy. Such findings are particularly relevant to the effort to prevent the atherosclerotic diseases, since they indicate the need for attention to improved life-styles beginning as early in life as possible, in order to prevent or ameliorate the mass emergence of hypercholesterolemia and the other established major risk factors.[37,47,48]

Thus, for at least a quarter of a century there have been sufficient data to cast serious doubt on the validity of standards commonly accepted in the United States for normal serum cholesterol concentration. They indicate that lifelong pattern of diet was inducing a chronic hypercholesterolemia in a majority of Americans, contributing decisively to widespread atherogenesis. They further suggested that optimal serum cholesterol levels, for optimal freedom from atherosclerotic disease over an optimal life span, are considerably lower than those common in the United States population, due to the "richness" of the diet.

Among the international studies of living population samples, those dealing with the effects of migration have also yielded important findings. In the 1950s, several reports were published indicating that changes in mode of life, particularly shift to a "richer" diet as a result of emigration from a less affluent part of the world to a more affluent western country, were associated with higher levels of serum cholesterol and higher CHD incidence and mortality rates. Studies of this type were done on Yemenite Jews in Israel, including comparisons with Ashkenazi and Sephardic Jews there; on Neapolitans in Naples and Boston; on Italians generally compared to Italian–Americans; and on Japanese compared to Japanese–Americans (in Hawaii, California, and in the United States overall).[21,22]

Among the most highly industrialized countries, as noted above, Japan stands out in stark contrast to all others by virtue of its low CHD mortality rates. Understandably, therefore, comparisons between population samples in Japan and western countries and between Japanese migrants to the United States and Japanese in Japan have been a primary focus of epidemiologic research. A major study of this kind was initiated in 1965 with middle-aged men of Japanese ancestry living in Hiroshima and Nagasaki, Japan; in Honolulu, Hawaii; and in the San

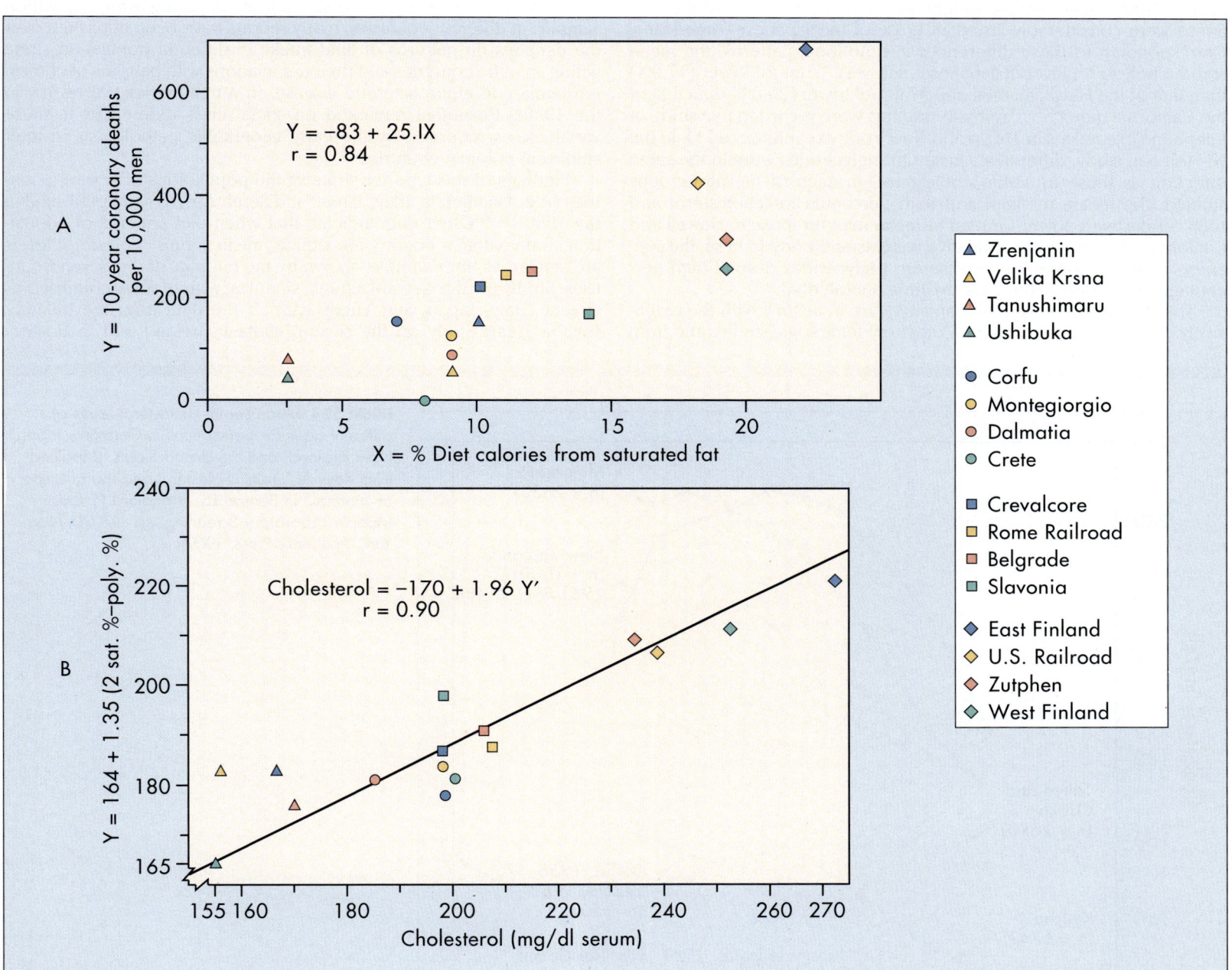

FIGURE 59.3 Results of the Seven Countries Study. **A.** Ten-year coronary death rates of the cohorts plotted against the percentage of dietary calories supplied by saturated fatty acids. **B.** Relation of mean serum cholesterol concentration of the cohorts at entry to fat composition of the diet expressed in the multiple regression equation derived from controlled dietary experiments in Minnesota. (Modified from Keys A (ed): Seven Countries—A Multivariate Analysis of Death and Coronary Heart Disease. Cambridge, Harvard University Press, 1980)

Francisco Bay Area (the Ni-Hon-San study). At baseline, nutritional patterns of the three populations were assessed by a 24-hour dietary recall, plus a dietary acculturation questionnaire designed to ascertain the traditional "Japaneseness" of each man's eating pattern. Eight foods (e.g., soybean curd, rice, seaweeds) were considered as indicators of traditional Japanese food habits; three (fish, meat, eggs) as neutral or common to all; nine (e.g., ice cream, bread, potatoes) as indicators of Americanization. Based on both methods, differences between the Japanese and the two Japanese–American population samples were striking. Whereas the great majority of the men in Hiroshima and Nagasaki were eating a diet made up chiefly of typically Japanese foods, this was not true for the men in Hawaii and California. Nutrient analyses indicated that group mean intakes of total fat, saturated fat, and animal protein were much lower in the Japanese than in the Japanese–American men.[52,65-70] Group mean intakes of dietary cholesterol, simple carbohydrate, total protein, and unsaturated fat were also lower in the Japanese. Group mean intakes of total carbohydrate, complex carbohydrate, alcohol, and salt were higher in the Japanese. Group mean relative weight and skinfold thickness of the Japanese were considerably less than those of the Japanese–Americans. Corresponding to these differences in nutritional patterns, the mean serum cholesterol level of Japanese men was 37 mg/dl lower (17.0%) than that of the Hawaiian men and 47 mg/dl lower (20.6%) than that of the California men.[52,65-70] (Similar findings were recorded in a study of telephone executives in Tokyo and New York; see reference 71). In the Ni-Hon-San study, differences in serum triglycerides were in the same direction as those in serum cholesterol. In each of the age groups studied, the mean, median, and 95th percentile for cholesterol and triglycerides were lower for men in Japan than for those in Hawaii and California. With their lower relative weights and body fatness, the Japanese men had lower levels of serum triglycerides despite high percentages of calories from carbohydrate and alcohol.

The data from the Ni-Hon-San study are in accord with the extensively documented findings from other epidemiologic studies and from interventional experiments in humans in controlled (institutionalized) and free-living circumstances that dietary lipids (saturated fat, cholesterol, polyunsaturated fat) play a key role in the long-term determination of human serum cholesterol patterns.

Data are now available from this study on CHD prevalence, incidence, and mortality.[68-70] Prevalence rates of the various forms of CHD at baseline were generally lower in the Japanese compared with the Japanese–American men, especially compared to the California group. Analyses of death certificates after 4 to 5 years of follow-up showed age-specific CHD death rates for all three groups to be lower than those for American whites. The CHD death rates were consistently and significantly lower for the Japanese than for the Japanese–American men. Correspondingly, marked differences were reported in incidence of myocardial infarction and CHD death for the three cohorts. The incidence rate was lowest for the Japanese. The Hawaiian men had an age-standardized rate 2.1 times that of the Japanese men; the California men, 1.5 times that of the Hawaiian men and 3.2 times that of the Japanese men.

In addition to the international studies comparing living population samples in different countries, many reports have been published over the decades on patterns of lipid intake in different population strata within specific countries and their associations with patterns of cholesterolemia and atherosclerotic disease. In a comprehensive review in the 1930s, Rosenthal remarked on social class differences in these variables, as recorded by the early geographic pathologists in their studies in colonial countries.[72]

Findings of this type for strata of the populations of several countries (e.g., Guatemala, Italy, Japan, and South Africa) were published in the 1950s.[21,22] Other data indicate that when diet patterns of population strata within a country are similar, mean serum cholesterol levels are similar, as, for example, shown by the findings of the Seven Countries Study on the several chunk samples within such countries as Greece, Italy, Japan, and Yugoslavia,[21,22] the data from the Ireland–Boston Heart Study on the several strata in Ireland and in Boston,

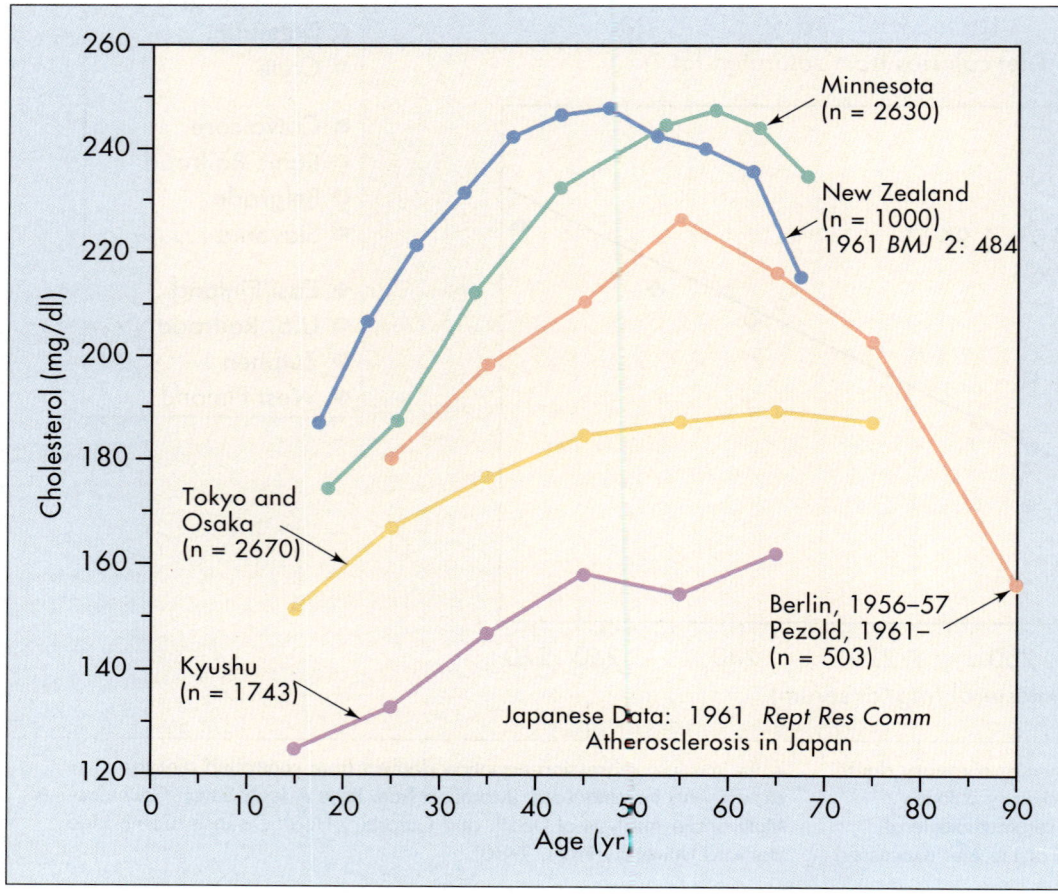

FIGURE 59.4 Mean serum cholesterol levels at different ages for populations in Germany, Japan, New Zealand, and the United States. (Modified from Keys A: Serum cholesterol and the question of "normal." In Benson ES, Strandjord PE (eds): Multiple Laboratory Screening, pp 147–170. New York, Academic Press, 1969)

respectively,[73,74] and the findings of the Ni-Hon-San Study of Japanese–Americans in Hawaii and the San Francisco Bay area.[52,65-70] Other reports, from Belgium, Israel, Italy, the Solomon Islands, and Yugoslavia, for example, have yielded further data along these lines.[10] The Solomon Islands data are also intriguing in terms of their much lower mean levels compared to values for Americans.[75]

Repeated studies of population samples of United States adults in the 1950s and 1960s yielded similar high mean serum cholesterol levels, reflecting similar group mean patterns of dietary lipid intake across the country, irrespective of region, income, urban or rural status, or occupation.[10,22] Therefore, to assess effects of diets of differing lipid composition on mean serum cholesterol of Americans, special groups had to be identified (e.g., Navajo Indians and Trappist monks). In accordance with their lower intake of saturated fat and cholesterol, mean serum cholesterol levels were lower for such groups than those of age-matched and sex-matched Americans from the general population.[10,21,22] Correspondingly, as intakes of saturated fat and cholesterol by Americans in general declined during the last 15 years, population mean serum cholesterol levels also fell (see below).

Within the general United States population, studies of vegetarians have also yielded meaningful and clear-cut data. An early study compared nutritional and serum cholesterol findings on groups of lacto-ovo-vegetarians, pure vegetarians, and groups eating usual American omnivorous diets.[76] The differences in serum cholesterol in the three groups were sizable and clear-cut. The pure vegetarians, eating no eggs, dairy foods, meats, or any other animal products, and therefore ingesting a cholesterol-free diet low in saturated fat (but with an average intake of 130 g vegetable fat per day, 35% of total calories), had a mean serum cholesterol 29% lower than the omnivores, and the lacto-ovo-vegetarians were 16% lower than the omnivores; an unequivocal indication of the capacity of Americans to have sizably lower serum cholesterol levels when ingesting diets different in lipid composition from usual ones.

Another such data set is available from a study comparing residents of a Boston commune (where a so-called macrobiotic diet was eaten) and age-matched people from Framingham, Massachusetts, ingesting usual American fare. The macrobiotic diet, relying principally on whole grains, beans, and fresh vegetables as staples, resembled a Japanese diet. Fish was reportedly consumed at least once a week by about 40% of the commune residents. Only 28% reported such frequent consumption of dairy products; 11%, eggs; and none, poultry or meat. Compared to the group of controls, the vegetarians' mean serum cholesterol as well as their LDL-cholesterol and VLDL-cholesterol were markedly and significantly lower.[77] These large differences, ranging from 31% to 38%, could not be accounted for by the lower weights of the vegetarians. Multiple regression analyses showed that for the vegetarians, avoidance of animal products in general, and specifically of eggs and dairy foods in the preceding week, was associated with low levels of serum cholesterol and cholesterol-bearing LDL and VLDL.

An additional comparison of this type also gives data on mortality for three groups of California Seventh Day Adventists (nonvegetarian, lacto-ovo-vegetarian, and pure vegetarian) compared to the general population in California. Seventh Day Adventists consuming habitual lacto-ovo-vegetarian diets had lower mean serum cholesterol levels than Americans generally. Long-term follow-up of the status of 47,000 Seventh Day Adventists in California revealed much lower age-standardized CHD mortality rates for the three groups of Adventists than those found in the general population. For men age 35 and over, CHD mortality rates were 34% lower for the nonvegetarians, 57% lower for the lacto-ovo-vegetarians, and 77% lower for the pure vegetarians.[78]

Seventh Day Adventists differ from the general population also in abstaining from both alcohol and tobacco, and tending to avoid coffee, other caffeine-containing beverages, hot condiments and spices, and highly refined foods. Instead, the Adventists use whole grains, vegetables, and nuts abundantly. Thus, it is likely that the superior prognosis of the Seventh Day Adventist population in regard to CHD is a result of multiple differences in life-style, including eating, smoking, and drinking habits. In any case, these and other data on American Seventh Day Adventists (see below) further confirm the etiologically significant relationship among habitual diet (particularly its lipid composition), population mean serum cholesterol levels, and CHD.

INTRAPOPULATION EPIDEMIOLOGIC RESEARCH
"RICH" DIET, PARTICULARLY HIGH DIETARY LIPID INTAKE AND CALORIE IMBALANCE, OF INDIVIDUALS AND THEIR SERUM CHOLESTEROL LEVELS.

In the foregoing section, extensive data were presented demonstrating that for population groups a significant relationship exists between mean intake of dietary lipid and mean serum cholesterol level. In particular, the higher the population mean intake of cholesterol and saturated fat, the higher the population mean serum cholesterol level. In addition, higher population mean polyunsaturated fat intake is associated with modestly lower population mean serum cholesterol levels.

However, epidemiologic studies on this matter in regard to individuals within a population have yielded inconsistent results, and this has been puzzling until recently. Thus, several studies reported either no association or only low-order, nonsignificant correlations between individual dietary lipids (e.g., dietary cholesterol, saturated fat) and serum cholesterol as measured for individuals within a population. In contrast, other investigations have found significant positive associations. The negative results have been puzzling given the data from several other lines of investigation showing that dietary lipid intakes of individuals do have a sizable effect on their serum cholesterol levels. Thus, the influence of dietary saturated and polyunsaturated fatty acids and of dietary cholesterol on level of serum cholesterol has been well established in controlled experimental studies under isocaloric conditions. Decreasing the proportion of calories from saturated fat, increasing the proportion from polyunsaturated fat, and decreasing the amount of cholesterol in the diet of individuals will, on the average, lower their serum cholesterol by predictable amounts. These results demonstrating the effect of dietary lipid on serum cholesterol in humans are consistent with those from interpopulation studies (see above), diet intervention programs (in both free-living and institutionalized populations), and animal-experimental research.[1,10,17-22,25-27,35-37,50,52,76,77,79]

In recent years, this paradox has been systematically explored, and several factors have been pinpointed as responsible for the reported negative or nonsignificant findings. First, cross-sectional correlations between dietary lipid and serum cholesterol are biased toward zero by differences between individuals in nondietary factors affecting level of serum cholesterol (e.g., genetic factors) not specifically quantifiable at present, hence not amenable to adjustment in statistical analyses. This bias can be avoided by correlating *change* in diet with *change* in serum cholesterol if the nondietary factors remain constant. Second, in cultures with a highly varied food supply, individual variation from day to day in consumption of a dietary factor (e.g., saturated fat) is usually as large as or larger than the variation between persons. Under such circumstances, a single 24-hour dietary recall or a brief dietary history cannot validly distinguish one person from another. The inevitable result again is to bias correlations toward zero. This bias cannot be avoided simply by increasing the sample size, but it can be controlled by increasing the number of measurements of diet for each person.[9,80] Third, other factors also tend to obscure the association between dietary lipid and serum cholesterol, for example, inaccuracies in the procedures for assessing diet in free-living populations; restricted variability of dietary factors within populations (as compared to variability among populations); use of analyses involving only one dietary lipid (e.g., saturated fat) without controlling for the others known to influence serum cholesterol; or selective change in diet among persons after learning that they are hypercholesterolemic.[81] The same prolems exist for studies attempting to assess the relationship between the dietary intake of individuals within a population and their risk of subsequent CHD.

In regard to this set of problems, it is instructive to note in greater detail the results of the two studies recently reporting positive results. One is unique in that it dealt with the Tarahumara Indians of northern Mexico, a population with little intraindividual variability in diet, that is, a diet for individuals that by usual American standards would be regarded as very monotonous. Under this circumstance, a large, significant correlation between dietary cholesterol and plasma total cholesterol was recorded ($r = 0.898$, $P < 0.01$).[82]

As to the second, among prospective epidemiologic investigations of western industrialized populations, the Western Electric Company study is unique in regard to nutritional data, since in-depth diet histories were taken on almost all men in the cohort at both the entry and first annual examinations in 1958 and 1959.[83] The standardized interview method yielded information on average daily intake of nutrients over the preceding 28 days. Trivariate analysis of the 1958 baseline data showed dietary cholesterol and percent of calories from saturated fat to be significantly related to serum cholesterol; the P value for percent of calories from polyunsaturated fat was nearly significant.[53,83] In the 5-factor analysis, the relationship between dietary saturated fat and serum cholesterol remained significant; body mass index (BMI) was also significantly related to serum cholesterol. Combined dietary lipid score, computed from the equation of Keys and associates, also was significantly related to serum cholesterol ($P < 0.001$), as was BMI.

At the first annual reexamination in 1959, sizable numbers of men with high baseline serum cholesterol reported changes in their dietary lipid intake, having been informed after the entry survey that they were hypercholesterolemic. For the whole cohort, change in dietary cholesterol, saturated fat, combined lipid score, and body mass index from entry to year 1 and change in serum cholesterol were significantly related.[53,83]

These and other recent data show that there is concordance in findings from all types of studies—interpopulation and interindividual epidemiologic investigations, interventional experiments on groups of people, and animal research—on the effects of dietary lipid and of calorie balance on serum cholesterol. The interventional studies in humans further show that while there are differences in responsiveness of serum cholesterol of individuals to change in dietary lipid, the overall finding for the human species as a whole is that serum total cholesterol responds significantly to changes in dietary lipid (i.e., to changes in both amount and type of neutral fat [saturates, polyunsaturates] and in dietary cholesterol). This is the case also for the main atherogenic fraction of serum TC: LDL-C.

"RICH" DIET, PARTICULARLY CALORIE IMBALANCE, HIGH SODIUM INTAKE, HEAVY ALCOHOL INTAKE OF INDIVIDUALS AND THEIR BLOOD PRESSURE LEVELS. Many epidemiologic studies all over the world have shown a significant association between overweight and prevalence of elevated blood pressure levels, in children, youth, young adults, middle-aged adults, and the elderly. This relationship is independent of other correlates of high blood pressure (HBP), including those that are related to life-style and diet (e.g., hyperuricemia, hyperglycemia, hypercholesterolemia, rapid pulse).[84] Prospective data show that both overweight at baseline and gain in weight by persons normotensive at baseline are significantly and independently related to risk of developing HBP. All these findings are concordant with clinical evidence on ability to lower HBP of obese people by weight reduction.

In contrast to the overwhelming mass of epidemiologic data relating calorie imbalance to blood pressure of individuals, the evidence from within-population studies on dietary sodium and blood pressure is limited and inconsistent. Exploration of this matter has been fraught with all the difficulties described above in regard to the dietary lipid–serum cholesterol relationship, plus one other, which is the virtual impossibility of estimating sodium intake in large numbers of free-living individuals by nutritional assessment methods, with the consequent need to rely on multiple timed urine collections (24-hour or overnight) properly done by each person.[85-87] Despite this major difficulty, recent studies using urine-collection methods have yielded significant positive findings of an independent association between excretion of sodium or sodium and potassium (as indicators of electrolyte intake) and blood pressure.[29,36,88,89] These data are concordant with those from anthropology, interpopulation epidemiologic research, physiologic and clinical investigation (including randomized controlled trials and therapeutics), and animal experimentation on the central role of dietary sodium and sodium metabolism in the etiology and pathogenesis of high-normal and high blood pressure levels.

In the last decade, several within-population studies have documented a significant independent association between level of habitual intake of alcohol by individuals and their likelihood of being hypertensive.[36,90] Table 59.10 presents representative data.[91,92] Prospective analyses for the two Chicago cohorts yield data indicating that for the men normotensive at baseline, risk of becoming hypertensive was markedly greater for heavy drinkers compared to others.[92] The likelihood that this association between drinking and HBP is etiologically significant is supported by investigations indicating that hypertensive problem drinkers become normotensive and remain normotensive when they stop drinking.[93] Clinical therapeutics and physiologic studies also have yielded data supporting this conclusion.

Epidemiologic research, both interpopulation and intrapopulation in focus, is at present actively exploring possible effects on blood pressure of several other aspects of present-day "rich" diet. Pending clarification of as yet unresolved issues (e.g., on influences on blood pressure of amount and type of dietary lipid, protein, carbohydrate, and fiber, and of such other electrolytes as calcium and magnesium), it is a reasonable judgment that established findings on the relationships of obesity, high sodium intake, and heavy alcohol consumption to HBP afford valuable approaches for the nonpharmacologic prevention and control of this established major CHD risk factor.[29,30]

"RICH" DIET, PARTICULARLY CALORIE IMBALANCE, OF INDIVIDUALS AND THEIR RISK OF DIABETES. Among middle-aged and elderly adults, non-insulin-dependent diabetes is far-and-away the most prevalent type. The one trait repeatedly shown in within-population studies to be related to occurrence of diabetes among such adults is overweight, particularly marked overweight.[43] It is a reasonable inference that prevention and correction of marked obesity can contribute importantly to reducing prevalence rates of diabetes in the population. Thus, this aspect of improved nutrition and life-style has significance in regard to prevention and control of all three diet-related established major CHD risk factors—hypercholesterolemia, high blood pressure, and diabetes.

"RICH" DIET, PARTICULARLY HIGH INTAKE OF CHOLESTEROL AND SATURATED FAT, OF INDIVIDUALS AND THEIR CORONARY HEART DISEASE RISK. Finally, in the last few years, several studies have reported data demonstrating a significant independent relationship between dietary lipid intake, particularly cholesterol, and long-term risk of CHD.[74,83,94-99] The findings are remarkable for their scope and consistency, particularly since all the methodologic difficulties described above in regard to assessing the relationship between dietary lipid intakes of individuals and their serum cholesterol levels are operative in regard to the dietary lipid–CHD risk issue, in aggravated form in view of the long follow-up needed to test the question.

The first within-population investigation to report such a significant positive relationship was the Western Electric Study. With use of the average for each man of the 1958 and 1959 dietary lipid, serum cholesterol, and body mass index data, analyses showed dietary cholesterol, combined dietary lipid scores, and serum cholesterol were all positively related to 19-year risk of CHD death, and dietary polyunsaturated fat was inversely related.[83,94] Multivariate analyses showed that these significant relationships were independent of the other major risk factors, such as entry blood pressure, cigarette use, and age, all also significantly related to 19-year risk of CHD death. The observation in the Western Electric Study that dietary cholesterol and polyunsaturated fatty acids (PUFA) were significantly associated with risk of CHD death after adjustment for serum cholesterol concentration at baseline supports the idea that these dietary factors may be related to atherosclerosis by other mechanisms in addition to the level of serum total cholesterol (*e.g.*, by effects on lipoprotein fractions and subfractions, on thrombogenic or antithrombogenic mechanisms).

Five other studies have recently reported similar findings, on Hawaiian Japanese–American men; men of Irish ethnic background in Boston and Ireland; men in Amsterdam and in Zutphen, The Netherlands; and Seventh Day Adventists in California.[74,83,94,96-99] The data from these several investigations are impressive in regard to the consistent finding of a significant independent relationship between dietary cholesterol or foods high in dietary cholesterol and long-term CHD risk. This is a finding entirely in keeping with the results of 80 years of animal research in this field, including findings in nonhuman primates, all demonstrating the key role of dietary cholesterol in atherogenesis. Thus, particularly in the context of the total literature, the recent epidemiologic findings on individuals lend strong support to the conclusion that dietary lipid (cholesterol, saturated fat, polyunsaturated fat), especially dietary cholesterol, relates significantly to risk of CHD not only through their important influence on serum cholesterol, but directly and independently as well.

Among the established major risk factors for CHD, "rich" diet—particularly high intake of cholesterol and saturated fat—is of pivotal and central importance in the causation of epidemic premature CHD in populations.[1,21,22] When such a diet is absent or rare in the population, epidemic CHD does not occur, even when there are high prevalence rates of hypertension and cigarette use (witness Japan). Correspondingly, HBP and products of tobacco smoke are not atherogenic *per se* in experimental animals when the diet is low in cholesterol and fat, but they significantly accelerate and intensify atherogenesis induced by feeding cholesterol and fat. Thus, hypertension and cigarette smoking are important adjuvant and supplementary causes of epidemic premature CHD. Population-wide habitual high intake of cholesterol-saturated fat is the primary and essential cause—the *sine qua non*—of the epidemic.

"RICH" DIET, PARTICULARLY CALORIE IMBALANCE, OF INDIVIDUALS AND THEIR CORONARY HEART DISEASE RISK.

Under American living conditions, long-term calorie imbalance with consequent overweight is an important factor accounting for high prevalence rates in the population of hypercholesterolemia, hypertension, and diabetes. Obesity continues to be a common trait in the United States, even in childhood and youth. This unprecedented mass social phenomenon is a consequence of the fact that for tens of millions of people the level of habitual physical activity is low, and foods of concentrated caloric content are readily available. A majority of the population gains weight during the years from young adulthood to middle age, to become obese (if not already obese in youth), with a sizable minority becoming grossly obese by middle age. This weight gain and obesity are associated not only with higher rates of hypertension, diabetes, and hypercholesterolemia in general, but also of hyperbeta- and hyperprebetalipoproteinemia (high LDL and VLDL), hypertriglyceridemia, and hypoalphalipoproteinemia (low HDL). That is, the whole serum lipid–lipoprotein profile is shifted in an atherogenic direction. Moreover, at least for persons under age 50 at entry into several long-term prospective epidemiologic studies, relative weight, that is, the ratio of observed weight to desirable weight for height and sex (from life insurance actuarial tables[22] or the body mass index [BMI] weight in kilograms divided by height in meters squared), is significantly related to risk of premature CHD over and above the influence of the major established risk factors.[44] In some studies, the relationship between

TABLE 59.10 PERCENT WITH HIGH BLOOD PRESSURE AMONG PROBLEM DRINKERS AND NON–PROBLEM DRINKERS

Chicago Peoples Gas Company: 1233 White Males Age 40 to 59 in 1958

Variable	Problem Drinkers (N = 38)	Non–Problem Drinkers (N = 1195)	t†	Adjusted* t
Systolic blood pressure ≥ 140	55.3	33.1	2.85	2.92
Systolic blood pressure ≥ 160	18.4	10.7	1.50	1.68
Diastolic blood pressure ≥ 90	34.2	20.4	2.06	2.66
Diastolic blood pressure ≥ 95	15.8	9.1	1.39	1.95

Chicago Western Electric Company: 1899 White Males Age 40 to 55 in 1957

Variable	Heavy Drinkers (N = 117)	Non–Heavy Drinkers (N = 1782)	t	Adjusted* t
Systolic blood pressure ≥ 140	59.0	36.9	4.75	4.30
Systolic blood pressure ≥ 160	28.2	11.7	5.18	4.66
Diastolic blood pressure ≥ 90	64.1	42.1	4.65	4.27
Diastolic blood pressure ≥ 95	40.2	20.4	5.02	4.75

* Adjusted by analysis of covariance for age, serum cholesterol, pulse, relative weight, and cigarettes per day.

† A t value of 1:96 or greater indicates a statistically significant difference in percent with HBP for the two groups.

(Data from Dyer A, Stamler J, Paul O et al: Alcohol consumption, cardiovascular risk factors, and mortality in two Chicago epidemiologic studies. Circulation 56:1067–1074, 1977; Dyer AR, Stamler J, Paul O et al: Alcohol, cardiovascular risk factors and mortality: The Chicago experience. Circulation 64(Suppl III):20–27, 1981)

relative weight or BMI and mortality, both from CHD and all causes, is U-shaped (*i.e.*, those at both the lower and highest ends of the distribution at baseline have higher death rates over the long term than those with intermediate levels, and therefore a quadratic model fits the data much better than a linear model).[100]

On the other hand, for some middle-aged male populations, univariate and multivariate analyses show no significant relationship between indices of relative weight and CHD risk, despite the correlation between relative weight and serum cholesterol, blood pressure, and so on. The reasons for this apparently paradoxical finding remain to be elucidated. The inverse relationship between relative weight indices and cigarette smoking does not seem to be an adequate explanation, since the lack of a significant association in these studies remains after controlling for this confounding factor. One new clue, needing careful exploration, is the recent finding in several studies that long-term CHD and all causes mortality rates are significantly higher for lean compared to overweight hypertensives.[101,102]

In any case, obesity, particularly marked obesity, in youth, young adulthood, and middle age is a common and important problem. Its prevention and control have a considerable potential for lowering CHD risk, first and foremost since they can contribute sizably to the achievement and maintenance of optimal blood pressure and plasma lipid–lipoprotein levels, and the avoidance and control of maturity-onset diabetes.

OTHER FACTORS

SEDENTARY LIFE-STYLE AND CORONARY HEART DISEASE RISK

In 1953, research findings were reported from England indicating CHD mortality rates were significantly higher in sedentary transport and post office workers compared to their physically active fellow employees serving as bus conductors and letter carriers.[10,21,22] Several other prospective epidemiologic studies, including some in the United States, yielded similar results. However, others found little or no association between habitual inactivity at work and CHD risk. Data on life expectancy and mortality patterns of athletes compared to nonathletes also suggest a less favorable prognosis for the physically inactive, particularly compared to athletes who remain active into middle age. An autopsy study in England also obtained supportive evidence, showing middle-aged decedents engaged in sedentary or light work had a higher frequency of coronary occlusion and myocardial fibrosis than those who had been involved in heavy activity in their occupations. An autopsy study of violent deaths in Finland reported more severe coronary atherosclerosis in those engaged in sedentary work compared to the active, but a United States study found no such difference.[10,36]

Subsequent investigations, such as the Framingham (Massachusetts), Health Insurance Plan (New York), San Francisco longshoremen, Harvard college entrants, and British civil servants studies, have collected data beyond job classification to characterize habitual physical activity of individuals in their cohorts. These studies all report data indicating a significant independent deleterious effect of sedentary life-style on coronary risk. An extensive literature also exists on possible mechanisms.

Several symposia proceedings and major reviews are available on this matter.[10,36] Its definitive resolution is rendered difficult for several reasons: effects of self-selection of individuals early in life into active versus inactive occupations and leisure time activity patterns; imprecision in classifying people by habitual physical activity and the related variable of possible major concern, cardiopulmonary fitness; and confounding by other relevant aspects of life-style and other risk factors. It is not likely that an unequivocal conclusion in this area will be forthcoming in the next few years. Clearly, the emergence of sedentary life-style as a mass phenomenon in the 20th century in the industrialized countries is a major departure from the living pattern of the human species set by millions of years of evolution. Given coexistent "rich" diet and cigarette smoking, plus stressful psychosocial behavior patterns (see below), it is a reasonable judgment, based on the evidence available, that the sedentary habit adds insult to injury (*i.e.*, is probably an independent CHD risk factor).

BEHAVIORAL–PSYCHOSOCIAL FACTORS AND CORONARY HEART DISEASE RISK

A body of research evidence exists indicating that given other aspects of life-style in the United States (habits of eating, drinking, smoking, and exercise), certain behavioral and psychosocial factors may also contribute independently to CHD risk. A major area of investigation has been the type A behavior pattern, common in modern competitive society.[10] While some prospective epidemiologic studies have obtained positive evidence on type A behavior and CHD risk, others have recorded negative findings. Therefore, it is a reasonable judgment at this juncture to designate this trait as a possible, but not established, CHD risk factor. Other psychosocial factors have also been implicated, such as job or marital dissatisfaction, social incongruities, movement into unfamiliar circumstances, low level of social contact and social support, and, nowadays in western industrialized countries, lower social class.

OTHER FACTORS AND CORONARY HEART DISEASE RISK

Many other traits have been implicated as CHD risk factors. These include aspects of "rich" modern diet in addition to those already discussed above (*e.g.*, high intake of refined and processed sugars, and of coffee; low intake of fiber, fish, polyunsaturated fish oils). Also implicated are rapid heart rate; hyperuricemia; abnormalities in circulating factors related to clotting and thrombosis; hormonal imbalances (hypoestrogenism in women, hyperandrogenism and hypoandrogenism in men, hypothyroidism, and so on); high white blood cell counts; infectious, autoimmune, and genetic mechanisms affecting the integrity of the coronary arterial wall; and familial factors over and above the established major risk factors. A review of current knowledge on such traits is beyond the scope of this chapter.

Use of oral contraceptives, a practice involving millions of women, merits separate and special mention, since it undoubtedly increases CHD risk. While relative risk is several-fold, absolute excess risk is low in the teens, 20s, and early 30s, given the generally low risk of CHD among women of this age. From age 35 on, absolute excess risks become sizable, particularly when other major risk factors are present, most especially cigarette use. Women, like men, should be counseled not to smoke, and explicit information about the high risks of smoking should be given to women taking oral contraceptives. Alternatively, at age 35 and above, other forms of contraception should be considered.

SIGNS OF SUBCLINICAL CORONARY HEART DISEASE

Extensive evidence exists demonstrating that persons with subclinical signs of possible or probable CHD, for example, abnormalities in the resting electrocardiogram (ECG) or in the ECG response to exercise, are at increased risk of CHD. This excess risk is over and above their risk status attributable to dietary lipid, serum cholesterol, blood pressure, or cigarette use, all of which relate to risk of major coronary events in persons both with and without evidence of subclinical CHD. Control of established major risk factors is therefore especially important and urgent for persons at very high risk due to both subclinical CHD and these traits.

Signs of subclinical CHD are, of course, not risk factors in the sense defined heretofore in this chapter. That is, they are not traits etiologically involved in the causation of severe atherosclerotic coronary heart disease, but rather relatively late consequences of the long-term operation of such traits. Once present, however, they may themselves reflect abnormalities related pathophysiologically and pathogenetically to risk of major coronary events; hence they may call for special interventions to break late links in the chain of causation.

PEDIATRIC ASPECTS OF LIFE-STYLES, MAJOR RISK FACTORS (INCLUDING FAMILIAL PATTERNS OF RISK), AND CORONARY HEART DISEASE

Primary habit formation begins in infancy and develops powerfully during childhood and youth. It is a truism that the primary establishment of healthy living habits early in life is preferable to, and easier than, changing habits in adulthood.

Data from several studies show that from the first decade of life, American children tend to have higher mean levels of relative weight, serum cholesterol, and blood pressure than children in many other countries. As already noted, gross obesity is now widely prevalent among children and youth in the United States. Sizable proportions of American youngsters are sedentary, are cigarette smokers, and are physically unfit. Clearly, population-wide, as well as among high-risk groups, strategies are needed to improve habits among children and youth, as well as among adults.

In regard to such risk factors as serum cholesterol and blood pressure, it has been shown in recent prospective studies that children tend over the years to stay close to their places in the distribution of these variables for their age and sex group. That is, a child in the upper range of blood pressure or serum cholesterol (e.g., above the 75th percentile) for his or her age and sex group on two successive annual or biennial examinations tends to remain in that position subsequently, and is on a collision course in terms of increased risk of frankly high levels from young adulthood on. As with adults, obese children are more likely to have high levels of these risk factors.

All these traits tend to aggregate in families. For at least some of these factors, particularly serum cholesterol and blood pressure, the familial linkage almost certainly has both genetic and environmental components, and in its common form it is polygenic, rather than monogenic, with biochemical pathways as yet totally or largely undefined.

The only decades-long study following teenagers into middle age has clearly established that obesity, blood pressure elevation, and cigarette use early in life relate strongly to risk of fatal CHD in middle age.[44] (No data on serum cholesterol were available in that study.)

Finally, as the analyses of the International Atherosclerosis Project and other autopsy studies have shown, atherogenesis begins early in life, with its more advanced forms already manifest by the third decade in sizable numbers of people living in western industrial societies.[19]

These facts all indicate the soundness of approaches to primary prevention of the atherosclerotic diseases beginning early in life with a two-pronged strategy, aimed at achieving improved life-styles and risk-factor status for the young generation overall, and with pinpointed special efforts directed to those known to be at especially high risk because of positive family history and high levels of the major risk factors.

DEVELOPMENT OF PUBLIC POLICY FOR THE PRIMARY PREVENTION OF CORONARY HEART DISEASE

The initial public statement calling for a coronary preventive effort apparently was the *Statement on Arteriosclerosis, Main Cause of "Heart Attacks" and "Strokes,"* co-authored in 1959 by a group of cardiologists and cardiovascular researchers, and supported by 106 members of the American Society for the Study of Arteriosclerosis (later the Council on Arteriosclerosis, American Heart Association).[103] This was an initiative of a group of individuals, not of an organization, voluntary or official. This brochure was circulated in hundreds of thousands of copies by the National Health Education Committee. This document, written over a quarter of a century ago, called attention to traits such as hypercholesterolemia, cigarette smoking, and hypertension that were later designated major risk factors, plus overweight and a positive family history of premature hypertensive and atherosclerotic disease.

A year later, in 1960, the American Heart Association (AHA) issued its first statement on cigarette smoking and cardiovascular disease.[104] Updates have been published periodically.

In 1961, the American Heart Association issued its first statement on diet and CHD, calling attention both to the matter of lipid composition of the diet (avoidance and correction of high intake of saturated fat and cholesterol) and caloric imbalance and consequent obesity.[105] This was the first statement enunciating a two-pronged strategy, that is, improved nutrition for the whole population and special efforts for its higher risk individuals and families. The AHA has at intervals updated this report, and has promulgated related special reports (*e.g.,* for children and for persons with hyperlipidemia).[47,48,106–108]

In 1964, the landmark *Report of the Advisory Committee to the Surgeon General on Smoking and Health* was published, probably the first clear lead from the federal government relating to the coronary prevention effort.[109] Mandated by the Congress, annual reports of the Surgeon General on smoking and health are valuable updates.[38,39]

In 1970, the Inter-Society Commission for Heart Disease Resources (ICHD) issued its *Report on the Primary Prevention of the Atherosclerotic Diseases*.[1] Like its predecessors, it was thoroughly documented with references to the research literature, delineating the scientific foundation of the prevention effort. Table 59.11 presents the succinct summary the ICHD distilled from its recommendations. The report also gave detailed recommendations on implementation. The Inter-Society Commission, established as a result of federal legislation and at the request of the Assistant Secretary for Health (the Surgeon General), was made up of representatives of all the key medical and health pro-

---

TABLE 59.11 RECOMMENDATIONS FOR PRIMARY PREVENTION OF THE ATHEROSCLEROTIC DISEASES, INTER-SOCIETY COMMISSION FOR HEART DISEASE RESOURCES, 1970

The Commission recommends that a strategy of primary prevention of premature atherosclerotic diseases be adopted as long-term national policy for the United States and to implement this strategy that adequate resources of money and manpower be committed to accomplish:
  Changes in diet to prevent or control hyperlipidemia, obesity, hypertension and diabetes.
  Elimination of cigarette smoking.
  Pharmacologic control of elevated blood pressure.

fessional organizations concerned with this challenge. A comprehensive update of this report was published in 1984.[35]

In 1971, both the White House Conference on Nutrition and the Task Force on Arteriosclerosis of the National Heart and Lung Institute also addressed these matters and made available to the health professions and the public similar summary recommendations, in agreement with those already noted.[110,111] In 1971 also, the ICHD published its *Guidelines for the Detection, Diagnosis, and Management of Hypertensive Populations*.[112]

In 1973, there was another important development: the official assumption of federal responsibility, at the cabinet level, for control of hypertension as a major unsolved mass public health problem, with the launching by the Secretary of Health, Education, and Welfare of the National High Blood Pressure Education Program (NHBPEP), under the aegis of the National Heart, Lung, and Blood Institute.[113] At intervals since, expert groups cooperating with and advising the NHBPEP have made available guidelines for the optimal nutritional–hygienic and pharmacologic care of persons with high blood pressure.[114,115]

In the late 1970s, the Select Committee on Nutrition and Human Needs of the United States Senate presented a set of *Dietary Goals for the United States*, emphasizing improvement in both the lipid and carbohydrate composition of the diet.[116] This report also called attention to the matter of avoiding and correcting caloric imbalance and consequent obesity, and high sodium intake. It also succinctly indicated reasonable approaches to food selection to achieve these dietary goals. Like all such recommendations, these were also concerned with aiding Americans to maintain and even to improve intake of all essential nutrients. Implicitly or explicitly, they were also dedicated to helping Americans to continue, in a healthier way, to enjoy one of life's pleasures: the pleasure of eating, for example, by taking tips from Mediterranean and Far Eastern eating styles (but without high sodium). In the course of this effort, the AHA produced a national best seller, the *American Heart Association Cook Book*, now in its third edition.[117]

In 1979, the American Diabetes Association updated its earlier reports, presented jointly with the American Dietetic Association, on principles of nutrition and dietary recommendations for individuals with diabetes.[118]

At the turn of the decade, the Report of the Surgeon General, *Healthy People—A Report on Health Promotion and Disease Prevention*, was published, dealing comprehensively with the major present-day challenges to the health of the American people at each stage of life, including those of better life-styles from childhood on, better habits in regard to eating, drinking, smoking, and exercise, to help control the coronary epidemic and other major chronic disease problems as well.[119] This was followed shortly by supplementary reports.[120-122] Subsequently, national goals were promulgated for the prevention effort into the 1990s, for example, in regard to serum cholesterol, obesity, and smoking.[123,124]

Early in 1980, the United States Department of Agriculture and of Health, Education, and Welfare (now Health and Human Services) published the colorful folder, *Nutrition and Your Health: Dietary Guidelines for Americans*.[125] This was updated in 1985 (Fig. 59.5).[126]

During the late 1970s, developments in federal regulatory agencies and in other parts of the national executive branch also were generally of a positive nature in regard to CHD preventive approaches.

Early in 1980 also, the Committee on Dietary Allowances, Food and Nutrition Board, National Academy of Sciences, in the ninth edition of its *Recommended Dietary Allowances*, presented guidelines on desirable intakes of dietary fat and carbohydrate.[127]

In March, 1981, the proceedings were published of the Eleventh Bethesda Conference on the Prevention of Coronary Heart Disease.[128] This conference, convened by the American College of Cardiology with the co-sponsorship of the American Heart Association, the Centers for Disease Control of the United States Public Health Service, and the National Heart, Lung, and Blood Institute (NHLBI), and with participation of major national medical and health professional organizations, focused on the role of physicians in CHD prevention. Later in 1981, the Working Group of Arteriosclerosis of NHLBI presented its

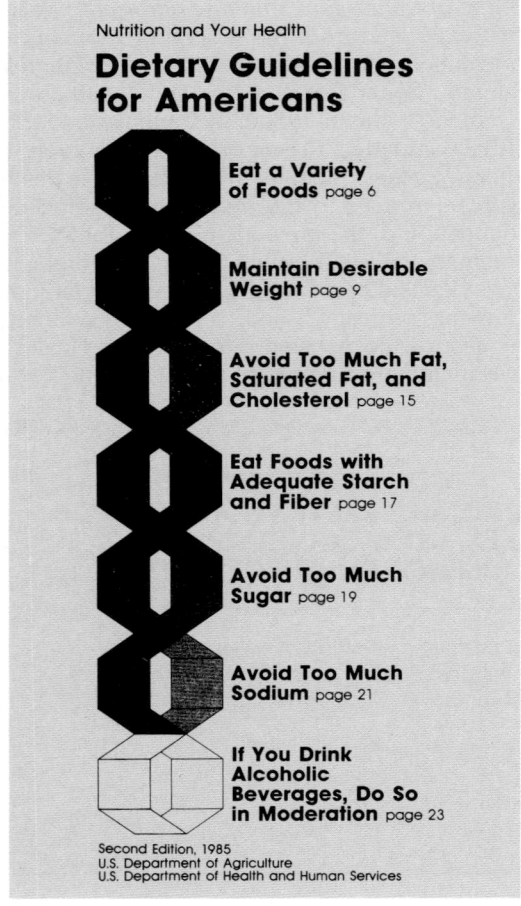

FIGURE 59.5 Reproduction of the cover of the brochure *Dietary Guidelines for Americans*. (United States Department of Agriculture and United States Department of Health and Human Services: Nutrition and Your Health: Dietary Guidelines for Americans, 2nd ed. Washington, DC, United States Department of Agriculture and United States Department of Health and Human Services, 1985)

report, in two volumes, the first a summary with conclusions and recommendations, the second a set of comprehensive reviews of knowledge on atherosclerosis.[129,130] The recommendations included proposals for a national cardiovascular nutrition education program and a national no smoking education program. Following the NIH Consensus Conference on Lowering Blood Cholesterol to Prevent Heart Disease in December, 1984,[131] NHLBI has launched a National Cholesterol Education Program.[132]

Clearly, while there are dissenting views,[133,134] effective consistent public policy leads are available, developed by expert groups and responsible organizations over almost three decades, reflecting a rich mine of research information and a broad consensus in the scientific, professional, voluntary, and official communities. And, in fact, similar position statements are available from expert groups in other countries experiencing the coronary epidemic, and from the World Health Organization, the International Society and Federation of Cardiology, and the European Atherosclerosis Society.[10,37,128,135-140]

RECENT CHANGES IN LIFE-STYLE AND LIFE-STYLE–RELATED RISK FACTORS BY THE AMERICAN PEOPLE

The development of public policy has been steady and progressive over these last 25 years, but the resources for dissemination have been modest. What about physicians, other health professionals, the American people? Have they been reached? Have they responded?

CHANGES IN EATING PATTERNS

Data are available on these matters from two United States Department of Agriculture (USDA) surveys, in 1976 and 1980, respectively.[141,142] They deal with whether Americans have recently changed their eating styles because of health or nutrition concerns. About half of the random sample of the population in 1976 replied in the affirmative, as did almost two thirds in 1980. Respondents indicated that they had done so either to alleviate existing health problems or to avoid potential ones. Some stated they had done so on advice of their physicians, others on their own. The reasons were as one would expect: identification of such problems as hyperlipidemia, obesity, hypertension, and diabetes, with diet change instituted to help control these. In addition, a substantial number of people reported modifying their diets for general public health and preventive medicine purposes. Such changes were made more frequently in households of higher educational and income levels and where the adults were younger. Changes frequently reported were reduced intake of calories, fat (particularly products high in animal fat), cholesterol, and salt. In accord with these findings, the National Ambulatory Medical Care Survey conducted by the United States Public Health Service reported that in 1979, 33,154,000 visits by patients to physicians were for diet counseling, representing 6% of all visits.[143] In terms of diagnostic categories, there were 8,348,000 visits for "obesity and other hyperalimentation" (1.5% of all visits).

All this is, of course, reporting of self-described behavior, but there are also hard data consistent with the USDA survey results. Thus, per capita consumption of eggs (the yolk is the single largest source of dietary cholesterol; see Table 59.1) has gone down steadily from its 1950 peak, down 33% by 1984.[6,144] Total milk fat solids per capita have declined by a like amount. At the same time, reflecting purchase at the supermarket of more and more fat-free and low-fat products (skim milk, 1% and 2% milk, low-fat yogurt, ice milk, and low-fat cottage cheese), consumption of nonfat milk solids has declined much less. And, over the decades, a remarkable change has occurred in the use of the visible fats (Fig. 59.6 and Table 59.12).[145] Since 1950, use of lard has gone down 85% per capita, and use of butter, down 55%, both reflecting continuation and acceleration of a decades-long downward trend. Margarine has come into increasing use, with a 67% increase in its per capita consumption since 1950 alone, and for years now a sizable proportion of the total margarine is of the "soft" variety, which is relatively low in saturated fats and high in unsaturated and polyunsaturated fats, a deliberate response of manufacturers and consumers to nutritional advice related to serum cholesterol reduction and coronary prevention. Use of vegetable shortening has also increased, by 91% since 1950, and again there has been a change in composition, with an increasing proportion liquid (*i.e.*, relatively low in saturates and high in unsaturates). And, of course, all these vegetable fats, like all vegetable products, contain no dietary cholesterol. Finally, there has been a marked increase in use of vegetable oils, most of them (with the exception of coconut and palm oils) also relatively low in saturates and high in polyunsaturates.

On the other hand, since World War II, mean per capita available

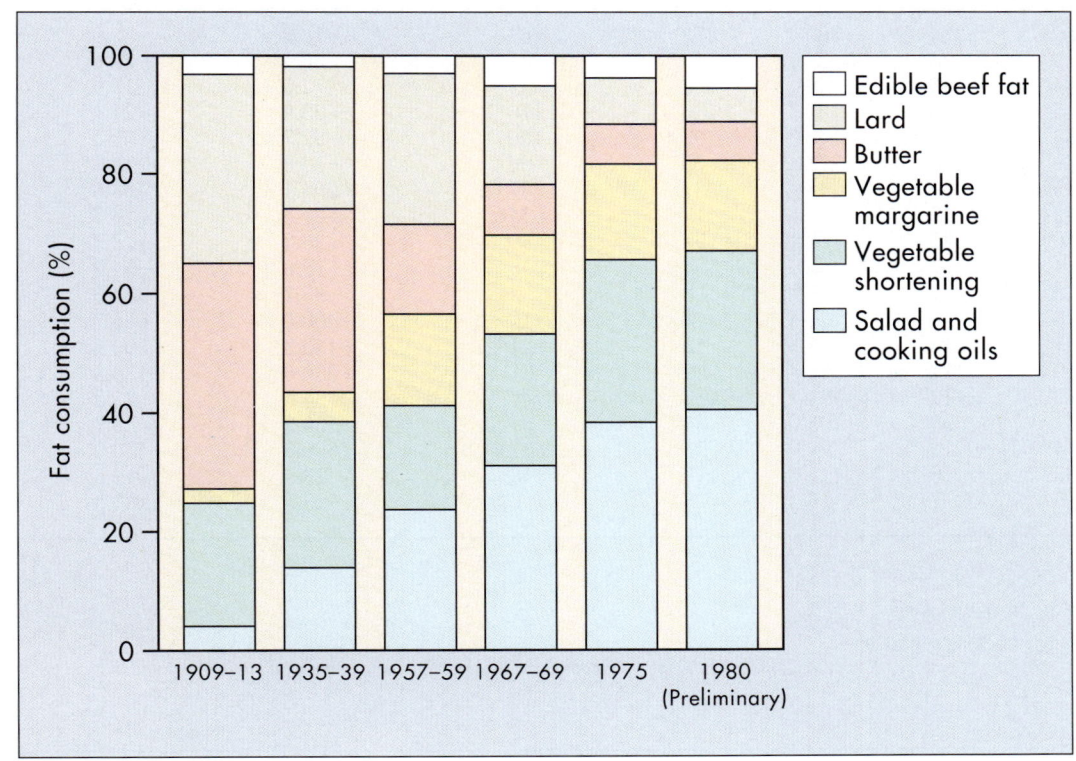

FIGURE 59.6 Nutrient fat from fats and oils (per capita civilian consumption), United States diet, 1909 to 1980. (Modified from US Department of Agriculture, Human Nutrition Information Service: Unpublished data on nutrient fat from fats and oils in the US food supply. Hyattsville, MD, US Department of Agriculture, 1981)

meat, particularly beef, has gone up sizably, peaking in 1970 (Table 59.12),[6,144] and the resultant increase in available saturated fat and cholesterol has in part, but only in part, compensated for the sizable declines in these dietary lipids due to the downward trends in egg yolk, dairy fat, and the visible fats high in these components. Note too the decline in meat, including beef, since 1970, reflecting the concern of millions of American families to cut down on intake of saturated fat and cholesterol.

Data are also available from the USDA 1977 to 1978 Nationwide Food Consumption Survey involving 30,000 households. These include a comparison of 1965 and 1977 findings (Table 59.13).[7] In general, these are in agreement with the overall national food disappearance trends (see Table 59.12).[6,144] However, note the trend in regard to beef, that is, decreased per capita intakes for young and middle-aged adults in the 1977 compared with the 1965 household survey, suggesting that at least for these age groups the downward trend may have begun earlier than indicated by the disappearance data. (The Food Consumption Survey findings show a sizable increase in per capita beef consumption from 1965 to 1977 for males age 15 to 18 and 19 to 22.) The household survey data indicate a considerable decline in percent of calories from total fat, from 45.1% in 1965 to 36.2% in 1977. The USDA data, therefore, indicate that there have been modest but significant decreases in saturated fat and cholesterol intake by the American people.

Compared to the 1965 household survey data, the 1977 data also indicate a decreased intake of total calories by young adult and middle-aged American men and women (see Table 59.13).[7] These data are intriguing in relation to the findings of the 1960 to 1962 and 1971 to 1974 Health Examination Surveys, which indicate no change in the early 1970s, possibly even a slight increase, in the sizable proportion of Americans who are grossly obese.[146] Perhaps by the late 1970s and the 1980s this situation was changed; this needs to be assessed.

One other trend merits attention here: until the 1980s, all the data indicated rises in per capita consumption of alcohol,[6] and the epidemiologic evidence indicates a direct proportionality between average per capita consumption and prevalence of heavy drinking. This last phenomenon is of direct concern, since research in recent years has shown that heavy drinking is associated with higher prevalence and incidence rates of hypertension, independent of other traits related to risk of high blood pressure. At this point, it is also appropriate to note that no data are available on trends of sodium consumption by the United States population.

Data from other sources indicate trends similar to those summarized above. Thus, comparison of the data on men volunteering for the Multiple Risk Factor Intervention Trial in the mid 1970s, and on men of the Framingham Study and the National Diet–Heart Study surveyed a decade or so earlier, indicates modest declines in the 1970s in total fat, saturated fat, and dietary cholesterol intake, and a modest rise in intake of polyunsaturated fats.[147-149]

CHANGES IN SERUM CHOLESTEROL

In agreement with all these sets of nutritional data, surveys of the population indicate declines in average serum cholesterol levels toward more desirable goals (Fig. 59.7).[150] Thus, repeated samplings in the late 1950s and early 1960s yielded average values for groups of middle-aged men ranging around 235 mg/dl. In the late 1960s and 1970s, the mean was 15 mg to 20 mg lower (about 215), a decrease of about 7%. Data on representative samples of the United States population indicate that the decline in serum cholesterol have been greater for the more educated than for the less educated.[151] These changes in serum cholesterol, almost certainly a result of the changes in patterns of food and nutrient ingestion noted above, have taken place despite the limited resources available for reaching the public on these matters, and

TABLE 59.12 TRENDS OF FOOD PRODUCTS AVAILABLE FOR PER CAPITA ANNUAL CONSUMPTION, UNITED STATES, 1940–1984

Product	Year						% Change	
	1940	1950	1960	1970	1980	1984 (Preliminary)	1940–1984	1950–1984
Eggs (number)	319	389	334	309	272	261	−18.2	−32.9
Milk fat solids*	33	29	24	21	20	21	−36.4	−27.6
Nonfat milk solids*	38	44	43	40	36	37	−2.6	−15.9
Meats (carcass weight)*	142	145	174	192	180	176	+23.9	+21.4
Beef	55	63	85	113	103	106	+92.7	+68.3
Pork	74	69	78	73	73	66	−10.8	−4.3
Chicken and turkey*	17	25	34	48	61	67	+294.1	+168.0
Fish*	11	12	10	12	13	14	+27.3	+16.7
Fats and oils, total†	46	46	45	53	57	59	+28.3	+28.3
Butter	17	11	7	5	4	5	−70.6	−54.5
Lard	14	13	7	5	2	2	−85.7	−84.6
Margarine	2	6	9	11	11	10	+400.0	+66.7
Shortening	9	11	13	17	18	21	+133.3	+90.9
Other	7	9	11	18	22	21	+200.0	+133.3
Refined sugars and syrups*	107	115	112	124	137	144	+34.6	+25.2
Refined sugar	96	101	98	103	84	67	−30.2	−33.7
Corn sweeteners‡	11	14	14	21	53	77	+600.0	+450.0
Wheat flour*	155	135	118	111	117	118	−23.9	−12.6
Dry beans*	8	9	7	6	5	6§	−25.0	−33.3

* lb/person/year

† Fats and oils; total is by fat content, individual items are by actual weight.

‡ Since 1980, the majority of the corn sweeteners are high fructose products.

§ 1983

TABLE 59.13 INTAKE OF FOODS AND NUTRIENTS PER PERSON BY AGE AND SEX, 1965 AND 1977, AND PERCENT CHANGE,* 1977 COMPARED TO 1965, UNITED STATES NATIONWIDE FOOD CONSUMPTION SURVEYS

	Food or Nutrient (g/day)											
	Milk and Milk Drinks	Cheese	Eggs	Beef	Pork	Poultry	Fish	Beef, Pork, Poultry, Fish	Fats, Oils	Calories	Protein	Fat
Age 25–34												
Men												
1965	318	11	55	110	98	32	14	254	42	2,917	118.6	146.1
1977	243	21	38	89	55	31	14	189	18	2,449	98.1	114.8
%Δ	−23.6	+90.9	−30.9	−19.1	−43.9	−3.1	0.0	−25.6	−57.1	−16.0	−17.3	−21.4
Women												
1965	204	10	27	64	54	21	9	148	23	1,803	72.3	86.5
1977	182	19	26	50	32	25	10	117	15	1,616	65.9	73.7
%Δ	−10.8	+90.0	−3.7	−21.9	−40.7	+19.0	+11.1	−20.9	−34.8	−10.4	−8.9	−14.8
Age 35–50												
Men												
1965	236	13	51	102	82	33	13	230	39	2,632	106.2	132.4
1977	203	18	41	79	52	32	17	180	19	2,314	95.6	109.3
%Δ	−14.0	+38.5	−19.6	−22.5	−36.6	−3.0	+30.8	−21.7	−51.3	−12.1	−10.0	−17.4
Women												
1965	152	13	31	57	50	25	13	145	23	1,652	68.3	80.2
1977	130	18	23	51	32	25	14	122	14	1,514	63.9	70.8
%Δ	−14.5	+38.5	−25.8	−10.5	−36.0	0.0	+7.7	−15.9	−39.1	−8.4	−6.4	−11.7
Age 51–64												
Men												
1965	203	14	51	81	91	28	18	218	35	2,422	98.0	121.3
1977	180	17	36	74	57	33	22	186	18	2,148	90.1	101.6
%Δ	−11.3	+21.4	−29.4	−8.6	−37.4	+17.9	+22.2	−14.7	−48.6	−11.3	−8.1	−16.2
Women												
1965	151	14	33	54	49	25	9	137	24	1,619	67.4	79.9
1977	139	19	24	54	30	27	12	123	15	1,522	65.2	71.2
%Δ	−7.9	+35.7	−27.3	0.0	−38.8	+8.0	+33.3	−10.2	−37.5	−6.0	−3.3	−10.9

* %Δ is percent change: $\frac{1965-1977}{1965}$

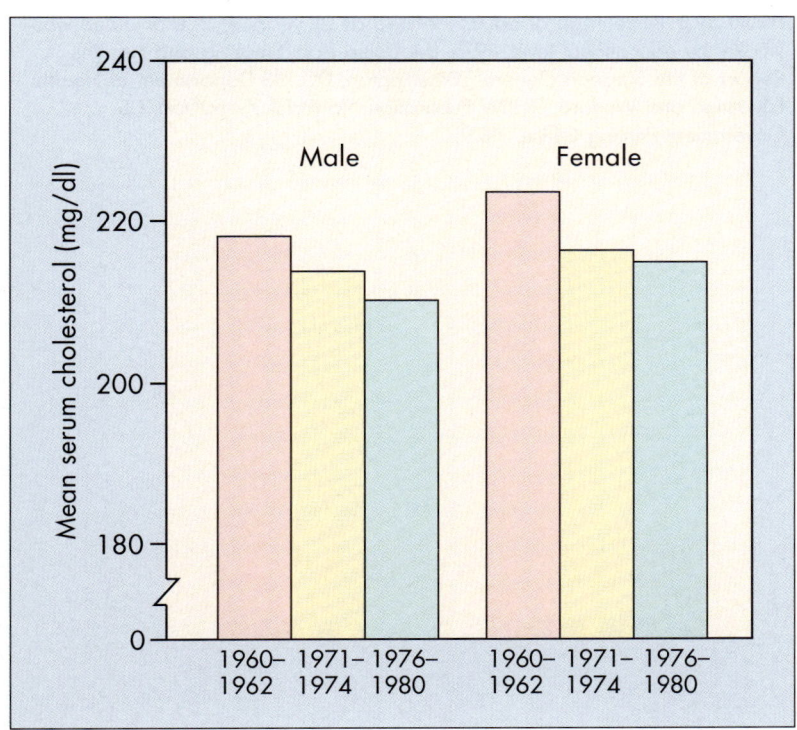

FIGURE 59.7 Mean serum cholesterol levels for persons 20 to 74 years of age, by sex, United States, selected periods, 1960 to 1980. *Note:* all values referenced to the Abell-Kendall method, J Biol Chem 195:357–366, 1952. (Modified from Charting the Nation's Health—Trends since 1960. Hyattsville, MD, US Department of Health and Human Services, Public Health Service, National Center for Health Statistics, DHHS Pub No [PHS] 85-1251, August, 1985).

despite the fact that the main content of food advertising on television runs counter to, rather than supports, the public education effort.[152] While the declines in serum cholesterol are relatively modest, indicating that much remains to be done, they are substantial enough to reach "critical mass" (*i.e.*, they are detectable in the population at large).

CHANGES IN CIGARETTE SMOKING

The situation is similar with respect to cigarette smoking among adults, particularly those in the coronary-prone years from the fourth decade of life on. The prevalence of smoking in the United States population, at least in regard to men, actually peaked in the early 1950s, and declined sizably even before the landmark *Report to the Surgeon General on Smoking and Health* in 1964. Thereafter, the decline accelerated, particularly for adult men. In 1965, a majority of men (51%) were still cigarette smokers; by 1983, this proportion was down to 35%, a fall of 31%.[153] For women, the 1965 and 1983 smoking prevalence rates were 33% and 29%, respectively; a fall of 12%. For both men and women, smoking is now a habit of a minority. Again, the higher the educational level, the more this is the case (Fig. 59.8).[154] These data clearly indicate that it is possible to affect the smoking situation, and that substantial progress has already been made, despite the limited resources for anti-smoking efforts, especially compared with the huge expenditures for advertising and lobbying by the tobacco companies. However, there are still big problems. Thus, the prevalence of heavy smoking (25 or more cigarettes per day) has apparently not yet decreased among adults.[153] There is still a big problem of smoking among teenagers, although data from the late 1970s indicate the beginnings of a decline. And there is the special problem of millions of women who are smoking cigarettes and using the contraceptive pill.

CHANGES IN PHYSICAL ACTIVITY

One transformation in behavior in the country has been the large-scale adoption of leisure time exercise. Direct trend data on this are lacking, although there are confirmatory data on sales of running shoes, tennis racquets, and so on. Survey findings also indicate that in this regard, as in all others, the change is more conspicuous among the more educated than among the less educated.[155] It is also greater among men than women.

PROGRESS IN THE CONTROL OF HIGH BLOOD PRESSURE

In the late 1960s and early 1970s, after publication of the landmark reports of the Veterans Administration (VA) antihypertensive drug trial,[156-158] it became increasingly a matter of concern that the great majority of the millions with high blood pressure in the population were undetected, untreated, or uncontrolled. This came to be known as the $\frac{1}{2} \times \frac{1}{2} \times \frac{1}{2}$ phenomenon: about half the hypertensives were detected; half of those detected were treated; and half of those treated were controlled (*i.e.*, only one in eight detected, treated, and controlled). The VA data on efficacy of treatment and the survey data on the low level of control were major foundations for the 1973 federal initiative establishing the National High Blood Pressure Education Program.

In the years since, the proportion of hypertensives detected, treated, and controlled has risen steadily. By the mid 1970s, it was approaching the 50% mark, and in the early 1980s it was still higher in many communities. However, a substantial number of people with high blood pressure remain to be detected.

In agreement with the data on progress in the control effort, the number of patient visits to physicians, both first and repeat visits, for care for hypertensive disease has risen steadily, much more so than visits to physicians for all causes. In 1979, there were 200,501,000 office visits by patients to physicians for a blood pressure check, and 23,607,000 for hypertension (36% and 4.2% of all visits, respectively).[143] Correspondingly, the number of filled prescriptions for antihypertensive medication and the expenditure for such prescriptions (after correction for inflation) have risen sizably.[159]

THE DECLINE IN CORONARY HEART DISEASE MORTALITY AND INCIDENCE

From at least 1940 into the 1960s, there was a steady rise in CHD mortality rates in the United States, particularly for men, both white and black. In the later 1960s, a break in the curve occurred, with a

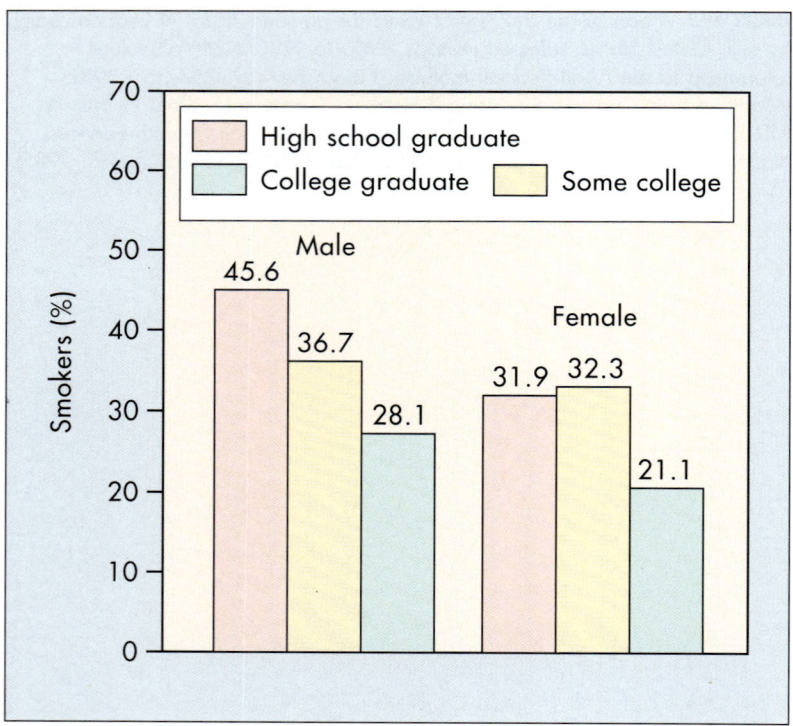

FIGURE 59.8 Percentage of adults (defined as 21 years of age or older) who smoke, by educational level, 1975. (Modified from Smoking and Health: Report of the Surgeon General. Washington, DC, US Department of Health, Education and Welfare, DHEW Publication No (PHS) 79-50066, US Government Printing Office, 1979)

steady decline from 1968 on, continuing through 1984, the year of latest record (Fig. 59.9).[160] For the decade 1969 to 1978, for persons age 35 to 74 (*i.e.*, the age group being victimized by the epidemic of *premature* CHD) the decline overall was 27%; 568,000 lives were saved.[129,130]

Stroke mortality rates have declined even more dramatically percentage-wise. Given the fall in coronary and stroke death rates, the "big two" among the major cardiovascular diseases, the death rate for that broad category has also fallen markedly, more so than for noncardiovascular diseases (see Fig. 59.9).[160] For the 35 to 74 age group, over 800,000 lives were saved from cardiovascular death over the decade 1969 to 1978, 74% of all lives saved during those years.

For the population overall, despite the absolute increase in total numbers, and, in its middle-aged and aging segment, despite an increase of almost 2 years in average age, there was an absolute decline in all cardiovascular deaths, which peaked at 1,037,000 in 1973 and decreased to 962,000 in 1978. But these deaths are still all too many, and still all too many in the prime of life. The task in prevention is clearly defined.

In regard to the mortality decline, the United States has set the pace among the nations, as it has in the development of public policy and in beginning to improve life-styles and control major risk factors (Fig. 59.10). In 1968, United States CHD mortality rates for middle-aged men were the second highest in the world, after Finland. As a result of the decline in mortality, by 1978 they were the eighth among 27 countries, the lowest but still all too high, still at epidemic levels. A large group of countries in eastern, northern, and western Europe were still registering increases in CHD mortality rates, trends related statistically to national trends of dietary lipid intake and cigarette use.[94,161]

As shown above, based on data from long-term prospective studies (the Pooling Project data collected in the late 1950s and 1960s and the MRFIT screenee data from the 1970s and 1980s), the estimate is that elevated levels of serum cholesterol, blood pressure, and cigarette use were responsible for about 70% to 85% of all major coronary events among the middle-aged American men in those cohorts. These are the excess cases, attributable to the major risk factors (see Tables 59.3 and 59.7).[3,13] A reasonable inference from these data is that a potential exists to lower coronary rates by 70%, or even 85%, if all American men were to achieve optimal levels for the major risk factors.

Over the last 15 years or so, Americans have been moving toward these more favorable goals, the more educated more so than the less educated, at least in regard to key aspects of life-style. And for American men age 35 to 74, the coronary rates have declined by about 40%. Moreover, for the more educated, data are available from three sources, studies of Metropolitan Life Insurance Company insurees,[162] Dupont Company employees (Table 59.14),[163] and California physicians (Table 59.15),[164] indicating that the decline is greater for the more educated than for the less educated. This is, of course, the expected finding, given the greater degree of change in life-styles and life-style–related risk factors of the more educated than the less educated—if these changes are playing an important role in the mortality decline.[165] That is, these data give further weight to the widely held estimate that the changes in life-style and life-style–related risk factors have made a key contribution to the decline in CHD mortality.

Given the trends from the late 1960s to the mid-1980s, it is reasonable to propose a goal: to continue to work to reduce the still high coronary and cardiovascular death rates by 3% a year into the 1990s, so that by the mid-1990s, compared with the peak in the late 1960s, the

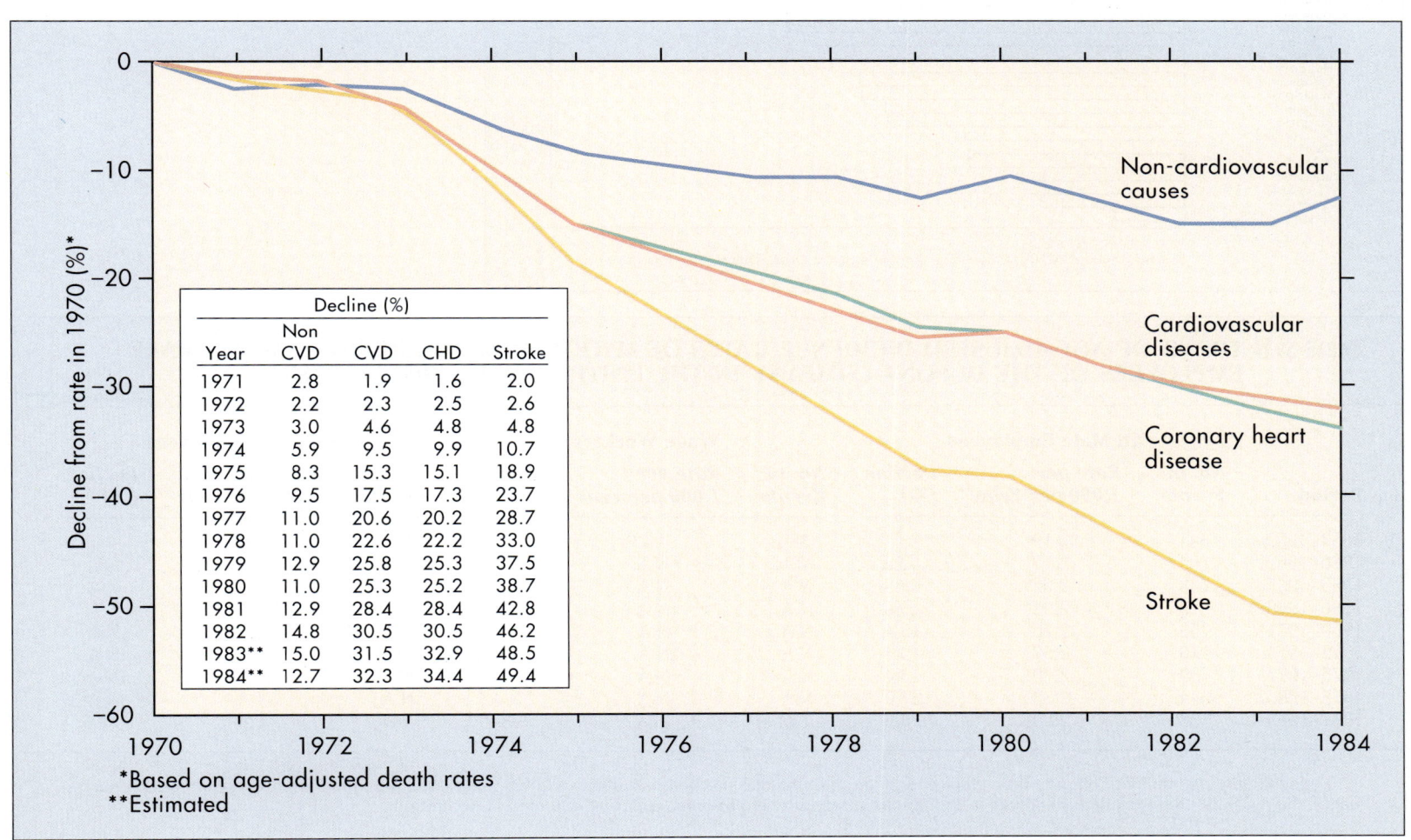

FIGURE 59.9 Decline in mortality for cardiovascular diseases and noncardiovascular causes of death, United States, 1970 to 1984. (Modified from National Heart, Lung, and Blood Institute. Vital Statistics of the United States. Rockville, MD, National Center for Health Statistics, 1986)

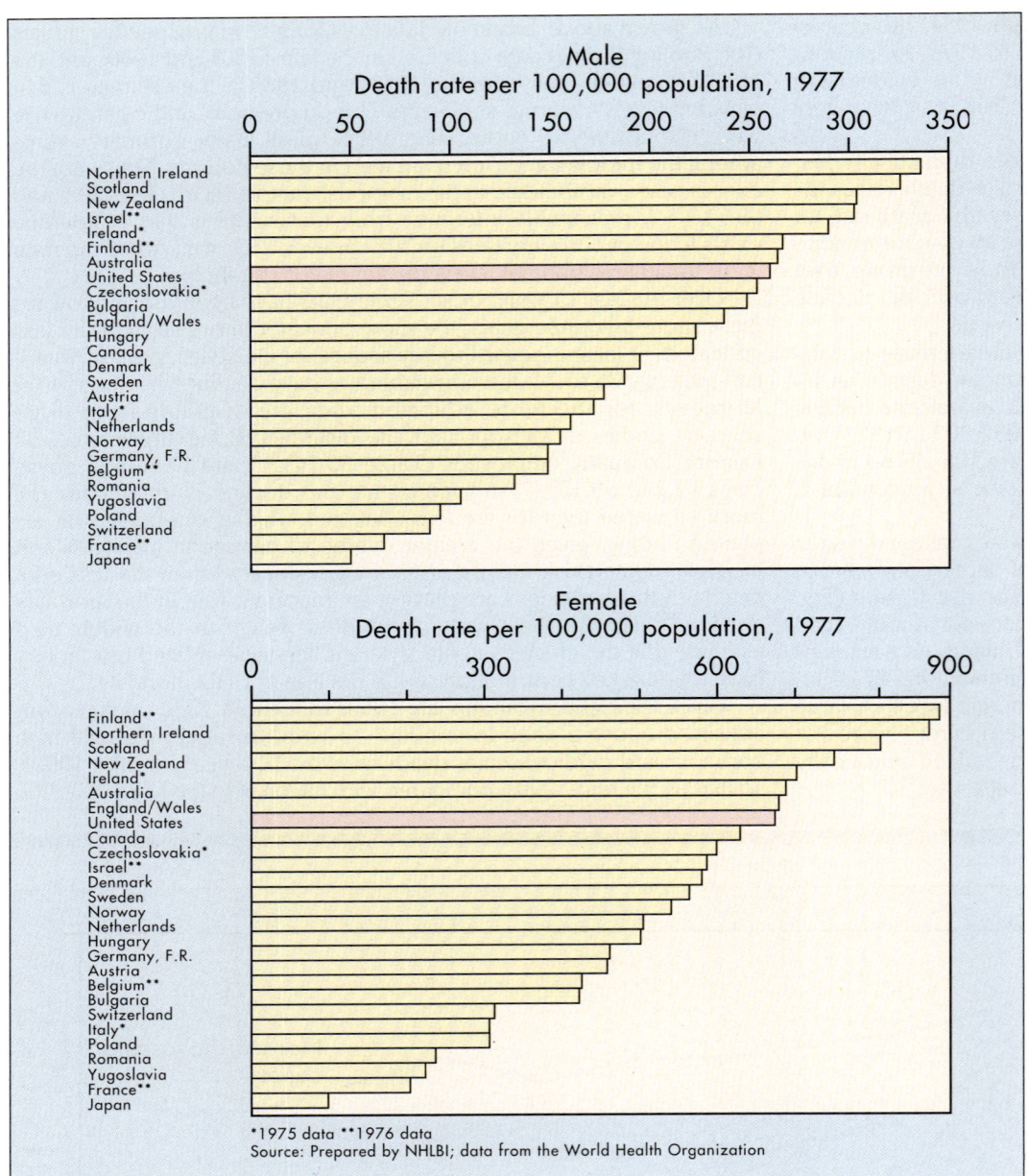

FIGURE 59.10 Death rates for coronary heart disease by country; **(A)** men and **(B)** women 35 to 74 years of age, 1969 to 1977. (Working Group on Arteriosclerosis of the National Heart, Lung, and Blood Institute: Report of the Working Group on Arteriosclerosis of the National Heart, Lung, and Blood Institute—Summary, Conclusions, and Recommendations, Vol 1. Bethesda, MD, US Department of Health and Human Services, Public Health Service, National Institutes of Health, NIH Publication No 81-2034, June, 1981)

TABLE 59.14 TREND OF AGE-ADJUSTED INCIDENCE RATES OF MYOCARDIAL INFARCTION AMONG MALE EMPLOYEES OF THE DUPONT COMPANY IN THE UNITED STATES, 1957 TO 1983*

	All Male Employees			Wage Workers			Salaried Employees		
Period	No. of Events	Rate per 1,000 per Year	Decline (%)	No. of Events	Rate per 1,000 per Year	Decline (%)	No. of Events	Rate per 1,000 per Year	Decline (%)
1957–1959	641	3.19		384	3.13		257	3.30	
1960–1962	704	3.12	2.2	N.A.	N.A.	N.A.	N.A.	N.A.	N.A.
1963–1965	733	2.92	8.5	N.A.	N.A.	N.A.	N.A.	N.A.	N.A.
1966–1968	819	2.98	6.6	N.A.	N.A.	N.A.	N.A.	N.A.	N.A.
1969–1971	758	2.70	15.4	N.A.	N.A.	N.A.	N.A.	N.A.	N.A.
1972–1974	710	2.57	19.4	N.A.	N.A.	N.A.	N.A.	N.A.	N.A.
1975–1977	739	2.70	15.4	N.A.	N.A.	N.A.	N.A.	N.A.	N.A.
1978–1980	644	2.33	27.0	N.A.	N.A.	N.A.	N.A.	N.A.	N.A.
1981–1983	538	2.29	28.2	272	2.56	18.2	266	2.06	37.6

* During these years, DuPont Company male employees in the United States numbered 75,000 to 94,000; 55% to 60% were production workers receiving hourly wages; the remainder were salaried employees in managerial, supervisory, professional, technical, and clerical occupations.

FIGURE 59.10 (continued)

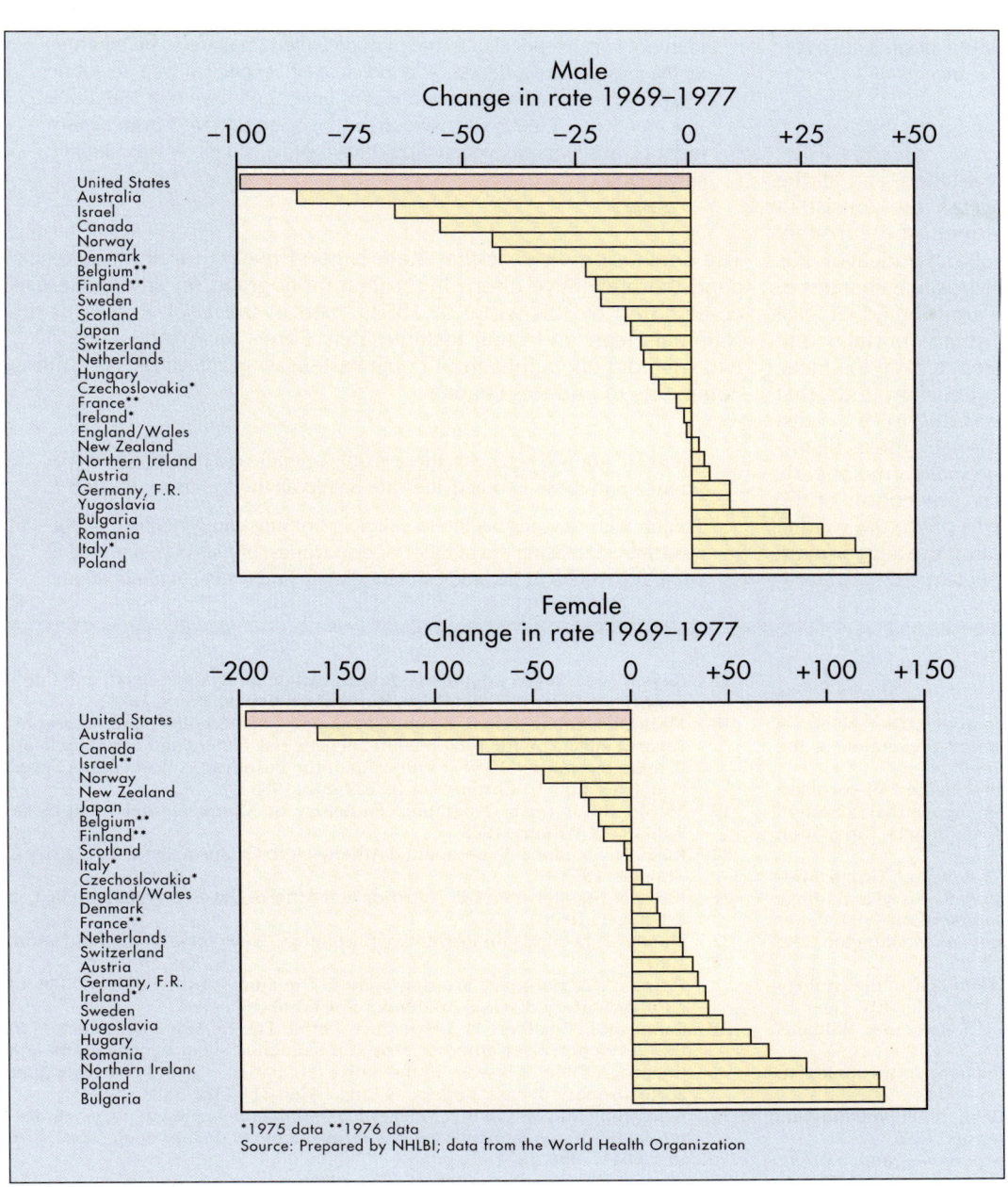

*1975 data **1976 data
Source: Prepared by NHLBI; data from the World Health Organization

TABLE 59.15 STANDARDIZED MORTALITY RATIOS, FIVE-YEAR PERIODS—CALIFORNIA MALE PHYSICIANS COMPARED TO AGE-MATCHED AMERICAN WHITE MEN

	Cause of Death		
Years	Coronary Heart Disease	Lung Cancer	All Causes
1950–1954	115	51	89
1955–1959	97	70	80
1960–1964	86	52	79
1965–1969	80	57	78
1970–1974	74	29	67
1975–1979	69	30	67
% Change: 1950–1954 → 1975–1979	−40.0%	−41.2%	−24.7%
% Change: 1965–1969 → 1975–1979	−13.7%	−47.4%	−14.1%

total decline will be over 60%. A second and related goal is to overcome the disparities among social strata in the decline.

CONCLUSIONS

These data, together with all the other scientific evidence, and all the findings on what has happened over the last 25 years, are consistent with the conclusion that undertaking and developing the coronary prevention effort over the last 25 years has been a sound endeavor. It is a reasonable inference, given all the facts, that the positive changes in life-styles and risk factors among Americans have contributed, at least in part, to the decline so far registered in the coronary mortality and incidence rates. This is not only a reasonable inference from the facts, it is a reasonable conclusion on fundamental theoretical grounds, that is, the basic generalization that epidemic disease is due to ". . . disturbances of human culture," so that amelioration of these disturbances breaks links in the chain of causation, especially crucial early links, and thereby contributes critically to primary prevention of the epidemic. Of course, it is very hard unequivocally to prove the validity of that inference. But in that regard, it is worth noting the sage remark of Darwin on the shortcomings of excessive scepticism[166]:

I am not very skeptical, a frame of mind which I believe to be injurious to the progress of science. A good deal of skepticism in a scientific man is advisable to avoid much loss of time, but I have met with not a few men, who, I feel sure, have often thus been deterred from experiment or observations which would have proved directly or indirectly serviceable.

The conclusion, then, is that there is good reason to continue to expand the preventive effort. In the first monograph on atherosclerosis co-authored by this writer in 1953,[20] and in the 1971 Report of the National Heart and Lung Institute Task Force on Arteriosclerosis,[111] two splendid quotations from Louis Pasteur were cited; they are fitting comments to end this chapter.

There are not two sciences, there is only science and the application of science and these two activities are linked as the fruit is to the tree.

To him who devotes his life to science, nothing can give more happiness than increasing the number of discoveries, but his cup of joy is full when the results of his studies immediately find practical applications.

REFERENCES

1. Inter-Society Commission for Heart Disease Resources. Atherosclerosis Study Group and Epidemiology Study Group: Primary prevention of the atherosclerotic diseases. Circulation 42:A55–A95, 1970
2. Coronary Drug Project Research Group: The natural history of coronary heart disease: Prognostic factors after recovery from myocardial infarction in 2789 men: The 5-year findings of the Coronary Drug Project. Circulation 66:401–414, 1982
3. Stamler J, Wentworth DN, Neaton JD, for the MRFIT Research Group: Middle-aged American men at very low risk of coronary death: Six-year findings on 356,222 screenees of the Multiple Risk Factor Intervention Trial. Paper presented at the Xth World Congress of Cardiology, at Washington, DC, September 16, 1986
4. Stamler J, Berkson DM, Lindberg HA: Risk factors: Their role in the etiology and pathogenesis of the atherosclerotic diseases. In Wissler RW, Geer JC (eds): The Pathogenesis of Atherosclerosis, pp 41–119. Baltimore, Williams & Wilkins, 1972
5. Ackerknecht EH: Rudolf Virchow—Doctor, Statesman, Anthropologist. Madison, University of Wisconsin Press, 1953
6. Statistical Abstract of the United States: 1986, 106th ed, p 121. Washington, DC, US Department of Commerce, Bureau of the Census, 1986
7. Rizek R, Jackson EM: Current food consumption practices and nutrient sources in the American diet. Hyattsville, MD, Consumer Nutrition Center—Human Nutrition Science and Education Administration, US Department of Agriculture, 1980
8. Block G, Dresser CM, Hartman AM, Carroll MD: Nutrient sources in the American diet: Quantitative data from the NHANES II Survey. II. Macronutrients and fats. Am J Epidemiol 122:27–40, 1985
9. Liu K, Stamler J, Stamler R et al: Methodological problems in characterizing an individual's plasma glucose level. J Chronic Dis 35:475–485, 1982
10. Working Group on Arteriosclerosis of the National Heart, Lung, and Blood Institute: Prevention. Report of the Working Group on Arteriosclerosis of the National Heart, Lung, and Blood Institute, Vol 2, pp 261–422. Bethesda, MD, US Department of Health and Human Services, Public Health Service, National Institutes of Health, NIH Publication No 81-2035, September, 1981
11. Feinleib M, Kannel WB, Tedeschi CG et al: The relation of antemortem characteristics to cardiovascular findings at necropsy. The Framingham study. Atherosclerosis 34:145–157, 1979
12. Rhoads GG, Blackwelder WC, Stemmermann GN et al: Coronary risk factors and autopsy findings in Japanese-American Men. Lab Invest 38:304–311, 1978
13. Stamler J, Wentworth D, Neaton JD, for the MRFIT Cooperative Research Group: Is the relationship between serum cholesterol and risk of death from coronary heart disease continuous and graded? Findings on the 356,222 primary screenees of the Multiple Risk Factor Intervention Trial (MRFIT). JAMA 256:2823–2828, 1986
14. Cornfield J: Joint dependence of risk of coronary heart disease on serum cholesterol and systolic blood pressure: A discriminant function and analysis. Fed Proc 21(Suppl II):58–61, 1962
15. Lipid Research Clinics Program: The Lipid Research Clinics Coronary Primary Prevention Trial results. I. Reduction in incidence of coronary heart disease. JAMA 251:351–364, 1984
16. Lipid Research Clinics Program: The Lipid Research Clinics Coronary Primary Prevention Trial results. II. The relationship of reduction in incidence of coronary heart disease to cholesterol lowering. JAMA 51:365–374, 1984
17. Keys A (ed): Seven Countries—A Multivariate Analysis of Death and Coronary Heart Disease. Cambridge, Harvard University Press, 1980
18. Mariotti S, Capocaccia R, Farchi G et al: Age, period, cohort and geographical area effects on the relationship between risk factors and coronary heart disease mortality—15-year follow-up of the European cohorts of the Seven Countries study. J Chronic Dis 39:229–242, 1986
19. McGill HC Jr (ed): Geographic Pathology of Atherosclerosis. Baltimore, Williams & Wilkins, 1968
20. Katz LN, Stamler J: Experimental Atherosclerosis. Springfield, IL, Charles C Thomas, 1953
21. Katz LN, Stamler J, Pick R: Nutrition and Atherosclerosis. Philadelphia, Lea & Febiger, 1958
22. Stamler J: Lectures on Preventive Cardiology. New York, Grune & Stratton, 1967
23. Pearson TA: Coronary arteriography in the study of the epidemiology of coronary artery disease. Epidemiol Rev 6:140–166, 1984
24. Campeau L, Enjalbert M, Lesperance J et al: The relation of risk factors to the development of atherosclerosis in saphenous-vein bypass grafts and the progression of disease in the native circulation—A study 10 years after aortocoronary bypass surgery. N Engl J Med 311:1329–1332, 1984
25. Armstrong ML, Megan MB, Warner ED: Intimal thickening in normocholesterolemic rhesus monkeys fed low supplements of dietary cholesterol. Circ Res 34:447–454, 1974
26. Wissler RW, Vesselinovitch D: The effects of various dietary fats on the development and regression of hypercholesterolemia and atherosclerosis. In Sirtori C, Ricci G, Gorini S (eds): Diet and Atherosclerosis, pp 65–76. New York, Plenum Press, 1975
27. Clarkson TB, Bond MG, Bullock BC, Marzetta CA: A study of atherosclerosis in regression in *Macaca mulatta*. IV. Changes in coronary arteries from animals with atherosclerosis induced for 19 months and then regressed for 24 to 48 months at plasma cholesterol concentrations of 300 or 200 mg/dl. Exp Mol Pathol 34:345–368, 1981
28. Stamler J: Metabolic factors related to prognosis and prevention post myocardial infarction. Paper presented at the Annual Meeting of the European Atherosclerosis Group, in Naples, Italy, June 20, 1986
29. Stamler J: Nutritional approaches to the primary prevention and treatment of hypertension. Sir George Pickering Lecture, presented at the British Hypertension Society meeting, Cambridge, England, September 17–18, 1985. Hypertension, in press
30. Stamler R, Grimm R, Gosch FC et al: Control of high blood pressure by nutritional therapy: Results of a 4-year randomized controlled trial—The Hypertension Control Program. JAMA 257:1484–1491, 1987
31. Cohen JD, Wentworth DN, Neaton JD, Kuller LH, Stamler J, for the MRFIT Cooperative Research Group: Comparative analysis of risk factors for death from stroke and from coronary heart disease: Six-year findings on 361,662 screenees of the Multiple Risk Factor Intervention Trial. Paper presented at the Xth World Congress of Cardiology, Washington, DC, September 15, 1986
32. Dyer AR, Stamler J, Shekelle RB et al: Hypertension in the elderly. Med Clin North Am 61:513–529, 1977
33. Rutan GH, Kuller LH, Neaton JD, Wentworth DN, Smith WM, for the MRFIT Cooperative Research Group: Isolated systolic hypertension, a powerful predictor of mortality in young people. Poster presentation at the Xth World Congress of Cardiology, Washington, DC, September 18, 1986
34. American Heart Association, Nutrition Committee: Coronary risk factor statement for the American public—A statement of the Nutrition Committee of the American Heart Association. Arteriosclerosis 5:678A–682A, 1985

35. Inter-Society Commission for Heart Disease Resources. Atherosclerosis Study Group: Optimal resources for primary prevention of atherosclerotic diseases. Circulation 70:153A–205A, 1984
36. Kaplan NM, Stamler J (eds): Prevention of Coronary Heart Disease: Practical Management of the Risk Factors. Philadelphia, WB Saunders, 1983
37. WHO Expert Committee on the Prevention of Coronary Heart Disease: Prevention of coronary heart disease. World Health Organization Technical Report Series No 678. Geneva, World Health Organization, 1982
38. The Health Consequences of Smoking—Cardiovascular Disease—A Report of the Surgeon General. Bethesda, MD, US Department of Health and Human Services, Public Health Service, DHHS (PHS) 84-50204, 1983
39. The Health Consequences of Smoking—The Changing Cigarette—A Report of the Surgeon General. Bethesda, MD, US Department of Health and Human Services, Public Health Service, DHHS (PHS) 81-50156, 1981
40. Byington R, Dyer AR, Garside D et al: Recent trends of major coronary risk factors and CHD mortality in the United States and other industrialized countries. In Havlik R, Feinleib M (eds): Proceedings of the Conference on the Decline in Coronary Heart Disease Mortality, pp 340–379. Washington, DC, US Department of Health, Education, and Welfare, Public Health Service, National Institutes of Health, NIH Publication No 79-1610, May, 1979
41. Pan W-H, Cedres LB, Liu K et al: Relationship of clinical diabetes and asymptomatic hyperglycemia to risk of coronary heart disease mortality in men and women. Am J Epidemiol 123:504–556, 1986
42. Stamler R, Stamler J (guest eds): Asymptomatic hyperglycemia and coronary heart disease: A series of papers by the International Collaborative Group, based on studies in fifteen populations. J Chronic Dis 32:683–837, 1979
43. Berkson DM, Stamler J: Epidemiology of the killer chronic diseases. Winick M (ed): Nutrition and the Killer Diseases, pp 17–55. New York, John Wiley & Sons, 1981
44. Paffenbarger RS, Notkin J, Krueger DE et al: Chronic disease in former college students. II. Methods of study and observations on mortality from coronary heart disease. Am J Public Health 56:962–971, 1966
45. Newman WP III, Freedman DS, Voors AW et al: Relation of serum lipoprotein levels and systolic blood pressure to early atherosclerosis—The Bogalusa Heart study. N Engl J Med 314:138–144, 1986
46. Berenson GS (ed): Cardiovascular Risk Factors in Children: The Early Natural History of Atherosclerosis and Essential Hypertension. New York, Oxford University Press, 1980
47. Ad Hoc Committee on Nutrition Education in the Young, American Heart Association Nutrition Committee: Nutrition education in the young—A statement for health professionals. Circulation 69:918A–921A, 1980
48. Weidman W, Kwiterovich P Jr, Jesse M, Nugent E: Diet in the healthy child—Task Force Committee of the Nutrition Committee and the Cardiovascular Disease in the Young Council of the American Heart Association. Circulation 67:1411A–1414A, 1983
49. Pooling Project Research Group: Relationship of blood pressure, serum cholesterol, smoking habit, relative weight and ECG abnormalities to incidence of major coronary events: Final report of the Pooling Project. J Chronic Dis 31:210–306, 1978
50. Stamler J: Improved life styles: Their potential for the primary prevention of atherosclerosis and hypertension in childhood. In Lauer RM, Shekelle RB (eds): Childhood Prevention of Atherosclerosis and Hypertension, pp 3–36. New York, Raven Press, 1980
51. Tao SC, Huang ZD, Tsai RS et al: Dietary patterns, serum lipids, urinary electrolytes, and blood pressure: Middle-aged male and female workers and farmers in North and South China. Paper presented at the Xth World Congress of Cardiology, at Washington, DC, September 16, 1986
52. Stamler J: Population studies. In Levy RI, Rifkind BM, Dennis BH, Ernst ND (eds): Nutrition, Lipids, and Coronary Heart Disease—A Global View, pp 25–88. New York, Raven Press, 1979
53. Stamler J: Does cholesterol change alter coronary artery disease risk? Epidemiologic evidence. In Proceedings of a Symposium on the Decline in Coronary Heart Disease Mortality—The Role of Cholesterol Change? pp 27–45. New York, Science and Medicine, 1983
54. Malmros H: The relation of nutrition to health—A statistical study of the effect of war-time on arteriosclerosis, cardiosclerosis, tuberculosis, and diabetes. Acta Med Scand (Suppl) 246:137–153, 1950
55. Keys A, Brozek J, Herschel A et al: The Biology of Human Starvation, Vol 1. Minneapolis, University of Minnesota Press, 1950
56. Cowdry EV: Arteriosclerosis. New York, Macmillan, 1933
57. Beitzke H: Zur Entsehung der Atherosklerose. Virchows Arch [A] 267:625–647, 1928
58. Schettler G: Atherosclerosis during periods of food deprivation following World Wars I and II. Prev Med 12:75–83, 1983
59. Kimura N: Analysis of 10,000 postmortem examinations in Japan. In Keys A, White PD (eds): World Trends in Cardiology: I. Cardiovascular Epidemiology, p 22. New York, Hoeber-Harper, 1956
60. White NK, Edwards JE, Dry TJ: The relationship of the degree of coronary atherosclerosis with age, in men. Circulation 1:645–654, 1950
61. Snapper I: Chinese Lessons to Western Medicine. New York, Interscience, 1941
62. West KM (ed): Epidemiology of Diabetes and Its Vascular Lesions. New York, Elsevier-North Holland, 1978
63. Tracy RE, Toca VT, Strong JP, Richards ML: Relationship of raised atherosclerotic lesions to fatty streaks in cigarette smokers. Atherosclerosis 38:347–357, 1981
64. Keys A: Serum cholesterol and the question of "normal." In Benson ES, Strandjord PE (eds): Multiple Laboratory Screening, pp 147–170. New York, Academic Press, 1969
65. Kato H, Tillotson J, Nichaman MZ et al: Epidemiologic studies of coronary heart disease and stroke in Japanese men living in Japan, Hawaii and California. Serum lipids and diet. Am J Epidemiol 97:372–385, 1973
66. Tillotson J, Kato H, Nichaman MZ et al: Epidemiology of coronary heart disease and stroke in Japanese men living in Japan, Hawaii, and California. Methodology for comparison of diet. Am J Clin Nutr 26:177–184, 1973
67. Kagan A, Harris BR, Winkelstein W Jr et al: Epidemiologic studies of coronary heart disease and stroke in Japanese men living in Japan, Hawaii and California. Demographic, physical, dietary and biochemical characteristics. J Chronic Dis 17:345–364, 1974
68. Marmot MG, Syme SL, Kagan A et al: Epidemiologic studies of coronary heart disease and stroke in Japanese men living in Japan, Hawaii and California. Prevalence of coronary and hypertensive heart disease and associated risk factors. Am J Epidemiol 102:514–525, 1975
69. Worth RM, Kato H, Rhoads GG et al: Epidemiologic studies of coronary heart disease and stroke in Japanese men living in Japan, Hawaii and California. Mortality. Am J Epidemiol 102:481–490, 1975
70. Robertson TL, Kato H, Rhoads GG et al: Epidemiologic studies of coronary heart disease and stroke in Japanese men living in Japan, Hawaii and California. Incidence of myocardial infarction and death from coronary heart disease. Am J Cardiol 39:239–243, 1977
71. Saikai Y, Comstock GW, Stone RW, Suzuki T: Cardiovascular risk factors among Japanese and American telephone executives. Int J Epidemiol 6:7–15, 1977
72. Rosenthal SR: Studies in atherosclerosis: Chemical, experimental and morphologic. Arch Pathol 18:473–506, 660–698, and 827–842, 1934
73. Brown J, Bourke GJ, Gearty GF et al: Nutritional and epidemiologic factors related to heart disease. In Bourne G (ed): World Review of Nutrition and Dietetics, Vol 12. pp 1–42. New York, Karger, 1970
74. Kushi LH, Lew RA, Stare FJ et al: Diet and 20-year mortality from coronary heart disease. N Engl J Med 312:811–818, 1985
75. Page LB, Damon A, Moellering RC Jr: Antecedents of cardiovascular disease in six Solomon Islands societies. Circulation 49:1132–1146, 1974
76. Hardinge MG, Stare JF: Nutritional studies of vegetarians. 2. Dietary and serum levels of cholesterol. Am J Clin Nutr 2:83–88, 1954
77. Sacks FM, Castelli WP, Donner A, Kass EH: Plasma lipids and lipoproteins in vegetarians and controls. N Engl J Med 292:1148–1151, 1975
78. Phillips RL, Lemon FR, Beeson WL, Kuzma JW: Coronary heart disease mortality among Seventh-Day Adventists with differing dietary habits—A preliminary report. Am J Clin Nutr (Suppl) 31:S191–S198, 1978
79. Working Group of Arteriosclerosis of the National Heart, Lung, and Blood Institute: Fundamental research—Laboratory and epidemiological. Report of the Working Group of Arteriosclerosis of the National Heart, Lung, and Blood Institute, Vol 2, pp 1–82. Bethesda, MD, US Department of Health and Human Services, Public Health Service, National Institutes of Health, NIH Publication No 81-2035, Sept 1981
80. Liu K, Stamler J, Dyer A et al: Statistical methods to assess and minimize the role of intra-individual variability in obscuring the relationship between dietary lipids and serum cholesterol. J Chronic Dis 31:399–418, 1978
81. Shekelle RB, Stamler J, Paul O et al: Dietary lipids and serum cholesterol level—Change in diet confounds the cross-sectional association. Am J Epidemiol 115:506–514, 1982
82. Connor WE, Cerqueira MT, Rodney MS et al: The plasma lipids, lipoproteins, and diet of the Tarahumara Indians of Mexico. Am J Clin Nutr 31:1131–1142, 1978
83. Shekelle RB, Shryock AM, Paul O et al: Diet, serum cholesterol, and death from coronary heart disease—The Western Electric study. N Engl J Med 304:65–70, 1981
84. Stamler J, Berkson DM, Dyer A et al: Relationship of multiple variables to blood pressure—Findings from four Chicago epidemiologic studies. In Paul O (ed): Epidemiology and Control of Hypertension, pp 307–356. Miami, Symposia Specialists, 1975
85. Liu K, Cooper R, McKeever J et al: Assessment of the association between habitual salt intake and high blood pressure: Methodological problems. Am J Epidemiol 110:219–226, 1979
86. Liu K, Cooper R, Soltero I, Stamler J: Variability in 24-hour sodium excretion in children. Hypertension 1:631–636, 1979
87. Liu K, Dyer AR, Cooper RS et al: Can overnight urine replace 24-hour urine collection to assess salt intake? Hypertension 1:529–536, 1979
88. Stamler J: Epidemiologic evidence on the role of nutrition in arterial hypertension. International Symposium on Nutritional and Metabolic Aspects of Arterial Hypertension, Anacapri, June 3–4, 1985. Journal of Clinical Hypertension, in press
89. Stamler J: Preventive cardiology. In Cheng TO (ed): International Practice of Cardiology, pp 1231–1255. Elmsford, NY, Pergamon Press, 1986
90. Glueck CT, Barboriak J (guest eds): Symposium on Alcohol and Cardiovascular Diseases. Circulation 64(Suppl III):1–84, 1981
91. Dyer A, Stamler J, Paul O et al: Alcohol consumption, cardiovascular risk factors, and mortality in two Chicago epidemiologic studies. Circulation 56:1067–1074, 1977

92. Dyer AR, Stamler J, Paul O et al: Alcohol, cardiovascular risk factors and mortality: The Chicago experience. Circulation 64(Suppl III):20–27, 1981
93. Saunders JB, Beevers DG, Paton A: Alcohol-induced hypertension. Lancet 2:653–656, 1981
94. Liu K, Stamler J, Trevisan M, Moss D: Dietary lipids, sugar, fiber, and mortality from coronary heart disease—Bivariate analysis of international data. Arteriosclerosis 2:221–227, 1982
95. Kromhout D, Bosschieter EB, Coulander CDL: The inverse relation between fish consumption and 20-year mortality from coronary heart disease. N Engl J Med 312:1205–1209, 1985
96. Yano K, Reed DM, McGee DL: Ten-year incidence of coronary heart disease in the Honolulu Heart Program: Relationship to biologic and lifestyle characteristics. Am J Epidemiol 119:653–666, 1984
97. Kahn HA, Phillips RL: Association between reported diet and all-cause mortality: Twenty-one-year follow-up on 27,530 adult Seventh-Day Adventists. Am J Epidemiol 119:775–787, 1984
98. Snowdon DA, Phillips RL, Fraser GE: Meat consumption and fatal ischemic heart disease. Prev Med 13:490–500, 1984
99. Nube M, Kok FJ, Vandenbroucke JP et al: Scoring of prudent dietary habits and its relation to 25 year survival. J Am Diet Assoc 87:171–175, 1987
100. Dyer AR, Stamler J, Berkson DM, Lindberg HA: Relationship of relative weight and body mass index to 14-year mortality in the Peoples Gas Company study. J Chronic Dis 28:109–123, 1975
101. Hypertension Detection and Follow-up Program Cooperative Group: Mortality findings for Stepped-Care and Referred-Care participants in the Hypertension Detection and Follow-up Program, stratified by other risk factors. Prev Med 14:312–335, 1985
102. Pan W-H, Liu K, Dyer A et al: Thin hypertensives and their cause-specific mortality risk. In press
103. White PD, Sprague HB, Stamler J et al: A Statement on Arteriosclerosis, Main Cause of "Heart Attacks" and "Strokes." New York, National Health Education Committee, Inc., 1959
104. American Heart Association, Ad Hoc Committee on Smoking and Cardiovascular Disease: Cigarette smoking and cardiovascular disease. Circulation 22:160–166, 1960
105. American Heart Association, Central Committee for Medical and Community Program: Dietary Fat and Its Relation to Heart Attacks and Strokes. New York, American Heart Association, EM 180, 1961
106. Grundy SM, Bilheimer D, Blackburn H et al: Rationale of the Diet–Heart Statement of the American Heart Association—Report of Nutrition Committee. Circulation 65:839A–854A, 1982
107. American Heart Association, Nutrition Committee and the Council on Arteriosclerosis: Recommendations for treatment of hyperlipidemia in adults. Circulation 69:1065A–1090A, 1984
108. American Heart Association, Nutrition Committee: Dietary guidelines for healthy adult Americans. Circulation 74:1465A–1468A, 1986
109. Smoking and Health: Report of the Advisory Committee to the Surgeon General of the Public Health Service, US Department of Health, Education, and Welfare, Public Health Service Publication No 1103. Washington, DC, Superintendent of Documents, US Government Printing Office, 1964
110. Keys A (Chairman), Page IH (Vice Chairman): Final Report to the President from the White House Conference on Food, Nutrition and Health. Washington, DC, The White House, 1970
111. Task Force on Arteriosclerosis of the National Heart and Lung Institute: Arteriosclerosis, Vol I. Washington, DC, US Department of Health, Education, and Welfare, Public Health Service, DHEW Publication No (NIH) 72-137, June 1971
112. Inter-Society Commission for Heart Disease Resources, Hypertension Study Group: Guidelines for detection, diagnosis and management of hypertensive populations. Circulation 44:A263–A272, 1971
113. National Conference on High Blood Pressure Education. Washington, DC, National Heart and Lung Institute, DHEW Publication No (NIH) 73-486, 1973
114. Joint National Committee on Detection, Evaluation, and Treatment of High Blood Pressure: The 1984 Report of the Joint National Committee on Detection, Evaluation, and Treatment of High Blood Pressure. Arch Intern Med 144:1045–1057, 1984
115. Subcommittee on Nonpharmacological Therapy of the 1984 Joint National Committee on Detection, Evaluation, and Treatment of High Blood Pressure: Nonpharmacological approaches to the control of high blood pressure. Final Report. Hypertension 8:444–467, 1986
116. Select Committee on Nutrition and Human Needs, US Senate: Dietary Goals for the United States, 2nd ed. Washington, DC, US Government Printing Office, Dec 1977
117. American Heart Association: The American Heart Association Cookbook, 3rd ed. New York, David McKay Co, 1980
118. American Diabetes Association and American Dietetic Association Committee on Food and Nutrition: Principles of nutrition and dietary recommendations for patients with diabetes mellitus: 1971. A special report. Diabetes 20:633–634, 1971
119. Healthy People: The Surgeon General's Report on Health Promotion and Disease Prevention. Washington, DC, US Department of Health, Education, and Welfare, Public Health Service, DHEW Publication No (PHS) 79-55071, 1970
120. Promotion Health/Preventing Disease—Objectives for the Nation. Washington, DC, Department of Health and Human Services, Public Health Service, Office of Disease Prevention and Health Promotion, Center for Disease Control, Health Resources Administration, Fall 1980
121. Institute of Medicine, National Academy of Sciences: Healthy People. The Surgeon General's Report on Health Promotion and Disease Prevention, Background Papers, 1979. Washington, DC, US Department of Health, Education, and Welfare, Public Health Service, Office of the Assistant Secretary for Health and Surgeon General, DHEW Publication No (PHS) 79-55071A, US Government Printing Office, 1979
122. Proceedings of Prospects for a Healthier America: Achieving the Nation's Health Promotion Objectives. Washington, DC, US Department of Health and Human Services, Public Health Service, Office of Disease Prevention and Health Promotion, Nov 1984
123. Health—United States, 1983, and Prevention Profile. Washington, DC, US Department of Health and Human Services, Public Health Service, National Center for Health Statistics, DHHS Pub No (PHS) 84-1232, US Government Printing Office, Dec 1983
124. The 1990 Health Objectives for the Nation: A Midcourse Review. Washington, DC, US Department of Health and Human Services, Public Health Service, Office of Disease Prevention and Health Promotion, Nov 1986
125. US Department of Agriculture and US Department of Health, Education, and Welfare: Nutrition and Your Health—Dietary Guidelines for Americans. Washington, DC, US Department of Agriculture, US Department of Health, Education, and Welfare, 1980
126. US Department of Agriculture and US Department of Health and Human Services: Nutrition and Your Health—Dietary Guidelines for Americans, 2nd ed. Washington, DC, US Department of Agriculture, US Department of Health and Human Services, 1985
127. National Academy of Sciences: Recommended Dietary Allowances, 9th ed. Washington, DC, National Research Council, National Academy of Sciences, 1980
128. Stamler J, Abelmann WH (eds): Bethesda Conference Report—Eleventh Bethesda Conference: Prevention of Coronary Heart Disease. Am J Cardiol 47:713–776, 1981
129. Working Group on Arteriosclerosis of the National Heart, Lung, and Blood Institute: Report of the Working Group on Arteriosclerosis of the National Heart, Lung, and Blood Institute—Summary, Conclusions, and Recommendations, Vol 1. Bethesda, MD, US Department of Health and Human Services, Public Health Service, National Institutes of Health, NIH Publication No 81-2034, June 1981
130. Working Group on Arteriosclerosis of the National Heart, Lung, and Blood Institute: Report of the Working Group on Arteriosclerosis of the National Heart, Lung, and Blood Institute, Vol 2. Bethesda, MD, US Department of Health and Human Services, Public Health Service, National Institutes of Health, NIH Publication No 81-2035, Sept 1981
131. Office of Medical Applications of Research, National Institutes of Health: Consensus Conference—Lowering blood cholesterol to prevent heart disease. JAMA 253:2080–2086, 1985
132. Lenfant C: A new challenge for America: The National Cholesterol Education Program. Circulation 73:855–856, 1986
133. Food and Nutrition Board, Division of Biological Sciences, Assembly of Life Sciences, National Research Council, National Academy of Sciences: Toward Healthful Diets. Washington, DC, National Academy of Sciences, 1980
134. Ahrens EH: Dietary fats and coronary heart disease: Unfinished business. Lancet 2:1345–1348, 1979
135. WHO Expert Committee on Smoking Control: Smoking and its effects on health. Report of the WHO Expert Committee on Smoking Control. Technical Report Series No 568, Geneva, World Health Organization, 1975
136. WHO Expert Committee on Smoking Control: Controlling the smoking epidemic. Report of the WHO Expert Committee on Smoking Control. Technical Report Series No 636, Geneva, World Health Organization, 1979
137. Community Prevention and Control of Cardiovascular Diseases—Report of a WHO Expert Committee. Technical Report Series No 732, Geneva, World Health Organization, 1986
138. Pyörälä K, Rapaport E, König K et al (eds): Secondary Prevention of Coronary Heart Disease—Workshop of the International Society and Federation of Cardiology, Titisee, October 21–24, 1983. New York, Thieme-Stratton, 1983
139. Fourth WHO/ISH Conference on Mild Hypertension: Mild Hypertension—From Trials to Practice. Konigstein, Federal Republic of Germany, December 6, 1985
140. Assmann G, Lewis B, Mancini M et al (Co-Chairmen) and other members of the European Study Group: Strategy for the prevention of coronary heart disease—A policy statement of the European Atherosclerosis Society. Eur Heart J 8:77–88, 1987
141. Jones JL: Are health concerns changing the American diet? National Food Situation, NFS-159, pp 27–28. Washington, DC, US Department of Agriculture, March, 1977
142. Jones J, Weimer J: A survey of health-related food choices. National Food Review, NFR-12, pp 16–19. Washington, DC, US Department of Agriculture, Fall, 1980
143. 1979 Summary, National Ambulatory Care Survey, pp 1–11. Hyattsville, MD, National Center for Health Statistics Advance Data No 66, March 2, 1981
144. Statistical Abstract of the United States: 1975, 96th ed, p 92. Washington, DC, US Department of Commerce, Bureau of the Census, 1975
145. US Department of Agriculture, Human Nutrition Information Service: Un-

published data on nutrient fat from fats and oils in the US food supply. Hyattsville, MD, US Department of Agriculture, 1981
146. Dietary Intake Source Data: United States, 1976–80. National Health Survey. Hyattsville, MD, National Center for Health Statistics, Series 11, No 231, March, 1983
147. Caggiula AW, Christakis G, Farrand M et al: The Multiple Risk Factor Intervention Trial (MRFIT). IV. Intervention on blood lipids. Prev Med 10:442–475, 1981
148. Kannel WB, Gordon T: The Framingham Study—An Epidemiological Investigation of Cardiovascular Disease. Section 24: The Framingham Diet Study: Diet and the Regulation of Serum Cholesterol. Washington, DC, US Department of Health, Education and Welfare, Public Health Service, National Institutes of Health, April, 1970
149. National Diet–Heart Study Research Group: The National Diet–Heart Study final report. Circulation 37(Suppl 1):1–428, 1968
150. Charting the Nation's Health—Trends since 1960. Hyattsville, MD, US Department of Health and Human Services, Public Health Service, National Center for Health Statistics, DHHS Pub No (PHS) 85-1251, August, 1985
151. National Center for Health Statistics, National Heart, Lung, and Blood Institute Collaborative Lipid Group: Trends in serum cholesterol levels among US adults aged 20 to 74 years. Data from the National Health and Nutrition Examination Surveys, 1960 to 1980. JAMA 257:937–942, 1987
152. Masover L: Television Food Advertising: A Positive or Negative Contribution to Nutrition Education? MPH Thesis, Department of Community Health and Preventive Medicine, Northwestern University Medical School, Chicago, 1977
153. Statistical Abstract of the United States: 1986, 106th ed, p 760. Washington, DC, US Department of Commerce, Bureau of the Census, 1986
154. Smoking and Health: Report of the Surgeon General. Washington, DC, US Department of Health, Education and Welfare, DHEW Publication No (PHS) 79-50066, US Government Printing Office, 1979
155. American Institute of Public Opinion: Gallup Poll on Exercise. Princeton, NJ, Gallup Poll, 1978
156. Veterans Administration Cooperative Study Group on Antihypertensive Agents: Effects of treatment on morbidity in hypertension—Results in patients with diastolic blood pressures averaging 115 through 129 mm Hg. JAMA 202:1028–1034, 1967
157. Veterans Administration Cooperative Study Group on Antihypertensive Agents: Effects of treatment on morbidity in hypertension. II. Results in patients with diastolic blood pressure averaging 90 through 114 mm Hg. JAMA 213:1143–1152, 1970
158. Veterans Administration Cooperative Study Group on Antihypertensive Agents: Effects of treatment on morbidity in hypertension. III. Influence of age, diastolic pressure, and prior cardiovascular disease; further analysis of side effects. Circulation 45:991–1004, 1972
159. National Disease and Therapeutic Index, 1965–1975. Ambler, PA, IMS American Ltd, 1977
160. National Heart, Lung, and Blood Institute. Vital Statistics of the United States. Rockville, MD, National Center for Health Statistics, 1986
161. Stamler J: The marked decline in coronary heart disease mortality rates in the United States, 1968–1981: Summary of findings and possible explanations. Cardiology 72:11–22, 1985
162. Recent trends in mortality from cardiovascular diseases. Stat Bull Metropol Life Ins Co 60(2):3–8, 1979
163. Pell S, Fayerweather WE: Trends in the incidence of myocardial infarction and in associated mortality and morbidity in a large employed population, 1957–1983. N Engl J Med 312:1005–1011, 1985
164. Enstrom JE: Trends in mortality among California physicians after giving up smoking: 1950–79. Br Med J 286:1101–1105, 1983
165. Stamler J: Editorial: Coronary heart disease: Doing the "right things." N Engl J Med 312:1053–1055, 1985
166. Darwin F (ed): The Life and Letters of Charles Darwin, Vol 1, p 83. New York, Appleton-Century-Crofts, 1896

LIPID ABNORMALITIES: MECHANISMS, CLINICAL CLASSIFICATIONS, AND MANAGEMENT

Robert W. Mahley • Thomas P. Bersot

One well-established risk factor that accelerates the development of coronary heart disease is an elevated plasma cholesterol level. The focus of this chapter is on the role of plasma cholesterol in atherogenesis. The mechanisms by which specific lipoproteins are involved in the process are discussed, along with the prevention and treatment of high plasma cholesterol levels. Hypertriglyceridemia, although not directly a risk factor, is also discussed because it must be considered in the effective management of patients with hypercholesterolemia.

Coronary heart disease is caused by atherosclerosis, the disease process in which the lumen of the coronary arteries is narrowed by plaques that are the stratum on which coronary artery thrombi are formed. Atherosclerosis is characterized by lipid deposition (primarily cholesterol and cholesteryl esters) in and around cells of the arterial wall. The earliest lesion may well be the appearance of cholesterol-laden macrophages that accumulate in the subintimal space immediately below the endothelial cells lining the artery. The process is further characterized by cellular proliferation and fibrosis. The key to unraveling the role of high plasma cholesterol levels in the process of accelerated atherogenesis involves both an understanding of those plasma lipoproteins that enhance the delivery of cholesterol to cells of the arterial wall and the identification of the cells that are responsible for the accumulation of the cholesterol.

The cholesterol–diet–heart hypothesis has been debated for many years. However, sufficient data are now available to establish that a direct relationship exists between high plasma cholesterol levels, diets high in fat and cholesterol, and accelerated coronary heart disease. All of the data gathered from diverse experimental disciplines consistently support this conclusion. No one study or scientific approach can be used to draw this conclusion, but when one looks at all of the pieces of this puzzle from the research laboratory, the metabolic ward, population studies, and clinical trials, the data overwhelmingly support the cholesterol–diet–heart hypothesis.

RELATIONSHIP BETWEEN PLASMA CHOLESTEROL LEVELS AND CORONARY HEART DISEASE

Evidence from a variety of studies has established a causal relationship between plasma cholesterol levels and coronary heart disease.[1-3] This conclusion is supported by a report of a National Institutes of Health Consensus Panel that considered much of the available data relating to the topic of plasma cholesterol and heart disease.[4,5] In this section, selected data supporting the causal relationship between elevated plasma cholesterol levels and coronary heart disease is summarized.

Epidemiologic evidence concerning plasma cholesterol levels and coronary heart disease risk in various populations of the world has demonstrated that the risk of developing coronary heart disease increases as the plasma cholesterol level increases. For example, several populations, specifically those of North America, Northern and Central Europe, New Zealand, and Australia, have average cholesterol levels of 220 mg to 280 mg/dl. In these areas, coronary heart disease is a major health problem. Furthermore, intermediate levels of cholesterol, averaging 180 mg to 200 mg/dl, are typical for people in the Mediterranean countries of Greece, Yugoslavia, and Italy, and in certain Latin American countries (values for 95% of the population studied in these countries ranged from 130 mg to 250 mg/dl). The incidence of coronary heart disease in the latter group of populations is about one-half that seen in the affluent Western countries. In contrast, populations in the Orient and Mediterranean Basin have mean cholesterol levels of approximately 160 mg/dl (with 95% of the population in these areas having values from 110 mg to 210 mg/dl). These populations have very low overall risk of coronary heart disease, and myocardial infarctions are rare.

The differences between populations can be dramatically illustrated by consideration of results obtained from surveys of Japanese in Kyushu and of Karelians in Finland. A 10-year coronary heart disease death rate for the Japanese was approximately 7 per 1000, as compared with approximately 70 per 1000 for the Finnish population. As shown in Figure 60.1, little overlap in plasma cholesterol levels is observed in a comparison of the Japanese (an average of <150 mg/dl) with the Finnish population (an average of >250 mg/dl).

The Ni-Ho-San study indicates that differences among populations are strongly influenced by environment, behavior, and culture. Although heritable factors provide a different background on which environment works, they are not the prime determinants of the differences in plasma cholesterol values. Japanese men on mainland Japan were shown to have a mean cholesterol level of approximately 180 mg/dl, whereas Japanese men and their offspring living in Hawaii and California had mean levels of 220 mg to 230 mg/dl. The differences in cholesterol levels among these three groups of Japanese were correlated with the incidence of mortality from coronary heart disease. Japanese men and their offspring living in California had a twofold to threefold greater incidence of coronary heart disease than Japanese men in Japan. Change in diet appears to play a key role in increasing the risk of coronary heart disease. Japanese people living in the United States altered their diet by adopting a Western diet high in saturated fat and cholesterol, forsaking the more traditional low-fat, low-cholesterol diet of Japan.[2]

Data from the Pooling Project, the Seven Countries Study, and the Framingham Study strongly suggest that risk increases at levels of cholesterol greater than 200 mg/dl and probably increases when cholesterol levels exceed 180 mg/dl. (Data from the Seven Countries Study are shown in Figure 60.2.) In addition, examination of certain data from these and other studies indicate that there is a sharp increase in coronary heart disease risk when cholesterol levels are above 200 mg to 220 mg/dl. These data not only help to establish the causal relationship between plasma cholesterol and coronary heart disease but are also important in defining "normal" plasma cholesterol levels.

Epidemiologic surveys of coronary disease incidence, plasma cholesterol concentrations, and dietary habits have demonstrated positive correlations between all three of these parameters. Furthermore, it has been demonstrated that cholesterol levels can be lowered by decreasing saturated fat and cholesterol intake. Metabolic ward studies have shown that reducing saturated fat and cholesterol intake and increasing polyunsaturated fat in the diet will reduce the concentration of plasma cholesterol and low-density lipoproteins (LDL).

Animal model studies have also established a causal relationship between plasma cholesterol levels, diets high in fat and cholesterol, and accelerated atherosclerosis.[6] Virtually every animal investigated develops a high blood cholesterol level and atherosclerosis when fed a diet high in fat and cholesterol. Even though many of these studies have used excessively high levels of saturated fat and cholesterol to induce accelerated atherosclerosis in a very short period of time, there are studies in which monkeys have been fed fat- and cholesterol-rich diets similar to those consumed by certain populations in the world. The development of accelerated atherosclerosis in these monkeys was clearly associated with diet-induced hyperlipidemia.

One of the clearest demonstrations of the relationship between plasma cholesterol and coronary heart disease comes from studies of the genetic lipid abnormalities in humans. For example, patients with homozygous familial hypercholesterolemia have high levels of plasma cholesterol (specifically, an elevation of LDL) and usually die of coronary heart disease in their second decade of life. Patients with type III hyperlipoproteinemia also have elevated cholesterol levels and develop accelerated peripheral and coronary artery disease.[7]

RELATIONSHIP BETWEEN THE REDUCTION OF PLASMA CHOLESTEROL LEVELS AND DECREASED RISK OF CORONARY HEART DISEASE

A National Institutes of Health Consensus Panel has agreed that available data demonstrate that a reduction of plasma cholesterol levels can be expected to have a beneficial effect on the incidence of coronary heart disease.[4] This conclusion was based on a review of several dietary trials.[1,2] Reduction of fat and cholesterol consumption resulted in lowered plasma cholesterol levels and a 23% to 35% reduction in the incidence of coronary heart disease. In addition, the Coronary Primary Prevention Trial (CPPT) completed in 1982 and the Helsinki Heart Study (HHS) completed in 1987 demonstrated that lowering plasma cholesterol levels resulted in significant reductions in the rate of coronary heart disease in hypercholesterolemic men.[8-10] In the CPPT, cholestyramine lowered total cholesterol an average of 9% and was associated with a 19% reduction in the combined rate of fatal and nonfatal coronary disease. The HHS participants received gemfibrozil, which reduced average total cholesterol levels by 11%. This resulted in a 34% reduction in the incidence of coronary heart disease, primarily nonfatal myocardial infarction. The greater reduction in coronary disease incidence observed in the HHS participants, despite similar lowering of cholesterol levels in both studies, may be attributable to the fact that high-density lipoprotein (HDL) cholesterol levels increased by 11% in HHS participants but only by 3% in the CPPT treatment group.

The Cholesterol-Lowering Atherosclerosis Study provides arteriographic evidence that lowering cholesterol concentrations retards and/or reverses the development of atherosclerosis in both the native vessels and in vein bypass grafts of coronary artery bypass surgery patients.[11] Drug treatment with colestipol and nicotinic acid resulted in a 26% reduction in total cholesterol compared with a 4% reduction in the placebo group. After 2 years of treatment, repeat arteriography revealed significantly improved coronary artery status in 16.2% of the drug-treated versus 2.4% of the placebo-treated patients. The National Heart, Lung, and Blood Institute Type II Coronary Intervention Trial, in which cholestyramine lowered total cholesterol levels by 17%, also demonstrated a significant lack of progression of coronary artery disease, as determined by arteriography.[12]

Results from these and other clinical trials suggest that for every 1% reduction in the plasma cholesterol level, there is a 2% reduction in the incidence of coronary heart disease. Clearly, at least a 5% to 10% reduction in plasma cholesterol can be achieved by adoption of a prudent (low-saturated fat, low-cholesterol) diet, and it is predicted that this modest life-style change alone could result in a 10% to 20% reduction in coronary heart disease (*i.e.*, up to 100,000 fewer deaths from myocardial infarction per year). For the small percentage of patients whose hypercholesterolemia is refractory to dietary intervention alone,

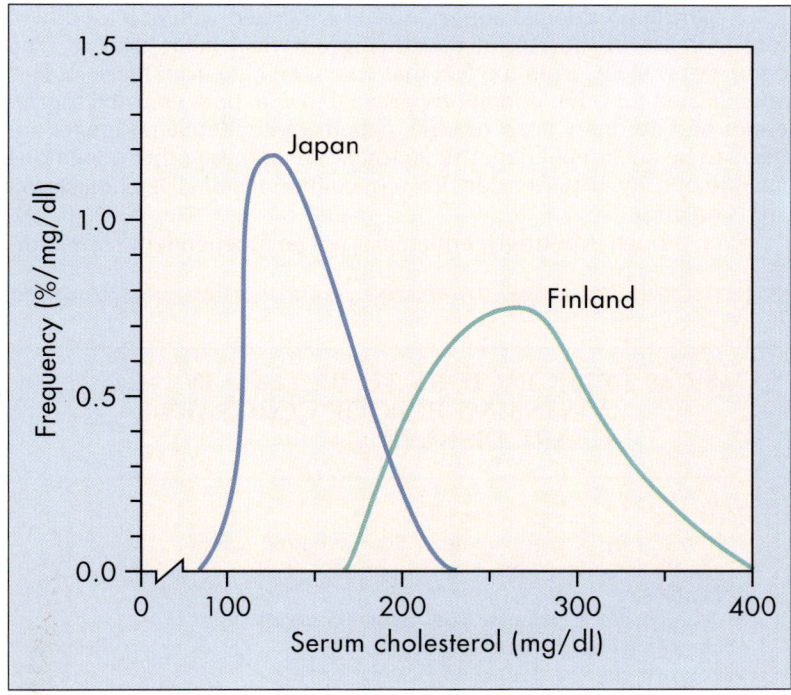

FIGURE 60.1 Distribution of serum cholesterol levels within Japanese and Finnish populations. (Modified from Blackburn H: Epidemiological evidence. In American Health Foundation (Wynder EL [ed]): Plasma Lipids: Optimal Levels for Health, pp 3–72. New York, Academic Press, 1980)

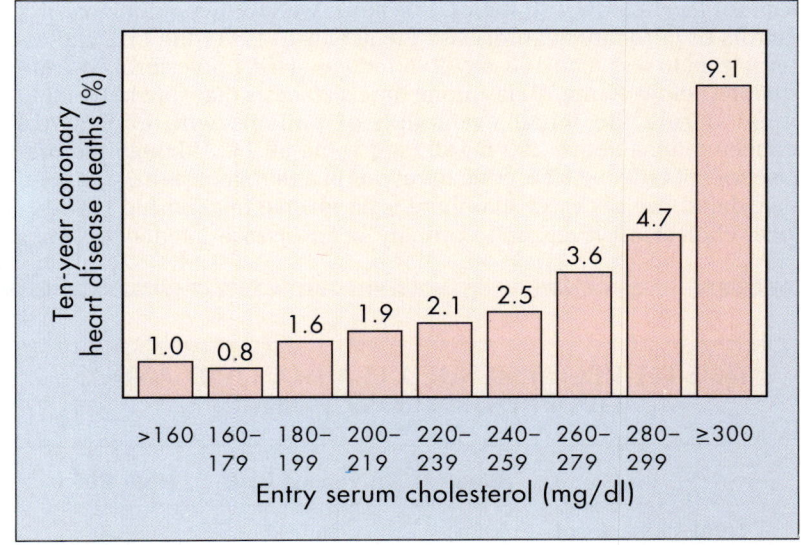

FIGURE 60.2 Correlation between the coronary heart disease deaths and the serum cholesterol levels at entry into the study. (Modified from Blackburn H: Epidemiological evidence. In American Health Foundation (Wynder EL [ed]): Plasma Lipids: Optimal Levels for Health, pp 3–72. New York, Academic Press, 1980)

pharmacologic normalization of cholesterol levels is now possible, especially since the advent of cholesterol biosynthesis inhibitors such as lovastatin.[13]

DEFINITION OF A "NORMAL" PLASMA CHOLESTEROL LEVEL

Normal levels of substances circulating in the blood usually represent values between the 5th and 95th percentiles in the population. However, the use of values for plasma cholesterol in excess of the 95th percentile (250 mg to 280 mg/dl for adults) to define the upper limits of "normal" is unreasonable in our population, which is suffering from an epidemic of coronary heart disease. In the United States, approximately 50% of the population has plasma cholesterol levels above 200 mg to 230 mg/dl, values that are associated with an increased risk of developing premature coronary heart disease. The definition of a "normal" plasma cholesterol level should be one that decreases the risk of developing premature coronary heart disease and yet is reasonably attainable. It may be desirable for all persons to have plasma cholesterol levels of 160 mg to 180 mg/dl; however, dietary changes necessary to achieve this goal may be too stringent in view of present-day dietary habits. It is essential for the health of Americans that the population be encouraged to adopt a diet that will lower plasma cholesterol levels to these desired levels.

The National Cholesterol Education Program Expert Panel on Detection, Evaluation, and Treatment of High Blood Cholesterol in Adults has redefined hypercholesterolemia into two categories: increased risk (200 mg to 240 mg/dl) and high risk (above 240 mg/dl; Table 60.1).[5] Recommendations for cholesterol-lowering therapy for specific patients are based on the magnitude of hypercholesterolemia and on the presence or absence of other risk factors or confirmed coronary heart disease. Total cholesterol or LDL cholesterol values in the range of increased risk (see Table 60.1) require more aggressive treatment in a patient with two or more other coronary heart disease risk factors (Table 60.2) or definite coronary heart disease. Diet therapy should be initiated in all persons with increased-risk or high-risk cholesterol levels (specific dietary therapy is discussed in the section on diagnosis of lipid abnormalities). The treatment goal for patients with two additional risk factors or established coronary heart disease is an LDL cholesterol level below 130 mg/dl. For those without two additional risk factors or coronary heart disease the goal is to lower the LDL cholesterol level to less than 160 mg/dl. A reduced HDL cholesterol concentration (below 35 mg/dl) is among the risk factors that should be identified during the initial evaluation of patients with cholesterol concentrations above 200 mg/dl (see Table 60.1). Although the precise role of reduced HDL concentrations in atherogenesis has not been elucidated, we do know that there is an inverse relationship between HDL cholesterol levels and coronary heart disease incidence. Drugs are added to a treatment regimen if a 6-month trial of diet therapy has not reduced the cholesterol concentration to below the desired level.

In most cases (with the exception of genetic lipid disorders), high plasma cholesterol levels can be lowered by dietary treatment. The rationale for this form of treatment is based on results of metabolic ward studies, which have demonstrated effective lowering of cholesterol levels with diet, as well as on results of clinical trials, which have shown that lowering cholesterol levels reduces the incidence of myocardial infarction. There is a reasonable expectation that dietary intervention alone will be effective in reducing plasma cholesterol levels and ultimately the risk of coronary heart disease. With this prospect in mind, the National Institutes of Health Consensus Panel recommended that adoption of a prudent diet by the entire population of the United States would begin to lower plasma cholesterol levels toward those found in populations that have much less coronary heart disease.

DEFINITION OF A "NORMAL" PLASMA TRIGLYCERIDE LEVEL

Hypertriglyceridemia in the absence of hypercholesterolemia has not been proven to be an *independent* risk factor for coronary heart disease. However, hypertriglyceridemia is often associated with other conditions that do impose increased risk of developing atherosclerosis. Thus, hypertriglyceridemia may serve as an indicator of an underlying problem requiring medical attention.

Normal values for plasma triglycerides have been established by the National Institutes of Health Consensus Conference on Treatment of Hypertriglyceridemia.[14] In patients who have fasted 12 hours, values below 250 mg/dl are normal and warrant no further evaluation. Patients with values between 250 mg and 500 mg/dl are designated as having "borderline hypertriglyceridemia," and those with values above 500 mg/dl are designated as having "definite hypertriglyceridemia."

Triglyceride values above 500 mg/dl are clearly associated with an increased risk of developing pancreatitis, a risk that is clearly decreased when the triglyceride levels are lowered in patients with such high levels. However, a relationship between hypertriglyceridemia and atherosclerotic vascular disease, which is the subject of continuing investigation, has not been established. Hypertriglyceridemia occurs frequently in patients with coronary disease, and in prospective studies, hypertriglyceridemia appears to be associated with at least a two-fold increase in the risk of developing coronary heart disease. The controversy stems from the fact that when the data from these studies are adjusted for other conditions associated with both elevated triglycerides and coronary heart disease, hypertriglyceridemia no longer appears to be an independent risk factor. Some of these other conditions include obesity, hypertension, low concentrations of HDL cholesterol, and smoking.

Even though hypertriglyceridemia is not an independent risk factor,

TABLE 60.1 RECOMMENDED PLASMA LIPID AND LIPOPROTEIN LEVELS (mg/dl)*

	Ideal	Increased Risk	High Risk
Total Cholesterol	<200	200–240	>240
LDL Cholesterol	<130	130–160	>160
Triglycerides	<250		
HDL Cholesterol	40–55	<35	

* Based on the recommendations of the National Cholesterol Education Program.[5] The three categories of risk have been definitely established only for total cholesterol and LDL cholesterol.

TABLE 60.2 RISK FACTORS TO BE USED IN ASSESSING RISK OF CORONARY HEART DISEASE

Male sex
Family history of coronary heart disease before age 55
Cigarette smoking (more than 10 per day)
Hypertension
HDL cholesterol concentration below 35 mg/dl
Diabetes mellitus
Cerebrovascular or peripheral vascular disease
Weight 30% or more above ideal

the presence of elevated levels of triglycerides should stimulate a careful search for other conditions or secondary disorders that may be associated with increased coronary heart disease risk. Obese persons frequently have elevated triglyceride concentrations, as do chronic alcohol users. Drugs such as estrogens (alone or in oral contraceptives), thiazide diuretics, and certain β-blockers also elevate triglyceride levels. Diabetes mellitus, hypothyroidism, and chronic renal disease frequently cause hypertriglyceridemia, as do less common disorders such as paraproteinemias, Cushing's syndrome, sepsis, the postmyocardial infarction state, and certain types of glycogen storage disease.

When borderline hypertriglyceridemia coexists with hypercholesterolemia, it is clear that an increased risk of developing coronary heart disease exists. Paradoxically, it is unclear whether this risk is increased in patients with severe hypertriglyceridemia (values above 500 mg/dl) and concomitant hypercholesterolemia. However, treatment to lower triglyceride levels is indicated in such patients to reduce the risk of developing pancreatitis.

BASIC INFORMATION NECESSARY TO UNDERSTAND LIPOPROTEIN-CHOLESTEROL METABOLISM

To appreciate how an elevated level of plasma cholesterol is involved in accelerating atherogenesis, a basic understanding of lipoproteins and their metabolism is necessary.[6,7,15,16] The major classes of plasma lipoproteins differ in their content of various lipids (cholesterol, cholesteryl esters, phospholipids, and triglycerides) and specific proteins, referred to as apolipoproteins (Fig. 60.3). The apolipoproteins direct the metabolism of the lipoproteins. A major role of two of the apolipoproteins, apo-B and apo-E, is to mediate the interaction of specific lipoproteins with cell-surface receptors on various cells. They mediate uptake of lipoproteins that provide cholesterol to cells; the cholesterol is used in membrane biosynthesis or as a precursor of steroid hormones in certain endocrine tissues. Furthermore, parenchymal cells of the liver play a key role in total body cholesterol metabolism and serve as the principal cells for the elimination of cholesterol from the body through the bile. Cholesterol cannot be degraded within the body and must be eliminated by excretion.

Cell-surface lipoprotein receptors play key roles in cholesterol homeostasis.[16-18] The apo-B,E(LDL) receptor is present on most extrahepatic cells as well as on parenchymal cells of the liver. This receptor is principally responsible for LDL uptake and catabolism, the process by which plasma LDL concentrations are regulated. The binding and uptake is mediated by apo-B. In addition to the apo-B,E(LDL) receptor, the liver may possess an additional receptor, postulated to be the chylomicron remnant (apo-E) receptor. This receptor, which does not recognize apo-B-containing LDL, appears to be responsible primarily for the uptake of chylomicron remnants that transport dietary fat from the intestine to the liver. Apolipoprotein E is responsible for mediating the uptake of remnants by this receptor. With this basic introduction, it is now possible to describe the role of the major lipoproteins in cholesterol transport (Fig. 60.4, Table 60.3).

Chylomicrons are synthesized by the intestine to transport dietary triglycerides and cholesterol. After entering the plasma compartment, the chylomicron triglycerides are hydrolyzed by the action of lipoprotein lipase, which is located on the surfaces of capillary endothelial cells. The triglyceride fatty acids are then taken up by the local tissues. This action of lipoprotein lipase results in the production of cholesterol-enriched chylomicron remnants. The chylomicron remnants are rapidly cleared from the plasma by the liver (see Fig. 60.4, ①); their cholesterol is converted to bile acids and excreted or used in membrane or hepatic lipoprotein biosynthesis. Very-low-density lipoproteins (VLDL) are triglyceride-rich particles synthesized by the liver. As the VLDL circulate, they are acted on by lipases, and fatty acids are liberated for storage or used as an energy source in various tissues. Thus the VLDL are converted to intermediate-density lipoproteins (IDL). The IDL are either removed from the plasma by the liver (see Fig. 60.4, ②) or are converted to LDL by further action of the lipases (see Fig. 60.4, ③). By virtue of the removal of triglyceride from the VLDL, the IDL and LDL become enriched in cholesterol. The LDL are the end-products of VLDL catabolism and are the major cholesterol-bearing lipoproteins in the plasma. They are catabolized by both the liver and extrahepatic tissues via the apo-B,E(LDL) receptor (see Fig. 60.4, ④). High-density lipoproteins are derived from several sources and appear to play a role in acquiring and redistributing cholesterol among cells (Fig. 60.5). The HDL are a heterogeneous class of lipoproteins. In the following section they are described in terms of their role as protective, or antiatherogenic, lipoproteins. However, one sub-

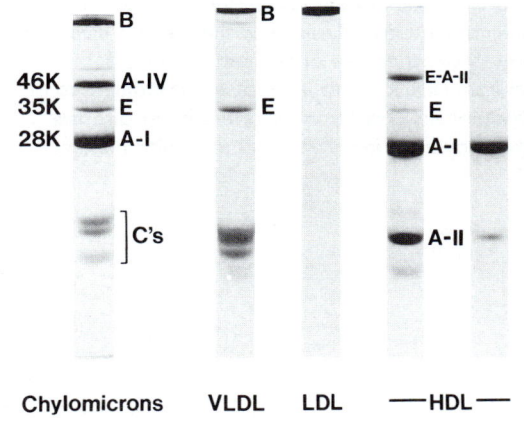

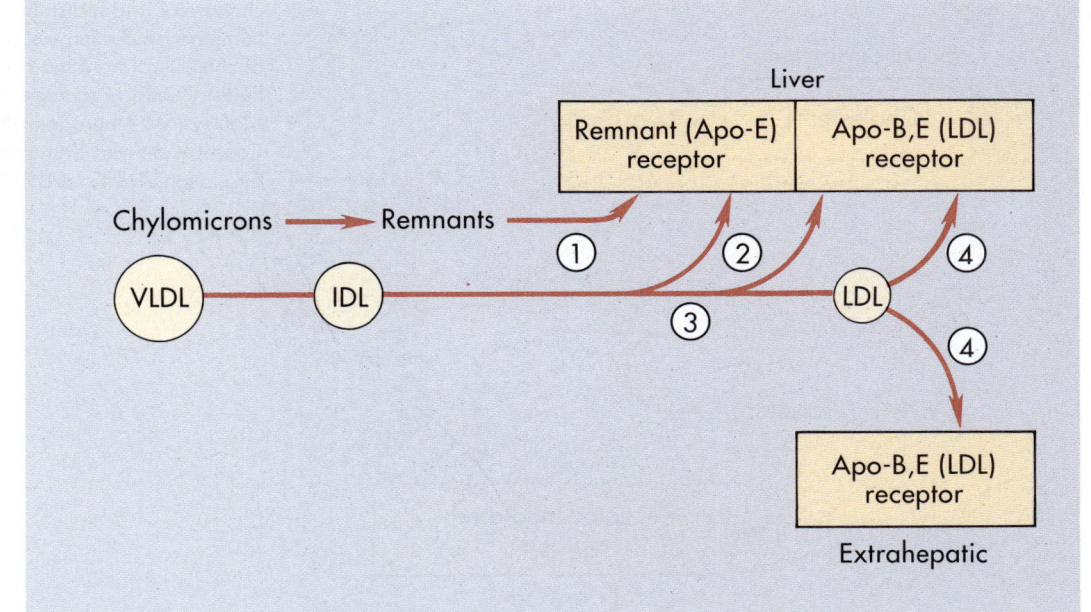

FIGURE 60.4 General scheme of lipoprotein metabolism. See text for details. (Modified from Mahley RW: Atherogenic lipoproteins and coronary artery heart disease: Concepts derived from recent advances in cellular and molecular biology. Circulation 72:943, 1985)

fraction, which accounts for a minor proportion of the total HDL, is enriched in apo-E (HDL-with apo-E) and is of metabolic importance in atherogenesis. Most HDL ("typical" HDL) lack apo-E.

MECHANISMS BY WHICH SPECIFIC LIPOPROTEINS CAUSE ATHEROSCLEROSIS

Genetic disorders in humans and specific dietary alterations in humans and animals result in changes in lipoproteins that have been most informative in establishing the identity of atherogenic (and antiatherogenic) lipoproteins. Type III hyperlipoproteinemia and familial hypercholesterolemia are two genetic diseases associated with accelerated atherosclerosis. Although relatively few cases of coronary artery disease are caused by these disorders, the study of these diseases has provided key insights into the role of specific lipoproteins in atherogenesis. The importance of understanding these genetic disorders lies in the close parallels between the lipoproteins seen in patients with these diseases and lipoproteins induced by the consumption of diets high in saturated fat and cholesterol. As discussed, diet-induced changes in lipoproteins appear to be responsible for the widespread hypercholesterolemia seen in the US population and the associated high incidence of coronary artery disease.

TYPE III HYPERLIPOPROTEINEMIA

Patients with type III hyperlipoproteinemia develop accelerated atherosclerosis that involves both coronary and peripheral arteries.[7,19,20] This disorder is associated with hypertriglyceridemia and hypercholesterolemia that is characterized by the accumulation in the plasma of cholesterol-rich remnants of chylomicrons and VLDL, which are referred to collectively as β-VLDL. These remnants have β-electrophoretic mobility rather than the pre-β-migration observed in normal VLDL. In considering the atherogenic potential of lipoproteins in this disorder, it is important to note that patients with type III disease usually have low levels of LDL and HDL and that the hyperlipidemia is associated exclusively with elevated levels of the β-VLDL. The underlying genetic defect responsible for the lipoprotein abnormalities is the synthesis of an abnormal form of apo-E, that is, a form that does

TABLE 60.3 CLASSIFICATION AND CHARACTERIZATION OF THE PLASMA LIPOPROTEINS

	Density (g/ml)	Electrophoretic Mobility	Major Lipid(s)	Origin	Function
Chylomicrons	<1.006	Origin	Triglyceride	Intestine	Transports dietary triglyceride and cholesterol
Chylomicron remnants	<1.006	Origin to β	Triglyceride, cholesterol	Derived from chylomicrons	Transports dietary cholesterol
VLDL	<1.006	Pre-β	Triglyceride	Liver	Transports endogenous triglyceride
IDL	1.006–1.02	β	Cholesterol	Derived from VLDL	Transports cholesterol
LDL	1.02–1.063	β	Cholesterol	Derived from VLDL	Transports cholesterol
HDL	1.063–1.21	α	Phospholipid, cholesterol	Liver, intestine	Transports cholesterol

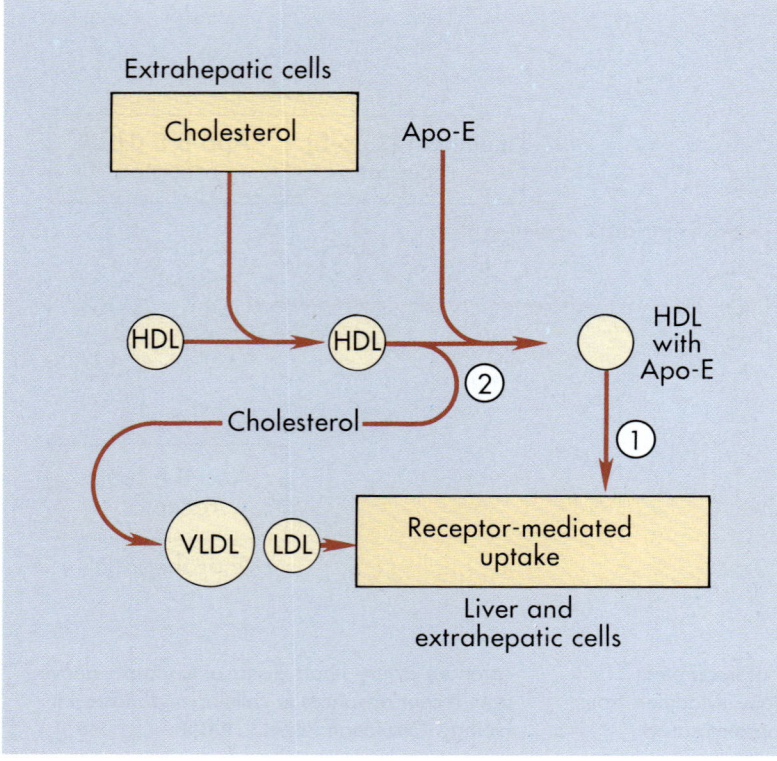

FIGURE 60.5 Role of HDL in acquiring cholesterol from cells containing excess cholesterol and redistributing it to cells requiring cholesterol for steroid hormone production and membrane biosynthesis or to the liver for elimination of cholesterol from the body. ① Direct uptake of HDL-with apo-E. ② Redistribution of cholesterol from HDL to other lipoproteins. (Modified from Mahley RW: Atherogenic lipoproteins and coronary artery heart disease: Concepts derived from recent advances in cellular and molecular biology. Circulation 72:943, 1985)

not bind normally to lipoprotein receptors. A brief description of apo-E and its role in lipoprotein metabolism will illustrate how this defect interferes with the catabolism of specific lipoproteins and how these lipoproteins contribute to the development of accelerated atherosclerosis.

The molecular defect that has been identified in type III hyperlipoproteinemia is the inheritance of genes coding for dysfunctional forms of apo-E. Multiple alleles in the population code for apo-E isoforms that differ in protein structure by single amino acid substitutions. The most common isoform of apo-E seen in the population is apo-E3 (about 60% of the population is homozygous for apo-E3). Type III hyperlipoproteinemia is most often associated with apo-E2 homozygosity. Four variant isoforms of apo-E have been identified in studies of patients with type III hyperlipoproteinemia. These variant forms of apo-E exhibit defective binding to lipoprotein receptors, which accounts for the delayed clearance and increased concentration of apo-E–containing, cholesterol-rich lipoproteins in patients with type III disease.[15,16,19-21]

The abnormal apo-E, defective in its ability to bind to the lipoprotein receptors, disrupts the normal metabolism of chylomicron and VLDL remnants (the β-VLDL) by preventing the normal, receptor-mediated uptake of these lipoproteins. In addition, the presence of the abnormal form of apo-E interferes with the normal formation of LDL from β-VLDL and IDL in type III disease, which could account for the low level of LDL seen in patients with type III hyperlipoproteinemia and could contribute further to the accumulation of β-VLDL in the plasma. The cholesterol-rich remnants (the β-VLDL) that accumulate must now be cleared from the plasma by an alternate pathway. The alternate route may well be through macrophages (scavenger cells), including macrophages of the arterial wall that participate in foam cell production in atherosclerotic lesions.

The β-VLDL and macrophages have been implicated in atherogenesis.[16,22] Both chylomicron and VLDL remnants cause massive cholesteryl ester accumulation in macrophages in tissue culture and convert them to cells closely resembling foam cells. It has been shown that foam cells within the arterial wall possess the ability to bind and take up the β-VLDL.

The postulated role of β-VLDL in atherogenesis has been further supported by the observation that lipoproteins very similar to β-VLDL are induced by fat and cholesterol feeding.[6,7] Animals fed diets high in fat and cholesterol have markedly elevated levels of β-VLDL (chylomicron and VLDL remnants) in their plasma and develop accelerated atherosclerosis. These diet-induced β-VLDL also cause cholesteryl ester accumulation in macrophages. Furthermore, lipoproteins resembling β-VLDL are seen in the plasma of humans after consumption of a single high-fat, high-cholesterol meal, and it is reasonable to speculate that these transiently present lipoproteins may contribute to the atherogenic risk seen in populations consuming such diets. Dietary intervention could be expected to alter the production of these potentially atherogenic lipoproteins.

Unlike type III hyperlipoproteinemia, in which the accumulation of β-VLDL is due to the presence of the defective-binding apo-E, the β-VLDL accumulation seen after fat and cholesterol feeding appears to be secondary to the down-regulation of expression of apo-B,E(LDL) receptors. Cholesterol feeding decreases the expression of apo-B,E(LDL) receptors in the liver. Presumably, chylomicron and VLDL overproduction induced by the dietary fat and cholesterol, in association with a decrease in apo-B,E(LDL) receptors, exceeds the ability of the remnant receptors to clear the excess particles from the plasma, resulting in the accumulation of both the chylomicron and VLDL remnants. Thus, either an impaired ability of apo-E-containing lipoproteins to interact with the receptors, as seen in type III hyperlipoproteinemia, or a decreased expression of the apo-B,E(LDL) receptor, as seen in fat and cholesterol feeding in animals, results in lipoprotein remnant accumulation. Both conditions are associated with accelerated atherosclerosis.

A careful study of the changes in HDL in both type III hyperlipoproteinemia and in animals fed high-fat and high-cholesterol diets suggests the mechanisms by which these lipoproteins may function as protective, or antiatherogenic, lipoproteins.[6,7,20] The changes include a reduction in the typical HDL (i.e., HDL-without apo-E) and an increase in HDL-with apo-E (HDL$_1$ or HDL$_c$). These changes appear to reflect the role of HDL in the process referred to as reverse cholesterol transport. Cholesterol deposited in extrahepatic tissues, including cells of the arterial wall, may be acquired by HDL, especially HDL-without apo-E (see Fig. 60.5). These HDL increase in size as their cholesteryl ester content increases and they acquire the apo-E. Because apo-E is synthesized by various cells, including macrophages, it is available within the interstitial fluid to become associated with the cholesterol-enriched HDL (i.e., HDL-with apo-E). The presence of the apo-E on these lipoproteins can now target the HDL-with apo-E to cells with either the apo-B,E(LDL) or remnant (apo-E) receptors. Alternatively, it has been postulated that the cholesterol in HDL can be transferred to other lipoproteins (e.g., VLDL or LDL) that are then taken up by the lipoprotein receptors. By either process, the HDL can participate in the redistribution of cholesterol from cholesterol-loaded cells to cells requiring cholesterol or to the liver for elimination of cholesterol from the body.

The decreased level of HDL-without apo-E in patients with type III disease (or in fat- and cholesterol-fed animals) could reflect the enhanced use of these particles as precursors in the formation of the cholesterol-loaded HDL-with apo-E. The association of low levels of HDL with an increased risk of coronary artery disease may well be due to the lack of sufficient quantities of HDL necessary to facilitate the egress of cholesterol from cells of the arterial wall in the face of large quantities of lipoproteins (e.g., β-VLDL), thus causing the deposition of cholesterol within these cells.

FAMILIAL HYPERCHOLESTEROLEMIA

Familial hypercholesterolemia dramatically illustrates the role of LDL in the development of accelerated atherosclerosis.[23] Patients with this disorder either lack or have defective apo-B,E(LDL) receptors (see Fig. 60.4, ④). Defective receptors prevent normal uptake and catabolism of LDL and IDL, thus increasing plasma LDL concentrations. Death from coronary artery disease often occurs in the second decade of life for patients homozygous for this disorder. In addition to the presence of extremely high levels of LDL, patients also have abnormally high levels of IDL, which resemble VLDL remnants and which could contribute to the atherogenic process through the mechanisms discussed previously.

Low-density lipoproteins also accumulate in the plasma of animals fed diets high in fat and cholesterol.[6,7,17,20] In the animal models, the increase in plasma LDL levels is very likely secondary to the down-regulation of the expression of the apoB,E(LDL) receptors, which would be expected to decrease LDL catabolism and to result in an elevation of the plasma LDL concentration. This may well be the mechanism by which the consumption of high-fat, high-cholesterol diets by humans results in elevated plasma cholesterol levels and predisposes humans to increased risk of developing coronary artery heart disease.

The precise mechanism that makes LDL atherogenic is not entirely clear.[16,22,24] High levels of LDL may lead to endothelial damage and subsequently to the increased flux of LDL into the arterial wall. The LDL do accumulate in the arterial wall in association with atherosclerotic lesions, and these lesions are associated with cholesterol accumulation in smooth muscle cells and macrophages. However, at the present time, it is difficult to explain how the smooth muscle cells could acquire excess cholesterol. In tissue culture, the apo-B,E(LDL) receptors are efficiently down-regulated by delivery of cholesterol to these cells and will not mediate excessive uptake and accumulation of cholesterol. Furthermore, *in vitro* studies show that macrophages also do not accumulate massive amounts of cholesteryl ester after incubation with even high concentrations of normal LDL.

However, there is an intriguing hypothesis that suggests how macrophages may become loaded with cholesterol in response to high levels of LDL. It has been shown that chemically modified (acetylated) LDL can be recognized by unique receptors on macrophages (referred to as the acetylated LDL receptor or the receptor for chemically modified LDL).[16,22] Low-density lipoproteins altered by acetylation, acetoacetylation, oxidation, or malondialdehyde modification in the laboratory can be recognized by this receptor and can cause massive cholesteryl ester accumulation within the macrophages. Such modifications of LDL could occur in the plasma as the lipoproteins circulate or in the arterial wall as they perfuse through the tissue. In addition, LDL complexed to glycosaminoglycans, such as dextran sulfate, can also be recognized and taken up by macrophages, causing cholesterol accumulation. Despite the attractiveness of these postulated mechanisms, more data are needed to establish their importance in the pathogenesis of atherosclerosis.

CLASSIFICATION OF PATIENTS WITH HYPERLIPIDEMIA

Two readily available clinical laboratory tests—measurement of plasma cholesterol and triglyceride concentrations—serve as the basic criteria for practical classification of patients with disorders of plasma lipoprotein metabolism. This classification system is also useful in determining a therapeutic regimen for the hyperlipidemic patient. In this system, patients are assigned to a "cholesterol problem" group if their plasma cholesterol concentration alone is elevated or if it is greater than the triglyceride concentration. Patients are considered to have a "triglyceride problem" if the triglyceride concentration is both elevated and greater than the cholesterol concentration.

HERITABLE DISORDERS OF PLASMA LIPOPROTEIN METABOLISM

The currently recognized heritable disorders of lipoprotein metabolism are listed in Table 60.4, and those that are associated with premature coronary atherosclerosis or pancreatitis are identified. Although an understanding of the underlying pathophysiology of these disorders is helpful in treating patients with hyperlipidemia, it is not usually necessary to know which disorder a given patient has in order to treat that patient. It is usually necessary to study the plasma lipids of a patient's relatives before the specific disorder can be identified with confidence.

HERITABLE DISORDERS ASSOCIATED WITH PLASMA CHOLESTEROL ELEVATIONS

FAMILIAL HYPERCHOLESTEROLEMIA. Patients with familial hypercholesterolemia usually seek medical help when they develop xanthomas of the extensor tendons or when they develop symptomatic premature coronary atherosclerosis.[23] The disorder may also be discovered in the course of screening relatives of patients with coronary disease. About 4% of patients under the age of 60 who have suffered a myocardial infarction have familial hypercholesterolemia.[25]

TABLE 60.4 CLASSIFICATION AND CHARACTERIZATION OF DISORDERS OF LIPOPROTEIN METABOLISM

Disorder	Biochemical Defect	Lipoprotein Phenotype	Major Lipoprotein Elevated	Cholesterol Levels (mg/dl)	Triglyceride Levels (mg/dl)	Coronary Heart Disease	Peripheral Disease	Xanthomas	Obesity	Hyperglycemia	Pancreatitis
Elevated Cholesterol Level											
Familial hypercholesterolemia	Defective apo-B,E(LDL) receptors	IIa, IIb	LDL	>300	Usually normal to slightly increased	+		Tendon, xanthelasma			
Familial combined hyperlipidemia	Unknown	IIa, IIb	LDL	>275	200–300	+			+	+	
Polygenic hypercholesterolemia	Unknown	IIa, IIb	LDL	>275	200–300	+					
Elevated Triglyceride Levels											
Familial hypertriglyceridemia	Unknown	IV	VLDL	Normal to slightly increased	250–500	+			+	+	
Familial combined hyperlipidemia	Unknown	IV, V	VLDL or VLDL and chylomicrons	Normal to slightly increased	250–500	+			+	+	
Familial type V hyperlipoproteinemia	Unknown	IV, V	Chylomicrons, VLDL	Normal to slightly increased	>500	unknown		Eruptive	+	+	+
Lipoprotein lipase (LPL) deficiency	Deficiency of LPL	I	Chylomicrons	Normal to slightly increased	>500			Eruptive			+
Apo-C-II deficiency	Deficiency of apo-C-II	I	Chylomicrons	Normal to slightly increased	>500			Uncommon			+
Type III hyperlipoproteinemia	Defective apo-E	III	β-VLDL	275–500	275–500	+	+	Palmar crease, tuberous, xanthelasma	+	+	

The incidence of heterozygous familial hypercholesterolemia is estimated to be 1 in 500. Homozygous patients are much rarer (1 in 1 million). The disorder is inherited as an autosomal dominant trait.

PATHOPHYSIOLOGY. The underlying defect in familial hypercholesterolemia is an absence of apo-B,E(LDL) receptors or the presence of defective receptors, as discussed in the previous section.[17,23] Fibroblasts from heterozygous familial hypercholesterolemic patients express about 50% as many apo-B,E(LDL) receptors as do fibroblasts from normal persons. The fibroblasts of homozygous patients usually have only 0% to 2% of the normal complement of cell-surface receptors, which results in a decreased clearance of LDL from the plasma. As a consequence of the inability to use LDL cholesterol, cells synthesize an increased amount of cholesterol, which in the liver results in an increased production of VLDL, the immediate precursor of LDL. Occasionally the oversynthesis of VLDL will cause an increase in the serum VLDL concentration as well as an increase in the LDL concentration. However, the elevated VLDL concentration is usually slight; as a consequence, the total cholesterol concentration is always greater than the triglyceride concentration. Cholesterol levels of 500 mg to 900 mg/dl and 300 mg to 500 mg/dl are seen in homozygous and heterozygous familial hypercholesterolemia, respectively.

CLINICAL COURSE. In both heterozygous and homozygous patients, the elevation of LDL cholesterol levels is apparent from the time of birth, and the diagnosis can be made by measuring the concentration of LDL cholesterol in umbilical cord blood samples (total cholesterol values of affected newborn patients are usually in excess of 92 mg/dl, and LDL cholesterol in cord blood exceeds 41 mg/dl[26]). Xanthomas in heterozygotes usually are apparent by age 20, and symptomatic coronary artery disease in male patients occurs on the average by age 45. Overt coronary heart disease usually occurs later in females, presumably due to their having higher HDL concentrations than men and to the possible protective influences of estrogens and progestins.

Homozygous persons are sometimes born with cutaneous tuberous xanthomas and develop clinically manifest coronary heart disease during childhood. In the absence of heroic therapeutic measures (*e.g.*, liver transplant or chronic plasma exchange) to lower LDL levels, these patients usually die of complications of this disorder before they reach 25 years of age.

PHYSICAL FINDINGS. The most common physical finding in familial hypercholesterolemia is xanthoma of the extensor tendons. Heterozygous patients are usually in the second decade of life before these xanthomas become obvious. The most common locations are the extensor tendons of the hands and the Achilles tendon. Casual palpation of the Achilles tendon will often suffice to establish that a tendon is thickened. If precise measurement is required, calipers or xerography can be used. Arcus juvenilis and palpebral xanthomas (xanthelasma) are also frequently encountered, but arcus and xanthelasma are not necessarily indicative of hypercholesterolemia when they appear after age 40.

DIAGNOSIS. Absolute confirmation of this diagnosis requires measurement of the number of apo-B,E(LDL) receptors expressed on fibroblasts grown from a skin biopsy. Measurements of apo-B,E(LDL) receptor numbers are not routinely available; consequently, the diagnosis of familial hypercholesterolemia usually depends on the finding of an elevated LDL cholesterol concentration, xanthomas of the extensor tendons, and a family history of premature (before age 50) coronary atherosclerosis. When a tentative diagnosis of familial hypercholesterolemia is made, an extensive evaluation of the plasma cholesterol levels of family members should be initiated.

FAMILIAL COMBINED HYPERLIPIDEMIA. Familial combined hyperlipidemia, also known as familial multiple lipoprotein-type hyperlipidemia, was first identified in 1972 during a survey of the incidence of hyperlipidemia in patients who had suffered a myocardial infarction and in their relatives.[25,27] This disorder occurred in about 11% of survivors of myocardial infarction under age 60. The designation "combined" refers to the fact that individual members of an affected kindred can have elevated concentrations of different lipoproteins. These include elevations of VLDL (type IV), VLDL and LDL (type IIb), LDL (type IIa), and chylomicrons plus VLDL (type V). The existence of these multiple lipoprotein types within the same family demonstrates the lack of utility of lipoprotein typing in genetic studies of hyperlipidemia. Efforts are now directed toward classifying disorders of plasma lipid metabolism according to the underlying pathophysiologic mechanism. However, the defect in familial combined hyperlipidemia has not yet been defined.

The natural history and physical findings in familial combined hyperlipidemia differ from those of familial hypercholesterolemia and can be used to distinguish the two disorders. Skin fibroblasts of familial combined hyperlipidemic patients have been shown to express normal numbers of apo-B,E(LDL) receptors.[28] Children in affected kindreds do not manifest hyperlipidemia, unlike familial hypercholesterolemic patients, whose hypercholesterolemia is present at birth. Xanthomas of the extensor tendons, common in familial hypercholesterolemia, do not occur in familial combined hyperlipidemic patients with similarly elevated LDL concentrations. Familial combined hyperlipidemia is believed to be inherited as an autosomal dominant trait; however, definitive proof of the single-gene mode of inheritance will require delineation of the underlying metabolic defect.

CLINICAL PRESENTATION AND DIAGNOSIS. In the absence of blood cholesterol screening, most patients with familial combined hyperlipidemia come to medical attention because of the onset of symptoms of atherosclerotic vascular disease. Definitive diagnosis requires that as many family members as possible undergo plasma lipid testing and that the multiple lipoprotein types, as described previously, be demonstrated within the patient's family. However, successful treatment does not require performance of this diagnostic exercise because the therapeutic maneuvers that are useful in treating familial combined hyperlipidemia are the same as those used in familial hypercholesterolemia.

POLYGENIC HYPERCHOLESTEROLEMIA. About 5% of patients who have suffered a myocardial infarction and are under the age of 60 have been found to have polygenic hypercholesterolemia, a disorder in which several genes, as well as environmental factors, interact to elevate plasma LDL concentrations.[25] Analysis of the distribution of cholesterol concentrations of the relatives of affected patients suggested that multiple cholesterol-elevating genes were operative in this disorder. This analysis demonstrated that cholesterol values of family members with polygenic hypercholesterolemia are distributed continuously, with no clear-cut separation between normal and affected family members; a bimodal distribution of cholesterol values would be expected for hyperlipidemia transmitted as an autosomal dominant trait. In addition to cholesterol-elevating genetic abnormalities in these patients, dietary and other environmental factors may contribute to the hyperlipidemia.

CLINICAL PRESENTATION. Hypercholesterolemia due to polygenic hypercholesterolemia cannot be distinguished from familial combined hyperlipidemia in the absence of extensive family screening studies. There are no peculiar physical findings that serve to identify this group. Treatment is the same as for hypercholesterolemic patients with familial hypercholesterolemia or familial combined hyperlipidemia.

HERITABLE DISORDERS ASSOCIATED WITH PLASMA TRIGLYCERIDE ELEVATIONS

Hypertriglyceridemia is the most frequent plasma lipid abnormality seen in patients who have suffered a myocardial infarction and in their relatives.[25] About 15% of patients under age 60 were hypertriglyceridemic in the Seattle Heart Study, and another 7% had hypertriglyceridemia and mild hypercholesterolemia as well.[25,27] The triglyceride levels are elevated when there is an increase in the concentration of VLDL, of chylomicrons, or of both. The VLDL are composed of about 60% triglyceride and 10% to 15% cholesterol. Thus, elevated levels of VLDL may elevate both the triglyceride and cholesterol concentrations. Chylomicrons consist of about 90% to 95% triglyceride and 5% to 10% cholesterol. Thus, chylomicronemia must be severe for the total cholesterol concentration to be elevated. Although severe chylomicronemia (triglyceride levels > 1000 mg/dl) can cause pancreatitis, elevated levels of this lipoprotein have not been associated with premature coronary heart disease.

Despite the increased frequency with which hypertriglyceridemia (without hypercholesterolemia) occurs in patients with coronary artery disease, it has not been established that it is an independent risk factor. This is because hypertriglyceridemic patients frequently have other disorders (diabetes mellitus, obesity, and/or hypertension) that are associated with increased risk for coronary heart disease. In such patients, the elevation of the triglyceride concentration may simply be an indicator of an underlying condition that promotes atherogenesis, which is independent of the hypertriglyceridemia.

The genetic disorders in which the plasma triglyceride concentration is increased are listed in Table 60.4. Three of these diseases, familial hypertriglyceridemia, familial combined hyperlipidemia, and type III hyperlipoproteinemia, are associated with accelerated atherosclerosis. In the others, pancreatitis, but not coronary heart disease, occurs with increased frequency as a result of chylomicronemia.

FAMILIAL HYPERTRIGLYCERIDEMIA. Familial hypertriglyceridemia is a disorder in which mild to moderate hypertriglyceridemia occurs owing to elevated levels of VLDL. The metabolic defect has not been established. The plasma triglyceride concentration is usually not greater than 500 mg/dl, and the cholesterol level is normal or slightly increased. This disorder is usually detected when a person presents with symptoms of vascular disease. In the Seattle Heart Study, about 5% of patients under age 60 were found to have this disorder.[25,27] In addition to hypertriglyceridemia, these patients have an increased incidence of obesity, type II diabetes mellitus, hyperuricemia, and hypertension.

Although the disorder is inherited as an autosomal dominant trait, hypertriglyceridemia usually does not become manifest until the third decade of life. Weight gain is often responsible for the appearance of the elevated triglyceride level, as is the regular consumption of alcohol. Because development of the hypertriglyceridemia is age dependent and affected by other factors as well, normolipidemic relatives of probands with this disorder cannot be confident that their triglyceride levels will remain normal. Thus, the plasma lipid levels of the family members should be measured at least every 5 years.

The triglyceride level usually does not exceed 1000 mg/dl in familial hypertriglyceridemia; thus, pancreatitis rarely, if ever, occurs. For the same reason, eruptive xanthomas and lipemia retinalis are not characteristics of these patients.

FAMILIAL COMBINED HYPERLIPIDEMIA. About one third of the affected members of kindreds with familial combined hyperlipidemia have elevated VLDL concentrations.[25] Concomitant chylomicronemia is occasionally seen in these patients. No distinctive clinical findings can be used to distinguish patients with elevated VLDL concentrations due to familial combined hyperlipidemia from those with hypertriglyceridemia due to familial hypertriglyceridemia. Extensive family screening is required to establish which disorder a given patient has, but establishing the genetic diagnosis is not a prerequisite for treatment. As noted in the discussion of this disorder in the section on hypercholesterolemia, patients with familial combined hyperlipidemia have an increased incidence of premature coronary atherosclerosis.

FAMILIAL TYPE V HYPERLIPOPROTEINEMIA. Type V hyperlipoproteinemia is characterized by elevated concentrations of chylomicrons and VLDL in the fasting state.[29,30] Although it is uncertain whether these patients are predisposed to accelerated atherosclerosis, it is clear that an increased incidence of pancreatitis exists because these patients often have triglyceride values above 1000 mg/dl.

Hypertriglyceridemia occurs in about 50% of the relatives of patients with type V hyperlipoproteinemia, but most of these relatives have only an elevation of VLDL. Only about 15% of the relatives have both elevated VLDL and chylomicronemia. For this reason, it is presumed that this disorder is inherited as an autosomal dominant trait. However, delineation of the genetic defect will be required before the precise mode of inheritance is understood. The prevalence of type V hyperlipoproteinemia is estimated to be 0.2% to 0.3% in males and even less in females; however, an accurate assessment of the true incidence of this genetic trait, which may be greater than these values indicate, will depend on the identification of a specific diagnostic marker.

PATHOPHYSIOLOGY. The underlying defect in type V hyperlipoproteinemia is unknown. This disorder may represent a syndrome caused by one of several different genetically or environmentally determined factors. Metabolic studies have determined that patients with type V disease usually have an increased production and a retarded clearance of both VLDL and chylomicrons. This delayed clearance may be explained by measurements of the lipoprotein lipase activity. Such studies have shown that the post-heparin lipase activity is about 70% of that observed in normolipidemic controls and that the adipose tissue and skeletal muscle lipase activities are 35% to 45% of those seen in controls.[30] Despite these reductions in lipase activity in type V disease, the reductions alone are probably not great enough to account for the hyperlipidemia. Overproduction of chylomicrons induced by eating a fat-enriched diet or overproduction of VLDL as is seen in obesity most likely exceeds the reduced capacity of the lipase system in these patients. The consequence is hyperlipidemia.

CLINICAL PRESENTATION. The development of hyperlipidemia in this disorder usually occurs after age 20. This later onset serves to distinguish type V hyperlipoproteinemia from two rare, but clinically similar, disorders: familial lipoprotein lipase deficiency and familial apolipoprotein C-II deficiency. In the latter two disorders, the hyperlipidemia and subsequent clinical complications are present from the time of birth.

In type V hyperlipoproteinemia, severe chylomicronemia and its clinical sequelae are often associated with weight gain, newly developed diabetes mellitus, oral contraceptive use, regular alcohol use, or pregnancy. More than 50% of these patients have episodic abdominal pain that may be due to pancreatitis, capsular distention of the liver and spleen due to fatty infiltration, or occult reasons. Eruptive xanthomas also occur in about half of the patients. Hypertension, diabetes mellitus, hyperuricemia, and hypertension are also frequently observed.

Patients with triglyceride levels above 2000 mg/dl often have eruptive xanthomas, lipemia retinalis, and hepatosplenomegaly. Triglyceride accumulation in macrophages accounts for the xanthomas and splenomegaly; however, in the liver, there is fat accumulation in both parenchymal cells (hepatocytes) and macrophages (Kupffer cells).

DIAGNOSIS. The finding of a triglyceride concentration in excess of 1000 mg/dl in the absence of underlying disorders that might cause chylomicronemia should arouse suspicion of the presence of type V hyperlipoproteinemia. The plasma triglyceride:cholesterol ratio nearly always exceeds 5:1 and approaches 10:1 as the concentration of chylomicrons increases.[29] Inspection of the plasma after undisturbed storage overnight reveals a layer of chylomicrons at the top of the sample and a turbid infranatant, reflecting the presence of an elevated concentration of VLDL. If a patient with type V disease has undergone treatment, the chylomicronemia may no longer be present, thus obscuring the diagnosis of this disorder.

FAMILIAL LIPOPROTEIN LIPASE DEFICIENCY (TYPE I HYPERLIPOPROTEINEMIA). Familial lipoprotein lipase deficiency (type I hyperlipoproteinemia) occurs as a consequence of an inherited deficiency of lipoprotein lipase activity.[30] This deficiency results in a markedly retarded clearance of chylomicrons and an impairment in VLDL clearance. The resulting hyperlipidemia is severe and is associated with recurrent abdominal pain and pancreatitis. There is no increased incidence of atherosclerotic vascular disease.

CLINICAL PRESENTATION. The severe hyperlipidemia associated with this disorder begins as soon as the affected infant begins to ingest whole milk. Abdominal pain, with or without pancreatitis, eruptive xanthomas, and hepatosplenomegaly are frequent findings in such children. For these reasons, most patients with type I disease are discovered shortly after birth. However, some parents learn empirically to reduce the fat in their child's diet, and a child so treated occasionally may not come to medical attention until later in life. Anemia, which occurs particularly in patients with splenomegaly, is rare. The life expectancy in these patients depends on the avoidance of dietary fat, which prevents pancreatitis. Unlike type V hyperlipoproteinemia, there is no increase in the incidence of obesity, hypertension, hyperuricemia, or type II diabetes mellitus.

PATHOGENESIS. It is not known whether the deficiency of lipoprotein lipase activity in these patients is due to the failure to synthesize this protein or whether it is due to the synthesis of a structurally altered protein. Assays presently in use depend on measuring the activity of the enzyme rather than the plasma enzyme concentration. Such assays suggest that the disorder is inherited as an autosomal recessive trait.

Dietary fat restriction, to usually less than 50 g/day, is the only successful mode of therapy for these patients. Because fatty acids with carbon chain lengths of 12 or less are absorbed directly into the portal circulation, medium-chain triglycerides are often used as a supplemental source of calories.

FAMILIAL APOLIPOPROTEIN C-II DEFICIENCY. Familial apolipoprotein C-II deficiency is a very rare disorder that is due to a deficiency or absence of normal apo-C-II, a cofactor of lipoprotein lipase.[30] The deficiency of apo-C-II prevents normal lipoprotein lipase-mediated catabolism of chylomicrons and VLDL. Four kindreds and 19 affected persons have been identified.

Although apo-C-II deficiency and lipoprotein lipase deficiency are similar in many respects, there are significant differences. Pancreatitis is more common in apo-C-II deficiency, but patients usually exhibit no symptoms until the second decade of life. Eruptive xanthomas, common in lipoprotein lipase deficiency, are not seen in patients with apo-C-II deficiency. Hepatosplenomegaly is also rare in apo-C-II deficiency.

Analyses of the available families to date suggest that the disorder is inherited as an autosomal recessive trait. Obligate heterozygotes have normal plasma lipid levels despite having lipoprotein lipase activity that is 50% of that observed in normal persons.

TYPE III HYPERLIPOPROTEINEMIA. In patients with type III hyperlipoproteinemia (also referred to as primary dysbetalipoproteinemia), both the triglyceride and cholesterol concentrations are elevated.[7,19,20] It is appropriate to consider this disorder among the hypertriglyceridemic states because the therapeutic measures employed in type III hyperlipoproteinemia are the same as for other hypertriglyceridemias. This is the only disorder in which the triglyceride and cholesterol concentrations are nearly equal.[19,20] The incidence of this disease in coronary heart disease patients under age 60 is estimated to be 0.2% to 1%.[31]

PATHOPHYSIOLOGY. Patients with this disorder are usually homozygous for one of several apo-E gene alleles that code for an isoform of apo-E that binds poorly to lipoprotein receptors.[7,19,20] This results in the accumulation of abnormal cholesterol-enriched chylomicron and VLDL remnants in the plasma. However, more than homozygosity for these structurally abnormal apo-E isoforms is required for a patient to become hyperlipidemic, as indicated by the following observations: Not all E2/2 homozygotes become hyperlipidemic. The incidence of E2 homozygosity in the population is estimated at about 1%; yet the incidence of patients with type III hyperlipoproteinemia is but a fraction of this. Development of the hyperlipidemia is age dependent. Although a few cases of children with type III hyperlipoproteinemia have been reported, the hyperlipidemia is almost always not discovered until patients are in the third decade of life or, in the case of E2 homozygous patients, until one of several other medical problems occurs. These problems include hypothyroidism and the development of obesity. In E2 homozygous females, menopause often aggravates or precipitates the development of hyperlipidemia. A discussion concerning the mechanisms by which these secondary factors precipitate the development of overt type III hyperlipoproteinemia is presented elsewhere.[7,19,20]

CLINICAL PRESENTATION. Patients come to medical attention when they seek treatment after developing xanthomas or symptomatic atherosclerotic vascular disease. Xanthomas usually occur no earlier than 25 to 35 years of age because hyperlipidemia and excessive β-VLDL concentrations do not usually occur until about 20 years of age. When examined, about half of the patients are found to have tuberoeruptive xanthomas and palmar crease xanthomas (xanthoma striata palmaris), a diagnostic hallmark of type III hyperlipoproteinemia. Xanthomas of the extensor tendons occur in about 10% of type III patients but usually occur in patients who have tuberous xanthomas as well. There is also an increased frequency of hyperuricemia and glucose intolerance; however, gout and clinical diabetes mellitus are relatively rare. Symptoms of vascular disease do not usually appear before age 35.

DIAGNOSIS. The occurrence of tuberoeruptive or palmar crease xanthomas is highly correlated with the presence of type III hyperlipoproteinemia and should strongly suggest this diagnosis. However, about 50% of affected patients have no xanthomas, and diagnosis of the disorder must be suggested by other findings. Chief among these is the existence of nearly equal elevations of triglyceride and cholesterol concentrations.

The diagnostic benchmark used to substantiate this diagnosis is the establishment of the E2/2 phenotype by isoelectric focusing of the patient's VLDL apolipoproteins. However, because this technique is not widely available, the diagnosis must be made by other means. If the techniques for VLDL, LDL, and HDL isolation by ultracentrifugation are available, then the VLDL cholesterol concentration in plasma can be determined. If the ratio of the VLDL cholesterol concentration to the total plasma triglyceride concentration is above 0.3, then the diagnosis of type III hyperlipoproteinemia is established.

SECONDARY HYPERLIPIDEMIA

Hyperlipidemia occurs frequently as a secondary manifestation of an underlying disorder. Hypertriglyceridemia is commonly seen in obesity, diabetes mellitus, chronic renal disease (nephrosis or chronic failure), hypothyroidism, and chronic alcohol use. Less common disorders that cause secondary elevations of triglycerides include dysgammaglobulinemia, certain glycogen storage diseases, and Cushing's syndrome. Certain drugs also elevate triglyceride levels and include estrogens, oral contraceptives, glucocorticoids, thiazide diuretics, and some β-blockers. Secondary hypercholesterolemia is encountered most commonly in hypothyroidism and in cholestatic liver disease. Successful treatment of the underlying disorder usually abolishes the hyperlipidemia, and specific therapy for the hyperlipidemia is usually not successful if the underlying disease is not well controlled.

DIAGNOSIS OF LIPID ABNORMALITIES

On initial examination, all adult patients should have their cholesterol measured (fasting not required); if the value is normal, the measurement should be repeated every 5 years. Patients with elevated values should have confirmatory cholesterol determinations as well as fasting (12 hours) triglyceride measurements at the same time. If patients have total cholesterol levels between 200 mg and 240 mg/dl and do not have two or more additional risk factors (see Table 60.2) or coronary heart disease, they should begin diet therapy to reduce the total cholesterol level and be retested annually. For those patients who have two or more additional risk factors or coronary heart disease, and cholesterol levels above 200 mg/dl, estimation of lipoprotein cholesterol levels should be done to guide therapy more accurately. This estimation involves measuring total cholesterol, total triglyceride, and HDL cholesterol concentrations from a blood sample obtained after the patient has fasted 12 hours. From these values the LDL cholesterol level can be calculated by the formula: LDL cholesterol = total cholesterol − HDL cholesterol − (triglyceride/5). The term (triglyceride/5) provides an estimate of the VLDL cholesterol concentration and is reasonably accurate if the triglyceride concentration is below 400 mg/dl. The HDL cholesterol level is also useful to exclude the possibility that the patient's hypercholesterolemia is due to an elevated HDL cholesterol concentration. Moderate hypercholesterolemia (240 mg to 280 mg/dl) can be caused by very high concentrations of HDL. Such elevations are rare and do not appear to increase the risk of developing coronary heart disease. Elevations of HDL can occur on a familial basis and in those who exercise vigorously. Such patients would probably not require any treatment to alter plasma lipids. The HDL cholesterol level should also be determined in patients who have atherosclerotic vascular disease but no other apparent risk factors, or in persons who have a family history of premature atherosclerosis in the absence of other risk factors. In men the normal HDL cholesterol concentration range is between 40 mg and 50 mg/dl, and in premenopausal women it is usually between 45 mg and 55 mg/dl.

Once the plasma cholesterol and triglyceride values are known, patients should be categorized for treatment according to the lipid concentration that is most elevated. Thus, there are two broad categories of patients: those with "cholesterol problems" and those with "triglyceride problems." Family screening should be done to identify others at risk of developing premature atherosclerosis. Family screening may also be helpful in identifying a specific heritable disorder of cholesterol metabolism. However, it is often quite difficult to screen enough family members to establish the genetic diagnosis of the hyperlipidemia, and treatment does not require a precise genetic diagnosis.

DIETARY TREATMENT OF HYPERLIPIDEMIA

At the present time, a single diet is used in the treatment of all hyperlipidemic patients. Diet therapy should be employed in all patients prior to drug therapy. Most patients respond well enough to diet so that drug treatment is not necessary. Those patients who require drugs will usually obtain better results if they comply with the dietary regimen as well. Dietary treatment should be tried for 6 months to 1 year (except in extreme cases of hyperlipidemia [i.e., when the LDL cholesterol concentration exceeds 225 mg/dl]) prior to the use of drugs. For the overweight patient, weight reduction should accompany any dietary treatment. Often, weight reduction has a profound effect on plasma lipids.

THE TWO-PHASE DIETARY PROGRAM

The approach with dietary treatment is to reduce the intake of saturated fat and cholesterol in two graded steps. Most Americans consume about 40% of their calories as fat, and saturated fat constitutes 18% to 20% of their total calories. Average cholesterol intake is between 350 mg and 500 mg/day. The National Cholesterol Education Program's dietary regimen reduces saturated fat, total fat, and cholesterol in a graded fashion.[5]

After a patient has followed each phase for at least 3 months, cholesterol and triglyceride determinations should be repeated to determine the effectiveness of the diet.

PHASE I

In phase I, calories are obtained as follows: 30% of total calories as fat, 50% to 60% as carbohydrate, and 15% to 20% as protein. The fat should contain no more than 10% saturated, 10% to 15% monounsaturated, and up to 10% polyunsaturated fatty acids. Complex carbohydrates should constitute the major source of total carbohydrates. Cholesterol intake should be below 300 mg/day.

PHASE II

In phase II, 30% of calories are as fat (but less than 7% as saturated, up to 10% as polyunsaturated, and 10% to 15% as monounsaturated fatty acids), 50% to 60% as carbohydrate, and 15% to 20% as protein, with cholesterol intake limited to 200 mg/day.

OTHER DIETARY OBJECTIVES IN HYPERTRIGLYCERIDEMIC PATIENTS

For hypertriglyceridemic patients, there are several other dietary objectives. The first of these is weight reduction, which often normalizes elevated triglyceride levels. Abstinence from alcohol is required in some patients, especially those with triglyceride levels above 500 mg/dl. Fat restriction more stringent than that called for in phase II may also be required in dietary fat-sensitive patients with type V hyperlipoproteinemia. Patients with familial lipoprotein lipase deficiency or apo-C-II deficiency must severely limit fat consumption.

EFFECTIVENESS OF FISH CONSUMPTION IN LOWERING LIPID LEVELS

The results of several studies have emphasized the importance of regular fish consumption in reducing plasma lipid levels and in preventing coronary heart disease. Large doses (20 g/day) of fish oils enriched in omega-3 fatty acids have been shown to reduce plasma lipid levels in hyperlipidemic persons.[32] An epidemiologic study also showed that inclusion of fish in the diet twice or more weekly correlated with a reduced incidence of coronary heart disease.[33] Although further information is required to define the mechanisms by which omega-3 fatty acids influence plasma lipid metabolism, it seems prudent to suggest including fish in the diet regularly.

OAT BRAN AND OTHER SOLUBLE FIBERS

The water-soluble portion of undigestible plant residue lowers LDL cholesterol by about 25% in patients with very high cholesterol levels (~265 mg/dl) and normal triglyceride concentrations. To achieve this, patients had to consume 100 g of oat bran daily (five muffins and a bowl of hot cereal) during the 3 weeks of the study.[34] Similar reductions (~20%) of LDL cholesterol have also been achieved with psyllium hydrophilic mucilloid (3.4 g [1 tsp] three times daily) in hypercholesterolemic men.[35] Normolipidemic individuals on such diets exhibited much less of a response.[36] Thus, soluble fiber appears to lower cholesterol levels in hypercholesterolemic patients in the short run, but the long-term efficacy and safety of such high-fiber diets have yet to be established.

REFERENCES

1. Blackburn H: Epidemiological evidence. In American Health Foundation: Plasma Lipids: Optimal Levels for Health, p 3. New York, Academic Press, 1980
2. Stamler J: Population studies. In Levy RI, Rifkind BM, Dennis BH et al (eds): Nutrition in Health and Disease, Vol 1, Nutrition, Lipids and Coronary Heart Diseases: A Global View, p 25. New York, Raven Press, 1979
3. Mahley RW: The role of dietary fat and cholesterol in atherosclerosis and lipoprotein metabolism. West J Med 134:34, 1981
4. National Institutes of Health Consensus Development Conference: Lowering blood cholesterol to prevent heart disease. JAMA 253:2080, 1985
5. Expert Panel, National Cholesterol Education Program: Report of the National Cholesterol Education Program Expert Panel on detection, evaluation, and treatment of high blood cholesterol in adults. Arch Intern Med 148:36, 1988
6. Mahley RW: Development of accelerated atherosclerosis: Concepts derived from cell biology and animal model studies. Arch Pathol Lab Med 107:393, 1983
7. Mahley RW: Atherogenic lipoproteins and coronary artery heart disease: Concepts derived from recent advances in cellular and molecular biology. Circulation 72:943, 1985
8. Lipid Research Clinics Program: The Lipid Research Clinics Coronary Primary Prevention Trial results. I. Reduction in incidence of coronary heart disease. JAMA 251:351, 1984
9. Lipid Research Clinics Program: The Lipid Research Clinics Coronary Primary Prevention Trial results. II. The relationship of reduction in incidence of coronary heart disease to cholesterol lowering. JAMA 251:365, 1984
10. Frick MH, Elo O, Haapa K et al: Helsinki Heart Study: Primary-prevention trial with gemfibrozil in middle-aged men with dyslipidemia: Safety of treatment, changes in risk factors, and incidence of coronary heart disease. N Engl J Med 317:1237, 1987
11. Blankenhorn DH, Nessim SA, Johnson RL et al: Beneficial effects of combined colestipol-niacin therapy on coronary atherosclerosis and coronary venous bypass grafts. JAMA 257:3233, 1987
12. Brensike JF, Levy RI, Kelsey SF et al: Effects of therapy with cholestyramine on progression of coronary arteriosclerosis: Results of the NHLBI Type II Coronary Intervention Study. Circulation 69:313, 1984
13. Vega GL, Grundy SM: Treatment of primary moderate hypercholesterolemia with lovastatin (mevinolin) and colestipol. JAMA 257:33, 1987
14. National Institutes of Health Consensus Development Conference: Treatment of hypertriglyceridemia. JAMA 251:1196, 1984
15. Mahley RW, Innerarity TL, Rall SC Jr et al: Plasma lipoproteins: Apolipoprotein structure and function. J Lipid Res 25:1277, 1984
16. Mahley RW, Innerarity TL: Lipoprotein receptors and cholesterol homeostasis. Biochim Biophys Acta 737:197, 1983
17. Brown MS, Goldstein JL: How LDL receptors influence cholesterol and atherosclerosis. Sci Am 251:58, 1984
18. Brown MS, Goldstein JL: A receptor-mediated pathway for cholesterol homeostasis. Science 232:34, 1986
19. Mahley RW, Rall, SC Jr: Type III hyperlipoproteinemia (dysbetalipoproteinemia): The role of apolipoprotein E in normal and abnormal lipoprotein metabolism. In Scriver CR, Beaudet AL, Sly WS et al (eds): The Metabolic Basis of Inherited Disease, 6th ed, p 1195. New York, McGraw-Hill, 1989
20. Mahley RW, Innerarity TL, Rall SC Jr et al: Lipoproteins of special significance in atherosclerosis: Insights provided by studies of type III hyperlipoproteinemia. Ann NY Acad Sci 454:209, 1985
21. Mahley RW: Apolipoprotein E: Cholesterol transport protein with expanding role in cell biology. Science 240:622, 1988
22. Brown MS, Goldstein JL: Lipoprotein metabolism in the macrophage: Implications for cholesterol deposition in atherosclerosis. Annu Rev Biochem 52:223, 1983
23. Goldstein JL, Brown MS: Familial hypercholesterolemia. In Stanbury JB, Wyngaarden JB, Fredrickson DS et al (eds): The Metabolic Basis of Inherited Disease, 5th ed, p 672. New York, McGraw-Hill, 1983
24. Steinberg D: Lipoproteins and atherosclerosis: A look back and a look ahead. Arteriosclerosis 3:283, 1983
25. Goldstein JL, Hazzard WR, Schrott HG et al: Hyperlipidemia in coronary heart disease. I. Lipid levels in 500 survivors of myocardial infaction. J Clin Invest 52:1533, 1973
26. Kwiterovich PO Jr, Levy RI, Fredrickson DS: Neonatal diagnosis of familial type II hyperlipoproteinemia. Lancet 1:118, 1973
27. Goldstein JL, Schrott HG, Hazzard WR et al: Hyperlipidemia in coronary heart disease. II. Genetic analysis of lipid levels in 176 families and delineation of a new inherited disorder, combined hyperlipidemia. J Clin Invest 52:1544, 1973
28. Goldstein JL, Dana SE, Brunschede GY et al: Genetic heterogeneity in familial hypercholesterolemia: Evidence for two different mutations affecting functions of low-density lipoprotein receptor. Proc Natl Acad Sci USA 72:1092, 1975
29. Greenberg BH, Blackwelder WC, Levy RI: Primary type V hyperlipoproteinemia: A descriptive study in 32 families. Ann Intern Med 87:526, 1977
30. Nikkilä EA: Familial lipoprotein lipase deficiency and related disorders of chylomicron metabolism. In Stanbury JB, Wyngaarden JB, Fredrickson DS et al (eds): The Metabolic Basis of Inherited Disease, 5th ed, p 622. New York, McGraw-Hill, 1983
31. Hazzard WR, Goldstein JL, Schrott HG et al: Hyperlipidemia in coronary heart disease. III. Evaluation of lipoprotein phenotypes of 156 genetically defined survivors of myocardial infarction. J Clin Invest 52:1569, 1973
32. Phillipson BE, Rothrock DW, Connor WE et al: Reduction of plasma lipids, lipoproteins, and apoproteins by dietary fish oils in patients with hypertriglyceridemia. N Engl J Med 312:1210, 1985
33. Kromhout D, Bosschieter EB, Coulander CdeL: The inverse relation between fish consumption and 20-year mortality from coronary heart disease. N Engl J Med 312:1205, 1985
34. Anderson JW, Story L, Sieling B et al: Hypocholesterolemic effects of oat-bran or bean intake for hypercholesterolemic men. Am J Clin Nutr 40:1146, 1984
35. Anderson JW, Zettwoch N, Feldman T et al: Cholesterol-lowering effects of psyllium hydrophilic mucilloid for hypercholesterolemic men. Arch Intern Med 148:292, 1988
36. Van Horn LV, Liu K, Parker D et al: Serum lipid response to oat product intake with a fat-modified diet. J Am Diet Assoc 86:759, 1986

EVALUATION OF THE PATIENT WITH SIGNS AND SYMPTOMS OF ISCHEMIC HEART DISEASE

Louis J. Dell'Italia • Robert A. O'Rourke

The pathophysiologic mechanism of myocardial ischemia includes not only fixed obstructive coronary artery disease due to atherosclerosis but also variable degrees of coronary artery stenosis due to increased coronary vascular tone with or without associated coronary atherosclerosis. Thus, a patient may present with a wide variety of clinical and laboratory manifestations of myocardial ischemia. Furthermore, with recent advances in technology, the evaluation to detect or exclude ischemic heart disease often is not initiated because of a patient's symptom of chest pain but emanates from an abnormal electrocardiogram or equivocal results during exercise testing, radionuclide ventriculography, or thallium-201 perfusion studies. The purpose of this chapter is to establish a rational diagnostic approach to the patient who presents with symptoms or laboratory signs of ischemic heart disease in light of the complex pathophysiologic mechanisms that may precipitate myocardial ischemia.

☐ HISTORY

Although there is no uniform presenting symptom for ischemic heart disease, chest pain or discomfort represents the most common reason for presentation to a physician. The term *angina*, which was originally described by Heberden in 1768, connoted a sense of strangling associated with anxiety and fear of death (angor animi) that accompanied this sensation in the chest.[1] However, as every clinician well knows, a patient's description of ischemic chest pain may take on many forms, which include, for example, burning, viselike tightness, squeezing, choking, heaviness, knifelike, and suffocating. To complicate matters further, the forms of discomfort may involve the epigastric rather than the mid-sternal area with the patient describing a "burning or indigestion feeling." Although the etiology of the various forms of discomfort is complex and not fully understood, there is an adequate explanation for the many patterns of referred pain that can be manifested in the neck, jaw, left shoulder, and left arm. The convergence–projection theory proposed by Foreman and Ohata[2] has a clear anatomical explanation in the spinal cord where impulses mediated by the sympathetic afferent pathway converge with impulses from somatic thoracic structures onto the same ascending spinal neurons. Thus, impulses reaching visceral afferent neurons may stimulate nearby intermediate neurons that are receptors for somatic impulses and subsequently may produce a sensation of discomfort in the various referred areas in the chest, neck, or arms.

Since the quality or character of the chest discomfort can be difficult to interpret, the duration, location, precipitating factors, and means of relief are very important in the overall assessment of the patient with chest pain (Table 61.1). Typical anginal chest pain usually comes on gradually and reaches its maximal intensity over a period of 2 to 3 minutes. If the pain is related to exertion, then relief should occur within 2 to 3 minutes after the cessation of exercise. Chest pain that lasts for hours or days is not consistent with angina pectoris. Chest discomfort that is described as a piercing knife, tingling sensation, or shocks that last for 2 to 3 seconds is also not due to myocardial ischemia. Ischemic chest pain usually has a deep visceral character, which does not permit the patient to localize the discomfort to a very specific region of the chest, for example, the left nipple. A discretely localized area of chest pain that is also associated with very atypical characteristics such as stabbing or shocklike sensations is not due to myocardial ischemia.

The assessment of chest pain is not complete without an evaluation of the precipitating factors that elicit chest discomfort. This evaluation not only is useful to the physician in the diagnostic assessment but also may aid in determining the stability of the anginal pattern or whether there are elements in the symptomatology suggesting fixed coronary artery stenosis vs. variable coronary artery obstruction. Classic angina is most frequently experienced during exercise, and effort angina is the usual reason for presentation in patients who have only fixed obstructive coronary artery stenoses.

During exercise there is an increase in heart rate, blood pressure, and myocardial contractility because of sympathetic stimulation that results in an increase in myocardial oxygen demand. This is balanced mainly by an augmentation of coronary blood flow because the coronary circulation does not have the capacity to increase its oxygen extraction, since myocardial oxygen extraction is already high at rest and at normal workloads. Thus, coronary blood flow and, subsequently, myocardial oxygen supply are limited by the degree of coronary artery narrowing. The double product (heart rate × blood pressure) has been used as a relatively reliable indirect marker of myocardial oxygen consumption in patients with fixed coronary artery disease because it incorporates two very important factors affecting the myocardial oxygen demand: (1) the tension or systolic pressure developed by the ventricular wall (in Laplace's law, tension = pressure × radius/wall thickness) and (2) the heart rate, which is directly related to myocardial oxygen demand and immensely affects the diastolic filling time when most of the coronary blood flow to the left ventricular endocardium occurs.[3] Because myocardial oxygen supply is highly dependent on the ability to increase coronary blood flow, the extent of physical activity (increase in heart rate × systolic blood pressure product) that precipitates angina appears to be related to the degree of fixed coronary arterial stenosis but not necessarily to the number of coronary arteries with severe obstructive lesions.

Other precipitating factors other than exercise may aid the physician in determining the etiology of chest pain. For example, some patients who may have a classic history for exertional angina may also experience angina at rest. When the patient is carefully questioned, the physician may find that these episodes of chest discomfort at rest may be associated with emotional lability such as occurs during anger, fright, or uncomfortable situations. Other patients may experience angina after ingesting a large meal. These symptoms may be due to augmented sympathetic tone, which increases heart rate, blood pressure, and coronary vascular tone. This pathophysiologic mechanism can also be invoked for patients who characteristically experience angina on exposure to cold weather.

Angina occurring at rest after a patient has retired to bed represents a specific type of rest angina often appearing in patients with chronic stable exertional angina. Angina may occur before sleep, soon after the patient reclines. This results from an increase in left ventricular wall stress (and, thus MVO_2) brought about by the increased left ventricular volume resulting from the augmentation of venous return in the supine position. Angina that occurs during sleep usually occurs in the early morning hours. This has been attributed to superimposed or isolated coronary artery spasm, since increased coronary vascular tone has been demonstrated to be common during this time of the day.

Coronary vasomotor tone is an extremely important determinant of coronary artery blood flow. It is now well established that coronary arterial tone is influenced by a multitude of factors, which include autonomic activity, metabolic products, and circulatory neurohumoral substances.[4] Although the precise mechanism of angina pectoris is unclear, one or a combination of the above factors is responsible for producing an acute decrease in myocardial oxygen supply in patients with fixed obstructive coronary artery disease and in patients with otherwise normal coronary artery anatomy. This added feature in the mechanism of myocardial oxygen supply produces the variable clinical manifestations of angina. Thus, patients may present with unpredictable and a variable threshold for angina ranging from pain at rest on certain days to pain that can only be elicited with maximal physical activity at other times. Most patients who demonstrate a vasospastic component to their anginal pattern also have fixed obstructive coronary artery disease of varying severity.

A few patients with classic angina pectoris have symptoms in the setting of normal coronary artery anatomy. Most of these have spontaneous or provokable coronary artery spasm. The triggering mechanism for variant or Prinzmetal's angina is usually unclear. Episodes of pain usually occur at rest without any precipitating factors and in the absence of exertion. The duration of chest discomfort may be longer than with classic exertion-induced angina pectoris, but relief is usually obtained within 1 to 2 minutes after administration of sublingual nitroglycerin. In addition, a cyclical anginal pattern may be elicited with symptoms occurring more frequently during early morning hours. However, the anginal pattern and characteristics of chest pain may vary in the same patient on different occasions. Electrocardiographic recordings taken during pain, when abnormal, most commonly demonstrate ST segment elevation, but ST segment depression or T wave changes may also be shown. Variant angina occurs in males and females at any age but appears to be more common in younger females, who may also demonstrate other forms of vasoreactivity such as migraine headaches or Raynaud's phenomenon. In addition, electrocardiograms recorded during chest pain may also demonstrate disturbances of atrioventricular conduction, bradyarrhythmias, and/or ventricular arrhythmias.[5]

Whether the etiology of myocardial ischemia is due to fixed obstructive disease, spasm superimposed on fixed obstructive coronary artery disease, or variant (Prinzmetal's) angina, the mode of the relief of chest pain with sublingual nitroglycerin is similar for all three clinical syndromes. Relief of chest pain after the administration of sublingual nitroglycerin usually occurs within 1 to 5 minutes and can be a helpful diagnostic clue to the presence of myocardial ischemic pain. However, pain due to esophageal spasm may also be relieved by sublingual nitroglycerin in a similar time frame.

The term *unstable angina* is used quite frequently in clinical practice and has also been referred to as "preinfarction angina." Based on the cooperative study definition of the National Institutes of Health, a diagnosis of unstable angina can be made when one or more of the following historical features are present: (1) angina pectoris of new onset (usually within the last month and brought on by minimal exertion); (2) development of more severe, prolonged, or frequent angina superimposed on a preexisting pattern of relatively stable, effort-related angina pectoris; or (3) angina pectoris at rest as well as with minimal exertion. Most patients with criterion 1 or 2 also have angina at rest.

Patients may present with symptoms other than chest pain that are manifestations of myocardial ischemia. Dyspnea without associated angina pectoris occurs infrequently, but this may be the only manifestation of myocardial ischemia in patients who have a defective anginal warning system, such as patients with diabetes mellitus. Shortness of breath results from ischemia-induced left ventricular dysfunction that increases left ventricular end-diastolic and pulmonary venous pressures. Palpitations, dizziness, and syncope due to ventricular tachyarrhythmias or ventricular fibrillation rarely occur in the absence of angina pectoris. However, frequent premature ventricular beats on a routine 12-lead electrocardiogram may be a harbinger of obstructive coronary artery disease in a patient who is relatively free of symptoms. In addition, lightheadedness or syncope may result from hypotension during ischemic episodes when left ventricular pump function is severely impaired, as in patients with severe left main coronary artery stenosis.

TABLE 61.1 CHARACTERISTICS OF ANGINA PECTORIS

Quality
Pressure of heavy weight on the chest
Burning
Tightness
Constriction about the throat
Visceral quality (deep, heavy, squeezing, aching)
Gradual increase in intensity followed by gradual fading away

Location
Over sternum or very near to it
Anywhere between epigastrium and pharynx
Occasionally limited to left shoulder and left arm
Rarely limited to right arm
Limited to lower jaw
Lower cervical or upper thoracic spine
Left interscapular or suprascapular area

Duration
0.5 to 30 minutes

Precipitating Factors
Relationship to exercise
Effort that involves use of arms above the head
Cold environment
Walking against the wind
Walking after a large meal
Emotional factors involved with physical exercise
Fright, anger, anxiety
Coitus

Nitroglycerin Relief
Relief of pain occurring within 45 seconds to 5 minutes of taking nitroglycerin

Radiation
Medial aspect of left arm
Left shoulder
Jaw
Occasionally right arm

Associated Symptoms
Shortness of breath
Dizziness, lightheadedness, syncope
Palpitations
Weakness

An evaluation of the patient who complains of chest pain is not complete without an assessment of the risk factors for coronary artery disease. Most of the data on this subject comes from epidemiologic studies that evaluate clinically healthy individuals and follow these groups prospectively to detect the development of coronary artery disease. Clearly, age represents a significant risk factor since numerous autopsy series have demonstrated a higher prevalence of coronary artery disease for both males and females over age 55. Although this disease is quite rare in young women, it is a major cause of death for young men between 35 and 44 years of age. The Framingham heart study has identified the presence of four major risk factors in both men and women for the presence of coronary artery disease: (1) hypertension, (2) elevated serum cholesterol level, (3) smoking, and (4) glucose intolerance.[6,7]

Despite the large body of data that links an elevated serum cholesterol level to coronary artery disease, it is well appreciated that no single level of cholesterol clearly separates those patients at risk from those who are not. Results of many recent investigations strongly suggest that the lipoprotein complexes that transport cholesterol in serum may affect atherogenesis independent of the total cholesterol level. The results of these studies show that an elevated serum low-density lipoprotein cholesterol level has a positive correlation with the prevalence of coronary artery disease, and the level of serum high-density lipoprotein cholesterol has an inverse correlation with the prevalence of coronary artery disease.[8] Therefore, it may be important to measure the serum lipoprotein cholesterol level in a patient who has a serum cholesterol value in the high normal range and other risk factors previously mentioned or a strongly positive family history for coronary artery disease. Other risk factors that have been associated with the presence of coronary artery disease include obesity, type A personality, use of oral contraceptives, and a sedentary life-style.

PHYSICAL EXAMINATION

The general physical examination of the patient with chronic ischemic heart disease may be entirely normal; however, a simple blood pressure determination and general inspection may reveal the following risk factors for coronary artery disease: systemic hypertension, xanthomas suggestive of hypercholesterolemia, and arcus senilis, which in patients under 50 years of age is also suggestive of hypercholesterolemia. A fundoscopic examination may reveal retinal changes that are common in patients with coronary artery disease even in the absence of diabetes mellitus and systemic hypertension. These findings include an abnormal light reflex, which is the most sensitive sign, and abnormal vessel tortuosity and decreased vessel caliber, which are less sensitive but more specific signs for the presence of coronary artery disease[9].

Palpation of the peripheral pulses may reveal a decreased pulse amplitude with bruits on auscultation thereby indicating generalized atherosclerosis. Inspection of the neck may reveal an elevated jugular venous pressure consistent with systemic venous hypertension. Closer inspection of the elevated venous pulsations may reveal equal amplitudes of the a and v wave, thereby suggesting either right ventricular dysfunction or tricuspid regurgitation, one of the possible causes being previous right ventricular infarction.[10] These findings in addition to Kussmaul's sign may be seen in other chronic conditions such as restrictive cardiomyopathy, constrictive pericarditis, and cor pulmonale.

Palpation of the precordium may reveal a sustained left parasternal impulse, which suggests right ventricular systolic hypertension. In addition, the point of maximal impulse of the left ventricle may be displaced lateral to the mid-clavicular line suggesting previous left ventricular infarction and subsequent chamber dilatation. However, Eilen and co-workers have demonstrated that the location of the apical impulse in relation to the mid-clavicular or mid-sternal line is not a reliable indicator of left ventricular end-diastolic volume, while an apical impulse diameter greater than 3 cm is a more accurate indicator of left ventricular chamber enlargement.[11] Assessment of the point of maximal impulse may reveal a palpable presystolic and/or diastolic rapid filling component(s) of the left ventricular impulse. The former usually is accompanied by an S_4 on auscultation and the latter with an S_3. If the patient is rotated into the left lateral decubitus position, the apical impulse may be examined more carefully and such abnormalities are more likely to be recognized. Also, in this position, a sustained and diffuse outward bulging during left ventricular systole indicates the likelihood of a dyskinetic myocardial segment or aneurysm.

Auscultation of the patient with chronic ischemic heart disease usually reveals a normal S_1, but it may be decreased in intensity in the presence of first-degree atrioventricular block. The S_2 occasionally exhibits paradoxic splitting with expiration during myocardial ischemia. This finding results from left ventricular dysfunction with a delayed and sometimes prolonged left ventricular ejection time during an ischemic episode. In the left lateral decubitus position an S_3 may be heard at the apex at rest or during isometric hand grip exercise. A fourth heart sound (S_4) frequently is heard in many patients over 40 years of age who have no evidence of ischemic heart disease. It is heard commonly in patients with systolic hypertension, cardiomyopathies, aortic stenosis, or degenerative cardiac disease. It usually indicates diminished left ventricular compliance and is common in the elderly, since left ventricular distensibility decreases with aging. Thus, the specificity of this finding for the presence of obstructive coronary artery disease is low; however, the absence of an S_4 both at rest and during exercise in a patient in sinus rhythm is a point against the diagnosis of acute or chronic myocardial ischemia.[12]

Apical systolic murmurs can be heard either at rest or during provocation with isometric hand grip exercise. These murmurs result from dysfunction of the papillary muscle and overlying left ventricular wall segments. They can be maximum in intensity in early, mid, or late systole and may also be associated with mid to late systolic clicks characteristic of mitral valve prolapse.[13] Generally, the murmur of anterior papillary muscle dysfunction radiates to the axilla while the murmur of posterior papillary muscle dysfunction radiates to the base of the heart. Thus, the latter is easily confused with the mid-systolic murmur due to flow across a normal or obstructed semilunar valve. In addition, tricuspid or mitral regurgitant murmurs may result from abnormal coaptation of the atrioventricular valves during systole owing to right or left ventricular infarction with subsequent chamber enlargement and/or annular dilatation. Often a murmur of mitral or tricuspid regurgitation presents only during episodes of chest pain and/or heart failure.

It should be emphasized that all of the physical findings discussed above are nonspecific for the presence of severe coronary artery stenosis, and many of these findings can be found in the patient with nonischemic cardiomyopathy. Furthermore, if the S_4 is discounted, more than 25% of patients with symptomatic obstructive coronary artery disease will have an entirely normal physical examination.

CHEST ROENTGENOGRAPHY

The chest roentgenogram is normal in many patients with chronic ischemic heart disease. However, the cardiac silhouette may be enlarged owing to previous myocardial infarction and impaired left ventricular systolic function. This results in left ventricular enlargement on the anteroposterior and lateral chest roentgenograms. Since left ventricular dysfunction is associated with an increase in diastolic filling pressures, the left atrium may also be enlarged. This may be readily appreciated by straightening of the left heart border on the anteroposterior film and associated widening of the angle between the right and left main-stem bronchus.

Since infarction of the right ventricle may result in significant chamber enlargement of both right atrium and right ventricle, the anteroposterior projection may demonstrate a prominent right heart border and the lateral projection may reveal an obliteration of the retrosternal air space. In addition, right ventricular enlargement may be seen as a result of chronic elevation of left ventricular filling pressure owing to extensive infarction of the left ventricle. In the latter case, the chest roentgenogram will reveal biventricular enlargement.

Infarcted myocardium can occasionally be visualized on the chest film when calcium is deposited in the area of infarction. This is usually visualized as a curvilinear thin radiodense line along the left ventricular border that can be seen when it is projected tangentially to the x-ray beam. A left ventricular aneurysm can be detected when an abnormal bulge projects outward from the cardiac silhouette. Occasionally these aneurysmal dilatations may have calcium deposits in their thin walls.

Calcium deposits within the coronary arteries are extremely difficult to visualize on the plain roentgenogram owing to normal heart motion. However, fluoroscopy allows adequate visualization of calcific deposits within the coronary arteries that are most commonly located in their proximal portions. Most studies have shown that the presence of calcium within the walls of the coronary arteries is a very specific finding for high-grade obstructive coronary artery disease in patients under 65 years of age. However, in older age-groups, this finding does not necessarily indicate severe obstructive coronary artery disease.[14,15]

In the majority of patients with chronic ischemic heart disease, the lung fields are clear without evidence of pulmonary venous hypertension. After a large amount of left ventricular myocardium is infarcted, pulmonary venous pressure rises owing to the elevation of left ventricular diastolic pressures. Increased pulmonary venous pressure results in an increase in interstitial fluid with a resultant haziness of the normally sharp lines of demarcation of the hilar vessels. In addition, pulmonary vessels contract in response to hypoxia, causing a reversal of pulmonary blood flow pattern from a caudal to a cephalad direction and thus producing the characteristic "antler pattern." The chest roentgenogram in chronic left ventricular failure may also demonstrate blunting of the costophrenic angles, right and left pleural effusions, Kerley B lines, and an interstitial pattern in the lung fields.

ELECTROCARDIOGRAPHY

The resting electrocardiogram has been reported to be normal in 25% to 50% of the patients who present for an evaluation of ischemic heart disease. A careful inspection for diagnostic Q waves, ST segment and T wave abnormalities, conduction disturbances, and premature ventricular beats can provide diagnostic clues and pitfalls when one attempts to predict the presence of obstructive coronary artery disease from the resting electrocardiogram.

The presence of diagnostic Q waves on the electrocardiogram obviously provides credence to the likelihood of severe obstructive coronary artery disease. However, electrocardiograms are often normal in patients who have severe three-vessel coronary artery disease or in patients who have totally occluded vessels on coronary arteriography with collateral circulation distal to the obstructed vessel. Other studies have demonstrated a low sensitivity of the resting electrocardiogram for diagnosing old myocardial infarction when compared with postmortem examination. This lack of sensitivity of the electrocardiogram for detecting previous myocardial infarction has been attributed to a scarring down of the infarcted zone, the presence of multiple infarctions involving several areas of the myocardium that neutralizes the abnormal electrocardiographic finding of any single infarction, and the presence of intraventricular conduction disturbances such as left anterior hemiblock and left bundle branch block, which may mask the presence of an inferior myocardial infarction and an anterior myocardial infarction, respectively.

Studies in which serial electrocardiograms were performed in a large number of patients with myocardial infarction have demonstrated that Q waves disappear in 6% to 7% of the patients studied.[16] Normalization of Q waves appears to be as high as 20% to 25% for patients with inferior myocardial infarction. Furthermore, nontransmural myocardial infarction is not associated with a diagnostic Q wave pattern and the electrocardiogram may revert to normal or to nonspecific ST and T wave abnormalities. Thus, it is quite clear that the electrocardiogram is a very insensitive marker for previous myocardial infarction.

The most common findings on the electrocardiogram in patients with chronic ischemic heart disease are nonspecific ST and T wave changes. These are defined as minor deviations of the ST segment, T wave flattening, or slight T wave inversions. However, there are numerous other factors that cause these common electrocardiographic findings. Other electrocardiographic signs of myocardial ischemia may be manifested as one of the following changes: (1) abnormally tall T waves, (2) symmetrically or deeply inverted T waves, (3) horizontal ST segment depression with or without T wave inversion, (4) normalization of previously abnormal T waves, and (5) inversion of U waves.

Peaked T waves in normal patients and in patients with hyperkalemia can be differentiated from the abnormally tall T waves in patients with myocardial infarction in that the QT interval is usually prolonged in the latter group. Other causes of prominent T waves include the secondary T wave changes of left ventricular hypertrophy and left bundle branch block and the bizarre peaked T waves that may be upright or inverted in patients with intracranial bleeding.

In the absence of QRS abnormalities, the presence of deep symmetrically inverted T waves is usually associated with acute or chronic myocardial ischemia. However, T wave inversions may be seen in the following conditions: persistent juvenile pattern in the early precordial leads and the normal electrocardiogram of young black males and trained athletes, usually in association with ST segment elevation. The differential diagnosis of deep T wave inversions is beyond the scope of this chapter; however, the clinician is commonly confronted with the patient who has longstanding hypertension and symptoms of chest pain. The classic repolarization abnormalities of left ventricular hypertrophy are ST segments that demonstrate an upward convexity with T wave inversions in the left precordial leads. Electrocardiographic findings in patients with left ventricular hypertrophy may demonstrate variations in these repolarization abnormalities without QRS voltage criteria of left ventricular hypertrophy and are often difficult to differentiate from primary myocardial ischemic changes. Serial electrocardiograms recorded during chest pain in patients with coincident left ventricular hypertrophy and myocardial ischemia may document further ST segment depression that returns to baseline after the chest discomfort has resolved.

With ST segment depression, T waves may be upright or inverted; however, isolated ST segment depression with upright T waves is more suggestive of myocardial ischemia. Digitalis therapy is one of the more common causes of ST segment depression. ST segments in patients receiving digitalis usually demonstrate a scooped-out or concave-upward appearance with a shortened QT interval that may help to differentiate these changes from myocardial ischemia.

Other less common repolarization findings associated with myocardial ischemia include pseudonormalization of the T wave pattern and U wave inversions. Premature ventricular beats are the most common arrhythmia in normal individuals, in the elderly, and in patients with chronic coronary artery disease. Further assessment may or may not be necessary after an evaluation of the history, risk factors, and physical examination. Conduction abnormalities are often present as a "normal variant," especially in the elderly population. However, the clinician should realize that an otherwise unexplained nonspecific intraventricular conduction defect or complete left bundle branch block in younger age-groups may be a harbinger of coronary artery disease or other organic heart disease.

After an evaluation of the history, physical examination, chest roentgenogram, and electrocardiogram, the physician must decide whether a patient is at high, medium, or low risk for the presence of coronary artery disease. At the present time there are many tests that may lead to the diagnosis of coronary artery disease. However, each test has variable sensitivities and specificities that are related to technical limitations and the nature of the patient population to which the test is applied. Taking these facts into consideration, the following sections will outline a rational approach for the selection of the optimal test that will provide the most definitive diagnostic information for detecting the presence of coronary artery disease.

EXERCISE ELECTROCARDIOGRAPHY

Exercise electrocardiography is extremely useful in detecting myocardial ischemia in patients with coronary artery disease. To apply this method appropriately the clinician must have a thorough understanding of the measurements to be obtained and the patient population being evaluated because there are many subtle clues and pitfalls in the diagnoses of coronary artery disease during exercise electrocardiography.

Myocardial ischemia on the electrocardiogram during exercise is commonly manifested by the following changes in the ST segments: (1) downsloping ST segment depression, (2) flat ST segment depression, and (3) slow upsloping ST segment depression. The most commonly used criterion for a positive electrocardiographic result during exercise treadmill testing is the appearance of greater than or equal to 1 mm of ST segment depression for 0.08 second after the J point of the QRS complex, with the PR segment serving as the baseline of reference (Fig. 61.1). This finding commonly results from inadequate perfusion of the subendocardium during exercise and represents a current of injury vector during diastole that is opposite in direction to the main QRS vector. Downsloping ST segment depression is highly specific for coronary artery disease, while horizontal or slowly upsloping ST segment depressions are less specific indicators of coronary artery disease. However, marked ST segment depression ($\geq$ 2 mm), ST segment depression occurring early (before 6 minutes) during exercise treadmill testing, and persistent ST segment depression for more than 8 minutes after the cessation of exercise are highly specific findings for the presence of severe obstructive coronary artery disease irrespective of the type of ST segment depression encountered.

Other changes in the stress electrocardiogram that may be consistent with myocardial ischemia include the following: development of left bundle branch block, appearance of inverted U waves, inversion of the T waves, appearance of a Q wave, increased R wave amplitude, and the appearance of ventricular arrhythmias during exercise. These abnormal responses during exercise are nonspecific and, therefore, are of questionable value in the diagnosis of coronary artery disease. However, the presence of ventricular premature beats during exercise warrants further discussion since this is a common finding in many normal patients and in patients with ischemic heart disease.

First, it has been shown that the statistical probability of developing coronary heart disease is approximately three times greater in otherwise healthy men with ominous exertional ventricular arrhythmias.[17] Second, in patients with known coronary artery disease this finding appears to portend a poor prognosis only in those patients who have had a myocardial infarction or who have accompanying ST segment depression.[18] The following guidelines are set forth by Koppes and co-workers in their comprehensive review of the literature concerning the significance of ventricular premature beats during stress electrocardiography[19]:

1. Patients with coronary artery disease usually manifest arrhythmias at lower heart rates, and these arrhythmias are somewhat more reproducible than those seen in normal subjects, who usually develop ventricular arrhythmias at heart rates greater than 130 beats per minute.
2. Premature ventricular beats at rest that abolish with exercise can occur in healthy patients as well as in patients with coronary artery disease.
3. The appearance of ventricular ectopic beats that occur only during the recovery phase is of questionable significance.
4. Ventricular tachycardia either at rest or during exercise usually rep-

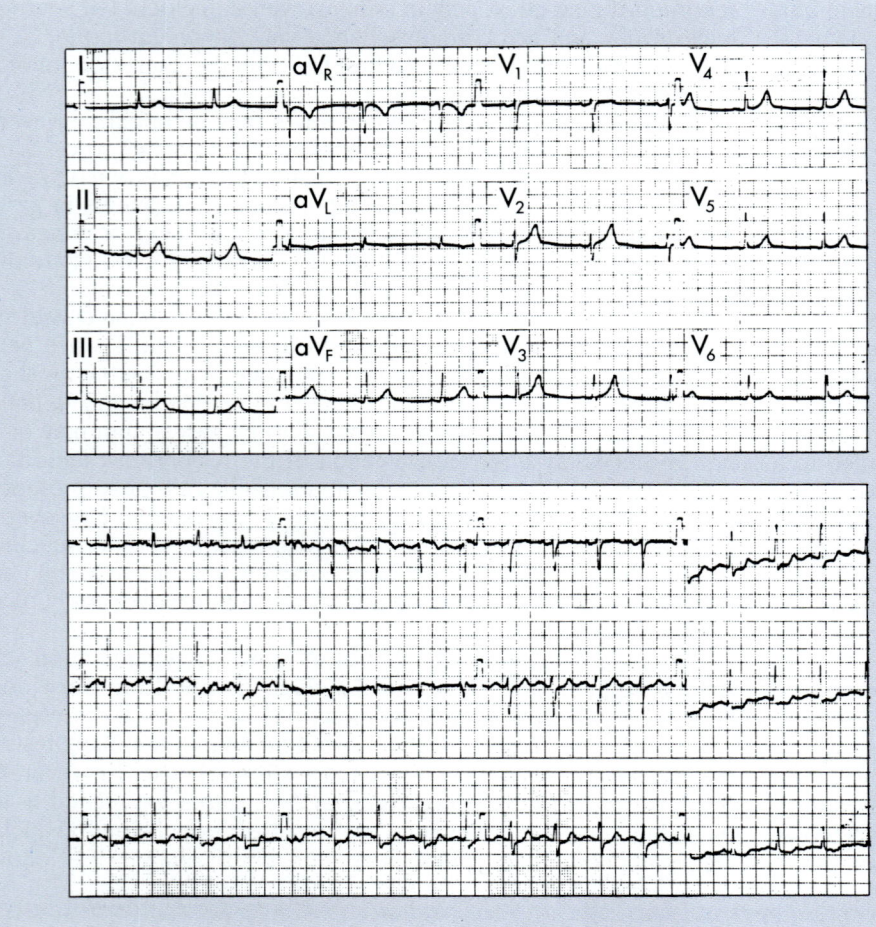

FIGURE 61.1 Upper panel displays a 12-lead electrocardiogram during hyperventilation. At 6 minutes of exercise a complaint of chest pain was accompanied by ST segment depressions in II, III, aV_F, V_4, V_5, and V_6, which was diagnostic of myocardial ischemia.

resents some form of underlying organic heart disease or myocardial ischemia.

5. The frequency of exercise-induced ventricular arrhythmias increases with advancing age in the absence of coronary artery disease.

There are a number of factors other than myocardial ischemia that can produce ST segment depression on stress electrocardiography and thereby lead to a false-positive diagnosis of coronary artery disease. These factors fall into the following etiologic groups: (1) physiologic (functional) factors; (2) organic, noncoronary heart disease; (3) altered ventricular conduction; and (4) metabolic factors (Table 61.2). These factors should be kept in mind or corrected before exercise electrocardiography is performed.

Other factors may be operating to produce false-negative results during stress electrocardiography. The ST segment elevation that occurs in the distribution of myocardial scar during exercise may neutralize the opposing ST segment depression in the distribution of a severely stenosed vessel. Consequently, ST segments will remain at baseline. In addition, an inadequate stress, one achieving less than 85% of the predicted maximal heart rate, may not be a sufficient increase in myocardial oxygen demand to produce ischemic ST segment changes on the electrocardiogram. This may occur for various reasons, including concomitant use of β-blockers, early leg fatigue, or "chronotropic insufficiency."

In a comprehensive review by Gibson and Beller of 16 studies in which the results of stress electrocardiography and coronary angiography were compared, the average sensitivity was 64% (range 47% to 81%) and the average specificity was 89% (range 69% to 96%) for stress electrocardiography.[20] The high false-negative rate in these patients with symptomatic coronary artery disease (angina pectoris) was attributed to the lack of sensitivity of stress electrocardiography in the diagnosis of single vessel disease. The average sensitivity of the test increased from 44% to 71% to 85% for one-, two-, and three-vessel disease, respectively. Thus, the test becomes more sensitive as the number of stenotic vessels increases. In addition, coronary angiography *per se* does not provide physiologic information concerning the presence or absence of myocardial ischemia due to the coronary artery stenoses. Among the studies in the literature, criteria for "significant" coronary stenosis vary between 50% and 75% reduction in luminal diameter. Elegant studies that evaluate the coronary flow response to a hyperemic stimulus have shown that the physiologic assessment of angiographically documented coronary stenoses of less than 60% is fraught with errors.[21] Therefore, coronary angiography may provide a faulty standard of reference for determining physiologically significant coronary artery disease when there is less than 60% reduction in luminal diameter.

Patients occasionally develop ST segment elevation with exercise, and this finding has two potential pathophysiologic mechanisms: (1) transmural ischemia due to coronary artery spasm and (2) left ventricular dyskinetic wall segments during exercise that behave like a ventricular aneurysm electrocardiographically. The former response usually distorts the QRS segment in addition to producing ST segment elevation while the latter response does not distort the QRS complex and is not associated with T wave inversions in the process of recovery from ischemia.

Findings on physical examination during exercise electrocardiography may provide important diagnostic clues to the presence of important left ventricular dysfunction, but their sensitivity and specificity are limited. The development of shortness of breath associated with rales and an S_3 represents severe left ventricular dysfunction brought about by exercise. In addition, the appearance of a mitral regurgitant systolic murmur or a precordial bulge could be due to left ventricular dysfunction. A fall of the systolic arterial blood pressure early during exercise can be observed in any cardiac condition that limits the increment in cardiac output, including cardiomyopathy, valvular heart disease, or coronary artery disease. When this occurs in the setting of coronary artery disease, it usually indicates the presence of extensive previous myocardial infarction or the development of widespread left ventricular ischemia due to left main or severe three-vessel coronary artery stenosis.

An abnormally low heart rate response at maximal exercise and an inappropriately high heart rate response at submaximal exercise may be encountered during exercise electrocardiography. The former response may be due to ischemic or nonischemic sinus node disease, drug effect, or physical conditioning. The latter response may be due to vasoregulatory asthenia, prolonged bed rest, anemia, or volume depletion or may represent a compensatory response of the left ventricle to maintain cardiac output in patients who have severe left ventricular dysfunction. The prognostic significance of relatively low or high heart rates during exercise testing has not been demonstrated.

In utilizing stress electrocardiography the physician attempts to distinguish correctly between those patients who do and those who do not have coronary artery disease. The sensitivity, specificity, and predictive value of this test collectively define the accuracy of exercise-induced ST segment depression for identifying patients with coronary artery disease that is documented by coronary angiography.[22] Sensitivity reflects the ability of the exercise stress test to identify the presence of coronary artery disease.

$$\text{Sensitivity} = \frac{\text{True positives}}{\text{True positives} + \text{false negatives}} \times 100$$

where, true positives are patients with both abnormal stress tests and abnormal angiograms and false negatives are patients with normal stress tests who have abnormal angiograms. Specificity is a measure of

---

TABLE 61.2 CAUSES OF FALSE-POSITIVE ST SEGMENT DEPRESSION DURING EXERCISE STRESS TESTING

Physiologic	Altered Ventricular Activation
Actual repolarization	Left bundle branch block (left precordial leads)
Hyperventilation	Right bundle branch block (right precordial leads)
Vasoregulatory lability	Wolff-Parkinson-White syndrome (and various pre-excitation syndromes)
Organic, Noncoronary Heart Disease	**Metabolic**
Aortic stenosis	Drug effect (*i.e.*, digitalis)
Cardiomyopathy	Electrolyte imbalance (*i.e.*, hypokalemia)
Left ventricular hypertrophy (caused by aortic stenosis, hypertension)	Hypoxemia
Mitral valve prolapse	Recent food intake
Pericardial disorders	Anemia
Idiopathic hypertrophic subaortic stenosis	

the reliability of the stress test for identifying those patients who do not have coronary artery disease.

$$\text{Specificity} = \frac{\text{True negatives}}{\text{True negatives} + \text{false positives}} \times 100$$

where, true negatives are patients with normal stress tests who have normal angiograms and false positives are patients with abnormal stress tests and normal angiograms. The positive predictive value for exercise electrocardiography in identifying those patients with coronary artery disease is defined as follows:

$$\text{Positive predictive value} = \frac{\text{True positives}}{\text{True positives} + \text{false positives}} \times 100$$

Thus, if a test has a positive predictive value of 90%, then 90% of the results are true positives and 10% represent false-positive results. In contrast, the negative predictive value of a test is as follows:

$$\text{Negative predictive value} = \frac{\text{True negatives}}{\text{True negatives} + \text{false negatives}} \times 100$$

In the diagnosis of coronary artery disease, the physician is most interested in the predictive value (positive and negative) of stress electrocardiography, which defines the accuracy of the test for detecting coronary artery disease.

Thus, a test that has a low positive predictive value incorrectly identifies patients with coronary artery disease and, therefore, subjects a large number of these patients to unneeded medications, cardiac catheterization, and restrictions in life-style. Alternatively, a test with a low negative predictive value has many false-negative results and misses many patients with coronary artery disease who may go on to myocardial infarction or sudden death if left untreated. In order to avoid these possibilities, the physician must understand that the predictive value of a test is directly related to the prevalence of the disease in the population being studied according to Bayes' theorem (Table 61.3). The prevalence of coronary artery disease is related to age, sex, type of chest pain, and many other factors. For example, a 40-year-old premenopausal woman with a typical chest pain probably has a 1% prevalence of coronary artery disease. Then exercise electrocardiography (a test with a 60% sensitivity and 90% specificity for identifying angiographically proven coronary artery disease) will produce a number of positive tests that suggest the presence of coronary artery disease. However, because of the low prevalence of this disease in this particular population, only 6% of the positive tests correctly identify the presence of disease (true positive) while 94% of the tests will be falsely positive. However, the predictive value of a negative test for ruling out coronary artery disease is 99% (true negatives). Thus, if the pretest likelihood of coronary disease is low (less than 10%), a normal test rules out coronary artery disease with a high degree of accuracy as long as an adequate stress is achieved but a positive test is not at all accurate in confirming the presence of coronary artery disease.

On the other hand, a 65-year-old man with exertional chest pain has a high probability of coronary artery disease, and, thus, diagnostic ST segment depression during stress electrocardiography has a positive predictive value of 98% and a negative predictive value of 20%. Since a negative test result does not exclude the diagnoses of coronary artery disease with great certainty, the physician is obligated to perform other diagnostic tests to rule out the presence of ischemic heart disease in this patient population with a high likelihood of disease. In addition, while the positive test is no surprise to the experienced clinician who performs a complete history and physical examination beforehand, valuable prognostic information may be obtained from a positive test when more than 2 mm of ST segment depression, hypotension, or ventricular arrhythmias with ST segment depression occur during exercise.

Between these two extremes of patient populations with low and high prevalence of coronary artery disease are those patients who represent a 50% chance of having disease. These patients represent a heterogeneous group since a 35-year-old man probably has a 5% to 10% chance of having coronary artery disease; however, a history of classic exertional chest pain and a strong family history may raise his probability to 50% to 60%. On the other hand, a 70-year-old man with very atypical chest pain represents a disease prevalence of probably 60%. In addition, the older patient may have many of the characteristics that confound the interpretation of stress electrocardiography, including β-blocker therapy, poor functional capacity, "chronotropic insufficiency," hypertension, and abnormal resting electrocardiogram. Nonetheless, the positive predictive value and negative predictive value of stress electrocardiography is relatively high in the patient population with a 50% pretest probability of disease. Furthermore, even though the incidence of false-negative test results is approximately 30%, an adequate maximum electrocardiographic stress test is unlikely to be normal in patients with significant fixed coronary artery disease, especially three-vessel or left main coronary artery disease. These examples underscore the importance of considering the prevalence of disease, the patient population, and the anticipated problems in achieving interpretable test results before ordering stress electrocardiography.

A final statement should be made concerning the use of exercise electrocardiography in assessing asymptomatic patients who come to evaluation for reasons other than chest pain. According to currently available literature, the prevalence of false-positive tests among asymptomatic patients is approximately 60%.[23,24] These values are reasonable, since it has been established that the prevalence of silent coronary artery disease in men over 50 years of age is approximately 5% in studies of large cohorts of patients. However, asymptomatic patients with other risk factors including increased age, smoking, and high serum cholesterol levels should be evaluated with another noninvasive procedure (i.e., thallium-201) or cardiac catheterization in order to rule out coronary artery disease.[25,26] Thus, stress electrocardiography is not very useful for evaluating individual asymptomatic patients owing to the high incidence of false-positive test results.

NUCLEAR STUDIES
MYOCARDIAL PERFUSION IMAGING WITH THALLIUM-201

Several agents have been investigated for myocardial perfusion imaging and certain physical and biologic properties make thallium-201 the best myocardial perfusion agent available for routine clinical use. This radioisotope has a 73-hour half-life and low photon energies that are easy to detect on existing collimator camera systems. Thallium-201 is

TABLE 61.3 PERFORMANCE OF EXERCISE TREADMILL TESTING WITH A SENSITIVITY OF 60% AND A SPECIFICITY OF 90% IN POPULATION WITH A VARIABLE PREVALENCE OF CORONARY ARTERY DISEASE

Actual Disease Prevalence	1%	10%	50%	90%
Predictive Value of a Positive Test	6%	40%	86%	98%
False-Positive Rate	94%	60%	14%	2%
Predictive Value of a Negative Test	99%	95%	70%	20%
False-Negative Rate	1%	5%	30%	80%

cleared from the myocardial blood pool rapidly with a half-life of 1 minute, and its uptake by myocardial cells has been demonstrated to correlate highly with coronary blood flow over a wide range of perfusion rates. In the normal individual, after intravenous injection of thallium-201 at peak exercise there is a homogeneous uptake of the radionuclide in the myocardium. However, as coronary flow decreases due to the presence of coronary artery stenoses, the percentage of thallium extracted by myocardial cells decreases in a linear fashion to the extreme point where an area of myocardial scar resulting from a totally occluded coronary artery demonstrates complete absence of thallium uptake.

Experimental evidence suggests that thallium-201 myocardial uptake is dependent on several factors, including myocardial blood flow, vascular permeability, and hypoxia and acidosis, which may impair the sodium–potassium ATPase pump. In addition, others have observed in cell culture that hyperkalemia severely reduces the amount of thallium uptake by viable myocytes. Therefore, in patients with coronary artery disease, myocardial blood flow is limited by fixed coronary artery stenoses, which results in distal hypoxemia, conversion from aerobic to anaerobic metabolism, and the production of localized acidosis and extracellular hyperkalemia, all of which reduce regional myocardial uptake of thallium. The imbalance between myocardial blood flow and myocardial oxygen demand during exercise causes regional ischemia in areas supplied by stenotic coronary arteries, thereby producing regional thallium defects relative to other areas of myocardium that have normal coronary arteries and normal coronary flow characteristics (Fig. 61.2). Three to 4 hours after exercise stress, redistribution or delayed uptake of thallium-201 occurs in the areas that were ischemic during exercise, while those areas that contain no viable myocardium demonstrate persistent absence of thallium-201 activity.

Thallium-201 myocardial scintigraphy is performed in conjunction with exercise electrocardiography. Intravenous injection of the radionuclide is usually performed approximately 60 seconds before the achievement of peak exercise. Peak thallium myocardial activity is achieved approximately 10 minutes after injection and persists for 25 to 30 minutes thereafter. Thus, immediate postexercise myocardial imaging should be performed during this time period and redistribution images should be obtained 3 to 4 hours after stress.

There are several important points that must be considered when performing stress myocardial scintigraphy with thallium-201. First, since myocardial uptake of thallium-201 is proportional to coronary blood flow, it is extremely important that adequate exercise stress (heart rate × blood pressure) is achieved. However, the sensitivity for detecting coronary artery disease is not as dependent on achievement of maximal stress (>85% predicted heart rate) as it is in exercise electrocardiography alone. Second, immediate postexercise myocardial scintigraphy should be completed within 40 minutes of injection of the radionuclide in order to obtain optimal images at peak thallium myocardial activity. Finally, care must be taken in the intravenous injection of thallium-201, since tissue infiltration may significantly affect immediate post-stress and delay-redistribution images. Thus, technically adequate thallium myocardial images require not only proper equipment but also a strong commitment to the precise acquisition of data by properly trained technicians.

A discussion of the several methods available for thallium-201 myocardial imaging is beyond the scope of this chapter. In simple terms these various methods include planar images or tomographic images, either of which can be evaluated in a simple qualitative manner by visual inspection or in a more sophisticated manner using quantitative analysis. This analysis evaluates sequential temporal reduction in myocardial thallium activity that is normalized to peak thallium activity in the immediate postexercise period.[27] When thallium myocardial activity is normalized to peak activity, sequential reduction with time is observed in normal subjects and either no change or an actual accumulation of thallium activity is observed in the patients with myocardial ischemia during exercise.

In a summary of 22 published studies involving more than 2000 patients, Gibson and Beller reported that overall sensitivity and specificity for the stress thallium-201 scintigram was superior to the exercise electrocardiogram for detecting coronary artery disease in patients with chest pain.[20] The sensitivity of stress thallium scintigraphy was 83% compared with 73% for stress electrocardiography and had a specificity of 90% compared with 82% for stress electrocardiography. In the majority of these studies where a simple qualitative analysis of planar thallium distribution was employed, myocardial scintigraphy was found statistically superior to exercise stress electrocardiography. This was especially true in patients with one-vessel coronary artery disease where the sensitivity of stress electrocardiography was particularly low. Work by Madahi and Garcia using quantitative analysis of thallium-201 myocardial activity has demonstrated a similar sensitivity and specificity for detecting coronary artery disease when compared with a simple qualitative analysis. However, detection of multivessel coronary artery disease and the location of coronary artery stenoses was significantly improved with quantitative analysis.[27,28] The best overall sensitivities for detecting significant stenoses in the left anterior descending artery, right coronary artery, and circumflex artery are approximately 85%, 80%, and 65%, respectively. The reasons for the low sensitivity for detection of circumflex artery stenosis at this time are unclear.

Recently, thallium-201 exercise imaging has provided information that correlates with the state of left ventricular contractility. Increased lung activity in the immediate postexercise anterior image has been shown to correlate with exercise-induced elevation of left ventricular filling pressures and appears to be a marker for left ventricular dysfunction. In addition, reversible thallium defects have correlated with improved regional wall motion observed after a postextrasystolic beat during cineventriculography and with improvement in wall motion after coronary artery bypass grafting.[29] In contrast, fixed defects that demonstrate no thallium uptake in the 4-hour delayed image do not demonstrate postextrasystolic potentiation or improvement in regional

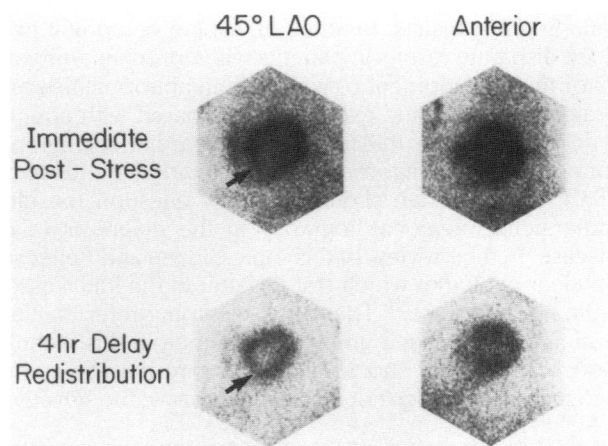

FIGURE 61.2 Unprocessed planar thallium-201 images in the 45° left anterior oblique (LAO) and anterior views taken 10 minutes after exercise (top) and 4 hours later (bottom). The arrows point to a relative decrease in count activity in the inferoapical and septal areas of the immediate post-stress LAO image, which is less apparent on the 4-hour delay redistribution image, thereby indicating ischemia.

wall motion after coronary artery bypass grafting. In summary, thallium-201 myocardial scintigraphy provides markedly improved sensitivity and specificity for the detection of coronary artery disease and superior ability for defining the location and extent of coronary artery stenosis when compared with exercise electrocardiography.

The reliability of any single test for detecting coronary artery disease using a Bayesian analytical approach has important limitations. However, the use of two tests in the same patient improves the reliability of the results because both tests are based on endpoints that are independent of one another. Combined stress electrocardiography and thallium-201 myocardial scintigraphy uses two independent endpoints (electrical events and myocardial distribution of a radionuclide) to identify the physiologic manifestations of myocardial ischemia. The combination of these two tests, therefore, provides enhanced diagnostic information when applied to patients with low, medium, and high probability of coronary artery disease.

When the prevalence of coronary artery disease is extremely low, a negative stress electrocardiogram along with normal myocardial perfusion of thallium-201 radionuclide excludes the presence of significant coronary artery disease as long as adequate stress is obtained. In contrast, if both tests are positive, the likelihood of significant coronary artery disease most likely exceeds 80%. Since exercise thallium-201 scintigraphy has a higher sensitivity and specificity for the detection of coronary artery disease, a normal electrocardiographic response accompanied by an abnormal distribution of thallium-201 would weigh heavily in favor of significant coronary artery disease even in a patient with very low pretest probability. Conversely, when stress electrocardiography is positive and thallium myocardial scintigraphy is negative, the physician may decide that the stress electrocardiogram represents a false-positive result, especially when the patient in question is in a very low probability category for the prevalence of coronary artery disease and adequate stress is achieved.

Those patients with intermediate risk for the presence of coronary artery disease receive the maximal diagnostic benefits from exercise electrocardiography. This effect is enhanced further when both exercise electrocardiography and thallium-201 myocardial scintigraphy are combined; thus, when both tests are abnormal, the diagnosis of significant coronary artery disease can be made with approximately 95% certainty and can be ruled out with the same degree of certainty when both tests are negative. Again, difficulty arises in older patients who may not achieve adequate stress due to "chronotropic insufficiency," impaired functional capacity, or the concomitant use of β-blocker therapy. This results in a low heart rate–blood pressure product and raises a number of diagnostic dilemmas in the interpretation of thallium images due to low coronary flow and inadequate uptake of the radionuclide by the myocardial cells. This results in a thallium image that simulates diffuse three-vessel coronary artery disease with both a diffuse decrease in myocardial thallium activity and an abnormal washout on quantitative analysis. Such a response in a patient who has a high pretest likelihood of disease leaves the physician and patient in an extremely uneasy situation, since significant coronary artery disease cannot be ruled out with a high degree of certainty. At this point further diagnostic tests are needed in order to exclude coronary artery disease. In this circumstance, we recommend coronary arteriography especially in patients whose age, sex, and history of chest pain suggest a greater than 50% prevalence of coronary artery disease.

RADIONUCLIDE ANGIOCARDIOGRAPHY

Radionuclide angiocardiography differs from thallium-201 myocardial imaging in that the radionuclide that is used (technetium-99m) has a shorter half-life (6 hours) and remains exclusively intravascular after injection. The two techniques commonly used employ the first-pass and equilibrium radionuclide angiocardiographic methods. Both techniques have been shown to correlate highly with contrast ventriculography for assessing left ventricular ejection fraction and regional wall motion.

An assessment of left ventricular systolic performance at rest is usually normal in patients who present with various chest pain syndromes for the first time. Radionuclide angiocardiography may identify wall motion abnormalities owing to severe myocardial ischemia or previous myocardial infarction that may not be apparent from the patient's clinical history or resting electrocardiogram. However, depression of left ventricular systolic performance or abnormalities of regional left ventricular wall motion can be seen in other cardiac conditions such as nonischemic cardiomyopathy, valvular heart disease, left bundle branch block, and severe hypertension.

Since radionuclide angiocardiography is limited in the detection of coronary artery disease in patients at rest, it has been used to evaluate left ventricular ejection fraction and regional wall motion in response to graded exercise. A failure to increase the left ventricular ejection fraction by more than five units above the resting value was initially reported to be a marker for significant coronary artery stenosis. However, it is now very clear that evaluation of the left ventricular ejection fraction alone is a nonspecific finding for detection of coronary artery disease and that many subgroups of patients without myocardial ischemia have an abnormal ejection fraction response to exercise. Austin and co-workers reported that the left ventricular ejection fraction frequently does not increase and may actually decrease in women with atypical chest pain and normal coronary arteriography.[30] Port and colleagues have also demonstrated a linear decline of the left ventricular ejection fraction response to exercise with increasing age.[31] In addition, many normal patients with resting left ventricular ejection fraction in the high normal range (>70%) may not demonstrate more than a five-unit increase in ejection fraction at peak exercise.[32] Other studies have reported poor specificity of the left ventricular ejection fraction response to exercise for detecting coronary artery disease.[33,34] In summary, this finding is particularly common with female sex, advanced age, high normal resting ejection fraction, and hypertension.[35]

Therefore, the combination of a deterioration in wall motion in any left ventricular wall segment and failure of the left ventricular ejection fraction to increase more than five units has been used as criteria for detection of coronary artery disease. Gibson and Beller, in a review of seven studies, reported that sensitivity and specificity were approximately 90% when both of these criteria were met.[20] As in thallium myocardial scintigraphy, the sensitivity of this test for detecting coronary artery disease is much improved over stress electrocardiography alone because regional wall motion abnormalities and a decrease in left ventricular ejection fraction with exercise can occur before the onset of symptoms or evidence of ischemic ST segment depression on the electrocardiogram.

Other problems relevant to the application of this technique are conflicting reports concerning the concomitant use of β-blocking drugs during exercise testing. Use of these drugs may preserve a normal exercise response of the left ventricular ejection fraction in patients with coronary artery disease and may blunt a normal ejection fraction response in patients with normal coronary artery anatomy. At this time it appears that the effect of these drugs on the left ventricular ejection fraction response to exercise is quite variable, and patients should be exercised off all β-blocker therapy in order to avoid confounding test results. In addition, supine vs. upright exercise may produce disparate results in patients with coronary artery disease that may favor the development of wall motion abnormalities owing to a higher preload when supine exercise is compared with upright exercise.

Since exercise thallium-201 myocardial scintigraphy can be performed with a similar sensitivity (90%) and a better specificity (90% vs. 80%), the physician should critically question the utility of exercise radionuclide angiocardiography in the diagnosis of coronary artery disease. In their review of this topic Gibson and Beller state that there is no clear choice of which test is better in the initial assessment of ischemic heart disease.[20] These investigators prefer thallium-201 exercise testing owing to their greater experience in this technique. In conclusion, the clinician should also be aware that the combination of the two techniques does not appear to improve the sensitivity or specificity for detecting coronary artery disease by thallium treadmill testing alone and the patient will achieve greater workloads during treadmill exercise than during upright or supine bicycle exercise. All of the above data weigh heavily in favor of thallium treadmill testing as the more specific radionuclide technique for detecting myocardial ischemia.

ECHOCARDIOGRAPHY

Regional dysfunction of left ventricular myocardial segments is an important and common manifestation of ischemic heart disease. The use of echocardiography to evaluate overall left ventricular performance and regional left ventricular wall motion is valuable in the diagnosis of coronary artery disease. Since many cardiac problems other than coronary disease also may present with global depression of left ventricular function, regional left ventricular wall motion abnormalities such as hypokinesis, akinesis, and dyskinesis are more specific findings for the presence of coronary artery disease. In patients who present with signs or symptoms suggestive of ischemic heart disease, the demonstration of such findings would confirm the diagnosis of segmental coronary artery disease with great certainty. However, such findings occur very infrequently on the resting echocardiogram in patients who present with chest pain syndromes and who have no electrocardiographic or historical evidence of myocardial infarction. Both M-mode and two-dimensional echocardiography are widely available to the clinician, and each has significant advantages and disadvantages in the overall assessment of left ventricular performance.

Since M-mode echocardiography provides a high level of temporal resolution of cardiac motion, it can be used to assess valvular function and left ventricular wall motion. An M-mode scan from the apex to the base of the heart in a patient with coronary artery disease is shown in Figure 61.3. The basal portion of the left side of the septum and posterior left ventricular wall contract normally, while septal wall motion becomes akinetic as the M-mode beam approaches the base of the heart. However, this technique, which employs a thin ultrasonic beam and provides a one-chord, one-plane view of the heart, is quite limited by its lack of spatial orientation. Many areas of the left ventricle, including the apex, lateral, and inferior walls, are not accessible to the M-mode echocardiographic examination. Furthermore, this technique is not useful for the accurate estimation of left ventricular volume in patients with segmental myocardial disease because the M-mode calculation of volumes assumes the left ventricle to be a prolate ellipse. In addition, methods that evaluate left ventricular systolic function, such as the percentage change in left ventricular transverse dimension from end-diastole to end-systole, are also inaccurate in the presence of coronary artery disease.

These significant disadvantages of the M-mode echocardiogram for evaluating left ventricular regional wall motion and overall systolic performance are overcome by the two-dimensional echocardiogram, which provides better spatial resolution by employing a wide-angle ultrasonic beam. Thus, this technique allows the visualization of multiple tomographic sections of the heart in the short- and long-axis planes, thereby providing a complete assessment of segmental left ventricular wall motion. In addition, accurate estimates of left ventricular volumes and ejection fraction can be obtained from apical biplane two-dimensional echocardiographic images using a modification of Simpson's rule.[36] Thus, it appears that two-dimensional echocardiography is ideally suited for the evaluation of the patient with ischemic heart disease.

Because left ventricular systolic function and regional wall motion at rest are frequently normal in patients who present with signs or symptoms of ischemic heart disease, exercise two-dimensional echocardiography has been used to detect regional wall motion abnormalities that may occur during various forms of exercise. Two-dimensional echocardiographic measurements can be performed on a beat-to-beat basis; therefore, this method offers significant advantages over equilibrium radionuclide angiocardiography, which summates radionuclide activity over a 2-minute period and, therefore, may not detect these transient changes in segmental wall motion. Furthermore, the commonly used biapical two-dimensional echocardiographic images provide a more extensive assessment of left ventricular regional wall motion than a single-plane left anterior oblique radionuclide angiocardiogram. In addition, studies that employ the first-pass technique for evaluating left ventricular systolic performance during exercise may obtain spurious data since resting studies are often obtained soon after exercise at a time when regional wall motion and left ventricular systolic performance may be improved.[37-39]

Despite the advantages of two-dimensional echocardiography during upright bicycle exercise, a significant limitation of this technique often precluding adequate images during exercise results from movement and respiratory artifacts at high workloads. Nonetheless, we have performed adequate studies in approximately 70% of patients with coronary artery disease and have demonstrated a variable response of the left ventricular ejection fraction from rest to peak exercise with some patients increasing their ejection fraction.[40] This ejection fraction response differs from previous reports and may be a reflection of the

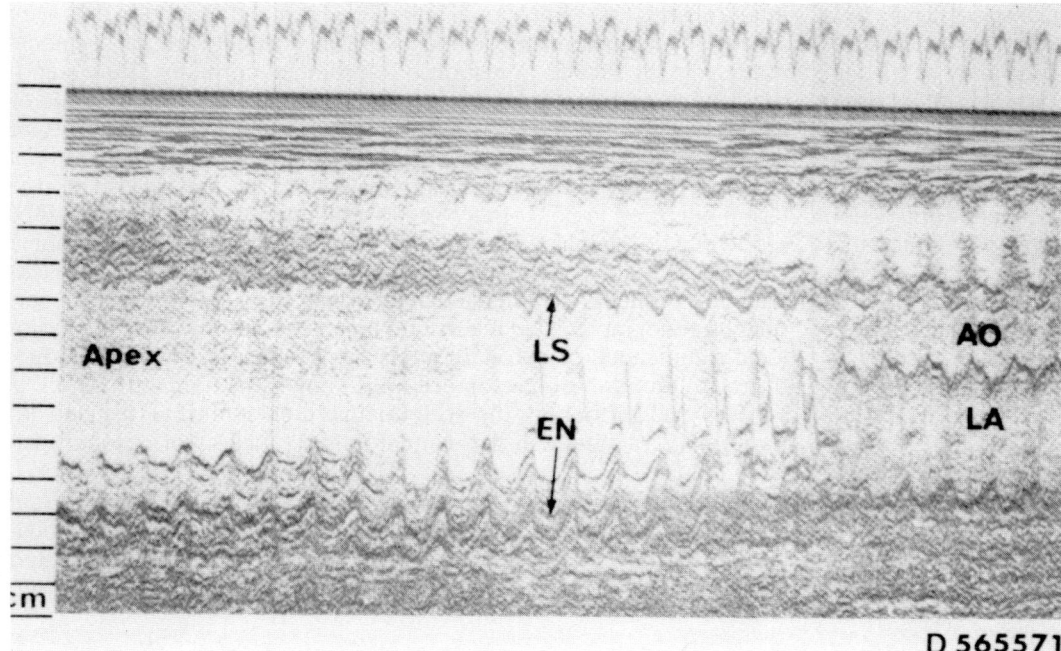

FIGURE 61.3 M-mode echocardiogram that scans the heart from the apex to the base demonstrates normal basal septal motion at the level of the mitral valve. As the ultrasonic beam is directed to the apex, septal motion becomes akinetic. Posterior wall moves normally. (LS, left septum; AO, aorta; LA, left atrium, EN, endocardium) (Dillon, Feigenbaum, Weyman et al: M-mode echocardiography in the evaluation of patients for aneurysmectomy. Circulation 53:657, 1976. By permission of the American Heart Association, Inc)

technical advantages of two-dimensional echocardiography over radionuclide angiocardiography that were discussed in the previous paragraph.

Morganroth and co-workers evaluated left ventricular wall motion at rest and during supine bicycle exercise in normal subjects and in patients with documented coronary artery disease and found a significant incidence of false-negative two-dimensional echocardiographic studies in the patients who had angiographically proven coronary artery disease.[41] This result most likely represents the failure of a single cross-sectional two-dimensional echocardiographic image to evaluate all left ventricular wall segments. Other investigators have evaluated biapical two-dimensional echocardiography at rest and immediately after treadmill exercise in patients who present with various chest pain syndromes. Limacher and Maurer and their associates have reported average sensitivity and specificity of 87% and 90% for detection of angiographically proven coronary artery stenosis.[42,43] This improved accuracy for detecting the presence of coronary artery disease can be attributed to the maximal workload that can be obtained on treadmill exercise and the improved ability of biapical two-dimensional echocardiographic images for evaluation of left ventricular wall motion.

In summary, exercise two-dimensional echocardiography at rest and at peak exercise is mainly a research tool that is reserved only for the very experienced technician. However, comparison of left ventricular wall motion at rest and immediately after treadmill exercise has potential for providing complementary information to exercise treadmill testing. Nonetheless, this enthusiasm must be tempered by the fact that adequate two-dimensional echocardiograms cannot be obtained in all patients and therefore there is significant limitation in its application.

AMBULATORY ELECTROCARDIOGRAPHY

Ambulatory electrocardiography has been successfully used in the detection and treatment of ventricular ectopic activity in patients with specific cardiac disorders. In addition, ST segment elevation during ambulatory electrocardiography in association with chest pain is a very specific indicator of transmural ischemia in patients with variant angina.

There have been reports of transient asymptomatic ST segment depression during daily activity in patients with angiographically documented coronary artery disease.[44,45] All patients met the standard criteria of more than 1 mm horizontal or downsloping ST segment depression that persisted for 0.08 second or longer and was clearly present in at least three consecutive beats in the electrocardiographic recording. It is of interest that in both of these studies diagnostic ST segment depression occurred at heart rates that were markedly lower than exercise-induced ischemia documented on treadmill stress tests. In a prospective analysis of patients with various chest pain syndromes, Crawford and co-workers demonstrated limited specificity of ST segment depression during ambulatory electrocardiographic monitoring in patients without coronary artery disease documented by coronary angiography.[46] This result is not surprising when one considers the problems associated with electrode stability, lead orientation, and variations in the QRS-T complex that may result from changes in position and from the effects of hyperventilation and recent food intake that may produce ST segment depression and thereby simulate myocardial ischemia.

An American Heart Association special report cautions against the interpretation of ST segment shifts as markers for myocardial ischemia in asymptomatic patients on ambulatory electrocardiography.[47] At this time the true sensitivity and specificity of ST segment depression for indicating myocardial ischemia in patients without symptoms on ambulatory electrocardiography are not known. Therefore, additional objective data from exercise treadmill testing or other noninvasive means of detecting coronary artery disease should always be available before attributing asymptomatic ST segment depression to myocardial ischemia during ambulatory electrocardiography.

CORONARY ANGIOGRAPHY

The definitive diagnosis of coronary artery disease can be made only by coronary arteriography. However, the therapeutic and prognostic information that can be gained from this procedure adds more to the proper management of patients than simply confirmation of the presence of coronary artery stenosis. Data from the European Coronary Surgery study showed that there was a significant improvement in survival rate for those patients randomized to surgery who had normal left ventricular function and three-vessel disease and for those patients who had two-vessel disease in which the proximal portion of the left anterior descending artery was involved (reduction in luminal diameter $\geq 75\%$).[48,49] In contrast, the results of the Coronary Artery Surgery study showed no improvement in long-term survival with surgery compared with medical therapy for patients with two- and three-vessel disease and normal ventricular function. However, survival was improved by surgery in those patients with three-vessel disease and reduced left ventricular ejection fraction.[50,51] Finally, all studies indicate that survival is significantly improved by surgical vs. medical therapy in patients with left main coronary artery stenosis.[48-52] As mentioned previously, the extent of physical activity that precipitates angina is inversely correlated with the degree of fixed coronary artery stenosis but not necessarily to the number of coronary arteries with severe obstructive lesions nor to the location of these lesions. Coronary angiography identifies severity, location, and extent of coronary artery disease, and, therefore, a case for cardiac catheterization can be made for all patients with stable angina pectoris, especially those with an early positive electrocardiographic exercise test before or after treatment with β-blocking drugs and/or calcium channel blocking agents.

Coronary arteriography also demonstrates the severity of coronary artery stenosis. In most clinical laboratories, the percent reduction in luminal diameter of the coronary artery is determined by visual inspection of the coronary cineangiogram in two orthogonal planes. The severity and location of stenosis provide valuable information concerning the amount of myocardium at risk in the area distal to the stenosis. However, the physiologic importance of any given stenosis cannot be assumed on the basis of coronary angiography alone, especially when the reduction in luminal diameter is less than 70%. Early methods for validating the angiographic interpretation of coronary stenosis used comparisons with postmortem pathologic studies.[53] Most of these studies concluded that coronary angiography usually underestimates the severity of the lesion. However, such comparisons may not be appropriate because the coronary arteriogram reflects the luminal geometry of a distended vessel whereas most pathologic studies examine the undistended vessel.

Experimental studies have demonstrated that progressive coronary artery obstruction in a normal vessel leads to a gradual diminution of reactive hyperemic response because distal coronary arterial segments are maximally dilated in response to proximal coronary artery stenosis.[54] White and co-workers applied a Doppler velocity flow probe to an epicardial coronary vessel at open heart surgery in order to measure the reactive hyperemic response after 20 seconds of coronary arterial occlusion.[21] They found that underestimation of the severity of the lesion occurred in 95% of the vessels examined with greater than 60% reduction in luminal diameter estimated by coronary arteriography. However, both overestimation and underestimation of lesions with less than 60% reduction in luminal diameter were very common. Thus, coronary arteriography is an inaccurate means of determining the physiologic significance of coronary artery stenosis especially when reductions in luminal diameter are less than 60%. This problem is confounded further by the well-documented interobserver and intraobserver variability in the standard visual analysis of coronary angiograms.

Therefore, although coronary arteriography provides important therapeutic and prognostic information concerning the severity, location, and extent of coronary artery stenosis, the physician is obligated to perform a physiologic assessment of the obstructive lesions before determining subsequent management and therapy when coronary stenosis is in the 60% range. This can be accomplished initially through a comprehensive history that may determine the anginal pattern as stable or unstable. In addition, a highly positive exercise test (greater than 2 mm ST segment depression) that occurs early during exercise with or without hypotension correlates highly with severe obstructive coronary artery disease. Finally, stress thallium-201 myocardial scintigraphy can determine the location and physiologic significance of obstructive coronary artery disease and can be an important adjunct to coronary angiography.

Once the physician has determined that a patient has physiologically significant coronary disease, he has the options of continued medical therapy, coronary angioplasty, or coronary artery bypass grafting. Coronary arteriography provides extremely important information concerning the latter two options. The feasibility of coronary artery bypass grafting is determined by the diameter of the coronary artery distal to the stenosis, and it is generally accepted that diameters in the range of 1.0 mm to 1.3 mm are suitable for grafting. Recent technologic advances in coronary angioplasty have expanded its application to certain patients with two- and three-vessel disease. Coronary arteriography provides important anatomical information that determines the feasibility of coronary angioplasty on the basis of location, contour, amount of calcium deposition, and extent of coronary artery stenoses.

Coronary arteriography also has the potential for detecting dynamic forms of obstruction due to alteration in vasomotion superimposed on either normal coronary arteries and/or those with coronary atherosclerosis. Ergonovine maleate, an ergot alkaloid and α-adrenergic agonist with a direct constrictive effect on vascular smooth muscle, has been used to induce coronary artery spasm in the patient in the coronary care unit or preferably in the catheterization laboratory. This provocative test is highly sensitive for producing coronary artery spasm in patients with variant (Prinzmetal's) angina in the absence of concomitant nitrate or calcium antagonist therapy. However, it has been our experience and that of others[55] that in the setting of normal coronary arteries the incidence of a positive provocative test is extremely low. Studies that review the experience of ergonovine in large numbers of patients demonstrate that a positive test is highly unlikely in patients who have exertional chest pain, both exertional and rest pain, and an absence of ST segment elevation, ST segment depression, or T wave changes during episodes of chest pain.[55,56] In addition, variant angina has been reported to be extremely uncommon in patients with valvular

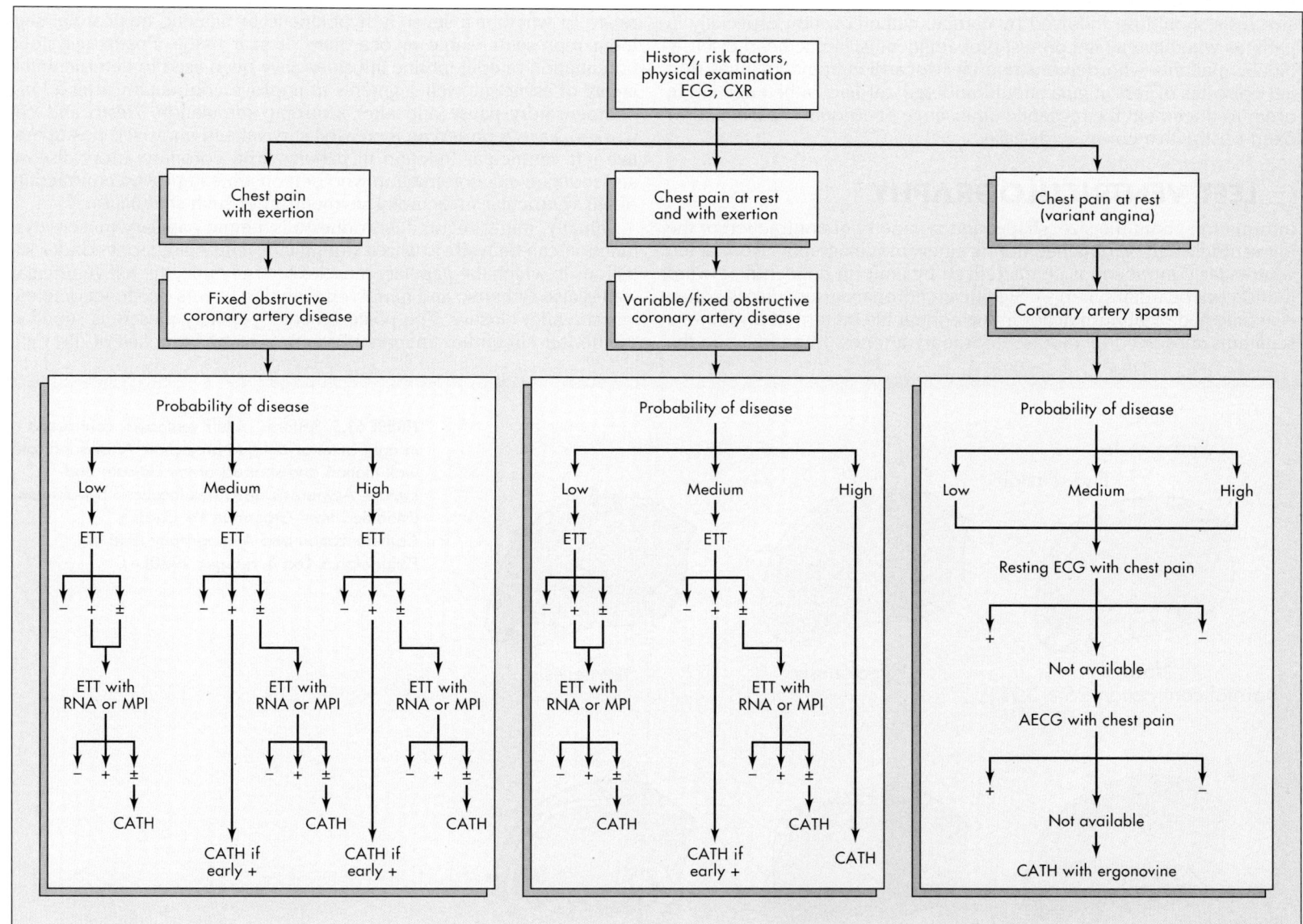

FIGURE 61.4 Indications for cardiac catheterization. (*ETT*, exercise tolerance test; −, absence of chest pain, MPI, RNA, or ST segment changes consistent with ischemia; +, presence of chest pain, MPI, RNA, or ST segment changes consistent with ischemia; ±, equivocal results; *RNA*, radionuclide angiocardiography; *MPI*, myocardial perfusion imaging with thallium-201; *CATH*, cardiac catheterization; *AECG*, ambulatory electrocardiography; *Early +*, Bruce ETT with chest pain and ST segment changes consistent with ischemia at less than 6 minutes.)

heart disease and various nonischemic cardiomyopathies. Ergonovine provocation is most frequently positive in patients who demonstrate angina at rest, a recent myocardial infarction, and insignificant coronary artery stenosis. Finally, it was concluded that when a patient presents with unexplained rest angina, coronary artery spasm could be safely ruled out if there are no electrocardiographic changes during episodes of pain; and although rest angina was a highly sensitive finding in patients with variant angina, it was very nonspecific.

In summary, because of the prognostic, physiologic, and therapeutic information that can be obtained from coronary arteriography we believe that the indications for this test go far beyond a simple diagnosis that rules in the presence of either fixed or variably obstructed coronary artery disease. Nonetheless, it may not always be clearly indicated when a patient with chest pain should undergo cardiac catheterization (Fig. 61.4). However, noninvasive testing, as outlined in previous sections, may identify patients at risk for the following: left main coronary artery stenosis due to an early positive exercise tolerance test with hypotension, severe three-vessel coronary disease demonstrated by exercise thallium-201 myocardial scintigraphy, and left ventricular dysfunction manifested by radionuclide angiography or two-dimensional echocardiography. Definitive information concerning coronary anatomy and left ventricular function in such patients is necessary before one can recommend bypass surgery rather than medical therapy in order to improve survival. Conversely, equivocal results on noninvasive tests should be followed by cardiac catheterization especially in patients who have a high pretest probability of ischemic heart disease. Finally, patients who demonstrate electrocardiographic changes during episodes of rest angina should undergo cardiac catheterization in order to document the presence or absence of coronary spasm and/or fixed obstructive coronary disease.

LEFT VENTRICULOGRAPHY

Information about the size, shape, and symmetry of contraction of the left ventricle can be obtained during cineventriculography. Normal left ventricular contraction is characterized by uniform concentric inward motion (myocardial synergy). Significant coronary artery disease often is manifested by abnormalities in the contractile pattern of myocardial segments subserved by diseased coronary arteries. Depending on the degree of motion impairment, each segment may be described as hypokinetic, akinetic, dyskinetic, or aneurysmal (Fig. 61.5). These wall motion abnormalities are most commonly found in patients with previous myocardial infarction but can occasionally be found in patients with angina and no history of myocardial infarction.

In addition to an assessment of the contractile patterns of left ventricular myocardial segments, one may also obtain information concerning overall left ventricular function through a calculation of the left ventricular ejection fraction (end-diastolic volume − end-systolic volume/end-diastolic volume) in a single-plane, right anterior oblique view. However, Cohn and co-workers have shown that biplane cineventriculography produces more accurate estimates of left ventricular volume and ejection fraction in patients with coronary artery disease.[57] For example, a single-plane, right anterior oblique projection may produce a spuriously low left ventricular ejection fraction in the presence of a proximal left anterior descending artery occlusion in which the majority of the anterior wall and apex may be rendered akinetic. When a left anterior oblique view is included, a normally contracting posterior wall significantly improves the calculation of ejection fraction. Therefore, left ventricular wall motion and systolic performance should be evaluated in two orthogonal views using biplane cineventriculography in order to obtain an accurate assessment of overall left ventricular performance in patients with coronary artery disease.

Other questions may be answered during cineventriculography that relate to whether a severely hypokinetic or akinetic myocardial segment represents viable myocardium or scar tissue. Postextrasystolic potentiation or epinephrine infusions have been used to determine the ability of asynergic wall segments to improve contractility after a long compensatory pause and after inotropic stimulation. Nesto and co-workers have reported an increased survival and improved postoperative left ventricular function in patients with coronary artery disease and reduced ejection fraction who demonstrate improved contractility of left ventricular myocardial segments after such stimulation.[58]

Finally, mitral regurgitation due to ischemic papillary muscle dysfunction can be well visualized during cineventriculography. Under situations in which the papillary muscles are ischemic, the left ventricular wall is also ischemic and mitral regurgitation occurs due to incomplete mitral leaflet closure. The posteromedial papillary muscle is supplied by the left circumflex marginal branches or by branches of the right

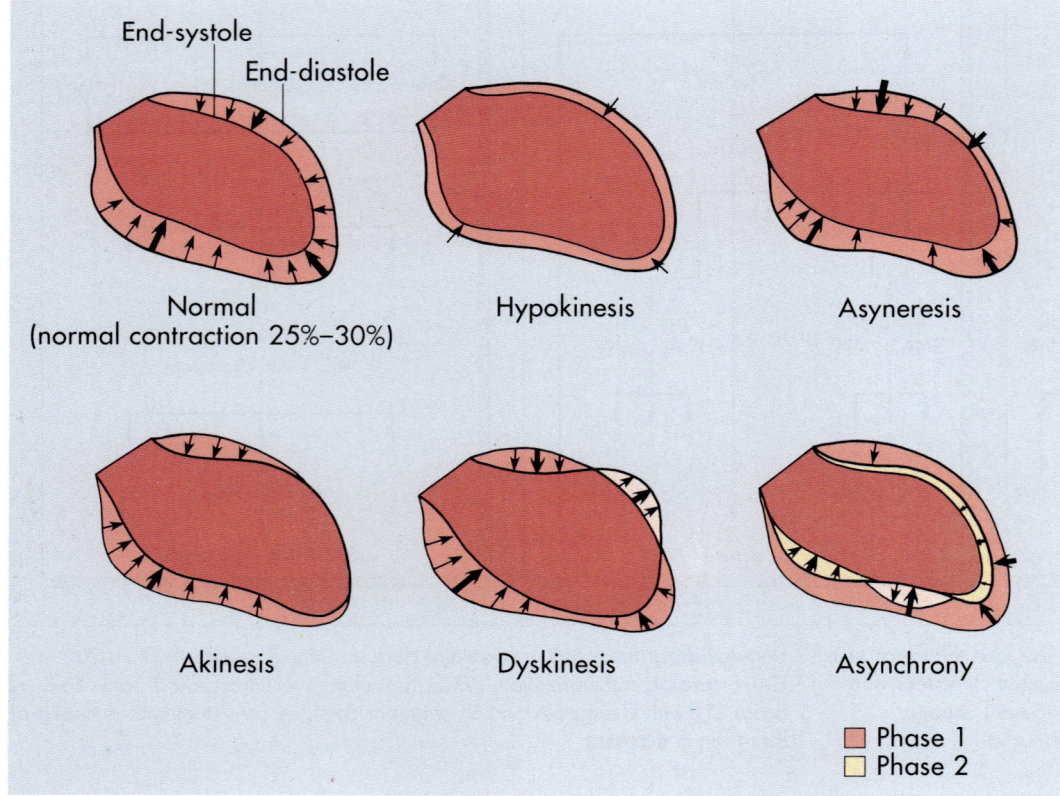

FIGURE 61.5 Patterns of left ventricular contraction in right anterior oblique projection. Arrows indicate wall motion and shaded areas indicate end-systole. Asyneresis describes localized hypokinesis. (Modified from Grossman W: Cardiac Catheterization and Angiography (2nd ed). Philadelphia, Lea & Febiger, 1980)

coronary artery distal to the posterolateral wall. The anterolateral papillary muscle receives blood mainly from the diagonal branches of the left anterior descending artery. Mild to moderate mitral regurgitation may occur in the presence of occlusion of these vessels or during an acute ischemic episode brought on by exertion or by isometric hand grip exercise.

REFERENCES

1. Heberden W: Some account of a disorder of the breast. Med Trans R Coll Phys Lond 2:59, 1786
2. Foreman RD, Ohata CA: Effects of coronary artery occlusion on thoracic spinal neurons receiving viscerosomatic inputs. Am J Physiol 238:H667, 1980
3. Bing RJ: Cardiac metabolism. Physiol Rev 45:2, 1965
4. Braunwald E, Sobel BE: Coronary blood flow and myocardial ischemia. In Braunwald E (ed): Heart Disease, p 1235. Philadelphia, WB Saunders, 1984
5. Hillis LD, Braunwald E: Coronary artery spasm. N Engl J Med, 299:695, 1978
6. Kannel WB, Castelli WP, Gordon T et al: Serum cholesterol, lipoproteins and the risk of coronary heart disease: The Framingham Study. Ann Intern Med 74:1, 1971
7. Kannel WB, McGee D, Gordon T: A general cardiovascular risk profile: The Framingham Study. Am J Cardiol 38:46, 1976
8. Gotto AM, Bierman EL, Connor WE et al: Recommendations for treatment of hyperlipidemia in adults: A joint statement of the Nutrition Committee and the Council on Arteriosclerosis. Circulation 69:1065A, 1984
9. Michelson EL, Morganroth J, Nichols CW et al: Retinal arteriolar changes as an indicator of coronary artery disease. Arch Intern Med 139:1139, 1979
10. Dell'Italia LJ, Starling MR, O'Rourke RA: Physical examination for exclusion of hemodynamically important right ventricular infarction. Ann Intern Med 99:608, 1983
11. Eilen SD, Crawford MH, O'Rourke RA: Accuracy of precordial palpation for detecting increased left ventricular volume. Ann Intern Med 99:628, 1983
12. Hill JC, O'Rourke RA, Lewis RP et al: The diagnostic value of the atrial gallop in acute myocardial infarction. Am Heart J 78:194, 1969
13. Steelman RB, White RS, Hill JC et al: Mid-systolic clicks arteriosclerotic heart disease: A new facet in the clinical syndrome of papillary muscle dysfunction. Circulation 44:503, 1971
14. Margolis JR, Chen JTT, Kong Y et al: The diagnostic and prognostic significance of coronary artery calcification: A report of 800 cases. Radiology 137:609, 1980
15. Rifkin RD: Coronary calcification: A neglected clue to coronary artery disease. J Cardiovasc Med 5:343, 1980
16. Goldberger AL: Myocardial infarction: Electrocardiographic Differential Diagnosis, 3rd ed, p 303. St. Louis, CV Mosby, 1984
17. Blackburn H, Taylor HL, Hamrell B et al: Premature ventricular complexes induced by stress testing. Am J Cardiol 31:441, 1973
18. Udall JA, Ellestad MH: Predictive implications of ventricular premature contractions associated with treadmill exercise testing. Circulation 56:985, 1977
19. Koppes G, McKiernan T, Bassan M et al: Treadmill exercise testing: II. Curr Prob Cardiol 7:1, 1977
20. Gibson RS, Beller GA: Should exercise electrocardiographic testing be replaced by radioisotope methods? In Rahimtoola SH (ed): Controversies in Cardiology, pp 1–31. Philadelphia, FA Davis, 1983
21. White CW, Wright CB, Doty DB et al: Does visual interpretation of the coronary arteriogram predict the physiologic importance of coronary stenosis? N Engl J Med 310:819, 1984
22. Galen RS: The predictive value of laboratory test. Am J Cardiol 36:536, 1975
23. Froelicher VF, Yanowitz FG, Thompson AJ: Correlation of coronary angiography and the electrocardiographic response to maximal treadmill testing in 76 asymptomatic men. Circulation 48:597, 1973
24. Borer JS, Brensike JF, Redwood DR et al: Limitations of the electrocardiographic response to exercise in predicting coronary artery disease. N Engl J Med 293:367, 1975
25. Cohn PF, Brown EJ, Cohn JK: Detection and management of coronary artery disease in the asymptomatic population. Am Heart J 108:1064, 1984
26. Giagnoni E, Secchi MB, Wu SC et al: Prognostic value of exercise EKG testing in asymptomatic normotensive subjects: A prospective matched study. N Engl J Med 309:1085, 1983
27. Garcia E, Madahi J, Berman D et al: Space/time quantitation of thallium-201 myocardial scintigraphy. J Nucl Med 22:309, 1981
28. Madahi J: Improved noninvasive assessment of coronary artery disease by quantitative analysis of regional stress myocardial distribution and washout of thallium-201. Circulation 64:924, 1981
29. Rozanski A, Berman DS, Gray R et al: Use of thallium-201 redistribution scintigraphy in the preoperative differentiation of reversible and nonreversible myocardial asynergy. Circulation 64:936, 1981
30. Austin EH, Cobb FR, Coleman E et al: Prospective evaluation of radionuclide angiocardiography for the diagnosis of coronary artery disease. Am J Cardiol 50:1212, 1982
31. Port S, Cobb FR, Coleman RE et al: Effect of age on the response of the left ventricular ejection fraction to exercise. N Engl J Med 303:1133, 1980
32. Gibbons RJ, Lee KL, Cobb F et al: Ejection fraction response to exercise in patients with chest pain and normal coronary arteriograms. Circulation 64:952, 1981
33. Osbakken MD, Boucher CA, Okada RD et al: Spectrum of global left ventricular responses to supine exercise: Limitation in the use of ejection fraction in identifying patients with coronary artery disease. Am J Cardiol 51:28, 1983
34. Rozanski A, Diamond GA, Berman D et al: The declining specificity of exercise radionuclide ventriculography. N Engl J Med 309:518, 1983
35. Wasserman AG, Katz RJ, Varghese PJ et al: Exercise radionuclide ventriculographic responses in hypertensive patients with chest pain. N Engl J Med 311:1276, 1984
36. Starling MR, Crawford MH, Sorensen SG et al: Comparative accuracy of apical biplane cross-sectional echocardiography and gated equilibrium radionuclide angiography for estimating left ventricular size and performance. Circulation 63:1075, 1981
37. Dell'Italia LJ, Amon KW, Crawford MH: Two-dimensional echo detection of improved wall motion and left ventricular function immediately after exercise in early post myocardial infarction patients (abstr). J Am Coll Cardiol 3:613, 1984
38. Rozanski A, Berman D, Gray R et al: Preoperative prediction of reversible myocardial asynergy by postexercise radionuclide ventriculography. N Engl J Med 307:212, 1982
39. Rozanski A, Elkayam U, Berman DS et al: Improvement of resting myocardial asynergy with cessation of upright bicycle exercise. Circulation 67:529, 1983
40. Crawford MH, Amon KW, Vance WS: Exercise 2-dimensional echocardiography: Quantitation of left ventricular performance in patients with severe angina pectoris. Am J Cardiol 51:1, 1983
41. Morganroth J, Chen CC, David D et al: Exercise cross-sectional echocardiographic diagnosis of coronary artery disease. Am J Cardiol 47:20, 1981
42. Limacher MC, Quinones MA, Poliner LR et al: Detection of coronary artery disease with exercise two-dimensional echocardiography: Description of a clinically applicable method and comparison with radionuclide ventriculography. Circulation 67:1211, 1983
43. Maurer G, Nanda NC: Two-dimensional echocardiographic evaluation of exercise-induced left and right ventricular asynergy: Correlation with thallium scanning. Am J Cardiol 48:720, 1981
44. Deanfield JE, Selwyn AP, Chierchia S et al: Myocardial ischaemia during daily life in patients with stable angina: Its relation to symptoms and heart rate changes. Lancet 2:753, 1983
45. Schang SJ, Pepine CJ: Transient asymptomatic ST segment depression during daily activity. Am J Cardiol 39:396, 1977
46. Crawford MH, Mendoza CA, O'Rourke RA et al: Limitations of continuous ambulatory electrocardiogram monitoring for detecting coronary artery disease. Ann Intern Med 89:1, 1978
47. Sheffield LT, Berson A, Bragg-Remschel D et al: Recommendations for standards of instrumentation and practice in the use of ambulatory electrocardiography. Circulation 71:626A, 1985
48. European Coronary Surgery Study Group: Long-term results of prospective randomized study of coronary artery bypass surgery in stable angina pectoris. Lancet 2:1173, 1982
49. European Coronary Surgery Study Group: Prospective randomized study of coronary artery bypass surgery in stable angina pectoris: A progress report on survival. Circulation 65:11, 1982
50. CASS Principal Investigators and their associates: Coronary Artery Surgery Study (CASS): A randomized trial of coronary artery bypass surgery: Survival data. Circulation 68:939, 1983
51. CASS Principal Investigators and their associates: Coronary Artery Surgery Study (CASS): A randomized trial of coronary artery bypass surgery: Quality of life in patients randomly assigned to treatment groups. Circulation 68:951, 1983
52. Takaro T, Hultgren H, Lipton M et al: VA Cooperative Randomized Study for coronary arterial occlusive disease: II. Left main artery disease. Circulation (Suppl III) 54:107, 1976
53. Arnett EN, Isner JM, Redwood DR et al: Coronary artery narrowing in coronary heart disease: Comparison of cineangiographic and necropsy findings. Ann Intern Med 91:350, 1979
54. Gould KL, Lipscomb K, Hamilton GW: Physiologic basis for assessing critical coronary stenosis: Instantaneous flow response and regional distribution during coronary hyperemia as measures of coronary flow reserve. Am J Cardiol 33:87, 1974
55. Carabello BA, Gash AK: Provocative ergonovine testing in patients without obstructive coronary disease. Cathet Cardiovasc Diagn 9:261, 1983
56. Bertrand ME, LaBlanche JM, Tilmant PY et al: Frequency of provoked coronary arterial spasm in 1089 consecutive patients undergoing coronary arteriography. Circulation 65:1299, 1982
57. Cohn PF, Gorlin R, Adams DF et al: Comparison of biplane and single plane left ventriculograms in patients with coronary artery disease. Am J Cardiol 33:1, 1974
58. Nesto RW, Cohn LH, Collins JJ et al: Inotropic contractile reserve: A useful predictor of increased 5 year survival and improved postoperative left ventricular function in patients with coronary artery disease and reduced ejection fraction. Am J Cardiol 50:39, 1982

STABLE ANGINA PECTORIS
Joel S. Karliner

There is a disorder of the breast, marked with strong and peculiar symptoms, considerable for the kind of danger belonging to it, and not extremely rare, of which I do not recollect any mention among medical authors. The seat of it, and sense of strangling and anxiety with which it is attended may make it not improperly be called Angina pectoris.

Those who are afflicted with it, are seized, while they are walking, and more particularly when they walk soon after eating, with a painful and most disagreeable sensation in the breast, which seems as if it would take their life away, if it were to increase or to continue: The moment they stand still, all this uneasiness vanishes. In all other respects the patients are at the beginning of this disorder perfectly well, and in particular have no shortness of breath, from which it is totally different.

The os sterni is usually pointed to as the seat of this malady, but it seems sometimes as if it was under the lower part of it, and at other times under the middle or upper part, but always inclining more to the left side, and sometimes there is joined with it a pain about the middle of the left arm. What the particular mischief is, which is referred to these different parts of the sternum, it is not easy to guess, and I have had no opportunity of knowing with certainty. It may be a strong cramp, or an ulcer, or possibly both.[1]

This classic description identifies many of the key elements in the clinical syndrome of angina pectoris. We shall turn first to a discussion of the pathogenesis of this disorder.

PATHOGENESIS
PATHOLOGY

In most instances, classic angina pectoris produced by exertion and relieved by rest is the result of atherosclerotic obstruction of the coronary arterial tree. Several anatomical sites of obstruction are possible: the major coronary arterial trunks and their epicardial branches, the coronary ostia at the aorta, and the small vessels that are located intramyocardially.[2] However, the most common sites by far are the major coronary arterial trunks and their epicardial branches.

Postmortem coronary angiographic studies and dissections of hearts of young individuals raised in the United States demonstrate that 45% have some evidence of atherosclerosis and 5% have gross evidence of severe coronary atherosclerosis.[3] Since the clinical manifestations of symptomatic heart disease usually occur in middle or later life, it seems evident that the process of atherosclerotic obstruction of the epicardial coronary arteries, at least in its early stages, is a relatively slow one, but numerous instances of rapid progression in symptomatic patients have also been documented. Necropsy studies indicate that clinically isolated, severe angina pectoris can be associated with advanced, diffuse luminal narrowing but with relatively little myocardial damage.[4] However, severe disease also can be present in the absence of symptoms or with only minimal symptoms. Clinically, hypertension is commonly associated with atherosclerotic obstruction of the large epicardial coronary vessels.

Coronary ostial narrowing results from various diseases of the aorta, including atherosclerosis, dissecting and saccular aneurysm, aortitis, calcification of the aorta in proximity to the origin of a coronary artery, and following radiation therapy. Diseases of the small coronary arteries are usually not associated with angina pectoris. Where such abnormalities can be demonstrated they tend to occur in the presence of a cardiomyopathy, either idiopathic or associated with heritable neuromuscular or musculoskeletal disease, such as Duchenne's muscular dystrophy or Friedreich's ataxia.[5] Vascular inflammation or infiltration of the small coronary arteries also occurs in diseases such as lupus erythematosus, rheumatoid arthritis, and amyloidosis. Small and medium-sized coronary arteries may also be involved in polyarteritis nodosa. Small-vessel coronary artery disease in patients with systemic sclerosis is associated with myocardial perfusion abnormalities, but angina pectoris is an uncommon complaint. Thrombotic microcirculatory cardiac lesions also occur in thrombotic thrombocytopenic purpura.

PHYSIOLOGIC CONSIDERATIONS
DETERMINANTS OF MYOCARDIAL OXYGEN DEMAND

Among the most important of the physiologic factors that determine the heart's demands for oxygen are the heart size, the left ventricular systolic pressure, the heart rate, and the level of myocardial inotropic state.[6] Both heart size and left ventricular pressure are important determinants of myocardial wall tension, which in turn is probably the major influence on myocardial oxygen demand. Although resting cardiac size has been conventionally related to preload and left ventricular pressure to "afterload" on the myocardium, these two measures, according to the law of Laplace, are directly related to left ventricular wall tension and hence to myocardial oxygen demand. The law of Laplace, a formula for thin-walled shells, states that wall force, or tension, is directly related to the product of intracavitary pressure and radius; in addition, myocardial wall stress usually is considered to be inversely related to ventricular wall thickness. Thus, an increased preload at a given level of left ventricular systolic pressure will augment wall tension, while a decline in preload will decrease wall tension. Conversely, an increase in afterload at any level of end-diastolic dimension or volume will raise wall tension and a decrease will diminish it. These considerations become particularly important when assessing the value of organic nitrates and blood pressure control in patients with angina pectoris.

The heart rate exerts an independent influence on myocardial oxygen requirements, tachycardia causing an increase and bradycardia a decrease. An increase in heart rate may also be associated with increased contractility. Drugs that affect the inotropic state of the left ventricle also alter myocardial oxygen demand, with agents that increase the inotropic state augmenting demand and drugs that decrease it diminishing demand. According to these considerations any therapeutic intervention that reduces heart size, left ventricular pressure, heart rate, and inotropic state will tend to decrease myocardial oxygen demand and hence should prevent or improve angina.

Many patients with chronic ischemic heart disease, especially those who have sustained a previous myocardial infarction, have abnormal left ventricular wall motion. The extent and severity of segmental wall motion abnormalities after myocardial infarction tend to correlate with reduced left ventricular performance. Thus, improvement in left ventricular asynergy produced by agents that ameliorate angina pectoris should benefit left ventricular performance, while worsening of asynergy could exacerbate angina. The latter is an important theoretic consideration for drugs that also tend to depress left ventricular performance, such as β-adrenergic antagonists and calcium channel blockers.

DETERMINANTS OF MYOCARDIAL OXYGEN SUPPLY

Under ordinary circumstances increases in myocardial oxygen demand, influenced by the factors discussed previously, are met by an appropriate increase in myocardial oxygen supply. However, in patients with coronary artery disease this is frequently not the case and the syndrome of angina pectoris ensues. The amount of oxygen used by the heart is directly related to coronary blood flow, the oxygen content of arterial blood and the amount of oxygen extracted from the blood by the heart. Of these two considerations only the first is of practical importance since the oxygen-carrying capacity of the blood cannot be significantly increased unless considerable hypoxemia is present. Furthermore, the heart extracts a high and relatively fixed amount of oxygen from the blood flowing through the coronary circulation. Therefore augmentation of coronary flow is the only practical mechanism by which increased metabolic demands can be met.

Coronary blood flow is markedly diminished during systole because the vascular tree is compressed by the myocardium. However, this phenomenon is not of major significance in the epicardial arteries, which extend primarily over the surface of the heart, as compared with the subendocardial vessels, which are compressed during systole. As a result of this compression systolic flow through these vessels is substantially reduced and aortic diastolic pressure becomes a major influence on coronary blood flow. Indeed, in the presence of hypotension and frank cardiogenic shock, aortic diastolic pressure is probably the major determinant of coronary flow. However, under ordinary circumstances the absolute level of aortic diastolic pressure is not the sole hemodynamic determinant responsible for driving blood through the coronary circulation. Because the coronary vessels are exposed to intramyocardial pressure during diastole as well as systole, it is clear that the net driving force responsible for maintaining coronary flow during diastole must be the difference between aortic diastolic pressure and intramyocardial diastolic pressure (the so-called transmural pressure). The latter is related to left ventricular diastolic pressure, and when this measure is elevated, as may occur during the episodes of angina pectoris, there may be significant diminution of subendocardial blood flow. This may be one of the reasons that lowering the left ventricular filling pressure may result in improvement of angina pectoris. It is also clear that a decrease in cardiac size will also reduce myocardial wall tension, thereby diminishing myocardial oxygen demand. Thus, appropriate treatment of angina pectoris should reduce demand while at the same time increasing supply.

LEFT VENTRICULAR DYSFUNCTION

Many patients with chronic ischemic heart disease complain of exertional dyspnea, often without chest pain.[7] This symptom could result from two possible mechanisms singly or in combination: (1) a reduction in cardiac output associated with a decline in ejection fraction and (2) an increase in left ventricular diastolic pressure associated with an increased heart rate. Thus, acute ischemia may lead to sufficient left ventricular dysfunction to produce symptoms of breathlessness, either with exertion or sometimes even at rest. Alterations in left ventricular diastolic pressure may result from changes in the diastolic properties of the myocardium or a shift in the diastolic pressure–volume curve that occurs with myocardial ischemia. This increase in diastolic pressure presumably is transmitted in a retrograde manner to the pulmonary capillaries, resulting in the symptom of dyspnea.

It is of course necessary to be aware of conditions that may be mistaken for dyspnea associated with ischemic heart disease. Many pathologic processes that cause breathlessness may produce such confusion. Among these are conditions that are not uncommon in patients with coronary heart disease, such as obesity, chronic obstructive pulmonary disease (which may lead to right-sided heart failure), hypothyroidism (which may be associated with pericardial effusion), and cirrhosis of the liver with ascites. Rarer afflictions include the nephrotic syndrome, vena caval obstruction, and severe nutritional deficiency with hypoproteinemia. These conditions may mimic congestive symptoms due to ischemic heart disease and should be excluded prior to initiating treatment.

METABOLIC ALTERATIONS

Studies in humans have indicated that myocardial blood flow is heterogeneous in patients with coronary artery disease, even at rest. This decrease in blood flow has generally been seen in the distribution of significantly obstructed coronary arteries. Radioisotope studies indicate that in patients with coronary disease studied at rest without clinical evidence of ischemia, lactic acid is released or produced by the myocardium even though chemical lactic acid studies show extraction.[8] The amount of lactic acid released appears to be related to the severity of the coronary artery disease. Such observations may explain, at least in part, the phenomenon of silent ischemia.

CORONARY VASOMOTION, COLLATERAL CIRCULATION, AND VASODILATOR RESERVE

In his second Lumleian lecture in 1910, Sir William Osler stated:

> Spasm or narrowing of the coronary artery, or even of one branch, may so modify the action of a section of the heart that it works with disturbed tension, and there are stretching and straining sufficient to arouse painful sensations. Or the heart may be in the same state as the leg muscles of a man with intermittent claudication, working smoothly when quiet, but instantly an effort is made, or a wave of emotion touches peripheral vessels, anything which heightens pressure and disturbs the normal contractions, brings on a crisis of pain. I do not know of any better explanation of anginal pain.[9]

This explanation of ischemia was disregarded for approximately 60 years, but evidence accumulated in the past 15 years has indicated that coronary vasomotion may indeed play an important role in the pathogenesis of ischemic chest pain and even of myocardial infarction in many patients.[10] There is now abundant evidence that the coronary arteries are not passive conduits for blood but exhibit active vasomotion under a variety of stimuli. These include catecholamines, prostaglandins, adenosine, histamine, calcium, serotonin, and cholinergic agonists. Even in the presence of advanced coronary arterial obstruction, the coronary vessels may show vasomotor activity.[11]

Under usual circumstances, the coronary vascular tree exhibits the phenomenon of autoregulation.[12] The large epicardial arteries act as conductance vessels while the intramyocardial arterioles act as resistance vessels because of their small diameter and well-developed media, which have the capacity to alter profoundly the resistance to coronary flow. Presumably, the resistance vessels dynamically alter their intrinsic tone in response to the heart's demands for oxygen. As a result, the delivery of oxygen and the demand for oxygen are tightly coupled. In the presence of fixed proximal obstruction in a large vessel, the resistance produced by such a narrowing becomes critical to flow once the vasodilator reserve capacity of the small vessels is reached.

However, this concept of autoregulation in the presence of fixed obstruction does not entirely explain a number of phenomena, including varying anginal threshold throughout the day and the occurrence of rest pain. The clear demonstration of coronary vasomotion has led to two important concepts: (1) that a primary decrease in coronary blood flow may occur as a result of excessive or abnormal vasomotion in a large epicardial artery and (2) that relatively modest degrees of vasoconstriction may induce ischemic chest pain in the presence of a coronary atherosclerotic lesion, while vasodilation tends to relieve pain. Such vasomotion tends to occur in the blood vessel immediately adjacent to an area of fixed obstruction, and the evolving concept of dynamic obstruction of coronary vessels has led to a better understanding of the pathophysiology of ischemic chest pain. Thus, in a vessel that has only mild to moderate coronary arterial obstruction, a modest amount of additional constriction produced by coronary vasomotion can lead to critical obstruction. Therapy directed at such vasomotion can produce dilatation either in the area of a critical obstruction or it can prevent the obstruction from becoming critical.

One anatomical factor potentially modifying both the fixed obstruction and alterations in coronary vasomotion is the functional importance of the coronary collateral circulation.[13] Thus it appears that the presence of adequate collateral vessels can significantly reduce the magnitude of exercise-induced ischemic left ventricular dysfunction in areas supplied by stenotic coronary arteries. However, there is little information regarding the ways in which such coronary arterial collateral circulation can be stimulated, nor is it possible to predict which patients have adequate collateral circulation on clinical grounds alone.

In addition to fixed coronary arterial obstruction and excessive coronary vasomotion, a third factor must also be considered in the pathogenesis of ischemic chest pain in some patients, particularly those with systemic arterial hypertension, those with left ventricular hypertrophy, and certain individuals with atypical chest pain. This phenomenon has been termed *reduced vasodilator reserve* and is thought to be particularly important in the small coronary vessels.[14,15] It is hypothesized that some patients have inappropriate coronary arteriolar or small coronary artery constriction that cannot be identified by standard angiographic assessment, since the vessels are too small to be visualized by angiography. Although measurements of coronary flow reserve using currently available techniques should be viewed with caution,[12] this concept may explain at least some instances of either atypical chest pain or of angina pectoris in patients with normal large coronary vessels in whom abnormal vasomotion cannot be demonstrated.

OTHER FACTORS

Finally, there are a variety of vascular factors that may play a role in the pathogenesis of myocardial ischemia. Among these are myocardial compression due to so-called muscle bridges; the phenomenon of coronary steal, in which a low resistance vessel siphons blood flow from the territory supplied by an obstructed vessel that has a high resistance to flow; and the intriguing observation that coronary vascular reserve is reduced in chronic smokers who have morphologically normal coronary vessels.[16]

CLINICAL RECOGNITION

The classic description of Heberden quoted at the beginning of this chapter contains nearly all the elements required for the clinical recognition of angina pectoris. We shall now consider the nature and differential diagnosis of precordial discomfort, the hallmark of angina pectoris.

Pain in the chest may arise from a variety of structures, including the heart, adjacent tissues such as the pericardium, and other thoracic structures such as the lungs and the pleura. Abnormalities of the great vessels may be a cause of chest pain as may other mediastinal structures such as the esophagus and those just below such as the stomach and gallbladder. Nonvascular neuromuscular disorders may also be a cause of chest pain. Thus, the astute physician will recognize that even a usually reliable patient may not provide a diagnostic history. Nevertheless, the history is the single most important feature in the evaluation of the nature and genesis of precordial discomfort. It is to the history that we must always turn before proceeding with diagnostic tests. A careful analysis of factors that precipitate chest pain is of critical importance since those characteristics are usually more specific than the intensity or character of the pain.

A literal definition of angina pectoris is "pain in the chest," but by common usage angina pectoris refers to precordial discomfort that is thought to be of cardiac origin. As Heberden noted, chest pain associated with coronary artery disease classically is produced by exertion and relieved by rest. Patients frequently describe the discomfort as a burning, pressing, tingling, heavy, or squeezing sensation. If it is severe, the patient may spontaneously clench his fist over the middle of the chest (positive Levine sign). The pain may radiate to the shoulders, neck, jaws, or arms. Usually the left arm or hand rather than the right is involved in such radiation. However, radiation is inconstant, and although extensive radiation has been associated with increased severity of coronary artery disease this is by no means always the case. Some patients never complain of chest pain or discomfort but only of shoulder, neck, jaw, or arm pain.

The pathogenesis of cardiac pain is uncertain, and the precise pathways are not well defined. Afferent fibers running in the cardiac sympathetic nerves are considered to be the major pathways for the transmission of cardiac pain.[17] From the heart these afferent fibers reach the spinal cord via the cardiac nerves, the upper five thoracic sympathetic ganglia, the white rami communicantes, and the upper five thoracic dorsal roots. Impulses mediated by these pathways converge with impulses from somatic thoracic structures into the same ascending spinal neurons. This convergence is thought to account for the projection of cardiac ischemic pain onto various dermatomes and provides the most likely explanation for referred pain. Other possible afferent sensory pathways include the ventral roots and vagal afferents. However, noxious stimuli (presumably hypoxia and acidosis) do not reliably and predictably produce pain. This may in part explain the common occurrence of silent ischemia, since pain may be perceived only when a sufficient level of afferent nerve traffic activates ascending neural pathways, thereby leading to the conscious perception of discomfort.

On occasion it is useful to prescribe sublingual nitroglycerin as a therapeutic test. Nitroglycerin takes approximately 10 or more seconds to be dissolved under the tongue, and its onset of action begins 45 to 60 seconds after dissolution. The peak action usually occurs about 2 minutes after dissolution, and its total duration of action may be up to 10 minutes or more. Thus, patients whose pain or discomfort is relieved within a few seconds after administration of sublingual nitroglycerin or those who take 30 minutes or more for pain relief may not have true angina pectoris caused by coronary artery disease. However, one should recognize that any therapeutic test employing sublingual nitroglycerin is at best only presumptive evidence for ischemic heart disease.

Among the many factors precipitating angina pectoris are physical exercise, emotional upset, and sometimes eating a meal. All of these raise myocardial oxygen demand by increasing both the heart rate and the systemic blood pressure. Indeed the product of these two measures is a useful index of myocardial oxygen demand. When measured, blood pressure usually rises before the onset of discomfort. If one encounters a patient during an episode of pain, physical findings may include an audible or intensified S_4, an S_3, and the emergence of an apical systolic murmur consistent with papillary muscle dysfunction. Other findings that have been described are transient paradoxic splitting of S_2, pulsus alternans, and a new area of palpable dyskinesis. Although these findings are useful, the historical analysis of precipitating factors remains the cornerstone on which the diagnosis of angina pectoris is largely based.

Usually, classic angina pectoris does not last longer than a few minutes and, as previously noted, is precipitated by exertion and relieved by rest. However, longer bouts of pain may occur at rest and in such individuals the possibility of more severe coronary artery disease must be considered. In such instances, hospitalization is often indicated and the possibility of coronary arteriography in preparation for balloon angioplasty or coronary artery bypass surgery may be considered. Patients who exhibit variant angina, that is, pain at rest associated with ST segment elevation, are definite candidates for urgent arteriography.

Left ventricular hypertrophy associated with aortic valvular stenosis should be considered as a cause of true angina pectoris even in the absence of obstructive coronary artery disease.[18] Clues to the diagnosis of hemodynamically significant valvular aortic stenosis are a harsh ejection systolic murmur at the base that often radiates to the apex and to the supraclavicular areas, a carotid arterial shudder, and a slow rising carotid arterial upstroke. In such patients, the major epicardial coronary arteries may be entirely normal but presumably the process of hypertrophy impairs the blood supply to subendocardial areas, leading to angina pectoris on exertion. Angina pectoris in association with suspected hemodynamically significant aortic valvular stenosis is an indication for cardiac catheterization and coronary arteriography since aortic valve replacement usually produces symptomatic relief. In addition, the occurrence of angina pectoris in such patients is an ominous prognostic sign and immediate hemodynamic study is indicated.

Precordial chest discomfort similar to that described in the preceding paragraphs that lasts for more than 20 to 30 minutes and is unrelieved by nitroglycerin may be a signal that a patient is having an acute myocardial infarction. Electrocardiographic changes may or may not accompany bouts of angina pectoris, and the same is true in the early stages of acute myocardial infarction. Patients who are suspected of having myocardial infarction should be hospitalized immediately and should be monitored if at all possible in a coronary care unit since during the early stages of acute myocardial infarction ventricular arrhythmias are probably the most common cause of sudden death. It is usually only later that frank pump failure occurs in some patients, but this does not usually lead to sudden death except when ventricular rupture and cardiac tamponade occur.

OTHER MANIFESTATIONS OF CHRONIC ISCHEMIC HEART DISEASE
REST PAIN

On occasion, rest pain may occur in patients with chronic stable angina pectoris, although if it is severe and prolonged, the diagnosis of unstable angina must be entertained. The genesis of rest pain may involve coronary vasoconstriction that occurs spontaneously in association with arteriosclerotic obstruction as described previously. An alternative mechanism that has been postulated is increased left ventricular size associated with augmented venous return that may occur in the recumbent position. This alteration in left ventricular size leads to an increase in myocardial oxygen demand because of an increase in wall tension. When this demand is not met by an adequate increase in oxygen supply, ischemic chest pain may ensue. A careful history may reveal that the patient wakes with chest pain when lying in one position, usually on the left side. This is analogous to the symptom of trepopnea, which is shortness of breath produced by a recumbency on one side, usually the left. The mechanism of angina produced in this way, as well as of trepopnea, is unknown, but presumably alterations in venous return and possibly restriction to left ventricular emptying may contribute to the pathogenesis of both.

A more severe manifestation of left ventricular dysfunction and resultant dyspnea in patients with angina pectoris is ischemic paralysis of the left ventricle, leading to acute pulmonary edema. This is a syndrome that usually does not occur in patients with chronic stable angina but in occasional individuals may be the only manifestation of ischemic heart disease and can even occur in the absence of ischemic pain. However, most such individuals will have severe underlying left ventricular dysfunction, usually following a myocardial infarction.

SILENT ISCHEMIA

Over the past decade it has become apparent that asymptomatic bouts of ischemia are more frequent than symptomatic episodes in patients with effort angina.[19] These observations have been made during ambulatory electrocardiographic monitoring in such individuals. Furthermore, it appears that in the same patient the severity of ischemia is generally the most important factor in determining the presence or absence of pain during an ischemic attack. The mean duration of ischemia appears to be longer during symptomatic episodes, which tend to be associated with greater alterations in the ST segment of the electrocardiogram. In patients monitored invasively, asymptomatic episodes are associated with an elevation of the left ventricular end-diastolic or pulmonary artery diastolic pressure in the majority of instances.[20] Since epidemiologic studies have estimated that 2% to 4% of middle-aged men have asymptomatic hemodynamically significant coronary artery disease,[21] the incidence of silent ischemia is probably even higher than studies in patients with documented ischemic heart disease indicate.

The pathogenesis of silent myocardial ischemia is not well understood. Such patients demonstrate significantly higher electrical pain thresholds and ischemic pain thresholds, as well as more tolerance to cold-induced ischemia, so that individual differences in sensibility to pain may partly explain the lack of symptoms in patients whose myocardial ischemia remains asymptomatic.[22] In addition, it has been suggested that differing endorphin levels among individuals may play a role in the perception of pain in general and specifically in angina pectoris. It has also been speculated but not proved that autonomic dysfunction, especially in patients with diabetes mellitus, may lead to a greater incidence of silent ischemia in these individuals.

DIFFERENTIAL DIAGNOSIS
ATYPICAL CHEST PAIN
ANXIETY AND HYPERVENTILATION

The typical anxious patient tends to complain of poorly localized, sometimes panprecordial discomfort. Moreover, anxious persons may localize pain to the area "over the heart," that is, over the left precordium, which is an unusual location for classic angina pectoris, and generally they do not describe radiation of pain. Complaints of a choking sensation or palpitations lasting for 30 minutes to an hour or more are common. Such individuals also may suffer from intermittent acute hyperventilation and have acute or chronic emotional problems. Occasionally symptoms can be reproduced if the patient is asked to hyperventilate in the office or hyperventilate during a treadmill exercise test. Some patients with anxiety and/or hyperventilation exhibit deep sighing or yawning respirations and complain of breathlessness without exertion.[23] However, it is obvious that patients with emotional problems and with anxiety may also develop ischemic heart disease, and often the diagnosis is not entirely clear when the patient is first seen.

BARLOW'S SYNDROME

Atypical chest discomfort is a common complaint of patients with the "click–murmur" syndrome associated with a billowing mitral leaflet.[24] This syndrome is exceedingly common, occurring in approximately 6% of normal women and in a much smaller percentage of normal men. In a small proportion of these individuals there are arrhythmias (both ventricular and supraventricular) and symptoms of chest discomfort that are highly atypical. The latter resemble those of the anxious patient, and indeed a high incidence of neurosis has been described in these patients. The pain may last for hours or even days, is unrelieved by nitroglycerin, and usually is localized either to one area of the precordium or radiates throughout many areas of the chest. However, it usually does not radiate to the arms, neck, or shoulders as does classic angina pectoris, although there are exceptions. Sometimes the chest discomfort is accompanied by either resting or exercise electrocardiographic abnormalities, including arrhythmias and ST segment depression. However, coronary arteriography almost always demonstrates normal vessels, although left ventricular dysfunction has been noted in severely symptomatic individuals. In the latter the pain may be associated with a cardiomyopathy of uncertain etiology. However, specific metabolic abnormalities or coronary arterial obstructive lesions in the smaller vessels have not been described. Clinical experience suggests that in the presence of arrhythmias and atypical chest pain therapy with propranolol may be helpful.

CHEST WALL PAIN

Chest wall pain or Tietze's syndrome is a common cause of chest discomfort. The latter involves tenderness of the costochondral or costosternal joints. In addition, discomfort of the xiphisternal joint may also mimic the pain of angina pectoris. The chest wall syndromes are frequently aggravated by movement, coughing, and deep breathing and can commonly be reproduced by local pressure. The pain is often relieved by infiltration with a local anesthetic. Tenderness of the chest muscles can also be reproduced by movements of the thoracic cage. Along with anxiety, chest wall pain is probably among the most common reasons for patients to complain of chest discomfort to the physician. However, patients with acute myocardial infarction may also complain of chest wall discomfort for reasons that are unclear. In general reassurance and possibly mild analgesia are all that is necessary for patients with chest wall pain.

PERICARDITIS

Pericarditis may occur at any age and is usually idiopathic, although it occurs often in association with uremia as well as following cardiothoracic operations (post-pericardiotomy syndrome). The stimulus for the pain in pericarditis presumably involves stretching of the receptors in the parietal pericardium and in the adjacent pleura by inflammation. Thus the pain of pericarditis may be pleuritic and is exacerbated by inspiration and coughing. The pain of pericarditis often mimics acute myocardial infarction and may be referred in a distribution typical of ischemic cardiac pain. However, it is usually worsened by recumbency and ameliorated by asking the patient to sit up and lean forward.

Patients with acute myocardial infarction, especially transmural infarction, frequently have some pericarditis during their course. Thus, if one encounters a patient several days after acute myocardial infarction (even a "silent" infarction), a pericardial friction rub may be heard in the presence of ST segment elevation on the electrocardiogram. Under these circumstances the differential diagnosis between pericarditis and myocardial infarction initially may not be clear. Of course the electrocardiogram is of considerable help in this regard since in pericarditis ST segment elevation tends to occur throughout virtually all leads and to change sequentially. Furthermore, T wave inversion and ST segment depression follow the acute ST segment elevation in a uniform fashion and significant Q waves do not appear in patients with pericarditis.

AORTIC DISSECTION

Dissecting aneurysm of the aorta is a potentially catastrophic event that may lead to chest pain. Unless the dissection becomes widespread the differential diagnosis among dissecting aneurysm, acute myocardial infarction, and a prolonged bout of angina pectoris may be virtually impossible. The pain usually begins in the anterior chest and radiates to the back or into the abdominal or lumbar areas and may involve the legs. Such radiation is extraordinarily rare in myocardial infarction or angina pectoris. Although abdominal pain may be severe, rebound tenderness, spasm, and guarding of the abdominal wall usually are not present. One should listen carefully for the murmur of aortic regurgitation; the latter is an immediate indication for angiographic study since the possibility of pericardial tamponade or dissection into one or both coronary arteries is a real one and can only be remedied by urgent surgical correction. Pericardial tamponade can also occur, and this is generally a terminal event. It is important to check the blood pressures in both the arms and the legs. Marked discrepancies in the pulses in the two arms or the absence of pulses in either the arms or one or both arms or legs are additional clues to the presence of dissecting aneurysm.

PULMONARY ARTERIAL HYPERTENSION

Pulmonary arterial hypertension may result from predominant right-to-left shunting such as occurs in congenital heart disease (Eisenmenger reaction), lung disease, left-sided heart disease such as mitral stenosis, and "primary" or unknown causes. Such patients may complain of chest pain resembling angina pectoris. The location, radiation, intensity, and quality of the pain may be identical to that occurring in patients with ischemic heart disease as may be the precipitating factors. However, nitroglycerin is often ineffective in such patients. Exertional syncope may also occur, presumably as the result of a low cardiac output. In general, the physical examination provides the clue to the diagnosis; a right ventricular lift and at times the murmur of pulmonic and/or tricuspid regurgitation are prominent features. In addition, the murmurs of mitral stenosis and mitral regurgitation should be sought. The electrocardiogram generally demonstrates a vertical or right axis in the frontal plane and evidence of right ventricular hypertrophy.

The pathogenesis of chest pain associated with pulmonary hypertension is unclear. It has been suggested that an increase of right ventricular pressure within the wall of that chamber may compromise myocardial blood flow resulting in ischemia and subsequent pain. In addition, the occurrence of low cardiac output with a reduced blood flow through the coronary arterial bed is another possibility.

PULMONARY INFARCTION

Acute pulmonary thromboembolism without pulmonary infarction usually does not cause chest discomfort. With massive pulmonary embolization, however, a reduction in cardiac output may lead to chest discomfort similar to that of angina pectoris. The pain associated with pulmonary infarction presumably is related to inflammation of the parietal pleura and is increased with inspiration. Predisposing factors are obesity, history of phlebitis, pregnancy, malignancy, congestive cardiac failure, and immobility. The latter is especially important in elderly patients. Thus, the clinical setting in which the chest pain occurs is often helpful in the differential diagnosis.

NONVASCULAR PULMONARY ABNORMALITIES: PNEUMONIA, PNEUMOTHORAX, AND MEDIASTINAL EMPHYSEMA

The nonvascular structures in the lungs and mediastinum may produce chest pain resembling the discomfort of angina pectoris. Among the most common of these is simple bacterial or viral pneumonia. These inflammatory processes are usually accompanied by fever, cough, pleuritic chest pain, and rales on auscultation. However, at times the chest may be free of adventitious sounds and the diagnosis is a roentgenographic one. In general acute inflammatory processes occurring in the lungs do not present a serious problem of differential diagnosis.

The development of spontaneous pneumothorax, however, may present a more difficult problem. Usually such an event is accompanied by the sudden onset of pain on either side of the chest. At times the pain is pleuritic and usually dyspnea is present. Tension pneumothorax may be accompanied by a sensation of substernal pressure or choking. This syndrome tends to recur in the same individuals and usually occurs in younger patients, especially those with a thin body habitus. Hypotension may complicate the picture, especially when a tension pneumothorax is present. Physical findings include tracheal and mediastinal displacement away from the side of pneumothorax and alterations in breath sounds that are usually diminished or absent on the affected side. The chest roentgenogram is usually diagnostic. The electrocardiogram may exhibit bizarre rotational patterns because of the shift of the heart in the mediastinum, but the clinical picture along with the roentgenogram usually clarifies the issue.

In mediastinal emphysema severe pain mimicking myocardial infarction may occur. At times, mediastinal emphysema may complicate spontaneous pneumothorax since the alveoli may rupture and air may dissect into the mediastinum. A systolic "crunch" (Hamman's sign) is present along the left sternal border and is common in mediastinal emphysema. Subcutaneous crepitations at the base of the neck are also common and indicate collections of air due to subcutaneous emphysema. Radiolucent areas consistent with this finding may be present on the chest roentgenogram, which is exceedingly helpful in the diagnosis of this syndrome.

GASTROINTESTINAL DISEASE: REFLUX ESOPHAGITIS, MOTILITY DISORDERS, PEPTIC ULCER, CHOLECYSTITIS, PANCREATITIS, ESOPHAGEAL RUPTURE

A variety of nonvascular intestinal diseases may cause precordial discomfort and are often important in the differential diagnosis of ischemic heart disease. It is common for patients with reflux esophagitis to complain of dull squeezing lower precordial discomfort shortly (30 minutes to 1 hour) after recumbency. This symptom may also occur after meals and is usually relieved by sitting upright. Nausea or regurgitation may occur, and the pain may also radiate to areas typical of ischemic heart disease. At times nitroglycerin seems to be useful, but antacids more commonly provide relief, as does raising the head of the bed 6 or more inches from the floor. It is sometimes helpful to perform a Bernstein test (perfusion of the esophagus with 0.1 N hydrochloric acid, which produces pain while perfusion with 0.9% sodium chloride does not). This condition may or may not be associated with a hiatal hernia; conversely the presence of a hiatal hernia does not indicate the inevitable presence of reflux esophagitis. Roentgenographic evaluation is often helpful in this condition. It should be emphasized that patients who awake with pain several hours after retiring should be suspected of having angina pectoris rather than reflux esophagitis.

Motility disorders of the esophagus may also produce precordial discomfort, particularly after meals. An important clue to the presence of esophageal spasm is that dysphagia may occur following intake of liquid as well as solid foods. A confounding factor is that precordial discomfort produced by abnormal esophageal motility may respond to sublingual nitroglycerin. Barium studies of the esophagus, provocation of pain by a Bernstein test, and esophageal manometric studies may all be necessary to confirm the diagnosis of abnormal esophageal motility.

Other abdominal conditions that may mimic the discomfort of ischemic heart disease include the pain of peptic ulcer disease. However, this discomfort is characteristically midepigastric rather than substernal and is generally relieved by antacids. The pain typical of complications of peptic ulcer disease such as perforation and obstruction may also mimic the discomfort of ischemic heart disease, but generally these complications lead to abdominal rather than chest findings.

The pain of cholecystitis usually is in the right upper quadrant of the abdomen but occasionally radiates to the epigastrium as well as into the lower chest. Again, precipitating factors are often helpful, such as relation to meals, nausea and vomiting, and pleuritic chest pain on the right often with radiation to the right shoulder. At times the differential diagnosis, however, may be difficult, and electrocardiographic changes may accompany acute attacks of cholecystitis. These changes usually represent repolarization abnormalities whose pathogenesis is uncertain; hyperventilation and dehydration may be factors. If the differential diagnosis is unclear, hospitalization may be required and it may be necessary to obtain serial electrocardiograms and serum enzyme studies.

Acute and chronic pancreatic disease may lead to precordial discomfort. The pain is usually epigastric and may radiate to the back, and it is not uncommon for a dissecting aneurysm to be considered in the differential diagnosis of acute pancreatitis. Serum enzyme determinations may be exceedingly useful in helping to make the proper diagnosis. Pancreatitis frequently occurs in the setting of alcoholism and in the presence of gallbladder or ulcer disease. Nevertheless such patients may also have ischemic heart disease and when the pain is acute the electrocardiogram may also demonstrate changes consistent with ischemic heart disease.

Esophageal rupture is a catastrophic event that may cause chest pain mimicking that of myocardial ischemia. Usually the patient gives a history of severe vomiting, perhaps associated with excess alcohol or food intake prior to the onset of the pain. Air is present in the mediastinum and extends upward into the neck.

NEUROVASCULAR AND NEUROMUSCULAR DISORDERS: CERVICAL DISK DISEASE, THORACIC OUTLET SYNDROME

A variety of neurovascular and neuromuscular diseases may also lead to chest discomfort. Among the more prominent of these is cervical disk disease in which herniation of an intervertebral disk causes nerve root compression and subsequent shoulder or arm pain. The pain of nerve root compression may last for several hours and even days and commonly occurs in one or both arms. In part the pain may be related to spasm in the muscle supplied by the nerve root. Pain due to compression of intervertebral disks is commonly aggravated by movement and by maneuvers that increase intraspinal pressure such as coughing, sneezing, or straining (Valsalva maneuver). Because the distribution of the pain may coincide with a dermatome often involved by the referred pain of ischemic heart disease, the differential diagnosis may not be immediately apparent. Again a careful history and a physical examination are often helpful, although at times an exercise test may be important in aiding the differential diagnosis.

Additional musculoskeletal disorders that may produce chest pain are grouped under the term *thoracic outlet syndrome*. This syndrome encompasses abnormalities that lead to compression of vessels and nerves as they exit from the thoracic spine in the cervical region. Among these are the presence of a cervical rib; the scalenus anticus syndrome (anomalous insertion or hypertrophy of the anterior scalene muscle, or an unusually large transverse process of one of the lower cervical vertebrae); the costoclavicular syndrome and the hyperabduction syndrome (neurovascular compression by the pectoralis minor tendon).

With a cervical rib, the shoulder on the affected side tends to droop and the trapezius muscle often exhibits some atrophy. The diagnosis is confirmed by roentgenography. Adson's maneuver may be helpful in diagnosing the scalenus anticus syndrome. This is accomplished with the patient seated and the head extended and turned to the side of the lesion. The patient is then instructed to breathe deeply, resulting in either diminution or total loss of the radial pulse on the affected side.

To reproduce costoclavicular compression, the patient stands, holds a deep inspiration, and braces the shoulders back in an exaggerated position of attention. The radial pulses are palpated before and during traction downward on the arm. If the pulse is not completely obliterated, a decrease in the cuff blood pressure should be sought.

To demonstrate neurovascular compression by the pectoralis minor tendon, the patient abducts and externally rotates his arm as if to throw a ball. The radial pulses and/or brachial blood pressure are checked for diminution. For all three maneuvers, bruits in the supraclavicular area during each maneuver should also be sought. The discomfort produced by these maneuvers can extend into the shoulder and neck and often produces parasthesias in the ulnar distribution (C8–T1). This distribution helps to separate thoracic outlet compression from the carpal tunnel syndrome, which usually involves the median nerve in the hand.

ADDITIONAL DIAGNOSTIC MEASURES
EXERCISE TOLERANCE TEST

The resting electrocardiogram is often normal in patients with angina pectoris, although it may reveal evidence of prior myocardial infarction or left ventricular hypertrophy. Repolarization abnormalities are common but tend to be nondiagnostic. Therefore, virtually all patients, except perhaps the very elderly and the disabled, should have an exercise tolerance test once the diagnosis of angina pectoris is suspected or confirmed on clinical grounds. This recommendation applies primarily to patients in whom the angina is stable and not to those who are having prolonged bouts of pain with ST segment deviations or to patients in whom myocardial infarction is suspected. Furthermore, in patients who are suspected of having hemodynamically significant aortic stenosis in association with angina pectoris an exercise tolerance test should not be performed. However, the vast majority of patients can undergo either a treadmill or bicycle exercise tolerance test without untoward effects. Such tests yield considerable information, both for the physician and for the patient, and are helpful in assessing the effects of therapy.[25]

Numerous studies have shown that the exercise electrocardiogram has a sensitivity of approximately 50% and a specificity of 90% when asymptomatic individuals are screened for coronary artery disease.[26] However, both of these figures are considerably higher when the prevalence of the disease in the population is taken into account. This type of test is extraordinarily useful in a population of middle-aged or older men who report symptoms suggestive of coronary artery disease. The exercise tolerance test may be particularly helpful in identifying a subgroup of patients at high risk for morbidity and mortality. The findings of severe exercise ischemia, such as ST segment depression of 2 mm or greater lasting more than 5 minutes involving three or more leads or a treadmill time of less than 3 minutes, portend an ominous prognosis and represent indications for further diagnostic studies, such as cardiac catheterization.[27] Exertional hypotension is another finding that is suggestive of left main coronary artery disease or three-vessel disease with associated left ventricular dysfunction and is an indication for prompt cardiac catheterization.[28]

It is important to recognize that the exercise test should not be interpreted as "positive" or "negative." Interpretation of the test should relate to the probability of the existence of ischemia or to its severity. Thus patients who exercise for longer times (e.g., 10 minutes or more) on the treadmill and who have minor ST segment alterations and a normal blood pressure response have a much better prognosis compared with patients who have the early onset of deep ST segment depression associated with a reduced treadmill exercise time and exertional hypotension. Most patients will fall somewhere in between these two extremes, and their risk can be judged accordingly. In addition the treadmill exercise test provides an index of how much exertion the patient can perform and is useful both to the physician and the patient himself. Such studies can also be a guide to therapy when repeated several weeks, several months, or a year later. Whether periodic yearly treadmill exercise testing is a useful diagnostic approach has not been definitively established, but such periodic studies can encourage the patient and the physician that no deterioration has occurred. The decision to perform serial tests in patients with chronic angina pectoris should be made on an individual basis.

So called false-positive exercise tolerance tests may occur in the presence of mitral valve prolapse, congenital heart disease, valvular heart disease, and left ventricular hypertrophy. If a patient reaches an ischemic endpoint, such as angina or ST segment depression during the course of exercise, it is extraordinarily difficult to use the exercise test to quantitate the amount and function of residual myocardium, since severe coronary stenosis producing ischemia can limit exercise capacity in a patient with normal left ventricular performance.[28] Despite the observation that exercise capacity does not correlate well with resting or exercise left ventricular function, it is nevertheless accepted that the amount of work performed during an exercise test importantly influences the prognosis. Indeed, some have suggested that exercise duration is more important than exertional ST segment depression as a prognostic indicator in patients with coronary heart disease.[29]

THALLIUM-201 SCINTIGRAPHY

Not infrequently, one is faced with a patient with atypical chest discomfort who has an equivocal exercise test or who has some other abnormality precluding accurate assessment of the exercise test, such as a conduction abnormality. The latter includes left bundle branch block, some instances of right bundle branch block, and left anterior hemiblock. Under these circumstances it may be useful to combine the exercise tolerance test with a nuclear study, particularly a thallium-201 perfusion study.[30] It has been found that a normal exercise thallium-201 myocardial perfusion study is a most useful predictor of normal coronary arteries in patients with chest pain, especially individuals with atypical chest discomfort.[31] With newer computer approaches for evaluation of myocardial clearance or washout of thallium-201 as well as the uptake of this isotope, the number of false-positive thallium-201 studies has been considerably reduced.[32] In patients who cannot undergo exercise, the thallium-201 scintigram following the infusion of dipyridamole may prove useful. Thus, thallium-201 scintigraphy provides particularly helpful independent diagnostic information when other findings are equivocal. Under these circumstances, an abnormal thallium-201 study is much more likely to prompt coronary angiography for definitive diagnosis.

Additionally, the thallium-201 perfusion scintigram may be of use in another subset of patients with chronic stable angina: those who have had a previous myocardial infarction or who have undergone previous coronary artery bypass surgery. In such individuals, the scintigram may identify areas of myocardium in considerable jeopardy, especially myocardium that may be the major source of residual left ventricular function following infarction. Scintigraphy may also identify areas of nonperfused myocardium after coronary artery bypass surgery indicating graft occlusion and is helpful in further assessing the need for repeat angiography and possible surgery. Thus thallium-201 scintigraphy should be used as an adjunct in selected patients in whom the diagnosis of chronic stable angina of ischemic heart disease is in doubt or in whom additional diagnostic information is deemed necessary.

CORONARY ANGIOGRAPHY

Finally cardiac catheterization and coronary angiography should be reserved for those patients with chronic stable angina in whom angioplasty or coronary artery bypass surgery is contemplated or in whom the diagnosis is in doubt. As indicated previously, minimally symptomatic or asymptomatic patients with chronic stable angina pectoris tend to have a good prognosis. Conversely, the prognosis worsens with increasing severity of angina, even when factors such as pain threshold are taken into account. In such patients, coronary angiography should be preceded by at least an exercise tolerance test and in some instances, as indicated above, by a thallium-201 scintigram. Age and life-style should also be considered since some individuals are willing to tolerate only very modest amounts of precordial discomfort, while others are more stoic. The decision to pursue invasive diagnostic measures is an individual one to be made mutually by the patient and physician. Whether coronary angiography should be performed in all patients with a diagnosis of ischemic heart disease to establish prognosis is controversial. The bulk of studies indicate that patients with good exercise tolerance who are easily controlled by medication will not benefit by coronary bypass surgery and hence do not require routine coronary angiography. By contrast, individuals who perform poorly on the treadmill and who have extensive symptoms with two- and three-vessel disease, especially with mild reduction of left ventricular function, should probably undergo coronary arteriography, even if they fall into the category of chronic stable angina. There remains a large group of patients between these two subsets in whom a combination of historical information, exercise testing with or without scintigraphy, and the response to drug therapy will determine the need for invasive studies.

NATURAL HISTORY AND THE EFFECTS OF TREATMENT

Data from the Framingham study obtained in the 1950s and 1960s indicate that one in four men with angina can expect to have a myocardial infarction within 5 years.[33] The risk is one half of this for women. In the Framingham cohort, about 30% of individuals over age

55 died within 8 years and almost half of these deaths were sudden. In men, almost half the angina occurred after myocardial infarction compared with only 15% in women, while only 23% of infarctions were preceded by angina. Almost one in four myocardial infarctions were silent or went unrecognized, but such infarctions were rare in persons with prior angina. Subsequent data from the Framingham study revealed that remission of new-onset angina present for at least 2 years occurred in 32% of the men and almost 50% of the women, but in angina that had persisted for several years the subsequent remission rates were lower (14% for men and 19% for women).[34] These generally high remission rates, while encouraging, raise the question as to the initial accuracy of the diagnosis of angina pectoris in these patients.[35]

Studies indicate that asymptomatic patients have a better prognosis than symptomatic individuals.[36] Earlier data suggested that if only one of the three major coronary arterial branches (left anterior descending, left circumflex, or right) has a significant stenosis (greater than 70%), the annual mortality rate is approximately 2%.[37] If two of the three major arteries are stenosed, the rate is approximately 7%; and if all three arteries are stenosed, it will be approximately 11% per year. These data were collected before therapy with either β-adrenergic antagonists or calcium channel blockers was available. More recent evidence indicates that when patients are asymptomatic or only mildly symptomatic, the annual mortality rate in patients with one- and two-vessel disease is about 1.5% but is 6% for those with three-vessel disease.[38] Thus the prognosis appears to be excellent in patients with no symptoms or those with only mild symptoms who have only one- or two-vessel coronary disease. Patients with three-vessel disease who have retained good exercise capacity documented with objective testing have an annual mortality rate of 4%. However, patients with three-vessel disease and poor exercise capacity have a higher annual mortality rate of approximately 9%, and these individuals should be considered for revascularization.

Data from the Coronary Artery Surgery Study (CASS) indicate that the prognosis progressively worsens with the number of coronary arteries diseased, the number of proximal arterial segments diseased, and worsening left ventricular performance.[39] In the CASS study, these three indices accounted for an estimated 84% of the prognostic information available and the 6-year survival varied between 16% and 93%, depending on the values of these three indices. These data suggest that extensive noninvasive information, and possibly invasive information in some patients, should be obtained in order to determine prognosis and to evaluate the effects of therapy.

The natural history of atypical chest pain that is often confused with angina pectoris, particularly in women, appears to be benign, especially in patients who have normal coronary arteriograms.[40] In such individuals chest discomfort can often be treated symptomatically with medication and reassurance. Furthermore, this type of discomfort often tends to disappear after 1 or 2 years. Except when frank coronary vasospasm and variant angina can be documented, myocardial infarction is highly unlikely to occur.

TREATMENT
GENERAL MEASURES

In considering the treatment of angina pectoris, it is helpful to refer to a standard classification that can aid in assessing the results of treatment as well as the naturally occurring spontaneous variability in this syndrome. Such a classification is that of the Canadian Heart Association, which is shown in Table 62.1. This classification is perhaps more useful than the previously employed New York Heart Association classification and is a convenient guide to the success or failure of a particular therapy.

Systemic arterial hypertension is often a precursor and frequently accompanies chronic angina pectoris. Mild hypertension not uncommonly soars to much higher levels on exercise, and control of both resting and exercise blood pressure is an important goal in the management of every patient with angina pectoris. Although many of the channel blockers, may affect systemic arterial blood pressure, concurrent treatment with one or more antihypertensive agents is an important approach to therapy in many patients. As part of blood pressure control, weight reduction and the avoidance of excess sodium is often helpful. A prudent diet should be prescribed. Although there is little evidence that reduction in serum cholesterol levels can cause regression of atherosclerotic lesions, nevertheless it seems wise to reduce serum cholesterol levels either by dietary means or, if necessary, with the addition of drugs in the hope of retarding the atherosclerotic process.

The use of tobacco is clearly associated with an increased risk of coronary heart disease, and every attempt should be made at advising patients to discontinue smoking. This is often difficult for chronic smokers, and adjunct psychological measures or smoking clinics may be helpful. Although "tobacco angina" (angina on inhalation of tobacco smoke) is a rare phenomenon, it is not generally appreciated that tobacco smoke can interfere with the efficacy of antianginal drugs.[41] Smoking itself causes a rise in heart rate, which in turn increases myocardial oxygen demand. In addition, components of tobacco smoke may act as systemic vasoconstrictors, thereby raising blood pressure. For all of these reasons, it is imperative that patients be advised in the strongest terms to discontinue the use of tobacco.

Although patients with chronic angina pectoris should be encouraged to exercise moderately, there is no evidence that a post-training increase in exercise tolerance in such patients results from augmented myocardial oxygen delivery.[42] Rather, it appears to be related to a reduction in the coronary flow requirement for a given workload. Exercise prescriptions should be based in part on the results of a treadmill exercise tolerance test. Patients should be cautioned about exercising in cold air, which often brings on angina for reasons that are not well understood.[43] Patients should be told the differences between arm and leg exercise, the former causing the anginal threshold to be reached more rapidly than the latter.[44] Patients should be aware of the existence of the "walk-through" phenomenon. This occurs when a patient has angina during exercise, but as the exertion continues the angina disappears. Proposed mechanisms for the relief of angina during exercise include vasodilatation with a decline in heart rate and systemic arterial blood pressure, relief of effort-induced coronary arterial spasm, or dilatation of functioning collateral vessels.[45]

Patients should also be advised regarding sexual activity. It has been found that there is no difference in heart rate and blood pressure response of the male during sexual intercourse when the male-on-top

TABLE 62.1 GRADING OF ANGINA OF EFFORT BY THE CANADIAN CARDIOVASCULAR SOCIETY

I	Ordinary physical activity does not cause . . . angina, such as walking and climbing stairs. Angina with strenuous or rapid or prolonged exertion at work or recreation.
II	Slight limitation of ordinary activity. Walking or climbing stairs rapidly, walking uphill, walking or stair climbing after meals, or in cold, or in wind, or under emotional stress, or only during the few hours after awakening. Walking more than 2 blocks on the level and climbing more than one flight of ordinary stairs at a normal pace and in normal conditions.
III	Marked limitation of ordinary physical activity. Walking one to two blocks on the level and climbing one flight of stairs in normal conditions and at normal pace.
IV	Inability to carry on any physical activity without discomfort—anginal syndrome *may be* present at rest.

(Campeau L: Letters to the editor: Grading of angina pectoris. Circulation 54:522, 1976. By permission of the American Heart Association, Inc.)

has been compared with the male-on-bottom position.[46] Mean maximal heart rates in either position varied between 114 and 117 beats per minute, representing no more than 61% of predicted maximum heart rate responses for younger men (ages 20 to 29). Thus, if patients can achieve a heart rate of up to 120 beats per minute during an exercise tolerance test without chest pain, it is unlikely that sexual activity will bring on precardial discomfort. In addition, patients should be encouraged to use nitrates prophylactically.

There appears to be good evidence that in some patients with ischemic central nervous system disease, particularly males suffering from transient ischemic attacks, aspirin may be of benefit. Similarly in patients with unstable angina, there appears to be a reduction in the subsequent incidence of death or acute myocardial infarction in patients taking aspirin as compared with placebo.[47] Whether patients with chronic stable angina pectoris should take one aspirin tablet daily (324 mg) has not been proved.

Finally, one must consider the placebo effect in dealing with angina pectoris. Physicians should not ignore the therapeutic value of the placebo, particularly since a variety of abandoned therapies, such as xanthines, khellin, vitamin E, ligation of the internal mammary artery, and implantation of the internal mammary artery into the myocardium (Vineberg operation), have been advocated in the past as good treatments for angina and excellent results were reported.[48] With the advent of more objective measures of evaluation, such as treadmill exercise testing, nuclear studies and coronary arteriography, such placebo effects can be quantitated but not entirely eliminated. The placebo is probably one of the physician's most important therapeutic assets and a good physician–patient relationship, as in all medical treatment, can enhance the value of any specific therapy that is prescribed.

ORGANIC NITRATES

The organic nitrates are the oldest type of drug therapy known for the relief of angina pectoris. The cellular mechanisms by which nitrates produce one of their principal effects, relaxation of smooth muscle, are as yet unknown. In the intact organism there are several different mechanisms whereby nitrates are believed to relieve myocardial ischemia. Each of these principal actions may predominate at different times, even in the same patient.[49] All of these mechanisms, however, are dependent on the ability of the nitrates to relax smooth muscle. Thus it is hypothesized that the nitrates directly affect abnormal vasomotion either occurring spontaneously or in the region of atherosclerotic narrowing. Nitrates may also help to dilate collateral vessels supplying an ischemic area when the principal vessels supplying that territory are narrowed. It is well known that the nitrates reduce systemic venous tone and result in venous pooling. This indirect effect on the heart is probably important when ventricular diastolic pressures are elevated and in some instances when cardiac size is increased as well. On occasion, nitrates are administered under circumstances that result in a reduction in systemic arterial pressure. This is particularly so when nitroglycerin is administered intravenously. Intravenous nitroglycerin also affects venous pooling and dilates coronary vessels. In any individual instance either the direct or indirect effects of the nitrates or combinations of these effects may be important.

These beneficial effects of the nitrates on the systemic veins, arterioles, and coronary arteries may be opposed by sympathetic reflexes and neurohumoral adaptations.[50] Such homeostatic mechanisms may tend to diminish the initial benefit of the nitrates and cause the antianginal effects of these drugs to vary considerably among patients. For example, some of the benefit of the nitrates may be blunted in patients who depend primarily on peripheral venous dilatation induced by these agents since the body does not tolerate vasodilatation without activating direct compensatory mechanisms that affect fluid transport at the capillary level or other homeostatic mechanisms (such as the autonomic nervous system, activation of antidiuretic hormone, and the renin–angiotensin–aldosterone system). By contrast, the patient who depends primarily on the direct coronary resistance vessel dilating effect of the nitrates may show only a minor decrease in his response to this type of agent. However, it seems clear that some patients receiving chronic oral nitrate therapy may develop tolerance and require increasing doses, but the mechanism of such nitrate tolerance is not understood. In addition, such patients may be less sensitive to the vasodilating properties of acutely administered sublingual nitroglycerin. Thus in a patient with "progressive" angina, nitrate tolerance as well as disease progression should be considered.[51]

Sublingual nitroglycerin is the mainstay of antianginal therapy. All patients should be instructed in its use in the office and asked to take a tablet in the presence of the physician, noting its time of dissolution, its taste, and other sensations, such as dizziness and flushing. These are particularly important, since the patient can then tell whether he is taking an active preparation. The patient should be instructed to store nitroglycerin in a dark bottle and to keep a supply in the refrigerator since this agent is both light and heat sensitive. This prescription should be renewed periodically, preferably every 6 to 9 months, depending on use. The patient should be instructed to use sublingual nitroglycerin prophylactically, that is, before an activity that is known to produce angina in that particular individual. This may include any activity, such as walking up a slight incline, shopping, sexual activity, and situations that may produce emotional distress. Side effects of the nitrates are usually the result of their therapeutic action, such as flushing and warmth produced by systemic vasodilatation. At times a slight to moderate headache may also occur. Under these circumstances a patient may require dose reduction. Occasional patients are unable to tolerate the organic nitrates at all because of headache.

The variety of nitrate preparations currently available and their duration of action and dosage are summarized in Table 62.2. There is ample evidence that the so-called long-acting nitrates such as oral isosorbide dinitrate and nitroglycerin paste are effective for between 4

TABLE 62.2 COMMONLY USED NITRATES IN ANGINA PECTORIS

Agent	Dosage	Duration of Action
Sublingual nitroglycerin	0.16–0.67 mg every 5–10 min*	15–20 min
Isosorbide dinitrate		
Oral	10–60 mg every 4–6 hr	4–6 hr
Sublingual	2.5–10 mg every 2–4 hr	1.5–4 hr
Chewable	5–10 mg every 2–4 hr	2–3 hr
2% Nitroglycerin ointment	½–2 inch (1.3–5 cm; 7.5–30 mg) every 4–6 hr	3–6 hr
Transdermal nitroglycerin	5–30 cm^2; 12.5–154 mg; every 12–24 hr	6–8 hr

* Most commonly prescribed sublingual nitroglycerin dose is 0.4 mg.

and 6 hours. These agents are frequently given with a β-blocker and/or calcium channel antagonist. Intravenous nitroglycerin is reserved for patients with unstable angina. The introduction of nitroglycerin patches that produce therapeutic blood levels for up to 24 hours has led to considerable controversy.[52,53] It appears that these agents are effective for perhaps 6 to 8 hours, but sustained efficacy for more than this period of time has not been proved. It is possible that some of the systemic adjustments described above may obviate the efficacy of sustained nitroglycerin blood levels.

Additional recommendations are that patients be started on low doses and thereafter the nitrates should be increased as tolerated over a period of several days or weeks to the maximum dose.[54] Oral isosorbide dinitrate has a longer half-life than the sublingual form and therefore may be more desirable in ambulatory patients. Nitroglycerin ointment is occasionally disliked by some patients for cosmetic reasons. Furthermore, the dosage and duration of its action cannot be precisely controlled. Clinically it is often useful to use this preparation before retiring for the night.

β-ADRENERGIC ANTAGONISTS

As a group, the β-adrenergic blockers share certain characteristics.[55] All of these agents can produce central nervous system effects and myocardial depression, and all except pindolol, which has intrinsic sympathomimetic activity, may blunt the heart rate response to exercise. All carry the potential danger of the withdrawal syndrome (increased sympathetic activity sometimes leading to accelerated angina and myocardial infarction after abrupt drug withdrawal). However, this class of drug is extraordinarily useful in the treatment of chronic ischemic heart disease, and with the proliferation of agents now available (Table 62.3) the clinician can at least partially tailor the drug to the patient.

Among the individual properties of the β-blockers to consider is the issue of selectivity of the agent. β-Adrenergic receptors are considered to be divided into two classes, β_1 and β_2.[56] β_1-Receptors are located in the myocardium, although recent evidence suggests that β_2-receptors may also be present in human cardiac tissue, particularly in the atria.[57] β_2-Receptors are located in lung tissue, particularly the bronchioles, and in peripheral arterial vessels. Thus, blockade of β_2-receptors may lead to unopposed bronchoconstriction as well as to peripheral vascular constriction, sometimes causing excessive claudication, especially in colder climates. Also the mechanism whereby insulin-induced hypoglycemia is countered by mobilization of liver glycogen is dependent on a β_2-receptor for activation of phosphorylase. For these reasons one may wish to choose a drug with relative β_1-selectivity, such as metoprolol or atenolol.[58] Thus patients with asthma, chronic obstructive pulmonary disease, diabetes, or intermittent claudication may benefit from administration of a β_1-selective agent in low dosage. However, as one increases the dosage of such agents, selectivity is lost and both types of β-receptors are blocked. For example, this occurs at a dose of metoprolol that exceeds 100 mg daily.

Many patients who take β-blockers complain of fatigue and depression and sometimes nightmares. These side effects occur in up to 20% of patients receiving this type of agent and disappear on their withdrawal. Propranolol is the most lipid soluble of these agents and readily enters the central nervous system, while of the available agents atenolol is the least lipid soluble and most water soluble. However, definitive proof that the more water-soluble agents produce fewer central nervous system side effects is lacking. Central nervous system complaints are often confusing to the clinician, since they may mimic some of the symptoms of congestive cardiac failure. Although the β-adrenergic blockers are unequivocal myocardial depressants, it is unlikely that patients receiving oral agents for chronic angina pectoris will exhibit signs or symptoms of congestive cardiac failure unless myocardial depression is severe. Indeed myocardial depression is often exacerbated by ischemia, which can be prevented by administration of β-adrenergic blockers. Nevertheless, one must be cautious and follow patients with left ventricular dysfunction carefully. Simple measures such as weighing the patient daily and paying attention to symptoms such as breathlessness are often useful to follow in such individuals.

Many patients with ischemic heart disease also have some element of chronic renal insufficiency. Propranolol, metoprolol, timolol, and pindolol do not require dose adjustment in such individuals. By contrast, nadolol and atenolol are eliminated unchanged by the kidney and doses of these drugs should be reduced in patients with even mild renal insufficiency. However, nadolol and atenolol are at least theoretically useful in patients with hepatic insufficiency since their elimination is primarily renal. Pindolol exhibits intrinsic sympathomimetic activity and tends not to slow the heart rate the way the other β-blockers do. This agent may be useful in occasional patients who have symptomatic sinus bradycardia as a response to other β-blockers or who have intrinsic sinus node disease. In general, however, its usefulness appears to be somewhat limited.

Although much has been written about the β-blocker withdrawal syndrome,[59] its incidence fortunately appears to be quite low. Nevertheless when discontinuing a β-blocker for any reason, it is prudent to taper the drug over a period of several days. In an older population, the incidence of adverse reactions to many drugs is higher and adverse

TABLE 62.3 PHARMACOLOGY OF β-BLOCKERS

	Atenolol	Metoprolol	Nadolol	Pindolol	Propranolol	Timolol
Absorption (%)	50	>95	30	>95	>90	90
Bioavailability (%)	40	50	30	100	30	75
Protein binding (%)	<5	12	30	57	93	10
Lipid solubility	Weak	Moderate	Weak	Moderate	High	Weak
Elimination half-life (hr)	6–9	3–4	14–24	3–4	3.5–6	3–4
Primary route of elimination	Renal	Hepatic	Renal	Hepatic, renal	Hepatic	Hepatic, renal
Active metabolites	No	No	No	No	Yes	No
Relative β_1-selectivity	+	+	–	–	–	–
Membrane-stabilizing activity	–	–	–	+	++	–
Intrinsic sympathomimetic activity	–	–	–	+	–	–
Dose	50–100 mg qd	50 mg qd–100 mg bid	40–240 mg qd	5 mg bid–20 mg tid	10–80 mg qid; 10–320 mg qd (long-acting preparation)	10–30 mg bid

responses to β-blockers, particularly central nervous system symptoms, may be correspondingly augmented, although objective information in this regard is lacking.

Because blood levels of β-adrenergic blockers are not clinically useful and are expensive and difficult to obtain, the heart rate response to these agents remains the best single clinical indicator of their effectiveness in an individual patient. Generally it is useful to target the resting heart rate below 60 beats per minute with a range of 45 to 55 beats per minute being ideal. Often the heart rate will decrease to 40 to 45 beats per minute during sleep. Unless there is sinus node disease, however, it is unlikely that the heart rate will slow further after β-blockade. In addition, a heart rate of 40 to 45 beats per minute generally poses no danger to patients. Other drugs prescribed for patients with cardiovascular disease, such as digoxin and verapamil, will also cause a reduction in heart rate, and on occasion, their combination with a β-blocker may produce profound bradycardia. Thus the clinician should review the patient's medication as well as his heart rate response to combinations of these drugs before prescribing additional agents.

Despite the many differences noted in Table 62.3, the β-blocking agents appear to have a similar spectrum of therapeutic activity. Thus it can be said that if one agent in adequate doses does not work, neither will another. It also does not appear to be useful to add one β-blocker to another in the hope of improving the therapeutic response. However, one may wish to switch one β-blocker to another because of side effects. The differences in bioavailability, interpatient variations in serum levels, and differences in potency make it difficult to recommend equivalent doses among β-blockers. However, Table 62.4 uses studies that investigated oral doses of different agents that produced a similar reduction in such measurements as exercise tolerance, heart rate, and blood pressure and provides an estimate of starting doses. Therapy can then be titrated according to the individual response.

The usual doses of β-blockers are listed in Table 62.3. However, these doses may be modified by individual patient responses. There appears to be a wide therapeutic range in the dose of β-blockers, particularly with propranolol where serum levels may vary over an order of magnitude. Consequently the effective therapeutic dose of propranolol may vary from as little as 10 mg or 20 mg in some patients to several hundred milligrams or more in others. The dose range of other β-blockers is considerably narrower, but their therapeutic effectiveness will be modified both by alterations in renal and hepatic function and by concurrent medication. It is common to use a long-acting nitrate preparation in association with a β-blocker; and of the calcium channel antagonists, nifedipine appears to be most useful in combination with a β-blocker. This is because nifedipine tends to cause an increase in heart rate as a result of its vasodilating properties; this relative tachycardia can be counteracted by use of a β-blocker.

The β-blockers are a mainstay in the therapy of chronic angina pectoris, but because of their side effects many clinicians have tended to use a calcium channel blocker as a drug of first choice. There are no studies that demonstrate the superiority of either type of agent in patients with chronic stable angina pectoris, so that the clinician must make the choice based on patient tolerance, ease of administration, potential adverse reactions, drug interactions, and cost.

CALCIUM CHANNEL BLOCKERS

The introduction of this class of agents into clinical use in patients with chronic angina pectoris has provided an important additional approach to the treatment of this disorder. These agents all share the properties of reducing the transmembrane flux of calcium via the "slow" calcium channel; they all produce some reduction in cardiac performance; and all are smooth muscle vasodilators.[60] It is this latter property that is of particular importance in patients with chronic ischemic heart disease, especially when an element of abnormal coronary vasomotion is a consideration. The pertinent characteristics of these agents are summarized in Table 62.5. Currently nifedipine, verapamil, and diltiazem are available for use in the United States, but numerous other agents are undergoing therapeutic trials.

Although these agents are classified in one group, they differ markedly in their chemical structures and they also have differing effects on various portions of the cardiovascular system. Thus nifedipine is the most potent vasodilator of these three agents and may produce a number of adverse reactions, including peripheral edema, headache, flushing, and reflex tachycardia. Although nifedipine may be useful in some patients with angina pectoris when given alone, it appears to be best given in conjunction with a β-adrenergic blocker to offset the resulting tachycardia. Conversely nifedipine will tend to prevent an excessive bradycardia produced by a β-blocker, thereby adding further rationale to the use of these two drugs in combination.

By virtue of its effects on the cardiac conduction system, verapamil tends to produce bradycardia in some patients; therefore caution must be exercised when it is given to patients receiving a β-blocker and digoxin. Verapamil raises serum digoxin levels by uncertain mechanisms. Diltiazem is intermediate between the other two agents: it has some modest effects on the sinus rate, is a moderate peripheral vasodilator, and appears to have relatively few side effects on long-term administration. Initially it was recommended that up to 240 mg daily in divided doses should be prescribed, but it has been found that optimal effects often require doses of 360 mg daily and in some patients even this dose may need to be augmented depending on the individual clinical response.[61,62]

As indicated earlier, there appears to be no definitive evidence that either the β-blockers or calcium channel antagonists are superior in the

TABLE 62.4 ESTIMATED EQUIVALENT TOTAL DAILY DOSE WHEN SWITCHING β-BLOCKING AGENTS*

Propranolol	120 mg
Atenolol	50–100 mg
Metoprolol	150 mg
Nadolol	80–120 mg
Timolol	20 mg
Pindolol	30 mg

*Since dose requirements may vary, the dose of a β-blocker should be titrated to individual patient response.

TABLE 62.5 CALCIUM CHANNEL BLOCKERS

	Nifedipine	Verapamil	Diltiazem
Dosage	10–30 mg tid	80–160 mg tid	90 mg tid–90 mg qid (or higher)
Absorption	>90%	>90%	>90%
Bioavailability	60–70%	10–22%	<20%
Protein binding	90%	90%	80%
Plasma half-life (β phase)	5 hr	3–7 hr	4 hr
Metabolism	Extensively metabolized to an inert free acid and lactone	Extensive first-pass hepatic extraction (70% of oral dose)	Extensively deacylated
Excretion			
Renal (%)	70, 1st day (80 total)	50, 1st day (70 total)	35 (total)
Fecal (%)	15	15	65

treatment of chronic stable angina pectoris. If one is to choose a calcium channel blocker as a first-line drug, diltiazem appears to be the agent that is most free of adverse reactions and best tolerated by patients. Also diltiazem depends least on renal excretion (see Table 62.5), and therefore its dose requires little if any adjustment in older patients.

As mentioned previously, all of these agents have a negative inotropic effect. This may be particularly important in patients who have borderline left ventricular function or who have a previous history of overt congestive cardiac failure. As with the β-blockers, prevention of ischemia that induces further cardiac dysfunction may be beneficial. However, patients with severe left ventricular dysfunction probably should not be given a calcium channel blocker except under very carefully controlled circumstances. Conversely, patients with only mild to moderate left ventricular dysfunction usually tolerate these agents extraordinarily well. Constipation is a commonly reported side effect of chronic verapamil therapy, but all of the agents may cause gastrointestinal upset. There is no evidence that any of the calcium channel blockers are associated with rebound phenomena on their withdrawal.

Each calcium channel blocker has a recommended dosing regimen (see Table 62.5). Because comparative trials among these agents are few, it is difficult to make recommendations regarding equivalent doses when switching from one drug to another. Therefore, it seems prudent to individualize the dose and to titrate to the desired clinical response.

GENERAL APPROACH TO THE PATIENT: CLINICAL POINTERS

In a patient suspected of having chronic angina pectoris by history it is generally useful to perform an exercise tolerance test to identify patients at high risk for early morbidity and mortality.[63] Marked early ST segment deviation, exercise-induced hypotension, or inability to walk on a treadmill for more than a few minutes all suggest that critical coronary artery disease is present, and such patients should have cardiac catheterization. Conversely, patients who are able to walk long distances on the treadmill without chest pain or fatigue tend to have a good prognosis. Some have advocated that it is more cost effective either to perform coronary arteriography directly to confirm the diagnosis or to perform a nuclear study, such as a thallium-201 scintigram, in conjunction with the exercise tolerance test. At present it is not possible to make firm recommendations, although noninvasive testing should generally precede the invasive approach. When the history and exercise tolerance test are unequivocal and the decision is to provide medical therapy to the patient, no further studies need be done. If the chest pain is atypical and the diagnosis is unclear, one should certainly perform a nuclear perfusion study, possibly in conjunction with the first exercise test. It is rarely necessary to go first to cardiac catheterization and coronary angiography to confirm the initial diagnosis of chronic angina pectoris except in the most unusual of circumstances.

Once the diagnosis is established, the patient should be counseled regarding diet and smoking and therapy should be begun. All patients should receive therapeutic and prophylactic sublingual nitroglycerin and in addition at least one other agent, either a β-blocker or a calcium channel antagonist. In conjunction with these, it is often useful to prescribe long-acting nitrates as well. Once the clinical response to this therapy has been determined and the blood pressure well controlled, the physician and the patient may wish to discuss further options. Depending on the patient's age, work or recreational habits, and tolerance to discomfort, the decision regarding angiography and possible coronary artery bypass surgery can be made. Because of recent observations that asymptomatic or minimally symptomatic patients with one- or two-vessel disease do as well without surgery, the decision should be taken with these data in mind. The vast majority of patients will have a good to excellent initial therapeutic response to currently available agents and recent advances have made medical treatment for chronic stable angina pectoris even more effective.

REFERENCES

1. Heberden W: Some account of a disorder of the breast. In White PD: The historical background of angina pectoris. Mod Concepts Cardiovasc Dis 43:109, 1974
2. Blodaver Z, Neufeld HN, Edwards JE: Pathology of angina pectoris. Circulation 46:1048, 1972
3. McNamara JJ, Molot MA, Stremple JF et al: Coronary artery disease in combat casualties in Vietnam. JAMA 216:1185, 1971
4. Roberts WC: The coronary arteries and left ventricle in clinically isolated angina pectoris: A necropsy analysis. Circulation 54:388, 1976
5. James TN: Diseases of the large and small coronary arteries. Arch Intern Med 134:163, 1974
6. Karliner JS: Congestive Heart Failure: Pathophysiology and Treatment. In Karliner JS, Gregoratos G (eds): Coronary Care, pp 449–470. New York, Churchill Livingstone, 1981
7. Sharma B, Taylor SH: Reversible left-ventricular failure in angina pectoris. Lancet 2:902, 1970
8. Gertz EW, Wisneski JA, Neese R et al: Myocardial lactate metabolism: Evidence of lactate release during net chemical extraction in man. Circulation 63:1273, 1981
9. Osler W: Lumelian lecture on angina pectoris. In White PD: The historical background of angina pectoris. Mod Concepts Cardiovasc Dis 43:109, 1974
10. Maseri A, L'Abbate A, Chierchia S et al: Significance of spasm in the pathogenesis of ischemic heart disease. Am J Cardiol 44:788, 1979
11. Pierce CD, Dodge HT: The mechanisms of nitroglycerin action: Stenosis vasodilation as a major component of the drug response. Circulation 64:1089, 1981
12. Hoffman JIE: Maximal coronary flow and the concept of coronary vascular reserve. Circulation 70:153, 1984
13. Goldberg HL, Goldstein J, Borer JS et al: Functional importance of coronary collateral vessels. Am J Cardiol 53:694, 1984
14. Cannon RO, Watson RM, Rosing DR et al: Angina caused by reduced vasodilator reserve of the small coronary arteries. J Am Coll Cardiol 1:1359, 1983
15. Opherk D, Mall G, Zebe H et al: Reduction of coronary reserve: A mechanism for angina pectoris in patients with arterial hypertension and normal coronary arteries. Circulation 69:1, 1984
16. Gorlin R: Dynamic vascular factors in the genesis of myocardial ischemia. J Am Coll Cardiol 1:897, 1983
17. Malliani A, Lombardi F: Consideration of the fundamental mechanisms eliciting cardiac pain. Am Heart J 103:575, 1982
18. Hancock EW: Aortic stenosis, angina pectoris, and coronary artery disease. Am Heart J 93:382, 1977
19. Cecchi AC, Dovellini EV, Marchi F et al: Silent myocardial ischemia during ambulatory electrocardiographic monitoring in patients with effort angina. J Am Coll Cardiol 1:934, 1983
20. Chierchia S, Lazzari M, Freedman B et al: Impairment of myocardial perfusion and function during painless myocardial ischemia. J Am Coll Cardiol 1:924, 1983
21. Cohn PF: Silent myocardial ischemia in patients with a defective anginal warning system. Am J Cardiol 45:697, 1980
22. Droste C, Roskamm H: Experimental pain measurement in patients with asymptomatic myocardial ischemia. J Am Coll Cardiol 1:940, 1983
23. Wheatley CE: Hyperventilation syndrome: A frequent cause of chest pain. Chest 68:195, 1975
24. Levine HJ: Difficult problems in the diagnosis of chest pain. Am Heart J 100:108, 1980
25. Weiner DA, Ryan TJ, McCabe CH et al: Prognostic importance of a clinical profile and exercise test in medically treated patients with coronary artery disease. J Am Coll Cardiol 3:772, 1984
26. Uhl GS, Froelicher V: Screening for asymptomatic coronary artery disease. J Am Coll Cardiol 1:946, 1983
27. Weiner DA, McCabe CH, Tryan TJ: Prognostic assessment of patients with coronary artery disease by exercise testing. Am Heart J 105:749, 1983
28. Young GY, Froelicher VE: Exercise testing: An update. Mod Concepts Cardiovasc Dis 52:25, 1983
29. Bruce RA, DeRouen TA, Hammermeister KE: Noninvasive screening criteria for enhanced 4-year survival post aortocoronary bypass surgery. Circulation 60:638, 1979
30. Hlatky M, Botvinick E, Brundage B: The independent value of exercise thallium scintigraphy to physicians. Circulation 66:953, 1982
31. Berger BC, Abramowitz R, Park CH et al: Abnormal thallium-201 scans in patients with chest pain and angiographically normal coronary arteries. Am J Cardiol 52:365, 1983
32. Massie BM, Hollenberg M, Wisneski JA et al: Scintigraphic quantification of myocardial ischemia: A new approach. Circulation 68:747, 1983
33. Kannel WB, Feinleib M: Natural history of angina pectoris in the Framingham study: Prognosis and survival. Am J Cardiol 29:154, 1972
34. Kannel WB, Sorlie PD: Remission of clinical angina pectoris: The Framingham study. Am J Cardiol 42:119, 1978

35. Ayres SM, Mueller HS: Remission of angina pectoris. Am J Cardiol 42:520, 1978
36. Cohn PF: Prognosis and treatment of asymptomatic coronary artery disease. J Am Coll Cardiol 1:959, 1983
37. Reeves TJ, Oberman A, Jones WB et al: Natural history of angina pectoris. Am J Cardiol 33:423, 1974
38. Kent KM, Rosing CR, Ewels CJ et al: Prognosis of asymptomatic or mildly symptomatic patients with coronary artery disease. Am J Cardiol 49:1823, 1982
39. Ringqvist I, Fisher LD, Mock M et al: Prognostic value of angiographic indices of coronary artery disease from the coronary artery surgery study (CASS). J Clin Invest 71:1854, 1983
40. Waxler EB, Kimbiris D, Dreifus LS: The fate of women with normal coronary arteriograms and chest pain resembling angina pectoris. Am J Cardiol 28:25, 1971
41. Deanfield J, Wright C, Krikler S et al: Cigarette smoking and the treatment of angina with propranolol, atenolol, and nifedipine. N Eng J Med 310:951, 1984
42. Ferguson RJ, Cote P, Gauthier P et al: Changes in exercise coronary sinus blood flow with training in patients with angina pectoris. Circulation 58:41, 1978
43. Hattenhauer M, Neill WA: The effect of cold air inhalation on angina pectoris and myocardial oxygen supply. Circulation 51:1053, 1975
44. Wahren J, Bygdeman S: Onset of angina pectoris in relation to circulatory adaptation during arm and leg exercise. Circulation 44:432, 1971
45. Gorlin R: Role of coronary vasospasm in the pathogenesis of myocardial ischemia and angina pectoris. Am Heart J 103:598, 1982
46. Nemec ED, Mansfield L, Kennedy JW: Heart rate and blood pressure responses during sexual activity in normal males. Am Heart J 92:274, 1976
47. Lewis HD, Davis JW, Archibald DG et al: Protective effects of aspirin against acute myocardial infarction and death in men with unstable angina. N Engl J Med 309:396, 1983
48. Benson H, McCallie DP: Angina pectoris and the placebo effect. N Engl J Med 300:1424, 1979
49. McGregor M: The nitrates and myocardial ischemia. Circulation 66:689, 1982
50. Hollenberg M, Go M: Clinical studies with transdermal nitroglycerin. Am Heart J 108:223, 1984
51. Dalal JJ, Yao L, Parker JO: Nitrate tolerance: Influence of isosorbide dinitrate on the hemodynamic and antianginal effects of nitroglycerin. J Am Coll Cardiol 2:115, 1983
52. Reicheck N, Priest C, Zimrin D et al: Antianginal effects of nitroglycerin patches. Am J Cardiol 54:1, 1984
53. Abrams J: The brief saga of transdermal nitroglycerin discs: Paradise lost? Am J Cardiol 54:220, 1984
54. Abrams J: Nitroglycerin and long-acting nitrates. N Engl J Med 302:1234, 1980
55. Conolly ME, Kersting F, Dollery CT: The clinical pharmacology of β-adrenoceptor blocking drugs. Prog Cardiovasc Dis 19:203, 1976
56. Motulsky HJ, Insel PA: Adrenergic receptors in man: Direct identification, physiologic regulation, and clinical alterations. N Engl J Med 307:18, 1982
57. Brodde O-E, Karad K, Zerkowski H-R et al: Coexistence of β_1- and β_2-adrenoceptors in human right atrium. Circ Res 53:752, 1983
58. Frishman WH: β-Adrenoceptor antagonists: New drugs and new indications. N Engl J Med 305:500, 1981
59. Shand DG, Wood AJJ: Propranolol withdrawal syndrome—why? Circulation 58:202, 1978
60. Henry PD: Comparative pharmacology of calcium antagonists: Nifedipine, verapamil and diltiazem. Am J Cardiol 46:1047, 1980
61. Subramanian BV, Khurmi NS, Bowles MJ et al: Objective evaluation of three dose levels of diltiazem in patients with chronic stable angina. J Am Cell Cardiol 1:1144, 1983
62. Go M Jr, Hollenberg M: Improved efficacy of high-dose versus medium- and low-dose diltiazem therapy for chronic stable angina pectoris. Am J Cardiol 53:669, 1984
63. Silverman KJ, Grossman W: Angina pectoris: Natural history and strategies for evaluation and management. N Engl J Med 310:1712, 1984

Acute and Chronic Ischemic Heart Disease: Unstable Angina

Carl J. Pepine

Treatment of patients with unstable angina continues to be a difficult challenge for the clinician. One of the problems contributing to this difficulty is lack of a precise and commonly accepted definition. Crescendo angina, preinfarction angina, spontaneous angina, progressive angina, acute coronary insufficiency, impending infarction, and intermediate syndrome have been used to describe patients with ischemic heart disease whose chest pain was due neither to chronic stable effort angina nor to acute myocardial infarction. Some insight into the historical background of this problem may be helpful. Osler was one of the first to recognize that in some patients with angina, pain became more severe and, at times, this change in severity preceded acute myocardial infarction.[1] Sampson was another early worker to observe that this entity may lead to acute myocardial infarction.[2] All 29 of his patients, however, developed infarction. Such retrospective observations supported misnomers such as *impending infarction* and *preinfarction*, which are still used. These terms imply an unwarranted prognosis, which in turn evokes biased therapeutic decisions. Fowler, in an editorial on "pre-infarctional angina," was one of the first to attempt to clarify the terminology of this condition.[3] He coined the term *unstable angina*, which was subsequently used in one of the first prospective series by Gazes and co-workers.[4] However, this term is also somewhat imprecise and without pathophysiologic basis.

A rational approach to treatment of patients with unstable angina requires a thorough understanding of the illness. In addition to the clinical findings, knowledge of the pathophysiology and natural history of unstable angina is essential. The clinician also must be thoroughly familiar with the various treatment modalities available.

Based on clinical criteria, there are two relatively distinct types of patients within the group called unstable angina. One type includes patients *without previous angina* who suddenly begin to experience repeated episodes of chest pain, often at rest, frequently at night or in the early morning, or with a very low level of effort. The other type of patient has a *long history of effort angina* which either increases in frequency, occurs with less effort, or progresses to rest angina. The assumption underlying these descriptions is that the patient has very severe, extensive, rapidly progressive coronary atherosclerosis. In retrospect, we recognize that this assumption was a misunderstanding of a much more complex pathophysiology, which hampered efforts at effective treatment. The common feature in both types of patients is that signs and symptoms of myocardial ischemia occur at rest or during ordinary activities of normal daily living. The onset of, or change to, angina at rest has pathophysiologic meaning.

PATHOPHYSIOLOGY

To manage patients with unstable angina effectively, it is important to briefly review the pathophysiology of the syndrome. Essential features are that (1) major determinants of myocardial oxygen demand, such as heart rate and systolic blood pressure, do not regularly increase before the onset of ischemia and (2) vascular factors, such as altered coronary vasomotor tone and thrombosis, are often present. These features set the syndrome of rest angina apart from the syndrome of effort angina. In other words, the pathophysiologic mechanism responsible for production of ischemia at rest in patients with unstable angina usually involves a change in processes influencing myocardial oxygen supply. An understanding of these "supply side" processes in any given patient is important in determining effective therapy (Table 63.1).

The *coronary arteries* of most patients with chronic stable effort angina show severe multivessel atherosclerosis as a rule. Although the clinical manifestations and pathophysiology of unstable rest angina differ from those associated with stable effort angina, the extent and distribution of coronary atherosclerotic obstructions are, in general, not different. The number of diseased vessels and degree of obstruction are remarkably similar.[5,6] What is responsible for the change in symptoms or onset of symptoms to include ischemia at rest?

Studies suggest that the *morphology* of the coronary lesion may be different in unstable angina. The qualitative appearance of the coronary stenosis at autopsy was described by Levin and Fallon.[7] On the basis of postmortem angiographic and histologic study of patients dying of complications of myocardial infarction or coronary bypass surgery, these workers found coronary artery lesions with intraluminal lucencies or irregular borders. Pathologic examination showed that the appearance of these lesions was due to plaque rupture or partially occlusive thrombi. The lesions were described as "complicated lesions." Study of these lesions indicates that thrombus develops at sites of plaque disruption that relate to tears in its overlying fibrous cap.[8,9] Falk has found that most thrombus is layered, suggesting development over an extended period, and has also provided evidence suggesting peripheral embolization to produce occlusion.[9]

Angiographic studies in living patients with unstable angina support the postmortem observations. Again, nonocclusive intraluminal filling defects and eccentric narrowings with irregular borders are frequent findings.[10,11] The lesions, identified during life, most likely contain components of both ruptured plaque and nonocclusive thrombi. These components probably explain the relatively high frequency (76%) of recent progression of coronary lumen obstruction in patients with

TABLE 63.1 CORONARY VASCULAR FACTORS INVOLVED IN UNSTABLE ANGINA

Condition	Causes
Coronary atherosclerosis	Multivessel disease
	Plaque rupture/disruption
Dynamic coronary artery changes	Coronary spasm (obstructive)
	Increased tone (nonobstructive)
	Microvascular spasm
	Increased arteriolar tone
	"Physiologic" tone
Intimal injury	Platelet deposition and nonocclusive thrombus
	Leukocytes (monocytes and macrophages)
	Thromboxane and leukotrienes

stable angina who developed unstable angina reported by Moise and colleagues.[12] Although the precise mechanism involved in the interrelation of chronic stable effort angina, unstable rest angina, and acute myocardial infarction is unknown, the coronary circulation of the patient with an unstable ischemic syndrome is likely to show evidence of relatively recent progression of obstruction. In many instances, progression is due to a complicated lesion containing elements of plaque rupture and nonocclusive thrombi.

DYNAMIC CORONARY ARTERY CHANGES

Spasm was suggested for years as the basis of various ischemic syndromes, but this was not proven until demonstrated at angiography in patients with Prinzmetal's variant angina. The term *Prinzmetal's variant angina* applies to a relatively specific subset of patients with unstable angina, which includes only patients with ST segment elevation accompanying rest pain (discussed in detail elsewhere). Maseri and

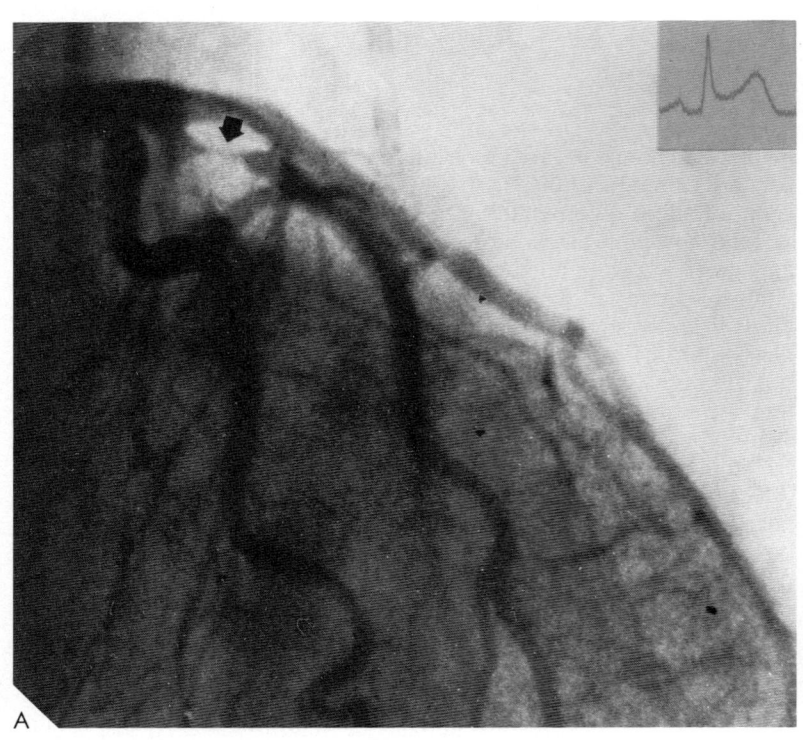
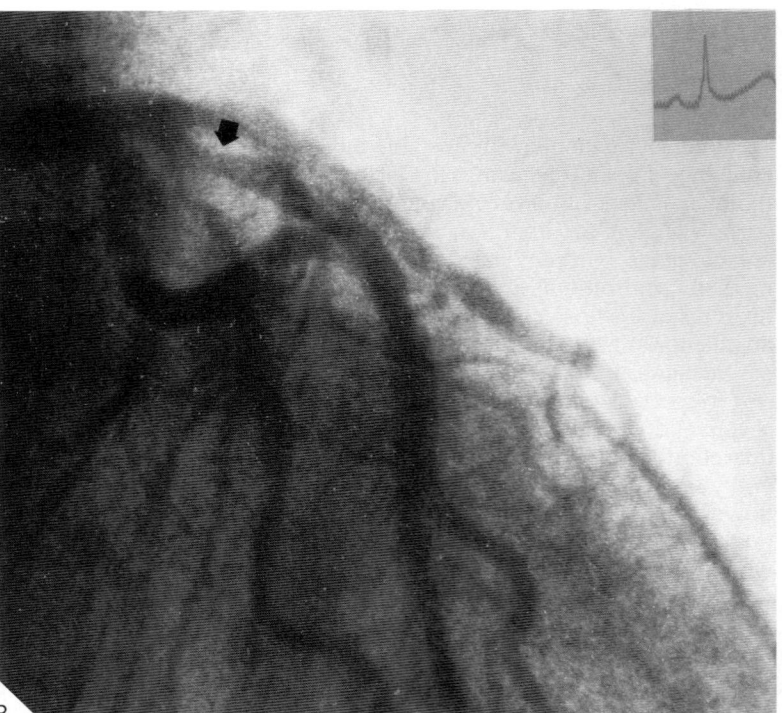
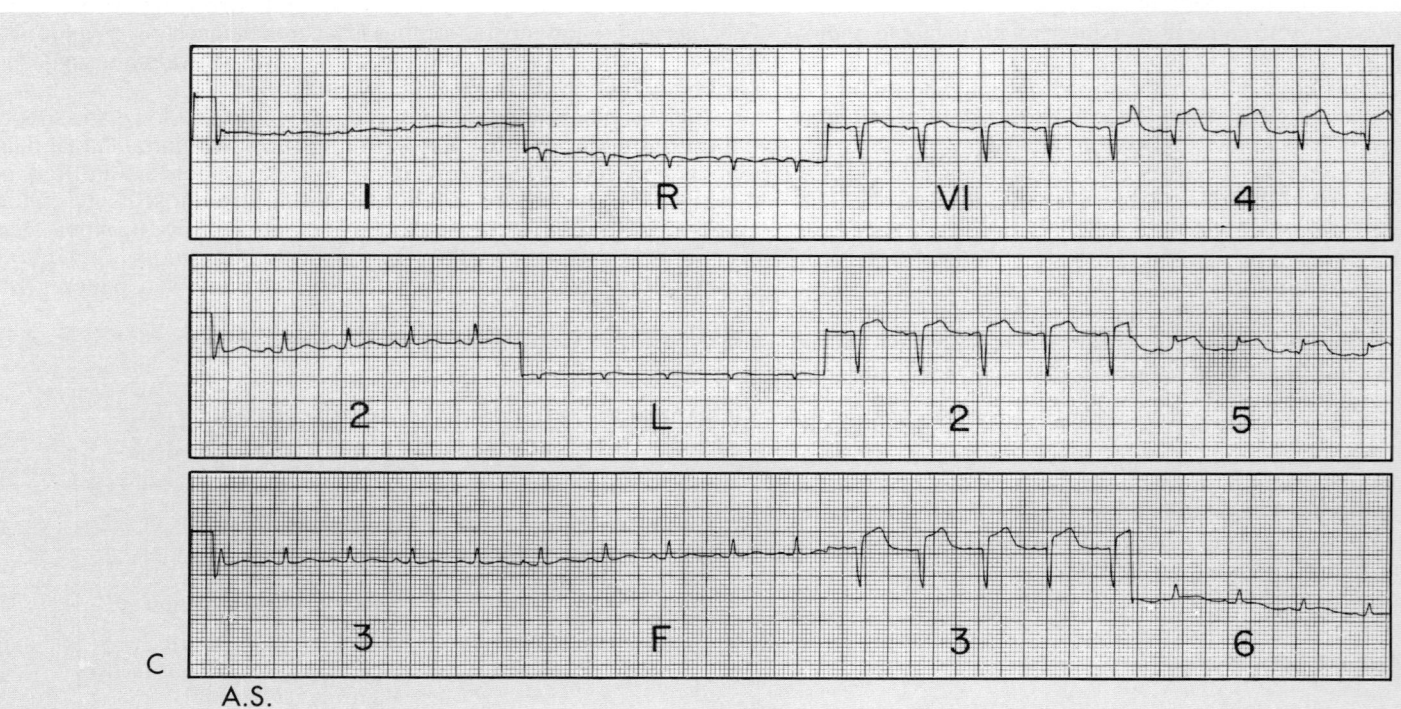

FIGURE 63.1 Coronary angiogram and electrocardiogram from a patient with unstable angina and coronary artery spasm who evolved an acute myocardial infarction. **A.** Anterior descending spasm (*arrow*) associated with ST segment elevation as detected by angiogram done during spontaneous rest angina. **B.** Relief of spasm occurred with intracoronary nitroglycerin (*arrow*). Spasm recurred despite large doses of intracoronary nitroglycerin, verapamil, nifedipine, and phentolamine, eventually resulting in anterior myocardial infarction as shown in the bottom panel of the electrocardiogram (**C**). (Lambert C, Pepine C: Acute myocardial infarction. In Cox RH (ed): Emerging Concepts of Pathogenesis and Treatment. Philadelphia, Praeger Publishing, 1986)

associates were among the first to recognize that Prinzmetal's angina represented only one aspect of a continuous spectrum of heterogeneous clinical findings associated with unstable angina at rest.[13] Many patients with rest angina and ST segment elevation during one episode have ST segment depression, T wave changes, or no electrocardiographic changes during other episodes. Some patients never have ST segment elevation but are otherwise clinically indistinguishable from those with ST segment elevation. Most have severe coronary atherosclerosis, but some have only minimal disease. A few patients have relatively normal coronary arteries. In most cases, regardless of the type of electrocardiographic change or coronary anatomy, determinants of myocardial oxygen demand do not increase just before the onset of rest angina. Coronary artery spasm, however, can be identified, if sought, in many of these cases. Evidence that spasm leads to intimal injury, thrombus formation, or plaque disruption is present in reports of unstable angina patients with spasm in one coronary artery who later develop myocardial infarction in the distribution of the same vessel (Fig. 63.1).[14]

It is generally agreed that intense arterial spasm reduces blood flow, resulting in ischemia or infarction in the distribution of the artery. Localized, large coronary artery vasomotor changes that do not completely occlude the vessel could affect the coronary artery in other ways. Vasomotor changes may account for morphologic changes (plaque rupture and nonocclusive thrombi) found in studies of the coronary circulation described above.[6,7,10,11] Other reports provide very strong evidence suggesting that focal arterial constriction, which does not reduce flow, may damage the arterial wall itself.[15-17] In one of these studies, vasoconstriction, which reduced the rabbit carotid artery diameter by 42% without change in blood flow, was associated with severe longitudinal folding of the luminal surface. Endothelial desquamation with extensive platelet deposition on the exposed subendothelium also occurred.[17] After 15 minutes, attached thrombus was seen with calcium deposits on the luminal side of the internal elastic lining.

After 24 hours, marked deposition of leukocytes was observed. Platelet and leukocyte-derived substances may in turn exert potent constrictor effects on vascular smooth muscle either at the site of endothelial injury or more distally. Platelets generate thromboxane A_2. Leukocytes trigger cell membranes to release arachidonic acid, which is metabolized by cyclo-oxygenase and lipoxygenase pathways to prostaglandins, thromboxanes, and leukotrienes.[18] Other experiments using a porcine preparation of arterial injury *in vivo* indicate that during arterial thrombosis platelets may contribute to vasoconstriction through release of prostanoids, serotonin, and platelet-derived growth factors.[19]

Platelets and other factors derived from eicosanoid metabolism may also play a role in dynamic coronary obstruction at sites of important coronary atherosclerosis. Experiments in dogs with coronary stenosis show that platelets adhere to exposed connective tissue of the coronary arterial wall and platelet aggregation occurs to produce cyclic reductions in blood flow.[20,21] Platelet aggregates may occlude the lumen, embolize, provide a site for fibrin thrombus formation, or stimulate generation of thromboxane A_2. Using the dog model, Bolli and co-workers showed that heparin did not alter these coronary flow reductions, but both aspirin and a platelet-active α-antagonist did.[22] These studies suggest that platelet aggregation causes the cyclic reductions in blood flow at sites of important stenosis. The beneficial effects of aspirin in patients with unstable angina, discussed in detail below,[23,24] support the suggestion that platelets and cyclo-oxygenase play an important role in coronary artery obstruction of these patients.

Intraluminal filling defects, representing thrombus, are seen in coronary angiograms of some patients with unstable angina. In my experience, these defects are usually discrete, often spherical radiolucencies seen at or just distal to sites of severe coronary stenosis (Fig. 63.2). They frequently are mobile; some stain with contrast material after repeated coronary injections. Most are surrounded by contrast material except for a narrow attachment site. Vetrovec and associates found

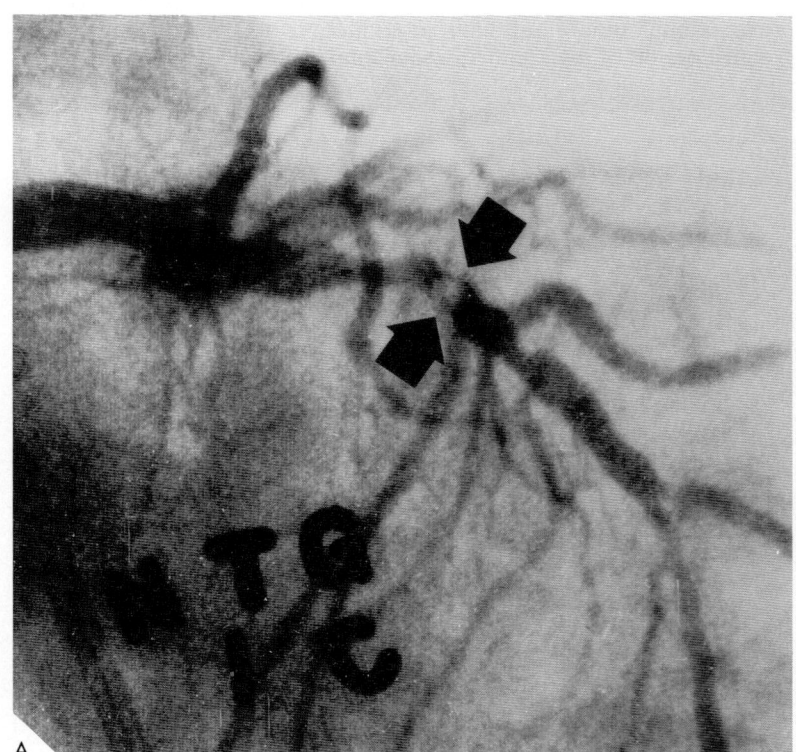
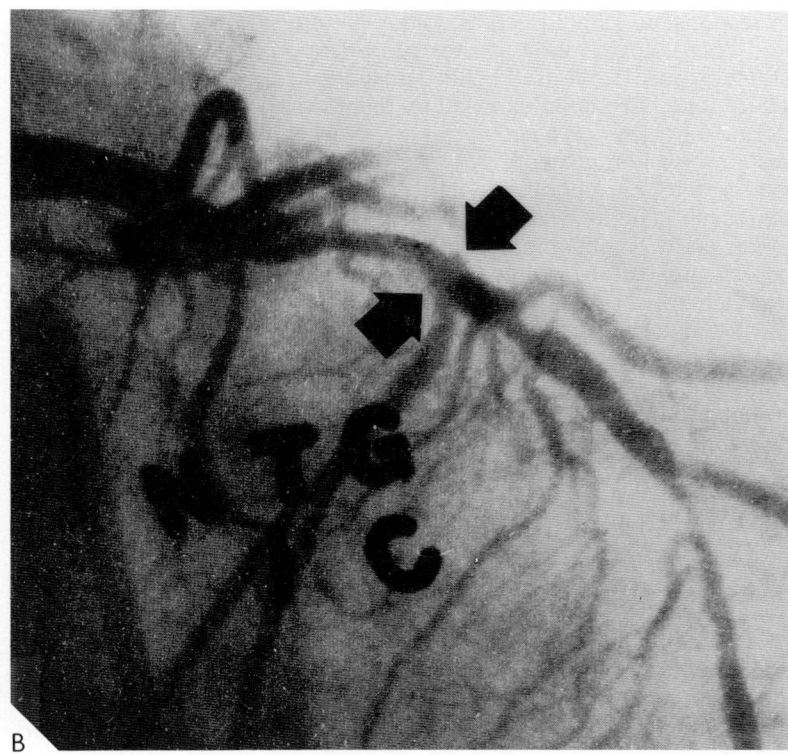

FIGURE 63.2 Coronary angiogram from a patient with unstable angina who had a nonocclusive thrombus. **A.** A radiolucent, spherical, filling defect (arrows) persists after intracoronary nitroglycerin in the proximal portion of the left anterior descending artery. This defect appeared mobile and is distal to areas of atherosclerotic obstruction. Other areas of coronary stenosis are present in the midportion of this vessel. **B.** Disappearance of the filling defect (arrows) followed intracoronary streptokinase administration, confirming that the defect was due to recent thrombus. (Lambert CR, Pepine CJ. Coronary artery spasm and pharmacology of coronary vasodilators. In El-Sherif N, Ramana CV (eds): The Pathophysiology and Pharmacotherapy of Myocardial Infarction. pp 117–154. Florida, Academic Press, 1986)

such defects in 11 of 13 patients within 5 days of the onset of an unstable ischemic syndrome.[25] In ten cases, the defect was localized to the ischemia related vessel. Evidence of complete or partial clearing was found after intracoronary streptokinase infusion, confirming the presence of recent thrombus. Mandelkorn and associates found similar results.[26] To determine the incidence of intracoronary thrombi in unstable angina, Capone and colleagues studied 119 consecutive patients within 14 days of the onset of rest angina.[27] None had evidence for acute myocardial infarction. A little over one third (37%) of the patients had intraluminal filling defects. However, the majority of those patients whose most recent rest pain episode had occurred within 1 day of angiography had filling defects, while a minority of those whose most recent episode of rest pain had occurred within 2 to 14 days of angiography had filling defects. Angioscopic examination of the coronary artery luminal surface by Sherman and co-workers in unstable angina patients during coronary bypass surgery frequently showed complex plaques and/or mural thrombi not necessarily apparent in the angiogram.[28] Ragged, ulcerated, hemorrhagic endothelium and thrombi characterized the coronary arteries of patients with unstable ischemic syndromes. Such lesions were not present in direct angioscopic examination of patients with stable ischemic syndromes undergoing bypass surgery. Other studies also suggest a close temporal relationship between rest pain episodes and intermittent thrombus formation.[29,30]

Evidence for both platelet activation,[29,30] assessed by urinary prostanoid measurements, and clotting activation,[30] assessed by plasma fibrinopeptide A measurements, has been found in unstable angina patients. These angiographic and angioscopic studies directly confirm the notion that intracoronary thrombus is another dynamic mechanism responsible for transient coronary flow reduction in patients with unstable angina at rest. It is also likely that the milieu (complex lesions, thromboxanes, leukotrienes, ischemia of vascular smooth muscle, thrombin, etc.) associated with intracoronary thrombus heightens coronary smooth muscle sensitivity to vasoconstricting factors.[31]

Some other dynamic coronary vascular factors could account for transient flow reduction in some patients with rest angina.[32] These factors include microvascular spasm; inappropriate arteriolar constriction in response to stimuli such as cold, cigarette smoke, or mental stress; and "physiologic" tone at sites of nonimportant atherosclerotic obstruction (see Table 63.1). Abnormalities in the control of coronary artery tone have been exposed by demonstration of vasoconstriction during intracoronary injection of low-dose acetylcholine.[33] Dilation in response to nitroglycerin, however, is intact. These observations suggest a defect in endothelial-derived vasodilation at sites of irregular lumens in patients with coronary artery disease. These factors, acting alone or in combination, could explain effects of such well-known aggravating factors as cold exposure, stress, and smoking on myocardial ischemia (Table 63.2).[34]

Blood itself may undergo alterations that contribute to the development of myocardial ischemia in patients with unstable angina. Possible platelet and leukocyte effects have been discussed previously. Effects of hematocrit and arterial Po_2 are well known as factors influencing myocardial oxygen delivery. Infrequently, anemia, polycythemia, or hypoxemia contributes to development of unstable angina. Rheologic factors such as viscosity, red cell flexibility, and fibrinogen may be important.[35] Plasma viscosity has been reported to be increased in unstable angina patients as compared with those with stable angina, those with myocardial infarction, and control subjects.[36] In one patient, waxing and waning angina over several days was associated with alternating increases and decreases in an abnormally elevated plasma viscosity. Following myocardial infarction, viscosity became normal. Plasma viscosity reflects the concentration of large asymmetric proteins in the blood, principally fibrinogen.[35] During ischemia, other factors in blood, such as thrombin and catecholamines, in physiologic concentrations, are potent local vasoconstrictors[37] and could influence large coronary artery size, microvascular resistance, or stenosis diameter.

Increased myocardial oxygen demand alone probably accounts for a *minority* of unstable angina episodes. Increases in heart rate and blood pressure, arising spontaneously or from other conditions in patients with limited coronary reserve, can cause myocardial ischemia. Conditions such as infection, tachyarrhythmia, hypertension, thyrotoxicosis, and drug exposure (see Table 63.2) increase myocardial oxygen demand disproportionate to oxygen delivery to cause unstable angina.

NATURAL HISTORY

An understanding of the natural history or prognosis of the unstable angina patient is important to planning effective treatment. Risks and benefits of various therapeutic modalities need to be weighed against assessment of the course of illness in any given patient. Unfortunately, the true natural course of unstable angina is unknown and probably not obtainable in today's setting. Data from reports employing "conventional" medical treatment (unnatural history) are widely variable, with the risk of myocardial infarction ranging from 0 to 34% over a follow-up period of 4 months.[38–41] The risk of death ranges from 0 to 29% in these trials. The general consensus, based on recent prospective studies using more uniform criteria, is that the clinical course of unstable angina is less frequently associated with either death or myocardial infarction than suggested from older reports. The course of various subgroups, summarized from data acquired by the National Heart Lung and Blood Institute cooperative study group to compare medical and surgical therapy in unstable angina, is illustrated in Figure 63.3. This study excluded patients with left main stenosis, prior treatment failures, and coronary anatomy or left ventricular function not suitable for surgery (i.e., those without important stenoses and those with extensive diffuse disease). The frequency of myocardial infarction during initial hospitalization was 8% and frequency of death was 3% in 147 patients receiving only medical treatment.[41] The course of medically treated patients followed for 30 months or more revealed that 14% had myocardial infarction and 6% died. Over this period of time, about 36% of medically treated patients developed unsatisfactory control of angina at rest or on effort and required rehospitalization for bypass surgery. Accordingly, initial and long-term therapy should be directed toward preventing infarction and death in addition to relieving ischemia. The greatest period of risk for myocardial infarction or death appears to be

TABLE 63.2 AGGRAVATING FACTORS IN UNSTABLE ANGINA

Factor	Examples
Environment	Smoking Stress (emotional) Cold exposure
Associated illness	Anemia Thyrotoxicosis Hypertension Arrhythmia Infection Polycythemia Hypoxemia
Vasoconstricting drugs	Nonprescription antihistamine and decongestant preparations Illegal drugs (e.g., cocaine, amphetamines)
Other drugs that rarely precipitate rest angina	Dihydropyridine calcium antagonists (nifedipine, nicardipine) Dipyridamole
Antianginal drugs abruptly withdrawn	Nitrates Nifedipine β-Blockers

early after presentation owing to a change in symptoms. Therapy should be instituted early and be particularly intense during the hours to days immediately after presentation in an attempt to prevent early ischemic events.

Identification of patients at high risk for ischemic events is important in determining appropriate therapy. As in other patients with ischemic heart disease, demographic features such as age, sex, and previous myocardial infarction are important to help predict outcome. Some characteristics of the ST segment shift may also be important. Patients with ST segment shifts that persist are at particularly high risk, but the type of ST segment change is not helpful as a predictor of events. In the NHLBI study, 79 of 288 patients had ST segment elevation, their initial infarction rate was 13%, and their death rate was 5%. There was no significant difference between initial event rates when patients with ST segment elevation were compared with either the entire group or those with ST segment depression.[41] Pre-existing evidence of severe coronary disease, in the form of a long history of angina or an old myocardial infarction, is a predictor of higher risk. Neither severity nor persistence of symptoms, however, seems to be an important risk factor. Hemodynamic changes such as blood pressure alterations, raised left ventricular filling pressure, and auscultatory findings such as gallop rhythm and so on do not appear to help predict the course of the patient with unstable angina. The status of left ventricular function (low ejection fraction or heart failure) is a potent, independent predictor of risk. Although not definitely proven, it is my view that the angiographic morphology of the coronary lesion may help to identify patients at high risk for subsequent cardiac events, such as myocardial infarction or sudden death. Patients with "complex lesions" appear to be at highest risk, while those with coronary spasm superimposed on minimal atherosclerosis are at lowest risk. The presence of left anterior descending coronary artery disease is not a useful predictor of such events.[41]

Important prognostic information has become available from studies of ST segment depression recorded by Holter monitoring in patients with unstable angina pectoris.[42–45] Taken collectively, these reports, which concern approximately 200 patients followed for 3 months to 2 years, provide strong evidence to suggest that the presence of recurrent ischemia documented by transient ST segment depression identifies a subgroup at high risk for events (Fig. 63.4).[44] Approximately 90% of these ischemic episodes were asymptomatic, and these observations were made during therapy with nitrates, β-blockers, and calcium antagonists, which controlled symptoms in the majority of

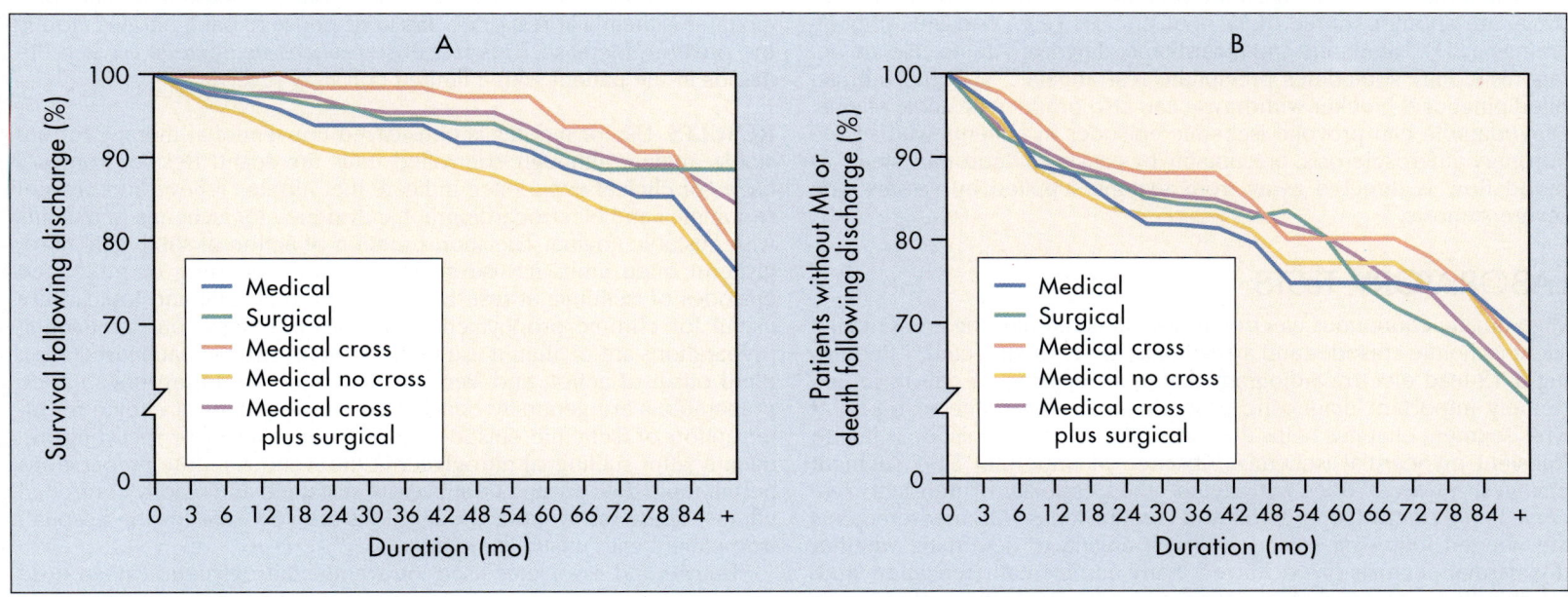

FIGURE 63.3 A. Survival of patients with unstable angina from various subgroups of the NHLBI cooperative trial. The 142 patients assigned to initial medical therapy (*blue line*) were not significantly different from any other subgroup over 7 years of follow-up. **B.** Percent of patients without myocardial infarction or death following discharge. The 142 patients assigned to initial medical therapy were not significantly different from any other group over 7 years of follow-up. (Modified from Conti CR: Unstable angina: Long-term follow-up of surgical and medical treatment. In Rafflenbeul W, Lichtlen PR, Balcon R (eds): Unstable Angina Pectoris, p 180. New York, Thieme-Stratton, 1981)

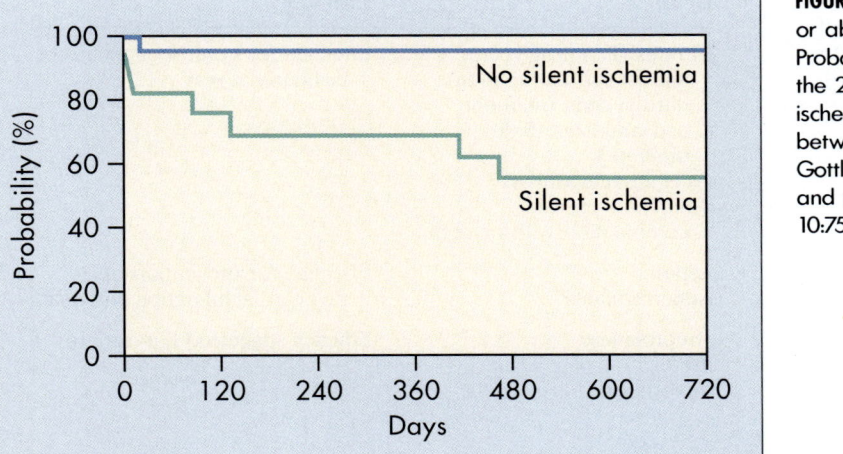

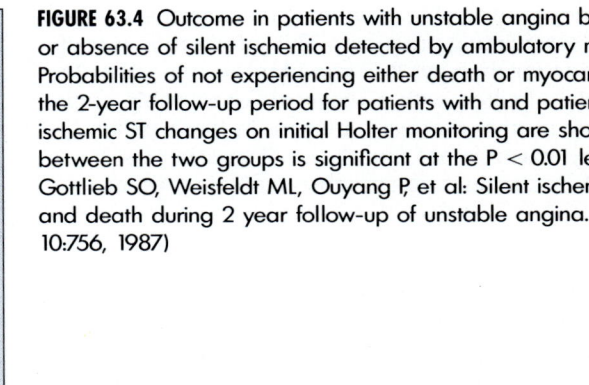

FIGURE 63.4 Outcome in patients with unstable angina based on the presence or absence of silent ischemia detected by ambulatory monitoring. Probabilities of not experiencing either death or myocardial infarction over the 2-year follow-up period for patients with and patients without silent ischemic ST changes on initial Holter monitoring are shown. The difference between the two groups is significant at the $P < 0.01$ level. (Modified from Gottlieb SO, Weisfeldt ML, Ouyang P, et al: Silent ischemia predicts infarction and death during 2 year follow-up of unstable angina. J Am Coll Cardiol 10:756, 1987)

cases. Those subjects who had prolonged ischemia (*e.g.*, greater than 60 minutes of silent ischemia per 24 hours of monitoring) were at highest risk.[43,45] Those with proximal coronary artery lesions appeared more likely to have prolonged ischemia.[45]

THERAPY
GENERAL MEASURES

The physician, patient, and family must appreciate that unstable angina is a serious illness. Those who care for these patients must be prepared to deal with potential consequences such as recurrent ischemia and acute myocardial infarction. General medical measures should include hospitalization with bed rest in a quiet environment. Evaluation should be aimed at confirming the diagnosis and identifying any possible aggravating factors, such as anemia, thyrotoxicosis, hypertension, arrhythmia, and infection. An independent precipitating factor may be noncompliance with taking medication. Treatment or removal of aggravating conditions should be initiated immediately when they are identified. Cessation of smoking and reduction of emotional stress are highly desirable. Some drugs frequently used in patients with ischemic heart disease may also contribute to an unstable angina syndrome (see Table 63.2). Vasoconstricting drugs are common in nonprescription antihistamine and decongestant preparations. Illegal psychoactive drugs are another source of vasoconstrictors (*e.g.*, cocaine, amphetamines, LSD). Nifedipine and nicardipine, dihydropyridine calcium antagonists, may sometimes precipitate rest angina.[46,47] Abrupt nitrate, nifedipine, or β-blocker withdrawal can also produce unstable angina. Dipyridamole can provoke ischemic episodes in patients with severe coronary atherosclerosis, presumably by causing a "coronary steal" as blood flow is directed away from regions supplied by vessels with severe stenosis.[48]

LABORATORY TESTS

High-quality continuous electrocardiographic monitoring is essential if silent ischemic episodes and arrhythmias are to be detected.[49] Recording a 12-lead electrocardiogram during an episode of pain is an extremely important diagnostic procedure. The presence of transient ST-T segment changes helps document that the pain episode is due to transient myocardial ischemia. Absence of important ST-T segment changes, however, does not exclude the possibility of transient ischemia. Serial electrocardiograms and creatine kinase MB measurements are needed following episodes of rest angina to determine whether myocardial necrosis has occurred. Early cardiac catheterization studies should be planned. More than any other test, these studies are important in defining coronary anatomy and in detecting coronary spasm, nonocclusive thrombus, and other dynamic coronary vascular factors. This is true particularly when coronary angiography is done during a spontaneous episode of chest pain or ST segment shift.[49] If coronary narrowings are found, the response to intracoronary nitroglycerin should aid in the identification of spasm.[50] Information from the catheterization study is invaluable in defining mechanisms involved in rest angina and in determining prognosis. This information is useful in suggesting directions for therapy. It is important to remember that 5% to 10% of patients admitted with a diagnosis of unstable angina have normal or nearly normal coronary arteries. In these patients, if evidence for coronary spasm is not found, the diagnosis must be revised. In another 10%, left main coronary obstruction is present.

GOALS

A major goal of therapy should be to relieve and prevent myocardial ischemia rather than only episodes of chest pain because of the relatively high frequency of asymptomatic transient ischemic episodes.[49] Because transient coronary flow reduction is the event initiating ischemia at rest in the majority of cases, therapy should be directed toward this event. The overall goals, however, must be to stabilize the clinical condition of the patient and prevent myocardial infarction and death. A number of therapeutic approaches can be used alone or in combination (Table 63.3).

PHARMACOLOGIC APPROACHES
NITRATES

RATIONALE. The rationale for use of nitrates in unstable angina is complex. Pharmacologically, nitrates relax vascular smooth muscle. In chronic stable effort angina, nitrates are effective in reducing myocardial oxygen requirements through reduction in myocardial wall tension mediated by reduced blood pressure and ventricular volumes. With the evidence that reduction in coronary flow initiates or perpetuates attacks of ischemia at rest in patients with unstable angina, other effects of nitrates become important. Nitrates dilate large coronary arteries and stenoses while enlarging collateral channels.[51] Nitrates also probably improve both the regional and transmural distribution of blood flow toward ischemic zones. These effects could improve regional blood flow in patients with important coronary obstruction due to atherosclerosis.[52] Nitrates relieve and prevent coronary artery spasm.[53] They also decrease platelet aggregability through stimulation of prostacyclin synthesis by endothelial cells and inhibitional thromboxane A_2 synthesis.[54,55] In patients who have a blood pressure increase that either precipitates ischemia at rest or occurs in response to pain, nitrates modify the pressure increase. This response reduces myocardial oxygen demands in the patient with a limited coronary reserve.

RESULTS. Use of nitrates is considered conventional therapy for unstable angina, although controlled trials are scant. Results from decades of clinical experience indicate that nitrates relieve and prevent rest angina and electrocardiographic evidence for ischemia in patients with unstable angina. The short duration of action of sublingual nitroglycerin often limits its use in patients with recurring or prolonged episodes of ischemia at rest. Long-acting forms (oral and topical) are useful for chronic prophylactic ambulatory therapy, but long-acting preparations are of limited use in the acutely unstable patient requiring rapid onset of action and frequent dose titration. Intravenous nitrate preparations are generally considered the treatment of choice for interruption of ischemic episodes at rest not relieved or recurring frequently after sublingual nitroglycerin. Intravenous nitrate preparations permit rapid delivery and titration with sustained and readily controlled effects. These intravenous preparations are very safe for the hospitalized patient with unstable angina.

Dauwe and associates used intravenous nitroglycerin (mean dose

TABLE 63.3 PHARMACOTHERAPY OF UNSTABLE ANGINA

Drug	Efficacy
Nitrates (IV nitroglycerin and isosorbide dinitrate; nitroglycerin ointment and oral isosorbide dinitrate)	Effective for control of recurrent ischemia at rest
Calcium antagonists	
β-Blockers used in combination with nitrates	
Aspirin	Effective for prevention of myocardial infarction and death
Anticoagulants	
Streptokinase	Efficacy suggested but not proven
rt-PA	
Amiodarone	

of 47 µg/min, range 9 µg to 180 µg) for 7 days (mean) in 14 patients with unstable rest angina despite propranolol and long-acting nitrates.[56] All 14 patients responded, and when intravenous nitroglycerin was discontinued in three, angina recurred. Mikolich and colleagues summarized data on 45 unstable angina patients who received intravenous nitroglycerin (mean dose 54 µg/min, range 5 µg to 267 µg), and 40 patients (89%) responded.[57] Twenty-four of the twenty-eight patients who had not responded to multiple sublingual tablets responded to intravenous nitroglycerin. Interestingly, there was only a 5 mm Hg decline in systolic blood pressure, without significant change in heart rate. Similar results were reported by DePace and co-workers in 20 patients who had three or more rest angina episodes a day while receiving other nitrate preparations.[58] With a mean dose of 72 µg/min (range 15 µg to 226 µg) 17 patients (85%) responded. Kaplan and co-workers treated 35 patients with rest angina who were unresponsive to oral or topical nitrates and β-blockers with intravenous nitroglycerin (mean dose 140 µg/min, range 50 µg to 350 µg).[59] A beneficial response was seen in 33 patients (94%), and morphine use also decreased significantly. Distante and associates demonstrated dramatic reduction or prevention of both symptomatic and asymptomatic ischemic episodes occurring at rest using continuous isosorbide dinitrate infusion.[60] This study used continuous electrocardiographic monitoring and a double-blind crossover placebo-controlled design in 12 patients with ischemia at rest.

Curfman and associates conducted a prospective randomized study comparing intravenous nitroglycerin to a combination of isosorbide dinitrate and nitroglycerin ointment in 40 consecutive patients with two or more episodes of spontaneous angina over a 48-hour period.[61] Some patients had asymptomatic ischemic episodes documented by electrocardiographic monitoring. The doses of intravenous nitroglycerin (10 µg to 200 µg/min) and isosorbide dinitrate (20 mg to 60 mg) plus nitroglycerin ointment (1 to 2 inches), both given every 6 hours, were adjusted so that mean blood pressure was reduced similarly. Both treatment groups received β-blockers titrated to maintain a resting heart rate of 45 to 60 beats per minute. Both nitrate treatment regimens significantly reduced the number of spontaneous ischemic episodes. Intravenous nitroglycerin, however, provided a more consistent and sustained beneficial effect over the first 2 days as ischemic episodes tended to recur in patients given isosorbide dinitrate and nitroglycerin ointment. Effects of long-term nitrate therapy on cardiac events in unstable angina are unknown.

RECOMMENDATIONS. From the foregoing, it is reasonable to conclude that nitrates in general are very beneficial in unstable angina, and intravenous preparations offer an advantage for initial therapy. After the patient's condition has stabilized, long-acting nitrates in the form of oral isosorbide dinitrate or nitroglycerin ointment are recommended to prevent recurrence of transient ischemic episodes. Continuous high-dose nitrate therapy, however, is likely to result in tolerance. While the clinical importance of nitrate tolerance in patients with unstable angina has not been determined, avoidance of high doses given "around the clock" by use of doses titrated to prevent ischemia and eccentric dosing schedules may minimize the development of tolerance.

β-ADRENERGIC BLOCKERS

RATIONALE. Like nitrates, β-blockers have also been considered part of "standard therapy" of unstable angina without adequately controlled trials. Unlike nitrates, however, the rationale for use of β-blockers is not clear. β-Blocker use evolved from a period before the pathophysiologic mechanisms responsible for the onset of transient ischemia in patients with rest angina were understood. Previously, unstable angina was thought to represent simply a severe form of chronic effort angina. Because β-blockers prevent the rise in heart rate, blood pressure, and contractility that causes effort-induced ischemia, these agents were also used in unstable angina. We now know that few patients with unstable angina have increases in the determinants of myocardial oxygen demand to precipitate rest angina. Accordingly, it might be expected that β-blockers would either not be beneficial or, if beneficial, act through some other mechanisms.

RESULTS. Results of uncontrolled observations by Papazogtov and Fischl and co-workers suggested that propranolol relieved rest pain in this syndrome.[62,63] Conti and colleagues reported 57 patients treated during initial hospitalization with β-blockers in addition to bed rest, nitrates, and anticoagulants.[64] Three patients died during initial hospitalization, and 14 continued to receive medical treatment alone. The authors concluded that initial improvement could be obtained with medical therapy. A controlled trial by Guazzi and associates found that β-blockers (practolol or propranolol) abolished spontaneous angina in patients with either ST segment depression or elevation as compared with placebo.[65] Substitution of placebo for active β-blocker caused prompt reappearance of symptoms. The mean dose of propranolol was 368 mg a day, and these patients were not taking long-acting nitrates. In patients with unstable angina, Cairns and colleagues and Yusuf and co-workers suggested that β-blockers produce a myocardial "protective" effect.[66,67] However, criteria for diagnosis of eventual infarction and follow-up of these patients did not include further chest pain. It is likely that many of these patients already had inevitable infarction when they were admitted before definitive electrocardiographic and enzyme changes developed.

Uncontrolled reports countering the favorable results reviewed above are numerous, and some relate to use of surgical therapy in patients whose angina recurred with β-blocker therapy. Gold and colleagues reported that propranolol, in combination with long-acting nitrates, failed to prevent recurrence of rest ischemia in nine patients.[68] There are case reports suggesting that spontaneously occurring Prinzmetal's angina may be aggravated by β-blockers.[69–71] A controlled trial done in patients with Prinzmetal's angina suggested that ischemic episodes, detected by continuous electrocardiographic recordings, were prolonged during propranolol treatment as compared with periods of placebo treatment.[71]

There are several controlled trials reported that assess the short-term effects of β-blockers compared with those of placebo in patients with unstable angina. A randomized double-blind crossover trial by Capucci and co-workers examined effects of propranolol, verapamil, and placebo in 18 patients with unstable angina associated with electrocardiographic changes (7 had elevation and 11 had depression of ST segments).[72] Thirteen of 14 patients undergoing angiography had severe coronary artery disease. Mean angina frequency was 3.0 and 2.3 episodes a day during two placebo periods and 1.7 episodes a day with propranolol (240 mg/day) (Fig. 63.5). Parodi and co-workers conducted a controlled trial using a double crossover protocol in ten patients with unstable angina.[73] Total ischemic episodes were counted from continuous electrocardiographic tape recordings. The response to propranolol (300 mg/day) was similar to the response observed with placebo (Fig. 63.6). In both the Capucci and the Parodi studies, verapamil was very effective (see below).

The value of the addition of propranolol to coronary vasodilators (nitrates and nifedipine) in 81 patients with unstable angina was assessed by Gottlieb and co-workers[74] in a randomized double-blind placebo-controlled 4-week trial. The incidences of cardiac death and myocardial infarction and the requirements for revascularization were no different when comparing those receiving the addition of propranolol with those receiving placebo. The propranolol group, however, had a significantly lower cumulative probability of experiencing recurrent rest angina and a reduced duration and frequency of painful (angina) and silent ischemic episodes by continuous electrocardiographic recording compared with the placebo group.

A longer-term trial comparing atenolol against placebo and heparin was performed by Telford and Wilson in patients with intermediate syndrome.[75] After one week, transmural myocardial infarction developed in 9 of 54 patients (17%) assigned placebo and eight of 60 (13%) assigned atenolol (P = NS). Two early deaths occurred in the placebo group, while no deaths occurred in the atenolol group. Between 1 and 8 weeks, myocardial infarction occurred in one placebo-treated patient, and readmission for increasing angina without infarction occurred in two additional patients. In the atenolol group, two patients had myocardial infarction while six were readmitted for increasing pain without infarction and three deaths occurred. Comparing all 109 patients who received atenolol with those who did not (Table 63.4) shows that atenolol did not change the infarction or death rate as compared with the 105 patients who did not receive the β-blocker. Heparin, however, appeared effective (see below).

Comparison trials have also been done without placebo controls. In one short-term controlled trial, Muller and co-workers randomly assigned either conventional therapy of propranolol plus isosorbide dinitrate or nifedipine to 133 patients with unstable angina.[76] They concluded that, overall, conventional therapy with propranolol and nitrates was equivalent to that achieved with nifedipine alone for controlling angina and preventing myocardial infarction or death. In the subgroup of 67 patients receiving propranolol prior to randomization, however, addition of nifedipine appeared more beneficial than increasing the propranolol dose in controlling pain. I presume that these were patients who had been receiving propranolol for chronic stable effort angina before admission for unstable angina. By contrast, the 59 patients not receiving prior propranolol, whom I presume were patients with relatively new-onset angina, appeared to benefit more from propranolol than from nifedipine for pain control. These results suggest clinically useful pathways for treatment of patients presenting with unstable angina. However, it could be argued that because this trial did not have a placebo control it is not possible to tell whether both regimens were equally effective or equally ineffective. A more recent multicenter, double-blind, placebo-controlled trial examined the effects of nifedipine, metoprolol, and their combination in 338 patients not pretreated with a β-blocker.[77] Nifedipine was evaluated in another 177 patients pretreated with a β-blocker. Recurrent ischemia or myocardial infarction within 48 hours was reduced by metoprolol in patients not previously taking a β-blocker. Combination of metoprolol with nifedipine, in fixed doses, provided no further benefit, and use of nifedipine

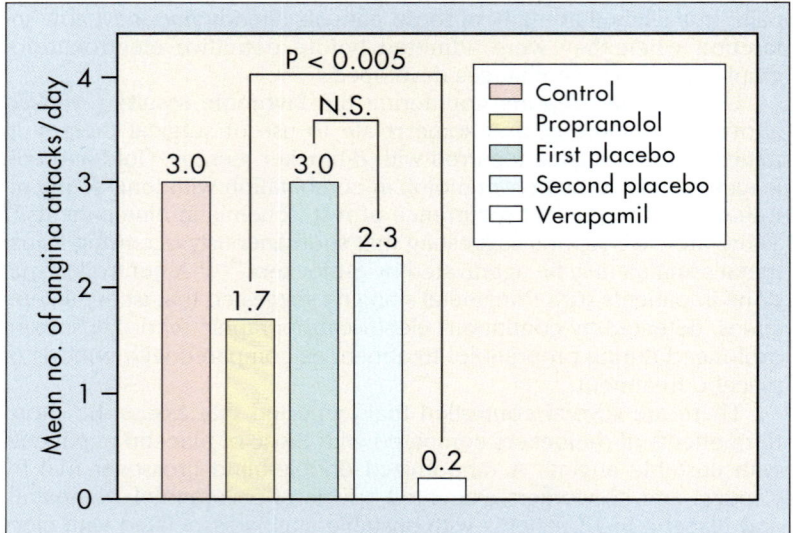

FIGURE 63.5 Results of a placebo-controlled trial examining effects of propranolol and verapamil in 18 patients with unstable angina. Mean angina frequency during the control period was similar to angina frequency observed during the first and second double-blind placebo periods. Propranolol decreased the frequency of angina minimally. However, verapamil caused a dramatic reduction in angina frequency compared with either propranolol or placebo-controlled periods. (Modified from Capucci di A, Bracchetti D, Carini G et al: Confronto in doppio cieco fra verapamil e propanololo nella terapia dell'angina instabile. Boll Soc Ital Cardiol 27:447, 1982)

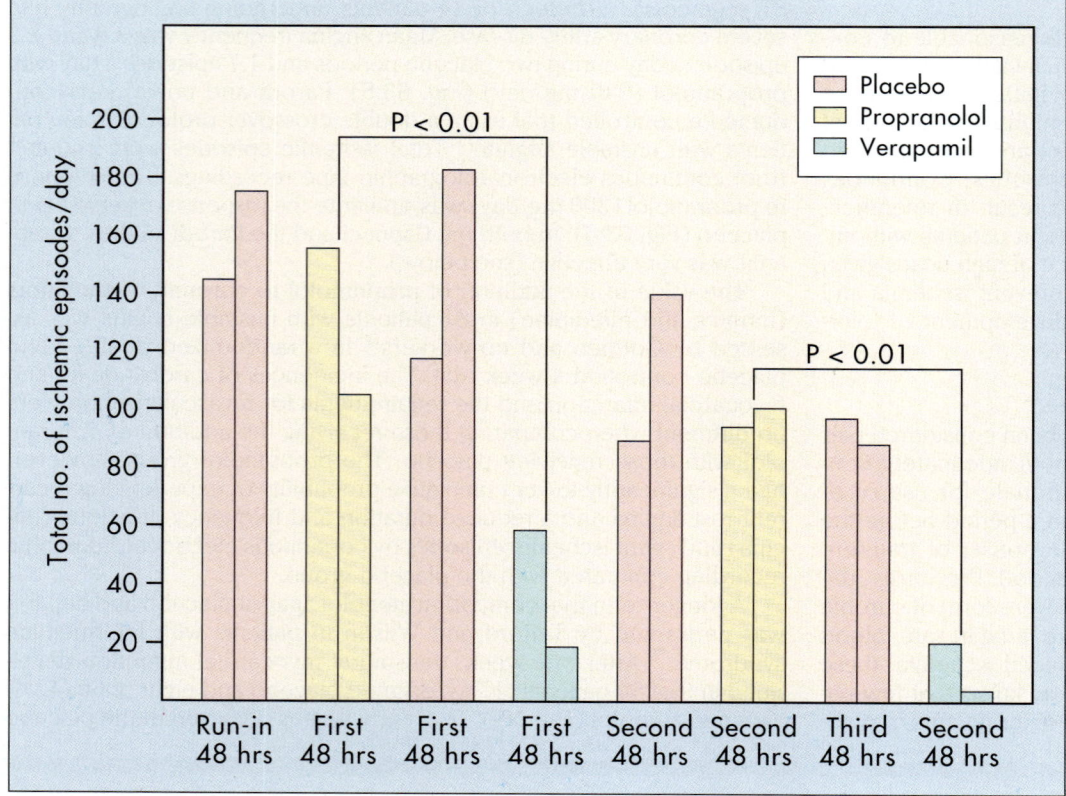

FIGURE 63.6 Results of a double-blind, placebo-controlled, double-crossover trial comparing effects of propranolol and verapamil with placebo in 12 patients with unstable angina. Total number of ischemic episodes (painful and silent) per 24-hour period tabulated from continuously recorded electrocardiograms is shown on the vertical axis. Propranolol treatment produced no significant change in the frequency of these episodes compared with adjacent placebo periods. Verapamil, however, caused a statistically significant reduction in the frequency of ischemic episodes compared with either the adjacent propranolol or placebo periods. (Modified from Parodi O, Simonetti I, L'Abbate A: Verapamil versus propranolol for angina at rest. Am J Cardiol 50:923, 1982)

alone was possibly detrimental. In patients receiving prior β-blockade, however, the addition of nifedipine was beneficial.

Fouet and associates compared propranolol and diltiazem using a single-blind trial in 70 patients with unstable angina.[78] Twenty-nine had ST segment elevation and forty-one had other repolarization changes. Treatment was randomized and considered successful when spontaneous pain was completely prevented. Overall, there was no difference between the response observed with propranolol and that seen with diltiazem. Among the 24 patients with only rest pain, however, 9 of 13 were successfully treated with diltiazem, while treatment of all 11 treated with propranolol failed. Eight of these 11 patients with propranolol failures were immediately successfully treated when crossed over to diltiazem. The authors concluded that diltiazem was preferable to propranolol. More recently, Theroux and associates compared propranolol and diltiazem in 100 patients with unstable angina after excluding all patients who either had ST segment elevation or were receiving β-blockers on admission.[79] All patients were also given isosorbide dinitrate (120 mg daily) concurrent with the study drug. Results of in-hospital 1-month and 5-month follow-up results with propranolol were not significantly different from those seen with diltiazem.

RECOMMENDATIONS. My interpretation of these trials is that initial treatment of unstable rest angina with β-blockers provides some possibly beneficial results. In most favorable reports, however, long-acting nitrates were also used and the beneficial result relates to combination therapy rather than therapy with a β-blocker alone. If β-blockers are beneficial, what is the mechanism responsible for improvement of rest angina? One possibility is that β-blockers interfere with neurologic pathways for pain transmission or alter central awareness of pain. Another possibility is that β-blockers depress myocardial contractility and slow resting heart rate minimally. Consequently, myocardial oxygen demands are more appropriately matched to the reduced coronary flow that occurs in unstable angina. Alternately, large doses of β-blockers may actually relieve spasm, dilate collaterals, or redistribute coronary blood flow. It is also possible that propranolol reverses abnormal platelet aggregability in patients with ischemia.[80]

CALCIUM ANTAGONISTS

RATIONALE. Calcium channel blockers are a relatively new class of drugs that is extremely effective in relieving and preventing coronary spasm through a mechanism different from that of nitroglycerin. Calcium blockers have the ability to dilate coronary arterioles and alter responses of large coronary arteries to certain stimuli, enhancing blood flow to jeopardized myocardial regions. These compounds reduce myocardial oxygen demands through peripheral vasodilatation and reduction of systolic wall tension and myocardial contractility. An effective coronary action can be achieved at doses that cause no or only minimal myocardial depression. Their peripheral vascular effects, acting to reduce ventricular loading, provide reflex cardiac stimulation counteracting the myocardial depression. In most persons with relatively normal or minimally depressed ventricular function, net depression in function is not observed. These agents also inhibit platelet aggregation. A comprehensive review of the pharmacology of calcium antagonists appears elsewhere in these volumes.

RESULTS. Results of calcium antagonist use in unstable angina from controlled and uncontrolled studies deal with both the subset of patients with Prinzmetal's angina and the more general group with unstable angina. Approximately 80% of Prinzmetal's angina patients become pain free over the short term with calcium channel blocker treatment.[81] Results dealing with only Prinzmetal's angina are reviewed in detail elsewhere in this volume. In the more common variety of unstable angina, that associated with ST segment depression or T wave changes and not limited to ST segment elevation, calcium antagonists are also extremely effective. Uncontrolled experiences indicate that addition of nifedipine (30 mg to 120 mg/day) prevents rest or spontaneous angina in about 80% of patients whose symptoms were unresponsive to nitrates and propranolol alone.[82-84] Improvement was maintained, in many cases, over short- and intermediate-term follow-up. Withdrawal from nifedipine resulted in recurrence of rest angina in many but not all patients in whom this maneuver was attempted.

There are a few controlled trials comparing calcium blockers with placebo. In the trials of Parodi and colleagues and Capucci and colleagues discussed under β-blocker therapy, the response to verapamil was also evaluated (Figs. 63.5 and 63.6).[72,73] Both groups found highly significant reduction in the frequency of ischemia at rest using verapamil as compared with either placebo or propranolol. Both symptomatic and asymptomatic ischemic episodes were prevented by verapamil. In another placebo-controlled trial, Mehta and co-workers found that verapamil (320 mg to 480 mg) was effective in 13 of 15 patients with unstable angina associated with ST segment shifts.[85] These patients were taking only sublingual nitroglycerin. Gerstenblith and associates randomly assigned either placebo or nifedipine to 138 patients with unstable angina who were receiving propranolol plus nitrates.[86] Early (4 months) and long-term results showed no differences between

TABLE 63.4 FREQUENCY OF ISCHEMIC EVENTS IN A CONTROLLED TRIAL COMPARING ATENOLOL, HEPARIN, AND PLACEBO

	No. of Patients	Transmural Myocardial Infarction	Deaths	Readmission for Cardiac Pain Without Infarction
First Week of Trial				
Placebo	54	9 (17%)	2	
Atenolol	60	8 (13%)	0	
Heparin	51	1 (2%)	0	
Heparin and atenolol	49	2 (4%)	0	
Between 1 and 8 Weeks				
Placebo	54	1	0	2
Atenolol	60	2	3	6
Heparin	51	1	0	2
Heparin and atenolol	49	3	0	2

(Data from Telford AM, Wilson C: Trial of heparin versus atenolol in prevention of myocardial infarction in intermediate coronary syndrome. Lancet 1:1225, 1981)

the treatments in the frequency of either death or myocardial infarction (Fig. 63.7).[87] Failure of treatment to prevent the need for bypass surgery due to recurrence of symptoms was reduced in patients taking nifedipine, but this effect was seen only in the subgroup with ST segment elevation. These results were similar to those found by Muller and colleagues.[76] In a multicenter, double-blind, placebo-controlled study,[77] nifedipine given without β-blockers was not beneficial and possibly detrimental but when unstable angina evolved while patients were receiving a β-blocker, the addition of nifedipine was beneficial. The comparison trials of diltiazem versus propranolol indicate that diltiazem is also effective in unstable angina.[78,79]

I reported results in the initial year of treatment with either nifedipine, verapamil, or diltiazem initiated as monotherapy in 45 patients with rest angina who were responders during short-term controlled trials (Table 63.5).[88] Approximately 50% of the patients required additional antianginal drugs to control rest angina during the year, and myocardial infarction and death continued to occur despite control of rest angina. These events, however, occurred only in the patients with severe coronary artery disease. Another trial by Blaustein and colleagues evaluated the adjunctive role of nifedipine in 47 patients whose unstable angina was refractory to nitrates and β-blockers.[89] Twenty-two (47%) improved significantly over an average follow-up of 12 months, but despite improvement 8 of these had cardiac events within the first 4 months. Eighteen other patients had no symptomatic improvement, and 7 of these had cardiac events within the first 4 months. In another 7 patients, relief was not sufficient to permit discharge, and 1 of these patients had an ischemic event. An early symptomatic response did not predict the subsequent incidence of cardiac events.

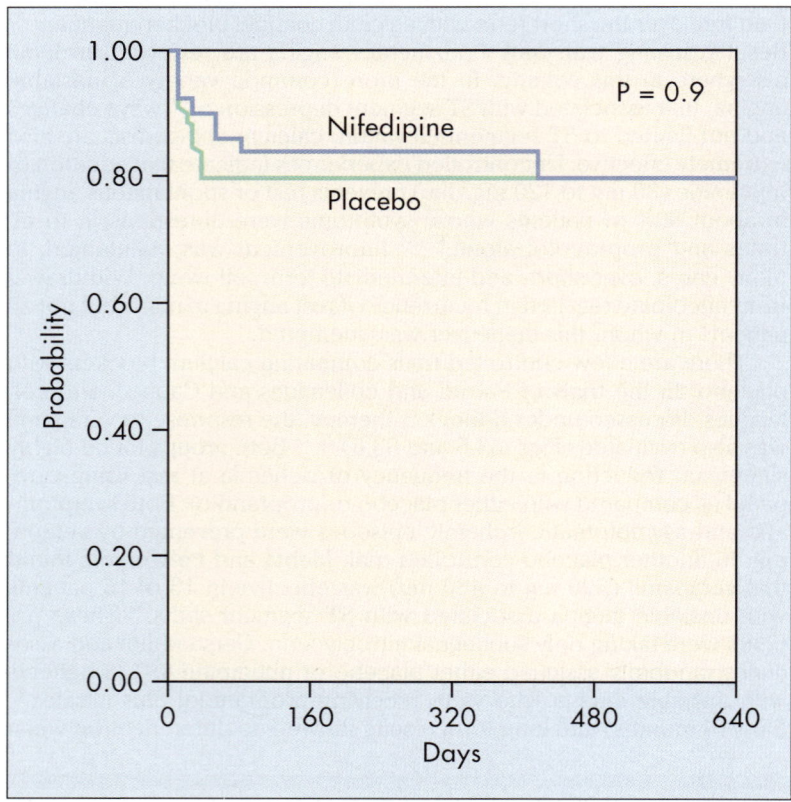

FIGURE 63.7 The effect of adding nifedipine or placebo to standard therapy consisting of a β-blocker and long-acting nitrates on morbidity and mortality in 138 unstable angina patients. The probability that therapy could prevent myocardial infarction or death is shown on the vertical axis. Over the course of follow-up of almost 2 years, addition of nifedipine had no important effect in prevention of myocardial infarction or death. (Modified from Ouyang P, Brinker J, Mellits ED et al: Variables predictive of successful medical therapy in patients with unstable angina: Selection by multivariate analysis from clinical, electrocardiographic, and angiographic evaluations. Circulation 70:367, 1984)

TABLE 63.5 CLINICAL OUTCOME FOR ALL PATIENTS DURING INITIAL YEAR OF THERAPY WITH A CALCIUM ANTAGONIST

	Total (n = 45)	Coronary Angiography		CAS (n = 35)
		CAD (n = 27)	No CAD (n = 18)	
Number of Patients				
"Good" response	29 (64%)	18 (67%)	11 (61%)	24 (69%)
"Fair" response	2 (4%)	0	2 (7%)	2 (6%)
"Unchanged"	1 (2%)	1 (4%)	0	1 (3%)
Coronary events	13 (29%)	9 (33%)	4 (22%)	9 (25%)
Number of Events by Type				
Sudden death	3	3	0	1
Myocardial infarction	5	5	0	2
Hospitalization (↑AP/ROMI/CAB)	8	4	4	6

↑AP, unacceptable increase in angina; ROMI, exclude myocardial infarction; CAB, coronary artery bypass surgery; CAD, coronary artery disease; CAS, coronary artery spasm either proven by angiography or suspected by transient ST.

Electrocardiographic changes occurring with rest pain did not identify a group either at higher risk or with a better response to nifedipine. The authors concluded that patients who are unresponsive to nitrates and β-blockers constitute a high-risk subset of unstable angina and that nifedipine, while controlling symptoms and the need for bypass surgery, does not prevent morbidity or mortality.

RECOMMENDATIONS. The information available strongly supports the view that calcium antagonists are very effective in the initial treatment of unstable angina. These drugs appear to control rest pain and verapamil also has been shown to control asymptomatic ischemic episodes. However, there is no evidence to suggest that either myocardial infarction or death is prevented in long-term follow-up. Use of nifedipine, without a β-blocker, however, may not be effective and is possibly detrimental in some patients. I suspect that this relates to potent reflex sympathetic stimulation in patients with severe stenosis who have minimal to no dynamic component to their coronary obstruction. Use of these drugs is discussed elsewhere in this volume.

ANTICOAGULANTS

RATIONALE. For decades, the rationale for use of anticoagulation in unstable angina was to prevent coronary thrombosis, which was believed to be the cause of acute myocardial infarction.[90,91]

RESULTS. Several uncontrolled or inadequately controlled studies suggested that anticoagulation may improve prognosis in unstable angina.[90,91] Because the presence of coronary thrombosis was not conclusively established as a factor in acute Q wave myocardial infarction until the report of DeWood and associates in 1980,[92] and because of unenthusiastic reports, anticoagulation for ischemic heart disease became unpopular. However, evidence supporting a role for intracoronary thrombus in unstable angina as well as acute transmural myocardial infarction has renewed interest in anticoagulation. Telford and Wilson reported a randomized double-blind placebo-controlled study comparing heparin (5000 units IV every 6 hours), atenolol (100 mg a day), a combination of both, and placebo in 214 patients with unstable angina.[75] Heparin was continued for 7 days, after which all patients under 65 years of age received warfarin for 8 weeks. After 1 week, myocardial infarction developed in 17% of patients receiving placebo (see Table 63.4) and 13% of those taking atenolol, but only 2% of patients receiving heparin alone and 4% of those receiving heparin plus atenolol developed infarction. These early results were highly significant and the benefit of anticoagulation was maintained for 8 weeks. These findings confirmed an earlier report by Wood, which suggested that 3% of unstable angina patients who were treated by anticoagulants had infarctions and 6% died, whereas 22% of patients not treated with anticoagulants had infarctions and 30% died.[91]

RECOMMENDATIONS. As Wood stated in 1961, these differences are clearly impressive.[91] Management of the unstable angina syndrome should include intravenous heparin when contraindications to anticoagulation are absent.

THROMBOLYTIC AGENTS

RATIONALE. The evidence demonstrating intracoronary thrombus in patients with unstable angina provides the basis for consideration of thrombolytic agents in this syndrome.[25-27,31]

RESULTS. Lawrence and associates randomized 40 unstable angina patients to either streptokinase (250,000 U over 30 minutes followed by 100,000 U/hr for 24 hours) or a control group.[93] Both groups received warfarin for 6 months. During this period, 8 of 20 patients (40%) not receiving streptokinase had events (four myocardial infarctions and four deaths), whereas only 1 of 20 (5%) given streptokinase had an event (death). Although there was no angiographic documentation that coronary thrombus was either present or altered by streptokinase in these cases, the results are encouraging. Streptokinase therapy is also known to reduce blood viscosity[94] and platelet adhesiveness,[95] both of which are increased in unstable angina patients.

Angiographic evidence for thrombolysis following intracoronary streptokinase was documented in five of seven unstable angina patients by Vetrovec and associates and four of nine patients by Mandelkorn and associates.[25,26] Narrowed coronary arteries improved following intracoronary administration of urokinase in 20 of 21 patients studied by Gotoh and associates.[96]

Gold and co-workers[97] examined effects of recombinant tissue plasminogen activator (rt-PA) in 24 patients with unstable rest angina associated with transient ST segment changes without recent myocardial infarction. All patients received nitrates, calcium antagonists, β-blockers, and heparin for 12 to 24 hours and were then randomized to receive a 12-hour intravenous infusion of either placebo or rt-PA (1.75 mg/kg). Thus, heparin was given to both groups. At coronary angiography most of the placebo-treated patients had intracoronary thrombus while none of the rt-PA–treated patients had intracoronary thrombus. A significant association was noted between the presence of intracoronary thrombus and recurrent angina. Bleeding, however, occurred in most of the rt-PA–treated patients. To determine if bleeding was related to combination rt-PA and heparin, 9 other patients were studied. Five received placebo while 4 received rt-PA without heparin. Bleeding still occurred in 3 of the 4 rt-PA–treated patients, and rt-PA alone failed to lyse intracoronary thrombus in 3 of these 4 patients.[98]

Evidence that suggested that development of acute myocardial infarction in patients hospitalized for unstable angina could be prevented by very early intervention with intracoronary streptokinase was presented by Davies and colleagues.[31] Eight patients hospitalized for unstable angina developed nine periods of chest pain persisting longer than 30 minutes and associated with anterior ST segment elevation, which was unresponsive to intravenous nitrates and verapamil. The left anterior descending artery was found to be totally occluded during seven periods, and it was reopened by intracoronary streptokinase (5000 U/min for 18 to 80 minutes) in five. No infarction developed in four of these instances.

RECOMMENDATIONS. These observations with thrombolytic therapy in unstable angina are exciting and merit further exploration, particularly with controlled trials. At present, the use of intracoronary thrombolytic agents may be warranted only in highly selected patients who develop symptoms in close proximity to demonstration of intracoronary thrombus.

ANTIPLATELET AGENTS

RATIONALE. Circumstantial evidence from animal studies implicating platelet aggregation and eicosanoids in myocardial ischemia and infarction forms the basis for use of antiplatelet agents.[20-22]

RESULTS. Prostaglandin E_1 infusion was evaluated in 19 patients with unstable angina by Siegle and associates.[99] This vasodilator and inhibitor of platelet aggregation significantly decreased the number of rest angina episodes and eliminated the need for intravenous nitroglycerin and morphine in ten patients. Adverse effects were generally minor. The authors concluded that this treatment may be of value.

Infusion of prostacyclin for 72 hours in an uncontrolled study by Szczeklik and colleagues in seven unstable angina patients reduced the frequency of angina.[100] This beneficial effect lasted for 2 to 3 months. Prostacyclin infusion failed to prevent induction of ST segment depression by atrial pacing in seven other patients with stable effort angina. Chierchia and co-workers compared prostacyclin with placebo in six patients with Prinzmetal's angina.[101] Although systemic vasodilation and reduction of platelet aggregation occurred, no effect on ischemic episodes was observed in five patients. In one patient, however, prostacyclin consistently abolished rest angina. In another study, this group administered intravenous aspirin to similar patients and found no effect on ischemic episodes recorded by continuous electrocardiographic monitoring, although thromboxane B_2 decreased dramatically.[102] In contrast, a thromboxane antagonist, phthalazinol, abolished rest angina in eight patients with Prinzmetal's angina.[103]

In the Veterans Administration Cooperative Trial,[23] 1266 men were randomized to receive either 324 mg/day buffered aspirin or placebo early after presentation for unstable angina. After 12 weeks, the frequencies of nonfatal myocardial infarction and death were significantly decreased (approximately 50%) in those receiving aspirin compared with placebo. These beneficial results were confirmed in a report by Cairns and associates of a randomized double-blind trial of aspirin (325 mg four times daily), sulfinpyrazone (200 mg four times daily), or placebo in 555 unstable angina patients of either sex.[24] After a mean follow-up of 19 months, the risk of nonfatal myocardial infarction and cardiac death was significantly reduced in those receiving aspirin but not sulfinpyrazone.

RECOMMENDATIONS. Aspirin appears to reduce the risk of myocardial infarction and death in patients with unstable angina. Its use is strongly recommended in patients of either sex for at least 2 years. Whether aspirin's beneficial effect is independent of that found with heparin has not been determined. Results relative to preventing rest angina due to coronary spasm by either aspirin or prostacyclin are mixed. Other drugs influencing platelet and prostaglandin pathways deserve further investigation in unstable rest angina.

OTHER POSSIBLY EFFECTIVE DRUGS

Alinidine, a sinus node inhibitor that does not interact with β-blockers, was given to 24 patients with unstable angina with heart rates exceeding 100 beats per minute by Simoons and Hugenholtz.[104] After doses up to 40 mg, alinidine decreased heart rate by 14 beats per minute (mean) and mean arterial pressure by 3 mm Hg. Signs of heart failure developed in three patients, although overall left ventricular filling pressure remained unchanged. The authors concluded that this potentially beneficial agent warranted further study. *Amiodarone*, originally introduced for angina and more recently shown effective for control of arrhythmias, has been used to control Prinzmetal's angina. This potent vasodilator, with α- and β-adrenergic antagonist activity, was evaluated for treatment of unstable angina by Bertholet and associates in a randomized controlled trial in 40 unstable-angina patients.[105] Initially, 20 patients received amiodarone (150 mg/day) intravenously plus 200 mg orally every 8 hours and 200 mg orally three times a day beginning on the fourth day). If angina recurred, nifedipine was added. In the other 20 patients, nifedipine was given as the initial drug. If nifedipine therapy failed, amiodarone was added according to the scheme described above. Initial treatment with amiodarone was successful within 8 hours in 12 of the 20 patients, while none of the 8 nonresponders improved

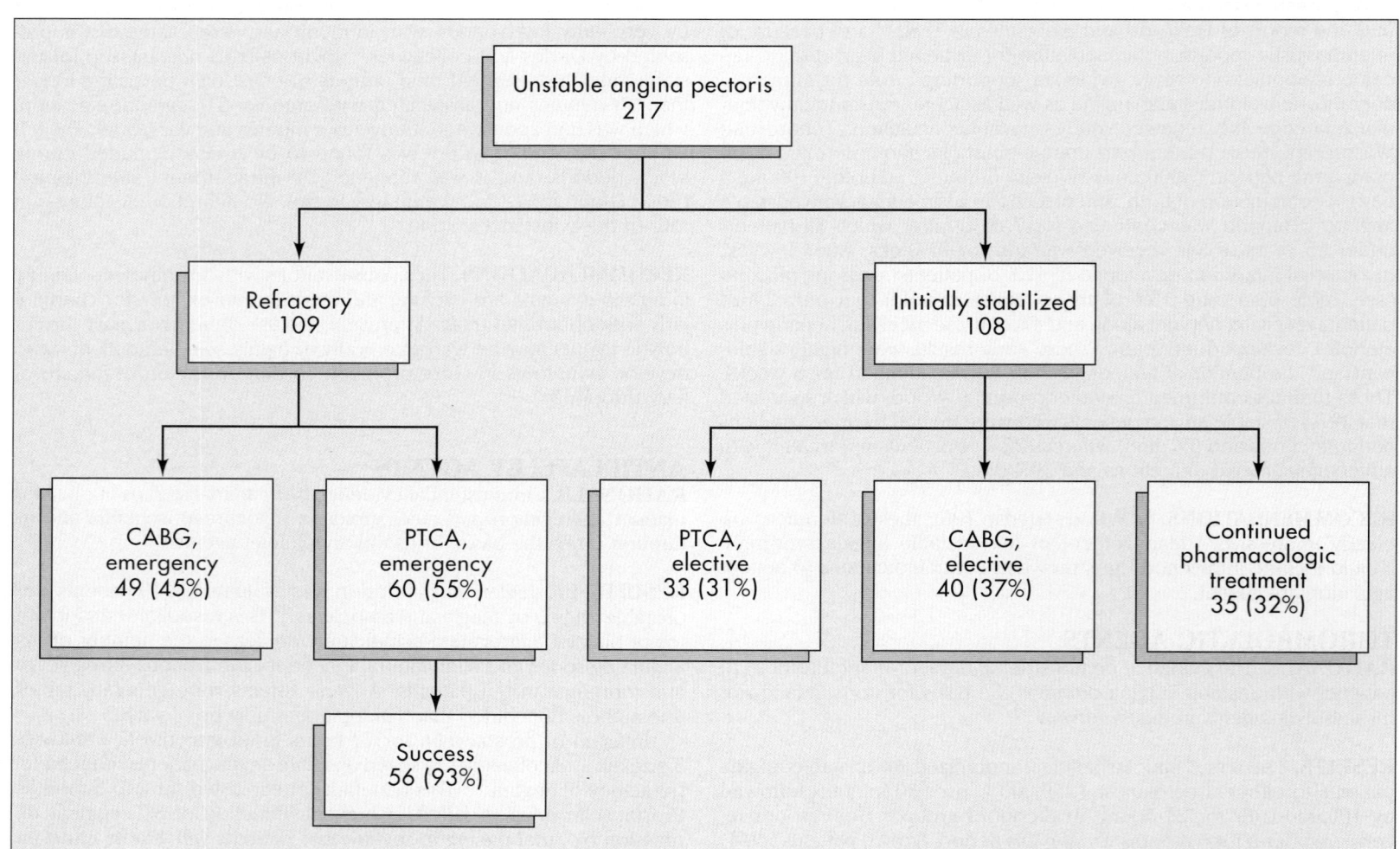

FIGURE 63.8 Emergency coronary angioplasty in refractory unstable angina. (CABG, coronary artery bypass graft; PTCA, percutaneous transluminal coronary angioplasty) (Data from De Feyter PJ, Serruys PW, Van Den Brand M et al: Emergency coronary angioplasty in refractory unstable angina. N Engl J Med 313:342, 1985)

with addition of nifedipine. Initial treatment with nifedipine was successful within 8 hours in 6 of 20 patients, but amiadarone controlled angina in 11 of the 14 nonresponders. The authors concluded that amiodarone has value for initial treatment of unstable angina. In my opinion, significant side effects will limit use of amiodarone in unstable angina.

NONPHARMACOLOGIC APPROACHES
PERCUTANEOUS TRANSLUMINAL CORONARY ANGIOPLASTY

RATIONALE. Knowledge that recent progression of severe coronary atherosclerosis frequently accompanies the onset of unstable angina then led to the use of percutaneous transluminal coronary angioplasty (PTCA) as treatment. Results with PTCA, in general, are known to be better with relatively recent onset of symptoms.

RESULTS. Several uncontrolled studies document a growing clinical experience with PTCA in unstable angina. Meyer and associates treated 47 patients with PTCA within 36 hours of admission for unstable rest angina.[106] The initial success rate was 72% compared with 68% in a parallel patient group with chronic stable angina. As noted previously, the location and severity of stenoses in the patients with chronic stable and unstable angina were similar. Likewise, complications after PTCA were similar in the stable and unstable angina groups. Williams and associates reported results in 17 patients with unstable angina initially treated with medical therapy followed by PTCA, which was successful in 13.[107] Faxon and associates summarized results of 442 patients from the National Heart, Lung, and Blood Institute (NHLBI)-PTCA Registry with unstable angina and one with vessel disease who underwent PTCA.[108] Both the immediate success rate and the complication rate were the same as the rates found in a parallel group of stable-angina patients with single vessel disease who underwent PTCA. Results of PTCA for unstable angina were also compared with results from 330 similar patients from the NHLBI coronary artery surgery study (CASS) who underwent coronary artery bypass grafting. Ninety-two percent of the PTCA patients reported improvement in angina, compared with 80% of those in the surgical group. The authors concluded that results from retrospective analysis suggest that PTCA can be performed safely and successfully in patients with unstable angina and that PTCA compares favorably with coronary bypass surgery.

De Feyter and co-workers reported results of emergency PTCA in patients with unstable angina (Fig. 63.8).[109] In a group of 217 patients with unstable angina pectoris, 109 were refractory to intensive medical therapy for 24 hours, and 60 were selected for emergency PTCA. The procedure was initially successful in 56 (93%); this initial success included six of seven patients with a totally occluded vessel (86%). In all of 47 patients followed after angioplasty with exercise electrocardiographic testing and thallium scintigraphy, the exercise capacity was virtually normal. The authors of the study concluded that emergency PTCA is very efficacious in selected patients with refractory unstable angina. This favorable experience has been confirmed by other centers.[110-112] Similar results have been found following PTCA in patients developing unstable angina in the early postinfarction period.[113-115] Also regional myocardial dysfunction, due to stunning of the myocardium in patients with unstable angina, frequently improves after successful PTCA.[116]

RECOMMENDATIONS. In unstable-angina patients who have angiographic characteristics appropriate for PTCA, PTCA is an acceptable alternative to bypass surgery.

INTRA-AORTIC BALLOON PUMPING

RATIONALE. Intra-aortic balloon pumping (IABP) increases the diastolic pressure gradient for coronary flow by increasing diastolic pressure in the aorta and decreasing left ventricular end-diastolic pressure while reducing systolic pressure. Thus, myocardial oxygen supply is improved relative to myocardial oxygen demand.

RESULTS. Results of uncontrolled clinical observations by Weintraub and colleagues indicate that in 82 patients with medically refractory unstable angina for 48 hours, IABP insertion was a technical failure in 11, while in 72 it was effective in controlling angina and permitting cardiac catheterization.[117] Serious complications occurred in five (6%) of their patients and consisted of dissection, sepsis, and myocardial infarction. Minor complications occurred in five others.

RECOMMENDATIONS. For the infrequent case with ischemia not initially controlled by combination medical therapy, IABP offers immediate but temporary control of the ischemia at rest. Coronary angiography and definitive revascularization therapy such as PTCA or coronary bypass surgery can then be completed before the patient is weaned from IABP.

SURGICAL THERAPY

RATIONALE AND RESULTS. Previous randomized trials in patients with unstable angina comparing initial surgical treatment with medical treatment have documented relatively low operative mortality and marked relief of symptoms.[39-41] Surgical therapy, however, showed no clear advantage in terms of survival or incidence of myocardial infarction in these trials. Patients with left main coronary artery stenosis were excluded from these randomized trials. Medical failure rates ranged between 20% and 40% over 3 to 5 years of follow-up (see Fig. 63.3), depending on the severity of coronary disease.[41] These results have led to the conclusion that emergency bypass surgery, as early treatment for the patient with unstable angina, offers no distinct advantage in terms of morbidity and mortality. Emergency or semiurgent surgical therapy is usually limited to those patients who have recurrent ischemia at rest during maximally tolerated medical therapy. Indeed, the addition of calcium antagonists, heparin, aspirin, IABP, and PTCA to the nitrate and β-blocker therapy used in these controlled trials has made the number of patients requiring emergency surgery extremely small.

Rankin and colleagues reviewed results of surgical management of 100 patients with persistent unstable angina despite nitrates, propranolol, and nifedipine.[118] Fifty-two of these patients had a myocardial infarction precipitating unstable angina within the preceding 30 days. After stabilization was achieved by addition of IABP, in patients with left main stenosis or triple-vessel disease coronary revascularization was completed. There were four hospital deaths (4%). The 2-year survival rate was 89%, and 81% of surviving patients had New York Heart Association class I or II disease. These excellent results are attributed to improved methods of myocardial protection.

Results of the most recent Veterans Administration cooperative study comparing medical and surgical treatment for unstable angina in general supported the results of the earlier studies summarized above.[119] This study, however, showed significant early improvement in survival in a subgroup of patients treated with coronary bypass. These patients were characterized by compromised left ventricular function reflected by a decreased ejection fraction. When the interaction between ejection fraction and treatment was examined, 2-year mortality for medically treated patients increased as expected when the ejection fraction was less than 0.60 (Fig. 63.9). The 2-year mortality for surgically treated patients, however, was relatively similar at all ejection fractions so that patients with ejection fractions less than 0.59 appeared to benefit from surgery. Thus, surgery seemed to eliminate the deleterious effect of low ejection fraction on mortality. This possibly beneficial result, however, was not supported by life-table analysis of all patients. It should also be noted that the protocol permitted 10 days between the last episode of angina and randomization and surgery was done 9 days (mean) after randomization. Therefore, these results should not be equated with emergency or semiurgent surgery.

RECOMMENDATIONS. Emergency surgical therapy is rarely required and limited to selected cases with continuing ischemic episodes on maximally tolerated medical therapy. Elective surgical therapy follows many of the same guidelines used for other coronary artery disease syndromes (*e.g.*, recurring ischemia or other factors suggesting high risk).

SUMMARY AND CONCLUSIONS

Following the general measures outlined above, all patients should receive a period of 3 to 5 days of intensive medical management (Table 63.6). Drug treatment should be directed toward improving or preventing reduction in myocardial oxygen supply. For patients who are having ongoing episodes of ischemia at rest, intravenous infusion of nitroglycerin should replace oral or transcutaneous nitrate preparations. If the patient is receiving β-blockers or calcium antagonists, it is probably wise to maintain these treatments in the early stage of management. An exception to this recommendation is any suggestion of aggravation of angina by a dihydropyridine calcium antagonist (*e.g.*, nifedipine, nicardipine).[46,47] If this possibility exists, a nondihydropyridine calcium antagonist (diltiazem or verapamil) should be substituted. The β-blocker should be maintained to avoid possible withdrawal phenomena that occasionally manifest as increased ischemia. The intravenous nitroglycerin dose should be titrated to relieve and prevent rest angina and electrocardiographic evidence for myocardial ischemia. I recommend adding a calcium antagonist or increasing the calcium antagonist dose if one is present. My choice is to use either diltiazem or verapamil orally if the patient is not receiving a β-blocker on admission. If the patient is receiving a β-blocker, concurrent use of verapamil should be avoided. If there is an increase in heart rate or blood pressure during therapy with nitrates and a calcium blocker, the dose of β-blocker should be increased. Aspirin and probably heparin should also be used when no contraindication to these agents is present. In patients who continue to have ischemic episodes on this regimen while receiving maximally tolerated doses of intravenous nitroglycerin, calcium antagonists, and β-blockers, IABP should be used. After performing coronary angiography followed by PTCA or coronary bypass surgery in patients with suitable anatomy, the balloon pump should be removed promptly to limit the possibility of complication.

After initial treatment, in my experience, 85% to 90% of patients have control of ischemia at rest with combination therapy using intravenous nitroglycerin, β-blockers, and calcium antagonists. At this stage, intravenous nitrates should be replaced by oral and topical nitrates and a decision should be made about continuation or discontinuation of the β-blocker. If the patient has another indication for a β-blocker (*e.g.*, effort angina, tachycardia, arrhythmias, hypertension, or previous infarction), it should be continued. If the patient has no other indication for β-blocker therapy or if he has side-effects, the decision to reduce or discontinue the β-blocker must be individualized. If withdrawal is attempted, it should be done slowly, preferably over several weeks. Early catheterization is strongly recommended in all patients presenting with unstable angina. Decisions relative to more definitive therapy such as PTCA and coronary bypass surgery must be individualized based on a complete assessment of all of the data on hand. In general, the decision for definitive therapy should rest on the demonstration of continuing episodes of ischemia at either rest or unacceptably low effort, provided, of course, that the patient does not have left main coronary disease, which dictates surgical therapy.

With our more complete understanding of the pathophysiology of unstable angina and the wide variety of treatments at hand, the outcome for these patients is considerably more favorable than it has been in the past.

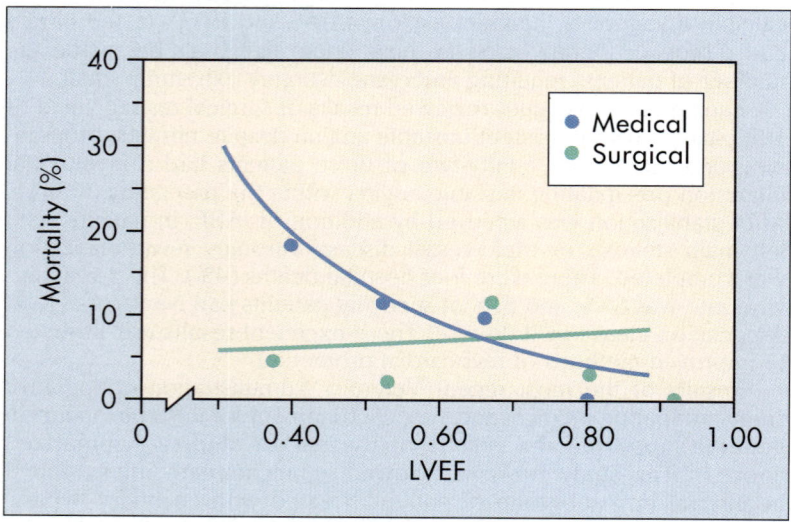

FIGURE 63.9 Influence of ejection fraction on mortality at 2 years following randomly assigned medical or surgical treatment in the Veterans Administration Cooperative Unstable Angina Study. Mortality among medically treated and surgically treated patients is shown for left ventricular ejection fraction (LVEF) intervals 0.30 to 0.44, 0.45 to 0.59, 0.60 to 0.74, 0.75 to 0.89, and ≥ 0.90. The slope of the curve for the medical group is significantly different from zero (P = 0.006) and indicates the predicted effect of ejection fraction on mortality. This effect appears to be modified in those receiving surgery as the slope for the surgical group is not significantly different from zero. (Modified from Luchi RJ, Scott SM, Deupree RH et al: Comparison of medical and surgical treatment for unstable angina pectoris. N Engl J Med 316:977, 1987)

TABLE 63.6 TREATMENT STRATEGY FOR UNSTABLE ANGINA PATIENTS

Initial Therapy
1. Hospitalization in CCU setting
2. Nitroglycerin infusion
3. Heparinization
4. Not taking β-blocker: Add β-blocker, diltiazem, or verapamil.
5. Taking β-blocker: Add either diltiazem or nifedipine.
6. Consider IABP and emergency coronary angiography if ischemia recurs with maximum tolerated doses of drugs in nos. 2, 4, and 5 above.
7. Add aspirin and schedule coronary angiography.

Subsequent Therapy
Medical, PTCA, or CABG is based on:
1. Clinical findings (*e.g.*, recurrent or prolonged ischemia, unacceptable effort tolerance)
2. Anatomical considerations (*e.g.*, left main coronary artery stenosis, reduced ejection fraction)

REFERENCES

1. Osler W: The Lumleian lectures on angina pectoris. Lancet 1:699, 1910; Lancet 2:839, 1910
2. Sampson J, Eliaser M: The diagnosis of impending acute coronary artery occlusion. Am Heart J 13:675, 1937
3. Fowler NO: Preinfarction angina: A need for an objective definition and for a controlled clinical trial of its management. Circulation 44:755, 1971
4. Gazes PC, Mobley EM Jr, Faris HM Jr et al: Preinfarctional (unstable) angina: A prospective study—ten year follow-up: Prognostic significance of electrocardiographic changes. Circulation 48:331, 1973
5. Alison HW, Russell RO Jr, Mantle JA et al: Coronary anatomy and arteriography in patients with unstable angina pectoris. Am J Cardiol 41:204, 1978
6. Fuster V, Frye RL, Connolly DC: Arteriographic patterns early in the onset of the coronary syndromes. Br Heart J 37:1250, 1975
7. Levin DC, Fallon JT: Significance of the angiographic morphology of localized coronary stenosis: Histopathologic correlations. Circulation 66:316, 1982
8. Davis MJ, Thomas A: Thrombus and acute coronary artery lesions in sudden cardiac death, ischemic death. N Engl J Med 310:1137, 1984
9. Falk E: Unstable angina with fatal outcome: Dynamic coronary thrombosis leading to infarction and/or sudden death: Autopsy evidence of recurrent mural thrombosis with peripheral embolization culminating in total vascular occlusion. Circulation 71:699, 1985
10. Vetrovec GW, Cowley MJ, Overton H et al: Intracoronary thrombus in syndromes of unstable myocardial ischemia. Am Heart J 102:1202, 1981
11. Ambrose JA, Winters SL, Stern A et al: Angiographic morphology and the pathogenesis of unstable angina pectoris. J Am Coll Cardiol 5:609, 1985
12. Moise A, Theroux P, Taeymans Y et al: Unstable angina and progression of coronary atherosclerosis. N Engl J Med 309:685, 1983
13. Maseri A, Chierchia S, L'Abbate A: Pathogenetic mechanisms underlying the clinical events associated with atherosclerotic heart disease. Circulation (Suppl V) 62:V-3, 1980
14. Maseri A, L'Abbate AL, Barold G et al: Coronary vasospasm as a possible cause of myocardial infarction: Conclusion derived from the study of "preinfarction" angina. N Engl J Med 299:1271, 1978
15. Gertz SD, Uretsky G, Wajnberg RS et al: Endothelial cell damage and thrombus formation after partial arterial constriction: Relevance to the role of coronary artery spasm in the pathogenesis of myocardial infarction. Circulation 63:476, 1981
16. Joris I, Majno G: Endothelial changes induced by arterial spasm. Am J Pathol 102:346, 1981
17. Kurgan A, Gertz SD, Wajnberg RS: Intimal changes associated with arterial spasm induced by periarterial application of calcium chloride. Exp Mol Pathol 39:176, 1983
18. Lewis RA, Austen KF: The biologically active leukotrienes: Biosynthesis, metabolism, receptors, functions & pharmacology. J Clin Invest 73:889, 1984
19. Lam JYT, Chesebro JH, Steele PM et al: Is vasospasm related to platelet deposition? Relationship in a porcine preparation of arterial injury in vivo. Circulation 75:243, 1987
20. Uchida Y, Yoshimoto N, Murao S: Cyclic fluctuations in coronary blood pressure and flow induced by coronary artery constriction. Jpn Heart J 16:454, 1975
21. Folts JD, Crowell EB Jr, Rowe GG: Platelet aggregation in partially obstructed vessels and its elimination with aspirin. Circulation 54:365, 1976
22. Bolli R, Ware JA, Brandon TA et al: Platelet-mediated thrombosis in stenosed canine coronary arteries: Inhibition by nicergoline, a platelet-active alpha-adrenergic antagonist. J Am Coll Cardiol 3:1417, 1984
23. Lewis HD, Davis JW, Archibald DG et al: Protective effects of aspirin against acute myocardial infarction and death in men with unstable angina. N Engl J Med 309:396, 1983
24. Cairns J, Gent M, Singer J et al: Aspirin, sulfinpyrazone, or both in unstable angina: Results of a Canadian Multicenter Trial. N Engl J Med 313:1369, 1985
25. Vetrovec GW, Leinbach RC, Gold HK et al: Intracoronary thrombolysis in syndromes of ischemia: Angiographic and clinical results. Am Heart J 104:946, 1984
26. Mandelkorn JB, Wolf NM, Singh S: Intracoronary thrombus in nontransmural myocardial infarction and in unstable angina pectoris. Am J Cardiol 52:1, 1983
27. Capone GJ, Wolf N, Meyer B: Frequency of intracoronary filling defects by angiography in angina pectoris at rest. Am J Cardiol 56:403, 1985
28. Sherman CT, Litvack F, Grundfest W et al: Coronary angioscopy in patients with unstable angina pectoris. N Engl J Med 315:913, 1986
29. Fitzgerald DJ, Roy L, Catella F et al: Platelet activation in unstable coronary disease. N Engl J Med 315:983, 1986
30. Theroux P, Latour JG, Leger-Gauthier C et al: Fibrinopeptide A and platelet factor levels in unstable angina pectoris. Circulation 75:156, 1987
31. Davies GJ, Chierchia S, Maseri A: Prevention of myocardial infarction by very early treatment. N Engl J Med 311:1488, 1984
32. Pepine CJ, Feldman RL: Dynamic coronary blood flow reduction: Supply side considerations. Int J Cardiol 3:3, 1983
33. Ludmer PL. Selwyn AP, Shook TL et al: Paradoxical vasoconstriction induced by acetylcholine in atherosclerotic coronary arteries. N Engl J Med 315:1046, 1986
34. Deanfield JE, Shea MJ, Wilson RA et al. Direct effects of smoking on the heart: Silent ischemic disturbances of coronary flow. Am J Cardiol 57:1005, 1986
35. Nicolaides AN, Bowers, Harbourne T: Blood viscosity, red cell flexibility, haematocrit and plasma fibrinogen in patients with angina. Lancet 2:943, 1977
36. Fuchs J, Weinberger I, Rotenberg Z: Plasma viscosity in ischemic heart disease. Am Heart J 108:435, 1984
37. Ku D: Coronary vascular reactivity after acute myocardial ischemia. Science 218:576, 1982
38. Bertolasi CA, Tronge JE, Mon GA et al: Clinical spectrum of "unstable angina." Clin Cardiol 2:113, 1979
39. Selden R, Neill WA, Ritzmann LW et al: Medical versus surgical therapy for acute coronary insufficiency: A randomized study. N Engl J Med 293:1329, 1975
40. Pugh B, Platt MR, Mills LJ et al: Unstable angina pectoris: A randomized study of patients treated medically and surgically. Am J Cardiol 41:1291, 1978
41. Conti CR. Unstable angina: Long-term follow-up of surgical and medical treatment. In Rafflenbeul W, Lichtlen PR, Balcon R (eds): Unstable Angina Pectoris, p 180. New York, Thieme-Stratton, 1981
42. Johnson SM, Mauritson DR, Winniford MD et al: Continuous electrocardiographic monitoring in patients with unstable angina pectoris: Identification of high-risk subgroup with severe coronary disease, variant angina, and/or impaired early prognosis. Am Heart J 103:4, 1982
43. Gottlieb SO, Weisfeldt ML, Ouyang P et al: Silent ischemia as a marker for early unfavorable outcomes in patients with unstable angina. N Engl J Med 314:1214, 1986
44. Gottlieb SO, Weisfeldt ML, Ouyang P et al: Silent ischemia predicts infarction and death during 2-year follow-up of unstable angina. J Am Coll Cardiol 10:756, 1987
45. Nademanee K, Intarachot V, Josephson MA et al: Prognostic significance of silent myocardial ischemia in patients with unstable angina. J Am Coll Cardiol 10:1, 1987
46. Lambert CR, Hill JA, Feldman RL et al: Myocardial ischemia during intravenous nicardipine administration. Am J Cardiol 55:844, 1985
47. Schanzenbacher P, Deeg P, Liebau G: Paradoxical angina after nifedipine: Angiographic documentation. Am J Cardiol 53:345, 1984
48. Feldman RL, Nichols WW, Pepine CJ et al: Acute effect of intravenous dipyridamole on regional coronary hemodynamic and metabolism. Circulation 64:333, 1981
49. Biagini A, Mazzei MG, Carpeggiani C et al: Vasospastic ischemic mechanism of frequent asymptomatic transient ST-T changes during continuous electrocardiographic monitoring in selected unstable angina patients. Am Heart J 103:13, 1982
50. Pepine CJ, Feldman RL, Conti CR: Action of intracoronary nitroglycerin in refractory coronary artery spasm. Circulation 65:411, 1982
51. Feldman RL, Pepine CJ, Conti CR: Magnitude of dilatation of large and small coronary arteries by nitroglycerin. Circulation 64:324, 1981
52. Mehta J, Pepine CJ: Effect of sublingual nitroglycerin on regional flow in patients with and without coronary disease. Circulation 58:803, 1978
53. Hill JA, Feldman RL, Pepine CJ et al: Randomized double-blind comparison of nifedipine and isosorbide dinitrate in patients with coronary artery spasm. Am J Cardiol 49:431, 1982
54. Levin RI, Jaffe EA, Weksler BB: Nitroglycerin stimulates synthesis of prostacyclin by cultured human endothelial cells. J Clin Invest 67:762, 1981
55. Schror K, Grodzinska L, Darius H: Stimulation of coronary vascular prostacyclin and inhibition of human platelet thromboxane A_2 after low-dose nitroglycerin. Thromb Res 23:59, 1981
56. Dauwe F, Affaki G, Waters DD et al: Intravenous nitroglycerin in refractory unstable angina. Am J Cardiol 43:416, 1979
57. Mikolich JR, Nicoloff NB, Robinson PH: Relief of refractory angina with continuous intravenous infusion of nitroglycerin. Chest 77:375, 1980
58. DePace NL, Herline IM, Kotler MN et al: Intravenous nitroglycerin for rest angina. Arch Intern Med 142:1806, 1982
59. Kaplan K, Davison R, Parker M et al: Intravenous nitroglycerin for the treatment of angina at rest unresponsive to standard nitrate therapy. Am J Cardiol 51:694, 1983
60. Distante A, Maseri A, Severi S et al: Management of vasospastic angina at rest by continuous infusion of isosorbide dinitrate: A double-blind crossover study in coronary care unit. Am J Cardiol 44:533, 1979
61. Curfman GD, Heinsimer JA, Lozner EC et al: Intravenous nitroglycerin in the treatment of spontaneous angina pectoris: A prospective, randomized trial. Circulation 67:276, 1983
62. Papazogtov NM: Use of propranolol in preinfarction angina. Circulation 44:303, 1971
63. Fischl SJ, Herman MVB, Gorlin R: The intermediate coronary syndrome: Clinical, angiographic, and therapeutic aspects. N Engl J Med 288:1193, 1973
64. Conti CR, Brawley RK, Griffith LSC et al: Unstable angina pectoris: Morbidity and mortality in 57 consecutive patients evaluated angiographically. Am

65. Guazzi M, Fiorentini C, Polese A: Treatment of spontaneous angina pectoris with beta blocking agents: A clinical, electrocardiographic, and haemodynamic appraisal. Br Heart J 37:1235, 1975
66. Cairns JA, Fantus IG, Klassen GA: Unstable angina pectoris. Am Heart J 92:373, 1976
67. Yusuf S, Ramsdale D, Peto R et al: Early intravenous atenolol treatment in suspected acute myocardial infarction. Lancet 2:273, 1980
68. Gold H, Leinbach R, Sanders C et al. Intra-aortic balloon pumping for ventricular septal defect or mitral regurgitation complicating acute myocardial infarction. Circulation 47:1191, 1973
69. Bodenheimer M, Lipski J, Donoso E et al: Prinzmetal's variant angina: A clinical and electrocardiographic study. Am Heart J 87:304, 1974
70. MacAlpin RN, Kattus AA, Alvaro AB: Angina pectoris at rest with preservation of exercise capacity: Prinzmetal's variant angina. Circulation 47:946, 1973
71. Robertson RM, Alastair MD, Wood JJ et al: Exacerbation of vasotonic angina pectoris by propranolol. Circulation 65:281, 1982
72. Capucci di A, Bracchetti D, Carini GC et al: Confronto in doppio cieco fra verapamil e propranololo nella terapia dell'angina instabile. Boll Soc Ital Cardiol 27:447, 1982
73. Parodi O, Simonetti I, L'Abbate A: Verapamil versus propranolol for angina at rest. Am J Cardiol 50:923, 1982
74. Gottlieb SO, Weisfeldt ML, Ouyang P et al: Effect of the addition of propranolol to therapy with nifedipine for unstable angina pectoris: A randomized, double-blind, placebo-controlled trial. Circulation 73:331, 1986
75. Telford AM, Wilson C: Trial of heparin versus atenolol in prevention of myocardial infarction in intermediate coronary syndrome. Lancet 1:1225, 1981
76. Muller JE, Turi ZG, Pearle DL et al: Nifedipine and conventional therapy for unstable angina pectoris: A randomized, double-blind comparison. Circulation 69:728, 1984
77. HINT: Early treatment of unstable angina in the coronary care unit: A randomised, double blind, placebo controlled comparison of recurrent ischaemia in patients treated with nifedipine or metoprolol or both: Report of the Holland Interuniversity Nifedipine/Metoprolol Trial (HINT) Research Group. Br Heart J 56:400, 1986
78. Fouet X, Usdin JP, Gayet CH et al: Comparison of short-term efficacy of diltiazem and propranolol in unstable angina at rest: A randomized trial in 70 patients. Eur Heart J 4:691, 1983
79. Theroux P, Taeymans Y, Morissette D et al: A randomized study comparing propranolol and diltiazem in the treatment of unstable angina. J Am Coll Cardiol 5:717, 1985
80. Gelman JS, Mehta J: Platelets and prostaglandins in sudden death: Therapeutic implications. In Josephson M (ed): Cardiovascular Clinics, Vol 15, No. 3, p 65. Philadelphia, FA Davis, 1985
81. Pepine CJ, Feldman RL, Whittle J et al: Effect of diltiazem in patients with variant angina: A randomized double blind trial. Am Heart J 101:719, 1981
82. Previtali M, Salerno J, Tavazzi L et al: Treatment of angina at rest with nifedipine: A short-term controlled study. Am J Cardiol 45:825, 1980
83. Hugenholtz PG, Michels HF, Serruys PW et al: Nifedipine in the treatment of unstable angina, coronary spasm, and myocardial ischemia. Am J Cardiol 47:163, 1981
84. Moses JW, Wertheimer JH, Bodenheimer MM et al: Efficacy of nifedipine in rest angina refractory to propranolol and nitrates in patients with obstructive coronary artery disease. Ann Intern Med 94:425, 1981
85. Mehta J, Pepine CJ, Day M et al: Short-term efficacy of oral verapamil in rest angina: A double-blind placebo controlled trial in CCU patients. Am J Med 71:977, 1981
86. Gerstenblith G, Ouyang P, Achuff SC et al: Nifedipine in unstable angina: A double-blind randomized trial. N Engl J Med 306:885, 1982
87. Ouyang P, Brinker J, Mellits ED et al: Variables predictive of successful medical therapy in patients with unstable angina: Selection by multivariate analysis from clinical, electrocardiographic, and angiographic evaluations. Circulation 70:367, 1984
88. Pepine CJ, Feldman RL, Hill JA et al: Clinical outcome after treatment of rest angina with calcium blockers: Comparative experience during the initial year of therapy with diltiazem, nifedipine, and verapamil. Am Heart J 106:1341, 1983
89. Blaustein AS, Heller GV, Kolman BS: Adjunctive nifedipine therapy in high-risk, medically refractory, unstable angina pectoris. Am J Cardiol 52:950, 1983
90. Smith KS, Papp C: The prevention of impending cardiac infarction by anticoagulant treatment. Br Heart J 13:467, 1951
91. Wood P: Acute and sub-acute coronary insufficiency. Br Med J 1:1779, 1961
92. De Wood MA, Spores MA, Notske R et al: Prevalence of total coronary occlusion during the early hours of transmural myocardial infarction. N Engl J Med 303:897, 1980
93. Lawrence JR, Shepherd JT, Bone I et al: Fibrinolytic therapy in unstable angina pectoris: A controlled clinical trial. Thromb Res 17:767, 1980
94. Benda L. Influence of streptokinase on blood rheology and coagulation. Postgrad Med J 49:129, 1973
95. Niewarowski S, Gurewich V, Senyi A et al: The effect of fibrinolysis on platelet function. Thromb Diathesis Haemost 47:99, 1971
96. Gotoh K, Minamino T, Katoh D et al: The role of intracoronary thrombus in unstable angina: Angiographic assessment and thrombolytic therapy during ongoing anginal attacks. Circulation 77:526, 1988
97. Gold HK, Johns JA, Leinbach RC et al: A randomized, blinded, placebo-controlled trial of recombinant human tissue-type plasminogen activator in patients with unstable angina pectoris. Circulation 75:1192, 1987
98. Gold HK, Johns JR, Leinbach RC et al: Thrombolytic therapy for unstable angina pectoris: Rational and results. J Am Coll Cardiol 10:91B, 1987
99. Siegle JS, Shah PK, Nathan M et al: Prostaglandin E-1 infusion in unstable angina: Effects on anginal frequency and cardiac function. Am Heart J 108:863, 1981
100. Szczeklik A, Szczeklik J, Nizankowski R et al: Prostacyclin for acute coronary insufficiency. Artery 8:7, 1980
101. Chierchia S, Patrono C, Crea F et al: Effects of intravenous prostacyclin in variant angina. Circulation 65:470, 1982
102. Chierchia S, deCaterina R, Crea F et al: Failure of thromboxane A_2 blockage to prevent attacks of vasospastic angina. Circulation 66:702, 1982
103. Shimamota T, Numano F, Motomiya T: Myocardial ischemic attacks induced experimentally by thromboxane A_2 antagonists, EG626 and its clinical trial. Jpn Circ 41:785, 1977
104. Simoons ML, Hugenholtz PG: Haemodynamic effects of alinidine, a specific sinus node inhibitor in patients with unstable angina or myocardial infarction. Eur Heart J 5:277, 1984
105. Bertholet M, Hastir F, Renier J et al: The value of amiodarone for the treatment of unstable angina. Acta Cardiol 38:503, 1983
106. Meyer J, Schmitz H, Erbel B et al: Transluminal angioplasty in patients with unstable angina pectoris. In Kaltenbach (ed): Transluminal coronary angioplasty and intracoronary thrombolysis, p 367. Berlin, Springer Verlag, 1982
107. Williams DO, Riley RS, Singh AK et al: Evaluation of the role of coronary angioplasty in patients with unstable angina pectoris. Am Heart J 102:1, 1981
108. Faxon DP, Detre K, McCabe CH et al: Role of percutaneous transluminal coronary angioplasty in the treatment of unstable angina. Am J Cardiol 53:131C, 1983
109. De Feyter P, Serruys PW, Van Den Brand M et al: Emergency coronary angioplasty in refractory unstable angina. N Engl J Med 313:342, 1985
110. Plokker HW, Ernst SM, Bal ET et al: Percutaneous transluminal coronary angioplasty in patients with unstable angina pectoris refractory to medical therapy: Long-term clinical and angiographic results. Cathet Cardiovasc Diagn 14:15, 1988
111. Wohlgelernter D, Cleman M, Highman HA et al: Percutaneous transluminal coronary angioplasty of the "culprit lesion" for management of unstable angina pectoris in patients with multivessel coronary artery disease. Am J Cardiol 58:460, 1986
112. Sharma B, Wyeth RP, Kolath GS et al: Percutaneous transluminal coronary angioplasty of one vessel for refractory unstable angina pectoris: Efficacy in single and multivessel disease. Br Heart J 59:280, 1988
113. Gottlieb SO, Walford GD, Ouyang P et al: Initial and late results of coronary angioplasty for early postinfarction unstable angina. Cathet Cardiovasc Diagn 13:93, 1987
114. Safian RD, Snyder LD, Synder BA et al: Usefulness of percutaneous transluminal coronary angioplasty for unstable angina pectoris after non-Q-wave acute myocardial infarction. Am J Cardiol 59:263, 1987
115. De Feyter PJ, Serruys PW, Soward A et al: Coronary angioplasty for early postinfarction unstable angina. Circulation 74:1365, 1986
116. De Feyter PJ, Suryapranata H, Serruys PW et al: Effects of successful percutaneous transluminal coronary angioplasty on global and regional left ventricular function in unstable angina pectoris. Am J Cardiol 60:993, 1987
117. Weintraub RM, Aroesty JM, Paulin S et al: Medically refractory unstable angina pectoris. I. Long-term follow-up of patients undergoing intra-aortic balloon counterpulsation and operation. Am J Cardiol 43:877, 1979
118. Rankin JS, Newton JR, Califf RM et al: Clinical characteristics and current management of medically refractory unstable angina. Ann Surg 200:457, 1984
119. Luchi RJ, Scott SM, Deupree RH et al: Comparison of medical and surgical treatment for unstable angina pectoris. N Engl J Med 316:977, 1987

SILENT ISCHEMIA

William W. Parmley

INTRODUCTION

Myocardial ischemia occurs whenever there is an imbalance between the oxygen supply and demand of the heart. The clinical manifestations of ischemia can be dramatic and unexpected, such as acute myocardial infarction; predictable, such as typical stable angina pectoris induced by exercise; or unrecognized, such as silent ischemia. Not uncommonly, ischemia is manifested by unusual or atypical symptoms such as dyspnea or abdominal discomfort. In silent ischemia, there are not even subtle clinical markers of its presence.

We generally recognize the potential for adverse effects associated with clinically manifest ischemia and treat patients accordingly. It is disconcerting, therefore, to realize that silent ischemia is the most common form of ischemia and yet often remains untreated because it is unrecognized. Current knowledge of silent ischemia is increasing rapidly, but many questions remain unanswered. The purpose of this chapter is to review current knowledge and explore the status of some of the unanswered questions. Future data may profoundly affect the way we screen and treat patients if it is possible to define subgroups of patients with silent ischemia who are at risk for myocardial infarction, serious arrhythmias, or sudden death.

DEFINITION AND CLASSIFICATION

By definition, silent ischemia occurs when there is objective evidence of ischemia in the absence of symptoms. Most studies of silent myocardial ischemia have employed ambulatory electrocardiographic monitoring.[1-5] It is important to recognize, however, that the most sensitive index of ischemia is a change in regional wall motion.[6,7] Thus, any invasive or noninvasive technique that can monitor a change in regional wall motion has the potential for detecting and quantitating silent ischemia. Because of the infrequent nature of these episodes, however, studies have relied heavily on continuous electrocardiographic recordings for their documentation. Changes in regional blood flow have also been used to document the presence of silent ischemia,[5,8] although these techniques cannot be used to monitor spontaneous events in everyday life. It is important to remember that because ischemia can be caused by either an increase in myocardial oxygen demand and/or a decrease in oxygen supply, it may be necessary to assess both sides of the equation carefully in order to understand all of the factors contributing to individual episodes.

Various subsets of patients with silent ischemia have been identified. One general classification of such individuals is that of Cohn and co-workers[9]:

Type 1. Individuals who have never experienced any cardiac symptoms. This might include, for example, an individual who has underlying coronary artery disease, a positive treadmill test, and no symptoms.
Type 2. Individuals who have had a myocardial infarction and subsequently exhibit painless ischemia as with an exercise test.
Type 3. Individuals who have recognized angina pectoris but in addition have episodes of silent ischemia. It is particularly in this group that the phrase "total ischemic burden"[10] has been applied to indicate the probability that the total number and duration of all ischemic episodes may be more important than just the clinically manifest episodes.

ASYMPTOMATIC CORONARY ARTERY DISEASE

In order to begin to define the numbers of people who have silent ischemia, it is important to first define individuals with asymptomatic coronary artery disease, recognizing that not all of them will have silent ischemia. Such individuals could also include those with silent or unrecognized myocardial infarction, arrhythmias, sudden death, or ischemic cardiomyopathy.

Several studies have attempted to estimate the prevalence of asymptomatic coronary artery disease. Eriksson did maximal treadmill tests in approximately 2000 middle-aged males in Norway (average age 50).[11] Those with positive tests underwent coronary arteriography, and about 2.5% of the entire group had asymptomatic coronary disease.

In healthy U.S. Air Force personnel (average age 42), Froelicher found approximately 10% with positive exercise treadmill tests.[12] In those individuals with positive tests undergoing cardiac catheterization, about 25% had significant coronary artery disease. Overall, therefore, the incidence of asymptomatic coronary artery disease in the total group was about 2.5%.

Diamond and Forrester reviewed data from approximately 24,000 autopsies.[13] In males not known to have coronary disease (age 30–69) the prevalence of significant coronary artery disease was 6.4%.

In summarizing these studies, it seems reasonable to assume that up to about 4% of middle-aged U.S. males have asymptomatic coronary artery disease. One of the challenges of the future will be to identify any high-risk subgroups in a cost-effective manner. At the moment, however, it does not appear reasonable to screen the population at large in an attempt to find patients with asymptomatic coronary disease. Potential candidates who could be considered are those with multiple risk factors, those in occupations with risk to the public (*e.g.*, pilots), or those who wish to change their lifestyle and undergo strenuous exercise.

The incidence of Type 2 patients with silent ischemia can be estimated from the numbers of patients with acute myocardial infarction and postinfarction patients with ischemia.[14] There are approximately 500,000 patients hospitalized for myocardial infarction in the United States each year. About 400,000 survive. Of those, about 100,000 will have persistent heart failure, arrhythmias, or angina. About one third of the remaining patients (100,000) would have a positive exercise treadmill test, but only about one half would have angina. That leaves an incidence of about 50,000 new postinfarction patients each year who have silent ischemia. As will be discussed later, this group of patients has a higher mortality than postinfarction patients without ischemia. Identification of this subgroup, therefore, assumes some importance.

The prevalence of Type 3 silent ischemia can be estimated from the number of patients with angina who are being treated in the United States.[14] Of the four million such patients, it is estimated that about three fourths, or three million patients, also have frequent episodes of silent ischemia. Studies of patients with angina and silent ischemia indicate that about three fourths of all ischemic episodes are silent. This makes silent ischemia the most common manifestation of coronary artery disease, albeit unrecognized.

DIAGNOSIS OF SILENT ISCHEMIA

Since information about silent ischemia continues to accumulate, it is unclear at present whether one should routinely employ noninvasive techniques to screen for silent ischemia. Nevertheless, it is important to review those techniques that are available to detect and quantitate episodes of silent myocardial ischemia. Although much of the current effort to collect data remains in the realm of clinical research, it appears that a knowledge of the frequency and duration of silent ischemia in individual patients may provide clinically important information. Furthermore, such information allows for the subsetting of patients according to risk. Table 64.1 lists the available techniques for diagnosing silent ischemia. Each one is discussed briefly below.

The electrocardiogram is a traditionally important technique for diagnosing episodes of transient ischemia. Beginning with a normal electrocardiogram, the development of flat or downsloping ST depression of one millimeter or more, particularly during a standardized exercise treadmill test, has been a reasonable standard for exercise-induced myocardial ischemia, although false-positives are not uncommon, particularly in a patient population at low risk for coronary artery disease.[15] A number of other factors can influence the electrocardiogram, including position, maneuvers such as hyperventilation, alterations in sympathetic tone, various drugs, electrolyte problems, and so forth. Thus, the specificity of this change in the electrocardiogram is less than ideal and must be considered in the context of an individual patient. In individuals who are at low risk for coronary disease, such ST changes must be considered with great caution as to their specificity for silent myocardial ischemia. In individuals with known coronary disease and angina pectoris, however, particularly those who have characteristic ST-T wave changes during exercise-induced angina, recordings of the electrocardiogram at other times appear to have more specificity in indicating the presence of silent myocardial ischemia. For example, in one study of 17 asymptomatic men with positive treadmill tests, 11 had silent ischemic episodes on prolonged ambulatory electrocardiographic recordings, and all had significant coronary artery disease.[16] Of the other 6, 5 did not have significant coronary artery disease on angiography and had no silent ischemia.

TABLE 64.1 TECHNIQUES FOR DIAGNOSING SILENT ISCHEMIA

Electrocardiogram
Standardized treadmill test
Ambulatory ECG

Coronary Blood Flow
Thallium-201
Rubidium-82 positron emission tomography

Hemodynamics
Regional wall motion
Rise in pulmonary capillary wedge pressure

Metabolism
Lactate production
Nuclear magnetic resonance spectroscopy
Positron emission tomography

Fluoroscopy

The most common tool used in studies of silent ischemia is the ambulatory electrocardiogram.[1-5] Episodes are considered to represent ischemia when a normal electrocardiogram undergoes a characteristic sequence of events over at least a one-minute period. This sequence includes characteristic flat or downsloping ST depression of at least 1 mm with a gradual onset and offset of the episodes, all of which last at least one minute. In patients with known coronary artery disease, it is probable that these changes are quite specific for episodes of silent ischemia, although there is not enough independent data during such episodes to be sure of their significance.

There is some controversy about the potential for "ischemic" ST changes in normal individuals undergoing ambulatory electrocardiography.[17] No flat ST depression was seen in 33 ambulatory individuals[18] or in 42 sleeping subjects.[19] However, Armstrong and co-workers[20] found a 30% incidence of ST depression in 50 asymptomatic men. Deanfield[21] studied 80 normal volunteers and found only 2 with transient ST depression. J-point depression with upsloping ST segments occurred in 36%. Thus, characteristic flat ST depression of 1 mm or more below an isoelectric baseline for at least one minute appears to be uncommon in the normal population. However, it is unlikely that the ambulatory electrocardiogram will be more specific than the exercise electrocardiogram in normal individuals. Thus caution must be used in interpreting results in normal people.[17] In patients with known coronary artery disease, such changes are far more specific for ischemia. Coy and co-workers[16] suggested that the optimal monitoring period to detect silent ischemia may be 72 hours.

A more direct noninvasive marker of coronary blood flow, such as thallium-201 or rubidium-82 positron emission tomography (PET), has been invaluable in determining the significance of painless ST segment depression. In particular, studies with rubidium-82 PET have shown that patients with known episodes of ischemia can have dramatic reductions in regional coronary blood flow with significant or even minimal electrocardiographic changes.[8] The spontaneous episodes of silent ischemia can also be provoked by maneuvers that produce generalized vasoconstriction,[22] such as mental stress (Fig. 64.1), immersion of the forearm in ice water, emotion, and so on. Where available, such additional independent evidence of silent myocardial ischemia appears to be of great importance in clarifying the significance of episodes of ST depression.

Since regional ischemia is always characterized by alterations in regional wall motion, the ability to detect such hemodynamic abnormalities can be of great importance in quantitating silent ischemia. To make such a diagnosis, wall-motion studies are needed under controlled conditions and during an episode of silent ischemia.[6] At present, this is not generally possible in the ambulatory setting, although, in patients undergoing technetium-99 wall-motion studies, cardiac catheterization, or other imaging procedures, it is possible to detect regional wall-motion changes during an episode of silent ischemia.[23,24] It is possible that ambulatory techniques might be adapted to evaluate this phenomenon which, in some sense, represents the gold-standard response to an inadequate coronary supply. Other hemodynamic effects are also characteristic of an episode of silent ischemia. For example, in patients with a balloon tip catheter in the pulmonary artery, there is usually a rise in pulmonary capillary wedge pressure with an ischemic episode. Levy and co-workers[25] studied 19 ambulatory men with episodes of silent ischemia. All but 3 of the 67 episodes of ST depression (32 silent) were accompanied by a significant increase in pulmonary artery diastolic pressure. This rise in left ventricular end-diastolic pressure is not specific for ischemia but is a good marker in an appropriate clinical setting. It is probably less specific than a change in regional wall motion.

There is some evidence that silent myocardial ischemia can be a more chronic phenomenon rather than just a transient event. For example, in some patients with coronary artery disease who are studied preoperatively, there is regional lactate production in the area supplied by the left anterior descending coronary artery.[26] After bypass grafting, there is reversal of this abnormal lactate metabolism. Studies of regional wall motion in some patients have shown that preoperative hypokinesis can be converted to normal wall motion following bypass surgery.[27] Interventional studies with nitroglycerin and paired electrical stimulation have also identified areas of regional hypokinesis that improve their wall motion acutely in response to these interventions.[24] These same areas show sustained improvement following revascularization. Thus, hypokinetic zones of "stunned" or "hibernating"[28] myocardium may be representative of more chronic silent ischemia, as compared to the transient and shorter episodes seen on ambulatory electrocardiography.

Metabolic changes can also be used as a marker of ischemia. The heart normally extracts lactate from the perfusing arterial blood so that the output of lactate in the coronary venous effluent is less than that in the arterial supply. During the onset of ischemia, however, where the heart is unable to use pyruvate as a substrate, there is additional conversion of pyruvate to lactate with an output of lactate in the coronary sinus flow.[29] Both global and regional measurements of lactate production have been made as a marker of ischemic episodes in individual patients.[26] Newer techniques, such as nuclear magnetic resonance imaging, provide the possibility of noninvasive measurements of high-energy phosphates, inorganic phosphate, and pH as sensitive markers of regional ischemia.[30] Such techniques, however, have been restricted primarily to global changes in the heart in small animal models but undoubtedly will be adapted in the future to the clinical situation. Certain metabolic studies with PET can also be useful.[31]

Another noninvasive technique includes use of fluoroscopy to look for coronary artery calcification as a marker of asymptomatic coronary artery disease. In a study by Langou and associates,[32] 129 asymptomatic males (average age 46) were screened with an exercise treadmill test and cardiac fluoroscopy to look for coronary artery calcification. Thirteen had both tests positive, and 12 of the 13 had significant coronary artery disease. This study emphasizes the principle that two or more positive noninvasive markers of coronary artery disease will be more specific in diagnosing patients with either asymptomatic coronary artery disease or silent myocardial ischemia.

☐ MECHANISMS FOR THE ABSENCE OF DISCOMFORT IN SILENT ISCHEMIA

Three major mechanisms have been proposed as to why silent ischemia does not manifest itself as a clinical symptom in some patients with coronary artery disease. These three mechanisms include (1) impaired neural pathways, (2) insufficient ischemia to produce discomfort, and (3) altered pain threshold. Each one of these will be reviewed briefly, since there is evidence in support of each one.

When one transplants the heart of one individual into another and severs all neural pathways, there is an absence of angina pectoris. This occurs because of the severance of those neural pathways that mediate this form of chest discomfort. The peripheral neuropathy of diabetes may contribute to silent ischemia in some patients. Data regarding the frequency of silent ischemia in diabetic patients are conflicting, but, in general, shows about the same prevalence in diabetic as in nondiabetic patients.[33] Some have postulated that acute myocardial infarction itself may damage neural pathways and thus interfere with the appreciation of ischemia from a closely related zone of myocardium.

Insufficient ischemia to reach the pain threshold is also a possible explanation in some patients. Figure 64.2 reviews the sequence of events occurring in patients who develop myocardial ischemia. Some of these data have been collected from patients undergoing balloon angioplasty, during which the balloon has occluded the coronary artery.[6] Within a few seconds of occluding the coronary artery, there is a change in the contractile pattern of the affected myocardium. Relaxation rate is affected first, and this is followed in a few seconds by a decrease in contraction. This occurs rapidly because of the continuing and immediate need of the myocardium for a supply of oxygen. At about 15 seconds or more, the left ventricular filling pressure is elevated, and electrocardiographic changes occur by 20 seconds. In other studies it is apparent that metabolic abnormalities, such as lactate production, can precede electrocardiographic changes. Angina pectoris may not develop until 20 or 30 seconds after the onset of the occlusion. One could postulate, therefore, that in some circumstances one has ischemia of insufficient magnitude or duration to reach the anginal threshhold. Even though electrocardiographic or regional wall-motion changes occur, the patient may be unaware of it. In a study by Cecchi and colleagues[34] of patients who underwent ambulatory electrocardiographic recording to detect episodes of ischemia, painful episodes were more likely to occur in association with more vigorous activities, whereas asymptomatic episodes were more likely to occur with less severe exertion. This effect of duration or severity of the episode, however, cannot be the sole factor, since marked abnormalities in perfusion and function can occur without pain, suggesting that other factors may be involved as well.

A third factor that may be involved is a differing pain threshold in different patients. It seems intuitive that some individuals must have different pain thresholds. This has been studied recently in two different reports, both of which reached the same conclusion.[35,36] In patients undergoing discomfort threshold testing, asymptomatic patients with myocardial ischemia tend to have higher pain thresholds than those with symptomatic myocardial ischemia. The overlap of the data, however, is considerable, suggesting that this cannot be the only explanation for the difference, although in some patients it may play a dominant role. Some workers have questioned whether pain-relieving substances such as endogenous endorphins might be responsible for the inability to perceive discomfort. The narcotic antagonist, naloxone,

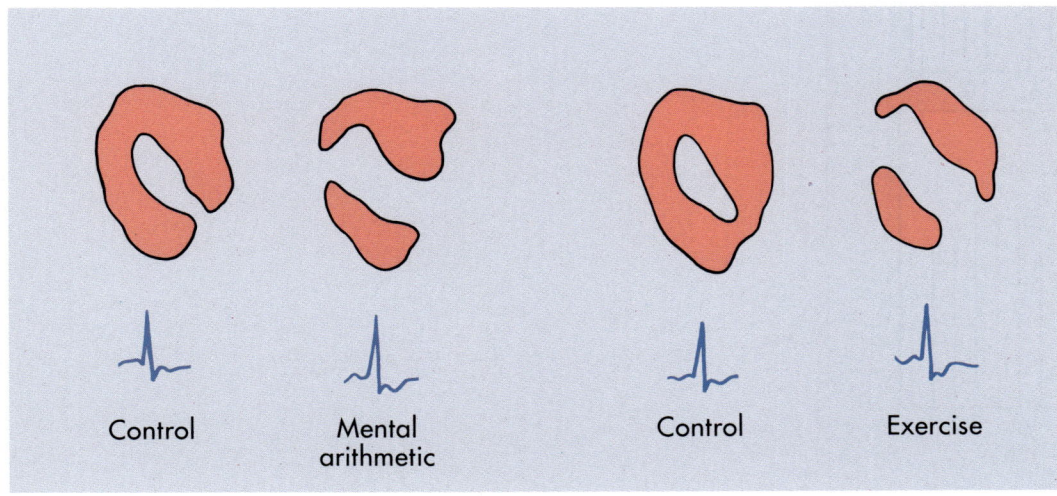

FIGURE 64.1 Representative PET scans showing the myocardial uptake of rubidium 82 and the accompanying electrocardiogram in a patient with chronic, stable angina and coronary disease, under controlled circumstances and following either mental arithmetic or exercise. Note the similar perfusion defect and ECG changes although the mental arithmetic was unaccompanied by chest pain. (Modified from Selwyn AP, Shea M, Deanfield JE et al: Character of transient ischemia in angina pectoris. Am J Cardiol 58:21B–25B, 1986)

had no effect, suggesting that this is an unlikely mechanism for silent ischemia.[37] In another study plasma β-endorphins were increased after exercise and were suggestively lower in patients with angina compared to those without angina.[38]

Overall, it is likely that several different mechanisms may play a role in silent ischemia in different episodes and in different individuals. These would include impairment of neural pathways, alterations in the severity and duration of ischemia, and alterations in pain threshold. It is likely that further knowledge will become available about these mechanisms as additional patient groups are analyzed.

SILENT ISCHEMIA IN PATIENTS WITH ANGINA PECTORIS

Several studies have confirmed that angina pectoris is commonly accompanied by additional episodes of silent ischemia. About three

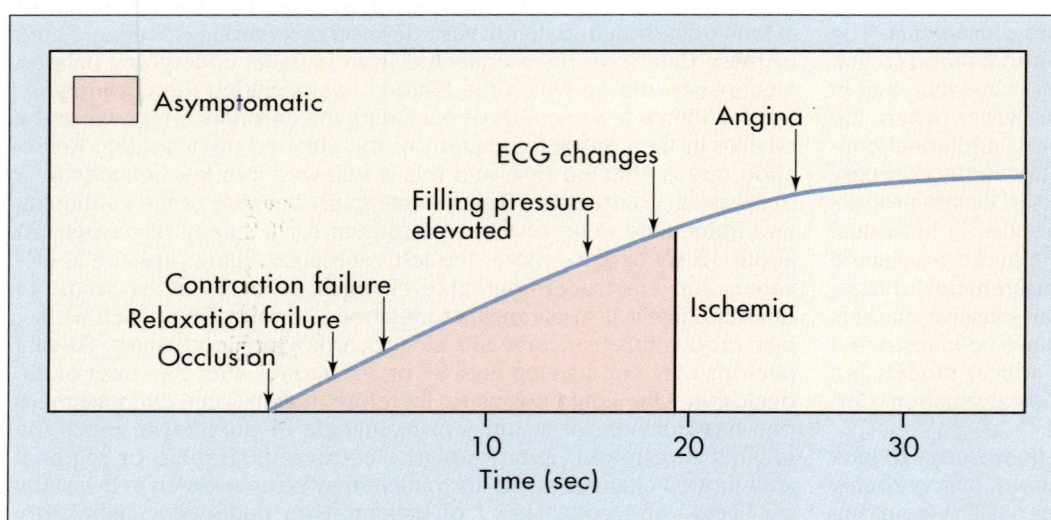

FIGURE 64.2 The sequence of events during an episode of angina produced by balloon occlusion of a coronary stenosis. Note that angina is the last in a sequence of events, indicating the possibility that silent ischemia may occur if the progression of events does not reach the anginal threshhold. (Modified from Sigwart V, Grbic M, Payot M et al: Ischemic events during coronary artery balloon obstruction. In Rutishauser W, Roskamm H (eds): Silent Myocardial Ischemia, pp 29–36. Berlin, Springer-Verlag, 1984)

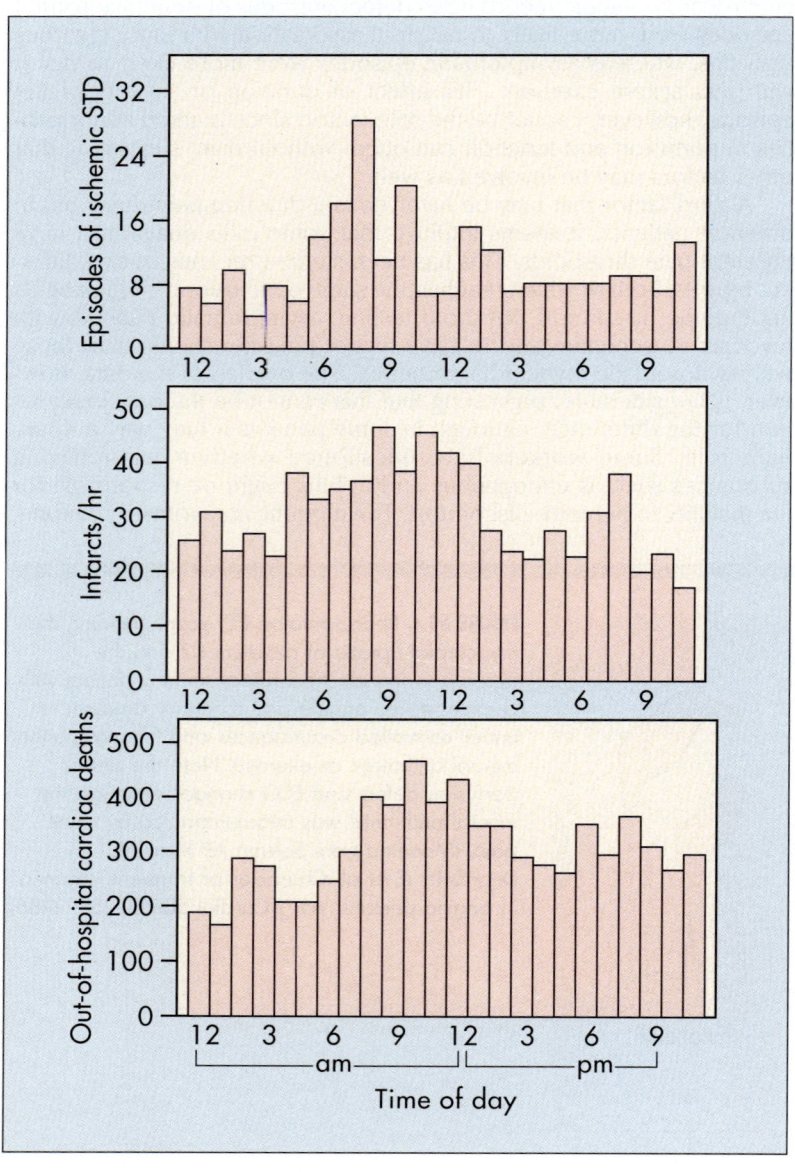

FIGURE 64.3 Twenty-four-hour distribution of coronary events as detected by ambulatory monitoring. Note the predominance of events in the morning hours for both silent ischemia, myocardial infarction, and out-of-hospital mortality. (Modified from Rocco MB, Nabel EG, and Selwyn AP: Circadian rhythms and coronary artery disease. Am J Cardiol 59:13C–17C, 1987)

fourths of patients with angina also have silent ischemia.[39,40] In those patients with both types of episodes, it appears that three fourths of all ischemic episodes are silent. Some, in fact, may be relatively long lasting in comparison to the usual duration of anginal episodes. An interesting circadian variation has also been noted with episodes of silent ischemia.[41] They tend to occur as a morning phenomenon, particularly after awakening in the early morning hours. This circadian variation is similar to the morning predominance of anginal pain in Prinzmetal's or variant angina, acute myocardial infarction, sudden death,[42] high blood pressure readings in patients with essential hypertension, and the occurrence of stroke (Fig. 64.3). There may be a common pathophysiologic connection that ties all of these vascular events together. Obvious candidates include vasoconstriction or platelet aggregation with subsequent vasoconstriction and/or thrombosis. This circadian variation, however, suggests that if one has elected to treat such patients, it would be wise to begin treatment early in the morning in order to decrease the large amount of silent ischemia occurring at that time.

The mechanism of presumed vasoconstriction that causes silent ischemia is unclear. It is likely that several mechanisms may be playing a role. An imbalance between vasoconstrictor and vasodilator influences may be important. When endothelium is damaged, there may be a reduction or loss of vasodilator influences such as prostacyclin or endothelial relaxing factor. Vasoconstrictive influences include α-adrenergic tone, platelet-produced thromboxane A_2, serotonin, and histamine. Recent studies suggest that endothelial damage can result in a vasodilator substance such as acetylcholine becoming a vasoconstrictor.[43] It is possible that multiple mechanisms may be playing a role. In particular, the concept of an imbalance between vasoconstricting and vasodilating factors is an attractive one. Since about 70% of human coronary lesions are felt to be eccentric,[44] vasoconstriction of the uninvolved vascular wall could be a common event. Alternatively, damage to downstream endothelium could occur in almost all lesions. These hypotheses need further clarification.

The other fact that is clear about silent ischemia is that there are large variations over weeks and months in the numbers of episodes of silent ischemia, even in patients who may have stable angina pectoris. Data are limited in this regard because of the need for multiple ambulatory electrocardiographic recordings over many months. Nevertheless, this variation is striking,[45] as seen in Figure 64.4. Another interesting sequence of events is illustrated in this figure. In this particular patient example, in addition to the marked variability in numbers of silent ischemic episodes, there appears to be a crescendo of silent ischemia just prior to myocardial infarction. This raises intriguing possibilities about the occurrence of platelet aggregation, thrombus formation, or vasoconstriction manifesting themselves as episodes of silent ischemia and as prodromes to acute myocardial infarction. Although this particular phenomenon may be restricted to a small percentage of patients who have myocardial infarction, it is an important pathophysiologic sequence that needs to be examined further.

Relative to the uncertainty regarding the incidence of acute myocardial infarction in patients with silent ischemia,[46] Assey and associates[47] compared two matched groups of patients—those with silent ischemia and those without. Of interest was the fact that over a follow-up of greater than 30 months, 6 of 27 patients with silent ischemia had a myocardial infarction compared with 1 of 28 in the angina group.

In considering the mechanisms of silent ischemia, there is considerable evidence that vasoconstriction is playing a role. In studies with rubidium-82 PET, there is evidence that an absolute decrease in blood flow occurs during silent ischemia.[48] This strongly suggests that coronary vasoconstriction is occurring in such episodes. When considering the relative importance of an increase in myocardial oxygen demand and a decrease in flow, it is important to note that the heart rate at which ischemia occurs appears to be less during episodes of silent ischemia monitored on the ambulatory electrocardiogram than the heart rate during exercise testing in the same patients. This phenomenon is noted in Figure 64.5, where a histogram distribution shows the lower heart rates at the time of ST depression during episodes of silent ischemia.[49] This information also tends to decrease the potential importance of increased myocardial oxygen demand in episodes of silent ischemia. It should be pointed out, however, that there are some episodes that are produced primarily by an increase in demand and other episodes that may be produced by a combination of both increased demand and decreased supply.

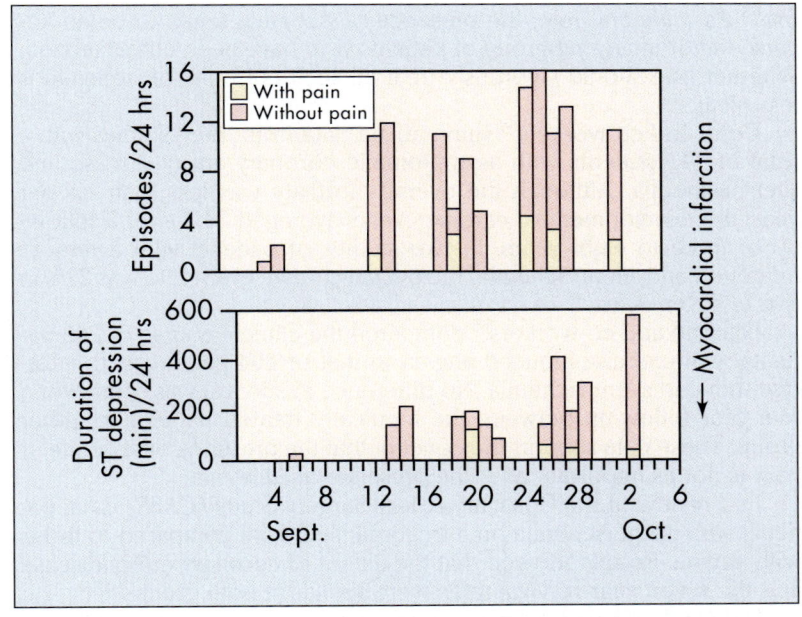

FIGURE 64.4 Serial ambulatory monitoring in a given patient done as part of a long-term research protocol. Note the considerable variability in silent ischemia, which did not have a given relationship to angina pectoris. In particular, the duration of episodes increased substantially, although angina remained constant and was followed shortly by a myocardial infarction. (Modified from Deanfield JE, Maseri A, Selwyn AP et al: Myocardial ischemia during daily life in patients with stable angina; its relation to symptoms and heart rate changes. Lancet ii: 753–758, 1983)

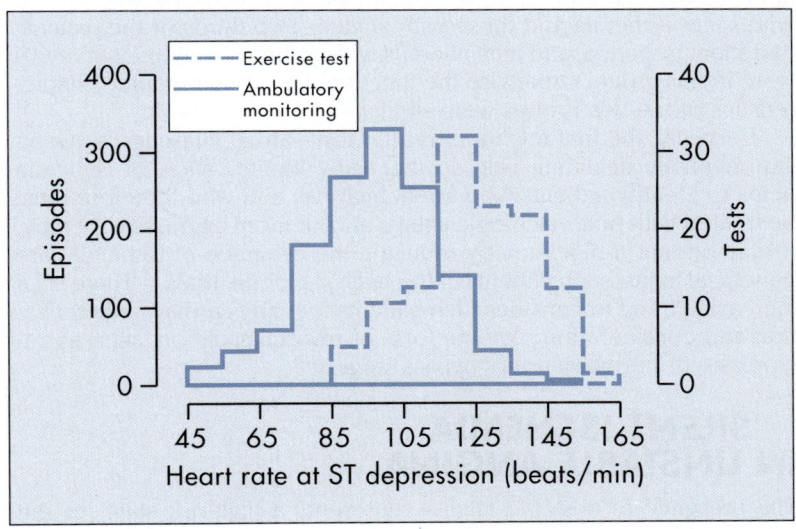

FIGURE 64.5 Two histograms show the distribution of heart rates at the onset of ST depression during an exercise test or ambulatory monitoring. In general, the heart rate at which ST depression occurred during ambulatory monitoring is less than the heart rate at which ST depression occurred during exercise. (Modified from Deanfield JE, Maseri A, Selwyn AP et al: Myocardial ischemia during daily life in patients with stable angina; its relation to symptoms and heart rate changes. Lancet ii:753–758, 1983)

SILENT MYOCARDIAL INFARCTION

The best data on the incidence of silent myocardial infarction come from the prospective Framingham Study.[50] In this study, data indicated that about 25% to 35% of myocardial infarctions are unrecognized by patient or physician. The Multiple Risk Factor Intervention Trial (MRFIT) confirmed these numbers.[51] Although some of these episodes may have been misinterpreted by the patient and/or physician, the data strongly suggest that about one out of three episodes of acute myocardial infarction are unrecognized and presumably silent. This frequency of silent myocardial infarction is probably higher in diabetic patients, which supports the hypothesis that involvement of neural pathways by diabetes alters the perception of pain in such individuals. The incidence of silent infarction in different age groups was relatively constant in the Framingham study, although there was some suggestion that it might be slightly more common at more advanced ages. There was a similar suggestion that it might be more common in women.[50] Although these trends were not striking, they should at least alert the physician to an enhanced possibility in certain patient groups such as elderly women.

SILENT ISCHEMIA AFTER MYOCARDIAL INFARCTION

One subset of patients where silent ischemia poses an increased risk is in patients soon after myocardial infarction. It is common practice to evaluate such patients with either a limited or maximal treadmill stress test at some defined time after acute myocardial infarction. In addition, such tests have been combined with thallium scintigraphy. In such studies, data suggest that patients who demonstrate ischemia on their postinfarction treadmill test are at higher risk than patients without ischemia. In a study by Theroux and associates,[52] patients were divided into two groups—those who demonstrated ST segment depression on a treadmill test and those who did not. The difference in one-year mortality was 27% in those with a positive test compared with 2% in those with a negative test. Although such striking differences have not been seen in all studies,[53] it is clear that the presence of silent myocardial ischemia does pose an additional risk to patients after myocardial infarction. In a study of 60 patients with a positive exercise test soon after myocardial infarction, a comparison was made between those with silent ischemia and those with angina. Two thirds of the patients had silent ischemia, and all 9 patients with diabetes mellitus (out of 60) were in this group. Otherwise the functional and angiographic characteristics of the two groups were similar.[54]

Certainly, the first few months after myocardial infarction show an exponentially declining risk, so that early identification of ischemia helps to identify patients who are at high risk and who therefore must be treated with pharmacologic agents and/or more aggressive therapy. It may be that β-blockers, by reducing the evidence of ischemia, are beneficial in just such patients in the large β-blocker trials.[55] There is an increasing trend to consider such patients for early cardiac catheterization and consideration of some form of revascularization, such as angioplasty or coronary artery bypass surgery.

SILENT ISCHEMIA IN UNSTABLE ANGINA

The presence of unstable angina represents a high-risk state for the patient with coronary artery disease. It is clear from a number of studies that the ischemia associated with unstable angina is associated with coronary vasoconstriction.[56,57] Studies have demonstrated an abrupt reduction in venous oxygen concentration in coronary sinus blood draining the heart, suggesting a marked reduction in flow with an increased arteriovenous oxygen difference.[56] Such changes occur spontaneously and in some instances are cyclical. There is evidence that this phenomenon might be mediated, in part, by platelet aggregation, both from studies in an animal model[58] and from the beneficial effect of aspirin in the Veterans' Administration study.[59] Vasoconstriction, platelets, and perhaps nonocclusive thrombi appear to play an important role in unstable angina and provide the setting for multiple episodes of silent myocardial ischemia. This sets the stage for appropriate antiplatelet therapy, such as aspirin, and for appropriate coronary vasodilators, such as the nitrates and calcium entry blockers. In general, such patients tend to have high-grade coronary artery disease and should generally be considered as candidates for coronary angiography and some revascularization procedure, such as angioplasty or coronary artery bypass surgery.

In a study by Gottlieb and co-workers,[60] of 70 patients with unstable angina, silent ischemia occurred in more than 50% and was a marker for an early unfavorable outcome.

PROGNOSIS OF SILENT ISCHEMIA

One of the more difficult aspects of silent ischemia is to determine its prognostic effects in patients who do not have an acute ischemic syndrome, such as unstable angina or myocardial infarction. In a study by Cohn and co-workers,[61] it was noted that patients with asymptomatic coronary disease appear to have a lesser mortality than those with manifest angina. In a more recent study,[62] it was noted that the follow-up mortality in patients with silent ischemia was approximately the same as those with manifest angina. Some arguments have been raised that patients may be at high risk for ischemic events and sudden death without an anginal warning system. Certainly, the substrate for sudden death is usually triple vessel coronary artery disease and ventricular dysfunction. In such patients with severe triple vessel disease and left ventricular dysfunction, silent ischemia may well trigger adverse events, such as sudden death, although it is unclear whether patients with silent ischemia are at greater risk than similar patients with angina. Additional data will be required to answer this important question.

One of the more interesting studies on long-term prognosis is that of Erikssen and co-workers.[11] In a group of middle-aged individuals who were screened for coronary artery disease with a treadmill test, approximately 2.5% had asymptomatic coronary artery disease. In follow-up there was a 0.5% incidence of sudden death, which occurred only in patients with three-vessel disease. The prognosis was worsened after an infarction or in the presence of left ventricular dysfunction. Other studies have suggested a yearly mortality in the range of 5% to 6%.[63] As a general rule, the presence of ischemia tends to be an adverse factor in any subgroup of patients who have been characterized. Whether one should vigorously treat all such episodes of ischemia is less clear.

Cohn and co-workers[64] summarized data from three studies with a total of 141 patients with asymptomatic coronary artery disease and silent ischemia. Although the overall mortality was less than 1% per year, the development of cardiac events averaged 34% over a follow-up of three to eight years. In two studies of patients with a remote infarction and silent ischemia, the overall cardiac event rate was 21% in five to seven years.

Falcone and co-workers[65] compared the clinical course of 269 patients with exercise-induced angina to that of 204 patients with exercise-induced silent ischemia. No difference in survival was seen over a four-year follow-up between the medically treated patients in either group. These data support the concept that the presence or absence of pain is not as important as is the presence of ischemia.

In a review of the Coronary Artery Surgery Study (CASS) data, patients with silent ischemia on a treadmill test were compared to those with angina. Results showed that the extent of coronary artery disease and the seven-year survival rates were similar in both groups.[62]

DeWood and co-workers[66] compared the survival curves of 26 patients with ST changes but no angina during an ambulatory electrocardiogram and 32 patients with no ischemia during an ambulatory electrocardiogram. All patients had coronary disease. The group exhibiting ischemia had a higher cardiac event rate (46%) and mortality (9%) over three years compared to an event rate of 23% and 6% in the nonischemic group. The presence of silent ischemia appeared to contribute to a worse outcome.

In 28 patients with exercise-induced thallium defects, Walters and co-workers[67] showed a worse prognosis in those without exercise-induced symptoms compared to those who developed angina during the stress test.

In patients with coronary artery disease who survive out-of-hospital ventricular fibrillation, silent ischemia is common and has been implicated as a pathophysiologic cause.[68]

There seems to be clear-cut evidence that the presence of ischemia has an adverse prognostic effect in every subset of patients with coronary artery disease. One important concept is that angina is not an independent risk factor: that is, ischemia is the risk factor, independent of the presence or absence of angina.[69] This concept is illustrated in the follow-up of patients in the medical arm of the CASS study (Fig. 64.6). Note that exercise-induced ischemia (ST depression) worsened the prognosis, whether or not angina was present.[70]

SURGERY FOR ASYMPTOMATIC CORONARY ARTERY DISEASE

Coronary artery bypass grafting is an important technique for relieving symptoms, and in some groups of patients it can prolong life. It is less clear what the potential role of surgery is in patients with asymptomatic coronary artery disease or silent ischemia. If a patient is truly asymptomatic, it will be difficult for bypass surgery to improve symptoms. The major role of such surgery, therefore, would appear to be in prolongation of life. Surgery can be done with low mortality and morbidity in patients who are asymptomatic. The potential effects on long-term mortality are less certain. In a study by Norris and colleagues,[71] high-risk patients with two to three previous myocardial infarctions were randomized to medical or surgical therapy. Although only 50 patients were randomized in each group, there was no difference in annual mortality between the two groups. In the CASS angina study,[72] patients with mild angina appeared to fare as well whether treated medically or surgically, at least over the first five years. In longer term follow-up, however, those patients with advanced coronary artery disease and left ventricular dysfunction had a better survival curve with surgical therapy. Similarly, in all studies, those patients with left main coronary artery disease do better with surgery than with medical therapy.[73] It would appear appropriate, therefore, to consider the possibility of surgery in patients with silent ischemia if they have either left main coronary artery disease or severe triple vessel disease with left ventricular dysfunction.

Blumenthal and co-workers[74] noted a number of patients who had markedly positive tests with minimal or no symptoms in a retrospective review of a large cohort of patients catheterized for coronary artery disease. In those patients with markedly positive exercise tests and minimal or no symptoms, there was a high incidence of left main coronary artery disease and triple vessel coronary artery disease. It appears reasonable, therefore, that a markedly positive test, even in the absence of symptoms, should alert the physician to the possibility of severe, high-grade coronary artery disease. Cardiac catheterization to rule out left main coronary artery disease seems to be the logical next step.

In a comparative study of surgical versus medical therapy in patients with mild angina, it was noted that patients with triple vessel disease and left ventricular dysfunction may also live longer with surgery, as compared to medical therapy.[75] Although most of the studies in the literature deal with symptomatic patients and, therefore, are difficult to extrapolate to the truly asymptomatic patient with silent ischemia, it still appears reasonable to consider that patients with left ventricular dysfunction and severe coronary artery disease are potential candidates for revascularization, even in the absence of usual anginal symptoms.

It is unclear what potential role balloon angioplasty might play in patients with silent ischemia. In patients who have undergone myocardial infarction and thrombolytic therapy, it appears that those patients who have also undergone balloon angioplasty following thrombolytic therapy have less ischemia on treadmill testing than those who have just had thrombolytic therapy.[76] Thus, although one can dissolve the clot that produced the infarction, the underlying severe lesion remained in the group treated only with thrombolytic therapy but was dilated in the patients treated with balloon angioplasty. Although there is a temptation to correct coronary lesions if they are found in patients with silent ischemia and asymptomatic coronary disease, this course of action remains unproven therapy at the present time. The role of balloon angioplasty in silent ischemia, therefore, remains to be determined, except for some obvious subsets where continuing ischemia places patients at higher risk.

MEDICAL THERAPY IN SILENT ISCHEMIA

In patients with manifest angina pectoris, all three classes of antianginal drugs—β-blockers, nitrates, and calcium entry blockers—appear to be beneficial in reducing the incidence of angina. Presumably all three classes of drugs are helpful in reducing myocardial oxygen demand, and the calcium blockers and nitrates are also effective in relieving vasoconstriction and thus improving supply in patients affected.[77,78] Studies in patients with angina have also suggested that combination drug therapy may be slightly more effective than any single class of drugs used alone. There are little data in patients with silent ischemia to judge the same effects. It would appear, however, that the

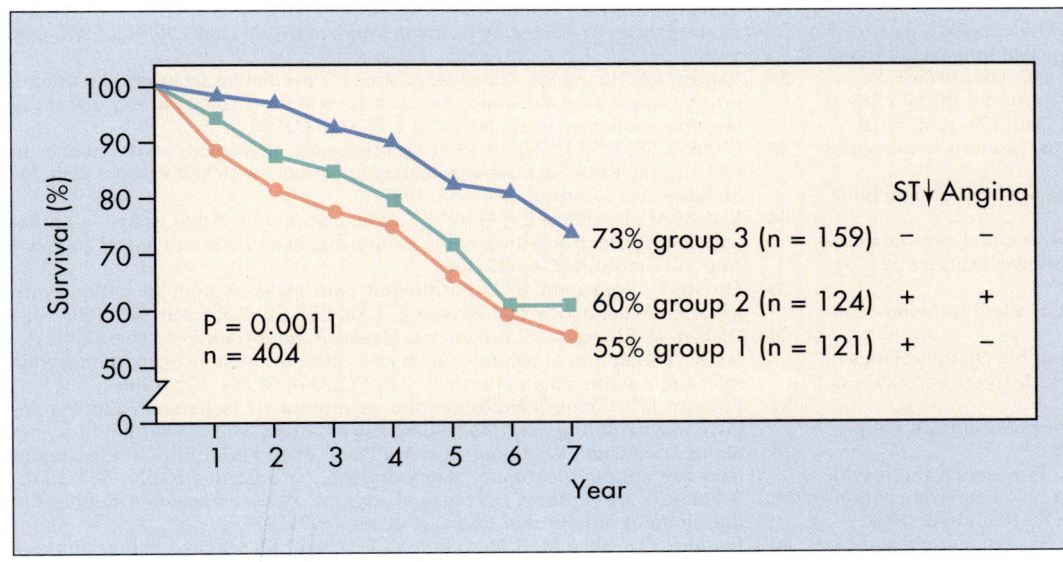

FIGURE 64.6 Cumulative survival in 404 medically treated patients from the CASS study. During exercise, group 1 had ischemic ST-segment depression without angina; group 2 had both ischemic ST depression and angina; and group 3 had neither ischemic ST depression nor angina.[70]

same principles may well apply and that all three classes of drugs appear to be beneficial in patients with episodes of silent ischemia. Because of the preponderance of evidence that silent ischemia may be associated with vasoconstriction,[79] it seems reasonable to consider that nitrates or calcium entry blockers might potentially play a more important role than β-blockers in this subset of patients. At the same time, however, it should be noted that the β-blockers have been effective in reducing morbidity and mortality in postmyocardial infarction patients in a way that the calcium blockers have not yet been proved effective. Since continuing ischemia may well be the substrate for adverse events in such patients, one cannot lightly dismiss the β-blockers. In the absence, therefore, of hard comparative data at this point in time, it would appear reasonable that all three classes of drugs can be considered as potential therapy for patients with silent ischemia, in a manner analagous to angina pectoris.

A more difficult question to answer is which patients should be considered for treatment. It seems logical that the greatest benefit will be achieved by treating high-risk patients. This group would include individuals seen soon after myocardial infarction or in association with unstable angina. It might also include individuals who have triple vessel disease and left ventricular dysfunction. It seems reasonable to consider such patients for pharmacologic treatment and, in some cases, for consideration of revascularization procedures. It is less clear whether totally asymptomatic patients with good exercise tolerance and silent ischemia need to be treated in an aggressive manner. Ongoing studies will help to answer such questions regarding these individuals who generally have a good prognosis with a less than 1% per year mortality.

CLINICAL IMPLICATIONS

This chapter has reviewed current knowledge of our understanding of the prevalence and importance of silent myocardial ischemia. Because this topic is of great current interest, ongoing and future clinical studies will help to answer many of the questions posed. Until hard facts are available, however, it appears reasonable to evaluate patients for the potential presence of silent ischemia if they fall in certain high-risk groups. If such patients are found to have silent ischemia, it also appears prudent to consider treatment with pharmacologic agents, or in cases of a perceived high risk, to consider more aggressive therapy such as angioplasty or coronary artery bypass surgery. On the other hand, it appears unjustified to routinely screen healthy individuals for the presence of silent myocardial ischemia. Studies are best reserved for those individuals with known coronary artery disease and especially for those individuals who are perceived to be at high risk because of other prognostic factors.

REFERENCES

1. Singh BN, Nademanee K, Figueras J, Josephson MA: Hemodynamic and electrocardiographic correlates of symptomatic and silent myocardial ischemia: Pathophysiologic and therapeutic implications. Am J Cardiol 58:3B–10B, 1986
2. Subramanian VB: Clinical and research applications of ambulatory holter ST-segment and heart rate monitoring. Am J Cardiol 58:11B–20B, 1986
3. Rocco MB, Nabel EG, Selwyn AP: Circadian rhythms and coronary artery disease. Am J Cardiol 59:13C–17C, 1986
4. Deanfield JE: Holter monitoring in assessment of angina pectoris. Am J Cardiol 59:18C–22C, 1987
5. Deanfield JA, Shea MJ, Selwyn AP: Clinical evaluation of transient myocardial ischemia during daily life. Am J Med (Suppl 3A) 79:18–24, 1985
6. Sigwart V, Grbic M, Payot M et al: Ischemic events during coronary artery balloon obstruction. In Rutishauser W, Roskamm H (eds): Silent Myocardial Ischemia, pp 29–36. Berlin, Springer-Verlag, 1984
7. Tomoda H, Parmley WW, Fujimura S, Matloff JM: Effects of ischemia and reoxygenation on the regional myocardial performance of the dog. Am J Physiol 221:1718–1721, 1971
8. Selwyn AP, Shea MJ, Deanfield JE et al: Clinical problems in coronary disease are caused by wide variety of ischemic episodes that affect patients out of hospital. Am J Med (Suppl 3A) 79:12–17, 1985
9. Cohn PF: Asymptomatic coronary artery disease. Modern Concepts of Cardiovascular Disease 50:55–60, 1981
10. Cohn PF: Total ischemic burden: Definition, mechanisms, and therapeutic implications. Am J Med (Suppl 4A) 81:2–11, 1986
11. Eriksen J, Thaulow E: Follow-up of patients with asymptomatic myocardial ischemia. In Rutishauser W, Roskamm H (eds): Silent Myocardial Ischemia, pp 156–164. Berlin, Springer-Verlag, 1984
12. Froelicher VF, Yanowitz FG, Thompson AJ Jr et al. The correlation of coronary angiography and the electrocardiographic response to maximal treadmill testing in 76 asymptomatic men. Circulation 48:597–604, 1973
13. Diamond GA, Forrester JS: Analysis of probability as an aid in the clinical diagnosis of coronary-artery disease. N Engl J Med 300:1350–1358, 1979
14. Cohn PF: Silent myocardial ischemia: Present status. Modern Concepts of Cardiovascular Disease 56:1–5, 1987
15. Ellestad MH: Stress-testing: Principles and Practices, 2nd Ed. Philadelphia, FA Davis, 1980
16. Coy KM, Imperi GA, Lambert CR, Pepine CJ: Silent myocardial ischemia during daily activities in asymptomatic men with positive exercise test responses. Am J Cardiol 59:45–49, 1987
17. Berman DS, Rozanski A, Knoebel SB: The detection of silent ischemia: Cautions and precautions. Circulation 75:101–105, 1987
18. Tzivoni D, Stern Z, Keren A, Stern S: Electrocardiographic characteristics of neurocirculatory asthenia during everyday activities. Br Heart J 44:426–432, 1980
19. Stern S, Tzivoni D: Dynamic changes in the ST-T segment during sleep in ischemic heart disease. Am J Cardiol 32:17–20, 1973
20. Armstrong WF, Jordan JW, Morris SN, McHenry PL: Prevalence and magnitude of S-T segment and T wave abnormalities in normal men during continuous ambulatory electrocardiography. Am J Cardiol 49:1636–1642, 1982
21. Deanfield JE, Ribiero P, Oakley K et al: Analysis of ST-segment changes in normal subjects: Implications for ambulatory monitoring in angina pectoris. Am J Cardiol 54:1321–1325, 1984
22. Selwyn AP, Shea M, Deanfield JE et al: Character of transient ischemia in angina pectoris. Am J Cardiol 58:21B–25B, 1986
23. Chatterjee K, Parmley WW, Marcus H et al: Depression of left ventricular function due to acute myocardial ischemia and its reversal following aortocoronary saphenous vein bypass. N Engl J Med 286:1117–1122, 1972
24. Klausner SC, Ratshin RA, Tyberg JV et al: The similarity of changes in segmental contraction patterns induced by post-extrasystolic potentiation and nitroglycerin. Circulation 54:615–623, 1976
25. Levy R et al: The haemodynamic significance of asymptomatic ST segment depression assessed by ambulatory pulmonary artery pressure monitoring. Br Heart J 56:526–530, 1986
26. Chatterjee K, Matloff JM, Swan HJC et al: Abnormal regional metabolism and mechanical function in patients with ischemic heart disease: Improvement after successful regional revascularization by aortocoronary bypass. Circulation 52:390–399, 1975
27. Chatterjee K, Swan HJC, Parmley WW et al: Influence of direct myocardial revascularization on left ventricular asynergy and function in patients with coronary heart disease: With and without previous myocardial infarction. Circulation 47:276–286, 1973
28. Braunwald E, Rutherford JD: Reversible ischemic left ventricular dysfunction: Evidence for the "hibernating myocardium." J Am Coll Cardiol 8:1467–1470, 1986
29. Gertz EW, Wisneski JA, Neese R et al: Myocardial lactate metabolism: Evidence of lactate release during net chemical extraction in man. Circulation 63:1273, 1981
30. Osbakken M, Briggs RW: NMR: Theory and review of cardiac applications. Am Heart J 108:574, 1984
31. Tillish J, Brunken R, Marshall R et al: Reversibility of cardiac wall motion abnormalities predicted by positron tomography. N Engl J Med 314:884–888, 1986
32. Langou RA, Huang EK, Kelley MJ, Cohen LS: Predictive accuracy of coronary artery calcification and abnormal exercise test for coronary artery disease in asymptomatic men. Circulation 62:1196–1203, 1980
33. Chipkin SR, Frid D, Alpert JS et al: Frequency of painless myocardial ischemia during exercise tolerance testing in patients with and without diabetes mellitus. Am J Cardiol 59:61–65, 1987
34. Cecchi AC, Dovellini EV, Marchi R et al: Silent myocardial ischemia during ambulatory electrocardiographic monitoring in patients with effort angina. J Am Coll Cardiol 1:934–939, 1983
35. Droste C, Roskamm H: Experimental pain measurement in patient with asymptomatic myocardial ischemia. J Am Coll Cardiol 1:940–945, 1983
36. Glazier JJ, Chierchia S, Brown MJ, Maseri A: Importance of generalized defective perception of painful stimuli as a cause of silent myocardial ischemia in chronic stable angina pectoris. Am J Cardiol 58:667–672, 1986
37. Ellestad MH, Kuan P: Naloxone and asymptomatic ischemia: Failure to induce angina during exercise testing. Am J Cardiol 54:982–984, 1984
38. Sheps DS, Adams KF, Hinderliter A, Price C et al: Endorphins are related to pain perception in coronary artery disease. Am J Cardiol 59:523–527, 1987
39. Schang SJ Jr, Pepine CJ: Transient asymptomatic ST-segment depression during daily activity. Am J Cardiol 39:396–402, 1977
40. Deanfield JE, Shea M, Ribiero P et al: Transient ST-segment depression as a

marker of myocardial ischemia during daily life. Am J Cardiol 54:1195–1200, 1984

41. Rocco MB, Nabel EG, Selwyn AP: Circadian rhythms and coronary artery disease. Am J Cardiol 59:13C–17C, 1987
42. Muller JE, Ludmer PL, Willich SN et al: Circadian variation in the frequency of sudden cardiac death. Circulation 75:131–138, 1987
43. Ludmer PL, Selwyn AP, Shook TL et al: Parodoxical acetylcholine-induced coronary artery constriction in patients with coronary artery disease. N Engl J Med 315:1045–1051, 1986
44. Freudenberg H, Lichtlen PR: The normal wall segment in coronary stenosis—post mortem study. Z Cardiol 70:863–870, 1971
45. Cohn PF: Total ischemic burden: Definition, mechanisms, and therapeutic implications. Am J Med 81:2–6, 1986
46. Deedwania P: Silent myocardial ischemia and its relationship to acute myocardial infarction. Cardiology Clinics 4:643–658, 1986
47. Assey ME, Walters GL, Hendrix GH et al: Incidence of acute myocardial infarction in patients with exercise-induced silent myocardial ischemia. Am J Cardiol 59:497–500, 1987
48. Selwyn AP, Allan RM, L'Abbate A et al: Relation between regional myocardial uptake of rubidium-82 and perfusion: Absolute reduction of cation uptake in ischemia. Am J Cardiol 50:112–121, 1982
49. Deanfield JE, Shea M, Ribiero P et al: Transient ST-segment depression as a marker of myocardial ischemia during daily life. Am J Cardiol 54:1195–1200, 1984
50. Kannel WB: Prevalence and clinical aspects of unrecognized myocardial infarction and sudden unexpected death. Circulation (Suppl II) 75:II 4–5, 1987
51. Grimm RH, Tillinghast S, Daniels K et al: Unrecognized myocardial infarction: Experience in the multiple risk factor intervention trial (MRFIT). Circulation (Suppl II) 75:II-6–II-11, 1987
52. Theroux P, Waters DD, Halpren C et al: Prognostic value of exercise testing soon after myocardial infarction. N Engl J Med 301:341–345, 1979
53. Starling MR, Cranford MH, Kennedy GT, O'Rourke RA: Exercise testing early after myocardial infarction: Predictive value for subsequent unstable angina and death. Am J Cardiol 46:909–914, 1980
54. Ouyang P, Shapiro EP, Chandra NC et al: An angiographic and functional comparison of patients with silent and symptomatic treadmill ischemia early after myocardial infarction. Am J Cardiol 59:730–734, 1987
55. May GS: A review of long-term Beta blocker trials in survivors of myocardial infarction. Circulation (Suppl II) 67:I-46–I-49, 1983
56. Chiercia S, Lazzari M, Freedman B et al: Impairment of myocardial perfusion and function during painless myocardial ischemia. J Am Coll Cardiol 1:924–930, 1983
57. Nademanee K, Intarachot V, Singh PN et al: Characteristics and clinical significance of silent myocardial ischemia in unstable angina. Am J Cardiol 58:26B–33B, 1986
58. Folts JD, Gallagher K, Rowe GC: Blood flow reduction in stenosed canine arteries: Vasospasm or platelet aggregation. Circulation 65:248, 1982
59. Lewis HD, Davis JW, Archibald DG et al: Protective effects of aspirin against acute myocardial infarction and death in men with unstable angina. N Engl J Med 309:396–403, 1983
60. Gottlieb SO, Weisfeldt ML, Ouyang P et al: Silent ischemia as a marker for early unfavorable outcomes in patients with unstable angina. N Engl J Med 314:214–219, 1986
61. Cohn PF, Harris P, Barry WH et al: Prognostic importance of anginal symptoms in angiographically defined coronary artery disease. Am J Cardiol 47:233, 1981
62. Weiner DA, Ryan TJ, McCabe CH et al: Significance of silent myocardial ischemia during exercise testing in patients with coronary artery disease. Am J Cardiol 59:725–729, 1987
63. Cohn PF: Silent Myocardial Ischemia and Infarction. New York, Marcel Dekker, 1986
64. Cohn PF: Silent myocardial ischemia, classification, prevalence, and prognosis. Am J Med (Suppl 3A) 79:2–6, 1985
65. Falcone C, De Servi S, Poma E et al: Clinical significance of exercise-induced silent myocardial ischemia in patients with coronary artery disease. J Am Coll Cardiol 9:295–299, 1987
66. Dewood MA: Long-term prognosis of patients with and without silent ischemia (abstr). Circulation 74:II–59, 1986
67. Walters GL, Assey ME, Hendrix GH et al: Increased incidence of myocardial infarction in patients with exercise induced silent myocardial ischemia (abstr). Circulation 74:II–58, 1986
68. Hodges M, Wyeth RP: Demonstration of exercise induced painless myocardial ischemia in survivors of out-of-hospital ventricular fibrillation. Am J Cardiol 59:740–745, 1987
69. Chatterjee K: Ischemia—silent or manifest: Does it matter? J Amer Coll Cardiol 13:1503–1505, 1989
70. Weiner DA, Ryan TJ, McCabe CH et al: The role of exercise-induced silent myocardial ischemia in patients with abnormal left ventricular function: A report from the Coronary Artery Surgery Study (CASS) Registry. Am Heart J 118:649–654, 1989
71. Norris RM, Agnew TM, Brandt PWT et al: Coronary surgery after recurrent myocardial infarction: Progress of a trial comparing surgical with non-surgical management for asymptomatic patients with advanced coronary disease. Circulation 63:785–792, 1981
72. Passamani E, Davis KB, Gillespie MJ et al: A randomized trial of coronary artery bypass surgery: Survival of patients with a low ejection fraction. N Engl J Med 312:1665–1671, 1985
73. Takaro T: The Veteran's Cooperative Randomized Study of surgery for coronary arterial occlusive disease: Subgroup with significant left main lesions. Circulation 54:III–107, 1976
74. Blumenthal DS, Weiss JL, Mellits ED, Gerstenblith G: The predictive value of a strongly positive stress test in patients with minimal symptoms. Am J Med 70:1005–1010, 1981
75. Hammermeister KE, DeRoven TA, Dodge HT: Comparison of survival of medically and surgically treated patients in Seattle Heart Watch. Circulation 65:535, 1982
76. Fung AY, Lai P, Junl JE: Prevention of subsequent exercise induced perinfarct ischemia by emergency coronary angioplasty in acute MI. J Am Coll Cardiol 8:496–503, 1986
77. Resnekov L: Silent myocardial ischemia, therapeutic implications. Am J Med (Suppl 3A) 79:30–34, 1985
78. Pepine CJ, Hill JA: Medical therapy for silent myocardial ischemia. Circulation (Suppl II) 75:II-43–46, 1987
79. Deanfield JE, Maseri A, Selwyn AP et al: Myocardial ischemia during daily life in patients with stable angina; its relation to symptoms and heart rate changes. Lancet ii:753–758, 1983

VARIANT ANGINA

John Speer Schroeder

The term *variant angina* was coined by Prinzmetal in 1959 when he and his co-workers published a description of three patients that varied from traditional exertional or Heberden's angina.[1,2] The prime "variant" features were typical of angina pectoris except that it occurred at rest or during sleep rather than during exertion and an electrocardiogram (ECG) during an episode of chest pain showed ST segment elevation suggestive of an acute myocardial infarction rather than ST segment depression. However, resolution of the pain by sublingual nitroglycerin spontaneously resulted in resolution of the abnormal ST segment elevation. The authors proposed that this syndrome was most likely due to temporary occlusion of a large diseased coronary artery due to increased tone or local spasm. Previous observers have also commented on the possibility of spasm of the coronary artery causing or contributing to the angina pectoris syndrome. Osler observed that angina pectoris was associated with changes in the arterial wall that were organic or functional.[3] Then, in 1941, Wilson and Johnston reported a patient with ST segment elevation in ECG leads II, III, and aV$_F$ during spontaneous episodes of chest pain and observed that "the attendant myocardial ischemia is due to a change in caliber of coronary arteries affected, rather than an increase in work of the heart."[4]

Variant angina pectoris was considered a relatively rare problem until the advent of coronary arteriography in the early 1970s, when it was observed that as many as 10% of patients with rest or unstable angina have a normal or relatively normal coronary arteriogram.[5] Subsequently, the introduction of a provocative test for Prinzmetal's angina allowed more precise definition, characterization, and understanding of the syndrome.[6] Many of Prinzmetal's theories about the pathophysiology of variant angina have turned out to be remarkably perceptive.

This chapter will focus on variant angina rather than discuss the multiple angina syndromes in which coronary artery spasm may play a role.

CLINICAL PRESENTATION

The typical patient with variant angina reports recurrent episodes of angina pectoris that are typical in their character, distribution, and responsiveness to nitroglycerin. The pain is substernal, with a tight, constricting pressure sensation in the chest that may radiate into the neck, jaw, teeth, or inner aspect of the left and/or right arm. Occasionally, patients report the pain occurring predominantly in the jaw or arm with minimal or no chest pain. The pain typically awakens the patients at night or in the early morning hours and can be very severe. Other episodes may occur after arising in the early morning or at other times of the day during rest. In addition to the unprovoked episodes, approximately 50% of patients also report at least some angina related to physical exertion or excitement but these episodes may occur after cessation of the activity rather than at its peak. Although the circadian nature of the attacks usually remains similar for a given patient, the frequency and severity of the episodes tend to be highly variable and cyclical. Many patients report general worsening of their symptoms during periods of emotional stress in their lives.

The angina usually resolves spontaneously after a few minutes but may last much longer. Response to sublingual nitroglycerin tends to be excellent; in fact, the diagnosis should be questioned if there is not a rapid response to either oral or sublingual nitrates. Patients may complain of anxiety or shortness of breath during the angina if the pain is prolonged and causes transient left ventricular dysfunction and pulmonary venous congestion. Patients with more severe episodes may present with complaints of syncope during or following their angina. It is believed that these syncopal episodes are related to either ischemia-induced ventricular arrhythmias or hypotension.

In addition to a careful history and characterization of the pain, one should look for other features of the variant angina syndrome and for manifestations of other vasospastic phenomena. Most patients present between the ages of 35 and 50 years. There is a female predominance and a frequent smoking history, and most patients acknowledge stress or tension either in their personal life or job. There is frequently a history of migraine headache in the patient or his or her family. Complaints of Raynaud's phenomenon are common, and some patients simply complain that their hands and feet have been cold all of their lives.

A high index of suspicion for variant angina is important since these patients may themselves attribute their chest pains to "nerves," and unless the diagnosis of variant angina is being considered many of these patients are diagnosed as having psychogenic chest pain. The report that the chest pain awakens them from sleep is one of the most important clues that this is a medical problem rather than a psychological one.

PATHOPHYSIOLOGY

In contrast to exertion-induced angina pectoris in which the pain and myocardial ischemia reflect an inadequate increase in coronary blood flow through the diseased coronary vessel as myocardial work and oxygen demand increase, variant angina occurs due to a transient reduction in coronary flow. Although this etiology has been proposed for many years, and repeatedly demonstrated experimentally, the first patient with documented spontaneous coronary spasm during coronary arteriography was reported by Oliva and co-workers in 1973.[7] Since that time, numerous investigators have observed and reported focal coronary artery spasm occurring either spontaneously or after provocation during coronary arteriography.[8–10] There is little doubt that this focal spasm is responsible for the reduction in coronary flow and causes transient transmural myocardial ischemia, resulting in the chest pain or variant angina. The coronary spasm tends to be focal and frequently occurs at an area of atherosclerotic plaque or abnormality in the vessel. MacAlpin and associates have reported that the focal spasm tends to occur in the same area on repeated occasions and in an area of atherosclerotic plaque during both spontaneous and provoked spasm.[11] The spasm can occur in any of the coronary arteries, although the right coronary artery and, to a lesser degree, the left anterior descending coronary artery are the ones most commonly involved. Patients with very severe coronary artery spasm have been observed to have spasm in more than one vessel or for the spasm to involve a greater length of the vessel. Incomplete occlusion of the vessel has been observed repeatedly. This may cause nontransmural myocardial ischemia in the area supplied by the vessel, resulting in ST segment depression or even silent ischemia in these patients. It is believed, however, that this nontransmural ischemia is simply part of the spectrum of coronary artery spasm and that causes for occasionally incomplete spasm are the same as those for complete occlusion of a vessel.

There are three questions regarding the pathophysiology of this coronary artery spasm: (1) Why does the spasm tend to occur in a localized area of the vessel? (2) What initiates or precipitates the spasm? (3) What are the underlying pathophysiologic causes?

First, the fact that the spasm tends to occur in areas of abnormality or atherosclerotic plaques suggests a local hyperreactivity in the wall of the coronary artery. It has been observed that patients with variant angina tend to have recurrent episodes in the same location, suggesting that this is a local abnormality or hyperreactivity to some vasoconstrictive influence rather than to a generalized hyperreactivity or abnormality in the innervation or level of sympathetic tone of the coronary vessels. Ginsburg and co-workers have reported that in human coronary arteries, areas containing atherosclerotic plaques tend to be more reactive to some vasoconstrictive influences such as histamine in comparison to areas that are not involved with the atherosclerotic process.[12] These studies have been confirmed by other investigators and suggest that a local abnormality may be responsible for the spasm. In addition, it has been recognized that varying provocative agents can precipitate coronary artery spasm in an individual patient. This would suggest that it is not the agent but an abnormality in vasoreactivity in the area where the spasm occurs that is responsible for the spasm and the clinical symptoms.

Second, what are the precipitating causes of this focal spasm in an area of local increased vasoreactivity? Many hypotheses have been proposed including increased vagal tone during sleep. This hypothesis has been supported by the use of methacholine inducing coronary spasm in some reports.[13,14] However, the mechanism for the actual vasoconstrictor triggering of the focal spasm during this period is not understood. Other authors have proposed that the focal spasm occurs at times of increased vagal tone when there is unopposed withdrawal of sympathetic tone such as during sleep or after exercise. Other hypotheses have centered around the general or local release of vasoconstrictive substances such as thromboxane A_2 or sympathomimetic amines; however, these theories would not explain the focality of the spasm.

It is most likely that two circumstances are required to have typical variant angina. One is a local hyperreactivity of a segment of coronary artery, and the other is abnormal release or triggering of the vasoconstrictive influence.

DIAGNOSIS
HISTORY AND PHYSICAL EXAMINATION

The hallmark of a patient with variant angina is the history of spontaneous or unprovoked episodes of typical angina pectoris. At times when the patient is not having variant angina, examination is usually normal or unrelated to the variant angina syndrome. During an episode of pain, the patient may manifest symptoms of pain, sweating, tachycardia, and increased blood pressure in response to the pain. Ventricular arrhythmias are common. The patient with right coronary spasm may have varying degrees of atrioventricular (AV) block. More severe or prolonged episodes of myocardial ischemia may result in manifestations of left ventricular dysfunction such as an S_3 or S_4 gallop rhythm, bibasalar rales or pulmonary congestion or a transient murmur of mitral insufficiency due to ischemic papillary muscle dysfunction. The diagnosis, however, although suspected on the basis of history and physical examination must be confirmed on the ECG and preferably during coronary arteriography.

ECG STUDIES

To establish the diagnosis of typical variant angina it is essential to observe transient ST segment elevation on an ECG during an episode of preferably spontaneous angina pectoris. The ECG abnormalities occur in the areas supplied by the artery that is undergoing coronary spasm and is transiently occluded. The ST segment elevation can be

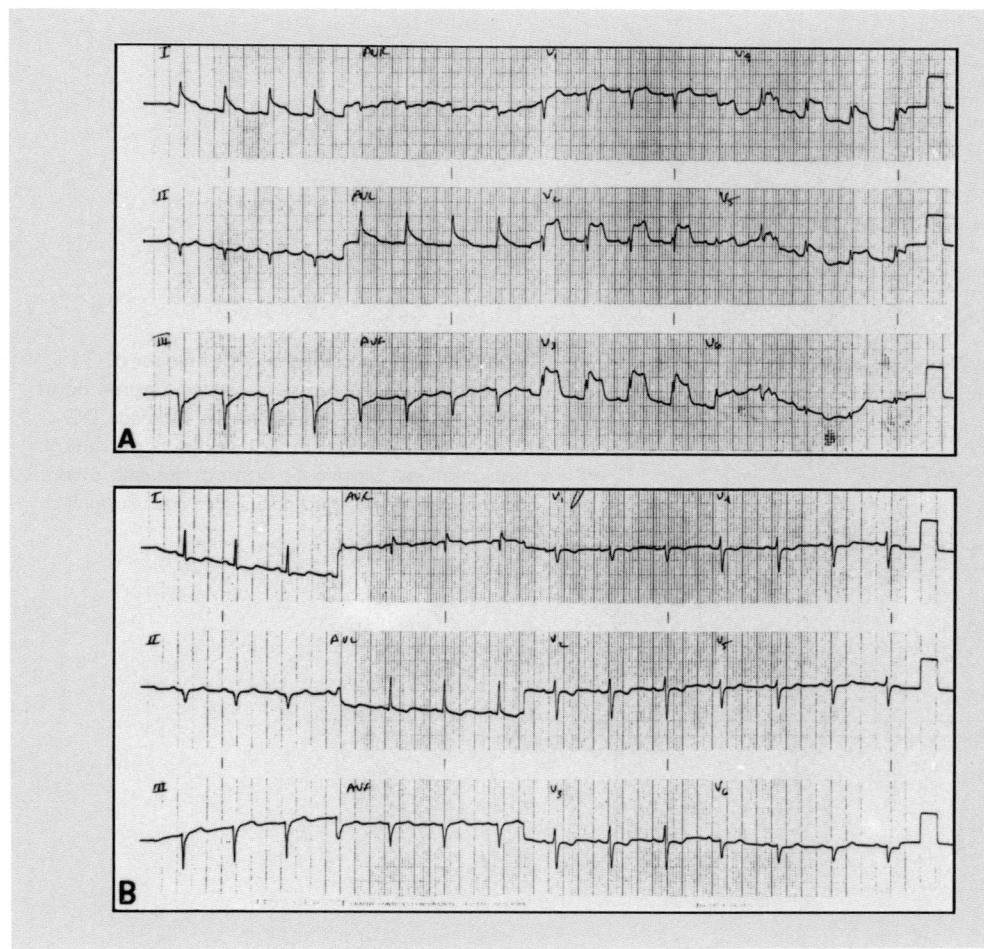

FIGURE 65.1 Marked ST segment elevation in the anterior leads of a 12-lead ECG during angina caused by spasm of the left anterior descending artery induced by 0.1 mg ergonovine maleate (**A**) and after nitroglycerin (**B**). (Schroeder JS (ed): Invasive Cardiology, pp 83–96. Philadelphia, FA Davis, 1984)

either minimal or at times very dramatic, nearly obscuring the QRS complex and appearing to be the initial ECG manifestations of an acute transmural myocardial infarction (Fig. 65.1). However, the ST segment elevation resolves with the administration of sublingual nitroglycerin. It is not unusual to see ventricular arrhythmias or even ventricular tachycardia or complete heart block during an episode of severe coronary artery spasm. Since the episodes of pain tend to occur at night and spontaneously, it may be difficult to record an ECG during a severe episode of pain. There are several alternative approaches to this in order to establish a diagnosis.

AMBULATORY ECG MONITORING

If the patient is having frequent or daily episodes of chest pain, ambulatory ECG recordings may be effective in establishing the diagnosis. A two-channel recorder with sufficiently low frequency response to detect 0.1 mV changes is essential. By recording two channels, that is, one inferior and one anterior lead, ST segment elevation reflecting spasm of either the right or left anterior descending coronary artery may be observed (Fig. 65.2). In addition, patients who complain of syncope or palpitations may have arrhythmias or heart block documented during chest pain as well (Fig. 65.3).

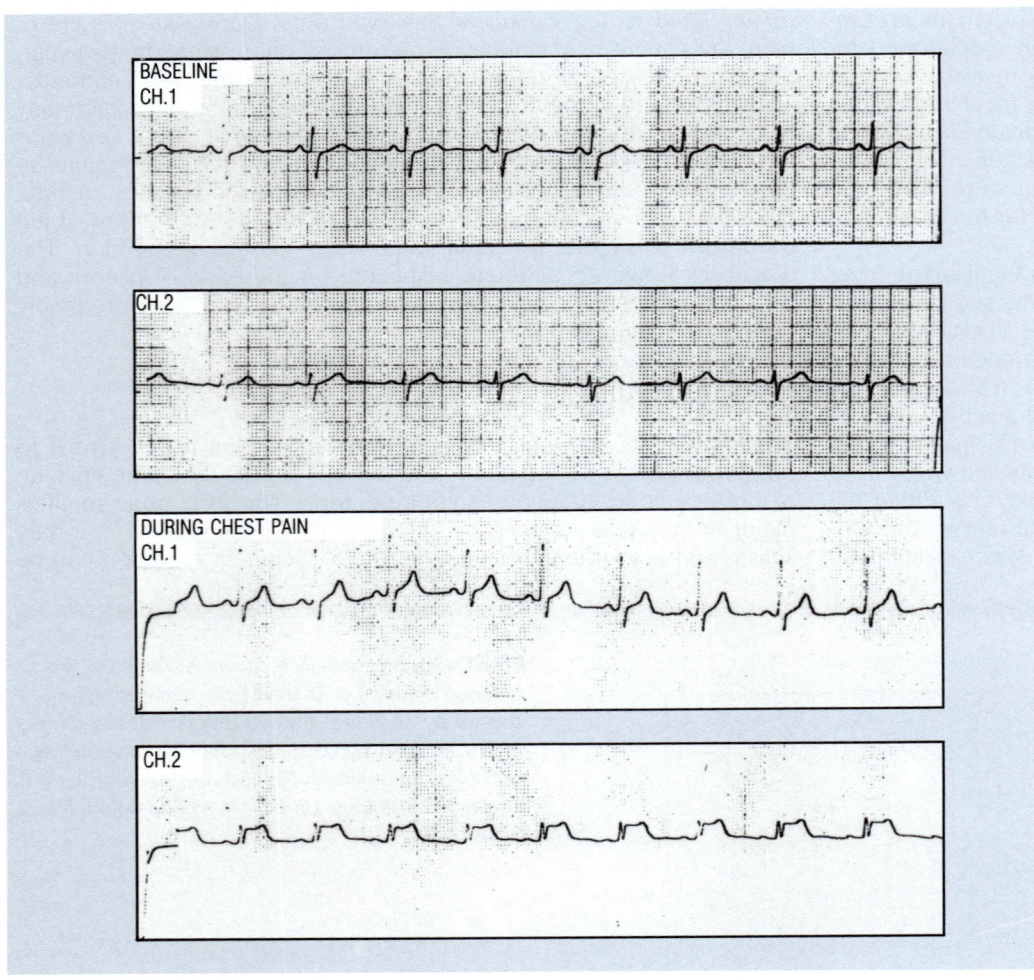

FIGURE 65.2 Two-channel ambulatory ECG recordings during pain-free period (*upper panel*) and during angina (*lower panel*). (Schroeder JS (ed): Invasive Cardiology. Philadelphia, FA Davis, 1984)

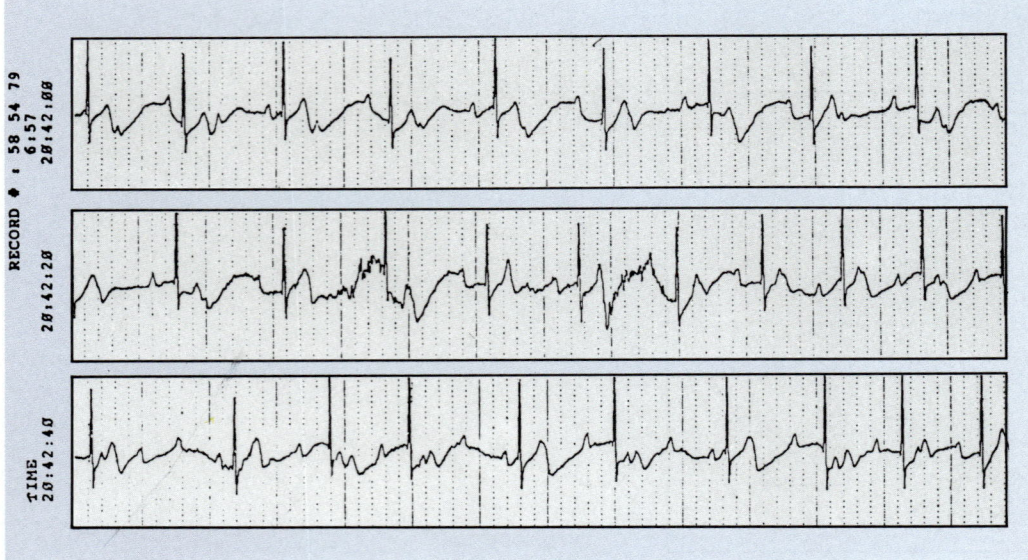

FIGURE 65.3 Computer printout of Holter ECG recording showing transient second-degree heart block. (Ginsburg R, Schroeder JS, Harrison DC: Coronary artery spasm: Pathophysiology, clinical presentations, diagnostic approaches and rational treatment. West J Med 136:398, 1982. Reprinted by permission)

At other times, patients may have minimal or no chest pain during the episode reflecting "silent ischemia" as detected on the ECG. In these patients there may be episodes of transient ST segment depression or even occasionally ST segment elevation that are brief and so do not come to clinical attention or result in complaints of angina. In order to establish a diagnosis of variant angina, it is preferable to have at least one episode of ST segment elevation in association with a complaint of or observed chest pain.

SELF-INITIATED TRANSTELEPHONIC ECG MONITORING

Since many patients with variant angina have infrequent or unpredictable chest pain that is not suitable for diagnosis by ambulatory ECG monitoring, Ginsburg and colleagues have reported the use of transtelephonic transmission of an ECG during symptomatic chest pain.[15] Here, a transtelephonic device such as the Cardiobeeper (Survival Technology), which is a bipolar lead system with low frequency response, can be used to transmit one or two leads of an ECG during chest pain. The episode can either be stored on certain units for subsequent transmission or be transmitted by telephone directly during chest pain and recorded for subsequent analysis. It is essential that a baseline transmission be taken for comparison owing to the highly variable nature of ST segment shifts. This system is quite helpful when it is positive, particularly if ST segment elevation is observed (Fig. 65.4). However, because of the single lead nature of the transmission system and the difficulty in ascertaining how severe the symptomatic episode of chest pain was, a negative test does not rule out a diagnosis of variant angina.

TREADMILL EXERCISE TESTING

Although the typical patient with variant angina who has relatively normal coronary arteries will have a negative treadmill exercise test and no exertional evidence of chest pain, there are several subgroups of patients who may have abnormalities during exercise testing. One group of patients may have coronary artery spasm that occurs shortly after cessation of exercise. The typical patient does very well during the treadmill test and has relatively normal exercise tolerance in the absence of any ST segment abnormalities. Once exercise has stopped, the onset of variant angina is noted within the first 5 minutes and at this time ST segment elevation is present. For this reason the ECG leads should be left on patients for at least 10 minutes post exercise. Another group of patients may have coronary artery spasm superimposed on a severely occlusive atherosclerotic lesion. These patients typically complain of effort-induced angina as well and can be identified by detecting either ST segment depression during low level exercise testing or poor exercise tolerance or even exercise-induced hypotension. It is essential that these patients who have ST segment depression plus a history of unprovoked and spontaneous angina undergo coronary arteriography to rule out severe proximal occlusive coronary artery disease.

IN-HOSPITAL ECG RECORDING

Despite multiple attempts some patients elude establishment of a diagnosis of variant angina as outpatients because of the difficulty in obtaining a suitable ECG during chest pain. In these patients, it may be feasible to establish the diagnosis by hospitalizing the patient and attaching a 12-lead ECG to monitor the patient overnight. The patient can be instructed to push the record button if chest pain occurs in order to record a 12-lead ECG during chest pain before nitroglycerin is administered or before the pain resolves spontaneously. This approach does not require support from other medical personnel or the availability of a telephone, and it can be useful in the difficult-to-diagnose patient.

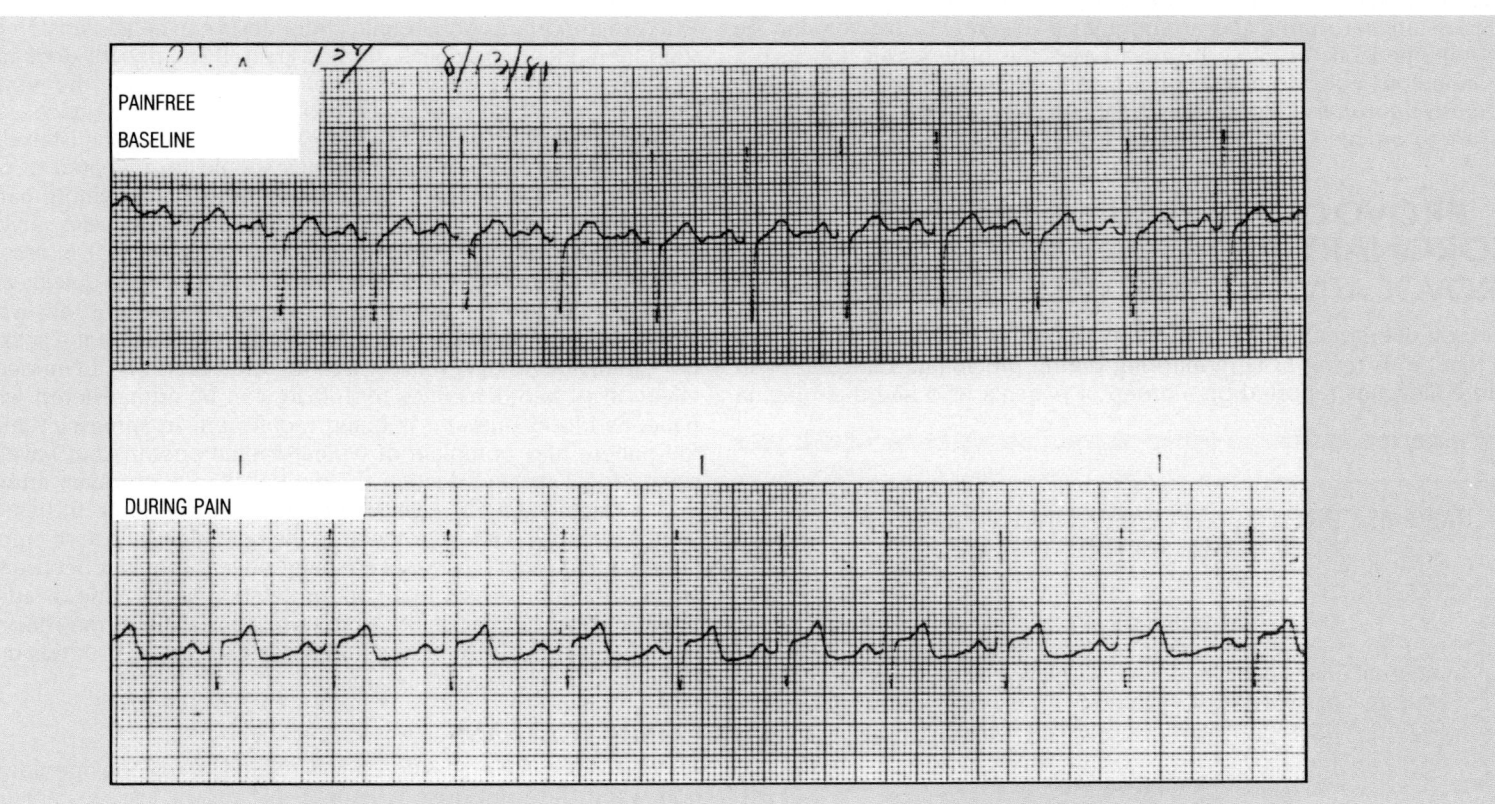

FIGURE 65.4 ST segment elevation compared with baseline, documented by transtelephonic ECG transmission during chest pain. (Schroeder JS (ed): Invasive Cardiology, Philadelphia, FA Davis, 1984)

CORONARY ARTERIOGRAPHY

Since unprovoked angina may be the first manifestation of unstable angina reflecting an extremely severe proximal coronary artery occlusion or early thrombotic occlusion, it is generally recommended that all patients with rest or unprovoked angina undergo coronary arteriography. This study allows definition of the severity of the coronary artery disease and assists in separating the severe occlusive coronary patient who may require angioplasty or surgery from the patient with variant angina who has normal coronary arteries and will respond to medical therapy.

Unless the patient gives a history suggestive of severe occlusive coronary disease, that is, either progressively severe effort angina or risk factors of coronary disease suggesting that this may not be variant angina, it is important to stop all antianginal medications for at least 24 hours prior to coronary arteriography. Nitroglycerin can be used for treatment of spontaneous episodes of pain until 1 hour prior to the procedure. It is particularly important that all long-acting nitrates, transcutaneously applied nitrates such as nitrate patches, and calcium antagonists be stopped. If the patient is having frequent episodes of pain, this should be done in the hospital under close medical observation.

In addition to cessation of any antianginal premedications, it is important to obtain informed consent for administration of ergonovine maleate during the arteriogram.

Routine coronary arteriography is first accomplished to determine whether the patient has severe coronary artery disease and unstable angina or whether he has mild disease or completely normal vessels and therefore falls into the suspect variant angina group. Occasionally a patient will have a spontaneous episode of angina during the arteriogram, and documentation of complete or incomplete focal spasm associated with the patient's typical chest pain will help establish the diagnosis. It is helpful to apply radiolucent electrode pads on the chest wall for a complete 12-lead ECG prior to start of the arteriogram if variant angina is suspected. A three-channel 12-lead ECG machine can then be attached, and if the patient has angina or has complaints that suggest angina during the arteriogram ST segment changes can be documented on the ECG. In most cases the patient will not have a spontaneous episode of chest pain, and after documentation of nonocclusive coronary disease or normal coronary arteries, it may be necessary to proceed with provocative testing (Table 65.1).

PROVOCATIVE TESTING DURING CORONARY ARTERIOGRAPHY
PROVOCATIVE TESTING WITH ERGONOVINE

The use of ergot alkaloids to induce angina pectoris was first reported in the 1950s using ECG monitoring during precipitated angina. Stein and colleagues reported on a group of patients who had their angina pectoris precipitated by 0.2 mg to 6.0 mg of ergonovine.[16] In nine of those patients there was ST segment depression, and this approach was proposed as a test for occlusive coronary artery disease. Scherf and co-workers also reported on provocative testing with ergonovine in 19 patients with coronary artery disease.[17] Unfortunately, 5 of their patients developed prolonged episodes of angina and one death occurred. Little provocative testing was done until the 1970s when coronary arteriography allowed more controlled evaluation of the response to provocation. Reports of my studies and those of others in the mid and late 1970s established the proper dosing and sequencing of ergonovine testing and its usefulness in the diagnosis of variant angina.[6,16,17]

TECHNIQUE

The Stanford University sequential protocol for administration of ergonovine maleate to provoke coronary artery spasm is outlined in Table 65.2. It is essential to anticipate the need for provocative testing so that informed consent, cessation of antianginal medications, and proper preparation of the patient can be accomplished prior to documentation of normal coronary vessels or insufficient coronary disease to explain the patient's rest angina.

Once the coronary arteriogram has been reviewed, preparation for ergonovine testing can begin. It is essential that a 12-lead ECG be obtained prior to and after each dose of ergonovine. The diagnosis of variant angina requires both observed focal spasm and either reproduction of the patient's typical chest pain or ST segment elevation on the ECG. Since the focal spasm may result in serious myocardial ischemia, it is essential to have intravenous nitroglycerin immediately available in a syringe and ready for administration to reverse the spasm.

The protocol sequence for the three doses of ergonovine is shown in Table 65.2. If the patient is having very frequent angina, a first dose of 0.025 mg should be given instead of the standard dose of 0.05 mg. It is also important to wait a full 3 minutes after each dose since the majority of patients will develop symptomatic coronary spasm within that time period. Prior to the administration of the subsequent dose, injection of the suspect coronary artery and recording of a 12-lead ECG are important. Additionally, these tests can be administered at any time the patient complains of chest pain. If the patient does not have documented focal spasm or symptomatic chest pain, the next higher dose of ergonovine is administered with a similar sequence.

After a total of 0.4 mg of ergonovine has been administered, visualization of both the coronary arteries should be repeated in order to document any significant spasm, whether or not symptomatic, and obtain a final ECG. If there is evidence of focal spasm, myocardial ischemia on the ECG, or complaints of chest pain, it is essential to document the coronary arteriographic abnormality as quickly as possible and then reverse the spasm. Coronary spasm can always be reversed by intravenous nitroglycerin, 50 μg to 200 μg. If the spasm does not rapidly begin to reverse within 30 to 60 seconds, an intracoronary injection of another 50 μg to 100 μg can be administered while the patient's blood pressure is being monitored. In some circumstances the patient may complain of typical angina pectoris but have no observed focal spasm on either the right or the left coronary arteriogram and no significant ST segment elevation on the ECG. In this circumstance one may wish to proceed to the next higher dose of ergonovine if the patient is not having severe pain, since this may reflect spasm of a small intramural vessel that cannot be seen at the time of arteriography. As discussed under interpretation, some patients may have typical pain that is thought to be due to esophageal spasm, but this has been difficult to document in humans.

COMPLICATIONS

There are few adverse side effects related to ergonovine administration when the total dose is kept to 0.4 mg or less, except for mild hypertension and occasional complaints of nausea. Heupler and co-workers reported on a total of 862 patients who had undergone ergonovine testing because of suspected variant angina or who had in-

TABLE 65.1 PROVOCATIVE TESTING FOR CORONARY ARTERY SPASM

Indications
Insufficient coronary artery disease to explain patient's rest, nocturnal or unprovoked angina
Uncertain response to nitrates and calcium blockers

Contraindications
Uncontrolled hypertension
Pregnancy
? Severe coronary artery disease

sufficient occlusive coronary disease to explain their symptoms.[18,19] A total of 110 ergonovine tests were positive, and no deaths or myocardial infarctions occurred. Heupler did report some prolonged episodes of angina and emphasized the requirement for early administration of nitroglycerin to reverse any spasm. Deaths have been reported related to ergonovine provocation. Buxton and associates reported on five patients who were "refractory to sublingual nitroglycerin."[20] Four of these patients had a cardiac arrest related to their myocardial ischemia, and three died during the procedure. The authors proposed that the ergonovine-induced coronary spasm was responsible and emphasized the dangers of provocative testing. On review of this report, however, the patients did not receive graded doses of ergonovine, which may have been related to the difficulty in reversing the spasm. It is important that strict adherence to the Stanford University or a similar protocol be observed, particularly if the patient is having frequent angina.

INTERPRETATION

Our original report of ergonovine testing in 1977 described 13 patients who had focal coronary spasm of 57 patients challenged with ergonovine maleate.[6] We require that the focal spasm be occlusive or near-occlusive and that there be a 50% reduction or more in lumen diameter. In addition, the patient must either have reproduction of the chest pain or ST segment elevation in the 12-lead ECG, which reflects myocardial ischemia due to spasm in the corresponding vessel. If these criteria are used, 9 of the 13 patients with focal coronary spasm had both chest pain and ST segment elevation similar to their spontaneous episodes. One additional patient had ST segment depression. Three patients whose history was consistent with typical variant angina had focal spasm that was more than 50% occlusive but did not have ST segment changes on the ECG or chest pain. The other 44 patients who did not demonstrate focal spasm represented a spectrum of patients with and without coronary artery disease. Approximately two thirds of these patients had normal coronary arteries, and many of these patients had underlying mitral valve prolapse. The other third of the patients had mild to moderate coronary artery disease but no severe atherosclerotic occlusions. A typical response to ergonovine testing and its reversal with nitroglycerin is shown in Figure 65.5.

Since the ergot alkaloids may result in physiologic narrowing of a vessel, it is important to require focal spasm of the coronary vessel in order to establish the diagnosis. Cipriano and co-workers reported that there is 20% or less diffuse narrowing of normal coronary vessels when a maximum dose of 0.4 mg of ergonovine is administered.[21] They also reported that a dose–response relationship does exist, demonstrating approximately 10% narrowing with a dose of 0.05 mg, 16% with 0.1 mg, and a total of 20% with the maximum total dose of 0.4 mg of ergonovine (Fig. 65.6). It is interesting to note that a small group of cardiac transplant patients with denervated hearts had a similar response, suggesting that the ergonovine acts directly rather than through the sympathetic nervous system. Although the nonspecific vasoconstrictor activity of ergonovine is of concern regarding the establishment of a diagnosis of coronary artery spasm, if focal spasm is required with reproduction of either the patient's chest pain or myocardial ischemia, very few false-positive tests have been reported. Curry and colleagues analyzed seven patients who developed spontaneous pain during arteriography and compared the results with ergonovine-induced episodes of spasm.[22] When they compared clinical, ECG, and left ventricular functional abnormalities as well as arterio-

TABLE 65.2 STANFORD UNIVERSITY PROTOCOL FOR ERGONOVINE PROVOCATION

Preparation
1. Stop all antianginal medications
2. Administer minimal premedication
3. Obtain informed consent
4. Prepare ergonovine
5. Prepare intravenous nitroglycerin
6. Place electrodes for 12-lead ECG

Protocol Sequence

Minimal Time Interval (min)	Dose of IV Ergonovine	12-lead ECG	Coronary Injection
0	0.05 mg		Right and left
1.5			Inject right or left at onset of chest pain or ST shift
3.0	0.1 mg		
4.5			
6.0	0.25 mg		
7.5			
9.0			
11.0			Right and left before completing procedure

At onset of pain or ST segment shift:
1. Inject suspicious coronary artery. If no spasm, inject other coronary artery. If no spasm, proceed to next dose if pain is mild to moderate.
2. As soon as focal spasm is documented, reverse spasm with intravenous or intracoronary nitroglycerin, 100 µg to 200 µg.

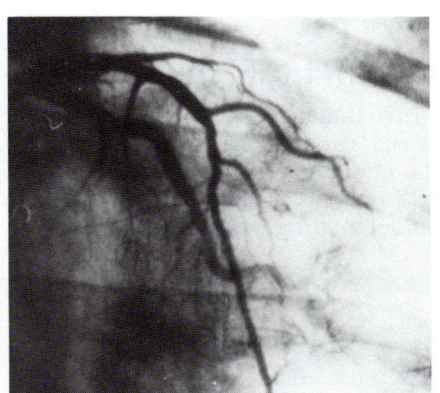
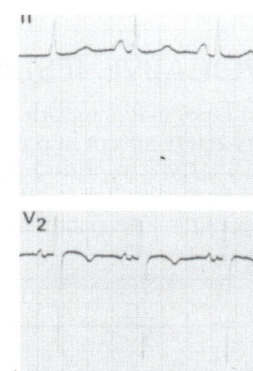
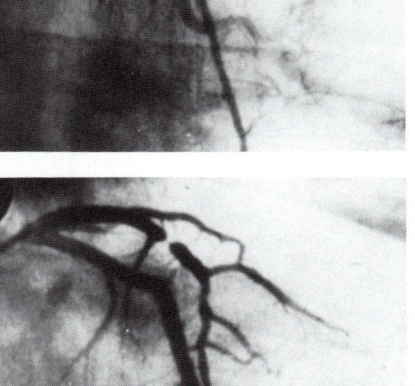
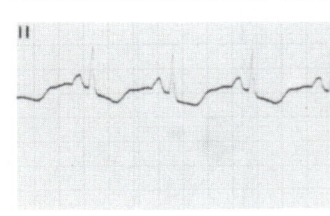
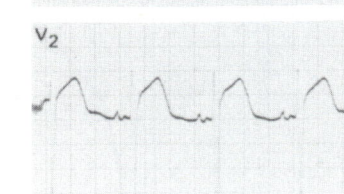

FIGURE 65.5 Left coronary arteriogram shows normal vessels in top panel and marked focal spasm of the left anterior descending artery with associated ST segment elevation in V₂ in the lower panel. (Ginsberg RG et al: Coronary spasm: Pathophysiology, clinical presentations, diagnostic approaches, and rational treatment. West J Med 136:398, 1982. Reprinted by permission)

graphic changes during the spontaneous episode versus ergonovine testing, the results were quite similar. ST segment elevation and focal spasm occurred in similar areas of the coronary arteriogram and resulted in similar abnormalities on the ECG. This is not only further evidence that ergonovine testing is helpful in establishment of a diagnosis of variant angina but also contributes to the idea that the disease is due to a local hyperreactive abnormality in the vessel wall.

Finally, how often does ergonovine testing precipitate coronary artery spasm in patients who do not have variant angina? Bertrand and colleagues reported on 134 patients who experienced focal spasm out of a total of 1,089 consecutive patients undergoing coronary arteriography for a wide range of indications.[23] Spasm was observed in 20% of patients who had had a recent myocardial infarction. The spasm was superimposed on a fixed atherosclerotic region in over 60% of these patients. No coronary artery spasm was observed in patients with normal coronary arteries if variant angina was not suspected. Thus it appears that the likelihood of a false-positive test in patients who do not have variant angina is low as long as the total dose of ergonovine is kept to less than 0.4 total mg.

PROVOCATION OF ESOPHAGEAL SPASM

In 1981, Eastwood and co-workers reported on the use of ergonovine to precipitate esophageal spasm in patients presenting with substernal chest pain.[24] They reported that during ergonovine testing five patients developed typical chest pain and esophageal manometric abnormalities consistent with esophageal spasm. Two of these nine patients denied any angina or chest pain. However, two of the five positive responders also showed marked ST segment elevation on the ECG; these two patients had previous negative ergonovine tests during nitrate administration. The role of esophageal manometry remains unclear owing to the difficulty in assessing a positive or negative response and the variable nature of the disease.

PROVOCATIVE TESTING WITH METHACHOLINE

Endo and associates reported in 1976 that methacholine may produce coronary artery spasm in patients with variant angina.[13] Stang and colleagues, in 1982, reported on the effects of 10 mg of methacholine administered subcutaneously in 13 patients with suspected coronary artery spasm.[14] Five patients developed coronary spasm, and three of these patients developed typical angina with ECG changes. The mechanism by which methacholine may precipitate coronary spasm is not clear. One theory is that the spasm results from direct stimulation of cholinergic muscarinic receptors on peripheral vascular smooth muscle, which then results in an abrupt fall in blood pressure with reflex-mediated increases in sympathetic tone, including α-adrenergic tone on the coronary arteries, precipitating spasm. However, Ginsburg and co-workers have shown that acetylcholine may directly precipitate coronary spasm *in vitro*, and therefore there may be a more direct influence of cholinergic agonism on the provocation of the spasm in these patients.[15]

HYPERVENTILATION TESTING

Yasue and associates reported that hyperventilation in combination with Tris-buffer infusion sufficient to raise the arterial blood pH to 7.65 precipitated angina.[25] Eight of nine patients tested had positive responses, although this was not documented by coronary arteriography. Girotti and colleagues performed hyperventilation 111 times in 10 patients with Prinzmetal's angina whose myocardial ischemia was induced by hyperventilation.[26] They demonstrated that treatment with antianginal medicines tend to decrease the frequency of a positive response to hyperventilation but also indicated that hyperventilation did not seem to be as sensitive as ergonovine testing for the typical patient with Prinzmetal's variant angina.

COLD PRESSOR TESTING

Raizner and colleagues reported on 35 patients undergoing coronary arteriography that was not necessary for diagnosis of chest pain syndromes due to coronary artery disease or variant angina.[27] The test consisted of immersion of the right hand in ice water for 1 minute, during which time there was a mean rise in systolic blood pressure of 17 mm Hg but no change in the heart rate. Seven of the patients had focal spasm induced, although only two showed any abnormality on the ECG. When the authors analyzed the arteriograms quantitatively, they demonstrated increased luminal narrowing of coronary segments in both groups, but it was more pronounced in the variant angina group ($-12.7 \pm 11.5\%$ compared with the control group $-5.1 \pm 1.2\%$). In order to compare the sensitivity of ergonovine exercise and cold pres-

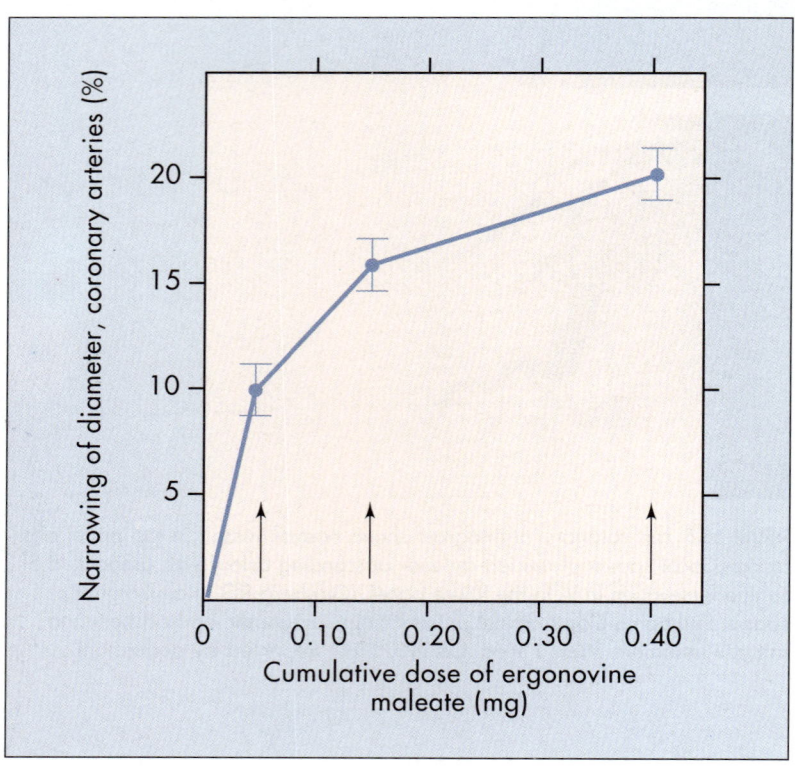

FIGURE 65.6 Dose–response curve that demonstrates narrowing of coronary arteries of $10 \pm 1.5\%$, $16 \pm 14\%$, and $20 \pm 1.3\%$ (mean $\pm$ SEM), after serial intravenous injections of 0.05 mg, 0.10 mg, and 0.25 mg ergonovine maleate. The increment of narrowing of coronary arteries decreases with successive injections of larger amounts of the drug. (Modified from Cipriano PR et al: The effects of ergonovine maleate on coronary artery size. Circulation 59:82, 1979)

sor testing in patients with documented variant angina, Waters and associates performed the three studies serially in 34 patients.[28] They also performed exercise testing in 17 patients. Using myocardial ischemia and ST segment elevation as signs of a positive test, ergonovine produced a positive test in 94% of patients, exercise testing in 29%, and cold pressor testing in 9% of patients. The authors concluded that the sensitivity of cold pressor testing was much too low to be useful in identifying patients with variant angina.

HISTAMINE PROVOCATION

Ginsburg and colleagues reported on the use of intravenous histamine, 0.05 mg to 0.1 mg/min, in the presence of a selective H_2 blocker in 12 patients with documented variant angina.[29] Coronary artery spasm was precipitated in 4 of these patients, confirmed by ECG changes as well as chest pain. The authors concluded that although there was a positive result, the side effects of headache and nausea limited the widespread usefulness of this procedure.

CLINICAL IMPLICATIONS

Ergonovine maleate administration to provoke spasm in patients with suspected variant angina continues to be the most reliable, sensitive, and specific approach to diagnosis. It is essential that the possibility of provocative testing be anticipated so that antianginal medications including nitrates can be stopped prior to the test and informed consent can be obtained from the patient. A positive test reflects a 50% or more focal narrowing of the coronary artery and/or ST segment elevation or depression of greater than 2 mm on a 12-lead ECG. Provocative testing requires immediate reversal of the spasm so that severe prolonged myocardial ischemia, which can lead to major complications and/or death during testing, does not occur. Other provocative agents that have been evaluated do not seem to be as useful at this time and may not be until better understanding of the pathophysiology of the underlying abnormality is understood.

DIFFERENTIAL DIAGNOSIS

The most important group of patients to consider in the differential diagnosis at the time that a patient presents with rest or nocturnal chest pain is those with unstable or crescendo angina due to severe underlying coronary artery disease (Table 65.3). Although most of these patients will have a history of known coronary artery disease or effort angina in the past, a few patients will present *de novo* with this syndrome. Factors that will be helpful in evaluating this patient are the presence of coronary artery disease risk factors, presence of an old myocardial infarction on the ECG, and persistent ECG evidence of ischemia, which would suggest a persistent occlusion or partial occlusion rather than a transient occlusion due to coronary spasm. In patients who have not had previous coronary arteriography, it is essential to proceed with this evaluation to rule out tight occlusion or preinfarction angina.

Most troublesome is the patient who develops typical chest pain in response to ergonovine testing but does not have demonstrable significant focal spasm on coronary arteriography or major ST segment changes on the ECG. The pathophysiology of chest pain in many of these patients is poorly understood. Esophageal spasm has been proposed as a cause, although results of studies with ergonovine provocation during esophageal manometry have been difficult to interpret. These patients may have spasm of intramural vessels or have small vessel coronary disease that is poorly understood at this time.

Finally, it is important to remember that the coronary spasm generally responds extremely well to either sublingual or intravenous nitroglycerin. In the patient with persistent ST segment elevation, the early phase of acute myocardial infarction must be considered and ruled out.

In the past it has been proposed that coronary artery spasm was responsible for the atypical chest pain of mitral valve prolapse. However, studies with ergonovine testing at Stanford University in large groups of such patients as well as studies at other institutions have conclusively ruled out coronary spasm as an important pathophysiologic mechanism for chest pain in this patient group.

TREATMENT
MEDICAL THERAPY

Acute treatment of the chest pain episode is generally sublingual nitroglycerin. This is highly effective treatment, which almost always reverses the spasm. In fact, the diagnosis of transient coronary spasm should be questioned if there is not an excellent response to the nitroglycerin. Other sublingual nitrate preparations may be useful as well in terminating the acute attack.

Long-acting oral nitrates have long been used for prophylaxis in patients with variant angina.[30] Oral agents such as isosorbide dinitrate, time suspension capsules, and nitroglycerin paste have all been reported to be effective. The primary limiting factor with use of prophylactic nitrate therapy is the suspected development of tolerance in these patients, although it has been poorly documented in long-term clinical trials. Another limiting factor is the fact that many patients require high doses of nitrates for prophylaxis, which may lead to a significant frequency of adverse side effects, particularly headache and hypotension at a dose level that will prevent the spontaneous episodes of chest pain and angina. Controlled trials of nitrate efficacy for prophylaxis have been limited. Hill and co-workers reported on a double-blind randomized crossover comparison of nifedipine versus isosorbide dinitrate in 19 patients with variant angina.[31] There was a 72% decrease in angina frequency during nifedipine therapy and a 63% de-

TABLE 65.3 CLINICAL CHARACTERISTICS OF ANGINA SUBTYPES

	Stable	Unstable	Variant
Chest Pain			
Character	Typical	Typical	Typical
Onset	Exertion	Rest/exertion	Rest
ECG during Pain	ST segment depression	ST segment depression Occasional ST segment elevation	ST segment elevation Occasional ST segment depression
Coronary Arteriogram	Coronary artery disease	Severe coronary artery disease	Normal or mild coronary artery disease

crease during isosorbide dinitrate therapy compared with placebo. The authors concluded that the two agents were approximately equally effective in this particular trial. Intravenous administration of isosorbide dinitrate at a dose of 1.25 to 5.0 mg/hr has been reported to be effective in patients in whom oral agents did not control recurrent episodes of angina. In addition, sodium nitroprusside has been reported to be effective, but the adverse side effects of hypotension must be monitored carefully in this patient group.

α-Adrenergic blockers such as phenoxybenzamine or phentolamine have also been reported to be effective in preventing repeated episode of coronary artery spasm in variant angina patients.[30] The mechanism proposed is simply blockade of coronary artery α-receptors, resulting in prevention of focal spasm. Although these agents have been reported to be effective, it was common to have to achieve doses that cause significant orthostatic hypotension before they were effective in preventing episodes of coronary spasm. For this reason, these treatments have generally been abandoned with the advent of demonstrated excellent efficacy of the calcium blockers.

TREATMENT OF ARRHYTHMIAS

Patients may either develop heart block due to spasm of the right coronary artery or ventricular arrhythmias, including sustained ventricular tachycardia, due to spasm of the right, circumflex, or left anterior descending coronary arteries. These arrhythmias generally occur in the setting of either myocardial ischemia or reperfusion when the spasm is broken or resolves spontaneously. For this reason antiarrhythmic drugs are not very effective and treatment should be directed at treatment or prevention of the focal coronary spasm. Patients who have episodes of second- or third-degree heart block and syncope who have not responded to prophylactic therapy with calcium blockers will benefit from a demand pacemaker.

CALCIUM ANTAGONISTS

The recent availability of a group of pharmaceutical agents called calcium antagonists has dramatically improved the success of therapy and most likely improved the long-term prognosis for patients with variant angina. The calcium antagonists block the influx of ionized calcium via slow channels during the plateau phase of the action potential. This blocking action is more potent at the calcium channel of the vascular smooth muscle cells than of the myocardial cell. This differential effect allows relaxation of vascular smooth muscle at therapeutic concentrations of the drug, which results in minimal negative inotropic activity. The calcium antagonists therefore cause a decrease in coronary vascular tone and reactivity, which results in increases in coronary flow. These agents also appear to block the abnormal hyperreactivity or spasm of coronary vessels, which is the cause of variant angina. Clinical trials with calcium antagonists have conclusively shown marked reduction in angina frequency during therapy with calcium antagonists.

Diltiazem, nifedipine, and verapamil are all effective for prophylaxis in variant angina. These agents have been proven efficacious in double-blind randomized placebo-controlled trials with 50% to 70% reduction in angina frequency and nitroglycerin consumption compared with a placebo control. Endo and colleagues first reported that diltiazem was effective for prophylaxis of variant angina in 1975.[32] After initial experience with this agent in Japan, subsequent studies in the United States have confirmed that diltiazem is not only efficacious but safe for short- and long-term efficacy in variant angina. Rosenthal and co-workers reported on a total of 13 patients with documented coronary spasm and variant angina who completed a prospective randomized dose-finding crossover study of diltiazem, 120 mg and 240 mg/day, versus placebo, each given for a 2-week period.[33] The 240-mg/day dose of diltiazem resulted in a decrease in pain of 79% to 50% (P = 0.03) and a significant decrease in angina frequency from 1.6 to 0.4 episodes per day, with similar reductions in nitroglycerin consumption. There was no evidence for a rebound phenomenon when the diltiazem was abruptly changed to placebo, and there were no significant adverse side effects. These findings were confirmed by other investigators, including Pepine and colleagues, who studied a similar group of patients in whom 64% had either complete or partial resolution of their angina during therapy with diltiazem.[34] Diltiazem has also been shown to be effective for long-term treatment of these patients without evidence of either tolerance or rebound. Rosenthal and co-workers reported in 1983 on the long-term efficacy of diltiazem in 16 patients with clinical variant angina.[35] This 44-week study involved eleven 28-day cycles with one random placebo period during the first five cycles and one during the last six cycles. There was a 73% decrease in angina frequency in phase I and a 55% decrease compared with placebo in phase II. In addition, marked disease attenuation was noted. Thus diltiazem is effective as long-term therapy without evidence of drug tolerance developing.

Open-label experience with the patients who have been on diltiazem shows similar results. My colleagues and I reported on 36 patients who were followed in the Stanford Coronary Artery Spasm Clinic for 6 months or more.[36] During a mean of 7.5 months of diltiazem therapy, angina frequency was reduced from 21.5 to 1.3 attacks per week on either 240 mg or 360 mg of diltiazem daily (Fig. 65.7). Pain breakthrough occurred a mean of 1.7 times during the 17.5-month follow-up and tended to be of short duration and related to episodes of stress in the patient's life. Six patients had trace to 1+ pedal edema, but no other adverse side effects were reported. Thus diltiazem appears to be effective for short- and long-term prophylaxis for variant angina.

Nifedipine for prophylaxis of Prinzmetal's variant angina was first reported by Hosoda and associates in 1975.[37] These uncontrolled studies reported a dramatic reduction in angina frequency. Testing of this agent in the United States was first reported by Antman and colleagues in 1980.[38] In an open-label study of 127 patients with documented coronary spasm and variant angina, doses of 40 mg to 160 mg/day resulted in a 63% of patients being completely relieved of their angina. Furthermore, a total of 87% of patients had 50% or more reduction in the frequency of angina. The authors reported that approximately 5% of patients had to terminate therapy because of adverse side effects. Although few controlled studies of this agent have been reported, it is clear that this is a highly effective drug for prophylaxis of variant angina. It has also been demonstrated in the cardiac catheterization laboratory to block spasm during provocation with ergonovine maleate. With regard to long-term responses, Hill and co-workers reported on 26 patients who had angina due to coronary spasm who completed a crossover study comparing nifedipine with isosorbide dinitrate.[39] Of the 18 patients who had a short-term beneficial response to nifedipine, 14 were followed for an average of 9.4 months on long-term nifedipine therapy. Overall, 80% of patients had a 50% or more decrease in angina frequency. Three patients did have a marked increase in angina at 9, 14, and 3 months after initiation of therapy, requiring hospitalization. In addition, nifedipine was discontinued in two patients and the dose was decreased in three additional patients because of significant adverse side effects. The authors reported that adverse side effects were common, but reduction of dosing usually diminished the unwanted effects of the drug.

Verapamil has also been reported to be effective in carefully controlled randomized trials. Johnson and colleagues reported in 1981 on prophylactic use of verapamil in 16 patients with variant angina over a 9-month period.[40] During the treatment period with verapamil, the angina frequency decreased from 12.6 to 1.7 pain episodes per week with similar decreases in nitroglycerin consumption. Holter monitoring showed marked reductions in episodes of ST segment deviation from 33.1 to 7.1 deviations per week while on active therapy.[41] The authors concluded that verapamil was an effective drug for therapy of variant angina, but it should be noted that 14 of the 16 patients were also receiving oral isosorbide dinitrate, mean dose 105 mg/day, with a range of 20 mg to 200 mg given in four to six divided doses.

There have been very few comparative studies of the efficacy of calcium blockers for treatment of variant angina. The only study that has attempted to compare these agents was a survey of 11 cardiology institutes in Japan where investigators were asked to comment on their impression of the efficacy of nifedipine, diltiazem, and verapamil.[42] Efficacy rates were assessed at 94% for nifedipine, 90.8% for diltiazem, and 85.7% for verapamil. These agents also tended to be more effective in patients with normal or nearly normal coronary arteries rather than in patients with coronary disease. It is interesting, however, that verapamil was reported as markedly effective in only 10.7% of patients compared with 80.5% for diltiazem and 77.2% for nifedipine. The authors also reported that in 15 patients on a combination of nifedipine and diltiazem that 73.3% had a markedly effective response. Waters and co-workers reported that nifedipine and diltiazem were approximately equally efficacious in preventing coronary spasm or markedly increasing the dose required to provoke coronary spasm during ergonovine testing in the coronary care unit.[43]

Other studies have attempted to compare calcium antagonists with long-acting nitrates. Ginsburg and co-workers reported on 12 patients who were entered into a randomized double-blind study comparing nifedipine, mean dose 82 mg/day, with isosorbide dinitrate, mean dose 66 mg/day. Treatment of the 12 patients resulted in a total of 161 patient-days that were available for analysis.[44] During baseline there was an average of 1.1 angina attacks per day on placebo, which fell to 0.28 per day during nifedipine treatment and to 0.39 per day during isosorbide dinitrate treatment (Fig. 65.8). There is no statistical difference between these two responses. A number of adverse side effects occurred, with headache being the most prominent during isosorbide dinitrate treatment in 81% of patients and dependent edema occurring in 33% of patients during nifedipine treatment. Significant adverse side effects requiring cessation of therapy occurred in two patients on nifedipine and in three patients on isosorbide dinitrate. The authors concluded that both of these agents were effective but that nifedipine was preferred by the majority of patients.

Patients who are refractory to treatment with oral calcium channel blockers will respond to intravenous isosorbide dinitrate or intrave-

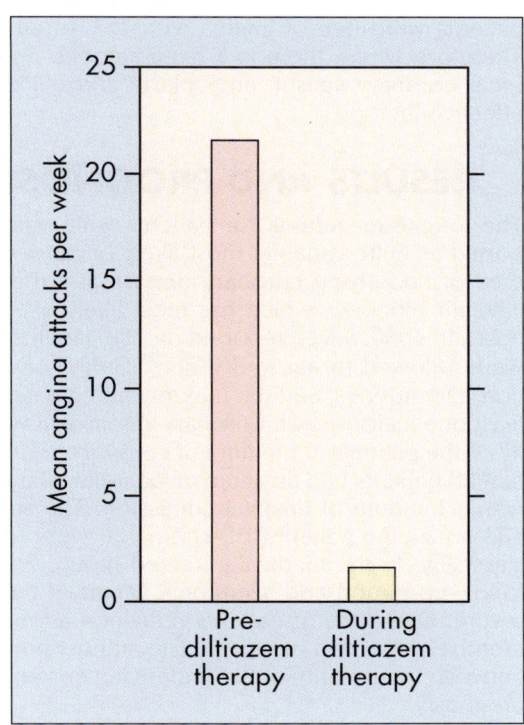

FIGURE 65.7 Response of 36 patients with angina due to documented coronary arterial spasm during medical therapy with long-acting nitrates (pre-diltiazem) and after therapy with 240 to 360 mg/day of diltiazem. (Modified from Schroeder JS, Lamb IH, Ginsberg R et al: Diltiazem for long-term therapy of coronary arterial spasm. Am J Cardiol 49:533, 1982)

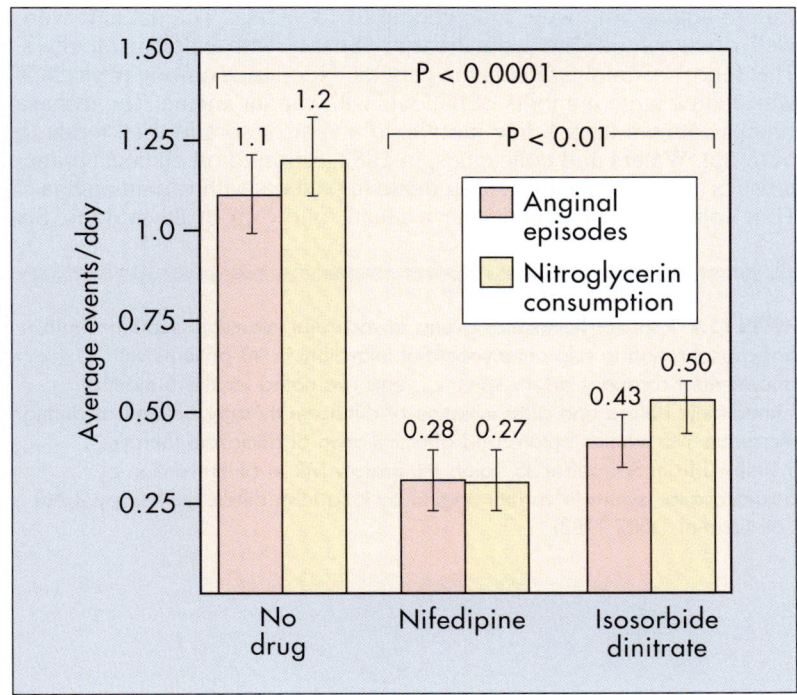

FIGURE 65.8 Comparison of nifedipine versus isosorbide dinitrate drug efficacy in variant angina therapy in terms of reduction of anginal episodes and sublingual nitroglycerin consumption. (Modified from Ginsburg R, Lamb IH, Schroeder JS et al: Randomized double-blind comparison of nifedipine and isosorbide dinitrate therapy in variant angina pectoris due to coronary artery spasm. Am Heart J 103:44, 1982)

nous nitroglycerin. However, in the medically refractory patient, consideration should be given to combining diltiazem and nifedipine, gradually increasing the combined dose to the limit of adverse effects.

β-Blockers have been reported to occasionally be detrimental or to aggravate variant angina. Robertson and colleagues reported in 1982 that both 160 mg and 640 mg of propranolol per day were associated with significantly prolonged angina episodes compared with findings in control groups.[45] Tilmant, in 1983, studied 11 patients on placebo, diltiazem, propanolol, or a combination.[46] Propranolol resulted in increased frequency and duration of angina attacks, but when diltiazem was added, this adverse effect disappeared. Therefore, β-blockers are generally not recommended for the patient with variant angina, although they can be used for demand-related angina in the setting of occlusive coronary artery disease if calcium antagonists are given concurrently.

Is there any evidence that long-term use of calcium antagonists may affect the long-term prognosis of these patients? My colleagues and I reported on 43 patients with variant angina and compared their cardiovascular event rate after beginning diltiazem therapy with that at an equal time prior to therapy.[47] Cardiovascular events defined as myocardial infarction, sudden death, and hospitalization for prolonged angina were decreased significantly during both the 6 and mean 19.6 months of therapy compared with a similar period prior to the initiation of therapy. When the data were analyzed by the binomial principle, 22 events occurred during the 19.6 months before therapy and 2 events on therapy (Fig. 65.9). No patient died during the follow-up period, and there were reports of a dramatic decrease in angina frequency of approximately 94%. The authors concluded that although this was a retrospective trial, that the marked reduction in events during drug therapy suggested a protective effect and that these patients should be maintained on long-term therapy with this drug. Because of the marked improvement in angina symptoms it is sometimes difficult to assess how long the patient should be treated with calcium antagonists. Most authors recommend that the patients be treated at least 1 year with gradual reduction in calcium antagonist therapy after that if the patient remains pain free. We have found that flares in angina frequency occur at times of emotional stress and the patients may need increases in their dosing.

SURGICAL THERAPY

Although the calcium antagonists are highly effective for prophylaxis in this patient group, an occasional patient has severe unrelenting spasm despite maximal medical therapy. Some authors have reported coronary bypass grafting in such patients with the hypothesis that the graft can bypass the area of focal spasm and result in sufficient perfusion even when spasm occurs.[48] However, those patients who have severe coronary spasm may have a more diffuse process. Subsequent reports indicate that the spasm may involve or propagate distal to the area of the insertion of the bypass graft, and this approach is generally no longer applied in this patient group. Nordstrom and co-workers reported on persistence of chest pain despite coronary bypass grafts and a relatively high occlusion rate or postoperative infarction rate.[49] Because of the possibility of sympathetic nervous system–induced spasm, plexectomy at the time of aortocoronary bypass grafting has been reported in an effort to more completely denervate the vessel.[50] Although many of these patients seem to improve, it has been difficult to assess the short- and long-term efficacy of these procedures. Prior to the introduction of calcium antagonists, Clark and colleagues reported on four patients who underwent cardiac denervation because of unrelenting coronary spasm with myocardial ischemia and/or ventricular arrhythmias.[51] Two of their four patients died, but the two survivors did have good short-term relief of the coronary spasm.

Percutaneous transluminal coronary angioplasty has also been proposed as effective therapy for variant angina.[52] Corcos and co-workers reported on 21 patients with variant angina of whom 17 also had effort-induced angina.[53] All patients had single-vessel disease with 60% to 95% stenotic lesions present. Angioplasty was successful in 19 patients, but only 8 remained free of angina. The re-stenosis rate appeared to be higher in those patients who had calcium antagonists discontinued after the procedure (80%) compared with those who continued the drug (21%). During a mean follow-up of 33 months, 20 patients were free of angina with 75% of all antianginal medication. Therefore where there is a fixed stenotic coronary lesion related to focal coronary spasm, angioplasty and calcium antagonists may be effective therapies.

RESULTS AND PROGNOSIS

The long-term outlook for patients with variant angina has been reported as quite variable, most likely because of differences in the degree of underlying coronary disease and the more recent advent of calcium blockers, which has most likely altered the long-term prognosis. In 1980, Severi reported on 138 patients with variant angina who were followed for up to 8 years.[54] Only 9 of 107 patients had normal coronary arteries, and the majority had greater than 50% stenosis of at least one major vessel. Coronary vasospasm was demonstrated in only 37 of the patients at the time of coronary arteriography. They reported that 28 patients had an acute myocardial infarction and 5 patients died within 1 month of hospital admission. The authors then followed the 133 remaining patients, of whom 120 were treated medically and 13 surgically. In the medically treated group, 7 patients died during the follow-up period and symptoms generally became less frequent and severe. Over 50% of patients remained asymptomatic for at least 12 months by the end of year 4. The authors noted a general correlation between the severity of the underlying coronary disease and the poor prognosis.

Girotti reported on spontaneous remission in four patients with variant angina who were followed up to 15 years.[55] The patients were well documented and were treated variably with calcium blockers. This report certainly reflects the general experience among physicians who follow large numbers of patients with variant angina. The disease process occurs from a few months to a year or so and then tends to burn out. Waters and colleagues, in 1982, reported on clinical characteristics associated with sudden death in patients with variant angina.[56] They followed 114 patients for a mean follow-up of 26 months. Six

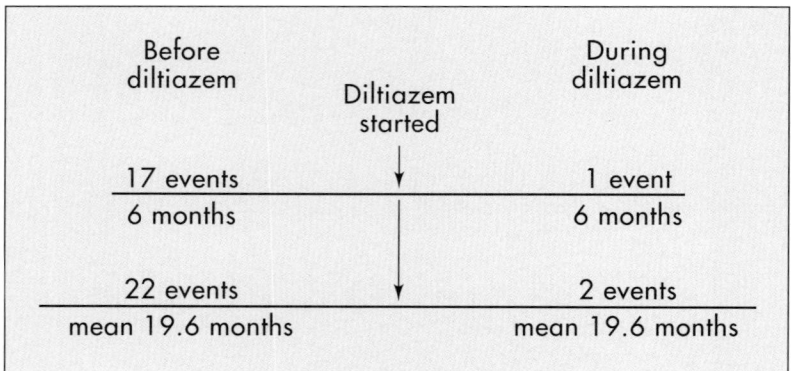

FIGURE 65.9 Total cardiovascular events (myocardial infarction, sudden death, or hospitalization to rule out myocardial infarction) in 43 patients with documented coronary artery spasm. Events are noted for the 6 months immediately before and after initiation of diltiazem therapy, as well as during the mean 19.6 months before and after initiation of dilitiazem therapy. (Modified from Schroeder JS, Lamb IH, Bristow MR et al: Prevention of cardiovascular events in variant angina by long-term diltiazem therapy. J Am Coll Cardiol 1:1507, 1983)

died suddenly, and 13 others were resuscitated during this period of time. The patients who died suddenly appeared to have more serious arrhythmias on Holter monitoring. In addition, patients with spontaneous attacks tended to differ from other survivors in the degree of ischemia during attacks as manifested by more severe ST segment elevation. Cipriano and co-workers reported on the clinical course of 25 patients who had been followed an average of 2.7 years at Stanford University Medical Center after having documented coronary artery spasm in the cardiac catheterization laboratory.[57] Seventeen patients received medical therapy, and 6 had cardiac surgery. Of the 23 survivors, 21 had either no chest pain or markedly reduced symptoms. The authors concluded that the clinical course was quite variable, with most patients improving but major cardiac complications being quite common (*i.e.*, 11 of 25 patients [44%]) and clinical coronary arteriographic features of limited use in predicting major problems.

More recently, Waters and associates reported that variant angina patients who did not have multivessel disease who were treated with a calcium blocker such as nifedipine, diltiazem, or verapamil had improved survival without infarction compared with treatment with either perhexiline or long-acting nitrates (92% vs. 67% at 1, 2, and 3 years; $P = 0.005$).[58] The authors concluded that the addition of a calcium channel blocker appears to reduce complications in patients with variant angina if they did not have significant coronary artery disease. Bott-Silverman and Heupler reported in 1983 on the experience from the Cleveland Clinic.[59] The authors commented that the natural history of medically treated patients with pure coronary spasm was characterized by recurrent episodes of frequent spontaneous remissions and a poor long-term response to long-acting nitrates but an excellent response to calcium channel blockers. Fifteen percent of their patients had a definite remission with no recurrence over at least 2 years. None of their patients died a cardiac death. These more recent experiences and reports are more consistent with our experience that patients who have coronary artery spasm and no or mild coronary disease do extremely well if they have long-term therapy with a calcium channel blocker. For this reason we recommend that patients continue medication for at least 1 to 2 years and then that it be tapered slowly and that medication be added at any time that there is a recurrence of symptoms.

REFERENCES

1. Prinzmetal M, Kennamer R, Merliss R et al: A variant form of angina pectoris. Am J Med 27:375, 1959
2. Prinzmetal M, Ekmekci A, Kennamer R et al: Variant form of angina pectoris. JAMA 174:1794, 1960
3. Osler W: Lumleian lectures on angina pectoris. Lancet 1:697, 1910
4. Wilson FN, Johnston FD: The occurrence in angina pectoris of electrocardiographic changes similar in magnitude and in kind to those produced by myocardial infarction. Am Heart J 22:64, 1941
5. Scanlon PJ, Niemichas R, Moran JF et al: Accelerated angina pectoris: Clinical, hemodynamic, arteriographic and therapeutic experience in 85 patients. Circulation 47:19, 1973
6. Schroeder JS, Bolen JL, Quint RA et al: Provocation of coronary spasm with ergonovine maleate: New test with results in 57 patients undergoing coronary arteriography. Am J Cardiol 40:487, 1977
7. Oliva PB, Potts DE, Pluss RG: Coronary arterial spasm causing Prinzmetal's variant angina. N Engl J Med 288:745, 1973
8. Schroeder JS, Silverman JF, Harrison DC: Right coronary artery spasm causing Prinzmetal's variant angina. Chest 65:573, 1974
9. Maseri A, Pesola A, Marzilli M et al: Coronary vasospasm in angina pectoris. Lancet 1:713, 1977
10. McAlpin R, Kattus A, Alvaro A: Angina pectoris at rest with preservation of exercise capacity: Prinzmetal's variant angina. Circulation 47:946, 1973
11. MacAlpin RN: Relation of coronary arterial spasm to sites of organic stenosis. Am J Cardiol 46:143, 1980
12. Ginsburg R, Bristow MR, Schroeder JS et al: Effects of pharmacologic agents on isolated human coronary arteries. In Santamore WP, Bove AA (eds): Coronary Artery Disease, pp 103–115. Baltimore, Urban & Schwarzenberg, 1982
13. Endo M, Hiroswaka K, Kancko N et al: Prinzmetal's variant angina: Coronary arteriogram and left ventriculogram during angina attack induced by methacholine. N Engl J Med 294:250, 1976
14. Stang JM, Kolibash AJ, Schorling JB et al: Methacholine provocation of Prinzmetal's variant angina pectoris: A revised perspective. Clin Cardiol 5:393, 1982
15. Ginsburg R, Lamb IH, Schroeder JS et al: Long-term transtelephonic monitoring in variant angina. Am Heart J 102:196, 1981
16. Stein I: The ergonovine test for coronary insufficiency. Angiology 14:23, 1963
17. Scherf D, Perlman A, Schlackman M: Effect of dihydroergotamine on heart. Proc Soc Exp Biol Med 71:420, 1949
18. Heupler FA, Proudfit WL, Razavi M et al: Ergonovine maleate provocative test for coronary artery spasm. Am J Cardiol 41:631, 1978
19. Heupler FA: Provocative testing for coronary artery spasm: Risk, method and rationale. Am J Cardiol 46:335, 1980
20. Buxton A, Goldberg S, Hirshfeld JW et al: Refractory ergonovine-induced coronary vasospasm: Importance of intracoronary nitroglycerin. Am J Cardiol 46:329, 1980
21. Cipriano PR, Guthaner DF, Orlick AE et al: The effects of ergonovine-induced maleate on coronary arterial size. Circulation 59:82, 1979
22. Curry RC, Pepine CJ, Sabom MB et al: Similarities of ergonovine-induced and spontaneous attacks of variant angina. Circulation 59:307, 1979
23. Bertrand ME, La Blanche JM, Tilmant PY et al: Frequency of provoked coronary arterial spasm in 1089 consecutive patients undergoing coronary arteriography. Circulation 65:1299, 1982
24. Eastwood GL, Weiner BH, Dickerson WJ et al: Use of ergonovine to identify esophageal spasm in patients with chest pain. Ann Intern Med 94:768, 1981
25. Yasue H, Nagao M, Omote S et al: Coronary arterial spasm and Prinzmetal's variant form of angina induced by hyperventilation and tris-buffer infusion. Circulation 56:56, 1978
26. Girotti LA, Crosatto JR, Messuti H et al: The hyperventilation test as a method for developing successful therapy in Prinzmetal's angina. Am J Cardiol 49:834, 1982
27. Raizner AE, Chahine RA, Ishimorei T et al: Provocation of coronary artery spasm by the cold pressor test. Circulation 62:925, 1980
28. Waters DD, Szlachcic J, Bonan R et al: Comparative sensitivity of exercise, cold pressor and ergonovine testing in provoking attacks of variant angina in patients with active disease. Cardiology 67(2):310, 1983
29. Ginsburg R, Bristow MR, Kantrowitz N et al: Histamine provocation of clinical coronary artery spasm: Implications concerning pathogenesis of variant angina pectoris. Am Heart J 102:819, 1981
30. Schroeder JS, Rosenthal S, Ginsburg R et al: Medical therapy of Prinzmetal's variant angina. Chest 78:231, 1980
31. Hill JA, Feldman RL, Pepine CJ et al: Randomized double-blind comparison of nifedipine and isosorbide dinitrate in patients with coronary arterial spasm. Am J Cardiol 49:431, 1982
32. Endo M, Kanda I, Hosoda S et al: Prinzmetal's variant form of angina pectoris. Circulation 52:33, 1975
33. Rosenthal SJ, Ginsburg R, Lamb I et al: The efficacy of diltiazem for control of symptoms of coronary arterial spasm. Am J Cardiol 46:1027, 1980
34. Pepine CJ, Feldman RL, Whittle J et al: Effects of diltiazem in patients with variant angina: A randomized double-blind trial. Am Heart J 101:719, 1981
35. Rosenthal SJ, Lamb IH, Schroeder JS et al: Long-term efficacy of diltiazem for control of symptoms of coronary arterial spasm. Circ Res 52:153, 1983
36. Schroeder JS, Lamb IH, Ginsburg R: Diltiazem for long-term therapy of coronary arterial spasm. Am J Cardiol 49:533, 1982
37. Hosoda S, Kasanuki H, Mityata K et al: Results of clinical investigation of nifedipine in angina pectoris with special reference to its therapeutic efficacy in attacks at rest. In Hishimoto K, Kimura E, Kobayshi T (eds): Proceedings of International Nifedipine "Adalat" Symposium: New Drug Therapy of Ischemic Heart Disease, pp 185–189. Tokyo, University of Tokyo Press, 1975
38. Antman E, Muller J, Goldberg S et al: Nifedipine therapy for coronary spasm: Experience in 127 patients. N Engl J Med 302:1269, 1980
39. Hill JA, Feldman RL, Pepine CJ et al: Randomized double-blind comparison of nifedipine and isosorbide dinitrate in patients with coronary arterial spasm. Am J Cardiol 49:431, 1982
40. Johnson SM, Mauritson DR, Hillis LD et al: Verapamil in the treatment of Prinzmetal's variant angina: A long-term, double-blind, randomized trial (abstr). Am J Cardiol 47:399, 1981
41. Johnson SM, Mauritson DR, Willerson JT et al: Verapamil administration in variant angina pectoris. JAMA 245:1849, 1981
42. Kimura E, Kishida H: Treatment of variant angina with drugs: A survey of 11 cardiology institutes in Japan. Circulation 63(4):844, 1981
43. Waters DD, Szlachcic J, Theroux P et al: Ergonovine testing to detect spontaneous remissions of variant angina during long-term treatment with calcium antagonist drugs. Am J Cardiol 47:179, 1981
44. Ginsburg R, Lamb IH, Schroeder JS et al: Randomized double-blind comparison of nifedipine and isosorbide dinitrate therapy in variant angina pectoris due to coronary artery spasm. Am Heart J 103:44, 1981
45. Robertson RM, Wood AJ, Vaughn WK et al: Exacerbation of vasotonic angina pectoris by propranolol. Circulation 65:281, 1982
46. Tilmant PY, La Blanche JM, Thieuleux FA et al: Detrimental effect of propranolol in patients with coronary arterial spasm countered by combination with diltiazem. Am J Cardiol 52:230, 1983
47. Schroeder JS, Lamb IH, Bristow MR et al: Prevention of cardiovascular events in variant angina by long-term diltiazem therapy. J Am Coll Cardiol 1:1507, 1983

48. Shubrooks SJ, Bete JM, Hutter AM et al: Variant angina pectoris: Clinical and anatomic spectrum and results of coronary bypass surgery. Am J Cardiol 36:142, 1975
49. Nordstrom LA, Lillehei JP, Adicoff A et al: Coronary artery surgery for recurrent ventricular arrhythmias in patients with variant angina. Am Heart J 89:236, 1975
50. Bertrand ME, LaBlanche JM, Tilmant PY: Treatment of Prinzmetal's variant angina. Am J Cardiol 47:174, 1981
51. Clark DA, Quint RA, Mitchell RL et al: Coronary artery spasm. J Thorac Cardiovasc Surg 73:332, 1977
52. Leisch F, Herbinger W, Brucke P: Role of percutaneous transluminal coronary angioplasty in patients with variant angina and coexistent coronary stenosis refractory to maximal medical therapy. Clin Cardiol 7:654, 1984
53. Corcos T, David PR, Bourassa MG et al: Percutaneous transluminal coronary angioplasty for the treatment of variant angina. J Am Coll Cardiol 5:1046, 1985
54. Severi S, Davies G, Maseri A et al: Long-term prognosis of "variant" angina with medical treatment. Am J Cardiol 46:226, 1980
55. Girotti Al, Rutitzky B, Schmidberg J et al: Spontaneous remission in variant angina. Br Heart J 45:517, 1981
56. Waters DD, Szlachcic J, Miller D et al: Clinical characteristics of patients with variant angina complicated by myocardial infarction or death within 1 month. Am J Cardiol 49:658, 1982
57. Cipriano PR, Koch FH, Rosenthal SJ et al: Myocardial infarction in patients with coronary artery spasm demonstrated by angiography. Am Heart J 105:542, 1983
58. Waters DD, Miller D, Szlachcic J et al: Factors influencing the long-term prognosis of treated patients with variant angina. Circulation 68:258, 1983
59. Bott-Silverman C, Heupler FA: Natural history of pure coronary artery spasm in patients treated medically. J Am Coll Cardiol 2:200, 1983

GENERAL REFERENCES

Higgins CB, Wexler L, Silverman JF et al: Clinical and arteriographic features of Prinzmetal's variant angina: Documentation of etiologic factors. Am J Cardiol 37:831, 1976
Hillis LD, Braunwald E: Coronary artery spasm. N Engl J Med 299:695, 1978
Luchi R, Chahine R, Raizner A: Coronary artery spasm. Ann Intern Med 52:972, 1975
Maseri A, Steveri S, De Nes M et al: "Variant" angina: Myocardial ischemia. Am J Cardiol 42:1019, 1978

ACUTE MYOCARDIAL INFARCTION: PATHOPHYSIOLOGY

Wilbur Y. W. Lew • Martin M. LeWinter

HISTORICAL PERSPECTIVES

The pathophysiology of acute myocardial infarction has been a source of controversy for years. A brief historical review[1] is therefore of interest in introducing this topic.

Hippocrates postulated that heart disease could cause sudden death. However, it was not until the 16th century that precordial chest pain and an irregular pulse were related to sudden death (in reports by Benivieni, Vesalius, Columbus, Lusitanus, and Diversus). In the late 17th and early 18th centuries, several investigators (Drelincourt, Bellini, Thesbesius, Crell, and Senac) found ossification of the coronary arteries on postmortem examinations. In 1761, Morgagni described myocardial scars (from prior infarction), which he postulated would interfere with myocardial force generation. In 1768, Heberden presented his classic clinical description of angina pectoris. Several British physicians (including Fothergill, Hunter, Jenner, Black, and Parry) proposed that angina pectoris and sudden death were related to coronary artery ossification. In 1809, Burns proposed that angina pectoris represented an imbalance between myocardial energy supply and expenditure. In contrast, Laennec, in 1826, attributed angina pectoris to an abnormality of the sympathetic nerves of the heart. In 1859, Malmsten and Duben described the microscopic features of myocardial necrosis and described a coronary artery with a recanalized clot. Vlupian (1866) and Payne (1870) examined the coronary arteries in the region of myocardial infarction. They found thrombi that formed at the site of atherosclerotic plaques. Hammer (1878) is credited with the first antemortem diagnosis of coronary thrombosis. During this period, experimental animal studies (by Panum, Bezold, and Cohnheim) demonstrated that interruption of coronary blood flow resulted in arrhythmias, hypotension, and death. Wiegert (1880) and Leyden (1884) proposed that if coronary occlusion occurs over a long period of time, coronary collateral blood flow will develop and limit the extent of damage. Leyden also noted that little or no necrosis occurred in cases of sudden coronary thrombosis, whereas extensive fibrosis and aneurysmal dilatation occurred in chronic cases. At the turn of the century, Dock (1896), Krehl (1901), and Osler (1901) suggested that the heart may continue to function for variable periods of time following acute infarction. This was followed by the important studies of Obrastzow and Straschesko (1910) and Herrick (1912),[2] who demonstrated that acute myocardial infarction can be diagnosed ante mortem, is not always immediately fatal, and is frequently associated with coronary thrombosis. Herrick also stressed the importance of collateral blood vessels and the function of the uninvolved myocardium.[2] Although it was several years before these findings were accepted, their results ultimately became so entrenched in medical thought that the terms *coronary thrombosis* and *myocardial infarction* became virtually interchangeable for decades. Furthermore, these studies were the beginning of a greater understanding of the distinction between angina pectoris and acute myocardial infarction.

CAUSES OF ACUTE MYOCARDIAL INFARCTION

Coronary blood flow provides oxygen and metabolic substrates to the heart. In addition, coronary flow allows for the efficient removal of metabolic end-products such as lactic acid, hydrogen ions, and carbon dioxide. Thus, a reduction in coronary blood flow not only reduces myocardial oxygen supply but also reduces the ability to remove the end-products of myocardial metabolism. This condition is termed *myocardial ischemia*. If oxygen delivery is reduced without a concomitant reduction in coronary blood flow, myocardial metabolic end-products are still removed. This condition is termed *hypoxia* or *anoxia*, depending on whether the oxygen in the coronary blood is reduced or absent, respectively. Any of these conditions (ischemia, hypoxia, or anoxia) can result in myocardial infarction if the derangements are severe and/or prolonged.

The causes of acute myocardial infarction can be separated into those that limit myocardial oxygen supply and those that increase myocardial oxygen demand. Aortic stenosis and thyrotoxicosis, for example, are associated with marked increases in myocardial oxygen demands, which occasionally cause acute myocardial infarction.[3] However, acute myocardial infarction more commonly occurs as a consequence of reduced myocardial oxygen supply, which is not adequate to meet myocardial oxygen demand.

Myocardial oxygen supply is reduced either when oxygen content of the coronary blood is reduced or when coronary blood flow is reduced. Severe anemia and carbon monoxide poisoning, for example, are associated with marked reductions in oxygen content, which can result in myocardial infarction.[3] However, myocardial oxygen supply more commonly is reduced because of reduced coronary blood flow. An atherosclerotic plaque in the coronary artery is by far the most common cause for reduced coronary blood flow. Other anatomical causes of coronary flow obstruction include thrombus formation, emboli (from vegetations in infective endocarditis, from intramural or valvular thrombus, or from neoplasms), coronary artery dissection, coronary artery aneurysms, trauma, congenital anomalies of the coronary arteries (e.g., anomalous origin of the left coronary artery), arteritis (lupus erythematosus, polyarteritis nodosa, rheumatoid arthritis, ankylosing spondylitis, syphilis), coronary mural thickening following radiation exposure (which also produces accelerated atherosclerosis), and diseases such as amyloidosis and the mucopolysacharridoses.[3] Coronary blood flow can be reduced by hemodynamic causes such as a fall in diastolic perfusion pressure below the autoregulatory range (e.g., hypotension, excessive vasodilation, aortic insufficiency) or inadequate diastolic perfusion time (e.g., rapid heart rates). Coronary blood flow can also be reduced by functional causes such as coronary artery spasm or increased blood viscosity (e.g., thrombocytosis, polycythemia vera, hypercoagulability). Severe or prolonged reductions in coronary blood flow by any of these anatomical, hemodynamic, or functional mechanisms can cause acute myocardial infarction.

The etiology of acute myocardial infarction may be multifactorial in some cases. Cocaine abuse, for example, is temporally associated with acute myocardial infarction in patients with both normal and abnormal coronary arteries.[4,5] Postulated mechanisms for acute infarction in this setting include an abrupt increase in myocardial oxygen consumption (cocaine blocks reuptake of norepinephrine in adrenergic nerve endings), coronary vasoconstriction, acute thrombosis, and/or reaction to the contaminants in cocaine.

Some patients with acute myocardial infarction do not have any obvious predisposing cause and the coronary arteries appear "normal" on coronary arteriography[6] or by postmortem examination.[7] In many of these reports the coronary arteries were examined days to months after acute myocardial infarction. Thus the "normal" appearance of the coronary artery does not rule out the possibility that acute myocardial infarction had been caused by a transient episode of coronary artery spasm or an episode of coronary artery thrombosis with subsequent thrombolysis and recanalization. Nevertheless, there are well documented cases of patients with acute myocardial infarction and normal coronary arteries seen by arteriography within hours of the onset of symptoms.[8] These cases may be related to coronary artery spasm and/or platelet aggregates.[8] Another potential cause is microvascular angina, a syndrome of chest pain with normal-appearing epicardial coronary arteries. This syndrome is related to an abnormal vasodilator reserve of small coronary arteries that are not visible by coronary arteriography. Although the prognosis is generally favorable, microvascular angina or other types of small-vessel disease may potentially contribute to myocardial infarction. Patients with acute myocardial infarction and normal coronary arteries have a favorable prognosis.[9] The prevalence of several risk factors for coronary artery disease (including family history, hyperlipidemia, hypertension, and glucose intolerance) is lower in patients with acute myocardial infarction and normal, as compared with abnormal, coronary arteries.[9]

Despite the diversity of causes, the vast majority of acute myocardial infarctions occur in the setting of atherosclerotic coronary artery disease. Thus, the remainder of this chapter focuses primarily on the pathophysiology of acute myocardial infarction as a complication of atherosclerotic coronary artery disease.

THE ATHEROSCLEROTIC PLAQUE IN ACUTE MYOCARDIAL INFARCTION

Atherosclerotic plaques reduce the cross-sectional area of the coronary artery lumen. Although coronary perfusion pressure falls distal to the site of stenosis, coronary blood flow remains constant because of vasodilation and a decrease in coronary resistance distal to the site of the plaque. This property of autoregulation allows coronary blood flow to remain constant over a wide range of coronary perfusion pressures.[10] However, when coronary perfusion pressure falls below approximately 60 mm Hg, the distal coronary bed becomes maximally vasodilated, autoregulation is lost, and coronary blood flow becomes directly dependent on the perfusion pressure.[10]

The coronary reserve, or the ability to increase coronary blood flow by vasodilation, is reduced when a stenotic lesion reduces the coronary artery lumen diameter by as little as 30%. When the coronary lumen is reduced by 90%, coronary reserve is minimal.[11] With this degree of stenosis, coronary blood flow is adequate at rest but cannot increase in response to acute increases in metabolic demands. Coronary reserve becomes limited in the subendocardium before the subepicardium.[12]

The most important factor that determines the hemodynamic significance of a stenotic lesion is the degree of luminal area reduction. Additional factors that influence the hemodynamic significance of an atherosclerotic plaque include the length and geometry of the lesion, the velocity and pattern of coronary blood flow, and the blood viscosity.[13] The degree of luminal obstruction is not necessarily fixed, particularly with eccentric lesions. Drug-induced or spontaneous relaxation and contraction of the vascular smooth muscle in the "normal" regions, adjacent to the atherosclerotic plaque, can cause dynamic changes in the severity of the stenosis.

Acute myocardial infarction usually occurs in an area supplied by a coronary artery with an atherosclerotic plaque. In advanced lesions, the atherosclerotic plaque is often "soft" (i.e., an atheroma), containing a necrotic core filled with cell debris, cholesterol crystals, and lipid-laden macrophages. The core is covered by a fibrous cap composed of a thin layer of smooth muscle cells, collagen fibers, and foam cells. Alterations in the integrity of the plaque appear to be important in the pathophysiology of acute myocardial ischemia and infarction.

Disruption of the atherosclerotic plaque is frequently observed on postmortem examination of patients who have died of acute myocardial infarction. The frequency of this finding ranges from 70% to 100% in several pathologic series.[14–17] Plaque disruption may occur in several forms, including intimal fissures, breaks, tears, rents, erosions, or ulcerations of the atherosclerotic plaque. Plaque disruption is seen more frequently in patients who die within a few days, rather than after a few weeks, following acute myocardial infarction.[14]

A disrupted atherosclerotic plaque may serve as the nidus for thrombus formation.[14] Most plaque disruptions are associated with overlying thrombus formation, and, conversely, most cases of coronary thrombosis occur at the site of a ruptured atheromatous plaque.[14–17] The thrombus frequently contains platelet aggregates or substances from the atherosclerotic plaque, such as cholesterol crystals, foam cells, and intimal collagen fibers. These findings support the concept that plaque rupture precedes (or leads to) thrombus formation.[15]

The precise mechanism for initiating plaque disruption is not known. It has been postulated that plaque disruption occurs as a consequence of chronic hemodynamic trauma, inflammatory or chemical injury to the endothelium, or coronary artery spasm.[16] The normal twisting and bending motions of the heart and its coronary arteries is another possible mechanism for tearing the thin fibrous cap of the atherosclerotic plaque.[17]

Disruption of the atherosclerotic plaque could lead to acute coronary artery occlusion and myocardial ischemia by several mechanisms. Injury to the endothelial barrier produces a communication between the coronary lumen and the atherosclerotic plaque, which allows blood, fibrin, and platelets to infiltrate into the plaque. This intraintimal thrombus formation increases the size of the plaque, resulting in further obstruction of the coronary lumen. Intraintimal thrombus formation also increases intraplaque pressure, leading to further plaque rupture. Another mechanism for initiating coronary artery occlusion occurs when the contents of the ruptured plaque are released into the coronary lumen and embolize into the distal coronary bed. The perfusion bed distal to the site of an acute thrombus often contains platelet and fibrin microemboli and microinfarcts.[18,19] Another possible mechanism for occluding blood flow involves local intraluminal thrombus formation. A rupture or break in the fibrous cap of the atherosclerotic plaque exposes the necrotic core and collagen fibers of the plaque to the overlying coronary blood flow. This serves as a nidus for thrombus formation, which can become occlusive. Occlusive thrombi occur more frequently when the underlying plaque already produces significant coronary artery stenosis.[17] Such plaques may be subjected to greater mechanical trauma because of the increased local turbulence associated with severe coronary artery stenosis.

Plaque fissures may play an important role in sudden death. In one study, plaque fissures were found in the vast majority of patients who died within 6 hours of the onset of acute ischemic symptoms.[20] Most of these plaque fissures were associated with either intraluminal or intraintimal thrombus formation. Interestingly, several cases of sudden death were associated with plaque fissures and thrombus formation in lesions that decreased the coronary artery diameter by less than 50%. Such lesions are not usually considered hemodynamically significant. It also should be noted that the high incidence of intraluminal thrombi (74%) reported in this study[20] is in contrast to the low incidence of thrombosis found in several other pathologic series of sudden death.[21,22]

Plaque ruptures are seen on pathologic examination of patients with unstable angina preceding fatal myocardial infarction.[18] The plaque ulcerations in patients with unstable angina demonstrate recurrent thrombus formation with intermittent fragmentation.[18,23]

In patients with acute myocardial infarction treated with thrombolytic therapy, the severity of the underlying coronary artery stenosis may be surprisingly mild or moderate.[24] The coronary artery lesion responsible for an acute myocardial infarction may not differ in severity from lesions in noninfarcted vessels.[25] Similarly, the severity of coronary artery stenosis may not differ between patients with stable and unstable angina pectoris. However, coronary artery lesions associated with acute myocardial infarction or unstable angina have a complex morphologic appearance on angiography that suggests ulceration related to plaque disruption and/or thrombus formation.[25,26] The presence of plaque disruptions in patients with myocardial infarction, unstable angina, and sudden death suggests a common pathophysiologic mechanism. Although the degree of luminal obstruction by an atherosclerotic plaque is important, the plaque morphology and likelihood for plaque disruption with occlusive thrombus formation may be of equal importance. The clinical sequelae depend on the magnitude and acuteness of the plaque disruption, the extent of thrombus formation, the initiation of local vasoconstriction, and the duration of reduced coronary flow.

CORONARY ARTERY THROMBOSIS

Disruption of atherosclerotic plaques occurs frequently in patients with unstable angina and acute myocardial infarction. Contact of circulating platelets with exposed subendothelial collagen fibers and microfibrils initiates platelet adhesion and aggregation. Adenosine diphosphate (ADP) and thromboxane A_2 are released, which enhances platelet aggregation. Intrinsic and extrinsic coagulation pathways are activated, leading to thrombin generation, fibrin deposition, thrombus growth, and stabilization. The incidence of coronary thrombosis has been examined extensively in autopsy studies and more recently by coronary arteriography during the acute phase of myocardial infarction. The incidence of coronary thrombosis differs between groups of patients with transmural myocardial infarction, subendocardial myocardial infarction, sudden death, or unstable angina.

The incidence of coronary artery thrombosis is very high in patients with transmural myocardial infarction. The incidence of coronary thrombi in patients with acute myocardial infarction is greater than 90% in the majority of several large autopsy series (greater than 50% in all studies).[16,27,28] Thrombus is most often found at the site of an atherosclerotic plaque, particularly if the plaque occludes 75% or more of the coronary lumen and/or if there is a long area of stenosis.[15,16,28,29] Intracoronary thrombi occur more frequently with larger infarcts.[28,29] Reports have been conflicting as to whether the incidence of coronary thrombi decreases,[15] increases,[29] or does not change[16,28] with increasing length of survival following the acute myocardial infarction.

The incidence of total coronary artery occlusion following acute myocardial infarction has been examined ante mortem with coronary arteriography. In patients studied 1 month after acute myocardial infarction, approximately half have total coronary artery occlusion and fewer than one third have subtotal (>90%) occlusions.[30] The incidence of total coronary artery occlusion is much higher in patients studied within the first 24 hours of acute myocardial infarction.[31] In patients undergoing emergency coronary revascularization within the first day of an acute myocardial infarction, intracoronary clots can be found at the site of a ruptured plaque in the involved coronary artery.[32]

DeWood and co-workers performed coronary arteriography in 322 patients within 24 hours of an acute myocardial infarction.[31] Among patients studied within 6 hours of the onset of symptoms, 86% had total and 10% had subtotal (>95%) occlusion of the coronary artery. The incidence of total coronary artery occlusion declined significantly to 67% among patients studied between 6 and 24 hours after onset of symptoms. In 70% of patients who underwent emergency coronary artery bypass surgery, coronary thrombus was recovered by a Fogarty catheter. Thus, the sensitivity and specificity of coronary arteriography for diagnosing coronary thrombus could be evaluated. Coronary arteriography demonstrated 88% true-positive results (i.e., 88% of coronary arteriograms diagnostic of coronary thrombus had the diagnosis confirmed during surgery), 12% false-positive results (thrombus not found during surgery), and 25% false-negative results (thrombus recovered during surgery but not diagnosed by angiography). These figures are comparable to postmortem angiogram studies that report an 88% sensitivity and 79% specificity for detecting complicated lesions (those with plaque rupture or hemorrhage and/or occlusive or recanalized thrombus).[26] Thus the incidence of occlusive coronary thrombosis is extremely high during the acute phase of acute myocardial infarction but decreases significantly within hours. The decrease in total coronary artery obstruction may be related to spontaneous thrombolysis and/or resolution of coronary artery spasm.[31]

In contrast to transmural infarctions, the incidence of coronary artery thrombosis is lower in patients with subendocardial myocardial infarctions. Most autopsy studies report that fewer than half of the patients with subendocardial infarcts have coronary artery thrombosis,[16,28,33] with some studies finding no evidence of coronary thrombosis in any patient.[29,34] Patients with subendocardial infarcts tend to have severe three-vessel coronary artery disease, suggesting that some subendocardial infarcts are caused by generalized hypoperfusion rather than local thrombosis.[33,34] These autopsy results have been confirmed with coronary arteriographic studies. The patency rate of the involved vessel is significantly higher in patients 11 days (mean) after a non–Q wave than a Q wave myocardial infarction (54% vs. 25%).[35] DeWood and co-workers performed coronary arteriography in 341 patients within the first week of a non–Q wave myocardial infarction.[36] Only 26% of patients studied within the first 24 hours had total coronary artery occlusion. This incidence increased significantly to 37% in patients studied between days 1 and 3 and to 42% for patients studied between days 3 and 7 of a non–Q wave infarction.[36] Patients with total coronary artery occlusion were more likely to develop collateral blood vessels. Thus, occlusive coronary artery thrombosis does not play as dominant a role in nontransmural as compared with transmural myocardial infarctions.

The incidence of coronary artery thrombosis in patients with sudden death is less clear. Most autopsy studies found coronary thrombosis in fewer than 20% of patients dying within the first hour of the onset of ischemic symptoms.[21,22] In patients who survive for several hours after the onset of symptoms, the incidence of coronary thrombosis increases to 30% or more.[21,22] In contrast, one study found a high (74%) incidence of coronary thrombosis in patients with sudden death but no difference between patients surviving for minutes and those surviving 1 to 6 hours after the onset of symptoms.[20] With the exception of this last study, coronary artery thrombosis does not appear to be common in patients with sudden death.

Coronary artery thrombosis occurs in patients with unstable angina. In patients with unstable angina who die within 6 hours of chest pain, plaque fissures were found at autopsy in 90%, occlusive thrombi in 36%, and platelet aggregates in the myocardium distal to the plaque in 30%.[37] The thrombus is often layered with materials of differing age, suggesting that recurrent or episodic thrombosis occurred with intermittent fragmentation leading to microemboli in the distal circulation.[18] Patients with unstable angina have complicated lesions on coronary arteriography that are consistent with plaque disruption.[25] Coronary thrombosis is seen by coronary arteriography in 50% to 60% of patients with unstable angina when examined within days[38-40] or during[41] episodes of angina. The low incidence of coronary thrombosis observed in earlier studies is likely related to the fact that coronary arteriography was performed weeks to months after the unstable angina. Coronary thrombi are particularly common in patients studied within hours of their angina[39,41] and in patients refractory to aggressive therapy.[38] Patients with unstable angina but without thrombus often have other angiographic findings that suggest an acute process (e.g., intraluminal filling defects or complex lesions).[40] The frequency of coronary thrombi diagnosed by coronary arteriography is not as high in patients with unstable angina as with acute myocardial infarction.[31] Part of this difference may reflect thrombus size. In unstable angina, thrombus formation may be smaller and occur in multiple episodes, making acute thrombus formation more difficult to diagnose by angiography. Sherman and associates examined ten patients with unstable angina with coronary angioscopy.[23] Although coronary thrombus was seen with angioscopy in all seven patients with rest angina, thrombus was diagnosed by coronary arteriography in only one patient. Although complex plaques were seen with angioscopy in the other three patients with accelerated angina, this was diagnosed by arteriography in only one patient. Thus, coronary thrombosis may be important in unstable angina but its frequency may be underestimated by coronary arteriography.

THE ROLE OF PLATELETS IN MYOCARDIAL ISCHEMIA AND INFARCTION

Platelets, which are important in the pathogenesis of atherosclerosis, also have been implicated in the pathophysiology of acute myocardial ischemia and infarction. Platelets can be activated by several mechanisms. The hemodynamic turbulence associated with coronary artery stenosis induces platelet aggregation in experimental models.[42,43] Catecholamines and stress, which commonly accompany (or precede) acute myocardial ischemia, also induce platelet aggregation.[44,45] Disruption of the atherosclerotic plaque (by any of the mechanisms discussed in the preceding section) exposes the subendothelial collagen and smooth muscle fibers, providing a nidus for platelet adhesion and aggregation.

The importance of platelet aggregates in myocardial ischemia is suggested by several observations in experimental animal studies. Following electrically induced damage to the coronary artery intima, platelet aggregates form at the site of intimal injury and occlude the coronary artery lumen.[46] Occlusive platelet aggregates also form in experimental models of mild coronary artery stenosis.[42,43] In these studies, the local turbulence and shear forces produced by the stenosis may activate platelets directly. Alternatively, local endothelial lesions could serve as a nidus for platelet adhesion and formation of occlusive platelet microthrombi.[43]

Platelet aggregates can be detected in the coronary sinus blood within minutes following experimental coronary artery occlusion.[47] Platelet trapping in the form of microthrombi is found in the microcirculation of the ischemic zone[48] and marginal areas.[49] Occlusive platelet aggregates and microthrombi do not form if platelet function is altered prior to the induction of myocardial ischemia (e.g., with aspirin).[42,46,47,49]

In clinical autopsy studies, platelet and fibrin microthrombi are found in patients with sudden death due to acute myocardial infarction.[50] Platelet aggregates are more common in patients with coronary artery disease who die suddenly due to cardiac rather than noncardiac causes.[51] Platelet aggregates are also found on postmortem examination of patients with unstable angina and acute infarction or sudden death.[18,19,37]

Platelet survival is shorter in patients with coronary artery disease.[52] Patients with coronary artery disease have lower platelet counts and lower platelet aggregates in the coronary sinus than aortic blood, a gradient that is reduced with aspirin therapy.[53] Such a gradient is not found in patients without coronary artery disease, suggesting that active platelets and platelet aggregates are removed as blood traverses the atherosclerotic coronary vasculature.[53]

Acute episodes of angina pectoris in patients with unstable angina are associated with platelet activation.[54] Increased platelet aggregates appear in the coronary sinus blood of patients with pacing-induced ischemia.[53] Platelet aggregability increases in the initial hours of acute myocardial infarction, then decreases over time.[27,55] Some but not all studies have found increased circulating platelet aggregates with acute myocardial ischemia and infarction.[27] Elevation of the platelet-specific proteins platelet factor 4 and β-thromboglobulin (released from α granules during platelet aggregation) occurs in patients with unstable angina and during acute myocardial infarction. However, this may reflect a generalized response to increased catecholamine levels. Although it is apparent that patients with acute myocardial ischemia and infarction have increased platelet activation, it is unclear if this represents a response of normal platelets to plaque disruption or if there are abnormally hyperreactive platelets that are more prone to aggregate and induce thrombosis.

There is a parallel between the circadian variation in platelet aggregability and the occurrence of acute myocardial ischemia and infarction.[56] This provides indirect clinical evidence for a role of platelets in the pathophysiology of acute myocardial ischemia. The onset of acute myocardial infarction has a circadian periodicity with a threefold higher frequency of events in the morning than late evening.[57] The circadian pattern and timing of peak events can be modified in subgroups of patients with congestive heart failure, prior myocardial infarction, or diabetes or in patients who use β-blockers.[58] A circadian pattern also occurs for sudden death[56] and transient myocardial ischemia.[59] In normal volunteers there is a morning increase in plasma norepinephrine, epinephrine, and platelet aggregability.[60] The morning increase in platelet aggregability is primarily related to the assumption of an upright position. Emotional stress may also increase platelet activation.[45] These findings do not prove a causal relation but are consistent with the hypothesis that alterations in platelet function may predispose to acute myocardial ischemia and infarction.

If platelets are important in the pathophysiology of acute myocardial infarction, then interference with platelet function might be beneficial in preventing or reducing the severity of acute myocardial ischemia. This rationale has led to several large randomized clinical trials to determine whether aspirin, dipyridamole, or sulfinpyrazone prevent recurrent cardiovascular events in patients following acute myocardial infarction (secondary prevention trials), provide protective effects in patients during an acute myocardial infarction or with unstable angina, or reduce acute cardiovascular events in healthy persons (primary prevention trials).

There have been seven large, prospective secondary prevention trials that have studied the effects of long-term aspirin therapy (300–1500 mg/day) initiated days to years after an acute myocardial infarction.[61-67] The enrollment for each study ranged from 700 to 4500 patients with clinical follow-up for 1 to 4 years. One study found no benefit of therapy,[65] and one study found a significant reduction in recurrent myocardial infarction in patients treated with a combination of aspirin and Persantine.[67] In the remaining five studies, there was a trend toward reduced total and cardiovascular mortality and reduced incidence of sudden death in patients treated with aspirin, although these beneficial trends did not reach statistical significance.[61-64,66] Two trials found significant beneficial effects of chronic sulfinpyrazone treatment following myocardial infarction.[68,69] However, the statistical methodology in one of these studies has raised several concerns.[68,70,71] Although most of these secondary prevention trials have not found statistically significant benefits of chronic antiplatelet therapy, an overview of these trials (combining results from over 18,000 patients) demonstrated that antiplatelet therapy significantly reduces nonfatal myocardial infarction by 31%, reduces vascular deaths by 13%, and reduces strokes by 42%.[72] This overview did not detect any difference between the different doses of aspirin or between the different antiplatelet drugs.[72]

The effects of aspirin therapy during the acute phase of myocardial infarction was examined in the Second International Study of Infarct Survival (ISIS-2) trial.[73] In 17,187 patients with suspected acute myocardial infarction, therapy was initiated within the first 24 hours (median 5 hours) with either 1.5 MU streptokinase (infused over 1 hour), aspirin (160 mg/day for 1 month), both, or neither. Both drugs significantly reduced vascular deaths at 5 weeks and 15 months, with additive benefits from the combination of both drugs. Aspirin reduced vascular deaths at 5 weeks by 23% and reduced the reinfarction rate by 50%.[73]

Three randomized trials found significant benefits of aspirin therapy (325 to 1300 mg/day) in patients with unstable angina.[74-76] Aspirin started within the first 24 hours reduced the in-hospital incidence of acute myocardial infarction from 12% to 3%.[76] Acute heparin therapy provided similar benefits during the acute phase. In two other studies, aspirin started within the first 8 days of hospitalization reduced the incidence of acute myocardial infarction and cardiac death by more than 50% during follow-up periods of 12 weeks to 2 years.[74,75] One of those studies failed to demonstrate any benefit of sulfinpyrazone therapy in patients with unstable angina.[75]

Two randomized, primary prevention trials have been performed in healthy male physicians followed for a mean of 5 to 6 years. Long-term aspirin therapy was administered to 5139 physicians in Great Britain (500 mg/day)[77] and to 22,071 physicians in the Physicians' Health Study in the United States (325 mg every other day).[78] Aspirin therapy did not alter the risk of acute myocardial infarction in the British study, although the number of events was low (resulting in wide confidence intervals for results).[77] In the Physicians' Health Study, aspirin significantly reduced the risk of acute myocardial infarction by 44% and reduced overall vascular events by 18%.[78] The benefits of aspirin therapy on acute myocardial infarction were limited to men 50 years or older.[78]

In summary, the concept that activation of platelets is important in the pathophysiology of acute myocardial ischemia and infarction is indirectly supported by observations that inhibition of platelets with aspirin provides significant protective effects in unstable angina[74-76] and during the acute phase of myocardial infarction.[73] However, a causal relationship between abnormal platelet activation and acute myocardial ischemia or infarction would be more difficult to establish. Although several large primary and secondary prevention trials have generally shown positive benefits of antiplatelet therapy, the lack of more strongly positive results may be related to the limited size, a low incidence rate, and the fact that initiation of acute myocardial ischemia or infarction is likely to be complex and multifactorial.

INTERACTIONS BETWEEN PLATELETS AND THE VASCULAR ENDOTHELIUM

The local balance between prostacyclin (PGI_2) and thromboxane A_2 (TXA_2) is a major determinant of platelet adhesion and aggregation.[79] Platelets do not normally adhere to the vessel wall because of the local production of PGI_2 by the vascular endothelium. PGI_2 is a potent vasodilator and inhibitor of platelet aggregation. There also is a circulating source of PGI_2, although its concentration is probably too low to contribute significantly to the inhibition of platelet aggregation.[80] The effects of PGI_2 are opposed by TXA_2, which is produced by platelets. TXA_2 is a potent vasoconstrictor and promotor of platelet aggregation.

Although PGI_2 and TXA_2 have opposing effects, both are derived from a common precursor, arachidonic acid.[79] Arachidonic acid is stored in the phospholipid layer of the cell membrane. A variety of chemical and mechanical stimuli activate phospholipase to release arachidonic acid into the cell. Arachidonic acid is converted by the enzyme cyclo-oxygenase into the cyclic endoperoxide intermediary compounds. These compounds are converted to either PGI_2 or TXA_2 depending on the cell type. In the vascular endothelium, the enzyme prostacyclin synthetase results in the preferential formation of PGI_2. In blood platelets, the enzyme thromboxane synthetase converts the endoperoxide compounds into TXA_2. Both PGI_2 and TXA_2 have short half-lives and are rapidly converted into the inert but stable compounds 6-ketoprostaglandin $F_{1\alpha}$ (6-keto-$PGF_{1\alpha}$) and thromboxane B_2 (TXB_2), respectively.

The coronary vasculature produces several other prostaglandins besides PGI_2, including PGE_2, $PGF_{2\alpha}$, and PGD_2.[81] PGE_2 is a vasodilator that promotes platelet aggregation. $PGF_{2\alpha}$ is a venoconstrictor. PGD_2 inhibits platelet aggregation. There are site-dependent differences for prostaglandin production. The major prostaglandin produced in large coronary arteries is PGI_2, whereas in coronary microvessels more PGE_2 than PGI_2 is produced.[81,82]

Platelets and the vascular endothelium produce several important products in addition to TXA_2 and PGI_2. Activated platelets also secrete vasoactive substances such as serotonin (5-hydroxytryptamine or 5-HT) and platelet activating factor (PAF). The vascular endothelium also produces endothelium-derived relaxing factor (EDRF) and contracting factors.[83] EDRF is released by mechanical factors (e.g., shear stress), by neurohumoral factors (e.g., norepinephrine or stimulation of α_2-adrenoreceptors), by local mediators (e.g., bradykinin or histamine), and by several of the products of coagulation and platelets (e.g., ADP, thrombin, and 5-HT).[83] Platelet-induced release of EDRF may provide a protective effect by inhibiting coronary contraction induced by aggregating platelets and by acting synergistically with PGI_2 in inhibiting platelet aggregation.[84,85] The vascular endothelium modulates the influence of platelet aggregates and its products. In the presence of an intact endothelium, the release of adenine nucleotides (ADP and adenosine triphosphate [ATP]) by platelets induces relaxation of coronary arteries through an endothelial-mediated process.[86] In the absence of an intact endothelium, release of TXA_2 and serotonin by aggregating platelets directly activates smooth muscle to contract coronary arteries.[86]

Although the vascular endothelium and platelets produce several important products, there has been particular interest in the local balance between PGI_2 and TXA_2. These compounds have extremely short half-lives but are converted to the stable compounds 6-keto-$PGF_{1\alpha}$ and TXB_2, respectively. Plasma measurements of the stable metabolites have been used to indirectly evaluate the activity of PGI_2 and TXA_2. However, methodologic problems and artifacts related to sampling may cause the PGI_2 and TXA_2 activity to be overestimated.[79] The intrinsic rates of PGI_2 and TXA_2 formation are extremely low.[80,87] It only requires minimal activation (*e.g.*, 0.1%) of platelets during or after specimen collection to produce erroneously high estimates of TXA_2 activity. Similarly, plasma or coronary sinus measurements of 6-keto-$PGF_{1\alpha}$ may overestimate cardiac PGI_2 activity since cardiac catheterization itself may produce a mild vascular trauma sufficient to increase prostacyclin formation.[88] Noninvasive estimates of PGI_2 and TXA_2 activity can be obtained by measuring the major urinary metabolites 2,3-dinor-6-keto-$PGF_{1\alpha}$ and 2,3-dinor-TXB_2, respectively. However, these measurements do not identify the source of cell or tissue production of PGI_2 and TXA_2.

The presence of atherosclerosis may produce abnormalities in PGI_2 and EDRF production. In animals with experimentally induced atherosclerosis, the coronary arteries have a reduced capacity for PGI_2 production.[89] This impairment may predispose to the development of platelet aggregation and thrombi formation in atherosclerotic arteries.[89] However, the significance of these findings is uncertain since the capacity for PGI_2 production (even if reduced) far exceeds the normal rate of PGI_2 biosynthesis.[80]

The rate of PGI_2 production has been measured in patients with atherosclerosis with conflicting results. Some investigators found reduced PGI_2 production in patients with ischemic heart disease,[90] while others report increased PGI_2 biosynthesis rates in patients with atherosclerotic peripheral artery disease.[91] In some studies, no difference in coronary sinus blood levels of 6-keto-$PGF_{1\alpha}$ and PGE_2 was found between patients with and without ischemic heart disease.[92] Thus, it remains unresolved whether patients with atherosclerotic coronary artery disease have an impairment in local PGI_2 production that predisposes them to platelet aggregation and acute myocardial ischemia.

Abnormalities in the vascular endothelium are found in experimental models of atherosclerosis. There is an impairment in endothelial-dependent relaxation with atherosclerosis that may decrease flow rates and predispose to platelet aggregation and/or coronary artery spasm.[93] EDRF production is improved in experimental models of atherosclerosis by dietary supplements of fish oils.[94] The inverse relation between high dietary fish consumption and the incidence of coronary heart disease[95] may be related to this enhancement in EDRF production, which produces vasodilator effects and inhibits platelet aggregation.

In experimental myocardial ischemia and hypoxia several prostaglandins are released, including prostaglandins E, A, and F.[96,97] In patients with pacing-induced ischemia, prostaglandins F and E are released into the coronary sinus blood.[98] The site of prostaglandin production under these conditions is not known. There is increased PGI_2 biosynthesis during acute myocardial ischemia that probably arises from the vascular endothelium. Coronary sinus blood levels of 6-keto-$PGF_{1\alpha}$ increases within minutes of experimental coronary artery occlusion.[99] Blood levels of 6-keto-$PGF_{1\alpha}$ are elevated in patients during the first week of an acute myocardial infarction. Urinary 2,3-dinor-6-keto-$PGF_{1\alpha}$, a more specific and reliable indicator of *in vivo* PGI_2 biosynthesis, is elevated modestly in patients with unstable angina coincident with episodes of chest pain and evidence of platelet activation.[54] In patients with acute myocardial infarction, urinary 2,3-dinor-6-keto-$PGF_{1\alpha}$ increases in direct proportion to the peak creatine kinase, peaks during the first 24 to 36 hours, and then returns to baseline levels.[54,100] It is postulated that the source of increased PGI_2 during acute myocardial infarction is the infarcted myocardium and necrotic vascular endothelium, whereas the increase in PGI_2 biosynthesis during episodes of chest pain in unstable angina is due to stimulation of the vascular endothelium by activated platelets.[54]

Alterations in TXA_2 production may also produce a local imbalance between PGI_2 and TXA_2, resulting in platelet adhesion and aggregation. Platelets from patients and animals with atherosclerosis produce increased amounts of TXA_2, suggesting a predisposition to platelet aggregation.[101,102] In animal studies, TXB_2 levels in the coronary sinus increase within 1 to 2 minutes of coronary artery ligation.[99,103] In clinical studies, venous and coronary sinus blood levels of TXB_2 are elevated during pacing-induced ischemia,[104,105] during episodes of chest pain in unstable angina,[92] and with acute myocardial infarction.[103,106] Urinary 2,3-dinor-TXB_2, a more reliable measurement of TXA_2 activity,[79,87] increases significantly in patients with unstable angina, postinfarction angina, and acute myocardial infarction.[38,54,100] Urinary 2,3-dinor-TXB_2 levels are particularly high in patients with unstable angina who do not respond to therapy and have angiographic evidence of thrombus formation.[38] Urinary 2,3-dinor-TXB_2 may increase in patients with unstable angina in the absence of chest pain, possibly indicating episodes of silent ischemia.[54]

Experimental animal models have proven useful for examining the interaction between platelets and the vascular endothelium. Folts and colleagues produced a 60% to 80% partial coronary artery stenosis in dogs to produce a model of local endothelial damage.[42,107] In this model, platelet aggregates form, enlarge, and then fragment, producing dynamic changes in the degree of flow obstruction and causing cyclic reductions in coronary flow. The cyclic reduction in flow is abolished by inhibiting platelet aggregation with aspirin, indomethacin, and ibuprofen.[42,107] Willerson and associates used this model in an extensive series of studies.[108] They found elevated TXB_2 and 6-keto-$PGF_{1\alpha}$ levels distal to the site of endothelial injury and coronary artery stenosis. The cyclic reductions in coronary flow were abolished in 70% of animals by inhibiting platelet TXA_2 production and inhibiting platelet aggregation with pharmacologic inhibition of the enzyme thromboxane synthetase or with a thromboxane receptor antagonist. A thromboxane-mimetic drug restored cyclic flow reductions. Increased concentrations of serotonin were found at the site of stenosis and endothelial injury. The cyclic flow reductions could be eliminated in some animals by a serotonin receptor antagonist. Combined inhibition of the thromboxane and serotonin effects eliminated cyclic flow reductions in nearly all animals.[108]

Clinical studies also suggest a potential role of serotonin. Coronary sinus blood from patients with coronary artery disease contains a vasoconstrictor activity that is directly related to the extent and severity of the coronary lesions and is blocked by a serotonin receptor antagonist.[109] This suggests that platelets are activated and release serotonin after passage through atherosclerotic vessels.[109] In some patients with coronary artery disease, particularly those with complex and eccentric lesions, there is a transcardiac gradient of serotonin with higher levels in the coronary sinus than aortic blood.[110] Thus, in some cases of ischemic heart disease, release of serotonin may have important modulating effects and produce local vasoconstriction.

If a local imbalance between PGI_2 and TXA_2 is important for platelet adhesion and aggregation preceding acute myocardial ischemia and infarction, then therapy aimed at increasing PGI_2 levels or inhibiting TXA_2 production should be beneficial. Experimental studies have examined the effects of direct infusions of prostaglandins. Occlusive thrombus formation with electrically induced damage to the coronary intima is prevented with PGI_2 infusions.[46] In experimental coronary artery occlusion, infusions of PGI_2, PGE_1, and PGE_2 all reduce the extent of myocardial ischemia and infarction, as reflected by the electrocardiogram, creatine kinase release, and pathologic examination of infarct size.[111-114] Although PGI_2 inhibits platelet aggregation, platelets are hyperaggregable during acute myocardial infarction and are more resistant to the antiaggregatory effects of PGI_2 than under normal conditions.[55] The beneficial effects of prostaglandins may be related to inhibition of platelet aggregation, vasodilation of the coronary and systemic circulation, increase in collateral blood flow,[113] and stabilization of lysosomal membranes, preventing the release of damaging proteases and phospholipases.[111,112] PGE_1 may also reduce infarct size by inhibiting neutrophil migration and activation at the site of tissue injury.[114]

The effects of PGI_2 infusions have been examined in patients with ischemic heart disease. In patients with stable angina pectoris, PGI_2 infusion prolongs the time required to induce angina by pacing.[115] In patients with unstable angina[116] and acute myocardial infarction,[117] PGI_2 infusion reduces the severity of ischemia, primarily as a result of the beneficial hemodynamic effects. In one study, PGI_2 infusions reduced the extent of injury if started within 6 hours of acute myocardial infarction.[118] However, others have not found PGI_2 infusions to be beneficial in patients with acute myocardial infarction.[119] Also, PGI_2 infusions do not decrease the frequency of angina in patients with variant angina.[120]

Inhibition of platelet activation and aggregation may be a useful adjunct for thrombolytic therapy during acute myocardial infarction. Streptokinase, urokinase, tissue-type plasminogen activator (t-PA), and recombinant-type t-PA (rt-PA) are all useful thrombolytic agents for producing reperfusion in patients with acute myocardial infarction. However, approximately 30% of patients do not achieve reperfusion, and even among the patients with successful reperfusion there is a significant incidence of reocclusion. These complications may be related to abnormal platelet activity. In patients with acute myocardial infarction there is an increase in urinary 2,3-dinor-TXB_2 following streptokinase that can be inhibited by pretreatment with aspirin.[121] The increase in TXA_2 production is related to *in vivo* activation of platelets by streptokinase rather than washout of metabolites with reperfusion.[121] In animal models, platelet-rich arterial thrombus is significantly more resistant than erythrocyte-rich thrombus to lysis with rt-PA.[122] *In vitro* lysis of combined platelet and fibrin thrombi with urokinase is enhanced with the addition of PGI_2 (due to platelet antiaggregatory effects) or with pretreatment with aspirin.[123] In animal models of coronary thrombosis, a monoclonal antibody directed against the glycoprotein GPIIb/IIIa receptor that inhibits platelet aggregation prevents reocclusion following reperfusion with rt-PA.[124] Inhibition of platelet activity with the combined use of a TXA_2-receptor antagonist and serotonin S_2-receptor antagonist reduces the time and dose of t-PA required for reperfusion and prevents or delays reocclusion.[125] Thus there is experimental evidence demonstrating that more effective thrombolysis can be achieved by the combination of fibrinolytic therapy with inhibition of platelet activation and aggregation. Clinical support for this concept is derived from the ISIS-2 trial, which demonstrates that the combination of streptokinase and aspirin therapy during an acute myocardial infarction provides additive benefits (over the benefits from either agent alone) for reducing vascular deaths at 5 and 15 months.[73]

In summary, the local balance between PGI_2 production by the vascular endothelium and TXA_2 production by platelets is a major determinant of platelet adhesion and aggregation. This balance is modified by other products of the vascular endothelium, including EDRF, and by other products of platelets, including serotonin. Atherosclerosis may produce alterations in PGI_2 and EDRF production by the vascular endothelium and in platelet function, which predisposes to platelet adhesion and aggregation. During acute myocardial ischemia and infarction there is evidence for both increased TXA_2 release from activated platelets and increased PGI_2 activity from stimulation of the vascular endothelium. In both experimental and clinical studies, inhibition of platelet activity (with PGI_2 infusions, aspirin, thromboxane synthetase inhibitors, thromboxane receptor antagonists, and serotonin receptor antagonists) can reduce the consequences of acute myocardial ischemia and infarction. This therapeutic approach (inhibition of platelet activation and aggregation) can be used in combination with fibrinolytic therapy to improve the success of reperfusion and reduce the rate of reocclusion and to reduce subsequent vascular mortality.

ROLE OF NEUTROPHILS

The role of neutrophils in the inflammatory response and healing phases of acute myocardial infarction has been appreciated for years. Evidence suggests that neutrophils also play an important role in mediating cell damage during the early hours of acute myocardial ischemia and with reperfusion.[126] Leukocytes accumulate progressively during the initial hours of acute myocardial ischemia.[127,128] Leukocytes plug capillaries in regions with low direct and low collateral blood flow, thus increasing coronary vascular resistance.[127,129] During reperfusion, leukocyte accumulation increases and the adherent leukocyte plug cannot be dislodged, preventing restoration of capillary flow (the no-reflow phenomenon).[127–129]

Several mechanisms contribute to leukocyte accumulation and activation during acute myocardial ischemia. Leukocytes are large, stiff cells that normally traverse capillaries at a slow velocity and are adherent to the vascular endothelium. The decrease in perfusion pressure during acute myocardial ischemia increases leukocyte adhesion and leads to accumulation.[127] Several mechanisms contribute to chemotaxis during acute myocardial ischemia. Platelets release platelet activating factor and 12-hydroperoxy-eicosatetraenoic acid (12-HPETE), which are chemotactic. The complement system is activated during acute myocardial ischemia with resultant chemotaxis. After 45 minutes of experimental ischemia, C1q (a subunit of the first component of complement) accumulates in direct proportion to the severity of reduced coronary blood flow and is associated with localized accumulation of leukocytes.[130] Other components of complement (C3, C5, C4) may accumulate during experimental myocardial ischemia.[131] Cobra venom factor administered 30 minutes following coronary artery occlusion depletes complement and eliminates C3 and C5 accumulation, reduces neutrophil infiltration, and reduces the extent of infarction by both neutrophil-dependent and neutrophil-independent mechanisms.[131]

Several products of arachidonic acid, including those from activated platelets and neutrophils, contribute to chemotaxis. Arachidonic acid is converted by the cyclo-oxygenase enzyme to produce PGI_2 and TXA_2 in the vascular endothelium and platelets. In platelets, the 12-lipoxygenase enzyme converts arachidonic acid to 12-HPETE, which has chemotactic properties. In neutrophils, the 5-lipoxygenase enzyme converts arachidonic acid into 5-HPETE, which then converts to either 5-hydroxy-eicosatetraenoic acid (5-HETE) or into the leukotrienes, including LTB_4, LTD_4, LTC_4, and LTE_4.[132,133] The major leukotriene product of neutrophils is LTB_4, which is a potent chemotactic agent. Several leukotrienes increase vascular permeability and induce coronary vasoconstriction.[132–134] During experimental myocardial infarction, leukocyte infiltration is associated with leukotriene release, which contributes to tissue damage.[128,134] Neutrophils from patients with stable angina pectoris have increased chemotactic activity and increased potential for LTB_4 production.[135] Patients with unstable angina and acute myocardial infarction have evidence of intense *in vivo* activation of neutrophils.[135]

Neutrophils accumulated at the site of acute myocardial ischemia may produce myocardial damage by producing oxidants and/or releasing a large number of proteolytic enzymes.[136] Inability to distinguish between foreign and host cells results in the inadvertent destruction of normal cells and tissues. The membrane of neutrophils contains the enzyme NADPH oxidase, which is activated to shuttle electrons from cytosolic NADPH to dissolved oxygen in the extracellular fluid to produce superoxide anion (O_2^-), hydroxyl radical ($OH\cdot$), and hydrogen peroxide (H_2O_2). Hydrogen peroxide and the enzyme myeloperoxidase (released by neutrophils) oxidizes chloride ions to form hypochlorous acid (HOCl), a cytotoxic compound. Some chelated forms of iron and iron-binding proteins, which are commonly found in damaged cells, may catalyze the formation of hydroxyl radicals by the Haber-Weiss or Fenton reactions.[137] Oxygen-derived free radicals are directly cytotoxic and induce additional damage by reacting with nonradicals to initiate a chain reaction of free radical production.

Neutrophils are only one of several potential sources of oxygen-derived free radicals. Additional major sources for oxygen-derived free radicals include the mitochondria, the enzyme xanthine oxidase, and degradation of catecholamines by monamine oxidase.[137,138] There is a significant leakage of the superoxide radical from electron transport in the mitochondria, particularly with injury (*e.g.*, ischemia). The enzyme xanthine oxidase is found in several organs, including the lung, liver, intestine, and heart. There are significant tissue and species differences with substantial amounts of xanthine oxidase in the myocardium of dogs and rats, but very low levels in rabbits and humans.[138] The relative contribution of these potential sources to the production of oxygen-derived free radicals during acute myocardial ischemia is not known.

Several antioxidant enzyme pathways provide the host protection against damage from oxygen-derived free radicals. Endogenous biological scavenger enzymes include superoxide dismutase (SOD), which catalyzes the dismutation of superoxide anion to hydrogen peroxide, and the intracellular enzymes catalase and glutathione peroxidase, which catalyze the conversion of hydrogen peroxide to water. Vitamins C (ascorbate) and E (α-tocopherol) are additional endogenous free radical scavengers. There are no known endogenous scavengers of hydroxyl radicals.

Free radicals are produced early during acute myocardial ischemia.[139] Oxygen-derived free radicals, or the products of the chain reaction of free radical production, cause extensive damage by peroxidation of membrane phospholipids, formation of radicals with lipids, denaturation of proteins, and inactivation of important enzymes. Cell integrity is lost with damage to the cell membrane. Oxygen-derived free radicals, particularly the hydroxyl radical, produce extensive structural alterations in the vascular endothelium and mitochondria.[140] Myocardial tension development is reduced.[141] Damage to the vascular endothelium is manifest by increased vascular permeability and increased coronary artery perfusion pressure.[142] In addition to direct damage, the superoxide anion can inactivate EDRF from the vascular endothelium.[143]

In experimental studies, treatment with free radical scavengers protects against some of the structural and functional alterations produced by oxygen-derived free radicals.[140-142] The oxygen tension is low during acute myocardial ischemia but is adequate to support production of oxygen-derived free radicals. Restoration of oxygen with reperfusion may exacerbate tissue damage (oxygen paradox) by accelerating the production of oxygen-derived free radicals. Since reperfusion therapy has become increasingly common, several studies have examined whether free radical scavengers (e.g., SOD) reduce reperfusion injury and limit infarct size with conflicting results.[144]

The production of oxygen-derived free radicals is but one mechanism by which neutrophils contribute to damage during acute myocardial ischemia and infarction, and activated neutrophils are but one source of oxygen-derived free radicals. Nevertheless, experimental studies with acute myocardial ischemia and reperfusion indicate that neutrophils have an important pathophysiologic role. Removal of granulocytes prior to reperfusion prevents the no-reflow phenomenon, decreases edema formation, reduces post-reperfusion arrhythmias, and reduces myocardial stunning.[145,146] Neutrophil depletion with neutrophil antiserum reduces infarct size, an effect that is enhanced with the addition of a free radical scavenger.[147,148] Depletion of neutrophils with hydroxyurea has similar benefits.[128] Drugs that inhibit neutrophil activity (e.g., block the lipoxygenase pathways, decrease chemotaxis, decrease adherence, and decrease production of superoxide anion) decrease leukocyte infiltration and decrease infarct size in experimental models of myocardial ischemia and reperfusion.[128,149,150]

In summary, neutrophils accumulate during acute myocardial ischemia and mediate myocardial damage by several mechanisms, including a mechanical obstruction to capillary flow, release of leukotrienes and proteases, and production of oxygen-derived free radicals. Thus, neutrophils are important in influencing the extent of ischemic damage as well as mediating the no-reflow phenomenon, reperfusion injury, and myocardial stunning.

CORONARY ARTERY SPASM

Latham (1876) and Osler (1910) suggested that coronary artery spasm was important in angina pectoris. In 1959, Prinzmetal and co-workers described a variant form of angina that occurred at rest rather than with exertion.[151] They suggested that alterations in coronary artery tone in the region of atherosclerotic narrowing was responsible for this variant form. Coronary arteriography studies document that coronary artery spasm occurs at the site of an atherosclerotic plaque[152] or may occur in a "normal" coronary artery without atherosclerotic narrowing.[153]

Acute myocardial infarction can occur as a consequence of coronary artery spasm. In several cases, reversible coronary artery spasm can be demonstrated in a "normal" coronary artery (without significant stenosis) and subsequent myocardial infarction can occur with obstruction of the coronary artery at the same site.[154,155] Maseri and co-workers reported on a large series of patients with variant angina and found acute myocardial infarction to be a frequent sequel.[155] Coronary artery spasm can be demonstrated in many patients with unstable or crescendo angina. These same vessels can subsequently occlude and produce acute myocardial infarction 1 to 5 days later.[154] The symptoms of myocardial infarction in these patients are indistinguishable from the symptoms during typical angina episodes. However, the coronary artery spasm in these patients tends to be resistant to intracoronary nitroglycerin, even if it is given in massive doses.

Although some patients with coronary artery spasm can develop acute myocardial infarction, the role of spasm in the broader spectrum of myocardial infarction is less clear. In one study, coronary artery spasm could be induced during cardiac catheterization in 20% of patients with a recent myocardial infarction (less than 6 months previously), but in only 6% of patients with infarcts that had occurred more than 6 months previously.[156] These findings suggest that coronary artery spasm could be a cause of acute myocardial infarction. One group studied 15 patients by coronary arteriography within 12 hours of the onset of symptoms of an acute myocardial infarction.[157] In 6 patients (40%), intracoronary nitroglycerin increased blood flow in the acutely occluded coronary artery. Reperfusion with intracoronary nitroglycerin was particularly successful in patients studied within 6 hours of the onset of symptoms.[157] However, in several subsequent large series, intracoronary nitroglycerin improved coronary blood flow in fewer than 5% of patients with acute myocardial infarction, even among patients studied within 3 hours of the onset of symptoms.[158]

Although the incidence of coronary artery spasm has been low in several catheterization studies, these results are difficult to interpret. Patients with coronary artery spasm who respond to nitroglycerin (given at the onset of chest pain, in the emergency department, or in the coronary care unit) are less likely to be taken to the cardiac catheterization laboratory. Even if coronary artery spasm is an initiating factor, subsequent stasis and thrombus formation may sustain the myocardial ischemia. By the time the patient undergoes coronary arteriography, treatment of coronary artery spasm is no longer effective because the primary problem is now coronary artery thrombosis. The transient nature makes it difficult to establish the precise role of coronary artery spasm in the pathophysiology of acute myocardial ischemia and infarction.

Coronary artery spasm may occur concomitantly with or lead to coronary artery thrombosis and acute myocardial infarction. In one report, a patient developed coronary artery spasm and died of an acute myocardial infarction.[154] Autopsy revealed early thrombus formation at the site of atherosclerotic narrowing, which was the same site where coronary artery spasm had occurred.[154] In another case, coronary artery spasm developed during coronary arteriography and thrombus formation was observed.[159] The obstruction was resistant to nitroglycerin and verapamil, but mechanical perforation followed by intracoronary streptokinase returned the coronary artery to a normal appearance.

Coronary artery spasm may be an important precursor of acute myocardial infarction in patients with variant angina. Several series have examined the long-term prognosis of patients with variant angina and found a 25% incidence of acute myocardial infarction during follow-up periods of 2 to 8 years.[160-162] The incidence of myocardial infarction was significantly lower (5%–13%) in two large Japanese series, which may be related to the more frequent use of calcium channel blocker therapy in their patients.[163,164] In all of these series, 50% to 90%

of the infarctions occurred during the initial hospitalization or within the first 3 months of follow-up. The extent of the coronary artery disease (degree of stenosis and number of vessels involved) was a major factor influencing the incidence of acute myocardial infarction. Medical treatment with calcium channel blocking agents significantly improved the rate of survival without myocardial infarction. These studies demonstrate the significant risk of cardiac death or acute myocardial infarction in patients with variant angina, particularly within the first 3 months of hospitalization or cardiac catheterization.

The mechanism(s) for coronary artery spasm is not known but may be multifactorial. It has been suggested that a local imbalance between TXA_2 and PGI_2 production may be a cause for coronary artery spasm. Coronary artery spasm frequently occurs at sites with atherosclerotic lesions, and vessels with atherosclerosis may have some impairment in PGI_2 production.[89] Patients with variant angina have increased venous and coronary sinus blood levels of TXB_2 during episodes of ischemia.[105,165] However, inhibition of platelet production of TXA_2 with aspirin or indomethacin does not reduce the frequency of angina in patients with vasospasm.[165,166] In animal models of coronary artery spasm, intracoronary infusion of a TXA_2 analogue does not provoke coronary artery spasm and intravenous PGI_2 infusion does not prevent histamine-induced coronary artery spasm.[167] In patients with variant angina, PGI_2 infusions fail to provide any consistent reduction in ischemic episodes.[168] Finally, coronary sinus levels of TXB_2 levels do not increase until well after the onset of ischemia, suggesting that TXA_2 production is the consequence, not the cause, of coronary vasospasm.[165] Thus a local imbalance between TXA_2 and PGI_2 is probably not the major cause for coronary artery spasm.

Coronary artery spasm may be related to vasoconstriction induced by humoral factors, such as histamine or serotonin (5-HT). Coronary arteries from patients dying of ischemic heart disease have higher histamine concentrations and greater sensitivity (tension development) to histamine and 5-HT than coronary arteries without disease.[169] In one report, a patient died of coronary artery spasm and autopsy revealed increased mast cells in the adventitia of the coronary artery with previously documented spasm.[170] This case of coronary artery spasm may have been caused by mast cell release of vasoconstrictors such as histamine, prostaglandin D_2, and leukotrienes C_4 and D_4.[170] Histamine provokes coronary artery spasm in approximately half of the patients with variant angina.[171] However, this is less than ergonovine, which provokes coronary artery spasm in over 90% of patients with variant angina.[171,172] Several observations suggest a potential role for 5-HT in coronary artery spasm. Vasoconstriction can develop in normal coronary arteries with 5-HT, and atherosclerotic vessels have increased sensitivity to 5-HT.[169] In addition, atherosclerotic vessels have increased sensitivity to ergonovine, which is mediated by a serotonergic mechanism.[173] However, the specific serotonin receptor antagonist, ketanserin, does not reduce the frequency or severity of spontaneous episodes of coronary artery spasm[174] nor the ability to induce ischemia with ergonovine[175] in patients with variant angina.

Autonomic abnormalities with increased α-adrenergic stimulation have been postulated to cause coronary artery spasm.[176] The cold pressor test produces a reflex sympathetic response and can precipitate coronary artery spasm in patients with variant angina.[177] The normal response to the cold pressor test is coronary vasodilation related to β-adrenergic stimulation and flow-mediated vasodilation.[178] In patients with stable angina and atherosclerotic lesions, the cold pressor test produces a paradoxical vasoconstriction.[178] However, several lines of evidence indicate that abnormal α-adrenergic stimulation is not the major mechanism of coronary artery spasm. Abnormalities in autonomic function cannot be demonstrated in patients with variant angina, even during episodes of coronary artery spasm.[179] Holter monitoring reveals that episodes of coronary spasm are not preceded by changes in heart rate or QT interval.[180] α_1-Adrenergic blockade with prazosin or combined α_1- and α_2-adrenergic blockade with phentolamine does not reduce the frequency of coronary artery spasm.[180,181] Finally, the cold pressor test provokes coronary artery spasm in only 10% of patients with variant angina.[171,172] The low sensitivity of the cold pressor test is in contrast to exercise, hyperventilation, and histamine, which provoke coronary spasm in approximately half of patients with variant angina, and ergonovine, which provokes coronary spasm in over 90% of patients with variant angina.[171,172] Thus, it is not likely that abnormal α-adrenergic stimulation is the primary mechanism for most cases of coronary artery spasm.

Attention has focused on the role of endothelial dysfunction and coronary artery spasm.[93] The vascular endothelium produces EDRF, which acts synergistically with PGI_2 to inhibit platelet aggregation and inhibit the vasoconstriction induced by platelet aggregates.[84,85] Endothelium-dependent relaxation is impaired,[93,94] and the vasoconstrictor response to vasoactive substances is augmented[173] in experimental atherosclerosis. These changes are related to reduced EDRF production by atherosclerotic vessels.[93] If the vascular endothelium is mechanically denuded (with a balloon) in animals with diet-induced atherosclerosis, then coronary artery spasm with regional ischemia can be induced at the same site with histamine or serotonin.[182] The coronary artery spasm in this model subsides with nitroglycerin or is prevented by calcium channel blockers or blockade of the histamine H_1 receptor.[182] Impaired endothelium-mediated relaxation may persist for weeks despite endothelial regeneration, and endothelium-derived constricting factors may be released.[183] Repeated episodes of coronary artery spasm may produce intramural hemorrhage and endothelial damage.[184] These findings suggest that recurrent coronary artery spasm may lead to progression of atherosclerotic lesions and/or trigger acute myocardial ischemia or infarction.[184]

Clinical studies also indicate a role for the vascular endothelium in coronary artery spasm. Coronary artery spasm can occur as a complication of balloon angioplasty,[185] which may be related to disruption of the vascular endothelium. In human coronary arteries (as with animals), platelet aggregates release the vasoconstrictors 5-HT and TXA_2 and stimulate EDRF release, resulting in a net vasodilation effect.[186] Acetylcholine induces coronary vasodilation by the release of EDRF.[83] Intracoronary acetylcholine infusions produce vasodilation in patients with normal coronary arteries but produce paradoxical vasoconstriction in coronary arteries with advanced (and occasionally mild) atherosclerotic lesions.[187] These results are consistent with animal studies demonstrating impaired endothelial-dependent relaxation in atherosclerotic vessels.[93,94] In patients with variant angina, intracoronary acetylcholine can induce coronary artery spasm and myocardial ischemia.[188] This is blocked by pretreatment with atropine, suggesting an interaction between local vascular hypersensitivity and the parasympathetic nervous system.[187] In patients with variant angina, impairments in endothelial function (particularly in atherosclerotic vessels) may be responsible for the exaggerated hypersensitivity of coronary arteries to neural, humoral, and mechanical factors that lead to coronary artery spasm.

METABOLIC CONSEQUENCES OF ACUTE MYOCARDIAL ISCHEMIA

The heart accounts for only 0.3% of the body weight but is responsible for 7% of the body's resting oxygen consumption. These high metabolic requirements are met primarily by oxidative phosphorylation of fatty acids to produce ATP.[189] Glucose is an important metabolic substrate when the myocardial oxygen supply is limited or when there are acute increases in cardiac workload.[189] The heart also can use other carbohydrates (glycogen, lactic acid, pyruvate) and amino acids as metabolic substrates. Under basal conditions, myocardial oxygen extraction is nearly maximal (approximately 75%) so that an increase in myocardial oxygen demand must be met by an increase in coronary blood flow rather than by increased oxygen extraction. The presence of significant coronary artery narrowing by an atherosclerotic plaque reduces the coronary reserve and limits the ability to adequately meet an increase in myocardial oxygen demand.

Within 30 to 60 seconds of abrupt coronary artery occlusion, myocardial oxygen tension in the ischemic zone falls to near-zero levels. There is a rapid shift from aerobic to anaerobic cardiac metabolism. The cardiac stores of high-energy phosphates are limited and are rapidly depleted. The only other significant source of high-energy phosphates is derived from anaerobic glycolysis. Lactic acid is produced during anaerobic metabolism. Lactic acid accumulates since it neither can be metabolized further nor removed adequately because of the decrease in coronary blood flow. The accumulation of lactic acid, hydrogen ions, and NADH inhibits glycolysis, thus limiting the only significant source of ATP generation under anaerobic conditions.[190,191] The anaerobic generation of high-energy phosphates is not sufficient to meet the energy demands of the ischemic myocardium, even though the myocardial oxygen demands are reduced because of the decrease in myocardial contractility.

Myocardial dysfunction appears in the ischemic zone within a few seconds following coronary artery occlusion.[192] The biochemical basis for this early ischemic dysfunction is unclear, but it may be multifactorial.[193] One possibility is a depletion of high-energy phosphates. Within 30 seconds of coronary artery occlusion, tissue content of creatine phosphate in the ischemic zone declines by over 50%, ATP levels fall 20%, and tissue lactic acid values increase threefold.[194] After 30 minutes of ischemia, both creatine phosphate and ATP are reduced by 80% and tissue lactic acid has increased tenfold.[194] During the early minutes of ischemia, creatine phosphate is depleted at a more rapid rate than ATP. This suggests that ATP is replenished from creatine phosphate stores. There is greater depletion of creatine phosphate and greater accumulation of lactic acid in the subendocardium than subepicardium, reflecting greater susceptibility of the subendocardium to ischemia.[195] This is also reflected by a transmural gradient in pH with greater acidosis in the subendocardium than subepicardium.[196] Myocardial contractile function declines as ATP stores are depleted[197] and tissue acidosis develops.[198] However, the early ischemic dysfunction develops before high-energy phosphate stores are depleted.[199] Indeed, the early fall in ventricular pressure occurs before any change in ATP level.[200] The early ischemic dysfunction may be related to decreased ATP in specific cellular compartments,[201] but this hypothesis is difficult to test. Although depletion of ATP does not explain early ischemic dysfunction, it is likely that the decrease in intracellular ATP contributes to the contracture and rigor that develop with prolonged hypoxia or ischemia.[193]

During graded coronary artery occlusion, inorganic phosphate increases and the ratio of phosphocreatine to inorganic phosphate decreases in direct proportion to the decrease in subendocardial blood flow.[202] During acute hypoxia there is a rapid fall in ventricular pressure (particularly if glycolysis is also inhibited) associated with a simultaneous early increase in inorganic phosphate.[200] Inorganic phosphate produces a marked decrease in myofilament sensitivity to calcium[203] and decreases peak force generation with hypoxia.[204] Thus, the early increase in inorganic phosphate (from hydrolysis of creatine phosphate and ATP) during acute myocardial ischemia may contribute to early ischemic dysfunction.

It has been postulated that local tissue acidosis may contribute to early ischemic dysfunction. Although intracellular acidosis develops with acute myocardial ischemia, the magnitude of acidosis and rate of development appear inadequate to explain the marked early decrease in tension.[193] In studies with combined hypoxia and inhibition of glycolysis, ventricular pressure may decrease markedly without any change in intracellular pH.[200] Intracellular acidosis may contribute to the subsequent decline in tension by decreasing myofilament sensitivity to calcium.[205]

Another mechanism for early ischemic dysfunction is a decrease in calcium availability and/or decreased myofilament sensitivity to calcium.[193] In isolated muscle models of ischemia (anoxia combined with inhibition of glycolysis), the rapid fall in tension is accompanied by a rapid decrease in action potential duration, which may decrease calcium release by the sarcoplasmic reticulum.[193] Calcium transients (measured with aequorin) reflect the magnitude and rate of transient changes in intracellular free calcium with each cardiac cycle. With severe hypoxia, tension falls and the magnitude of the calcium transient does not change, suggesting a decrease in myofilament sensitivity to calcium.[206] When hypoxia is combined with inhibition of glycolysis, there is a more marked fall in tension with a parallel fall in the calcium transient.[206] Thus calcium delivery is limited and myofilament sensitivity to calcium may be reduced as well. Both intracellular acidosis and accumulation of inorganic phosphate may contribute to a decrease in myofilament sensitivity to calcium. Metabolic blockade leads to an increase in diastolic calcium and increase in resting tensions or contracture.[207,208] Some investigators have attributed contracture primarily to the fall in ATP since increases in diastolic calcium occur only after resting tensions increase.[193,207] However, others have found an increase in diastolic calcium preceding contracture.[208]

If ischemia is reversed during the early stages, all alterations in biochemical processes and myocardial function are fully reversible. However, if ischemia is prolonged, cardiac myocytes undergo irreversible damage even if coronary perfusion is restored. This irreversible stage of injury is characterized by ultrastructural alterations, including marked glycogen depletion, diffuse mitochondrial swelling, accumulation of amorphous densities in the matrix of the mitochondria, peripheral aggregation of nuclear chromatin, and small breaks in the plasmalemma of the sarcolemma.[209]

There are several potential causes of irreversible myocyte injury. Irreversible cell death has been correlated with severe (greater than 90%) depletion of ATP content and an inability to resynthesize creatine phosphate when reoxygenated.[210] Cells with depleted energy stores are unable to maintain ionic gradients across the cell membrane or to control cell volume.[211] Damage to the mitochondrial membranes further impairs energy production, which in turn increases the ionic defects across the membrane and creates a vicious cycle of damage.[212] Some investigators suggest that the inability of irreversibly damaged cells to regenerate ATP is not due to irreversible mitochondrial damage but rather due to the net loss of total adenine nucleotides.[197,213]

Calcium ions may play an important role in irreversible cell damage. As extracellular calcium concentrations increase, it requires a longer time to recover ventricular function following reperfusion. The extent of functional recovery is also less complete when calcium levels are elevated.[214] This effect is independent of the ATP level. It has been postulated that intracellular calcium accumulation and calcium overloading in the mitochondria decrease ATP production, contributing to irreversible cell damage.[215] Acute myocardial ischemia may activate phospholipases, which accelerate phospholipid degradation in the sarcoplasmic reticulum and plasma membranes, resulting in a breakdown of the calcium permeability barrier.[215]

Calcium overload during reperfusion may be related to increased Na^+-Ca^{2+} exchange.[193,216] The intracellular acidosis of ischemia increases H^+-Na^+ exchange, leading to intracellular Na^+ accumulation. Acidosis inhibits Na^+-Ca^{2+} exchange. Reperfusion reverses the acidosis and ATP depletion, which restores Na^+-Ca^{2+} exchange, leading to intracellular Ca^{2+} accumulation. Calcium entry via calcium channels is probably not an important mechanism since calcium channel inhibition during reperfusion does not prevent calcium overload.[217] Although calcium channel blockade provides some protective effects, this is likely due to decreases in contractility and myocardial oxygen demands.[218] Thus, the experimental evidence does not support the theoretical use of calcium channel blockers to prevent calcium overload. Some experimental studies suggest that calcium channel blocking agents reduce infarct size, possibly related to the secondary effects on hemodynamics and collateral blood flow.[219] The results from several large clinical trials have been generally disappointing, with calcium channel blocking agents providing no significant reduction in infarct size, morbidity, or mortality from acute myocardial infarction.[219]

Several products that are produced during myocardial ischemia can contribute to myocardial dysfunction and permanent damage. If lactic acid accumulates during myocardial ischemia, recovery of ventricular function following reperfusion requires a longer time and is less complete than when lactic acid does not accumulate.[214] Circulating catecholamine levels increase in patients with acute myocardial infarction.[220] Increased catecholamines produce arrhythmias, increase myocardial oxygen consumption, and cause oxygen wasting due to mitochondrial uncoupling. Each of these alterations can increase the severity and extent of myocardial ischemia and damage.

Catecholamines also activate triglyceride lipase in adipose tissue and suppress insulin secretion. As a result, circulating free fatty acid levels increase during acute myocardial ischemia.[221] Catecholamines also promote intramyocardial lipolysis.[222] Nonesterified fatty acids accumulate in the ischemic region, particularly in the subendocardium.[223] The elevated fatty acids have several detrimental effects. Fatty acids increase myocardial oxygen consumption by an oxygen wasting effect.[224] Fatty acids exert a negative inotropic effect on the heart.[225] Fatty acids also may influence metabolic pathways, causing depletion of intracellular glycogen, alterations in membrane permeability (leading to cell damage), and inhibition of calcium transport in the sarcoplasmic reticulum. These alterations contribute to the functional impairments and arrhythmias during acute myocardial ischemia.[221,226]

Finally, oxygen-derived free radicals produced during acute myocardial ischemia may contribute to myocardial damage, particularly with reperfusion (reperfusion injury and the oxygen paradox).[139,140] Oxygen-derived free radicals and their products cause peroxidation of membrane phospholipids, denature proteins, inactivate enzymes, and damage mitochondria. Structural damage to the vascular endothelium increases vascular permeability, and EDRF is inactivated by oxygen-derived free radicals.[142,143] As discussed previously in the section on the role of neutrophils, oxygen-derived free radicals may play an important role in the pathophysiology of acute myocardial ischemia and infarction and of reperfusion injury.

FUNCTIONAL CONSEQUENCES OF ACUTE MYOCARDIAL ISCHEMIA
SYSTOLIC ALTERATIONS

Acute myocardial ischemia is associated with characteristic alterations in regional ventricular function. Within seconds of total coronary artery occlusion, systolic shortening in the ischemic region decreases.[192] After 30 seconds of ischemia, the ischemic region performs little or no effective work.[227] Gradually, systolic shortening is replaced by late systolic then holosystolic lengthening or bulging. After 3 to 5 minutes of ischemia, the ischemic region demonstrates marked bulging during isovolumic systole and akinesis during the ejection phase.[192,228] Shortening in the ischemic region occurs paradoxically during isovolumic relaxation and early diastole.

The paradoxic systolic bulging indicates that work is being performed on, rather than by, the ischemic region.[227] Regional work in the ischemic region is estimated to be near or below zero.[229] Lengthening of the ischemic region during systole and shortening during isovolumic relaxation suggest that the ischemic region is behaving in a primarily passive manner, with lengthening or shortening due to load changes in the passive tension-length relation.[230] Indeed, an increased preload reduces the extent of systolic bulging as the ischemic region operates on a steeper (stiffer) portion of its passive tension-length curve.[230,231] The acutely ischemic myocardium is not entirely passive but may retain some initial residual contractile function.[232] During acute myocardial ischemia, acute inotropic stimulation with isoproterenol[233] and postextrasystolic potentiation[234] decreases the paradoxic systolic bulging in the ischemic region. Paradoxic systolic bulging of the ischemic region does not necessarily indicate purely passive behavior. Paradoxic systolic lengthening is observed when any weakly contracting muscle is placed in series with a more strongly contracting muscle.[235] Thus, a disparity in the rate or extent of tension development between any two regions (i.e., asynchronous force generation) is sufficient to produce paradoxic systolic bulging. The late (postsystolic) shortening in the ischemic region may represent active contraction with a delay in relaxation.[236] In experimental ischemia, the extent of postsystolic shortening during ischemia is predictive of the extent of recovery in function 2 to 3 weeks following reperfusion.[236]

The magnitude of the functional impairment in the ischemic region is directly related to the severity of the coronary blood flow reduction.[237-239] With mild degrees of ischemia, as induced with partial coronary artery stenosis, coronary blood flow is reduced in the subendocardium but remains normal in the subepicardium.[237,239] Such mild degrees of ischemia are associated with a mild decrease in systolic function (as measured by segment shortening or wall thickening) or hypokinesis. As coronary blood flow is more severely reduced, the degree of hypokinesis worsens until the ischemic region becomes akinetic. With severe transmural reductions in coronary blood flow, as induced by total coronary artery occlusion, paradoxic systolic bulging or dyskinetic wall motion occurs in the ischemic region.[237,238] Thus, there is a direct relationship between regional myocardial blood flow and function in the ischemic region. The flow-function relation is modified with reperfusion. For a comparable degree of myocardial infarction, regional blood flow in the ischemic region is significantly higher if reperfusion occurs than with permanent occlusions.[240]

Functional abnormalities are detected in nonischemic areas directly adjacent to the ischemic region. For example, with mild myocardial ischemia there is a decrease in subendocardial blood flow and function.[237,238] Functional impairments also occur in the overlying nonischemic subepicardium, even though subepicardial blood flow is normal.[239] The functional alterations in normally perfused nonischemic areas may be due to mechanical "tethering" to the abnormally contracting ischemic region. A similar phenomenon occurs in nonischemic areas that are laterally adjacent to the ischemic region. The lateral nonischemic border is subjected to increased wall stress because of its location adjacent to an abnormally functioning ischemic region.[241] Functional alterations in adjacent lateral border areas occur despite normal coronary perfusion.[242]

The lateral extent of the functional border zone can be defined by comparing regional blood flow and wall thickening measurements.[243] The perfusion boundary that separates ischemic from nonischemic myocardium is sharply demarcated. Systolic wall thickening is normal or increased in nonischemic myocardium more than 10 mm from the perfusion boundary. Although nonischemic myocardium within 10 mm of the perfusion boundary has normal myocardial blood flow, there are functional impairments that are more severe with increasing proximity to the perfusion boundary. Although the extent of functional impairment overestimates ischemic region size, the error may be small since the lateral extent of the functional border zone is relatively narrow and severe functional impairments are limited to nonischemic regions directly adjacent to the perfusion boundary.[243]

Nonischemic areas that are remote from the ischemic region may display functional alterations. Augmented shortening or "hyperfunction" of nonischemic areas occurs in experimental studies[228,243,244] and in patients[245,246] with acute myocardial ischemia and infarction. Increased nonischemic area shortening is due to a combination of increased use of the Frank-Starling mechanism (secondary to an ischemia-induced increase in left ventricular end-diastolic pressure) and a regional intraventricular unloading effect.[228,231] Although increased sympathetic stimulation may contribute, acute myocardial ischemia in the presence of β-blockade[228] and in isolated hearts (which lack reflex neurohumoral responses) still produces hyperkinesis in nonischemic regions.[247]

Hyperfunction of nonischemic areas has been considered as a compensatory mechanism. However, a significant portion of the increase in nonischemic area shortening is expended in paradoxically stretching the ischemic region during isovolumic systole, thus reducing the amount of effective shortening by nonischemic areas available for ventricular ejection.[228] Although hyperkinesis develops, regional work in nonischemic areas decreases because of the regional intraventricular unloading effect.[247] If left ventricular end-diastolic pressure does not change with acute myocardial ischemia, there is no increased use of the Frank-Starling mechanism and ejection phase shortening in nonischemic areas actually decreases.[231] Thus, the ischemic region imposes a mechanical disadvantage on nonischemic areas that is directly related to the amount of paradoxic systolic bulging in the ischemic region. The magnitude of this mechanical disadvantage is directly proportional to the size and inversely proportional to the stiffness of the ischemic region.[231,248]

An increase in coronary blood flow may accompany the hyperkinesis of nonischemic areas.[249] However, if a stenosis is present in the coronary artery supplying the nonischemic area, coronary blood flow to the nonischemic area may decrease with acute myocardial ischemia and nonischemic shortening fails to increase, that is, acute myocardial ischemia produces a relative hypoperfusion to nonischemic areas supplied by a coronary artery with stenosis.[249] Acute coronary artery occlusion also may interrupt collateral blood supply to distal sites and induce myocardial dysfunction at sites remote from the area of acute myocardial ischemia.

Patients with acute myocardial infarction and hyperkinesis in nonischemic areas are more likely to have single rather than multivessel coronary artery disease.[245,246] In contrast, patients with acute myocardial infarction and asynergy at remote sites are more likely to have three-vessel disease and a higher mortality rate.[245] The presence of a 50% or greater stenosis in the noninfarct vessel is associated with an absence of hyperkinesis in the nonischemic area.[246] Patients with hyperkinesis in nonischemic areas have a higher ejection fraction and a lower in-hospital mortality than patients with poorer function in nonischemic areas.[246] Thus, function of nonischemic areas during acute myocardial ischemia and infarction has important prognostic implications.

ALTERATIONS DURING ISOVOLUMIC RELAXATION

Characteristic alterations in regional ventricular function are seen in both ischemic and nonischemic regions during isovolumic relaxation. The ischemic region shortens paradoxically during isovolumic relaxation and early diastole. This paradoxic shortening has been attributed to elastic recoil of the passively stretched ischemic region or to persistent late systolic active shortening.[192,230,236,250] Lengthening of nonischemic areas during isovolumic relaxation (segmental early relaxation) occurs in acute myocardial ischemia[251] and in patients with chronic ischemic heart disease.[252] Early lengthening of nonischemic areas may reflect a mechanical interaction between ischemic and nonischemic areas during isovolumic relaxation.[253] The importance of segmental early relaxation is uncertain, since it occurs with increased asynchrony in the absence of ischemia[254] and in patients without coronary artery disease and without regional alterations in ventricular function.[252,253]

Asynchronous wall motion during isovolumic relaxation slows the rate of left ventricular pressure fall, as reflected by a decrease in peak $-dP/dt$ (to less negative values) and an increase in τ, the time constant of left ventricular pressure fall.[255,256] Peak $-dP/dt$ falls within 5 seconds of acute coronary artery occlusion.[256] With graded coronary artery occlusion, the fall in peak $-dP/dt$ may precede any other hemodynamic change.[255] Peak $-dP/dt$ decreases and τ increases with acute myocardial ischemia (produced by pacing, exercise, or occurring spontaneously) in both clinical[257-259] and animal studies.[255,260-262] Although peak $-dP/dt$ has been used as an index of ventricular relaxation, its use is limited because it is extremely sensitive to acute changes in afterload and inotropic state.[263] A decrease in peak $-dP/dt$ during acute myocardial ischemia may reflect ischemia-induced alterations in loading rather than a primary effect of ischemia on ventricular relaxation.

Tau (τ), the time constant of left ventricular pressure fall, is a more useful index of the rate of left ventricular pressure fall, although τ is also influenced by loading conditions.[263] The mechanisms for a slower rate of left ventricular pressure fall during acute myocardial ischemia are multifactorial.[254,263] Ischemia directly impairs myocardial relaxation processes and indirectly slows the rate of left ventricular pressure fall by altering loading conditions, decreasing contractility, and increasing asynchrony. Asynchrony of regional ventricular function slows the rate of left ventricular pressure fall even in the absence of ischemia.[254] Thus, acute myocardial ischemia alters ventricular relaxation processes by both direct and indirect mechanisms.

DIASTOLIC ALTERATIONS

Acute myocardial ischemia induces alterations in early diastolic filling related to asynchronous wall motion during early diastole,[264] incomplete ventricular relaxation, and/or alterations in left ventricular chamber or myocardial stiffness. Incomplete relaxation results in higher ventricular diastolic pressures, which retards diastolic filling and decreases diastolic filling time.[265] Reduced systolic emptying and higher end-systolic volumes impair diastolic filling by increasing inflow impedance.[250] Acute myocardial ischemia increases myocardial stiffness, which slows diastolic filling.

Patients with acute and chronic ischemia have abnormal diastolic filling. Peak filling rates are reduced in patients with exercise-induced ischemia.[266,267] Peak filling rates may fail to increase (the normal response) or may decrease in patients with pacing-induced ischemia.[268] These diastolic abnormalities may precede systolic abnormalities.[268] In some studies, peak filling rates do not change (including rates normalized for stroke volume and end-diastolic volume) in patients with post pacing-induced ischemia, despite a slower rate of left ventricular pressure fall and increased asynchrony during early diastole.[269] Global peak filling rates were maintained in these patients because peak lengthening rates in nonischemic areas tended to increase and offset the decrease in peak lengthening rates in the ischemic region.[269] The apparent discrepancies in different studies reflect the difficulties in clinically evaluating diastolic function.[270] For example, a decrease in peak filling rate can be related to an ischemia-induced decrease in the rate of left ventricular pressure fall, asynchronous wall motion during early diastole, and/or an increase in ventricular stiffness. However, an abnormal decrease in filling rate may be masked by the increase in left atrial pressure with ischemia.[270]

Abnormalities in diastolic filling are potentially reversible. In patients with acute myocardial infarction, peak filling rates increase following successful reperfusion.[271] Revascularization eliminates some of the abnormalities that develop with exercise-induced ischemia, including exercise-induced asynergy, decrease in ejection fraction and increase in end-diastolic pressure.[272] Following revascularization, patients have more rapid rates of left ventricular pressure fall and a greater increase in peak filling rate in response to exercise.[272]

Left ventricular filling pressures are frequently elevated in patients with acute myocardial infarction[273,274] and in animals with experimental myocardial ischemia.[228,233,275-278] Mild elevations in ventricular filling pressure improve ventricular function by increasing use of the Frank-Starling mechanism in nonischemic areas.[228] However, marked elevations in left ventricular filling pressure are associated with pulmonary venous congestion, low stroke volume, and, in severe cases, the clinical syndrome of cardiogenic shock.[273] The mortality rate increases sharply when patients with acute myocardial infarction have such severe hemodynamic complications.

There is an "optimal" left ventricular filling pressure, which maximizes stroke volume while minimizing adverse hemodynamic complications in patients with acute myocardial infarction.[273,279] Generally, this corresponds to mean pulmonary capillary wedge pressures in the 15- to 20-mm Hg range. The major mechanism for improving regional and global ventricular function at these "optimal" filling pressures is due to the maximal use of the Frank-Starling mechanism in nonischemic areas.[231] In addition, there is a reduction in the mechanical disadvantage imposed by the ischemic region at high as compared with low ventricular filling pressures.[231] Most likely, this is due to movement of the ischemic region to a steeper (stiffer) position on its passive length–tension curve, thus increasing its resistance to passive systolic bulging. Therefore at "optimal" left ventricular filling pressures, less shortening by nonischemic areas is "wasted" in stretching the ischemic region during isovolumic systole, that is, the ischemic zone imposes less of a mechanical disadvantage on the nonischemic areas.[231]

In patients with coronary artery disease or experimental coronary artery stenosis, pacing tachycardia or exercise induces acute myocardial ischemia with an upward shift in the diastolic pressure–volume (P-V) or pressure–length (P-L) relation.[260–262,272,280–282] Similar shifts occur in animals with global hypoxia[283] or when global ischemia is combined with an increase in myocardial oxygen demands.[284] The increase in left ventricular diastolic pressure at a matched diastolic volume or length indicates an ischemia-induced decrease in left ventricular distensibility. In contrast, there is no shift in left ventricular diastolic P-V or P-L relations in some experimental studies with global ischemia, suggesting that left ventricular distensibility or compliance (or its inverse, stiffness) does not change.[285,286] In still other experimental studies, acute ischemia with coronary artery occlusion[275,281,282,287] or global ischemia[283] produces a rightward shift in diastolic P-V or P-L relations. In these studies, the increase in left ventricular volume or length at a matched diastolic pressure suggests that left ventricular compliance increases (or stiffness decreases). However, it has been noted that despite an ischemia-induced rightward shift, the end-diastolic P-V or P-L relation is steeper after ischemia, indicating an increase (rather than decrease) in myocardial stiffness.[275,281]

The issue of whether ischemia alters left ventricular distensibility has important implications for left ventricular filling dynamics, systolic function, and symptoms (*e.g.*, pulmonary venous congestion). It is important to consider whether the ischemic myocardium has an intrinsic change in stiffness (*e.g.*, an upward shift to a new diastolic P-V or P-L relation) or whether the ventricle is merely operating on a higher, steeper (stiffer) portion of a single passive P-V or P-L relation (*i.e.*, an upward and rightward shift to a new position on the same curve). Some of the apparent discrepancies in whether stiffness in the ischemic ventricle increases, decreases, or does not change can be resolved by considering strain rather than volume or length measurements. Strain measures the extent of deformation relative to a reference configuration with zero stress. In practice, the zero stress reference configuration for volume (V_0) or length (L_0) is approximated by measuring the passive left ventricular volume or length when transmural pressure is zero. With acute myocardial ischemia, a significant portion of the rightward shift in diastolic P-V and P-L relations is due to an increase in V_0 and L_0 (*e.g.*, L_0 increases approximately 16%).[287–289] An increase in volume or length over time under a constant load is termed *creep*. Ischemia induces creep, as reflected by an increase in V_0 or L_0, which can be reversed with reperfusion.[289] Although ischemia produces a rightward shift in diastolic P-V or P-L relations, normalization of the volumes or lengths to the appropriate V_0 or L_0, respectively, indicates that there is an increase in slope of the pressure–strain relation, that is, a true increase in stiffness. Such changes would be missed without proper normalization.[288]

Acute ischemia produces structural and functional changes consistent with ischemia-induced creep. There is a marked increase in both diastolic and systolic sarcomere lengths in the ischemic region.[290] The ischemia-induced increase in unstressed volume and segment lengths (V_0 and L_0, respectively) may be due to systolic overstretch of sarcomeres. Consistent with this hypothesis, there is a parallel between the impairment in systolic function and the magnitude of the rightward shift in diastolic P-V and P-L relations. Both abnormalities are more severe when acute myocardial ischemia is produced by a decrease in myocardial oxygen supply (coronary artery occlusion) rather than by an increase in myocardial oxygen demand.[282]

Global measurements of left ventricular function may not accurately reflect the effects of regional ischemia. In patients with coronary artery disease and pacing-induced angina, the left ventricular diastolic P-V relation may shift upward to a new P-V curve in some patients and may shift up and to the right to a higher position on the same P-V curve in other patients.[291] Analysis of regional P-L relations, however, demonstrates an upward shift to a new P-L curve in the ischemic region in all cases (indicating an increase in regional myocardial stiffness), whereas nonischemic areas only shift to a higher position along a single P-L relation. Global measurements represent a hybrid of the disparate regional responses (in ischemic and nonischemic areas) and thus may give seemingly conflicting results.[291]

The diastolic alterations produced by acute myocardial ischemia depend on the experimental model.[280] When acute myocardial ischemia is produced by a primary increase in myocardial oxygen demand (*e.g.*, pacing-induced ischemia in the presence of coronary artery stenosis) there is an upward shift in the diastolic P-V or P-L relation.[260–262,272,280–282,284] In contrast, acute myocardial ischemia produced by a primary decrease in myocardial oxygen supply (*e.g.*, coronary artery occlusion) shifts the diastolic P-V or P-L relation rightward.[275,281,282,287] Several mechanisms have been proposed to explain these differences. Acute myocardial ischemia produces concomitant alterations in right ventricular loading, which may influence left ventricular diastolic function by ventricular interaction effects.[281] However, ventricular interaction effects may not be a major mechanism since the ischemia-induced shifts in left ventricular diastolic P-V or P-L relations are not duplicated by right-sided heart volume overload alone[260] and persist even with large changes in right-sided heart loading conditions.[262] Furthermore, similar shifts in the left ventricular diastolic P-V relation occur with acute ischemia in the absence of an intact pericardium or when the right side of the heart is vented.[260,284] Ischemia may shift the diastolic P-V relation by increasing the asynchrony in left ventricular diastolic wall motion. However, similar shifts in diastolic P-V relations can be produced with global ischemia in the absence of discrete asynchrony.[283,284]

The influence of the model of ischemia on the shift in diastolic P-V and P-L relations may be related to the extent of impairment in systolic function. Systolic function is more severely impaired when acute myocardial ischemia is produced by a primary decrease in supply rather than a primary increase in myocardial oxygen demand.[282] This difference may be related to differences in creep. In acute myocardial ischemia produced by a primary increase in myocardial oxygen demand there is an inverse relation between the magnitude of decrease in segment stroke work and the upward shift in diastolic P-L relation.[292] The upward shift of the diastolic P-L relation with demand ischemia is greatest when systolic function is well preserved.[292] Thus, differences in the shift in diastolic P-V or P-L relations may reflect differences in the magnitude of systolic function abnormalities.

The model of acute myocardial ischemia influences the metabolic alteration and coronary "turgor" effects. Decreased supply ischemia (coronary artery occlusion) reduces the coronary blood volume and collapses the coronary vasculature. This decrease in coronary "turgor" contributes to the initial increase in diastolic compliance.[283] Depletion of subendocardial creatine phosphate (with accumulation of inorganic phosphate) and myocardial tissue acidosis are greater with acute myocardial ischemia produced by a decrease in supply rather than an increase in myocardial oxygen demand.[282] The upward shift in the diastolic P-V relation with demand ischemia is greater following caffeine, suggesting that calcium reuptake by the sarcoplasmic reticulum (which is inhibited by caffeine) may be impaired and contribute to incomplete relaxation and persistent diastolic tone.[261] However, such an interpretation should be made cautiously since caffeine also increases myofilament sensitivity to calcium and other mechanisms such as Na^+–Ca^{2+} exchange may produce rapid relaxation even in the presence of impaired sarcoplasmic reticulum function[293] (although ischemia also impairs Na^+–Ca^{2+} exchange).

In summary, both diastolic filling and passive diastolic properties are altered with acute myocardial ischemia. The direct effects of ischemia are difficult to determine because diastolic filling also is altered by the secondary effects of ischemia on systolic function, ventricular relaxation, loading conditions, and asynchrony. Acute myocardial ischemia increases diastolic filling pressure by several mechanisms. Mild elevations in filling pressure are beneficial by improving function in nonischemic areas and reducing the mechanical disadvantage of the ischemic region. Marked elevations in filling pressure are associated with symptoms of pulmonary venous congestion and a significant increase in morbidity and mortality. Acute ischemia increases left ventricular stiffness, a finding complicated by ischemia-induced creep, the model of ischemia (increased demand vs. decreased supply, regional vs. global ischemia), and coronary turgor effects. The structural and metabolic basis for these changes is being actively investigated.

FUNCTIONAL AND NEURAL CONSEQUENCES OF SIZE AND SITE

The size and site of the ischemic region are important determinants of the functional consequences and the reflex neural changes with acute myocardial ischemia and infarction. In experimental studies, there is a direct correlation between infarct size and the severity of reduction in peak cardiac output, pressure generating capacity, and ejection fraction.[294-296] The mechanical disadvantage imposed by the ischemic region on nonischemic areas is directly related to the size of the ischemic region.[248] Although total collateral blood flow increases with an increase in ischemic area at risk, the normalized collateral flow (flow per gram of ischemic myocardium) is lower with large risk areas because of a higher collateral resistance per mass of tissue.[297] As ischemic region size increases, there is a corresponding decrease in the amount of nonischemic myocardium available to compensate for the loss of systolic function. In addition, the mechanical disadvantage imposed on nonischemic regions increases with ischemic region size. Thus, the ability of the remaining nonischemic myocardium to provide effective compensation decreases with an increase in ischemic region size.[248]

In patients with acute myocardial infarction there is a progressive decrease in left ventricular ejection fraction as the size of the infarct or the extent and severity of abnormally contracting segments increase.[274,298] Left ventricular filling pressures increase in direct proportion to the size of the ischemic region. Both early and late mortality are directly related to myocardial infarct size.[299-301] Patients surviving large myocardial infarctions have a worse functional class and shorter duration of survival than survivors of small infarcts.[299,300] Early thrombolytic therapy in patients with acute myocardial infarction reduces infarct size and improves left ventricular function.[302,303]

The site of myocardial infarction also is important. Both early and late mortality rates are higher in patients with anterior as compared with inferior wall infarctions.[300,304,305] The major reason for greater functional impairment with anterior wall infarction is due to the larger infarct size with anterior as compared with inferior wall infarcts.[274,300,305] When patients with anterior and inferior wall infarctions of similar size are compared, the functional impairment[274,306] and survival curves[300] are similar. However, these studies are difficult to interpret since the accuracy of clinical estimates of infarct size differs for anterior and inferior wall myocardial infarctions. Patients with inferior wall infarctions frequently have concomitant occult involvement of the right ventricle. Thus, enzymatic estimates of the extent of left ventricular infarct, or infarct size, are less reliable with inferior than with anterior wall infarctions.[298,304]

Experimental studies demonstrate greater functional impairment with anterior than inferoposterior wall infarctions. Collateral blood flow is lower with anterior than inferoposterior infarcts.[307] For a similar extent of ischemia or infarct size, ejection fraction falls more with left anterior descending than left circumflex coronary artery occlusions.[308,309] The mechanical disadvantage imposed by the ischemic region on nonischemic areas is greater with anterior than posterior wall ischemia.[310] There are site-dependent differences in function of remote nonischemic areas. For a comparable ischemic region at risk or similar extent of hypoperfusion, there is greater hyperkinesis in remote nonischemic areas with posterior than anterior wall myocardial ischemia.[310,311] These findings may be related to differences in geometry (of the ischemic anterior as compared with ischemic posterior wall) and/or regional differences in loading.

Reflex cardiovascular responses depend on the size and site of acute myocardial ischemia. Acute myocardial ischemia simultaneously stimulates cardiac vagal and sympathetic afferents, with the predominant reflex response determined by the extent or size of the ischemic region.[312] There are transmural differences in neural pathways that influence the response to ischemia. The primary ventricular pathway for sympathetic nerves is in the subepicardial layer, whereas vagal nerves are in the subendocardial layer. Transmural myocardial infarction and ischemia interrupt both afferent and efferent pathways for sympathetic and vagal fibers producing local denervation of the ischemic region and distal apical nonischemic areas.[313-315] Subendocardial ischemia produces vagal denervation in the ischemic region and overlying nonischemic epicardium because of the subendocardial course of vagal nerves.[315,316] However, subendocardial ischemia does not produce sympathetic denervation unless there is a significant reduction in epicardial blood flow.[315] The denervation produced by acute myocardial ischemia occurs within minutes and becomes more severe over the first 3 hours.[315,317] The denervation is reversible with early reperfusion[315] but persists for days to weeks following chronic occlusion.[313,314]

In addition to transmural differences, there are regional differences in receptor location. The cardiac receptors that activate vagal afferents to induce the cardioinhibitor and vasodepressor Bezold-Jarisch reflex are preferentially located in the inferoposterior wall of the left ventricle.[318,319] Accordingly, acute myocardial ischemia of the inferoposterior wall produces a reflex bradycardia and vasodepressor response.[318,319] The reflex response to changes in cardiac filling pressures is mediated by mechanoreceptors with vagal afferents. The reflex response to a decrease in filling pressure is impaired 1 month after an inferoposterior, but not anterior, wall myocardial infarction.[320] One explanation for these results is that acute myocardial infarction of the inferoposterior wall damaged the sensory endings responsible for this reflex because these endings are located preferentially in the inferoposterior wall.[320]

Clinical studies confirm the importance of the site of myocardial infarction on the reflex cardiovascular response. There is preferential activation of vagal afferents with acute myocardial ischemia of the inferoposterior wall. Bradycardia and hypotension occur more frequently in patients with acute posterior than anterior wall myocardial infarction.[321-323] A transient bradycardia and hypotension occur in patients with acute myocardial infarction and reperfusion of the right, but not left anterior descending, coronary artery.[324] Coronary artery spasm of vessels supplying the inferior ventricle produces bradycardia, whereas spasm of vessels supplying the anterior wall produces tachycardia.[325] Sensory endings in the inferior wall may be damaged during acute myocardial infarction.[320] In this regard there is greater depression in baroreflex sensitivity (which reflects an impairment in the vagal efferent response) in patients 1 month after an acute inferior as compared with an anterior wall myocardial infarction.[326]

In summary, the size and site of acute myocardial ischemia and infarction have important implications with regard to the extent of functional impairment (in both ischemic and nonischemic areas), collateral blood flow, reflex cardiovascular response, and morbidity and mortality.

TIME COURSE OF FUNCTIONAL ALTERATIONS

The functional consequences of acute myocardial ischemia are fully reversible if coronary blood flow is reestablished early. If the ischemic myocardium is reperfused within 5 minutes of acute experimental ischemia, systolic function promptly returns to normal, whereas diastolic abnormalities may require 30 to 45 minutes to resolve fully.[275] If the ischemic myocardium is reperfused after 15 minutes of ischemia, abnormalities in subendocardial blood flow and function may persist for over 3 hours before returning to normal.[327] If reperfusion occurs after 1 hour of ischemia, it may require up to 1 month for full recovery of ventricular function.[278] This prolonged impairment in myocardial function despite adequate coronary blood flow has been termed *stunned myocardium*. If ischemia persists for 2 or more hours before reperfusion, complete functional recovery of the ischemic region may never occur, particularly if the initial period of ischemia was severe and/or extensive.[277,278] These experimental studies demonstrate the nonlinear relationship between the duration of myocardial ischemia and the recovery of function. A modest increase in the duration of ischemia can markedly decrease the extent and prolong the time required for functional recovery. The times described in these studies are not absolute but rather provide a relative time frame for the relation between the duration of ischemia and the time course for recovery. Clinical studies show significant benefits of reperfusion therapy well beyond 2 hours of acute myocardial ischemia. The ischemic region is likely heterogeneous with a central core of severely ischemic myocardium surrounded by areas of less severe ischemia. This heterogeneity is dependent on the shape and size of the ischemic region and presence of collateral blood flow. Although "late" reperfusion therapy may not salvage a central core of severely ischemic myocardium, there may be significant amounts of less severely ischemic myocardium that can be salvaged.

The mortality from an acute myocardial infarction is reduced with thrombolytic therapy, particularly if initiated early.[73,328] Regional and global ventricular function improve with reperfusion therapy, particularly in patients with anterior wall myocardial infarctions.[329-331] Early changes in global ventricular function may be difficult to interpret because initial improvements in ischemic region function may be offset by a decrease in hyperkinesis in nonischemic areas, resulting in no net change in global ejection fraction. Furthermore, there can be a spontaneous improvement in regional and global ventricular function secondary to spontaneous recanalization and reperfusion of occluded vessels early during the myocardial infarction.[31,332,333] Assessment of ventricular function early after an acute myocardial infarction may overestimate the full extent of damage because additional improvements in function may occur months after myocardial infarction.[330] This delayed improvement may be related to recovery of function in stunned myocardium.

Improvements in ventricular function following reperfusion may require weeks if there is stunned myocardium.[278] The mechanisms for myocardial stunning are not certain. Although it has been proposed that there is inadequate energy supply, the stunned myocardium demonstrates a normal contractile reserve.[334] Experimental studies indicate that the myofilament sensitivity to calcium is reduced in stunned myocardium.[335] Some of the functional impairments in stunned myocardium may be related to structural changes with disruption of the myocardial collagen matrix.[336]

If coronary blood flow is not reestablished, the ischemic myocardium undergoes necrosis. The extent of ischemic damage is influenced by the presence of functioning coronary collateral blood vessels.[337,338] Coronary collaterals develop in regions with moderately severe coronary artery stenosis.[339] If the coronary artery stenosis progresses to total occlusion slowly, coronary collaterals develop that will limit the extent of myocardial infarction.[340] Patients who have functioning collateral vessels tend to have less extensive infarcts,[341,342] milder functional impairment,[30] and a longer time period during which reperfusion will salvage ischemic myocardium and improve regional function.[343]

In experimental studies there is a characteristic evolution of alterations in regional ventricular function as the acutely ischemic myocardium undergoes necrosis and subsequent healing. The majority of the changes in regional function in the ischemic region occur within the first 5 minutes of coronary artery occlusion.[233,244] The aneurysmal bulging of the ischemic region remains stable for the first 24 hours of myocardial infarction.[233,244] However, some studies do demonstrate either a mild decrease[344] or increase[276] in aneurysmal bulging over the first few hours. Regional and global ventricular function improve in the days to weeks following an acute myocardial infarction.[345-347] This improvement in function has been attributed to an increase in stiffness of the ischemic myocardium,[348] scar contraction,[349] and hypertrophy in marginal and nonischemic regions of the ventricle.[244,276,350] Hypertrophy of nonischemic myocytes may begin within days of acute infarction.[351] Improvements in ventricular function weeks after acute myocardial infarction also may reflect recovery of stunned myocardium.

The time course of functional changes also has been examined in patients with acute myocardial infarction. The left ventricular ejection fraction varies widely in the same patient during the first 24 hours of infarction.[352] Over the first several weeks following acute myocardial infarction, most patients either demonstrate no change or have an increase in ejection fraction.[353,354] Cardiac index increases during the first few weeks, particularly in patients who had only mild hemodynamic impairment during the acute phase of infarction.[346,355] In contrast, patients with markedly elevated filling pressures during the acute phase of infarction have little improvement or deterioration in ventricular function during the healing phase.[353,355] Patients with acute myocardial infarction with severe hemodynamic complications have a particularly poor prognosis. After the first few weeks of recovery there is little further improvement in ventricular function over the next few months.[346]

REMODELING AND SHAPE CHANGES

Significant remodeling of the left ventricle occurs following acute myocardial infarction.[356] Infarct expansion is an acute dilation and thinning of the infarct zone that typically occurs after 1 week but may begin as soon as 24 hours after an acute myocardial infarction. Infarct expansion occurs in approximately one-third of patients with acute myocardial infarction, particularly in patients with anterior wall infarcts, transmural infarcts, and infarcts above a critical size ($\geq 10\%$ of the left ventricular mass). A significant amount of the infarct expansion is related to a structural rearrangement with cell slippage.[357] Although there is no additional necrosis, infarct expansion increases the functional size of the infarct and the ventricular dilation may increase wall stress and myocardial oxygen consumption. Remodeling changes may be generalized and involve dilation of nonischemic regions as well.[358,359] Patients may have remodeling changes with progressive ventricular dilation months after myocardial infarction.[359,360]

Several factors influence the extent of infarct expansion. Corticosteroids and nonsteroidal anti-inflammatory agents result in thinner infarcts and may promote infarct expansion, possibly by increasing cell slippage.[356] Infarct expansion is promoted by an increase in systolic load, whereas a decrease in load or the presence of hypertrophy has protective effects. In both experimental and clinical studies, chronic captopril therapy significantly attenuates the extent of ventricular dilation following acute myocardial infarction.[360,361] Although the benefits of early reperfusion are well known, "late" reperfusion that does not limit infarct size may inhibit infarct expansion and aneurysm formation.[362]

Infarct expansion may lead to several complications, including congestive heart failure, mural thrombus, cardiac rupture, chronic aneurysm formation, and increased mortality.[356] Infarct expansion should be distinguished from infarct extension, which is the infarction of additional myocardium, typically within the first 2 weeks following an acute myocardial infarction.[356] Infarct extension occurs more commonly with subendocardial and non–Q wave myocardial infarction. Patients with congestive heart failure, hypertension, diabetes, and transient episodes of hypotension during acute myocardial infarction are more likely to have infarct extension. Infarct extension is associated with an increase in morbidity and mortality.

Left ventricular aneurysms are an important complication of acute myocardial infarction. In the Coronary Artery Surgery Study (CASS), left ventricular aneurysms were found in 7.6% of patients with significant ($\geq 50\%$ stenosis) coronary artery disease.[363] Left ventricular aneurysms may develop in approximately one-fifth of patients with their first acute myocardial infarction.[364] Most aneurysms form within 3 months of an acute anterior wall infarction and are associated with a significant increase in mortality.[364] Functional aneurysms may develop as early as the first 2 to 3 days of an acute myocardial infarction and early aneurysms are associated with an even greater increase in mortality.[364,365] Collateral blood flow to the ischemic region and successful reperfusion decrease the likelihood of ventricular aneurysm formation.[366,367] Left ventricular aneurysms can produce several complications, including congestive heart failure, mural thrombus formation, ventricular arrhythmias, and angina pectoris.

Mural thrombus formation in the left ventricle is a common complication of acute myocardial infarction, particularly in the presence of infarct expansion or aneurysm formation. Mural thrombi typically develop within the first week of a transmural anterior wall myocardial infarction.[368] Mural thrombi are more common if there are severe and extensive wall motion abnormalities or marked changes in left ventricular shape and contour.[369] Hemostasis of blood in the ventricular apex predisposes to thrombus formation.[370] In patients with anterior wall myocardial infarction, mural thrombi occur more frequently with β-blocker therapy (due to the negative inotropic effects and/or more severe reduction in apical wall motion) and less frequently with anticoagulant therapy.[371,372]

CONCLUSIONS

Acute myocardial infarction occurs as a complication of atherosclerotic coronary artery disease in most cases. Disruption of the atherosclerotic plaque leads to platelet adhesion, activation, aggregation, and formation of an occlusive thrombus. Platelet activation may be related to a local imbalance between prostaglandin I_2 and thromboxane A_2 (produced by the vascular endothelium and platelets, respectively), platelet release of serotonin, impaired endothelium-dependent relaxation (in the presence of atherosclerotic lesions), and coronary artery spasm. Neutrophils accumulate with acute myocardial ischemia and mechanically obstruct capillary flow, inducing myocardial damage by the release of proteases and leukotrienes and the production of oxygen-derived free radicals. Coronary artery spasm may initiate acute myocardial ischemia or may occur as a secondary factor that sustains and/or exacerbates myocardial ischemia.

The importance of platelets in acute myocardial ischemia and infarction is suggested by several large clinical trials. Inhibition of platelet function with aspirin reduces the infarction rate in patients with unstable angina. Aspirin therapy during the early hours of acute myocardial infarction reduces mortality and reinfarction rates. Long-term aspirin therapy may reduce acute myocardial infarction in some subgroups of healthy persons (primary prevention) and tends to reduce reinfarctions in patients with prior myocardial infarction (secondary prevention). Finally, there is a circadian variation in the incidence of acute myocardial infarction (peak incidence in the morning) that may be related to a similar circadian variation in platelet aggregability.

Functional impairments develop within seconds following coronary artery occlusion. The metabolic basis for early ischemic dysfunction is unknown but may involve an increase in inorganic phosphate, intracellular acidosis, and/or alterations in myofilament sensitivity to calcium. Prolonged ischemia leads to irreversible cell damage that may be related to severe ATP depletion, membrane damage that impairs cell integrity, and intracellular calcium overload. Cell damage is exacerbated by acidosis, catecholamines, fatty acids, and oxygen-derived free radicals that accompany acute myocardial ischemia.

Impairments in systolic and diastolic function develop rapidly with acute myocardial ischemia in direct relation to the severity and extent of decreased coronary blood flow. The ischemic region develops a paradoxic systolic bulge as it is passively stretched, although there is some residual contractile function. Mild functional impairments occur in nonischemic areas (functional border zone) tethered to the abnormally contracting ischemic region. Remote nonischemic areas develop hyperkinesis due to increased use of the Frank-Starling mechanism, a regional intraventricular unloading effect, and shape changes.

Acute myocardial ischemia slows the rate of left ventricular pressure fall due to a direct impairment of ventricular relaxation, as well as secondary alterations in loading conditions and asynchrony. The slower rate of left ventricular pressure fall, increase in myocardial stiffness, and increased asynchrony contribute to higher diastolic filling pressures and slower rates of diastolic filling.

The functional consequences, morbidity, and mortality of acute myocardial infarction are directly related to the size of the ischemic region or infarct. The severity of ischemia and infarct size are reduced by the presence of coronary collaterals. The site of acute myocardial ischemia influences the extent of functional impairment and mortality, largely due to differences in infarct size. The transmural extent and site of acute myocardial ischemia determine the nature of the reflex cardiovascular response. As an example, reflex bradycardia and vasodepressor effects occur primarily with acute myocardial ischemia of the inferoposterior wall.

Early reperfusion produces significant salvage of myocardial function and improved survival. A delay in reperfusion may still produce functional recovery, although it may require days to weeks for function to improve in stunned myocardium. The left ventricle undergoes significant remodeling and shape changes during the recovery phase. Infarct expansion and ventricular aneurysm formation occur commonly with large, transmural, anterior wall myocardial infarctions. These remodeling changes may lead to several complications, including congestive heart failure, mural thrombus formation, cardiac rupture, and ventricular arrhythmias.

REFERENCES

1. Liebowitz JO (ed): The History of Coronary Heart Disease. London, William Clowes & Sons, 1970
2. Herrick JB: Clinical features of sudden obstruction of the coronary arteries. JAMA 59:2015, 1912
3. Cheitlin MD, McAllister HA, de Castro CM: Myocardial infarction without atherosclerosis. JAMA 231:951, 1975
4. Isner JM, Estes M III, Thompson PD et al: Acute cardiac events temporally related to cocaine abuse. N Engl J Med 315:1438, 1986
5. Smith HWB III, Liberman HA, Brody SL et al: Acute myocardial infarction temporally related to cocaine use: Clinical, angiographic, and pathophysiologic observations. Ann Intern Med 107:13, 1987
6. Khan AH, Haywood LJ: Myocardial infarction in nine patients with radiologically patent coronary arteries. N Engl J Med 291:427, 1974
7. Eliot RS, Baroldi G, Leone A: Necropsy studies in myocardial infarction with minimal or no coronary luminal reduction due to atherosclerosis. Circulation 49:1127, 1974
8. Oliva PB, Breckinridge JC: Acute myocardial infarction with normal and near normal coronary arteries: Documentation with coronary arteriography within 12½ hours of the onset of symptoms in two cases (three episodes). Am J Cardiol 40:1000, 1977
9. Raymond R, Lynch J, Underwood D et al: Myocardial infarction and normal coronary arteriography: A 10-year clinical and risk analysis of 74 patients. J Am Coll Cardiol 11:471, 1988
10. Mosher P, Ross J Jr, McFate PA et al: Control of coronary blood flow by an autoregulatory mechanism. Circ Res 14:250, 1964
11. Gould, KL, Lipscomb K, Hamilton GW: Physiologic basis for assessing critical coronary stenosis: Instantaneous flow response and regional distribution during coronary hyperemia as measures of coronary flow reserve. Am J Cardiol 33:87, 1974
12. Ball RM, Bache RJ: Distribution of myocardial blood flow in the exercising dog with restricted coronary artery inflow. Circ Res 38:60, 1976
13. Lipscomb K, Hooten S: Effect of stenotic dimensions and blood flow on the hemodynamic significance of model coronary artery stenoses. Am J Cardiol 42:781, 1978
14. Ridolfi RL, Hutchins GM: The relationship between coronary artery lesions and myocardial infarcts: Ulceration of atherosclerotic plaques precipitating coronary thrombosis. Am Heart J 93:468, 1977
15. Horie T, Sekiguchi M, Hirosawa K: Coronary thrombosis in pathogenesis of acute myocardial infarction: Histopathological study of coronary arteries in 108 necropsied cases using serial section. Br Heart J 40:153, 1978
16. Buja LM, Willerson JT: Clinicopathologic correlates of acute ischemic heart disease syndromes. Am J Cardiol 47:343, 1981
17. Falk E: Plaque rupture with severe pre-existing stenosis precipitating coronary thrombosis: Characteristics of coronary atherosclerotic plaques underlying fatal occlusive thrombi. Br Heart J 50:127, 1983
18. Falk E: Unstable angina with fatal outcome: Dynamic coronary thrombosis

leading to infarction and/or sudden death: Autopsy evidence of recurrent mural thrombosis with peripheral embolization culminating in total vascular occlusion. Circulation 71:699, 1985
19. Frink RJ, Rooney PA Jr, Trowbridge JO et al: Coronary thrombosis and platelet/fibrin microemboli in death associated with acute myocardial infarction. Br Heart J 59:196, 1988
20. Davies MJ, Thomas A: Thrombosis and acute coronary-artery lesions in sudden cardiac ischemic death. N Engl J Med 310:1137, 1984
21. Spain DM, Bradess VA: Sudden death from coronary heart disease: Survival time, frequency of thrombi, and cigarette smoking. Chest 58:107, 1970
22. Baroldi G, Falzi G, Mariani F: Sudden coronary death. A postmortem study in 208 selected cases compared to 97 "control" subjects. Am Heart J 98:20, 1979
23. Sherman CT, Litvack F, Grundfest W et al: Coronary angioscopy in patients with unstable angina pectoris. N Engl J Med 315:913, 1986
24. Brown BG, Gallery CA, Badger RS et al: Incomplete lysis of thrombus in the moderate underlying atherosclerotic lesion during intracoronary infusion of streptokinase for acute myocardial infarction: Quantitative angiographic observations. Circulation 73:653, 1986
25. Wilson RF, Holida MD, White CW: Quantitative angiographic morphology of coronary stenoses leading to myocardial infarction or unstable angina. Circulation 73:286, 1986
26. Levin DC, Fallon JT: Significance of the angiographic morphology of localized coronary stenoses: Histopathologic correlations. Circulation 66:316, 1982
27. Oliva PB: Pathophysiology of acute myocardial infarction. Ann Intern Med 94:236, 1981
28. Silver MD, Baroldi G, Mariani F: The relationship between acute occlusive coronary thrombi and myocardial infarction studied in 100 consecutive patients. Circulation 61:219, 1980
29. Baroldi G, Radice F, Schmid G et al: Morphology of acute myocardial infarction in relation to coronary thrombosis. Am Heart J 87:65, 1974
30. Betriu A, Castaner A, Sanz GA et al: Angiographic findings 1 month after myocardial infarction: A prospective study of 259 survivors. Circulation 65:1099, 1982
31. DeWood MA, Spores J, Notske R et al: Prevalence of total coronary occlusion during the early hours of transmural myocardial infarction. N Engl J Med 303:897, 1980
32. Phillips SJ, Kongtahworn C, Zeff RH et al: Emergency coronary artery revascularization: A possible therapy for acute myocardial infarction. Circulation 60:241, 1979
33. Davies MJ, Woolf N, Robertson WB: Pathology of acute myocardial infarction with particular reference to occlusive coronary thrombi. Br Heart J 38:659, 1976
34. Geer JC, Crago CA, Little WC et al: Subendocardial ischemic myocardial lesions associated with severe coronary atherosclerosis. Am J Pathol 98:663, 1980
35. Gibson RS, Beller GA, Gheorghiade M et al: The prevalence and clinical significance of residual myocardial ischemia 2 weeks after uncomplicated non-Q wave infarction: A prospective natural history study. Circulation 73:1186, 1986
36. DeWood MA, Stifter WF, Simpson CS et al: Coronary arteriographic findings soon after non–Q wave myocardial infarction. N Engl J Med 315:417, 1986
37. Davies MJ, Thomas AC, Knapman PA et al: Intramyocardial platelet aggregation in patients with unstable angina suffering sudden ischemic cardiac death. Circulation 73:418, 1986
38. Hamm CW, Lorenz RL, Bleifeld W et al: Biochemical evidence of platelet activation in patients with persistent unstable angina. J Am Coll Cardiol 10:998, 1987
39. Capone G, Wolf NM, Meyer B et al: Frequency of intracoronary filling defects by angiography in angina pectoris at rest. Am J Cardiol 56:403, 1985
40. Cowley MJ, DiSciascio G, Rehr RB et al: Angiographic observations and clinical relevance of coronary thrombus in unstable angina pectoris. Am J Cardiol 63:108E, 1989
41. Gotoh K, Minamino T, Katoh O et al: The role of intracoronary thrombus in unstable angina: Angiographic assessment and thrombolytic therapy during ongoing anginal attacks. Circulation 77:526, 1988
42. Folts JD, Crowell EB Jr, Rowe GG: Platelet aggregation in partially obstructed vessels and its elimination with aspirin. Circulation 54:365, 1976
43. Gertz SD, Uretsky G, Wajnberg RS et al: Endothelial cell damage and thrombus formation after partial arterial constriction: Relevance to the role of coronary artery spasm in the pathogenesis of myocardial infarction. Circulation 63:476, 1981
44. Haft JI, Kranz PD, Albert FJ et al: Intravascular platelet aggregation in the heart induced by norepinephrine: Microscopic studies. Circulation 46:698, 1972
45. Levine SP, Towell BL, Suarez AM et al: Platelet activation and secretion associated with emotional stress. Circulation 71:1129, 1985
46. Romson JL, Haack DW, Abrams GD et al: Prevention of occlusive coronary artery thrombosis by prostacyclin infusion in the dog. Circulation 64:906, 1981
47. Vik-Mo H: Effects of acute myocardial ischaemia on platelet aggregation in the coronary sinus and aorta in dogs. Scand J Haematol 19:68, 1977
48. Moschos CB, Lahiri K, Lyons M et al: Relation of microcirculatory thrombosis to thrombus in the proximal coronary artery: Effect of aspirin, dipyridamole, and thrombolysis. Am Heart J 86:61, 1973
49. Ruf W, McNamara JJ, Suehiro A et al: Platelet trapping in myocardial infarct in baboons: Therapeutic effect of aspirin. Am J Cardiol 46:405, 1980
50. El-Maraghi N, Genton E: The relevance of platelet and fibrin thromboembolism of the coronary microcirculation, with special reference to sudden cardiac death. Circulation 62:936, 1980
51. Haerem JW: Platelet aggregates in intramyocardial vessels of patients dying suddenly and unexpectedly of coronary artery disease. Atherosclerosis 15:199, 1972
52. Steele PP, Weily HS, Davies H et al: Platelet function studies in coronary artery disease. Circulation 48:1194, 1973
53. Mehta J, Mehta P, Pepine CJ et al: Platelet function studies in coronary artery disease: VII. Effect of aspirin and tachycardia stress on aortic and coronary venous blood. Am J Cardiol 45:945, 1980
54. Fitzgerald DJ, Roy L, Catella F et al: Platelet activation in unstable coronary disease. N Engl J Med 315:983, 1986
55. Mueller HS, Rao PS, Greenberg MA et al: Systemic and transcardiac platelet activity in acute myocardial infarction in man: Resistance to prostacyclin. Circulation 72:1336, 1985
56. Muller JE, Tofler GH, Stone PH: Circadian variation and triggers of onset of acute cardiovascular disease. Circulation 79:733, 1989
57. Muller JE, Stone PH, Turi ZG et al: Circadian variation in the frequency of onset of acute myocardial infarction. N Engl J Med 313:1315, 1985
58. Hjalmarson A, Gilpin EA, Nicod P et al: Differing circadian patterns of symptom onset in subgroups of patients with acute myocardial infarction. Circulation 80:267, 1989
59. Rocco MB, Barry J, Campbell S et al: Circadian variation of transient myocardial ischemia in patients with coronary artery disease. Circulation 75:395, 1987
60. Tofler GH, Brezinski D, Schafer AI et al: Concurrent morning increase in platelet aggregability and the risk of myocardial infarction and sudden cardiac death. N Engl J Med 316:1514, 1987
61. Elwood PC, Cochrane AL, Burr ML et al: A randomized controlled trial of acetyl salicylic acid in the secondary prevention of mortality from myocardial infarction. Br Med J 1:436, 1974
62. The Coronary Drug Project Research Group: Aspirin in coronary heart disease. J Chronic Dis 29:625, 1976
63. Breddin K, Loew D, Lechner K et al: The German-Austrian Aspirin Trial: A comparison of acetylsalicylic acid, placebo and phenprocoumon in secondary prevention of myocardial infarction. Circulation 62:V-63, 1980
64. Elwood PC, Sweetnam PM: Aspirin and secondary mortality after myocardial infarction. Lancet 2:1313, 1979
65. Aspirin Myocardial Infarction Study Research Group: A randomized, controlled trial of aspirin in persons recovered from myocardial infarction. JAMA 243:661, 1980
66. The Persantine-Aspirin Reinfarction Study Research Group: Persantine and aspirin in coronary heart disease. Circulation 62:449, 1980
67. Klimt CR, Knatterud GL, Stamler J et al: Persantine-aspirin reinfarction study: II. Secondary coronary prevention with persantine and aspirin. J Am Coll Cardiol 7:251, 1986
68. The Anturane Reinfarction Trial Research Group: Sulfinpyrazone in the prevention of sudden death after myocardial infarction. N Engl J Med 302:250, 1980
69. The Anturan Reinfarction Italian Study Group: Sulphinpyrazone in postmyocardial infarction. Lancet 1:237, 1982
70. The FDA's critique of the Anturane Reinfarction Trial. N Engl J Med 303:1488, 1980
71. The Anturane Reinfarction Trial: Reevaluation of outcome. N Engl J Med 306:1005, 1982
72. Antiplatelet Trialists' Collaboration: Secondary prevention of vascular disease by prolonged antiplatelet treatment. Br Med J 296:320, 1988
73. ISIS-2 (Second International Study of Infarct Survival) Collaborative Group: Randomized trial of intravenous streptokinase, oral aspirin, both, or neither among 17,187 cases of suspected acute myocardial infarction: ISIS-2. Lancet 2:349, 1988
74. Lewis HD Jr, Davis JW, Archibald DG et al: Protective effects of aspirin against acute myocardial infarction and death in men with unstable angina: Results of a Veterans Administration Cooperative Study. N Engl J Med 309:396, 1983
75. Cairns JA, Gent M, Singer J et al: Aspirin, sulfinpyrazone, or both in unstable angina: Results of a Canadian Multicenter Trial. N Engl J Med 313:1369, 1985
76. Theroux P, Ouimet H, McCans J et al: Aspirin, heparin, or both to treat acute unstable angina. N Engl J Med 319:1105, 1988
77. Peto R, Gray R, Collins R et al: Randomised trial of prophylactic daily aspirin in British male doctors. Br Med J 296:313, 1988
78. Steering Committee of the Physicians' Health Study Research Group: Final report on the aspirin component of the ongoing Physicians' Health Study. N Engl J Med 321:129, 1989
79. Oates JA, FitzGerald GA, Branch RA et al: Clinical implications of prostaglandin and thromboxane A_2 formation: I. N Engl J Med 319:689, 1988
80. FitzGerald GA, Brash AR, Falardeau P et al: Estimated rate of prostacyclin secretion into the circulation of normal man. J Clin Invest 68:1272, 1981

81. Gerritsen ME, Printz MP: Sites of prostaglandin synthesis in the bovine heart and isolated bovine coronary microvessels. Circ Res 49:1152, 1981
82. Gerritsen ME, Cheli CD: Arachidonic acid and prostaglandin endoperoxide metabolism in isolated rabbit and coronary microvessels and isolated and cultivated coronary microvessel endothelial cells. J Clin Invest 72:1658, 1983
83. Furchgott RF, Vanhoutte PM: Endothelium-derived relaxing and contracting factors. FASEB J 3:2007, 1989
84. Azuma H, Ishikawa M, Sekizaki S: Endothelium-dependent inhibition of platelet aggregation. Br J Pharmacol 88:411, 1986
85. Radomski MW, Palmer RMJ, Moncada S: Comparative pharmacology of endothelium-derived relaxing factor, nitric oxide, and prostacylin in platelets. Br J Pharmacol 92:181, 1987
86. Houston DS, Shepherd JT, Vanhoutte PM: Aggregating human platelets cause direct contraction and endothelium-dependent relaxation of isolated canine coronary arteries: Role of serotonin, thromboxane A_2, and adenine nucleotides. J Clin Invest 78:539, 1986
87. Patrono C, Ciabattoni G, Pugliese F et al: Estimated rate of thromboxane secretion into the circulation of normal humans. J Clin Invest 77:590, 1986
88. Roy L, Knapp HP, Robertson RM et al: Endogenous biosynthesis of prostacyclin during cardiac catheterization and angiography in man. Circulation 71:434, 1985
89. Dembinska-Kiec A, Gryglewska T, Zmuda A et al: The generation of prostacyclin by arteries and by the coronary vascular bed is reduced in experimental atherosclerosis in rabbits. Prostaglandins 14:1025, 1977
90. Neri Serneri GG, Masotti G, Poggesi L et al: Reduced prostacyclin production in patients with different manifestations of ischemic heart disease. Am J Cardiol 49:1146, 1982
91. FitzGerald GA, Smith B, Pedersen AK et al: Increased prostacyclin biosynthesis in patients with severe atherosclerosis and platelet activation. N Engl J Med 310:1065, 1984
92. Hirsh PD, Hillis LD, Campbell WB et al: Release of prostaglandins and thromboxane into the coronary circulation in patients with ischemic heart disease. N Engl J Med 304:685, 1981
93. Vanhoutte PM, Shimokawa H: Endothelium-derived relaxing factor and coronary vasospasm. Circulation 80:1, 1989
94. Shimokawa H, Vanhoutte PM: Dietary cod-liver oil improves endothelium-dependent responses in hypercholesterolemic and atherosclerotic porcine coronary arteries. Circulation 78:1421, 1988
95. Kromhout D, Bosschieter EB, de Lezenne Coulander C: The inverse relation between fish consumption and 20-year mortality from coronary heart disease. N Engl J Med 312:1205, 1985
96. Kraemer RJ, Phernetton TM, Folts JD: Prostaglandin-like substances in coronary venous blood following myocardial ischemia. J Pharmacol Exp Ther 199:611, 1976
97. Berger HJ, Zaret BL, Speroff L et al: Regional cardiac prostaglandin release during myocardial ischemia in anesthetized dogs. Circ Res 38:566, 1976
98. Berger HJ, Zaret BL, Speroff L et al: Cardiac prostaglandin release during myocardial ischemia induced by atrial pacing in patients with coronary artery disease. Am J Cardiol 39:481, 1977
99. Coker SJ, Parratt JR, Ledingham IM et al: Thromboxane and prostacyclin release from ischaemic myocardium in relation to arrhythmias. Nature 291:323, 1981
100. Hendriksson P, Wennmalm A, Edhag O et al: In vivo production of prostacyclin and thromboxane in patients with acute myocardial infarction. Br Heart J 55:543, 1986
101. Zmuda A, Dembinska-Kiec A, Chytkowski A et al: Experimental atherosclerosis in rabbits: Platelet aggregation, thromboxane A_2 generation and antiaggregatory potency of prostacyclin. Prostaglandin 14:1035, 1977
102. Szczeklik A, Gryglewski RJ, Musial J et al: Thromboxane generation and platelet aggregation in survivals of myocardial infarction. Thromb Haemost 40:66, 1978
103. Walinsky P, Smith JB, Lefer AM et al: Thromboxane A_2 in acute myocardial infarction. Am Heart J 108:868, 1984
104. Lewy RI, Wiener L, Walinsky P et al: Thromboxane release during pacing-induced angina pectoris: Possible vasoconstrictor influence on the coronary vasculature. Circulation 61:1165, 1980
105. Tada M, Kuzuya T, Inoue M et al: Elevation of thromboxane B_2 levels in patients with classic and variant angina pectoris. Circulation 64:1107, 1981
106. Friedrich T, Lichey J, Nigam S et al: Follow-up of prostaglandin plasma levels after acute myocardial infarction. Am Heart J 109:218, 1985
107. Folts JD, Gallagher K, Rowe GG: Blood flow reductions in stenosed canine coronary arteries: Vasospasm or platelet aggregation. Circulation 65:248, 1982
108. Willerson JT, Golino P, Eidt J et al: Specific platelet mediators and unstable coronary artery lesions: Experimental evidence and potential clinical implications. Circulation 80:198, 1989
109. Rubanyi GM, Frye RL, Holmes DR Jr et al: Vasoconstrictor activity of coronary sinus plasma from patients with coronary artery disease. J Am Coll Cardiol 9:1243, 1987
110. van den Berg EK, Schmitz JM, Benedict CR et al: Transcardiac serotonin concentration is increased in selected patients with limiting angina and complex coronary lesion morphology. Circulation 79:116, 1989
111. Ogletree ML, Lefer AM: Prostaglandin-induced preservation of the ischemic myocardium. Circ Res 42:218, 1978
112. Araki H, Lefer AM: Role of prostacyclin in the preservation of ischemic myocardial tissue in the perfused cat heart. Circ Res 47:757, 1980
113. Jugdutt BI, Hutchins GM, Bulkley BH et al: Dissimilar effects of prostacyclin, prostaglandin E_1, and prostaglandin E_2 on myocardial infarct size after coronary occlusion in conscious dogs. Circ Res 49:685, 1981
114. Simpson PJ, Mickelson J, Fantone JC et al: Reduction of experimental canine myocardial infarct size with prostaglandin E_1: Inhibition of neutrophil migration and activation. J Pharmacol Exp Ther 244:619, 1988
115. Bergman G, Daly K, Atkinson L et al: Prostacyclin: Haemodynamic and metabolic effects in patients with coronary artery disease. Lancet 1:569, 1981
116. Siegel RJ, Shah PK, Nathan M et al: Prostaglandin E_1 infusion in unstable angina: Effects on anginal frequency and cardiac function. Am Heart J 108:863, 1984
117. Popat KD, Pitt B: Hemodynamic effects of prostaglandin E_1 infusion in patients with acute myocardial infarction and left ventricular failure. Am Heart J 103:485, 1982
118. Henriksson P, Edhag O, Wennmalm A: Prostacyclin infusion in patients with acute myocardial infarction. Br Heart J 53:173, 1985
119. Kiernan FJ, Kluger J, Regnier JC et al: Epoprostenol sodium (prostacyclin) infusion in acute myocardial infarction. Br Heart J 56:428, 1986
120. Chierchia S, Patrono C, Crea F et al: Effects of intravenous prostacyclin in variant angina. Circulation 65:470, 1982
121. Fitzgerald DJ, Catella F, Roy L et al: Marked platelet activation *in vivo* after intravenous streptokinase in patients with acute myocardial infarction. Circulation 77:142, 1988
122. Jang I-K, Gold HK, Ziskind AA et al: Differential sensitivity of erythrocyte-rich and platelet-rich arterial thrombi to lysis with recombinant tissue-type plasminogen activator: A possible explanation for resistance to coronary thrombolysis. Circulation 79:920, 1989
123. Terres W, Beythien C, Kupper W et al: Effects of aspirin and prostaglandin E_1 on the *in vitro* thrombolysis with urokinase: Evidence for a possible role of inhibiting platelet activity in thrombolysis. Circulation 79:1309, 1989
124. Yasuda T, Gold HK, Fallon JT et al: Monoclonal antibody against the platelet glycoprotein (GP) IIb/IIIa receptor prevents coronary artery reocclusion after reperfusion with recombinant tissue-type plasminogen activator in dogs. J Clin Invest 81:1284, 1988
125. Golino P, Ashton J, NcNatt et al: Simultaneous administration of thromboxane A_2- and serotonin S_2-receptor antagonists markedly enhances thrombolysis and prevents or delays reocclusion after tissue-type plasminogen activator in a canine model of coronary thrombosis. Circulation 79:911, 1989
126. Mehta JL, Nichols WW, Mehta P: Neutrophils as potential participants in acute myocardial ischemia: Relevance to reperfusion. J Am Coll Cardiol 11:1309, 1988
127. Engler RL, Schmid-Schönbein GW, Pavelec RS: Leukocyte capillary plugging in myocardial ischemia and reperfusion in the dog. Am J Pathol 111:98, 1983
128. Mullane KM, Read N, Salmon JA et al: Role of leukocytes in acute myocardial infarction in anesthetized dogs: Relationship to myocardial salvage by anti-inflammatory drugs. J Pharmacol Exp Ther 228:510, 1984
129. Engler RL, Dahlgren MD, Peterson MA et al: Accumulation of polymorphonuclear leukocytes during 3-h experimental myocardial ischemia. Am J Physiol 251:H93, 1986
130. Rossen RD, Swain JL, Michael LH et al: Selective accumulation of the first component of complement and leukocytes in ischemic canine heart muscle: A possible initiator of an extra myocardial mechanism of ischemic injury. Circ Res 57:119, 1985
131. Crawford MH, Grover FL, Kolb WP et al: Complement and neutrophil activation in the pathogenesis of ischemic myocardial injury. Circulation 78:1449, 1988
132. Lewis RA, Austen KF: The biologically active leukotrienes: Biosynthesis, metabolism, receptors, functions, and pharmacology. J Clin Invest 73:889, 1984
133. Feuerstein G, Hallenbeck JM: Leukotrienes in health and disease. FASEB J 1:186, 1987
134. Evers AS, Murphree S, Saffitz JE et al: Effects of endogenously produced leukotrienes, thromboxane, and prostaglandins on coronary vascular resistance in rabbit myocardial infarction. J Clin Invest 75:992, 1985
135. Mehta J, Dinerman J, Mehta P et al: Neutrophil function in ischemic heart disease. Circulation 79:549, 1989
136. Weiss SJ: Tissue destruction by neutrophils. N Engl J Med 320:365, 1989
137. McCord JM: Free radicals and myocardial ischemia: Overview and outlook. Free Radical Biol Med 4:9, 1988
138. Downey JM, Hearse DJ, Yellon DM: The role of xanthine oxidase during myocardial ischemia in several species including man. J Mol Cell Cardiol 20 (Suppl II):55, 1988
139. Rao PS, Cohen MV, Mueller HS: Production of free radicals and lipid peroxides in early experimental myocardial ischemia. J Mol Cell Cardiol 15:713, 1983
140. Burton KP, McCord JM, Ghai G: Myocardial alterations due to free-radical generation. Am J Physiol 246:H776, 1984
141. Blaustein AS, Schine L, Brooks WW et al: Influence of exogenously generated oxidant species on myocardial function. Am J Physiol 250:H595, 1986

142. Jackson CV, Mickelson JK, Pope TK et al: O₂ free radical–mediated myocardial and vascular dysfunction. Am J Physiol 251:H1225, 1986
143. Gryglewski RJ, Palmer RMJ, Moncada S: Superoxide anion is involved in the breakdown of endothelium-derived vascular relaxing factor. Nature 320:454, 1986
144. Engler R, Gilpin E: Can superoxide dismutase alter myocardial infarct size? Circulation 79:1137, 1989
145. Engler RL, Dahlgren MD, Morris DD et al: Role of leukocytes in response to acute myocardial ischemia and reflow in dogs. Am J Physiol 251:H314, 1986
146. Engler R, Covell JW: Granulocytes cause reperfusion ventricular dysfunction after 15-minute ischemia in the dog. Circ Res 61:20, 1987
147. Romson JL, Hook BG, Kunkel SL et al: Reduction of the extent of ischemic myocardial injury by neutrophil depletion in the dog. Circulation 67:1016, 1983
148. Mitsos SE, Askew TE, Fantone JC et al: Protective effects of N-2-mercaptopropionyl glycine against myocardial reperfusion injury after neutrophil depletion in the dog: Evidence for the role of intracellular-derived free radicals. Circulation 73:1077, 1986
149. Bednar M, Smith B, Pinto A et al: Nafazatrom-induced salvage of ischemic myocardium in anesthetized dogs is mediated through inhibition of neutrophil function. Circ Res 57:131, 1985
150. Bajaj AK, Cobb MA, Virmani R et al: Limitation of myocardial reperfusion injury by intravenous perfluorochemicals: Role of neutrophil activation. Circulation 79:645, 1989
151. Prinzmetal M, Kennamer R, Merliss R et al: Angina pectoris I: A variant form of angina pectoris: Preliminary report. Am J Med 27:375, 1959
152. Dhurandhar RW, Watt DL, Silver MD et al: Prinzmetal's variant form of angina with arteriographic evidence of coronary arterial spasm. Am J Cardiol 30:902, 1972
153. Oliva PB, Potts DE, Pluss RG: Coronary arterial spasm in Prinzmetal angina: Documentation by coronary arteriography. N Engl J Med 288:745, 1973
154. Maseri A, L'Abbate A, Baroldi G et al: Coronary vasospasm as a possible cause of myocardial infarction: A conclusion derived from the Study of "Preinfarction" Angina. N Engl J Med 299:1271, 1978
155. Maseri A, Severi S, De Nes M et al: "Variant" angina: One aspect of a continuous spectrum of vasospastic myocardial ischemia: Pathogenetic mechanisms, estimated incidence and clinical and coronary arteriographic findings in 138 patients. Am J Cardiol 42:1019, 1978
156. Bertrand ME, LaBlanche JM, Tilmant PY et al: Frequency of provoked coronary arterial spasm in 1089 consecutive patients undergoing coronary arteriography. Circulation 65:1299, 1982
157. Oliva PB, Breckinridge JC: Arteriographic evidence of coronary arterial spasm in acute myocardial infarction. Circulation 56:366, 1977
158. Ganz W, Geft I, Maddahi J et al: Nonsurgical reperfusion in evolving myocardial infarction. J Am Coll Cardiol 1:1247, 1983
159. Vincent GM, Anderson JL, Marshall HW: Coronary spasm producing coronary thrombosis and myocardial infarction. N Engl J Med 309:220, 1983
160. Severi S, Davies G, Maseri A et al: Long-term prognosis of "variant" angina with medical treatment. Am J Cardiol 46:226, 1980
161. Mark DB, Califf RM, Morris KG et al: Clinical characteristics and long-term survival of patients with variant angina. Circulation 69:880, 1984
162. Walling A, Waters DD, Miller DD et al: Long-term prognosis of patients with variant angina. Circulation 76:990, 1987
163. Nakamura M, Takeshita A, Nose Y: Clinical characteristics associated with myocardial infarction, arrhythmias, and sudden death in patients with vasospastic angina. Circulation 75:1110, 1987
164. Yasue H, Takizawa A, Nagao M et al: Long-term prognosis for patients with variant angina and influential factors. Circulation 78:1, 1988
165. Robertson RM, Robertson D, Roberts LJ et al: Thromboxane A₂ in vasotonic angina pectoris: Evidence from direct measurements and inhibitor trials. N Engl J Med 304:998, 1981
166. Chierchia S, de Caterina R, Crea F et al: Failure of thromboxane A₂ blockade to prevent attacks of vasospastic angina. Circulation 66:702, 1982
167. Shimokawa H, Tomoike H, Nabeyama S et al: Histamine-induced spasm not significantly modulated by prostanoids in a swine model of coronary artery spasm. J Am Coll Cardiol 6:321, 1985
168. Chierchia S, Patrono C, Crea F et al: Effects of intravenous prostacyclin in variant angina. Circulation 65:470, 1982
169. Kalsner S, Richards R: Coronary arteries of cardiac patients are hyperactive and contain stores of amines: A mechanism for coronary spasm. Science 223:1435, 1984
170. Forman MB, Oates JA, Robertson D et al: Increased adventitial mast cells in a patient with coronary spasm. N Engl J Med 313:1138, 1985
171. Kaski JC, Crea F, Meran D et al: Local coronary supersensitivity to diverse vasoconstrictive stimuli in patients with variant angina. Circulation 74:1255, 1986
172. Waters DD, Szlachcic J, Bonan R et al: Comparative sensitivity of exercise, cold pressor and ergonovine testing in provoking attacks of variant angina in patients with active disease. Circulation 67:310, 1983
173. Henry PD, Yokoyama M: Supersensitivity of atherosclerotic rabbit aorta to ergonovine: Mediation by a serotonergic mechanism. J Clin Invest 66:306, 1980
174. De Caterina R, Carpeggiani C, L'Abbate A: A double-blind, placebo-controlled study of ketanserin in patients with Prinzmetal's angina: Evidence against a role for serotonin in the genesis of coronary vasospasm. Circulation 69:889, 1984
175. Freedman SB, Chierchia S, Rodriguez-Plaza L et al: Ergonovine-induced myocardial ischemia: No role for serotonergic receptors? Circulation 70:178, 1984
176. Yasue H, Touyama M, Shimamoto M et al: Role of autonomic nervous system in the pathogenesis of Prinzmetal's variant form of angina. Circulation 50:534, 1974
177. Raizner AE, Chahine RA, Ishimori T et al: Provocation of coronary artery spasm by the cold pressor test: Hemodynamic, arteriographic and quantitative angiographic observations. Circulation 62:925, 1980
178. Nabel EG, Ganz P, Gordon JB et al: Dilation of normal and constriction of atherosclerotic coronary arteries caused by the cold pressor test. Circulation 77:43, 1988
179. Robertson D, Robertson RM, Nies AS et al: Variant angina pectoris: Investigation of indexes of sympathetic nervous system function. Am J Cardiol 43:1080, 1979
180. Chierchia S, Davies G, Berkenboom G et al: Alpha-adrenergic receptors and coronary spasm: An elusive link. Circulation 69:8, 1984
181. Winniford MD, Filipchuk N, Hillis LD: Alpha-adrenergic blockade for variant angina: A long-term, double-blind, randomized trial. Circulation 67:1185, 1983
182. Shimokawa H, Tomoike H, Nabeyama S et al: Coronary artery spasm induced in atherosclerotic miniature swine. Science 221:560, 1983
183. Shimokawa H, Aarhus LL, Vanhoutte PM: Porcine coronary arteries with regenerated endothelium have a reduced endothelium-dependent responsiveness to aggregating platelets and serotonin. Circ Res 61:256, 1987
184. Nagasawa K, Tomoike H, Hayashi Y et al: Intramural hemorrhage and endothelial changes in atherosclerotic coronary artery after repetitive episodes of spasm in x-ray–irradiated hypercholesterolemic pigs. Circ Res 65:272, 1989
185. Dorros G, Cowley MJ, Simpson J et al: Percutaneous transluminal coronary angioplasty: Report of complications from the National Heart, Lung, and Blood Institute PTCA Registry. Circulation 67:723, 1983
186. Förstermann U, Mügge A, Bode SM et al: Response of human coronary arteries to aggregating platelets: Importance of endothelium-derived relaxing factor and prostanoids. Circ Res 63:306, 1988
187. Ludmer PL, Selwyn AP, Shook TL et al: Paradoxical vasoconstriction induced by acetylcholine in atherosclerotic coronary arteries. N Engl J Med 315:1046, 1986
188. Yasue H, Horio Y, Nakamura N et al: Induction of coronary artery spasm by acetylcholine in patients with variant angina: Possible role of the parasympathetic nervous system in the pathogenesis of coronary artery spasm. Circulation 74:955, 1986
189. Neely JR, Rovetto MJ, Oram JF: Myocardial utilization of carbohydrate and lipids. Prog Cardiovasc Dis 15:289, 1972
190. Rovetto MJ, Lamberton WF, Neely JR: Mechanisms of glycolytic inhibition in ischemic rat hearts. Circ Res 37:742, 1975
191. Neely JR, Feuvray D: Metabolic products and myocardial ischemia. Am J Pathol 102:282, 1981
192. Tennant R, Wiggers CJ: The effect of coronary occlusion on myocardial contraction. Am J Physiol 112:351, 1935
193. Allen DG, Orchard CH: Myocardial contractile function during ischemia and hypoxia. Circ Res 60:153, 1987
194. Braasch W, Gudbjarnason S, Puri PS et al: Early changes in energy metabolism in the myocardium following acute coronary artery occlusion in anesthetized dogs. Circ Res 23:429, 1968
195. Dunn RB, Griggs DM Jr: Transmural gradients in ventricular tissue metabolites produced by stopping coronary blood flow in the dog. Circ Res 37:438, 1975
196. Watson RM, Markle DR, Ro YM et al: Transmural pH gradient in canine myocardial ischemia. Am J Physiol 246:H232, 1984
197. Reibel DK, Rovetto MJ: Myocardial ATP synthesis and mechanical function following oxygen deficiency. Am J Physiol 234:H620, 1978
198. Steenbergen C, Deleeuw G, Rich T et al: Effects of acidosis and ischemia on contractility and intracellular pH of rat heart. Circ Res 41:849, 1977
199. Kanaide H, Yoshimura R, Makino N et al: Regional myocardial function and metabolism during acute coronary artery occlusion. Am J Physiol 242:H980, 1982
200. Allen DG, Morris PG, Orchard CH et al: A nuclear magnetic resonance study of metabolism in the ferret heart during hypoxia and inhibition of glycolysis. J Physiol 361:185, 1985
201. Hearse DJ: Oxygen deprivation and early myocardial contractile failure: A reassessment of the possible role of adenosine triphosphate. Am J Cardiol 44:1115, 1979
202. Schaefer S, Camacho SA, Gober J et al: Response of myocardial metabolites to graded regional ischemia: ^{31}P NMR spectroscopy of porcine myocardium in vivo. Circ Res 64:968, 1989
203. Kentish JC: The effects of inorganic phosphate and creatine phosphate on force production in skinned muscles from rat ventricle. J Physiol 370:585, 1986
204. Kusuoka H, Weisfeldt ML, Zweier JL et al: Mechanism of early contractile failure during hypoxia in intact ferret heart: Evidence for modulation of maximal Ca^{2+}-activated force by inorganic phosphate. Circ Res 59:270, 1986

205. Blanchard EM, Solaro RJ: Inhibition of the activation and troponin calcium binding of dog cardiac myofibrils by acidic pH. Circ Res 55:382, 1984
206. Allen DG, Orchard CH: Intracellular calcium concentration during hypoxia and metabolic inhibition in mammalian ventricular muscle. J Physiol 339:107, 1983
207. Smith GL, Allen DG: Effects of metabolic blockade on intracellular calcium concentration in isolated ferret ventricular muscle. Circ Res 62:1223, 1988
208. Eisner DA, Nichols CG, O'Neill SC et al: The effects of metabolic inhibition on intracellular calcium and pH in isolated rat ventricular cells. J Physiol 411:393, 1989
209. Jennings RB, Reimer KA: Lethal myocardial ischemic injury. Am J Pathol 102:241, 1981
210. Jennings RB, Hawkins HK, Lowe JE et al: Relation between high energy phosphate and lethal injury in myocardial ischemia in the dog. Am J Pathol 92:187, 1978
211. Reimer KA, Jennings RB, Hill ML: Total ischemia in dog hearts, in vitro: II. High energy phosphate depletion and associated defects in energy metabolism, cell volume regulation, and sarcolemmal integrity. Circ Res 49:901, 1981
212. Trump BF, Mergner WJ, Kahng MW et al: Studies on the subcellular pathophysiology of ischemia. Circulation 53(Suppl I):I-17, 1976
213. Vary TC, Angelakos ET, Schaffer SW: Relationship between adenine nucleotide metabolism and irreversible ischemic tissue damage in isolated perfused rat heart. Circ Res 45:218, 1979
214. Neely JR, Grotyohann LW: Role of glycolytic products in damage to ischemic myocardium: Dissociation of adenosine triphosphate levels and recovery of function of reperfused ischemic hearts. Circ Res 55:816, 1984
215. Farber JL, Chien KR, Mittnacht S Jr: The pathogenesis of irreversible cell injury in ischemia. Am J Pathol 102:271, 1981
216. Tani M, Neely JR: Role of intracellular Na^+ in Ca^{2+} overload and depressed recovery of ventricular function of reperfused ischemic rat hearts: Possible involvement of H^+-Na^+ and Na^+-Ca^{2+} exchange. Circ Res 65:1045, 1989
217. Watts JA, Koch CD, LaNoue KF: Effects of Ca^{2+} antagonism on energy metabolism: Ca^{2+} and heart function after ischemia. Am J Physiol 238:H909, 1980
218. Cheung JY, Leaf A, Bonventre JV: Mechanism of protection by verapamil and nifedipine from anoxic injury in isolated cardiac myocytes. Am J Physiol 246:C323, 1984
219. Skolnick AE, Frishman WH: Calcium channel blockers in myocardial infarction. Arch Intern Med 149:1669, 1989
220. McAlpine HM, Morton JJ, Leckie B et al: Neuroendocrine activation after acute myocardial infarction. Br Heart J 60:117, 1988
221. Katz AM, Messineo FC: Lipid-membrane interactions and the pathogenesis of ischemic damage in the myocardium. Circ Res 48:1, 1981
222. Simonson S, Kjekshus JK: The effect of free fatty acids on myocardial oxygen consumption during atrial pacing and catecholamine infusion in man. Circulation 58:484, 1978
223. van der Vusse GJ, Roemen ThHM, Prinzen FW et al: Uptake and tissue content of fatty acids in dog myocardium under normoxic and ischemic conditions. Circ Res 50:538, 1982
224. Mjos OD: Effect of free fatty acids on myocardial function and oxygen consumption in intact dogs. J Clin Invest 50:1386, 1971
225. Liedtke A, Nellis S, Neely JR: Effects of excess free fatty acids on mechanical and metabolic function in normal and ischemic myocardium in swine. Circ Res 43:652, 1978
226. Corr PB, Gross RW, Sobel BE: Amphipathic metabolites and membrane dysfunction in ischemic myocardium. Circ Res 55:135, 1984
227. Tyberg JV, Forrester JS, Wyatt HL et al: An analysis of segmental ischemic dysfunction utilizing the pressure-length loop. Circulation 49:748, 1974
228. Lew WYW, Chen Z, Guth B et al: Mechanisms of augmented segment shortening in nonischemic areas during acute ischemia of the canine left ventricle. Circ Res 56:351, 1985
229. Goto Y, Igarashi Y, Yasumura Y et al: Integrated regional work equals total left ventricular work in regionally ischemic canine heart. Am J Physiol 254:H894, 1988
230. Akaishi M, Weintraub WS, Schneider RM et al: Analysis of systolic bulging: Mechanical characteristics of acutely ischemic myocardium in the conscious dog. Circ Res 58:209, 1986
231. Lew WYW, Ban-Hayashi E: Mechanisms of improving regional and global ventricular function by preload alterations during acute ischemia in the canine left ventricle. Circulation 72:1125, 1985
232. Yoran C, Sonnenblick EH, Kirk ES: Contractile reserve and left ventricular function in regional myocardial ischemia in the dog. Circulation 66:121, 1982
233. Roan P, Scales F, Saffer S et al: Functional characterization of left ventricular segmental responses during the initial 24 hr and 1 wk after experimental canine myocardial infarction. J Clin Invest 64:1074, 1979
234. Boden WE, Liang C, Hood WB Jr: Postextrasystolic potentiation of regional mechanical performance during prolonged myocardial ischemia in the dog. Circulation 61:1063, 1980
235. Weigner AW, Allen GJ, Bing OHL: Weak and strong myocardium in series: Implications for segmental dysfunction. Am J Physiol 235:H776, 1978
236. Takayama M, Norris RM, Brown MA et al: Postsystolic shortening of acutely ischemic canine myocardium predicts early and late recovery of function after coronary artery reperfusion. Circulation 78:994, 1988
237. Gallagher KP, Kumada T, Koziol JA et al: Significance of regional wall thickening abnormalities relative to transmural myocardial perfusion in anesthetized dogs. Circulation 62:1266, 1980
238. Vatner SF: Correlation between acute reductions in myocardial blood flow and function in conscious dogs. Circ Res 47:201, 1980
239. Gallagher KP, Osakada G, Hess OM et al: Subepicardial segmental function during coronary stenosis and the role of myocardial fiber orientation. Circ Res 50:352, 1982
240. Chu A, Cobb FR: Reperfusion alters the relation between blood flow and the remaining myocardial infarction. Circulation 79:884, 1989
241. Bogen DK, Rabinowitz SA, Needleman A et al: An analysis of the mechanical disadvantage of myocardial infarction in the canine left ventricle. Circ Res 47:728, 1980
242. Cox DA, Vatner SF: Myocardial function in areas of heterogeneous perfusion after coronary artery occlusion in conscious dogs. Circulation 66:1154, 1982
243. Gallagher KP, Gerren RA, Stirling MC et al: The distribution of functional impairment across the lateral border of acutely ischemic myocardium. Circ Res 58:570, 1986
244. Theroux P, Ross J Jr, Franklin D et al: Regional myocardial function and dimensions early and late after myocardial infarction in the unanesthetized dog. Circ Res 40:158, 1977
245. Jaarsma W, Visser CA, Eenige Van MJ et al: Prognostic implications of regional hyperkinesia and remote asynergy of noninfarcted myocardium. Am J Cardiol 58:394, 1986
246. Grines CL, Topol EJ, Califf RM et al: Prognostic implications and predictors of enhanced regional wall motion of the noninfarct zone after thrombolysis and angioplasty therapy of acute myocardial infarction. Circulation 80:245, 1989
247. Goto Y, Igarashi Y, Yamada O et al: Hyperkinesis without the Frank-Starling mechanism in a nonischemic region of acutely ischemic excised canine heart. Circulation 77:468, 1988
248. Lew WYW: Influence of ischemic zone size on nonischemic area function in the canine left ventricle. Am J Physiol 252:H990, 1987
249. Homans DC, Sublett E, Elsperger J et al: Mechanisms of remote myocardial dysfunction during coronary artery occlusion in the presence of multivessel disease. Circulation 74:588, 1986
250. Hess OM, Osakada G, Lavelle JF et al: Left ventricular geometry during partial and complete coronary occlusion in the conscious dog. Int J Cardiol 1:387, 1982
251. Van Houten FX, Serur JR, Borkenhagen DM et al: Experimental myocardial ischemia: IV. Shape and volume changes during "isovolumetric relaxation" in normal and ischemic ventricles. Circulation 62:350, 1980
252. Ludbrook PA, Byrne JD, Tiefenbrunn AJ: Association of asynchronous protodiastolic segmental wall motion with impaired left ventricular relaxation. Circulation 64:1201, 1981
253. Gaasch WH, Blaustein AS, Bing OHL: Asynchronous (segmental early) relaxation of the left ventricle. J Am Coll Cardiol 5:891, 1985
254. Lew WYW, Rasmussen CM: Influence of nonuniformity on rate of left ventricular pressure fall in the dog. Am J Physiol 256:H222, 1989
255. Waters DD, Da Luz P, Wyatt HL et al: Early changes in regional and global left ventricular function induced by graded reductions in regional coronary perfusion. Am J Cardiol 39:537, 1977
256. Kumada T, Karliner JS, Pouleur H et al: Effects of coronary occlusion on early ventricular diastolic events in conscious dogs. Am J Physiol 237:H542, 1979
257. Mann T, Goldberg S, Mudge GH Jr et al: Factors contributing to altered left ventricular diastolic properties during angina pectoris. Circulation 59:14, 1979
258. Carroll JD, Hess OM, Hirzel HO et al: Exercise-induced ischemia: The influence of altered relaxation on early diastolic pressures. Circulation 67:521, 1983
259. Sharma B, Behrens TW, Erlein D et al: Left ventricular diastolic properties and filling characteristics during spontaneous angina pectoris at rest. Am J Cardiol 52:704, 1983
260. Serizawa T, Carabello BA, Grossman W: Effect of pacing-induced ischemia on left ventricular diastolic pressure-volume relations in dogs with coronary stenoses. Circ Res 46:430, 1980
261. Paulus WJ, Serizawa T, Grossman W: Altered left ventricular diastolic properties during pacing-induced ischemia in dogs with coronary stenoses: Potentiation by caffeine. Circ Res 50:218, 1982
262. Momomura S, Bradley AB, Grossman W: Left ventricular diastolic pressure-segment length relations and end-diastolic distensibility in dogs with coronary stenoses: An angina physiology model. Circ Res 55:203, 1984
263. Brutsaert DL, Rademakers FE, Sys SU et al: Analysis of relaxation in the evaluation of ventricular function of the heart. Prog Cardiovasc Dis 28:143, 1985
264. Bonow RO, Vitale DF, Bacharach SL et al: Asynchronous left ventricular regional function and impaired global diastolic filling in patients with coronary artery disease: Reversal after coronary angioplasty. Circulation 71:297, 1985
265. Weisfeldt ML, Armstrong P, Scully HE et al: Incomplete relaxation between beats after myocardial hypoxia and ischemia. J Clin Invest 53:626, 1974
266. Reduto LA, Wickemeyer WJ, Young JB et al: Left ventricular diastolic per-

267. Poliner LR, Farber SH, Glaeser DH et al: Alteration of diastolic filling rate during exercise radionuclide angiography: A highly sensitive technique for detection of coronary artery disease. Circulation 70:942, 1984
268. Aroesty JM, McKay RG, Heller GV et al: Simultaneous assessment of left ventricular systolic and diastolic dysfunction during pacing-induced ischemia. Circulation 71:889, 1985
269. Nakamura Y, Sasayama S, Nonogi H et al: Effects of pacing-induced ischemia on early left ventricular filling and regional myocardial dynamics and their modification by nifedipine. Circulation 76:1232, 1987
270. Lew WYW: Evaluation of left ventricular diastolic function. Circulation 79:1393, 1989
271. Bonow RO, Kent KM, Rosing DR et al: Improved left ventricular diastolic filling in patients with coronary artery disease after percutaneous transluminal coronary angioplasty. Circulation 66:1159, 1982
272. Carroll JD, Hess OM, Hirzel HO et al: Left ventricular systolic and diastolic function in coronary artery disease: Effects of revascularization on exercise-induced ischemia. Circulation 72:119, 1985
273. Forrester JS, Diamond G, Chatterjee K et al: Medical therapy of acute myocardial infarction by application of hemodynamic subsets. N Engl J Med 295:1356 (part I), 1404 (part II), 1976
274. Bertrand ME, Rousseau MF, Lablanche JM et al: Cineangiographic assessment of left ventricular function in the acute phase of transmural myocardial infarction. Am J Cardiol 43:472, 1979
275. Theroux P, Ross J Jr, Franklin D et al: Regional myocardial function in the conscious dog during acute coronary occlusion and responses to morphine, propranolol, nitroglycerin, and lidocaine. Circulation 53:302, 1976
276. Roan PG, Buja LM, Izquierdo C et al: Interrelationships between regional left ventricular function, coronary blood flow, and myocellular necrosis during the initial 24 hours and 1 week after experimental coronary occlusion in awake, unsedated dogs. Circ Res 49:31, 1981
277. Bush LR, Buja LM, Samowitz W et al: Recovery of left ventricular segmental function after long-term reperfusion following temporary coronary artery occlusion in conscious dogs: Comparison of 2- and 4-hour occlusions. Circ Res 53:248, 1983
278. Lavallee M, Cox D, Patrick TA et al: Salvage of myocardial function by coronary artery reperfusion 1, 2, and 3 hours after occlusion in conscious dogs. Circ Res 53:235, 1983
279. Crexells C, Chatterjee K, Forrester JS et al: Optimal level of filling pressure in the left side of the heart in acute myocardial infarction. N Engl J Med 289:1263, 1973
280. Apstein CS, Grossman W: Opposite initial effects of supply and demand ischemia on left ventricular diastolic compliance: The ischemia-diastolic paradox. J Mol Cell Cardiol 19:119, 1987
281. Hess OM, Osakada G, Lavelle JF et al: Diastolic myocardial wall stiffness and ventricular relaxation during partial and complete coronary artery occlusions in the conscious dog. Circ Res 52:387, 1983
282. Momomura S, Ingwall JS, Parker A et al: The relationships of high energy phosphates, tissue pH, and regional blood flow to diastolic distensibility in the ischemic dog myocardium. Circ Res 57:822, 1985
283. Vogel WM, Apstein CS, Briggs LL et al: Acute alterations in left ventricular diastolic chamber stiffness: Role of the "erectile" effect of coronary arterial pressure and flow in normal and damaged hearts. Circ Res 51:465, 1982
284. Isoyama S, Apstein CS, Wexler LF et al: Acute decrease in left ventricular diastolic chamber distensibility during simulated angina in isolated hearts. Circ Res 61:925, 1987
285. Palacios I, Johnson RA, Newell JB et al: Left ventricular end-diastolic pressure volume relationships with experimental acute global ischemia. Circulation 53:428, 1976
286. Wong BYS, Toyama M, Reis RL et al: Sequential changes in left ventricular compliance during acute coronary occlusion in the isovolumic working canine heart. Circ Res 43:274, 1978
287. Edwards CH II, Rankin JS, McHale PA et al: Effects of ischemia on left ventricular regional function in the conscious dog. Am J Physiol 240:H413, 1981
288. Visner MS, Arentzen CE, Parrish DG et al: Effects of global ischemia on the diastolic properties of the left ventricle in the conscious dog. Circulation 71:610, 1985
289. Glower DD, Schaper J, Kabas JS et al: Relation between reversal of diastolic creep and recovery of systolic function after ischemic myocardial injury in conscious dogs. Circ Res 60:850, 1987
290. Crozatier A, Ashraf M, Franklin D et al: Sarcomere length in experimental myocardial infarction: Evidence for sarcomere overstretch in dyskinetic ventricular regions. J Mol Cell Cardiol 9:785, 1977
291. Sasayama S, Nonogi H, Miyazaki S et al: Changes in diastolic properties of the regional myocardium during pacing-induced ischemia in human subjects. J Am Coll Cardiol 5:599, 1985
292. Paulus WJ, Grossman W, Serizawa T et al: Different effects of two types of ischemia on myocardial systolic and diastolic function. Am J Physiol 248:H719, 1985
293. Bers DM, Bridge JHB: Relaxation of rabbit ventricular muscle by Na-Ca exchange and sarcoplasmic reticulum calcium pump: Ryanodine and voltage sensitivity. Circ Res 65:334, 1989
294. Pfeffer MA, Pfeffer JM, Fishbein MC et al: Myocardial infarct size and ventricular function in rats. Circ Res 44:503, 1979
295. Fletcher PJ, Pfeffer JM, Pfeffer MA et al: Left ventricular diastolic pressure-volume relations in rats with healed myocardial infarction: Effects on systolic function. Circ Res 49:618, 1981
296. Schneider RM, Chu A, Akaishi M et al: Left ventricular ejection fraction after acute coronary occlusion in conscious dogs: Relation to the extent and site of myocardial infarction. Circulation 72:632, 1985
297. Gumm DC, Cooper SM, Thompson SB et al: Influence of risk area size and location on native collateral resistance and ischemic zone perfusion. Am J Physiol 254:H473, 1988
298. Rogers WJ, McDaniel HG, Smith LR et al: Correlation of angiographic estimates of myocardial infarct size and accumulated release of creatine kinase MB isoenzyme in man. Circulation 56:199, 1977
299. Sobel BE, Bresnahan GF, Shell WE et al: Myocardial infarct size in man and its relation to prognosis. Circulation 46:640, 1972
300. Geltman EM, Ehsani AA, Campbell MK et al: The influence of location and extent of myocardial infarction on long-term ventricular dysrhythmia and mortality. Circulation 60:805, 1979
301. Thompson TL, Fletcher EE, Kotavatis V: Enzymatic indices of myocardial necrosis: Influence on short- and long-term prognosis after myocardial infarction. Circulation 59:113, 1979
302. van der Laarse A, Kerkhoff PLM, Vermeer F et al: Relation between infarct size and left ventricular performance assessed in patients with first acute myocardial infarction randomized to intracoronary thrombolytic therapy or to conventional therapy. Am J Cardiol 61:1, 1988
303. Ritchie JL, Cerqueira M, Maynard C et al: Ventricular function and infarct size: The Western Washington Intravenous Streptokinase in Myocardial Infarction Trial. J Am Coll Cardiol 11:689, 1988
304. Strauss HD, Sobel BE, Roberts R: The influence of occult right ventricular infarction on enzymatically estimated infarct size, hemodynamics and prognosis. Circulation 62:503, 1980
305. Thanavaro S, Kleiger RE, Province MA et al: Effect of infarct location on the in-hospital prognosis of patient with first transmural myocardial infarction. Circulation 66:742, 1982
306. Fox R, Hakki A, Iskandrian AS et al: Location of myocardial necrosis as an independent determinant of left ventricular performance: Analysis of 96 patients. Am J Cardiol 53:483, 1984
307. Becker LC, Schuster EH, Jugdutt BI et al: Relationship between myocardial infarct size and occluded bed size in the dog: Difference between left anterior descending and circumflex coronary artery occlusions. Circulation 67:549, 1983
308. Schneider RM, Chu A, Akaishi M et al: Left ventricular ejection fraction after acute coronary occlusion in conscious dogs: Relation to the extent and site of myocardial infarction. Circulation 72:632, 1985
309. Schneider RM, Morris KG, Chu A et al: Relation between myocardial perfusion and left ventricular function following acute coronary occlusion: Disproportionate effects of anterior vs. inferior ischemia. Circ Res 60:60, 1987
310. Hoit BD, Lew WYW: Functional consequences of acute anterior vs. posterior wall ischemia in canine left ventricles. Am J Physiol 254:H1065, 1988
311. Marino PN, Kass DA, Becker LC et al: Influence of site of regional ischemia on nonischemic thickening in anesthetized dogs. Am J Physiol 256:H1417, 1989
312. Lombardi F, Casalone C, Bella PD et al: Global versus regional myocardial ischaemia: Differences in cardiovascular and sympathetic responses in cat. Cardiovasc Res 18:14, 1984
313. Barber MJ, Mueller TM, Henry D et al: Transmural myocardial infarction in the dog produces sympathectomy in noninfarcted myocardium. Circulation 67:787, 1983
314. Barber MJ, Mueller TM, Davies BG et al: Interruption of sympathetic and vagal-mediated afferent responses by transmural myocardial infarction. Circulation 72:623, 1985
315. Inoue H, Skale BT, Zipes DP: Effects of ischemia on cardiac afferent sympathetic and vagal reflexes in dog. Am J Physiol 255:H26, 1988
316. Martins JB, Lewis R, Wendt D et al: Subendocardial infarction produces epicardial parasympathetic denervation in canine left ventricle. Am J Physiol 256:H859, 1989
317. Inoue H, Zipes DP: Time course of denervation of efferent sympathetic and vagal nerves after occlusion of the coronary artery in the canine heart. Circ Res 62:1111, 1988
318. Thames MD, Kloppfenstein HS, Abboud FM et al: Preferential distribution of inhibitory cardiac receptors with vagal afferents to the inferoposterior wall of the left ventricle activated during coronary occlusion in the dog. Circ Res 43:512, 1978
319. Walker JL, Thames MD, Abboud FM et al: Preferential distribution of inhibitory cardiac receptors in left ventricle of the dog. Am J Physiol 235:H188, 1978
320. Minisi AJ, Thames MD: Effect of chronic myocardial infarction on vagal cardiopulmonary baroreflex. Circ Res 65:396, 1989
321. George M, Greenwood TW: Relation between bradycardia and the site of myocardial infarction. Lancet 2:739, 1967
322. Adgey AAJ, Allen JD, Geddes JS et al: Acute phase of myocardial infarction. Lancet 2:501, 1979
323. Webb SW, Adgey AAJ, Pantridge JF: Autonomic disturbance at onset of

323. acute myocardial infarction. Br Med J 3:89, 1972
324. Wei JY, Markis JE, Malagold M et al: Cardiovascular reflexes stimulated by reperfusion of ischemic myocardium in acute myocardial infarction. Circulation 67:796, 1983
325. Perez-Gomez F, De Dios M, Rey J et al: Prinzmetal's angina: Reflex cardiovascular response during episode of pain. Br Heart J 42:81, 1979
326. La Rovere MT, Specchia G, Mortara A et al: Baroreflex sensitivity, clinical correlates, and cardiovascular mortality among patients with a first myocardial infarction: A prospective study. Circulation 78:816, 1988
327. Heyndrickx GR, Baig H, Nellens P et al: Depression of regional blood flow and wall thickening after brief coronary occlusions. Am J Physiol 234:H653, 1978
328. Gruppo Italiano per lo Studio della Streptochinasi nell'infarto miocardico (GISSI). Effectiveness of intravenous thrombolytic treatment in acute myocardial infarction. Lancet 1:397, 1986
329. Martin GV, Sheehan FH, Stadius M et al: Intravenous streptokinase for acute myocardial infarction: Effects on global and regional systolic function. Circulation 78:258, 1988
330. Sheehan FH, Doerr R, Schmidt WG et al: Early recovery of left ventricular function after thrombolytic therapy for acute myocardial infarction: An important determinant of survival. J Am Coll Cardiol 12:289, 1988
331. Bassand J-P, Machecourt J, Cassagnes J et al: Multicenter trial of intravenous anisoylated plasminogen streptokinase activator complex (APSAC) in acute myocardial infarction: Effects on infarct size and left ventricular function. J Am Coll Cardiol 13:988, 1989
332. Ong L, Reiser P, Coromillas J et al: Left ventricular function and rapid release of creatine kinase MB in acute myocardial infarction: Evidence for spontaneous reperfusion. N Engl J Med 309:1, 1983
333. De Feyter PJ, van Eenige MJ, van der Wall EE et al: Effects of spontaneous and streptokinase-induced recanalization on left ventricular function after myocardial infarction. Circulation 67:1039, 1983
334. Ito BR, Tate H, Kobayashi M et al: Reversibly injured, postischemic canine myocardium retains normal contractile reserve. Circ Res 61:834, 1987
335. Kusuoka H, Porterfield JK, Weisman HF et al: Pathophysiology and pathogenesis of stunned myocardium: Depressed Ca^{2+} activation of contraction as a consequence of reperfusion-induced cellular calcium overload in ferret hearts. J Clin Invest 79:950, 1987
336. Zhao M, Zhang H, Robinson TF et al: Profound structural alterations of the extracellular collagen matrix in postischemic dysfunctional ("stunned") but viable myocardium. J Am Coll Cardiol 10:1322, 1987
337. Gregg DE, Patterson RE: Functional importance of the coronary collaterals. N Engl J Med 303:1404, 1980
338. Newman PE: The coronary collateral circulation: Determinants and functional significance in ischemic heart disease. Am Heart J 102:431, 1981
339. Levin DC: Pathways and functional significance of the coronary collateral circulation. Circulation 50:831, 1974
340. Schaper W, Flameng W, Winkler B et al: Quantification of collateral resistance in acute and chronic experimental coronary occlusion in the dog. Circ Res 39:371, 1976
341. Williams DO, Amsterdam EA, Miller RR et al: Functional significance of coronary collateral vessels in patients with acute myocardial infarction: Relation to pump performance, cardiogenic shock and survival. Am J Cardiol 37:345, 1976
342. Nohara R, Kambara H, Murakami T et al: Collateral function in early acute myocardial infarction. Am J Cardiol 52:955, 1983
343. Rogers WJ, Hood WP Jr, Mantle JA et al: Return of left ventricular function after reperfusion in patients with myocardial infarction: Importance of subtotal stenoses or intact collaterals. Circulation 69:338, 1984
344. Pirzada FA, Ekong EA, Vokanas PS et al: Experimental myocardial infarction: XIII. Sequential changes in left ventricular pressure-length relationships in the acute phase. Circulation 53:970, 1976
345. Kumar R, Hood WB Jr, Joison J et al: Experimental myocardial infarction: II. Acute depression and subsequent recovery of left ventricular function: Serial measurements in intact conscious dogs. J Clin Invest 49:55, 1970
346. Kupper W, Bleifeld W, Hanrath P et al: Left ventricular hemodynamics and function in acute myocardial infarction: Studies during the acute phase, convalescence and late recovery. Am J Cardiol 40:900, 1970
347. Gibbons EF, Hogan RD, Franklin TD et al: The natural history of regional dysfunction in a canine preparation of chronic infarction. Circulation 71:394, 1985
348. Hood WB Jr, Bianco JA, Kumar R et al: Experimental myocardial infarction: IV. Reduction of left ventricular compliance in the healing phase. J Clin Invest 49:1316, 1970
349. Choong CY, Gibbons EF, Hogan RD et al: Relationship of functional recovery to scar contraction after myocardial infarction in the canine left ventricle. Am Heart J 117:819, 1989
350. Sasayama S, Gallagher KP, Kemper WS et al: Regional left ventricular wall thickness early and late after coronary occlusion in the conscious dog. Am J Physiol 240:H293, 1981
351. Anversa P, Loud AV, Levicky V et al: Left ventricular failure induced by myocardial infarction: I. Myocyte hypertrophy. Am J Physiol 248:H876, 1985
352. Wackers FJ, Berger HJ, Weinberg MA et al: Spontaneous changes in left ventricular function over the first 24 hours of acute myocardial infarction: Implications for evaluating early therapeutic interventions. Circulation 66:748, 1982
353. Schelbert HR, Henning H, Ashburn WL et al: Serial measurements of left ventricular ejection fraction by radionuclide angiography early and late after myocardial infarction. Am J Cardiol 38:407, 1976
354. Reduto LA, Berger HJ, Cohen LS et al: Sequential radionuclide assessment of left and right ventricular performance after acute transmural myocardial infarction. Ann Intern Med 89:441, 1978
355. Rahimtoola SH, DiGilio MM, Ehsani A et al: Changes in left ventricular performance from early after acute myocardial infarction to the convalescent phase. Circulation 46:770, 1972
356. Weisman HF, Healy B: Myocardial infarct expansion, infarct extension, and reinfarction: Pathophysiologic concepts. Prog Cardiovasc Dis 30:73, 1987
357. Weisman HF, Bush DE, Mannisi JA et al: Cellular mechanisms of myocardial infarct expansion. Circulation 78:186, 1988
358. McKay RG, Pfeffer MA, Pasternak RC et al: Left ventricular remodeling after myocardial infarction: A corollary to infarct expansion. Circulation 74:693, 1986
359. Warren SE, Royal HD, Markis JE et al: Time course of left ventricular dilation after myocardial infarction: Influence of infarct-related artery and success of coronary thrombolysis. J Am Coll Cardiol 11:12, 1988
360. Pfeffer MA, Lamas GA, Vaughan DE et al: Effect of captopril on progressive ventricular dilatation after anterior myocardial infarction. N Engl J Med 319:80, 1988
361. Pfeffer JM, Pfeffer MA, Braunwald E: Influence of chronic captopril therapy on the infarcted left ventricle of the rat. Circ Res 57:84, 1985
362. Hochman JS, Choo H: Limitation of myocardial infarct expansion by reperfusion independent of myocardial salvage. Circulation 75:299, 1987
363. Faxon DP, Ryan TJ, Davis KB et al: Prognostic significance of angiographically documented left ventricular aneurysm from the Coronary Artery Surgery Study (CASS). Am J Cardiol 50:157, 1982
364. Visser CA, Kan G, Meltzer RS et al: Incidence, timing and prognostic value of left ventricular aneurysm formation after myocardial infarction: A prospective, serial echocardiographic study of 158 patients. Am J Cardiol 57:729, 1986
365. Meizlish JL, Berger HJ, Plankey M et al: Functional left ventricular aneurysm formation after acute anterior transmural myocardial infarction: Incidence, natural history, and prognostic implications. N Engl J Med 311:1001, 1984
366. Forman MB, Collins HW, Kopelman HA et al: Determinants of left ventricular aneurysm formation after anterior myocardial infarction: A clinical and angiographic study. J Am Coll Cardiol 8:1256, 1986
367. Hirai T, Fujita M, Nakajima H et al: Importance of collateral circulation for prevention of left ventricular aneurysm formation in acute myocardial infarction. Circulation 79:791, 1989
368. Gueret P, Dubourg O, Ferrier A et al: Effects of full-dose heparin anticoagulation on the development of left ventricular thrombosis in acute transmural myocardial infarction. J Am Coll Cardiol 8:419, 1986
369. Lamas GA, Vaughan DE, Pfeffer MA: Left ventricular thrombus formation after first anterior wall acute myocardial infarction. Am J Cardiol 62:31, 1988
370. Beppu S, Izumi S, Miyatake K et al: Abnormal blood pathways in left ventricular cavity in acute myocardial infarction: Experimental observations with special reference to regional wall motion abnormality and hemostasis. Circulation 78:157, 1988
371. Johannessen K-A, Nordrehaug JE, von der Lippe G: Increased occurrence of left ventricular thrombi during early treatment with timolol in patients with acute myocardial infarction. Circulation 75:151, 1987
372. Turpie AGG, Robinson JG, Doyle DJ et al: Comparison of high-dose with low-dose subcutaneous heparin to prevent left ventricular mural thrombosis in patients with acute transmural anterior myocardial infarction. N Engl J Med 320:352, 1989

MEASUREMENT OF MYOCARDIAL INFARCTION SIZE

L. Maximilian Buja ▪ James T. Willerson

The extent of myocardial necrosis associated with myocardial infarction is of primary importance in determining whether left ventricular dysfunction develops, including the "power failure" complications of cardiogenic shock, congestive heart failure, and/or recurrent and medically refractory arrhythmias (Fig. 67.1).[1] This observation has led to extensive efforts to develop sensitive and noninvasive methods for sizing myocardial infarcts,[2-19] and it has also been a stimulus for efforts to reduce infarct size.[20-30] In this review we will describe current methods used to estimate infarct size in humans, emphasizing the current abilities and limitations in the measurement of infarct size.

The methods used presently vary from enzymatic measurements to imaging techniques. Each of the current methods has certain limitations, but several provide good means of estimating the relative extent of myocardial necrosis.

ENZYMATIC ESTIMATES OF INFARCT SIZE

Measurements of creatine kinase (CK) and its myocardial specific isoenzyme, CK-MB, are currently the most sensitive and specific enzymatic estimates for diagnosing acute myocardial infarction.[2-4,6] Myocardial CK depletion is proportional to infarct size in experimental animals.[5,6] Sobel and co-workers have demonstrated that quantitative estimates of infarct size may be obtained not only by measurements of tissue CK but also by analysis of CK in systemic venous blood.[5,6] They developed a mathematical model based on the rate of release of myocardial CK into the circulation, its volume and distribution, and its clearance rate, and they estimated infarct size as CK lost from 1 g of myocardium undergoing homogeneous infarction (CK-gram equivalent). This method provides accurate estimates of the extent of infarction in animals[31] and in patients.[32] It has been demonstrated that enzymatically estimated infarct size predicts the risk of subsequent death from pump failure and arrhythmias and the functional class of survivors of infarction.[33,34] CK-MB estimates of infarct size also correlate with the percentage of abnormally contracting left ventricular segments and left ventricular ejection fraction measured by radionuclide ventriculography[35] and by bi-plane angiography.[36]

The CK method for estimating infarct size has certain limitations. First, large infarcts are underestimated by this technique because less CK is released from areas of severely reduced blood flow at the center of the infarct.[37] Coronary reperfusion during evolving infarction causes a greater and earlier release of CK per gram of infarcted tissue than does permanent coronary occlusion.[38] This is a potentially important limitation when one considers that thrombolytic therapy is used frequently in patients seen within the first few hours of the onset of symptoms with clinical evidence of an acute transmural (Q wave) myocardial infarction. In addition, there is a certain incidence of drug-induced and spontaneous reperfusion associated with coronary arterial spasm or coronary thrombosis. CK drainage from the heart is from venous and lymphatic flow; thus, increases in either may alter the amount of CK that appears in the systemic circulation, resulting in an overestimation of infarct size by this approach. Propranolol, sedatives, and anesthetics may alter the rate of CK removal from the circulation,

---

Supported in part by NHLBI Ischemic SCOR HL-17669 and the Moss Heart Fund, Dallas, Texas.

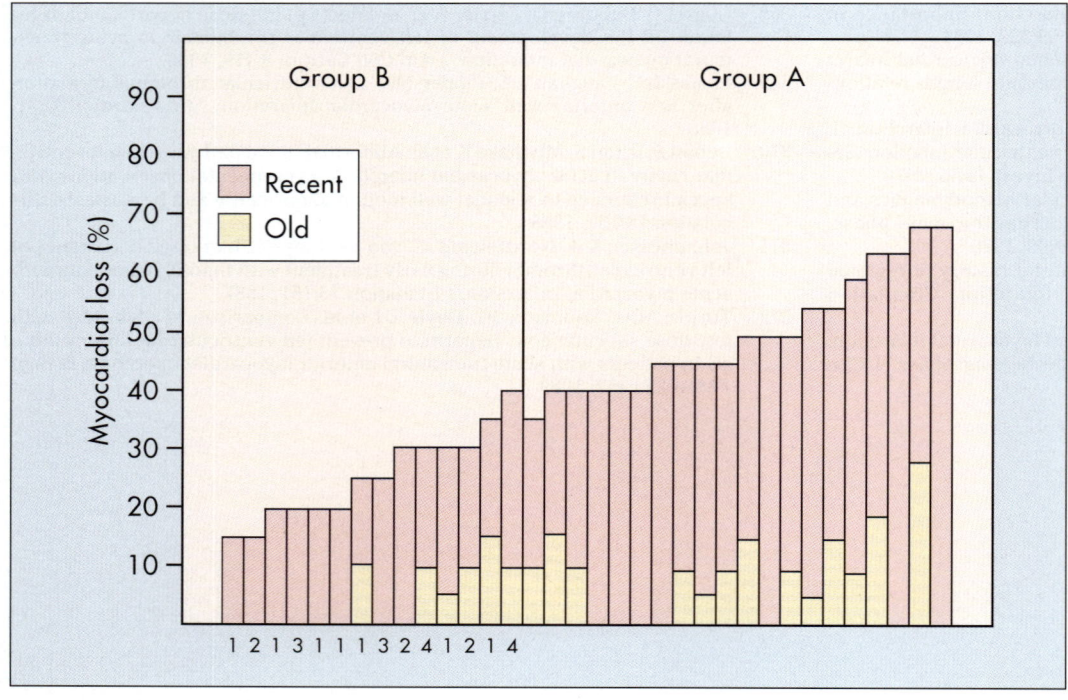

FIGURE 67.1 Relationship between infarct size in patients dying after myocardial infarction with (group A) and without cardiogenic shock (group B). Patients dying with cardiogenic shock generally had greater than or equal to 40% of their ventricular muscle mass irreversibly damaged. (Modified from Page DL, Caulfield JB, Kastor JA et al: Myocardial changes associated with cardiogenic shock. N Engl J Med 285:133, 1971)

thus influencing the estimation of infarct size by this method.[39] The plasma disappearance rate (Kd) for CK varies among individuals and, thus, some investigators believe that Kd should be calculated from the descending limb of the CK time–activity curve for every subject who is studied, to ensure the most accurate estimate of infarct size. Using CK alone as a marker of myocardial damage may result in overestimation of infarct size, too, especially in patients who are hypotensive, have skeletal muscle injury, or are in shock, since some of the CK may come from organs other than the heart. More accurate estimates of infarct size are obtained by measuring CK-MB, especially when this is done by quantitative measurement of CK-MB concentration, such as by radio-immunoassay.[40,41] Estimates of infarct size using CK or CK-MB measurements require hours to several days for their completion. Typically, one needs to identify the upstroke and descending limb of the CK time–activity curve for an accurate measurement and frequent sampling of CK-MB (*i.e.*, every 4 to 6 hours is ordinarily necessary for a period of 24 hours to 36 hours). Thus, a rapid estimate of infarct size is generally not available using this approach. However, recent work suggests that analysis of isoforms of CK-MM or CK-MB in plasma holds promise for rapid detection of myocardial infarction and coronary revascularization, although estimation of infarct size with isoforms involves problems similar to those discussed above.[42,43]

INFARCT-AVID IMAGING FOR MEASURING INFARCT SIZE
TECHNETIUM-99m STANNOUS PYROPHOSPHATE IMAGING

Technetium-99m stannous pyrophosphate has been the most widely used imaging agent to detect myocardial infarction. In animals, increased uptake of pyrophosphate requires cell necrosis, increases in intracellular calcium, and some residual blood flow to the area of cell necrosis.[10,14] The delivery of pyrophosphate to the area of infarction is dependent on coronary blood flow, and maximal pyrophosphate uptake generally occurs in regions where coronary blood flow has been reduced to 10% to 40% of control values.[10,14] The pyrophosphate scintigrams generally become abnormal within 12 hours of the appearance of symptoms suggestive of infarction, increase in positivity over the first 24 to 72 hours, and become negative by approximately 1 week after infarction (Fig. 67.2).[10–12,14] The sensitivity of this technique for the diagnosis of acute myocardial infarction is approximately 90%[44,45] when serial myocardial imaging is used and the studies are interpreted by experienced observers. Substantial evidence exists that pyrophosphate accumulation occurs primarily in irreversibly damaged cells (Fig. 67.3).[10–12,14,44,46] Single photon emission tomography (SPECT imaging) has proved useful in allowing a three-dimensional estimate of infarct presence and size with pyrophosphate (Fig. 67.4).[47,48] SPECT imaging with pyrophosphate allows the detection of infarcts less than 3 g in size in animals,[49] improves the specificity and sensitivity of pyrophosphate imaging in the detection of small myocardial infarcts in patients,[47,48] and allows an accurate estimate of infarct size independent of infarct location in animal models (Fig. 67.5).[49] Furthermore, SPECT imaging with pyrophosphate estimates of infarct size correlate closely with CK estimates of infarct size in patients.[50]

There are also some problems encountered with pyrophosphate in identifying new myocardial infarction and sizing infarcts in patients.[51] Included are the differentiation of bone and myocardial uptake in some scintigrams; distinguishing blood pool activity from increased pyrophosphate uptake with some infarcts; and the need for serial imaging over 3 to 4 days to identify a new myocardial infarct in some patients. SPECT imaging with pyrophosphate and blood pool overlay helps to eliminate potential difficulty in differentiating blood pool uptake from increased myocardial uptake of pyrophosphate, in identifying infarcts under 3 g in size, and in differentiating bone from increased myocardial uptake of pyrophosphate.[47,48] However, some patients retain persistently positive scintigrams after an earlier infarct,[52,53] and other patients with unstable angina pectoris have abnormal pyrophosphate scintigrams in the absence of other evidence of myocardial infarction.[54] In both of these circumstances, clinicopathologic correlations have often demonstrated the presence of irreversible cellular injury correctly identified by pyrophosphate imaging, even if there were no enzymatic or electrocardiographic evidence indicative of a new myocardial infarction.[44] False-positive results occur rarely in some patients with calcified left ventricular aneurysm or calcific valvular heart disease.

OTHER INFARCT-AVID IMAGING AGENTS

An antibody to myosin has been developed, and it appears to identify irreversibly damaged myocardium in animal models.[55] It may also prove useful in both infarct detection and infarct sizing in patients. Other infarct-avid imaging approaches have been used but, thus far, none appears equal or superior to pyrophosphate scintigraphy.

COMPUTED TOMOGRAPHY

Computed transverse axial tomography (CT scanning) has been used to detect and estimate the size of myocardial infarcts in animals.[56] *In vitro* and *in vivo* studies of canine hearts after experimental myocardial infarction have demonstrated that infarcted myocardium has re-

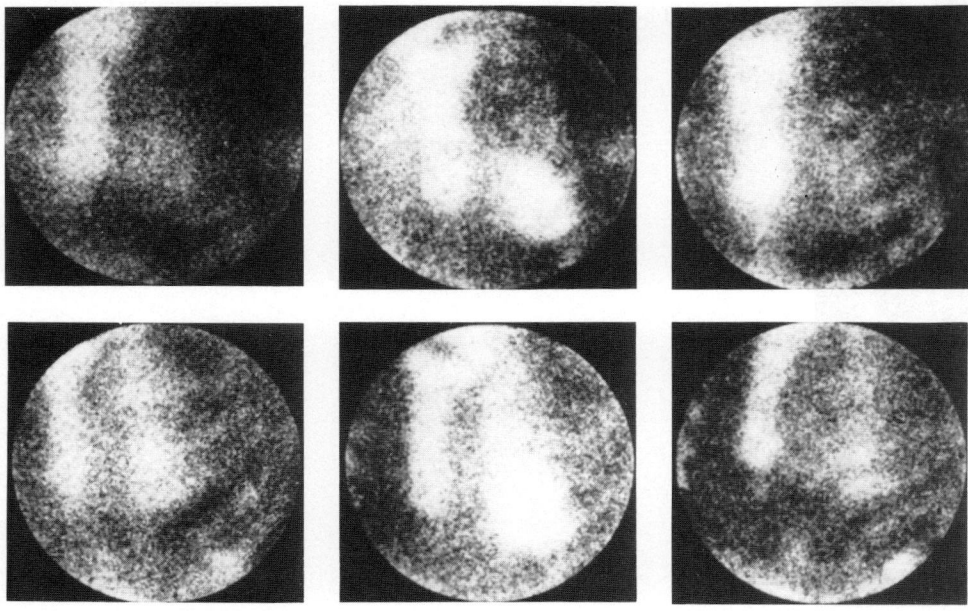

FIGURE 67.2 Increase in intensity of a technetium-99m pyrophosphate myocardial scintigram that occurs with time in most patients with acute transmural myocardial infarction. The left panels demonstrate the faintly positive radioisotope uptake approximately 10 hours after myocardial infarction, the center panels the increased uptake 3 days after infarction, and the right panels the marked resolution in Tc-99m-PPi uptake approximately 7 days after infarction.

duced attenuation, apparently because of edema associated with infarction.[57-61] The intravenous injection of contrast material before sacrifice allows good delineation of the area of infarction and an accurate estimate of infarct size (Fig. 67.6).[56] This technique may have major value in patients because of the recent development of rapid-speed CT scanning with gating capability. This approach should allow relatively accurate measurements of infarct size.

CT scanning is associated with at least moderate radiation exposure. Furthermore, the time after myocardial infarction is a critical issue regarding whether contrast material that is injected is excluded from or actually enters and helps to delineate the region of infarction.[57,58] When more than a few hours elapse after infarction (i.e., more than 14 to 15 hours), collateral blood flow increases to the region of damage, and the area of infarction may be delineated as a region with a slow clearance of the contrast material.[57,58] In patients with renal insufficiency, the need to inject contrast material is a problem since it may lead to further deterioration in renal function. Finally, the need to have rapid-speed CT scanning for optimal resolution and sensitivity in cardiac evaluation makes the expense of this imaging system an important factor in its general availability.

MAGNETIC RESONANCE IMAGING

Studies have indicated that magnetic resonance imaging (MRI) allows the detection of myocardial infarction in animals[62-64] and patients (Fig. 67.7).[65-67] The resolution of this technique is excellent, and MRI imag-

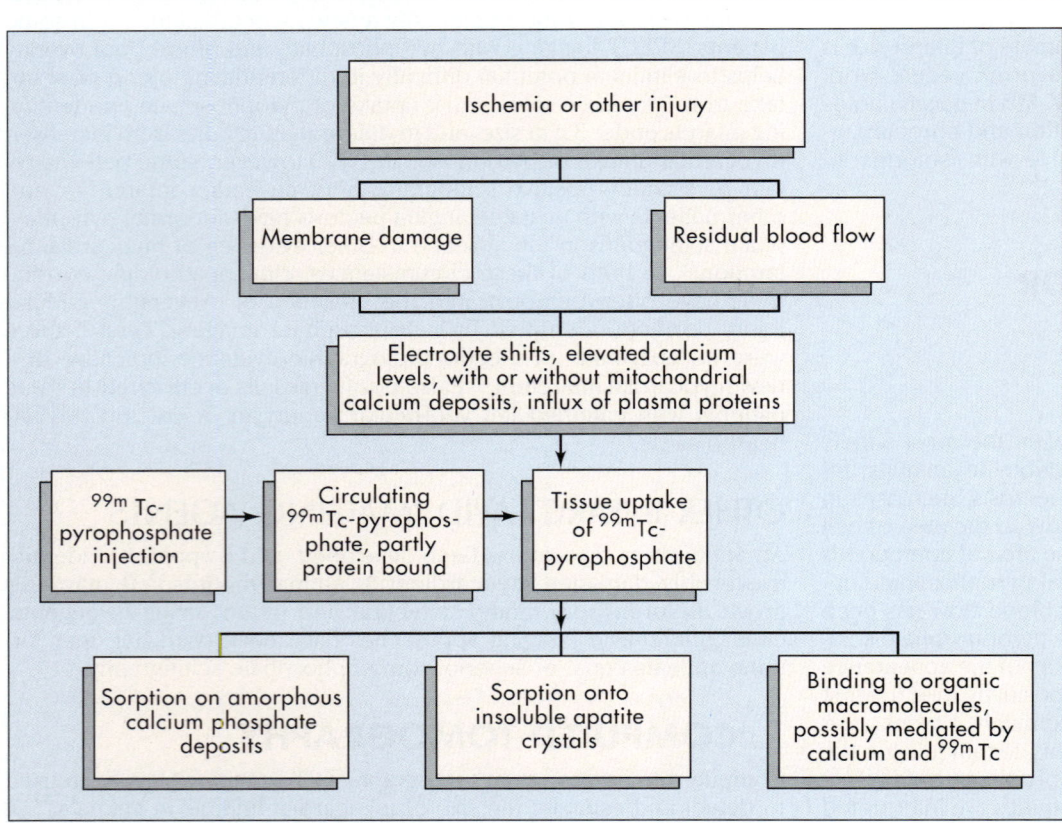

FIGURE 67.3 Pathophysiologic scheme explaining pyrophosphate incorporation in irreversibly damaged myocardium. (Modified from Buja LM, Tofe AJ, Kulkarni PV et al: Sites and mechanisms of localization of technetium-99m phosphorus radiopharmaceuticals in acute myocardial infarcts and other tissues. J Clin Invest 60:724, 1977)

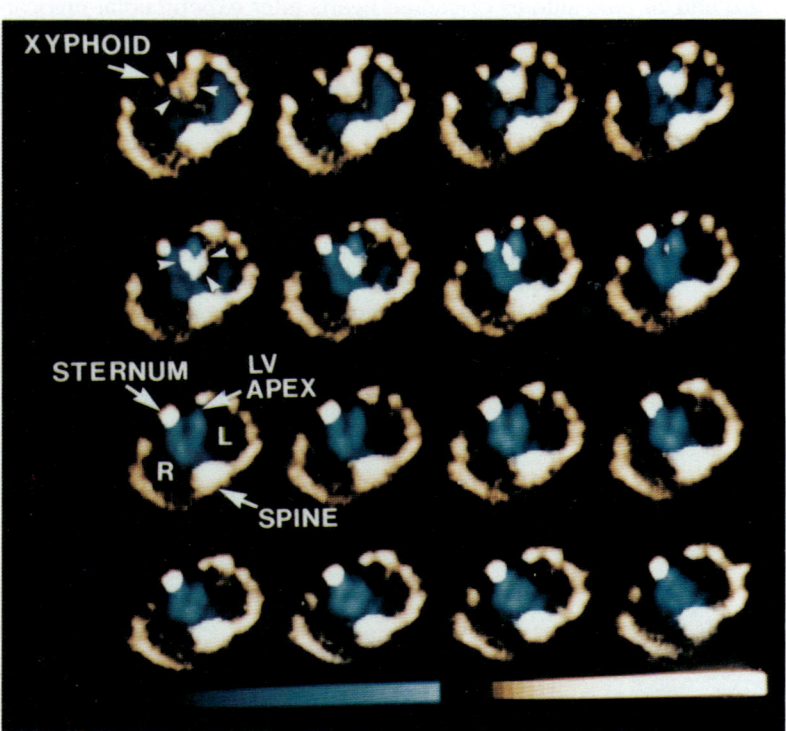

FIGURE 67.4 An overlay of a single photon tomographic emission study (SPECT) of a technetium-99m pyrophosphate scintigram (*gold color*) on the radionuclide ventriculogram (*blue*). Study demonstrates an anterolateral and septal myocardial infarct. This technique allows more accurate localization of infarcts and better estimates of their size.

ing coupled with the injection of a paramagnetic contrast material allows good delineation of regions of experimental infarction in animals.[64,68] A major advantage of this method is that it does not produce any radiation to the patient. However, extensive experience in infarct sizing in animals and patients is still being obtained.

The full potential of MRI in infarct sizing is not yet clear. However, it seems likely that it will be necessary to inject either a perfusion marker or an agent that accumulates selectively in the region of irreversible damage, to allow accurate delineation of the extent of myocardial infarction by MRI. The selection of an ideal agent for infarct delineation and sizing has not yet been accomplished.

QRS PRECORDIAL MAPPING

QRS mapping has also been used to assess directional changes in infarct size.[7,23] This technique is an outgrowth of original efforts that used epicardial ST segment elevation recorded 15 minutes after the onset of permanent coronary artery occlusion in animal models[20] and that demonstrated epicardial ST segment elevation to be a good predictor of the subsequent development of Q waves and the loss of R waves at the same sites 6 and 24 hours later. Furthermore, acute reduction in ST segment elevation following a beneficial pharmacologic intervention correlates with preservation of R wave height and reduction in myocardial CK depletion and infarct size. Changes in the height of the R wave or the development of Q waves at precordial sites of initial ST segment elevation have been used to detect alterations in infarct size in animal models and more recently in patients. With the use of this technique, precordial electrocardiograms are recorded from at least 35 sites on the anterior chest as soon after suspected myocardial infarction as possible. A second precordial map is recorded approximately 1 week later to evaluate changes in the QRS complex at sites initially at risk (i.e., those sites demonstrating ST segment elevation initially).

The major disadvantage of precordial mapping and measuring R wave loss and Q wave development as an estimate of infarct size is that

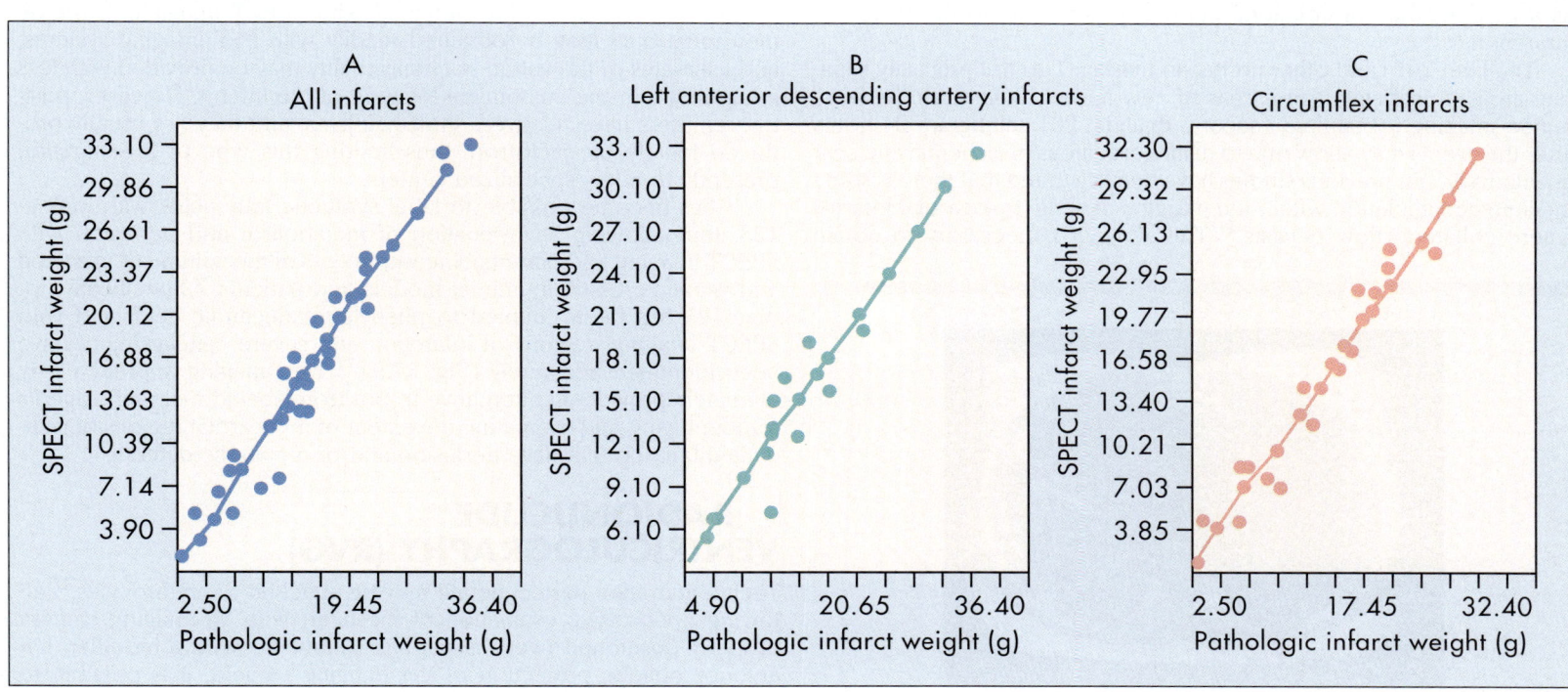

FIGURE 67.5 Ability of technetium-99m pyrophosphate and SPECT imaging to allow accurate measurements of experimentally created canine myocardial infarcts. (Modified from Lewis SE, Devous MD, Sr, Corbett JR et al: Measurement of infarct size in acute canine myocardial infarction by single photon emission computed tomography with technetium-99m pyrophosphate. Am J Cardiol 54:193, 1984)

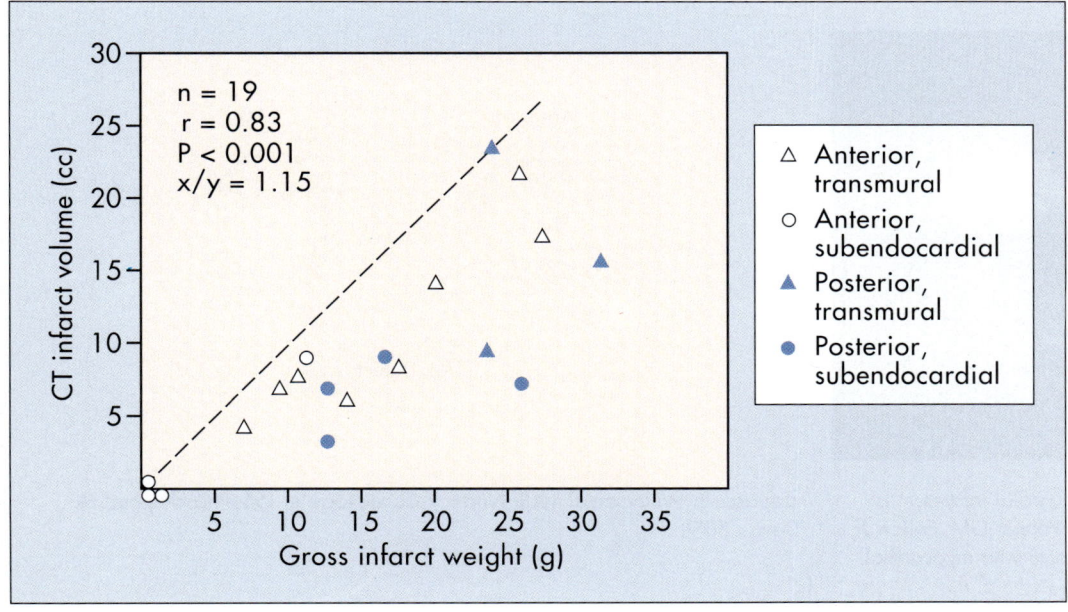

FIGURE 67.6 CT imaging with the injection of contrast allows accurate measurements of infarct size in dog hearts with left anterior descending or circumflex coronary artery occlusion. CT measurements were made *in vitro* after *in vivo* coronary arterial occlusion. The CT estimates underestimated morphologic infarct size as shown. (Modified from Gray WR, Buja LM, Hagler HL et al: Computed tomography for localization and sizing of experimental acute myocardial infarcts. Circulation 58:497, 1978)

it is applicable only to patients with transmural (Q wave) anterior or lateral infarction. Furthermore, for the most accurate assessment, patients should be without intraventricular conduction defects, pericarditis, cardioversion injury to the heart, and previous extensive myocardial infarction. In addition, this approach provides only a qualitative estimation of the extent of infarction. Furthermore, a spontaneous reduction in ST segment elevation occurred within 6 to 12 hours of infarction without being associated with decreased infarct size.

PERFUSION IMAGING DETECTION OF MYOCARDIAL INFARCTION AND ISCHEMIA

Thallium-201 is used widely for myocardial perfusion imaging.[69] It has also been used to detect myocardial infarction[15,16] and to estimate its size for prognostic purposes (Fig. 67.8).[70] Thallium-201 defects identify and provide an opportunity to measure the total area of ischemia, including the infarction and poorly perfused regions. Thallium-201 myocardial scintigraphy is most sensitive in infarct detection within 6 hours of the event, and it becomes less sensitive 24 hours later, presumably as a consequence of collateral perfusion increasing to the region of infarction.[15,16]

Thallium-201 (and other perfusion markers) do not precisely separate areas of ischemia from areas of new and old infarction. Redistribution imaging (obtaining a second thallium-201 scintigram 24 hours after the event) may allow one to distinguish areas of ischemia and scar qualitatively, but previous studies have demonstrated that there is some thallium accumulation within the margins of acute myocardial infarcts where collateral flow persists.[14] Therefore, it is necessary to obtain thallium-201 scintigrams relatively acutely to afford an estimate of infarct size (and the extent of ischemia) in patients and to allow a prediction of prognosis.[70]

METABOLIC PERFUSION IMAGING

Positron emitters have been used to assess metabolism and perfusion in animals[71] and in patients[17] with evolving myocardial infarction. Specifically, ^{13}N ammonia and ^{11}C-labeled fatty acids (^{11}C palmitate) have been used for these purposes. Hypoxic or ischemic myocardium does not extract ^{11}C-labeled palmitate normally, and the area of reduced myocardial uptake can be detected with positron emission tomographic (PET) imaging systems noninvasively. The volume of tissue demonstrating decreased uptake of the fatty acid correlates closely with infarct size in dogs studied 48 hours after infarction,[71] and in patients has shown qualitative comparison with the location and estimates of the area of infarction.[17]

Neither of the position emitters distinguishes ischemic and infarcted tissue or acute and old infarcts, but PET imaging has intrinsic resolution superior to that obtained with SPECT imaging. Three-dimensional data may be obtained readily with PET imaging systems, and estimates of the volume of abnormality may be provided with less concern about the anatomical location of the infarct. However, positron emitters have relatively short half-lives, and they are usually produced locally by cyclotron, thus limiting this type of investigation presently to a few specialized centers.

It has become possible to label synthetic fatty acids with iodine-123, thus allowing an evaluation of metabolism and perfusion with SPECT imaging and potential measurements of the volume of infarcted and ischemic tissue in animal models and patients.[72] Specifically, iodine-123 has been coupled to phenylpentadecanoic acid, and with SPECT imaging, regions of infarction and severe cellular injury have been identified accurately (Fig. 67.9).[72] This imaging approach may ultimately provide an alternative to positron-labeled metabolic agents for identifying and estimating the extent of myocardial regions of ischemia-infarction that have perfusion and/or metabolic defects.

RADIONUCLIDE VENTRICULOGRAPHY (RVG)

Technetium-99m pertechnetate may be attached to erythrocytes,[73] allowing noninvasive evaluation of the heart with an imaging camera properly positioned over the cardiac silhouette. With a modified left anterior oblique projection of the imaging camera, it is possible to separate the left and right ventricles and to measure accurately ejection fraction and ventricular volumes at rest and during exercise (Fig. 67.10).[74-78] In addition, regional wall motion alterations may be esti-

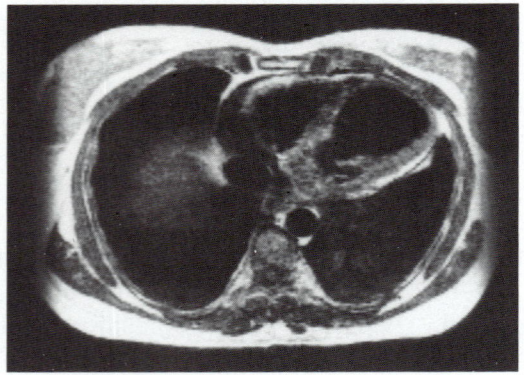

FIGURE 67.7 Magnetic resonance image of a chronic myocardial infarction. The infarct is evidenced by the marked wall thinning in the inferior and apical aspects of the left ventricle.

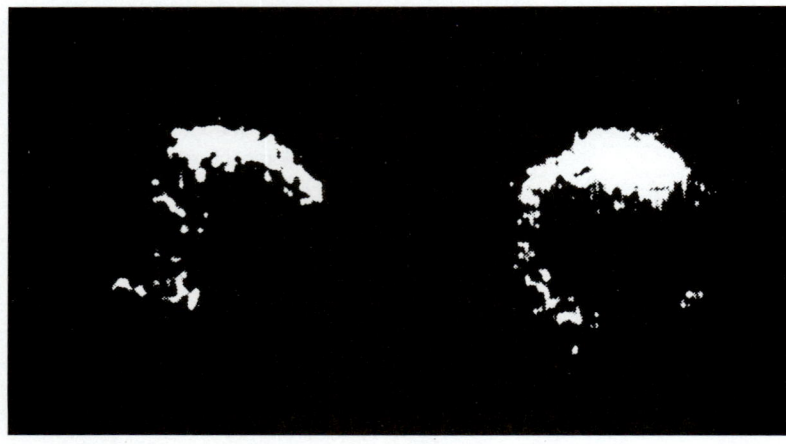

FIGURE 67.8 Perfusion defect associated with recent myocardial infarction is demonstrated by thallium-201 myocardial scintigraphy. (Pohost GM, Fallon JT, Strauss HW: The role of radionuclide techniques in patients with myocardial disease. In Willerson JT (ed): Nuclear Cardiology, p 154. Philadelphia, FA Davis, 1979)

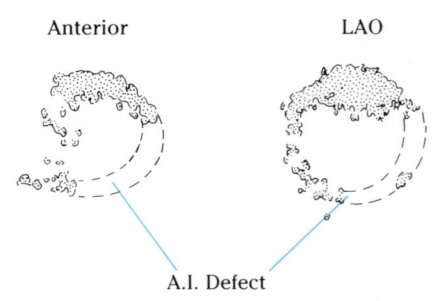

mated with this approach. Thus, one may make noninvasive measurements of global and regional ventricular function, and thereby establish the functional impact of myocardial infarction on ventricular performance. Such measurements include an estimate of the impact of ischemia-infarction (old and new) on ventricular performance. Using this approach, one may determine whether interventions designed to limit infarct size and consequently protect ventricular function have that effect by performing radionuclide ventriculography soon after myocardial infarction and repeating this test 10 days and 6 weeks later. Improvement in global and/or segmental function in properly controlled evaluations suggests a protective effect of a specific intervention.

Decreases in global and/or segmental ventricular function may be caused by old or new myocardial infarction, myocardial ischemia, or some nonischemic independent cause (*i.e.*, myocardial dysfunction associated with viral injury, alcohol abuse, valvular heart disease, or

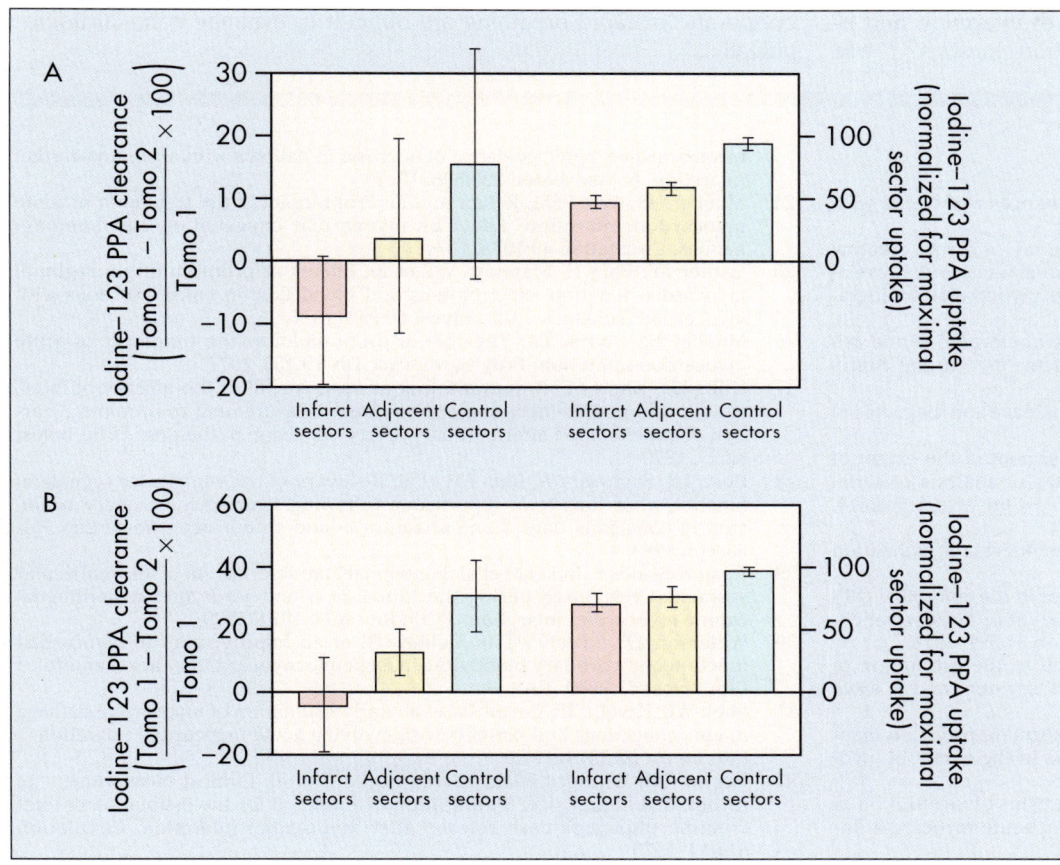

FIGURE 67.9 A: Mean values for iodine-123–phenylpentadecanoic acid (PPA) uptake (*right*) and clearance (*left*) in infarct sectors, sectors adjacent to myocardial infarction, and control left ventricle in experimentally created canine myocardial infarcts. Permanent left anterior descending coronary occlusion was used in this evaluation. Mean ± standard deviations are shown. **B.** Iodine-123 PPA uptake (*right*) and clearance (*left*) in left ventricular sectors in dogs with temporary left anterior descending coronary occlusion and reperfusion. The format is similar to that described in the upper panel. (Modified from Rellas JS, Corbett JR, Kulkarni P et al: Iodine-123 phenylpentadecanoic acid: Detection of acute myocardial infarction and injury using an iodinated fatty acid and single photon emission tomography. Am J Cardiol 52:1326, 1983)

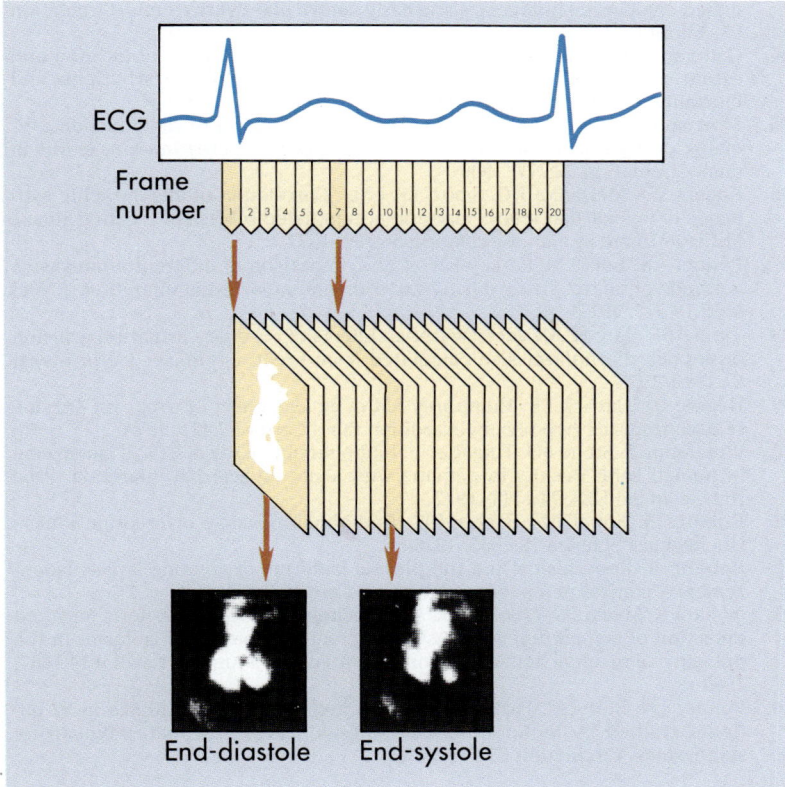

FIGURE 67.10 Technique used for obtaining radionuclide ventriculograms and gated imaging (MUGA imaging). Radionuclide counts are obtained during various portions of the cardiac cycle and are summed and played back so that one may evaluate global and segmental function.

systemic arterial hypertension). Therefore, one needs to distinguish the presence of other nonischemic causes of ventricular dysfunction and use this method in patients with myocardial infarction as the sole cause for altered ventricular function.

TWO-DIMENSIONAL ECHOCARDIOGRAPHY

Two-dimensional echocardiography provides another relatively noninvasive means for repeated evaluation of wall motion in the left ventricle and for determining the functional impact of infarction and ischemia on global and segmental ventricular function. In dogs[79,80] and humans,[81,82] two-dimensional echocardiographic measurements of the extent of infarction usually overestimate infarct size. However, regional systolic wall thickening may provide good identification of the extent of infarction.[80]

Regions of ischemia and infarction will be detected using this approach. In addition, regions of old infarction will not be separated from areas of new infarction. Nevertheless, echocardiography provides a qualitative means of estimating the extent of ischemia-infarction and of identifying alterations in regional and global function. However, not all patients are suitable for echocardiographic evaluation; in particular, those patients with severe intrinsic lung disease, obesity, inability to cooperate, or rapid breathing are difficult to evaluate echocardiographically.

REFERENCES

1. Page DL, Caulfield JB, Kastor JA et al: Myocardial changes associated with cardiogenic shock. N Engl J Med 285:133, 1971
2. Rude RE, Rubin HS, Stone MJ et al: Radioimmunoassay of serum creatine kinase B isoenzyme in the diagnosis of acute myocardial infarction: Correlation with technetium-99m stannous pyrophosphate myocardial scintigraphy. Am J Med 68:405, 1980
3. Roberts R, Gowda KS, Ludbrook PA et al: Specificity of elevated serum MB creatine phosphokinase activity in the diagnosis of acute myocardial infarction. Am J Cardiol 36:433, 1975
4. Roberts R, Sobel BE: Isoenzymes of creatine phosphokinase and diagnosis of myocardial infarction. Ann Intern Med 79:741, 1973
5. Shell WE, Kjekshus JK, Sobel BE: Quantitative assessment of the extent of myocardial infarction in the conscious dog by means of analysis of serial changes in serum creatine phosphokinase activity. J Clin Invest 50:2614, 1971
6. Roberts R, Henry PD, Sobel BE: An improved basis for enzymatic estimation of infarct size. Circulation 52:743, 1975
7. Hillis LD, Askenazi J, Braunwald E et al: Use of changes in the epicardial QRS complex to assess interventions which modify the extent of myocardial necrosis following coronary artery occlusion. Circulation 54:591, 1976
8. Henning H, Hardarson T, Francis G et al: Approach to the estimation of myocardial infarct size by analysis of precordial ST segment and R wave maps. Am J Cardiol 41:1, 1978
9. Maroko PR, Libby P, Covell JW et al: Precordial ST segment elevation mapping: An atraumatic method for assessing alterations in the extent of myocardial ischemic injury. Am J Cardiol 29:223, 1972
10. Buja LM, Tofe AJ, Kulkarni PV et al: Sites and mechanisms of localization of technetium-99m phosphorus radiopharmaceuticals in acute myocardial infarcts and other tissues. J Clin Invest 60:724, 1977
11. Stokely EM, Buja LM, Lewis SE et al: Measurement of acute myocardial infarcts in dogs with 99m-Tc-stannous pyrophosphate scintigrams. J Nucl Med 17:1, 1975
12. Willerson JT, Parkey RW, Stokely EM et al: Infarct sizing with technetium-99m stannous pyrophosphate scintigraphy in dogs and man: Relationship between scintigraphic and precordial mapping estimates of infarct size in patients. Cardiovasc Res 11:291, 1977
13. Lewis M, Buja LM, Saffer S et al: Experimental infarct sizing using computer processing and a three-dimensional model. Science 197:167, 1977
14. Buja LM, Parkey RW, Stokely EM et al: Pathophysiology of technetium-99m stannous pyrophosphate and thallium-201 scintigraphy of acute anterior myocardial infarcts in dogs. J Clin Invest 57:1508, 1976
15. Wackers FJ, Becker AE, Samson G et al: Location and size of acute transmural myocardial infarction estimated from thallium-201 scintiscans: A clinicopathologic study. Circulation 56:72, 1977
16. Wackers FJT, Sokole EB, Samson G et al: Value and limitations of thallium-201 scintigraphy in the acute phase of myocardial infarction. N Engl J Med 295:1, 1976
17. Sobel BE, Weiss ES, Welch MJ et al: Detection of remote myocardial infarction in patients with positron emission transaxial tomography and intravenous ^{11}C-palmitate. Circulation 55:853, 1977
18. Gray WR Jr, Parkey RW, Buja LM et al: Computed tomography: In vitro evaluation of myocardial infarction. Radiology 122:511, 1977
19. Weiss JL, Bulkley BH, Hutchins GM et al: Two-dimensional echocardiographic recognition of myocardial injury in man: Comparison with postmortem studies. Circulation 63:401, 1981
20. Maroko PR, Kjekshus JK, Sobel BE et al: Factors influencing infarct size following experimental coronary artery occlusions. Circulation 43:67, 1971
21. Maroko PR, Braunwald E: Modification of myocardial infarct size after coronary occlusion. Ann Intern Med 79:720, 1973
22. Hillis LD, Fishbein MC, Braunwald E et al: The influence of the time interval between coronary artery occlusion and the administration of hyaluronidase on salvage of ischemic myocardium in dogs. Circ Res 41:26, 1977
23. Maroko PR, Hillis LD, Muller JE et al: Favorable effects of hyaluronidase on electrocardiographic evidence of necrosis in patients with acute myocardial infarction. N Engl J Med 296:898, 1977
24. Mueller HS, Ayres SM, Religa A et al: Propranolol in the treatment of acute myocardial infarction: Effect on myocardial oxygenation and hemodynamics. Circulation 49:1078, 1974
25. Vatner SF, Baig H, Manders WT et al: Effects of propranolol on regional myocardial function, electrograms and blood flow in conscious dogs with myocardial ischemia. J Clin Invest 60:353, 1977
26. Mueller HS, Ayres SM: The role of propranolol in the treatment of acute myocardial infarction. Prog Cardiovasc Dis 19:405, 1977
27. Hillis LD, Khuri SF, Braunwald E et al: Assessment of the efficacy of interventions to limit ischemic injury by direct measurement of intramural carbon dioxide tension after coronary artery occlusion in the dog. J Clin Invest 63:99, 1979
28. Bush LR, Samowitz W, Buja LM et al: Recovery of left ventricular segmental function after long-term reperfusion following temporary coronary occlusion in conscious dogs: Comparison of 2- and 4-hour occlusions. Circ Res 53:248, 1983
29. Roan P, Scales F, Buja LM et al: Functional characterization of left ventricular segmental responses during the initial 24 h and 1 wk after experimental canine myocardial infarction. J Clin Invest 64:1074, 1979
30. Willerson JT, Powell WJ Jr, Guiney TE et al: Improvement in myocardial function and coronary blood flow in ischemic myocardium after mannitol. J Clin Invest 51:2989, 1972
31. Shell WE, Lavelle JF, Covell JW et al: Early estimation of myocardial damage in conscious dogs and patients with evolving acute myocardial infarction. J Clin Invest 52:2579, 1973
32. Norris RM, Whitlock RML, Barratt-Boyes C et al: Clinical measurement of myocardial infarct size: Modification of a method for the estimation of total creatine phosphokinase release after myocardial infarction. Circulation 51:614, 1975
33. Cox J, Jr, Roberts R, Ambos HD et al: Relations between enzymatically estimated myocardial infarct size and early ventricular dysrhythmia. Circulation 53 (Suppl I):150, 1976
34. Geltman EM, Ehsani AA, Campbell MK et al: The influence of location and extent of myocardial infarction on long-term ventricular dysrhythmia and mortality. Circulation 60:805, 1979
35. Morrison J, Coromilas J, Munsey D et al: Correlation of radionuclide estimates of myocardial infarction size and release of creatine kinase-MB in man. Circulation 62:277, 1980
36. Rogers WJ, McDaniel HG, Smith LR et al: Correlation of angiographic estimates of myocardial infarct size and accumulated release of creatine kinase MB isoenzyme in man. Circulation 56:199, 1977
37. Poliner LR, Buja LM, Parkey RW et al: Comparison of different noninvasive methods of infarct sizing during experimental myocardial infarction. J Nucl Med 18:517, 1977
38. Vatner SF, Baig H, Manders WT et al: Effects of coronary artery reperfusion on myocardial infarct size calculated from creatine kinase. J Clin Invest 61:1048, 1978
39. Hearse DJ, Garlick PB, Humphrey SM et al: The effect of drugs on enzyme release from the hypoxic myocardium. Eur J Cardiol 7:421, 1978
40. Willerson JT, Stone MJ, Ting R et al: Radioimmunoassay of CPK-B isoenzyme in human sera: Results in patients with acute myocardial infarction. Proc Natl Acad Sci USA 74:1711, 1977
41. Roberts R, Sobel BE, Parker CW: Radioimmunoassay of creatine kinase isoenzymes. Science 194:855, 1976
42. Roberts R: Reperfusion and the plasma isoforms of creatine kinase isoenzymes: A clinical perspective. J Am Coll Cardiol 9:464, 1987
43. Nohara R, Myears DW, Sobel BE, Abendschein DR: Optimal criteria for rapid detection of myocardial reperfusion by creatine kinase MM isoforms in the presence of residual high grade coronary stenosis. J Am Coll Cardiol 14:1067, 1989
44. Poliner LR, Buja LM, Parkey RW et al: Clinicopathologic findings in 52 patients studied by technetium-99m stannous pyrophosphate myocardial scintigrams. Circulation 59:257, 1979

45. Rutherford JD, Roberts R, Muller JE et al: Electrocardiographic, enzymatic, and scintigraphic criteria of acute myocardial infarction as determined from study of 726 patients (A MILIS Study). Am J Cardiol 55:1463, 1985
46. Izquierdo C, Devous M, Nicod P et al: A comparison of infarct identification with 99m-technetium pyrophosphate and triphenyl tetrazolium chloride staining. J Nucl Med 24:492, 1983
47. Corbett JR, Lewis M, Willerson JT et al: Technetium-99m pyrophosphate imaging in patients with acute myocardial infarction: Comparison of planar images with single-photon tomography with and without blood pool overlay. Circulation 69:1120, 1984
48. Corbett JR, Lewis SE, Wolfe CL et al: Measurement of myocardial infarct size in patients by technetium pyrophosphate single photon tomography. Am J Cardiol 54:1349, 1984
49. Lewis SE, Devous MD Sr, Corbett JR et al: Measurement of infarct size in acute canine myocardial infarction by single photon emission computed tomography with technetium-99m pyrophosphate. Am J Cardiol 54:193, 1984.
50. Jansen DE, Corbett JR, Lewis SE et al: Quantification of myocardial infarction: A comparison of single photon emission computed tomography with pyrophosphate to serial plasma MB-creatine kinase measurements. Circulation 72:327, 1985
51. Willerson JT, Parkey RW, Bonte FJ et al: Pathophysiologic considerations and clinicopathological correlates with technetium-99m stannous pyrophosphate myocardial scintigraphy. Semin Nucl Med 10:54, 1980
52. Nicod P, Lewis SE, Corbett JR et al: Increased incidence of "persistently abnormal" technetium pyrophosphate myocardial scintigrams following myocardial infarction in patients with diabetes mellitus. Am Heart J 103:822, 1982
53. Croft C, Rude RE, Lewis SE et al: Comparison of left ventricular function in infarct size in patients with and without persistently positive technetium-99m pyrophosphate myocardial scintigrams after myocardial infarction: Analysis of 357 patients. Am J Cardiol 53:421, 1984
54. Donsky MS, Curry GE, Parkey RW et al: Unstable angina pectoris: Clinical, angiographic, and myocardial scintigraphic observations. Br Heart J 38:257, 1976
55. Khaw BA, Beller GA, Haber E et al: Localization of cardiac myosin-specific antibody in myocardial infarction. J Clin Invest 58:439, 1976
56. Gray WR, Buja LM, Hagler HL et al: Computed tomography for localization and sizing of experimental acute myocardial infarcts. Circulation 58:497, 1978
57. Adams DF, Hessel SJ, Judy PF et al: Computed tomography of the normal and infarcted myocardium. AJR 126:786, 1976
58. Higgins CB, Siemers PT, Schmidt W: Detection, quantitation and contrast enhancement of myocardial infarction utilizing computerized axial tomography. Am J Cardiol 41:361, 1978
59. Powell WJ Jr, Wittenberg J, Maturi RA et al: Detection of edema associated with myocardial ischemia by computerized tomography in isolated, arrested canine hearts. Circulation 55:99, 1977
60. Slutsky RA, Mattrey RF, Long SA et al: *In vivo* estimation of myocardial infarct size and left ventricular function by prospectively gated computerized transmission tomography. Circulation 67:759, 1983
61. Higgins CB, Siemers PT, Schmidt W et al: Evaluation of myocardial ischemic damage of various ages by computerized transmission tomography. Circulation 60:284, 1979
62. Pflugfelder PW, Wisenberg G, Prato FS et al: Early detection of canine myocardial infarction by magnetic resonance imaging *in vivo*. Circulation 71:587, 1985
63. Johnston DL, Brady TJ, Ratner AV et al: Assessment of myocardial ischemia with proton magnetic resonance: Effects of a three-hour coronary occlusion with and without reperfusion. Circulation 71:595, 1985
64. Rehr RB, Peshock RM, Malloy C et al: Improved *in vivo* magnetic resonance imaging of acute myocardial infarction after intravenous paramagnetic contrast agent administration. Am J Cardiol 57:864, 1986
65. Wesby G, Higgins CB, Lanzer P et al: Imaging and characterization of acute MI *in vivo* by gated NMR. Circulation 69:125, 1984
66. Herfkeus RJ et al: NMR imaging of the cardiovascular system: Normal and pathologic findings. Radiology 147:749, 1983
67. Hawkes RC et al: NMR tomography of the normal heart. J Comput Assist Tomogr 5:605, 1981
68. Schaefer S, Malloy CR, Katz J et al: Gadolinium-DTPA-enhanced nuclear magnetic resonance imaging of reperfused myocardium: Identification of the myocardial bed at risk. J Am Coll Cardiol 12:1064, 1988
69. Pohost GM, Zir LM, Moore RH et al: Differentiation of transiently ischemic from infarcted myocardium by serial imaging after a single dose of thallium-201. Circulation 55:294, 1977
70. Silverman KJ, Becker LC, Bulkley BH et al: Value of early thallium-201 scintigraphy for predicting mortality in patients with acute myocardial infarction. Circulation 61:996, 1980
71. Weiss ES, Ahmed SA, Welch MJ et al: Quantification of infarction in cross sections of canine myocardium *in vivo* with positron emission transaxial tomography and ^{11}C-palmitate. Circulation 55:66, 1977
72. Rellas JS, Corbett JR, Kulkarni P et al: Iodine-123 phenylpentadecanoic acid: Detection of acute myocardial infarction and injury using an iodinated fatty acid and single photon emission tomography. Am J Cardiol 52:1326, 1983
73. Stokely EM, Parkey RW, Bonte FJ et al: Gated blood pool imaging following technetium-99m phosphate scintigraphy. Radiology 120:433, 1976
74. Rigo P, Murray M, Strauss HW et al: Left ventricular function in acute myocardial infarction evaluated by gated scintiphotography. Circulation 50:678, 1974
75. Reduto LA, Berger HJ, Cohen LS et al: Sequential radionuclide assessment of left and right ventricular performance after acute transmural myocardial infarction. Ann Intern Med 89:441, 1978
76. Dehmer GJ, Lewis SE, Hillis LD et al: Nongeometric determination of left ventricular volumes from equilibrium blood pool scans. Am J Cardiol 45:293, 1980
77. Dehmer GJ, Lewis SE, Hillis LD et al: Exercise induced alterations in left ventricular volumes in man: Usefulness in predicting the relative extent of coronary artery disease. Circulation 63:1008, 1981
78. Slutsky R, Karliner J, Ricci D et al: Left ventricular volumes by gated equilibrium radionuclide angiography: A new method. Circulation 60:556, 1979
79. Wyatt HL, Meerbaum S, Heng MK et al: Experimental evaluation of the extent of myocardial dyssynergy and infarct size by two-dimensional echocardiography. Circulation 63:607, 1981
80. Lieberman AN, Weiss JL, Jugdutt BI et al: Two-dimensional echocardiography and infarct size: Relationship of regional wall motion and thickening to the extent of myocardial infarction in the dog. Circulation 63:739, 1981
81. Farcot JC et al: Two-dimensional echocardiographic visualization of ventricular septal rupture after acute myocardial infarction. Am J Cardiol 45:370, 1980
82. Heger J et al: Cross-sectional echocardiography in acute myocardial infarction: Detection and localization of regional left ventricular asynergy. Circulation 60:531, 1979

Management of Uncomplicated Acute Myocardial Infarction

Gabriel Gregoratos

The components of management of an uncomplicated acute myocardial infarction (AMI) are several:

1. Adequate prehospital care including immediate entry of the patient into a life support environment and transfer to a coronary care unit (CCU)
2. Relief of pain and apprehension as well as institution of a variety of general measures designed to promote patient comfort and myocardial repair
3. Establishment of diagnosis and quantitation of the extent of myocardial damage
4. Prevention and therapy of complications of AMI including arrhythmias, thromboembolic problems, hemodynamic aberrations, and hypoxemia
5. Myocardial salvage whether by pharmacologic means or by reperfusion techniques
6. Physical and psychological rehabilitation and establishment of prognosis

PREHOSPITAL AND CORONARY CARE

Acute myocardial infarction is a common cardiac event in the United States. It is estimated that between 1.2 and 1.5 million Americans may develop an AMI annually and between 0.5 and 0.6 million of them will not survive the event.[1] Several studies have reported a 40% to 60% mortality rate within the first hour of the onset of symptoms with the majority of patients dying before they could reach the hospital.[2,3] Furthermore, it has been well documented that most deaths from AMI occurring within the first hour after the onset of symptoms are due to ventricular fibrillation.[4]

A major factor contributing to the large prehospital mortality from AMI is the delay between the onset of symptoms and initiation of intensive care therapy. Major variables resulting in this delay include a prolonged "decision time," defined as the interval between the onset of symptoms and the patient's or family's decision to seek medical help, delays resulting from the patient-physician encounter in a nonhospital environment, delays due to transportation problems to the hospital and, finally, emergency department and admitting procedure delays.[5,6] It is therefore readily apparent that to reduce prehospital mortality a significant reduction in the time interval between the onset of symptoms and institution of intensive care therapy is necessary.

PUBLIC AND PHYSICIAN EDUCATION

Although the presenting symptoms of AMI are classically believed to appear suddenly, careful questioning of patients often will yield evidence of a symptomatic prodromal phase. It has been variously estimated that 44% to 70% of patients with AMI experience premonitory symptoms in the weeks prior to infarction.[7,8] Frequently these premonitory symptoms are quite atypical. Instead of the classic substernal constriction, patients often report midepigastric distress believed to represent indigestion, pain in the interscapular region believed to represent musculoskeletal pain, and occasionally pain in the mandible or teeth, prompting them to seek the attention of a dentist. Studies suggest that up to 25% of AMIs are unrecognized initially either because they are "silent" or because symptoms are atypical.[9] Public education has been attempted by the American Heart Association and its affiliates[1] and other organizations. Nevertheless, a great deal remains to be accomplished in this area.

PHYSICIAN–PATIENT INTERACTION

Several studies have reported that only 16% to 26% of patients seeking medical attention for a presumed AMI go directly to the hospital without seeking prior medical advice.[8] Frequently the attitude and index of suspicion of the physician are directly responsible for delaying the patient at this stage. Patients instructed by their physicians to proceed directly to a hospital emergency department had hospital arrival times similar to those who went to the hospital directly without seeking medical advice. However, a significant delay occurred when the physician's advice included an office visit, trial of medication, or consultation with a cardiovascular specialist. Education of physicians to avoid these relatively ineffective out-of-hospital encounters with patients presumed to be suffering an AMI is clearly necessary.

TRANSPORTATION AND MOBILE CORONARY CARE

The private automobile is still the primary method of transportation of patients with AMI to a hospital.[10] In addition to prolongation of arrival time due to traffic congestion, inadequate directions, or automobile breakdowns, transportation by private automobile has the major disadvantage that should a patient suffer a cardiac arrest during transportation, delivery of effective therapy is difficult. The desirability of delivering immediate intensive care to patients with a suspected AMI has been known for many years. Pantridge and Geddes implemented the first mobile coronary care unit in Belfast in 1966.[11] Mobile coronary care units are well-equipped ambulances staffed by paramedics or other personnel trained in the care of the infarct patient and able to deliver definitive therapy while the patient is in transit.[12] These units are equipped with monitoring oscilloscopes and direct-writing electrocardiographs, defibrillators, oxygen, endotracheal tubes, laryngoscopes and suction apparatus, and all commonly used cardiovascular drugs. Ideally these units should be equipped with a radiotelemetry system that allows transmission of the electrocardiogram to the base station. Furthermore, radio communication must be available with the base station to allow the mobile CCU personnel to obtain information and advice from physicians and nurses at the base station.

Mobile CCU systems have been implemented in several areas, including Belfast, Ireland, Seattle, Washington, and Columbus, Ohio. The effectiveness of these units has been well documented, and the frequency of death during transportation of the patient can be reduced significantly. In at least one study, a reduction of in-transit mortality from 22% to 9% was recorded when defibrillation equipment and trained paramedical personnel were available.[13,14]

CORONARY CARE UNITS

In conjunction with the development of CCUs during the past 2 decades, the in-hospital mortality of patients with AMI has declined significantly. In the Minnesota Heart survey a 35% improvement in 4-year survival was documented for men with AMI hospitalized in 1980 compared with those hospitalized in 1970 and a similar 27% improvement occurred in women. Reduced hospital mortality for AMI patients accounted for 70% of the overall gain in survival between 1970 and 1980 in men and for virtually all of the gain in women.[15] This reduction of acute mortality is primarily due to the elimination of primary arrhythmias as a cause of death. Prevention of arrhythmic deaths is the result of continuous rhythm monitoring in the CCU by specially trained nurses who have the capability under specific protocols to administer immediate treatment and prophylaxis of arrhythmias even in the absence of physicians. In addition, the clustering of patients with AMI in one intensive care unit improves greatly the efficient use of trained personnel and highly specialized equipment (*e.g.*, defibrillators, ventilators, pacemakers). An excellent historical review of the development of coronary care units has been published.[16]

In order for a CCU to function effectively, specific policies and procedures must be in effect (Fig. 68.1). These policies must cover all the usual contingencies expected in the care of a patient with an AMI and allow the nurses and other paramedical personnel to intervene immediately even in the absence of a physician.[17]

As mentioned previously, the major reason for the efficacy of CCUs is the early detection and treatment of arrhythmias. This is accomplished by means of continuous electrocardiographic monitoring with electronic monitoring equipment of progressively increasing technologic sophistication. Most commonly the rhythm monitoring is carried out by means of an integrated hard-wire bedside and central station system.[17] The specific lead being monitored can vary, depending on the morphology of the patient's electrocardiogram (Fig. 68.2). Most often, a modified lead V_1 (MCL_1) is employed since this lead usually provides good P waves for dysrhythmia analysis as well as QRS complexes that can be easily analyzed for the presence of intraventricular conduction defects.[18] Monitoring is usually carried out by a member of the nursing staff seated at the central station. However, several studies indicate that continuous monitoring surveillance is nearly impossible even in the best organized and staffed CCUs. Estimates of effective visual monitor surveillance range from 20% to 50% of monitoring time. For these reasons and in conjunction with the development of sophisticated algorithms for the recognition of arrhythmias, computerized monitoring systems are being used with increasing frequency. The recent emphasis on hemodynamic monitoring for the treatment of serious hemodynamic complications of AMI as well as the currently expanding indications for acute intervention in AMI have further consolidated the important role of CCUs.

Questions have been raised regarding the efficacy and cost-effectiveness of CCUs[19] especially in patients with uncomplicated AMI.[20] In a randomized trial comparing home management and hospital management of groups of AMI patients, the 6-week mortality rates were 13% and 11%, respectively. Although these mortality rates are very similar, the significance of the study is not clear, since approximately 25% of patients with serious arrhythmias or hemodynamic complications were excluded. Because prediction of early complications is difficult and because current medical practice in the United States is not conducive to prompt intensive care at home, it is recommended that all patients with documented or suspected AMI should be admitted to a CCU. Early discharge may be appropriate for the patient with an uncomplicated AMI and is discussed later in this chapter.

STEP-DOWN (INTERMEDIATE) UNITS

Following the initial development of CCUs and demonstration of a definite reduction in early AMI mortality, several observers reported the persistence of significant mortality rates during the post-CCU phase of hospitalization of AMI patients.[21,22] Many of these deaths occurred suddenly and unexpectedly and were therefore presumed to be due to sudden tachyarrhythmias or bradyarrhythmias.[23,24] These observations led to the development of step-down or intermediate CCUs, which allow continuous rhythm monitoring of ambulatory patients. Monitoring is carried out by means of radiotelemetry at a central station by trained personnel, computer analysis, or both. Additional advantages of step-down units occupied entirely by post-AMI patients include facilitation of patient education, patient rehabilitation, and the psychological support that patients derive from one another.

GENERAL PRINCIPLES OF MANAGEMENT
RELIEF OF PAIN AND APPREHENSION

Immediate relief of pain and anxiety associated with acute myocardial infarction is essential. Most patients experience intense anxiety resulting both from their symptoms and from their recognition of the implications of the suspected diagnosis. It is crucial to remember that in many patients early during the course of AMI there exists a state of autonomic nervous system imbalance.[25] This imbalance may take the form either of parasympathetic overactivity associated with bradycardia and hypotension or of sympathetic overactivity characterized by tachycardia and hypertension. The choice of analgesic will depend to some extent on the presence or absence of these autonomic nervous system syndromes. It is now well documented that pain and anxiety can produce coronary arterial spasm and stimulate catecholamine release that further increase heart rate, cardiac output, and cardiac work and in fact may precipitate lethal arrhythmias.[26]

Morphine sulfate remains the drug of choice for the treatment of pain and anxiety in most patients with AMI despite the availability of other drugs such as meperidine, pentazocine, and nalbuphine. Morphine is remarkably well tolerated by patients with coronary artery disease. In fact, large doses of intravenous morphine have been widely used to provide profound analgesia during cardiac surgery precisely because of the relative lack of circulatory depression from this drug.[27] On the other hand, morphine often decreases alveolar ventilation and increases right-to-left shunting with subsequent decrease in arterial oxygen tension.[28] Furthermore, this agent may produce hypotension because of peripheral and splanchnic vasodilatation and especially pooling of blood in the venous system.[29] Although reductions in ventricular preload may play some role in myocardial salvage, as discussed subsequently, morphine is not the ideal drug to effect preload reduction. For these reasons it should be administered in small doses that can be repeated as necessary in preference to a single large dose. It is important to remember that in AMI the minimal dose of morphine that will produce the desired analgesic effect should be used. Current recommendations are to administer several small increments of morphine in doses of 2 to 4 mg intravenously. Since the peak effect of intravenously administered morphine occurs within 15 to 20 minutes,[30] the dose may be titrated to the appropriate level of analgesia with reduced risk of respiratory depression or hypotension. Some patients may require up to 15 mg for pain relief.

In the presence of parasympathetic nervous system overactivity with bradycardia and hypotension, morphine sulfate, a parasympathomimetic agent, should be given with great caution, if at all. In this clinical setting, it has been recommended that atropine be administered in conjunction with morphine or that meperidine, a vagolytic agent, be substituted. When this drug is administered parenterally, it is important to remember that a dose of 75 mg provides analgesia approximately equivalent to 8 to 10 mg of morphine.

The most bothersome side effects of morphine relate to the nauseant and emetic actions it produces by stimulating the chemoreceptor trigger zone. Drug-induced nausea and vomiting may be minimized by the concomitant administration of 0.4 to 0.6 mg of atropine intravenously or prescription of a phenothiazine compound. Great care, however, should be exercised because of the synergistic effects of phenothiazines and narcotic analgesics. Another side effect of morphine is increased urinary bladder sphincter tone, which may result in urinary retention requiring catheterization for relief.

Certain patients are particularly sensitive to morphine, and special care must be exercised in administering this drug. This is particularly true of those with severe chronic obstructive pulmonary disease who may prove to be highly sensitive to the respiratory depressant action of the drug. Also, older patients and especially those taking diuretics chronically may develop significant hypotension after intravenous morphine. In patients with hepatocellular dysfunction, the duration of action of morphine may be prolonged, since inactivation of the drug occurs by conjugation in the liver.

If the patient remains restless and anxious following relief of chest pain, mild sedation during the first 24 to 48 hours after admission is indicated and often required. A benzodiazepine drug is useful in this setting. Currently, diazepam is preferred to barbiturates because of its lesser central nervous system depressant action and the fact that it does not interact as commonly with other cardiovascular drugs. Hemodynamic studies have demonstrated that diazepam reduces left ventricular filling pressure and systemic arterial pressure, thus exerting a minor, but beneficial, effect on depressed left ventricular function.[30] Other studies have concluded that diazepam given intravenously reduces release of catecholamines and may in fact diminish the incidence of ventricular arrhythmias in the setting of AMI.[31] In the absence of hypotension, depression, and mental confusion, diazepam given in doses of 2.5 to 5 mg orally three times daily has proven to be an effective sedative and tranquilizer. Older patients and those with a significant psychologic depressive reaction may do better if given alprazolam, 0.25 mg two to three times daily. This is a newer benzodiazepine with reportedly fewer depressant side effects. Many patients in the CCU develop a disturbed sleep pattern and require a hypnotic at bedtime. Flurazepam, 15 to 30 mg orally, and triazolam, 0.125 to 0.25 mg orally, are effective temporary aids in this situation.

Nitrous oxide administered by inhalation has been shown to be an effective analgesic and antianxiety agent in AMI that is well tolerated without the limiting side effects of opiates.[32] However, this agent has not gained wide acceptance in AMI, probably because of complexity of administration.

Patients with a completed AMI usually become free of pain with effective analgesic therapy within 6 to 12 hours of admission to the CCU. Some of these patients may complain of a vague, residual, mild precordial discomfort that generally does not require additional analgesic therapy. However, recurrences of severe anginal pain indicate ongoing myocardial ischemia and treatment should be directed toward relief of this problem with nitrates, calcium inhibitors, and/or β-blockade.

DIET

During the first 24 hours after admission, it is customary to limit oral intake to clear liquids containing no more than 1 g of sodium. Total fluid intake is limited to between 1500 and 2000 ml for the first 24 hours, sufficient to maintain a urinary output of 800 to 1000 ml. The

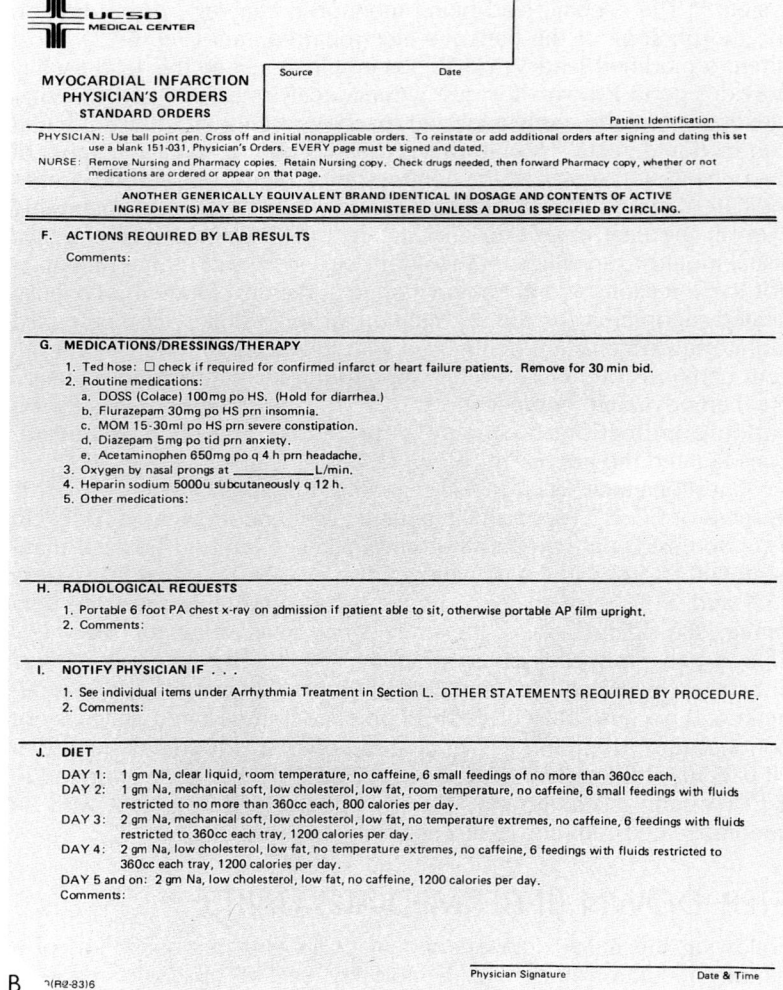

FIGURE 68.1 A–C. Example of standing admission orders to a coronary care unit. The orders set forth recommended policies for the initial care of patients with AMI and give nursing personnel the authority to treat life-threatening arrhythmias. (Courtesy of the University of California Medical Center, San Diego)

main purpose of prescribing clear liquids initially is to minimize the risk of aspiration should a cardiac arrest occur and resuscitation be required. Over the years it has become customary to allow the patient only tepid liquids, avoiding extremes of temperature. However, studies have shown that hot or cold liquids in the immediate postinfarction period do not produce deleterious effects.[33] If the patient is nauseated, as is often the case following an inferior AMI or as a result of narcotic analgesic administration, oral intake of fluids is withheld and an intravenous infusion of 1500 ml of 5% glucose in half-normal saline is substituted.

In the patient with an uncomplicated AMI, diet is advanced to a soft, low-sodium, low-cholesterol balanced polyunsaturated/saturated fat diet on the second day. Patients with coronary atherosclerosis are almost always in need of dietary re-education. Their initial stay in the CCU provides the necessary motivation to learn and adhere to a more appropriate diet. Good dietary instructions are essential in order for the patient to accept a diet that he will be able to follow after discharge. Elderly patients sustaining a second or a third AMI or patients who are not overweight and whose lipid profile is in the normal range probably need not adhere to a rigid diet. By the fourth postinfarction day, if the patient's course is uncomplicated, the diet should be advanced to a regular one with sodium and fat restrictions as outlined previously. Lipid profiles should not be measured on admission to the CCU since such values are often altered during the acute phase of AMI; reliable measurements cannot be made until the convalescent phase. A recent study, however, indicated that the reduction in serum lipid levels, which is often seen in the early phase of AMI, occurred approximately 36 hours after the onset of symptoms.[34] According to this study, serum lipid levels obtained the morning after the development of the AMI correlated well with those 3 months later. It appears reasonable therefore to obtain the patient's lipid phenotype soon after hospital admission in order to tailor the diet accordingly.

Coffee and tea are usually excluded from the diet of patients with AMI because of the positive chronotropic and inotropic effects of methylated xanthines and their potential for the production of arrhythmias.[35] The use of tobacco in the CCU is strictly prohibited because of the acute circulatory responses to cigarette smoking that commonly result in catecholamine release. Furthermore, strenuous efforts are indicated to re-educate patients in the long-term risks of cigarette smoking. Cigarettes have been clearly implicated as an important risk factor in the development of atherosclerotic vascular disease[36] especially in patients younger than age 45.[37] Since most patients with AMI are receiving narcotic analgesics and/or tranquilizers during the early phase of their hospitalization, there is little tendency to complain about the lack of cigarettes. The immediate postinfarction period while the patient is confined in the CCU may be the ideal time to eliminate the tobacco habit. Alcoholic beverages are usually denied to patients in the CCU and during subsequent convalescence. However, there is no clear medical reason why small amounts of alcohol should not be allowed for carefully selected patients. A common sense approach must be used.

BED REST AND PHYSICAL ACTIVITY

The patient with an uncomplicated AMI should not be totally confined to bed for more than 24 to 36 hours and should be able to use a

UCSD MEDICAL CENTER

MYOCARDIAL INFARCTION PHYSICIAN'S ORDERS STANDARD ORDERS

Source Date

Patient Identification

PHYSICIAN: Use ball point pen. Cross off and initial nonapplicable orders. To reinstate or add additional orders after signing and dating this set use a blank 151-031, Physician's Orders. EVERY page must be signed and dated.

NURSE: Remove Nursing and Pharmacy copies. Retain Nursing copy. Check drugs needed, then forward Pharmacy copy, whether or not medications are ordered or appear on that page.

ANOTHER GENERICALLY EQUIVALENT BRAND IDENTICAL IN DOSAGE AND CONTENTS OF ACTIVE INGREDIENT(S) MAY BE DISPENSED AND ADMINISTERED UNLESS A DRUG IS SPECIFIED BY CIRCLING.

K. ACTIVITY/AMBULATION/STIMULATION

1. Activity: (Physician should check appropriate items in 1b.)
   a. Admission Day: Bedrest, commode for BM only. No commode privileges if patient is hypotensive, has a temporary pacemaker or uncontrolled ventricular ectopy.
   b. Day 1: ☐ (1) Same as admission day.
   ☐ (2) Exercise Step ___ ADL Step ___ Ambulation Step ___
2. Stimulation:
   a. Day 1: No TV, radio, reading.
   Visitors: Immediate family only - maximum of two at a time for 10 minutes x 4, from 1PM to 8PM.
   b. Day 2 & 3: May read or listen to radio.
   Visitors: Immediate family only - maximum of two at a time for 15 minutes x 4, from 1PM to 8PM.
   c. Day 4 on: At patient's and nurses' discretion.
3. Bathe patient first 3 days, then assist (except as outlined in activity protocol).
4. No electric shavers to be used if patient has a pacemaker.
5. Patient not allowed to comb hair or shave face days 1-3.
6. Comments:

L. ARRHYTHMIA TREATMENT

1. Prophylactic Lidocaine therapy: All patients with documented or suspected AMI or with unstable angina (except patients over age 70 years and patients with cardiac or hepatic failure)
   a. Lidocaine bolus 1mg/kg.
   b. Licocaine infusion 2mg/min (start concurrently).
   c. Repeat Lidocaine bolus 0.5mg/kg 20 min after first bolus.
2. ☐ Physician check here to cancel above order.
3. Ventricular fibrillation: counter shock immediately with 250 watt/sec (stored), repeat if necessary; then give 100mg of Lidocaine IV push (50mg if patient on Lidocaine) and follow with IV drip of 4mg/min; if ventricular fibrillation persists 45 seconds, begin CPR; then call House Officer.
4. Ventricular tachycardia with rate greater than 120: deliver a hard blow over the precordium and give Lidocaine as directed above; if it persists, counter shock with 250 watts/sec and call House Officer.
5. "Slow" ventricular tachycardia with rate less than 120: call House Officer.
6. Ventricular premature beats greater than 6/min, multifocal, R on T of preceding beat or coupled: give Lidocaine as directed above (item 1) and call House Officer.
7. Ventricular premature beats less than 6/min: call House Officer.
8. Asystole: begin cardiopulmonary resuscitation immediately.
9. Severe sinus bradycardia HR less than 40: give 0.6mg Atropine IV push and call House Officer.
10. All other arrhythmias: call House Officer.
11. Comments:

Physician Signature Date & Time

C 32-83)6

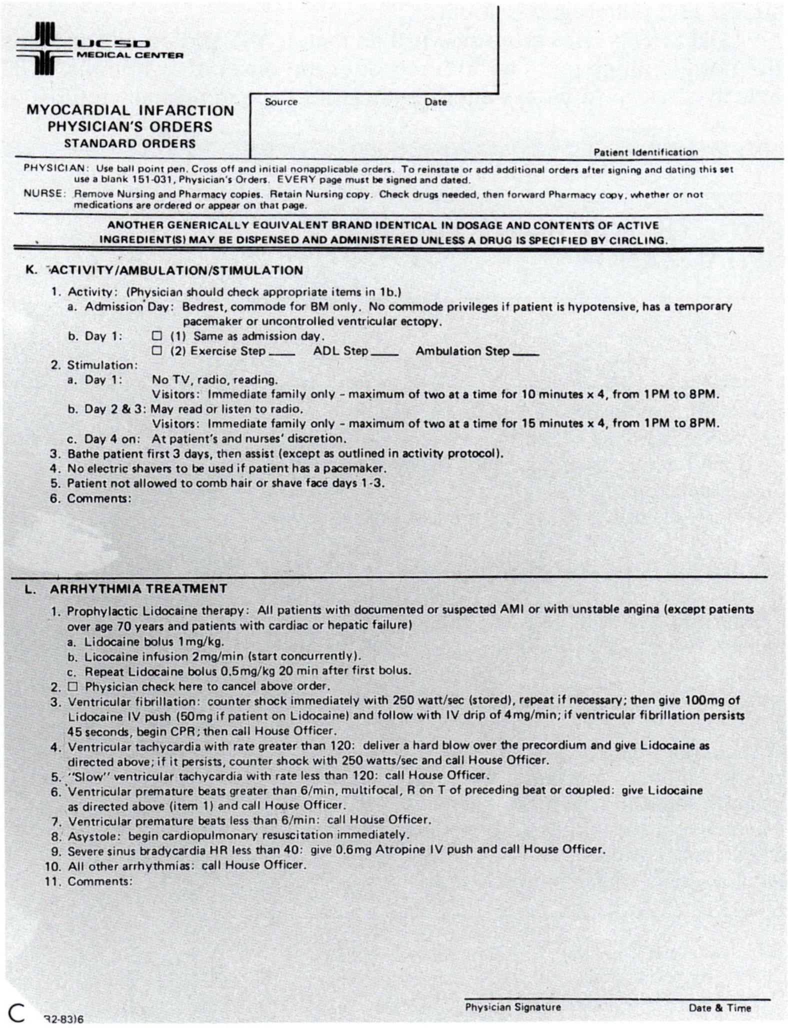

FIGURE 68.1 (continued).

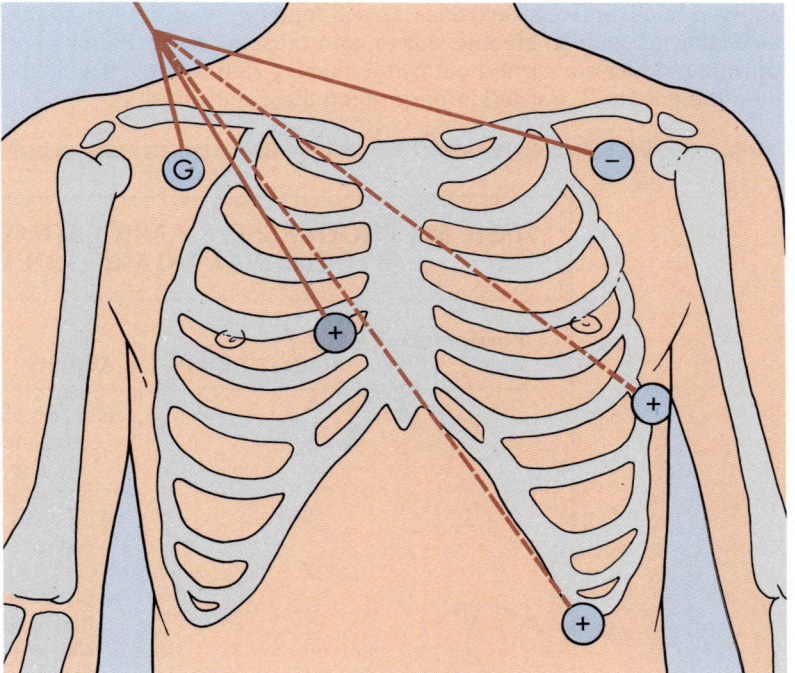

FIGURE 68.2 ECG lead configuration for continuous rhythm monitoring in the CCU. MCL_1 (modified V_1) is indicated by the solid lines and alternative leads MCL_6 or M_{111} by the dashed lines as proposed by Marriott and Fogg. (Modified from Marriott HJL, Fogg E: Constant monitoring for cardiac dysrhythmias and blocks. Mod Concepts Cardiovasc Dis 39:103, 1970)

bedside commode from the time of admission. This approach is in direct contrast to the strict limitation of activity regimens practiced until recently. The abuse of absolute bed rest was emphasized over 30 years ago by Levine and Lown in their classic paper on the chair treatment of coronary thrombosis.[38] In the absence of complications (arrhythmias and heart failure), patients with AMI are kept in the CCU for 2 to 3 days. On the second and third day they are helped out of bed and allowed to sit in a comfortable chair by the bedside for two 30-minute periods on the second day and two 1-hour periods on the third day. On transfer to the intermediate CCU, patients are assigned to a progressive ambulation protocol (Table 68.1). Patients with uncomplicated courses may be discharged as early as 1 week after AMI with a low incidence of serious late complications at 6 months.[39] In general it is customary to discharge patients from the hospital 7 to 10 days after the occurrence of an uncomplicated AMI. Prolonged hospitalization and especially prolonged bed rest are deleterious and often lead to complications, such as constipation, thrombophlebitis and pulmonary embolism, urinary retention, stress ulcers, and physical deconditioning. Elderly patients are particularly susceptible to these complications and should therefore benefit the most from implementation of an early supervised ambulation program following AMI.

Measures to prevent some of the complications of bed rest should be initiated on admission to the CCU. Constipation is combated by the administration of a stool softener, such as dioctyl sodium sulfosuccinate, 100 mg once or twice daily. Venous thromboembolic complications can be avoided by instructing the patient to perform active range of motion exercises of the lower extremities. If the patient is too ill or unable to do so himself, the nursing staff performs passive exercises for the patient. Antiemboli stockings should be applied and removed for 30 minutes twice daily.

From day 2 onward, the patient with an uncomplicated AMI is allowed such personal activities as self-feeding, washing hands and face, shaving with an electric shaver, and brushing teeth. Bathing and brushing of hair are carried out by the nursing staff through day 3, and then the patient is assisted in performing these activities.

DIAGNOSIS OF ACUTE MYOCARDIAL INFARCTION

Classically, AMI is diagnosed as a syndrome of chest pain, serial electrocardiographic changes, and elevated serum enzymes. Unfortunately, chest pain in AMI is often atypical and as many as 10% to 15% of AMI cases may be silent. Similarly, electrocardiographic changes are often nondiagnostic and limited to repolarization abnormalities (nontransmural or non-Q wave AMI). The definitive diagnosis, therefore, of AMI is often dependent on the demonstration of biochemical and mechanical cardiac abnormalities.

SERIAL ENZYME CHANGES

Myocardial cells undergoing necrosis release a number of enzymes into the circulation where they can be detected by specific chemical reactions. Diagnostic criteria for AMI have been formulated dependent on the increase in the serum activity levels of these enzymes. Determinations of serum activity of aspartate aminotransferase (AST), lactic dehydrogenase (LDH), and creatine kinase (CK) have been used extensively in the laboratory diagnosis of AMI.

AST was the first enzyme used in the diagnosis of AMI and LDH was the second. Despite the historical importance of AST, this enzyme has been shown to be nonspecific and relatively insensitive and today plays a limited role in the diagnosis of AMI.[40] In general, AST activity in the serum exceeds normal values within 8 to 12 hours after the onset of symptoms of chest pain and peaks at approximately 24 to 36 hours after infarction, returning to normal levels within 3 to 4 days. AST activity in the serum can be falsely elevated in a variety of conditions, including primary hepatocellular disease, hepatic congestion due to heart failure, skeletal muscle injury (*e.g.*, intramuscular injections), shock, and pulmonary embolism.[41]

LDH activity rises more slowly than that of AST and usually exceeds the normal range in 24 to 36 hours after the onset of symptoms. LDH activity peaks 3 to 5 days after the onset of pain and usually returns to

TABLE 68.1 PROGRESSIVE AMBULATION PROTOCOL FOR 10-DAY ACUTE MYOCARDIAL INFARCTION HOSPITALIZATION

Postinfarct Day	Stage	Date	Activity
	1		Bed rest all of day. Use of bedside commode once with assistance. May bathe face and arms. Passive exercise to feet and legs twice a day. Avoid crossing ankles or legs, since it limits the blood circulation.
	2		With chair near bed, begin sitting in chair for short periods twice a day.
	3		Sit in chair 1 hour three times a day. Shave self while sitting in chair. Walk to bathroom with help twice a day. While in chair, may exercise arms and legs with swinging motion.
	4		Walk slowly 1 minute twice a day with help. Sit in chair 1 hour five times a day.
	5		Walk slowly 1 minute one to four times a day. Bathe self using sink in room.
	6		Walk in hall as before but going at a quicker pace.
	7		Walk in hall 2 minutes three to four times a day. May shower.
	8		Walk in hall 3 minutes three to four times a day.
	9		Walk in hall 4 minutes four to six times a day. Climb down one flight of stairs with supervision.
	10		Climb up one flight of stairs with supervision only.

(Modified from Gregoratos G, Gleeson E: Initial therapy of acute myocardial infarction. In Karliner JS, Gregoratos G [eds]: Coronary Care, p 155. Edinburgh, Churchill Livingstone, 1981, by permission)

normal levels 8 to 10 days after infarction. It is thus a useful test for patients coming to the physician's attention several days following an episode suggestive of AMI. Like the AST determination, total LDH determination in the serum is not a specific test for AMI. Probably the most common false-positive elevation is the result of hemolysis. Other causes of false-positive tests include hepatocellular disease, hepatic congestion, pulmonary embolism, skeletal muscle injury, shock, and a variety of neoplasms.

Serum CK activity begins to rise earlier than either AST or LDH activity following the onset of AMI. Peak CK values are usually seen 24 to 30 hours following the onset of symptoms and return to normal within 3 to 4 days. Elevation of serum CK is the most sensitive clinical enzyme test for AMI.[42] However, false-positive results are seen in patients with skeletal muscle disorders, diabetes mellitus, or alcoholism; following vigorous exercise or convulsions; and after intramuscular injections. In contrast to AST and LDH, serum CK activity does not rise in patients with heart failure or hepatocellular disease.

The development of clinical assays for the determination of the isoenzymes of LDH and CK in the serum has been a significant advance in the biochemical diagnosis of AMI. Five LDH isoenzymes have been separated electrophoretically and are numbered LD1 through LD5 depending on the speed of their migration toward the anode of the electrophoretic field. The myocardium contains mainly LD1, whereas skeletal muscle and liver LDH is composed primarily of LD4 and LD5. Therefore, noncardiac causes of total serum LDH elevation can be readily distinguished from AMI by analysis of the LDH isoenzyme pattern. Increased serum LD1 activity occurs in 8 to 24 hours after AMI and precedes the elevation of total serum LDH.[40-42] However, since red blood cells also possess significant LD1 activity, special care must be taken during blood specimen withdrawal to avoid hemolysis. The sensitivity and specificity of the LD1/LD2 ratio of 0.9 or higher in the diagnosis of AMI exceeds 90%.

CK activity can be separated electrophoretically into three isoenzymes (MB, MM, and BB). CK-BB isoenzyme usually predominates in brain and kidney extracts. Skeletal muscle contains primarily CK-MM, whereas both CK-MM and CK-MB isoenzymes are present in the myocardium. Although small amounts of CK-MB isoenzyme are found in other organs (diaphragm, uterus, tongue, and prostate), in practical clinical terms serum CK-MB elevations must be considered as the most specific biochemical marker today for AMI. However, it should be kept in mind that other forms of myocardial injury, such as trauma, cardiac surgery, and myocarditis, may also produce elevated serum CK-MB activity. Similarly, in patients with severe skeletal muscle trauma large amounts of both CK-MM and CK-MB isoenzyme are released in the circulation even in the absence of AMI. The time course and magnitude of serum enzyme changes in AMI are illustrated in Figure 68.3.

With the advent of serum enzyme assays, it has become customary for patients admitted to a CCU for a suspected AMI to have serial determinations of serum CK, LDH, and AST every 6 to 8 hours. The development of CK-MB assays has improved significantly the speed and specificity of biochemical diagnosis of AMI. Studies have demonstrated that CK-MB elevations in the serum are both more sensitive and more specific markers of AMI, and it is therefore recommended that standard enzyme determinations be replaced by CK-MB determinations that provide faster and safer diagnosis of AMI and reduce hospitalization time for patients without infarction.[43] In one study, peak CK-MB levels were recorded at 10 ± 2 hours following the onset of symptoms in patients with non–Q wave (nontransmural) infarction as opposed to 16.2 ± 5 hours in patients with classic Q wave (transmural) infarcts.[44] These findings are consistent with early spontaneous reperfusion in patients with non–Q wave myocardial infarction and support data obtained from thrombolytic trials that also show early peak CK-MB levels in the serum of patients achieving reperfusion. Elevation of serum myoglobin occurs in patients with AMI, and the sensitivity and specificity of myoglobin release appear to be similar to that of CK-MB. However, its relative advantage over detection of CK-MB has not been demonstrated.

Current concepts hold that AMI is a dynamic process that may be influenced favorably by therapeutic interventions to limit its extent. Since the ultimate size of AMI is probably the most important determi-

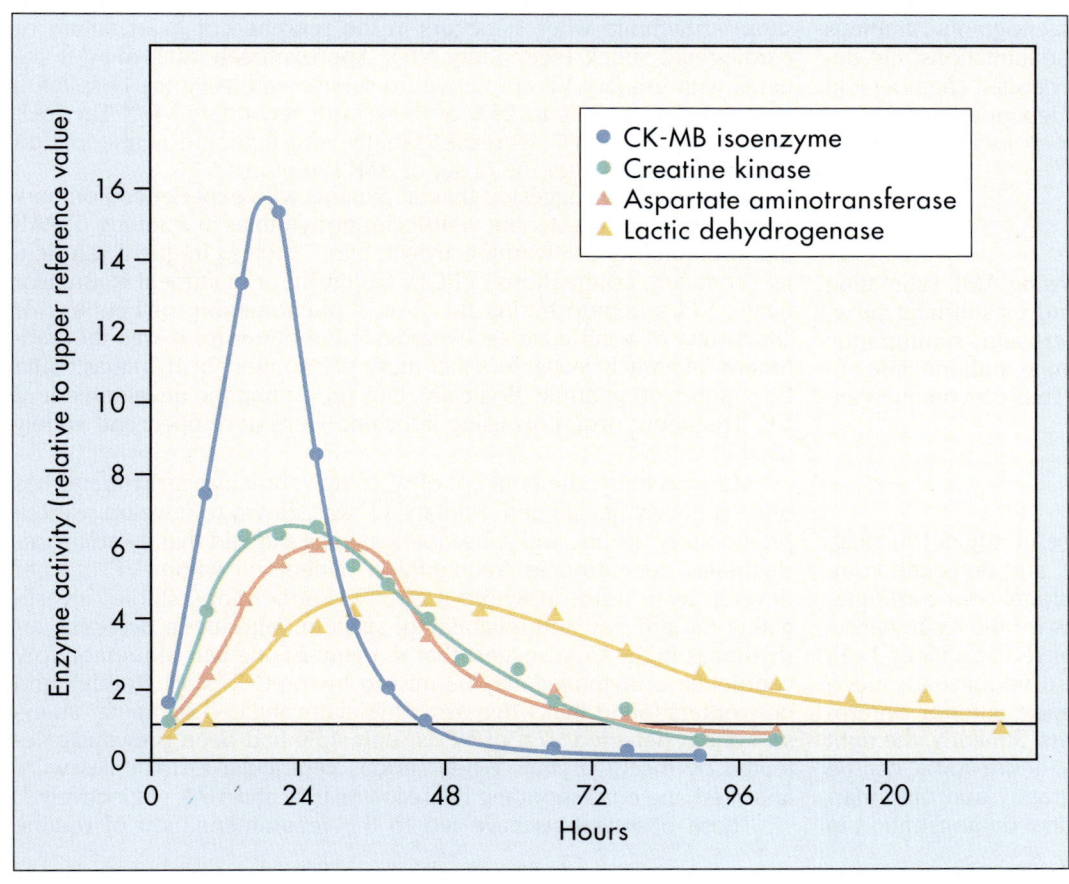

FIGURE 68.3 Time course and activity level of various enzymes in the serum following the onset of AMI symptoms. (Modified from Grande P, Christiansen C, Pedersen A et al: Optimal diagnosis in acute myocardial infarction. Circulation 61:723, 1980)

nant of long-term prognosis,[45] quantification of the extent of myocardial necrosis has been a major focus of investigation. AMI size has been estimated by analysis of serum CK time activity curves and more recently from curves obtained by the quantitative assay of serum MB-CK activity.[40,46,47] Work by Ryan and co-workers suggests that peak serum CK activity also correlates well with infarct size.[48] It must be kept in mind, however, that serum enzyme activities are influenced by a variety of factors other than infarct size *per se,* such as changes in regional myocardial perfusion, clearance of the enzyme from the serum, exchange of enzyme between vascular and extravascular compartments, and inactivation of the enzyme locally in the myocardium and in lymph. These complex considerations regarding infarct size estimation are covered in more detail elsewhere in this volume.

CHEST ROENTGENOGRAPHY

In uncomplicated AMI the chest roentgenogram usually provides little diagnostic help. The common findings of cardiomegaly and pulmonary congestion may well be absent on the initial chest roentgenogram, which is almost invariably a portable film obtained either in the emergency department or in the CCU. Cardiomegaly in this setting usually signifies previous infarct or an additional form of heart disease (*e.g.,* hypertensive cardiovascular disease) with chronic left ventricular (LV) dilatation. The presence of true cardiomegaly (a difficult assessment on a portable film) usually suggests significant impairment of LV function. Conversely, the LV end-diastolic volume may be significantly increased, but the cardiac silhouette may remain in the normal range. Increased pulmonary vascular markings, especially redistribution of pulmonary blood flow to the apices on an upright chest film, generally reflect elevated LV end-diastolic pressure. It is important to recognize the limitations of this observation. First, LV end-diastolic pressure may become elevated in acute ischemia primarily as a result of decreased LV diastolic compliance. Therefore, pulmonary congestion cannot be interpreted as indicative of LV failure (systolic ventricular dysfunction) without corroboration by other studies. Second, there may be important discrepancies between the chest roentgenogram and the level of LV end-diastolic pressure because of the time required for pulmonary edema fluid to accumulate after the LV pressure has risen. It is not unusual for 12 hours to elapse before the roentgenographic findings reflect the true hemodynamic state. Despite these limitations, the degree of pulmonary congestion and size of the left cardiac chambers on the initial chest film appear to be highly useful independent predictors in defining groups of patients with AMI who are at increased risk of death within the first year after the acute event.[49]

RADIONUCLIDE STUDIES

Radionuclide techniques may be useful in diagnosing AMI, estimating infarct size, determining ventricular function, and establishing prognosis. These techniques include myocardial perfusion scintigraphy with thallium-201 or technetium-99m pyrophosphate, radionuclide angiography, and positron emission tomography. These techniques are discussed elsewhere in this volume.

ECHOCARDIOGRAPHY

Echocardiography has become an extremely useful adjunct in diagnosing AMI, quantitating the extent of infarction, and detecting complications. This is particularly true of two-dimensional echocardiography. This technique is superior to M-mode studies for the examination of regional LV wall motion abnormalities because it provides both longitudinal and transverse views of the LV and visualizes a much larger portion of the LV chamber, including the apex, anterior, anterolateral, septal, inferior, and posterior wall segments. Similarly, the right ventricle, which is frequently involved in inferoposterior AMIs, can be visualized well by two-dimensional echocardiography and only marginally so by M-mode techniques. Since the original demonstration in 1974 that wall motion abnormalities that accompany AMI can be visualized noninvasively with cross-sectional echocardiography, many studies have shown that the extent of circumferential abnormal wall motion correlates well with infarct size.[50-52] Efforts have been directed to extend these observations to more quantitative measurements.[53]

Abnormalities of regional LV wall motion can be observed almost universally in patients with AMI.[54] Several studies have concluded that important prognostic information can be derived from early two-dimensional echocardiography.[55,56] Wall motion abnormalities found in areas remote from the area of infarction seem to correlate with higher serum CK activity and identify patients at high risk for the development of subsequent complications.

In addition to the detection and quantification of ventricular wall motion abnormalities, two-dimensional echocardiography is useful in identifying early potential complications of AMI, such as LV thrombus, which is a common post-AMI finding. Not only can LV thrombus be easily identified by this technique, but the configuration of the thrombus also seems to be predictive of subsequent systemic embolization.[57] These and other relevant considerations are discussed elsewhere. Because of the relative ease, low cost, and high yield of important information obtained by this technique, it is reasonable to recommend at this time that all patients admitted with an infarction should have an early two-dimensional echocardiographic study.

PREVENTION AND TREATMENT OF COMPLICATIONS
VENTRICULAR TACHYARRHYTHMIAS

Even patients with an uncomplicated AMI are at high risk for the sudden development of ventricular tachyarrhythmias. Ventricular fibrillation (VF) occurs in 8% to 15% of patients with AMI.[58] In over one half of these patients, VF develops in the absence of heart failure or cardiogenic shock and is therefore called primary VF. The majority of instances of primary VF occur within the first few hours after the onset of AMI symptoms. Although this is a potentially lethal arrhythmia, evidence from many studies suggests that when properly treated, primary VF has totally different prognostic implications compared with the same arrhythmia when it occurs in the presence of heart failure or cardiogenic shock (secondary VF). Approximately 80% of AMI patients with primary VF are known to survive and leave the hospital in contrast to only 20% to 25% of those with secondary VF.[58] The incidence of primary VF decreases rapidly with time and is uncommon beyond 48 hours after the onset of AMI symptoms.[59,60]

It was initially suggested that all patients who experienced primary VF or other life-threatening ventricular arrhythmias in a setting of AMI had premonitory or "warning arrhythmias," such as frequent ventricular premature contractions (VPCs), multiform or multifocal ventricular beats, VPCs demonstrating the R-on-T phenomenon, or couplets or short runs of ventricular tachycardia.[61] Furthermore, it was the contention of early investigators that these premonitory arrhythmias could be suppressed pharmacologically, thus preventing the development of VF. Treatment protocols using lidocaine were developed and widely used in CCUs.[62]

More recently, the concept of warning ventricular arrhythmias has been seriously questioned. Primary VF was shown to develop without premonitory events, and subsequent studies showed that "warning arrhythmias" occurred as frequently in patients in whom VF did not develop as in those in whom it did.[60,63] Furthermore, studies investigating the efficacy and reliability of visual monitoring in detecting arrhythmias in the CCU suggest that as many as one half of premonitory ventricular arrhythmias may be missed by the CCU staff. Romhilt and co-workers found that whereas a physician-validated computer analysis system detected 97% of VPCs, only 45% had been previously detected by the CCU staff. When serious ventricular arrhythmias were analyzed, the corresponding figures were 93% and 16%, respectively.[64]

These observations have led to the recommendation of routine lidocaine prophylaxis in patients hospitalized with AMI.[65] In a double-blind, randomized study of 212 consecutive patients, Lie and co-workers supported this view by demonstrating a definite reduction in the incidence of primary VF in patients treated prophylactically with adequate doses of lidocaine when compared with those not so treated.[66] If lidocaine prophylaxis is to be administered, it is given to all patients with a history suggestive of AMI since the highest risk of primary VF is in the earliest hours after the onset of symptoms. A natural consequence of this approach is that therapy will be administered to a substantial group of patients not at risk for primary VF (*i.e.*, those without AMI). In addition, the side effects of lidocaine therapy must be taken into account. In the study of Lie and co-workers, side effects occurred in 16 of 107 patients receiving lidocaine. The adverse reactions were limited to central nervous system symptoms including drowsiness, numbness of the tongue and lips, speech disturbances, and dizziness. Other investigators have reported focal and grand mal seizures and even respiratory arrest occurring as complications of lidocaine therapy, especially when the plasma levels exceeded 9 μg/ml with the usual therapeutic level being 1.4 to 6 μg/ml.[67]

Despite numerous studies, there is no general agreement as to when lidocaine should be administered in the setting of AMI.[68] Three different methods of administration are recommended and supported by different authorities:

1. Administration of lidocaine prophylactically to all patients with a documented or strongly suspected AMI who are seen within the first 24 hours after the onset of symptoms
2. Administration only to those patients who demonstrate "warning arrhythmias"
3. Administration only to those patients who have experienced one or more episodes of ventricular tachycardia or VF

Therefore, in the absence of general agreement it is best to reserve decision as to the use of prophylactic lidocaine based on local policy and personnel considerations. It has been stated that the need for prophylactic antiarrhythmic drug administration is inversely proportional to the sophistication of the therapeutic environment.[69] In many large CCUs where adequate staffing and large numbers of highly trained personnel including house officers and critical care nurses are available, it may not be necessary or even prudent to use prophylactic lidocaine routinely in the treatment of uncomplicated AMI. However, when staffing is marginal and computerized arrhythmia monitoring systems and house staff are absent, current information suggests that prophylactic lidocaine should be administered to all patients with documented or strongly suspected AMI. The Bethesda Task Force (on critical care) recommends prophylactic lidocaine for 24 hours in patients with AMI.

Whether lidocaine is administered prophylactically or therapeutically for documented arrhythmias, it is important to administer the drug correctly. A therapeutic blood level (1.4 to 6.4 μg/ml) should be achieved as quickly as possible and maintained during the high-risk period or until another effective antiarrhythmic agent is started. A loading dose of 75 to 100 mg (1 to 1.3 mg/kg for an average adult) is administered intravenously as a bolus over several minutes. Concurrently, a continuous infusion of 50 μg/kg/min (3 mg/min for a 60-kg patient) is started. The purpose of the constant infusion initiated at the time of the bolus injection is to maintain the plasma concentration of lidocaine in the therapeutic range. However, because of the short half-life and the two-compartment distribution of lidocaine, plasma levels may transiently fall below the therapeutic range even with this technique. Therefore, a second lidocaine bolus of 0.5 to 0.75 mg/kg should be administered 8 to 10 minutes after the initial bolus. If significant ventricular ectopy persists, additional lidocaine may be given in 50-mg bolus injections to a total of 225 mg and the infusion may be increased to a maximum of 4 mg/min. If the ventricular ectopy is controlled and after a steady state has been achieved for 3 to 4 hours, it is generally recommended that the lidocaine infusion rate be reduced to 40 μg/kg/min (2.4 mg/min for a 60-kg patient). This dosage schedule should maintain adequate therapeutic plasma levels in most patients and avoid toxicity. In the presence of congestive heart failure, shock, or significant hepatocellular disease, the lidocaine dosage described here should be reduced by one half.

Recently, interest has developed in the role of hypomagnesemia in the development of ventricular tachyarrhythmias. In a small, double-blind, placebo-controlled pilot study, 200 patients received either 65 ml of magnesium sulfate intravenously over a 24-hour period or a placebo saline infusion. The 24-hour mortality was lower in the patients receiving magnesium, but the reduction was not statistically significant. Ventricular arrhythmias requiring treatment were less frequent in the magnesium-treated group. The total number of deaths and episodes of ventricular arrhythmias was significantly less in the magnesium-treated patients than in the placebo group. No adverse reactions were reported by the investigators.[70] Although this and other similar small studies are provocative, the precise role of intravenous magnesium infusion in patients with AMI remains to be determined and cannot be recommended as routine therapy, unless documented hypomagnesemia is present.

VENTRICULAR FIBRILLATION

If VF occurs as a witnessed event, immediate electrical defibrillation is indicated. The longer VF persists, the less likely it is to respond to defibrillation. Current recommendations are that electrical defibrillation be carried out as soon as possible after the onset of witnessed VF that does not respond to a single precordial "thump." If defibrillation cannot be instituted within 2 minutes of the development of the arrhythmia, then full basic life support should be initiated prior to electrical defibrillation.[71]

The delivered energy during the initial defibrillatory attempt should be 200 to 300 joules for an adult patient. Since transthoracic resistance drops with successive electrical countershocks, if the first countershock is unsuccessful, a second electrical defibrillation should be carried out immediately by delivering the same energy of 200 to 300 joules.[72] If the second countershock is also unsuccessful, basic life support must be instituted, appropriate drugs administered, and then further attempts at defibrillation with countershocks up to 360 joules of delivered energy should be attempted.

If repeated episodes of VF occur despite adequate lidocaine therapy, bretylium tosylate treatment should be initiated. The antiarrhythmic action of bretylium is poorly understood. It has been shown to raise the VF threshold and to increase the duration of both the action potential and effective refractory period. In VF, bretylium should be administered at a dose of 5 mg/kg rapidly intravenously in the undiluted form. Electric defibrillation then should be performed as described. If VF persists, the dose of bretylium can be increased to 10 mg/kg and repeated as necessary.

VENTRICULAR TACHYCARDIA

Ventricular tachycardia (VT) is a wide QRS (>120 msec) regular or slightly irregular rhythm of ventricular origin. VT may occur within the first few days after the onset of AMI or may not appear until later. Several studies support the concept that the pathophysiologic mechanisms of early and late post-AMI VT are different.[58] In the setting of AMI, VT is usually of left ventricular origin and will often have the configuration of a monophasic R or qR complex in right precordial leads such as MCL_1. However, in patients with Q waves in V_1 and V_2 due to an anteroseptal myocardial infarction, supraventricular tachycardia with aberrancy and right bundle branch block configuration will resemble the qR configuration of VT of left ventricular origin. If the configuration of the wide QRS tachycardia is identical to the configuration of previously recorded isolated VPCs, this can be an important diagnostic clue. Other clues that help make the diagnosis of VT are the slight irregularity, the presence of atrioventricular dissociation with independent atrial activity (seen in approximately 50% of episodes of VT), the presence of fusion (Dressler) beats, and the presence of a very wide QRS complex exceeding 140 msec in duration.[73] Bedside clues can be helpful in establishing the difficult differential diagnosis between VT and supraventricular tachycardia with aberrant intraventricular conduction. These clues include the presence of irregular cannon waves in the jugular venous pulse caused by contraction of the right atrium against a closed tricuspid valve, variation in the intensity of the first heart sound, and variation in the intensity of the Korotkoff sounds recorded during blood pressure determination.

In treating a wide QRS tachycardia in a setting of AMI, immediate assessment of the hemodynamic consequences is essential. If the tachycardia is causing circulatory collapse and inadequate organ perfusion, immediate synchronized direct-current countershock using relatively low energies of 25 to 50 joules should be employed. However, if the ventricular rate is very rapid and synchronization not possible, electrical defibrillation as for ventricular fibrillation should be carried out beginning with 100 joules of delivered energy. Although precordial thumps have been shown to be effective in restoring sinus rhythm in early onset VT, they have also been shown to cause ventricular fibrillation when used in this setting.[76] Therefore, a precordial thump should never be administered for VT unless an electrical defibrillator is immediately available.

When the ventricular rate is 150 beats per minute or less and the arrhythmia is well tolerated hemodynamically, a brief trial of pharmacologic therapy is in order. The drug of choice is lidocaine, and it should be administered in amounts similar to those described for VF. An initial bolus of 100 mg intravenously given over 2 or 3 minutes is the usual starting point, followed by an intravenous infusion of 3 or 4 mg/min with a second bolus of 50 mg given intravenously 8 to 10 minutes later.

If lidocaine does not produce reversion of the VT and the patient is still hemodynamically compensated, procainamide is the next drug of choice. In order to produce a therapeutic level of 5 μg/ml, the intravenous loading dose of procainamide is 10 mg/kg. However, the maximum rate of procainamide administration is only 100 mg intravenously over a 2-minute period. This dose is usually repeated every 5 minutes until the tachycardia is abolished or until a maximum of 1 g has been given. Careful monitoring of the blood pressure for hypotension and of the electrocardiogram for evidence of intraventricular conduction defects is necessary. After the loading dose of procainamide has been given, maintenance intravenous infusion at a dose of 1 to 5 mg/min should be started to prevent recurrent VT. If this schedule is followed, it is evident that for an average-sized adult patient 30 to 40 minutes will be required to administer the loading dose of procainamide. This is clearly too long for acute therapy of VT. However, it is my impression that if VT will respond to procainamide, it will do so after 200 to 300 mg. Rarely will patients require the full loading dose of 1 g before sinus rhythm is restored. In general, even with maintenance of reasonable hemodynamics it is best not to allow patients with a recent AMI to remain in VT for longer than 10 to 15 minutes. Following sinus rhythm restoration, it is important to investigate and correct underlying abnormalities, such as hypoxia, hypotension, acid-base disturbances, and electrolyte abnormalities. In this connection, studies have suggested an inverse correlation between serum potassium levels at the time of admission and the occurrence of ventricular arrhythmias in patients with AMI.[75]

If both lidocaine and procainamide are unsuccessful in restoration of sinus rhythm and/or prevention of recurrent attacks of VT, therapy with bretylium tosylate should be initiated. In this setting, 500 mg of bretylium is usually diluted to 50 ml and 5 to 10 mg/kg is infused intravenously over a period of 10 minutes. In the alert and conscious patient nausea and vomiting may follow a more rapid injection. If VT persists, this dose is repeated in 1 to 2 hours, and if necessary the same dose may be administered every 6 to 8 hours for prevention of recurrent VT. Alternately, the drug is administered as a continuous infusion at the rate of 2 mg/min. It must be remembered that whereas the action of bretylium in VF is rapid, in VT its effects may be delayed for 20 minutes or more. VT refractory to lidocaine, procainamide, and bretylium may respond to intravenous amiodarone. Amiodarone, 5 mg/kg, should be infused within 1 hour, and then a 1-g infusion should be given in 24 hours.

Patients with recurrent VT refractory to electrical cardioversion and pharmacologic therapy as outlined previously may be successfully treated with overdrive atrial or ventricular pacing. Finally, emerging evidence suggests that the early administration of β-adrenergic blocking drugs may be useful in preventing episodes of ventricular arrhythmias after AMI. In Hjalmarson's study, 41 episodes of VF occurred in placebo-treated patients, whereas only six episodes were recorded in the metroprolol-treated patients ($P < 0.05$).[76] However, additional confirmatory studies must be obtained regarding this point before β-blocking drugs can be recommended for the prophylaxis against ventricular arrhythmias in AMI.

ACCELERATED IDIOVENTRICULAR RHYTHM

Accelerated idioventricular rhythm (AIVR) is recognized when three or more wide QRS (ventricular) complexes occur in sequence at a rate between 50 and 100 beats per minute. Idioventricular rhythm (IVR) is similar to AIVR except that its rate is slow (usually below 45 beats per minute) and it usually occurs in the presence of complete heart block. In the majority of cases the AIVR rate tends to be very close to the sinus rate and AIVR frequently emerges in a setting of sinus bradycardia or during the slow phase of sinus arrhythmia.[77] Since the AIVR rate and sinus node rate are frequently very close, it is common to observe competition and development of fusion beats.

The incidence of AIVR in AMI is between 9.5% and 23%.[77] AIVR occurs more commonly in patients with inferior AMI and generally is believed to have a benign prognosis.[78] Primary VF has been reported in 12% of patients with AIVR, an incidence similar to that of primary VF in all patients with AMI. Although the occurrence of AIVR has not been associated with increased mortality or a greater incidence of VF, studies have reported an increased incidence of VT in association with AIVR occurring at rates over 75 beats per minute.[79]

AIVR in a setting of an inferior AMI and at rates of less than 75 beats per minute frequently presents as a paroxysmal, self-limited arrhythmia without hemodynamic consequences. If the patient is asymptomatic and blood pressure is maintained, treatment of AIVR is not indicated. In the occasional patient who becomes hypotensive, AIVR may be easily overdriven by increasing the sinus rate with atropine. Dosage and precautions to be observed in using atropine in the setting of AMI are discussed in the section dealing with sinus bradycardia. When the AIVR rate approaches 100 beats per minute or when AIVR occurs in anterior infarction and especially when the rate is variable, treatment with lidocaine is indicated in an effort to suppress the arrhythmia and prevent the development of VT.

VENTRICULAR PREMATURE CONTRACTIONS

Suppression of VPCs in patients with AMI is based on the concept of "warning arrhythmias" proposed by Lown and others in the early days of the CCU era.[61] This concept stated that the occurrence of primary VF is more common in patients with VPCs that have specific characteristics. These characteristics are frequency of more than six VPCs per minute, occurrence of ventricular couplets, multifocal or multiform configuration, and a prematurity index of less than 0.85 (prematurity index equals VPC coupling interval/normal QT interval). As discussed previously, the concept of "warning arrhythmias" did not withstand the test of time. Furthermore, a number of studies report no reduction in mortality despite the administration of antiarrhythmic agents and suppression of VPCs as well as primary VF.[80] Despite these findings, however, it still appears reasonable to treat complex ventricular ectopy in the early post-AMI period in an effort to reduce the incidence of VF.

Therapy for complex VPCs is probably best carried out with a lidocaine regimen as described for VF and VT. Patients over age 70 and those who are admitted to the CCU more than 6 hours after the onset of AMI symptoms are less likely to develop VF and are at high risk of developing lidocaine toxicity. Such patients should probably not receive prophylactic lidocaine therapy.

In patients with sinus tachycardia who are seen very early (less than 1 hour) after the onset of symptoms of AMI, complex ventricular ectopy is probably the result of augmented sympathoadrenal stimulation. In this setting β-adrenergic blockade is usually effective in controlling both the sinus tachycardia and the ventricular ectopy. Dosage and mode of administration as well as contraindications to the administration of β-blocking drugs in AMI are discussed below.

SUPRAVENTRICULAR TACHYARRHYTHMIAS

Supraventricular tachyarrhythmias are relatively uncommon (except for sinus tachycardia) in patients with uncomplicated AMI. When they occur they impose a significant rate burden that may be intolerable because of several different mechanisms:

1. Since myocardial oxygen consumption is directly related to heart rate, tachycardia increases myocardial oxygen requirements and areas of myocardium with borderline coronary perfusion may be rendered more ischemic.
2. During rapid heart rates, the time available for diastolic coronary perfusion of the ischemic myocardium is further decreased and coronary blood flow may suffer.
3. Reduction in the duration of diastole may result in inadequate ventricular filling and reduced cardiac output.

It therefore becomes obvious that even in an uncomplicated AMI the occurrence of a supraventricular tachycardia with rapid ventricular response can be deleterious and requires prompt attention and treatment.

SINUS TACHYCARDIA

In general, sinus tachycardia is said to be present in adults when the sinus rate exceeds 100 beats per minute. The upper limit varies depending on the patient's age and physical condition, but in adults it rarely exceeds 150 to 160 beats per minute. In patients with AMI an increase in sinus node rate may be due either to inhibition of vagal suppression or to excessive sympathetic discharge. Frequently, this is due to fear, continuing pain, or anxiety. It may also result from concurrent occult complications, which include infection, pericarditis, pulmonary embolism, heart failure, hypovolemia, and fever.

Persistent sinus tachycardia at rates of over 120 beats per minute must be treated promptly. Adequate relief of pain with intravenous morphine sulfate is the first therapeutic step if the patient is not totally pain free. Similarly, apprehension must be dealt with by reassurance and, as necessary, sedation with a benzodiazepine drug. Relief of pain and anxiety will almost always result in slowing of the sinus rate. Older patients who have been receiving chronic diuretic therapy prior to the development of AMI are often hypovolemic. This diagnosis can be difficult and may require measurement of the pulmonary artery wedge pressure by means of a balloon flotation catheter. If the patient is hypovolemic, treatment with intravenous fluid is required. If the patient is in pump failure with markedly elevated left ventricular filling pressures, treatment with diuretics, vasodilators, and positive inotropic agents singly or in combination is necessary.

Occasionally, despite reassurance and pain relief and in the absence of hypovolemia, fever, or pump failure, a hyperdynamic circulatory state is produced by excessive sympathetic nervous system discharge. In this setting, the careful administration of small doses of a short-acting, preferably cardioselective, β-blocking drug is indicated. Metoprolol may be given in doses of 2.5 to 5 mg intravenously and repeated if necessary to a total of 15 mg over a period of 30 minutes while the patient is kept under strict observation. Alternatively, propranolol may be given in doses of 1 to 2 mg intravenously every 5 minutes until the sinus tachycardia is controlled with a total dose not exceeding 0.1 mg/kg.

Esmolol is an ultrashort-acting, recently released β-blocker with a half-life of approximately 9 minutes. This short half-life offers definite advantages over other β-blockers in the treatment of sinus tachycardia and other supraventricular arrhythmias in patients with AMI. Since its half-life is so short, undesirable side effects are minimized. It is administered as a loading dose of 0.5 mg/kg intravenously over 1 minute followed by 0.05 mg/kg/min over 4 minutes. Maintenance infusion ranges from 0.05 to 0.2 mg/kg/min.[81]

PREMATURE ATRIAL CONTRACTIONS

Premature atrial contractions (PACs) are frequently observed after infarction, but seldom require specific therapy. However, the presence of PACs often indicates the development of atrial dilatation due to occult heart failure and may precede more serious forms of supraventricular tachyarrhythmias. Therefore, the occurrence of PACs merits attention, and if occult heart failure is present, prompt treatment of this condition is indicated.

When PACs are frequent, resulting in atrial bigeminy or brief runs of supraventricular tachycardia, they should be treated promptly. PACs usually respond well to a class I antiarrhythmic agent (e.g., quinidine or procainamide) as well as digitalis therapy. My preference is to establish responsiveness of the PACs by administering a class I agent intravenously. For example, procainamide may be administered in incremental intravenous doses of 50 mg/min until the PACs are eliminated or until 500 mg of the drug has been given. If this initial therapy is successful, it may be followed by oral procainamide in doses of 500 mg orally every 4 hours or 750 mg of the sustained-release form every 6 hours.

SUPRAVENTRICULAR TACHYCARDIA

Supraventricular tachycardia (SVT) is an uncommon rhythm disturbance in AMI. Most often it represents a reentrant tachycardia that uses the atrioventricular junction or a concealed accessory pathway. In general, because of the rapid ventricular rate seen in this arrhythmia (rates of 180 to 220 beats per minute are common), SVT is not well tolerated and immediate therapy is essential. A variety of treatments are available. However, if the patient is not hypotensive, the treatment of choice is intravenous verapamil in incremental doses of 2.5 mg to a maximum of 10 mg. The commonly used vagal maneuvers for SVT are frequently unsuccessful in the setting of AMI. Similarly, the administration of α-adrenergic pressor agents to increase arterial pressure and stimulate the carotid sinus baroreceptors, a common form of therapy for SVT ordinarily, may be hazardous in patients with AMI and should be avoided.[82] If the patient becomes hypotensive or develops angina with or without associated ST segment changes on the electrocardiogram as a result of rapid VT, immediate termination of this arrhythmia by means of low-energy, direct-current synchronized countershock should be carried out. Alternatively, if the facilities for rapid insertion of a catheter electrode are available, rapid atrial stimulation will often terminate SVT.[83]

ATRIAL FLUTTER

Atrial flutter (AF) is characterized by regular atrial depolarizations most often at a rate of 300 beats per minute. The electrocardiogram characteristically demonstrates inverted atrial depolarization waveforms in leads II, III, and aV$_F$ with a continuously active baseline imparting the characteristic "sawtooth" appearance in these leads. It is noteworthy that in precordial leads, such as monitor lead MCL$_1$, the flutter waves appear as fairly normal P waves and lack the characteristic "flutter pattern." AF is also believed to be a reentrant arrhythmia primarily involving the right atrium. In the absence of atrioventricular node disease, AF results in 2:1 atrioventricular conduction and therefore a ventricular rate of 150 beats per minute. In the setting of AMI, this rate often imposes an unacceptable burden on the heart and must be treated promptly.

Treatment of AF, if urgent, should be either by overdrive atrial pacing or by low-energy (10 to 20 joules) direct-current countershock. Verapamil intravenously may also be tried in doses similar to those described for SVT. In contrast to the effects of this agent in SVT, sinus rhythm will be restored in the minority of patients with AF. However, verapamil will often increase the degree of atrioventricular block and slow the ventricular response with consequent hemodynamic improvement.

ATRIAL FIBRILLATION

According to present concepts, atrial fibrillation (AFib) is the result of multiple "micro reentry" circuits in the atria. It is characterized by irregular baseline activity on the electrocardiogram and an irregularly irregular ventricular response. Atrial rates are usually between 400 and 700 beats per minute. When AFib occurs in a setting of AMI, its hemodynamic consequences are usually severe, not only because of the resultant rapid ventricular rate but also because of loss of atrial transport function. Usually there is associated hypotension, recurrent or persistent angina, congestive failure, and increasing myocardial ischemia. Under these circumstances, immediate reversion to sinus rhythm using direct-current synchronized countershock is a simple and effective mode of therapy. Following the reversion to sinus rhythm, therapy should be directed toward the underlying cause (usually congestive heart failure) and to the prevention of recurrences by the administration of an antiarrhythmic agent, such as quinidine or procainamide.[84] If the situation is less urgent, therapy with incremental intravenous doses of digoxin to increase the atrioventricular block and reduce ventricular rate is a reasonable alternative. If, despite therapy, the patient is experiencing recurrent episodes of paroxysmal AFib, anticoagulant therapy should be instituted in an effort to prevent catastrophic systemic embolization.

BRADYARRHYTHMIAS

Bradyarrhythmias in patients with AMI fall in two major categories: sinus bradycardia and atrioventricular block. In general, bradyarrhythmias are undesirable in patients with a recent AMI for several reasons:

1. Slow heart rates may enhance the appearance of ectopic pacemakers, which in turn may precipitate additional arrhythmias.
2. Slow heart rates increase the inhomogeneity of repolarization of the myocardium, thus promoting conditions for the development of reentrant tachycardias.
3. Ectopic pacemakers developing as a result of slow heart rate may be ill timed and, therefore, ineffective in producing ventricular excitation.
4. Ectopic foci developing as a result of slow heart rate may in fact be "escape mechanisms," for example, junctional escape rhythm resulting in loss of atrial transport function.
5. Cardiac output may be significantly lowered by slow heart rates and, in the setting of AMI, produce hypoperfusion and further ischemic damage of border zones.

Only sinus bradycardia occurs commonly in uncomplicated AMI, and, therefore, only this bradyarrhythmia will be discussed in this section.

Sinus bradycardia (SB) is found most frequently in a setting of inferior myocardial infarction. Excess vagal tone is responsible for most instances of SB although ischemic injury of the sinoatrial node may also have the same effects. The origin of the excess vagal discharge is debated, but there is evidence to suggest that stimulation of cardiac vagal afferent receptors in the inferoposterior wall of the left ventricle near the crux of the heart as a result of inferior wall ischemic injury may be responsible.

Many patients will be completely stable with adequate blood pressure, cardiac output, and organ perfusion at heart rates of less than 60 beats per minute. Patients who tolerate the SB well should be observed and monitored carefully and not necessarily treated with drugs.

Patients who do not tolerate the slow heart rate hemodynamically should be treated with atropine, 0.4 to 0.6 mg intravenously every 5 to 10 minutes with a total dose not exceeding 2 mg. Sufficient atropine should be administered to increase the sinus rate to approximately 60 beats per minute. Often, when atropine is given and the sinus rate accelerates, the VPCs seen in association with SB will disappear and systemic arterial pressure will be restored toward normal.[85,86] It is important to avoid giving patients large, single doses of atropine since there is a potential for marked sinus tachycardia to develop, creating an undesirable increase in myocardial oxygen requirements. It has been amply documented that the injudicious use of atropine may provoke serious ventricular arrhythmias.[87] On the other hand, when atropine is given in incremental doses as described previously, exceeding the desired heart rate goal is uncommon.

Occasionally symptomatic SB will be unresponsive to atropine in full doses (2 mg total). In this situation, a temporary transvenous electronic pacemaker is the therapy of second choice. Pacemaker therapy is both safer and more reliable than the administration of isoproterenol that had been previously recommended. Because isoproterenol may promote ventricular ectopy and uniformly increases myocardial oxygen requirements, it should be reserved only for the patient who is severely bradycardic and hypotensive as a result of having received large amounts of β-adrenergic blocking drugs.

In general the prognosis of sinus bradycardia in a patient with otherwise uncomplicated AMI is good. Common experience indicates that after a successful initial treatment with atropine, it is unusual for the sinus rate to slow again.

THROMBOEMBOLIC COMPLICATIONS

The potential thromboembolic complications of an AMI fall into four categories:

1. Development of peripheral venous thrombosis and pulmonary embolization
2. Formation of mural thrombus overlying the area of infarction with systemic embolization a potential hazard
3. Progression of the coronary arterial thrombus responsible for the AMI to other coronary vessels, thus causing infarct extension
4. Reocclusion of the infarct-related artery following successful reperfusion either by thrombolytic therapy or angioplasty

Despite clinical trials dating back to the landmark study of Wright and co-workers in 1948,[88] the benefits of anticoagulant therapy in AMI have only recently been conclusively documented. In general, most studies have suggested that although infarct-related mortality has not been significantly reduced by the use of anticoagulant therapy, clinically recognized thromboembolic complications are reduced by conventional full-dose anticoagulation.[89,90]

The current widespread use of two-dimensional echocardiography has been of great value in determining the incidence of ventricular mural thrombi in patients with AMI. In a recent prospective study of 261 patients with AMI, mural thrombi were found in 34% of anterior wall infarctions and 1.5% of inferior wall infarctions. An apical wall motion abnormality was found in all patients with ventricular thrombus formation.[91] In this study, none of the 25 patients who received full-dose anticoagulant therapy had a systemic embolic event whereas embolization occurred in 7 of 18 patients who had not received anticoagulant treatment. Similarly, in the Veterans Administration Cooperative Clinical Trial, anticoagulant therapy decreased the incidence of cerebral emboli resulting from ventricular mural thrombi from 10% to 4%.[90]

More recently, it has been clearly shown that the administration of "mini-dose" heparin in doses sufficient to inactivate factor Xa without affecting conventional laboratory tests substantially reduces the incidence of deep venous thrombosis and pulmonary embolism.[92,93] Mini-dose heparin therapy, however, has not been shown to reduce the high incidence of left ventricular mural thrombi.[94] A recent, prospective, double-blind, randomized trial compared the efficacy of high-dose subcutaneous heparin (12,500 units every 12 hours) with low-dose heparin (5,000 units every 12 hours) in the prevention of LV mural thrombus in 221 patients with AMI. Mural thrombus was identified by two-dimensional echocardiography in 11% of patients in the high-dose group and 32% of those in the low-dose group.[95]

CURRENT PRACTICE

In view of the continuing controversy[96] regarding the efficacy of anticoagulant drugs in AMI and the risk of hemorrhagic complications, proper selection of patients appears to offer the most reasonable current approach.

In general, all patients admitted to a CCU with documented or strongly suspected AMI should be started on low-dose heparin therapy consisting of 5,000 units subcutaneously every 12 hours. Contraindications to low-dose heparin therapy are active bleeding diathesis, active gastrointestinal or genitourinary bleeding, and recent central nervous system or eye surgery. Low-dose heparin therapy should be continued until the patient is actively ambulating, usually about the seventh day after admission.

Full-dose anticoagulation usually consists of 5,000 to 10,000 units of heparin given intravenously as a bolus and followed by a continuous infusion of heparin starting at 1,000 units/hr. The rate of the infusion is adjusted to maintain the activated partial thromboplastin time between two and three times normal. After a period of 5 to 10 days of intravenous heparin therapy, patients are usually changed to oral warfarin in doses sufficient to maintain the prothrombin time at approximately twice normal.

Full-dose anticoagulation should be administered to all "poor risk" patients with documented or suspected AMI, those with extensive anterior wall infarction, and those who are believed to be at an increased risk for thromboembolic complications (Table 68.2).[96,97] The rationale and indications for full-dose anticoagulant therapy following reperfusion (whether by thrombolytic drug or angioplasty) are discussed in Chapters 69 and 73.

In general, it is customary to continue full-dose anticoagulation until the patient is ambulatory, but depending on the initial indications, such therapy may be continued for a variable period of time following hospital discharge. In the presence of compelling contraindications to full-dose anticoagulant therapy (Table 68.3), these patients should be placed on low-dose heparin therapy.

ANTIPLATELET THERAPY

Like anticoagulants, antiplatelet agents have been used clinically as interventional therapy for AMI. Most trials to date have studied the efficacy of antiplatelet agents as secondary prevention therapy for recurrent myocardial infarction and cardiac death.[98] Recent large-scale, randomized, placebo-controlled clinical trials have clearly demonstrated that aspirin administered to patients with unstable angina significantly reduces mortality and development of AMI.[99,100] Of great interest are the results of the Second International Study of Infarct Survival (ISIS-2) trial. In this trial, 17,187 patients entering 417 hospitals up to 24 hours after the onset of suspected AMI were randomized between the following: intravenous infusion of 1.5 million units of streptokinase; 160 mg/day of enteric-coated aspirin administered for 1 month; both active treatments; or neither active treatment. Both streptokinase alone and aspirin alone each produced a highly significant reduction in 5-week vascular mortality. Mortality in the aspirin-treated group was 9.4% compared with mortality of those given placebos of 11.8%, whereas mortality in subjects given streptokinase was 9.2% compared with the 12% of those receiving placebo. The combination of streptokinase and aspirin was significantly better than either agent alone (mortality 8% for combined treatment versus 13.2% for no treatment).[101]

Although the precise mechanism of the beneficial action of aspirin in AMI is not completely understood, in view of the ISIS-2 data, it seems prudent to recommend the administration of aspirin to every patient admitted with this diagnosis. Dosage recommendations range from 160 to 650 mg daily, with most investigators agreeing that a single adult tablet (325 mg) daily is the appropriate dose at our current level of knowledge.

Of great interest regarding the mechanism of action of aspirin in AMI is preliminary experimental evidence that seems to suggest that aspirin can directly protect the ischemic or reperfused myocardium through a mechanism associated with improved energy metabolism independent of any antiplatelet activity.[102]

HYPOXEMIA AND OXYGEN THERAPY

Patients with AMI are commonly hypoxemic, especially when LV failure complicates the AMI. Even in the absence of LV failure, however, hypoxemia occurs due to several pathophysiologic mechanisms: (1) ventilation-perfusion abnormalities in the lung[103]; (2) collapse of small airways with resulting right-to-left intrapulmonary shunting; (3) preex-

---

TABLE 68.2 INDICATIONS FOR FULL-DOSE ANTICOAGULATION IN ACUTE MYOCARDIAL INFARCTION

Chronic anticoagulant therapy
History of previous pulmonary or systemic embolization
Active venous thrombosis
Massive cardiac enlargement
Left ventricular aneurysm
Presence of mural thrombus
Cardiogenic shock
Congestive heart failure
Atrial fibrillation
Massive obesity
Inability to ambulate
Extensive varicosities of lower extremities
Following thrombolytic reperfusion therapy
Following angioplasty of infarct-related artery

(Modified from Gregoratos G, Gleeson E: Initial therapy of acute myocardial infarction. In Karliner JS, Gregoratos G [eds]: Coronary Care, p 142. Edinburgh, Churchill Livingstone, 1981, by permission)

TABLE 68.3 CONTRAINDICATIONS TO FULL-DOSE ANTICOAGULATION IN ACUTE MYOCARDIAL INFARCTION

Active bleeding problem (e.g., gastrointestinal, genitourinary)
Hemorrhagic diathesis (congenital, hepatic, or drug-induced)
Active peptic ulcer disease
Recent neurosurgery or ocular surgery
Presence of purpura
Hepatic or renal insufficiency (severe)
Severe hypertension (sustained blood pressure > 190/110 mm Hg)
Open wounds
Sepsis, especially infective endocarditis
Lack of adequate laboratory support
Anticipated invasive bedside procedures (e.g., thoracentesis, subclavian vein puncture, Swan-Ganz insertion)

(Gregoratos G, Gleeson E: Initial therapy of acute myocardial infarction. In Karliner JS, Gregoratos G [eds]: Coronary Care, p 143. Edinburgh, Churchill Livingstone, 1981, by permission)

isting chronic pulmonary disease; (4) atelectasis and hypoventilation due to enforced bed rest; and (5) interstitial and alveolar pulmonary edema. In addition, recent experimental and clinical evidence suggests that increased oxygen (O_2) tension in the inspired air protects and may salvage ischemic myocardium.[104,105] Because of the above, it has become common practice to administer supplemental oxygen therapy to all patients admitted with an AMI. Clinical experience indicates that oxygen will reverse hypoxemia more readily in uncomplicated AMI than in cases with associated LV failure or cardiogenic shock. Therapy with oxygen may increase systemic vascular resistance slightly, and systemic arterial pressure and cardiac output may decline slightly. However, these hemodynamic changes are not believed to be clinically relevant. Furthermore, oxygen therapy may cause redistribution of blood flow to the relatively ischemic myocardium. Studies by Loeb and associates have failed to document significant effects on LV performance when patients with AMI were given oxygen at 6 liters/min through a nasal cannula or a face mask.[106]

Arterial oxygen tension should be measured at the time a patient with a documented or suspected AMI is admitted to the CCU. Although supplemental oxygen therapy may theoretically be omitted in the presence of normal arterial oxygen tension, widespread practice indicates that low flow oxygen (2 to 4 liters/min by nasal cannula) is given all patients during the initial phase of their hospitalization irrespective of arterial oxygen tension. The rationale for this approach is that hypoxemia may develop gradually because of occult LV failure or because of one of the pathophysiologic mechanisms mentioned previously. Since it may be several hours before hypoxemia becomes clinically obvious and since the adverse effects of low flow oxygen therapy are clinically negligible, current practice is to administer low-flow oxygen to all patients with AMI.[17] Patients who are severely hypoxemic will benefit from intermittent positive-pressure breathing with 40% to 100% oxygen-enriched mixtures. Patients in pulmonary edema may require endotracheal intubation and mechanical ventilation with or without positive end-expiratory pressure. Patients who are moderately or severely hypoxic should have their oxygen tension measured serially. A satisfactory noninvasive substitute for multiple arterial punctures is the continuous monitoring of hemoglobin oxygen saturation by means of an ear or pulse oximeter.

HEMODYNAMIC COMPLICATIONS

The management of the major hemodynamic complications of AMI is covered elsewhere. In this section consideration will be given to three problems only: (1) hypovolemic hypotension, (2) persistent hypertension, and (3) right ventricular infarction.

HYPOVOLEMIC HYPOTENSION

Patients receiving chronic diuretic therapy, especially in the older age-groups, are frequently hypovolemic. When such a patient is admitted with an AMI, he is frequently found to have a tachycardia and be mildly to moderately hypotensive. At this point it may not be clinically possible to decide whether the tachycardia and hypotension are due to hypovolemia or to incipient LV failure. The detection of a ventricular diastolic gallop rhythm (S_3) may not be easy, and the appearance on the chest roentgenogram frequently lags 8 to 12 hours behind the hemodynamic changes. If hypovolemia is suspected, a judicious "challenge" with a small fluid load is indicated. Sequential 50-ml intravenous bolus infusions of normal saline may be administered and their effects judged clinically. Preferably, a balloon flotation catheter should be inserted, since this will allow the measurement of pulmonary artery wedge pressure (LV filling pressure) and provide precise guidelines for the administration of fluid. It must be remembered that because LV compliance is reduced in AMI, LV filling pressures of 8 to 12 mm Hg, although in the normal range, may represent a preload that is inadequate for the maintenance of normal cardiac output.

HYPERTENSION

Many patients with AMI will be hypertensive on admission to the CCU. In general, mild to moderate hypertension with systolic blood pressure up to 180 mm Hg will frequently respond to pain relief and sedation alone. More resistent cases of hypertension will often subside when a mild vasodilator such as nitroglycerin is administered either sublingually or transcutaneously.[28] When hypertension is associated with sympathetic overactivity and tachycardia,[107] β-adrenergic blockade is the treatment of choice. Propranolol and other β-adrenergic blocking agents, however, must be administered cautiously since the tachycardia and mild hypertension noted may in fact represent responses to LV failure rather than sympathetic overactivity. The presence of a loud S_1, wide pulse pressure, and absence of tachypnea are clinical clues that the tachycardia and hypertension are not due to LV dysfunction.[108] If the cause of persistent tachycardia and hypertension cannot be resolved clinically with certainty, measurement of LV filling pressure by means of a balloon flotation catheter should be undertaken before β-adrenergic blocking agents are administered.

Severely hypertensive patients with levels in excess of 180/110 mm Hg despite adequate sedation, analgesia, and administration of sublingual nitroglycerin require prompt pharmacologic intervention. Intravenous infusion of nitroglycerin should be tried first. Nitroglycerin infusion is started at a dose of 15 to 20 µg/min and increased by 10 µg/min every 5 minutes until the desired effect is obtained. Dosages of 200 to 400 µg/min may be required and are well tolerated in the presence of severe hypertension. It should be noted that the above-mentioned doses of nitroglycerin are far in excess of those usually administered for preload reduction in LV failure. If nitroglycerin is ineffective, a sodium nitroprusside infusion should be substituted despite reports that this agent may cause extension of infarction when given to moderately hypertensive patients.[109] This recommendation is based on the rationale that treatment of severe hypertension with nitroprusside will result in greater reduction of myocardial oxygen requirements than any reduction of myocardial oxygen supply stemming from the potential "coronary steal" occasionally associated with the use of this agent.[110]

Although the classic prognostic studies of Peel and colleagues[111] and Norris and co-workers[112] did not include hypertension as a definite adverse prognostic factor, other studies indicate that mortality after AMI is significantly higher in hypertensive patients (37%) than in a normotensive group (24%).[113] A possible exception to the practice of aggressively treating post-AMI hypertension involves the patients with bradycardia and hypertension. It has been shown, in at least one study, that in the presence of bradyarrhythmias, patients with normal or elevated blood pressures had improved survival rates when compared with patients with bradycardia and hypotension.[113]

RIGHT VENTRICULAR INFARCTION

Previously believed to be uncommon, right ventricular (RV) infarction occurs in approximately 40% of patients with LV inferior wall AMI. In the majority of patients, the extent of RV infarction is limited and clinically obvious RV failure is uncommon. However, occult RV dysfunction may be demonstrated in many patients with an inferior AMI when the RV is examined by means of two-dimensional echocardiography or radionuclide angiography.

The diagnosis of RV infarction remains difficult. Since it is almost always associated with an inferior AMI, the first step toward making the diagnosis is to suspect its presence. Clinical clues include elevation of jugular venous pressure (reflecting raised RV filling pressure) and the presence of right-sided S_3 or S_4 gallop rhythms. Kussmaul's sign, in the presence of inferior AMI, is very suggestive of RV infarction. Recording right-sided precordial leads (V_{3R} through V_{6R}) may be helpful in making the diagnosis of RV AMI. The most consistent electrocardiographic finding associated with RV infarction in one study was the presence of ST segment elevation of 1 mm or more in lead V_{4R}.[114] When RV infarction is extensive, hypotension and low cardiac output may result. In this setting, the diagnosis of AMI in the RV is confirmed by the much greater level of RV filling pressure when compared with LV filling pressure (right atrial pressure exceeds pulmonary artery wedge pressure). Occasionally RV dysfunction is of such severity that cardiogenic shock may develop even in the face of only moderate impairment of left ventricular systolic function. Severe RV dysfunction may produce a hemodynamic pattern that mimics cardiac tamponade or constrictive pericarditis.[115]

The management of RV infarction will depend on the severity of the hemodynamic derangements. When the only hemodynamic aberration is elevation of central venous pressure, expectant therapy is indicated. When hypotension and low cardiac output develop as a result of RV infarction, volume expansion is the initial treatment of choice. If this intervention is unsuccessful, treatment with positive inotropic agents such as dobutamine or with vasodilator drugs has been found to be helpful. If the low output state is associated with bradyarrhythmia, atrial or atrioventricular sequential pacing has been reported to improve cardiac output in cases in which ventricular pacing was ineffective.[116]

MYOCARDIAL SALVAGE

Convincing evidence has accumulated in recent years that ultimate prognosis following AMI is directly related to the size of the infarct (*i.e.*, the amount of damaged myocardium).[117] The early experimental studies of Maroko and co-workers,[118] subsequently confirmed by other investigators, indicate that the development of myocardial necrosis is a dynamic event, and therapeutic interventions that favorably alter the relationship between oxygen supply and demand in the ischemic area may result in salvage of viable myocardium and minimize ultimate infarct size. The estimation of infarct size remains at this time a difficult and imprecise process. Interventions that are believed to alter favorably the myocardial oxygen supply-demand ratio in the ischemic zone include mechanical and pharmacologic reperfusion and the administration of pharmacologic agents, such as β-adrenergic blocking drugs and nitrate vasodilators. Whether these interventions should be employed in the management of the uncomplicated AMI remains unclear at this time.

β-ADRENERGIC BLOCKADE

It has been known for many years that myocardial infarction is an acute physiologic and psychological stress during which sympathetic nervous system activity increases with a consequent increase in plasma and urinary catecholamine levels.[119] Furthermore, Mueller demonstrated that in experimental myocardial infarction the norepinephrine content of coronary venous blood is increased, indicating catecholamine release by the ischemic myocardium.[120] This high local catecholamine environment may be expected to exert positive chronotropic and inotropic effects that wastefully increase myocardial oxygen requirements and may lead to extension of the infarct. Additionally, it has been shown that increased local catecholamine concentrations enhance the potential for the induction of reentrant ventricular arrhythmias.[121] At least in part this is probably the result of increased circulating levels of free fatty acids produced by the lipolytic effects of catecholamines. Based on the above observations, it appears reasonable to expect that pharmacologic blockade of β-adrenoreceptors in the acutely infarcted and ischemic myocardium may be beneficial both in decreasing myocardial oxygen requirements and limiting infarct size and in providing a degree of protection against ventricular arrhythmias.[122,123]

Clinical studies reported to date are not in full agreement regarding the efficacy of β-adrenergic blockade in the early stages following AMI. In a nonrandomized study, Snow was the first to report reduction in mortality from AMI in patients treated with propranolol.[124] Several other investigators, however, were unable to detect differences in mortality between β-blocker-treated and placebo-treated groups of AMI patients when treatment was started as soon as possible after the onset of symptoms.[125-127] In one double-blind, randomized study from Göteborg, Sweden, patients were given the selective β_1-blocker metoprolol or placebo beginning as soon as possible after their arrival to the hospital. There was a documented 36% reduction in mortality at 90 days among the metoprolol-treated patients when compared with the placebo-treated patients.[128] On 12-month follow-up, all patients who survived the initial 90-day period were still alive. Further analysis of the metoprolol data shows that only 6 metoprolol-treated patients had episodes of VF during hospitalization versus 17 placebo-treated patients. Furthermore, the 17 placebo-treated patients had a total of 41 episodes of VF whereas only 1 episode of this arrhythmia occurred in each of the 6 metoprolol-treated patients.[129] The Göteborg investigators further report that among patients receiving metoprolol within the first 12 hours after the onset of pain, there was evidence of myocardial infarct size limitation, thus favorably influencing both short- and long-term prognosis.[130,131]

Although the findings of the Göteborg study are impressive, a subsequent much larger, multicenter international study failed to duplicate the original results.[132] In the Metoprolol in Acute Myocardial Infarction (MIAMI) trial, 5,778 patients were randomized to placebo and an intravenous metoprolol loading dose (three 5-mg injections at 2-minute intervals) or to placebo followed by an oral regimen of 200 mg metoprolol or placebo daily. After 15 days, the mortality was 4.9% in the placebo group and 4.3% in the metoprolol group. This difference was not statistically significant.[133] However, when patients were divided into high-risk (three or more risk factors) and low-risk (two or less risk factors) groups, a 29% difference in mortality in favor of the metoprolol-treated group emerged. Overall, there was no significant difference in incidence of ventricular fibrillation or recurrent myocardial infarction between the treatment and placebo groups. Conversely, the First International Study of Infarct Survival (ISIS-1) trial reported a 15% reduction in 7-day mortality of patients treated with intravenous followed by oral atenolol when compared with placebo. This was a large, multicenter trial in which 16,027 patients entering 245 CCUs were randomized to the atenolol or placebo groups.[134]

Preliminary results from the Thrombolysis in Myocardial Infarction (TIMI-IIB) trial are also relevant. In this large trial sponsored by the National Heart, Lung, and Blood Institute (NHLBI), a subgroup of 1,390 patients who were eligible for acute intravenous β-blockade therapy were randomized to receive either 15 mg intravenous metoprolol followed by oral β-blockade on entry to this study or to receive oral β-blockade therapy beginning on day 6 after infarction.[135] Among the group receiving intravenous metoprolol, 16 patients sustained nonfatal reinfarctions and 107 patients had recurrent ischemic episodes by 6 days after study entry, compared with 31 and 147 patients, respectively, among those randomized to receive delayed oral blockade (P = 0.02 and 0.005, respectively).

Despite these encouraging results, the routine administration of β-blocking drugs in patients with uncomplicated AMI cannot be recommended at this time. It must be remembered that during the initial 24 to 48 hours after the onset of infarction, deterioration of LV function may develop rapidly and unexpectedly. Treatment with β-blocking drugs under these circumstances may be hazardous. Until further evidence accumulates, current recommendations for β-blockade therapy in AMI are limited to patients with evidence of excess sympathetic discharge (hypertension and sinus tachycardia) and to those previously receiving chronic β-blockade therapy. Additionally, β-blockade is indicated in patients with AMI who experience persistent or recurrent ischemic pain, progressive or recurrent serum enzyme elevations suggesting infarct extension, and ventricular tachyarrhythmias refractory to lidocaine or other antiarrhythmics early after the onset of AMI. Whether β-blocking drugs should be administered in the totally uncomplicated AMI patient is an unresolved question at this time. Similarly, the efficacy of β-blocking drugs administered in conjunction with thrombolytic therapy remains to be confirmed. It is unlikely that β-blockade will reduce infarct size significantly if it is started more than 6 hours after the onset of symptoms since by this time the extent of infarction has been established in most patients.

Contraindications to the administration of β-blocking drugs in patients with AMI include sinus bradycardia below the rate of 50 beats per minute, hypotension with a systolic arterial pressure consistently below 100 mm Hg, clinical or hemodynamic evidence of LV failure (moist rales of more than minimal extent), and broncho-obstructive disease with documented history of expiratory wheezing.

The beneficial effects of β-blocking agents on mortality following acute myocardial infarction has now been well documented in several prospective, double-blind secondary prevention trials. This topic is discussed later in this chapter.

NITRATES AND OTHER VASODILATORS

Nitroglycerin (NTG) in AMI was initially believed to be contraindicated because of the risk of hypotension that in turn might increase the area of infarction.[136] In recent years, however, vasodilators have been used with increasing frequency in this clinical setting. In patients with AMI, NTG and other nitrates (e.g., isosorbide dinitrate) have been shown to exert several potentially beneficial effects:

1. Reduction of systemic vascular resistance with consequent reduction of impedance to ejection by the LV and improved efficiency of the heart as a pump
2. Peripheral venodilatation with consequent reduction in the pulmonary capillary wedge pressure, and reduction in left ventricular end-systolic and end-diastolic volumes
3. Increase in collateral coronary flow to the subendocardial areas of the myocardium
4. Dilatation of the epicardial coronary arteries
5. Reduction in LV wall motion asynergy to the extent that such asynergy is due to reversible myocardial ischemia and not to completed infarction.[137]

Because of the above actions, vasodilators may in fact decrease myocardial ischemic injury and limit infarct size.[138] In addition, vasodilator therapy benefits patients with AMI and LV failure.[139] In this setting vasodilators diminish the elevated LV filling pressure and increase cardiac output. When vasodilators are administered to patients with normal LV filling pressure, cardiac output consistently declines.[140] In terms of myocardial salvage, initial experimental and human studies suggested that although NTG alone is of minor value in decreasing myocardial ischemic injury, this effect could be greatly enhanced if the reflex tachycardia and hypotension that accompany the use of this agent were eliminated by the simultaneous administration of a pressor agent, such as methoxamine or phenylephrine.[141,142] However, this type of pharmacologic intervention remains even today too complex and too aggressive for the patient with uncomplicated AMI. Not only does it require continuous monitoring of systemic arterial and LV filling pressures, but it also increases the risk for extension of ischemic injury if perfect balance between vasodilator and pressor effects is not achieved.

More recent studies suggest that NTG alone may be beneficial in protecting ischemic myocardium in the patient with uncomplicated AMI when given early. Flaherty and co-workers performed a randomized prospective trial in which NTG was given continuously by the intravenous route for 48 hours after the onset of symptoms of AMI.[143] The mean infusion rate of NTG was 90 μg/min, and the endpoint was a reduction of the mean arterial pressure by 10%. Treatment with NTG starting less than 10 hours after the onset of symptoms was associated with fewer infarct complications in the first 10 days. The incidence of congestive heart failure, infarct extension, or cardiac death was 15% in patients treated early and 39% in the other patients. Mortality at 3 months was reported as 15% for the early treatment group and 25% in others. In addition to significant improvement in LV ejection fraction in the treatment group, improvement in thallium-201 perfusion was also documented in patients treated with NTG.

Similar results were observed in a well-controlled trial by Jugdutt and Warnica.[144] These investigators administered NTG infusion sufficient to lower mean arterial pressure by 10% in normotensive and 30% in hypertensive patients, but not to a level below 80 mm Hg, and maintained the infusion for 39 hours. Compared with the control group, patients receiving NTG infusion had a lower CK infarct size, and this difference held for both anterior and inferior AMI. Other indices of infarct size were also improved with NTG compared with controls. At 10 days after AMI, LV asynergy was 40% less, LV ejection fraction 22% greater, and Killip Class score 41% less. In addition, infarct expansion and thinning were less in the NTG-treated group than in the controls. Infarct-related major complications (LV thrombus, cardiogenic shock, and infarct extension) were less frequent in the NTG group than in the control group, and mortality was less in hospital, at 3 months and at 12 months, although this advantage was only present in the anterior AMI subgroup.[144]

In view of these encouraging reports, it is my practice to administer intravenous NTG to patients with AMI who have no contraindications to this form of therapy. This is true even for patients with uncomplicated AMI. Intravenous NTG is titrated to lower mean arterial pressure by 10% if patients are normotensive, or by 30% in the presence of hypertension. At no time should mean arterial pressure decline below 80 mm Hg. Careful blood pressure monitoring is essential, but in the patient with an uncomplicated infarct this can be carried out noninvasively and the insertion of an arterial monitoring line is not recommended.

Because NTG is a potent vasodilator, it may cause profound hypotension in the patient who is hypovolemic or in the patient with borderline hypotension. Furthermore, in the normotensive patient with a normal cardiac output and normal or slightly low LV filling pressures, NTG will often reduce both cardiac output and ventricular filling pressure and cause serious hypotension. Paradoxic responses to sublingual NTG have been reported, such as the occurrence of severe hypotension and associated bradycardia in patients with AMI.[145] Treatment of these complications includes increasing venous return to the heart by elevating the lower extremities, administration of parenteral fluids and atropine, and cessation of NTG administration. However, intravenous NTG may be of great value in patients with complicated AMI and especially those with persistent ischemic pain and evidence of progressive myocardial injury. Although Kim and Williams reported that large and frequent doses of NTG sublingually during the first 4 hours after the onset of AMI symptoms limited the electrocardiographic signs of myocardial necrosis,[146] it is preferable that, in this setting, NTG be administered by a continuous intravenous infusion. When AMI is complicated by LV failure, if the decision is made to treat the patient with a vasodilator agent, NTG should be considered as the initial drug of choice in preference to sodium nitroprusside. This latter agent primarily affects nondilated resistance vessels, thus generating the appropriate conditions for increasing the area of myocardial injury by producing a "steal" phenomenon away from the ischemic area.[147,148] NTG on the other hand, dilates the conductance vessels, especially the larger coronary epicardial arteries, increasing coronary blood flow and myocardial perfusion homogeneously.[149,150]

If one elects not to administer intravenous NTG in patients with uncomplicated AMI, intermittent small doses of sublingual or transcutaneous NTG designed to produce mild venodilatation with little or no arterial dilatation may reduce ventricular volume and pressure and thus benefit the ischemic myocardium. Evidence to this effect is suggestive, but no well-documented studies are available to indicate that the administration of small doses of NTG (or other nitrates) in fact reduces myocardial damage and mortality rates in patients with uncomplicated AMI.

CALCIUM CHANNEL BLOCKERS

Calcium channel blockers have been shown to be effective in the treatment of chronic stable angina, unstable angina, and vasospastic angina.[151–153] Several pharmacologic actions of these agents suggest that they may be beneficial in the setting of AMI. These actions include coronary vasodilatation and reversal of coronary spasm, improvement of collateral coronary flow to the ischemic area, reduction in myocardial oxygen requirements, and protection of ischemic cells by decreasing calcium ion accumulation in the mitochondria of ischemic myocytes.[154]

Despite these theoretic considerations, the results of both experimental and clinical studies on the effects of calcium blockers in AMI are conflicting. Muller and co-workers reported the first large clinical study on the use of nifedipine in AMI.[155] The results were disturbing in that there was no significant difference in the extent of infarction (as determined by MB-CK analysis) in the treated and untreated groups and in that mortality was greater in the nifedipine-treated group than in the placebo-treated patients (8% vs. 0). Similarly, the Danish Multicenter Study Group on the effects of verapamil in AMI found no significant difference in mortality or reinfarction rates between the verapamil-treated and placebo groups.[156]

Studies reported by the Diltiazem Reinfarction Group provide additional insight into the use of calcium channel blocking drugs in acute myocardial infarction. In a multicenter, double-blind, randomized study, the effects of diltiazem on reinfarction and postinfarction angina were evaluated. In 576 patients with non–Q wave myocardial infarction, diltiazem decreased the incidence of reinfarction by 51% and the incidence of refractory postinfarction angina by 50% during the first 14 days after AMI when compared with placebo.[157] There was no difference in mortality between those patients receiving diltiazem or placebo, and the primary endpoint of the study was reduction in recurrent myocardial infarction and frequency of postinfarction angina, rather than improvement in survival. In a subsequent study, the long-term effect of diltiazem on mortality and reinfarction in a much larger randomized, double-blind, multicenter trial was examined. Total and cumulative mortality rates were nearly the same for both diltiazem-treated and placebo-treated groups. A significant bidirectional relationship between diltiazem and pulmonary congestion was recorded. In patients without pulmonary congestion, diltiazem was associated with a reduced number of cardiac events, whereas in patients with pulmonary congestion it was associated with an increased number of cardiac events. Similarly, in patients with an ejection fraction of more than 40%, diltiazem reduced the number of cardiac events whereas in patients with LV ejection fraction of less than 40%, administration of this agent was associated with an increased risk of death and nonfatal reinfarction.[158]

In view of these findings, there is no good evidence to recommend the use of calcium channel blockers to all patients with uncomplicated AMI. However, patients with a non–Q wave myocardial infarction and patients with preserved LV ejection fraction may well benefit from the administration of diltiazem. Similarly, patients with persistent post-AMI angina, particularly when vasospasm is implicated, may well benefit from combined therapy of a nitrate and calcium channel blocker. It always should be kept in mind, however, that all calcium channel blockers are myocardial depressants and should, therefore, be administered with caution in a setting of AMI. Furthermore, verapamil and, to a lesser extent, diltiazem depress conduction through the atrioventricular node and may promote atrioventricular nodal block, especially in the presence of ongoing myocardial ischemia.

OTHER PHARMACOLOGIC INTERVENTIONS
LIMITATION OF INFARCT SIZE

Early experimental studies demonstrated that in the ischemic myocardium, fatty acid oxidation is impaired and glucose becomes the principal source of energy. It was subsequently determined that oxidative phosphorylation and myocardial performance in the ischemic dog heart were improved by the infusion of glucose–insulin–potassium (GIK).[159] Other investigators found that either glucose alone or GIK increased myocardial contractility due to the hyperosmolar action of glucose,[160] reduced the myocardial uptake of circulating free fatty acids, and restored intracellular potassium concentration, stabilizing membrane potential and reducing the incidence of serious ventricular arrhythmias.[161,162]

As a result of these and similar experimental observations, several small clinical studies have been reported on the use of GIK in AMI. GIK is a solution of 300 g glucose, 50 units of regular insulin, and 80 mEq of potassium chloride in 1,000 ml of water administered at the rate of 1.5 ml/kg/hr. Clinical observations include reduction of plasma concentration of free fatty acids and improvement of ventricular stroke work[163,164] and reduction of VPCs.[165] Nonrandomized clinical studies suggest that mortality from AMI may be reduced by GIK infusion,[166] and Rogers and co-workers noted hemodynamic improvement with an increase in global ejection fraction and reduction of ischemic segment asynergy.[167]

To date, however, there have been no reports of prospective randomized trials demonstrating definite reduction in AMI mortality or reduction in infarct size. As a result, the administration of GIK in AMI patients cannot be recommended, except as an investigative procedure.

Another approach to the treatment of patients with AMI resulted from observations that cobra venom factor, glucocorticoids, and hyaluronidase were shown to limit the inflammatory/immune response and reduce myocardial necrosis in the experimental animal.[168–170] In clinical AMI, however, the administration of corticosteroids has had variable effects. Whereas an initial study reported that a single large dose of methylprednisolone administered to patients with AMI decreased infarct size,[171] other studies showed an increase in infarct size with persistent elevation of plasma MB-CK and the suggestion of increased mortality, perhaps due to impairment of healing and an excessively high incidence of ventricular rupture.[172,173] In view of the above and despite the discrepancies noted between experimental and clinical studies, the administration of corticosteroids to patients with AMI is not recommended.

Hyaluronidase has been shown in some small, prospective trials to diminish the development of Q waves, suggesting that ischemic myocardium is protected and that evolution of infarction is partially aborted.[174] In one study, hyaluronidase administered intravenously in doses of 500 NF units/kg every 6 hours for 48 hours was associated with a small reduction in mortality.[175] However, given the lack of convincing evidence and large-scale prospective trials, the administration of hyaluronidase must still be considered an investigational procedure.

Oxygen-derived free radicals (superoxide anion, hydrogen peroxide, the hydroxyl radical, and others) have been recognized as cytotoxic, unstable, and highly reactive byproducts of oxidative metabolism. Evidence suggests that the production of oxygen-derived free radicals increases in a variety of pathophysiologic conditions, including ischemia and especially ischemia followed by reperfusion. The hypothesis that free radicals represent the final common pathway of tissue destruction has been advanced.

Recent experimental studies have demonstrated myocardial protection and reduction in infarct size by the administration of free radical scavengers, such as superoxide dismutase and catalase.[176,177] It is not clear at this time whether free radical scavengers are equally effective if given prior to the initiation of the ischemic process or just prior to reperfusion. This is probably so because the relative contribution and importance of free radicals produced during ischemia versus those formed at the time of reperfusion have not been clearly demonstrated. Clinical studies are underway to ascertain the role of free radical scavengers in patients with AMI. The efficacy of these agents in human AMI remains to be evaluated, although results from experimental studies are encouraging for their potential application in myocardial ischemia and reperfusion.

PREVENTION OF LEFT VENTRICULAR DYSFUNCTION

Following extensive anterior wall AMI, patients frequently experience progressive cardiac dilatation, congestive heart failure, and ultimately death. Experimental animal data following coronary artery ligation have shown that both cardiac dilatation and death can be decreased by the administration of angiotensin-converting enzyme (ACE) inhibitors.[178] A double-blind, placebo-controlled study was undertaken to determine if captopril can reduce ventricular dilatation and improve exercise tolerance in patients with anterior wall AMI. All patients received β-blockers and, as required, digitalis, diuretics, and antiarrhythmic drugs. No other vasodilators were administered. All patients were observed over a period of 1 year. Captopril-treated patients demonstrated a decline in pulmonary artery wedge pressure and a lesser increase in end-diastolic LV volume than the placebo group. These changes were not statistically significant, however. Exercise duration was significantly improved in the captopril-treated group at 3, 9, and 12 months after initiation of this study. The conclusions reached by the investigators were that captopril administration attenuates LV enlargement, reduces LV filling pressures, and improves exercise tolerance after anterior wall AMI.[179] Although these results are encouraging, further evidence is needed before the routine use of ACE inhibitors following AMI can be recommended. A large multicenter trial is currently underway to examine the effects of ACE inhibition on the development of congestive heart failure and survival following AMI.

REHABILITATION AND PROGNOSIS

Preparation of the patient with AMI for discharge and home care should begin as soon as possible after his condition has stabilized in the CCU. Early progressive ambulation and exercise therapy are now commonly employed and minimize the adverse physiologic effects of prolonged bed rest. As part of the post-CCU therapy, intensive educational efforts are necessary. Before discharge from the hospital, the patient should be instructed regarding progressive physical activity, proper diet, use of medications, and vocational rehabilitation. Group sessions afford psychological support and facilitate rehabilitation. Attempts at behavior modification are useful and may be successful in this setting.[180]

The length of hospitalization following AMI has progressively decreased in the past several years. Convincing evidence is now available supporting patient discharge after an uncomplicated AMI within 7 days. Eight studies involving nearly 900 patients discharged after 7 to 14 days have shown the practice of early discharge to be feasible and without adverse effects on short-term mortality or morbidity.[181]

Even earlier discharge appears to be feasible. In a very small randomized study, patients with uncomplicated AMI underwent submaximal exercise treadmill testing on day 3 and those with no evidence of provocable ischemia were randomized to early (3-day) or conventional (7- to 10-day) timing of hospital discharge. Follow-up at 6 months revealed no deaths or new ventricular aneurysms, and the early discharge and conventional discharge groups had similar numbers of hospital admissions, reinfarctions, and development of postinfarction angina.[182] It was concluded that in carefully selected patients with uncomplicated AMI, hospital discharge after 3 days is feasible. However, before this strategy can be recommended, its safety and desirability must be confirmed in much larger prospective clinical trials. It is my practice to discharge patients with an uncomplicated AMI 6 to 8 days after admission. Patients who have suffered complications are kept in the hospital for a longer period of time until their condition has stabilized for several days and they are responding to appropriate treatment.

In recent years, the practice of performing a low-level exercise stress test on all patients with uncomplicated AMI prior to discharge from the hospital has evolved. The safety of exercise studies early after AMI has been well documented. In 634 submaximal exercise tests carried out 11 to 21 days after AMI, there were no serious complications.[183] Early low-level exercise stress tests are useful both in prescribing an exercise rehabilitation program for the patient and in providing important prognostic information. In the study of Theroux and colleagues, 210 patients were studied by submaximal treadmill testing an average of 11 days after AMI. The 1-year mortality rate was 2.1% in patients without exercise-induced ST segment depression and 27% in patients manifesting ischemic ST segment response to exercise.[184]

Six to 8 weeks after AMI, patients who have no angina, heart failure, or other complications should be tested with a maximal or near-maximal exercise test. These tests will uncover a higher percentage of existing abnormalities than submaximal testing 2 to 3 weeks after infarction. In one study, 35% of patients with normal low-level exercise test responses showed an abnormality on a more vigorous 6-week post-AMI stress test.[185]

Additional predischarge investigation frequently includes a 24-hour ambulatory rhythm monitoring and coronary arteriography. The prognostic significance of late post-AMI ventricular arrhythmias detected on Holter monitoring is now well documented. In the study of Moss and co-workers, 193 patients underwent 6-hour predischarge Holter monitor recordings. Patients with fewer than 20 uniform VPCs per hour subsequently were found to have an 8% post-hospital complication rate. Patients with 20 or more uniform VPCs per hour, those with multiform VPCs, or those with a bigeminal pattern experienced a 31% incidence of complications.[186] It is generally believed that the presence of complex ventricular ectopy during the late post-AMI hospital phase helps identify patients with three-vessel coronary artery disease. Schulze and co-workers reported 38 patients who had both a 24-hour Holter monitor and coronary arteriography 10 to 24 days after AMI. None of the 14 patients with one-vessel disease demonstrated complex VPCs, whereas 10 of 14 patients with three-vessel disease had complex ventricular ectopy on the Holter monitor.[187] In addition, the presence of complex VPCs in the late hospital phase after AMI identifies patients with more extensive myocardial damage. In one study only 3 of 29 patients with complex VPCs had ejection fractions of more than 40%, whereas 33 of 52 without complex ventricular ectopy had an ejection fraction of more than 40%.

Thus, patients with complex, late, post-AMI ventricular ectopy should undergo further investigation, since such ectopy is frequently associated with three-vessel coronary artery disease and sudden cardiac death. In deciding whether to treat patients who exhibit late post-AMI ventricular ectopy with antiarrhythmic agents, one must keep in mind the numerous adverse reactions associated with antiarrhythmic therapy (especially Class IA and IC drugs). Evidence suggests that all antiarrhythmic drugs have to some extent a proarrhythmic action. Data from a retrospective study suggest that the survival rate for a group of patients receiving antiarrhythmic drugs was in fact lower than that of a similar group of patients who were not actively treated.[188] Preliminary (1989) as yet unpublished data from the NHLBI-sponsored Cardiac Arrhythmia Suppression Trial (CAST) are in accord with this viewpoint.

Given the available information, it is my practice not to administer antiarrhythmic drugs routinely in post-AMI patients who demonstrate ventricular ectopy. Rather, I treat such patients with β-blocking agents because of their documented protective effects and their relative safety. Patients with complex ventricular ectopy are referred for complete noninvasive and invasive studies (including electrophysiologic assessment) in an effort to treat reversible myocardial ischemia and eliminate mechanical causes of ectopy, such as a ventricular aneurysm.

Another important prognostic factor is the number of coronary arteries with significant obstructive disease. Taylor and co-workers found a 27% mortality rate over a period of 30 months in patients with three-vessel coronary artery disease, but only 4% and 6% mortality rates over the same period of time in patients with one- and two-vessel disease, respectively, among patients who underwent coronary arteriography within 21 days after AMI.[189] Numerous studies have confirmed these results, and for this reason in many centers cardiac catheterization and coronary arteriography are now being carried out more or less routinely in survivors of AMI even if they have no late symptoms. This applies especially to patients with "non–Q wave" AMIs, since it has been well documented that such patients have an increased late mortality, in part due to a higher reinfarction rate.[190]

Most studies found similar anatomical findings independent of the patient's clinical course. Approximately one third of patients each were found to have serious obstruction in one, two, or three vessels, and 10% were found to have significant left main coronary artery disease.[191] Of equal importance is the finding that two thirds of these patients had residual viable myocardium that was seriously jeopardized being perfused by critically narrowed vessels.[192] Despite these findings, the question of routine coronary arteriography in survivors of AMI is not resolved. In general, I believe that it is possible to identify high-risk patients from their clinical course and from noninvasive studies including early and late post-AMI exercise testing (probably in conjunction with myocardial perfusion scintigraphy) as well as ambulatory Holter monitoring. Patients identified by these procedures to be at high risk and patients with critical occupations should then undergo cardiac catheterization and coronary arteriography even in the absence of symptoms. Patients identified as having significant three-vessel coronary artery disease and those with hemodynamically significant left main coronary artery stenosis may then be recommended for aortocoronary bypass graft surgery.[183] Patients with single-vessel or two-vessel disease generally are treated medically and expectantly.

During the past 2 decades, the concept of secondary prevention of reinfarction and death following an AMI has been actively investigated. Antiplatelet agents, antiarrhythmic drugs, anticoagulants, lipid-lowering drugs, and even β-blockers until recently had not been shown to improve long-term survival conclusively. Three large randomized trials employing β-blockers (timolol, propranolol, and metoprolol) have been reported.[76,193,194] All three studies documented that β-blocking agents improve survival in a wide spectrum of postinfarction patients by reducing the incidence of sudden death and reinfarction. Since neither intrinsic sympathomimetic activity, cardioselectivity, nor membrane-stabilizing activity appear to be necessary, it is likely that the beneficial effects of this class of drugs is secondary to β-adrenergic blockade. Long-term survival is improved in all age-groups for all types of infarcts and most risk groups. However, patients with no electrical or mechanical complications from AMI derived the least benefit from propranolol in the β-blocker heart attack trial.[195] Therefore, stratification of patients into appropriate post-AMI risk groups is necessary. Patients at high risk for late post-AMI mortality should be afforded the benefit of prophylactic treatment with β-adrenergic blockers provided there are no contraindications (overt congestive heart failure, asthma, or bradyarrhythmias). Therapy should start 7 to 10 days after the infarct, and the dose of the β-blocking drug should be sufficient to reduce the heart rate response to exercise. Current evidence suggests that therapy should be continued for at least 2 years. Investigation continues into the effectiveness of secondary prevention with other agents, such as calcium channel blockers, anticoagulants, antiplatelet drugs, lipid-lowering drugs, and antiarrhythmic agents.

REFERENCES

1. Heart Facts 1983. Dallas, American Heart Association, 1982
2. Kannel WR, Barry P, Dawber T: Immediate mortality in coronary heart disease: Framingham Study. Proceedings of the 4th World Congress on Cardiology, vol IVB, p 176. Mexico, Impresona Galve, S.A., 1963
3. McNeilly RH, Pemberton J: Duration of last attack in 998 fatal cases of coronary artery disease and its relation to possible cardiac resuscitation. Br Med J 3:139, 1968
4. Pantridge JF, Webb SW, Adgey AAH et al: The first hour after the onset of acute myocardial infarction. In Yu PN, Goodwin JF (eds): Progress in Cardiology, p 173. Philadelphia, Lea & Febiger, 1974
5. Moss AJ, Wynár B, Goldstein S: Delay in hospitalization during the acute coronary period. Am J Cardiol 24:659, 1969
6. Simon AB, Feinleib M, Thompson HK Jr: Components of delay in the prehospital phase of acute myocardial infarction. Am J Cardiol 30:476, 1972
7. Goldstein S, Moss AJ, Greene W: Sudden death in acute myocardial infarction: Relationship to factors affecting delay in hospitalization. Arch Intern Med 129:720, 1972
8. Solomon HA, Edwards AL, Killip T: Prodromata in acute myocardial infarction. Circulation 40:463, 1969
9. Kannel WB, Abbot RD: Incidence and prognosis of unrecognized myocardial infarction: An update on the Framingham Study. N Engl J Med 311:1144, 1984
10. Oscherwitz M, Edlavitch SA, Grenough K: Patient and system delay in prehospital coronary care: Proceedings of the national conference on standards for cardiopulmonary resuscitation and emergency cardiac care. Am Heart Assoc 139, 1973
11. Pantridge JF, Geddes JS: A mobile intensive care unit in the management of myocardial infarction. Lancet 2:271, 1967
12. Pantridge JF, Geddes JS: Diseases of the cardiovascular system: Management of acute myocardial infarction. Br Med J 2:168, 1976
13. Crampton RS, Aldrich FR, Gascho JA et al: Reduction of prehospital, ambulance and community coronary death rates by the community-wide emergency cardiac care system. Am J Med 58:151, 1975
14. Lewis RP, Lanese RR, Stang JM et al: Reduction of mortality from prehospital myocardial infarction by prudent patient activation of mobile coronary care system. Am Heart J 103:123, 1982
15. Gomez-Marin O, Folsom AR, Kotke TE et al: Improvement in long-term survival among patients hospitalized with acute myocardial infarction, 1970 to 1980. N Engl J Med 316:1353, 1987
16. Julian DG: The history of coronary care units. Br Heart J 57:497, 1987
17. Gregoratos G, Gleeson E: Initial therapy of acute myocardial infarction. In Karliner JS, Gregoratos G (eds): Coronary Care, p 127. Edinburgh, Churchill Livingstone, 1981
18. Marriott HJL, Fogg E: Constant monitoring for cardiac dysrhythmias and blocks. Mod Concepts Cardiovasc Dis 39:103, 1970
19. Bloom BS, Peterson OL: End results, costs and productivity of coronary care units. N Engl J Med 228:72, 1973
20. Morris AL, Nernberg V, Roos NP et al: Acute myocardial infarction: Survey of urban and rural hospital mortality. Am Heart J 105:44, 1983
21. Gotsman MS, Schrire V: Acute myocardial infarction—an ideal concept of progressive coronary care: South Afr Med J 42:829, 1968
22. Grace WJ, Yarvote PM: Acute myocardial infarction: The course of the illness following discharge from the coronary care unit. Chest 59:15, 1971
23. Bigger JT, Dresdale RJ, Heissenbutel RH et al: Ventricular arrhythmias in ischemic heart disease. Prog Cardiovasc Dis 19:255, 1977
24. Lie KI, Liem KL, Schnilemburg RM et al: Early identification of patients developing late in-hospital ventricular fibrillation after discharge from the coronary care unit. Am J Cardiol 41:674, 1978
25. Webb SW, Adgey AAJ, Pantridge JF: Autonomic disturbances at onset of acute myocardial infarction. Br Med J 3:89, 1972
26. Lown B, Verrier RL, Rabinowitz SH: Neural and psychologic mechanisms and the problem of sudden cardiac death. Am J Cardiol 39:890, 1977
27. Lowenstein E: Morphine "anesthesia"—a perspective. Anesthesiology 35:563, 1971
28. Gazes PC, Gaddy JE: Bedside management of acute myocardial infarction. Am Heart J 97:782, 1979
29. Vasco JS, Henney RP, Oldham HM et al: Mechanism of action of morphine in the treatment of experimental pulmonary edema. Am J Cardiol 18:876, 1966
30. Cote P, Cameau L, Bourassa MG: Therapeutic implications of diazepam in patients with elevated left ventricular filling pressure. Am Heart J 91:747, 1976
31. Melsom M, Andreassen P, Melsom H et al: Diazepam in acute myocardial infarction. Br Heart J 38:804, 1976
32. Thompson PL, Lown B: Nitrous oxide as an analgesic in acute myocardial infarction. JAMA 235:924, 1976
33. Cohen IM, Alpert JS, Francis GS et al: Safety of hot and cold liquids in patients with acute myocardial infarction. Chest 71:450, 1977
34. Fyfe T, Baxter RH, Cochran KM et al: Plasma-lipid changes after myocardial infarction. Lancet 2:997, 1971
35. Ritchie JM: Central nervous system stimulants: II. The xanthines. In Goodman LS, Gilman A (eds): The Pharmacological Basis of Therapeutics, 3rd ed, p 354. New York, Macmillan, 1965
36. Doyle JT: Tobacco and the cardiovascular system. In Hurst JW (ed): The Heart, 4th ed, p 1820. New York, McGraw-Hill, 1978
37. Hoit BD, Gilpin EA, Ross J Jr: Myocardial infarction in young patients: A discrete clinical entity. J Am Coll Cardiol 5(2, part 2):422, 1985
38. Levine SA, Lown B: The "chair" treatment of coronary thrombosis. Trans Assoc Am Physicians 64:316, 1951
39. McNeer JF, Wagner GS, Ginsburg PB et al: Hospital discharge one week after acute myocardial infarction. N Engl J Med 298:229, 1978
40. Roberts R: Serum enzyme determinations in the diagnosis of acute myocardial infarction. In Karliner JS, Gregoratos G (eds): Coronary Care, p 218. Edinburgh, Churchill Livingstone, 1981
41. Sobel BE, Shell WE: Serum enzyme determinations in the diagnosis and assessment of myocardial infarction. Circulation 45:471, 1972
42. Goldberg DM, Windfield DA: Diagnostic accuracy of serum enzyme assays for myocardial infarction in a general hospital population. Br Heart J 34:597, 1972
43. Grande P, Christiansen C, Pedersen A et al: Optimal diagnosis in acute myocardial infarction. Circulation 61:723, 1980
44. Sharkey SW, Apple FS, Elsperger KJ et al: Early peak of creatine kinase–MB

in acute myocardial infarction with a nondiagnostic electrocardiogram. Am Heart J 116:1207, 1988
45. Maroko PR, Kjekshus JK, Sobel BE et al: Factors influencing infarct size following experimental coronary artery occlusion. Circulation 43:67, 1971
46. Sobel BE, Markam J, Karlsberg RP et al: The nature of disappearance of creatine kinase from the circulation and its influence on enzymatic estimation of infarct size. Circ Res 41:836, 1977
47. Roberts R, Gowda KS, Ludbrook PA et al: Specificity of elevated serum MB creatine phosphokinase activity in the diagnosis of acute myocardial ischemia. Am J Cardiol 36:433, 1975
48. Ryan W, Karliner JS, Gilpin EA et al: The creatine kinase curve area and peak creatine kinase after acute myocardial infarction: Usefulness and limitations. Am Heart J 101:162, 1981
49. Battler A, Karliner JS, Higgins CB et al: The initial chest x-ray in acute myocardial infarction: Prediction of early and late mortality and survival. Circulation 61:1004, 1980
50. Weyman AE, Peskoe SM, Williams ES et al: Detection of left ventricular aneurysms by cross-sectional echocardiography. Circulation 54:936, 1976
51. Weiss JL, Bulkley BH, Hutchins GM et al: Two-dimensional echocardiographic recognition of myocardial injury in man: Comparison with post mortem studies. Circulation 63:401, 1981
52. Wyatt HL, Meerbaum S, Heng MK et al: Experimental evaluation of the extent of myocardial dyssynergy and infarct size by two-dimensional echocardiography. Circulation 63:607, 1981
53. Gillam LD, Hogan RD, Foale RA et al: A comparison of quantitative echocardiographic methods for delineating infarct-induced abnormal wall motion. Circulation 70:113, 1984
54. Visser CA, Lie KI, Becker AE et al: Apex two-dimensional echocardiography: Alternative approach to quantification of acute myocardial infarction. Br Heart J 47:461, 1982
55. Horowitz RS, Morganroth J: Immediate detection of early high-risk patients with acute myocardial infarction using two-dimensional echocardiographic evaluation of left ventricular regional wall motion abnormalities. Am Heart J 103:814, 1982
56. Gibson RS, Bishop HL, Stamm RB et al: Value of early two-dimensional echocardiography in patients with acute myocardial infarction. Am J Cardiol 49:1110, 1982
57. Haugland JM, Asinger RW, Mikell FL et al: Embolic potential of left ventricular thrombi detected by two-dimensional echocardiography. Circulation 70:588, 1984
58. Bigger JT Jr, Dresdale RJ, Heissenbuttel RH et al: Ventricular arrhythmias in ischemic heart disease: Mechanism, prevalence, significance and management. Prog Cardiovasc Dis 19:255, 1977
59. Adgey AAJ, Allen JD, Geddes JS et al: Acute phase of myocardial infarction. Lancet 2:501, 1971
60. Lawrie DM, Higgins MR, Godman MJ et al: Ventricular fibrillation complicating acute myocardial infarction. Lancet 2:523, 1968
61. Lown B, Fakhro AM, Hood WB et al: The coronary care unit: New perspectives and directions. JAMA 199:188, 1967
62. Grace WJ: Protocol for the management of arrhythmias in acute myocardial infarction. Crit Care Med 2:234, 1974
63. Lie KI, Wellens HJJ, Downar E et al: Observations on patients with primary ventricular fibrillation complicating acute myocardial infarction. Circulation 52:755, 1975
64. Romhilt DW, Bloomfield SS, Chou TC et al: Unreliability of conventional electrocardiographic monitoring for arrhythmia detection in coronary care units. Am J Cardiol 31:457, 1973
65. Harrison DC: Should lidocaine be administered routinely to all patients after acute myocardial infarction? Circulation 58:581, 1978
66. Lie KI, Wellens HJ, Van Kapelle FJ et al: Lidocaine in the prevention of primary ventricular fibrillation. N Engl J Med 291:1324, 1974
67. Harrison DC, Meffin PJ, Winkle RA: Clinical pharmacokinetics of antiarrhythmic drugs. Prog Cardiovasc Dis 20:217, 1977
68. Kertes P, Hunt D: Prophylaxis of primary ventricular fibrillation in acute myocardial infarction. The case against lignocaine. Br Heart J 52:241, 1984
69. Koch-Weser J: Antiarrhythmic drugs for ischemic heart disease. Postgrad Med 59:168, 1976
70. Smith LF, Heagerty AM, Bing RF et al: Intravenous infusion of magnesium sulphate after acute myocardial infarction: Effects on arrhythmias and mortality. Int J Cardiol 12:175, 1986
71. McIntyre KM, Lewis AJ (eds): Textbook of Advanced Cardiac Life Support. Dallas, American Heart Association, 1981
72. Dahl CF, Ewy GA, Ewy MD et al: Transthoracic impedance to direct current discharge: Effects of repeated countershocks. Med Instrum 10:151, 1976
73. Wellens HJ, Bar FW, Lie KI: The value of the electrocardiogram in the differential diagnosis of a tachycardia with a widened QRS complex. Am J Med 64:27, 1978
74. Zoll PM, Belgard AH, Weintraub MJ et al: External mechanical cardiac stimulation. N Engl J Med 294:1274, 1976
75. Cooper WD, Kuan P, Reuben SR et al: Cardiac arrhythmias following acute myocardial infarction. Eur Heart J 5:464, 1984
76. Hjalmarson A: Early intervention with a beta-blocking drug after acute myocardial infarction. Am J Cardiol 54:11E, 1984
77. Norris RM, Mercer CJ: Significance of idioventricular rhythms in acute myocardial infarction. Prog Cardiovasc Dis 16:455, 1974
78. Talbot S, Greaves M: Association of ventricular extrasystoles and ventricular tachycardia with idioventricular rhythm. Br Heart J 38:457, 1976
79. deSoyza N, Bissett JK, Kane JJ et al: Association of accelerated idioventricular rhythm and paroxysmal ventricular tachycardia in acute myocardial infarction. Am J Cardiol 34:667, 1974
80. May GS, Furberg CD, Eberlein KA et al: Secondary prevention after myocardial infarction. Prog Cardiovasc Dis 25:335, 1983
81. Ahmad S, Giles TD: Managing supraventricular arrhythmias during acute MI. J Crit Illness 4:78, 1989
82. Zipes DP, Troup PJ: New antiarrhythmic agents: Amiodarone, aprindine, disopyramide, ethmozin, mexiletene, tocainide, verapamil. Am J Cardiol 41:1005, 1978
83. Vergara GS, Hildner FJ, Schoenfeld CB et al: Conversion of supraventricular tachycardias with rapid atrial stimulation. Circulation 46:788, 1972
84. Sodermark J, Jonsson B, Olsson A et al: Effects of quinidine on maintaining sinus rhythm after conversion of atrial fibrillation or flutter. Br Heart J 37:986, 1975
85. Warren JV, Lewis RP: Beneficial effects of atropine in the pre-hospital phase of coronary care. Am J Cardiol 37:68, 1976
86. Pantridge JF, Webb SW, Adgey AAJ et al: The first hour after the onset of acute myocardial infarction. In Yu PN, Goodwin JF (eds): Progress in Cardiology. Philadelphia, Lea & Febiger, 1974
87. Dauchot P, Gravenstein JS: Bradycardia after myocardial ischemia and its treatment with atropine. Anesthesiology 44:501, 1976
88. Wright IS, Marple CK, Beck DF: Report of the committee for the evaluation of anticoagulants in the treatment of coronary thrombosis. Am Heart J 36:801, 1948
89. Report of the Working Party on Anticoagulant Therapy in Coronary Thrombosis to the Medical Research Council: Assessment of short-term anticoagulant administration after cardiac infarction. Br Med J 1:335, 1969
90. Veterans Administration cooperative clinical trial: Anticoagulants in acute myocardial infarction. JAMA 225:724, 1973
91. Weinreich DJ, Burke JF, Pauletto FJ: Left ventricular mural thrombi complicating acute myocardial infarction: Long-term follow-up with serial echocardiography. Ann Intern Med 100:789, 1984
92. Pitt A, Anderson ST, Habersberger PG et al: Low dose heparin in the prevention of deep vein thrombosis in patients with acute myocardial infarction. Am Heart J 99:574, 1980
93. Hull R, Delmore T, Carter C et al: Adjusted subcutaneous heparin versus warfarin sodium in the long-term treatment of venous thrombosis. N Engl J Med 306:189, 1982
94. Asinger RW, Mikell FL, Elsperger J et al: Incidence of left ventricular thrombosis after acute transmural myocardial infarction: Serial evaluation by two-dimensional echocardiography. N Engl J Med 305:297, 1981
95. Turpie AG, Robinson JG, Doyle DJ et al: Comparison of high-dose with low-dose subcutaneous heparin to prevent left ventricular mural thrombosis in patients with acute transmural anterial myocardial infarction. N Engl J Med 320:352, 1989
96. Russek HI: Anticoagulants should not be used routinely for acute myocardial infarction. Cardiovasc Clin 8:123, 1977
97. Selzer A: Principles of Clinical Cardiology, pp 355–356. Philadelphia, WB Saunders, 1975
98. Frishman WH, Miller KP: Platelets and antiplatelet therapy in ischemic heart disease. Curr Prob Cardiol 11:73, 1986
99. Lewis HD Jr, Davis JW, Archibald DG, et al: Protective effects of aspirin against acute myocardial infarction and death in men with unstable angina: Results of a Veterans Administration cooperative study. N Engl J Med 309:396, 1983
100. Cairns JA, Gent M, Singer J, et al: Aspirin, sulfinpyrazone, or both in unstable angina. N Engl J Med 313:1369, 1985
101. ISIS-2 (Second International Study of Infarct Survival) Collaborative Group: Randomized trial of intravenous streptokinase, oral aspirin, both or neither among 17,187 cases of suspected acute myocardial infarction: ISIS-2. Lancet 2:349, 1988
102. Karmazyn M, Neely JR: Evidence for a direct protective effect of aspirin on the ischemic and reperfused heart. Circulation 78(Pt II):II–16, 1988
103. Pace JB, Gunnar RM: Influence of coronary occlusion on pulmonary vascular resistance in anesthetized dogs. Am J Cardiol 39:60, 1977
104. Madias JE, Hood WB Jr: Reduction of precordial ST-segment elevation in patients with anterior myocardial infarction by oxygen breathing. Circulation 53(suppl I):198, 1976
105. Maroko PR, Radvany P, Braunwald E et al: Reduction of infarct size by oxygen inhalation following acute coronary occlusion. Circulation 52:360, 1975
106. Loeb HS, Chuquimia R, Sinno MZ et al: Effects of low-flow oxygen on the hemodynamics and left ventricular function in patients with uncomplicated acute myocardial infarction. Chest 60:352, 1971
107. Chatterjee K, Swan HJC: Hemodynamic profile of acute myocardial infarction. In Corday E, Swan HJC (eds): Myocardial infarction, p 51. Baltimore, Williams & Wilkins, 1973
108. Gunnar RM, Loeb HS, Scanlon PJ et al: Management of acute myocardial infarction and accelerating angina. Prog Cardiovasc Dis 22:1, 1979
109. Chiarello M, Gold HK, Leinbach RC et al: Comparison between the effects of nitroprusside and nitroglycerin on ischemic injury after acute myocardial infarction. Circulation 54:766, 1976

110. Mann T, Holman BL, Green LH et al: Effect of nitroprusside on regional myocardial blood flow and comparison with nitroglycerin in patients with coronary artery disease. Circulation 55–56(suppl III):33, 1977
111. Peel AAF, Semple T, Wang I et al: A coronary prognostic index for grading the severity of infarction. Br Heart J 24:745, 1962
112. Norris RM, Brandt PWT, Caughey DE et al: A new coronary prognostic index. Lancet 1:274, 1969
113. Beck AO, Hochrein H: Clinical course and prognosis of myocardial infarction in hypertensives. Dtsch Med Wochenschr 99:815, 1974
114. Braat SH, Brugada P, de Zwaan C et al: Value of the electrocardiogram in diagnosing right ventricular infarction in patients with an acute inferior wall myocardial infarction. Br Heart J 49:368, 1983
115. Lorell B, Leinbach RC, Pohost GM et al: Right ventricular infarction: Clinical diagnosis and differentiation from cardiac tamponade and pericardial constriction. Am J Cardiol 43:465, 1979
116. Topol EJ, Goldschlager N, Ports TA et al: Hemodynamic benefit of atrial pacing in right ventricular myocardial infarction. Ann Intern Med 96:594, 1982
117. Alonso DR, Scheidt S, Post M et al: Pathophysiology of cardiogenic shock. Circulation 48:588, 1973
118. Maroko PR, Kjekshus JK, Sobel BE et al: Factors influencing infarct size following experimental coronary artery occlusions. Circulation 43:67, 1971
119. Klein RF, Troyer WG, Thompson HK et al: Catecholamine excretion in myocardial infarction. Arch Intern Med 86:470, 1968
120. Mueller H: Propranolol in acute myocardial infarction in man: Effects on hemodynamics and myocardial oxygenation. Acta Med Scand Suppl 587:17, 1976
121. Wit AL, Hoffman BF, Rosen MR: Electrophysiology and pharmacology of cardiac arrhythmias: IX. Cardiac electrophysiologic effects of beta adrenergic stimulation and blockade. Am Heart J 90:521, 1975
122. Lee RJ: Beta adrenergic blockade in acute myocardial infarction. Life Sci 23:2539, 1978
123. Gold HK, Leinbach C, Maroko PR: Propranolol-induced reduction of signs of ischemic injury during acute myocardial infarction. Am J Cardiol 38:689, 1976
124. Snow PJD: Effect of propranolol in myocardial infarction. Lancet 2:551, 1965
125. Balcon R, Jewitt DE, Davies JPH et al: A controlled trial of propranolol in acute myocardial infarction. Lancet 2:917, 1966
126. Clausen J, Felsby M, Schonau-Jorgensen F et al: Absence of prophylactic effect of propranolol in myocardial infarction. Lancet 2:920, 1966
127. Wilcox RG, Rowley JM, Hampton JR et al: Randomized placebo-controlled trial comparing oxprenolol with disopyramide phosphate in immediate treatment of suspected myocardial infarction. Lancet 2:765, 1980
128. Hjalmarson A, Herlitz J, Malek I et al: Effect on mortality of metroprolol in acute myocardial infarction: A double-blind randomised trial. Lancet 2:823, 1981
129. Ryden L, Ariniego R, Arnman K et al: A double-blind trial of metoprolol in acute myocardial infarction: Effects on ventricular tachyarrhythmias. N Engl J Med 308:614, 1983
130. Herlitz J, Elmfeldt D, Hjalmarson A et al: Effect of metoprolol on indirect signs of the size and severity of acute myocardial infarction. Am J Cardiol 51:1281, 1983
131. Herlitz J, Hjalmarson A, Holmberg S et al: Effect of metoprolol on chest pain in acute myocardial infarction. Br Heart J 51:438, 1984
132. The MIAMI trial research group: Metroprolol in acute myocardial infarction (MIAMI). A randomized placebo-controlled international trial. Eur Heart J 6:199, 1985
133. The MIAMI Trial Research Group: Mortality. Am J Cardiol 56:15G, 1985
134. ISIS-1 (First International Study of Infarct Survival) Collaborative Group: Randomized trial of intravenous atenolol among 16,027 cases of suspected acute myocardial infarction: ISIS-1. Lancet 1:57, 1986
135. The TIMI Study Group: Comparison of invasive and conservative strategies after treatment with intravenous tissue plasminogen activator in acute myocardial infarction. Results of the thrombolysis in myocardial infarction (TIMI) phase II trial. N Engl J Med 320:618, 1989
136. Nitroglycerin in acute myocardial infarction. Med Lett 18:37, 1976
137. Shah R, Bodenheimer MM, Banda VS et al: Nitroglycerin and ventricular performance: Differential effect in the presence of reversible and irreversible asynergy. Chest 70:473, 1976
138. Epstein SE, Kent KM, Borer JS et al: Vasodilators in the management of acute myocardial infarction. Adv Cardiol 22:138, 1978
139. Flaherty JT, Reid PR, Kelly DT et al: Intravenous nitroglycerin in acute myocardial infarction. Circulation 51:132, 1975
140. Chatterjee K, Parmley WW, Ganz W et al: Hemodynamic and metabolic responses to vasodilator therapy in acute myocardial infarction. Circulation 48:1183, 1973
141. Hirshfeld JW Jr, Borer JS, Goldstein RE et al: Reduction in severity and extent of myocardial infarction when nitroglycerin and methoxamine are administered during coronary occlusion. Circulation 49:291, 1974
142. Borer JS, Redwood DR, Levitt B et al: Reduction in myocardial ischemia with nitroglycerin or nitroglycerin plus phenylephrine administered during acute myocardial infarction in man. N Engl J Med 293:1008, 1975
143. Flaherty JT, Becker LC, Bulkley BH et al: Randomized prospective trial of intravenous nitroglycerin in patients with AMI. Circulation 68:576, 1983
144. Jugdutt BI, Warnica JW: Intravenous nitroglycerin therapy to limit myocardial infarct size, expansion and complications. Effect of timing, dosage and infarct location. Circulation 78:906, 1988
145. Come PA, Pitt B: Nitroglycerin induced severe hypotension and bradycardia in patients with acute myocardial infarction. Circulation 54:624, 1976
146. Kim YI, Williams JF Jr: Large dose sublingual nitroglycerin in myocardial infarction: Relief of chest pain and reduction of Q wave randomized perspective study. Circulation 64(suppl 4):195, 1981
147. Chiarello M, Gold HK, Leimbach RC et al: Comparison between the effects of nitroprusside and nitroglycerin on ischemic injury after acute myocardial infarction. Circulation 54:766, 1976
148. Mann T, Holman BL, Green LH et al: Effect of nitroprusside on regional myocardial blood flow and comparison with nitroglycerin in patients with coronary artery disease. Circulation 55–56(suppl 3):33, 1977
149. Cohen MV, Kirk ES: Differential response of large and small coronary arteries to nitroglycerin and angiotensin: Autoregulation and tachycardias. Circ Res 33:445, 1973
150. Miller RR, Vismara LA, Williams DO et al: Pharmacologic mechanisms for left ventricular unloading in clinical congestive heart failure: Differential effects of nitroprusside, phentolamine and nitroglycerin on cardiac function and peripheral circulation. Circ Res 39:127, 1976
151. Moskowitz RM, Piccini PA, Nacarelli GV et al: Nifedipine therapy for stable angina pectoris: Preliminary results of effects on angina frequency and treadmill exercise response. Am J Cardiol 44:811, 1979
152. Muller JE, Turi ZG, Pearle DL et al: Nifedipine and conventional therapy for unstable angina pectoris: A randomized, double-blind comparison. Circulation 69:728, 1984
153. Antman E, Muller JE, Goldberg S et al: Nifedipine therapy for coronary artery spasm: Experience in 127 patients. N Engl J Med 302:1269, 1980
154. Clark RE, Christlieb IY, Henry PD et al: Nifedipine: A myocardial protective agent. Am J Cardiol 44:825, 1979
155. Muller JE, Morrison J, Stone PH et al: Nifedipine therapy for patients with threatened and acute myocardial infarction: A randomized, double-blind, placebo-controlled comparison. Circulation 69:740, 1984
156. Verapamil in acute myocardial infarction. Danish multicenter study group on verapamil in myocardial infarction. Am J Cardiol 54:24E, 1984
157. Gibson RS, Boden WE, Theroux P et al: Diltiazem and reinfarction in patients with non-Q-wave myocardial infarction: Results of a double blind, randomized, multicenter trial. N Engl J Med 315:423, 1986
158. The Multicenter Diltiazem Postinfarction Trial Research Group: The effect of diltiazem on mortality and reinfarction after myocardial infarction. N Engl J Med 319:385, 1988
159. Calva E, Mujica A, Bisteni A et al: Oxidative phosphorylation in cardiac infarct: Effect of glucose-KC-insulin solution. Am J Physiol 209:371, 1965
160. Wildenthal K, Mierzwiak DS, Mitchell JH: Acute effects of increased serum osmolality on left ventricular performance. Am J Physiol 216:898, 1969
161. Regan TJ, Harman MA, Lehan PH et al: Ventricular arrhythmias, and K^+ transfer during myocardial ischemia and intervention with procainamide, insulin or glucose solution. J Clin Invest 46:1657, 1967
162. Sodi-Pallares D, Bisteni A, Medrano GA et al: The polarizing treatment of acute myocardial infarction: Possibility of its use in other cardiovascular conditions. Dis Chest 43:424, 1963
163. Rackley CE, Russell RO Jr, Rogers WJ et al: Glucose–insulin–potassium infusion: Review of clinical experience. Postgrad Med 65:93, 1979
164. Mantle JA, Rogers WJ, McDaniel HG et al: Metabolic support of mechanical performance in myocardial infarction in man: A randomized clinical trial of glucose–insulin–potassium. Am J Cardiol 43:395, 1979
165. Rogers WJ, Segall PH, McDaniel HG et al: Prospective randomized trial of glucose–insulin–potassium in acute myocardial infarction. Am J Cardiol 43:801, 1979
166. Heng MK, Norris RM, Singh BN et al: Effects of glucose and glucose–insulin–potassium on hemodynamics and enzyme release after acute myocardial infarction. Am J Cardiol 49:811, 1982
167. Rogers WJ, McDaniel HG, Mantle JA et al: Prospective randomized trial of glucose–insulin–potassium infusion in acute myocardial infarction: Effects of hemodynamics, short- and long-term survival. J Am Coll Cardiol 1:628, 1983
168. Maroko PR, Carpenter CB, Chiariello M et al: Reduction by cobra venom factor of myocardial necrosis following coronary artery occlusion. J Clin Invest 61:661, 1978
169. Masters TN, Harbold NB Jr, Hall DG et al: Beneficial metabolic effects of methylprednisolone sodium succinate in acute myocardial ischemia. Am J Cardiol 37:557, 1976
170. Maroko PR, Libby P, Bloor CM et al: Reduction by hyaluronidase of myocardial necrosis following coronary artery occlusion. Circulation 46:430, 1972
171. Morrison J, Redutto L, Pizzarello R et al: Modification of myocardial injury in man by corticosteroid administration. Circulation 53(suppl I):200, 1976
172. Roberts R, DeMello V, Sobel BE et al: Deleterious effects of methyl prednisolone in patients with myocardial infarction. Circulation 53(suppl I):204, 1976
173. Bulkley BH, Roberts WC: Steroid therapy during acute myocardial infarction: A cause of delayed healing and of ventricular aneurysm. Am J Med 56:244, 1974.
174. Henderson A, Campbell RWF, Julian DG: Effect of a highly purified hyaluronidase preparation (GL enzyme) on electrocardiographic changes in

acute myocardial infarction. Lancet 1:874, 1982

175. Flint EJ, Cadigan PJ, De Giovanni J et al: Effect of GL enzyme (a highly purified form of hyaluronidase) on mortality after myocardial infarction. Lancet 1:871, 1982
176. Jolly SR, Kane WJ, Bailie MB et al: Canine myocardial infarction reperfusion injury: Its reduction by the combined administration of superoxide dismutase and catalase. Circulation 54:277, 1984
177. Tamura Y, Driscoll EM, Senyshyn JC et al: Effects of polyethylene glycol-superoxide dismutase on myocardial infarct size and scar formation in the canine heart. Circulation 76(suppl IV):IV-200, 1987
178. Pfeffer MA, Pfeffer JM, Steinberg C et al: Survival after an experimental myocardial infarction: Beneficial effects of long-term therapy with captopril. Circulation 72:406, 1985
179. Pfeffer MA, Lamas GA, Vaughan DE et al: Effect of captopril on progressive ventricular dilatation after anterior myocardial infarction. N Engl J Med 319:80, 1988
180. Ewart CK, Taylor CB, Reese L et al: Effects of early postinfarction exercise testing on self perception and subsequent physical activity. J Am Coll Cardiol 1:662, 1983
181. Pryor DB, Hindman MC, Wagner GS et al: Early discharge after acute myocardial infarction. Ann Intern Med 99:528, 1983
182. Topol EJ, Burek K, O'Neill WW et al: A randomized controlled trial of hospital discharge three days after myocardial infarction in the era of reperfusion. N Engl J Med 318:1083, 1988
183. Spann JF: Changing concepts of pathophysiology, prognosis and therapy in acute myocardial infarction. Am J Med 74:877, 1983
184. Theroux P, Waters DD, Halphen C et al: Prognostic value of exercise testing soon after myocardial infarction. N Engl J Med 301:341, 1979
185. Starling MR, Crawford MH, Gemma TK et al: Treadmill exercise tests predischarge and six weeks post-myocardial infarction to detect abnormalities of known prognostic value. Ann Intern Med 94:727, 1981
186. Moss A, DeCamilla J, Mietlowski W et al: Prognostic grading and significance of ventricular premature beats after recovery from myocardial infarction. Circulation 49:460, 1974
187. Schulze RA, Humphries JO, Griffith LSC et al: Left ventricular and coronary angiographic anatomy: Relationship to ventricular irritability in the late hospital phase of acute myocardial infarction. Circulation 55:839, 1977
188. Rapaport E, Remedios P: The high risk patient after recovery from myocardial infarction: Recognition and management. J Am Coll Cardiol 1:391, 1983
189. Taylor G, Humphries JO, Mellits ED et al: Predictors of clinical course, coronary anatomy and left ventricular function after recovery from acute myocardial infarction. Circulation 62:960, 1980
190. Goldberg RK, Fenster PE: Significance of the Q wave in acute myocardial infarction. Clin Cardiol 8:40, 1985
191. Rackley CE, Russell RO, Mantle JA: Modern approach to myocardial infarction: Determination of prognosis and therapy. Am Heart J 101:75, 1981
192. Turner JD, Schwartz KM, Logic JR: Detection of residual jeopardized myocardium three weeks after myocardial infarction by exercise testing with thallium 201 myocardial scintigraphy. Circulation 61:729, 1980
193. The Norwegian Multicenter study group: Timolol-induced reduction in mortality and reinfarction in patients surviving acute myocardial infarction. N Engl J Med 304:801, 1981
194. Beta blocker heart attack study group: The beta-blocker heart attack trial. JAMA 246:2073, 1981
195. Lichstein E, Furberg C, Hawkins CM: Do all post myocardial infarction patients benefit from propranolol therapy? Analysis of subgroups with electrical and mechanical complications. J Am Coll Cardiol 3:576, 1984

GENERAL REFERENCES

Dell'Italia LJ, Starling MR: Right ventricular infarction: An important clinical entity. Curr Probl Cardiol 9:6, 1984

Frishman WH, Furberg CD, Friedewald WT: The use of β-adrenergic blocking drugs in patients with myocardial infarction. Curr Probl Cardiol 9:9, 1984

Hillis LD, Braunwald E: Myocardial ischemia. N Engl J Med 296:971, 1034, 1093, 1977

Humphries JO: Acute myocardial infarction: Pharmacologic treatment in the coronary care unit. Cardiovasc Clin 14:119, 1984

Reperfusion in Acute Myocardial Infarction

David W. Muller • Eric J. Topol

Approaches to the management of acute myocardial infarction have changed significantly during the past 2 decades. The desirability of minimizing the extent of myocardial injury during infarction has long been recognized. Initial efforts to achieve this goal by improving the imbalance between myocardial supply and demand consisted primarily of pharmacologic interventions to reduce myocardial work. The use of β-adrenergic blocking agents, for example, to reduce heart rate and myocardial contractility has been extensively studied and a number of large, randomized trials have demonstrated the efficacy of these agents in reducing infarct size, early mortality, and subsequent reinfarction, albeit to a limited extent.[1-3]

More aggressive approaches have attempted to reestablish blood flow to the ischemic myocardium with the aim of salvaging some or all of the jeopardized cardiac muscle. The feasibility of performing coronary angiography in the early hours of acute infarction and of mechanically reestablishing coronary patency was reported by Rentrop and co-workers in 1979.[4] Among others, this study prompted further investigation and the search for both pharmacologic and mechanical interventions to dissolve or disrupt occlusive thrombus.

RATIONALE FOR REPERFUSION

These changes in therapeutic approach have paralleled changes in the understanding of the pathophysiology of acute infarction. Although recognized pathologically during the last century, thrombotic occlusion was for many years believed to lead inevitably to sudden death. Following the description by Herrick in 1912 of the clinical features of sudden obstruction of the coronary arteries,[5] the pathophysiology of acute infarction and, in particular, the role of coronary thrombosis was much debated. Based on autopsy studies showing a relatively low incidence of thrombotic occlusion in persons dying of acute infarction, some authors considered it to be a result rather than a cause of infarction.[6,7] This view was challenged by DeWood and colleagues,[8] who performed coronary angiography on 517 patients during the first 24 hours of acute infarction to document the prevalence of complete coronary occlusion. These investigators noted an 87% incidence of complete, presumably thrombotic occlusion in patients studied within 4 hours of the onset of symptoms and a 65% incidence in patients studied between 12 and 24 hours. They argued that this falling incidence of coronary occlusion was inconsistent with coronary thrombosis being secondary to acute infarction. Instead, this observation and the low prevalence of coronary occlusion in autopsy studies were postulated to result from spontaneous thrombolysis. These findings, the subsequent success of intracoronary thrombolytic therapy in reestablishing vessel patency,[4,9] and direct observations of intraluminal thrombus at the time of emergency coronary surgery during evolving myocardial infarction[8] led to the unequivocal implication of thrombus as the principal cause of acute coronary occlusion.

In addition, the findings of DeWood and colleagues emphasized the importance of an underlying flow-limiting atherosclerotic narrowing of the vessel. More recently, the concept of the initiation of thrombus formation by rupture or fissuring of these atherosclerotic plaques has been proposed[10] and validated by angioscopic observations[11] and by correlating angiographic appearances with postmortem pathologic findings.[12] Although the factors responsible for triggering plaque rupture are poorly understood, the central importance of thrombus formation on a complicated atherosclerotic plaque is now generally accepted and forms the basis for the current approaches to reperfusion therapy.

A second fundamental premise on which this approach is based is that there is a finite time-frame during which myocardial damage occurs. This damage was shown in an animal model by Reimer and associates[13] to proceed with time in a "wavefront" from the subendocardial region, supplied by nutrient end-arteries, to the subepicardium. Whereas reestablishment of coronary flow within 2 hours resulted in full functional recovery of the ischemic myocardium, reperfusion as late as 6 hours after the onset of ischemia resulted in subendocardial necrosis but preservation of myocardial cell biochemistry, histology, and function in the subepicardium. Although the time-frame may not necessarily be extrapolated from the animal model directly to the human situation in which slowly developing coronary stenoses encourage the development of a collateral circulation, the principle of myocardial salvage by reperfusion remains the same.

In an era in which mortality from arrhythmias during acute infarction has been dramatically reduced by sophisticated monitoring facilities, antiarrhythmic drug therapy, and cardiac defibrillation, the extent of myocardial dysfunction has become the predominant determinant of both early and late mortality and morbidity. Therapies such as myocardial reperfusion, which have the potential to minimize the extent of myocardial damage, have therefore been rigorously pursued.

THROMBOLYTIC THERAPY

Historically, the first approach to myocardial reperfusion therapy was the use of thrombolytic therapy. The presence of a naturally occurring substance (urokinase) that was capable of dissolving fibrin in urine was recognized toward the end of the past century. In 1933, Tillett and Garner[14] observed that an extract of a culture of group C streptococci could lyse thrombus and subsequently the fibrinolytic enzyme streptokinase was isolated and characterized. Its clinical use began in 1954 with the successful lysis of pleural thrombus.[15] Early studies[16-18] using intravenous streptokinase in the setting of acute infarction, however, were disappointing and met with little enthusiasm, in part because of lingering doubts about the pathologic basis for its use. The widely varying efficacy reported (which related to the use of inadequate doses of streptokinase and the often delayed time of its administration) and concerns about the potential bleeding complications prevented its widespread acceptance for many years.

After this prolonged initial lull in enthusiasm, interest in the use of thrombolytic therapy was again generated following reports by Chazov and colleagues[9] in 1976 and Rentrop and associates[4] in 1979 documenting the success of intracoronary streptokinase in reestablishing vessel patency. These pivotal papers heralded the beginnings of the so-called reperfusion era.

THROMBOGENESIS AND FIBRINOLYSIS

The integrity of the vascular tree relies on the interaction of circulating platelets and plasma coagulation factors at sites of breaches in the vessel wall. Following platelet adhesion and aggregation, activation of the coagulation cascade results ultimately in the formation of fibrin, an insoluble monomeric protein, from circulating fibrinogen. Clot stability requires the polymerization of fibrin, a process that strengthens it and increases its resistance to degradation.

Opposing this thrombotic process and maintaining blood flow under normal conditions are a number of circulating proteolytic enzymes. These include antithrombin III (which inactivates thrombin and the serine protease coagulating factors), α_2-macroglobulin, and the plasminogen fibrinolytic system.

Plasminogen, an inactive plasma protein, is synthesized in the liver and becomes bound to fibrin during thrombus formation. It is converted to its active form, plasmin, by kallikrein (formed during the activation of the intrinsic coagulation pathway) and by vascular endothelial activating factors (Fig. 69.1). These factors include tissue-type plasminogen activator (t-PA) and urokinase-type plasminogen activator (u-PA). Plasmin nonspecifically degrades fibrin, fibrinogen, prothrombin, and clotting Factors V and VIII and is itself regulated by the very rapidly acting circulating protein α_2-antiplasmin. This enzyme prevents systemic defibrination by neutralizing circulating plasmin. Fibrin-bound plasmin, on the other hand, is relatively protected from the proteolytic action of α_2-antiplasmin.

Both endogenous and exogenous thrombolytic agents have been used in clinical trials to achieve vascular reperfusion. They include indirectly acting plasminogen activators such as streptokinase and those that directly activate plasminogen such as urokinase, t-PA, and u-PA.

STREPTOKINASE

Streptokinase is an exogenous, indirect activator of the fibrinolytic system. It combines with circulating plasminogen in a 1:1 ratio to form a streptokinase–plasmin activator complex. A conformational change in the plasminogen molecule then exposes enzymatic sites capable in turn of activating additional circulating plasminogen molecules. Unlike the "clot selective" thrombolytic agents such as t-PA, streptokinase has no particular affinity for fibrin-bound plasminogen (see Fig. 69.1). It causes activation of circulating plasmin, resulting in systemic depletion of fibrinogen and the formation of fibrinogen degradation products (FDPs), which have antiplatelet and anticoagulant activity.[19]

A foreign bacterial protein, streptokinase is also antigenic and its use is therefore not uncommonly associated with allergic reactions. Previous exposure to streptococci is almost universal in the adult population and antibodies to the organism are frequently present in low titers. Unless recent streptococcal infection has caused elevated antibody titers (a relative contraindication to streptokinase administration), allergic reactions are usually mild and include a low-grade fever, urticarial rash, nausea, and occasionally a serum-sickness–like illness. Life-threatening anaphylactic reactions occur rarely. Of 5905 patients given intravenous streptokinase in one study,[20] anaphylactic reactions requiring cessation of drug administration were reported in only 7 patients (0.1%). Prior administration of intravenous corticosteroids and antihistamines does not appear to prevent anaphylaxis but may reduce the frequency of less significant allergic reactions.

Following streptokinase administration, antibodies rise rapidly from the end of the first week to peak at levels up to 1000 times initial titers within several weeks.[21] They return to basal levels approximately 6 months later. During this period, administration of a second dose of streptokinase is inadvisable because of the increased likelihood of allergic reactions and the possibility of secondary resistance to its therapeutic actions.

ADMINISTRATION

Standard regimens for the administration of streptokinase have included low-dose, prolonged infusions for the treatment of pulmonary embolism and deep venous thrombosis (typically a loading dose of 250,000 units over 20 to 30 minutes followed by 100,000 units/hr for 24 hours) and higher-dose, brief-duration infusions for acute myocardial infarction. Intracoronary therapy is most commonly given as a loading dose of 20,000 to 50,000 units followed by 2000 to 6000 units/hr. The preferred dose for intravenous streptokinase in recent clinical trials has been 1.5 million units over 30 to 60 minutes. Because adequate dose-response curve studies have not yet been performed, however, it remains uncertain whether this is the optimal dose or whether higher doses may have greater therapeutic efficacy without necessarily having a higher incidence of side effects.

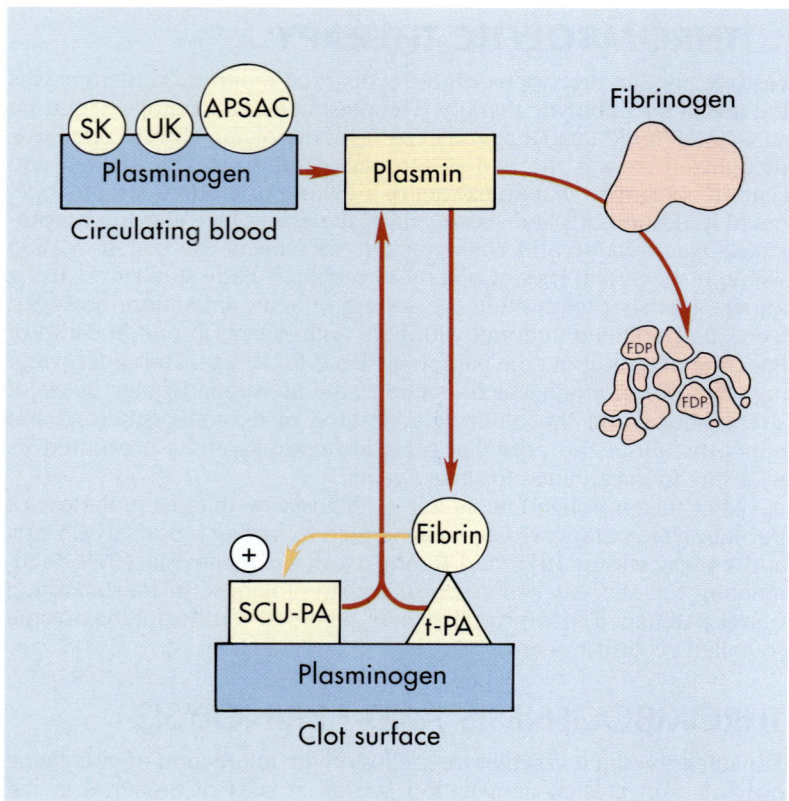

FIGURE 69.1 Schematic representation of the action of fibrinolytic enzymes. Streptokinase (SK), urokinase (UK), and acylated plasminogen-streptokinase activator complex (APSAC) work predominantly on circulating plasminogen; tissue-type plasminogen activator (t-PA) and single-chain urokinase plasminogen activator (SCU-PA) are relatively clot selective. (FDP, fibrinogen degradation product) (Modified from Topol EJ: Clinical use of streptokinase and urokinase therapy for acute myocardial infarction. Heart Lung 16:760, 1987)

The pharmacologic half-life for streptokinase is 18 minutes, and both intracoronary and intravenous administration result in a systemic lytic state that lasts for 18 to 24 hours until hepatic synthesis of fibrinogen returns clotting parameters to normal.

SIDE EFFECTS

The major hazard of thrombolytic therapy is potentially life-threatening hemorrhage. Minor bleeding episodes are common. Periaccess bleeding frequently follows invasive procedures such as cardiac catheterization and results in a substantially higher requirement for blood transfusion. The most devastating side effect is intracranial hemorrhage, which occurred in 9 of 8377 (0.1%) patients receiving intravenous streptokinase.[22]

Other side effects include hypotension and reperfusion arrhythmias. Hypotension occurs in approximately 15% of patients treated by intravenous infusion[23] and is believed to result from activation of the vasodilator bradykinin. The most common rhythm disturbance is accelerated idioventricular rhythm, a benign rhythm that also occurs frequently in patients treated with conventional therapy. Sinus bradycardia and varying degrees of atrioventricular block may also occur, particularly following reperfusion of the inferior wall. Both ventricular fibrillation and ventricular tachycardia[24] have been reported to occur with increased frequency compared with conventional therapy and a combined incidence of 12% to 15%.

ASSESSMENT OF EFFICACY

In assessing the efficacy of streptokinase and other thrombolytic agents, several endpoints need to be considered (Table 69.1). First, the frequency with which vessel patency is reestablished is clearly of fundamental importance. Recanalization *per se,* however, may not necessarily result in increased event-free survival. Late spontaneous reperfusion occurs during the normal course of acute infarction in 20% to 25%.[8] Whether this or late, pharmacologically mediated reperfusion provides significant short- or long-term survival advantage is unclear and is the subject of ongoing investigations. Once reperfusion has been achieved, the frequency of infarct vessel reocclusion during the early postinfarction period becomes an important additional determinant of clinical outcome.

The second endpoint is left ventricular function. Comparison of regional wall motion abnormalities by radionuclide or contrast ventriculography is a sensitive index of myocardial preservation. On the other hand, while evaluation is limited by the compensatory hyperkinesis of noninfarcted myocardium, measurement of global left ventricular function gives useful prognostic and clinically relevant information. Alternatively, assessment of infarct size has some merit but is limited by currently available techniques. Measurement of cardiac enzyme profiles, analysis of 12-lead surface electrocardiograms and myocardial uptake of radionuclide isotopes, for example, are imprecise and, at best, semiquantitative. Assessment of regional metabolic integrity by positron emission tomography[25] has, perhaps, the greatest potential for quantifying the success of coronary reperfusion by identifying viable myocardial tissue. At present, this modality is limited by its lack of widespread applicability and will, for some time, remain predominantly a research tool.

The most definitive endpoint is mortality. Reduction in early and late mortality is the primary aim of each reperfusion strategy. Unless this reduction is substantial, however, a very large sample size (in excess of 10,000 patients) is required and, to date, few clinical trials with this statistical power have been performed.

CLINICAL TRIALS

INTRACORONARY. Since the initial descriptions of Chazov and coworkers[9] and Rentrop and associates,[4] there have been numerous randomized, controlled trials of intracoronary streptokinase in acute myocardial infarction. In a cumulative analysis by Topol[26] of the pooled data of 1175 patients in nine such trials, the recanalization rate documented by sequential coronary angiography was 76.5%. The 30-day mortality was 13.3% in the placebo group and 9.8% in the streptokinase-treated group, a difference that did not achieve statistical significance.

The two largest trials of intracoronary streptokinase have been the Western Washington Intracoronary Streptokinase Study[27] and the Dutch Inter-University Study.[28] The Western Washington study randomized 250 patients to receive either intracoronary streptokinase or conventional therapy. The mean time to the initiation of therapy was 4.6 hours, and to reperfusion it was in excess of 6 hours. No difference in global or regional ejection fraction was demonstrated, but, in spite of this, a decrease in early mortality (3.7% vs. 11.2%; $P = 0.02$) was observed. In addition, a substantial difference in 1-year mortality was noted between those in whom early reperfusion was successfully achieved and those in whom it failed (2.5% vs. 14.6%; $P = 0.008$).

The lack of improvement in left ventricular function noted in this study in patients receiving intracoronary streptokinase more than 4 hours from the onset of symptoms has been confirmed in many studies.[29,30] In contrast, other randomized trials have shown significant improvement in left ventricular function in those patients treated within 4 hours.[24,28,31,32] One such study was the Dutch Inter-University trial in which 269 patients received either intracoronary streptokinase, intravenous and intracoronary streptokinase, or streptokinase and coronary angioplasty to achieve early recanalization. The mean time to treatment in the streptokinase group was 3.2 hours. When data were compared with those of a conventionally treated group, a significant difference was noted in 28-day mortality (5.9% vs. 11.7%; $P = 0.018$), in 1-year mortality (9% vs. 16%; $P = 0.01$), and in both regional and global left ventricular function.

This apparent time-dependent difference in clinical efficacy of intracoronary streptokinase has highlighted important logistic considerations and has resulted in its virtual abandonment as a primary therapy. Not only is it impractical to treat all patients presenting to primary and secondary care institutions in this manner, but the delays associated with performing coronary angiography prior to administering intracoronary streptokinase limit the potential number of patients being treated to a small percentage of the total population.

On the other hand, direct comparisons of the efficacy of intravenous and intracoronary streptokinase[33] have shown no significant dif-

---

TABLE 69.1 THROMBOLYTIC THERAPY FOR ACUTE MYOCARDIAL INFARCTION: ASSESSMENT OF EFFICACY

Infarct vessel recanalization:
  Early vs. late (?"cosmetic")
  Initial vs. sustained patency
  Pretreatment angiography (?initial subtotal occlusion)
Left ventricular function:
  Contrast ventriculography vs. radionuclide angiography
  Global vs. regional wall motion
Infarct size:
  CK-MB curve analysis
  ECG: Q wave, R wave, ST segment mapping
  Radionuclide: SPECT, PET
    Technetium pyrophosphate
    Thallium
    Antimyosin antibodies
Mortality:
  In-hospital vs. long-term
  Does not account for quality of life, recurrent ischemia, or infarction

SPECT, Single-photon emission computed tomography; PET, positron emission tomography.

(Adapted from Topol EJ: Clinical use of streptokinase and urokinase therapy for acute myocardial infarction. Heart Lung 16:760, 1987)

ference in clinical outcome, ventricular function, or complications. Furthermore, intravenous therapy can be administered an average of 1.5 to 2 hours earlier than intracoronary thrombolytic therapy[33] and can be given by trained medical or paramedical staff[34,35] at the site of first contact or in transit to a health care center. For these reasons, intracoronary thrombolytic therapy has gradually given way to the more convenient and thus more widely applicable intravenous route of administration.

INTRAVENOUS STREPTOKINASE. The increasing popularity of intravenous streptokinase in acute infarction provided the impetus for a large number of clinical trials of varying magnitude and complexity. Only two of these, the Gruppo Italiano per lo Studio della Streptochinasi nell'Infarcto Miocardio (GISSI) study[20] and the Second International Study of Infarct Survival Collaborative Group (ISIS-2),[22] have been large enough to show statistically significant differences in survival. The GISSI study, reported in 1986, randomized 11,806 patients presenting within 12 hours of the onset of symptoms. Of these, 5905 patients received an infusion of 1.5 million units intravenous streptokinase over 60 minutes. When compared with a control group, the overall 21-day mortality was reduced by 18%. Subgroup analyses again emphasized the importance of early treatment. Those treated within 3 hours had a 23% reduction in mortality and those within 1 hour, a striking 47% reduction. No significant difference was apparent for those receiving streptokinase more than 6 hours from the onset of symptoms.

In contrast, an improvement in 5-week vascular mortality was apparent in all subgroups of patients in the ISIS-2 study, including those treated between 13 and 24 hours. In this very large, multicenter study, 17,189 patients presenting within 24 hours of suspected acute myocardial infarction were randomized to receive (1) 1.5 million units intravenous streptokinase, (2) 160 mg/day enteric-coated aspirin for 1 month, (3) both streptokinase and aspirin, or (4) neither therapy. The reduction in 5-week mortality was 21% for patients treated with aspirin, 26% for those treated with streptokinase, and 42% for those receiving both active treatments (Fig. 69.2). These differences were maintained in each group during a median follow-up period of 15 months.

Importantly, the incidence of nonfatal reinfarction, although higher in the group treated with streptokinase alone, was not significantly different from the control group in those patients treated with streptokinase and aspirin. The incidence of side effects was no greater with this combination. These findings suggest that early initiation of antiplatelet therapy may play an important synergistic role with streptokinase in achieving reperfusion and in subsequently maintaining infarct vessel patency.

Several smaller studies have examined the effect of intravenous streptokinase on left ventricular function. In the Intravenous Streptokinase in Acute Myocardial Infarction trial (ISAM)[36] in which 1741 patients received 1.5 million units streptokinase or placebo, global and regional left ventricular ejection fractions were significantly higher in the actively treated group and analysis of cardiac enzyme profiles suggested a reduction in infarct size in patients receiving streptokinase within 3 hours, regardless of infarct site. No significant difference was apparent in the in-hospital or 21-day mortality of the two groups. These findings are supported by similar observations reported by the Western Washington Intravenous Streptokinase in Myocardial Infarction Trial[37] and by the Auckland study group.[38]

STREPTOKINASE ANALOGUES

Although it is an effective thrombolytic agent, streptokinase is far from optimal. Ideally, the administration of a thrombolytic agent would result in rapid and complete reperfusion in all patients without risk of hemorrhagic complications, allergic reactions, or infarct vessel reocclusion. It should also be inexpensive.

Modification of the streptokinase molecule by the addition of acyl groups has yielded a number of compounds with improved pharmacokinetic profiles. One of these, anisoylated plasminogen–streptokinase activator complex (APSAC), has been made available for clinical use. The addition of an acyl group to the serine residue of the catalytic site of the enzyme protects the streptokinase–plasminogen complex from degradation by α_2-antiplasmin and limits its activation in the systemic circulation. Because fibrin-binding sites are not affected, binding of the complex at sites of thrombus formation occurs before its activation by spontaneous hydrolytic deacylation.

In addition, the more gradual onset of its action results in less significant systemic hypotension. This allows the administration of APSAC by rapid infusion, thus achieving an earlier therapeutic effect and greater likelihood of successful reperfusion. The preferred dosage regimen is 30 mg given by intravenous infusion over 2 to 5 minutes. The plasma half-life, determined primarily by the rate of its deacylation, is 95 minutes, considerably longer than that of streptokinase (Table 69.2).

Since its introduction, APSAC has been the subject of a number of placebo-controlled and comparative clinical trials. Not all of the pre-

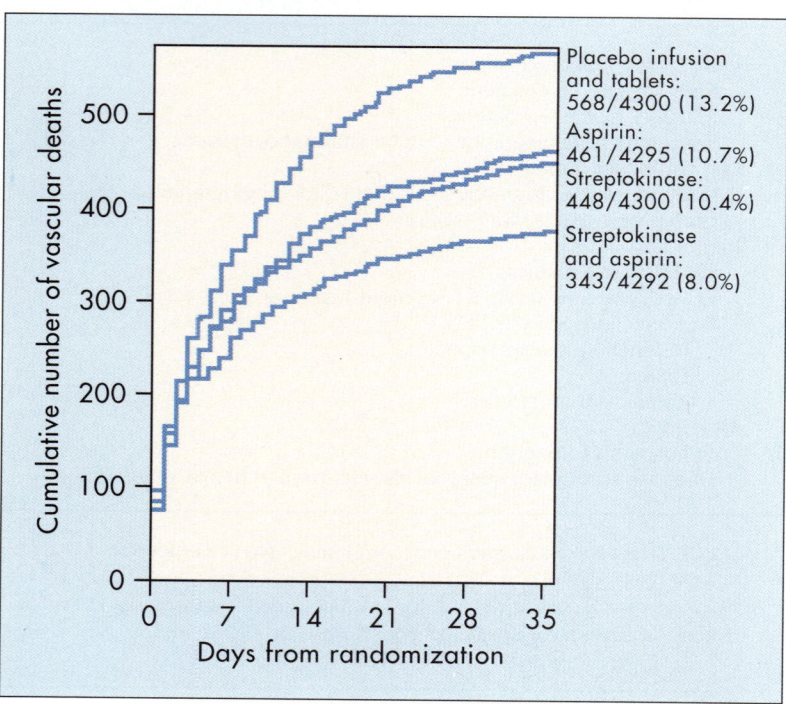

FIGURE 69.2 Cumulative vascular mortality in days 0–35. All patients allocated placebo therapy compared with aspirin alone, streptokinase alone, and the combination of aspirin and streptokinase. (Modified from ISIS-2 Collaborative Group: Randomized trial of intravenous streptokinase, oral aspirin, both, or neither among 17,187 cases of suspected acute myocardial infarction: ISIS-2. Lancet 2:349, 1988)

dicted advantages of APSAC over streptokinase have been confirmed. Whereas doses of less than 10 mg do appear to be relatively fibrin selective, for example, the larger doses required to achieve an acceptable reperfusion rate cause systemic fibrinolysis to an extent comparable to that of streptokinase.[39] Similarly, the incidence of hypotension following intravenous administration of APSAC is not insignificant. Nevertheless, it has proven to be a well-tolerated, effective, and easily administered thrombolytic agent. Anderson and associates[40] reported the results of an angiographically controlled comparative study in which 240 patients presenting within 6 hours of the onset of symptoms of acute myocardial infarction were randomized to receive either 30 mg intravenous APSAC over 2 to 4 minutes or 160,000 units intravenous streptokinase over 60 minutes. Reperfusion rates were comparable (51% for APSAC vs. 60% for streptokinase; $P < 0.18$) at 90 minutes. Mean time to reperfusion was 43 minutes for intravenous APSAC and 31 minutes for intracoronary streptokinase.

As has previously been demonstrated for streptokinase therapy, the reperfusion rate for intravenous APSAC in this study was highly time dependent (60% if given less than 4 hours from symptom onset compared with 33% if more than 4 hours, $P = 0.001$) and its efficacy was also dependent on the completeness of coronary occlusion at initial angiography (43% if TIMI grade 0 flow compared with 78% if TIMI grade 1 flow). The frequency of infarct vessel reocclusion was low and not significantly different between the two groups.

These results are similar to those reported by other investigators.[39,41] Following analysis of the pooled mortality data from studies reported up to February 1987, which showed a trend toward a substantial reduction in 30-day mortality from 12.3% in the conventionally treated group to 6.1% in those treated with APSAC,[42] a large, multicenter mortality study of APSAC in acute myocardial infarction (AIMS) was initiated in the United Kingdom. The trial enrolled 1004 patients presenting within 6 hours of the onset of acute myocardial infarction and was terminated prematurely following an interim analysis of the 30-day mortality data.[43] This analysis showed an almost identical reduction in mortality from 12.2% in the placebo group to 6.4% in those treated with intravenous APSAC. This striking 47% reduction in mortality was minimally affected by time to administration from symptom onset and applied to patients both younger than and older than 65 years of age. These results confirm the findings of the GISSI and ISIS-2 studies of an unequivocal survival advantage in patients treated with intravenous thrombolytic therapy during the early hours of evolving myocardial infarction. The relative benefits of APSAC over streptokinase appear to be small but definite. It is not clear at this stage whether these advantages will be translated into clinical practice.

UROKINASE AND PROUROKINASE

Urokinase and its precursor, single-chain urokinase plasminogen activator (scu-PA or prourokinase), also have a number of theoretical advantages over streptokinase. To date, however, clinical experience with these agents in acute myocardial infarction is relatively limited. Originally isolated from urine, urokinase is a naturally occurring, circulating enzyme formed *in vivo* by epithelial cells and for clinical use by tissue culture of human fetal kidney cells. The active enzyme is a double-chain glycoprotein with a molecular weight of 55,000 daltons. It has the advantage of being nonantigenic and therefore not subject to allergic reactions or to attenuation of its action by endogenous neutralizing antibodies. Unlike streptokinase, urokinase has a direct, dose-dependent action on circulating plasminogen, but like streptokinase, it has no clot specificity and activates plasminogen equally well in the presence and absence of fibrin.

Single-chain urokinase plasminogen activator (scu-PA) is the single-chain proenzyme and is inactive when administered. It binds preferentially to fibrin-bound plasminogen and, on the fibrin surface, is converted to the active double-chain form by plasmin-mediated proteolytic cleavage. Accordingly, it has greater clot selectivity than urokinase or streptokinase. It is cleared quickly from the circulation by hepatic metabolism with a plasma half-life of 7 minutes.

TABLE 69.2 SELECTION OF THROMBOLYTIC AGENT FOR ACUTE MYOCARDIAL INFARCTION

	SK	t-PA	APSAC	UK
Thrombolytic Efficacy (90 min)	50–55%	75–80%	50–55%	55–65%
Time Dependent (>3 hr)	Yes	No	Yes	Yes
Hemostatic Breakdown	4+	1–2+	3+	3+
Hypotension	Yes	No	Yes	No
Half-life	18 min	4 min	95 min	14 min
Allergic Reactions	Yes	No	Yes	No
Mortality Reduction	GISSI (18%↓) ISIS-2 (26%↓)	ASSET (26%↓) ECSG (51%↓)	AIMS (47%↓)	
LV Function Improvement	New Zealand WWIVST* ISAM	TICO NHF Johns Hopkins ECSG		
Stand Alone Without PTCA (Immediate)	?	Yes	?	?
Useful in Rescue PTCA	Yes	Not alone	?	Yes
Approximate Cost/Dose	$200/1.5 million units	$2200/100 mg	$1200/30 mg	$2200/3 million units

* Anterior infarction only.

AIMS, APSAC in Myocardial Infarction Study; APSAC, Anisoylated Plasminogen Streptokinase Activator Complex; ASSET, Anglo-Scandinavian Study of Early Thrombolysis; ECSG, European Cooperative Study Group; ISAM, Intravenous Streptokinase in Acute Myocardial Infarction; ISIS-2, International Study of Infarct Survival-2; NHF, National Heart Foundation (Australia); SK, Streptokinase; TICO, Thrombolysis in Coronary Occlusion; t-PA, Tissue plasminogen activator; UK, Urokinase; WWIVST, Western Washington Intravenous Streptokinase Trial.

Both urokinase and scu-PA may be given rapidly without causing hypotension. Doses of 6000 units/hr for intracoronary urokinase and 2 to 3 million units by intravenous infusion are considered equipotent to the standard streptokinase regimens.

CLINICAL USE

INTRACORONARY UROKINASE. Several small studies of intracoronary urokinase have shown comparable efficacy to that of intracoronary streptokinase.[44-46] Reperfusion rates ranged from 60% to 90%. In 1984, for example, Tennant and co-workers[47] compared the efficacy of intracoronary streptokinase and urokinase in 80 patients presenting within 12 hours of the onset of symptoms. The reperfusion rate was 60% for urokinase and 57% for streptokinase (P = NS). Streptokinase therapy was associated with a greater fall in fibrinogen levels and a higher incidence of hemorrhagic complications (29% vs. 11%; P = 0.001).

INTRAVENOUS UROKINASE. In 1985, Mathey and associates reported the results of a trial of intravenous urokinase for acute myocardial infarction.[44] Fifty patients presenting within 3 hours of the onset of chest pain were given a bolus dose of 2 million units of urokinase. The reperfusion rate was 60% after 1 hour. Analysis of regional left ventricular wall motion by contrast angiography performed at presentation and 2 weeks later showed significant improvement in patients in whom reperfusion was successfully achieved compared with those in whom thrombolytic therapy failed. As with streptokinase, the likelihood of preserving left ventricular wall motion appeared to be time dependent with little apparent benefit beyond 2 hours.

In this study, assessment of hematologic parameters showed evidence of a significant systemic fibrinolytic effect. Fibrinogen levels dropped from 370 ± 142 mg/dl to 79 ± 68 mg/dl and plasmin levels remained elevated for 6 hours. In spite of this, no significant bleeding complications were reported.

Very similar findings were reported more recently by Califf and colleagues[48] and by the German Activator Urokinase Study (GAUS) group.[49] In the latter study, 70 mg intravenous tissue-type plasminogen activator (t-PA) was compared with 3.0 million units intravenous urokinase in 245 patients presenting within 6 hours of symptom onset. The reperfusion rate for urokinase was 64% at 90 minutes, and the 24-hour reocclusion rate and in-hospital reinfarction rate were 11% and 15%, respectively. These findings were not significantly different from those of t-PA. Although fibrinogen levels were significantly lower in the urokinase group, the incidence of hemorrhagic complications was comparable and low in both groups.

INTRAVENOUS SCU-PA. Clinical studies with scu-PA have been greatly facilitated by gene cloning and expression of the recombinant protein by *Escherichia coli,* but, to date, little published data are available for comparison with other thrombolytic agents. Preliminary investigations using doses of 30 mg to 50 mg have shown comparatively low reperfusion rates and a relatively long time to reperfusion.[50]

More recently, evidence has been presented that suggests that the combination of scu-PA with other thrombolytic agents may be complementary. Early data from a multicenter, dose-finding pilot study, for example, suggest an augmentation of the efficacy of scu-PA by the initial administration of a small bolus of intravenous urokinase. In 18 patients treated with a combination of 50 mg scu-PA and 200,000 units urokinase, the reperfusion rate was increased from 65% for scu-PA alone to 83% and the time to reperfusion was reduced from 60 to 30 minutes.[51] Clinical trials currently in progress comparing the combination of urokinase and scu-PA with urokinase alone will provide additional information about this potentially highly effective strategy.

Urokinase and its precursor scu-PA seem, therefore, to be safe and effective thrombolytic agents. Their widespread use has not yet been endorsed, however, principally because of the far greater cost of these agents. A 3-million-unit dose of urokinase currently costs $2200, more than ten times the $200 cost of an equivalent 1.5 million unit dose of streptokinase. If the combination of urokinase and scu-PA is shown to significantly reduce the doses required, these agents may then become cost-effective alternatives to streptokinase.

TISSUE-TYPE PLASMINOGEN ACTIVATOR

Structurally related to scu-PA, t-PA is also an endogenous activator of plasminogen and is secreted by vascular endothelium. It is a serine protease with a molecular weight of 70,000 daltons. Its single-chain form is proteolytically converted by plasmin to a two-chain molecule linked by a disulfide bond. In contrast to the urokinase enzyme system, both the single- and double-chain forms are actively fibrinolytic and both have a low affinity for circulating plasminogen.

In the presence of fibrin, both forms of t-PA bind with high affinity to specific fibrin-binding sites. In so doing, the t-PA molecule undergoes a conformational change that facilitates the activation of adjacent plasminogen molecules incorporated into fibrin during polymerization. The resulting conversion of plasminogen to plasmin on the fibrin surface is augmented by a factor of several hundred compared with the rate and efficiency of its activation in the absence of fibrin.

Although the presence of t-PA was recognized more than 40 years ago, low-yielding techniques prevented its clinical application until 1982 when Collen and co-workers[52] isolated and purified t-PA from human melanoma cell culture fluid. The subsequent cloning of the gene responsible for its production allowed much greater yields of the enzyme and its use in clinical trials. Apart from a few early investigations using melanoma cell–derived t-PA, all subsequent studies have used recombinant t-PA (rt-PA).

Initial preparations of rt-PA consisted principally of the double-chain molecule. Since the adoption of the suspension culture method of production in late 1985, the preparation used is predominantly the single-chain form. Although their fibrinolytic activities are comparable, the more rapid hepatic clearance and shorter plasma half-life of the latter (5 vs. 8 minutes) necessitates the use of higher doses than originally used.

The short half-life of t-PA has both advantages and predictable disadvantages. Whereas the rapid offset of its action is desirable in the event of unwanted hemorrhagic complications or the unexpected need for invasive surgical procedures, it also results in a significantly higher reocclusion rate. The incidence of infarct vessel reocclusion reported in clinical trials of intravenous t-PA has varied considerably, ranging from 10%[53] to 33%.[54] This problem was addressed by Gold and associates,[55] who showed a significant reduction in reocclusion rate using a prolonged low-dose infusion.

Early open-label dose ranging studies noted a significant reduction in the incidence of hemorrhagic complications and transfusion requirements without compromising efficacy of reperfusion when doses of 80 mg to 100 mg were compared with doses up to 150 mg.[56] It is usual now, therefore, to give a total dose of approximately 100 mg t-PA by infusion over 3 to 6 hours, 60 mg of which is given in the first hour. Using this regimen, allergic reactions and hemodynamic deterioration have not been encountered.

CLINICAL TRIALS

In 1984, Collen and co-workers reported the first results of intravenous rt-PA in acute myocardial infarction.[57] In this randomized, placebo-controlled trial, 33 patients received 0.5 mg to 0.75 mg/kg rt-PA over 30 to 120 minutes. Angiographically confirmed recanalization was evident in 24 patients (75%) 90 minutes after the initiation of therapy.

Since these encouraging initial results, a number of larger studies have been performed. The Thrombolysis in Myocardial Infarction (TIMI) study and the European Cooperative Study evaluated the relative efficacies of intravenous t-PA and streptokinase with vessel patency as the primary end-point. Phase 1 of the TIMI Study Group trial was reported in 1985.[58] After baseline angiography, 214 patients with occluded infarct-related arteries were randomized to receive either 80 mg of intravenous rt-PA over 3 hours or 1.5 million units of streptokinase at a mean of 4.8 hours from the onset of symptoms. Repeat angiography at 90 minutes showed a 60% patency rate for rt-PA compared with 35% for streptokinase, a difference that was highly significant ($P < 0.001$).

This difference has been attributed to the relatively late time of administration of the thrombolytic agents. Whereas the efficacy of streptokinase is highly time dependent, t-PA is less affected by this factor. Although the difference was less apparent and not statistically significant in those receiving t-PA or streptokinase within 4 hours, t-PA achieved a higher reperfusion rate at each time interval.

In spite of the relative fibrin specificity of t-PA, bleeding complications were comparable in the two groups. Fibrinogen levels fell by 58% in the streptokinase-treated group and by 33% in those treated with t-PA. These changes were accompanied by a more significant fall in plasminogen level and rise in FDPs in patients receiving streptokinase. Although major life-threatening hemorrhage was not reported in either group, periaccess hemorrhage was common (t-PA, 43%; streptokinase, 47%) and a relatively high proportion required transfusion of 2 or more units of blood (t-PA, 25%; streptokinase, 21%).

This increased incidence of bleeding in both treatment groups was attributed to the concomitant use of aggressive anticoagulation regimens to minimize reocclusion and reinfarction. In spite of this, angiographically documented infarct vessel reocclusion occurred in 11% in the streptokinase group and 14% in the t-PA group.

Also published in 1985 was the report of the European Cooperative Study Group comparative trial of intravenous streptokinase and t-PA.[59] In this study, 0.75 mg/kg double-chain t-PA given over 90 minutes was compared with 1.5 million units streptokinase given over 60 minutes at a mean of 2.8 hours from the onset of symptoms. Ninety-minute coronary patency was 70% for those receiving rt-PA and 55% for the streptokinase treated group ($P = 0.054$). These findings support those of the TIMI trial, which found t-PA to be superior to streptokinase even when given within 4 hours of the onset of symptoms.

Several studies[60,61] have shown an improvement in left ventricular function following the administration of t-PA (see Table 69.2), but to date the only intravenous t-PA–placebo mortality study is the Anglo-Scandinavian Study of Early Thrombolysis (ASSET)[62] in which 5011 patients with suspected acute myocardial infarction received either t-PA or placebo within 5 hours of symptom onset. Thirty-day mortality was reduced from 9.7% in the placebo group to 7.2% in the treated group. This 26% reduction is comparable to the streptokinase-mediated reduction in early mortality noted in the GISSI and ISIS-2 studies.

More recently, preliminary data from the very large International t-PA/Streptokinase Mortality trial have shown no apparent difference in the mortality of acute myocardial infarction following t-PA therapy when compared with the much less expensive agent streptokinase. In this study, 20,749 patients were randomly assigned to either intravenous t-PA or streptokinase and, subsequently, to either subcutaneous heparin or no heparin. Each patient received oral aspirin, and the early use of intravenous β-adrenergic blocking therapy was encouraged. More than 98% of the patients received thrombolytic therapy within 6 hours of the onset of symptoms; approximately 23% of the patients were >70 years old. The mortality rates for each of the therapeutic regimens were very similar (Fig. 69.3). The mortality rates without heparin were 8.7% for t-PA, compared with 9.2% for streptokinase, and with combined thrombolysis and heparin the mortality rates were 9.2% and 7.9%, respectively.[63] However, in this study the heparin was given subcutaneously rather than intravenously, and it was not commenced until 12 hours after the thrombolytic infusion. Recent studies have suggested that optimal reperfusion rates are not achieved with t-PA therapy if anticoagulation with heparin is delayed. Thus, although it is unlikely that there are substantial differences in the impact of these two agents on the early mortality of acute myocardial infarction, it is possible that small differences may have been masked by a suboptimal heparinization regimen. Further studies are currently planned to address this question specifically.

COMBINATION THERAPY

Although t-PA does achieve more rapid reperfusion with fewer side effects than earlier generation thrombolytic agents, it, too, is far from optimal. Attention has therefore been focused first on the use of combinations of currently available lytic agents and second on the design and synthesis of more effective compounds by manipulation of their molecular structure.

The differing modes of action of the various plasminogen activators offer the potential for synergistic activity between combinations of these agents. Although the results of *in vitro* studies have been somewhat conflicting, *in vivo* observations in animal models have sup-

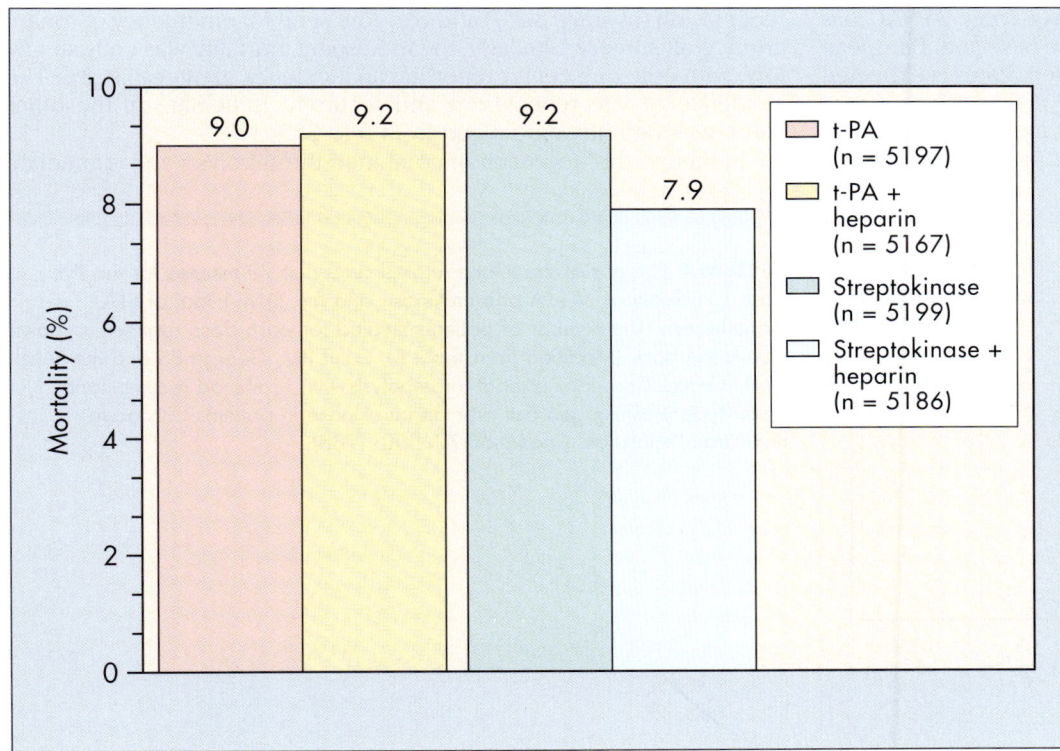

FIGURE 69.3 Comparison of the early mortality following t-PA or streptokinase therapy, with or without subcutaneous heparin, in the International t-PA/Streptokinase Mortality Trial.

ported this concept.[64] Similarly, preliminary studies in patients with acute myocardial infarction[65] have shown the combination of small doses of t-PA and scu-PA to achieve a high rate of reperfusion with minimal reduction in systemic fibrinogen levels.

Combinations of other thrombolytic agents have also been used. The TAMI Study group[66] reported a study of 146 patients treated with five different combinations of intravenous t-PA and urokinase (Fig. 69.4). Unlike the initial pilot studies, however, reperfusion rates were suboptimal in those patients treated with low doses of each agent. On the other hand, coronary patency rates were uniformly high in those patients treated with 1 mg/kg intravenous t-PA and not increased by progressively higher doses of urokinase. When compared with the previously reported efficacy of t-PA alone[53] given as a dose of 150 mg over 6 to 8 hours, the coronary patency rate was not significantly augmented by any combination of urokinase and t-PA (see Fig. 69.4).

Of the five dosage regimens compared, no combination achieved a coronary patency rate greater than 75%. The authors postulated that this may represent a plateau of efficacy for thrombolytic therapy. At this time, the factors responsible for this consistently observed 25% failure rate are unknown. The possible mechanisms are multiple and include too extensive a burden of thrombus for adequate penetration by the thrombolytic agent, the presence of neutralizing antibodies to antigenic lytic agents, plasminogen deficiency or dysplasminogenemia, and heightened α_2-antiplasmin activity. In addition, arterial occlusion may be nonthrombotic and due, for example, to obstructive intimal dissection or subintimal hemorrhage.

Although the addition of urokinase to t-PA did not appear to augment coronary patency in the TAMI study, it was noted that the combination of t-PA and urokinase resulted in a relatively low reocclusion rate of 9%, a rate that compares favorably with the previously reported rates for t-PA alone.

It was concluded from this study, therefore, that no evidence of synergism between these agents was demonstrated but that the combination of urokinase and t-PA may avoid the need for prolonged infusions of t-PA to minimize infarct vessel reocclusion and, in doing so, may minimize the risk of hemorrhagic complications. Several multicenter studies currently in progress have been designed to further examine this question.

NEW APPROACHES

Many attempts have been made to modify known thrombolytic agents to reduce their antigenicity, to slow the rate of their inactivation, and to increase their fibrin specificity. To date, however, only APSAC has been released for clinical use and is now available in several European countries. Approval for its general use in the United States is expected soon.

The potential of bioengineering techniques of molecular manipulation to create more specific and more effective thrombolytic agents has been reviewed by Verstraete[67] and Collen.[68] Streptokinase, for example, has been conjugated with polyethylene glycol, a nonantigenic polymer, to reduce its immunogenicity and to prolong the duration of its action. Similarly, binding streptokinase to soluble activated dextran has been shown to substantially prolong its half-life without affecting its fibrinolytic activity.

Alternative approaches have included the conjugation of urokinase to a fibrin-specific monoclonal antibody to "target" the thrombolytic agent. Similarly, genetically designed mutants and hybrids of t-PA, which have a promising degree of fibrin specificity and affinity, have been produced by amino-acid additions, deletions, and substitutions. It is very likely, therefore, that in the near future thrombolytic agents with much improved pharmacokinetic profiles will be available for clinical testing. It is not yet clear, however, whether the augmented potency of these newer agents will be achieved at the expense of clinical safety and an increased incidence of hemorrhagic complications.

PERCUTANEOUS TRANSLUMINAL CORONARY ANGIOPLASTY

The demonstration of significant improvement in left ventricular function and in the early mortality of acute myocardial infarction following successful thrombolysis[27,28] drew attention to the potential for intervention by mechanical means to achieve comparable or superior results.

Percutaneous transluminal coronary angioplasty (PTCA) was introduced by Grüntzig and associates in 1977[69] and soon became widely available for patients with stable angina and fixed coronary stenoses. The successful application of this technique in the setting of acute infarction was first described in 1982 by Meyer and associates, who successfully dilated residual coronary stenoses following initial reperfusion of the infarct vessel using intracoronary streptokinase.[70]

INTRACORONARY THROMBOLYSIS AND PTCA

During the subsequent period in which intracoronary thrombolytic therapy enjoyed considerable popularity, balloon dilatation of the underlying coronary stenosis became a logical extension of the procedure in those centers in which it was feasible. The findings of 16 clinical studies reported between 1982 and 1986 have been summarized in a recent review.[71] For the pooled population of 483 patients, the average technical success rate was 82%. Most studies reported a low rate of reocclusion (average 3.2%) and very low need for emergency coronary artery graft surgery. Similarly, the in-hospital mortality was consistently low, with only one center reporting an incidence greater than 8%. The incidence of late reocclusion and recurrent ischemia, on the other hand, was variable and ranged from 0 to 33%.

In theory, this approach of combined thrombolysis and immediate

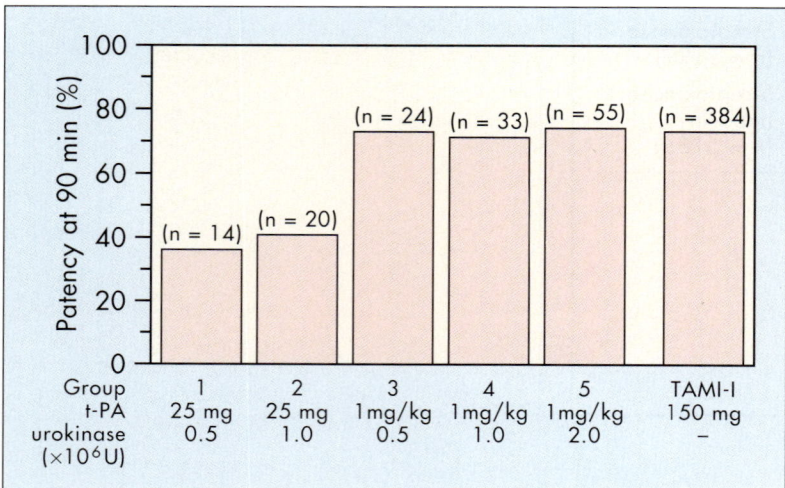

FIGURE 69.4 Patency of the infarct-related artery at 90 minutes for the five dose combinations of t-PA and urokinase and the TAMI-1 trial of t-PA monotherapy. The number of patients studied for each dose regimen is shown above the bars. (Modified from Topol EJ, Califf RM, George BS and the TAMI Study Group: Coronary arterial thrombolysis with combined recombinant tissue-type plasminogen activator and urokinase in patients with acute myocardial infarction. Circulation 77: 1100, 1988)

PTCA has a number of attractive advantages over thrombolysis alone. First, to date no thrombolytic agent or combination of agents has consistently achieved reperfusion rates in excess of 75% to 80% when evaluated at up to 90 minutes after administration.[66] Thrombolytic therapy alone, therefore, appears to fail in at least 25% of all patients treated and, at present, no clinical criteria accurately identify this subgroup.[72] Coronary angiography, on the other hand, allows this group to be readily identified and treated by immediate PTCA.

Second, the use of thrombolytic therapy does little to alter the pathophysiologic conditions responsible for initiating acute coronary occlusion. In the majority of patients, coronary thrombosis is precipitated by rupture or fissuring of an atheromatous plaque at the site of a high-grade stenosis in the infarct-related artery.[12] This site remains a nidus for platelet aggregation and thrombogenesis, particularly when coronary flow remains compromised. It is not surprising, therefore, that reocclusion and reinfarction are common following successful thrombolysis-mediated reperfusion, often in spite of full-dose antiplatelet and anticoagulant therapy. In 1984, Harrison and associates[73] correlated the incidence of rethrombosis with the severity of the residual coronary stenosis. In a group of 24 patients with successful streptokinase-mediated reperfusion, the incidence of angiographically confirmed rethrombosis was 54% in patients with a minimal luminal area of the residual stenosis of 0.4 mm^2 compared with 0% in those with a greater luminal area. It could be expected from this study that the altered coronary hemodynamics following successful PTCA should reduce the likelihood of recurrent thrombosis. More recently, however, Ellis and associates[74] found that none of 29 clinical and angiographic variables, including residual coronary stenosis severity, cross-sectional area, and lesion morphology, were predictive of recurrent ischemic events in a population of 95 patients with successful t-PA–mediated thrombolysis. Clearly, therefore, although the severity of the residual stenosis is an important variable, the clinical outcome following successful thrombolysis will be determined by the interaction of multiple factors.

The third potential advantage of thrombolysis and subsequent coronary angioplasty is that following thrombolysis alone the presence of a flow-limiting, residual stenosis may inhibit or impede full functional recovery of the jeopardized myocardium. This concept was supported by the findings of O'Neill and associates[75] and Topol and colleagues,[76] which demonstrated greater augmentation of left ventricular function following successful PTCA than following successful thrombolysis.

Finally, an ill-defined proportion of patients presenting during the early hours of acute infarction will be ineligible for thrombolytic therapy because of relative or absolute contraindications such as advanced age, bleeding diathesis, or recent surgery or trauma. In this group, immediate coronary angioplasty has the potential to achieve reperfusion with a much reduced risk. The feasibility of performing PTCA as a primary treatment for acute infarction was reported by Hartzler and co-workers[77] in 1986 and has been confirmed in several other studies.[78,79]

Although this approach is sound in theory, the predicted benefits of immediate PTCA were not consistently apparent in early studies. In 1986, Erbel and associates[80] reported the results of a randomized, controlled trial comparing intracoronary streptokinase with intracoronary streptokinase followed by immediate PTCA. In this study, the technical angioplasty success rate of 65% was unusually low and the incidence of early reocclusion a disappointing 14%. This incidence was not significantly different from the 20% noted in the group treated with streptokinase alone. Similarly, global left ventricular ejection fraction was not significantly different between the two groups and in only the subgroup of patients with anterior myocardial infarction was any difference in regional wall motion apparent. Interestingly, however, a recently published 2.5-year follow-up of these patients[81] noted an 8.6% reduction in mortality and an 11.2% reduction in the incidence of reinfarction in those patients treated with intracoronary streptokinase and angioplasty in spite of the absence of detectable short-term benefit.

DIRECT CORONARY ANGIOPLASTY

An alternative to intracoronary thrombolysis followed by PTCA is the direct approach of PTCA as the first and only treatment for acute infarction. This has a number of potential advantages over both intracoronary and intravenous thrombolysis. Not only does it avoid the risks of hemorrhagic complications associated with thrombolytic therapy, but it also achieves a consistently higher recanalization rate and improves left ventricular function to a greater extent than intracoronary thrombolysis.[75] Its application is limited, however, by the same factors that contributed to the eventual displacement of intracoronary thrombolysis by intravenous thrombolytic therapy. Few centers have the facilities or the skilled manpower to perform emergency coronary angioplasty on all patients with acute myocardial infarction at the time of presentation.

INTRAVENOUS THROMBOLYSIS AND PTCA

Since the recognition of the delays and logistic difficulties inherent in giving thrombolytic therapy by the intracoronary route and in performing direct coronary angioplasty, attention has turned to the use of initial intravenous thrombolytic therapy followed by immediate or delayed PTCA. This combination of medical and mechanical intervention has been the subject of a number of major clinical trials. Stack and associates, for example, reported the results of a study in which 216 patients were treated initially with an intravenous infusion of 1.5 million units of streptokinase followed by immediate PTCA.[82] Coronary patency was achieved in 90%. In those patients in whom infarct vessel patency was maintained with minimal residual stenosis, significant improvement was noted in global ejection fraction (44% vs. 49%; $P < 0.0001$). Similarly, regional infarct zone wall motion, calculated using the centerline method[83] and expressing abnormal wall motion as standard deviation (SD) from the normal mean, was also significantly enhanced (-3.0 to -2.4 SD/chord; $P < 0.0001$).

Three other published clinical trials have aimed to determine the optimal timing of coronary angioplasty following initial intravenous thrombolysis. This factor clearly has important implications for the management of the majority of patients presenting with acute infarction. Immediate PTCA could be expected to have the greatest impact on overall patency rate, improvement in left ventricular function, the incidence of recurrent ischemia, and mortality. It, too, requires immediate angiography, however, and therefore has all the disadvantages and limitations of intracoronary thrombolysis combined with PTCA.

The alternative strategies include deferring angiography and angioplasty for 18 to 48 hours (*i.e.*, until the earliest practical time), for at least 7 to 10 days (which allows time for stabilization with antiplatelet and anticoagulant therapy and transportation of the patient from outlying centers to centers with facilities for PTCA), or indefinitely if stress testing shows no evidence of provocable ischemia.

The three large, randomized clinical studies that have investigated these alternatives have been dissimilar in design but quite concordant in their conclusions (Table 69.3). The agent used in each case was t-PA because of evidence of its superior lytic potency.[58,59] In the Thrombolysis and Angioplasty in Myocardial Infarction study, patients were randomized after successful t-PA–mediated reperfusion to either immediate PTCA or to a deferred strategy of PTCA 7 to 10 days later.[84] Both the TIMI 2A and the European Cooperative Study Group (ECSG) trial, on the other hand, randomized patients prior to angiography. Coronary angiography was then performed, with PTCA when feasible, either immediately or at 18 to 48 hours in TIMI 2A[85] or at 10 to 20 days in the ECSG trial.[86]

The findings in each of these studies led the authors to conclude that immediate PTCA offers no particular advantage but potentially several disadvantages over the deferred, elective strategy. These conclusions were based on the following observations. The primary end point for each study was predischarge left ventricular function (Fig. 69.5). In contrast to previous studies, no significant difference in global or regional left ventricular function was apparent between the two groups. Global left ventricular function did not improve significantly in either, and regional infarct zone wall motion improved to the same extent in the immediate and deferred PTCA patients. Second, in-hospital mortality was higher in the immediate PTCA group (Fig. 69.6). Although this reached statistical significance only in the ECSG trial (7% vs. 3%), a similar trend was noted in the other two studies (TAMI, 4% vs. 1%; TIMI, 8% vs. 5%). Third, although the procedural success rate and incidence of post-PTCA infarct vessel reocclusion were comparable in the two groups, emergency coronary artery graft surgery was required more commonly during immediate PTCA (TAMI, 7% vs. 2%; TIMI, 6% vs. 2%). Finally, the need to perform invasive angiographic procedures following fibrinolytic therapy in all patients in the TAMI trial and in the immediate PTCA groups of the TIMI and the ECSG trials resulted in a substantially higher incidence of hemorrhagic complications and requirement for blood transfusion compared with those patients in whom angiography was deferred for at least 18 hours.

The one important difference between the two strategies that did favor immediate PTCA was in the incidence of recurrent ischemic events. In the TAMI study, recurrent ischemia necessitating emergency angiography followed by either PTCA or coronary artery bypass surgery occurred in 5% of those treated by immediate PTCA compared with 19% of those awaiting the deferred procedure.

Several other observations from the TAMI trial are of note. First, of those patients in the deferred PTCA group believed initially to have hemodynamically significant residual stenoses in the infarct-related artery, at repeat angiography 14% had substantial reduction in the severity of the stenosis, obviating the need for PTCA. This suggests that angiography 90 minutes after the administration of t-PA may be too early to assess the severity and hemodynamic importance of the residual stenosis. These findings are consistent with those of Harrison and associates[73] in which the minimal luminal cross-sectional area of the residual stenosis more than doubled in 7 of 17 patients at repeat coronary angiography 8 to 14 days after initial streptokinase reperfusion.

TABLE 69.3 TRIALS OF INTRAVENOUS t-PA AND IMMEDIATE PTCA

	TAMI	ECSG	TIMI 2A
Patients (n)	386	367	389
No. Patients Randomized	197	367	389
Dose of Tissue Plasminogen Activator (mg)	150 mg	100 mg	100 mg*, 150 mg†
Randomization Without/With Angiography	With	Without	Without
Patients Undergoing Immediate PTCA of Those Randomized or Eligible (%)	68%	92%	70%
Immediate PTCA			
In-Hospital Mortality	4/99 (4%)	12/183 (7%)	15/195 (8%)
LVEF (7–20 d)	0.53	0.51	0.50
Reocclusion	11%	12.5%	NR
Deferred Approach			
In-Hospital Mortality	1/98 (1%)	5/184 (3%)	10/194 (5%)
LVEF (7–20 d)	0.56	0.51	0.49
Reocclusion	13%	11%	NR

* The last two thirds of patients entered in TIMI 2A received 100 mg.

† The first one third of patients entered in TIMI 2A received 150 mg.

ECSG, European Cooperative Study Group; LVEF, left ventricular ejection fraction; NR, not reported; PTCA, percutaneous transluminal coronary angioplasty; TAMI, Thrombolysis and Angioplasty in Myocardial Infarction; TIMI, Thrombolysis in Myocardial Infarction; t-PA, tissue plasminogen activator
(Topol EJ: Coronary angioplasty for acute myocardial infarction. Ann Intern Med 109:974, 1988)

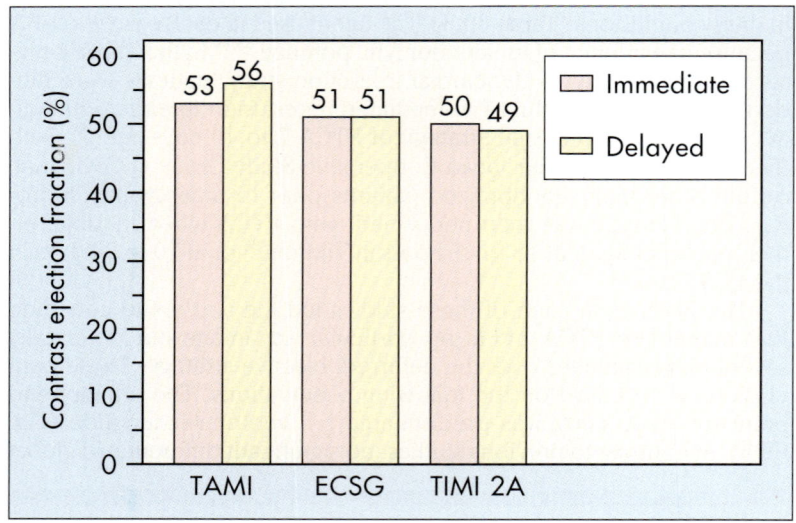

FIGURE 69.5 Left ventricular function in the immediate coronary angioplasty trials. No differences were observed in predischarge ejection fraction for the immediate vs. deferred strategies. (ECSG, European Co-operative Study Group; TAMI, Thrombolysis and Angioplasty in Myocardial Infarction Study Group; TIMI 2A, Thrombolysis in Myocardial Infarction Study Group. (Modified from Topol EJ: Coronary angioplasty for acute myocardial infarction. Ann Intern Med 109:974, 1988)

The likely mechanisms of the further improvement in angiographic appearance are continued lysis of residual thrombus and/or resolution of associated coronary artery spasm. In a significant proportion of this population, therefore, an immediate PTCA strategy would unnecessarily expose the patient to the potential hazards of coronary angioplasty.

An important subgroup in the TAMI study was the 25% of the original population of 386 patients in whom lytic therapy failed to reestablish luminal patency. In this group, "rescue" PTCA was attempted and was successful in 86%, increasing the overall reperfusion rate to 94%. In spite of this, however, the in-hospital mortality for this group was considerably higher (10.4% vs. 5.2%; $P = 0.06$) than in those patients with a patent infarct vessel following t-PA alone. Similarly, the reocclusion rate following successful PTCA in this group was a disappointing 29% and the subsequent course notable for a high rate of ventricular arrhythmias and hemodynamic instability. Not surprisingly, recovery of left ventricular function was minimal.

Whether these poor results will be applicable to all patients failing thrombolytic therapy remains to be determined. A small pilot study has offered some hope that other combinations may be more successful.[87] "Rescue" PTCA was performed on a group of patients with persisting occlusion of the infarct-related artery after the administration of a combination of intravenous t-PA and urokinase. In this study of 27 patients, no in-hospital deaths were reported, the reocclusion rate was only 4% and left ventricular function improved significantly between baseline and 1 week follow-up. It is possible, therefore, that emergency PTCA following failed thrombolytic therapy may yet prove to be an important strategy.

INTRAVENOUS THROMBOLYSIS AND DEFERRED PTCA

A final strategy that is under investigation may prove to be the most practical, most economical, and most widely applicable. It is clear that, when appropriate, intravenous thrombolysis is the preferred initial management for acute infarction and can be initiated in community hospitals without expertise in coronary angiography. What remains unclear, however, is whether all patients receiving thrombolytic therapy require angiographic evaluation. It is possible that predischarge, submaximal stress testing will identify those patients at risk of recurrent ischemia or infarction. For this group and for those with early postinfarction angina, transfer to a center with facilities for coronary angiography and, if necessary, coronary angioplasty or bypass graft surgery is appropriate. Those with no evidence of provocable ischemia, on the other hand, may be best treated medically with careful clinical observation for evidence of recurrent ischemia, thus reducing the workload of tertiary referral centers and avoiding unnecessary and potentially hazardous invasive procedures. Several ongoing randomized, controlled clinical trials have been designed to determine the optimal management of this group of relatively low risk patients.

EMERGENCY SURGICAL REVASCULARIZATION

The most definitive and time-honored method of achieving myocardial revascularization is coronary artery bypass graft surgery. Although some centers have been able to institute surgical revascularization as a primary strategy for the management of acute myocardial infarction, this approach is neither logistically nor economically applicable to the majority of centers with cardiac surgical facilities.

Nevertheless, data have been accumulated to support the notion that emergency surgical revascularization is a safe and effective form of therapy either as a primary strategy or when thrombolytic therapy and angioplasty have failed or are inappropriate. Several studies have shown a significant improvement in left ventricular function and long-term survival following emergency coronary surgery.[88–90] A number of factors are likely to contribute to this improvement. The early implementation of cardiopulmonary bypass rapidly and almost completely reduces myocardial work. Similarly, hypothermic cardiac arrest minimizes cellular metabolic requirements and myocardial perfusion with an appropriately buffered, low calcium, high amino-acid cardioplegic solution may minimize cellular injury associated with reperfusion.[91] In addition, the application of coronary artery grafts to all compromised vessels ensures a more complete revascularization than can be achieved with either thrombolytic therapy or emergency coronary angioplasty.

Two large, uncontrolled clinical series have been reported in which emergency surgical revascularization was the primary strategy for acute myocardial infarction. In 1983, DeWood and colleagues[88] reported a series of 701 patients on whom coronary surgery was performed within 24 hours of the onset of symptoms. The overall in-hospital mortality was 5.2% for the group of 440 patients with transmural infarction and 3.0% of 261 patients with nontransmural infarction. Although these mortality rates compare favorably with historical controls of medically treated patients, the outcome was highly dependent on the duration of symptoms, on the severity of the underlying coronary artery disease, and on the presence or absence of presurgical hemodynamic compromise. A significantly higher mortality was noted in those revascularized more than 6 hours from the onset of symptoms (3.8% vs. 8%; $P = 0.05$). Similarly, in-hospital mortality rose from 2.3% in those patients with single-vessel disease to 9% in those with three-vessel disease and 28% in those with presurgical evidence of Killip Class 3 clinical status.

A second nonrandomized study was reported by Phillips and associates[89] in 1986. In a subgroup of 189 patients with multivessel disease, emergency coronary artery graft surgery was performed with an in-hos-

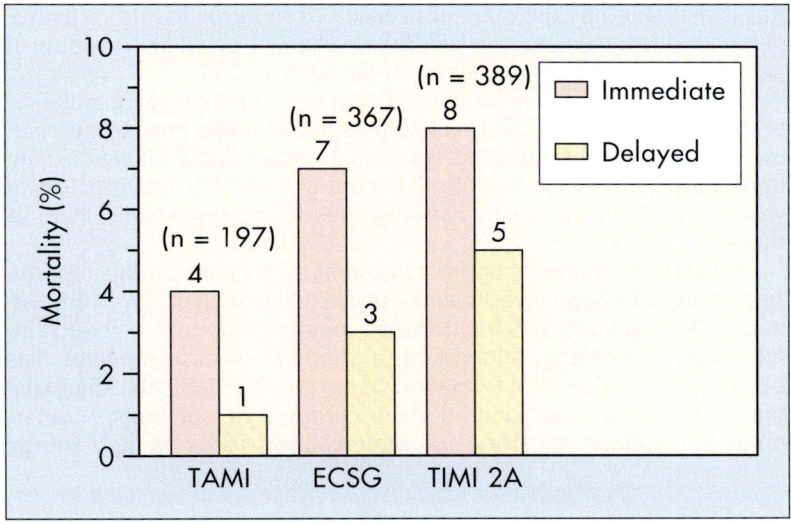

FIGURE 69.6 In-hospital mortality in the immediate coronary angioplasty trials. Differences between immediate and deferred strategies reached statistical significance only in the ECSG trial. Abbreviations as in Figure 69.5. (Data adapted from references 83–85)

pital mortality of 3.7%. The time to reperfusion was again an important determinant of outcome as were the presence of a collateral vascular supply and whether the infarct vessel was completely or subtotally occluded.

POST-THROMBOLYSIS SURGICAL REVASCULARIZATION

Although the studies of DeWood and colleagues[88] and Phillips and associates[89] have demonstrated the feasibility and efficacy of immediate surgical revascularization, coronary surgery is more commonly reserved for those patients in whom thrombolytic therapy and angioplasty have failed to adequately reperfuse a substantial segment of jeopardized myocardium and in whom there is evidence of ongoing ischemia.

Several studies have demonstrated the safety of surgical revascularization following thrombolytic therapy. Kereiakes and co-workers[90] reported the outcome of 24 patients on whom emergency coronary surgery was performed following intravenous t-PA at a mean of 7.3 hours from the onset of symptoms. In 11 of these patients coronary anatomy was considered unsuitable for PTCA, and in 13 patients the attempted coronary angioplasty was complicated by reclosure of the infarct-related artery due to intimal dissection and rethrombosis.

Comparison of preoperative and predischarge contrast left ventriculograms showed a striking improvement in global left ventricular ejection fraction from $49 \pm 6\%$ to $56 \pm 6\%$ ($P = 0.008$) and in infarct zone wall motion from -2.6 ± 0.5 to -1.5 ± 1.1 SD/chord ($P = 0.001$). There were no intraoperative deaths. Three of eight patients (38%) with preoperative cardiogenic shock died in the early postoperative period, and three patients required surgical reexploration because of significant postoperative hemorrhage.

It is likely, therefore, that emergency surgical revascularization will continue to play an important adjunctive role in the management of acute infarction particularly in situations in which suboptimal revascularization is achieved by thrombolysis and/or coronary angioplasty.

UNRESOLVED ISSUES

The enthusiasm with which thrombolytic therapy has been embraced over the past decade and the numerous studies that have followed its widespread use during this period have allowed many of the questions raised to be satisfactorily answered. Several important issues remain unresolved, however, and require further investigation. These include the importance of achieving infarct vessel recanalization beyond the period during which significant improvement in myocardial function can be expected, the extent to which reperfusion injury mitigates against the salutary effects of reperfusion therapy, the desirability of fibrin specificity, and whether reperfusion therapy is economically justifiable.

LATE REPERFUSION

Although it has been unequivocally established that thrombolytic therapy achieves reperfusion, that early reperfusion preserves left ventricular function, and that improvement in left ventricular function is associated with increased survival, it is not clear whether this is the only mechanism by which mortality is reduced. Several studies[27,81] have shown improvement in survival without an apparent improvement in left ventricular function in patients treated with thrombolytic therapy more than 4 hours from the onset of symptoms. In addition, the findings of the ISIS-2 study support the premise that reperfusion as late as 24 hours may improve event-free survival. Several of possible mechanisms have been postulated to account for these observations. It is known, for example, from animal models of acute infarction, that late reperfusion may prevent or at least minimize the severity of infarct zone expansion and late aneurysm formation.[92] Systolic bulging of the infarct zone occurs very early after the onset of acute infarction and is followed by infarct expansion due to thinning and dilatation of this region. Preservation of an epicardial rim of viable tissue may reduce the likelihood of this occurring. In addition, the decrease in compliance due to interstitial and cellular edema following reperfusion may increase myocardial resistance to expansion. Because infarct zone expansion has been correlated with an increase in both sudden death and congestive heart failure,[93,94] it is conceivable that this may be one mechanism by which late reperfusion improves survival.

A second possibility is that myocardial reperfusion may impede the development of a substrate for ventricular arrhythmias. Kersschot and co-workers[95] performed programmed ventricular stimulation at a mean of 26 days from presentation in 36 consecutive patients randomized to receive either intravenous and intracoronary streptokinase or conventional therapy. Sustained monomorphic ventricular tachycardia was inducible in 67% of the control group compared with 29% of those receiving reperfusion therapy. Similar findings were reported by Sager and colleagues,[96] who studied 32 patients with transmural anterior myocardial infarcts complicated by left ventricular aneurysm formation. Sixteen of these patients received thrombolytic therapy, and the remainder received conventional medical therapy. Although there were no differences in left ventricular function between the two groups, of the 20 patients with no sustained clinical ventricular arrhythmias, ventricular tachycardia was inducible in 88% of those who had received thrombolytic therapy compared with 8% of those treated conventionally. It is possible, therefore, that reperfusion therapy may minimize myocardial electrical instability following recent infarction.

Finally, blood and plasma viscosity fall significantly with the reduction in concentration of plasma fibrinogen.[97] The associated change in resistance to flow has two important effects. First, it improves perfusion in the myocardial microcirculation and second, by decreasing afterload, it reduces myocardial work. In addition, activation of platelet-bound plasminogen results in impaired adhesion and decreased aggregation responses, thus inhibiting platelet activation and reducing clot stability.[98] Whether these rheologic and antiplatelet effects play important roles in reducing mortality remains to be established.

REPERFUSION INJURY

The potential for revascularization of the acutely ischemic myocardium to accelerate cellular injury rather than enhance cellular viability has been recognized for more than a decade.[99] Several factors contribute to this detrimental effect. The onset of cellular ischemia is followed rapidly by the cessation of aerobic oxidative phosphorylation, the depletion of high-energy phosphate stores, and the accumulation of hypoxanthine from the degradation of adenosine triphosphate. Restoration of blood flow and oxygen supply results in the oxidation of hypoxanthine, catalyzed by the enzyme xanthine oxidase, and in the generation of superoxide anions. These highly reactive oxygen-free radicals have the potential to cause severe tissue injury by peroxidation of lipid membranes and mitochondria. Under normal circumstances, this is prevented by the rapid conversion of superoxide ions to hydrogen peroxide by the enzyme superoxide dismutase, but in the setting of acute ischemia the cellular levels of this enzyme fall.

The accelerated cellular damage that accompanies myocardial reperfusion is associated with characteristic histologic changes, including explosive cellular swelling, lysosomal rupture, intracellular calcium deposition, and tetanic myofibrillary contraction.[100] In addition, loss of vascular endothelial integrity predisposes to intramyocardial hemorrhage.

Several experimental approaches aiming to minimize this reperfusion injury have been investigated. Superoxide dismutase given intravenously, for example, has been shown in animal models to reduce infarct size.[101] Similarly, allopurinol, a xanthine oxidase inhibitor, has been used to reduce the formation of oxygen-free radicals. Manipulation of amino-acid concentrations in cardioplegic solutions to determine the optimal substrate for replenishing stores of high-energy phosphate pathway intermediates has also been attempted and is believed to influence postischemic myocardial recovery following surgical revascularization.[91]

FIBRIN SPECIFICITY

The proposition that fibrin specificity endows thrombolytic therapy with greater efficacy and safety has been challenged.[102,103] Although some studies have shown a greater lytic potency of the naturally occurring, more fibrin-selective plasminogen activators, their impact on the incidence of bleeding and rethrombosis and their overall clinical benefit have been less apparent.

This may well be explained by the multifactorial effects of thrombolytic therapy on coagulation pathways and platelet function. Initial therapy is characterized by the generation of plasmin, variable depletion of coagulation factors, and impairment of platelet function. This is followed by a period of relative hypercoagulability due first to the activation of newly formed platelets and release of thromboxane A_2[104] and second to the activation of Factor V and subsequent conversion of prothrombin to thrombin.[105] In the absence of systemic fibrinolysis, these changes may result in thrombus formation and infarct vessel reocclusion. Fibrin-specific thrombolytic agents, therefore, might be expected to have a higher incidence of rethrombosis following successful reperfusion without necessarily having a lower incidence of hemorrhagic complications. The GISSI-II trial, which is directly comparing streptokinase and t-PA prospectively, may provide some answers to this question.

COST-EFFECTIVENESS

As a relatively new but already widely applied technology, myocardial reperfusion using thrombolytic therapy with or without coronary angioplasty has not yet been carefully examined to determine its cost-effectiveness. One study by Topol and co-workers[106] has suggested that coronary reperfusion therapy may allow early mobilization of patients with uncomplicated myocardial infarcts and discharge from the hospital as early as 3 days after admission. In this study, the early discharge protocol was associated with no greater incidence of recurrent isch-

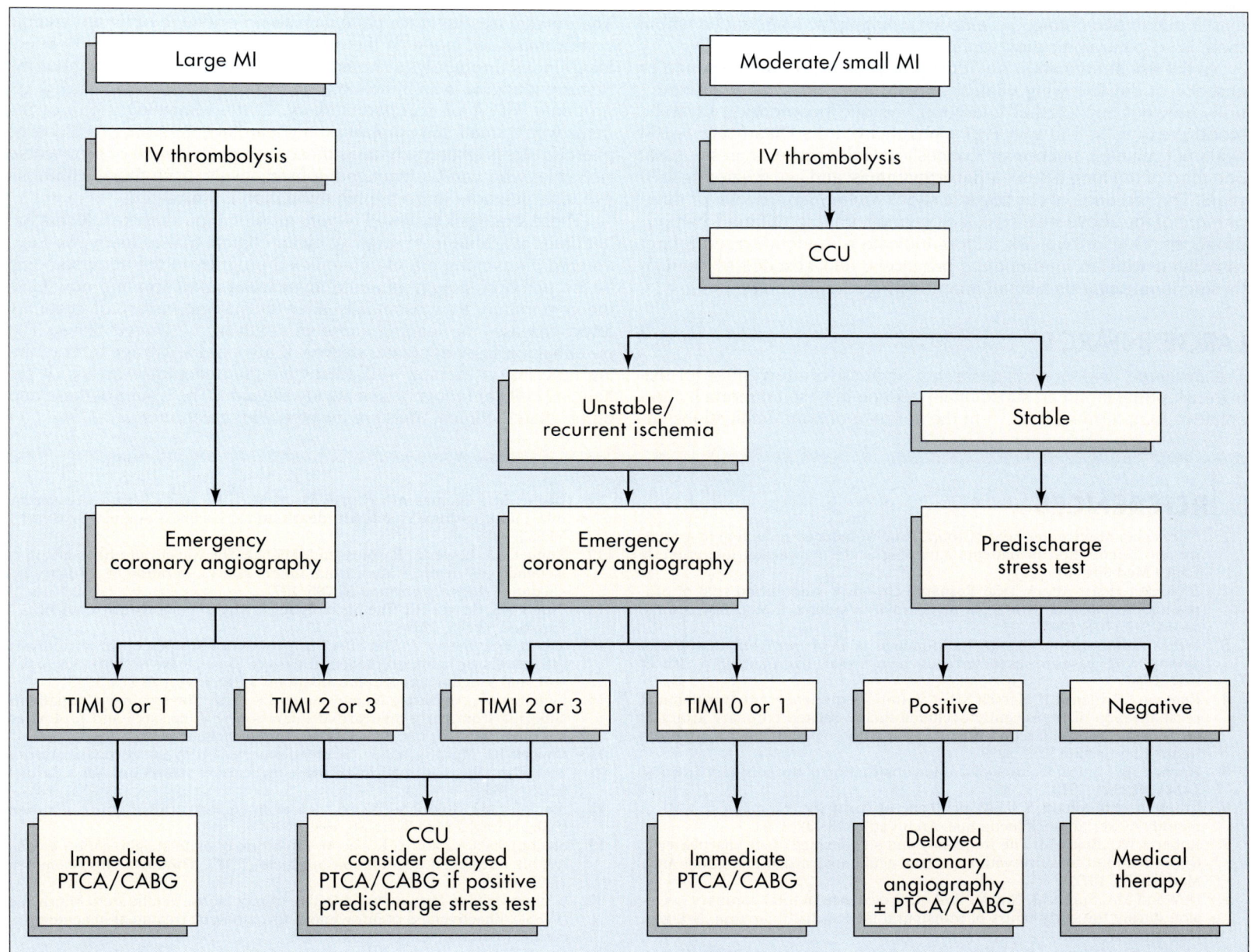

FIGURE 69.7 Proposed strategy for the management of acute myocardial infarction in patients presenting within the first 6 to 8 hours in whom there is no contraindication to thrombolytic therapy. (TIMI, Thrombolysis in Myocardial Infarction study; PTCA, percutaneous transluminal coronary angioplasty, CABG, coronary artery bypass graft)

emia, sudden death, or aneurysm formation. Cumulative hospital and professional charges were reduced by 30% compared with the conventionally treated group. Although these results are encouraging, the population studied represents only 15% of the total infarct population screened. Continuing close scrutiny of the escalating costs of medical care is therefore required and may ultimately influence which subgroups of patients receive reperfusion therapy.

OPTIMAL STRATEGY

The optimal strategy for the management of patients presenting during the early hours of acute myocardial infarction is at present unknown. Similarly, it is not yet clear whether fibrinolytic therapy is of benefit to patients with unstable, preinfarction syndromes. Because the incidence of misdiagnosis in populations of patients presenting with chest pain and nonspecific ST segment changes is not insignificant, we consider it prudent at this stage to limit the use of such therapy to patients with unequivocal electrocardiographic changes of acute infarction. Based on currently available information, the following is offered as an outline for the management of those patients presenting within 6 to 8 hours of the onset of symptoms who have chest pain unrelieved by sublingual nitroglycerin associated with ST segment elevation of at least 1 mm in two contiguous electrocardiographic leads and in whom there is no contraindication to thrombolytic therapy (Fig. 69.7).

Initial risk stratification on admission is based on the presence or absence of the following clinical criteria: anterior myocardial infarction, previous myocardial infarction, systolic hypotension (systolic blood pressure < 100 mm Hg), sinus tachycardia (heart rate > 100 beats per minute), pulmonary congestion (rales higher than the basal one third of the lung fields), atrial arrhythmias, and age greater than 70 years. The presence of cardiogenic shock, pulmonary edema, or three or more of the above seven risk factors implies a large infarct with poor prognosis. One or two risk factors indicate a moderate-sized infarct associated with an intermediate prognosis, and absence of each of these criteria suggests a small infarct with good prognosis.

LARGE INFARCT

The available evidence suggests that aggressive intervention in this high-risk population can substantially reduce in-hospital mortality and enhance long-term survival.[107] In the absence of contraindications, intravenous thrombolytic therapy should be given and followed by emergency coronary angiography. If flow in the infarct-related artery remains suboptimal, immediate PTCA or coronary artery surgery should then be performed (see Fig. 69.5). In those patients with contraindications to thrombolytic therapy or in whom immediate coronary angiography and angioplasty can be performed with minimal delay, this is the alternative and preferable course.

MODERATE-SIZED INFARCT

Those patients with moderate-sized infarcts also warrant intravenous thrombolytic therapy. The bias in our institution is to then perform early angiography. Preliminary data from the TIMI study group, however, suggest that this may be unnecessary in patients with uncomplicated infarcts in whom predischarge exercise stress testing may identify those requiring further intervention. Indications for urgent coronary angiography include the development of recurrent chest pain or hemodynamically significant complications.

SMALL, LOW RISK INFARCT

The optimal treatment for patients with no evidence of hemodynamic compromise and none of the above risk factors is not well defined. Intravenous thrombolysis should be considered but is not mandatory. Recurrent angina is an indication for coronary angiography and, if appropriate, PTCA or coronary surgery. In the remaining group of patients with a small, uncomplicated myocardial infarction, predischarge exercise stress testing separates those with no evidence of provocable ischemia, who can be managed conservatively, from those with positive tests in whom angiographic evaluation is warranted.

These strategies may well require modification as more information becomes available from ongoing major clinical trials. Clearly, we have entered an exciting era of unparalleled progress in the understanding of the pathophysiology of acute myocardial infarction and now have the opportunity to substantially alter the natural history of coronary artery disease, the leading cause of death in the United States. The potential for an even greater degree of myocardial salvage by combining reperfusion therapy with adjunctive pharmacologic means of enhancing cellular recovery is being investigated. The results of these and other related clinical trials are awaited with great interest.

REFERENCES

1. Norwegian Multicenter Study Group: Timolol-induced reduction in mortality and reinfarction in patients surviving acute myocardial infarction. N Engl J Med 304:801, 1981
2. β-Blocker Heart Attack Trial Research Group: A randomized trial of propranolol in patients with acute myocardial infarction. I. Mortality results. JAMA 247:1707, 1982
3. ISIS-1 Collaborative Group: Randomized trial of intravenous atenolol among 16,027 cases of suspected acute myocardial infarction: ISIS-1. Lancet 2:57, 1986
4. Rentrop KP, Blanke H, Karsch KR et al: Initial experience with transluminal recanalization of the recently occluded infarct-related coronary artery in acute myocardial infarction: Comparison with conventionally treated patients. Clin Cardiol 2:92, 1979
5. Herrick JB: Clinical features of sudden obstruction of the coronary arteries. JAMA 59:2015, 1912
6. Erlich JC, Shinohara Y: Low incidence of coronary thrombosis in MI: A restudy by serial block technique. Arch Pathol 78:432, 1964
7. Roberts WC, Buja LM: The frequency and significance of coronary arterial thrombi and other observations in fatal acute myocardial infarction. Am J Med 52:425, 1972
8. DeWood MA, Spores J, Notske R et al: Prevalence of total coronary occlusion during the early hours of transmural myocardial infarction. N Engl J Med 303:897, 1980
9. Chazov EI, Mateeva LS, Mazaev AV et al: Intracoronary administration of fibrinolysin in acute myocardial infarction. Ter Arkh 48:8, 1976
10. Falk E: Plaque rupture with severe pre-existing stenosis precipitating coronary thrombosis. Br Heart J 50:127, 1983
11. Morice MC, Marco J, Fajadet J et al: Percutaneous coronary angioscopy before and after angioplasty in acute myocardial infarction: Preliminary results (abstr). Circulation (Suppl IV)76:IV-282, 1987
12. Davies MJ, Thomas AC: Plaque fissuring: The cause of acute myocardial infarction, sudden ischaemic death and crescendo angina. Br Heart J 53:363, 1985
13. Reimer KA, Lowe JE, Rasmussen MM et al: The wavefront phenomenon of ischemic cell death. I. Myocardial infarct size vs. duration of coronary occlusion in dogs. Circulation 56:786, 1977
14. Tillett WS, Garner RL: The fibrinolytic activity of hemolytic streptococci. J Exp Med 58:485, 1933
15. Tillett WS, Sherry S: The effect in patients of streptococcal fibrinolysin (streptokinase) and streptococcal desoxyribonuclease on fibrinous, purulent, and sanguinous pleural exudations. J Clin Invest 28:173, 1949
16. Fletcher AP, Alkjaersig N, Smyrniotis FE et al: The treatment of patients suffering from early myocardial infarction with massive and prolonged streptokinase therapy. Trans Assoc Am Physicians 71:287, 1958
17. Boucek RJ, Murphy WP Jr: Sequential perfusion of the coronary arteries with fibrinolysis in man following a myocardial infarction. Am J Cardiol 6:525, 1960
18. Stampfer MJ, Goldhaber SZ, Yusuf S et al: Pooled results from randomized trials. N Engl J Med 307:1180, 1982
19. Stachurska J, Latallo Z, Kopec M: Inhibition of platelet aggregation by dialysable fibrinogen degradation products (FDP). Thromb Diath Haemorrh 23:91, 1970
20. Gruppo Italiano Per Lo Studio Della Streptochinasi Nell'Infarcto Miocardio (GISSI): Effectiveness of intravenous thrombolytic treatment in acute myocardial infarction. Lancet 1:397, 1986
21. Spottl F, Kaiser R: Rapid detection and quantitation of precipitating streptokinase antibodies. Thromb Diath Haemorrh 32:608, 1974
22. ISIS-2 Collaborative Group: Randomized trial of intravenous streptokinase, oral aspirin, both, or neither among 17,187 cases of suspected acute myocardial infarction: ISIS-2. Lancet 2:349, 1988
23. Lew AS, Laramee P, Cercek B et al: The hypotensive effect of intravenous streptokinase in patients with acute myocardial infarction. Circulation

24. Mathey DG, Kuck KH, Tisner V et al: Nonsurgical coronary artery recanalization in acute transmural myocardial infarction. Circulation 63:489, 1981
25. Sobel BE, Geltman EM, Tiefenbrunn AJ: Improvement of regional myocardial metabolism after coronary thrombolysis induced with tissue-type plasminogen activator or streptokinase. Circulation 69:983, 1984
26. Topol EJ: Clinical use of streptokinase and urokinase therapy for acute myocardial infarction. Heart Lung 16:760, 1987
27. Kennedy JW, Ritchie JL, Davis KB et al: The western Washington randomized trial of intracoronary streptokinase in acute myocardial infarction. N Engl J Med 312:1073, 1985
28. Simoons ML, Brand M, de Zwaan C et al: Improved survival after early thrombolysis in acute myocardial infarction. Lancet 2:578, 1985
29. Rentrop KP, Feit F, Blanke H et al: Effects of intracoronary streptokinase and intracoronary nitroglycerin infusion on coronary angiographic patterns and mortality in patients with acute myocardial infarction. N Engl J Med 311:1458, 1984
30. Khaja F, Walton JA Jr, Brymer JF et al: Intracoronary fibrinolytic therapy in acute myocardial infarction. N Engl J Med 308:1305, 1983
31. Neuhaus KL, Tebbe U, Sauer G et al: High dose intravenous streptokinase in acute MI. Clin Cardiol 6:426, 1983
32. White HD, Norris RM, Brown MA et al: Effect of intravenous streptokinase on left ventricular function and early survival after acute myocardial infarction. N Engl J Med 317:850, 1987
33. Anderson JL, Marshall HW, Askins JC et al: A randomized trial of intravenous and intracoronary streptokinase in patients with acute myocardial infarction. Circulation 70:606, 1984
34. Topol EJ, Fung AY, Kline E et al: Safety of helicopter transport and out-of-hospital intravenous fibrinolytic therapy in patients with evolving myocardial infarction. Cathet Cardiovasc Diag 13:151, 1986
35. Topol EJ, Bates ER, Walton JA Jr et al: Community hospital administration of intravenous tissue plasminogen activator in acute myocardial infarction: Improved timing, thrombolytic efficacy, and ventricular function. J Am Coll Cardiol 10:1173, 1987
36. The I.S.A.M. Study Group: A prospective trial of intravenous streptokinase in acute myocardial infarction (I.S.A.M.). N Engl J Med 314:1465, 1986
37. Ritchie JL, Cerqueira M, Maynard C et al: Ventricular function and infarct size: The Western Washington Intravenous Streptokinase in Myocardial Infarction Trial. J Am Coll Cardiol 11:689, 1988
38. White HD, Norris RM, Brown MA et al: Effect of intravenous streptokinase on left ventricular function and early survival after acute myocardial infarction. N Engl J Med 317:850, 1987
39. Marder VJ, Rothbard RL, Fitzpatrick PG et al: Rapid lysis of coronary artery thrombi with anisoylated plasminogen: Streptokinase activator complex. Ann Intern Med 104:304, 1986
40. Anderson JL, Rothbard RL, Hackworthy RA et al: Multicenter Reperfusion Trial of Intravenous Anisoylated Plasminogen Streptokinase Activator Complex (APSAC) in acute myocardial infarction: Controlled comparison with intracoronary streptokinase. J Am Coll Cardiol 11:1153, 1988
41. Bounier JJRM, de Swart JBRM, Hoffman JJML: Intravenous (IV) APSAC vs intracoronary (IC) streptokinase in the treatment of acute myocardial infarction (abstr). J Am Coll Cardiol 9:62A, 1987
42. Johnson ES, Creegan RJ: An interim report of the efficacy and safety of anisoylated plasminogen streptokinase activator complex in acute myocardial infarction. Drugs 33:261, 1987
43. AIMS Trial Study Group: Effect of intravenous APSAC on mortality after acute myocardial infarction: Preliminary report of a placebo-controlled clinical trial. Lancet 1:545, 1988
44. Tennant SN, Dixon J, Venable TC et al: Intracoronary thrombolysis in patients with acute myocardial infarction: Comparison of the efficacy of urokinase with streptokinase. Circulation 69:756, 1984
45. Sato I, Yamagata T, Sueda T et al: Effects of intracoronary thrombolysis therapy on left ventricular function after acute myocardial infarction. Jpn Circ J 49:616, 1985
46. Cernigliaro C, Sansa M, Campi A et al: Efficacy of intracoronary and intravenous urokinase in acute myocardial infarction. G Ital Cardiol 14:927, 1984
47. Mathey DG, Schofer J, Sheehan FH et al: Intravenous urokinase in acute myocardial infarction. Am J Cardiol 55:878, 1985
48. Califf RM, Wall T, Tcheng JE et al: High dose urokinase for acute myocardial infarction: Results in high rate of sustained infarct artery patency (abstr). Circulation 78(II):304, 1988
49. Neuhaus KL, Tebbe U, Gottwick M et al: Intravenous recombinant tissue plasminogen activator (rt-PA) and urokinase in acute myocardial infarction: Results of the German Activator Urokinase Study (GAUS). J Am Coll Cardiol 12:581, 1988
50. Muller JE for the Prourokinase for Myocardial Infarction Study Group: Clot selective coronary thrombolysis with prourokinase. Circulation (Suppl IV)76:IV-121, 1987
51. Gurewich V: Experiences with pro-urokinase and potentiation of its fibrinolytic effect by urokinase and by tissue plasminogen activator. J Am Coll Cardiol 10:16B, 1987
52. Collen D, Rijken DC, Van Damme J et al: Purification of human tissue-type plasminogen activator in centigram quantities from human melanoma cell culture fluid and its conditioning for use in vivo. Thromb Haemost 48:294, 1982
53. Topol EJ, Califf RM, Kereiakes DJ et al: Thrombolysis and Angioplasty in Myocardial Infarction (TAMI) trial. J Am Coll Cardiol 10:65B, 1987
54. Williams DO, Borer J, Braunwald E et al: Intravenous recombinant tissue-type plasminogen activator in patients with acute myocardial infarction: A report from the NHLBI thrombolysis in myocardial infarction trial. Circulation 73(2):338, 1986
55. Johns JA, Gold HK, Leinbach RC et al: Prevention of coronary artery reocclusion and reduction in late coronary artery stenosis after thrombolytic therapy in patients with acute myocardial infarction. Circulation 78:546, 1988
56. Mueller HS, Rao AK, Forman SA, and the TIMI Investigators: Thrombolysis in Myocardial Infarction (TIMI): Comparative studies of coronary reperfusion and systemic fibrinogenolysis with two forms of recombinant tissue-type plasminogen activator. J Am Coll Cardiol 10:479, 1987
57. Collen D, Topol EJ, Tiefenbrunn AJ et al: Coronary thrombolysis with recombinant human tissue-type plasminogen activator: A prospective, randomized, placebo-controlled trial. Circulation 70:1012, 1984
58. Chesebro JH, Knatterud G, Roberts R et al: Thrombolysis in Myocardial Infarction (TIMI) Trial, Phase I: A comparison between intravenous tissue plasminogen activator and intravenous streptokinase. Circulation 76:142, 1987
59. Verstraete M, Brower RW, Collen D et al: Double-blind randomised trial of intravenous tissue-type plasminogen activator versus placebo in acute myocardial infarction. Lancet 2:965, 1985
60. National Heart Foundation of Australia Coronary Thrombolysis Group: Coronary thrombolysis and myocardial salvage by tissue plasminogen activator given up to 4 hours after onset of myocardial infarction. Lancet 1:203, 1988
61. O'Rourke M, Baron D, Keogh A et al: Limitation of myocardial infarction by early infusion of recombinant tissue-type plasminogen activator. Circulation 77:1311, 1988
62. Wilcox RG, Olsson CG, Skene AM et al for the ASSET Study Group: Trial of tissue plasminogen activator for mortality reduction in acute myocardial infarction: Anglo-Scandinavian Study of Early Thrombolysis (ASSET). Lancet 2:525, 1988
63. Tognoni G. Personal communication, 1990.
64. Ziskind AA, Gold HK, Yasuda T et al: Coronary thrombolysis in dogs with synergistic combinations of human tissue-type plasminogen activator (t-PA) and single chain urokinase-type plasminogen activator (scu-PA) (abstr). Clin Res 35:337A, 1987
65. Collen D, Van de Werf F: Coronary thrombolysis with low dose synergistic combinations of recombinant tissue-type plasminogen activator (rt-PA) and recombinant single chain urokinase-type plasminogen activator (scu-PA) in man. Am J Cardiol 60:431, 1987
66. Topol EJ, Califf RM, George BS and the TAMI Study Group: Coronary arterial thrombolysis with combined recombinant tissue-type plasminogen activator and urokinase in patients with acute myocardial infarction. Circulation 77:1100, 1988
67. Verstraete M: The search for the ideal thrombolytic agent. J Am Coll Cardiol 10:4B, 1987
68. Collen D: Molecular mechanism of action of newer thrombolytic agents. J Am Coll Cardiol 10:11B, 1987
69. Gruntzig AR, Myler RK, Hanna ES et al: Transluminal angioplasty of coronary artery stenosis (abstr). Circulation 56:84, 1977
70. Meyer J, Merx W, Schmitz H et al: Percutaneous transluminal coronary angioplasty immediately after intracoronary streptolysis of transmural myocardial infarction. Circulation 66:905, 1982
71. Topol EJ: Coronary angioplasty for acute myocardial infarction. Ann Intern Med 109:970, 1988
72. Kircher RJ, Topol EJ, O'Neill WW et al: Prediction of infarct coronary artery recanalization after intravenous thrombolytic therapy. Am J Cardiol 59:513, 1987
73. Harrison DG, Ferguson DW, Collins SM et al: Rethrombosis after reperfusion with streptokinase: Importance of geometry of residual lesions. Circulation 69:991, 1984
74. Ellis SG, Topol EJ, Debowey D et al: Recurrent ischemia without warning: Inability to predict ischemic events from residual stenosis after successful coronary thrombolysis (abstr). J Am Coll Cardiol 11:105A, 1988
75. O'Neill W, Timmis G, Bourdillon P et al: A prospective randomized clinical trial of intracoronary streptokinase versus coronary angioplasty therapy of acute myocardial infarction. N Engl J Med 314:812, 1986
76. Topol EJ, Weiss JL, Brinker JA et al: Regional wall motion improvement after coronary thrombolysis with recombinant tissue plasminogen activator: Importance of coronary angioplasty. J Am Coll Cardiol 6:426, 1985
77. Hartzler GO, Rutherford BD, McConahay DR et al: Percutaneous transluminal coronary angioplasty with and without thrombolytic therapy for treatment of acute myocardial infarction. Am Heart J 106:965, 1983
78. Rothbaum DA, Linnemeier TJ, Landin RJ et al: Emergency percutaneous transluminal coronary angioplasty in acute myocardial infarction: A 3-year experience. J Am Coll Cardiol 10:264, 1987
79. Kimura T, Nosaka H, Ueno K et al: Role of coronary angioplasty in acute myocardial infarction. Circulation 74:II-22, 1986
80. Erbel R, Pop T, Henrichs K-J et al: Percutaneous transluminal coronary angioplasty after thrombolytic therapy: A prospective controlled random-

ized trial. J Am Coll Cardiol 8:485, 1986
81. Erbel R, Pop T, Treese N et al: Long-term follow-up after thrombolysis therapy with and without PTCA in myocardial infarction (abstr). Circulation (Suppl IV)76:IV-181, 1987
82. Stack RS, O'Connor CM, Mark DB et al: Coronary perfusion during acute myocardial infarction with a combined therapy of coronary angioplasty and high-dose intravenous streptokinase. Circulation 77:151, 1988
83. Sheehan FH, Bolson EL, Dodge HT et al: Advantages and applications of the centerline method for characterizing regional ventricular function. Circulation 74:293, 1986
84. Topol EJ, Califf RM, George BS et al: A randomized trial of immediate versus delayed elective angioplasty after intravenous tissue plasminogen activator in acute myocardial infarction. N Engl J Med 317:581, 1987
85. TIMI Research Group: Immediate vs. delayed catheterization and angioplasty following thrombolytic therapy for acute myocardial infarction: TIMI IIA results. JAMA 260:2849, 1988
86. Simoons ML, Arnold AER, Betriu A et al: Thrombolysis with rt-PA in acute myocardial infarction: No beneficial effects of immediate PTCA. Lancet 1:197, 1988
87. Topol EJ, Califf RM, George BS et al: Insights derived from the Thrombolysis and Angioplasty in Myocardial Infarction (TAMI) trials: J Am Coll Cardiol 12:24A–31A, 1988
88. DeWood MA, Heit J, Spores J et al: Anterior transmural myocardial infarction: Effects of surgical coronary reperfusion on global and regional left ventricular function. J Am Coll Cardiol 1:1223, 1983
89. Phillips SJ, Zeff RH, Skinner JR et al: Reperfusion protocol and results in 738 patients with evolving myocardial infarction. Ann Thorac Surg 41:119, 1986
90. Kereiakes DJ, Topol EJ, George BS et al and the TAMI Study Group: Emergency coronary artery bypass surgery preserves global and regional left ventricular function after intravenous tissue plasminogen activator therapy for acute myocardial infarction. J Am Coll Cardiol 11:899, 1988
91. Allen B, Buckberg G: Studies of controlled reperfusion after ischemia. XVI. Early recovery of regional wall motion in patients following surgical revascularization after eight hours of acute coronary occlusion. Thorac Cardiovasc Surg 92:636, 1986
92. Hochman JS, Choo H: Limitation of myocardial infarct expansion by reperfusion independent of myocardial salvage. Circulation 75:299, 1987
93. Merzlish JL, Berger HJ, Plankey M et al: Functional left ventricular aneurysm formation: Incidence, natural history and prognostic implications. N Engl J Med 311:1001, 1984
94. Erlebacher JA, Weiss JL, Kallman C et al: Late effects of acute infarct dilation of heart size. Am J Cardiol 49:1120, 1982
95. Kersschot IE, Brugada P, Ramentol M et al: Effects of early reperfusion in acute myocardial infarction on arrhythmias induced by programmed stimulation: A prospective, randomized study. J Am Coll Cardiol 7:1234, 1986
96. Sager PT, Perlmutter RA, Rosenfeld LE et al: Electrophysiologic effects of thrombolytic therapy in patients with a transmural anterior myocardial infarction complicated by left ventricular aneurysm formation. J Am Coll Cardiol 12:19, 1988
97. Jan KM, Reinhart W, Chien S et al: Altered rheological properties of blood following administration of tissue plasminogen activator and streptokinase in patients with acute myocardial infarction (abstr). Circulation (Suppl III)72:III-417, 1985
98. Stricker RB, Wong D, Shin DT et al: Activation of plasminogen by tissue plasminogen activator on normal and thromboasthenic platelets: Effects on surface proteins and platelet aggregation. Blood 68:275, 1986
99. Bulkley BH, Hutchins GM: Myocardial consequences of coronary artery bypass graft surgery. The paradox of necrosis in areas of revascularization. Circulation 56:906, 1977
100. Jennings RB, Reimer KA: Factors involved in salvaging ischemic myocardium: Effect of reperfusion of arterial blood. Circulation (Suppl I)68:I-25, 1983
101. Ambrosio G, Becker LC, Hutchins GM et al: Reduction in experimental infarct size by recombinant human superoxide dismutase: Insights into the pathophysiology of reperfusion injury. Circulation 74:1424, 1986
102. Sherry S: Unresolved clinical pharmacological questions in thrombolytic therapy for acute myocardial infarction. J Am Coll Cardiol 12:519, 1988
103. Pitt B: Cost-specific thrombolytic agents: Is there an advantage? J Am Coll Cardiol 12:588, 1988
104. Ohlstein EH, Shebuski RJ: Tissue-type plasminogen activator (t-PA) increases plasma thromboxane levels which is associated with platelet hyperaggregation (abstr). Circulation (Suppl IV)76:IV-153, 1987
105. Lee CD, Mann KG: The activation of human coagulation factor V by plasmin (abstr). Blood (Suppl I)70:361a, 1987
106. Topol EJ, Burek K, O'Neill WW et al: A randomized controlled trial of hospital discharge three days after myocardial infarction in the era of reperfusion. N Engl J Med 318:1083, 1988
107. O'Neill WW: Management of cardiogenic shock. In Topol EJ (ed): Acute Coronary Intervention. New York, Alan R. Liss, 1987

COMPLICATIONS OF ACUTE MYOCARDIAL INFARCTION

Prediman K. Shah ▪ H. J. C. Swan

CHAPTER 70
VOLUME 2

Nearly one-half million patients are hospitalized annually in the United States with a diagnosis of acute myocardial infarction.[1] Although a substantial number of deaths related to acute myocardial infarction occur prior to admission of the patient to the hospital, the in-hospital course of 2 to 4 weeks is associated with a 10% to 15% mortality. Effective recognition and management of serious ventricular arrhythmias by modern coronary care units has allowed emergence of pump failure to be the leading cause of in-hospital mortality as well as a major contributor to post-discharge morbidity and mortality.[2]

Although many important complications can occur following myocardial infarction (Table 70.1), the discussion here will be restricted to complications not primarily related to disturbances of heart rate, rhythm, or conduction.

PATHOPHYSIOLOGY OF ACUTE MYOCARDIAL INFARCTION

The primary role of coronary thrombosis in the pathogenesis of acute myocardial infarction has now been firmly established. The high incidence (80% to 90%) of intracoronary thrombosis in evolving acute myocardial infarction has been confirmed by *in vivo* angiographic studies, meticulous autopsy studies, and recovery of coronary thrombus from the artery of infarction in patients undergoing emergency coronary artery bypass surgery.[3]

Disruption or ulceration of an underlying atherosclerotic plaque with subsequent exposure of subintimal connective tissue to circulating platelets appears to initiate the process of coronary thrombosis. Coronary thrombus may produce a total and permanent coronary occlusion, or, alternatively, in 15% to 25% of cases, it may result in subtotal or intermittent occlusion.

The dynamic and temporal dependence of myocardial necrosis following coronary artery occlusion has been demonstrated experimentally in animals.[4] Following acute coronary occlusion, and within the myocardial area at risk, necrosis begins within 15 to 20 minutes near the subendocardium and progresses toward the epicardium in a "wave front" of cell death such that it involves 57% of risk area at 3 hours and 71% at 6 hours. The rate of progression of myocardial necrosis is inversely related to the magnitude of residual perfusion to the area at risk, being slower when coronary occlusion is subtotal rather than total or where there are well-developed collaterals to the area at risk.

Studies of myocardial perfusion, viability, and function suggest that the pattern and time sequence of myocardial necrosis in humans may be similar to that in dogs and primates, with nearly complete necrosis of the area at risk occurring with 4 to 6 hours of persistent and total occlusion of the coronary artery. Hemodynamic factors may also influence the rate of myocardial necrosis in as much as hypotension, tachycardia, and increased left ventricular filling pressures may further jeopardize perfusion to the ischemic area, accelerating the process of necrosis. These pathophysiologic considerations have led to a concept of phases of acute myocardial infarction: (1) phase of ischemia, (2) phase of necrosis, (3) phase of compensation, and (4) phase of healing. These temporal phases allow the clinician to relate his diagnostic and therapeutic evaluations and interventions in accord with the underlying pathology and pathophysiology. Severely ischemic myocardium is incapable of mechanical contraction. In addition, necrotic myocardium is deprived of the viable mechanical elements to prevent passive stretch during systole and hence is vulnerable to "materials creep," which is described as the thinning and stretching phase of necrosis. The phase of compensation is associated with adjustments in cardiopulmonary, metabolic, and endocrine functions. The phase of healing is characterized by cellular infiltration and reabsorption, the

TABLE 70.1 IMPORTANT COMPLICATIONS OF ACUTE MYOCARDIAL INFARCTION

Electrical disturbances
  Dysrhythmias
    Bradycardia: sinus, atrioventricular junctional, idioventricular
    Premature beats: atrial, ventricular
    Tachyarrhythmias (supraventricular): atrial tachycardia, atrial fibrillation, atrial flutter, A-V junctional
    Tachyarrhythmias (ventricular): ventricular tachycardia, accelerated idioventricular rhythm, ventricular fibrillation
  Conduction abnormalities
    Atrioventricular nodal: first-degree, second-degree, and third-degree block
    Intraventricular: hemiblocks (left anterior left posterior), bundle branch block, third-degree atrioventricular block

Pump dysfunction
  Contractile dysfunction: left ventricular, right ventricular and biventricular failure, true ventricular aneurysm, infarct expansion
  Mechanical disruption: Acute mitral regurgitation (papillary muscle dysfunction or rupture), ventricular septal rupture, free wall rupture, pseudoaneurysm
  Electromechanical dissociation
Ischemia
  Postinfarction ischemia: ischemia in the infarct; ischemia at a distance
  Early recurrent infarction or infarct extension
Pericarditis
  Early (episternopericarditis)
  Late (Dressler's syndrome)
Thromboembolic
  Mural thrombosis with systemic embolism
  Deep vein thrombosis with pulmonary embolism

laying down of primitive collagen, and scar formation and maturation. For complete maturation, 4 to 6 months or more may be required if the infarct is large.

PATHOPHYSIOLOGY OF PUMP FAILURE

The clinical syndrome of pump failure in acute myocardial infarction (Fig. 70.1) results from the effects of one or more of the following: alterations in contractile function of the myocardium; abnormalities of diastolic pressure–volume relationship of the ventricles; and superimposed mechanical complications such as mitral regurgitation, left-to-right shunt secondary to interventricular septal rupture, cardiac free wall rupture leading to cardiac tamponade, or pseudoaneurysm formation. In any given patient pump failure may be precipitated, worsened, or perpetuated by additional factors, including sustained or recurrent supraventricular or ventricular arrhythmias, persistent severe bradyarrhythmias such as complete heart block, use of potent negative inotropic drugs, and relative or absolute hypovolemia.

DISTURBANCES OF SYSTOLIC CONTRACTILE FUNCTION

Severe reduction or total cessation of coronary blood flow, the proximate cause of acute myocardial infarction, results in a series of abnormalities in regional contractile function ranging from hypokinesis (reduction in extent of shortening) to akinesis (loss of contraction) to dyskinesis (systolic expansion).[5] Depending on the extent of myocardium involved as well as on the type of regional contractile dysfunction, there is a variable net alteration in left ventricular volumes and global ejection fraction as shown schematically in Figure 70.2. Without compensatory mechanisms, progressive abnormalities of regional contractile function result in increasing end-systolic left ventricular volumes with a consequent decrease in stroke volume and left ventricular ejection fraction. Similarly, for any given pattern of regional contractile dysfunction, an increasing extent of abnormally functioning left ventricular myocardium results in a progressively larger end-systolic volume and a lower stroke volume and ejection fraction. Reduced stroke volume, in turn, results in reduced cardiac output. A good relationship between the extent of regional contractile dysfunction and alterations in overall pump function in acute myocardial infarction has been demonstrated.[5,6] Thus, when contractile dysfunction involves 10% of the left ventricular perimeter, the left ventricular ejection fraction declines with minimal decrease in stroke volume, whereas fatal cardiogenic shock is usually associated with involvement of 40% or more. Clinical evidence of heart failure is generally observed when contractile dysfunction involves 25% to 40% of the left ventricular perimeter.

COMPENSATORY MECHANISMS

Compensatory mechanisms that may limit the degree of decline in cardiac output and blood pressure include the following:

1. Increased sympathoadrenal activity with increased circulating catecholamines results in tachycardia and an increase in systemic vas-

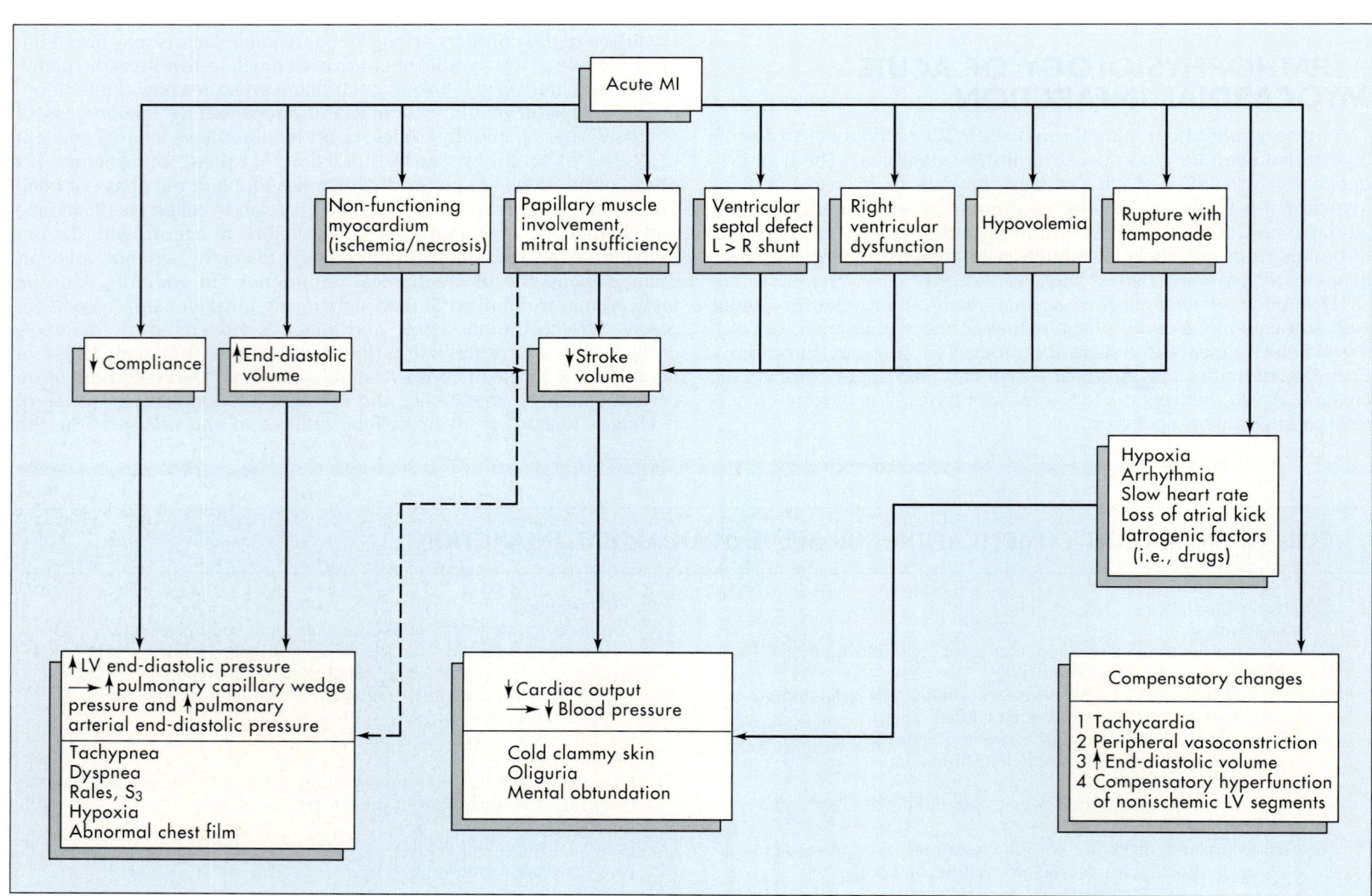

FIGURE 70.1 Pathogenesis of pump failure following acute myocardial infarction. (RV, right ventricular; LV, left ventricular)

cular resistance. Sympathoadrenal stimulation, however, may increase the risk of arrhythmias, exacerbate myocardial ischemia by increasing myocardial oxygen consumption, and increase left ventricular afterload by producing systemic vasoconstruction.

2. Increase in left ventricular end-diastolic volume allows the heart to use the Frank-Starling mechanism to minimize decreases in stroke volume despite a reduction in ejection fraction. Left ventricular dilatation, on the other hand, increases wall tension and myocardial oxygen demand and also predisposes to pulmonary venous congestion because of an associated increase in left ventricular end-diastolic pressure. Furthermore, papillary muscle dysfunction with mitral regurgitation may also result from left ventricular dilatation.

3. Hyperfunction of the noninfarcted, normally perfused remote myocardial segments occurs in order to reduce end-systolic volume and to preserve global ejection fraction and minimize decreases in stroke volume. Such compensatory hyperfunction may not be possible if the non-infarct-related myocardial segments demonstrate ischemia and dysfunction when their blood supply is dependent on an artery with significant stenosis and/or collaterals from the infarct-related occluded artery.

COMPLICATING MECHANISMS

Complicating additional factors contributing to a reduction in cardiac output and hypotension in acute myocardial infarction include the following:

1. Mitral regurgitation, a consequence of papillary muscle ischemia, infarction, or rupture, results in a decrease in forward stroke volume at the expense of regurgitation into the left atrium.
2. Intracardiac left-to-right shunt, from ventricular septal rupture, results in a proportionate decrease in left ventricular forward stroke volume.
3. Right ventricular ischemia and infarction results in decreases in left ventricular filling and a reduction in left ventricular end-diastolic volume.
4. Cardiac tamponade, usually from transmural rupture of an infarcted area, results in impedance to right and left ventricular filling and a decrease in end-diastolic volume and stroke volume.
5. Bradyarrhythmias or heart block reduces cardiac output because of a slow heart rate or by eliminating atrial contribution to ventricular filling.
6. Frequent or sustained atrial or ventricular tachyarrhythmias contribute to low cardiac output state by limiting ventricular filling, accentuating valvular regurgitation, or worsening myocardial ischemia.
7. Hypovolemia may complicate acute myocardial infarction and result in inadequate left ventricular filling and a decline in stroke volume. Hypovolemia is often secondary to injudicious diuresis, blood loss, or severe vomiting, diarrhea, and diaphoresis.
8. Primary decreases in peripheral vascular tone, triggered by neural reflexes originating from ischemic or infarcted segments of myocardium, may result in peripheral vasodilation and hypotension.

DISTURBANCES OF DIASTOLIC VENTRICULAR FUNCTION

Abnormalities in diastolic function occur frequently following acute myocardial infarction and include increases in left ventricular end-diastolic volume and changes in ventricular diastolic pressure–volume relationship or compliance. Since pulmonary capillary wedge pressure closely approximates the left ventricular mean diastolic filling pressure in absence of mitral valve disease, an elevated left ventricular filling pressure results in increases in pulmonary capillary wedge pressure. Elevations of left ventricular filling pressure result from an increased end-diastolic volume or a reduced diastolic compliance or both (Fig. 70.3). The mechanisms responsible for increasing left ventricular end-diastolic volume in acute myocardial infarction remain unclear but may involve the process of infarct-expansion.[7,8] Infarct-expansion results from stretching, lengthening, and thinning of the segment of transmural necrosis, probably reflecting disruption of the connective tissue framework of the myocardium with consequent slippage of myofibrils.

Alterations in left ventricular diastolic compliance occur frequently in acute myocardial infarction and may be detectable with even a limited extent of infarction. Although initially there may be an increase in compliance, most studies suggest that the overall compliance is generally reduced, probably reflecting alterations in viscoelastic properties of the ischemic and necrotic tissue due to cellular and interstitial edema in the acute phase and healing with fibrosis in the subacute and chronic phases.[9,10] Right ventricular dilatation and dysfunction accompanying ischemia or infarction of the right ventricle may also contribute to the decreased left ventricular compliance, resulting from leftward bulging of the interventricular septum into the left ventricle as well as an increase in intrapericardial pressures.

CONCEPTUAL MODEL

A conceptual model of interrelationships among infarct size, compliance, and systolic ventricular function proposed by Swan and colleagues[11] is useful in understanding the complex interrelationship between the extent of infarction, alterations in infarct compliance, ventricular volumes, and overall pump function as assessed by stroke volume and ejection fraction (Figs. 70.4 and 70.5). Although invasive hemodynamic monitoring has greatly expanded our understanding of the pathophysiology of acute myocardial infarction, such measurements as left ventricular filling pressure, cardiac output, arterial pressure, and derived parameters cannot fully describe altered ventricular function without consideration of changes in regional wall motion, ventricular compliance, chamber volume, and shape associated with acute myocardial infarction.

The model consists of a totally noncontractile infarct of variable

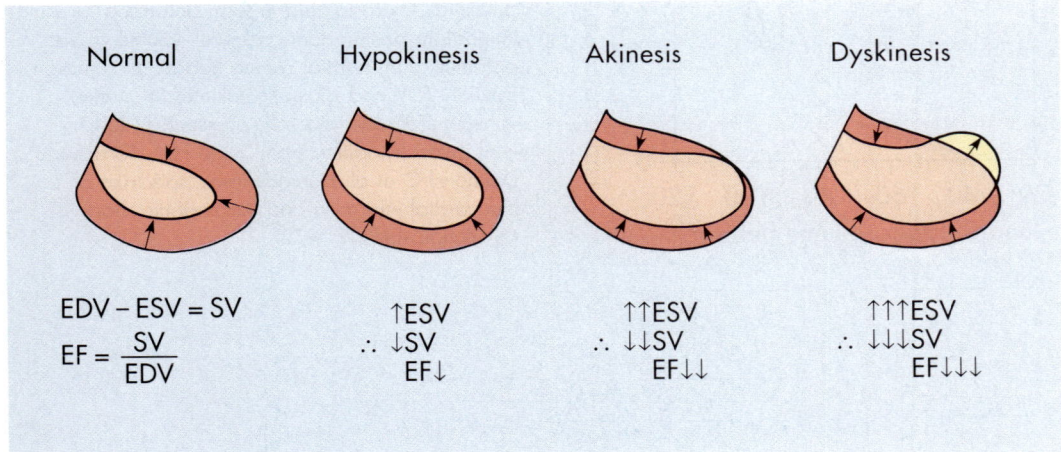

FIGURE 70.2 Patterns of left ventricular regional contractile dysfunction and their influence on end-diastolic volume (*EDV*), end-systolic volume (*ESV*), stroke volume (*SV*), and ejection fraction (*EF*). Note progressive declines in EF with increasing ESV consequent to increasing gradation of contractile dysfunction.

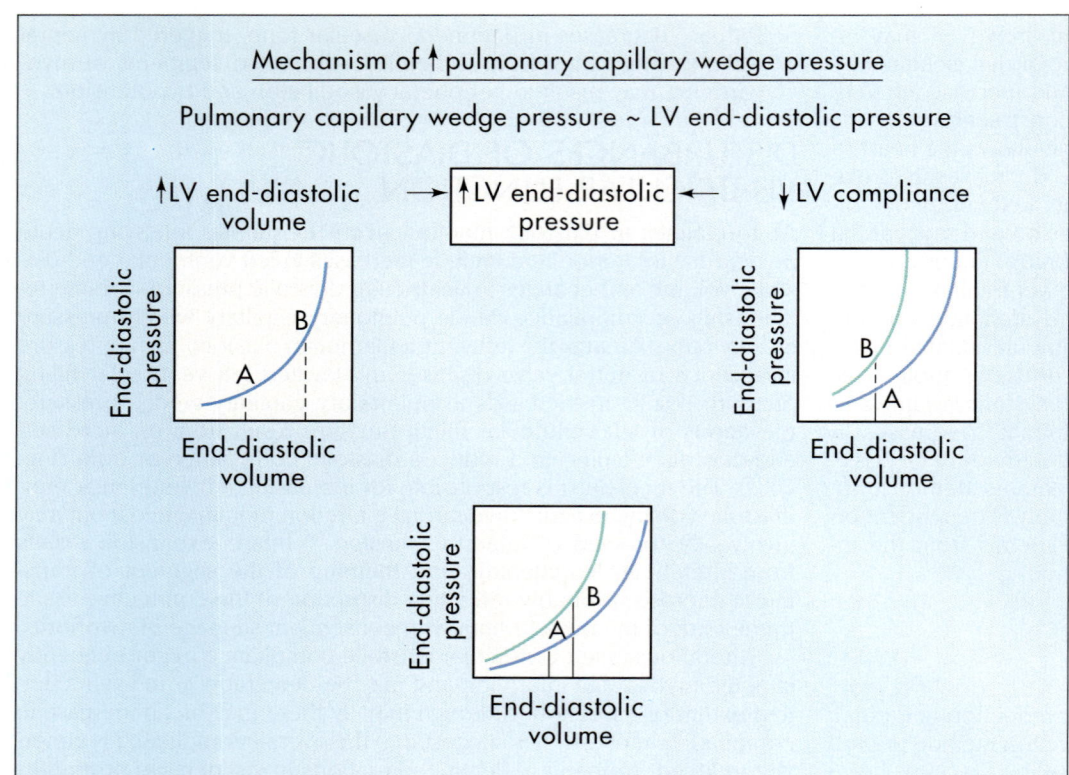

FIGURE 70.3 Two different mechanisms contributing to elevation of left ventricular end-diastolic pressure (*EDP*) (and consequently the pulmonary capillary wedge pressure [*PCW*]) are illustrated on the pressure–volume plots. **Top left.** Elevation of EDP secondary to increase in end-diastolic volume (*EDV*) as patient moves from A to B. **Top right.** Leftward and upward displacement of pressure–volume curve with an increase in EDP without a change in EDV, reflecting a reduced compliance, as patient moves from A to B. **Bottom.** Composite of increased EDV and reduced compliance as patient moves from A to B. Note that mitral regurgitation can raise PCW without involving any of these mechanisms by directly increasing left atrial pressure.

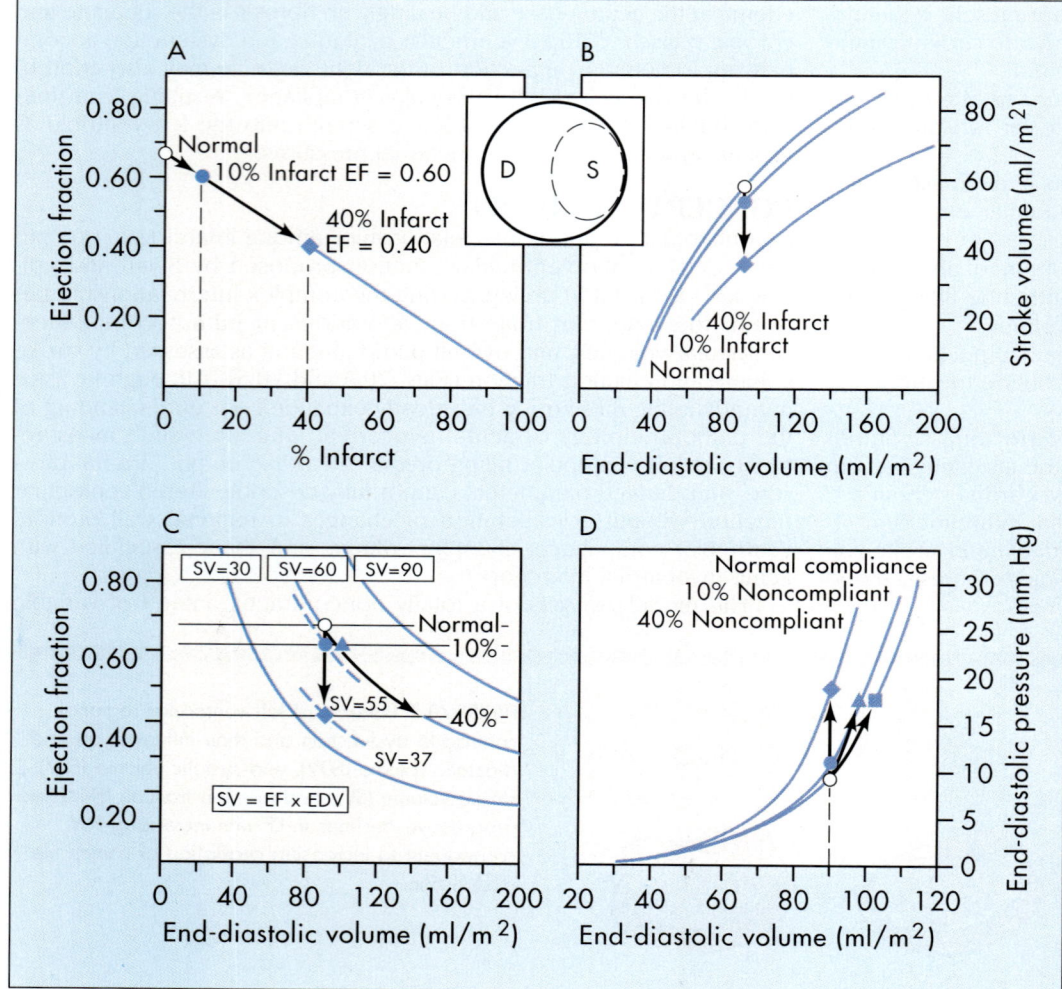

FIGURE 70.4 Hemodynamics of a noncompliant infarct. **A.** Relationship of EF, EDV, and SV to infarct size. The schematic diagram represents the heart in systole and diastole, and the infarct segment is assumed to be totally noncontractile and nondistensible. The resulting EF is a linear function of the remaining quantity of normally contracting myocardium (see text). Thus, with an infarct of 10% (*circle*), EF would fall from 0.67 to 0.60, and with a 40% infarct it would fall to 0.40 (*diamond*). **B.** Left ventricular function curves. Ten percent and 40% nondistensible infarct segments are associated with reductions in EF and SV at a constant EDV of 90 ml/m², and hence a downward shift in function curve representing the left ventricle as a whole. **C.** Relationship among EF, EDV, and SV. When EF is reduced by acute myocardial infarction, this may result in either a decreased SV at an unchanged EDV or a compensatory increase in EDV to maintain SV (see text). **D.** The obligatory changes in the pressure–volume relationships consequent on a noncompliant infarct. It is assumed that the infarct is rigid in the contracted state. The normal pressure–volume curve is based on values for normal heart volumes and normal diastolic pressures, extrapolated in form according to acute immediate postmortem pressure–volume curves obtained from normal canine hearts. (*EF*, ejection fraction; *EDV*, end-diastolic volume; *SV*, stroke volume; *EDP*, end-diastolic pressure; *LV*, left ventricular) (Modified from Swan HJC, Forrester JS, Diamond G et al: Hemodynamic spectrum of myocardial infarction and cardiogenic shock. Circulation 45:1097, 1972)

size, possessing an altered compliance, the temporal and directional course of which remains to be defined in detail, and a residual noninfarcted area with normal compliance. It is assumed, for simplicity, that left ventricular function is independent of the anatomical location of similarly sized infarcted segments. Since we are concerned primarily with the function of the heart as a pump, the ratio of stroke volume to end-diastolic volume—the ejection fraction—is used as the index of cardiac performance most appropriate to the purpose.

INFARCT SIZE

The immediate mechanical alterations following acute coronary occlusion are illustrated schematically in Figure 70.4. This analysis assumes normal myocardial contractility prior to infarction and, therefore, an ejection fraction of 0.67 for the normal noninfarcted ventricle. Such a ventricle would have an end-diastolic volume of 90 ml/m^2, an end-systolic volume of 30 ml/m^2, and a stroke volume of 60 ml/m^2. The area of infarct is considered to be completely noncontractile and, for

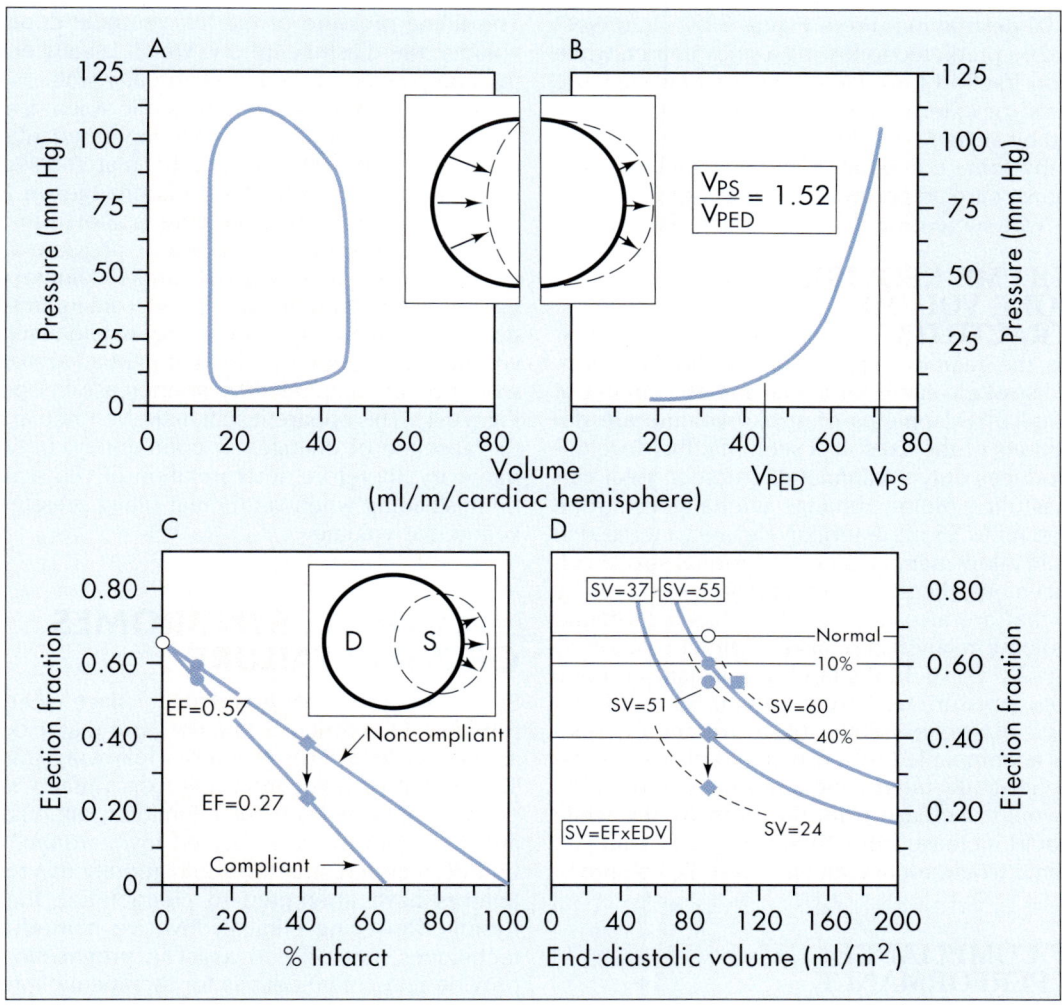

FIGURE 70.5 Hemodynamics of a compliant infarct. **A.** Assuming that one half of the spherical model is infarcted, the left ventricular pressure–volume relationship during systole and diastole in the noninfarcted cardiac hemisphere illustrates a normal pressure–volume loop and results in a V (or SV) of 30 ml/m^2. **B.** If the noncontractile infarct segment (right panel) exhibits normal compliance, it will stretch during ventricular systole, according to its passive pressure–volume curve with resultant paradoxical expansion, so that for normal pressure ranges the increase in volume during systole will be approximately equal to the decrease in volume of the contracting hemisphere. If the pressure–volume curve is less steep, the penalty is even greater. Forward SV can only be maintained with an increased end-diastolic and a reduced peak systolic pressure. In this model a forward SV of 15 ml/m^2 is possible at an EDP of 25 mm Hg and a peak systolic pressure of 70 mm Hg. **C.** Effect of normal compliance characteristics with paradoxical pulsations on EF. With outward movement of the infarct segment during systole, a portion of the potential systemic SV will be delivered into this segment. Thus, EF will be further reduced in the presence of a compliant infarct segment (circles for 10% infarct, diamonds for 40% infarct). The values are estimated for peak systolic pressures at the low range of normal. **D.** Interrelationship of EF, SV, and EDV. In the presence of paradoxical pulsation, reduction in EF is associated with a decrease in SV exceeding that predicted for a noncompliant infarct as shown in Figure 70.4A. When EDV remains unchanged in the presence of normal overall ventricular compliance, LVEDP is also unchanged (Figure 70.4D, open circle). The SV of 51 shown here may be returned to normal levels by compensatory ventricular dilatation only if the infarct is small (10% infarct). This rise in EDV produces a concomitant rise in LVEDP (Figure 70.4D, square). (EF, ejection fraction; EDV, end-diastolic volume; SV, stroke volume) (Modified from Swan HJC, Forrester JS, Diamond G et al: Hemodynamic spectrum of myocardial infarction and cardiogenic shock. Circulation 45:1097, 1972)

the present, absolutely nondistensible (noncompliant or stiff). If the model is considered as an infinite number of cones, each based on the surface of the sphere and with its apex at the center, the ejection fraction is reduced in direct relation to the size of the infarct (Fig. 70.4, A).

If end-diastolic volume remains constant, the overall performance of the ventricle, depicted in the form of a classic ventricular function curve, is depressed; however, the contractile state of the noninfarcted myocardial fibers has remained unchanged.

For purposes of comparison, a small infarct will be considered as equivalent to destruction of 10% of left ventricular mass, while a large infarct corresponds to 40% destruction. From Figure 70.4, A an ejection fraction of 0.60 would be predicted following a small infarct, while the corresponding ejection fraction for a large infarct would be 0.40. To maintain a normal level of external cardiac performance, stroke volume must be increased by an increase in end-diastolic volume, by a decrease in afterload, or by some combination of these mechanisms. Failing these compensations, cardiac performance must, of necessity, decrease proportionately with increasing infarct size (Fig. 70.4, B).

PRESSURE AND VOLUME REQUIREMENTS TO MAINTAIN STROKE VOLUME AT NORMAL CONTRACTILITY

Figure 70.4, C describes the relationship among ejection fraction, end-diastolic volume, and stroke volume for a 10% and 40% infarct of infinite stiffness (noncompliant). Isopleths of stroke volume are depicted as hyperbolic functions of the axes. It is seen that the development of a 10% infarct produces only a minimal decrease in total cardiac function. If end-diastolic volume remains unchanged, stroke volume is reduced from 60 ml to 55 ml. Alternatively, a 9% increase in end-diastolic volume would allow maintenance of a normal stroke volume. However, the replacement of contractile compliant elements by noncontractile elements that are also noncompliant has a profound effect on the pressure–volume relationship, also in direct relation to the infarct size (Fig. 70.4, D). For a 10% infarct at constant end-diastolic volume, end-diastolic pressure rises from 10 mm Hg to 12 mm Hg, although maintenance of stroke volume by increasing end-diastolic volume to 100 ml is accompanied by a rise in end-diastolic pressure. With the development of 40% infarct and a normal end-diastolic volume, stroke volume would decrease from 60 ml to 37 ml, while end-diastolic pressure would increase from 10 mm Hg to 20 mm Hg. Restoration of stroke volume would require an end-diastolic volume of 140 ml/m^2.

RELATIONSHIP OF COMPLIANCE TO VENTRICULAR PERFORMANCE

Since the infarcted segment does not participate in the process of contraction, it is subjected to repetitive passive stretch during each systole as intraventricular pressure rises (Fig. 70.5, B). Hence, this segment will lengthen to a degree dependent on its intrinsic length–tension characteristics and the level of systolic pressure. The parallel elastic elements of the healthy myocardium are protected from stretch by the intrinsic shortening of their contracting sarcomeres (Fig. 70.5, A). If the fibers of the infarcted segment follow the normal passive length–tension curve, then left ventricular function is further compromised as infarct size increases. Assuming normal compliance to be represented by a ratio of segment length at peak systolic pressure divided by segment length at end-diastole of 1.15 (15% increase in length), then the equivalent change in volume would be 1.15^3 or 1.52. On this basis, the ejection fraction would decrease further to 0.57 and 0.27 for a small and large infarct, respectively, in the presence of normal compliance. In the presence of normal heart size, such ejection fractions will permit stroke volumes of 51 ml and only 24 ml, respectively (Fig. 70.5, D). Although the 10% infarct heart is capable of further adjustment as outlined above (end-diastolic volume = 100 ml/m^2; end-diastolic pressure = 17 mm Hg) (see Fig. 70.4, D), the consequence of a compliant in contrast to a noncompliant diseased segment becomes substantial with infarcts in excess of 30% of left ventricular mass. With a 40% infarct, the stroke volume decreases to 24 ml at an end-diastolic pressure and end-diastolic volume identical to the noninfarcted heart and cannot be improved significantly without substantial increase in end-diastolic volume. Even if end-diastolic volume is increased to the level associated with a filling pressure of 20 mm Hg, stroke volume would rise only from 24 ml to 29 ml, in comparison to 37 ml when the infarct remains noncompliant.

FILLING PRESSURE AND VENTRICULAR FUNCTION CURVES

The filling pressure of the left ventricle depends on the end-systolic volume; the diastolic inflow, which usually equals stroke volume; and the compliance of the left ventricular wall.

Assuming a normal end-diastolic volume, a change in end-diastolic pressure will occur in relation to increased infarct size according to the compliance characteristics of the infarcted segment and of the normal myocardium. The effect of this change on left ventricular function curves based on filling pressure is shown in Figure 70.4, D. If a 40% infarct fails to stiffen, end-diastolic pressure and end-diastolic volume would remain unaltered but stroke volume would be reduced to a greater extent than that predicted from infarct size alone, as previously discussed. Stiffening of the infarct would result in true improvement in ventricular function by elimination of an area of systolic expansion but would be accompanied by an increase in end-diastolic pressure (see Fig. 70.4). This apparent shift in the ventricular function curve occurs in the absence of changes in contractility. In states where compliance may vary, therefore, interpretation of ventricular function curves may be misleading when ventricular filling pressure is used as an index of ventricular volume.

CLINICAL SYNDROMES OF PUMP FAILURE

Studies over the past two decades have clearly demonstrated the importance of ventricular function as a major determinant of short-term as well as long-term prognosis following myocardial infarction.[2,12,13] The extent of myocardial necrosis (infarct size) is one of the chief determinants of ventricular function, although alterations in compliance, function of noninfarcted myocardium, and mechanical disruption of infarcted structures may modify this relationship.[11] Thus investigators have attempted to characterize the severity of ventricular dysfunction using clinical, invasive hemodynamic and noninvasive techniques, not only to assist in prognostic assessment but also to provide rational guidelines for therapeutic interventions.[14–16]

CLINICAL SUBSETS (TABLE 70.2)

Killip and Kimball[14] characterized patients with acute myocardial infarction into four subsets based on admission physical findings:

Class I: No signs of left ventricular failure
Class II: S$_3$ gallop and/or pulmonary congestion limited to basal lung segments
Class III: Acute pulmonary edema
Class IV: Shock syndrome

Forrester and colleagues also classified patients with acute myocardial infarction into four subsets[15,16]:

I: No evidence of pulmonary congestion or systemic hypoperfusion
II: Evidence of pulmonary congestion without evidence of systemic hypoperfusion
III: Evidence of systemic hypoperfusion without evidence of pulmonary congestion
IV: Evidence of pulmonary congestion and systemic hypoperfusion

Although such clinical categorization is conceptually useful, several drawbacks should be recognized. For example, the magnitude of ventricular dysfunction determined by more objective invasive or noninvasive means often shows considerable overlap between various clinical classes and subsets of patients. Such discrepancies arise since patients exhibit clinical "phase lags" as pulmonary congestion develops or resolves; when symptoms and signs secondary to coexistent chronic obstructive lung disease are mistakenly interpreted as pulmonary congestion; when patients pass from one subset to another with or without therapy; or when changes in ventricular compliance alter left ventricular diastolic function. This type of categorization fails to account for specific causes of pump dysfunction, such as predominant right or left ventricular dysfunction, mitral regurgitation, and ventricular septal or free-wall rupture.

HEMODYNAMIC SUBSETS (TABLE 70.2)

Physiologic assessment of left ventricular function in acute myocardial infarction using invasive hemodynamic variables was made possible by the introduction of the balloon-flotation pulmonary artery thermodilution catheter by Swan, Ganz, and colleagues in the early 1970s.[16] Based on invasive hemodynamic evaluation of pulmonary capillary wedge pressure and cardiac index in 200 patients, Forrester and co-workers[15] classified patients with acute myocardial infarction into four subsets with differing mortalities and suggested that such a classification could be used to guide the selection of appropriate therapeutic interventions. Clinical evidence of pulmonary congestion is frequently observed when the pulmonary capillary wedge pressure is 18 mm Hg to 20 mm Hg or higher, whereas clinical evidence of systemic hypoperfusion is often present when the cardiac index is less than 2 to 2.2 liters/min/m^2. However, in 20% to 30% of cases, discrepancies between clinical findings and hemodynamic variables may be found. Various reasons for such discrepancies have already been alluded to.

INVASIVE HEMODYNAMIC MONITORING (SWAN-GANZ CATHETERIZATION AND INTRA-ARTERIAL PRESSURE MONITORING) (TABLE 70.3)

Patients with clinically uncomplicated acute myocardial infarction do not generally benefit from routine invasive monitoring. Such patients can be well assessed by carefully and meticulously performed clinical assessment, which takes into account for example the overall appearance of the patient, heart rate and rhythm, systemic blood pressure, careful repeated cardiac examination for gallops or murmurs, careful pulmonary auscultation for rales, assessment of pulmonary vasculature on a chest roentgenogram and assessment of adequacy of vital organ perfusion (*e.g.*, urine output, mental status). However, invasive hemodynamic monitoring is useful in hemodynamically complicated patients with acute myocardial infarction in order to clarify the role of hypovolemia, left ventricular failure, valvular regurgitation, septal rupture, right ventricular infarction, and cardiac tamponade in producing a state of hypotension, low-output syndrome, or pulmonary congestion and edema and to assist in the selection of appropriate therapeutic intervention and to follow the response to the intervention. Thus hemodynamic monitoring should be considered in those patients with acute myocardial infarction who demonstrate clinical evidence of severe pulmonary congestion, low-output state, persistent hypotension and shock unrelated to correctable bradycardia, persistent unexplained sinus tachycardia, or appearance of a new systolic murmur. In addition, noninvasive studies such as two-dimensional echocardiography, Doppler flow studies, and radionuclide scintigraphy can be used to complement clinical and hemodynamic assessment of patients with acute myocardial infarction as summarized in Table 70.4.

From a practical clinical standpoint, acute myocardial infarction complicated by pump dysfunction can be discussed under specific clinical categories or syndromes, outlined in Table 70.5.

PULMONARY CONGESTION WITHOUT A LOW-OUTPUT STATE

Mild degrees of pulmonary congestion are common in patients with acute myocardial infarction, resulting from an elevation of pulmonary capillary wedge pressure to the 18 mm Hg to 25 mm Hg range. The elevation of pulmonary capillary wedge pressure generally results from an increased left ventricular filling pressure due to decreased diastolic compliance, increased end-diastolic volume, or both, but it may also be due to mitral regurgitation. The patient may complain of dyspnea and orthopnea, whereas findings on examination include tachypnea, bibasilar post-tussive pulmonary rales and/or a palpable or audible S_3 gallop, mild to moderate hypoxemia, and radiologic evidence of mild to moderate pulmonary venous hypertension.

The object of therapy in such patients is to ensure adequate arterial oxygenation with the help of supplemental oxygen and to relieve pul-

TABLE 70.2 CLINICAL AND HEMODYNAMIC SUBSETS IN ACUTE MYOCARDIAL INFARCTION

Killip Class	Clinical Features	Hemodynamic Features	Approximate Proportion of Patients	Hospital Mortality
1	No signs of congestive heart failure		40–50%	6%
2	S_3 gallop, bibasilar rales		30–40%	17%
3	Acute pulmonary edema		10–15%	38%
4	Cardiogenic shock		5–10%	81%
Cedars-Sinai Clinical Subsets				
1	No pulmonary congestion or tissue hypoperfusion		25%	1%
2	Pulmonary congestion only		25%	11%
3	Tissue hypoperfusion only		15%	18%
4	Pulmonary congestion and tissue hypoperfusion		35%	60%
Cedars-Sinai Hemodynamic Subsets				
1		PCW ≤ 18; CI > 2.2	25%	3%
2		PCW > 18; CI > 2.2	25%	9%
3		PCW ≤ 18; CI ≤ 2.2	15%	23%
4		PCW > 18; CI ≤ 2.2	35%	51%

(PCW, Pulmonary capillary wedge pressure (mm Hg); CI, cardiac index (liters/min/m^2))

TABLE 70.3 INVASIVE HEMODYNAMIC MONITORING IN ACUTE MYOCARDIAL INFARCTION

Useful for
Clarifying role of hypovolemia, left ventricular failure, mitral regurgitation, interventricular septal rupture, right ventricular infarction, and cardiac tamponade in the genesis of pump failure
Selection of appropriate therapy for pump failure (*e.g.*, inotropes, vasodilators, volume)
Rapid assessment of response to therapy
Prognostic assessment (see Fig. 70.1)

Indications
Persistent low-output state, hypotension, or shock
Recurrent or refractory pulmonary congestion or edema
Appearance of a new systolic murmur
During the use of intravenous vasoactive drugs or intra-aortic balloon counterpulsation
Unexplained persistent sinus tachycardia

TABLE 70.4 ROLE OF NONINVASIVE TECHNIQUES FOR ASSESSMENT OF COMPLICATED ACUTE MYOCARDIAL INFARCTION WITH PUMP DYSFUNCTION

Technique	Useful in Diagnosis of
Echocardiography	Papillary muscle rupture
	Ventricular septal rupture
	Pseudoaneurysm
	True aneurysm and mural thrombus
	Infarct expansion
	Right ventricular infarction
	Pericardial effusion and tamponade
Doppler echocardiography	Acute mitral regurgitation
	Ventricular septal rupture
Radionuclide techniques	
Radionuclide ventriculography	Ventriculopenic state
	Right ventricular infarction
	Ventricular septal rupture (first-pass method)
	Pseudoaneurysm and true aneurysm
	Mural thrombus
	Subacute cardiac rupture with intrapericardial bleeding
Rest and redistribution thallium-201 scintigraphy	Differentiation of ischemic and viable from infarcted myocardium
Technetium-99m pyrophosphate scintigraphy	Diagnosis of right ventricular infarction
	Assessment of extent of infarction

TABLE 70.5 CATEGORIES OF PUMP DYSFUNCTION IN ACUTE MYOCARDIAL INFARCTION

Clinical Category	Pathophysiologic Basis	Equivalent Clinical Subsets — Killip	Equivalent Clinical Subsets — Cedars-Sinai	Equivalent Cedars-Sinai Hemodynamic Subset
Subclinical	Compensated ventricular dysfunction or normal or near-normal ventricular function	I	I	I
Clinically Overt				
Pulmonary congestion	Systolic and/or diastolic left ventricular dysfunction	II	II	II
	Mitral regurgitation			
	Ventricular septal rupture			
Acute pulmonary edema	As above but more severe	III	II	II
Low-output state, hypotension and shock				
With pulmonary congestion and edema				
Ventriculopenic state	Severe systolic and diastolic left ventricular dysfunction	IV	IV	IV
Mechanical lesions	Acute mitral regurgitation	IV	IV	IV
	Septal rupture			
Without pulmonary congestion or edema	Hypovolemia	IV	III	III
	Dominant right ventricular dysfunction			
	Cardiac rupture			
	Cardiac tamponade			
	Electromechanical dissociation			
	Severe bradyarrhythmias			

monary venous congestion by reducing left ventricular filling pressure and pulmonary capillary wedge pressure. This can usually be accomplished by judicious use of small doses of intravenous furosemide (20 mg to 40 mg). Reduction of left ventricular filling pressure and consequently the pulmonary capillary wedge pressure not only relieves pulmonary congestion but may also reduce left ventricular volume, wall tension, and myocardial oxygen demand while at the same time facilitating subendocardial myocardial perfusion. Measurements of venous capacitance in acute myocardial infarction have suggested that the diuretic effect of intravenous furosemide may be preceded by a venodilator action, contributing to its preload reducing effect.[17] A more recent study, however, has demonstrated a vasoconstrictor effect of intravenous furosemide preceding its diuretic effects in patients with chronic congestive heart failure.[18] Excessive diuresis should be avoided since that may result in electrolyte depletion (notably hypokalemia) as well as hypotension and a low-output state from underfilling of the left ventricle.

Vasodilators such as nitrates or sodium nitroprusside may also be used as an alternative or adjunct to diuretics in this subset of patients, particularly when pulmonary congestion is accompanied by evidence of mitral regurgitation or systemic hypertension. Vasodilators produce their beneficial effects in pulmonary congestion by producing venodilation, improving ventricular compliance, and decreasing ventricular afterload by arteriolar dilator effects, resulting in improvement in left ventricular function and reduction in mitral regurgitation or the degree of left-to-right shunt across a ventricular septal rupture. Long-acting nitrate preparations, such as sublingual isosorbide dinitrate (in doses of 2.5 mg to 10 mg every 3 to 4 hours) or 2% nitroglycerin ointment (½- to 1-inch applied cutaneously every 4 to 6 hours) are useful in providing mild to moderate vasodilator effects. Although hemodynamic monitoring is not generally necessary in this group of patients, objective documentation of effects of vasodilators may be appropriate when clinical assessment of efficacy is ambiguous. (Specifics of the use of intravenous vasodilators are considered later in this chapter.)

Use of cardiac glycosides in such patients remains a subject of controversy since hemodynamic benefit has not been consistently demonstrated.

ACUTE PULMONARY EDEMA WITHOUT SHOCK

Acute pulmonary edema is characterized by patients with more severe manifestations of acute pulmonary congestion (*i.e.*, severe respiratory distress, sometimes accompanied by expectoration of pink frothy sputum and often accompanied by cool, clammy, diaphoretic skin, increased heart rate, and elevated blood pressure indicative of a hyperactive sympathoadrenal system). This syndrome may be precipitated by extensive left ventricular systolic dysfunction secondary to massive acute myocardial infarction or cumulative effects of previous and new myocardial infarction. Acute pulmonary edema may also result from severe decrease in diastolic compliance with only relatively modest systolic contractile dysfunction (stiff heart); severe, acute, persistent, or intermittent mitral regurgitation, which can be independent of the size of left ventricular infarction, resulting from papillary muscle dysfunction or rupture; or profound global myocardial ischemia in association with relatively small or modest degree of myocardial necrosis. In all three of these situations, left ventricular systolic function, as assessed by ejection fraction, may be less depressed than suggested by the severity of the clinical state of the patient. Such patients are frequently severely hypoxemic and may exhibit some degree of retention of carbon dioxide and a decrease in arterial pH. Physical examination may show tachypnea, cyanosis, tachycardia, elevated blood pressure, cool and moist skin, and extensive bilateral pulmonary rales, occasionally accompanied by wheezing (cardiac asthma), or even diminished breath sounds, due to poor respiratory efforts. Acute pulmonary edema in myocardial infarction is usually caused by a rapid and marked elevation of pulmonary capillary wedge pressure (exceeding 25 mm Hg), although in some patients a decrease in capillary colloid oncotic pressure may play a contributory role. This has been suggested as a mechanism contributing to pulmonary edema precipitated by rapid infusion of crystalloid volume, which results in dilution of serum proteins and a fall in intravascular oncotic pressure. Acute pulmonary edema complicating myocardial infarction is associated with a high mortality, ranging from 30% to 50%.

The principles of management of acute cardiogenic pulmonary edema complicating myocardial infarction are outlined in Table 70.6. Maintenance of adequate gas exchange, a stable rhythm, and blood pressure and rapid reduction of pulmonary capillary wedge pressure are the primary short-term therapeutic objectives.

MAINTENANCE OF ADEQUATE GAS EXCHANGE

Maintenance of adequate gas exchange requires immediate assessment, using arterial blood gases, and administration of high concentrations (60% to 100%) of oxygen via a face mask. Endotracheal intubation should be considered in patients who appear moribund, are unable to maintain an arterial Po_2 of at least 60 mm Hg on face mask ventilation, and develop progressively rising Pco_2 or declining arterial pH. Mechanical ventilation, after endotracheal intubation, may need to be supplemented with addition of positive end-expiratory pressure

---

TABLE 70.6 PRINCIPLES IN THE MANAGEMENT OF POSTINFARCTION ACUTE PULMONARY EDEMA

1. Immediate objectives
   a. Maintain adequate gas exchange (supplemental O_2, intubation, PEEP)
   b. Convert persistent non-sinus tachyarrhythmias (cardioversion, appropriate drugs)
   c. Retard lung fluid filtration and promote fluid clearance by rapidly lowering PCW by
      1) Redistributive interventions (nitrates, other vasodilators, morphine, tourniquets)
      2) Depletive interventions (diuretics, ultrafiltration, phlebotomy)
      3) Improving LV function (vasodilators, inotropes, and IABP in hypotensive patients)
      4) Decreasing mitral regurgitation (vasodilators, IABP in severe cases)
2. Identify and treat precipitating factors (recurrent or persistent ischemia,* extensive necrosis, acute mitral regurgitation,* ventricular septal rupture,* arrhythmias)
3. Definitive surgery when appropriate
4. Avoid routine use of aminophylline, digitalis (exception: supraventricular arrhythmias), and intermittent positive-pressure breathing.

(PCW, pulmonary capillary wedge pressure; LV, left ventricular; PEEP, positive end-expiratory pressure; IABP, intra-aortic balloon pumping; *, conditions in which early cardiac surgery may be lifesaving)

(PEEP) in order to maintain adequate systemic oxygenation and allow the use of relatively safe concentrations of oxygen (*i.e.*, $FIO_2 \leq 60\%$). When using PEEP, physicians should be aware of potential complications associated with its use (*e.g.*, lung barotrauma and a decline in cardiac output secondary to reduced left ventricular preload and increase in right ventricular afterload). Hemodynamic and arterial blood gas monitoring is useful in determining the effects of PEEP on tissue oxygen delivery (a product of cardiac output and arterial oxygen content) and in the selection of optimal amounts of PEEP.

RAPID REDUCTION OF PULMONARY CAPILLARY WEDGE PRESSURE

At the present time, we recommend the use of nitrates to rapidly lower an elevated pulmonary capillary wedge pressure in acute pulmonary edema.[19,20] Nitrates produce a pharmacologic phlebotomy by their peripheral venodilator effects, shifting blood volume away from the intrathoracic to the extrathoracic compartment and thus rapidly lowering pulmonary venous and capillary pressure. A direct vasodilator effect of nitrates on pulmonary vasculature may contribute in some patients to unloading of the right ventricle, resulting in improved left ventricular compliance. Improvement in left ventricular function resulting from reduction in afterload and improved function of ischemic segments and a decrease or elimination of mitral regurgitation consequent to reduction of afterload may be additional important acute effects of nitrates. The effects of nitrates may be supplemented by administration of small intravenous doses of morphine sulfate, which often calms the agitated patient and has modest venodilator and arteriolar dilator actions. Although diuretics, especially intravenous furosemide, are frequently used as the primary treatment, their effect is slower and their use should be considered secondary to nitrates. In severely hypertensive patients or in those with significant mitral regurgitation, sodium nitroprusside may be extremely useful. Acute digitalization, intermittent positive-pressure ventilation, and routine use of aminophylline are generally not beneficial. In some patients use of rotating tourniquets or phlebotomy is recommended, but in our experience this is rarely necessary. Role of inotropic-vasopressor therapy and intra-aortic balloon pumping in acute pulmonary edema in selected patients is discussed later in this chapter. After successful emergency therapy of acute pulmonary edema, patients should be assessed for the presence of intermittent or persistent severe mitral regurgitation, ventricular septal rupture, and intermittent ischemia. Recognition of these complications is important since surgical intervention may be highly desirable for such patients.[21]

LOW-OUTPUT, HYPOTENSIVE SYNDROME OR SHOCK (TABLE 70.7)

Shock can be defined as a syndrome characterized by evidence of acute, severe, and prolonged tissue hypoperfusion, usually associated with a low arterial blood pressure (≤ 90 mm Hg systolic) and a markedly reduced cardiac output. In addition to hypotension and tachycardia, other clinical manifestations may include a variable blend of findings of cool clammy skin, diaphoresis, mental obtundation, and oliguria. Depending on the dominant pathophysiologic event precipitating shock, additional clinical findings may also be present. Hemodynamic findings in shock depend on the pathophysiologic state resulting in the shock syndrome. Shock syndrome can best be considered under two main categories: (1) shock with pulmonary congestion or edema and (2) shock without pulmonary congestion and edema.

SHOCK WITH EVIDENCE OF PULMONARY CONGESTION OR EDEMA

This particular type of shock syndrome may result from extensive left ventricular dysfunction (ventriculopenic state) and/or mechanical complications (*i.e.*, acute mitral regurgitation and ventricular septal rupture).

VENTRICULOPENIC SHOCK. This type of shock syndrome occurs in 10% to 15% of patients with acute myocardial infarction and results from severe left ventricular contractile dysfunction due to extensive acute myocardial infarction, acute myocardial infarction of less severe nature in patients with prior loss of myocardial function from old infarction, and, less commonly, large areas of ischemic nonfunctioning but viable myocardium along with only modest areas of myocardial infarction. Several pathologic studies have indicated that patients succumbing to this type of shock invariably demonstrate a cumulative involvement of at least 35% to 40% of total left ventricular mass.[22,23] In addition, patients frequently demonstrate marginal extension of recent areas of necrosis and focal necrotic areas remote from the major location of recent infarction.[24] Profound impairment of ventricular function results in perpetuation of ischemia and the process of necrosis because of systemic hypotension and coronary artery underperfusion. This vicious cycle is responsible for the progressive nature of myocardial damage found in this syndrome as reflected by stuttering and progressive elevation of plasma levels of myocardial specific enzymes.[24] Nearly 70% of patients succumbing to this type of shock demonstrate extensive and severe multivessel coronary obstructive disease with a high prevalence of left anterior descending coronary artery involvement.[25] It is tempting to suggest that early thinning, lengthening, and stretching of transmurally necrotic myocardium (infarct expansion) may contribute to acute ventricular dilatation and precipitation of pump failure in some patients.[26,27]

Severe hypoperfusion of various body organs owing to low cardiac and hypotension causes impairment of their function (*i.e.*, renal failure, hepatic dysfunction, pancreatic and gastrointestinal ischemia, enhanced anaerobic metabolism, and lactic acidosis). In addition pulmonary congestion and edema frequently result in varying degrees of hypoxemia and atelectasis and eventually may culminate into a syndrome indistinguishable from that of acute respiratory distress syndrome. Cardiac arrhythmias, both supraventricular as well as ventricular, are frequent accompaniments, whereas secondary complications such as systemic or pulmonary sepsis, renal failure, and gastrointestinal hemorrhage further contribute to the poor overall outlook of the patient. This type of shock is most likely to occur in older patients, in those with diabetes, in patients with prior infarction, and in those with anterior myocardial infarction. It is not yet completely clear whether the specific location of infarction is an independent contributor to development of shock beyond the extent of necrosis and the propensity for involvement of the conduction system and the valvular apparatus.

The clinical features of ventriculopenic shock include cool and clammy skin, peripheral cyanosis, oliguria with a urine output of less than 20 ml to 30 ml/hr, impaired mentation associated with a systolic blood pressure less than 90 mm Hg or 60 mm Hg below the previous basal level, and a thready rapid pulse with a narrow pulse pressure. In severe cases lactic acidosis is present as well. Arterial blood pressure should preferably be determined directly from an intra-arterial line since indirect cuff pressures may be 10 mm Hg to 20 mm Hg lower in the presence of intense peripheral vasoconstriction. Some patients may have recurrent episodes of ischemic cardiac pain, while others remain moribund. Depending on the severity of pulmonary congestion, patients may demonstrate varying degrees of respiratory distress, hypoxemia, and carbon dioxide retention. Cerebral underperfusion and use of narcotic analgesics, particularly in elderly patients, may result in Cheyne-Stokes respirations. Cardiac arrhythmias of various types occur frequently. As described previously, other clinical features of organ dysfunction may also become evident. Cardiac examination may demonstrate diminished intensity of sounds, atrial and/or ventricular gallops, pericardial friction rub, and dyskinetic apical impulse, whereas pulmonary examination reveals rales of varying distribution. Some patients may demonstrate frank hypothermia.[28]

Hemodynamic findings demonstrate a low arterial pressure, severely depressed cardiac and stroke work indices, elevated pulmonary

TABLE 70.7 LOW-OUTPUT STATE AND SHOCK FOLLOWING ACUTE MYOCARDIAL INFARCTION

Underlying Abnormality	Recognition — *Clinical*	Recognition — *Hemodynamic*	Others	Guides to Management	Prognosis
Ventriculopenic shock	Shock syndrome Rales, S_3 Abnormal chest film	Elevated PCW Depressed CI High SVR Low BP	Markedly depressed LVEF (i.e., $\sim \leq 0.30$)	Inotropes-pressors to maintain systemic BP ~ 90 mm Hg and cardiac index of >2 liters/m^2 Vasodilators added to keep PCW 12 to 15 mm Hg. IABP if no response to above General supportive care	Poor; mortality >80% Outlook better if CABG can salvage major areas of ischemic myocardium. Early nonsurgical reperfusion may salvage myocardium and improve outlook.
Acute severe mitral regurgitation	Shock syndrome Rales, S_3, abnormal chest film Holosystolic murmur; occasionally murmur not heard or soft and brief	Elevated PCW with tall v waves Depressed CI High SVR Low BP	LVEF may be normal, elevated, or variably depressed depending on extent of necrosis of LV Echo shows flail leaflet Doppler shows regurgitation	Vasodilators plus inotropes to maintain systolic BP ~ 90 and PCW 12 to 15 mm Hg and CI >2 liters/m^2 IABP followed by early catheterization and surgery General supportive care	Medically treated: poor (mortality $\sim 80\%$) Surgically treated: better (mortality 30–40%)
Acute VSD	Shock syndrome Rales, S_3 Holosystolic murmur with precordial thrill in 50%	O_2 step up from RA to RV or PA Thermodilution curve shows evidence of L > R shunt	First-pass radionuclide study shows L > R shunt LV and RVEF are variable as in mitral regurgitation and depend on extent of necrosis. 2D echocardiogram visualizes defect Shunt seen on Doppler	Same as above General supportive care	Same as above Outlook better for anterior defects and in those with normal RV function
Hypovolemia	Shock syndrome Lungs and chest film do not show signs of LV failure (but in some patients may show persistent signs of LV failure if hypovolemia is superimposed on a patient with prior LV failure, generally from over diuresis) Orthostatic ↑ in HR and/or ↓ in BP	PCW generally <12 to 15 mm Hg CI depressed SVR may be high. BP may be low. Some patients with this profile have RV infarction.		If patient has clinical evidence for hypoperfusion then rapid but careful volume expansion until PCW is ~ 15 mm Hg but no higher than 18 mm Hg	Good especially if response to volume infusion is good
Predominant acute right ventricular infarction	Shock syndrome in a patient with inferior infarction JVD or HJR in 70% cases Lungs and chest film generally clear with minimal or no signs of LV failure Occasionally pulsus paradoxus and Kussmaul sign Rarely severe hypoxia from R > L shunt across a PFO	RA pressure $\geq$ PCW Reduced PA and RV pulse pressure Depressed CI 30% may have normal-RA pressure (Volume challenge may bring out occult findings)	Dilated RV with ↓RVEF (<0.39) LVEF generally >0.45% Some patients have severely depressed LV and such patients should be categorized differently. Steep RA y' descent CG signs of RV infarction	Volume if PCW <15 mm Hg till PCW is ~ 15 mm Hg. If no improvement add inotropic agent and/or vasodilator depending on BP. (Most patients do not respond to volume alone.) Maintain atrial kick	Generally good barring intercurrent complications (i.e., concomitant severe LV dysfunction, mitral regurgitation or septal rupture)

(PCW, pulmonary capillary wedge pressure; CI, cardiac index; SVR, systemic vascular resistance; BP, blood pressure; LVEF, left ventricular ejection fraction; IABP, intra-aortic balloon pumping; CABG, coronary artery bypass graft; LV, left ventricle; VSD, ventricular septal defect; RA, right atrium; RV, right ventricle; PA, pulmonary artery; RVEF, right ventricular ejection fraction; HR, heart rate; JVD, jugular venous distension; HJR, hepatojugular reflex; PFO, patent foramen ovale)

arterial and capillary wedge pressures, elevated systemic vascular resistance, and a widened arteriovenous oxygen difference. The cardiac index is below 2.2 liters/min/m^2 and generally averages 1.6 liters/min/m^2, whereas the pulmonary capillary wedge pressure exceeds 18 mm Hg and generally averages 25 mm Hg. Some patients may actually have a relatively lower systemic vascular resistance, although in the majority it exceeds 2000 dyne·sec·cm^{-5}. The left ventricle is often dilated with severe and extensive regional contractile dysfunction and a global ejection fraction generally less than 0.30. A resting thallium-201 myocardial scan often demonstrates left ventricular dilatation, extensive nonreversible decrease in thallium-201 uptake, and increased lung uptake. An occasional patient demonstrates large areas of reversible thallium-201 defects, in addition to the irreversible defects in uptake, due to nonfunctioning but ischemic and viable myocardial segments. If perfusion is restored to such segments, their function could recover and contribute to survival of the patient.

The prognosis of this type of "cardiogenic shock" is extremely poor, with 80% to 100% in-hospital mortality. The small number of hospital survivors often live with continued heart failure and dysrhythmias and are faced with a low-probability of long-term survival. Prognosis appears to be more favorable in young patients, in those with single-vessel coronary disease, and in that subgroup of patients in which subsequent coronary artery revascularization salvages substantial amounts of jeopardized nonfunctioning but viable myocardium.

The chief objectives of management of ventriculopenic cardiogenic shock are to improve ventricular performance and cardiac output and maintain adequate systemic arterial pressure in order to sustain perfusion to vital organs and reduce pulmonary congestion; to preserve the viability and function of ischemic and jeopardized myocardium; and to limit the ultimate infarct size.

Appropriate management of the seriously ill patient with shock requires skilled physicians and nurses working in a well-equipped coronary care unit. General supportive measures are essential and include relief of pain and discomfort with judicious use of small doses of analgesics such as morphine, maintenance of adequate oxygenation and ventilation, which may require endotracheal intubation in some patients, prompt correction of electrolyte and acid–base abnormalities, control of fever, treatment of nausea and vomiting, control of cardiac dysrhythmias, and maintenance of an adequate heart rate with atrioventricular synchrony. It should be recognized that a severely damaged and ischemic ventricle is more susceptible to myocardial depressant effects of drugs, particularly the antiarrhythmic agents that are frequently used in such patients. The need for administration of drugs and their dosage must be carefully reviewed and monitored in order to avoid adverse effects.

Specific therapy of "cardiogenic shock" (Tables 70.7 and 70.8) requires not only careful clinical assessment but, in addition, virtually mandates the use of bedside hemodynamic monitoring using a Swan-Ganz thermodilution catheter as well as an indwelling intra-arterial cannula. Such invasive monitoring is useful not only to exclude the presence of other types of pump failure or shock (*i.e.*, mitral regurgitation, septal or free-wall rupture, hypovolemia, right ventricular infarction) but is also extremely useful in guiding the selection of specific drugs and other therapeutic interventions (see Table 70.6). Recent refinements in noninvasive techniques such as two-dimensional echocardiography, Doppler flow techniques, and radionuclide scintigraphy have made it possible to expand and refine the information obtained by clinical and invasive hemodynamic monitoring, in particular with reference to mechanical complications, right ventricular infarction, and extensive reversible ischemia. In most modern cardiac intensive care units, bedside assessment of critically ill patients is made with a combination of clinical and laboratory techniques, which considerably

TABLE 70.8 BENEFICIAL AND ADVERSE EFFECTS OF THERAPEUTIC INTERVENTIONS FOR POSTINFARCTION PUMP DYSFUNCTION

	Potential Effects	
Intervention	*Beneficial*	*Adverse*
↑Heart rate	May ↑ depressed CO and BP if HR is slow	↑MVO$_2$ and possible increase in ischemia; loss of atrial contribution if ventricular pacing is performed
Diuretics	Decrease PCW; improve pulmonary congestion	Hypovolemia; low CO and BP; azotemia; hypokalemia
Volume loading	May ↑ depressed CO and BP in presence of hypovolemia or rare cases of RV infarction	↑MVO$_2$ by increasing preload and possible ↑ in ischemia; pulmonary edema if PCW is not carefully monitored

Inotropic agents
  Digitalis
  Dopamine
  Norepinephrine
  Dobutamine
	May ↑ depressed CO and BP in presence of LV failure	May ↑ MVO$_2$ by ↑ HR (dopamine, dobutamine, norepinephrine); ↑ contractility (all agents); ↑ SVR (norepinephrine, digitalis, dopamine); may worsen LV failure and produce tissue hypoperfusion if SVR increased markedly or tachyarrhythmias occur

Vasodilators
  Nitroprusside
  Nitroglycerin
	May decrease elevated PCW and SVR; reduce MR; reduce L > R shunt; and elevate depressed cardiac output	May ↑ BP and compromise myocardial and other organ perfusion; may produce hypoxia, may produce toxic effects

IABP	Similar as above with maintenance and/or augmentation of diastolic coronary perfusion pressure	Complications related to IABP insertion and stay in the vascular compartment (*i.e.*, vascular insufficiency, infection)
Early reperfusion (thrombolysis, anticoagulants, PTCA)	May stop ischemia, limit infarction, improve LV function, restore inotropic responsiveness, prevent ischemia-related arrhythmias, reverse conduction abnormalities, prevent mural thrombus formation	Bleeding complications, hypotension, allergy (with thrombolytic-anticoagulant drugs)

(CO, cardiac output; BP, blood pressure; HR, heart rate; LV, left ventricular; PCW, pulmonary capillary wedge pressure; SVR, systemic vascular resistance; MR, mitral regurgitation; L > R, left to right; MVO$_2$, myocardial O$_2$ demand; HR, heart rate; IABP, intra-aortic balloon pumping; PTCA, percutaneous transluminal angioplasty) facilitate the correct and comprehensive diagnosis and therapy (Tables 70.3 and 70.6).

Specific therapeutic interventions include pharmacologic agents (inotropic and vasopressor drugs, vasodilators, diuretics), mechanical circulatory assist devices (intra-aortic balloon pumping, left heart assist device), reperfusion (thrombolysis, percutaneous transluminal angioplasty, coronary artery bypass graft surgery), and surgery for correction of mechanical complications. The true value of any of these therapeutic modalities has never been conclusively proven or disproven with proper controlled trials; therefore the discussion to follow must be considered in the light of personal experiences and individual patient "successes."

One of the objectives of management is to maintain peripheral tissue perfusion by improving cardiac output and maintaining an adequate systemic blood pressure (usually in the range of at least 90 mm Hg to 100 mm Hg systolic). These objectives may be accomplished by using inotropic and/or vasopressor agents in some patients.

DIGITALIS. Digitalis glycosides have been used in the management of both acute and chronic left ventricular failure. Acute digitalization is relatively ineffective or only marginally effective in severe pump failure following acute myocardial infarction. Ischemic myocardium appears to be more susceptible to arrhythmogenic effects of digitalis, and the coronary as well as peripheral vasoconstrictor effects of rapid intravenous administration of digitalis have produced deleterious consequences.[29] Therefore, the use of digitalis in cardiogenic shock is quite limited. However, digitalis is useful in the management of atrial arrhythmias (e.g., fibrillation, flutter) complicating myocardial infarction, which should be its chief indication in this setting.

CATECHOLAMINES (TABLE 70.9). Catecholamines are the most often used agents in cardiogenic shock for their inotropic and vasoactive effects. Dopamine and dobutamine are the most frequently used agents, whereas norepinephrine is used in fewer patients.

DOPAMINE. Intravenous dopamine exerts its cardiovascular effects by direct stimulation of α, β, and dopaminergic specific receptors as well as by release of endogenous norepinephrine from sympathetic nerve endings.[30,31] At relatively low doses of 2 μg to 5 μg/kg/min, a majority of patients demonstrate a significant increase in stroke volume and cardiac output mediated by β_1-adrenergic stimulant effects on myocardial contractility as well as an increase in renal blood flow with redistribution toward the inner third of renal cortex, an effect mediated by interaction with dopaminergic-specific receptors. Importantly, at this dosage chronotropic and peripheral vasoconstrictor effects are relatively minimal and deleterious effects on myocardial ischemia are not generally observed. With increasing doses, there are dose-dependent increases in chronotropic, arrhythmogenic, and α-adrenergically mediated vasoconstrictor and vasopressor effects that may result in a decrease in tissue perfusion and an increase in pulmonary arterial and left ventricular filling pressures secondary to elevated afterload. At large doses (>15 μg to 20 μg/kg/min) myocardial ischemia may be provoked due to inotropic, chronotropic, and vasopressor effects.

The use of an intravenous dopamine infusion in "cardiogenic shock" requires careful individual titration beginning with a low dose (2 μg to 5 μg/kg/min), to improve cardiac output, and renal and other organ perfusion and to maintain a systolic blood pressure of 90 mm Hg to 100 mm Hg without permitting excessive increases in heart rate (>110 to 115/min), emergence of supraventricular or ventricular arrhythmias, or excessive peripheral vasoconstriction. Because of marked individual variations in dose response, it is crucial to use the lowest dose that produces optimal hemodynamic and clinical improvement with the least adverse effects. Adverse effects include sinus tachycardia, atrial and ventricular arrhythmias, excessive peripheral vasoconstriction and compromise of tissue blood flow, precipitation or worsening of myocardial ischemia, gangrene at the infusion site especially when extravascular extravasation occurs, nausea and vomiting, and increased heart rate in the presence of supraventricular arrhythmias resulting from facilitation of atrioventricular conduction.

DOBUTAMINE. Dobutamine is a synthetic catecholamine that differs from dopamine in several respects. Dobutamine has predominantly β-adrenergic agonist actions accounting for its positive inotropic and chronotropic effects with only minimal α-adrenergic agonist effects accounting for its lack of appreciable vasoconstrictor effects even at large doses.[32] Furthermore, dobutamine does not release endogenous norepinephrine and has no direct renal vasodilator effects.[32] Dose-related increases in stroke volume, cardiac output, and reduction in left ventricular filling pressures are notable effects of intravenous dobutamine infusion in acute as well as chronic heart failure with inappropriate increases in heart rate being uncommonly observed at infusion rates under 15 μg to 20 μg/kg/min.[33]

Dobutamine is generally preferred over dopamine because it tends to produce equivalent increases in cardiac inotropy but with lesser

TABLE 70.9 CATECHOLAMINE RECEPTORS

Receptor	$\alpha 1$	$\alpha 2$	$\beta 1$	$\beta 2$	DA_1	DA_2
Epinephrine	+++	+++	+++	0	0	0
Norepinephrine	+++	+++	+++	0	0	0
Isoproterenol	0	0	+++	+++	0	0
Dopamine	++	++	+++	+	+++	0
Dobutamine	+	0	+++	+	0	0

Receptor Types

- α_1—Postsynaptic: Peripheral vasoconstriction
- α_2—Mostly presynaptic: Inhibition of norepinephrine release from sympathetic nerves
- β_1—Mostly cardiac: ↑ Contractility, ↑ rhythmicity, and ↑ conduction velocity
- β_2—Mostly smooth muscle: Peripheral vasodilation
  Bronchodilatation
- DA_1—Postsynaptic: Vasodilation in renal, splanchnic, cerebral, and coronary vasculature
- DA_2—Presynaptic: Inhibition of norepinephrine release from sympathetic nerves, induction of emesis, and inhibition of prolactin release

(DA, dopaminergic receptors; +, stimulation; 0, no effect)

increments in heart rate, a lower risk of arrhythmias, no vasoconstrictor effects, and more consistent reduction in left ventricular filling pressures. However, lack of direct renal vasodilator effects and relatively modest pressor effect, compared with the effects of dopamine, make dobutamine, as the sole agent, inappropriate when systemic blood pressure is very low (e.g., <70 mm Hg). The optimal use of dobutamine in cardiogenic shock should follow guidelines similar to those of dopamine (i.e., begin with a low dose (2 μg to 5 μg/kg/min) and increase the dose rapidly (every 5 to 10 minutes) under careful clinical, electrocardiographic, and hemodynamic monitoring until there is an improvement in cardiac output and the clinical status of the patient without adverse effects. Adverse effects include an excessive increase in heart rate, emergence of serious or frequent arrhythmias, provocation of myocardial ischemia, nausea, headache, and acceleration of atrioventricular conduction in the presence of supraventricular arrhythmias.

NOREPINEPHRINE. Norepinephrine is a naturally occurring catecholamine with potent arteriolar and venous constrictor effects mediated through α-adrenergic receptor stimulation with relatively modest β_1-adrenergically mediated myocardial inotropic and chronotropic effects. The peripheral vasoconstrictor effects of norepinephrine make it a very potent pressor agent with much less overall positive chronotropic effects compared with dopamine or dobutamine. Although such effects may temporarily maintain adequate arterial pressure in severely hypotensive patients, little increase or an actual decrease in cardiac output and compromise of peripheral organ blood flow results in later deterioration.[34] However, in patients with cardiogenic shock with a low systemic arterial pressure (≤70 mm Hg) and a normal or reduced systemic vascular resistance in whom pressor doses of dopamine produce serious adverse effects (tachyarrhythmias), small doses of norepinephrine may be used to maintain systemic arterial pressure around 90 mm Hg systolic with improvement in cardiac output in some patients.[35] Combined use of norepinephrine with an α-adrenergic blocking drug such as phentolamine, or direct vasodilators, such as nitroglycerin or sodium nitroprusside, is preferred since such combined therapy minimizes peripheral vasoconstrictor effects and helps unmask positive inotropic effects.[36] As with dopamine and dobutamine, norepinephrine is started at a low dose (1 μg to 4 μg/min) and increased to an optimal clinical and hemodynamic effect before excessive peripheral vasoconstriction or arrhythmias occur. Adverse effects are mostly related to excessive vasoconstriction and compromise of organ blood flow, worsening of ventricular function due to increased afterload, tissue necrosis and sloughing if extravascular extravasation occurs, increases in heart rate, and emergence of cardiac arrhythmias. In some patients, excessive increase in blood pressure may produce a slowing of heart rate through baroreceptor-mediated reflex increase in vagal tone.

VASODILATORS. The use of vasodilators in cardiogenic shock and heart failure is predicated on their ability to reduce ventricular afterload by dilating the systemic arteriolar bed and to reduce ventricular preload by dilating the peripheral venous or capacitance bed. Reduction in ventricular afterload results in a decreased outflow impedance to left ventricular ejection, thereby increasing forward stroke volume and cardiac output. In the presence of mitral regurgitation and ventricular septal rupture, decreased impedance to ejection into the aorta reduces the degree of regurgitation and left-to-right shunt while increasing forward output into the aorta. Preload reduction contributes to the reduction of ventricular filling pressures, thereby reducing pulmonary capillary wedge pressure, pulmonary arterial pressure, and right atrial pressure. While favorably influencing ventricular function, these afterload and preload reducing effects also tend to decrease myocardial oxygen demand and may favor subendocardial perfusion in diastole. Vasodilators may also influence the left ventricular diastolic pressure–volume relationship, shifting this relationship down and to the right owing to right ventricular unloading and reduction in the degree of pericardial restraint.

The major drawback of short-term vasodilator therapy in this clinical setting relates to excessive hypotension. Blood flow through coronary arteries with severe flow-limiting stenosis and impairment of autoregulatory reserve is highly dependent on arterial pressure. Thus vasodilator-induced hypotension may decrease coronary blood flow and increase oxygen demand when hypotension provokes reflex tachycardia. Hypotension may also compromise perfusion to other organs (i.e., brain, kidney, splanchnic bed). Excessive reduction of left ventricular filling pressures or use of vasodilators in patients with low or normal filling pressures predisposes to hypotension and tachycardia. These considerations demand caution and care in the use of vasodilators in critically ill patients and make frequent clinical and hemodynamic evaluation essential.

The effects of vasodilator therapy on the outcome of patients with cardiogenic shock have never been examined in properly controlled studies. Chatterjee and colleagues reported an apparent improvement in short-term survival of close to 50% in a small group of patients with severe pump failure complicating acute myocardial infarction treated with vasodilators; however, the 1-year survival was 20% and most survivors continued to have severe heart failure.[37]

Currently, the most commonly used vasodilators in patients with severe heart failure and shock are intravenous sodium nitroprusside and intravenous nitroglycerin. Intravenous agents such as these are preferred since they have a rapid onset of action (1 to 2 minutes) and a short half-life (2 to 4 minutes) and their effects rapidly dissipate within 10 to 15 minutes of cessation of infusion.

SODIUM NITROPRUSSIDE (TABLE 70.10). Sodium nitroprusside infusion produces prompt peripheral vasodilator effects on both arterial as well as venous circulation and produces hemodynamic and short-term clinical improvement in severe heart failure with or without shock accompanying acute myocardial infarction.[37,38] The beneficial effects are more pronounced in patients with markedly elevated left ventricular filling pressures and those with mitral regurgitation or septal rupture. Therapy should begin with a low dose (10 μg to 20 μg/min) with rapid increases, every 10 to 15 minutes until left ventricular filling pressure is lowered to the 15 mm Hg to 20 mm Hg range without permitting systolic arterial pressure to drop below 90 mm Hg. In patients with cardiogenic shock, vasodilator therapy alone may produce unacceptable degrees of arterial hypotension unless combined with an inotropic drug (dopamine or dobutamine) or mechanical circulatory assist with intra-aortic balloon counterpulsation.

Adverse effects of nitroprusside therapy include excessive hypotension, reflex tachycardia, potential for worsening of myocardial ischemia, accumulation of thiocyanate (particularly in presence of renal insufficiency and prolonged infusions) with thiocyanate toxicity, accumulation of cyanide with cyanide toxicity, worsening of arterial hypoxemia due to increasing intrapulmonary ventilation–perfusion mismatch, and, rarely, methemoglobinemia and vitamin B_{12} deficiency.[39,40] Limiting the dose and duration of therapy, frequent monitoring of serum thiocyanate levels to avoid exceeding levels of 6 mg/dl, and the prophylactic use of a cyanide chelating agent (i.e., hydroxycobalamin), have been recommended to avoid cyanide intoxication.[41]

INTRAVENOUS NITROGLYCERIN (TABLE 70.10). Intravenous nitroglycerin is also a rapid-acting vasodilator that tends to produce a greater reduction in ventricular filling pressures with variable degrees of increases in stroke volume and cardiac output in patients with severe left ventricular failure.[42] These differential effects have been attributed to preferential venodilation particularly at lower doses, but significant arteriolar dilation is also observed with increasing doses. Some studies have suggested that nitroglycerin may have a more favorable effect on the distribution of coronary blood flow to ischemic myocardium than nitroprusside, but careful comparative studies in cardiogenic shock have not been performed to confirm or refute the superiority of one over the other.

The adverse effects of nitroglycerin, like those of nitroprusside, include hypotension with reflex tachycardia, headaches from cerebral vasodilation and possibly increased intracranial tension, increasing intraocular pressure in patients with glaucoma, methemoglobinemia, Wernicke's encephalopathy, and ethanol intoxication (ethanol is the vehicle for many intravenous nitroglycerin preparations).[42,43] Hypotension and paradoxic profound bradycardia are rare but generally respond to administration of atropine and cessation of nitroglycerin therapy.[44] As in nitroprusside therapy, the intravenous use of nitroglycerin in cardiogenic shock frequently requires concomitant use of an inotropic drug (dopamine or dobutamine) or intra-aortic balloon counterpulsation in order to maintain or elevate a low systemic arterial pressure.

PHENTOLAMINE. Phentolamine is one of the earliest agents to have been used as a vasodilator. It is a nonselective α-adrenergic blocking agent and has direct smooth muscle relaxant and mild direct inotropic and chronotropic properties.[45] In comparison to nitroprusside and nitroglycerin, phentolamine produces a relatively greater increase in heart rate (and cardiac output) and a lesser decrease in filling pressures and is considerably more expensive. It is mainly used to minimize

TABLE 70.10 GUIDELINES FOR USE OF INTRAVENOUS CATECHOLAMINES AND VASODILATORS IN PUMP FAILURE FOLLOWING MYOCARDIAL INFARCTION

I. Catecholamines
  A. Begin with a low dose and titrate every 10 to 15 minutes to a therapeutic endpoint without provoking unacceptable adverse effects.
    1. Dopamine: Begin with 1 μg to 3 μg/kg/min and increase by 50-μg to 75-μg increments.
    2. Dobutamine: Begin with 2 μg to 5 μg/kg/min and increase by 50-μg to 75-μg increments.
    3. Norepinephrine: Begin with 1 μg to 3 μg/min and increase by 0.5-μg to 2-μg increments. Preferably use in combination with α-blocker (e.g., phentolamine).
  B. Use acidic solutions as diluents.
  C. Observe for adverse effects.
    1. Sinus tachycardia (rarely bradycardia may occur with norepinephrine-induced hypertension)
    2. Accelerated atrioventricular conduction and increased ventricular response in supraventricular arrhythmias
    3. Atrial and ventricular premature beats and tachyarrhythmias
    4. Worsening or provocation of ischemia or ventricular dysfunction
    5. Tissue hypoperfusion from excessive vasoconstriction and necrosis (from extravascular extravasation) may result from use of dopamine or norepinephrine
    6. Nausea and vomiting
II. Vasodilators
  A. Begin with low doses and titrate every 10 to 15 minutes to a therapeutic endpoint without provoking adverse effects.
    1. Sodium nitroprusside: Begin with 10 μg to 20 μg/min and increase by 10-μg to 20-μg/min increments.
    2. Intravenous nitroglycerin: Begin with 10 μg to 20 μg/min and increase by 10-μg to 20-μg/min increments.
    3. Intravenous phenotolamine: Begin with 0.5 mg/min and increase by 0.25-mg/min increments.
    4. Use freshly prepared solutions of nitroprusside (<6 to 8 hours old), and shield the reservoir from light.
  B. Preferably use nonabsorbent plastic tubings while using intravenous nitroglycerin to avoid adherence of nitroglycerin to plastic tubing.
  C. Observe for adverse effects.
    1. Flushing, headaches, hypotension
    2. Reflex tachycardia; rarely reflex bradycardia occurs from nitroglycerin.
    3. Worsening or precipitation of ischemia due to excessive hypotension and tachycardia and, possibly, maldistribution of coronary nutrient flow
    4. Arterial desaturation from intrapulmonary shunting
    5. Methemoglobinemia (nitroglycerin and nitroprusside)
    6. Thiocyanate and cyanide intoxication (nitroprusside)
    7. Precipitation of increased intracranial and intraocular pressure (nitrates)
    8. Ethanol intoxication during prolonged high dose infusions of intravenous nitroglycerin containing ethanol as a vehicle
III. Miscellaneous
  A. Infuse these potent drugs through free-flowing non-posture-dependent, large-bore, intravenous, preferably central, lines using well-calibrated constant-infusion pumps.
  B. Avoid abrupt cessation of infusion (unless serious adverse effects occur) and preferably wean off gradually.
  C. Avoid flushing infusion lines through which catecholamines or vasodilators are infusing, without first clearing the infusion line by withdrawing blood through it.
  D. If cardiac outputs are being performed using a Swan-Ganz catheter then avoid infusing drugs through right atrial port of Swan-Ganz catheters.

vasoconstrictor effects of norepinephrine infusion and the deleterious effects of extravascular extravasation of norepinephrine or dopamine.

COMBINED VASODILATOR AND CATECHOLAMINE THERAPY. Several studies have demonstrated the superior hemodynamic effects of combined vasodilator and inotropic drug therapy in chronic or acute low-output state and congestive heart failure.[46,47]

Afterload and preload reducing effects of vasodilators improve cardiac output and lower ventricular filling pressures, but systemic arterial hypotension remains a potential drawback. Inotropic drugs may improve ventricular function and cardiac output but may have inconsistent effects on ventricular filling pressures and potentially deleterious, excessive peripheral vasoconstrictor effects. Thus by using lower doses of more than one agent, combined therapy may offset each drug's adverse effects while augmenting overall ventricular function. Vasodilators frequently used for this purpose include α-adrenergic blockers such as phentolamine and direct vasodilators such as nitroglycerin and sodium nitroprusside. The principal advantage of adding a vasodilator to dopamine or dobutamine is that increments in cardiac output are achieved at much lower left ventricular filling pressures and systemic vascular resistance. Combined use of dopamine and dobutamine has also been suggested in the treatment of cardiogenic shock as a means of achieving better acute hemodynamic response at lower doses.[48]

Guidelines for use and adverse effects of cathecholamines and vasodilators are described in Table 70.10.

In addition to pharmacologic agents, mechanical circulatory assist devices, of which intra-aortic balloon pumping (Table 70.11, Fig. 70.6) is the most common, are used in the management of cardiogenic shock. The recent development of a percutaneous insertion technique has made it easier to accomplish balloon counterpulsation; however, a small number of patients require insertion of the device through a surgical femoral arteriotomy.[49] Intra-aortic balloon counterpulsation decreases left ventricular work and oxygen demand because of its afterload reducing effect while at the same time increased diastolic aortic pressure helps to maintain or improve coronary perfusion pressure and subendocardial blood flow.[50] The combined systolic unloading and diastolic augmentation tend to reduce myocardial ischemia, left ventricular filling pressures, mitral regurgitation, and left-to-right shunt across a ventricular septal rupture while the forward stroke volume and cardiac output shows a modest improvement. Phased pulsation synchronized with the electrocardiogram is used to begin balloon inflation at the time of aortic valve closure to produce diastolic pressure augmentation and to initiate deflation just prior to the onset of systole to produce systolic unloading. The beneficial hemodynamic effects of balloon counterpulsation may be further augmented by concomitant use of vasodilator and/or inotropic drugs.

Although patients with cardiogenic shock frequently demonstrate temporary clinical and hemodynamic improvement during intra-aortic balloon counterpulsation, short- and long-term mortality remain high unless intra-aortic balloon pumping is used for short-term stabilization of the patient in preparation for salvage of jeopardized nonfunctioning but still viable ischemic myocardium with coronary revascularization or correction of severe mechanical complications (e.g., mitral regurgitation and ventricular septal rupture).[50,51] The patients least likely to benefit from intra-aortic balloon pumping are those with multiple previous infarctions, those with large areas of myocardial scarring with massive irreversible necrosis, those with late and advanced stages of cardiogenic shock, and elderly patients with peripheral vascular disease who are most likely to experience morbidity from insertion of the device.[50,51] Initiation of balloon counterpulsation within a few hours after development of shock, evidence of large areas of ischemic but viable myocardium, and presence of mechanical complications (both amenable to definitive surgical therapy) offer the best prospects of benefits from intra-aortic balloon counterpulsation when subsequent surgical intervention is combined.[50,52]

From a practical vantage point, balloon counterpulsation should be considered for relatively young patients, free of severe aortoiliac disease or aortic regurgitation, who develop cardiogenic shock after their first infarction and have failed to improve with a trial of pharmacologic therapy given for 30 to 60 minutes. Every attempt should be made to determine the presence of surgically remediable lesions as described earlier, using noninvasive and invasive techniques. We recommend early cardiac catheterization, usually within 48 to 96 hours of onset of balloon counterpulsation, and surgical intervention for suitable patients. Those patients who are unsuitable for surgery or those in whom surgery must be delayed because of intercurrent complications should undergo weaning from balloon counterpulsation after a period of stabilization of 2 to 4 days.

Complications may occur in up to 30% of patients subjected to intra-aortic balloon counterpulsation regardless of whether the percu-

TABLE 70.11 INDICATIONS FOR INTRA-AORTIC BALLOON COUNTERPULSATION IN ACUTE MYOCARDIAL INFARCTION

Recurrent or persistent myocardial ischemia
Severe left or biventricular failure with or without shock
Intermittent or persistent severe mitral regurgitation
Ventricular septal rupture
Refractory recurrent and life-threatening ventricular dysrhythmias

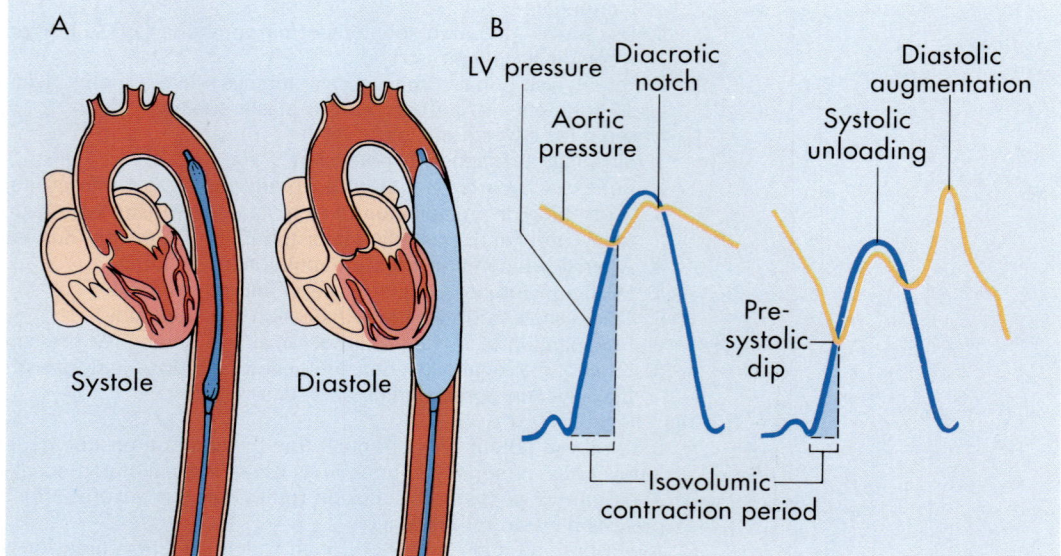

FIGURE 70.6 A. Schematic illustration of intra-aortic balloon pump. B. Principle of intra-aortic balloon counterpulsation. Initiation of balloon inflation is timed to the arterial dicrotic notch producing diastolic augmentation in arterial pressure whereas deflation of balloon prior to next ventricular systole contributes to systolic unloading.

taneous or surgical methods of insertion are employed.[50,51,53] The complications are mostly vascular (*e.g.*, vascular compromise of extremities and abdominal viscera, damage to femoral artery, and aortic dissection) but also include infection, hemolysis, thrombocytopenia, gas leak, and embolism. In our experience, complications are particularly likely with percutaneous insertion in older individuals (>70 years), especially older females, and in those with aortoiliac vascular disease.[51]

Since ventriculopenic shock results from large areas of nonfunctioning left ventricular myocardium, early restoration of myocardial blood flow during the evolutionary phase of myocardial infarction (phases of ischemia and mixed pathology), when substantial amounts of nonfunctioning myocardium are still viable, may be the most rational and effective therapy in preventing severe disability or death. Early reperfusion can relieve ischemia of jeopardized myocardium, restore its contractile function immediately or over time, render reperfused, salvaged, but nonfunctioning myocardium more responsive to inotropic agents, limit the eventual degree of necrosis, preserve ventricular function, and dramatically improve the outlook of these patients. Preliminary and mostly anecdotal reports of reperfusion by thrombolytic therapy, percutaneous transluminal coronary angioplasty, or both in selected patients with cardiogenic shock are encouraging and warrant further study.[54-56]

Cardiac surgery may (Table 70.12) improve the long-term survival of selected patients with shock following acute myocardial infarction. These patients may benefit from coronary revascularization and or corrective repair of a potentially lethal mechanical complication (*e.g.*, severe mitral regurgitation, ventricular septal or subacute free-wall rupture).[57] The potential value of myocardial revascularization in absence of mechanical complications depends on existence of ischemic but viable myocardium with impaired function, which would gain sufficient function from revascularization to sustain global ventricular function. After stabilization of the patient with general supportive, specific pharmacologic, and, in many cases, balloon counterpulsation therapy, prompt cardiac catheterization is recommended to define the presence and feasibility of cardiac surgery. Survival rates of 50% to 75% may be accomplished, with this approach, in properly selected cases.[57]

MECHANICAL COMPLICATIONS. Mechanical complications following myocardial infarction include acute mitral regurgitation (papillary muscle dysfunction and rupture) and septal or free wall rupture.

Cardiac rupture contributes to approximately 15% of all fatalities related to acute myocardial infarction. Cardiac rupture may present as papillary muscle rupture, ventricular septal rupture, or free wall rupture.

ACUTE MITRAL REGURGITATION. Acute mitral regurgitation following myocardial infarction can result from ischemia or necrosis of left ventricular papillary muscles and contiguous portions of the left ventricular wall from where the papillary muscles originate (papillary muscle dysfunction), from rupture of the tip or, less commonly, the trunk of a papillary muscle, and, rarely, from rupture of chordae tendineae.

PAPILLARY MUSCLE DYSFUNCTION. The mitral valve complex consists of the annulus, mitral leaflets (anterior and posterior), papillary muscles (anterolateral and posteromedial), 120 chordae tendineae, left ventricular wall where the two papillary muscles are attached, and the left atrial wall. An intricate balance of geometry and function of the components of the mitral valve complex is necessary for normal competent function of the mitral valve, failure of which can result in varying degrees of malfunction and regurgitation. The anterolateral papillary muscle has a relatively generous blood supply from the left anterior descending coronary artery or its diagonal branches and from the marginal termination of the left circumflex coronary artery. The posteromedial papillary muscle, on the other hand, has a relatively poorer and less reliable perfusion coming predominantly from the posterior descending branch of the angiographically dominant coronary artery (commonly the right but occasionally the left circumflex) with a few twigs from the nondominant artery. The anterolateral papillary muscle originates from the midportion of the anterolateral left ventricular wall and receives its chordal attachment from both mitral leaflets. The bulkier posteromedial papillary muscle originates from the junction of the lower or middle third of the ventricular septum and the posterior left ventricular wall and receives its chordal attachment from the medial half of both mitral leaflets. The high propensity of papillary muscles for ischemia and infarction in coronary disease is related partly to their disadvantaged blood supply from inconstant and tenuous sources and their innermost cardiac location at the terminus of cardiac arterial circulation and is subject to exiguous perfusion as well as to a relatively high degree of tension development during systole and its attendant high metabolic oxygen cost similar to that of subendocardial myocardium. Posteromedial papillary muscle ischemia, infarction, or rupture is five to ten times more common than that of anterolateral papillary muscle, possibly because of more inconsistent and tenuous blood supply coming predominantly from a single artery.

Papillary muscle ischemia or infarction is rarely sufficient to result in mitral regurgitation unless there is deranged contractile function of the left ventricular myocardium contiguous to the base of the papillary muscle.[58] It is likely that in many cases mitral regurgitation resulting from papillary muscle dysfunction occurs when papillary muscle contraction fails to occur or occurs along an abnormal axis, shifted inappropriately by coexistent ventricular dilatation and dyssynergy, resulting in inability of the mitral leaflets to coapt appropriately in systole.

Recognition of papillary muscle dysfunction complicating acute myocardial infarction requires demonstration of intermittent or persistent mitral regurgitation either by auscultation of a new systolic apical murmur of variable intensity, duration, pitch, and radiation or hemodynamic signs of disproportionately large v waves on pulmonary capillary wedge pressure or by left ventricular angiography. However, the systolic murmur may be ephemeral or lingering, soft or loud, high- or low-pitched, holosystolic or early systolic, or even completely absent despite severe mitral regurgitation.[59,60] Depending on the concomitant severity of left ventricular dysfunction and the degree of acute mitral regurgitation, the patient may develop clinical evidence of persistent or intermittent pulmonary congestion, pulmonary edema, hypotension, or shock state. Recognition of severe mitral regurgitation, persistent or intermittent, requires a high index of clinical suspicion and is aided by bedside Swan-Ganz right-sided heart catheterization (Fig. 70.7). Echocardiography coupled with Doppler flow study is also valuable in mak-

---

TABLE 70.12 INDICATIONS FOR CARDIAC CATHETERIZATION AND SURGERY IN THE "ACUTE PHASE" OF MYOCARDIAL INFARCTION

Acute severe intermittent or persistent mitral regurgitation
Acute ventricular septal rupture
Subacute cardiac rupture with tamponade
Refractory, recurrent, or continuing peri-infarction ischemia
Following thrombolysis, in presence of critical multivessel coronary artery disease
In selected patients with ventriculopenic shock, after a period of stabilization
Routinely, during early evolutionary phase to achieve revascularization and limit infarct size (controversial)

ing the correct diagnosis. Such patients should be subjected to prompt cardiac catheterization followed by surgery for the coronary artery disease with mitral valve repair or replacement. In preparation for cardiac catheterization and surgery, the condition of a severely symptomatic patient may require stabilization with pharmacologic unloading with intravenous vasodilators or with mechanical circulatory assist using the intra-aortic balloon pumping, as discussed earlier.

PAPILLARY MUSCLE RUPTURE. Rupture of left ventricular papillary muscle, a serious complication of acute myocardial infarction, occurs in approximately 1% of infarct cases and accounts for up to 5% of infarcts resulting in death.[61,62] Papillary muscle rupture tends to occur between 2 and 7 days after infarction, but up to 20% of cases may occur within 24 hours of onset of infarction. The majority of the ruptures involve the posteromedial papillary muscle, a complication of inferior or posterior infarction resulting from occlusive disease of the circumflex or the right coronary artery. The degree of left ventricular myocardial necrosis is variable with nearly 50% of patients demonstrating relatively small or subendocardial infarction.[62] Likewise the extent of coronary artery disease is also variable with nearly 50% of patients having single-vessel disease.[61] The most frequent form of papillary muscle rupture involves one of the smaller heads of the papillary muscle, whereas rupture of the main trunk of the papillary muscle is less common and generally incompatible with more than brief survival.[61]

The clinical presentation is dominated by relatively sudden development of severe pulmonary congestion and pulmonary edema with many patients rapidly progressing to hypotension and shock. This clinical picture is associated with and is a direct consequence of severe acute mitral regurgitation. A loud holosystolic apical murmur with widespread radiation may be detected. However, the systolic murmur may be brief (due to rapid equilibration of left atrial and left ventricular pressures in late systole), nondescript, and even completely absent (silent mitral regurgitation) in some patients.[60] The severe respiratory distress and adventitious pulmonary sounds caused by pulmonary edema may make it difficult to hear a murmur even when it is present. A palpable thrill is distinctly rare in papillary muscle rupture, occurring in about 2% of cases only. The electrocardiogram often shows evidence of inferior or posterior infarction, which in many cases may be limited to seemingly minor ST-T changes and a deceptively benign appearance despite the catastrophic clinical deterioration.[62] The chest film shows pulmonary congestion or edema, which may be preferentially distributed to upper lung lobes particularly on the right side, simulating pulmonary infiltrates. This preferential location may be the outcome of the mitral regurgitant jet being directed toward the orifice of the right upper lobe pulmonary veins. The left ventricular ejection fraction may be variably depressed, normal, or super normal depending upon the extent of left ventricular myocardial necrosis and the unloading effect of mitral regurgitation. Right ventricular ejection fraction may also be depressed owing to associated acute pulmonary arterial hypertension or coexistent right ventricular ischemic damage.

The diagnosis can be made noninvasively in the presence of the appropriate clinical context. Echocardiography, particularly the two-dimensional approach, may show a flail mitral leaflet. When a Doppler study is performed, the presence and severity of mitral regurgitation can be gauged at the bedside. Even when the characteristic mitral valve echo of papillary muscle rupture is not observed on echocardiography, relatively preserved left ventricular wall ejection fraction in a postinfarction patient with pulmonary edema and shock should suggest the diagnosis. Hemodynamic evaluation shows elevated pulmonary capillary wedge pressure with tall v waves, which may sometimes be reflected onto the pulmonary arterial tracing as well (see Fig. 70.7). Papillary muscle rupture can be differentiated from ventricular septal rupture by several features listed in Table 70.13.

The prognosis of patients with postinfarction papillary muscle rupture is poor, with a 50% mortality within 24 hours and a 94% mortality within 8 weeks.[61-63] Although some patients may appear to stabilize

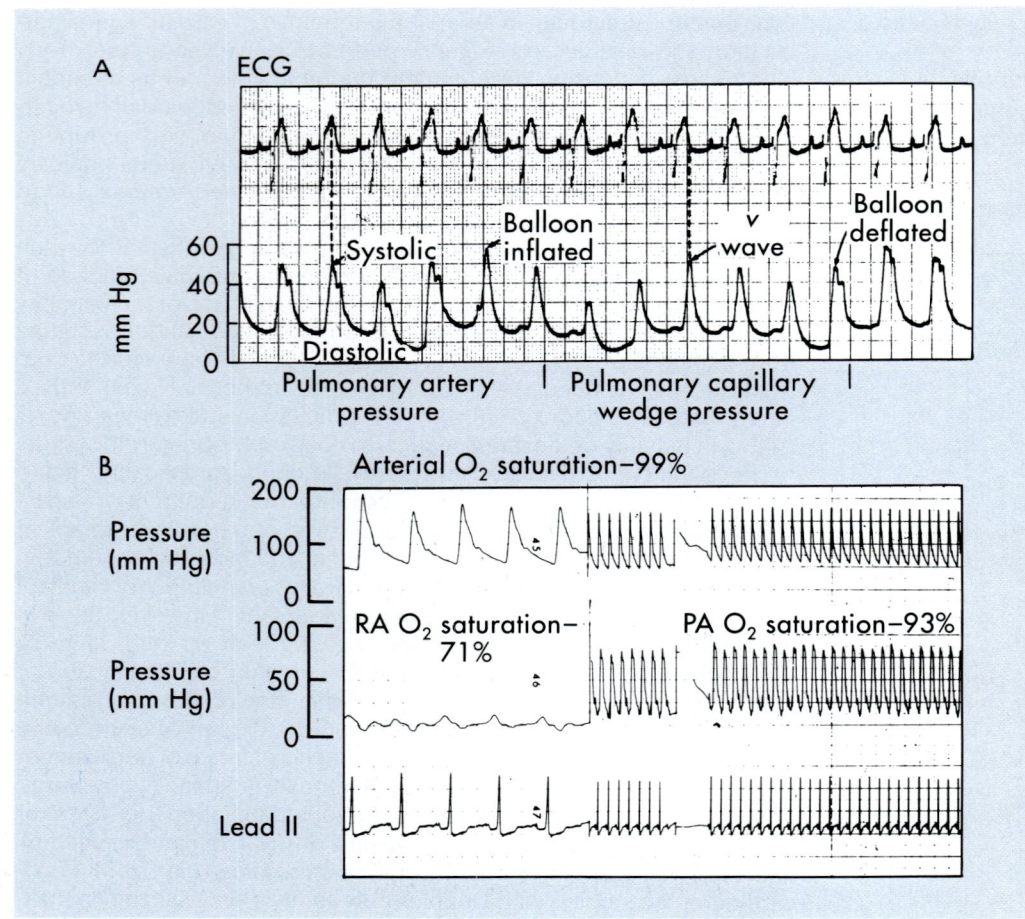

FIGURE 70.7 A. Pulmonary arterial and capillary wedge pressure tracing illustrating large v waves in a patient with acute postinfarction mitral regurgitation. B. Step-up of oxygen saturation from RA (right atrium) to PA (pulmonary artery) in a patient with postinfarction ventricular septal rupture.

and improve with supportive medical therapy, such improvement is invariably transitory and almost always followed by deterioration. Early surgical correction of the mitral leak by valve replacement or repair can salvage 60% to 70% of patients. The catastrophic clinical course, the frequent evidence of relatively limited extent of myocardial necrosis and obstructive coronary artery disease, and good surgical results provide an impetus and rationale for early recognition and early surgery in papillary muscle rupture.[61,62] In preparation for urgent cardiac catheterization and subsequent surgery, patients frequently require intra-aortic balloon pumping and additional diuretic, vasodilator, and/or inotropic therapy for temporary stabilization. Papillary muscle rupture is one of the few causes of pulmonary edema or shock complicating myocardial infarction in which aggressive and early surgical correction can result in a high short- and long-term survival rate in comparison to the natural history.

VENTRICULAR SEPTAL RUPTURE. Rupture of the interventricular septum is also a catastrophic and serious complication of acute myocardial infarction, which occurs in 0.5% to 2% cases of infauptraction and is responsible for 1% to 5% of all infarct-related deaths.[64] Septal rupture occurs equally frequently in anterior and inferior or posterior infarction and is associated with infarction of the interventricular septum as well as a variable extent of the left and/or right ventricular myocardium. Although multivessel obstructive coronary artery disease is common, septal rupture may complicate single-vessel disease. Rupture of the septum may occur as early as within the first 24 hours of onset of infarction or as late as 2 weeks later; however, most cases tend to occur between 3 and 7 days following infarction. Rupture of the septum results in a left-to-right interventricular shunt, producing right ventricular volume overload, increased pulmonary blood flow, and reduced systemic blood flow. Reduction in systemic blood flow results in a low-output hypotensive syndrome, which frequently progresses to shock. Similar to the situation in acute papillary muscle rupture, the left ventricular ejection fraction is variably depressed or normal, depending on the magnitude of infarction. The unloading effect of the left-to-right shunt results in a higher left ventricular ejection fraction relative to the extent of myocardial necrosis. The right ventricular ejection fraction may be depressed secondary to right ventricular volume overload and increased pulmonary arterial pressure, particularly in patients with concomitant ischemic damage of the right ventricle.

Ventricular septal rupture is associated with the development of a new harsh and loud holosystolic precordial murmur with widespread radiation. This is accompanied by a palpable thrill in about 50% of the cases. Clinically, the patient may have recurrence of chest pain and dyspnea followed by signs and symptoms of a low-output state, hypotension, or shock. Right ventricular volume overload secondary to the shunt, concomitant right ventricular ischemic damage, and tricuspid regurgitation may produce signs of systemic venous congestion out of proportion to those of pulmonary venous congestion. The diagnosis can be confirmed rapidly at the bedside using two-dimensional echocardiography, which demonstrates the site and approximate size of septal rupture.[65,66] The diagnosis can be further refined by using echo-bubble contrast or Doppler echocardiography. First-pass radionuclide ventriculography may also demonstrate an intracardiac left-to-right shunt. Bedside right-sided heart catheterization is useful in confirming the diagnosis and permits an approximate calculation of the degree of left-to-right shunt. An increase in oxygen saturation ($\geq$10%) from right atrium to right ventricle or proximal pulmonary artery in the appropriate clinical setting is virtually diagnostic of ventricular septal rupture (Fig. 70.7, B).

The clinical course of septal rupture is ominous, with a 24% mortality within 24 hours, a 46% mortality at 1 week, 67% to 82% mortality at 2 months, and only a 5% to 7% survival at 1 year.[57,64] Conservative medical therapy of septal rupture is generally ineffective. Afterload reduction by vasodilators may decrease left ventricular systolic pressure and reduce the degree of left-to-right shunt but more pulmonary than sys-

TABLE 70.13 COMPARISON OF PAPILLARY MUSCLE RUPTURE AND VENTRICULAR SEPTAL RUPTURE

	Papillary Muscle Rupture with Acute Mitral Regurgitation	Ventricular Septal Rupture
Clinical Findings	Occurs in 1% of all infarcts Peak incidence 3 to 5 days after infarction More frequent in inferoposterior infarcts (posterior papillary more frequently involved) Murmur usually loud and holosystolic but may be soft and nonholosystolic or completely absent Palpable precordial thrill rare	Occurs in 1% to 2% of all infarcts Peak incidence 3 to 5 days after infarct Equally frequent in anterior and inferior infarcts Murmur loud and holosystolic with widespread radiation 50% have palpable precordial thrill
Diagnostic Techniques		
Two-dimensional echocardiography	Flail or prolapsing leaflet	Visualization of defect in septum (with or without contrast echocardiography)
Doppler flow studies	Systolic regurgitant jet into left atrium	Detection of transseptal left-to-right shunt
Radionuclide ventriculography	Normal, increased, or reduced LV ejection fraction with abnormal stroke count ratio	Normal, increased, or reduced LV ejection fraction with abnormal stroke count ratio Left-to-right shunt on a first-pass study
Pulmonary artery catheterization	Prominent v waves on PCW tracing, reflected v waves on PA tracing. (Prominent v waves may also occur without mitral regurgitation)	Oxygen saturation in RV and PA shows a step-up compared with RA (PA > RA by $\geq$10% saturation)
Left ventricular angiography	Mitral regurgitation visualized	Ventricular septal defect visualized

(PCW, pulmonary capillary wedge pressure; PA, pulmonary artery; RV, right ventricle; RA, right atrium)

temic vasodilation could actually increase the shunt. Furthermore, severe systemic hypotension frequently precludes their use. Inotropic and vasopressor drug therapy may be necessary to sustain arterial blood pressure but could produce tachyarrhythmias, systemic vasoconstriction with increase of the left-to-right shunt, and myocardial ischemia. Transient stabilization can be achieved with intra-aortic balloon counterpulsation alone or in conjunction with vasodilator and inotropic drug therapy, but such stabilization is often temporary and should only be used in preparation for urgent cardiac catheterization to confirm the diagnosis and define coronary anatomy, mitral valve competence, and left ventricular function. This should be followed by prompt cardiac surgery involving repair of the defect and, when necessary, coronary bypass surgery and aneurysmectomy. Such an aggressive surgical approach results in 48% to 75% short-term survival.[57] Follow-up over 17 to 91 months has shown a late mortality of 5% to 14% in one series.[57] Cardiogenic shock, right ventricular infarction, and evidence of end organ failure (pulmonary, renal) appear to indicate a higher perioperative mortality.[57] The results of surgery appear more favorable for anteriorly located septal ruptures compared with posteriorly located defects, possibly due to technical problems encountered during repair of posteriorly located defects, coexistent mitral regurgitation, and ischemic right ventricular dysfunction.

FREE WALL RUPTURE. Free wall rupture is another catastrophic complication of acute myocardial infarction that may account for 8% to 24% of infarction-related deaths.[68] Free wall rupture occurs in 1.5% to 8% of all myocardial infarcts. Although about 30% of ruptures may occur within 24 hours of onset of infarction, the peak incidence appears to be on the 2nd to the 8th day post infarction.[67] The infarction is transmural, the infarct-related coronary artery is generally totally occluded with a thrombus, and collateral circulation is sparse or absent.[67,68] The rupture occurs mainly in the left ventricle, complicating anterior and inferior infarcts equally frequently, but rarely right ventricular rupture may complicate right ventricular infarction. Free wall rupture occurs more frequently after a first infarction, during and after the 7th decade, in females, and in those with history of systemic hypertension or hypertension complicating myocardial infarction.[68] Early ambulation and short-term use of anti-inflammatory drugs (corticosteroids, indomethacin) and anticoagulants might play a role in precipitating cardiac rupture, but this remains unproven. There is no convincing evidence to suggest that early thrombolytic-anticoagulant therapy initiated before transmural infarction is complete actually increases the risk of cardiac rupture. In fact, early reperfusion therapy may halt transmural spread of myocardial necrosis and reduce the risk of free wall rupture by preserving a viable shell of epicardial tissue. On the other hand, it is conceivable that thrombolytic anticoagulant therapy, if administered too late in the course of myocardial infarction when transmural necrosis and possibly pericarditis has already occurred, may be associated with an increased risk of cardiac rupture or hemopericardium.

Clinically, cardiac rupture often presents as a catastrophic syndrome characterized by sudden tearing pain rapidly followed by hypotension, distention of neck veins, and electromechanical dissociation and often accompanied by a vagally mediated junctional or sinus bradycardia. In some patients, this scenario may be preceded or accompanied by intense agitation and mental confusion, while in others intermittent chest pain may precede the full-blown catastrophic syndrome. Death often ensues rapidly because of hemopericardium and tamponade. Few cases with this mode of presentation can be salvaged by anything short of heroic measures (i.e., immediate pericardiocentesis, emergency thoracotomy, and surgical repair).

An occasional patient may present a more subacute course with progressively increasing signs of cardiac tamponade over hours or days. Only a high index of suspicion can lead to the proper investigation, diagnosis, and appropriate surgery.[69] Since the extent of myocardial necrosis can vary from small to large, it is particularly important to recognize this subacute entity since surgery can lead to gratifying long-term results.[58,70]

PSEUDOANEURYSM. Pseudoaneurysm is a rare complication of transmural myocardial infarction that results from rupture of the infarcted area, most often in the left ventricle, followed by containment of the resulting hemopericardium by circumferential adhesions between the pericardium and the epicardium (Fig. 70.8). Nearly 75% of cases of pseudoaneurysms reported in the literature have resulted from complications of cardiac surgery, chest trauma, and bacterial endocarditis.[70] The precise incidence is not known, but in a retrospective review Catherwood and colleagues detected a pseudoaneurysm in 0.5% of 1050 patients referred for cardiac catheterization.[71] The pseudoaneurysm tends to communicate with the body of the left ventricle through a narrow neck (diameter of neck being less than 50% of the diameter of fundus) and may remain small or enlarge progressively to become larger than the main left ventricle and is frequently lined by a mural thrombus. Unlike a true aneurysm the wall of the pseudoaneurysm is composed of pericardium and adhesions and is devoid of myocardial tissue and coronary arteries. Pseudoaneurysm may be clinically silent and only discovered during routine investigation, or it may present with clinical manifestations similar to those of a true aneurysm (i.e., progressively worsening congestive heart failure, recurrent ventricular arrhythmias, cardiomegaly with an abnormal bulge on the cardiac border, and persistent elevation of the ST segment overlying an area of infarction on the electrocardiogram). Systolic and diastolic

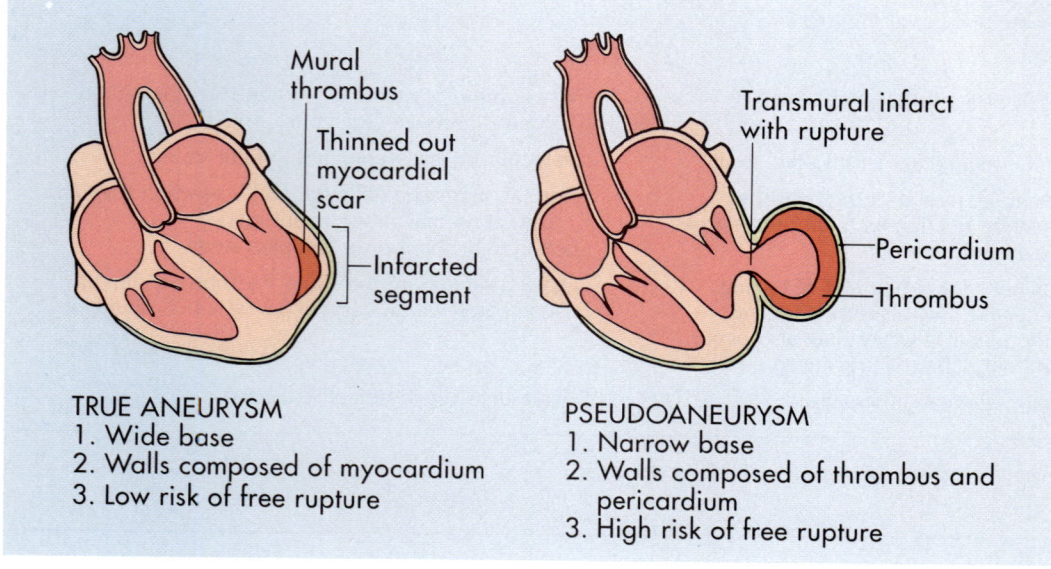

FIGURE 70.8 Schematic drawing of differences between a pseudoaneurysm and a true aneurysm.

murmurs, presumably related to a to-and-fro movement of blood across the narrow neck of the aneurysm may be present, thus simulating valvular heart disease.[72] Unlike a true aneurysm, the pseudoaneurysm is prone to free rupture with an invariably fatal outcome.[70] The diagnosis can be made by two-dimensional echocardiography or radionuclide ventriculography, magnetic resonance imaging or by contrast left ventricular angiography. Surgical resection is strongly recommended in symptomatic as well as asymptomatic patients irrespective of the size of the pseudoaneurysm to prevent a catastrophic outcome from rupture. Differentiation of pseudoaneurysm from true aneurysm is illustrated in Figure 8.

TRUE VENTRICULAR ANEURYSM. A true aneurysm occurs in 10% to 38% of patients surviving acute transmural myocardial infarction and is most frequently observed with anterior infarction, involving the left ventricular apex, the anterolateral wall, and the septum.[73] Less than 5% of clinically significant aneurysms involve the posterobasal part of the left ventricle, occurring after an inferoposterobasal infarction. The aneurysm is generally a circumscribed, noncontractile outpouching of the left ventricle, which probably forms when the necrotic tissue stretches, thins, and expands. Initially the aneurysm contains necrotic tissue, but with time its walls become more densely fibrotic and may even calcify. The aneurysms vary in size, have a wide base, and are frequently lined by thrombus.

A ventricular aneurysm puts the entire ventricle at a mechanical disadvantage by splinting adjacent normal myocardium, predisposing to malalignment of papillary muscles with consequent mitral regurgitation, thereby wasting contractile energy expended by normal myocardium that is used up by the aneurysm during its passive systolic outward bulging. These factors often result in progressive congestive heart failure and cardiomegaly. In spite of the high frequency of associated mural thrombosis (15% to 77% at necropsy or surgery) the frequency of clinically recognized systemic embolism is low (2% to 5%).[74] Ventricular aneurysm predisposes to recurrent ventricular arrhythmias and sudden death, and the arrhythmias are thought to originate from reentry circuits in the junction of aneurysm and the normal myocardium. Unlike a pseudoaneurysm, rupture of a true aneurysm is rare.

The diagnosis of ventricular aneurysm should be considered when a patient develops early or late severe heart failure, embolic events, or recurrent ventricular arrhythmias and has a diffuse or dyskinetic left ventricular apical impulse, a bulge on the left heart border on a chest film and ST segment elevation persisting beyond 2 weeks following acute infarction. A two-dimensional echocardiogram and a radionuclide ventriculogram can confirm the diagnosis and differentiate it from a pseudoaneurysm.[73]

Surgical resection of the aneurysm, often combined with coronary artery bypass grafting (since more than 50% have multivessel disease) and mitral valve repair or replacement if the papillary muscles are involved, is indicated when there is refractory heart failure and can lead to gratifying results, particularly when there is good contractile function of the noninvolved myocardium. Surgical resection is also performed when an aneurysm produces refractory and recurrent life-threatening arrhythmias but the results are better when sophisticated electrophysiologic mapping is used as a guide to delineate the site of origin of the arrhythmia. Systemic emboli of clinical significance appear to occur in 2% to 5% of patients with mural thrombus and ventricular aneurysm,[74] and anticoagulant therapy or surgical removal may be advised in such cases. However, there are no controlled studies documenting the efficacy of any treatment in the prevention of embolic events.

SHOCK SYNDROME WITHOUT PULMONARY CONGESTION OR PULMONARY EDEMA

HYPOVOLEMIA. Invasive hemodynamic studies in acute myocardial infarction have demonstrated that in some patients with shock, the left ventricular filling pressure is low or only minimally elevated and rapid volume expansion may improve the clinical and hemodynamic state.[75] The precise reasons for the hypovolemic state are not clear, but overdiuresis, excessive use of vasodilators, possible reflexly mediated inappropriate peripheral vascular pooling, and in some cases diaphoresis and vomiting resulting in dehydration contribute to volume depletion. These patients can be recognized when the low-output state or shock is associated with collapsed neck veins, lack of signs of pulmonary congestion on physical examination and chest film, and absence of an S_3 gallop. In others, the diagnosis can only be made with certainty using invasive hemodynamic monitoring. The hemodynamic profile of these patients is typified by the Cedars-Sinai subset III (*i.e.*, a cardiac index $\leq$ 2.2 liters/min/m^2 with a pulmonary capillary wedge pressure less than or equal to 18 mm Hg but usually considerably lower. It is also important to recognize that some patients with predominant right ventricular dysfunction complicating an acute inferior infarction may have a similar hemodynamic profile.

The treatment of hypovolemic shock requires rapid volume infusion using aliquots of 50 ml to 100 ml of fluid (colloid or crystalloid) under close clinical and hemodynamic observation until the pulmonary capillary wedge pressure is elevated to a maximum of 15 mm Hg to 18 mm Hg. Further volume infusion may precipitate pulmonary congestion or edema and should be avoided. In some patients, particularly those receiving crystalloid infusions, pulmonary congestion and edema may occur at lower pulmonary wedge pressure, possibly due to dilutional hypoalbuminemia that results in a reduction in intracapillary oncotic pressure. For these reasons, careful clinical assessment must be made in addition to hemodynamic monitoring when administering volume to these patients. Some patients fail to improve their pump function despite restoration of pulmonary capillary wedge pressure to seemingly adequate levels. Such patients generally have severely reduced left ventricular systolic function (ejection fraction) with the ventricle operating along a flat Starling curve. Alternatively, volume loading may elevate pulmonary capillary wedge pressure without a real increase in left ventricular preload or end-diastolic volume when left ventricular compliance is abnormal.

RIGHT VENTRICULAR ISCHEMIC DYSFUNCTION. Ischemia and infarction of the right ventricle (Fig. 70.9) may occur in as many as 30% to 40% of patients with acute inferior or posterior myocardial infarction.[76,77] It is generally associated with posterior septal infarction and variable degrees of inferoposterior left ventricular infarction since all these areas share a common blood supply from the right coronary artery.[77] Although right ventricular dysfunction due to ischemia and/or infarction may be clinically silent in many patients, in 30% to 40% of cases it is associated with a low-output, hypotensive syndrome simulating cardiogenic shock. Diagnosis of hemodynamically significant predominant right ventricular dysfunction in acute myocardial infarction should be considered in any patient with acute inferior or posterior myocardial infarction complicated by a low-output or hypotensive syndrome. Elevated jugular venous pressure or increased jugular venous pressure during inspiration (Kussmaul sign) or during abdominal compression (abdominojugular reflux) with little evidence of pulmonary congestion is present in nearly 70% of cases. In about 30% of patients, however, jugular venous pressure may not show any detectable abnormalities. A murmur of tricuspid regurgitation secondary to right ventricular papillary muscle dysfunction is rarely heard. Some patients also demonstrate pulsus paradoxus simulating cardiac tamponade.[78] The electrocardiogram, in addition to the changes of acute inferior infarction, frequently shows ST segment elevation in right-sided precordial leads (V_{3R} or V_{4R}) or less commonly over V_1 through V_5. Such precordial ST segment elevations may create confusing electrocardiographic patterns simulating concomitant left anterior descending coronary occlusion.[79] A wide spectrum of hemodynamic abnormalities may be observed with elevation of right atrial and right ventricular end-diastolic pressure equal to or above the pulmonary capillary wedge pressure, which may be low, normal, or only modestly elevated. Other hemodynamic findings may include a steep right atrial Y descent, with paradoxic increase in right atrial pressure during inspiration (Kussmaul sign), dip and plateau during diastole in the right ventricular pressure tracing, pulmonary arterial and right ventricular pulsus alternans, and diminished pulse pressure in the right ventricle and pulmonary artery. Many of these hemodynamic findings overlap with those of cardiac tamponade, constrictive pericarditis, or restrictive myocardial disease.[78] In nearly 30% of patients, however, abnormalities of right atrial pressure may not be evident initially but may appear later in the course of illness or be unmasked by volume infusion. Rarely, elevated right atrial pressure may create a right-to-left shunt through a stretched patent foramen ovale, resulting in severe arterial desaturation.[80] Echocardiography and radionuclide ventriculography demonstrate disproportionate right ventricular dilation, dyssynergy, and a depressed ejection fraction (<0.39) compared with the left ventricle, which generally demonstrates an ejection fraction greater than or equal to 0.45. However, severe left ventricular global and regional dysfunction may coexist in some cases of right ventricular infarction, and such patients should be considered to have severe biventricular dysfunction.[81] A technetium-99m pyrophosphate scan may demonstrate uptake in the right ventricle in some cases.

The low-output hypotensive syndrome results predominantly from reduced left ventricular filling and consequently a low left ventricular end-diastolic volume. However, bradyarrhythmias, which are frequently observed in this syndrome, in particular when associated with loss of appropriately timed atrial contraction, may aggravate or even precipitate the low-output syndrome. The reduction in left ventricular volume results from reduced right ventricular systolic function and a consequent decrease in pulmonary blood flow and left ventricular inflow as well as an increase in intrapericardial pressure secondary to right ventricular dilation, producing in effect, tamponade of the left ventricle.[76,78,82]

It is important to emphasize that volume infusion alone is rarely successful in improving the hemodynamic or clinical state, which frequently requires concomitant use of inotropic or vasoactive drug therapy.[76] The overall hospital outcome is favorable in this subset of patients, owing probably to spontaneous improvement that occurs in right ventricular function over time.[76] However, when severe left ventricular dysfunction (hemodynamic evidence of which may remain masked) coexists, and/or papillary muscle, free wall, or ventricular septal rupture occurs, the outlook becomes grave.[76,81] Rarely, tricuspid valve replacement for shock and severe tricuspid regurgitation and closure of a patent foramen ovale for refractory right-to-left shunt and life-threatening hypoxemia has been necessary.

RECURRENT EARLY POSTINFARCTION ISCHEMIA AND EXTENSION OF INFARCTION

EARLY POSTINFARCTION ISCHEMIA

Evidence of recurrent ischemia at rest or with minimal effort occurring within the first 7 to 10 days following an acute myocardial infarction is of particular concern since it represents evidence of additional myocardium at risk beyond the myocardium already lost in the process of initial infarction. The precise incidence of early recurrent ischemia is not well known but the reported incidence has varied between 23% and 60%.[83] Postinfarction ischemia may present as recurrent chest pain after a variable pain-free period following the onset of acute myocardial infarction with or without reversible ST-T wave changes on the electrocardiogram; episodic painless ST-T wave changes; recurrent bouts of left ventricular failure, mitral regurgitation from papillary muscle ischemia, conduction disturbances, or arrhythmias accompanied by ST-T changes with or without chest pain; or pain continuing for several hours following the onset of acute myocardial infarction without a truly pain-free interval. Recurrent ischemia has been reported to be more prevalent in nontransmural myocardial infarction, although that has not been confirmed.[83,84]

Postinfarction ischemia could represent a nontransmural and incomplete infarction that is threatening to extend to its transmural extent (ischemia in infarct zone) or is due to ischemia of remote myocardial segments (ischemia at a distance).[85,86] Ischemia in the infarct zone could result when there is preservation of some residual flow to the infarct zone because of subtotal thrombotic occlusion of the infarct-related artery or from neighboring collaterals, and this residual flow is intermittently jeopardized by platelet aggregation, change in size of thrombus, or alterations in vasomotor tone. When remote myocardial segments are perfused by coronary arteries with flow-limiting stenoses, they may become ischemic (ischemia at a distance) when systemic hypotension occurs, when myocardial oxygen demand is increased secondary to ventricular dilation and increased sympathoadrenal activity and heart rate, or when collateral inflow coming from the infarct-related artery is jeopardized by coronary occlusion. Schuster and Bulkley[85] have demonstrated that the long-term prognosis of patients with postinfarction angina due to "ischemia at a distance" is less favorable in comparison with that of patients with "ischemia in the infarct."

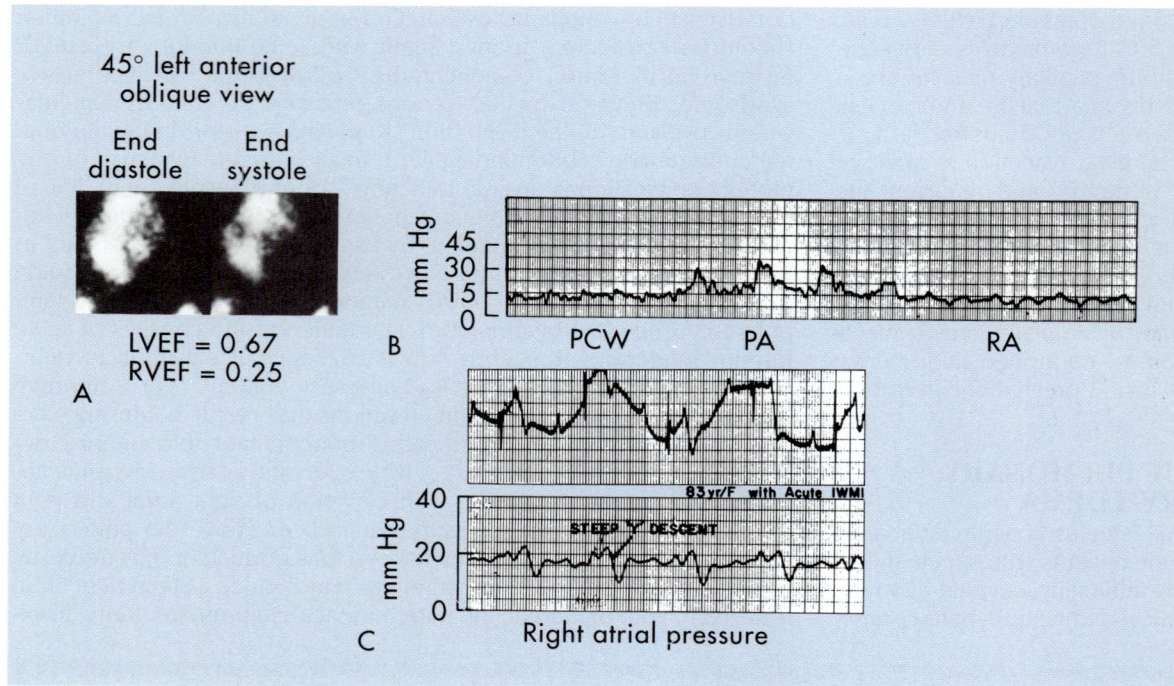

FIGURE 70.9 A. Radionuclide ventriculogram in 45° left anterior oblique projection demonstrating predominant right ventricular dysfunction in a patient with acute inferior infarction. (LV, left ventricle; RV, right ventricle; EF, ejection fraction). **B.** Hemodynamic findings of equalization of right atrial and pulmonary capillary wedge pressure (PCW) in a patient with postinfarction predominant right ventricular dysfunction. **C.** Abnormal right atrial pressure waveform showing steep y descent in a patient with postinfarction predominant right ventricular dysfunction.

Differentiation of recurrent postinfarction chest pain from that of pericarditis or impending cardiac rupture is crucial in order to institute appropriate therapy (see sections on pericarditis and cardiac rupture). A careful history, physical examination, and 12-lead electrocardiogram should be obtained immediately in a patient in whom recurrent ischemia is suspected. In some cases, 24-hour Holter monitoring to document ST-T changes may be valuable.

The management of such patients is predicated on the potential mechanisms of recurrent ischemia outlined previously. Nitrates, β-blockers, and calcium channel blockers are frequently used in the hope of preventing coronary vasospasm, of decreasing heart rate, preload, and afterload, of reducing myocardial oxygen demand, and of improving collateral flow to the potentially ischemic zone. However, more definitive methods of improving or maintaining adequate perfusion to the ischemic zone should be considered. Since early recurrent ischemia may presage infarct extension with its attendant complications, urgent cardiac catheterization to define coronary anatomy in preparation for nonsurgical percutaneous transluminal angioplasty or surgical revascularization may be indicated in some patients. It should, however, be pointed out that there are no large-scale clinical trials specifically addressing this issue and so the recommendations are based on clinical experience rather than proven data. Intra-aortic balloon pumping should be considered in the interim for patients who are unstable with frequent or prolonged episodes of ischemia poorly responsive to conservative therapy, especially when left ventricular failure, serious arrhythmias, or hypotension coexist. The primary role of coronary thrombosis as the proximate cause of severe flow reduction in acute myocardial infarction raises intriguing possibilities that thrombolytic-antithrombotic therapy may be a rational therapy in patients with early recurrent ischemia. Preliminary and uncontrolled reports suggest the potential usefulness of this approach, but further information is needed to put the role of such therapy in proper perspective.[87]

POSTINFARCTION EXTENSION

Extension of the original infarction has been reported to occur in 6% to 86% of patients depending on the criteria used. When strict criteria are used (i.e., recurrent chest pain 24 hours or more after original infarction with new persistent electrocardiographic changes and reelevation of plasma creatine kinase), the incidence is between 6% and 17%.[88] The pathophysiologic basis of extension is likely to be similar to the one described for recurrent postinfarction ischemia. The incidence of extension has been reported by some to be higher in nontransmural than transmural infarcts, while others have failed to find a significant difference.[83] The higher incidence in nontransmural infarction has been suggested to be due to the relatively higher prevalence of subtotal coronary occlusion in this subset of patients, creating a potentially unstable situation. Female gender and obesity have also been reported to increase risk of infarct extension by Marmor and co-workers[83] but not by Maisel and colleagues.[88]

Since infarct extension results in further left ventricular dysfunction and increases both the in-hospital as well as the long-term mortality, particularly among patients with initial nontransmural myocardial infarction, aggressive management of early postinfarction ischemia is recommended.[88]

POSTINFARCTION PERICARDITIS

Pericardial involvement following myocardial infarction occurs in three distinct forms: (1) an early episternopericarditis, (2) a delayed form called the postmyocardial infarction or Dressler's syndrome, and (3) pericardial involvement during cardiac rupture.

EARLY POSTINFARCTION PERICARDITIS

This complication has been reported to occur in 6% to 42% of patients (average incidence of 10%) with acute myocardial infarction, with a higher incidence being reported from autopsy studies and a lower incidence from clinical studies with stringent diagnostic criteria.[89] The majority of patients develop clinical evidence of pericarditis between 24 and 96 hours after infarction. The myocardial infarction is generally anatomically transmural, and in the vast majority of cases pericardial inflammation is localized to the area overlying the necrotic segment. Pericarditis tends to occur more frequently with large infarctions, and thus congestive heart failure and atrial and ventricular arrhythmias frequently coexist. Early pericarditis may be asymptomatic and only recognized when the characteristic pericardial friction rub is heard; however, in many patients, recurrent chest pain following acute infarction raises the initial suspicion of pericarditis. The pain of pericarditis is often reported by the patient to be different from the pain of infarction. It tends to be duller and is generally accentuated by breathing, coughing, sneezing, deglutition, truncal movement, and supine posture. The pain may also radiate to the shoulder and the left trapezius muscle ridge (trapezius ridge sign). The patient may have a low-grade fever. The diagnostic hallmark is a scratchy two- or three-component (early diastolic, presystolic, and systolic) pericardial friction rub heard along the left sternal border. The friction rub is notoriously evanescent and should be sought for several times a day. When the rub has a single component, usually systolic, it may be confused with a systolic murmur. Substantial pericardial effusion rarely occurs with early postinfarction pericarditis, and therefore an echocardiogram may not necessarily be helpful. Unlike the situation in acute viral pericarditis, the electrocardiogram is seldom helpful since ST-T segments have already been distorted by the process of infarction, making it difficult to detect additional ST-T changes of pericarditis.[90]

The correct identification of pericarditis as a cause of recurrent chest pain is important because its treatment differs substantially from that of recurrent ischemia or threatened extension of infarction. Furthermore, recurrent chest pain often alarms both the patient and medical staff, and the establishment of the diagnosis of pericarditis is reassuring to both. The symptoms of pericarditis show a prompt salutary response to analgesic anti-inflammatory medications (i.e., acetylsalicylic acid, indomethacin, or ibuprofen).[93] One of these drugs may be used three or four times a day in severely symptomatic patients, and the treatment can generally be stopped within 3 to 5 days. In rare cases, when severe symptoms persist despite the use of nonsteroidal anti-inflammatory drugs, a single large intravenous dose of a corticosteroid may relieve the symptoms. Experimental studies have suggested that indomethacin may provoke coronary vasoconstriction and interfere with infarct healing, but no persuasive clinical data suggest a major deleterious effect of its short-term use for the treatment of early postinfarction pericarditis. The use of anticoagulants in acute myocardial infarction complicated by early pericarditis has been considered to increase the risk of intrapericardial bleeding, although with careful anticoagulation this rarely happens. Such patients require close clinical surveillance for evidence of increasing pericardial effusion, and serial echocardiograms may be valuable in this regard.

POSTINFARCTION OR DRESSLER'S SYNDROME

This clinical syndrome, first described by Dressler in 1955, has been reported to occur in 1% to 3% of myocardial infarction patients 1 week to several months after the initial infarction,[92] although it is likely that the true incidence is much lower. The clinical picture is characterized by constitutional disturbances such as fever, malaise, anorexia, and manifestation of pleurisy, pericarditis, pleuropericardial effusions, pulmonary infiltrates with dyspnea, arthralgia or arthritis, and an elevated sedimentation rate and leukocyte count. Unlike early postinfarction pericarditis, this syndrome tends to run a more prolonged course of weeks to months with remissions and recurrences.

The etiology and pathogenesis of Dressler's syndrome are not well known. Demonstration of antimyocardial antibodies in 56% to 83% of patients with Dressler's syndrome has been presented as an argument in favor of an immunologic or autoimmune mechanism by some, while others have questioned such an etiologic relationship. A possible role of coxsackievirus B infection has also been suggested in view of a rising titer of antibodies against this agent found in some patients.

It is important to make the correct diagnosis of Dressler's syndrome since appropriate therapy is dramatically effective. Several other disorders including recurrent infarction, congestive heart failure (which may coexist), pneumonia, pulmonary embolism, viral pericarditis, and right ventricular infarction may present with a clinical picture similar to Dressler's syndrome.

The treatment of Dressler's syndrome is similar to that of early postinfarction pericarditis (*i.e.*, the use of nonsteroidal anti-inflammatory analgesic agents).[91] In severely symptomatic cases and in patients who do not respond to nonsteroidal agents, a course of oral corticosteroid therapy produces dramatic resolution.[91] The corticosteroids can generally be tapered over several weeks, although recurrences of symptoms are common, requiring a further reinstitution of corticosteroids followed by a slower tapering regimen. Cardiac tamponade is rare but may be precipitated by anticoagulant therapy, thereby requiring pericardiocentesis. Chronic constrictive pericarditis following Dressler's syndrome is also exceedingly rare. Prolonged use of corticosteroids, particularly when initiated early in the course of evolution of infarction, and possibly other anti-inflammatory drugs may delay infarct healing and result in infarct thinning, with the possible risk of aneurysm formation and cardiac rupture.

THROMBOEMBOLIC COMPLICATIONS

Deep vein thrombosis occurs in 30% to 40% of cases of acute myocardial infarction and is more common in patients older than 70 years and in those with obesity, varicose veins, congestive heart failure, shock, or previous history of thromboembolism. A hypercoagulable state and venous stasis secondary to bed rest and congestive heart failure are generally considered to be responsible for the high incidence of deep vein thrombosis. Deep vein thrombosis poses a threat to the patient by predisposing to pulmonary embolism. Prophylactic anticoagulant therapy, using low-dose subcutaneous heparin, has been shown to reduce the incidence of deep vein thrombosis as well as the risk of clinically significant pulmonary embolism.[93] Unless contraindications exist, patients with acute myocardial infarction, particularly those at high risk for deep vein thrombosis, should receive low-dose subcutaneous heparin (5000 units every 12 hours) until they are fully ambulatory. Full anticoagulant doses of intravenous heparin (20,000 to 30,000 units/day) should be used once deep vein thrombosis and/or pulmonary embolism has already occurred.

Mural left ventricular thrombi form frequently after acute myocardial infarction, being present in 18% to 68% of patients at autopsy and in nearly 50% of patients coming to cardiac surgery after acute myocardial infarction.[94,95] Mural thrombi tend to form mainly in patients with acute anterior myocardial infarction complicated by the formation of an aneurysm or apical dyssynergy.[95] These thrombi can be detected as early as 36 hours after infarction and may resolve spontaneously in some patients. Although mural left ventricular thrombi can be detected with contrast or radionuclide ventriculography, platelet-imaging modalities, and computed tomography, two-dimensional echocardiography has emerged as an excellent, sensitive, and specific noninvasive diagnostic tool suitable for practical and repeated clinical use in the diagnosis of mural thrombus.

Despite the high frequency of mural thrombus, clinically recognized systemic embolic events occur relatively infrequently (*i.e.*, in 5% to 10% of the cases). The appropriate management of patients with mural thrombi remains unclear, since no controlled studies involving various therapeutic regimens have been conducted. However, in view of the potentially catastrophic sequelae of systemic embolism (which tends to involve the central nervous system most frequently) and uncontrolled data suggesting a beneficial effect of long-term anticoagulation, anticoagulant therapy should be considered when a mural thrombus is detected and no contraindications to anticoagulant therapy exist. This may be particularly indicated in patients with protruding or freely mobile mural thrombi, which appear to be more vulnerable to systemic embolization.[95] High-dose thrombolytic and anticoagulant therapy given during evolving anterior myocardial infarction has been reported to reduce the incidence of mural thrombus formation.[95] One study has demonstrated the safety and usefulness of intravenous urokinase infusion in dissolving already formed mural left ventricular thrombi despite the theoretic fear that such therapy may predispose to clot fragmentation and systemic embolic events.[96]

REFERENCES

1. May GS, Furberg CD, Eberlein KA et al: Secondary prevention after myocardial infarction: A review of short-term acute phase trials. Prog Cardiovasc Dis 25:335, 1983
2. Multicenter Postinfarction Research Group: Risk stratification and survival after myocardial infarction. N Engl J Med 309:331, 1983
3. DeWood MA, Spore J, Notske R et al: Prevalence of total coronary occlusion during the early hours of transmural myocardial infarction. N Engl J Med 303:897, 1981
4. Reimer KA, Lowe JE, Rasmussen MM et al: The wave-front phenomenon of ischemic cell death. Circulation 56:786, 1977
5. Herman MV, Heinle RA, Klein MD et al: Localized disorders in myocardial contraction. N Engl J Med 227:222, 1967
6. Rackley CE, Russell RO Jr, Mantle JA et al: Modern approach to the patient with acute myocardial infarction. Curr Probl Cardiol 1:49, 1977
7. Eaton LW, Bulkley BH: Expansion of acute myocardial infarction: Its relationship to infarct morphology in a canine model. Circ Res 49:80, 1981
8. Erlebacher JA, Weiss JL, Eaton LW et al: Late effects of acute infarct dilation on heart size: A two-dimensional echocardiographic study. Am J Cardiol 49:1120, 1982
9. Bertrand M, Rousseau MF, LaBlanche JM et al: Cineangiographic assessment of left ventricular function in the acute phase of transmural myocardial infarction. Am J Cardiol 43:472, 1979
10. Bardet J, Rocha P, Rigaud M et al: Left ventricular compliance in acute myocardial infarction in man. Cardiovasc Res 11:122, 1977
11. Swan HJC, Forrester JS, Diamond G et al: Hemodynamic spectrum of myocardial infarction and cardiogenic shock. Circulation 45:1097, 1972
12. Shah PK, Pichler M, Berman DS et al: Left ventricular ejection fraction determined by radionuclide ventriculography in early stages of first transmural myocardial infarction: Relation to short term prognosis. Am J Cardiol 45:542, 1980
13. Bigger JT, Fleiss JL, Kleiger R et al: The relationship among ventricular arrhythmias, left ventricular dysfunction, and mortality in the 2 years after myocardial infarction. Circulation 69:250, 1984
14. Killip T, Kimball JT: Treatment of myocardial infarction in a coronary care unit: A two year experience with 250 patients. Am J Cardiol 20:457, 1967
15. Forrester JS, Diamond GA, Chatterjee K et al: Medical therapy of acute myocardial infarction by application of hemodynamic subsets: I. N Engl J Med 295:1356, 1976
16. Swan HJC, Ganz W, Forrester J et al: Catheterization of the heart in man with use of a flow-directed balloon-tipped catheter. N Engl J Med 283:447, 1970
17. Dikshit K, Vyden JK, Forrester JS et al: Renal and extrarenal hemodynamic effects of furosemide in congestive heart failure after acute myocardial infarction. N Engl J Med 288:1087, 1973
18. Francis GS, Siegel RM, Goldsmith SR et al: Acute vasoconstrictor response to intravenous furosemide in patients with chronic congestive heart failure. Ann Intern Med 103: I, 1985
19. Bussman WD, Kaltenbach M: Sublingual nitroglycerin in the treatment of left ventricular failure and pulmonary edema. Eur J Cardiol 4:327, 1976
20. Shah PK: Buccal nitroglycerin ointment in acute cardiac pulmonary edema. Ann Intern Med 103:153, 1985
21. Warnavicz MA, Parker H, Cheitlin MD: Prognosis of patients with acute pulmonary edema and normal ejection fraction after acute myocardial infarction. Circulation 67:330, 1983
22. Page DL, Caulfield JB, Kastor JA et al: Myocardial changes associated with cardiogenic shock. N Engl J Med 285:133, 1971
23. Alonso DR, Scheidt S, Post M et al: Pathophysiology of cardiogenic shock: Quantification of myocardial necrosis, clinical, pathologic and electrocardiographic correlation. Circulation 48:588, 1973
24. Gutovitz AL, Sobel BE, Roberts R: Progressive nature of myocardial injury in selected patients with cardiogenic shock. Am J Cardiol 41:469, 1978
25. Wackers FJ, Lie KI, Becker AE: Coronary artery disease in patients dying from cardiogenic shock or congestive heart failure in the setting of acute myocardial infarction. Br Heart J 38:906, 1976
26. Eaton LW, Weiss JL, Bulkley BH et al: Regional cardiac dilatation after acute myocardial infarction: Recognition by 2-D echocardiography. N Engl J Med 300:57, 1979
27. Meizlish JL, Berger HJ, Plankey M et al: Functional left ventricular aneurysm formation after acute anterior transmural myocardial infarction: Incidence, natural history and prognostic implications. N Engl J Med 311:1001, 1984
28. Doherty NE, Ades A, Shah PK et al: Hypothermia as a consequence of acute

myocardial infarction: Reversal with intra-aortic balloon counterpulsation. Ann Intern Med 101:863, 1984
29. Cohn JN, Tristani FE Khatri IM: Cardiac peripheral vascular effects of digitalis in clinical cardiogenic shock. Am Heart J 78:318, 1969
30. Goldberg LO: Cardiovascular and renal actions of Dopamine: I. Potential clinical applications. Pharmacol Rev 21:1, 1972
31. Mueller HS, Evans R, Ayres SM: Effects of dopamine on hemodynamics and myocardial metabolism in shock following acute myocardial infarction in man. Circulation 57:361, 1978
32. Sonnenbllilck EH, Frishman WH, Lejemtel TH: Dobutamine: A new synthetic cardioactive sympathetic amine. N Engl J Med 300:17, 1979
33. Gillespie TA, Ambos HD, Sobel BE et al: Effects of dobutamine in patients with acute myocardial infarction. Am J Cardiol 39:588, 1977
34. Mueller H, Ayres S, Giarinelli S Jr et al: Effect of isoproterenol, L-norepinephrine and intra-aortic counterpulsation on hemodynamics and myocardial metabolism in shock following myocardial infarction. Circulation 55:325, 1972
35. Kuhn LA: Shock in myocardial infarction: Medical treatment. Am J Cardiol 26:578, 1970
36. Gray RJ, Shah PK, Singh BN et al: Low cardiac-output states following open heart surgery: Comparative hemodynamic effects of dobutamine, dopamine and norepinephrine plus phentolamine. Chest 80:16, 1981
37. Chatterjee K, Swan HJC, Kaushik VS et al: Effects of vasodilator therapy for severe pump failure in acute myocardial infarction on short term and late prognosis. Circulation 53:797, 1976
38. Franciosa JB, Buiha NM, Limas CJ et al: Improved left ventricular function during nitroprusside infusion in acute myocardial infarction. Lancet 1:650, 1972
39. Palmer RP, Lasseter KC: Sodium nitroprusside. N Engl J Med 292:294, 1975
40. Davis DW, Kadar D, Steward DJ et al: A sudden death associated with the use of sodium nitroprusside for induction of hypotension during anaesthesia. Can Anaesth Soc J 22:547, 1975
41. Cottrell JE, Casthely P, Brodie JD et al: Prevention of nitroprusside-induced cyanide toxicity with hydroxycobalamin. N Engl J Med 298:809, 1978
42. Jaffe AS, Roberts R: The use of intravenous nitroglycerin in cardiovascular disease. Pharmacotherapy 2:273, 1982
43. Shook TL, Kirshenbaum JM, Hundley RF et al: Ethanol intoxication complicating intravenous nitroglycerin therapy. Ann Intern Med 101:498, 1984
44. Nemerowski M, Shah PK: Syndrome of severe bradycardia and hypotension following sublingual nitroglycerin administration. Cardiology 67:180, 1981
45. Majid PA, Sharma B, Taylor SH: Phentolamine for vasodilator therapy of severe heart failure. Lancet 2:719, 1971
46. Mickulic E, Cohn JN, Franciosa JA: Comparative hemodynamic effects of inotropic and vasodilator drugs in severe heart failure. Circulation 56:528, 1977
47. Miller RR, Awan NA, Joye JA et al: Combined dopamine and nitroprusside therapy in congestive heart failure. Circulation 55:881, 1977
48. Richard C, Ricome JL et al: Combined hemodynamic effects of dopamine and dobutamine in cardiogenic shock. Circulation 67:620, 1983
49. Bregman D, Nichols AB, Weiss MB et al: Percutaneous intra-aortic balloon insertion. Am J Cardiol 46:261, 1980
50. Leinbach RC, Gold HK: Intra-aortic balloon pumping: Use in treatment of cardiogenic shock and acute myocardial ischemia. In Karliner JS and Gregoratos G (eds): Coronary Care. Edinburgh, Churchill Livingstone, 1981
51. Goldberger M, Tabak SW, Shah PK: Clinical experience with intra-aortic balloon counterpulsation in 112 consecutive patients. Am Heart J 111:497, 1986
52. Dewood MA, Notske RN, Hensley GR et al: Intra-aortic balloon counterpulsation with or without reperfusion for myocardial infarction shock. Circulation 61:1105, 1980
53. Isner JM, Cohen SR, Vermani R et al: Complications of intra-aortic balloon counterpulsation device, clinical and morphological observations in 45 necropsy patients. Am J Cardiol 45:260, 1980
54. Lew AS, Weiss AT, Shah PK et al: Extensive myocardial salvage and reversal of cardiogenic shock after reperfusion of the left main coronary artery by intravenous streptokinase. Am J Cardiol 54:450, 1984
55. Mathey DG, Kuck KH, Tilsner V et al: Nonsurgical coronary artery recanalization in acute transmural myocardial infarction. Circulation 63:489, 1981
56. Meyer J, Marx W et al: Successful treatment of acute myocardial infarction shock by combined percutaneous transluminal coronary artery recanalization and angioplasty. Am Heart J 103:132, 1982
57. Gray RJ, Sethna D, Matloff JM: The role of cardiac surgery in acute myocardial infarction with mechanical complications. Am Heart J 106:723, 1983
58. Shelburne JC, Rubinstein D, Gorlin R: A reappraisal of papillary muscle dysfunction: Correlative clinical and angiographic study. Am J Med 46:862, 1969
59. Heikkila J: Mitral incompetence complicating acute myocardial infarction. Acta Med Scand 176:287, 1967
60. Forrester JS, Diamond G, Freedman S et al: Silent mitral insufficiency in acute myocardial infarction. Circulation 44:877, 1971
61. Nishimura RA, Schaff HV, Shuh C et al: Papillary muscle rupture complicating acute myocardial infarction: Analysis of 17 patients. Am J Cardiol 51:373, 1983
62. Wei JY, Hutchins GM, Bulkley BH: Papillary muscle rupture in fatal acute myocardial infarction. Ann Intern Med 90:149, 1979
63. Clements SD, Story WE, Hurst JW et al: Ruptured papillary muscle, a complication of acute myocardial infarction: Clinical presentation, diagnosis and treatment. Clin Cardiol 8:93, 1985
64. Fox AC, Glassman E, Isom OW: Surgically remediable complications of myocardial infarction. Prog Cardiovasc Dis 21:461, 1979
65. Farcot JC, Borsante L, Rigaud M et al: Two-dimensional echocardiographic visualization of ventricular septal rupture after acute anterior myocardial infarction. Am J Cardiol 45:370, 1980
66. Richards KL, Hoekenga DE, Leach JK et al: Doppler cardiographic diagnosis of interventricular septal rupture. Chest 76:101, 1979
67. Rasmussen S, Leth A, Kjoller E et al: Cardiac rupture in acute myocardial infarction: A review of 72 consecutive cases. Acta Med Scand 205:11, 1979
68. Bates RJ, Beutler S, Resnekov L et al: Cardiac rupture: Challenge in diagnosis and management. Am J Cardiol 40:1231, 1977
69. O'Rourke MF: Subacute heart rupture following myocardial infarction: Clinical features of a correctable condition. Lancet 2:124, 1973
70. Knowlton AA, Grauer J, Plehn JF et al: Ventricular pseudoaneurysm: A rare but ominous condition. Cardiovasc Rev Rep 6:508, 1985
71. Catherwood E, Mintz GS, Kotler MN et al: Two-dimensional echocardiographic recognition of left ventricular pseudoaneurysm. Circulation 62:294, 1980
72. Lopez-Martinez JI: Pulsatory and auscultatory phenomena in pseudoaneurysm of the heart. Am J Cardiol 15:422, 1965
73. Visser CA, Kan G, David GK et al: Echocardiographic cineangiographic correlation in detecting left ventricular aneurysm. Am J Cardiol 50:337, 1982
74. Froehlich RT, Falsetti HL, Doty DT et al: Prospective study of surgery for left ventricular aneurysm. Am J Cardiol 45:923, 1980
75. Russell RO Jr, Rackley CE, Pambo J et al: Effects of increasing left ventricular filling pressure in patients with acute myocardial infarction. J Clin Invest 49:1539, 1970
76. Shah PK, Maddahi J, Berman DS et al: Scintigraphically detected predominant right ventricular dysfunction in acute myocardial infarction: Clinical, hemodynamic correlates and implications for therapy and prognosis. J Am Coll Cardiol 6:1264, 1985
77. Isner JM, Roberts WC: Right ventricular infarction complicating left ventricular infarction complicating coronary artery disease. Am J Cardiol 42:885, 1978
78. Lorrell B, Leinbach RC, Pohost GM et al: Right ventricular infarction: Clinical diagnosis and differentiation from cardiac tamponade and pericardial constriction. Am J Cardiol 43:465, 1979
79. Geft IL, Shah PK, Rodriguez L et al: ST elevations in leads V_1 to V_5 may be caused by right coronary occlusion and acute right ventricular infarction. Am J Cardiol 53:991, 1984
80. Morris AL, Donen N: Hypoxia and intracardiac right to left shunt complicating inferior myocardial infarction with right ventricular extension. Arch Intern Med 138:1405, 1978
81. Shah PK, Maddahi J, Staniloff HM et al: The variable spectrum and prognostic implications of left and right ventricular ejection fractions determined early in the course of acute myocardial infarction associated with clinical evidence of no or mild heart failure. Am J Cardiol 58:387, 1986
82. Goldstein JH, Blahaker GJ, Verriez ED et al: The role of right ventricular systolic dysfunction and elevated intrapericardial pressure in the genesis of low cardiac output in experimental right ventricular infarction. Circulation 65:513, 1981
83. Marmor A, Sobel B, Roberts R: Factors presaging early recurrent myocardial infarction extension. Am J Cardiol 48:603, 1981
84. Madigan NP, Rutherford DB, Frye RL: The clinical course, prognosis and coronary anatomy of subendocardial infarction. Am J Med 60:634, 1976
85. Schuster EH, Bulkley BH: Early post-infarction angina: Ischemia at a distance and ischemia in the infarct zone. N Engl J Med 305:1101, 1981
86. Schuster EH, Bulkley BH: Ischemia at a distance after acute myocardial infarction: A cause of early postinfarction angina. Circulation 62:509, 1980
87. Shapiro EP, Brinker JA, Gottlieb SO et al: Intracoronary thrombolysis 3 to 13 days after acute myocardial infarction for postinfarction angina. Am J Cardiol 55:1453, 1985
88. Maisel AM, Ahnve S, Gilpin E et al: Prognosis of extension of myocardial infarct: The role of Q waves or non-Q wave infarction. Circulation 71:211, 1985
89. Lichstein E: Early postmyocardial infarction pericarditis. Pract Cardiol 8:60, 1982
90. Krainin FM, Flessas AP, Spodich DH: Infarction-associated pericarditis rarity of diagnostic electrocardiogram. N Engl J Med 311:1211, 1984
91. Berman J, Haffajee CI, Alpert JS: Therapy of symptomatic pericarditis after myocardial infarction: Retrospective and prospective studies of aspirin, indomethacin, prednisone and spontaneous resolution. Am Heart J 101:750, 1981
92. Dressler W: A complication of myocardial infarction resembling idiopathic, recurrent benign pericarditis. Circulation 12:697, 1955
93. Gallus AS, Hirsch J, Tuttle RJ et al: Small subcutaneous doses of heparin in prevention of venous thrombosis. N Engl J Med 288:545, 1973
94. Visser CA, Kau G, Meltzer RS et al: Embolic potential of left ventricular thrombus after myocardial infarction: A 2 dimensional echocardiographic study of 119 patients. J Am Coll Cardiol 5:1276, 1985
95. Eigler N, Maurer G, Shah PK: Effect of early systemic thrombolytic therapy on left ventricular mural thrombus formation in acute anterior myocardial infarction. Am J Cardiol 54:261, 1984
96. Kremer P, Rainer F, Tilsner V et al: Lysis of left ventricular thrombi with urokinase. Circulation 72:112, 1985

CARDIAC REHABILITATION

Victor F. Froelicher

Cardiac rehabilitation is the process of restoring psychological, physical, and social functions to optimal levels in persons who have sustained a cardiac event. Much of what was considered in the past to be cardiac rehabilitation has been accepted today as complete, proper patient care. The team approach, led by the physician, should include professionals with formal training in nursing, occupational and physical therapy, vocational rehabilitation, social work, dietetics, psychology, and exercise physiology. Objectives for the patients include reversal of the effects of hospitalization, education regarding their heart disease, assistance in returning to activities, and reduction of psychological problems. Objectives for society include reduction of the cost of health care by shortening treatment time and reducing medications and prevention of premature disability, thus maintaining individual productivity and lessening the need for societal support.

Although it encompasses much more, the primary thrust of cardiac rehabilitation is exercise; therefore, this chapter begins with a discussion of the basic concepts of exercise physiology. In recent years a complete shift from the conservative approach previously used to the prescription of safe, individualized levels of activity has both enhanced and hastened the recovery process.

BASIC EXERCISE PHYSIOLOGY

The cardiorespiratory response to exercise depends on the type of work the body is performing, the environmental circumstances, and the physiologic status of the individual.[1] Changes that occur with a single bout of acute exercise are called responses and are temporary. Adaptations are long-lasting changes in structure and/or function that occur with training (chronic exercise) and improve the body's response to subsequent exercise.

DYNAMIC VS. ISOMETRIC EXERCISE

Dynamic exercise (bicycling, walking, running, cross-country skiing, swimming) involves the movement of large muscle masses, a high blood flow, and increased cardiac output. Because this movement is rhythmic, there is a drop in total peripheral resistance and a "milking" action that returns blood to the heart. Dynamic exercise evokes a series of cardiovascular adjustments designed to (1) supply the active muscles with a sufficient blood supply, (2) dissipate the heat generated by the active muscles, and (3) maintain the blood supply to the heart and brain. There is an immediate dilation of the arteries and arterioles in active muscle because of the sudden increase in metabolites. This results in a decrease in systemic vascular resistance proportional to the muscle mass involved. For arterial blood pressure to be maintained there is an increase in sympathetic activity that causes constriction of the resistance vessels in the splanchnic bed, kidneys, and nonworking muscles. The generalized vasoconstriction in inactive tissues as well as the increased venous return result in maintenance of the heart's filling volume and pressure. As cardiac output increases, there is an increase in systemic arterial pressure. The increase in pulmonary blood flow causes a moderate increase in mean pulmonary artery pressure.

Isometric work (lifting weights, forceful squeezing or pressing) involves a constant muscular contraction that limits blood flow. Instead of a marked increase in cardiac output and blood flow, blood pressure must be increased to force blood into the active, contracting muscles. Dynamic exercise can be graded to gradually increase myocardial oxygen consumption, whereas isometric exercise is more difficult to grade and increases myocardial work very quickly without as great an increase in cardiac output. Although isometric exercise is good for peripheral muscle tone and function, it does not result in the beneficial cardiac and hemodynamic effects associated with dynamic exercise. Furthermore, it can be dangerous for heart disease patients with a dilated left ventricle because of the excessive level of myocardial pressure work associated with it and, therefore, should be used with caution.

RESPONSES TO ACUTE EXERCISE

HEART RATE

With the onset of dynamic exercise, heart rate increases very rapidly. If the workload is relatively light, a plateau is seen in 30 to 60 seconds and the rate remains relatively constant until the exercise is increased or terminated. The elicited heart rate response is proportional to the workload but dependent on the individual's age and physical condition. If the workload is heavy, the heart rate increases linearly until the point of exhaustion. In the first minutes of recovery, the heart rate decreases rapidly and then continues to decline slowly at a rate relative to the intensity and duration of the exercise. Isometric exercise does not increase heart rate as much as dynamic exercise but increases it out of proportion to the level of exercise.

BLOOD PRESSURE

The systolic and diastolic blood pressure response to exercise varies with the type and intensity of the exercise and age of the subject. In dynamic exercise of moderate to heavy intensity there is a gradual linear increase in systolic pressure and usually a decrease in diastolic pressure. The heart rate and blood pressure response to progressive treadmill exercise in normal persons is illustrated in Figure 71.1. An increase in diastolic blood pressure of greater than 15 mm Hg can be an indication of a tendency toward sustained hypertension. During isometric exercise there is an immediate increase in both systolic and diastolic pressure.

BLOOD FLOW

The control of blood flow during exercise is critical. Blood must be rapidly directed to working muscles to meet their demands for oxygen and fuels. At rest, a large portion of the cardiac output is directed to the spleen, liver, kidneys, brain, and heart, with only about 20% going to skeletal muscles. During exercise, skeletal muscles can receive more than 85% of cardiac output. A surprising portion of the cardiac output goes to the muscle groups supporting respiration.

The regulation of the circulation during exercise involves the following adaptations[2]:

1. Local. The resistance vessels dilate in the active muscle, owing to the products of muscle metabolism, which block the constriction in the muscle vessels caused by the sympathetic nervous system.
2. Mechanical. The muscle pump returns blood from the legs to the central circulation.
3. Neural. The sympathetic outflow is increased, and the vagal outflow is decreased. This causes tachycardia, increased contractility, and constriction of the resistance vessels in the kidneys and gut. Most of the increase in cardiac output during exercise is due to an increase

in heart rate. As exercise continues and body temperature rises, the sweat glands are activated and skin vessels dilate.

4. Humoral. If exercise is severe, epinephrine is released into the bloodstream. Sensors within skeletal muscle detect small changes in the local chemical environment, providing the feedback to maintain adequate muscle perfusion.

OXYGEN CONSUMPTION

It is important to distinguish between total body oxygen consumption and myocardial oxygen consumption as they are distinct in their determinants and in the way they are measured or estimated. Total body, or ventilatory, oxygen consumption ($\dot{V}O_2$) is the amount of oxygen that is extracted from inspired air as the body performs work.[3] Accurate measurement of $\dot{V}O_2$ requires gas analysis equipment, but it can be estimated from the workload performed as there is a relatively small variation in the oxygen cost of a given workload. The most common method for measuring $\dot{V}O_2$ involves treadmill or bike exercise with progressively increasing workloads. When an increase in workload fails to elicit a significant increase in $\dot{V}O_2$, the highest value attained represents the "max $\dot{V}O_2$". Maximal $\dot{V}O_2$ is equal to maximal cardiac output times maximal arteriovenous oxygen difference. The maximal arteriovenous oxygen difference during exercise has a physiologic limit that cannot be exceeded. $\dot{V}O_2$ is best estimated by the workload performed rather than by total exercise time because the latter depends on the protocol used as well as on endurance and muscular strength. Table 71.1 gives the oxygen cost of the stages of many of the commonly used exercise testing protocols.

Workload is measured in terms of the oxygen requirements for its performance, and values are given in METs. One MET is the *met*abolic oxygen requirement under basal conditions. Rather than accounting for differences in basal oxygen consumption as was first advocated, one MET is now an abbreviation for the average basal metabolic value: 3.5 ml of oxygen per kilogram of body weight per minute. It is important to become very familiar with the relative values of the MET because it is widely used in both exercise testing and in prescribing levels of activity to patients. The specific activity scale is one clinical tool for using these relationships to assess a patient's exercise capacity by just asking questions relating to normal activities performed (Table 71.2).[4]

Certain factors such as emotional stress, skill and coordination, and body mechanics can alter the oxygen cost of an activity. Although $\dot{V}O_2$max is affected by age, sex, exercise status, illness, genetics, and other factors, in general a $\dot{V}O_2$max of less than 5 METs carries a poor prognosis, 10 METs is considered a level of fitness, and 24 METs can be achieved by exceptional athletes. Over a walking speed range on the level of 2 mph to 5 mph, the respective speed equals the METs expended (*i.e.*, 2 mph = 2 METs, etc.). Thirteen METs is a level that indicates low risk in coronary heart disease patients regardless of abnormal exercise test responses, and, patients able to perform 10 METs do not gain survival benefit with coronary artery surgery over medical treatment.

Myocardial oxygen consumption is the amount of oxygen required by the heart to perform work. Accurate measurement of myocardial oxygen consumption requires the placement of catheters in a coronary artery and in the coronary venous sinus to measure oxygen content. The determinants of myocardial oxygen consumption include intramyocardial wall tension (left ventricular pressure times end-diastolic volume), contractility, and heart rate. Myocardial oxygen consumption is best estimated by the product of heart rate and systolic blood pressure (double product). Angina usually occurs at the same double product rather than at the same workload. When this is not the case, the influence of other factors should be suspected, such as a recent meal, adverse ambient temperature, or changes in coronary artery tone.

Considerable interaction takes place during exercise between the manifestations of abnormalities in myocardial perfusion and function.[5,6] The electrocardiographic response and angina are closely related to myocardial ischemia and coronary artery occlusion while the exercise capacity, systolic blood pressure response, and the heart rate response to exercise can be determined either by myocardial ischemia or dysfunction, as well as by reactions in the periphery. Exercise-induced ischemia can cause cardiac dysfunction, which results in exercise impairment and an abnormal blood pressure response. Often it is difficult to separate the impact of ischemia from the impact of left ventricular dysfunction on exercise responses. This complicates the interpretation of exercise test findings and makes it difficult to assess

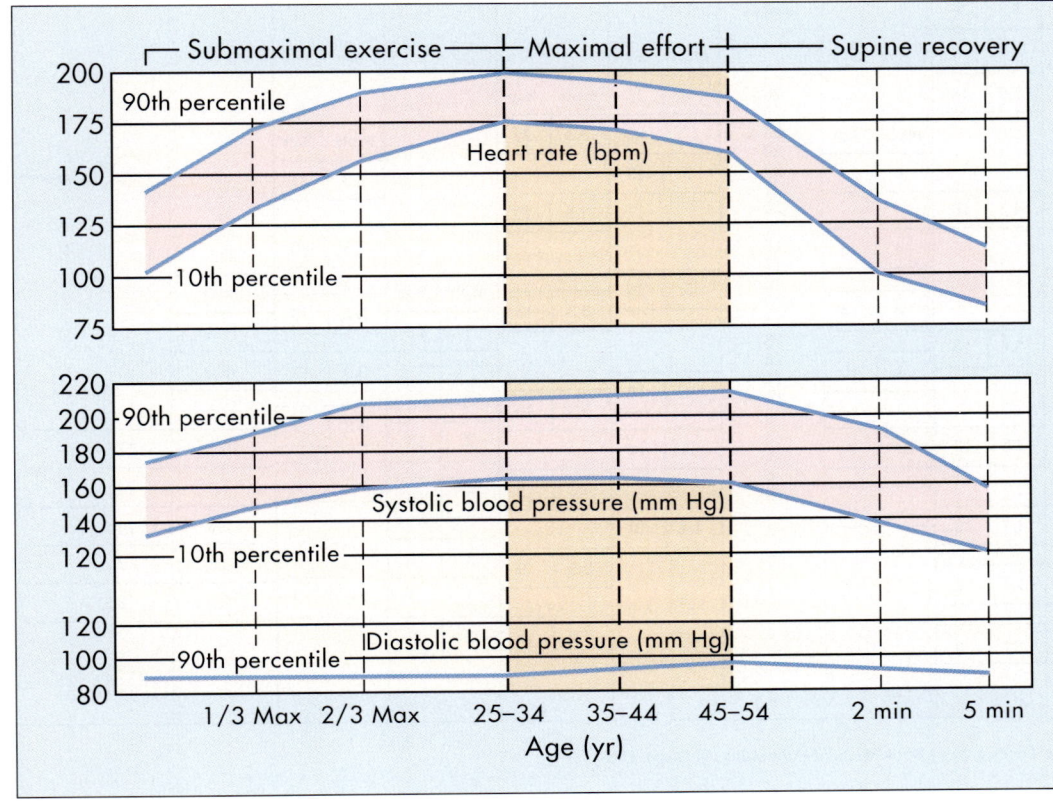

FIGURE 71.1 Blood pressure and heart rate response to a progressive treadmill protocol in healthy men.

the cause of symptoms. The severity of ischemia or the amount of myocardium in jeopardy is inversely related to the heart rate, systolic blood pressure, and exercise level achieved.

ADAPTATIONS TO CHRONIC EXERCISE (TRAINING)

Application of an appropriate recurring stimulus will result in adaptation; the greater the stimulus, the greater the adaptation. The adaptation tends to be specific to the type of stimulus provided and will occur only in the tissues and organs stressed.[7] This emphasizes the importance of a well-rounded exercise program designed to progressively increase workload until an optimal level of fitness can be reached and then properly maintained.

The benefits gained from an exercise program depend on a number of factors, including initial level of fitness, physical endowment, previous training, age, sex, and health of the individual. Greater changes are seen in previously sedentary persons as compared with those who are somewhat physically fit prior to beginning a program.

Animal studies strongly support the benefits of regular exercise on the heart. These studies clearly document significant cardiac morphologic changes in animals (more so in younger than older animals [Table 71.3]). Myocardial ischemia is a necessary stimulus for the development of collateral vessels, but exercise appears to enhance their development. Also, atherosclerotic lesions are less of a threat to myocardium supplied by coronary arteries that have been enlarged by exercise.

Hemodynamic results of an exercise program include the following: resting bradycardia, decrease in heart rate and systolic blood pressure at any matched submaximal workload, increase in maximal oxygen consumption and maximal cardiac output, increase in total blood volume, and more rapid return toward normal in recovery. Metabolic adaptations include improved glucose metabolism, decreased adrenergic hormone release, increased fat metabolism, and decrease in percent body fat.

EXERCISE PROGRAM DESIGN

The structure of an exercise program is very important.[7] The following should be included: aerobic activities for developing and maintaining cardiorespiratory fitness and proper body weight; strength and muscular endurance activities, which are low-level exercises to help maintain a degree of muscle tone and protect against injury; and flexibility exercises to improve joint range of motion and posture and to lessen fatigue and injuries. With this in mind, a variety of activities not only provides for a higher level of fitness but also gives the patient the opportunity to choose several that are enjoyable, a factor that can greatly affect adherence.

EXERCISE PRESCRIPTION

The exercise prescription should be on an individual basis, with consideration of patient attitude and motivation, and must address the mode, frequency, duration, and intensity of the exercise.

TABLE 71.1 EXERCISE TESTS AND VENTILATORY OXYGEN COST

Functional Class	Clinical Status	O$_2$ Cost (ml/kg/min)	METs	Bicycle Ergometer	Treadmill Protocols							
					Bruce 3-min stages mph %gr	Kattus mph %gr	Balke Ware % grade at 3.3 mph 1-min stages	Ellestad 3/2/3-min stages mph %gr	USAFSAM 2- or 3-min stages mph %gr	"Slow" USAFSAM mph %gr	McHenry mph %gr	Stanford % grade at 3 mph / % grade at 2 mph
Normal and I	Healthy, dependent on age, activity	56.0	16	1 watt = 6 kpds For 70-kg body weight	5.0 18		26 / 25	6 15	3.3 25			
		52.5	15			4 22	24 / 23					
		49.0	14	kpds			22 / 21	5 15			3.3 21	
		45.5	13	1500	4.2 16		20 / 19		3.3 20			
		42.0	12	1350		4 18	18 / 17				3.3 18	22.5
		38.5	11	1200			16 / 15	5 10	3.3 15		3.3 15	20.0
		35.0	10	1050	3.4 14	4 14	14 / 13			2 25		17.5
		31.5	9	900		4 10	12 / 11	4 10		2 20	3.3 12	15.0
	Sedentary healthy	28.0	8	750			10 / 9		3.3 10		3.3 9	12.5
		24.5	7		2.5 12	3 10	8 / 7	3 10		2 15		10.0 / 17.5
II		21.0	6	600		2 10	6 / 5		3.3 5	2 10	3.3 6	7.5 / 14
		17.5	5	450	1.7 10		4 / 3	1.7 10				5.0 / 10.5
	Limited Symptomatic	14.0	4	300	1.7 5		2 / 1		3.3 0	2 5		2.5 / 7
III		10.5	3	150							2.0 3	0.0 / 3.5
		7.0	2		1.7 0				2.0 0	2 0		
IV		3.5	1									

(Adapted from Froelicher V, Marcordes G: A Manual of Exercise Testing, Year Book Medical Publishing, Chicago, 1989)

Many different exercise modalities can be used to develop and maintain cardiorespiratory fitness. The types of exercise most commonly used are walking, jogging, cycling, swimming, cross-country skiing, dance, and roller-skating. These activities are rhythmical, involve a large proportion of total muscle mass, and maximize the use of large muscles. Continuous exercise of moderate intensity improves aerobic capacity through the cardiovascular changes described above and by increasing levels of myoglobin, mitochondrial enzymes (both size and number), glycogen stores, blood volume, and the oxidative capacity of muscle fibers.

For strength and muscular work, light weights are recommended, with a gradual but limited increase in workload, or one's own body weight (push-ups, sit-ups) is adequate resistance to develop and maintain a degree of muscle tone. There are exercises designed especially for flexibility (including special exercises for the elderly), or stretching exercises can be routinely performed as part of warm-up and cool-down for endurance activities.

Frequency of training should be 3 to 5 days per week spread through the week. Duration should be between 15 and 60 minutes, depending on the intensity of the activity. Previously sedentary and deconditioned subjects may require progressive development to reach even a 15-minute level. Both sporadic and more frequent participation may result in an increased risk of injury. In general, injury rates are most directly related to intensity. The level of intensity, on the other hand, appears to be more important for maintenance than frequency or duration.

Intensity should be at 50% to 80% of maximal ventilatory oxygen uptake, with most of the exercise in the mid to upper end of this range. This level, usually determined by treadmill testing, is most easily monitored by heart rate, which is linearly related to ventilatory oxygen consumption. The Karvonen technique for determining training heart rate most closely approximates the exercise intensity determined by gas analysis techniques.[8] It is calculated by subtracting basal heart rate from the maximal value, multiplying by 50% to 80%, depending on the intensity desired, and adding this product to the basal value. Levels of perceived exertion on the Borg scale of 13 to 15 approximate a training effect. The Borg scale (Table 71.4) correlates well with heart rate and the relative intensity of exercise.[9] For cardiac patients on β-blockers or with symptoms or signs that are maximal end points, an exercise effect can be achieved by subtracting 5 to 10 beats from the heart rate at the end point (*i.e.*, at angina) and thus training below their pain threshold. A warm-up and cool-down are very important. After a short warm-up (walking or light jogging for several minutes), the major muscles that will be used (depending on type of activity) can be stretched, possibly to lessen the chance of an injury. One should always begin slowly, gradually increase intensity, and avoid rapid movements that can stress joints. Stretching routines are more ritualistic than based in science.

PHASES OF CARDIAC REHABILITATION AFTER MYOCARDIAL INFARCTION

The typical phases included in the program are phase I, coronary care unit and inpatient care during the acute event; phase II, convalescence,

TABLE 71.2 ACTIVITIES THAT CORRESPOND TO CLASSES I TO IV OF THE SPECIFIC ACTIVITY SCALE

Class I (≥ 7 METs)	A patient can perform any of the following activities: Carrying 24 pounds up eight steps Carrying an 80-pound object Shoveling snow Skiing Playing basketball, touch football, squash, or handball Jogging/walking 5 mph
Class II (≥ 5 METs)	A patient does not meet class I criteria but can perform any of the following activities to completion without stopping: Carrying anything up eight steps Having sexual intercourse Gardening, raking, weeding Walking 4 miles per hour
Class III (≥ 2 METs)	A patient does not meet class I or class II criteria but can perform any of the following activities to completion without stopping: Walking down eight steps Taking a shower Changing bed sheets Mopping floors, cleaning windows Walking 2.5 mph Pushing a power mower Bowling Dressing without stopping
Class IV (≤ 2 METs)	None of the above

(Adapted from Goldman L, Hashimoto B, Cook EF et al: Comparative reproducibility and validity of systems for assessing cardiovascular functional class: Advantages of a new specific activity scale. Circulation 64:1227, 1981)

TABLE 71.3 BENEFICIAL CARDIAC CHANGES SECONDARY TO AN EXERCISE PROGRAM DOCUMENTED IN ANIMAL STUDIES

Myocardial hypertrophy
Increase in myocardial capillary-to-fiber ratio
Increase in coronary artery size
Improved myocardial function

TABLE 71.4 BORG SCALE: PERCEIVED LEVEL OF EXERTION

Perceived Level of Exertion	Description
6	
7	Very, very light
8	
9	Very light
10	
11	Light
12	
13	Somewhat hard
14	
15	Hard
16	
17	Very hard
18	
19	Very, very hard
20	

outpatient, or home program; and phase III, recovery or long-term community-based or home program. The time course and needs for each program must be individualized.

A critical issue is whether cardiac rehabilitation is going to become superfluous with the application of the new interventions, such as percutaneous transluminal coronary angioplasty (PTCA) and thrombolysis for acute myocardial infarction.[10] Multicenter trials have confirmed that mortality from acute myocardial infarction can be decreased by approximately 25% with thrombolysis and that the beneficial effects of aspirin may be additive. Depending on population selection, 20% of patients presenting with an acute myocardial infarction will meet the indications and contraindications for thrombolysis. Thrombolysis is most effective in patients with large anterior infarcts who are admitted to the hospital within 3 hours after the onset of symptoms. The place for acute PTCA during myocardial infarction appears to be rather limited. The need for PTCA after thrombolysis appears to be best determined by exercise testing as early PTCA attempts carry a high complication rate. There are no data showing that PTCA can prolong life or avert myocardial infarction although it is highly effective in the treatment of angina pectoris. Thus, in spite of these advances in therapy, there remain a large number of patients who will need cardiac rehabilitation.

PHASE I: CARDIAC REHABILITATION IN HOSPITAL AFTER ACUTE MYOCARDIAL INFARCTION

Prior to 1960, patients with acute myocardial infarction were believed to require prolonged restriction of physical activity. Patients were often kept at strict bed rest for 2 months, which resulted in deconditioning. The concern was that physical activity could lead to complications such as ventricular aneurysm formation, cardiac rupture, congestive heart failure, dysrhythmias, reinfarction, or sudden death.

Cain and colleagues, in 1961, were the first to report the safety and effectiveness of early ambulation.[11] They studied early ambulation of patients within 2 weeks after the infarction with electrocardiographic and blood pressure monitoring. Blackburn coordinated an important study in which patients at a Swiss hospital were randomized either to prolonged bed rest or early ambulation.[12] This study showed no increase in complications in those patients who underwent early ambulation. Sivarajan and colleagues, in Seattle, helped to promulgate the use of the early exercise test prior to discharge after myocardial infarction.[13] They also performed a randomized trial of early ambulation.[14] The progressive medical community in Seattle adopted many of the research methods these investigators used, and consequently there was not much difference between their intervention group and controls. Wenger has promoted the step approach to in-hospital cardiac rehabilitation.[15] This approach included early mobilization, range of motion activities, and progressive activity and was widely adopted across the United States. At first, these activities were performed by nursing staff; however, more recently, occupational and physical therapists have become primarily involved in the early ambulation of patients. This has been more for reasons of additional reimbursement because these health care professionals can bill for their services, while nursing services are included as part of the hospital charges.

Patient education activities during the acute phase usually consist of explanations about the coronary care unit, cardiac rehabilitation program, symptoms, and the delivery of routine diagnostic and therapeutic modalities. The patient should be educated as to the limitations imposed by the disease, potential for improvement, and precautions to be observed. The program must be individualized for the patient depending on his psychosocial and medical status. The medical status is determined largely by the severity of the myocardial infarction, but the medical history must also be considered.

SEVERITY OF THE MYOCARDIAL INFARCTION

The electrocardiographic pattern predicts the clinical course and outcome surprisingly well. The greater the number of areas with Q waves and the greater the R wave loss, the larger the myocardial infarction. Non–Q wave myocardial infarctions are usually less frequently associated with congestive heart failure or shock, but they can be complicated particularly when prior myocardial infarction has taken place. The concept that an initial subendocardial myocardial infarction is "uncompleted" and poses an increased risk has not been substantiated. However, an increased risk is associated with postinfarction angina and/or a history of prior myocardial infarction. Inferior infarcts are usually smaller, result in less of a decline in ejection fraction, and are less likely to be associated with shock or congestive heart failure. Anterior infarcts are more likely to cause aneurysms and a greater decrease in ejection fraction.

The size of a myocardial infarction can be judged by the creatine kinase (CK) levels, particularly by the amount of MB band released. Creatine kinase has improved the laboratory diagnosis of myocardial infarction because it is highly specific for myocardium. In general, the higher the amount of CK-MB released and the longer the creatine kinase level stays elevated, the larger the myocardial infarction. The occurrence of congestive heart failure, shock, or pericarditis is also an indicator of a relatively large myocardial infarction.

COMPLICATED VS. UNCOMPLICATED MYOCARDIAL INFARCTIONS

Morbidity and mortality in postinfarction patients who have complicated courses are much higher than in those with uncomplicated myocardial infarctions. The criteria for a complicated myocardial infarction are presented in Table 71.5. The most important clinical predictors have been prior myocardial infarction and the presence of congestive heart failure and/or cardiogenic shock. The progressive ambulation program should be delayed until such patients reach an uncomplicated status and then should proceed at a slower than normal pace.

It is possible to assess risk at different temporal points from presentation in the emergency department, through the coronary care unit and predischarge time, and during later follow-up. However, the clinical picture changes over time and a low risk patient can become a high-risk patient and vice versa. This changing risk is partially due to the vicissitudes of the atherosclerotic process, re-formation of thrombus, interventions, and disease–host interactions. For instance, a patient may present with premature ventricular contractions that then can disappear or worsen, chest pain may come and go, the electrocardiogram

TABLE 71.5 CRITERIA FOR CLASSIFICATION OF A COMPLICATED MYOCARDIAL INFARCTION*

Continued cardiac ischemia (pain, late enzyme rise)
Left ventricular failure (congestive heart failure, new murmurs, roentgenographic changes)
Shock (blood pressure drop, pallor, oliguria)
Important cardiac dysrhythmias (premature ventricular contractions greater than six per minute, atrial fibrillation)
Conduction disturbances (bundle branch block, atrioventricular block, hemiblock)
Severe pleurisy or pericarditis
Complicating illnesses
Marked creatine kinase rise without a noncardiac explanation or after thrombolysis

* One or more criteria classify a myocardial infarction as complicated.

may change, or the enzymes may have a late peak. This makes it difficult to classify a patient strictly at high or low risk: it is only the patient's physician who can determine the relative risk, aided by the nursing staff. However, this can lead to a great deal of frustration for the patient and the nurses. Often promises by the physician of discharge from the coronary care unit or other changes signifying progress must be superseded by the day's findings. The progressive steps very often must be adjusted, sometimes even several times in a day.

THE EFFECTS OF BED REST VS. BODY POSITION RELATIVE TO GRAVITY

Are the deleterious hemodynamic effects of bed rest, including decreased exercise capacity, due to inactivity or to the loss of the upright exposure to gravity?[16] Four reasons support the concept that many of these alterations are due to loss of the upright exposure to gravity: (1) supine exercise does not prevent the deconditioning effects of being in bed; (2) there is both less and a slower decline in maximal oxygen consumption with chair rest than with bed rest; (3) there is a greater decrease in maximal oxygen consumption after a period of bed rest measured during upright exercise versus supine exercise; and (4) a lower body positive pressure device decreases the deconditioning effect of bed rest. Thus, early sitting and walking may obviate much of the deterioration in cardiovascular performance, which in the past was iatrogenic secondary to the conservative approach.

EARLY AMBULATION. Patient activity should be regulated according to protocol. Table 71.6 lists the step approach used at Long Beach Veterans Administration Medical Center. The protocol should begin with range of motion exercises and sitting with legs dangling and progress to ambulation and calisthenics. Before the patient is allowed to exercise, the disease process must be stable. There should be no evidence of congestive heart failure, dangerous arrhythmias, or unstable

TABLE 71.6 POST–MYOCARDIAL INFARCTION PROTOCOL: EIGHT LEVELS OF ACTIVITY

Level	Activities	Nursing	Exceptions
I CCU	Strict bed rest Commode vs. bedpan Feed self if can sit up	Complete bed bath (pt. may wash genitalia) *Exercises:* 5 × each bid: exercises 1–4 (see below)	Chest pain DOE Frequent PVCs HR greater than 100 Dizziness Diaphoresis

<2 METs
Teaching: simple explanations of equipment and procedures. Reassurance!

Level	Activities	Nursing	Exceptions
II CCU	Bed rest, up in chair 1 × vs. dangle Bedside commode Feed self	Bed bath; pt. may wash hands, face, genitalia *Exercises:* Passive ROM bid 5 × each bid: exercises 1–5	Chest pain, DOE Frequent PVCs HR greater than 100 Dizziness Diaphoresis

<2 METs
Teaching: if diagnosis known—simple explanation, "You had a heart attack," and the role cardiac rehabilitation team will play in education and increasing activity.

Level	Activities	Nursing	Exceptions
III CCU or Ward	Bed rest—up in chair 20 min tid Bedside commode Meals in chair	Bed bath—pt. may wash hands, face, genitalia *Exercises:* Active ROM all extremities 5 × each bid: Exercises 1–6	Chest pain, DOE Frequent PVCs HR greater than 100 Dizziness Diaphoresis

2 METs
Teaching: restate diagnosis with healing time: 3 months. Activity progression to be slow and steady with attention to pacing convalescence.
Stress: report any cardiac symptoms (*e.g.*, chest, neck, jaw, arm, or abdominal discomfort).

Level	Activities	Nursing	Exceptions
IV Ward	Bed rest—bathroom privileges Up in chair as desired Walk about room	Partial bath (in bed or at sink)—Pt. not to wash back, legs, or feet *Exercises:* Active ROM bid 10 × each bid: 1–6 Add 5 × each bid: 7	Chest pain, DOE HR greater than 110 Frequent PVCs Dizziness Diaphoresis

<3 METs
Teaching: rehabilitation group discussion—family invited.
1. Anatomy and physiology of heart in relation to MI.
2. Convalescent care, activity progression and risk factor management—HBP, diet, activity, smoking, stress reduction.
3. Diet class low sodium and low cholesterol.
Reexplain class information on one-to-one level. Begin medication teaching including use of nitroglycerin.

Level	Activities	Nursing	Exceptions
V Ward	Up in room Walk to TV room and back after warm-up exercises Up in chair	Chair shower *Exercises:* Active ROM bid 10 × each bid 1–7 5 × each bid: exercise 8	Chest pain DOE HR greater than 110 Frequent PVCs Dizziness Diaphoresis

4 METs
Teaching: taking pulse. Explain medications, β-blockers and digitalis (if applicable), action of medications. Reasons for slow, steady activity increase over 3-month period. Report any problems noted as activity increases—(*e.g.*, [1] chest, neck, jaw, arm, abdominal pain, and/or pressure or discomfort; [2] shortness of breath).

Level	Activities	Nursing	Exceptions
VI Ward	Ward ambulation Work toward walking around floor square nonstop (1/6 mile) Start with 1 leg of square—gradually increase pace before distance (12 × around = mile)	Chair shower *Exercises:* 10 × each bid: exercises 1–8	Chest pain DOE HR greater than 110 Frequent PVCs Dizziness Diaphoresis

(Continued on p. 7.210)

angina. Blood pressure should remain within 20 mm Hg of the resting level during exercise, and heart rate should stay within 20 beats per minute of the resting level. If complications arise, the activity should be stopped and later restarted at a lower level. The patient should be able to walk stairs prior to discharge and by the time of discharge should be able to perform activities of daily living independently (3–4 MET level).

A consideration often forgotten when dealing with an older patient or one with complicating illnesses is the level of activity that was maintained prior to the myocardial infarction. If a patient was physically limited prior to the event, the plan for progressive ambulation must be modified. It is unlikely that a patient will be more physically active after myocardial infarction than before, unless activity was previously limited by angina that disappeared.

In addition to the oxygen cost and heart rate achieved during activity, the duration of the activity must be considered. The effect of prolonged exercise on myocardial scar formation has not been carefully studied, but it is known that during prolonged steady-state dynamic exercise heart rate increases, myocardial contractility declines, and left ventricular volume increases. Even though certain levels of exercise can be achieved by a patient, they should not be maintained for long periods of time. Probably the safest recommendation is to tell patients to avoid causing fatigue and to limit the duration of exercise by their fatigue level and perceived exertion.

EXERCISE TESTING BEFORE HOSPITAL DISCHARGE. The exercise test after an acute myocardial infarction has been shown to be safe. When performed prior to discharge, it should be submaximal (5 METs or less and not exceeding a Borg Scale level of 16). Later, when return to full activities is intended, it can be symptom and sign limited. This test has many benefits, including clarification of the response to exercise, determination of an exercise prescription, and recognition of the need for medications or interventions. It can have a beneficial psychological impact on recovery and begins the rehabilitation process. The treadmill test is considered the first step in the out-of-hospital cardiac rehabilitation exercise program. It helps the physician determine whether the patient is adequately medicated and helps in setting the exercise level. If untoward responses are noted, either the medication dosages are adjusted or the patient is considered for cardiac catheterization. In most hospitals, a submaximal target is used for this test although others have used a maximal test in uncomplicated patients. Whether or not this test has prognostic value has been questioned. Meta-analysis has shown that an abnormal exercise capacity or systolic blood pressure response is more predictive of increased risk than 1 mm of ST segment depression (Table 71.7).[17] However, ST segment depression probably indicates increased risk in men not taking digoxin whose resting electrocardiograms do not show extensive damage. The criterion of 2 mm or more of ST segment depression along with symptoms or abnormal hemodynamic responses appears to be useful for identifying high-risk patients who should be considered for cardiac catheterization and revascularization.

RETURN TO WORK AND SEXUAL ACTIVITY. Postdischarge activity recommendations have had little basis for their enforcement. The patient's return to work, driving, and sexual activity have been based on clinical judgments rather than physiologic assessments. These decisions should be based on the consequence of the coronary event (ischemia, symptoms of congestive failure, or dysrhythmias) and the nature of the activities (manual labor vs. desk work, light driving vs.

TABLE 71.6 POST–MYOCARDIAL INFARCTION PROTOCOL: EIGHT LEVELS OF ACTIVITY (Continued)

Level	Activities	Nursing	Exceptions
<5 METs			
Teaching: reinforce activity progression. Do not leave ward unless pushed in a wheelchair (needs ward nurse knowledge to leave ward). No heart patient is to push another patient!			
VII Ward	Ambulate off ward Walk up one flight of stairs with team member	Shower *Exercises:* 10 × each bid: exercises 1–9	Chest pain DOE Frequent PVCs HR greater than 120 Dizziness Diaphoresis
5 METs			
Teaching: review any questions. Stress: treadmill test is not a pass/fail situation.			
VIII	Submaximal treadmill test (5 MET or sign/symptom limited) for discharge. If held in hospital for problems, return to level as indicated. If held in hospital for elective procedure (*i.e.*, angiogram), stress the need to continue warm-up exercises and increase number of times around floor for training walk as in Level VI.		
5 METs			

Exercises for Post-MI Protocols (numbers used above in "Nursing" column)
1. Foot circles
2. Ankle pumps
3. Toe flexion and extension
4. Neck exercises
   a. Head nod, chin on chest, then look to sky
   b. Head tilt: lean left ear to left shoulder, then right ear to right shoulder
   c. Head turn: look to left, then right with chin over shoulder
   d. Five complete head circles, both right and left
5. Quadriceps setting, thigh press with knee locked
6. Shoulder exercises
   a. Shrug both shoulders up toward ears
   b. Move each shoulder in a circle forward and then backward
   c. Lift arms straight up over head until elbow is straight; alternate arms
7. Bring alternate knee to chest
8. Straight leg lifts, alternate legs
9. Side bends

Primary physician is to draw a line down through levels, date, and initial order. Patient may be held at any level. MI Date _____ Highest CK _____

(Composite develped by Barbara Kellerman, RN.)

ROM—range of motion, DOE—dyspnea on exertion, HR—heart rate.

congested freeway driving, sex with an established partner vs. other relationships) as well as the response to the exercise test.

Factors influencing return to work include age, severity of cardiac damage, financial compensation for illness, employer ignorance, termination of employment, and, very importantly, the patient's perception of his health status. Programs that develop a positive attitude and a sense of well-being may facilitate appropriate vocational adjustment in the coronary patient. The physician's attitude also greatly affects return to work; encouragement can be very beneficial.

In regard to sexual activity, the energy expenditure is related to the phase of involvement, the partner, and the position. In general, 4 to 5 METs are required during the orgasmic phase. The safest way to determine the patient's ability to maintain this level is with an exercise test. If a 5- to 6-MET level is achieved without difficulty, sexual activity should be safe to resume. Others believe that once the patient can safely perform the activities of daily living completely and without problem, sexual activity is safe to resume. Restrictions of sex, particularly in the older patient, can lead to a loss of function.

PHASE II: OUT-OF-HOSPITAL CARDIAC REHABILITATION

Hospital admission for an acute myocardial infarction is a stressful experience with a powerful impact. However, hospital discharge can be equally stressful after the patient has relied on the highly protective hospital support systems. Discharge into an uncertain future and to a home and work setting in which one is considered a helpless invalid can be as damaging to one's self-esteem as the acute event itself. The physician is faced with the difficult task not only of supervising the physical recovery of the patient but also of maintaining morale, providing education, helping the family cope and provide support, and facilitating the return to a gratifying life-style.

MEDICAL EVALUATION FOR THE EXERCISE COMPONENT

Not all patients need a formal exercise program, but most patients can benefit in some way from it. Some patients benefit from exercising with a group while others do better by themselves. The approach to each patient must be individualized as each patient's reaction to problems and needs will differ. The following is one approach to assess patients, placing them in a "niche" so one knows how to react to their symptoms, to them, and to their test results.[18] For every clinical situation there are exceptions: there is the high-risk patient who outlives his physician, the patient with barely any myocardium remaining who can run a marathon, and the low-risk patient who dies. Biological systems are complex, and we all continue to learn with each patient we treat.

HISTORY AND PHYSICAL EXAMINATION. The tools for assessment begin with the history and physical examination. The first step in evaluating patients for cardiac rehabilitation is to determine whether their coronary heart disease is stable. The manifestations of the disease that must be considered to be stable or not are myocardial ischemia, congestive heart failure, and dysrhythmias. Patients with ischemia can be symptomatic with classic angina pectoris or anginal variants or their equivalents or be asymptomatic.

The hallmark symptom of ischemia is chest pain. Remember that everyone has chest pains and usually ignores them. Once told about heart disease, the patient's routine pains become very frightening. It is important to separate nonischemic from ischemic chest pains. All chest pains should *not* be called angina pectoris. Angina becomes unstable when it changes its pattern (*i.e.*, occurs more frequently, at rest, or at lower workloads).

Increasing symptoms of congestive heart failure include sudden weight gain, edema in the lower extremities, dyspnea on exertion, and paroxysmal nocturnal dyspnea. Combinations of both ischemia and congestive heart failure are difficult to manage. Ischemia can cause transient congestive heart failure.

If the patient is stable, further assessment can proceed. In general, patients can be divided into those with limited myocardial reserve, those with myocardial ischemia, or those with combinations of both. First, find the ischemic threshold as determined by the onset of angina pectoris or ST segment depression at a particular heart rate, double product, or workload. Once this is clarified, the next evaluation is to determine the amount of mechanical reserve. Mechanical reserve relates to the amount of viable myocardium remaining after ischemic changes. Clinical clues that suggest the patient may not have much myocardial reserve include a history of congestive heart failure, cardiogenic shock, multiple prior myocardial infarctions, a large anterior myocardial infarction, cardiomegaly, a large creatine kinase elevation, multiple Q waves, or underlying problems such as cardiomyopathy or valvular heart disease. These patients must be watched for signs and symptoms of congestive heart failure while ischemic patients usually do not require such observation. They are limited by their maximal cardiac output, which usually cannot be improved. Rather than chest pain, they are limited by fatigue and pulmonary symptoms. However, the symptoms of low output or congestive heart failure should never be left unexplained. In the myocardial infarction patient they could be due to mitral valve insufficiency secondary either to papillary muscle dysfunction or rupture or to a dilated mitral annulus. A rare explanation is a ventricular septal defect due to septal infarction. A second process could be having an effect such as a cardiomyopathy or valvular defect.

In addition to myocardial ischemia and dysfunction, the other key features of heart disease to consider are arrhythmias, valvular function,

TABLE 71.7 RESULTS OF META-ANALYSIS OF THE 24 POST–MYOCARDIAL INFARCTION EXERCISE TEST STUDIES THAT USED FOLLOW-UP FOR CARDIAC EVENTS TO DETERMINE WHICH EXERCISE TEST RESPONSES INDICATE HIGH RISK

	Abnormal Exercise Test Responses				
	Systolic Blood Pressure	Premature Ventricular Contractions	Exercise Capacity	Angina	Segment Changes
No. With Reported Results	14	19	12	15	18
No. With Positive Results*	12	13	12	11	11

* Positive = exercise test response associated with an increased risk ratio for predicting cardiac events.
Adapted from Froelicher V, Marconder G: Manual of Exercise Testing, Year Book Medical Publishers, Chicago, 1989

and exercise capacity. These five features are important because they determine the prognosis as well as the manifestation of symptoms. Patients should be evaluated for these five features for optimal management as well as individualization of their rehabilitation program.

The electrocardiogram, chest roentgenogram, and exercise test are next in importance after a careful history and physical examination. The exercise test is the key to prescribing exercise. Specialized tests including echocardiography, radionuclides, and cardiac catheterization can be used to confirm impressions, clarify incongruous clinical situations, or identify coronary pathoanatomical patterns requiring revascularization. Table 71.8 provides an assessment of the key features of heart disease and the relative value of the various means of assessment.

CONTRAINDICATIONS TO EXERCISE TRAINING

Absolute contraindications are those known or suspected conditions that eliminate the patient from participating in exercise programs. Some of the absolute contraindications are unstable angina pectoris, dissecting aortic aneurysm, complete heart block, uncontrolled hypertension, congestive heart failure, or dysrhythmias, thrombophlebitis, and other complicating illnesses. In some conditions, contraindications are relative; that is, the benefits outweigh the risks involved if the patient exercises cautiously. The relative contraindications include frequent premature ventricular contractions, controlled dysrhythmias, intermittent claudication, metabolic disorders, and moderate anemia or pulmonary disease. If these contraindications are followed, studies show that the incidence of exertion-related cardiac arrest in cardiac rehabilitation programs is small and, because of the availability of rapid defibrillation, death rarely occurs.

OUT-OF-HOSPITAL CARDIAC REHABILITATION

The out-of-hospital programs have taken multiple approaches. In the late 1960s, the Cardiopulmonary Research Institute (CAPRI) program in Seattle was one of the earliest to develop a successful gymnasium-based program. Patients were referred by their private physicians, and community physicians volunteered their time to supervise patients while they exercised. The main thrust of this program was exercise although lectures were given to patients regarding risk factors. The CAPRI program is still very active and has been very successful in the Seattle community.[19] It is partially funded by public donations through the United Fund. The YMCA has been involved in similar programs throughout the United States.

Another approach was taken by Kasch and Boyer in San Diego in conjunction with the physical education program at San Diego State College. In coordination with several nearby hospitals, they launched a "grassy field" exercise program for cardiac patients. Local physicians volunteered their time to supervise the exercise. In both of these programs, defibrillators and drug boxes were available. Local ambulance teams were alerted to when patients would be exercising. Heart rates were monitored along with the electrocardiogram using defibrillators with see-through paddles. Patients were taught to take their own heart rate.

A very successful program using both approaches has been functioning for nearly 20 years at Wake Forest University in North Carolina.[20] This program has been the coordinated effort of an MD–PhD team. Many of these programs began to take advantage of individuals trained in exercise physiology. Coordinating with physicians and nurses, these health care professionals have made a strong contribution to the use of exercise as a therapy for cardiac patients.

In 1972, the publication of the results of the Arley House meeting had a great impact on cardiac protocols.[21] This international cardiac rehabilitation meeting was directed by Hellerstein and Naughton, who were also the principal investigators of the National Exercise and Heart Disease Project. Their protocol included electrocardiographic monitoring during all exercise sessions. This approach spread throughout the United States and has been promoted by commercial companies, which have franchised units either in hospitals or clinics where physicians were readily available. Either telemetry or hard-wiring of patients in groups of 4 to 12 was accomplished via a central station. Bicycles and treadmills were principally used though upper arm devices, and rowing devices have been used as well.

Pollock and colleagues worked closely with surgeons and cardiolo-

TABLE 71.8 EVALUATING THE KEY FEATURES OF HEART DISEASE

Key Features	History	Physical Examination	Chest Radiograph	ECG	Exercise Test	Echocardiogram	Nuclear Cardiology Thallium/RNV		Holter Monitoring	Cardiac Catheterization
Myocardial dysfunction	++++	+++	+++	++	++	+++	++	+++	+	++++
Myocardial ischemia	++++	++	+	+++	++++	+	+++ (with exercise)	++	+	++++
Functional capacity	+++	+++	++	+	++++	++	+	+	+	++
Atrial fibrillation and ventricular dysrhythmias	+++	+++	+	+++	++	+++	+	+	++++	+ (EP for VT +++)
Valvular function	++++	++++	++	+++	++	++++	+	+	+	++++
Cost	*	*	*	*	**	***	***	**	**	****
Risk	*	*	**	*	***	*	**	*	*	****

EP, electrophysiology studies; VT, sustained ventricular tachycardia; RNV, radionuclide ventriculography.

++++, very helpful part of assessment (high yield of information) or high benefit

+, least helpful (low yield of information) or low benefit

****, high cost or risk

*, low cost or risk

Need for test determined by physician assessment of ratio of benefit to cost and risk.

(Adapted from Froelicher VF, Atwood JE: Cardiac Disease. A Logical Approach Considering DRGS. Chicago, Year Book Medical Publishers, 1986)

gists and demonstrated the advantages of exercise training in patients after coronary artery bypass surgery.[7]

DeBusk and colleagues from Stanford University have proposed a totally different approach for the patient with uncomplicated myocardial infarction.[22] These investigators have been advocates of home exercise that is either unmonitored or monitored via telephone. Similar results with this program were reported as compared with more conventional programs. Dennis has now completed a work evaluation study in which patients were randomized to either usual care or to work evaluation, showing that it is cost-effective and safe to return patients to work early after myocardial infarction.[23]

SAFETY

The safety of cardiac rehabilitation has been well documented in the United States. In 1986, Van Camp and Peterson sent questionnaires to 167 randomly selected cardiac rehabilitation centers.[24] These centers reported over 51,000 patients exercised over 2 million hours from January 1980 to December 1984. During this time there were only 21 cardiac resuscitations (three fatal) and eight myocardial infarctions. This amounts to 8.9 cardiac arrests, 3.4 myocardial infarctions, and 1.3 fatalities per million hours of patient exercise. Surprisingly, electrocardiographic monitoring had little influence on complications, suggesting that perhaps this added expense is not necessary. However, appropriate medical personnel must be available to resuscitate the patients who do suffer an untoward event.

MONITORING THE EXERCISE COMPONENT

Only a percentage of patients will require supervised continuous electrocardiographically monitored exercise programs in addition to the counseling services. The major expense of rehabilitation programs is the supervised electrocardiographically monitored exercise portion, which requires trained personnel and expensive equipment. However, programs can take various forms. The program could be informal, involving patient counseling by the primary physician with or without an exercise prescription to be carried out without supervision at home or in a health facility. It could also involve patient counseling by a specialist in the absence of a primary physician. Formal programs can include patient counseling by a primary physician or counseling services plus a supervised exercise prescription without continuous electrocardiographic monitoring, or they can include counseling plus supervised continuous electrocardiographically monitored exercise. The stratification of patients into these groups can be performed using the means described in the patient evaluation. Table 71.9 is a list of the criteria for electrocardiographic monitoring advocated by the American College of Cardiologists/American Heart Association Subcommittee on Cardiac Rehabilitation.[25]

DURATION OF PROGRAM

The exercise prescription and education programs can usually be achieved over a 12-week period and are based on a 3 day per week frequency for 25 to 30 minutes per session at an appropriate intensity. Those identified as high-risk patients should be supervised and/or monitored as prescribed by the physician.

PHASE III: MAINTENANCE OF BEHAVIOR MODIFICATION TO DECREASE RISK

The purpose of phase III of a cardiac rehabilitation program is to prevent recurrence of cardiac events or symptoms and to maintain working capacity. Exercises include activities such as walking, jogging, cycling, or swimming and isotonic arm exercises. The intensity of training is based on the patient's medical and physical status and on the results of an exercise test. The patient can monitor himself during the phase III program through checks of heart rate, rhythm, and symptoms.[10] In many cases, intensity can be adequately monitored by subjective personal assessment including the Borg Scale, but patients should be instructed on how to palpate their pulse. When behavior modification is performed as part of a group with medical supervision, funding for this phase often must be borne by the patient because most types of health insurance do not cover it.

CURRENT CARDIAC REHABILITATION PRACTICED

Hlatky has completed a survey of over 1000 physicians nationwide, including family practitioners, internists, and cardiologists. This survey was similar to surveys accomplished in 1970 and 1979 (Table 71.10).[26] As is evident from these results, the length of hospitalization for an uncomplicated myocardial infarction has decreased. In 1970 approximately 20% of patients had a predischarge exercise test and by 1987 its use had increased to approximately 72%. Coronary angiography is used more often and β-blockers are prescribed in over half the post–

TABLE 71.9 AMERICAN HEART ASSOCIATION/AMERICAN COLLEGE OF CARDIOLOGISTS CRITERIA FOR ELECTROCARDIOGRAPHIC MONITORING DURING CARDIAC REHABILITATION

In the event that the following patients are selected for an exercise program, electrocardiographic monitoring should be included:
1. Severely depressed left ventricular function (Ejection fraction under 30)
2. Resting complex ventricular arrhythmia (Lown type 4 or 5)
3. Ventricular arrhythmias appearing or increasing with exercise
4. Decrease in systolic blood pressure with exercise
5. Survivors of sudden cardiac death
6. Patients following myocardial infarction complicated by congestive heart failure, cardiogenic shock, and/or serious ventricular arrhythmias
7. Patients with severe coronary artery disease and marked exercise-induced ischemia
8. Inability to self-monitor intensity due to physical or intellectual impairment

TABLE 71.10 PERCENTAGE OF PATIENTS UNDERGOING SELECTED PROCEDURES FROM A SURVEY OF OVER 1000 US PHYSICIANS

	Year Performed		
	1970	1979	1987
Myocardial Infarction			
Length of hospital stay for uncomplicated myocardial infarction (days)	21 Hospital 4.5 CCU	14 Hospital 3.5 CCU	9 Hospital 2.5 CCU
Procedure			
Predischarge exercise test	20%		72%
Coronary angiography on patients under 45 years of age		45%	82%
Holter monitoring			43%
Radionuclide exercise test			25%
β-Blockers		35%	72%
Return to activities/work	4 months		2 months

myocardial infarction patients. The time for return to work and full activities has decreased from 4 months after an event in 1970 to 2 months after an event in 1987.

SCIENTIFIC BASIS FOR EXERCISE PROGRAMS IN PATIENTS WITH CORONARY HEART DISEASE

Support for exercise programs in patients with coronary heart disease can be found in the intervention studies evaluating prognosis and changes in pathophysiology.

EFFECT ON MORTALITY AFTER MYOCARDIAL INFARCTION

As shown in Table 71.11, of the 12 studies that have either randomized patients to an exercise program after a myocardial infarction or considered controls, on the average there has been a 23% reduction in death in those patients who were in the exercise program.[27] These results are comparable to other interventions after infarction and give support to exercise as a therapy for patients with coronary heart disease.

CARDIAC CHANGES IN CORONARY HEART DISEASE PATIENTS

An important question has been whether regular exercise as part of cardiac rehabilitation can cause beneficial cardiac changes. Even in severe forms of heart disease, exercise can be effective in improving exercise capacity. The techniques for assessing change during exercise should be effective, since the effects of exercise are most likely to be subtle and only apparent during the stress of exercise. Compliance and adherence continues to be a problem in all exercise programs.

The exercise prescription has been standardized; however, recently a higher intensity has been advocated. The problem with this is that a higher intensity program has a higher complication rate. More impressive results have been reported, but higher intensity levels of training were used in highly selected patients. It would be difficult or dangerous to generalize this approach. The length of programs has been questioned. Reimbursement currently is for 3 months of training after a coronary event. Most likely, it takes longer than that to produce cardiac changes.

MEASURING CARDIAC CHANGES WITH AN EXERCISE PROGRAM

Measurement techniques have included invasive and noninvasive techniques.[27] There have been coronary angiographic studies before and after cardiac rehabilitation, but no changes have been seen in lesions. Respiratory gas analysis techniques have been used to evaluate cardiac rehabilitation. In addition to maximal oxygen consumption, cardiac output can be estimated. These studies have shown an increase in cardiac output at matched submaximal workloads after a training program. Systolic time intervals have been used and supposedly have improved; however, they are such an indirect measurement of myocardial contractility that it is not certain what the changes actually mean. The electrocardiogram has been assessed, and some studies have shown an increase in R wave amplitude, suggesting hypertrophy. This has not been a consistent finding. Studies have looked at ST segment depression during exercise before and after cardiac rehabilitation. There has not been a consistent finding of less ST segment depression at a matched submaximal double product. Echocardiographic studies have been done before and after exercise training, and in general these have only shown an improvement in younger persons with intensive levels of training.

Radionuclide exercise testing has been performed to evaluate cardiac rehabilitation. Its advantages are that myocardial perfusion and ventricular function can be assessed during exercise. Radionuclide ventriculography requires technetium-tagged red blood cells while thallium scintigraphy has been performed to assess perfusion. Newer techniques that have not yet been used to evaluate the changes due to an exercise program include computed tomography, magnetic resonance imaging, and positron emission tomography.

PERFEXT (PERFUSION PERFORMANCE EXERCISE TRIAL)

A randomized trial of the effects of exercise on patients with stable heart disease was performed at the University of California in San Diego.[28] As shown in Figure 71.2, 161 patients agreed to randomiza-

TABLE 71.11 TEN STUDIES COMPARING PATIENTS AFTER MYOCARDIAL INFARCTION IN AN EXERCISE PROGRAM WITH A CONTROL GROUP

Study	No. Patients Studied	Time Post Myocardial Infarction (months)	Years of Follow-up	Mortality (%) Control	Mortality (%) Exercise
Kentala (1972)	298	2	1	22	17
Wilhelmsen and Sanne (1977)	280	3	4	22	18
Kallio (1979)	370	3	2.5	30	22
NEHDP* (1981)	651	12.0	3	7.3	4.6
Ontario (1982)	733	6	4	7.3	9.5
Benysston (1983)	171	1.5	1	6.7	10
Carson (1983)	303	1.5	5	14	8
Vermeulen (1983)	51	1.5	5	10	4
Roman (1983)	193	2	9	5.8	3.6
Marta (1986)	167	1.5	4.5	6.3	7.4
Totals	3217			13.1% (overall average of 23% reduction in mortality)	10.4%

* National Exercise Heart Disease Project

(Froelicher VF: Exercise and The Heart: Clinical Concepts. Chicago, Year Book Medical Publishers, 1987)

tion and then underwent three exercise tests: (1) a treadmill test with maximal oxygen consumption and computerized exercise electrocardiogram, (2) a treadmill test with thallium scintigraphy, and (3) supine bike radionuclide ventriculography. Of 159 patients tested, 11 were found to have normal studies and 2 became unstable. That left 146 patients who were randomized to either training or controls. The exercise prescription was three times a week at 70% to 75% maximal heart rate. After 1 year, both groups returned for repeat testing. Thallium scintigraphy was measured in a meticulous fashion, both visually and by computer. At a double product matched to the pretest maximal double product, there was an improvement in thallium scintigrams only in patients with angina. The radionuclide ventriculography studies were relatively disappointing. There was no change in resting or exercise ejection fraction or percent change in ejection fraction. Fortunately, during the test the legs were kept straight out rather than elevated, so changes in end-systolic volume and end-diastolic volume were detected. In the training group there was less of an increase in end-systolic volume during the exercise test, suggesting that contractility was improved.

Schuler and co-workers, using a low-fat diet and an exercise program for 1 year in 18 patients with stable angina, found the results of the thallium scintigrams to be improved in over half the patients.[29] Cobb and colleagues at Duke University found an increase in ejection fraction at the pretraining maximal workload but no other changes in ejection fraction.[30]

Ehsani and associates have reported more dramatic results in a highly selected group of patients. In 1982, they first presented ten patients, all with asymptomatic exercise-induced ST segment depression.[31] These patients underwent a 12-month intense interval exercise program. The levels of training were higher than those normally used in cardiac rehabilitation. There was a 35% increase in maximal oxygen consumption, less ST segment depression, an increase in R wave amplitude, and echocardiographic changes. These investigators have also reported improvement in radionuclide ventriculography.[32] In addition, they recently reported the amelioration of exercise-induced hypertension in patients with coronary heart disease. However, they defined exertional hypotension as a 10-mm Hg drop in systolic blood pressure. Although there was a control group, it is surprising that such a drop would be reproducible.

CONCLUSIONS

Much of what began under the label of cardiac rehabilitation has now been assimilated into routine care. Indeed, hospital accreditation guidelines specify a multidisciplinary approach, including progressive ambulation for the cardiac patient. Cardiac rehabilitation has redirected interest to humanistic concerns, providing a balance to the emphasis on high technology. The average patient does not require all components of cardiac rehabilitation, but the usual patient can benefit from some of them. There is much scientific information to support the exercise component of cardiac rehabilitation. Analysis of controlled trials reveals similar efficacy to the best medical intervention after myocardial infarction. Physiologic studies support the occurrence of

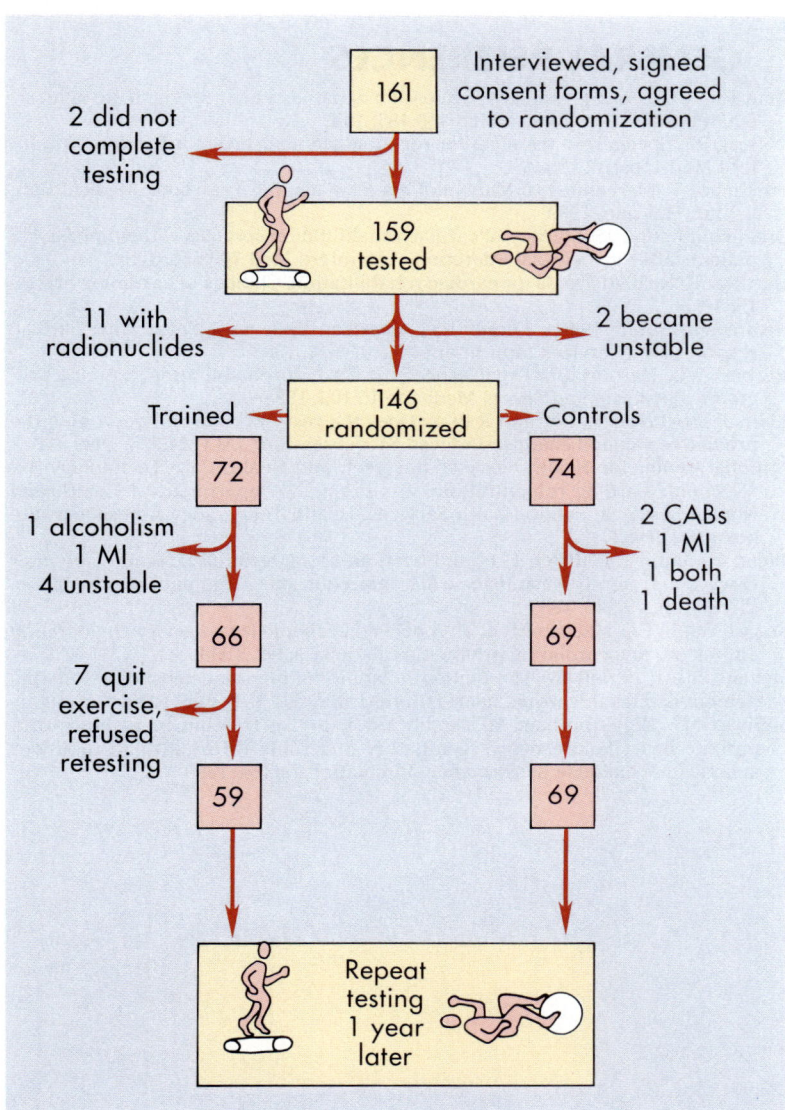

FIGURE 71.2 The design and patient flow in the randomized trial of the effect of exercise on myocardial perfusions and performance in patients with coronary artery disease.

beneficial cardiac changes in a wide range of cardiac patients. The modern physician should consider an exercise program as one viable option in the patient's therapeutic regimen.

There is much evidence to suggest that regular exercise is important for the primary and secondary prevention of coronary heart disease.[33] Unfortunately, this preventive modality is not as widespread as it should be. Fewer than 50% of Americans exercise three times a week for at least 20 minutes, which is the minimal amount confirming a health benefit. It is important that programs designed to increase physical activity document their benefit so that they are appropriately funded. Innovative attempts to increase the use of and compliance to exercise programs should be attempted.[34]

REFERENCES

1. Astrand P, Rodahl K: Textbook of Work Physiology, 2nd ed. New York, McGraw-Hill, 1977
2. Rowell LB, Sheriff DD, Wyss CR et al: The nature of the exercise stimulus. Acta Physiol Scand 128:7, 1986
3. Wasserman K: Anaerobiosis, lactate, and gas exchange during exercise: The issues. Fed Proc 45:2904, 1986
4. Goldman L, Hashimoto B, Cook EF et al: Comparative reproducibility and validity of systems for assessing cardiovascular functional class: Advantages of a new specific activity scale. Circulation 64:1227, 1981
5. Hammond KH, Kelly TL, Froelicher VF: Noninvasive testing in the evaluation of myocardial ischemia: Agreement among tests. J Am Coll Cardiol 5:59, 1985
6. McKirnan DM, Sullivan M, Jensen D et al: Treadmill performance and cardiac function in selected patients with coronary heart disease. J Am Coll Cardiol 3:253, 1984
7. Pollock ML, Schmidt DH (eds): Heart Disease and Rehabilitation, 2nd ed. New York, John Wiley & Sons, 1986
8. Davis JA, Convertino VA: A comparison of heart rate methods for predicting endurance training intensity. Med Sci Sports Exerc 7:295, 1975
9. Borg GA: Psychophysical bases of perceived exertion. Med Sci Sports Exerc 14:377, 1982
10. Gleichmann U: Will there be less need for cardiac rehabilitation programmes when acute treatment is intensified and shortened? Eur Heart J 8:29, 1987
11. Cain HD, Frasher WG, Stivelman R: Graded activity program for safe return to self-care after myocardial infarction. JAMA 117:111, 1961
12. Bloch A, Maeder J, Haissly J et al: Early mobilization after myocardial infarction: A controlled study. Am J Cardiol 34:152, 1974
13. Sivarajan ES, Snydsman A, Smith B et al: Low-level treadmill testing of 41 patients with acute myocardial infarction prior to discharge from the hospital. Heart Lung 6:975, 1977
14. Sivarajan ES, Bruce RA, Aimes MJ et al: In-hospital exercise after myocardial infarction does not improve treadmill performance. N Engl J Med 305:357, 1981
15. Wenger NK, Hellerstain HK, Blackburn H et al: Uncomplicated myocardial infarction. JAMA 224:511, 1973
16. Convertino VA: Effect of orthostatic stress on exercise performance after bed rest: Relation to inhospital rehabilitation. J Cardiac Rehabil 3:660, 1983
17. Froelicher VF, Perdue S, Pewen W et al: Application of meta-analysis using an electronic spread sheet to exercise testing in patients after myocardial infarction. Am J Med 83:1045, 1987
18. Froelicher VF, Atwood JE: Cardiac Disease. A Logical Approach Considering DRGs. Chicago, Year Book Medical Publishers, 1986
19. Hartwig R: Cardiopulmonary research institute—CAPRI. J Cardiac Rehab 2:481, 1982
20. Miller HS, Ribisl PM: Cardiac rehabilitation program at Wake Forest University. J Cardiac Rehab 2:503, 1982
21. Naughton JP, Hellerstein HK, Mohler IC: Exercise testing and exercise training in coronary heart disease. New York, Academic Press, 1973
22. DeBusk RF, Haskell WL, Miller NH et al: Medically directed at-home rehabilitation soon after clinical uncomplicated acute myocardial infarction: A new model for patient care. Am J Cardiol 55:251, 1985
23. Dennis CA, Houston-Miller N, Schwartz RG et al: Early return to work after uncomplicated myocardial infarction: Results of a randomized trial. JAMA 260:214, 1988
24. Van Camp SP, Peterson RA: Cardiovascular complications of outpatient cardiac rehabilitation programs. JAMA 256:1160, 1986
25. Parmley WW: President's page: Position report on cardiac rehabilitation. J Am Coll Cardiol 7:451, 1986
26. Hlatky MA, Cotugno HE, Mark DB et al: Trends in physician management of uncomplicated acute myocardial infarction, 1970 to 1987. Am J Cardiol 61:515, 1988
27. Froelicher VF: Exercise and the Heart: Clinical Concepts, 2nd ed. Chicago, Year Book Medical Publishers, 1987
28. Froelicher VF: The effect of exercise on myocardial perfusion and function in patients with coronary heart disease. Eur Heart J (Suppl G)8:1, 1987
29. Schuler G, Shlierf G, Wirth A et al: Low-fat diet and regular, supervised physical exercise in patients with symptomatic coronary artery disease: Reduction of stress-induced myocardial ischemia. Circulation 77:172, 1988
30. Cobb FR, Williams RS, McEwan P et al: Effects of exercise training on ventricular function in patients with recent myocardial infarction. Circulation 66:100, 1982
31. Ehsani AA, Martin WH III, Heath GW et al: Cardiac effects of prolonged and intense exercise training in patients with coronary artery disease. Am J Cardiol 50:246, 1982
32. Hagberg JM, Ehsani AA, Holloszy JO: Effect of 12 months of intense exercise training on stroke volume in patients with coronary artery disease. Circulation 6:1194, 1983
33. Powell KE, Thompson TD, Caspersen CJ et al: Physical activity and the incidence of coronary heart disease. Ann Rev Public Health 8:253, 1987
34. King AC, Taylor CB, Haskell WL et al: Strategies for increasing early adherence to and long-term maintenance of home-based exercise training in healthy middle-aged men and women. Am J Cardiol 61:628, 1988

GENERAL REFERENCES

American College of Physicians: Evaluation of patients after recent acute myocardial infarction. Ann Intern Med 110:485, 1989
DeBusk RF: Specialized testing after recent acute myocardial infarction. Ann Intern Med 110:470, 1989
Froelicher V, Marcondes G: Manual of exercise testing. Year book Medical Publishing, Chicago, 1989
Greenland P, Chu JS: Efficacy of cardiac rehabilitation services with emphasis on patients after myocardial infarction. Ann Intern Med 109:650, 1988
Hartley LH: Realistic goals for cardiac rehabilitation. Choices in Cardiology 2:214, 1988
Health and Public Policy Committee, American College of Physicians: Cardiac rehabilitation services. Ann Intern Med 15:671, 1988
Herbert WG, Herbert DL: Legal aspects of cardiac rehabilitation exercise programs. Physician and Sports Medicine 16:105, 1988
Klein J, Froelicher V, Detrano R et al: Does the rest ECG after MI determine the predictive value of exercise-induced ST depression? JACC 14:325, 1989
National Center for Health Services Research and Health Care Technology Assessment: Cardiac rehabilitation services. U.S. Department of Health and Human Services, Public Health Services. Health Technology Assessment Reports, 6:1, 1987
Nicod P, Gilpin E, Dittrich H et al: Short- and long-term clinical outcome after Q-wave and non-Q-wave myocardial infarction in a large patient population. Circulation 79:528, 1989
Ross J, Gilpin EA, Madsen EB et al: A decision scheme for coronary angiography after acute myocardial infarction. Circulation 79:292, 1989
Stevenson LW, Perloff JK: The limited reliability of physical signs for estimating hemodynamics in chronic heart failure. JAMA 261:884, 1989
Sullivan MJ, Higginbotham MB, Cobb FR: Exercise training in patients with chronic heart failure delays ventilatory anaerobic threshold and improves submaximal exercise performance. Circulation 79:324, 1989

CHAPTER 72

MANAGEMENT OF THE POSTMYOCARDIAL INFARCTION PATIENT

Nora Goldschlager

Survivors of acute myocardial infarction may be classified into three clinically definable groups with respect to postinfarction course and prognosis: (1) high risk, (2) low risk, and (3) moderate risk. Patients at high risk for cardiac events are those with evidence of left ventricular dysfunction during the acute phase of infarction, continuing myocardial ischemia demonstrated on an exercise test performed prior to hospital discharge, and complex ventricular extrasystolic activity (multiform and/or R-on-T ventricular complexes, bursts, or sustained ventricular tachycardia) demonstrated at the time of hospital discharge by ambulatory electrocardiographic monitoring. This high-risk group of patients constitutes about 20% of all patients admitted to the hospital with acute myocardial infarction, but has a mortality in the first postinfarction year of 20% to 50%.[1-3] Patients at low risk for postinfarction cardiac events in the first 1 to 2 subsequent years are survivors of a first infarction and no evidence of ongoing myocardial ischemia or complex ventricular extrasystolic activity at the time of hospital discharge. These patients comprise about 25% of all patients hospitalized with myocardial infarction and have an annual mortality of only 2% to 5%.[2,3] The remainder, 55% of all patients hospitalized with myocardial infarction, constitute an intermediate group at moderate risk. These patients usually have one or more of the above described features; their mortality in the first postinfarction year is about 10%. In recent years, identification and risk stratification of these clinical groups has received a great deal of attention, with emphasis being placed on reduction of postinfarction morbidity and mortality. The methods by which risk is stratified and the management of the postinfarction patient are described in this chapter.

EXERCISE TESTING

Exercise testing is being used with increasing frequency in patients recovering from myocardial infarction in order to identify those at high risk for subsequent cardiac events so that selection of patients for coronary arteriography and possible myocardial revascularization can have a rational basis. "Cardiac events" have generally been defined as recurrent myocardial infarction, cardiac death (sudden or nonsudden), and the development of unstable angina requiring myocardial revascularization. Exercise testing is a valuable method of assessing "ischemic risk"[4] in survivors of myocardial infarction.

ADVANTAGES

Both patient and physician benefit from the performance of an exercise test at the time of hospital discharge. The first of several advantages is that direct observation of the patient's response to an incremental workload is made by the supervising physician and the degree of patient comfort at a given work level assessed. The development of pallor, sweating, and unsteadiness of gait can be correlated with clinical events such as anginal pain, breathlessness, hypertension, or hypotension, and with electrocardiographic abnormalities, such as ST segment depression or arrhythmias. Correlative data of this nature are not available from other techniques of evaluation of the postinfarction patient: during ambulatory electrocardiographic monitoring, workloads of known intensity are not provided, detailed diaries of activities are not kept, electrocardiographic tracings are often suboptimal for accurate interpretation of ST segment deviations, and blood pressure is not recorded. Blood pressures can be evaluated during various activities by patient-activated portometric techniques; however, complete diaries are required and recording capabilities are often suboptimal, making this a rarely performed procedure.

The motor-driven treadmill is the form of exercise most widely employed in this clinical setting. The test allows the physician the opportunity to analyze 12 electrocardiographic leads. The increased sensitivity for the detection of multivessel coronary artery disease in patients with past myocardial infarction that is gained by multiple, rather than single, electrocardiographic lead monitoring has been documented.[5] Sensitivity can be increased from 55% to over 70% in patients with inferior myocardial infarction and from 40% to about 55% in patients with anterior myocardial infarction.[5] However, the use of multiple electrocardiographic leads for the enhancement of sensitivity for detection of multivessel coronary disease is attended by a decline in both specificity and predictive accuracy of the test. Specificity declines from 96% to 83% in patients with inferior myocardial infarction and from 94% to 67% in patients with anterior myocardial infarction.[5] Predictive accuracy falls from about 97% to 90% in patients with inferior infarction and from 91% to 70% in patients with anterior infarction. Thus, the presence of ST segment deviation alone (specifically ST segment depression) is insufficient to predict a future cardiac event; additional techniques, such as thallium-201 scintigraphy or radionuclide ventriculography, are required to improve predictive capability.

CANDIDATES FOR TREADMILL TESTING

The safety of treadmill exercise testing prior to hospital discharge is well established[6-9] and relates in part to careful selection of patients for the test. Patients who are generally excluded from predischarge exercise testing (Table 72.1) are those who have continuing evidence of myocardial ischemia manifested by anginal pain within a prior 3-day period,[10-12] systolic hypertension equaling or exceeding 150 mm Hg,[12-14] congestive heart failure manifested by an S_3 gallop rhythm and/or pulmonary rales, uncontrolled or poorly controlled atrial or ventricular arrhythmias, and an unstable resting electrocardiogram. Sinus tachycardia at rest and advanced age or sedentary life-style in an elderly patient may also constitute reasons for exclusion. The use of medications, such as digitalis preparations, nitrates, diuretics, β-blocking or calcium channel blocking agents, and antiarrhythmic drugs, does not constitute sufficient reason for exclusion from exercise testing. Similarly, a depressed ejection fraction unassociated with the aforementioned exclusion criteria does not preclude the performance of the test.

It is clear, in view of the above, that stress testing is performed predominantly in patients who are in New York Heart Association Functional Class I or II at the time of hospital discharge. Exclusion from predischarge treadmill testing *per se*, therefore, by virtue of the exclusion criteria, defines a group of patients at high risk for a future cardiac event. In some studies, exclusion from exercise testing has been found to be the strongest predictor of subsequent mortality,[2] correctly predicting 58% of nonsurvivors.

Depending on the particular hospital population, from 40% to 75% of all postinfarction patients are candidates for exercise testing.[9,11,15] Similar percentages of patients with inferior and anterior wall myocardial infarctions, and with transmural and nontransmural myocardial infarctions, are represented in published reports, suggesting that neither the site nor the electrocardiographic extent of myocardial infarction has significant import for functional class at the time of discharge. On the other hand, prior myocardial infarction with consequent left ventricular dysfunction undoubtedly does result in some patient selection bias, since such patients may be more likely to have congestive heart failure, thus excluding them from exercise.

The indications for termination of exercise (Table 72.2) include development of anginal pain, dyspnea, light-headedness, marked fatigue, three or more consecutive ectopic ventricular complexes, systolic hypertension (equal to or exceeding 180 mm Hg), and hypotension (fall in systolic pressure of 10 mm Hg or more). The attainment of a heart rate of 120 to 130 beats per minute and occurrence of significant ST segment depression (2 to 5 mm) have served as indications to terminate exercise in some,[9] but not all, laboratories.[6,11,16]

When these criteria are employed for patient selection and for the indications to stop exercise, serious complications, such as extension of infarction, development of postinfarction unstable angina, and/or sustained ventricular tachycardia or ventricular fibrillation, occur only rarely.

The recently reported results of a large survey of 193 facilities performing over 150,000 submaximal and symptom-limited exercise tests within 1 month of infarction included 41 (0.03%) fatal and 141 (0.09%) major nonfatal (resuscitated cardiac arrest and new myocardial infarction) complications, attesting to the very low risk of this procedure.[17] The overall complication rate was 0.02%, with nonfatal nonsustained ventricular tachycardia being the most commonly encountered problem, occurring in 1,788 of 2,306 complications.[17]

EXERCISE TEST PROTOCOLS

The exercise test protocols employed in patients recovering from acute myocardial infarction vary with the laboratory, but most are designed to provide incremental workloads, whether the exercise involves treadmill or upright or supine bicycle ergometry. The duration of each stage of incremental exercise is usually 2 to 3 minutes.

Exercise test protocols fall into four general categories: heart-rate-limited, workload limited, sign limited, and symptom limited. Heart-rate-limited tests are those that are terminated when a preselected heart rate is reached, regardless of whether electrocardiographic signs and/or symptoms suggesting myocardial ischemia have occurred. In the postinfarction patient, target heart rates are usually in the range of 120 to 130 beats per minute, equivalent to about 70% of age-predicted maximum. Heart-rate-limited stress tests have not been reported to result in complications; however, they are of questionable value in patients who have sinus tachycardia at rest, since such patients often achieve the target heart rate early in the exercise period, leading to test termination at a low workload.

Workload limited stress tests are stopped when a preselected workload (speed and/or grade, or given number of metabolic equivalents [METs]) is achieved, provided that signs or symptoms of myocardial ischemia have not already occurred. In general, the selected workload is low enough to preclude the development of heart rates exceeding 130 beats per minute, yet is high enough to ensure that the patient who is able to achieve it will be able to function reasonably well after hospital discharge. Both heart-rate-limited and workload-limited exercise tests are "submaximal," in that exercise is terminated before a clinical endpoint is achieved.

Sign-limited tests are terminated when signs suggesting the development of myocardial ischemia or significant left ventricular dysfunction occur. These signs include the development of marked ST segment depression; effort-related hypotension; and/or frequent, multiform, or bursts (three or more) of ventricular premature complexes. ST segment depression considered to indicate myocardial ischemia is defined as 1 mm or more of J point depression, with a downsloping or horizontal ST segment configuration (Fig. 72.1). In patients who have ST segment abnormalities at rest, the usual criterion for the ischemic response is an additional 1 mm of downsloping or horizontal depression[11,18]; in patients receiving digitalis preparations, an additional 2 mm is generally required.[13] Despite the widespread use of these criteria, their specificity and predictive accuracy in the clinical setting of recent myocardial infarction are unknown. As discussed subsequently, the low predictive accuracy of ST segment depression for future cardiac events suggests that this electrocardiographic abnormality may in some cases reflect reciprocal changes rather than myocardial ischemia.

A substantial amount of evidence suggests that exercise-induced ST segment elevation occurring in electrocardiographic leads displaying infarct-related Q waves reflects underlying infarct-related ventricular dyssynergy rather than myocardial ischemia (Fig. 72.2).[19–22] Some

TABLE 72.1 CRITERIA FOR EXCLUSION FROM EXERCISE TESTING IN THE POSTINFARCTION PATIENT

Anginal pain within preceding 3 days
S_3 gallop rhythm
Pulmonary rales
Poorly controlled hypertension (systolic blood pressure exceeding 150 mm Hg)
Poorly controlled arrhythmia
Limiting obstructive pulmonary disease
Limiting musculoskeletal disease

TABLE 72.2 INDICATIONS FOR TERMINATION OF EXERCISE TESTING IN THE POSTINFARCTION PATIENT

Symptoms
Anginal pain
Breathlessness
Fatigue
Dizziness
Claudication

Signs
Hypotension (10 mm Hg or greater fall in systolic blood pressure at any time)
Complex ventricular ectopy (doublets, bursts, sustained tachycardia, multiform complexes)
Marked ST segment depression (3 mm or greater ST segment depression compared with baseline electrocardiogram)

Other
Workload of 5 METs achieved
70% of age-predicted maximum heart rate achieved

investigators, however, include ST segment elevation as a criterion of myocardial ischemia in patients with recent myocardial infarction, thus potentially confounding the prognostic information provided by the exercise test results. Yet another type of electrocardiographic response consists of normalization during exercise of baseline T wave inversion. Since the precise meaning of this response is not known, its development does not constitute reason to stop exercise.

Effort-related hypotension is defined as a fall in systolic blood pressure of at least 10 mm Hg. Hypotension can develop after a flat or even a normal blood pressure response has occurred during the early minutes of exercise. Its appearance constitutes reason to terminate exercise immediately, since severe left ventricular dysfunction is a possible underlying cause.[23] Effort hypotension is not infrequently due to excessive preload reduction accompanying antianginal, diuretic, and antihypertensive regimens. In these cases the hypotension is not due to ischemic ventricular dysfunction, but since the differential diagnosis is often difficult, exercise test termination is the safest course; a repeat test may then be performed after medications have been temporarily discontinued.

Finally, the stress test protocol may be a symptom-limited one, in which exercise is continued until limiting symptoms occur, regardless of heart rate or magnitude of ST segment depression. Symptom-limited tests have been safely performed in large numbers of postinfarction patients.[11,15-17] The advantage of a symptom-limited exercise test lies in the potential ability to obtain the greatest diagnostic yield from the test, in terms of maximum achieved heart rate, greatest magnitude of ST segment depression, and highest frequency and complexity of ventricular ectopic activity. Serious ventricular extrasystolic activity and substantial magnitudes of ST segment depression have occurred with equal frequencies in patients achieving heart rates both below and above 130 beats per minute, suggesting that heart rate alone is an insufficient reason to stop the exercise test.[16] Despite these observa-

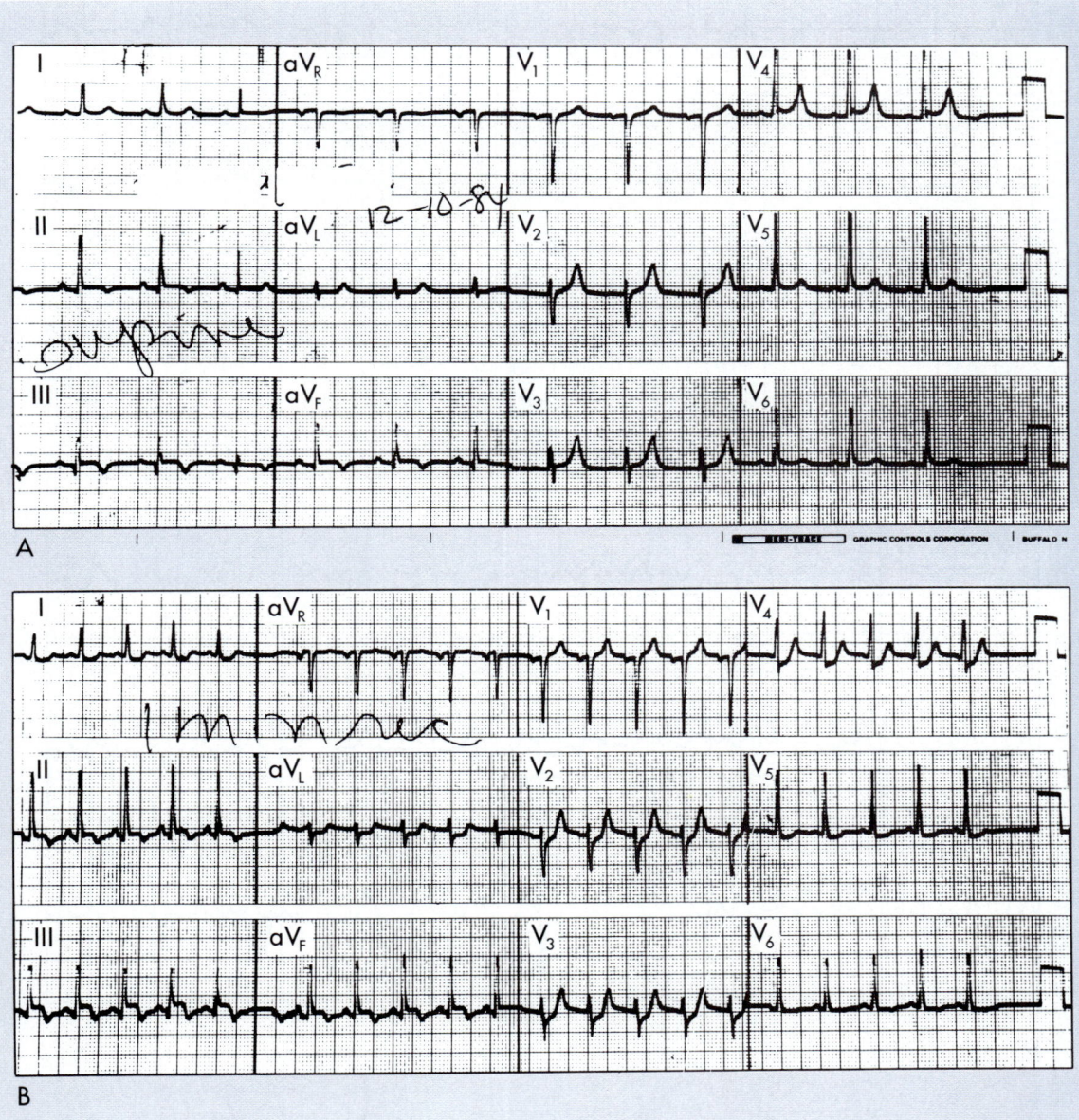

FIGURE 72.1 Resting and exercise 12-lead electrocardiograms from a 63-year-old man recovering from an uncomplicated inferior wall myocardial infarction. **A.** Resting electrocardiogram displays the Q waves and ST segment elevation of the recent inferior infarction. Anterior leads are within normal limits. **B.** At peak exercise, the ST segment elevation in the inferior leads is more pronounced and ischemic-appearing ST segment depression is present in leads I, aV$_L$, and V$_2$ through V$_4$. The patient was asymptomatic throughout the test. Although coronary arteriography (performed because of the abnormal exercise test result) showed significant three-vessel coronary artery disease, scintigraphy using thallium-201 failed to demonstrate myocardial ischemia in areas remote from the infarction. This illustrates the value of scintigraphic methods to enhance the predictive value of the exercise electrocardiogram for postinfarction morbidity and mortality.

tions, it remains to be demonstrated in long-term follow-up studies that symptom-limited tests in fact provide more accurate prognostic information than submaximal exercise test protocols.

From one third to four fifths of patients performing the predischarge exercise test are able to achieve a heart rate equal to 70% of their age-predicted maximum, and 20% to 60% can perform a workload of 5 METs. In symptom-limited tests, angina pectoris occurs in 6% to 15% of patients, hypotension in about 10%, and fatigue in about 30%. That fatigue is not more commonly observed may in part reflect the success of inpatient hospital rehabilitation programs. The most common symptom requiring test termination is breathlessness, which occurs in 60% to 100% of patients. The large range in percentages of patients in each of these categories reflects both the use of different exercise test protocols, in particular symptom-limited versus submaximal tests, and the different subsets of patient populations undergoing the test. For example, patients in functional Class II who are receiving cardioactive medications may be more likely to experience symptoms or to develop signs of myocardial ischemia during exercise, compared with patients in functional Class I who require no medications and who may be more likely to complete the exercise test protocol without problems. In one study,[12] 85% of functional Class I patients who required no medications at the time of hospital discharge were able to perform 9 minutes of exercise, in contrast to the data reported in most other series that include both medicated and unmedicated patients.

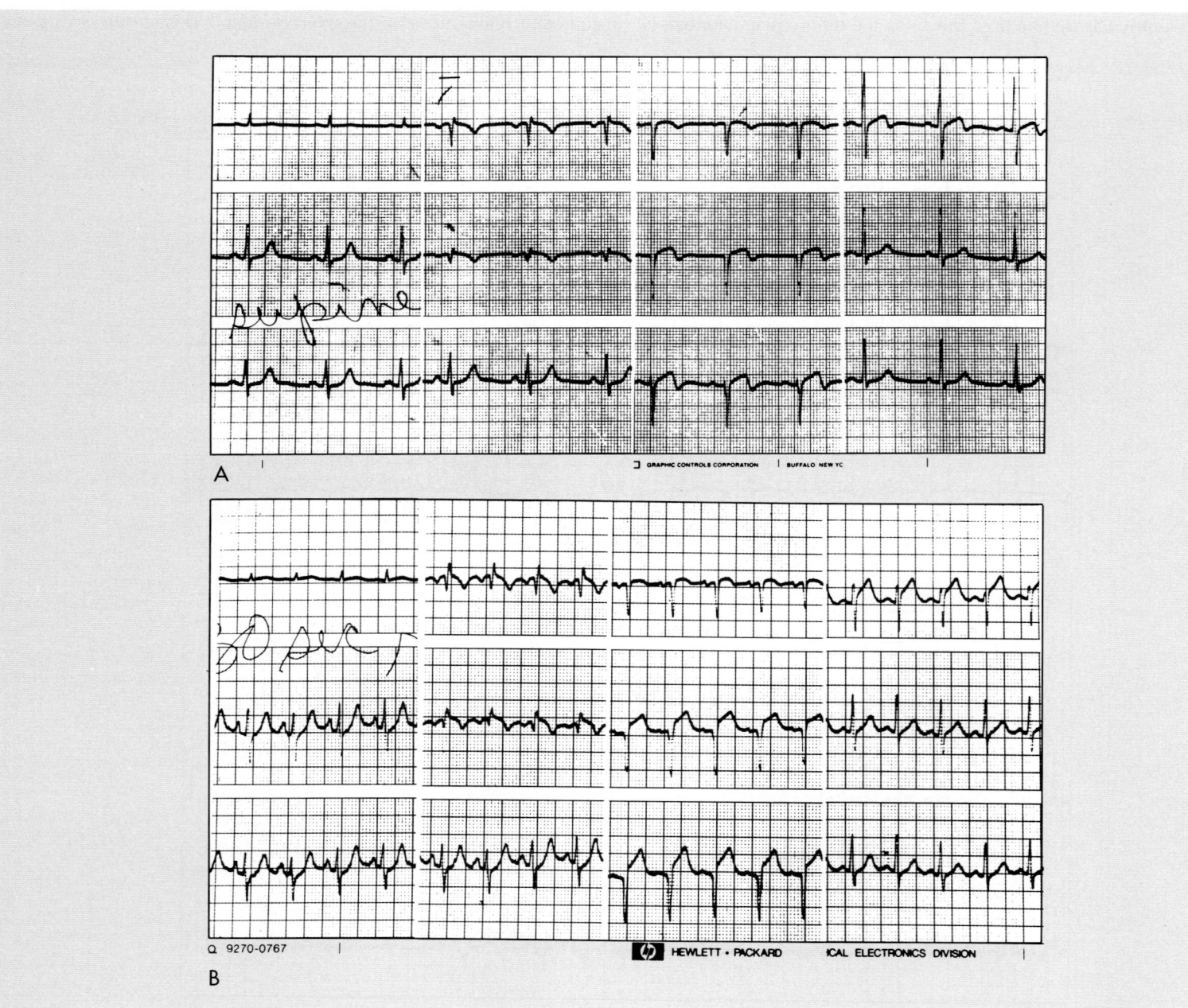

FIGURE 72.2 A. Resting 12-lead electrocardiogram obtained from a 56-year-old man recovering from an acute anterolateral wall myocardial infarction. Q waves and ST segment elevation are present in leads aV_L, V_1, and V_2; ST segment elevation is also present in lead V_3. **B.** A 12-lead electrocardiogram recorded 30 seconds into the postexercise recovery period. The patient completed 9 minutes of treadmill exercise, without developing signs or symptoms suggesting myocardial ischemia. The ST segment elevation in those electrocardiographic leads displaying Q waves of the anterolateral wall myocardial infarction is accentuated, and the T waves have normalized. ST segment depression is not present. Thallium-201 scintigraphy revealed evidence of the anterior wall myocardial infarction but no reversible perfusion defects suggesting remote ischemia. This patient is considered to have a "normal" predischarge exercise test.

The fact that most investigators state that the reasons for stopping exercise are similar in these patient subgroups suggests that some patients receive medications that are not needed.

Electrocardiographic abnormalities, specifically ST segment depression, occur in 25% to 30% of patients. In current practice, many physicians terminate exercise tests if marked (3 to 5 mm) ST segment depression occurs. This prevalence will be increased by performing symptom-limited tests rather than submaximal heart-rate-limited or workload-limited ones. Since both the presence and absence of ST segment depression have importance for the prediction of extent and severity of angiographically demonstrable coronary artery disease and for prognosis, an argument may be made for the routine performance of symptom-limited tests.

Ventricular arrhythmias are observed in 20% to 60% of patients[6,12,24]; salvoes (three or more consecutive ventricular extrasystoles) and multiform ventricular extrasystoles occur infrequently (1% to 2% of patients). Sustained ventricular tachycardia has not been reported. Ventricular fibrillation is extremely rare.[17] It is noteworthy that the frequency of ventricular ectopic activity is similar in heart-rate-limited and symptom-limited exercise tests,[16] suggesting that use of the latter protocol does not reduce the safety of the postinfarction exercise test. On the other hand, in one large survey it was found that nonfatal complications, including ventricular arrhythmias, were significantly greater during symptom-limited tests compared with submaximal tests (0.15% vs. 0.07%); however, the overall complication rate remained extremely low[17] and fatal complication rates were no different using the two protocols.

PROGNOSTIC VALUE OF THE EXERCISE TEST RESPONSE

THE NORMAL TEST

In assessing 1- and 2-year postinfarction prognosis, a normal low level exercise test is as important as an abnormal one. In the original study of Theroux and colleagues,[9] 62% of 210 patients did not develop ST segment depression, angina, hypotension, or significant ventricular arrhythmias. Of these, 54% had a benign postinfarction course over the first year of follow-up; 35% developed stable angina, and 3% had unstable angina; 6% had recurrent myocardial infarction; and 3.2% died. Thus, only 12% of patients with normal predischarge treadmill tests developed serious postinfarction problems (death, recurrent infarction, and unstable angina). This low risk (12% to 15%) for serious postinfarction complications in patients without abnormalities during predischarge treadmill testing has been confirmed by virtually all investigators,[8,10–12] despite the fact that patients are variably managed at the time of exercise and that the results of the test do not always influence subsequent medical management. Especially noteworthy is the low incidence of death from cardiac causes (less than 5%) in the first postinfarction year.[8,9–12,15,25,26]

The proportion of persons undergoing treadmill testing who do not develop abnormalities varies with the patient population and ranges from 40%[11] to over 80%[12]; a higher percentage of "normal" exercise responses may also result from the performance of submaximal, rather than symptom-limited, tests. Nevertheless, the consistency in prognostic capability among various published reports is remarkable; it may be explained by the lesser degree of severity and extent of coronary artery disease that is usually present.

ST SEGMENT DEPRESSION

The prognostic value of ST segment depression developing during treadmill testing after acute myocardial infarction was recognized in the late 1970s; virtually all subsequently published studies have confirmed the initial observations, with rare exceptions.[25] Theroux and colleagues[9] found that 30% of 210 patients undergoing predischarge exercise testing developed ST segment depression. Ten percent of these patients died in an average 1-year follow-up period; 85% of patients who died and 91% who died suddenly had developed exercise ST segment depression. One-year mortality in patients with ST segment depression was 27%, in contrast to a 2% mortality in patients without ST segment depression. The development of angina during stress testing did not add to the prognostic value of ST segment depression alone, an observation that has also been made by other investigators.[27] Sami and co-workers[10] followed 144 patients after myocardial infarction, of whom 33% developing ST segment depression died and 11% had recurrent infarction, compared with 0% and 6% incidences of these complications, respectively, in patients who did not develop ST segment abnormalities.

Since major morbidity (specifically, recurrent myocardial infarction) and mortality are not especially frequent in the early follow-up of post-infarction patients who qualify for predischarge exercise testing on the basis of their low risk, the development of ST segment depression has a low overall predictive accuracy for these events. Nevertheless, patients with ST segment abnormalities occurring in this clinical setting warrant close attention. The issue of whether to treat such patients with nitrates and/or β-blocking agents in order to prevent or reduce the ischemic response is unresolved, and no standard management regimens are currently employed. Similarly, the roles of early coronary angiography and myocardial revascularization in this patient group are not defined.

The use of a symptom-limited treadmill test protocol,[16] rather than a submaximal heart-rate-limited one, has demonstrated the value of marked ST segment depression (equal to or exceeding 2 mm) as having greater predictive value for major cardiac events than ST segment depression of less than 2 mm; the risk for recurrent infarction or death in the first 2 postinfarction follow-up years has been reported at 40% in the former and at 25% in the latter electrocardiographic category. In view of these observations, and in contrast to earlier studies, there appears to be a trend toward allowing postinfarction patients to complete the treadmill test protocol regardless of the magnitude of ST segment depression that develops.

Since the predictive accuracy of an abnormal ST segment response developing during exercise for major cardiac events is at most only about 25% and is considerably less in some series,[11,25,28] it seems rational to attempt to refine exercise test responses in order to achieve a higher predictive accuracy, enabling attention to be focused on the patient at higher risk. To this end, nuclear imaging techniques have been used along with exercise electrocardiography to assess the relationship between ST segment deviation and amount and location of "jeopardized" myocardium, that is, myocardium that is supplied by a stenosed coronary artery and is therefore at risk for ischemia or infarction.

VENTRICULAR ARRHYTHMIAS

The significance of exercise-induced ventricular arrhythmias in postinfarction patients is not entirely clear and remains controversial. The reported incidence of any ventricular arrhythmias (complex and noncomplex) developing during predischarge stress testing ranges from 15% to 56%; many patients developing ventricular arrhythmias are receiving antiarrhythmic (including β-blocking) medications at the time of the treadmill test, and others are placed on these agents as a direct consequence of the test results.[24] Thus, the natural postinfarction course of these patients might be altered significantly. The highest reported prevalence of exercise-related ventricular arrhythmias (56%) occurred in a group of asymptomatic patients who were receiving no medications at hospital discharge and thus represented a patient population free of peri-infarction complications.[12] It is reasonable to assume that either these patients achieved a higher workload than others or that the prognostic significance of ventricular arrhythmias varies with functional class.

As indicated previously, cardiac death within a short follow-up period is not especially common in patients qualifying for postinfarction exercise tests. Thus, the predictive accuracy for any one, or combination of, exercise test variable(s), including ventricular arrhythmias, is necessarily low. However, it does seem that exercise-induced ventricular arrhythmias are not closely associated with subsequent death, in contrast to the occurrence of ST segment depression. It is not surprising that a poor correlation between exercise ventricular arrhythmias and cardiac death exists when one considers that candidates for treadmill exercise after myocardial infarction do not have evidence of significant left ventricular dysfunction. In contrast, a much clearer relationship between ventricular arrhythmias and subsequent cardiac death has been established in patients with poor left ventricular function (who are excluded from predischarge exercise testing) using both ambulatory electrocardiographic monitoring and radionuclide techniques.[27]

In view of the uncertain predictive ability of exercise-related ventricular arrhythmias for subsequent cardiac events, the issue of whether to administer antiarrhythmic agents to patients in whom they occur may legitimately be raised. Although common sense might dictate antiarrhythmic treatment, recognition should be given to the ongoing controversy surrounding the issue of reproducibility of exercise-related ventricular arrhythmias, as well as to the problems in establishing valid criteria by which to assess response to such therapy. Finally, the relationship (or lack thereof) between the presence and type of ventricular arrhythmia and the threshold for sustained ventricular tachycardia or ventricular fibrillation must be appreciated, since therapeutic serum levels of antiarrhythmic agents may raise the latter without appreciably influencing the former.

BLOOD PRESSURE ABNORMALITIES

Effort-related hypotension in the postinfarction patient (≥ 10 mm Hg fall in systolic blood pressure or failure of systolic pressure to increase by at least 10 mm Hg) is an ominous finding that suggests the presence of underlying left main, severe left anterior descending, and/or three-vessel coronary artery disease, with significant left ventricular dysfunction.[23] It often occurs in patients who have reduced effort tolerance and who develop anginal pain, dyspnea, and/or ST segment depression during exercise. Asymptomatic patients requiring no medication at the time of hospital discharge have not been reported to develop exercise hypotension. Effort-induced hypotension occurs in predischarge exercise tests with a frequency of 10% to 25%.[11,15,28] Its relative rarity might reflect the good functional class of the patients undergoing postinfarction treadmill testing, despite the fact that severe multivessel coronary disease is often present in such patients.

Starling and colleagues[11] have addressed the prognostic value of an "inadequate" blood pressure response to postinfarction stress testing, defined as less than or equal to 10 mm Hg increase or greater than or equal to 20 mm Hg decrease in systolic-pressure or failure to achieve a peak systolic pressure during exercise exceeding 140 mm Hg. Of 130 patients exercised, 13% had an inadequate blood pressure response. Subsequent cardiac death, recurrent infarction, or development of unstable angina occurred in 38% of the 130 patients, of whom over 60% had an abnormal blood pressure response to exercise. The prediction of cardiac death during a 6- to 20-month follow-up period was enhanced by adding the abnormal blood pressure response to other manifestations of myocardial ischemia (ST segment depression and angina); however, cardiac death occurred so infrequently that the combination of variables failed to improve the predictive accuracy for death above 30%.

Fioretti and co-workers[2] found that failure to achieve a rise in systolic blood pressure of at least 45 mm Hg during exercise was the most sensitive predictor of mortality among all measured exercise test variables in 167 patients undergoing predischarge exercise testing, occurring in all nonsurvivors of infarction followed to 14 months. Risk stratification for mortality was developed by these investigators on the basis of exercise blood pressure response, with 13% and 2% mortality, respectively, in patients achieving less than or more than 30 mm Hg rise in systolic pressure. Similarly, Krone and colleagues[25] described incidences of death or recurrent infarction of 18% and 16%, respectively, in patients unable to achieve an exercise systolic pressure of at least 110 mm Hg, compared with 3% and 7% incidences, respectively, of these events in patients with higher achieved blood pressures.

In evaluating blood pressure response to exercise testing, the potential contributing role of long-acting nitrate preparations, of β-blocking and calcium channel blocking medication, and of antihypertensive therapy must be taken into account. In such patients, valid prognostic statements cannot be made from blood pressure response alone, but should be reserved for patients demonstrating other criteria for myocardial ischemia.

Whereas exercise hypotension has definite importance for postinfarction course and prognosis, hypertension developing during the stress test does not appear to have similar prognostic value. However, the demonstration of effort hypertension is of great clinical value in that antihypertensive therapy may be begun in an effort to lower myocardial oxygen demand in postinfarction patients performing a given level of work.

ANGIOGRAPHIC CORRELATIONS

Since exercise test responses after myocardial infarction have prognostic significance for major cardiac events, and since major cardiac events reflect underlying coronary artery anatomy and extent of left ventricular dysfunction, treadmill test results not unexpectedly have predictive value for coronary arteriographic findings. Coronary and left ventricular cineangiography have been performed around the time of hospital discharge by several laboratories, and the findings have been related to the exercise test responses.[13,14,29,30] In some series, a "normal" exercise test was associated with a very high prevalence of single-vessel coronary disease,[13,29] whereas in others the prevalence of single-vessel disease was essentially the same as that for multivessel disease.[14,30] However, patients developing symptoms or signs of myocardial ischemia virtually all have been found to have severe multivessel coronary artery disease.[13,29,30] The ability to define noninvasively the patient who, despite being in functional Class I or II, has a high probability of severe coronary disease and might therefore be at risk for subsequent cardiac death or recurrent infarction validates the use of the predischarge exercise test as a prelude to further investigative studies, such as coronary angiography.

OTHER EXERCISE RESPONSES

Although ST segment depression, hypotension, and ventricular arrhythmias have received the greatest attention as variables that have prognostic power for postinfarction course, other predictive responses that deserve mention include inability to complete 6 minutes of exercise[28] and inability to complete a given workload. Observations such as these are protocol dependent, however, since only in symptom-limited tests will such data be valid.

REPRODUCIBILITY OF TEST RESULTS

A paucity of information exists evaluating the reproducibility of exercise test results in postinfarction patients, despite the fact that decisions as to whether to proceed with coronary arteriography and possible myocardial revascularization are made on the basis of these results.[31,32]

In one study of patients exercised at the time of hospital discharge and again 6 weeks later,[31] ST segment depression was a reproducible finding, whereas ST segment elevation, abnormal blood pressure response, ventricular arrhythmias, and anginal pain were not. These observations can perhaps be explained by the fact that half the patients were receiving changing regimens of cardioactive medications during the specified time period and perhaps also by the natural history of the exercise response in postinfarction patients, which is only now beginning to be appreciated.

In another study,[32] unmedicated patients were exercised in the morning and in the evening over a 2-day period. For similar workloads and achieved rate-pressure products, ST segment depression was reproducible in only 57% of patients, ST segment elevation in 71%, anginal pain in 40%, and both ventricular arrhythmias and inadequate blood pressure response in none. The reasons for the lack of reproducibility of results of exercise tests performed within such a short period of time are not immediately clear but might reflect changes in coronary vasomotor arterial tone.

Senaratne and colleagues, in their study of 518 patients undergoing low-level bicycle exercise testing at hospital discharge followed by maximal exercise testing 6 to 8 weeks later, found that absence of symptoms and/or abnormal ST segment responses and blood pressure changes predicted continued absence in over 90% of patients (Fig. 72.3)[33]; in contrast, presence of these abnormalities during the predischarge test did not predict their continued presence 2 months later. Thus, patients at risk for a cardiac event will be identified at the predischarge exercise test. In this report, combining the results of the two exercise tests to assess the occurrence or nonoccurrence of a cardiac event in the first postinfarction year enhanced predictive value of the initial test by only 5%, to 75%. These investigators suggested that the predischarge exercise test alone provides the capability for prognostic stratification in most postinfarction patients, unless new clinical circumstances or work-related requirements dictate otherwise.

It should be recognized that some authorities now advocate that symptom-limited exercise testing be performed 3 weeks after infarction.[34] The risk of waiting seems to be small, particularly in low-risk patients.

APPLICATIONS OF NUCLEAR IMAGING TECHNIQUES

THALLIUM-201 SCINTIGRAPHY

The predictive value of stress electrocardiography for death or recurrent infarction in the first 1 or 2 postinfarction years is only about 25%. The addition of nuclear imaging techniques to the predischarge stress test can enhance the sensitivity for the diagnosis of myocardial ischemia and can localize ischemia to areas of myocardium subserved by specific coronary arteries, information that is not available from stress electrocardiography. Of equal importance to identifying and localizing myocardial ischemia, myocardial imaging techniques can improve the clinician's ability to define patients at low risk for a subsequent cardiac event even if the exercise electrocardiogram is abnormal.

Currently, only thallium-201 can be used reasonably easily in conjunction with treadmill testing. The measurement of rest and exercise ejection fractions, ventricular end-diastolic and end-systolic volumes, and regional wall motion disorders using intravascular isotopes can be performed easily only in patients performing supine or upright bicycle ergometry, a form of exercise not comparable to upright walking exercise.

The use of predischarge thallium-201 stress scintigraphy in postinfarction patients has been evaluated by Turner and colleagues[14] in patients subsequently having coronary arteriography. In this study, the sensitivity of scintigraphy for detecting multivessel coronary disease was found to vary with the severity of luminal obstruction, being only 20% for vessels with less than 70% obstruction, but 63% for vessels with more than 70% luminal narrowing.[14] Similar dependency of sensitivity on the severity of coronary disease was found for stress electrocardiography, in which sensitivities of 40% and 56% were present in patients having less or more than 70% luminal obstruction, respectively. In addition to these correlations, the ability of stress scintigraphy to detect presence and location of "jeopardized" myocardium (areas of noninfarcted myocardium supplied by stenotic coronary arteries) was assessed, rather than the presence of multivessel coronary disease per se. The sensitivity of an "ischemic" electrocardiographic response to the stress test and/or a reversible perfusion defect for both detection of multivessel coronary disease and jeopardized myocardium exceeded 80%. The specificity of stress scintigraphy for detecting multivessel coronary disease was 84%. Although this investigation did not assess postinfarction prognosis, it did demonstrate that stress scintigraphy is capable of identifying postinfarction patients who have normal or equivocal electrocardiographic responses to exercise who nevertheless have severe multivessel coronary disease that caused ischemia in areas of myocardium remote from the infarction. These findings have been corroborated by others.[35] The capability of defining subgroups of patients who are at differing risk for postinfarction complications is especially important, since by design the predischarge treadmill test is usually submaximal. Stress scintigraphy might be particularly recommended in patients receiving digitalis preparations and/or β-blocking agents, as in the one case valid electrocardiographic interpretation for myocardial ischemia is precluded, and in the other, target heart rate, albeit submaximal, is often not achievable.

In addition to demonstrating fixed (infarction) and reversible (ischemia) perfusion defects in areas of myocardium supplied by significantly stenosed coronary arteries, thallium-201 stress scintigraphy may also suggest the presence of clinically unsuspected left ventricular dysfunction by demonstrating increased pulmonary uptake of the isotope during exercise.[36] Gibson and co-workers[37] found that patients recovering from acute myocardial infarction who exhibited lung uptake during exercise had greater impairment of effort tolerance; higher prevalences of exercise-related fatigue, dyspnea, angina,

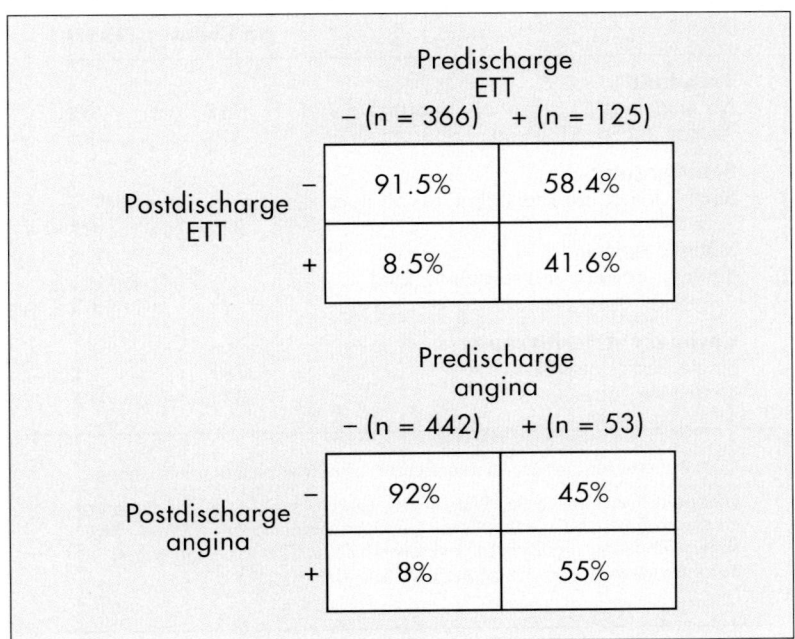

FIGURE 72.3 Comparison of results of submaximal (bicycle) exercise tolerance tests (ETTs) performed around the time of hospital discharge and maximal, symptom-limited tests performed 6 to 8 weeks later in patients after myocardial infarction. **A.** Comparison of ST segment and T wave abnormalities. The vast majority (91.5%) of patients who did not develop these electrocardiographic abnormalities on the predischarge test did not develop them during the maximal test. In contrast, 58.4% of patients with an ischemic response on the predischarge test had a normal response during the maximal test. **B.** Comparison of frequency of angina. The majority (92%) of patients not manifesting angina on the predischarge test remained free of angina on the maximal test, whereas almost half of those developing this symptom during the low-level test failed to demonstrate it during the maximal test. The diagrams indicate that patients with a "normal" predischarge exercise test are not likely to develop an abnormal one and that a single predischarge exercise test is adequate to identify this low-risk group. They also indicate that roughly half the patients with an "ischemic" response to predischarge exercise will have a normal test at a future date. Thallium-201 scintigraphy could perhaps better identify these subgroups. (Modified from Senaratne MPH, Hsu L, Rossall RE, Kappagoda T: Exercise testing after myocardial infarction: Relative values of the low level predischarge and the postdischarge exercise test. J Am Coll Cardiol 12:1416, 1988)

and/or ST segment depression; greater numbers of perfusion defects; and lower resting ejection fraction than those not demonstrating this phenomenon.

The ability of stress scintigraphy to localize areas of jeopardized myocardium remote from the site of the infarction has direct import for the meaning of the electrocardiographic criteria for myocardial ischemia in the postinfarction patient. The low predictive value of the electrocardiographic "ischemic response" for subsequent cardiac events based on exercise-induced ST segment depression alone must result from the lack of specificity of this abnormality for actual ongoing ischemia. ST segment depression in electrocardiographic leads remote from the acute infarction may therefore represent a reciprocal change rather than continuing ischemia, thus accounting for the benign postinfarction course in most patients with this electrocardiographic response. Stress scintigraphy is a method by which the actual significance of exercise-induced ST segment depression can be assessed: if reversible regional perfusion defects in areas remote from the infarction are demonstrated, ongoing ischemia is present; if reversible perfusion defects are absent, the electrocardiographic abnormalities are likely to represent reciprocal changes. Thus, stress scintigraphy should not only enhance the ability to detect ongoing ischemia but also should document its absence, thus refining the criteria for low-risk subgroups within the postinfarction population undergoing predischarge stress testing.

Gibson and co-workers[37] have addressed this issue by prospectively relating postinfarction course over an average follow-up period of 15 months to the results of treadmill testing (heart rate limited at 120 beats per minute), quantitative thallium-201 scintigraphy, and coronary angiography, with the specific intent of defining patients at high and low risk for subsequent death, recurrent infarction, or development of severe angina (Table 72.3). The study results clearly suggested that patients at low risk for these events were those with only a single regional perfusion defect, no redistribution of isotope over time, and absence of lung uptake, whereas patients at high risk for a subsequent event had multiple perfusion defects and/or pulmonary uptake of thallium-201.[37] Importantly, thallium-201 scintigraphy discriminated between low- and high-risk subgroups of patients better than did either stress electrocardiography or coronary arteriography, owing to the imperfect specificity of the former and to the anatomical, rather than the functional, nature of the latter (see Table 72.3); thus, the correct classification of low-risk patients may be enhanced without failing to identify those at higher risk.

Although this approach is more costly than exercise electrocardiography alone, the potential benefits to the long-term management of the postinfarction patient may justify this additional procedure. At the present time, the value of thallium-201 scintigraphy in submaximal exercise tests is not established in all laboratories and further studies are clearly warranted.

Unlike stress electrocardiography the relationship of stress scintigraphy performed at the time of hospital discharge to a maximal exercise test performed later in the postinfarction course has not been explored in depth. It is possible that serial stress scintigrams might improve the predictive accuracy for events, such as postinfarction angina and recurrent myocardial infarction, but not necessarily for development of congestive heart failure or arrhythmia-related sudden death.

EXERCISE RADIONUCLIDE VENTRICULOGRAPHY

The role of radionuclide ventriculography as an adjunct to exercise (supine or upright bicycle ergometry) has been evaluated as a method of improving the predictive accuracy for cardiac events in postinfarction patients.[38-41] Radionuclide ventriculography provides direct information on right and left ventricular function at rest and during exercise by measurements of end-diastolic and end-systolic volumes and ejection fractions at various stages of exercise. The appearance of reversible regional wall motion abnormalities reflecting areas of myocardium that are ischemic during exercise ("jeopardized") provides indirect evidence of perfusion abnormalities. The ratio of arterial pressure to end-systolic volume, a measurement considered to represent an index of myocardial function independent of loading conditions on the ventricle, can also be obtained.

Corbett and colleagues[39] assessed the sensitivity, specificity, and predictive value of predischarge exercise radionuclide ventriculography for the occurrence of death, recurrent infarction, congestive heart failure, and/or angina severe enough to require myocardial revascularization (Table 72.4). They found a substantially enhanced predictive value of this technique over exercise alone, especially for death and recurrent infarction. Significant differences between patients sustaining a major cardiac event and those remaining event free were (1) a lower resting ejection fraction (44% vs. 66%); (2) a lower peak exercise ejection fraction (37% vs. 76%), the exercise endpoint being ischemia, arrhythmias, angina, or attainment of a heart rate of 130 beats per minute; (3) a greater number of regional wall motion abnormalities; (4) higher resting end-diastolic and end-systolic volumes; (5) higher peak exercise end-systolic volume; and (6) subnormal increase in pressure-volume index with exercise. In general, therefore, patients who remained event free had a higher ejection fraction and more normal ventricular volumes, whereas patients who suffered a cardiac event had more severely compromised left ventricular function. The most severely depressed left ventricular performance during exercise was generally found in patients with anterior transmural myocardial infarction[40] compared with inferior transmural infarction or nontransmural infarction of either anterior or inferior walls, although exceptions were common and ventricular performance was not entirely predictable from location or extent of infarction. Importantly, predischarge left ventricular function during exercise was not predicted from clinical variables, such as prior myocardial infarction or congestive heart failure or by exercise test variables widely used to indicate myocardial ischemia (ST segment depression, angina, and achieved workload). Similar overall results have been reported by others[41] performing exercise radionuclide ventriculography 1 month after hospital discharge, rather than prior to it.

Experience with exercise radionuclide ventriculography has been somewhat limited, despite the improvement in predictive accuracy for

TABLE 72.3 COMPARISON OF EXERCISE ELECTROCARDIOGRAPHY, STRESS SCINTIGRAPHY, AND CORONARY ARTERIOGRAPHY IN ASSESSMENT OF POSTINFARCTION PROGNOSIS

	No Event	Event*
Treadmill		
No angina or ST segment abnormalities	74%	26%
Angina and/or ST segment abnormalities	51%	49%
Scintigraphy		
Single defect, no redistribution, no lung uptake	94%	6%
Multiple defects	38%	62%
Multiple defects, redistribution, lung uptake	14%	86%
Coronary Arteriography		
Single vessel disease	78%	22%
Multivessel disease	53%	47%

* Death, recurrent myocardial infarction, or severe postinfarction angina.

(Adapted from Gibson RS, Watson DD, Craddock GB et al: Prediction of cardiac events after uncomplicated myocardial infarction: A prospective study comparing predischarge exercise thallium-201 scintigraphy and coronary angiography. Circulation 68:321, 1983)

occurrence of subsequent cardiac events. This is due in part to logistical considerations. However, other considerations include the fact that myocardial ischemia as the cause of abnormal ventriculographic responses to exercise must be inferred, rather than directly ascertained; moreover, the patient must perform sufficient cardiopulmonary stress to result in myocardial ischemia, a requirement that may not be met during bicycle exercise.

RIGHT ATRIAL PACING

The percentage of postinfarction patients who are not candidates for exercise testing ranges from 30% to 70%, depending on the specific patient population.[7,8,10,11,42] In order to identify the ischemic response as well as to develop criteria for postinfarction rehabilitation and/or further diagnostic study in this group of patients, right atrial pacing has been employed[43-45]; its predictive value for recurrent myocardial infarction or death is reported to be similar to that of treadmill exercise testing. Perhaps the best use of postinfarction atrial pacing is in patients who for various reasons cannot or should not perform exercise (see Table 72.1). However, since these patients constitute a high-risk group in which mortality in the first postinfarction year exceeds 20%[1-3] and the annual mortality exceeds 10%, the use of any form of exercise test to identify such persons is possibly redundant.

Recently, thallium-201 imaging in combination with intravenous dipyridamole has been employed in postinfarction patients[46]; results are encouraging but are preliminary.

RESTING EJECTION FRACTION

Prognosis after myocardial infarction is directly related to the degree of left ventricular dysfunction, which reflects the extent of myocardial necrosis, and to the amount and functional state of remaining myocardium. It has been recognized for some years that clinical signs suggesting left ventricular dysfunction, such as congestive heart failure and an S_3 gallop, indicate a poor postinfarction prognosis. However, the predictive power of the presence of such signs for a cardiac event is variable, and, more importantly, the predictive power of the absence of such signs for a benign postinfarction course is poor.

The development of radionuclide ventriculography has allowed assessment of left ventricular ejection fraction at the time of hospital discharge and is considered by some to represent the variable most predictive of survival in patients with ischemic heart disease.[47] The resting ejection fraction is reasonably well correlated with clinical and radiologic evidence of congestive heart failure, but is poorly correlated with radiographic estimation of heart size, especially if heart size appears normal. Importantly, significant pulmonary congestion or pulmonary edema occurring in the coronary care unit during the acute phase of myocardial infarction does not predict a markedly depressed predischarge ejection fraction; up to 30% of such patients may have a normal ejection fraction at the time of hospital discharge.[48] The relationship of ejection fraction to electrocardiographic and enzymatic indices of infarct size is variable and depends on whether prior myocardial infarction has occurred; whether right ventricular myocardial infarction, contributing to enzyme rise, but not necessarily to size of left ventricular infarction, is present; and whether the myocardial infarction is transmural or nontransmural (which itself may be masked by prior infarction). In this regard, most transmural infarctions associated with Q waves on the electrocardiogram produce segmental wall motion abnormalities; the extent and severity of these areas of regional dyssynergy contribute directly to overall, or global, ejection fraction. Most major wall motion disorders (akinesis or dyskinesis) are associated with anterior wall myocardial infarction, and in patients with such abnormalities the ejection fraction usually does not change over time.

A subgroup of patients with myocardial infarction has been identified in whom pulmonary edema is present initially, but in whom the ejection fraction determined at the time of hospital discharge is normal.[48,49] Patients with these disparate findings are not rare and may constitute up to one third of all patients presenting with pulmonary edema and acute myocardial infarction.[48] The first-year mortality in this patient group is about 20%, lower than the 25% to 45% first-year mortality in patients with both pulmonary edema and depressed ejection fraction, but considerably higher than the 5% mortality in patients with no pulmonary edema and a normal predischarge ejection fraction. The explanation offered for these observations is that large amounts of myocardium are ischemic at the time of infarction; these areas then recover sufficiently to result in a normal ejection fraction. Recurrent ischemia in these jeopardized areas of myocardium is the cause of the poor prognosis.

Nicod and co-workers in a study of 972 patients[50] have extended these observations by dividing patients with and without clinical and radiographic signs of left ventricular failure during hospitalization into

TABLE 72.4 EXERCISE RADIONUCLIDE VENTRICULOGRAPHY IN POSTINFARCTION PATIENTS: RELATIONSHIP TO SUBSEQUENT CARDIAC EVENTS*

Finding	Sensitivity	Specificity	Predictive Accuracy
Stress electrocardiogram indicating ischemia	46%	67%	26%
No increase in ejection fraction with exercise	97%	90%	56%
New area of myocardial dyssynergy during exercise	80%	90%	46%
Increase in end-systolic volume with exercise	94%	93%	54%
Less than 35% increase in ratio of arterial pressure to end-systolic volume with exercise	100%	87%	57%

* Death, recurrent myocardial infarction, congestive heart failure, refractory angina.
(Data from Corbett JR, Dehmer GJ, Lewis SE et al: The prognostic value of submaximal exercise testing with radionuclide ventriculography before hospital discharge in patients with recent myocardial infarction. Circulation 64:535, 1981. Number of patients = 61, number of patients with cardiac events = 35)

groups having resting left ventricular ejection fractions of less than 40%, of 41% to 50%, and of greater than 50% and assessing mortality in the first postinfarction year. For each category of ejection fraction, the presence of either clinical or radiographic heart failure conferred additional substantial mortality (Table 72.5).[50] The increase in mortality was not due to recurrent myocardial infarction, nor could it be related to postinfarction angina or an abnormal exercise test; it did occur more often in older patients, in those with prior myocardial infarction, and in those with a large infarction (estimated by peak creatine kinase enzyme levels). These findings suggest that the ejection fraction provides somewhat limited, albeit valuable, information about ventricular function. Assessment of end-diastolic and end-systolic volumes and of diastolic function might be expected to provide better prognostic data; indeed, the report of Nicod and colleagues[50] suggests that ischemic diastolic dysfunction is perhaps the major determinant of the study results.

The influence of age and of presence or absence of prior myocardial infarction on postinfarction mortality for a given resting left ventricular ejection fraction have been confirmed in a large series.[51] In this study, an ejection fraction of less than 40% in patients aged 51 to 70 was associated with mortalities of 8% and 23%, respectively, in patients without and with prior infarction. Recent investigations in this and other areas in postinfarction patients have included patients older than age 70, in contrast to earlier studies in which elderly patients were excluded owing to assumed reduction in length of follow-up time. Inclusion of older patients should allow more precise analysis of the use of any given risk variable in the postinfarction patient.

As indicated earlier, many patients with depressed left ventricular ejection fraction at the time of hospital discharge have contraindications to exercise testing (see Table 72.1). In some studies,[2,52] therefore, exclusion from exercise testing is of great predictive power in assessing postinfarction mortality and morbidity, especially from congestive heart failure. Moreover, if ejection fraction is severely depressed at rest, its response during exercise adds no additional prognostic information.

Epstein and co-workers[53] have summarized the role of determination of ejection fraction at the time of hospital discharge by suggesting that about 50% of patients with clinical congestive failure in the hospital and that about 10% of patients without it will have ejection fractions of less than 30%; the first-year mortality in such patients ranges from 25% to 45%. Identification of these patients at high risk from severe ventricular functional impairment warrants aggressive medical management of associated problems, such as ventricular arrhythmias and recurrent congestive heart failure.

VENTRICULAR ARRHYTHMIAS

Observations made early in the 1970s indicated that ventricular extrasystolic activity in survivors of myocardial infarction could be indicated as a cause of subsequent cardiac mortality, including sudden cardiac death. Initial studies[54-57] analyzed the relationship between any and all ventricular extrasystolic activity and total and sudden cardiac death using ambulatory electrocardiographic monitoring performed well after the myocardial infarction had occurred. However, by their very design, these studies did not include the patients who had died within the first 2 to 3 postinfarction months, when risk of death is likely to be the highest.[39,54] Ambulatory electrocardiographic monitoring was therefore subsequently used around the time of hospital discharge in patients recovering from myocardial infarction in order to stratify more accurately survivors into subsets at different risk in the postinfarction period. Criteria for "simple" or "benign" and "complex" ventricular arrhythmias were derived in order to define more clearly the patients at highest risk.[55]

Although several large studies clearly show a relationship of complex ventricular arrhythmias to subsequent cardiac mortality, especially in the first postinfarction year,[2,54-64] the predictive value for total cardiac mortality and for sudden cardiac death is variable. This variability can be explained in part by differences among the reports in study design: there are substantial differences in (1) numbers of patients studied and numbers of men and women comprising the study group; (2) exclusion of patients over a certain age (usually the mid 60s) to ensure an adequate number of years of follow-up; (3) numbers of hours of ambulatory electrocardiographic monitoring performed; (4) definition of sudden cardiac death; and (5) an unclear, but potentially influential, role of the use of antiarrhythmic therapy, β-blockade medication as antianginal treatment or myocardial infarction prophylaxis, and digitalis.

A study[65] of 1,650 patients enrolled in the Beta Blocker Heart Attack Project (BHAT) who received propranolol and underwent 24-hour ambulatory electrocardiographic monitoring, and whose ventricular ectopy was categorized by frequency and complexity, found that propranolol did not confer a reduction in presumed arrhythmic mortality (sudden death) that was independent of the overall reduction in mortality.[65] This observation indicates that β-blocking agents may not abolish the relationship between postinfarction arrhythmias and subsequent death and suggests that trials of antiarrhythmic agents can be undertaken in patients receiving β-blocking medication without confounding the results.

Despite methodologic problems there is sufficient evidence to suggest strongly that patients with complex ventricular arrhythmias at the time of hospital discharge do constitute a higher risk subgroup than those without such rhythm disturbances. This risk is especially operative in the first postinfarction year[60,61] but may carry over into subsequent years. Moreover, risk assessment appears to be best defined by ambulatory electrocardiographic monitoring carried out at the time of hospital discharge, rather than later in the postinfarction course, when prognostic capability has declined or is not useful.[61]

VENTRICULAR TACHYCARDIA

Although it is acknowledged that complex ventricular extrasystolic activity documented on predischarge ambulatory electrocardiographic monitoring has predictive importance for mortality in the first postinfarction year, it is less clear that ventricular tachycardia *per se* carries the same prognostic information.

Most investigators who have addressed this specific issue have defined ventricular tachycardia as consisting of three or more consecutive ventricular extrasystoles occurring at rates exceeding 100 or 120 beats per minute.[66-68] Defined as such, several noteworthy observations have been made. First, episodes of ventricular tachycardia occur in patients who also have frequent and complex ventricular ectopy (multiform complexes, doublets, and R-on-T phenomena),[67,68] but in many patients they occur only once in a 24-hour period. Second, the

TABLE 72.5 ONE-YEAR MORTALITY IN PATIENTS WITH AND WITHOUT LEFT VENTRICULAR FAILURE: RELATIONSHIP TO EJECTION FRACTION

	LV Ejection Fraction		
	40% (n = 265)	41%–50% (n = 241)	50% (n = 466)
Clinical LV Failure			
Present (n = 400)	26%	19%	8%
Absent (n = 572)	12%	6%	3%
Radiographic LV Failure			
Present (n = 192)	36%	24%	14%
Absent (n = 771)	13%	9%	3%

(Adapted from Nicod P, Gilpin E, Dittrich H et al: Influence on prognosis and morbidity of left ventricular ejection fraction with and without signs of left ventricular failure after acute myocardial infarction. Am J Cardiol 61:1165, 1988)

overall incidence of ventricular tachycardia in a 24-hour monitoring period at the time of hospital discharge is only 1% to 3%,[66,67] but the incidence will vary with the duration of recording. Third, the number of ventricular complexes in each episode of ventricular tachycardia is extremely variable, but rarely exceeds 20 consecutive complexes. Fourth, most, but not all, episodes are unaccompanied by symptoms, presumably due to their brevity.[67] Fifth, R-on-T premature ventricular extrasystoles do not lead to ventricular tachycardia. Sixth, the ventricular tachycardia does not degenerate into ventricular fibrillation. Seventh, neither the occurrence nor the rate of the ventricular tachycardia are closely related to the underlying or immediately preceding sinus rate, although some investigators suggest that a slightly faster sinus rate may precede many episodes.[67] The tachycardia episodes are also not accompanied by post-tachycardia increase in sinus rate, suggesting that perhaps they are not hemodynamically compromising. Finally, ventricular tachycardia may not unequivocally predict either total or sudden cardiac death or recurrent myocardial infarction, despite data indicating that the arrhythmia often occurs in patients with worse functional classification, prior infarction, and history of congestive heart failure. The point is controversial, however, since 2-year mortality in patients with ventricular ectopy at the time of hospital discharge has recently been reported at 8%, 16%, and 37%, respectively, in patients with fewer than three ventricular extrasystoles per hour, those with more than three extrasystoles per hour *or* at least three consecutive extrasystoles, and those with more than three extrasystoles per hour *and* at least three consecutive extrasystoles.[4] The number of patients with ventricular tachycardia, as well as the number of deaths in a given follow-up period, is relatively small (around 5%), making interpretation of its significance unclear. Similarly, the role of antiarrhythmic therapy, use of digitalis, and use of β-blockade therapy as treatment for postinfarction angina or prophylaxis against recurrent infarction (rather than as antiarrhythmic therapy) is difficult to delineate.

The foregoing observations suggest that vigorous antiarrhythmic therapy to suppress ventricular tachycardia may not be warranted; however, treatment of complex ventricular arrhythmias (which include ventricular tachycardia) does appear to have a rational basis.

CONTRIBUTION OF RESTING EJECTION FRACTION TO PROGNOSTIC IMPORTANCE OF VENTRICULAR ARRHYTHMIAS

Early investigations of the prognostic import of predischarge ventricular arrhythmias on total and sudden cardiac death in survivors of myocardial infarction indicated that ventricular function had to play an important associated role, since it was recognized that prior infarction, past anterior wall myocardial infarction, and congestive heart failure were co-variables in the prediction of mortality.

One of the initial studies that used radionuclide ventriculography to determine left ventricular ejection fraction as a measure of postinfarction left ventricular function clearly demonstrated the interplay between ventricular arrhythmias of different grades of complexity and underlying ventricular performance in predicting sudden death (see Fig. 72.3).[27] In the study of Schultze and associates,[27] 81 patients had determination of left ventricular ejection fraction and 24-hour ambulatory electrocardiographic monitoring 10 to 21 days after acute infarction and were observed from 2 to 16 months (mean of 7 months). Ten percent of the patients died suddenly: their left ventricular ejection fraction was significantly lower than that of survivors (28% vs. 43%) as was the percent of the ventricle that was akinetic. In addition, all patients who died suddenly had significant (Lown grade 3 to 5[55]) ventricular arrhythmias; most of these were the same patients with depressed ejection fraction (see Fig. 72.4). The sudden cardiac death rates of patients with complex ventricular arrhythmias at 6 and 12 months were 31% and 66%, respectively, and the death rates in patients with ejection fractions less than and greater than 40% were 20% and 31%, respectively. The subgroup of patients with ejection fractions less than 40% and Lown grade 3 to 5 of arrhythmia complexity had the highest sudden death mortality (8 of 26, 31%), whereas no sudden deaths occurred in patients with depressed ejection fraction and uncomplicated (Lown class 0 to 2) ventricular arrhythmia, or with ejection fraction greater than 40%, regardless of any degree of arrhythmia complexity. Since publication of these data, virtually all studies have included both variables in the assessment of prognosis in survivors of myocardial infarction, since it appears that degree of complexity of ventricular arrhythmias confers on a given ejection fraction additional predictive importance, and vice versa. Nevertheless, two studies of large numbers of patients totaling 1146 did conclude that complex ventricular arrhythmias were related to high risk of death independently of left ventricular dysfunction.[69,70]

Several unresolved issues remain with regard to the information obtained from predischarge ambulatory electrocardiographic monitoring. Should patients with any frequency of complex ventricular arrhythmias receive antiarrhythmic medication or only those with a certain frequency of ectopy? Should treatment be given only to patients with complex ventricular arrhythmias and depressed ejection fractions? What is the endpoint of therapy: serum drug level or suppression of ventricular extrasystolic activity? Is total suppression of all ventricular arrhythmias a rational goal, or is suppression of only complex forms reasonable (and attainable)? What is the effect of thrombolytic treatment on frequency and prognostic importance of ventricular arrhythmias? In one study[71] it was suggested that thrombolysis is indeed associated with a lower frequency of ventricular ectopy; its effect on prognosis is not clear since the patients were not randomized and the control group not strictly comparable to the group successfully treated and long-term follow-up was not provided. For what length of time should antiarrhythmic medication be continued? Few studies provide a framework for rational decision making on this question, although the survival curves reported by Moss and co-workers[61] and the data of Rehnqvist and colleagues[62] suggest that ventricular ectopy present after the first postinfarction year continues to exert prognostic influence on subsequent mortality. What criteria should be applied for termination of antiarrhythmic therapy, and are yearly 24-hour monitoring periods sufficient? Finally, what is the relationship between complex ventricular arrhythmias and ventricular fibrillation? Does antiarrhythmic therapy that suppresses ventricular ectopy protect against ventricular fibrillation? Does the presence of one predict the other, as has been suggested in some studies?[72] And conversely, is a "therapeutic" serum level of an antiarrhythmic agent sufficient to protect against ventricular fibrillation while having minimal overall effect on ventricular arrhythmias?[73]

The recently terminated Cardiac Arrhythmia Pilot Study (CAPS) was specifically designed to address some of these issues.[74–77] This multicenter study assessed the effect of antiarrhythmic therapy (using flecainide, encainide, imipramine, and moricizine) on over 500 high-risk postinfarction patients observed for 1 year. In order to qualify for entry into the study, patients had to have more than 10 premature ventricular complexes per hour, more than five "runs" of three to nine consecutive ventricular extrasystoles at rates exceeding 100 beats per minute, and a left ventricular ejection fraction exceeding 20%; patients with postinfarction angina or congestive heart failure were excluded. Arrhythmia suppression was defined as greater than 70% reduction in ventricular ectopic activity and a greater than 90% reduction in ventricular "runs." The study results indicated that although flecainide and encainide were highly efficacious in reducing ventricular ectopic activity, a substantial incidence of new or worsening congestive heart failure accompanied the use of flecainide, regardless of entry ejection fraction. Younger patients with a first myocardial infarction and normal or near-normal ejection fraction derived the most benefit from antiarrhythmic therapy,[77] whereas those at presumed highest risk (older subjects with remote infarction and depressed ventricular ejection fraction) were the least well "protected" and the least likely to maintain suppression of their arrhythmia.

Interestingly, the CAPS study[76] identified a 37% "efficacy" rate using placebo, confirming and underscoring the substantial degree of spontaneous variability in frequency of ventricular arrhythmias. Since the death rate from cardiac arrest was relatively low in this study (45 of 502 patients, 9%) despite the inclusion of patients with significant left ventricular dysfunction, conclusions as to its prevention by these antiarrhythmic agents are not definitive. It is noteworthy, however, and perhaps somewhat unexpected, that antiarrhythmic therapy was not associated with worsening of preexisting arrhythmias ("proarrhythmia") in this patient population. Since completion of the CAPS study, the Cardiac Arrhythmia Suppression Trial (CAST) results have been published.[78] In this large study of 2309 patients, none of whom had drug-resistant ventricular arrhythmias, those receiving encainide or flecainide had a higher all-cause and arrhythmic death rate (7.7% and 4.5%, respectively) than did those receiving placebo (3.0% and 1.2%, respectively). These results led to termination of that portion of the trial that involved these antiarrhythmic agents, and to the recommendation that postinfarction patients without symptomatic ventricular arrhythmias should not receive them. Answers to the many unresolved issues concerning the role of antiarrhythmic agents in the prevention of sudden death may yet become apparent from future controlled investigations in large numbers of patients. At the present time, the roles of electrophysiologic investigation and signal-averaged electrocardiography in the postinfarction patient have been evaluated as affording an approach to these questions.

RELATIONSHIP OF EXTENT OF INFARCTION (Q WAVE AND NON–Q WAVE) TO THE PROGNOSTIC IMPORTANCE OF VENTRICULAR ARRHYTHMIAS

Most early studies of the prognostic role of ventricular arrhythmias in postinfarction patients did not take the type of infarction—Q wave or non–Q wave—into consideration, mainly because their respective differing clinical courses had not been clearly defined. Maisel and colleagues[79] analyzed 191 patients with non–Q wave infarction and 586 patients with Q wave infarction in order to determine the significance of complex ventricular arrhythmias in the two populations. Whereas 1-year survival was similar in the two groups if complex ventricular arrhythmias were not found on predischarge 24-hour ambulatory electrocardiographic monitoring, a substantial negative impact on prognosis could be demonstrated for the non–Q wave, but not the Q wave, groups, if these rhythm disturbances were found. Only 76% of patients with non–Q wave infarction and complex ventricular arrhythmias survived the first postinfarction year, compared with 90% of patients with Q wave infarction and complex ectopy. Moreover, the prevalence of complex ventricular ectopy in nonsurvivors of non–Q wave infarction was 62%, compared with a 32% prevalence in survivors.[79] Interestingly, the location of the Q wave infarction to anterior or inferior walls did not confer any additional risk for death.

The contribution of left ventricular ejection fraction to the prognostic significance of complex ventricular arrhythmias in patients with non–Q wave infarction is not as clear cut as it is in all survivors of infarction, a finding that could be explained by inclusion of a preponderance of patients with Q wave or prior infarction in previous series.[79] This lack of clear relationship of ejection fraction to mortality in patients with non–Q wave infarction can be explained by the observation that a normal or near-normal ejection fraction is found in most survivors of non–Q wave infarction, regardless of their arrhythmic risk category.

The basis for the observed enhanced arrhythmic risk in patients surviving non–Q wave infarction is likely the presence of underlying regions of ischemia[80] resulting from a possibly unstable coronary circulation, as well as from a juxtaposition of anatomic areas of viable and

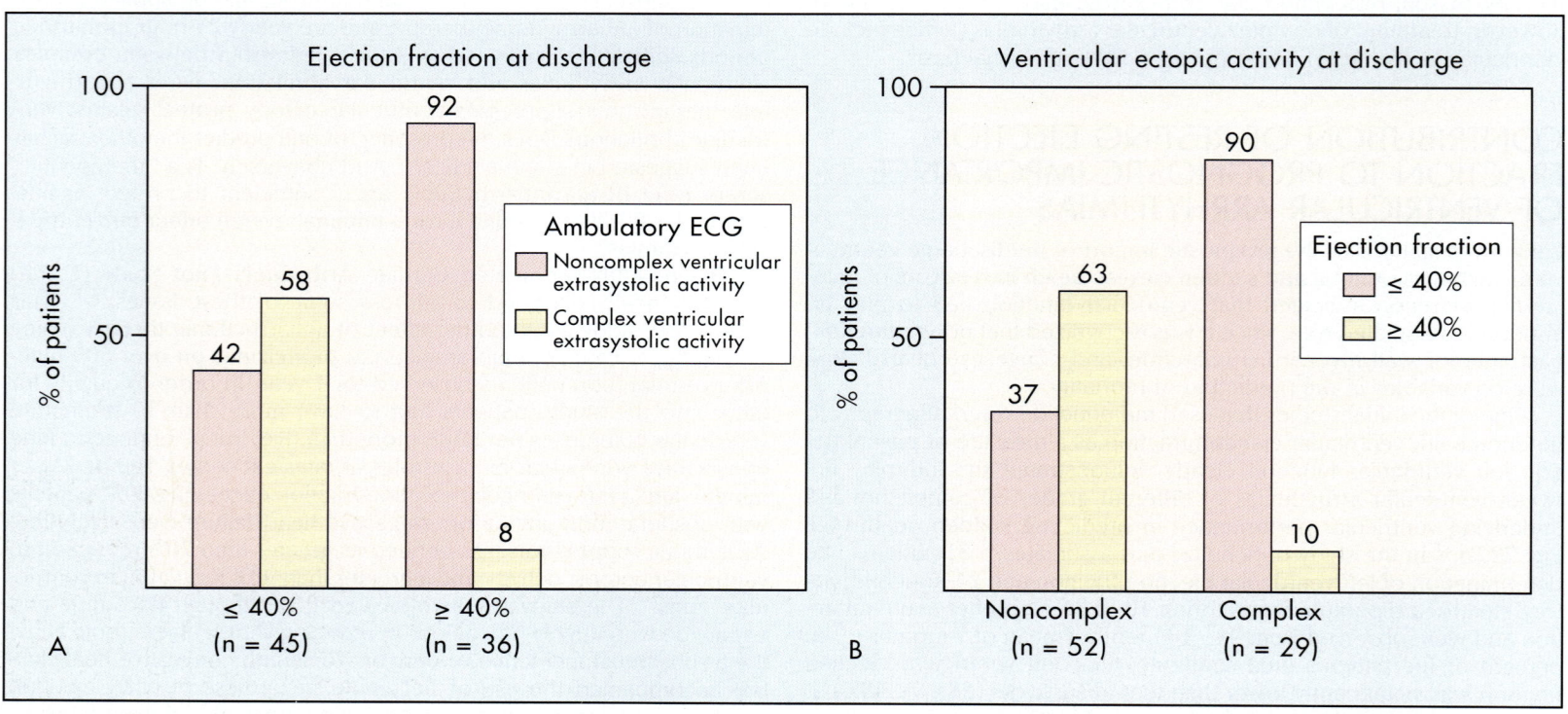

FIGURE 72.4 Relationship of ventricular arrhythmias and left ventricular ejection fraction determined at the time of hospital discharge in survivors of myocardial infarction. **A.** In patients with a depressed ejection fraction (less than 40%), 42% and 58%, respectively, have noncomplex and complex ventricular arrhythmias. (Complex ventricular arrhythmias include multiform complexes, doublets, bursts, and sustained runs of ventricular tachycardia and also R-on-T extrasystoles.) Thus, a depressed ejection fraction *per se* does not predict the presence of complex ventricular ectopy. In contrast, the majority of patients with a more normal ejection fraction who have ventricular arrhythmias have noncomplex forms (92% vs. 8%). **B.** Of patients with noncomplex ventricular arrhythmias, 37% have depressed ejection fraction and 63% have more normal ejection fraction; thus, the presence of noncomplex ventricular extrasystolic activity does not accurately predict the presence of normal left ventricular function. In contrast, of patients with complex ventricular arrhythmias, the majority (90%) have depressed ejection fraction. (Adapted from the data of Schultze RA Jr, Strauss HW, Pitt B: Sudden death in the year following myocardial infarction: Relation to ventricular premature contractions in the late hospital phase and left ventricular ejection fraction. Am J Med 62:192, 1977)

nonviable myocardium and of fibrosis (scar). These and other observations indicate that therapeutic strategies aimed at altering postinfarction prognosis must consider patients with Q wave and non–Q wave infarction separately.

ELECTROPHYSIOLOGIC STUDIES

In view of the rather compelling data that indicate that complex ventricular extrasystolic activity in the postinfarction patient has prognostic importance for subsequent cardiac death,[54-64] there has been much recent interest in identifying these patients with greater certainty than can be achieved from ambulatory electrocardiographic monitoring alone. As a result, the role of electrophysiologic testing prior to hospital discharge has been evaluated as a diagnostic and prognostic tool.

In an early report,[81] 48 clinically stable, non-high-risk survivors of acute myocardial infarction underwent electrophysiologic study within 8 to 85 days of their infarction and were followed for at least 1 year. The study protocol involved atrial pacing with introduction of a single ventricular pacing stimulus at varying times after a QRS complex; a "repetitive ventricular response" was defined as two or more ventricular premature beats resulting from the single coupled ventricular stimulus. Although no patient developed sustained ventricular tachycardia, 19 of the 48 (40%) developed a repetitive ventricular response; of these 19, 15 (79%) had ventricular tachycardia or sudden death in the ensuing 1-year follow-up period. In the postinfarction patients who did not develop the repetitive ventricular response, only 4 (8%) had ventricular tachycardia or death in the follow-up period, representing a significantly lower incidence. The predictive value of the repetitive ventricular response for subsequent ventricular tachycardia or sudden death was a very high 79%, whether or not the patients were receiving antiarrhythmic medications. It was observed in this study that the results of electrophysiologic testing in these stable patients without congestive heart failure or chest pain were not related to predischarge ejection fraction, extent of angiographically determined coronary artery disease, location of myocardial infarction, or prior myocardial infarction; they were, however, independent predictors of subsequent life-threatening arrhythmia or death.

This initial investigation engendered a great deal of controversy regarding methodology and reproducibility of results and was followed by several other studies[82-84] that attempted to validate this approach in defining prognosis in postinfarction patients. In the study of Hamer and associates,[85] 70 patients with myocardial infarction complicated by congestive heart failure, hypotension, and/or ventricular arrhythmias were studied prior to hospital discharge, in the absence of antiarrhythmic medication. Using a more aggressive stimulation protocol than in earlier studies, 29% developed either sustained or nonsustained ventricular tachycardia. Importantly, several of these patients had had no arrhythmia demonstrated by 24-hour ambulatory electrocardiographic monitoring. In the 1-year follow-up period in this study, only 25% (5 of 20) of patients with inducible ventricular tachycardia at the time of electrophysiologic study died; and in all but one case death was sudden. This outcome compared with a 15% incidence of death (most of which were also sudden) in patients in whom ventricular tachycardia was not induced at the time of electrophysiologic study. During the follow-up period, 37% of the patients received some form of antiarrhythmic therapy, thus precluding accurate calculation of the predictive value of the electrophysiologic study; however, it must be emphasized that some of the deaths occurred in patients receiving such medications.

Richards and co-workers,[84] using yet another stimulation protocol, investigated 165 non-high-risk postinfarction patients between 6 and 28 days following the acute event. *Ventricular electrical instability* was defined as the occurrence of ventricular tachycardia or ventricular fibrillation as a result of electrophysiologic study; repetitive ventricular responses and nonsustained ventricular tachycardia were not classified as electrical instability. Of the 165 patients, 38 (23%) developed ventricular tachycardia or fibrillation; 8 of the 38 (21%) died suddenly during an average 8-month follow-up period, compared with only 1 of 127 (0.07%) of patients who did not have electrical instability. One-year survival for the latter patients was 91%, compared with 65% in patients with inducible life-threatening ventricular arrhythmias. The predictive value of electrical instability for all deaths was calculated to be 26%, and for sudden death or development of spontaneous ventricular tachycardia in the follow-up period it was 32%. Importantly, the predictive value of the inability to demonstrate electrical instability was 98% for the absence of sudden death or development of spontaneous ventricular tachycardia. This finding is in contrast to other reported series[81,83] in which a negative electrophysiologic study did not predict absence of subsequent cardiac mortality and probably reflects the nature of the stimulation protocol as well as the rigid criteria for "electrical instability" (ventricular tachycardia or fibrillation). In the report of Richards and associates,[84] outcome did seem to be influenced to some degree by left ventricular ejection fraction determined during hospitalization.

In distinct contrast to these reports, the study of Marchlinski and colleagues[83] failed to show that the results of electrophysiologic testing could predict subsequent cardiac death. In this investigation, again employing a different stimulation protocol, 46 patients were evaluated 8 to 60 days following myocardial infarction; high-risk patients (congestive heart failure, unstable angina) were excluded. Twenty-two percent of patients developed sustained or nonsustained ventricular tachycardia during electrophysiologic stimulation; these rhythms had not been seen on predischarge ambulatory electrocardiographic monitoring, although patients with inducible ventricular tachycardia did demonstrate more complex extrasystolic activity than those without. In an 18-month follow-up period, cardiac death could not be related to inducibility of ventricular arrhythmias, but was more closely related to left ventricular ejection fraction, a finding that might be explained, at least in part, by the exclusion of patients with clinical congestive failure and evidence of continuing ischemia.

The marked discrepancies among these investigations no doubt relate to the use of different cardiac stimulation protocols; nonuniformity of definitions of sustained and nonsustained ventricular tachycardia, "electrical instability," and "repetitive ventricular response"; different and noncomparable patient populations; concomitant antiarrhythmic drug therapy or drug therapy initiated during the follow-up period; use of β-blocking medication not specifically as antiarrhythmic medication, but for hypertension, angina, or as prophylaxis against recurrent infarction; intercurrent cardiac events; and myocardial revascularization procedures. Notwithstanding these problems, the results reported to date are sufficiently provocative to suggest the need for a large-scale, carefully designed study of the role of electrophysiologic testing in the postinfarction patient. Randomized prospective studies of the effect of antiarrhythmic medications in "electrically unstable" patients are in progress.[84]

The effect of thrombolysis in patients undergoing electrophysiologic studies has been evaluated in several investigations[86-88]; the prevalence of inducible ventricular tachycardia in these patients ranges from 22% to 50%. In one randomized controlled study of 36 patients studied 1 month after infarction and followed to 15 months, inducibility of sustained ventricular tachycardia (defined as having a duration exceeding 30 seconds or requiring urgent cardioversion) was significantly less common (2 of 17) in a streptokinase-treated group compared with a group not receiving thrombolytic treatment (14 of 19); importantly, ventricular arrhythmias assessed by conventional bedside or ambulatory monitoring techniques did not differ in frequency or complexity between these groups.[86] The induction of any sustained ventricular arrhythmia (monomorphic or polymorphic tachycardia) was possible in all patients in whom reperfusion was not achieved, but in only 35% (6 of 17) of patients with successful reperfusion, a difference that has been confirmed in some,[87] but not all,[88] studies. Despite these findings, the predictive value of inducible ventricular tachycardia in patients receiving thrombolytic therapy in this and other studies remains low due to a low subsequent mortality.

Thrombolysis with reperfusion of the infarct-producing artery can effect the ability to induce ventricular arrhythmias by reducing the size of the infarction and thus potentially preserving a normal or near-normal ejection fraction, by creating a peri-infarction ischemic border zone that provides an anatomical and electrophysiologic substrate for arrhythmia production and maintenance, or by abolishing such a zone due to effects of the hemorrhagic reflow phenomenon. These developments are time dependent, suggesting that the optimal time for performing electrophysiologic studies needs to be clarified. Subsequent healing (scarring) of infarcted areas, stabilization or destabilization of ischemic zones, and remodeling of the ventricle, each one of which is time dependent, can all contribute to variable proclivity to arrhythmic events, as can the common clinical practice of performing myocardial revascularization procedures after thrombolytic therapy.

SIGNAL-AVERAGED ELECTROCARDIOGRAPHY

Signal-averaged electrocardiography is a technique that is being applied in the postinfarction patient in order to assess noninvasively the risk for an arrhythmic event. The signal-averaged electrocardiogram displays waveforms within the terminal portion of the QRS complex and ST segment that have too low an amplitude and too low a frequency to be detected by ordinary electrocardiographic equipment (Fig. 72.5). The presence of these waveforms, termed *late potentials*, together with a filtered QRS duration exceeding 120 msec, reflect areas in the underlying myocardium in which conduction of the cardiac electrical impulse is slowed and fragmented; such areas could serve as substrates for ventricular arrhythmogenesis. The underlying histopathology of these areas is currently not known with certainty in patients with acute myocardial infarction, although they have been related to areas of fibrosis interspersed with areas of viable myocardium in patients undergoing electrophysiologic mapping. Whereas the relationship between late potentials and other abnormalities of the signal-averaged electrocardiogram and inducibility of ventricular tachycardia in patients with recurrent clinical ventricular tachycardia is reasonably good, it is much less definite in postinfarction patients at the present time.

Abnormal late potentials have been recorded in 15% to over 50% of patients with acute myocardial infarction[89,90] and as early as 6 hours after presentation in some patients, but as late as 8 days in others.[90,91] Their prevalence may increase with time after hospital admission; in some patients they disappear during the hospitalization or shortly thereafter.[92] In one study,[92] the abnormal signal-averaged electrocardiogram returned to normal in 42% of patients by 2 months after the acute event. This variability in and unpredictability of evolution and natural history within the hospitalization period has been noted by several investigators,[89-91] but not all,[93] and has been ascribed to changing electrophysiologic conditions in the infarcted and ischemic myocardial milieu.

Several investigators[89,90,94] have failed to find a relationship between the early development of late potentials and the site and extent of infarction (Q wave vs. non–Q wave or as measured by peak creatine kinase enzyme levels) or use of thrombolytic agents, whereas others[92,95,96] have identified relationships with extensive infarcts and with those involving the inferior wall. In one study of the early course of myocardial infarction, McGuire and co-workers found that late potentials were common in patients who developed ventricular arrhythmias during hospitalization (8 of 10), but rare in those who did not (2 of 35).[90] This high sensitivity and specificity have not been confirmed in all studies, however,[89,91,92] and the predictive value of this technique for the development of in-hospital ventricular arrhythmias or sudden death remains uncertain (Table 72.6). Certain trends are suggested by a higher mortality in patients with late potentials compared with those without; however, the effect of concomitant therapy with β-blocking agents, antiarrhythmic drugs, and antiplatelet medication or anticoagulation could confound the interpretation of such trends.

The predictive capability of late potentials for long-term prognosis has been assessed in several prospective studies.[92-99] Usually, a single signal-averaged electrocardiogram is recorded around the time of hospital discharge and related to the occurrence of sustained symptomatic ventricular tachycardia or sudden death in the follow-up period. In the study of Cripps and co-workers,[97] both ischemic events (recurrent myocardial infarction and clinical requirement for myocardial revascularization) and arrhythmic events were assessed using a combination of both signal-averaged electrocardiography and submaximal and symptom-limited exercise testing. Not unexpectedly, occurrence or nonoccurrence of arrhythmic events was more accurately predicted by the presence or absence of late potentials (positive and negative predictive accuracies of 22% and 99%, respectively) than by exercise test results. Conversely, occurrence or nonoccurrence of ischemic events was predicted by exercise test results (positive and negative predictive accuracies of 30% and 97%, respectively), but not by the findings on signal-averaged electrocardiography. The study raises the issue of the nature of the trigger for postinfarction arrhythmias and suggests that the myocardial ischemia that is identified by exercise testing is not operative.

Kuchar and colleagues evaluated left ventricular ejection fraction, ventricular ectopy assessed by 24-hour ambulatory electrocardiographic monitoring, and the signal-averaged electrocardiogram in a

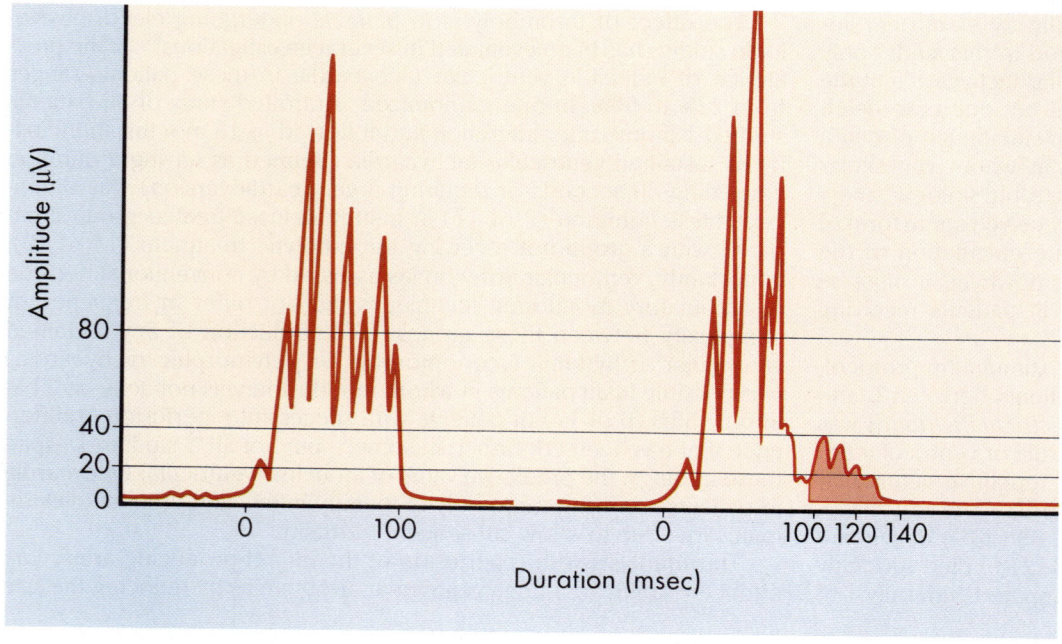

FIGURE 72.5 A. The normal signal-averaged QRS complex has a duration less than 120 msec and absence of low amplitude (less than 40 μV) deflections in its terminal portion. **B.** The abnormal signal-averaged complex is of prolonged duration (greater than 120 msec) and has late low amplitude potentials (*shaded area*) exceeding 40 msec in duration. An additional abnormality would consist of a calculated root mean square voltage of the terminal 40 msec that was less than 25 μV, at specific frequency filter settings.

large series of postinfarction patients (see Table 72.6).[95] In their study, the predictive value of an abnormal signal-averaged electrocardiogram of 28% (odds ratio 23.6) was somewhat greater than that of a left ventricular ejection fraction less than 40% (odds ratio 17.6) and the presence of complex ventricular ectopy on ambulatory electrocardiography (odds ratio 7.6). The high predictive accuracy of a normal signal-averaged electrocardiogram for the absence of postinfarction arrhythmic events was confirmed in this study (see Table 72.6). Importantly, these investigators found that an abnormality of only one of these tests yielded a probability of an arrhythmic event within their entire postinfarction population of less than 6%, whereas a combination of an abnormal signal-averaged electrocardiogram with an abnormality of either additional test increased this probability to about 33%. Similarly, Cripps and co-workers[93] found that combining an abnormal signal-averaged electrocardiogram with either clinical indices of congestive heart failure or frequent ventricular extrasystoles recorded on 24-hour ambulatory electrocardiographic monitoring improved the positive predictive accuracy for arrhythmic events from 25%, using an abnormal signal-averaged electrocardiogram alone, to 62% using the combination.

At the present time, the routine use of signal-averaged electrocardiography to predict postinfarction course and prognosis is not generally recommended, in part because of methodologic problems. These include uncertainty as to when to perform the signal-averaged electrocardiogram for optimum yield, questions as to which specific criteria for abnormality other than the presence of late potentials *per se* should be used, and uncertainty as to the best level of filtering of the QRS signal. Other information that must be known more precisely in order to apply the technique with confidence are the time course of development of late potentials and their natural history over time, their association with anterior and inferior infarction and the role of remote infarction, and their interaction with other, acknowledged, prognostic variables, such as ischemia, ventricular dysfunction, and complex ventricular ectopy, as assessed by ambulatory electrocardiographic monitoring. In this regard, it is noteworthy that the results of at least one investigation[92] suggest that the findings of serially performed signal-averaged electrocardiograms have no relationship to those of serially performed ambulatory electrocardiograms. The routine use of signal-averaged electrocardiography as a "screening test" for electrophysiologic studies in the postinfarction patient is also not uniformly recommended, in part because of the poor predictive capability of "positive" electrophysiologic studies themselves. Notwithstanding these considerations, the technique appears extremely promising as a method of noninvasively defining an area of myocardium that could serve as a nidus for electrical instability in both acute and remote myocardial infarction.

ANALYSIS OF RISK AFTER ACUTE MYOCARDIAL INFARCTION

Risk stratification of the postinfarction patient can be achieved using variables that reflect (1) extent of myocardial infarction, (2) potential life-threatening arrhythmias, (3) extent of postinfarction left ventricular dysfunction, and (4) continuing myocardial ischemia (Table 72.7).

Since in survivors of myocardial infarction most of the cardiac deaths and two thirds of all nonfatal cardiac events occur within the first 6 postinfarction months,[58,63,99-101] with stabilization in incidence thereafter, risk stratification determined at the time of hospital discharge could result in major impact on subsequent morbidity and mortality if appropriate interventions are made in properly selected moderate- to high-risk patient groups (see Fig. 72.6). Conversely, deliberate nonintervention in patients in low-risk groups becomes a rational and desirable approach to postinfarction management.

Both univariate and multivariate discriminant function analyses have been applied in assessing prognosis in survivors of myocardial infarction, with the result that different variables, alone and in combination, have different predictive values for postinfarction fatal and nonfatal events.[100,102-104] In addition, "postinfarction events" have focused primarily on mortality rather than on morbidity and the relationship of morbidity to mortality. The differences in predictive ability of selected variables for different cardiac events no doubt reflect, at least in part, differences in patient populations, differences in expression of

TABLE 72.6 RELATION OF ABNORMAL SIGNAL-AVERAGED ELECTROCARDIOGRAPHIC FINDINGS TO POSTINFARCTION VENTRICULAR ARRHYTHMIAS AND SUDDEN DEATH

Study	N	Time of Signal-Averaged ECG After Admission	Prevalence	Follow-up (yr)	Sensitivity	Specificity	Predictive Accuracy Positive	Predictive Accuracy Negative	Comment
Cripps et al[97]	176	12 ± 19	24%	2	82%	81%	22%	99%	Included patients with QRS duration exceeding 120 msec as only signal-averaged ECG abnormality
Kuchar et al[95]	200	11 ± 6	39%	0.5–2	50%	90%	28%	99%	Both late potentials and QRS duration exceeding 120 msec required
Gomes et al[99]	115	10 ± 6	44%	1.2	56%–75%	61%–84%	40% (anterior MI) 21% (inferior MI)		Higher prevalence of abnormal signal-averaged ECG in inferior MI compared with anterior MI. Sensitivity and specificity varied with filtering ranges used.

TABLE 72.7 SOME VARIABLES THAT HAVE BEEN CITED AS BEING PREDICTIVE OF SUBSEQUENT MORBIDITY AND MORTALITY IN POSTINFARCTION PATIENTS

Clinical Variables
Angina
Left ventricular dysfunction
   S_3 gallop rhythm
   Congestive heart failure
   Cardiothoracic ratio exceeding 0.50
   Digitalis therapy
   Diuretic therapy
Advanced age
Past myocardial infarction
ST segment depression in resting electrocardiogram

Exercise Test Variables
Inability to complete 4 METs workload
Ischemic electrocardiographic response
Angina during exercise
Abnormal blood pressure response
Ischemia in area(s) remote from infarction, as assessed by thallium scintigraphy
Exercise duration less than 3 minutes
Exclusion from exercise testing

Ambulatory Electrocardiography Variables
Complex ventricular extrasystoles
Nonsustained ventricular tachycardia
Sustained ventricular tachycardia

Angiographic Variables
Ejection fraction less than 40%
Multivessel coronary artery disease

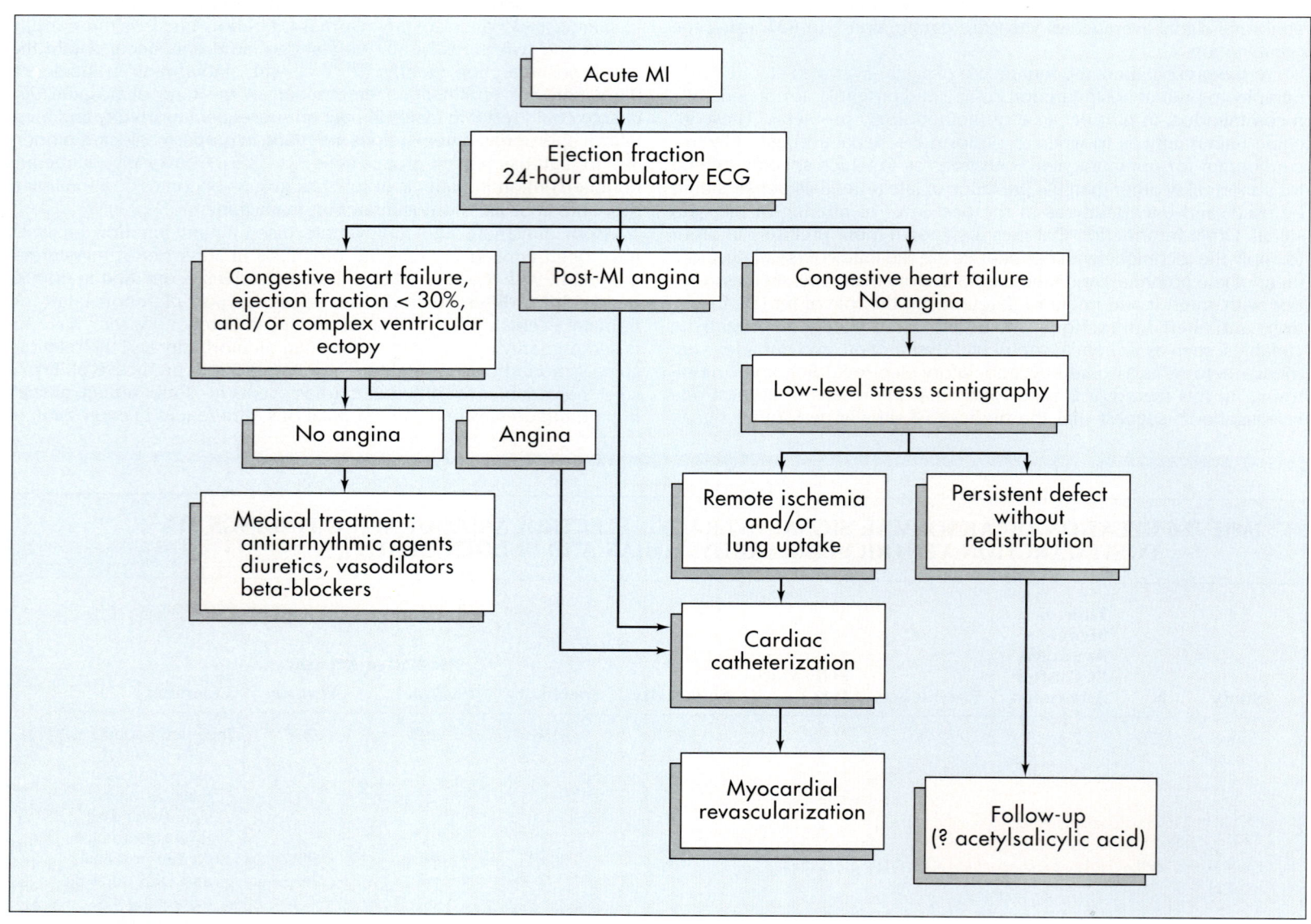

FIGURE 72.6 Approach to the post-myocardial infarction patient according to category of risk.

the underlying disease pattern within that population, and different statistical methodologies. The very selection of specific variables for univariate or multivariate analysis may bias the results. However, although this realization helps to explain sometimes disparate observations, it does little to unify the subject.

There are few investigations using coronary arteriographic findings in risk stratification of the postinfarction patient, nor is this procedure routine in the evaluation of such patients. Most of the available studies address the predictive value of angiographic findings in patients who have undergone predischarge exercise testing, but univariate and mutivariate analysis of risk has not been applied. Sanz and co-workers[104] and Taylor and colleagues[105] have prospectively analyzed postinfarction prognosis in patients who underwent coronary and left ventricular cineangiography. In the study of Sanz and co-workers,[104] involving 300 men followed up to 60 months, ejection fraction, extent of coronary disease, and occurrence of congestive heart failure in the coronary care unit were independent predictors of survival. Importantly, in patients with normal ejection fraction, good prognosis was not affected by the number of diseased coronary arteries. In contrast, in patients with ejection fractions of between 21% and 49%, long-term survival was influenced by extent of coronary disease, with 95% of patients with one-vessel disease, but 78% of patients with three-vessel disease surviving at 60 months after infarction. Of patients with ejection fractions below 20%, survival was poor regardless of the number of coronary arteries diseased; in general, coronary disease was extensive in these patients. From this study, it appears that adding coronary arteriographic findings to analysis of risk may help to define a subgroup of patients with depressed ejection fractions who might benefit from myocardial revascularization.

In contrast to these observations, the data of Taylor and associates[105] in 106 survivors of myocardial infarction followed up to 30 months indicate that only past acute myocardial infarction and ejection fraction less than 40% predict mortality, whereas the extent of coronary artery disease or presence of congestive heart failure in the coronary care unit made no further contribution to predictive ability.

The use of potentially predictive variables in a stepwise multivariate, rather than univariate, discriminant function analysis may not classify some variables that have prognostic capability when considered as univariate predictors. This indicates only that they provide no new or further information, not that they are not useful predictors when considered independently.

USE OF PROPHYLACTIC β-ADRENERGIC BLOCKING AGENTS

Since β-adrenergic stimulation plays a role both in myocardial ischemia and in the development and maintenance of arrhythmias in patients with ischemic heart disease, the possible protective role of β-adrenergic blocking medications, particularly in survivors of myocardial infarction, has received wide attention. The potential mechanisms of protective action by β-blocking agents have been summarized[106,107] and include reduction in myocardial oxygen consumption by decreases in heart rate, blood pressure, and myocardial contractility; modulation of sympathetically mediated arrhythmias; and favorable alterations in myocardial substrate utilization. Experimental evidence suggests that β-blockade can raise the threshold for ventricular fibrillation[108] and can increase or redistribute coronary artery blood flow to areas of ischemic myocardium,[109] both of which have direct relevance in the clinical setting of myocardial infarction.

Over 20 long-term trials of the use of β-blocking agents in over 17,000 survivors of acute myocardial infarction have been carried out in the past 2 decades.[110-123] The studies have used various β-blocking agents, differing protocols, varying times of entry into the postinfarction study, and different lengths of follow-up, making interpretation of the resulting data difficult. However, several larger series of improved study design are available (Tables 72.8 and 72.9) that do suggest that some benefit accrues to the postinfarction patient in terms of prevention of reinfarction and both sudden and nonsudden cardiac death.

There are many unresolved issues with regard to the use of β-blocking medications after myocardial infarction: Is there an advantage of one agent over another, or do they all confer equal protection? When is the optimum time to begin therapy? How long after myocardial infarction should the drug be continued? Is there an optimum dose of medication, and if so, how may it be assessed clinically? Should all

TABLE 72.8 DESIGN OF LONG-TERM β-BLOCKER TRIALS IN SURVIVORS OF MYOCARDIAL INFARCTION

Trial	Patients Randomized	β-Blocker	Daily Dose (mg)
Wilhelmsson et al[110]	230	Alprenolol	400
Ahlmark et al[111]	393	Alprenolol	400
Barber et al[112]	500	Practolol	600
Multicentre International Study[119]	3053	Practolol	400
Andersen et al[120]	480	Alprenolol	400
Baber et al[113]	720	Propranolol	120
Norwegian Multicenter Study[121]	1884	Timolol	20
β-Blocker Heart Attack Trial[122]	3738	Propranolol	180–240
Hansteen et al[114]	560	Propranolol	160
Julian et al[116]	1456	Sotalol	320
Taylor et al[115]	1103	Oxprenolol	80
Pindolol Study Group[117]	529	Pindolol	15
European Infarction Study[118]	1741	Oxprenolol	160–320
Lopressor Intervention Study[123]†	2397	Metoprolol	200

* P values computed for χ^2 test comparing the proportion of deaths in each group.

† Results pending.

(Frishman WH: Pharmacology of the β-Adrenoceptor Blocking Drugs, 2nd ed. New York, Appleton-Century-Crofts, 1984)

survivors of myocardial infarction receive these agents, or only those at higher risk of subsequent events? The last issue has recently been addressed.[124] In a low-risk group of survivors of infarction, the annual mortality is less than 1% to 2% per year, with a cumulative 1- to 2-year mortality of 3% to 7% or less.[121,123,125] In this patient group, therefore, the value (and expense) of using β-blockade therapy as a preventive measure may reasonably be questioned and is perhaps even undesirable in view of the recognized side-effects of these agents.[126]

Not all survivors of myocardial infarction are candidates for prophylactic β-blocking therapy. Patients with disturbances of sinus node function, sinoatrial conduction, or atrioventricular conduction are at risk for development of hemodynamically significant bradycardia. Patients with left ventricular failure who require sympathetic stimulation for maintenance of optimum ventricular function should not be treated with β-adrenergic blockade. In this connection, it should be recognized that a depressed resting left ventricular ejection fraction is not a contraindication *per se* to β-blocker therapy provided that clinical congestive failure is not present. Other contraindications to β-adrenergic blockade are coronary artery spasm, claudication, and bronchial asthma.

ROLE OF ASPIRIN THERAPY

The role of daily aspirin in the prevention of recurrent myocardial infarction or death in patients recovered from myocardial infarction has been evaluated in six large randomized, placebo-controlled studies[65,126-132] (see Table 72.10) and summarized in an excellent review.[130] There appears to be some beneficial effect of aspirin on survivors of myocardial infarction; however, it has been pointed out that there is an associated 28% increase in mortality from noncardiovascular causes, suggesting that aspirin therapy is not entirely benign.[131]

Unanswered questions regarding aspirin use in survivors of myocardial infarction are the optimum dose and schedule of administration

TABLE 72.9 DESIGN AND RESULTS OF LONG-TERM β-BLOCKER TRIALS IN SURVIVORS OF MYOCARDIAL INFARCTION

Trial	Mean Entry Time After MI (days)	Mean Length of Follow-up (months)	Mortality (%) Control	Mortality (%) Intervention	P*
Wilhelmsson et al[110]	7–21 after discharge	24	12.1	6.1	0.18
Ahlmark et al[111]	14 after diagnosis	24	11.8	7.2	0.48
Barber et al[112]	1.0	24	31.3	27.2	0.51
Multicentre International Study[119]	13.2	14	8.2	6.3	0.051
Andersen et al[120]	1.0	12	26.2	25.2	0.92
Baber et al[113]	8.5	9	7.4	7.9	0.91
Norwegian Multicenter Study[121]	11.5	17	16.2	10.4	0.0003
β-Blocker Heart Attack Trial[122]	13.8	25	9.8	7.2	0.005
Hansteen et al[114]	4–6	12	13.1	9.0	0.16
Julian et al[116]	8.3	12	8.9	7.3	0.32
Taylor et al[115]	14 mo	48	10.2	9.5	0.78
Pindolol Study Group[117]	1–21	24	17.7	17.1	0.36
European Infarction Study[118]	14–36	12	5.1	6.6	0.14

* P values computed for χ^2 test comparing the proportion of deaths in each group.

(Frishman WH: Pharmacology of the β-Adrenoceptor Blocking Drugs, 2nd ed. New York, Appleton-Century-Crofts, 1984)

TABLE 72.10 ASPIRIN IN SURVIVORS OF ACUTE MYOCARDIAL INFARCTION

Study	Aspirin No. Patients	% Mortality	% Cardiovascular Mortality	% Nonfatal MI	Placebo No. Patients	% Mortality	% Cardiovascular Mortality	% Nonfatal MI
Elwood and co-workers (1974)[125]	615	8.0	8.0		624	10.7	10.0	
Elwood and Sweetnam (1979)[127]	832	12.3	11.5		850	14.8	14.2	
Breddin and co-workers (1979)[128]	317	8.5	5.7		309	10.4	8.4	
Coronary Drug Project (1976)	758	5.8	5.4	3.7	771	8.3	7.8	4.2
Persantine-Aspirin Reinfarction Study (1980)[129]	810	10.5	9.3	6.9	406	12.8	11.1	9.9
Aspirin Myocardial Infarction Study (1980)[130]	2267	10.9	9.3	6.3	2960	9.7	8.7	8.1

of the drug and the length of time that therapy should be continued in patients at varying degrees of continued risk. General recommendations for aspirin therapy in all postinfarction patients without contraindications to use of the drug cannot be made with any degree of certainty as to outcome. Similar caveats can be made for the use of oral anticoagulants[132] and persantine.

REFERENCES

1. Davis HT, DeCamilla J, Bayer LW et al: Survivorship patterns in the posthospital phase of myocardial infarction. Circulation 60:1252, 1979
2. Fioretti P, Brower RW, Simoons ML et al: Prediction of mortality in hospital survivors of myocardial infarction: Comparison of predischarge exercise testing and radionuclide ventriculography at rest. Br Heart J 52:292, 1984
3. Kirk ES, Sonnenblick EH: Newer concepts in the pathophysiology of ischemic heart disease. Am Heart J 103:756, 1982
4. Moss AJ: Update of postinfarction-risk stratification: Physiologic variables. In Greenberg HM, Kulbertus HE, Moss AJ et al (eds): Clinical aspects of life-threatening arrhythmias. Ann NY Acad Sci 427:280, 1984
5. Tubau JF, Chaitman BR, Bourassa MG et al: Detection of multi-vessel coronary disease after myocardial infarction using exercise stress testing and multiple ECG lead systems. Circulation 61:44, 1980
6. Ericsson M, Granath A, Ohlsson P et al: Arrhythmias and symptoms during treadmill testing three weeks after myocardial infarction in 100 patients. Br Heart J 35:787, 1973
7. Ibsen G, Kjoller E, Styperek J et al: Routine exercise ECG three weeks after acute myocardial infarction. Acta Med Scand 198:463, 1975
8. Markiewicz H, Houston N, DeBusk RF: Exercise testing soon after myocardial infarction. Circulation 56:26, 1977
9. Theroux P, Waters DD, Halphen C et al: Prognostic value of exercise testing soon after myocardial infarction. N Engl J Med 301:341, 1979
10. Sami M, Draemer H, DeBusk RF: The prognostic significance of serial exercise testing after myocardial infarction. Circulation 60:1238, 1979
11. Starling MR, Crawford MH, Kennedy GT et al: Exercise testing early after myocardial infarction: Predictive value for subsequent unstable angina and death. Am J Cardiol 46:909, 1980
12. Koppes GM, Kruyer W, Beckmann CH et al: Responses to exercise early after uncomplicated myocardial infarction in patients receiving no medication: Long-term follow-up. Am J Cardiol 46:764, 1980
13. Dillahunt PH, Miller AB: Early treadmill testing after myocardial infarction. Chest 76:150, 1979
14. Turner JD, Schwartz KM, Logic JR et al: Detection of residual jeopardized myocardium 3 weeks after myocardial infarction by exercise testing with thallium-201 myocardial scintigraphy. Circulation 61:729, 1980
15. Davidson DM, DeBusk RF: Prognostic value of a single exercise test 3 weeks after uncomplicated myocardial infarction. Circulation 61:236, 1979
16. DeBusk RF, Haskell W: Symptom-limited vs heart-rate-limited exercise testing soon after myocardial infarction. Circulation 61:738, 1980
17. Hamm LF, Crow RS, Stull AG, Hannan P: Safety and characteristics of exercise testing early after acute myocardial infarction. Am J Cardiol 63:1193, 1989
18. Pulido JI, Doss J, Twieg D et al: Submaximal exercise testing after acute myocardial infarction: Myocardial scintigraphic and electrocardiographic observations. Am J Cardiol 42:19, 1978
19. Waters DD, Chaitman BR, Bourassa MG et al: Clinical and angiographic correlates of exercise-induced ST-segment elevation: Increased detection with multiple ECG leads. Circulation 61:286, 1980
20. Weiner DA, McCabe C, Klein MD et al: ST segment changes postinfarction: Predictive value for multivessel coronary disease and left ventricular aneurysm. Circulation 58:887, 1978
21. Paine TD, Dye LE, Roitman DI et al: Relation of graded exercise test findings after myocardial infarction to extent of coronary artery disease and left ventricular dysfunction. Am J Cardiol 42:716, 1978
22. Kramer N, Susmano A, Shekelle RB: The "false negative" treadmill exercise test and left ventricular dysfunction. Circulation 57:763, 1978
23. Thompson PD, Keleman MH: Hypotension accompanying the onset of exertional angina. Circulation 42:28, 1975
24. Smith JW, Dennis CA, Gassman A et al: Exercise testing three weeks after myocardial infarction. Chest 75:1, 1979
25. Krone RJ, Gillespie JA, Weld FM et al: Low-level exercise testing after myocardial infarction: Usefulness in enhancing clinical risk stratification. Circulation 71:80, 1985
26. Waters DD, Bosch X, Bouchard A et al: Comparison of clinical variables and variables derived from a limited predischarge exercise test as predictors of early and late mortality after myocardial infarction. J Am Coll Cardiol 5:11, 1985
27. Schultze RA Jr, Strauss HW, Pitt B: Sudden death in the year following myocardial infarction: Relation to ventricular premature contractions in the late hospital phase and left ventricular ejection fraction. Am J Med 62:192, 1977
28. Weld FM, Chu KL, Bigger JT et al: Risk stratification with low level exercise testing 2 weeks after acute infarction. Circulation 64:306, 1981
29. Fuller CM, Raizner AE, Verani MS et al: Early postmyocardial infarction treadmill stress testing: An accurate discrimination of multi- and single vessel coronary disease (abstr). Am J Cardiol 45:421, 1980
30. Schwartz KM, Turner JD, Sheffield LT et al: Limited exercise testing soon after myocardial infarction. Ann Intern Med 94:727, 1981
31. Starling MR, Crawford MH, Kennedy GT et al: Treadmill exercise tests predischarge and six weeks post myocardial infarction to detect abnormalities of known prognostic value. Ann Intern Med 94:721, 1981
32. Handler CE, Sowton E: Diurnal variation and reproducibility of predischarge submaximal exercise testing after myocardial infarction. Br Heart J 52:299, 1984
33. Senaratne MPJ, Hsu L, Rossall R, Kappagoda CT: Exercise testing after myocardial infarction: Relative values of the low level predischarge and the postdischarge exercise test. J Am Coll Cardiol 12:1416, 1988
34. DeBusk RF, Dennis CA: "Submaximal" predischarge exercise testing after acute myocardial infarction: Who needs it? Am J Cardiol 55:499, 1985
35. Buda AJ, Dubbin JD, MacDonald IL et al: Spontaneous changes in thallium-201 myocardial perfusion imaging after myocardial infarction. Am J Cardiol 50:1272, 1982
36. Bingham JB, McKusick KA, Strauss HW et al: Influence of coronary artery disease on pulmonary uptake of thallium-201. Am J Cardiol 46:821, 1980
37. Gibson RS, Watson DD, Craddock GB et al: Prediction of cardiac events after uncomplicated myocardial infarction: A prospective study comparing predischarge exercise thallium-201 scintigraphy and coronary angiography. Circulation 68:321, 1983
38. Corbett J, Dehmer GJ, Lewis SE et al: The prognostic value of submaximal exercise testing with radionuclide ventriculography in patients with recent myocardial infarction. Circulation 62:111, 1980
39. Corbett JR, Dehmer GJ, Lewis SE et al: The prognostic value of submaximal exercise testing with radionuclide ventriculography before hospital discharge in patients with recent myocardial infarction. Circulation 64:535, 1981
40. Corbett JR, Nicod PH, Huxley RL et al: Left ventricular functional alterations at rest and during submaximal exercise in patients with recent myocardial infarction. Am J Med 74:577, 1983
41. Dewhurst NG, Muir AL: Comparative prognostic value of radionuclide ventriculography at rest and during exercise on 100 patients after first myocardial infarction. Br Heart J 49:111, 1983
42. DeBusk RF, Houston N, Haskell W et al: Exercise training soon after myocardial infarction. Am J Cardiol 44:1223, 1979
43. Tzivoni D, Keren A, Gottlieb S et al: Right atrial pacing soon after myocardial infarction. Circulation 64:330, 1982
44. Tzivoni D, Gottlieb S, Keren A et al: Early right atrial pacing after myocardial infarction: I. Comparison with early treadmill testing. Am J Cardiol 53:414, 1984
45. Tzivoni D, Gottlieb S, Keren A et al: Early right atrial pacing after myocardial infarction: II. Results in 77 patients with predischarge angina pectoris, congestive heart failure, or age older than 70 years. Am J Cardiol 53:418, 1984
46. Leppo JA, O'Brien J, Rothendler JA et al: Dipyridamole–thallium-201 scintigraphy in the prediction of future cardiac events after acute myocardial infarction. N Engl J Med 310:1014, 1984
47. Hammermeister KE, DeRouen TA, Dodge HT: Variables predictive of survival in patients with coronary disease. Circulation 59:421, 1979
48. Greenberg H, McMaster P, Dwyer EM Jr et al: Left ventricular dysfunction after acute myocardial infarction: Results of a prospective multicenter study. J Am Coll Cardiol 4:867, 1984
49. Warnowicz MA, Parker H, Cheitlin MD: Prognosis of patients with acute pulmonary edema and normal ejection fraction after acute myocardial infarction. Circulation 67:330, 1983
50. Nicod P, Gilpin E, Dittrich H et al: Influence on prognosis and morbidity of left ventricular ejection fraction with and without signs of left ventricular failure after acute myocardial infarction. Am J Cardiol 61:1165, 1988
51. Ahnve S, Gilpin E, Dittrich H et al: First myocardial infarction: Age and ejection fraction identify a low-risk group. Am Heart J 116:925, 1988
52. DeBusk RF, Kraemer HC, Nash E: Stepwise risk stratification soon after myocardial infarction. Am J Cardiol 52:1161, 1983
53. Epstein SE, Palmeri ST, Patterson RE: Evaluation of patients after acute myocardial infarction: Indications for cardiac catheterization and surgical intervention. N Engl J Med 307:1487, 1982
54. Kotler M, Tabatznik B, Mower M et al: Prognostic significance of ventricular ectopic beats with respect to sudden death in the later postinfarction period. Circulation 47:959, 1973
55. Lown B, Wolf M: Approaches to sudden death from coronary heart disease. Circulation 44:130, 1971
56. Vismara L, Amsterdam E, Mason D: Relation of ventricular arrhythmias in the late hospital phase of acute myocardial infarction to sudden death after hospital discharge. Am J Med 59:6, 1975
57. Ruberman W, Weinblatt E, Goldberg JD et al: Ventricular premature com-

plexes and sudden death after myocardial infarction. Circulation 64:297, 1981
58. Moss AJ, DeCamilla J, Davis H et al: The early post-hospital phase of myocardial infarction: Prognostic stratification. Circulation 54:58, 1976
59. Moss AJ, DeCamilla J, Engstrom F et al: The post-hospital phase of myocardial infarction: Identification of patients with increased mortality risk. Circulation 49:460, 1974
60. Moss AJ, DeCamilla JJ, Davis HP et al: Clinical significance of ventricular ectopic beats in the early post-hospital phase of myocardial infarction. Am J Cardiol 39:635, 1977
61. Moss AJ, Davis HT, DeCamilla J et al: Ventricular ectopic beats and their relation to sudden and nonsudden cardiac death after myocardial infarction. Circulation 70:998, 1979
62. Rehnqvist N, Lundman T, Sjögren A: Prognostic implications of ventricular arrhythmias registered before discharge and one year after acute myocardial infarction. Acta Med Scand 204:203, 1978
63. Bigger JT Jr, Heller CA, Wenger TL et al: Risk stratification after acute myocardial infarction. Am J Cardiol 42:202, 1978
64. Bigger JT Jr, Weld FM: Analysis of prognostic significance of ventricular arrhythmias after myocardial infarction: Shortcomings of Lown grading system. Br Heart J 45:717, 1981
65. Kostis JB, Wilson AC, Sanders MR, Byington RP: Prognostic significance of ventricular ectopic activity in survivors of acute myocardial infarction who receive propranolol. Am J Cardiol 61:975, 1988
66. Anderson KP, DeCamilla J, Moss AJ: Clinical significance of ventricular tachycardia (3 beats or longer) detected during ambulatory monitoring after myocardial infarction. Circulation 57:890, 1978
67. Moller M, Nielsen BL, Fabricus J: Paroxysmal ventricular tachycardia during repeated 24-hour ambulatory electrocardiographic monitoring of post-myocardial infarction patients. Br Heart J 43:447, 1980
68. deSoyza N, Bennett FA, Murphy ML et al: The relationship of paroxysmal ventricular tachycardia complicating the acute phase and ventricular arrhythmia during the late hospital phase of myocardial infarction to long-term survival. Am J Med 64:377, 1978
69. Bigger JT Jr, Fleiss JL, Kleiger R et al: Multicenter post-infarction research group: The relationship among ventricular arrhythmias, left ventricular dysfunction, and mortality in the 2 years after myocardial infarction. Circulation 69:250, 1984
70. Mukharji J, Rude RE, Poole WK et al: MILIS Study Group: Risk factors for sudden death after acute myocardial infarction: Two year follow-up. Am J Cardiol 54:31, 1984
71. Theroux P, Morissette D, Juneau M et al: Influence of fibrinolysis and percutaneous transluminal coronary angioplasty on the frequency of ventricular premature complexes. Am J Cardiol 63:797, 1989
72. Kowey PR, Khuri S, Josa M et al: Vulnerability to ventricular fibrillation in patients with clinically manifest ventricular tachycardia. Am Heart J 108:88, 1984
73. Ezri MD, Huang SK, Denes P: The role of Holter monitoring in patients with recurrent sustained ventricular tachycardia: An electrophysiologic correlation. Am Heart J 108:1229, 1984
74. Greene HL, Richardson DW, Hallstrom AP et al: Congestive heart failure after acute myocardial infarction in patients receiving antiarrhythmic agents for ventricular premature complexes (Cardiac Arrhythmia Pilot Study). Am J Cardiol 63:393, 1989
75. Greene HL, Richardson DW, Barker AH: Classification of deaths after myocardial infarction as arrhythmic or nonarrhythmic (the Cardiac Arrhythmia Pilot Study). Am J Cardiol 63:1, 1989
76. Cardiac Arrhythmia Pilot Study (CAPS) Investigators: Effects of encainide, flecainide, imipramine and moricizine on ventricular arrhythmias during the year after acute myocardial infarction: The CAPS. Am J Cardiol 61:501, 1988
77. Anderson JL, Hallstrom AP, Griffith LS et al: Relation of baseline characteristics to suppression of ventricular arrhythmias during placebo and active antiarrhythmic therapy in patients after myocardial infarction. Circulation 79:610, 1989
78. The Cardiac Arrhythmia Suppression Trial Investigators. Preliminary report: effect of encainide and flecainide on mortality in a randomized trial of arrhythmia suppression after myocardial infarction. N Engl J Med 321:406, 1989
79. Maisel AS, Scott N, Gilpin E et al: Complex ventricular arrhythmias in patients with Q wave versus non-Q wave myocardial infarction. Circulation 72:963, 1985
80. Gibson RS, Beller GA, Gheorghiade M et al: The prevalence and clinical significance of residual myocardial ischemia 2 weeks after uncomplicated non-Q wave infarction: A prospective natural history study. Circulation 73:1186, 1986
81. Greene HL, Reid PR, Schaeffer AH: The repetitive ventricular response in man: A predictor of sudden death. N Engl J Med 299:729, 1978
82. Hamer A, Vohra J, Sloman G et al: Electrophysiologic studies in survivors of late cardiac arrest after myocardial infarction. Am Heart J 105:921, 1983
83. Marchlinski FE, Buxton AE, Waxman HL et al: Identifying patients at risk of sudden death after myocardial infarction: Value of the response to programmed stimulation, degree of ventricular ectopic activity and severity of left ventricular dysfunction. Am J Cardiol 52:1190, 1983
84. Richards DA, Cody DV, Denniss AR et al: Ventricular electrical instability: A predictor of death after myocardial infarction. Am J Cardiol 51:75, 1983
85. Hamer A, Vohra J, Hunt D et al: Prediction of sudden death by electrophysiologic studies in high risk patients surviving acute myocardial infarction. Am J Cardiol 50:223, 1982
86. Kersschot IE, Brugada P, Ramentol M et al: Effects of early reperfusion in acute myocardial infarction on arrhythmias induced by programmed stimulation: A prospective, randomized study. J Am Coll Cardiol 7:1234, 1986
87. Sager PT, Perlmutter AB, Rosenfeld LE et al: Electrophysiologic effects of thrombolytic therapy in patients with a transmural anterior myocardial infarction complicated by left ventricular aneurysm formation. J Am Coll Cardiol 12:19, 1988
88. McComb JM, Gold HK, Leinbach RC et al: Electrically induced ventricular arrhythmias in acute myocardial infarction treated with thrombolytic agents. Am J Cardiol 62:186, 1988
89. Grimm M, Billhardt RA, Mayerhofer KE, Denes P: Prognostic significance of signal-averaged ECGs during acute myocardial infarction: A preliminary report. J Electrocardiol 21:283, 1988
90. McGuire M, Kuchar D, Ganis J et al: Natural history of late potentials in the first ten days after acute myocardial infarction and relation to early ventricular arrhythmias. Am J Cardiol 61:1187, 1988
91. Lewis SJ, Lander PT, Taylor PA et al: Evolution of late potential activity in the first six weeks after acute myocardial infarction. Am J Cardiol 63:647, 1989
92. Turitto G, Caref EB, Macina G et al: Time course of ventricular arrhythmias and the signal-averaged electrocardiogram in the post-infarction period: A prospective study of correlation. Br Heart J 60:17, 1988
93. Cripps T, Bennett E, Camm AJ, Ward DE: High gain signal-averaged electrocardiogram combined with 24-hour monitoring in patients early after myocardial infarction for bedside prediction of arrhythmic events. Br Heart J 60:181, 1988
94. Gomes JA, Mehres R, Barreca P et al: Quantitative analysis of the high-frequency components of the signal-averaged QRS complex in patients with acute myocardial infarction: A prospective study. Circulation 72:105, 1985
95. Kuchar DL, Thorburn CW, Sammel NL: Prediction of serious arrhythmic events after myocardial infarction: Signal-averaged electrocardiogram, Holter monitoring and radionuclide ventriculography. J Am Coll Cardiol 9:531, 1987
96. Denniss AR, Richards DA, Ross DL, Uther JB: Comparison of prognostic significance of delayed potentials and inducible ventricular tachycardia in 206 survivors of acute myocardial infarction. Br Heart J 54:609, 1985
97. Cripps T, Bennett D, Camm J, Ward D: Prospective evaluation of clinical assessment, exercise testing and signal-averaged electrocardiogram in predicting outcome after acute myocardial infarction. Am J Cardiol 62:995, 1988
98. Kuchar DL, Thorburn CW, Sammel NL: Late potentials detected after myocardial infarction: Natural history and prognostic significance. Circulation 74:1280, 1986
99. Gomes JA, Winters SL, Martinson M et al: The prognostic significance of quantitative signal-averaged variables relative to clinical variables, site of myocardial infarction, ejection fraction and ventricular premature beats: A prospective study. J Am Coll Cardiol 13:377, 1989
100. DeFeyter PJ, vanEenige MJ, Dighton DH et al: Prognostic value of exercise testing, coronary angiography and left ventriculography 6-8 weeks after myocardial infarction. Circulation 66:527, 1982
101. Dwyer EM Jr, McMaster P, Greenberg H et al: Nonfatal cardiac events and recurrent infarction in the year after acute myocardial infarction. J Am Coll Cardiol 4:695, 1984
102. Gazes PC, Kitchell JR, Meltzer LE et al: Death rate among 795 patients in the first year after myocardial infarction. JAMA 197:906, 1966
103. The Multicenter Postinfarction Research Group: Risk stratification and survival after myocardial infarction. N Engl J Med 309:331, 1983
104. Sanz G, Castaner A, Betriu A et al: Determinants of prognosis in survivors of myocardial infarction. N Engl J Med 306:1065, 1982
105. Taylor GJ, Humphries JO, Mellits ED et al: Predictors of clinical course, coronary anatomy and left ventricular function after recovery from acute myocardial infarction. Circulation 62:960, 1980
106. Bigger JT Jr, Coromilas J: How do beta-blockers protect after myocardial infarction? Ann Intern Med 101:256, 1984
107. Frishman WH, Furberg CD, Friedewald WT: The use of β-adrenergic blocking drugs in patients with myocardial infarction. Curr Prob Cardiol 9:25, 1984
108. Pratt C, Lichstein E: Ventricular antiarrhythmic effects of beta-adrenergic blocking drugs: A review of mechanism and clinical studies. J Clin Pharmacol 22:335, 1982
109. Braunwald E, Muller JE, Kloner RA: Role of beta-adrenergic blockade in the therapy of patients with myocardial infarction. Am J Med 74:113, 1983
110. Wilhelmsson C, Vedin JA, Wilhelmsen L et al: Reduction of sudden deaths after myocardial infarction by treatment with alprenolol: Preliminary results. Lancet 2:1157, 1974
111. Ahlmark G, Saetre H: Long-term treatment with beta-blockers after myocardial infarction. Eur J Clin Pharmacol 10:77, 1976
112. Barber JM, Boyle DMc, Chaturvedi NC et al: Practolol in acute myocardial infarction. Acta Med Scand 587(suppl):213, 1976
113. Baber NS, Wainwright ED, Howitt G et al: Multicentre postinfarction trial of propranolol in 49 hospitals in the United Kingdom, Italy and Yugoslavia. Br

114. Hansteen V, Moinichen E, Lorentsen E et al: One year's treatment with propranolol after myocardial infarction: Preliminary report of Norwegian Multicentre Trial. Br Med J 284:155, 1982
115. Taylor SH, Silke B, Ebbutt A et al: A long-term prevention study with oxprenolol in coronary heart disease. N Engl J Med 307:1293, 1982
116. Julian DG, Prescott RJ, Jackson FS et al: A controlled trial of sotalol for one year after myocardial infarction. Lancet 1:1142, 1982
117. Australian and Swedish Pindolol Study Group: The effect of pindolol on the two years mortality after complicated myocardial infarction. Eur Heart J 4:367, 1983
118. European Infarction Study Group: European Infarction Study (E.I.S.): A secondary beta-blocker prevention trial after myocardial infarction. Circulation 68(Suppl III):III-394, 1984
119. Multicentre International Study: Reduction in mortality with long-term beta-adrenoceptor blockade: A multicentre international study. Br Med J 2:419, 1977
120. Andersen MP, Bechsgaard P, Frederiksen J et al: Effect of alprenolol on mortality among patients with definite or suspected acute myocardial infarction: Preliminary results. Lancet 2:865, 1979
121. Norwegian Multicenter Study Group: Timolol-induced reduction in mortality and reinfarction in patients surviving myocardial infarction. N Engl J Med 304:801, 1981
122. β-Blocker Heart Attack Trial Research Group: A randomized trial of propranolol in patients with acute myocardial infarction: I. Mortality results. JAMA 247:1707, 1982
123. Cutler JA: A review of ongoing trials of beta-blockers in the secondary prevention of coronary heart disease. Circulation 67(suppl I):I-62, 1983
124. Ahumada GG: Identification of patients who do not require beta antagonists after myocardial infarction. Am J Med 76:900, 1984
125. Elwood PC, Cochrane AL, Burr ML et al: A randomized controlled trial of acetylsalicylic acid in the secondary prevention of mortality from myocardial infarction. Br Med J 1:436, 1974
126. Koppes GM, Beckman CH, Jones FG: Propranolol therapy for ventricular arrhythmias 2 months after myocardial infarction. Am J Cardiol 46:322, 1980
127. Elwood PC, Sweetnam PM: Aspirin and secondary mortality after myocardial infarction. Lancet 2:1313, 1979
128. Breddin K, Loew D, Lechner K et al: Secondary prevention of myocardial infarction: Comparison of acetylsalicylic acid, phenprocoumon and placebo: A multicenter two-year prospective study. Thromb Haemost 40:225, 1979
129. Persantine-Aspirin Reinfarction Study Research Group: Persantine and aspirin in coronary heart disease. Circulation 62:449, 1980
130. Aspirin Myocardial Infarction Study Research Group: A randomized controlled trial of aspirin in persons recovered from myocardial infarction. JAMA 243:661, 1980
131. Canner PL: Aspirin in coronary heart disease: Comparison of six clinical trials. Isr J Med Sci 19:413, 1983
132. EPSIM Research Group: A controlled comparison of aspirin and oral anticoagulants in prevention of death after myocardial infarction. N Engl J Med 307:701, 1982

CHAPTER 73

TRANSLUMINAL CORONARY ANGIOPLASTY AND NEWER CATHETER-BASED INTERVENTIONS

Paul G. Yock

The term *angioplasty* was coined by Dotter, who pioneered the procedure in the early 1960s using diagnostic catheters to tunnel through occluded leg arteries.[1] Over the next several years Dotter, Judkins, and others refined the technique to include a guide wire over which progressively larger, tapered dilating catheters could be introduced. Although the success rates in the periphery were encouraging, the method was limited by vascular trauma caused by introducing the large-caliber, stiff dilators.

Investigators in both the United States and Europe recognized that a balloon catheter would offer the ideal combination of low-profile vascular entry in the deflated position with the capability for high-pressure expansion of the lesion. Although balloon catheters had already been developed for the treatment of urethral strictures, technical problems were encountered in designing a system for vascular applications. Dotter and colleagues initially experimented with latex balloons but found that the highly elastic balloon assumed the shape of the lesion, stretching the normal segments and not dilating the plaque. In 1974, Gruentzig introduced a new type of balloon catheter constructed of polyvinylchloride that could be expanded to a predetermined diameter beyond which very little stretching occurred, even at high pressures. The balloon system proved successful in extensive trials in the periphery and was subsequently miniaturized for coronary applications. The first human percutaneous transluminal coronary angioplasty (PTCA) was performed by Gruentzig[2,3] in September 1977 on a young Swiss man with a tight proximal left anterior descending artery stenosis (Fig. 73.1).

Several centers in Europe and the United States began PTCA programs in the subsequent year, and in 1979 the National Heart, Lung, and Blood Institute sponsored the first international PTCA registry. The registry closed in 1982 after enrollment of more than 3000 patients, most of whom had single-vessel disease, stable angina, and normal left ventricular function. In this group the primary success rate, defined as a 20% or greater improvement in luminal diameter, was 61%.[4,5] A significant learning curve was also documented, with operators who performed more than 50 cases having substantially lower rates of complications.[6]

During the early 1980s, advances in catheter technology and increased operator experience led to major improvements in the procedure. The use of a separate, movable coronary guide wire with a coaxial balloon catheter, introduced by Simpson and co-workers,[7] provided a safer and more effective means for subselective cannulation of coronary vessels. Improved guide wires were developed with flexible tips that could be shaped by the operator to the optimal configuration for a particular case. Better visualization was provided both by improved x-ray imaging equipment and by enhanced radiopacity of guide wires and catheters. In recognition of these changes, the PTCA registry was reopened in 1985–1986 with the enrollment of 2500 additional patients. Selection criteria were more liberal, with over half of the patients having multivessel disease and many with prior infarcts or impaired left ventricular function. Despite the more challenging case distribution, the primary success rate improved substantially to 78% with an overall decrease in emergency bypass surgery and nonfatal infarction.[8]

In the late 1980s, the use of angioplasty has increased dramatically;

it is estimated that as many as 400,000 PTCA procedures will be performed in 1990. Multivessel angioplasty has become routine in most centers, and increasingly complex lesions are being successfully treated with balloon catheters. Primary success rates have continued to improve, now averaging 90% or greater in most centers. In parallel, there has been explosive development in second-generation interventional devices including laser angioplasty catheters, "atherectomy" (plaque extraction) catheters, and intravascular stents. New pharmacologic approaches to the problems of abrupt reclosure and restenosis are being developed. Better visualization techniques are undergoing testing, including fiberoptic angioscopy and catheter-based ultrasound.

MECHANISMS OF ANGIOPLASTY

Dotter and Judkins originally conceptualized the process of balloon angioplasty as involving a compression and remolding of plaque, like a footprint in the snow.[1] Postmortem studies, however, have demonstrated that plaque compression contributes minimally to the net effect of angioplasty.[9] The major mechanism for lumen enlargement appears to be a combination of plaque splitting, separation of the plaque from the media, tearing of intima and media, and stretching of adventitia to accomodate the increased lumen size (Figs. 73.2 and 73.3).[10,11] As the balloon is inflated, high radial forces cause an initial splitting of the plaque-laden intima, usually at a point where the plaque is relatively thin. This splitting typically extends under the plaque, lifting it away from the media and producing an irregular lumen contour (see Fig. 73.3). The resultant tear can extend to the internal elastic lamina or may continue into media. Once the "skeleton" of plaque is split, further enlargement of the lumen can occur with stretching of the media and adventitia. In cases with eccentric deposits of plaque, stretching of the plaque-free wall segment can occur preferentially and the plaque may not undergo substantial splitting or remodeling. If the normal segment of vessel wall is highly elastic, it may not be possible to achieve a

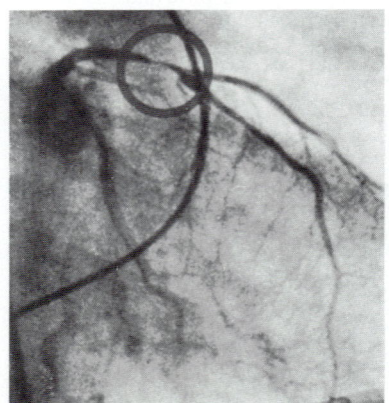
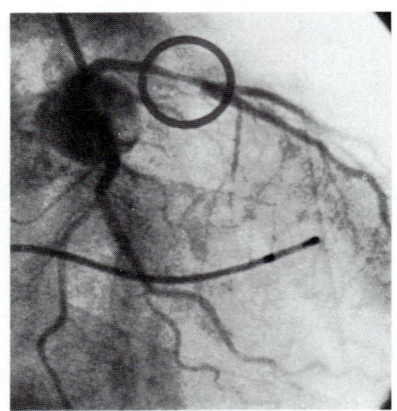
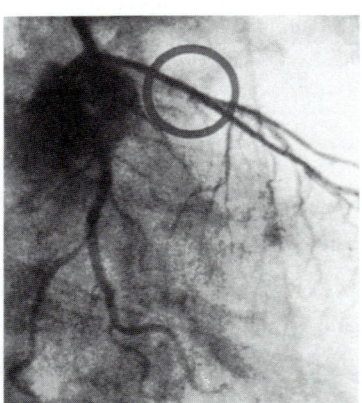

FIGURE 73.1 Angiograms from the first patient to undergo coronary angioplasty (performed by Andreas Gruentzig on September 16, 1977). The predilatation study is shown in the left panel, the immediate postdilatation angiogram in the middle panel, and the 1-month follow-up study on the right. (Courtesy of USCI, Division of C.R. Bard, Billerica, MA)

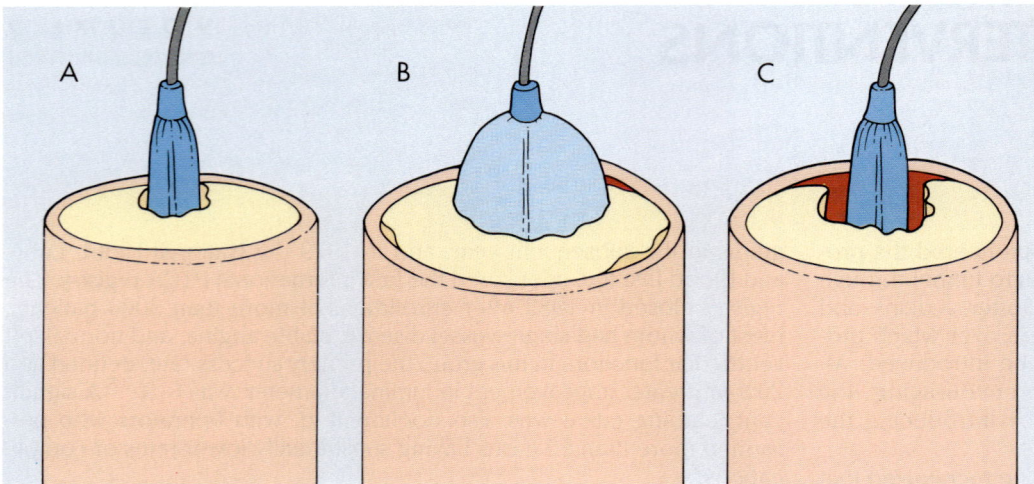

FIGURE 73.2 Schematic representation of the mechanism of balloon angioplasty. **A.** Deflated balloon across a tight, typically eccentric stenosis. **B.** Balloon inflation exerts high radial forces, causing tearing of the plaque away from the vessel wall and stretching of the remaining media and adventitia. Compression of plaque is minimal. **C.** Following balloon deflation there is rebound of the elastic vessel wall but the lumen remains substantially enlarged. Dissection planes have been created between the plaque and vessel wall. Repeat inflations, or inflations with a larger balloon, would further stretch the vessel wall and create a still larger lumen.

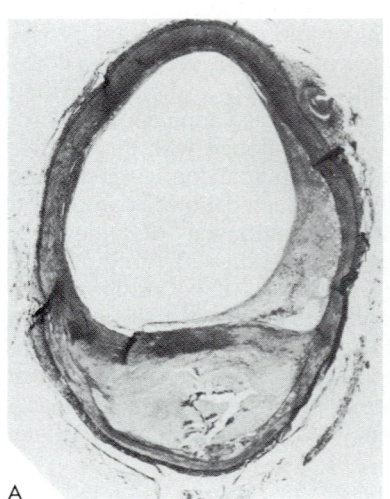
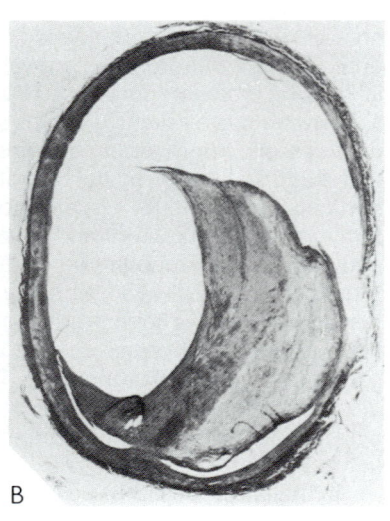

FIGURE 73.3 Demonstration of angioplasty effect on a pathologic femoral artery specimen. **A.** Undilated artery with an eccentric plaque. **B.** Postdilatation view. The plaque has dissected free from the underlying media and is protruding into the lumen of the vessel. The lumen area has increased by means of the dissection and stretching of the media and adventitia. (Zarins CK, Lu ET, Lewertz BL et al: Arterial disruption and remodeling following balloon dilatation. Surgery 92:1086, 1982)

long-lasting angioplasty result because the segment will return to its preinflation profile once the balloon is deflated. Embolization of significant amounts of plaque material is uncommon in native vessel angioplasty and does not contribute to lumen enlargement.

Evidence of disruption of plaque and arterial wall is seen angiographically in the majority of cases following PTCA.[12,13] The most common angiographic appearance is a haziness in the region of inflation, which may reflect entry of contrast medium into intimal or medial tears or the plaque substance itself. Specific intimal flaps or dissections can frequently be visualized (Fig. 73.4) and, if not extensive, may have an innocent or even positive prognostic implication.[14] Long or spiral dissections can lead to abrupt closure of the lumen. Although stretching of the media and adventitia appears to be an essential component of balloon angioplasty, evidence of aneurysm formation is rare by angiography.

The mechanism of angioplasty in saphenous vein grafts is essentially similar to that in native vessels, although stretching of the graft may play a relatively more significant role. Extensive deposits of "cheesy" atheroma occur in older grafts, and embolization during instrumentation of the artery is a significant risk. Dilatation of the anastomotic site has a marginally higher primary success rate than angioplasty of the body or ostium of the graft, perhaps because plaque splitting is more effective in the native vessel portion of the anastomosis, where the plaque has a more brittle character and the vessel is less likely to stretch.

INDICATIONS FOR PTCA

Both clinical and angiographic criteria are considered in selecting patients for PTCA (Tables 73.1 and 73.2). Because angioplasty is associated with a small but significant risk of infarction, emergency surgery, and death, the clinical selection criteria are generally similar to those for bypass surgery. In patients with stable angina, objective demonstration of ischemia by electrocardiogram or exercise testing is an essential condition for consideration. Patients with stable angina that is controlled with medications may still be candidates for PTCA if their angina significantly impairs their life style or they experience major side-effects from their medications. Patients with evidence for extensive myocardium at risk on treadmill testing—a markedly positive test at low levels of exercise—should also be considered for PTCA. Similar general guidelines for PTCA in stable angina patients have been published by the joint American Heart Association/American College of

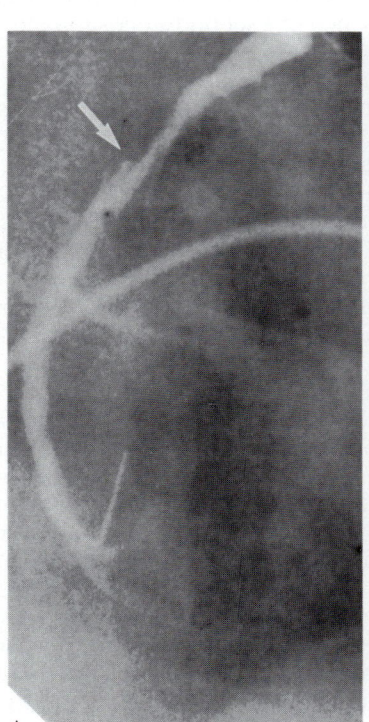
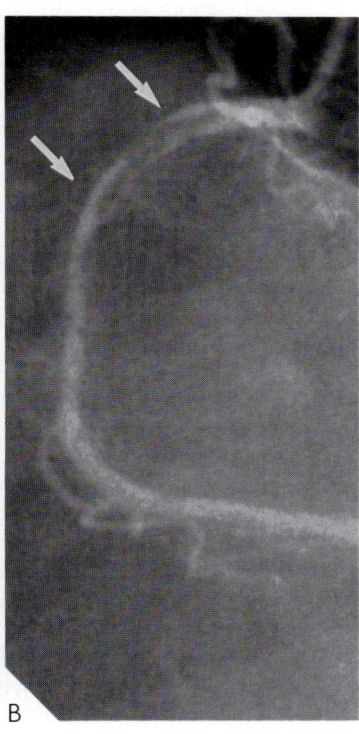

FIGURE 73.4 Angiograms from two patients showing proximal right coronary artery dissections following PTCA. **A.** Localized, minor dissection at the point indicated by the arrow. **B.** Long, spiral dissection in the region of the arrows. This artery closed completely a short time after the injection shown here.

TABLE 73.1 GENERAL CLINICAL INDICATIONS FOR PTCA
Stable Angina Failed medical therapy Ischemia at low level of exercise Substantial myocardium at risk
Unstable Angina Refractory to conventional pharmacotherapy "Culprit lesion" identified
Acute Myocardial Infarction Thrombolytic therapy contraindicated Failure to reperfuse with thrombolysis Reocclusion post thrombolysis Cardiogenic shock

TABLE 73.2 RISK FACTORS FOR ABRUPT RECLOSURE
Clinical Variables Unstable angina Female gender
Angiographic Variables Lesion on bend point or on branch point Lesion associated with thrombus Long lesion Other stenoses in same vessel
Procedural Variables Gradient greater than 20 mm Hg post PTCA Stenosis greater than 35% post PTCA Intimal tear or dissection

Cardiology Task Force on Angioplasty[15] and the Joint International Society and Federation of Cardiology and World Health Organization Task Force on Coronary Angioplasty.[16]

In patients with unstable angina, several studies have demonstrated the usefulness of PTCA in improving symptomatic status.[17-20] Primary success rates (defined variously as 20% to 40% improvement in luminal diameter, or less than 50% residual diameter narrowing) are in the 80% to 90% range, equal to or very slightly less than those in stable angina. In one study, symptomatic status at 1 year was better in unstable angina patients treated with PTCA versus bypass surgery.[17] In patients with variant angina (coronary spasm) and minimal or no fixed atherosclerotic disease, the risks of PTCA generally outweigh the benefits. With a combination of significant stenoses and spasm, angioplasty is technically feasible, but symptoms of spasm may recur and restenosis rates tend to be high.[21-23]

The use of PTCA combined with thrombolytic agents in acute myocardial infarction is reviewed elsewhere in this volume. At present the role of direct angioplasty (angioplasty without thrombolytic therapy) remains undefined. Initial studies suggest that primary recanalization rates with direct angioplasty are in the 80% to 90% range, exceeding the rates for thrombolytic therapy alone.[24,25] The reported incidence of abrupt reclosure and the rate of emergency bypass surgery have been only slightly higher than for stable angina patients, and in-hospital mortality rates have been low, 6% to 7%. The principal barrier to widespread application of this approach to treatment of acute infarction is the availability of trained operators and catheterization/surgical facilities on an emergent basis.

Other clinical variables influence the choice of patients for PTCA. Data from the first NHLBI registry indicated that in patients aged 65 years or older the primary success rate was significantly lower (53% vs. 63%) and the complication rates higher (55% vs. 34%) than in younger patients.[5] On the other hand, the 2.2% in-hospital mortality rate for these patients compared favorably with series on coronary bypass surgery for the elderly.[26] In addition, recent improvements in angioplasty equipment appear to have increased the success and safety of PTCA in this patient group.[27] A second independent predictor of lower success and increased mortality from the registry data was female sex. The major difference between women and men in mortality was contributed by a greater than fivefold increment in mortality for women undergoing emergency bypass surgery in the setting of failed PTCA. Women with a successful PTCA had a lower rate of restenosis, however, and fewer required bypass surgery. The symptomatic improvement following PTCA was similar for men and women.[5] Subsequent studies have not consistently shown a statistically significant difference for women in primary success rate, complication rate, or mortality.[28] Other clinical variables identified from the registry data as independent predictors of poor outcome for PTCA were prior coronary bypass surgery and duration of angina for more than 6 months. Prior coronary bypass surgery does not influence the primary success rate but does increase mortality because of the greater risks of repeat bypass grafting for failed PTCA. Patients with angina of longer duration may have harder, more calcific plaque that is less likely to dilate without complication.

ANATOMICAL CRITERIA

Angiographic variables influencing patient selection for PTCA include the number and location of diseased vessels, the specific morphologic features of the lesion, and the presence of complicating technical features such as extreme tortuosity or side branches. In patients with single-vessel disease, dilatation should be performed only if the vessel supplies a major portion of myocardium and the stenosis is clearly significant. In patients with 60% or less diameter stenosis, complication and restenosis rates are not significantly different than in patients with high-grade lesions.[29] In fact, an aggressive restenosis response may replace a pre-PTCA subcritical narrowing with a tighter, critical lesion.

With current equipment, primary success rates are generally independent of the coronary artery involved (left anterior descending, circumflex, right) and position in the vessel (proximal, mid, distal). An exception to this rule is the ostial stenosis of the left main or right coronary artery.[30,31] Here the elasticity of the vessel may be higher by virtue of attachment to the aortic wall, so that transient stretching rather than splitting of the plaque occurs. Lesions at bifurcations in the coronary tree are at risk for occlusion of the branch vessel if it arises from the lesion.[32] Current practice is to protect branch vessels by passing a second guide wire and balloon into the branch; dilatation of the branch vessel may be performed either simultaneously ("kissing balloon" technique) or sequentially.[33] Lesions located at acute bends in vessels are more likely to dissect, perhaps because the straightening of the balloon at high pressures exerts an unequal, tearing force on the vessel wall. Angled balloons have been introduced in the attempt to minimize this complication. Specific lesion morphology appears to have an impact on primary success rates but is difficult to characterize precisely with angiography. Eccentricity of the lesion correlated with adverse short-term effects in the registry analysis[5] but not in a more recent restrospective study from Emory University of abrupt reclosure.[34] The appearance of thrombus associated with the lesion is a negative prognostic factor for PTCA.[34,35] Other morphologic features that have been correlated with poor initial outcome include length of the lesion, calcification, and presence of a second stenosis in the same vessel.

Although chronic total occlusion was initially considered to be a contraindication for PTCA, recent data indicate that these lesions can be dilated with primary success rates of 50% to 75%. Viable myocardium may be present in these cases by virtue of collateral filling, and patients may have marked symptomatic benefit from revascularization of the primary vessel. The main determinant of successful PTCA in occlusions is the duration of the occlusion, judged from the patient's history. If the occlusion is older than 2 to 3 months, the likelihood of opening the vessel is substantially diminished.[36-38] Even if the procedure is successful initially, restenosis rates are high, reaching 55% at 8 months in one study.[39]

Multivessel angioplasty accounts for an increasing share of PTCA procedures currently performed and represents the majority of cases in many centers. For experienced operators, the primary success rate for multivessel dilatation appears to be comparable to that for single-vessel angioplasty.[40,41] The term *culprit lesion* angioplasty has been applied to the strategy of selectively dilating those lesions in multivessel disease that are responsible for ischemia. Identification of the culprit lesions is based on angiographic appearance of the stenosis,[42] localizing electrocardiographic evidence, and the results of exercise testing. This strategy has the potential advantage of less acute risk than an attempt at complete revascularization by PTCA and has been shown to provide excellent short-term symptomatic benefit. Patients with partial revascularization, however, are more likely to have recurrence of angina and to require a second revascularization procedure.[43,44] Staged angioplasty, in which a multivessel dilatation is performed in two or more sessions on different days, is one method for reducing the acute risk associated with dilatations in multiple territories.

PTCA is playing an increasingly important role in patients with previous bypass grafting (Fig. 73.5), as reoperation is associated with both increased perioperative mortality and less satisfactory long-term symptomatic benefit. Primary success rates in vein graft dilatation are excellent, in the 80% to 95% range.[45-48] Restenosis rates in these studies have been high, however, with overall values of 40% to 50%. Restenosis is much more likely to occur in dilatations involving the proximal anastomosis or graft body than the distal anastomosis to the coronary artery. Embolization of graft atheroma into the native circulation occurs occasionally, particularly in older grafts. In some cases, dilatation of the native vessel supplied by the graft may be more favorable than attempting PTCA of the graft itself; occasionally, dilatation of both the graft and the native vessel is performed. PTCA of the left main coronary artery, which is generally considered to have too great a risk for elective angioplasty, may be performed relatively safely in patients with a graft to the anterior descending and/or circumflex systems.[30]

PTCA VERSUS BYPASS SURGERY

At present, there are no data from randomized trials comparing catheter and surgical therapies for coronary disease. Several retrospective studies have analyzed different aspects of the comparison between PTCA and bypass surgery. Acutely, there is a higher incidence of infarction with PTCA than surgery, the bulk of which occurs in patients with failed angioplasty who require salvage surgery. In general, patients undergoing PTCA and bypass surgery have similar early symptomatic improvement.[49,50] PTCA patients leave the hospital earlier, on average, than bypass patients and also return to work earlier.[51] On a per-procedure basis, the costs of angioplasty are substantially less than for bypass surgery, but this advantage is diminished by the problem of restenosis, which demands additional expense in surveillance testing as well as repeat revascularization in 25% to 30% of cases.[52,53]

Long-term clinical benefits of angioplasty surgery are also difficult to compare using currently available data. Because of the problem of restenosis, a significantly smaller proportion of patients remain symptom free following a single PTCA than is the case with coronary bypass surgery. Nevertheless, the long-term results of PTCA-based management, including repeat dilatation as indicated, appear to be relatively favorable. In follow-up data from the first PTCA Registry, 70% of patients remained pain free at an average of 4 years.[54] At 5-year mean follow-up in a study from Emory University, the event-free rate was 79% (no death, infarction, or surgery).[55] Further insight into the relative roles of PTCA and surgery awaits completion of two large-scale, randomized clinical trials: the NHLBI-sponsored Bypass Angioplasty Revascularization Intervention (BARI) Trial and the Emory University Angioplasty vs. Surgery Trial (EAST).

TECHNIQUE

Once a patient is selected for PTCA, the preprocedure evaluation is conducted along similar lines as for cardiac catheterization. Preliminary laboratory data should include a recent chest roentgenogram, electrocardiogram, renal and electrolyte panel, prothrombin time, and hematocrit. Because of the possibility of salvage bypass grafting, additional screening tests such as pulmonary function tests may be advisable, depending on the patient. A specimen should be sent to the blood bank for type and screen. Informed consent must involve a careful discussion of the possibility of urgent surgery.

Although there is no standard medical regimen in preparation for angioplasty, many operators administer antiplatelet agents and calcium channel blockers prior to the procedure. Aspirin and dipyridamole, given beginning 24 hours prior to PTCA, have been shown to reduce the rate of early infarction.[56] A typical regimen consists of 325 mg of aspirin once daily and 75 mg of dipyridamole three times a day, beginning at least the day before the procedure. Some operators advocate the use of intravenous dextran infusion beginning before the procedure, although there is no definitive support for this practice in the literature.[57] Calcium channel blockers (usually either nifedipine or diltiazem) may be started in the hope of diminishing procedure-induced coronary spasm, although evidence for long-term benefit is lacking. Preprocedure sedation should be light, comparable to that for cardiac catheterization. Intramuscular atropine is administered prior to PTCA in some centers.

In the catheterization laboratory, patient preparation and vascular entry are similar to the procedure in routine angiography. PTCA may be performed from either a femoral or brachial approach, using standard Judkins or Sones cannulation techniques. A transvenous pacemaker should be placed in any patient with pre-existing conduction system disease and in all patients undergoing right and dominant left circumflex coronary angioplasty. In many centers pacemakers are inserted for all PTCA cases. Some operators favor a combined pacing/pulmonary artery catheter to allow simultaneous monitoring of pulmonary artery pressures.

Predilatation angiography may be performed using either standard diagnostic catheters or the larger angioplasty guiding catheters. These angiograms are used to make a final selection of equipment for the angioplasty and to provide a "road map" for the procedure. Heparin is administered prior to angiography; typically 5000 to 10,000 units is given as an initial bolus injection, and additional bolus injections are administered hourly.

The selection of an appropriate balloon catheter is based on a number of considerations. In general, two types of balloon systems are available: fixed guide wire catheters, in which the balloon is mounted directly on a guide wire, and movable guide wire catheters, in which the balloon is on a separate catheter that rides coaxially on a guide wire (Fig. 73.6). The fixed guide wire systems have the advantage of lower profiles (smaller deflated balloon diameters) and therefore cross a tight stenosis more easily. The movable guide wire systems are more readily steered down the branching coronary tree by virtue of the free torque (turning) of the guide wire within the balloon catheter lumen. These systems also allow the operator to leave a guide wire in place across the lesion as a track on which other catheters (e.g., larger balloons) can be introduced. With either system, balloons are provided in a range of inflated diameters from 1.5 mm to 4.5 mm. The appropriate balloon size is estimated from the angiogram by studying the diameter of the normal segments proximal and distal to the region of stenosis.

Guiding catheters are 8 or 9 F, large-lumen catheters that have three important functions: (1) they serve as conduits for the balloon/guide wire system into the coronary artery and provide relatively rigid

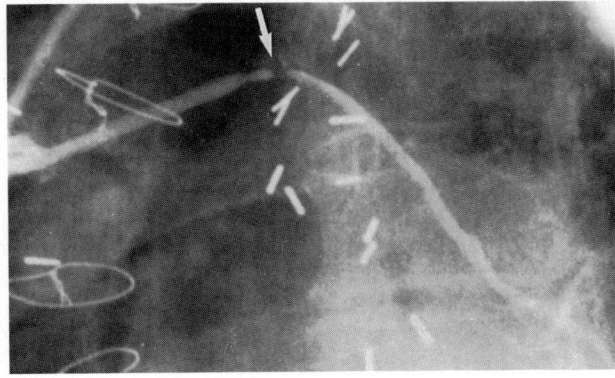
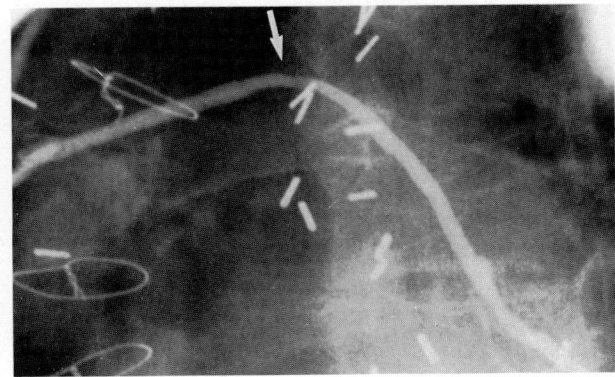

FIGURE 73.5 Pre-PTCA (left) and post-PTCA (right) angiograms showing successful dilation of a graft to an obtuse marginal coronary artery. Arrows indicate region of angioplasty.

support for forcing the deflated balloon across a stenosis; (2) they allow for the injection of contrast medium around the balloon catheter into the coronary arteries for visualization; and (3) they allow measurement of pressure at the ostium of the coronary artery by means of the fluid column around the balloon catheter. This last feature is extremely important, because too tight a fit between the guiding catheter and coronary ostium leads to occlusion of blood flow, which can be detected only by a low pressure at the tip of the guide. Like angiographic catheters, the guiding catheters are preshaped to optimize seating in the coronary ostium. Choice of the right type of guiding catheter is critical to the success of the procedure: lack of support by the guide is a common cause of failure, where attempts to pass the balloon catheter result only in pushing the guiding catheter out of the coronary ostium (the equal and opposite reaction).

Once a guiding catheter is securely in place, the balloon/guide wire system is advanced to the ostium (Fig. 73.7). With either a fixed or movable guide wire system, the next step is to direct the guide wire tip down the appropriate branch of the coronary tree and across the stenosis. The guide wire tip is highly flexible and can be shaped by the operator to a "J" configuration to facilitate making turns in the coronary tree. The guide wire is intensely radiopaque so that progress of the wire down the coronary vessel can be easily visualized. To pass the guide wire, the operator advances it while gently rotating it, keeping the tip of the wire free and negotiating any branches or curves. The guide wire is moved across the lesion, taking care not to catch the tip in the wall of the lesion. In the fixed guide wire systems, the catheter is then advanced until the balloon is centered in the lesion. With a movable guide wire system, the wire is advanced as far distally into the coronary artery as possible in order to provide maximum support for the balloon catheter. With the wire secured in place, usually by a second operator, the balloon catheter is advanced across the lesion. Often deeper seating of the guiding catheter in the coronary artery is necessary at this stage to provide extra support to the balloon.

When the balloon is centered in the lesion, the inflation sequence is begun. The characteristics of this sequence (*e.g.*, rate of inflation, maximal pressure, duration of inflation, number of inflations) vary among operators and are based on largely empiric considerations. Typically, pressures in the balloon are brought up to an initial range of 5 to 7 atmospheres (75–105 psi) within a few seconds. The imprint of the lesion on the balloon will often be seen as an indentation in the inflated balloon. Pressures are increased until the deformity disappears, signaling a successful "cracking" of the plaque. Studies on the pressure–volume characteristics of balloon inflation suggest that once this cracking is accomplished, the vessel will be substantially more compliant during subsequent inflations.[58] Some operators therefore regard abrupt disappearance of the balloon deformity as the end point of the inflation sequence, no matter how low the pressure. In other cases, there is no clear deformity in the balloon and the operator must judge the appropriate pressure and duration of inflation. Evidence from nonrandomized clinical trials suggests that longer inflations may provide better long-term angioplasty results, and many operators currently prefer inflations of at least 1 minute. In some cases ischemic symptoms are minimal during balloon inflation, and dilatations of several minutes or longer are well tolerated. In other patients, typically those without good collateral flow, hemodynamic instability may occur shortly after the balloon is inflated.

The most widely used index of a successful dilatation is the angiographic appearance of the lesion following the inflations. Frequently the balloon catheter must be removed from the guiding catheter to provide enough contrast medium flow for good visualization. A typical angiographic result in a successful case involves reduction in the percent of diameter stenosis to 10% to 20%, a smooth appearance to the wall, minimal angiographic evidence of dissection and a qualitatively brisk rate of contrast run-off into the distal coronary bed.

In addition to the angiographic appearance of the lesion, many operators measure a pressure gradient across the stenosis, as originally advocated by Gruentzig.[3] The measurement requires a balloon catheter with a fluid-filled pressure lumen and can be made by subtracting the distal pressure recorded at the tip of this catheter (with the balloon deflated) from the proximal pressure at the tip of the guiding catheter in the coronary ostium. Initial mean crossing gradients, prior to inflation, are in the 40-mm to 80-mm range; following a successful dilatation the gradients drop to the 0 to 15-mm range. Higher residual gradients have been associated with abrupt reclosure and restenosis and are used in some centers to determine whether further balloon inflations are necessary for a given lesion. The pressure gradients are subject to a number of artifacts, however, including the presence of the balloon catheter across the area of stenosis.[59] In addition, the push for

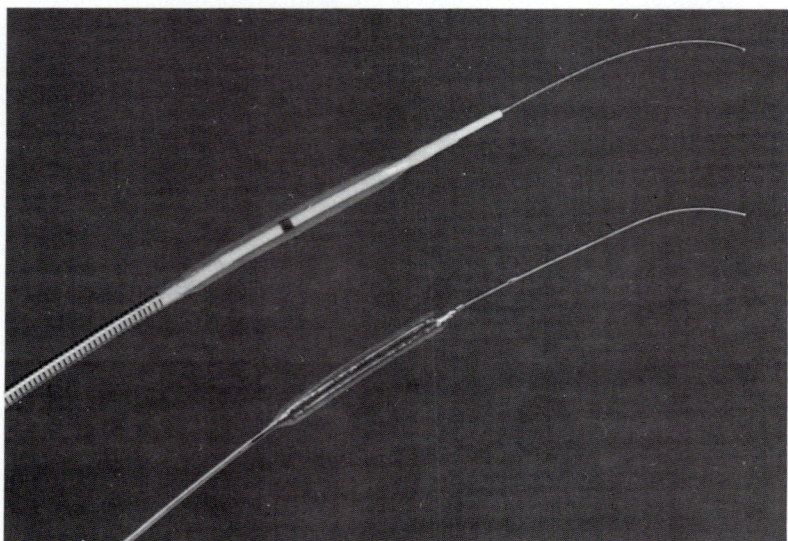

FIGURE 73.6 Examples of the two major types of balloon dilatation systems. The top catheter rides on a movable guide wire that can be advanced ahead of the catheter and torqued (turned) freely. The bottom catheter has a fixed guide wire tip, a configuration that sacrifices independent torque of the guide wire for the benefit of lower deflated balloon profile.

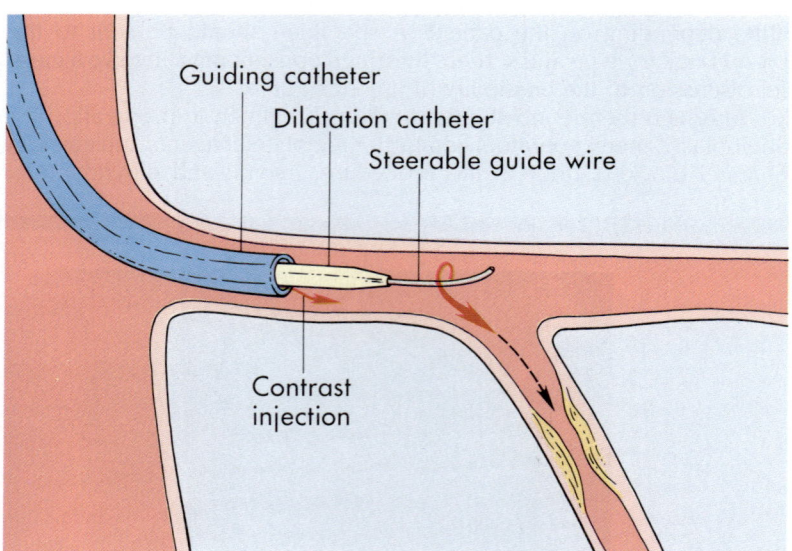

FIGURE 73.7 Schematic representation of the basic angioplasty procedure. The three major components of the system (guiding catheter, dilatation catheter, and guide wire) are shown. Contrast medium is injected through the guiding catheter to provide a "map" for passage of the guide wire and balloon catheter. (Modified from Baim DS, Faxon DP: Coronary angioplasty. In Grossman W (ed): Cardiac Catheterization and Angiography, 3rd ed. Philadelphia, Lea & Febiger, 1986)

development of lower profile catheters has led to sacrifice of the pressure lumen in many newer catheters.

Once the angioplasty has been successfully completed, the guide wire and catheter are removed and a final set of angiograms may be obtained. In the brachial cases, the arteriotomy is closed; in the femoral cases, the sheath is typically left in place for a few hours until the heparin effect is diminished. In patients with a suboptimal angiographic result, sheaths may be left overnight with the patient on a heparin drip, to allow easy access in case of abrupt reclosure of the coronary artery. In most centers, patients are routinely monitored for 4 to 12 hours following PTCA. Discharge typically occurs on the day following PTCA for most patients with uncomplicated procedures; in some centers, a maximum exercise test is performed as a screening procedure prior to discharge. Outpatient angioplasty, with the patient leaving the hospital later on the same day as the procedure, is being performed on selected patients in some centers.

ACUTE COMPLICATIONS

Coronary flow is interrupted during balloon inflation, and patients frequently experience some degree of chest discomfort during the period of balloon occlusion. The effects of coronary occlusion on ventricular performance are profound but transient. Significant regional wall motion abnormalities occur within 20 seconds of inflation and progress to segmental akinesis and dyskinesis within 1 minute.[60,61] Systolic volumes increase during the period of inflation, without any concomitant increase in diastolic volumes. Diastolic pressures rise markedly, however, resulting in an upward displacement of the pressure–volume curve with a corresponding increase in regional stiffness.[62] Following balloon deflation and resumption of flow, return of wall motion begins within 20 seconds and is generally back to normal within 60 to 90 seconds. During this period there is reactive hyperemia in coronary flow, as measured by the Doppler catheter technique.[63] The reactive hyperemia may be associated with a transient "overshoot" in segmental systolic function. Regional diastolic dysfunction may persist for 10 minutes or longer following resumption of flow and normal systolic function.

Six to 8% of patients will experience prolonged angina following balloon deflation.[64] In 4% to 5% of patients, prolonged angina is caused by abrupt reclosure of the vessel, owing to a combination of dissection, spasm, and/or thrombus formation.[34,35] Clinical and angiographic predictors of abrupt reclosure are discussed previously; in general, more complex lesions, particularly those associated with thrombus or at branch or bend points, are more likely to close. Abrupt reclosure often occurs during the first 30 minutes following dilatation. Accordingly, it is standard practice in many laboratories to observe patients with a guide wire in place across the lesion for at least 5 minutes following PTCA. If occlusion occurs, attempts to redilate the artery with a balloon catheter will be successful in 50% or more of the cases. In the situation of a dissection, longer, low-pressure inflation cycles are often used in the attempt to tack the flap back to the vessel wall. If thrombus is suspected as the primary mechanism of abrupt reclosure, intracoronary injection of lytic agents such as streptokinase or urokinase may be beneficial.[65]

If attempts to redilate the stenosis are unsuccessful and a significant territory of myocardium is at risk, the patient must be sent urgently for bypass surgery. At present, salvage bypass grafting is performed in 2% to 3% of patients undergoing PTCA. In optimal circumstances, patients can be placed on bypass within 30 minutes of vessel closure. Even with minimal delay, however, approximately one third of patients undergoing surgery will sustain some degree of myocardial infarction.[66-70] Use of the autoperfusion catheter (Fig. 73.8) provides marked stabilization of some patients with abrupt reclosure en route to the operating room.[71-73] This catheter is placed across the occlusion and provides a temporary conduit for blood flow by means of inlet and outlet holes located proximally and distally. Several other experimental catheter devices are being developed for management of acute occlusion, including laser and thermal welding catheters and intravascular stents (see Fig. 73.8). Placement of an intra-aortic balloon pump[74,75] or coronary sinus retroperfusion device[76] may help stabilize patients in whom direct intra-arterial reperfusion cannot be established.

The morbidity and mortality of bypass surgery in the setting of failed PTCA is significantly higher than in elective surgical cases. Operative mortality in the first PTCA registry was 6.4%,[66] but more recent reports suggest that appropriate mortality figures are in the 1% to 3%

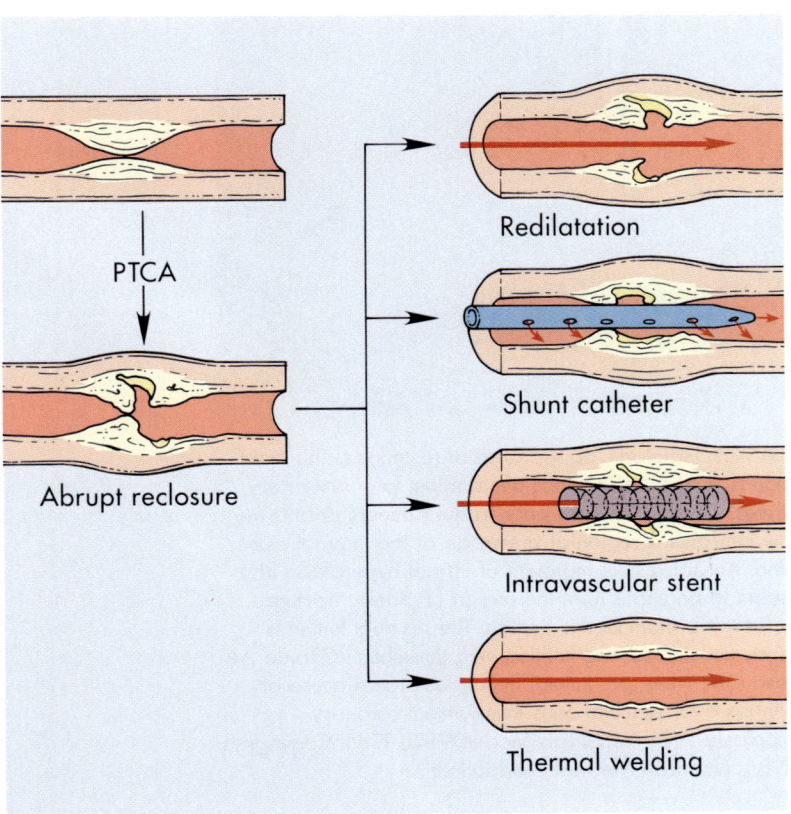

FIGURE 73.8 Options in the management of abrupt reclosure during PTCA. Repeat dilatation, usually with prolonged, low-pressure inflations, is successful in approximately half of cases; the autoperfusion or shunt catheter provides blood flow through the catheter to the distal vessel, allowing perfusion during transfer to the operating room; an intravascular stent can be placed in the region of dissection; thermal welding using a balloon heated by laser or other source may provide sealing of the dissection plane. (Modified from Baim DS: Interventional catheterization techniques. In Braunwald E (ed): Heart Disease: A Textbook of Cardiovascular Medicine, 3rd ed. Philadelphia, WB Saunders, 1988)

range.[69,70,77] Patients who survive salvage bypass surgery generally have an uncomplicated course, with excellent functional status in late follow-up.[78]

Other complications besides abrupt closure may contribute to refractory angina in the context of PTCA. Spasm is relatively common during instrumentation of the coronary arteries and can usually be treated by removing the balloon catheter or by infusing intracoronary nitroglycerin. Occlusion of side branches at the site of dilatation may cause chest discomfort and, in some cases, significant myocardial damage.[79] Embolization of plaque material or thrombus can occur and cause angina; this complication is usually detectable on the angiogram. Low-level, constant chest discomfort may arise from trauma to the vessel ("bruising" pain) and can last for 1 to 2 days following the procedure.

Patients who leave the catheterization laboratory with an open artery (less than 50% diameter stenosis) will generally have a favorable course, although abrupt reclosure can occur 24 hours or later following PTCA. Local hematoma formation is more common than in routine angiography because of the larger caliber sheaths and more rigorous anticoagulation, but significant bleeding is uncommon.

FOLLOW-UP POST PTCA: RESTENOSIS

The large majority of patients who undergo successful PTCA will have relief of symptoms and improvement in exercise capacity. Predischarge, or early postdischarge functional testing is performed in some centers in order to assess residual stenosis, provide an exercise prescription for the patient, and generate baseline information for follow-up.

Restenosis, a recurrence of narrowing in the area dilated, is the key concern in postdischarge management. The majority of patients who restenose will do so in the first 3 to 4 months following angioplasty; after 18 months a recurrence of angina is more likely due to progression of atherosclerosis at another site or in another vessel.[80,81] Although most patients with restenosis experience a recurrence of their typical chest discomfort, 15% to 25% of patients with angiographically proven restenosis are asymptomatic. For this reason, exercise testing is routinely performed in many centers once or more during the 4-month vulnerable period. Positive exercise electrocardiography,[78] and thallium[82-84] or radionuclide ventriculography studies[85] have been shown to correlate closely with angiographically proven restenosis. Patients with recurrence of angina or markedly positive functional tests in follow-up after PTCA should undergo repeat angiography.

Angiographic definitions of restenosis vary in the literature but generally are based on either a certain loss of the original gain in lumen size by PTCA (e.g., a 30% increase in diameter stenosis since PTCA) or a return of the stenosis to a certain level of significance (e.g., 70% diameter narrowing). Using these definitions, the 1-year rate of restenosis in most studies falls in the 25% to 35% range.[80,81,86-89] Primary success rates for repeat dilatation of restenosis lesions are comparable to those for first-time PTCA. Although initial studies suggested that the

TABLE 73.3 RISK FACTORS FOR RESTENOSIS

Clinical Variables
Male gender
Unstable angina
Diabetes
Previous restenosis
?Smoking
?Hypercholesterolemia

Anatomical Variables
Left anterior descending coronary artery (especially proximal)
Ostial lesion of left main or right arteries
Ostium or body of saphenous vein graft
Complete occlusion

Procedural Variables
Residual gradient greater than 15 mm Hg
Residual stenosis greater than 30%
?Absence of angiographically evident dissection

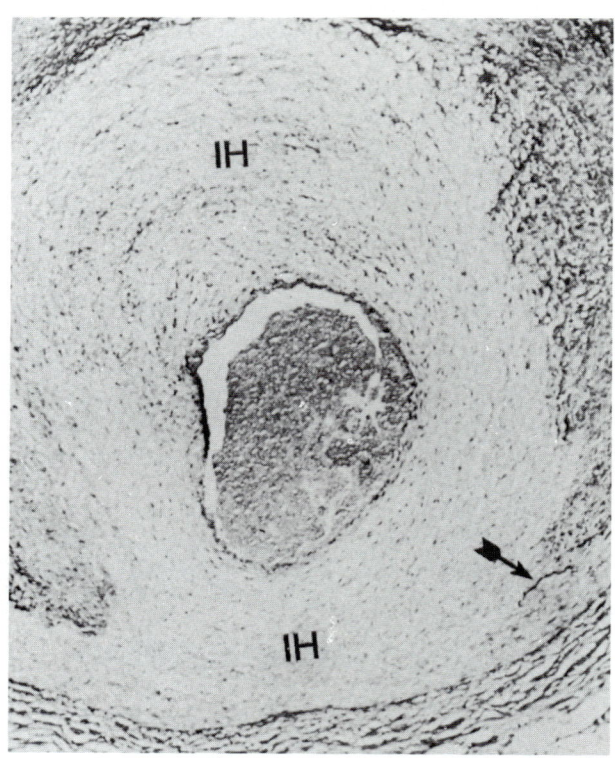

FIGURE 73.9 Histologic appearance of restenosis. This cross-section is from a left anterior descending coronary artery that was dilated 3 months prior to the patient's death. The arrow indicates a region of breakage of the internal elastic lamina. An aggressive ingrowth of intimal hyperplasia (IH) appears to originate from the region of plaque fracture seen at the bottom of this section. The residual lumen is severely constricted and is filled with thrombus. (Giraldo AA, Esposo OM, Meis JM: Intimal hyperplasia as a cause of restenosis after percutaneous transluminal coronary angioplasty. Arch Pathol Lab Med 109:173, 1985. Copyright © 1985, American Medical Association)

rate of restenosis was lower after a second PTCA procedure, more recent data suggest that restenosis rates are similar or even higher in the setting of multiple dilatations of the same lesions. In multivessel dilatation, restenosis rates are higher than in single-vessel PTCA on a per-patient basis but are approximately the same on a per-lesion basis.[90,91]

Clinical factors predictive of restenosis include male gender, unstable angina or recent onset of angina, and diabetes mellitus (Table 73.3). The significance of smoking and hypercholesterolemia is less clear. The single most powerful predictor of restenosis is the severity of the post-PTCA residual lesion, defined either angiographically (remaining stenosis greater than 30%) or in terms of pressure gradient (greater than 15 mm Hg). Location of the lesion also influences rates of restenosis: proximal lesions in general, particularly in the left anterior descending coronary artery, are associated with higher restenosis rates, as are lesions in the ostium or body of bypass grafts.[46] In the registry data, angiographically detectable dissection was a predictor of restenosis; however, in a more recent study dissection in the presence of a low pressure gradient was actually a favorable prognostic variable.[14] Various procedural factors are believed to be associated with restenosis, largely on an anecdotal basis. Undersizing of the balloon, shorter inflation times, and greater number of inflations have all been implicated.

The pathophysiologic mechanisms of restenosis appear to be substantially different from the atherosclerotic process. In autopsy studies the restenosis lesion is typically a proliferative, fibrocellular growth originating at the site of disruption of the plaque and extending into the lumen (Fig. 73.9).[92–94] The fibrocellular process consists primarily of smooth muscle cells and collagen; usually it is devoid of lipid. Organized thrombus is also seen in some lesions. Studies in animal models of angioplasty have suggested that restenosis may be initiated by aggressive platelet deposition, which occurs particularly in regions of deep dissection where there is exposed media. Platelet aggregation leads to release of potent vasoactive agents and mitogens, including platelet-derived growth factor, thromboxane B_2, adenosine diphosphate, and platelet factor 4. These agents serve as stimuli for proliferation and migration of smooth muscle cells from media to the neointima of the restenosis lesion.[95–97]

Although platelet/thrombus deposition appears to have a central role in the initiation of restenosis, the therapeutic implications have not been straightforward. Antiplatelet agents have been shown to inhibit restenosis in animal models,[98] but clinical studies with coumadin and with aspirin/dipyridamole have not shown any significant impact on the rate of restenosis in humans.[56,99] Studies are in progress with other antiplatelet agents (omega-3 fatty acids, prostacyclin analogues), pharmacologic blockers of platelet-derived growth factors, and other receptor blockers. Calcium channel blockers have become standard therapy after PTCA, although there are studies suggesting that neither diltiazem nor nifedipine has an impact on restenosis.[100,101]

NEW CATHETER-BASED THERAPIES

Although balloon dilatation is a relatively simple and effective approach to vascular disease, the problems of abrupt reclosure and restenosis have prompted a search for still better catheter technologies. Various types of mechanical catheter devices have been designed to extract or emulsify plaque. The Simpson atherectomy catheter (Fig. 73.10) is an example of a mechanical catheter that uses a rotating cutter to shave and remove layers of plaque.[102] In initial clinical trials in coronary arteries, the primary success rate is high in carefully selected lesions.[103] An important theoretical advantage of the atherectomy catheter is that by cutting and extracting plaque, the lumen left after the procedure is large and smooth so that the platelet adhesion/thrombosis sequence associated with restenosis may be less likely to occur. Other mechanical catheters are designed to drill through complete occlusions or enlarge an existing channel by abrading or cutting the walls with successively larger diameter systems.[104,105] Because embolization of particulate atheroma is a potential problem with these devices, extraction of the fragmented plaque by suction through the catheter is being investigated.

Another promising mechanical approach is stenting of arterial lesions using an expandable, tubular prosthesis that can be inserted by a catheter. The lattice-like stents become covered with a neointimal lining layer and can be placed across branch lesions without significant compromise of flow (Fig. 73.11). Preliminary clinical experience with metal stents has been encouraging, although thrombosis and intimal hyperplasia appear to be significant problems.[106–109] Plastic and absorbable stents are under development. The potential for application of stenting is great, both in the setting of failed angioplasty and as a

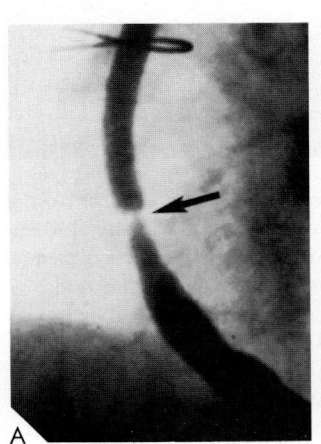
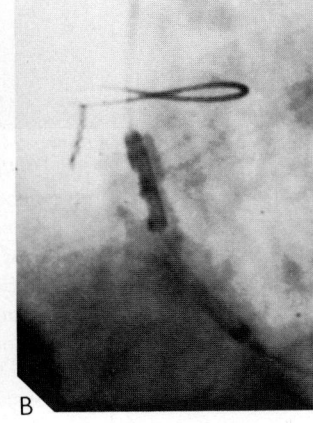
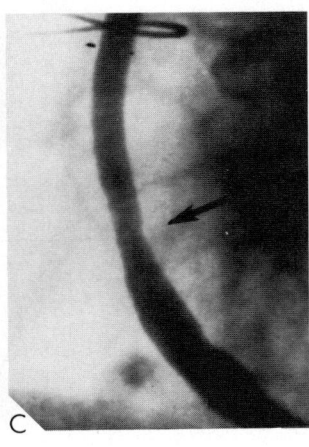
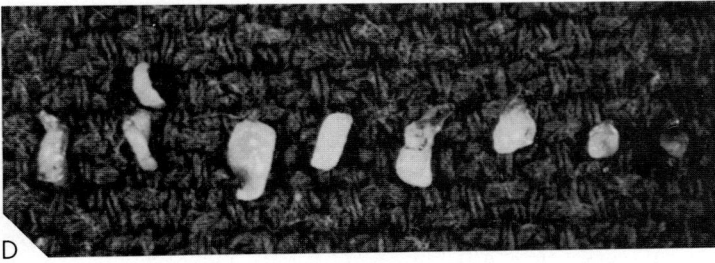

FIGURE 73.10 Example of percutaneous atherectomy of a right coronary artery bypass graft. **A.** Tight narrowing preatherectomy; this was a restenosis lesion following two previous balloon angioplasty procedures. **B.** The Simpson Atherocath is shown positioned across the lesion. **C.** Postatherectomy result, showing minimal residual stenosis and a smooth-appearing lumen. The bottom panel (**D**) is a photograph of pieces removed from the lesion (in the 1- to 2-mm diameter range), representing a combination of myointimal proliferation, atheroma, and thrombus. (Courtesy of T. Hinohara, MD; adapted with permission from Moore WS, Ahn SS (eds): Endovascular Surgery. Philadelphia, WB Saunders, 1988)

primary treatment for complex lesions that are unlikely to respond favorably to balloon dilatation.

LASER ANGIOPLASTY

On a theoretic basis, laser energy is uniquely well suited for application to angioplasty in several respects: laser energy can partially vaporize plaque, potentially reducing the problem of having to redistribute or remove it; over a range of wavelengths laser energy tends to be selectively absorbed by plaque, giving a degree of specificity to laser ablation; laser beams can travel down extremely thin optical fibers, which can be incorporated into low-profile catheter delivery systems.[110] Early animal experimentation with laser angioplasty confirmed the feasibility of laser ablation of atheroma but found high rates of perforation with the bare fiber systems.[111,112] Several strategies were developed to circumvent this problem, including capping the fiber tip with a metal ball that could be heated by the laser and provide thermal ablative energy. The so-called hot-tip laser has undergone clinical testing in the peripheral circulation, which has demonstrated that the device can cross totally occluded lesions with a perforation rate of less than 5%.[113] Initial testing in the coronary arteries has been limited by problems with mechanical engagement of the plaque and thermal damage to the artery, resulting in thrombosis.[114,115]

An alternative approach to the problem of perforation is the development of a guiding system to direct laser energy selectively toward atheroma. Direct visualization of plaque can be achieved using fiber-optic angioscopy[116,117]; this method has promise for guiding laser therapy based on recognition of surface plaque morphology. A second strategy involves fluorescence detection of plaque at the catheter tip. In one dual-laser system[118] a diagnostic laser first samples the fluorescence spectrum at the tip of the catheter. If the signal is compatible with plaque, the therapeutic laser is activated and allowed to fire. The system operates in a continuous "probe and treat" feedback loop. The accuracy in discriminating plaque versus normal wall in this system appears to be good in both *in vitro* and *in vivo* testing (Fig. 73.12). A third potential guiding technology is endovascular ultrasound, which has the theoretical advantage of providing information about the distribution of plaque below the endothelial surface.[119] High-energy ultrasound has also been shown to have potential application as a therapeutic modality.[120]

Laser energy is also being applied in a balloon system designed to weld the components of the disrupted arterial wall together, thus smoothing the lumen and inhibiting elastic recoil.[121] Data on restenosis following coronary laser balloon angioplasty are not yet available.

Testing of these various second-generation angioplasty devices is actively underway, and it is reasonable to expect that significant clinical impact will begin to occur in the next 1 to 2 years. If the problems of abrupt reclosure and restenosis can be minimized, the proportion of coronary procedures done using catheter techniques will increase substantially.

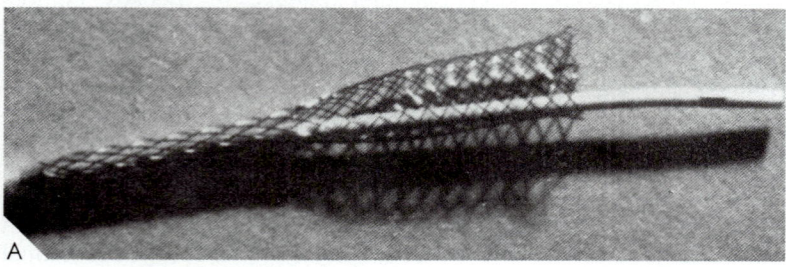
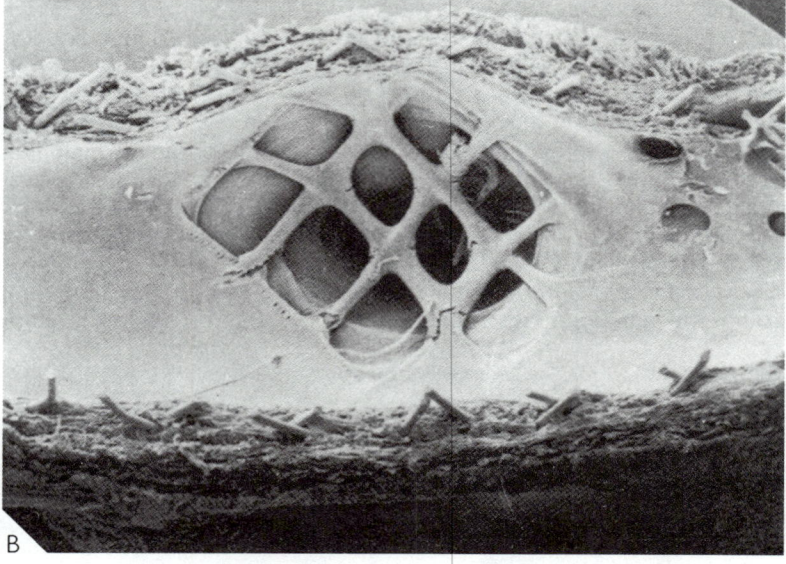

FIGURE 73.11 Intravascular stent. **A.** Catheter delivery system showing stent in the partially deployed (expanded) configuration. **B.** Scanning electron micrograph of a stented section of canine femoral artery. The vessel is sectioned parallel to the plane of the photograph. The smooth exposed surface is neoendothelium that has covered the stent in the main trunk of the vessel. The open lattice structure in the middle is an endothelialized section of stent that spans the opening of a major branch of the vessel. (Sigwart U, Puel J, Mirkovitch V et al: Intravascular stents to prevent occlusion and restenosis after transluminal angioplasty. N Engl J Med 316:701, 1987 Copyright © 1987, Massachusetts Medical Society)

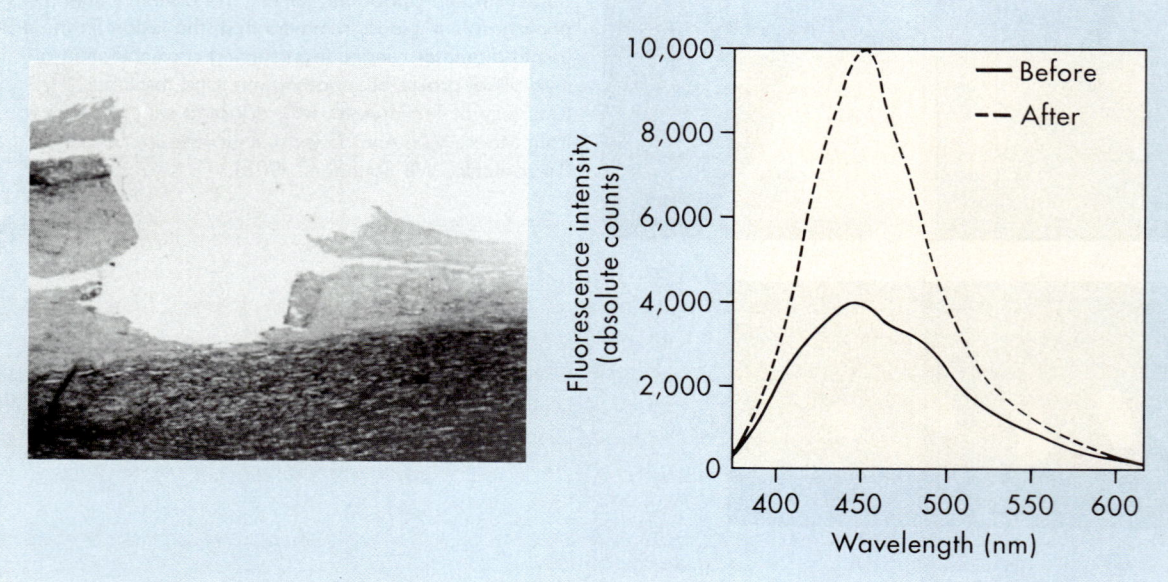

FIGURE 73.12 *In vitro* demonstration of fluorescence guidance system for laser angioplasty. The laser system was activated in the "probe and treat" sequence with the fiber directed perpendicular to the wall of a diseased section of aorta, shown in the histolic section on the left. The system automatically stopped when the detected spectrum changed from a characteristic signal for plaque (*solid line on the spectrum on the right*) to a signal typical for media (*dotted line*). As the pathologic section shows, the laser fiber penetrated the layer of plaque (*lighter, fragmented layer on top*) but stopped short of entering the media (*darker layer on bottom*). (Photo provided by MCM Laboratories with permission of M. Leon, MD)

REFERENCES

1. Dotter CT, Judkins MP: Transluminal treatment of arteriosclerotic obstruction: Description of a new technique and a preliminary report of its application. Circulation 30:654, 1964
2. Gruentzig AR, Myler RK, Hanna ES et al: Coronary transluminal angioplasty (abstr). Circulation (Suppl 3)56:84, 1977
3. Gruentzig A, Senning A, Siegenthaler WE: Nonoperative dilatation of coronary artery stenosis: Percutaneous transluminal coronary angioplasty (PTCA). N Engl J Med 301:61, 1979
4. Williams DO: When coronary angioplasty succeeds, when it fails: NHLBI PTCA Registry: Results to date. Cardiovasc Med 10:31, 1985
5. Proceedings of the National Heart, Lung and Blood Institute workshop on the outcome of percutaneous transluminal coronary angioplasty. Am J Cardiol 53:1C, 1984
6. Kelsey SF, Mullin SM, Detre KM et al: Effect of investigator experience on percutaneous transluminal coronary angioplasty. Am J Cardiol 53:56C, 1984
7. Simpson JB, Baim DS, Robert EW et al: A new catheter system for coronary angioplasty. Am J Cardiol 49:1216, 1982
8. Detre K, Holubkov R, Kelsey S et al: Percutaneous transluminal coronary angioplasty in 1985–1986 and 1977–1981: The National Heart, Lung, and Blood Institute Registry. N Engl J Med 318:265, 1988
9. Kinney TB, Chin K, Rurik GW et al: Transluminal angioplasty: A mechanical-pathophysiological correlation of its physical mechanisms. Radiology 153:85, 1984
10. Zarins CK, Lu CT, Gewertz BL et al: Arterial disruption and remodeling following balloon dilatation. Surgery 92:1086, 1982
11. Waller BF: Pathology of transluminal balloon angioplasty used in the treatment of coronary heart disease. Hum Pathol 18:476, 1987
12. Block PC, Myler RK, Stertzer S et al: Morphology after transluminal angioplasty in human beings. N Engl J Med 305:382, 1981
13. Holmes DR Jr, Vlietstra RE, Mock MB et al: Angiographic changes produced by percutaneous transluminal coronary angioplasty. Am J Cardiol 51:676, 1983
14. Leimgruber PP, Roubin GS, Anderson HV et al: Influence of intimal dissection on restenosis after successful coronary angioplasty. Circulation 72:530, 1985
15. Ryan TJ, Faxon DP, Gunnar RM et al: Guidelines for percutaneous transluminal coronary angioplasty: A report of the American College of Cardiology/American Heart Association Task Force on Assessment of Diagnostic and Therapeutic Cardiovascular Procedures (Subcommittee on Percutaneous Transluminal Coronary Angioplasty). Circulation 78:486, 1988
16. Bourassa MG, Alderman EL, Bertrand M et al: Report of the Joint ISFC/WHO Task Force on Coronary Angioplasty. Circulation 78:780, 1988
17. Faxon DP, Detre KM, McCabe CH et al: Role of percutaneous coronary angioplasty in the treatment of unstable angina: Report from the National Heart, Lung and Blood Institute, Percutaneous Transluminal Coronary Angioplasty and Coronary Artery Surgery Study Registries. Am J Cardiol 53:131C, 1984
18. DeFeyter PJ, Serruys PW, Van Den Brand M et al: Emergency coronary angioplasty in refractory unstable angina. N Engl J Med 313:342, 1985
19. Wohlgelernter D, Cleman M, Highman HA et al: Percutaneous transluminal coronary angioplasty of the "culprit lesion" for management of unstable angina pectoris in patients with multivessel coronary artery disease. Am J Cardiol 58:460, 1986
20. Steffenino G, Meier B, Finci L et al: Follow up results of treatment of unstable angina by coronary angioplasty. Br Heart J 57:416, 1987
21. David PR, Waters DD, Scholl JM et al: Percutaneous transluminal coronary angioplasty in patients with variant angina. Circulation 66:695, 1982
22. Corcos T, David PR, Bourassa MG et al: Percutaneous transluminal coronary angioplasty for the treatment of variant angina. J Am Coll Cardiol 5:1046, 1985
23. Bertrand ME, LaBlanche JM, Thieuleux FA et al: Comparative results of percutaneous transluminal angioplasty in patients with dynamic versus fixed coronary stenosis. J Am Coll Cardiol 8:504, 1986
24. Hartzler GO, McConahay DR, Johnson WL: Direct balloon angioplasty in acute myocardial infarction: Without prior use of streptokinase (abstr). J Am Coll Cardiol 7:149A, 1986
25. O'Neill W, Timmis G, Bourdillon P et al: A prospective randomized clinical trial of intracoronary streptokinase versus coronary angioplasty for acute myocardial infarction. N Engl J Med 314:812, 1986
26. Gersh BJ, Kronmal RA, Frye RL et al: Coronary arteriography and coronary artery bypass surgery: Morbidity and mortality in patients ages 65 years or older: A report from the Coronary Artery Surgery Study. Circulation 67:483, 1983
27. Raizner AE, Hust RG, Lewis JM et al: Transluminal coronary angioplasty in the elderly. Am J Cardiol 57:29, 1986
28. McEniery PT, Hollman J, Knezinek V et al: Comparative safety and efficacy of percutaneous transluminal coronary angioplasty in men and in women. Cathet Cardiovasc Diagn 13:364, 1987
29. Ischinger T, Gruentzig AR, Hollman J et al: Should coronary arteries with less than 60% diameter stenosis be treated by angioplasty? Circulation 68:148, 1983
30. Stertzer SH, Myler RK, Insel H et al: Percutaneous transluminal coronary angioplasty in left main stem coronary stenosis: A five-year appraisal. Int J Cardiol 9:149, 1985
31. Topol EJ, Ellis SG, Fishman J et al: Multicenter study of percutaneous transluminal angioplasty for right coronary artery ostial stenosis. J Am Coll Cardiol 9:1214, 1987
32. Meier B, Gruentzig AR, King SB III et al: Risk of side branch occlusion during coronary angioplasty. Am J Cardiol 53:10, 1984
33. Meier B: Kissing balloon coronary angioplasty. Am J Cardiol 54:918, 1984
34. Ellis SG, Roubin GS, King SB III et al: Angiographic and clinical predictors of acute closure after native vessel coronary angioplasty. Circulation 77:372, 1988
35. Mabin TA, Holmes DR Jr, Smith HC et al: Intracoronary thrombus: Role in coronary occlusion complicating percutaneous transluminal coronary angioplasty. J Am Coll Cardiol 5:198, 1985
36. Dervan JP, Baim DS, Cherniles J et al: Transluminal angioplasty of occluded coronary arteries: Use of a movable guide wire system. Circulation 68:776, 1983
37. Holmes DR Jr, Vlietstra RE, Reeder GS et al: Angioplasty in total coronary artery occlusion. J Am Coll Cardiol 3:845, 1984
38. Kereiakes DJ, Selmon MR, McAuley BJ et al: Angioplasty in total coronary artery occlusion: Experience in 76 consecutive patients. J Am Coll Cardiol 6:526, 1985
39. Melchior JP, Meier B, Urban P et al: Percutaneous transluminal coronary angioplasty for chronic total coronary arterial occlusion. Am J Cardiol 59:535, 1987
40. Hartzler GO: Percutaneous transluminal coronary angioplasty in multivessel disease. Cathet Cardiovas Diagn 9:537, 1983
41. Dorros G, Stertzer SH, Cowley MJ et al: Complex coronary angioplasty: Multiple coronary dilatations. Am J Cardiol (Suppl C)53:126, 1984
42. Ambrose JA, Winters SL, Stern A et al: Angiographic morphology and the pathogenesis of unstable angina pectoris. J Am Coll Cardiol 5:609, 1985
43. Vandormael MG, Chaitman BR, Ischinger T et al: Immediate and short-term benefit of multilesion coronary angioplasty: Influence of degree of revascularization. J Am Coll Cardiol 6:983, 1985
44. Vliestra RE, Holmes DR Jr, Reeder GS et al: Balloon angioplasty in multivessel coronary artery disease. Mayo Clic Proc 58:563, 1983
45. Douglas JS Jr, Gruentzig AR, King SB III et al: Percutaneous transluminal coronary angioplasty in patients with prior coronary bypass surgery. J Am Coll Cardiol 2:745, 1983
46. Dorros G, Johnson WD, Tector AJ et al: Percutaneous transluminal coronary angioplasty in patients with prior coronary artery bypass grafting. J Thorac Cardiovasc Surg 87:17, 1984
47. El Gamal M, Bonnier H, Michels R et al: Percutaneous transluminal angioplasty of stenosed aortocoronary bypass grafts. Br Heart J 52:617, 1984
48. Block PC, Cowley MJ, Kaltenbach M et al: Percutaneous angioplasty of stenoses of bypass grafts or of bypass graft anastomotic sites. Am J Cardiol 53:666, 1984
49. Jones EL, Murphy DA, Craver JM: Comparison of coronary artery bypass surgery and percutaneous transluminal coronary angioplasty including surgery for failed angioplasty. Am Heart J 107:830, 1984
50. Acinapura AJ, Cunningham JN Jr, Jacobowitz IJ et al: Efficacy of percutaneous transluminal coronary angioplasty compared with single-vessel bypass. J Thorac Cardiovasc Surg 89:35, 1985
51. Holmes DR Jr, Van Raden MJ, Reeder GS et al: Return to work after coronary angioplasty: A report from the National Heart, Lung, and Blood Institute Percutaneous Transluminal Coronary Angioplasty Registry. Am J Cardiol (Suppl C)53:48, 1984
52. Kelly ME, Taylor GJ, Moses HW et al: Comparative cost of myocardial revascularization: Percutaneous transluminal angioplasty and coronary artery bypass surgery. J Am Coll Cardiol 5:16, 1985
53. Reeder GS, Krishan I, Nobrega FT et al: Is percutaneous coronary angioplasty less expensive than bypass surgery? N Engl J Med 311:1157, 1984
54. Kent KM, Bentivoglio LG, Block PC et al: Long-term efficacy of percutaneous transluminal coronary angioplasty (PTCA): Report from the National Heart, Lung, and Blood Institute PTCA Registry. Am J Cardiol (Suppl C)53:27, 1984
55. Talley JD, Hurst JW, King SB et al: Clinical outcome 5 years after attempted percutaneous coronary angioplasty in 427 patients. Circulation 77:820, 1988
56. Schwartz L, Bourassa MG, Lesperance J et al: Aspirin and dipyridamole in the prevention of restenosis after percutaneous transluminal coronary angioplasty. N Engl J Med 318:1714, 1988
57. Swanson KT, Vliestra RE, Holmes DR Jr et al: Efficacy of adjunctive dextran during percutaneous transluminal coronary angioplasty. Am J Cardiol 54:447, 1984
58. Jain A, Demer LL, Raizner AE et al: *In vivo* assessment of vascular dilatation during percutaneous transluminal coronary angioplasty. Am J Cardiol 60:988, 1987
59. Leiboff R, Bren G, Katz R et al: Determinants of transstenotic gradients observed during angioplasty: An experimental model. Am J Cardiol 52:1311, 1983
60. Hauser AM, Gangadharan V, Ramos RG et al: Sequence of mechanical, electrocardiographic and clinical effects of repeated coronary artery occlusion in human beings: Echocardiographic observations during coronary angioplasty. J Am Coll Cardiol 5:193, 1985
61. Wohlgelernter D, Cleman M, Highman HA et al: Regional myocardial dysfunction during coronary angioplasty: Evaluation by two-dimensional echocardiography and 12 lead electrocardiography. J Am Coll Cardiol 7:1245,

62. Wijns W, Serruys PW, Slager CJ et al: Effect of coronary occlusion during percutaneous transluminal angioplasty in humans on left ventricular chamber stiffness and regional diastolic pressure-radius relations. J Am Coll Cardiol 7:455, 1986
63. Wilson RF, Johnson MR, Marcus ML et al: The effect of coronary angioplasty on coronary flow reserve. Circulation 77:873, 1988
64. Dorros G, Cowley MJ, Simpson J et al: Percutaneous transluminal coronary angioplasty: Report of complications from the National Heart, Lung, and Blood Institute PTCA registry. Circulation 67:723, 1983
65. Schofer J, Krebber H-J, Bleifeld W et al: Acute coronary artery occlusion during percutaneous transluminal coronary angioplasty: Reopening by intracoronary streptokinase before emergency coronary artery surgery to prevent myocardial infarction. Circulation 66:1325, 1982
66. Cowley MJ, Dorros G, Kelsey SF et al: Emergency coronary bypass surgery after coronary angioplasty: The National Heart, Lung and Blood Institute's Percutaneous Transluminal Coronary Angioplasty Registry experience. Am J Cardiol 53:22C, 1984
67. Reul GJ Jr, Cooley DA, Hallman GL et al: Coronary artery bypass for unsuccessful percutaneous transluminal coronary angioplasty. J Thorac Cardiovasc Surg 88:685, 1984
68. Killen DA, Hamaker WR, Reed WA: Coronary artery bypass following percutaneous transluminal coronary angioplasty. Ann Thorac Surg 40:133, 1985
69. Mabin TA, Holmes DR Jr, Smith HC et al: Follow-up clinical results in patients undergoing percutaneous transluminal coronary angioplasty. Circulation 71:754, 1985
70. Pelletier LC, Pardini A, Renkin J et al: Myocardial revascularization after failure of percutaneous transluminal coronary angioplasty. J Thorac Cardiovasc Surg 90:265, 1985
71. Hinohara T, Simpson JB, Phillips HR et al: Transluminal catheter reperfusion: A new technique to reestablish blood flow after coronary occlusion during percutaneous transluminal coronary angioplasty. Am J Cardiol 57:684, 1986
72. Turi BG, Campbell CA, Gottimukkala MV et al: Preservation of distal coronary perfusion during prolonged balloon inflation with an autoperfusion angioplasty catheter. Circulation 75:1273, 1987
73. Stack RS, Quigley PJ, Collins G et al: Perfusion balloon catheter. Am J Cardiol 61:77G, 1988
74. Alcan KE, Stertzer SH, Wallsh E et al: The role of intra-aortic balloon counterpulsation in patients undergoing percutaneous transluminal coronary angioplasty. Am Heart J 105:527, 1983
75. Murphy DA, Craver JM, Jones EL et al: Surgical management of acute myocardial ischemia following percutaneous transluminal coronary angioplasty: Role of the intra-aortic balloon pump. J Thorac Cardiovasc Surg 87:332, 1984
76. Beatt KJ, Serruys PW, De Feyter P et al: Haemodynamic observations during percutaneous transluminal coronary angioplasty in the presence of synchronised diastolic coronary sinus retroperfusion. Br Heart J 59:159, 1988
77. Brahos GJ, Baker NH, Ewy HG et al: Aortocoronary bypass following unsuccessful PTCA: Experience in 100 consecutive patients. Ann Thorac Surg 40:7, 1985
78. Meier B, Gruentzig AR, Siegenthaler WE et al: Long-term exercise performance after percutaneous transluminal coronary angioplasty and coronary artery bypass grafting. Circulation 68:796, 1983
79. Meier B, Gruentzig AR, King SB III et al: Risk of side branch occlusion during coronary angioplasty. Am J Cardiol 53:10, 1984
80. Roubin GS, King SB III, Douglas JS Jr: Restenosis after percutaneous transluminal coronary angioplasty: The Emory University experience. Am J Cardiol 60:39B, 1987
81. Rosing DR, Cannon RO III, Watson RW et al: Three year anatomic, functional and clinical follow-up after successful percutaneous transluminal coronary angioplasty. J Am Coll Cardiol 9:1, 1987
82. Harzel HO, Nuesch K, Gruentzig AR et al: Short- and long-term changes in myocardial perfusion after percutaneous transluminal coronary angioplasty assessed by thallium-210 exercise scintigraphy. Circulation 63:1001, 1981
83. Scholl J-M, Chaitman BR, David PR et al: Exercise electrocardiography and myocardial scintigraphy in the serial evaluation of the results of percutaneous transluminal coronary angioplasty. Circulation 66:380, 1982
84. Wijns W, Serruys PW, Reiber JHC et al: Early detection of restenosis after successful percutaneous transluminal coronary angioplasty by exercise-redistribution thallium scintigraphy. Am J Cardiol 55:357, 1985
85. DePuey EG, Leatherman LL, Leachman RD et al: Restenosis after transluminal coronary angioplasty detected with exercise-gated radionuclide ventriculography. J Am Coll Cardiol 4:1103, 1984
86. Holmes DR Jr, Vlietstra RE, Smith HC et al: Restenosis after percutaneous transluminal coronary angioplasty (PTCA): A report from the PTCA Registry of the National Heart, Lung and Blood Institute. Am J Cardiol 53:77c, 1984
87. Val PG, Bourassa MG, David PR et al: Restenosis after successful percutaneous transluminal coronary angioplasty: The Montreal Heart Institute experience. Am J Cardiol 60:50B, 1987
88. Gruentzig AR, King SB III, Schlumpf M et al: Long-term follow-up after percutaneous transluminal coronary angioplasty: The early Zurich experience. N Engl J Med 316:1127, 1987
89. Serruys PW, Luijten HE, Beatt KJ et al: Incidence of restenosis after successful coronary angioplasty: A time-related phenomenon. Circulation 77:361, 1988
90. Cowley MJ, Vetrovec GW, DiSciascio G et al: Coronary angioplasty of multiple vessels: Short-term outcome and long-term results. Circulation 72:1314, 1985
91. Mata LA, Bosch X, David PR et al: Clinical and angiographic assessment 6 months after double vessel percutaneous coronary angioplasty. J Am Coll Cardiol 6:1239, 1985
92. Essed CE, Van Den Brand M, Becker AE: Transluminal coronary angioplasty and early restenosis: Fibrocellular occlusion after wall laceration. Br Heart J 49:393, 1983
93. Austin GE, Ratliff NB, Hollman J et al: Intimal proliferation of smooth muscle cells as an explanation for recurrent coronary artery stenosis after percutaneous transluminal coronary angioplasty. J Am Coll Cardiol 6:369, 1985
94. Giraldo AA, Esposo OM, Meis JM et al: Intimal hyperplasia as a cause of restenosis after percutaneous transluminal coronary angioplasty. Arch Pathol Lab Med 109:173, 1985
95. Chesebro JH, Lam JYT, Badimon L et al: Restenosis after arterial angioplasty: A hemorrheologic response to injury. Am J Cardiol 60:10B, 1987
96. Faxon DP, Sanborn TA, Haudenschild CC: Mechanism of angioplasty and its relation to restenosis. Am J Cardiol 60:5B, 1987
97. Harker LA: Role of platelets and thrombosis in mechanisms of acute occlusion and restenosis after angioplasty. Am J Cardiol 60:20B, 1987
98. Faxon DP, Sanbord TA, Haudenschild CC et al: Effect of antiplatelet therapy on restenosis after experimental angioplasty. Am J Cardiol 53:72c, 1984
99. Thornton MA, Gruentzig AR, Hollman J et al: Coumadin and aspirin in prevention of recurrence after transluminal angioplasty: A randomized study. Circulation 69:721, 1984
100. Corcos T, David PR, Val PG et al: Failure of diltiazem to prevent restenosis after percutaneous transluminal coronary angioplasty. Am Heart J 109:926, 1985
101. Whitworth HB, Roubin GS, Hollman J et al: Effect of nifedipine on recurrent stenosis after percutaneous transluminal coronary angioplasty. J Am Coll Cardiol 8:1271, 1986
102. Simpson JB, Selmon MR, Robertson GC et al: Transluminal atherectomy for occlusive peripheral vascular disease. Am J Cardiol 61:96G, 1988
103. Simpson JB, Robertson GC, Selmon MR et al: Percutaneous coronary atherectomy (abstr). J Am Coll Cardiol 11:110A, 1988
104. Fourrier JL, Auth D, Lablanche JM et al: Human percutaneous coronary rotational atherectomy: Preliminary results (abstr). Circulation 78:II-82, 1988
105. Perez JA, Hinohara T, Quigley PJ et al: In vitro and in vivo experimental results using a new wire-guided concentric atherectomy device (abstr). J Am Coll Cardiol 11:109A, 1988
106. Palmaz JC, Sibbitt RR, Reuter ST et al: Expandable intraluminal graft: A preliminary study. Radiology 73:156, 1985
107. Sigwart U, Puel J, Mirkovitch V et al: Intravascular stents to prevent occlusion and restenosis after transluminal angioplasty. N Engl J Med 316:701, 1987
108. Serruys PW, Juilliere Y, Bertrand ME et al: Additional improvement of stenosis geometry in human coronary arteries by stenting after balloon dilatation. Am J Cardiol 61:71G, 1988
109. Schatz RA, Palmaz JC: Balloon expandable intravascular stents (BEIS) in human coronary arteries: Report of initial experience (abstr). Circulation 78:II-408, 1988
110. Abela GS: Laser arterial recanalization: A current perspective. J Am Coll Cardiol 12:103, 1988
111. Crea F, Abela GS, Fenech A et al: Transluminal laser irradiation of coronary arteries in live dogs: An angiographic and morphologic study of acute effect. Am J Cardiol 57:171, 1986
112. Ginsburg R, Wexler L, Mitchell R et al: Percutaneous transluminal laser angioplasty for treatment of peripheral vascular disease: Clinical experience with sixteen patients. Radiology 155:619, 1985
113. Sanborn TA, Cumberland DC, Greenfield AJ et al: Percutaneous laser thermal angioplasty: Initial results and 1-year follow-up in 129 femoropopliteal lesions. Radiology 168:121, 1988
114. Sanborn TA, Faxon DP, Kellett MA et al: Percutaneous coronary laser thermal angioplasty. J Am Coll Cardiol 8:1437, 1986
115. Crea F, Davis GM, McKenna WJ et al: Laser recanalization of coronary arteries by metal-capped optical fibres: Early clinical experience in patients with stable angina pectoris. Br Heart J 59:168, 1988
116. Sherman CT, Litvack F, Grundfest W et al: Coronary angioscopy in patients with unstable angina pectoris. N Engl J Med 315:913, 1986
117. Forrester JS, Litvack F, Grundfest W et al: A perspective of coronary disease seen through the arteries of living man. Circulation 75:505, 1987
118. Leon MB, Lu DY, Prevosti LG et al: Human arterial surface fluorescence: Atherosclerotic plaque identification and effects of laser atheroma ablation. J Am Coll Cardiol 12:94, 1988
119. Yock P, Linker D, Saether O et al: Intravascular two-dimensional catheter ultrasound: Initial clinical studies (abstr). Circulation 78:II-21, 1988
120. Segal RJ, DeCastro E, Forrester JS et al: In vivo ultrasonic recanalization of arterial occlusions (abstr). Circulation 78:II-270, 1988
121. Spears JR: Percutaneous transluminal coronary angioplasty restenosis: Potential prevention with laser balloon angioplasty. Am J Cardiol 60:61B, 1987

CORONARY ARTERY BYPASS SURGERY

Joel S. Karliner

Direct myocardial revascularization is currently performed routinely in thousands of patients in most cardiovascular centers around the world. Based on the pioneering work of Favaloro and his colleagues at the Cleveland Clinic in the 1960s, saphenous vein bypass grafting for the relief of angina pectoris was quickly accepted and by the early 1970s became an important therapeutic approach in the treatment of chronic ischemic heart disease.[1] Subsequent technical advances, including the use of the internal mammary artery as a conduit, better methods of myocardial protection, and improved medical therapy, particularly for patients with unstable angina, have made surgical myocardial revascularization an accepted procedure with relatively low but well-defined morbidity and mortality. More recently, older patients with more complex vascular disease, both in the coronary vessels and other vascular beds, have benefited from this procedure, albeit with a somewhat higher morbidity and mortality.

It was recognized early on that this new surgical procedure would have to be subjected to rigorous analysis to define both its benefits and its adverse effects. Consequently, a number of studies were undertaken, some of which were randomized, to define the utility of this relatively new procedure. Because randomized studies by necessity exclude large numbers of patients and thereby may not reflect practice in the community at large or may not include specific subgroups of patients at high risk, observational or database studies have also been carried out. In considering the results of coronary artery bypass surgery, it is therefore useful to review the largest of these studies with respect both to their randomized and observational or registry components.

RANDOMIZED STUDIES
STABLE ANGINA

In 1970, the Veterans Administration (VA) undertook a cooperative, prospective, randomized study to determine the potential benefits of coronary artery bypass surgery using saphenous vein grafts. In an early report, Takaro and co-workers noted a statistically significant survival difference in favor of surgery in the subgroup of patients with left main coronary artery obstruction.[2] Early follow-up data on patients without left main coronary artery obstruction did not demonstrate any statistically significant difference between medically and surgically treated patients.[3] The latter result was criticized by many observers because of the relatively high operative mortality reported in the VA Cooperative Study.

A long-term follow-up of this study has now been reported.[4] For all patients and for the 595 patients without left main coronary artery disease, cumulative survival did not differ significantly at 11 years according to treatment. However, the study did identify a statistically significant difference in survival that suggested benefit from surgical treatment in patients without left main coronary disease who were subdivided into high-risk subgroups defined angiographically, clinically, or by a combination of angiographic and clinical factors as follows: (1) high angiographic risk (three-vessel disease and impaired left ventricular function); (2) clinically defined high risk (at least two of the following: resting ST segment depression, a history of previous myocardial infarction, or a history of previous hypertension); or (3) combined angiographic and clinical high risk. Among these patients there was both a higher risk of dying and of benefit from surgical treatment at 7 years, but beyond 7 years the survival benefit gradually tended to diminish. By contrast, surgical treatment resulted in a nonsignificant survival disadvantage throughout the 11 years in subgroups of patients with normal left ventricular function, low angiographic risk, and low clinical risk and a statistically significant disadvantage at 11 years in patients with two-vessel disease. A possible explanation for the diminution of favorable results between 7 and 11 years may be late graft occlusion. Thus, in a randomized, prospective investigation, both the short-term and long-term VA Cooperative Study results have identified two groups of patients who appear to benefit from coronary artery revascularization: patients with left main coronary artery disease and those with extensive coronary artery disease and reduced left ventricular function who are at high risk as judged either by clinical or historical factors.

The European Coronary Surgery Study began recruiting patients in 1973 and completed patient entry in March 1976.[5-8] A total of 768 patients were recruited, all of whom were men younger than 65 years of age who had mild-to-moderate angina pectoris, at least two-vessel disease, and "good" left ventricular function. Of these, 373 were randomized to medical and 395 to surgical treatment. Although 83 medical patients subsequently underwent surgery and 27 surgical patients did not undergo surgery, these patients were not excluded from the analysis, and the group randomized to coronary bypass surgery was compared with the group randomized to medical treatment. In the total population, surgery improved survival significantly compared with conventional medical treatment after 8 years of follow-up (89% vs. 80%, P = 0.0013); survival was also improved in the subgroup with three-vessel disease (92% vs. 77%, P = 0.00015).[8] In patients with two-vessel disease in which one of these vessels was the proximal segment of the left anterior descending coronary artery, survival was greater with surgical treatment (90% vs. 79%, P < 0.013). There was no significant difference in survival between the two treatments in patients with one-vessel disease and in those with two-vessel disease without proximal left anterior descending artery obstruction. The incidence of recurrent myocardial infarction did not differ between the surgical and medical groups and surgery did not influence the gradually increasing rate of retirement from work.

Based on these results, Varnauskas and associates[8] suggested the following guidelines for decision making in selecting symptomatic patients for prophylactic surgery: coronary angiography should be performed when two or more of four noninvasive high-risk predictors are identified, that is, ischemic abnormalities on the resting electrocardiogram (ECG), marked ST segment depression during exercise, peripheral arterial disease, and age over 50 years. Surgery was advised for patients who show a 50% or greater stenosis in the left main coronary artery, or at least three major coronary arteries, or those who have greater than 75% stenosis in two major vessels, one of which is the proximal segment of the left anterior descending coronary artery.

These clinical and angiographic observations do not differ markedly from those of the VA Cooperative Study except that a major difference between the two conclusions was inherent in the study design because only patients with good left ventricular function were accepted into the European study. Otherwise, the recommendations regarding left main coronary artery disease, three-vessel disease, and clinical characteristics are quite similar. The European study did identify an additional risk factor, that is, proximal left anterior descending coronary artery obstruction.

The third major study was the Coronary Artery Surgery Study (CASS), which was divided into two major components: a randomized portion and a much larger registry portion (see below). The randomized study was designed to test the hypothesis that coronary artery bypass surgery significantly reduces the mortality rate and the myocardial infarction rate in patients with mild angina and in those who are asymptomatic after infarction but who have angiographically documented coronary artery disease.[9] It consisted of 780 patients who were considered operable and who had either mild stable angina pectoris or were free of angina after myocardial infarction. The major conclusions of this study were that in this specific subgroup of patients coronary artery bypass surgery neither prolonged life nor prevented myocardial infarction after a period of 5 years.[9] However, the quality of life was significantly improved, as manifested by relief of chest pain, improvement of both subjective and objective measurements of functional status, and a diminished requirement for drug therapy.[10] However, as in many other studies, no significant effect on employment or recreational status was observed. Similar observations regarding quality of life were made after a 5-year follow-up in the VA Cooperative Study.[11] However, at 10 years, symptoms increased and exercise tolerance decreased to levels similar to those of medically treated patients.

In the randomized CASS study, survival data continued to show no difference after 8 years between medical and surgical groups: 87% of patients assigned to surgical and 84% of those assigned to medical treatment were still alive.[12] However, as with the VA Cooperative Study, the randomized CASS data did demonstrate a significant advantage favoring surgical treatment in patients with triple-vessel disease and a reduced ejection fraction (less than 50% but greater than 35%) after 7 years of follow-up: 88% of the patients in the surgical group and 65% of those in the medical group were alive ($P = 0.009$).[12,13] By contrast, survival curves for patients with normal resting ejection fraction values were identical after 7 years.

Thus, analyses of three major randomized studies begun in the 1970s seem to lead to similar conclusions despite major differences in surgical mortality (which progressively declined with time), study design, and patient recruitment. Both the VA and the CASS studies showed improved survival with triple-vessel disease and a reduced ejection fraction. Both the European study and the VA study identified patients with left main coronary disease as being at major risk. And finally, the European study identified patients with triple-vessel disease and normal left ventricular function and patients with two-vessel disease and proximal obstruction of the left anterior descending coronary artery as being at higher risk. What is striking about these studies is not the differences in their conclusions, but rather the remarkable similarity of the data that these randomized studies provide.

A number of other randomized studies were also reported during this time. These tended to be smaller and some of their conclusions may therefore be subject to a type II error (i.e., an insufficient number of patients may have been included to identify differences between the groups). Thus, Norris and colleagues reported the results of surgical vs. medical treatment in 100 randomized patients and concluded that in the absence of disabling angina or left main coronary artery stenosis, coronary artery surgery need not be advised.[14] In another study of 100 patients with stable disabling angina randomized to medical (49 patients) or surgical (51 patients) therapy, coronary artery bypass surgery resulted in greater functional improvement and less unstable angina than medical therapy, but the likelihood of death from myocardial infarction was unchanged by operation.[15]

UNSTABLE ANGINA

In patients with unstable angina pectoris, a National Cooperative Study Group reported in 1978 that this syndrome can be managed acutely with intensive medical therapy and that elective surgery can be performed later with a low risk and good clinical results if the patient's angina fails to respond to medical treatment.[16] This early study was in part the basis for the current approach to the treatment of unstable angina that is accepted in most centers. Recently, Luchi and co-workers reported a multicenter, randomized, prospective study comparing medical therapy alone with coronary artery bypass surgery plus medical therapy in 468 men with unstable angina pectoris treated from 1976 through 1982.[17] This study, sponsored by the VA, demonstrated that patients with unstable angina had a similar outcome after 2 years regardless of whether they received medical therapy alone or coronary bypass surgery plus medical therapy. However, as with the randomized studies in chronic stable angina discussed earlier, patients with a reduced left ventricular ejection fraction tended to have a better 2-year survival rate after coronary artery bypass surgery. Furthermore, both this study and the National Cooperative Study Group noted a strikingly similar crossover rate from medical to surgical therapy: in the National Cooperative Study Group, after a follow-up period of 30 months, there was a 36% crossover rate to surgery;[16] the figure for the VA study after 2 years was 34%.[17]

OBSERVATIONAL STUDIES
METHODOLOGIC CONSIDERATIONS

As indicated above, nonrandomized observational studies may contribute a great deal of information beyond randomized clinical trials. This has been emphasized by Califf and colleagues,[18] who made the following points:

1. Only a small minority of patients seen in clinical practice for suspected coronary artery disease would have been eligible for any of the randomized trials. Women and those patients with severe symptoms have been underrepresented and the trials have evaluated few patients over the age of 65 years and no patients with marked impairment of left ventricular function (ejection fraction < 0.34). The latter two populations are those likely to derive greater benefit from coronary artery bypass grafting than patients included in the studies. Thus, Califf and associates point out that only 13%, 8%, and 4%, respectively, of the patients referred for cardiac catheterization to Duke University would have been eligible for the VA Cooperative Study, the European Coronary Artery Surgery Study, or CASS.[18] Since clinical databases have the advantage of enrolling all patients, the entire spectrum of illness can be studied.

2. Medical and other types of interventional therapy for patients with coronary artery disease have changed exceedingly rapidly. Since the last patient randomized in a major trial for the surgical treatment of coronary artery disease was enrolled in 1979, such individuals did not receive calcium channel antagonists and did not have the benefit of intravenous nitroglycerin for unstable angina. In addition, these patients were not routinely treated with antiplatelet agents to maintain graft patency, and the option of percutaneous balloon angioplasty was not available to them. For these reasons, Califf and colleagues have suggested that these changes in patient management have resulted in greater longevity in the 1980s than for equally sick patients cared for in the 1970s.[18]

3. Because randomized controlled trials are performed in selected centers, Califf and co-workers suggest that it is not altogether clear whether the results from such trials can be generalized to the practice setting of an individual physician.[18] As an example, they present a hypothetical patient 64 years of age with triple-vessel disease, frequent angina, resting ST segment depression, peripheral vascular disease, previous myocardial infarction, and an ejection fraction of 51%, with 95% proximal stenosis of the left anterior descending coronary artery. This patient has a 5-year medical survival of 42%, while his surgical survival is 82%. In contrast is a 51-year-old man with infrequent angina, triple-vessel disease, a normal resting ECG, no peripheral vascular disease, no previous myocardial infarction, and an ejection fraction of 64%, with a 75% distal stenosis of the same vessel. That individual's 5-year medical survival is 92% and his

surgical survival is 97%. Using data published from two of the randomized control trials, the clinician would necessarily place both patients in the same category, that is, triple-vessel disease with normal left ventricular function, and expect their medical and surgical survival to be similar, whereas it clearly differs markedly.

4. It should be noted that a major problem of the database is the nonrandom nature of the treatment received, and there is always the possibility that an unrecognized imbalance in baseline characteristics could explain any observed differences in outcome among therapies being compared. However, statistical methods can be used to reduce such bias from nonrandom treatment allocation. Nevertheless, it should be appreciated that there is such a need for sophisticated analytical ability when such databases are used to answer therapeutic questions.[18]

The CASS study is an important illustration of the issues outlined above. The CASS randomized prospective study reported only about 5% of the patients enrolled in the observational study (CASS registry).[19] Thus, data on 24,959 patients have been entered into the data bank and the outcome of numerous subsets of patients have been the subject of important reports. Selected aspects of these observational data are discussed below.

OPERATIVE MORTALITY

Multivariate discriminate analysis of the clinical and angiographic predictors of operative mortality in the CASS registry have indicated that the clinical variables most predictive of mortality are age, female sex, increased heart size, and congestive heart failure.[20,21] The operative mortality in 8,971 patients was 2.3%. Patients with left main coronary artery disease had an operative mortality of 3.84%. Mortality increased with age, from 0 in the 20- to 29-year-old group to 7.9% in the group 70 years of age and older. Operative mortality was higher for women in each age group, ranging from 2.8% for ages 30 to 39 years to 12.3% from age 70 years and older (0.8% and 5.8% for men). Clinical manifestations of congestive heart failure were associated with increased operative mortality. Mortality was 1.4% in one-vessel disease, 2.1% in two-vessel disease, and 2.8% in three-vessel disease. Among 1,019 patients with left main coronary artery stenosis, operative mortality ranged from 1.6% in patients with mild stenosis and a right dominant system to 25% in patients with severe (more than 90%) stenosis and left dominance. Operative mortality also varied with the ejection fraction (1.9% for an ejection fraction > 50% vs. 6.7% for an ejection fraction < 19%) and left ventricular wall motion score (1.7% for least abnormal and 9.1% for most abnormal).

There appears to be a general agreement from the CASS and other studies that there is an excess risk for coronary bypass surgery in women, which has been attributed to their smaller stature and the smaller diameter of the coronary vessels in this group of patients.[22-24] Douglas and associates reported that women not only had smaller distal coronary arteries, but more diabetes and hypertension and a higher rate of incomplete vascularization with subsequent reduced graft patency compared with men.[22]

PREDICTORS OF LONG-TERM SURVIVAL

In the CASS registry the 5-year survival rate among 8,971 operated patients was 90%.[25] Patients with left main coronary artery disease had a 5-year survival rate of 85%, while patients with lesions in other vessels had a 5-year survival rate of 91%. Among patients without left main coronary artery disease, the 5-year survival was 93% in those with single-vessel disease, 92% in those with double-vessel disease (both with operative mortalities under 2%), and 88% in patients with triple-vessel disease, where the operative mortality was 2.62% ($P = 0.009$ vs. single- and double-vessel disease). Patients with normal or nearly normal left ventricular function (i.e., left ventricular segmental wall motion scores ranging from 5 through 11) had a 5-year survival of 92% and an operative mortality under 2%. Patients with moderate left ventricular functional impairment had a 5-year survival of 80% and an operative mortality of 4.21%. In those with poor left ventricular function, the 5-year survival was 65% and the operative mortality was 6.21%. The difference in survival among these three groups was significant ($P < 0.0001$).

In the CASS registry data, good predictors of survival from angiographic data alone could be obtained from a combination of left ventricular function and the arteriographic extent of disease.[26] Three simple indices yielded the most information: the number of vessels diseased, the number of proximal arterial segments diseased, and the left ventricular wall motion score. These three indices accounted for an estimated 84% of the prognostic information available. Six-year survival varied between 93% and 16% depending on the value of these three indices.

Adler and associates reported a total 5-year survival of 89% among 2,004 patients who underwent their first coronary artery bypass graft operation between January, 1970 and December, 1980 without concomitant valve replacement or aneurysmectomy.[27] The 8-year survival rate was 80%. A multivariate Cox model regression analysis showed that the independent correlates of long-term survival were emergent operation with cardiogenic shock, use of a postoperative intra-aortic balloon, ejection fraction less than 50%, preoperative history of congestive heart failure, cardiopulmonary bypass time, uncorrected mitral regurgitation, left main coronary artery narrowing, and diabetes. After controlling for these factors, age, sex, and the percentage of narrowings that were bypassed were not independent correlates of long-term survival. Similar long-term survival rates have been reported by Hall and associates.[28]

Mock and co-workers reported on the survival of medically treated patients in the CASS registry.[29] Patients with good left ventricular function had a 4-year survival of 94%, 91%, and 79%, for one-, two-, and three-vessel disease, respectively. The 4-year survival rates of the patients with one- and two-vessel disease and poor left ventricular performance were 67% and 61%, respectively, while the 4-year survival of patients with three-vessel disease and poor left ventricular performance was only 42%. The latter is significantly lower than the survival for one- and two-vessel disease groups with poor left ventricular performance ($P = 0.001$).

Table 74.1 lists the comparison from the CASS randomized study of the 4-year medical and 5-year surgical survivorship based on left ven-

TABLE 74.1 COMPARISON OF MEDICAL AND SURGICAL SURVIVAL BASED ON LEFT VENTRICULAR PERFORMANCE AND NUMBER OF VESSELS INVOLVED

	Medical Therapy (4-Year Survival)	Surgical Therapy (5-Year Survival)
Left Ventricular Function		
Normal	90%	92%
Moderately depressed	71%	80%
Poor	53%	65%
Extent of Disease		
Single vessel	92%	93%
Double vessel	84%	92%
Triple vessel	68%	88%
Left main	63%	85%

(Data from Myers WO, Davis K, Foster ED et al: Surgical survival in the Coronary Artery Surgery [CASS] registry. Ann Thorac Surg 40:246, 1985; Mock MB, Ringqvist I, Fisher LD et al: Survival of medically treated patients in the Coronary Artery Surgery Study [CASS] registry Circulation 66:562, 1982; Chaitman BR, Davis KB, Kaiser SG et al: The role of coronary bypass surgery for left main equivalent coronary disease: The Coronary Artery Surgery Study Registry. Circulation [Supp III] 74:17, 1986)

tricular performance and number of vessels involved. As can be seen, these nonrandomized data indicate that medical treatment and surgical treatment are roughly equivalent for individuals with single-vessel disease exclusive of left main coronary artery obstruction and normal left ventricular function, but for any other combination surgical treatment appears to be superior. These observations are consistent both with clinical experience and the randomized studies described previously. It is highly unlikely that today patients with single-vessel lesions amenable to balloon angioplasty and normal left ventricular function would undergo bypass surgery. Further, Table 74.1 indicates that left ventricular function is probably a more important predictor of survival than the number of diseased vessels alone.

These observational data have been confirmed and extended by recent reports from Duke University.[30,31] Among 5,125 patients referred for cardiac catheterization between 1969 and 1984, 2,261 underwent surgery and 2,864 received medical therapy. In the entire population, surgical treatment was associated with improved survival compared to medical therapy, whether or not the analysis was adjusted for baseline variables ($P < 0.001$). This difference in survival increased progressively throughout the study period, such that survival after coronary revascularization in 1984 was significantly better than after medical therapy in most categories except single-vessel disease.[30] The rate of improvement in survival over time was much greater in surgical patients and the difference compared to medical therapy was highly significant (treatment interaction with time, $P < 0.0001$). Estimates of 5-year survival adjusted for baseline risk factors for a patient in 1977 with one-, two-, or three-vessel disease and an ejection fraction of 40% were, for medical therapy, 88%, 80%, and 64%, and for surgical therapy, 88%, 87%, and 80%. Corresponding projected estimates for 1984 were unchanged for medical patients but improved for surgical patients—93%, 92%, and 90%.[31] These survival data are very close to those noted in Table 74.1. Patients at risk due to nonanatomical factors such as age, anginal severity, or reduced ejection fraction had an absolute increment in survival that was a constant function of baseline medical risk.[30] Because of a differential improvement in surgical therapy over time, contemporary coronary revascularization is associated with improved longevity in the majority of patients with ischemic heart disease, especially in those with adverse prognostic indicators.[30,31]

Other observational studies in small groups of patients are consistent with these data. Hammermeister and associates noted that the greatest benefit of coronary artery bypass surgery in the Seattle Heart Watch Study occurred in patients with triple-vessel disease and reduced or moderately abnormal left ventricular function who were older than 48 years.[32] A previous study from the same group indicated improved survival for the surgically treated subgroup with two-vessel disease.[33]

It should be noted that most patients with coronary artery disease are operated on for symptoms that are often disabling. Such symptoms usually include chest pain, but exertional dyspnea (which may be an "anginal equivalent") may also be disabling in some patients. Most studies do not address the issue of the asymptomatic patient with known severe coronary disease or the asymptomatic patient in whom severe coronary disease may be unrecognized because of silent ischemia. Some of the former group were included in the randomized portion of the CASS study,[9] but to date there are no randomized prospective data on revascularization in patients with silent ischemia. Current practice in many centers dictates that when severe asymptomatic ischemia is identified by noninvasive testing (exercise tolerance test, thallium-201 scintigraphy, Holter monitoring) and anatomical abnormalities are confirmed by coronary arteriography, patients should be advised to undergo revascularization.

LEFT MAIN EQUIVALENT DISEASE

Observational studies have also addressed the question of left main equivalent disease. This has been described as combined disease of the left anterior descending and left circumflex coronary arteries proximal to the origin of their major branches. The mortality of patients with this combination of lesions is not as high as with disease of the left main coronary artery alone. The CASS and other observational studies have suggested that this combination of lesions identifies a high-risk group (as determined by angiography),[34,35] although it is not prognostically equivalent to left main coronary artery disease. The most important lesion is probably proximal left anterior descending coronary disease, as shown by the European Coronary Artery Surgery Study.[8,36] Nevertheless, such patients should be evaluated (as probably should almost all patients) using physiologic testing (see below). As Hutter has pointed out, left main equivalent disease is probably not the simple presence of obstructive disease in the left anterior descending coronary artery and circumflex–marginal system, but is in reality an anatomical situation that places a large proportion of cardiac muscle at risk from one event.[37] The CASS registry data confirm that survival and quality of life are enhanced by surgery in this subset of patients save for that small proportion who are asymptomatic after myocardial infarction or who have mild chronic stable angina and are under age 65 with well-preserved left ventricular function.[38]

UNSTABLE ANGINA

Other important observations of the CASS registry have related to both unstable angina and severe stable angina pectoris. Although a recent VA cooperative study (not the original VA Coronary Bypass Study) of unstable angina showed a trend in favor of increased survival in patients with reduced left ventricular function,[17] there are no other randomized data to examine the issue of unstable angina save for a small study of 40 patients published in 1975, which showed no advantage of urgent coronary bypass surgery.[39] However, the CASS registry has supplied information on 3,311 patients who underwent surgical therapy for unstable angina. Overall operative mortality was 3.9% and logistic regression analysis indicated that as with other predictors of mortality in the CASS experience, age, left ventricular score, and the presence of left main stenosis and a left dominant circulation affected operative mortality.[40] The 7-year cumulative survival rate was 79% and the long-term outcome included predictors similar to the larger cohort of patients with stable angina by Cox proportional hazards analysis; these were the left ventricular score, congestive heart failure score, other illness, extent of coronary disease, and cardiomegaly. Rahimtoola and associates reported favorable long-term results of coronary bypass surgery for unstable angina in 1,282 patients operated on from 1970 to 1982: survival rates were 92% at 5 years and 83% at 10 years.[41] There were no significant differences in the survival for any of the three clinical subgroups of patients with unstable angina: angina at rest, angina after recovery from acute myocardial infarction, and progressive angina of recent onset. Patients with unstable angina who have undergone previous bypass surgery do not do as well as other patients with unstable angina who require revascularization; their cumulative adverse events (death, myocardial infarction, and recurrent unstable angina) are greater, presumably because they are less amenable to revascularization.[42]

In the CASS registry there were 4,209 patients who met the criteria used in the randomized trial except for the degree of angina pectoris and the method of treatment selection.[43] The 5-year survival rate was greater than 93% in patients with Canadian Cardiovascular Society Class II angina pectoris and normal left ventricular function, regardless of the number of vessels involved or treatment received. Late survival of surgically treated patients with Class III and IV angina pectoris and normal left ventricular function was similar, regardless of the number of vessels involved (greater than 90% at 5 years). However, nonoperatively treated patients with Class III and IV angina pectoris and normal left ventricular function had poorer 5-year survival rates, with the lowest (74%) in patients with three-vessel disease ($P < 0.0001$). This difference was also observed in patients with abnormal left ventricular function, three-vessel disease, and Class III and IV angina pectoris; the 5-year survival rates were 82% for the operated group and 52% for the nonoperated group (P < 0.0001). These data are similar to the observations shown in Table 74.1 for patients with stable milder angina and indicate that surgical therapy for severe angina pectoris seems to be superior to medical therapy.

SUDDEN DEATH

It is not well appreciated that observational studies have also indicated that coronary bypass surgery may have a beneficial effect on the risk of sudden death. In the Seattle Heart Watch Study, the sudden death rate for subgroups of medically treated patients was 1.8 to 10.9 times higher than rates in subgroups of surgically treated patients with a comparable ejection fraction and extent of coronary artery disease.[44] These observations were confirmed by the CASS registry in which sudden death occurred in 257 (4.9%) of 5,258 medically treated and 101 (1.6%) of 6,250 surgically treated patients.[45] In a high-risk patient subset with three-vessel disease and a history of congestive heart failure, 91% of surgically treated patients had not suffered sudden death compared with 69% of medically treated patients. After Cox analysis was used to correct baseline variables, surgical treatment had an independent beneficial effect on sudden death (P < 0.0001). This reduction was most pronounced in high-risk patients.

AGE

As indicated above, Cox regression analysis in observational studies indicates that age is another factor contributing to operative mortality and to long-term morbidity and mortality.[20,21,25,46] Although coronary artery bypass surgery has been successfully performed in patients aged 65 years and older,[47-51] long-term survival, as might be expected, is not as favorable.[49] Operative mortality tends to be somewhat higher but survival clearly is improved with surgery when medical and surgical groups are compared. Thus, analysis of the CASS registry data in 1,491 nonrandomized patients 65 years of age or older indicated a cumulative survival rate at 6 years (adjusted for major differences in important baseline characteristics) of 79% in the surgical group and 64% in the medical group (P < 0.0001).[50] At 5 years, chest pain was absent in 62% of the surgical group and 29% of the medical group (P < 0.0001). Similar favorable results have been reported by others.[47,51] In the CASS registry, surgical benefit was greatest in the high risk patients and the prognosticators of high risk were similar to those described above.[48,49] Thus, age, while not an absolute contraindication to coronary bypass surgery, does carry an increased risk of morbidity and mortality, and certainly, where possible, other approaches should be considered, including medical therapy and balloon angioplasty. Nevertheless, many older patients may be good candidates for coronary bypass surgery, and as the population ages, this consideration will certainly become an increasingly important one.

REOPERATION

As disease progresses in native vessels with time and as progressive occlusion of saphenous vein bypass grafts occurs (see below), the number of reoperations for coronary artery disease will likely continue to increase,[52] although as other methods of therapy, particularly the use of the internal mammary artery and antiplatelet measures are more extensively used, this problem may diminish somewhat. The only large group of patients so far studied emerged from the data in the CASS registry.[53] After 60.5 months of follow-up, repeat coronary artery bypass grafting was required in 283 of 9,369 patients (3.0%). The mean interval between operations was 39.3 months. Patients needing reoperation tended to be young and female and have less extensive coronary artery disease, less left ventricular impairment, less evidence of congestive heart failure, and fewer coronary vessels bypassed at the first operation. Repeat operation carried an increased risk of death compared with initial surgery (5.3% vs. 3.1%, P < 0.05). However, the rates of perioperative myocardial infarction and of all surgical complications combined were not significantly different compared to those of initial bypass surgery. Although the investigators in this study found no significant differences in the frequency of the major cardiac complications of perioperative myocardial infarction, arrhythmia (except for atrial fibrillation), cardiogenic shock, conduction defects, or congestive heart failure occurring with initial as compared with repeat coronary artery bypass grafting, these cardiac events appear to be more lethal following reoperation; they accounted directly for or contributed to all the deaths among the patients in this series undergoing repeat surgery. Further, symptomatic relief of angina is not as effective after repeat bypass surgery, with only half the patients being angina-free 5 years after operation.[52]

DEPRESSED LEFT VENTRICULAR PERFORMANCE

Other considerations may play a role in the decision to perform coronary bypass surgery. These include the presence of depressed left ventricular performance and the possibility that in selected patients the myocardium might be "hibernating." The latter has been defined as the presence of left ventricular dysfunction that may be amenable to revascularization.[54] Although there are anecdotal reports of successful myocardial revascularization in patients with an ejection fraction of 20% or less,[55] improvement in left ventricular performance and long-term clinical status are more likely to occur in individuals with less severely impaired left ventricular performance at rest and evidence of exercise-induced ischemic dysfunction.[56] Objective documentation of immediate improvement of dysfunctional myocardial segments after coronary revascularization has been provided by intraoperative transesophageal echocardiography,[57] and long-term improvement has been documented using rest and exercise radionuclide ventriculography.[58]

SIZE OF RECURRENT INFARCTION

Another benefit of coronary artery bypass surgery appears to be the favorable effect of this procedure on the size of recurrent myocardial infarction. Thus, patients with previous bypass surgery tend to have a smaller myocardial infarction with fewer complications compared with patients who have not had surgery.[59] A possible explanation of this observation is that such individuals have better residual left ventricular function due to the presence of less jeopardized myocardium lying distal to the infarct-producing lesions.[60]

URGENT REVASCULARIZATION

With improvements in medical therapy, most patients with unstable angina can be controlled, and both angiography and, if necessary, myocardial revascularization can be performed electively. Although patients who have angina early during recovery from myocardial infarction can be operated on with morbidity and mortality rates approaching those seen with surgery for stable angina,[41,61,62] special considerations apply to this group of patients. Hochberg and associates reported 174 patients who underwent myocardial revascularization within 7 weeks of myocardial infarction.[63] The total hospital mortality was 16%; however, mortality fell from 46% for individuals within 1 week of infarction to 6% for those operated on 7 weeks after infarction. All 50 patients operated on at any time with an ejection fraction exceeding 50% survived their hospitalization. Among 124 patients with an ejection fraction of less than 50% operated on during this 7-week period, there were 17 (22%) hospital deaths, but in this latter group, survival rates steadily improved if revascularization was performed at a time more removed from infarction. Presumably, recovery of stunned myocardium and development of firm scar tissue contributed to improved later survival. Based on these data, Hochberg and colleagues recommended that if the ejection fraction is less than 50%, operation after myocardial infarction should be delayed at least 4 weeks.[63]

Another special consideration is the patient requiring emergency surgery after failed coronary angioplasty. In such individuals, surgery can be performed with low mortality but with a higher incidence of major postoperative complications. In the series of Golding and co-workers, the principal indications for emergency surgery were acute occlusion, dissection, unstable angina, ventricular arrhythmias, and unsuccessful dilatation.[64] Among 81 patients, there were two early deaths and 35 patients who had a postoperative myocardial infarction as evidenced by new Q waves and increases in serum glutamic-oxaloacetic transaminase (SGOT) and creatine kinase (CK)-MB activities. This high postoperative infarction rate has been noted by others.[65–67] The incidences of postoperative hemorrhage and respiratory failure were also higher.[63] Patients should be apprised of this information when providing informed consent for elective percutaneous transluminal angioplasty.

CRITIQUES

A number of critical appraisals of the randomized trials and the CASS registry studies described above have appeared.[19,54,68–75] As indicated previously, the CASS registry consists of a very large number of patients (24,959 patients undergoing coronary arteriography at 15 centers) and a controlled, randomized, prospective study involving 780 patients. Weinstein and Levin have pointed out that the randomized CASS data do not apply to patients with unstable angina, patients with angina more severe than Class II (Canadian Cardiovascular Society classification), congestive heart failure Class III or IV (New York Heart Association classification), age greater than 65 years, asymptomatic patients who have a positive exercise stress test, patients with left main coronary artery narrowing greater than 70% luminal diameter, an ejection fraction of less than 35%, a ventricular aneurysm likely to require resection, and valvular disease likely to require valve replacement.[68] However, it should be noted that several of these subgroups are included in the CASS registry (see discussion above). Weinstein and Levin have suggested that since the CASS randomized study applies only to a small minority of patients with coronary artery disease, attempts to extend the conclusions of this study to the vast majority of patients with coronary artery disease are unjustified.[68] They point out that the high percentage of crossover of the medical group to surgery made it impossible for the CASS randomized study to accomplish its primary goal of contrasting medical and surgical treatment. Despite the fact that crossover of medically assigned patients created a bias against surgical treatment, the observed mortality in the surgical group was still 31% lower than that in the medical group. Failure of the CASS randomized study to find this difference to be statistically significant must take into account the fact that the statistical power of the CASS randomized study was so low that a real difference was likely to be overlooked.[68]

Many of these criticisms are dealt with in the CASS registry, and the remarkable agreement in the conclusions of the three large randomized studies (which are extended by the registry data) render these valid criticisms less important than they might otherwise seem. Gunnar and Loeb have pointed out that in the CASS randomized study, 2,095 patients met both the clinical and angiographic criteria for randomization.[72] However, a significant number of patients with angiographic features of higher risk were offered and accepted surgical treatment (the nonrandomized surgical group). After the exclusion of many such higher-risk patients, the remaining patients, including those actually undergoing the randomization process, might be expected to have a favorable prognosis regardless of whether they received medical or surgical therapy. Rahimtoola has emphasized that all three randomized studies failed to define optimum medical therapy, and the effectiveness of medical therapy that was actually delivered was also largely undocumented.[54] He points out that the current data suggest that pharmacologic therapy for unstable angina has had little or no effect on cardiac morbidity and mortality and there have been no prospective randomized trials demonstrating that medical therapy of patients with chronic stable angina results in better survival rates compared with no specific medical therapy at all. He also notes that one third of the operative deaths in the European Coronary Artery Surgery Study occurred after randomization but before the performance of surgery. As indicated earlier, there is also considerable controversy regarding the assignment of crossover patients to medical and surgical therapy. Rahimtoola has suggested that there are no data to prove at what point the crossover rate compromises a randomized trial.[54] He has also emphasized the randomized CASS trial does not apply to the evaluation of patients soon after myocardial infarction who should be subjected to appropriate risk stratification.[71]

Despite these criticisms, the randomized trials and the CASS registry, along with other registry data, have had an important impact on our knowledge of the natural history of coronary artery disease and have also defined the "natural history" of surgical therapy. It has also been pointed out that these studies represent the results of surgical therapy performed in the late 1970s and do not necessarily apply to either medical or surgical therapy in the late 1980s.[19] Indeed, since these studies have been completed, physiologic evaluation in the assessment of patients with coronary artery disease has become a standard approach to care.[76] As Plotnick has emphasized, patients with multivessel disease do not constitute a homogeneous population.[77] Clinical decision making based only on the number of vessels with high-grade obstructive lesions is a one-dimensional approach to a multidimensional problem. Patients who develop ischemia in a large area of myocardium with minimal stress appear to be at highest risk for mortality during follow-up, and recent reports demonstrate that mortality correlates better with the total amount of myocardium that becomes ischemic during exercise testing than with the number of obstructed coronary arteries demonstrated angiographically.[78–80]

Thus, in patients with chronic stable angina, exercise testing, often with thallium-201, has become a standard approach to the assessment of jeopardized myocardium and has markedly influenced the decision-making process with regard to the choice of medical versus surgical therapy. All three large randomized studies did, in retrospect, identify criteria for high-risk groups based in part on history and exercise or resting ECG evaluation. Weiner and associates reported on the role of exercise testing in identifying patients with improved survival after coronary bypass surgery derived from 5,339 randomized patients entered into the CASS registry who underwent exercise testing.[76] These investigators concluded that by using physiologic testing, one can identify high- and low-risk groups among patients with triple-vessel disease. They found that the high-risk group of patients with triple-vessel disease exhibited improved survival with surgery whereas the low-risk group did not. The high-risk group was defined as those patients developing greater than 1-mm ST segment depression at stage I of the Bruce protocol. The 7-year survival rate was 81% for the 278 surgically treated patients versus 50% of the 120 medically treated patients ($P < 0.0001$). Among patients with triple-vessel disease who fit into the low-risk group by their definition (exercise into stage III or greater without ST segment depression), the surgical cohort did not survive longer than the medical cohort.

It seems apparent then that a variety of factors will influence survival among patients with chronic stable angina. These include the degree of left ventricular dysfunction, the number of vessels involved, the location and severity of lesions, and the response to physiologic testing. Using this information as well as historical factors (history of hypertension, previous myocardial infarction, age, and sex), it is now possible to identify high- and low-risk patients and to evolve an approach to treatment based on each patient's individual characteristics. Thus, despite their obvious limitations, the randomized studies along with their larger registry counterparts have contributed enormously to our current knowledge of surgical revascularization.

GRAFT OCCLUSION

Among the technical advances that have led to the superiority of surgical treatment over medical therapy in many of the selected circumstances described above are improved methods of myocardial protection employing blood or crystalloid cardioplegia with local hypothermia, conduit selection and preservation, blood conservation, anesthetic management, arrhythmia control, and, where necessary, pulmonary arterial catheter monitoring, pharmacologic unloading, intra-aortic balloon conterpulsation, and cardiac assist devices.[81] Despite these advances, long-term follow-up studies of patients after coronary artery bypass surgery employing the saphenous vein have noted a progressive decrease in benefit from this procedure with time, especially after 7 years. In 1978, Seides and associates suggested that most grafts patent several months after operation remain so for at least 4½ years and that symptomatic deterioration in the succeeding years is most often due to progression of disease in ungrafted vessels.[82] In addition to progression of atherosclerosis in ungrafted arteries, however, progression of obstruction was also described in grafts by Campeau and co-workers in 1979.[83] Pathologic changes in saphenous veins used as aortocoronary bypass grafts include endothelial damage, medial hypertrophy, medial necrosis, graft-wall fibrosis (media and adventitia), intimal fibrous thickening, intimal lipid deposition, and aneurysmal dilatation.[84] Native vessels initially free of disease appear to be at relatively low risk for development of disease within 5 years, but in surgically treated patients both grafted and nongrafted vessels show similar rates of progression.[85] Elevated blood lipids appear to be a major risk factor for progression in saphenous vein bypass grafts and are associated with progressive intimal fibromuscular proliferation or atheroma formation in the implanted vein;[86,87] atheromatous plaque rupture with superimposed occlusive thrombosis also occurs.[88] Frequency of the return of anginal symptoms correlates significantly with the degree of graft patency[89] and there appears to be accelerated progression of atherosclerosis in coronary vessels with minimal lesions that are bypassed.[90]

The most extensive studies of changes in grafts and coronary arteries after saphenous vein aortocoronary bypass surgery have been provided by the group at the Montreal Heart Institute. In their first 600 patients, patency rates were 87% to 92% within 1 month and 74% to 85% approximately 1 year after surgery.[91] Between 1 year and 6 years, the attrition rate of grafts averaged 2.2% per year. Early occlusion was due to thrombosis, whereas occlusion at 1 year was caused by fibrous intimal proliferation, which also led to a variable reduction in caliber and to a greater than 50% segmental stenosis in 5% to 15% of patent grafts. Bourassa and associates concluded that the most important determinant of graft patency at 1 year was the runoff capacity of the recipient artery followed by the quality of the surgical technique.[91] Late occlusion was related to atherosclerosis that became manifest only after at least 2 years. During the first year, only 10% of preexisting stenoses in nongrafted arteries showed progression of disease, and progression in these vessels increased to 46% at 6 years and was no longer different for preexisting lesions greater than 50% from that of grafted arteries. In a subsequent study, Campeau and co-workers reported that graft closure increased 2.5-fold from the interval between 1 year and 5 to 7 years to the following period between 7 and 12 years (10.2%–26.1%, $P < 0.02$).[92] Thus, the mean yearly attrition rate was augmented from 2% to 5.3%. Overall graft closure in their series was 63.3% at 10 to 12 years. Almost half of the patent grafts showed evidence of relatively severe atherosclerosis.

These observations regarding graft closure are consistent with the clinical observations from the VA randomized study, which showed reduced benefit from coronary artery surgery between 7 to 11 years in patients with triple-vessel disease and a reduced ejection fraction,[4] and with the CASS angiographic registry data.[93] It seems evident, then, that long-term follow-up of a large number of patients who have undergone aortocoronary bypass surgery using saphenous vein grafts has demonstrated a substantial number of graft occlusions in addition to progression of disease in native vessels. These findings emphasize the palliative nature of aortocoronary bypass surgery and, although they do not diminish its value in individual patients, have prompted the search for specific therapy to prevent such progression and for alternative surgical and other approaches to the treatment of these lesions.

ANTIPLATELET AGENTS

Both anticoagulation and antiplatelet agents have been utilized to reduce the incidence of acute graft occlusions. Gohlke reported that oral anticoagulation begun 7 days after surgery resulted in improved graft patency 2 months after surgery (90.4% of the treatment group vs. 84.6% of the control group, $P < 0.015$).[94] These investigators found that all anastomoses were patent in 81% of the treatment group and in 61% of the control group ($P < 0.02$). Flow measurement in 279 grafts suggested that grafts with a flow of less than 90 ml/min benefit from oral anticoagulation since no graft with a flow of more than 90 ml/min was occluded. The results of a large number of clinical trials were summarized by Gitler and Gitler.[95] All reported studies except those of Chesebro and colleagues[96] began treatment 1 to 3 days following surgery. The agents employed included aspirin, dipyridamole, and sulfinpyrazone.

The most impressive studies demonstrating the benefit of perioperative antiplatelet therapy are those of Chesebro and associates.[96,97] In their initial report, these investigators compared dipyridamole instituted 2 days before surgery plus aspirin added 7 hours after operation with placebo in 407 patients. They performed vein graft angiography in 360 of these patients within 6 months of operation (median, 8 days). Within 1 month of operation, 3% of vein graft distal anastomoses (10 of 351) were occluded in the treated patients, whereas 10% (38 of 362) were occluded in the placebo group. The proportion of patients with one or more distal anastomoses occluded was 8% (10 of 130) in the treated group and 21% (27 of 130) in the placebo group. This benefit in graft patency, which was highly statistically significant, persisted in each of over 50 subgroups. Chesebro and co-workers reported that early postoperative bleeding was similar in the two groups.

In a subsequent follow-up study, these investigators performed repeat vein graft angiography in 343 patients (84% of the original treated group) 11 to 18 months (median, 12 months) after operation.[97] Of 478 vein graft distal anastomoses, 11% were occluded in the treated group and 25% of 486 were occluded in the placebo group. The proportion of patients with one or more distal anastomoses occluded was 22% of 171 patients in the treated group and 47% of 172 in the placebo group. The late development of occlusions was reduced from 27% in the placebo group to 16% in the treated group. They interpreted their data to show that dipyridamole and aspirin continue to be effective in preventing vein graft occlusion after operation and recommended that such treatment should be continued for at least 1 year.

A recent VA Cooperative Study confirmed and extended these results.[98] In this study, Goldman and associates compared aspirin, 325 mg daily, with aspirin, 325 mg three times daily; aspirin plus dipyridamole, 325 mg and 75 mg, respectively, three times daily; sulfinpyrazone, 267 mg three times daily; and placebo, three times daily. Therapy was started 48 hours before surgery except for aspirin. When aspirin was a treatment, one 325-mg dose was given 12 hours before surgery and maintained thereafter according to the assigned regimen. Angiographic patency data were obtained 1 week after surgery. Analysis of early graft patency in 539 patients (1,736 grafts) revealed graft patency of greater than 90% (range, 90.6%–94%) for all antiplatelet regimens. All aspirin-containing therapeutic regimens improved graft patency compared to placebo (84.7%, $P < 0.03$). However, chest tube drainage measured within the first 35 hours after surgery revealed that the median loss with the aspirin-containing regimens exceeded that of placebo (800 ml, $P < 0.05$), whereas that with sulfinpyrazone did not. The reoperation rate was greater in all the treatment groups that received aspirin (5.9% vs. 1.8% for nonaspirin groups, $P < 0.01$). The overall operative mortality was 2.2%, without significant differences among treatment groups. Transient renal insufficiency occurred in 6.3% of patients taking sulfinpyrazone. Goldman and co-workers concluded that while vein graft patency was improved 1 week after coronary bypass surgery with all the antiplatelet drug regimens tested, the three aspirin regimens increased blood loss after coronary bypass surgery. All aspirin regimens were associated with increased rates of reoperation.[98]

Thus, at the present time it appears that the regimen proposed by Chesebro and associates,[96,97] in which dipyridamole is begun before operation and aspirin shortly following surgery, may be a more acceptable approach while providing an equivalent degree of graft patency. The VA Cooperative Study is being extended to a long-term follow-up study for at least 3 years. Although Chesebro and co-workers remained within the confines of their data by recommending that antiplatelet therapy should be continued for at least 1 year after saphenous vein bypass grafting,[97] in the absence of adverse reactions, it may be prudent to continue such therapy indefinitely until information from longer-term follow-up studies such as the VA Cooperative Study is available.

LIPID-LOWERING REGIMENS AND SMOKING

As indicated above, hyperlipidemia is an important risk factor for the development of atherosclerotic obstruction of saphenous vein aortocoronary bypass grafts.[86,87] In patients developing both saphenous vein occlusion and progression of disease in the native circulation, very low-density lipoproteins (VLDLs) and low-density lipoproteins (LDLs) are higher, and high-density lipoprotein (HDL) levels are lower compared with those without disease progression.[87] There is now direct evidence from the Cholesterol-Lowering Atherosclerosis Study (CLAS) that reduction of total plasma cholesterol with increased HDL and reduced LDL levels can result in less atherosclerosis in saphenous vein bypass grafts and actual regression of atherosclerosis in native vessels.[99] Passamani's accompanying editorial places both the dangers of continued hyperlipidemia and smoking in their proper perspective[100]:

> During the course of the NHLBI Coronary Artery Surgery Study, levels of risk factors did not change in the interval between entry and five-year follow-up in either the medically or surgically assigned patients. Generally, smokers continued to smoke; the proportion of patients with elevated blood pressure and elevated cholesterol level at entry and at five years was similar. The dangers of uncontrolled hypertension and continued smoking were clear during the Coronary Artery Surgery Study follow-up period. Perhaps patients and their physicians believed that bypass would deliver very long-term palliation, even with no changes in life-style. The lack of successful reduction in cholesterol levels among these patients with advanced vascular disease might have been due to reluctance on the part of physicians and their patients to undertake major life-style change and begin long-term, expensive, difficult-to-take drug therapy in the absence of clearcut proof that reduction of cholesterol levels is effective....
>
> Careful refinement of the details of perioperative management of coronary artery bypass graft patients in the 1970s resulted in substantial improvement in the rates of hospital mortality and morbidity. The CLAS data identify a posthospital management refinement, aggressive lowering of cholesterol levels, which promises further substantial improvement in the quality and quantity of life in bypass patients.

Based on these observations, every effort should be made to encourage the post-bypass patient to discontinue the use of tobacco and to embark on a lipid-lowering regimen, which may include drug therapy.

INTERNAL MAMMARY ARTERY GRAFTS

The use of the internal mammary artery as a bypass graft was introduced by a Russian surgeon, Professor Kolessov.[101] Subsequently, surgeons in this country, including Green and associates and Edwards and colleagues, performed similar operations on an increasingly larger number of patients.[101] The internal mammary artery is now used commonly to bypass the left anterior descending coronary artery and indeed is the current method of choice for this approach in most large surgical centers. Reasons for the better results obtained with the use of this vessel include the fact that its pedicle is retained with intact vasa vasorum and lymphatic drainage, and it is generally free of native atherosclerosis and makes an excellent size match with the native left anterior descending coronary artery.[102] Technical innovations include the use of the internal mammary artery as a free graft, bilateral grafting, bypass to the circumflex and right coronary arteries, and even sequential internal mammary artery grafts.[101] In addition, it is usually combined with saphenous vein bypass grafting to other vessels where indicated. The internal mammary artery also appears to exhibit the physiologic phenomenon of autoregulation in that the size of its lumen can with time adapt to variable flow requirements.[101] Thus, when the demand in the recipient coronary bed is low, such as in mild occlusions or with poor distal runoff, the distal portion of the internal mammary artery may actually narrow, particularly if the resistance to flow is elevated in a long graft. By contrast, when the demand is high, the internal mammary artery graft may dilate. These reactive changes may serve to maintain flow velocity and presumably help to maintain graft patency.

Use of the internal mammary artery appears to be contraindicated in the presence of vascular disease of the upper extremities, disease of the carotid or subclavian arteries, and if a blood pressure differential greater than 15 mm Hg exists between the arms.[102] The internal mammary artery is also generally not used in a markedly hypertrophied ventricle with a large native coronary artery or for emergency operation for unstable patients. Use of the internal mammary artery bypass requires a longer preparation time and is technically more difficult because of the smaller size of this vessel. One concern has been an increased incidence of sternal wound infection with this approach.

Results with the use of the internal mammary artery have been uniformly superior to those of the saphenous vein bypass graft, as reported in 1976 by Siegel and Loop in an early series.[103] Tector and colleagues concluded that the properly prepared internal mammary artery graft has the longest lasting patency and recommended its routine use for bypassing proximal left anterior descending coronary artery lesions.[104] Other large series have confirmed this approach.[105-109] Grondin and co-workers compared late changes in internal mammary artery and saphenous vein grafts in two consecutive series of patients 10 years after operation.[106] They detected atheromatous alterations in 44% of 66 patent saphenous vein grafts and in only 5.2% (1/19) of internal mammary artery grafts. Furthermore, they reported that patients who received internal mammary artery grafts had a better survival rate after 10 years (84.3% vs. 70%) than those who underwent saphenous vein bypass grafting. In a 15-year follow-up study, Cameron and associates compared 532 patients with one or two internal mammary artery grafts with or without additional saphenous vein grafts to 216 patients with saphenous vein grafts alone.[107] The patients who received at least one internal mammary artery bypass graft had better cumulative survival, less early recurrence of angina, fewer myocardial infarctions, fewer reoperations, and better cumulative event-free survival than the 216 patients with vein grafts alone. In young individuals (age 35 years or younger), mammary artery grafts have been recommended as the approach of choice.[108] Lytle and associates have also documented the low and decreasing perioperative risk of internal mammary artery bypass grafting.[109]

Despite the advantages outlined above, it must be recognized that internal mammary artery stenosis and sometimes complete occlusion do occur. Mechanical factors such as angulation at the anastomotic site, stretching, and other inadvertent injury during the procedure may account for such adverse results.[101] Diffuse stenosis involving the distal portion of the graft may result from stretching of a short graft, inadvertent ligation of the internal mammary vein, cautery-related heat injury, hematoma of the pedicle, competitive flow with coronary arteries that are not critically stenosed, and severe left ventricular hypertrophy.[101] Nevertheless, the high degree of patency of these grafts (well over 90% at 7–10 years) continues to make this approach the treatment of choice for revascularization of the left anterior descending coronary artery.

Despite these favorable results, Lefrak recently reported a survey of

750 surgeons performing myocardial revascularization who had done a total of over 122,000 coronary bypass operations annually, which suggested that the use of the internal mammary artery is more praised than practical.[110] Of these surgeons, 84% (649) listed the internal mammary artery as the graft of choice for bypassing the left anterior descending coronary artery, whereas 15% listed the saphenous vein. Only about half of the surgeons actually used the internal mammary artery, however, and only 30% used it in at least 90% of their operations. Lefrak concluded that in actual practice the internal mammary artery is often avoided in situations where it could be used as a coronary artery bypass graft. Thus, a substantial proportion of the population undergoing coronary bypass surgery in this country in the late 1980s can be expected not to have optimal results.

PERIOPERATIVE MYOCARDIAL INFARCTION

Perioperative myocardial infarction may contribute both to early and late morbidity and mortality after coronary artery surgery. However, acute myocardial infarction under these circumstances may be more difficult to detect than in the usual patient admitted to a coronary care unit. Conventional criteria for myocardial infarction have a low diagnostic performance in the setting of coronary bypass surgery.[111] Raabe and associates concluded that a newly positive postoperative pyrophosphate scintigram is more sensitive and specific than development of new postoperative Q waves for the diagnosis of hemodynamically significant postoperative myocardial infarction.[112] They also observed that CK-MB isoenzyme activity is highly sensitive but too nonspecific to be useful in the diagnosis of perioperative infarction.

In one early CASS report of 1,340 patients operated on in 1978, long-term survival was adversely affected by the appearance of new postoperative Q waves. Thus, the hospital mortality was 9.7% in the 62 patients who had new postoperative Q waves and 1.0% in the 1,278 patients who did not ($P < 0.001$).[113] The 3-year cumulative survival rates were 85% and 95%, respectively ($P < 0.001$). However, in patients who survived to hospital discharge, the presence of new postoperative Q waves did not adversely effect 3-year survival (94% and 96%, respectively). The survival rates were generally worse in patients who had a previous history of myocardial infarction or who had impaired left ventricular function preoperatively.

In the larger CASS registry study, myocardial infarction was determined by the presence of a localized depolarization abnormality (Q wave or loss of R wave), abnormal ST-T waves on the electrocardiogram, and changes in serum activity of myocardial enzymes.[114] In the perioperative infarction group, 51% of patients had new Q waves, 63% had evolution of regional ST-T wave changes, and 67% had a diagnostically significant elevation of serum enzyme activity. All three criteria were present in 32% of patients, and two of the three were present in 33%. Among these 9,777 patients who underwent operation between 1974 and 1979, definite or probable perioperative myocardial infarction using these criteria was diagnosed in 5.7% (561 patients). The incidence decreased from 6.6% in 1974 to 4.1% in 1979 ($P < 0.005$). In contrast to the early, smaller CASS study referred to above, this study in a much larger number of patients demonstrated that actuarial survival, including hospital deaths, at 1, 3, and 5 years, was significantly greater in patients without infarction than in patients with infarction (96%, 94%, and 90% vs. 78%, 74%, and 69%; $P < 0.001$). The difference persisted among patients dismissed from the hospital. Reduction of late survival among patients with perioperative infarction was due to the poor outcome of those who had complications (5-year survival rates 40% overall and 73% for patients dismissed from the hospital). Multivariate analysis identified perioperative myocardial infarction as an important independent predictor of late survival after bypass grafting. This predictor was surpassed only by left ventricular function, age, and number of associated medical diseases. Data from the Seattle Heart Watch Study confirm these CASS registry observations.[115]

The pathogenesis of perioperative myocardial infarction does not appear to be due to bypass graft occlusion. Bulkley and Hutchins reported an autopsy series of patients who died early after coronary bypass surgery and found that most perioperative infarctions occurred in the distribution of bypassed arteries and were usually associated with patent grafts and native vessels.[116] Utilizing contrast-enhanced computed tomography, Brindis and associates reported 14 patients with patent grafts and perioperative myocardial infarction in the distribution of the grafted vessel.[117] Four additional patients had an occluded graft and infarction in the distribution of the grafted vessels. These researchers concluded that the majority of perioperative myocardial infarctions associated with bypass surgery are not caused by graft occlusion. They suggested that the severity of coronary obstruction in the grafted vessel and the lack of collateral vessels to the region of the perioperative infarction in patients with patent grafts indicate that there is a portion of jeopardized myocardium that is subject to inadequate intraoperative preservation. This obviously represents an area that will require further study and perhaps merits additional improvements in myocardial preservation or antithrombotic therapy because of the clear adverse impact of perioperative myocardial infarction on both short- and long-term patient survival. With improved methods of myocardial preservation, including cold potassium cardioplegia, the incidence of perioperative myocardial infarction has undoubtedly been diminished. However, given the difficulty of making an accurate diagnosis, the true incidence of this complication and its precise impact on long-term morbidity and mortality are not known, but it clearly represents an important contribution to the adverse results of coronary bypass surgery.

VALVE DISEASE AND REPLACEMENT

If mitral valve insufficiency is due to coronary artery disease, concurrent replacement of the mitral valve combined with coronary artery bypass surgery carries a high morbidity and mortality. A ruptured papillary muscle or torn chordae tendineae with a dilated annulus is the usual pathology. In an early series, an 80% survival at 5 years in such patients was reported.[118] In 28 patients with ischemic mitral regurgitation who underwent a combined mitral valve replacement and coronary bypass surgery, Kay and associates noted a 5-year survival of only 43%.[119] When coronary artery bypass grafting is combined with mitral valve replacement for primary mitral valve (nonischemic) disease, the mortality rate was still high (7.3%) in the series reported by Lytle and co-workers.[120] Follow-up of 278 hospital survivors at a mean interval of 48 months (range, 2–165 months) documented survival of 85%, 66%, and 31% and an event-free survival of 65%, 46%, and 21% at 2, 5, and 10 years postoperatively. Thus, the combination of mitral valve dysfunction, whether ischemic or nonischemic, combined with coronary atherosclerosis requiring coronary bypass grafting, even when performed on an elective basis, has a high immediate morbidity and mortality and a long-term poor prognosis for survival.

By contrast, combined aortic valve replacement and myocardial revascularization carry a lower morbidity and mortality. In the series of Richardson and colleagues, early (30-day) mortality was 5.4% (12/220) of patients operated on during a 7.5-year period ending in June, 1977.[121] A similar operative mortality was reported by Lytle and associates between 1967 and 1981 (5.9%), with an operative mortality in later years (1978–1981) of 3.4%.[122] Richardson and co-workers reported a mean duration of follow-up of 22.5 months with a cumulative survival of 88% at 1 year and 77% at 3 years; these figures did not differ significantly from those for patients without coronary disease having isolated aortic valve replacement at their institution.[121] Lytle and associates reported a follow-up of 471 patients who survived hospitalization for 1 month to 135 months (mean, 41 months) after surgery.[122] Survival rates were 87%, 80%, and 55%, and event-free survival rates were 80%, 65%, and 39% at 2, 5, and 10 years after surgery, respectively. The late survival rate was unfavorably influenced by the presence of moderately or severely impaired left ventricular function and double-vessel coronary artery disease. Patients with bioprostheses who did not receive any anticoagulants had higher survival and event-free survival rates than did either patients with bioprostheses who received anticoagulants or patients with mechanical valves, whether they received any anticoagulants or not. Thus, aortic valve replacement, whether for an aortic stenosis or aortic insufficiency, when combined with myocardial revascularization carries a considerably lower morbidity and mortality than a similar operation with mitral valve replacement and is probably equivalent to isolated aortic valve replacement without concurrent bypass surgery.[123]

MANAGEMENT OF ASSOCIATED CEREBROVASCULAR AND OTHER PERIPHERAL VASCULAR DISEASE

Patients with coronary artery disease who require revascularization often have concurrent cerebrovascular or peripheral vascular disease, which may or may not be symptomatic. Conversely, many patients with the latter disorders who require either carotid endarterectomy, peripheral vascular bypass surgery, or abdominal aortic aneurysmectomy have coronary arterial obstructive disease of sufficient severity to increase the morbidity and mortality of these operations significantly.

For patients about to undergo coronary bypass surgery, routine evaluation should include an attempt to identify those with an increased risk for stroke during or following surgery. In general, patients with asymptomatic carotid bruits and lesions below well-defined limits are not considered to be candidates for routine carotid endarterectomy. Berkoff[124,125] has suggested an approach to such patients (Fig. 74.1). He considers the carotid lesion to be significant if the patient has greater than 85% unilateral carotid stenosis, greater than 75% bilateral stenosis, or severe unilateral stenosis and contralateral carotid obstruction. In these instances, the operative plan must take into consideration which lesion, coronary or carotid, presents the most risk to the patient and which combination of procedures offers the most benefit.

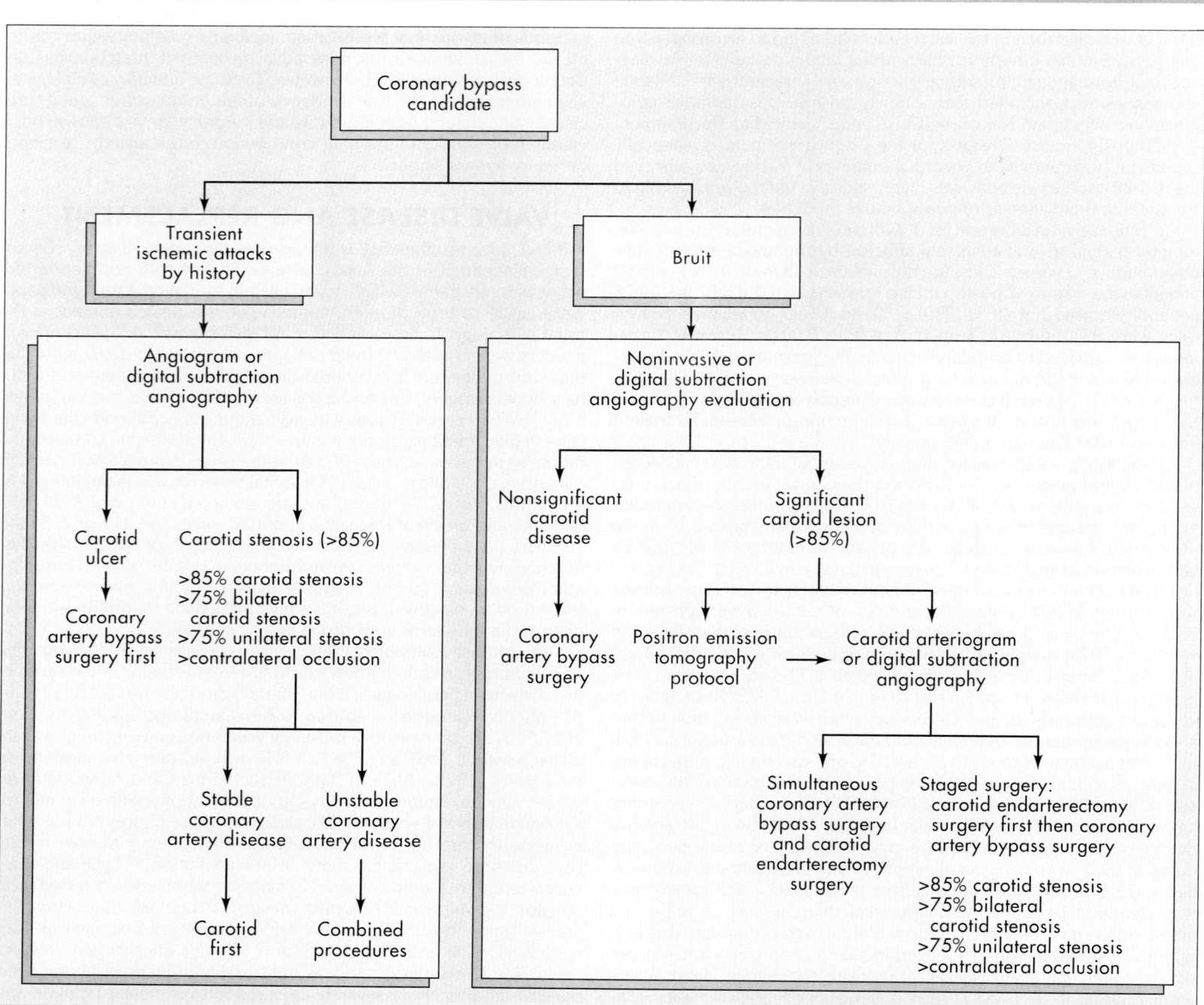

FIGURE 74.1 Sequential evaluation of patients with coronary artery disease. (Modified from Berkoff HA and Levine RL: Management of the vascular patient with multi-system atherosclerosis. Progress in Cardiovascular Diseases. 29:347–368, 1987)

Conversely, patients who require either carotid endarterectomy or peripheral vascular surgery, including abdominal aortic aneurysm repair, should have a screening evaluation for coronary artery disease. The usual history, physical examination, and resting ECG may be insufficiently revealing and a physiologic study, such as an exercise tolerance test, using thallium-201 if necessary, should be performed. Since many patients with peripheral vascular disease cannot exercise on a treadmill or a bicycle, a dipyridamole–thallium-201 study may be substituted.

When peripheral vascular disease surgery or abdominal aneurysmectomy is contemplated, the presence of severe coronary artery disease, as evidenced by noninvasive evaluation and confirmed by coronary arteriography, will lead to the performance of coronary artery bypass surgery or balloon angioplasty first. Among the indications for attacking the coronary disease first are left main stem disease >75%, left main equivalent disease, high-grade (>75%) proximal left anterior coronary obstruction, and severe double- or triple-vessel disease with documented reperfusion defects on thallium-201 scintigraphy.

When carotid obstruction is at issue, Berkoff recommends that this vessel be done first as a staged procedure if the disease is characterized by high-grade stenosis (>85%) and coronary artery disease is clinically stable without lesions as described in the preceding paragraph (Table 74.2).[124,125] When carotid endarterectomy is done first, careful attention must be paid to intraoperative cardiac monitoring. Berkoff advocates the use of arterial monitors, continuous ECG recording, and Swan-Ganz cathetization if indicated, and continued use of preoperative medications, particularly β-blockers.[124]

RETURN TO WORK AND OTHER ACTIVITIES

Despite the clear benefits conferred by coronary bypass surgery on relief of angina pectoris and under certain circumstances on increased longevity, it has been the experience of almost all investigators that employment status is not enhanced by this procedure. In the Seattle Heart Watch Study, surgical therapy was not more effective than medical treatment in maintaining full-time employment.[126] Johnson and coworkers reported that the main reason for not working was physical disability, with doctor's advice a distant second.[127] Older patients showed a trend of accelerated retirement after surgery. In the Mayo Clinic portion of the CASS registry, postoperative angina was the most powerful factor reducing return to work.[128] Postoperative employment also was lower if the patient was not working before surgery, was a laborer, or was older than 55 years (all $P < 0.01$). Although the level of nonwork physical activity was generally increased after bypass surgery, there was no relationship between physical activity and employment. Thus, preoperative work status, nonwork income, occupation, relief of symptoms, age, perception of health, education, and severity of disease appear to be important for estimating the likelihood of employment after surgery. Oberman and associates noted that other influences, such as attitudes of the family, employers, and physicians, undoubtedly alter the probability of return to the work force, but they are less well documented.[129] Thus, unless constructive approaches toward work rehabilitation are made, the possibility of return to gainful employment should not be considered an indication for or a necessary consequence of coronary artery bypass surgery. Although employment is not increased, coronary artery bypass surgery does appear to lead to substantial improvements in the quality of life, including general pleasure, reduction of anxiety and depression, and subjective improvement in job and family roles. However, sexual adjustment appears to improve the least and the frequency of sexual relations tends to decrease.[130]

TABLE 74.2 OPERATIVE PLAN WHEN BOTH OBSTRUCTIVE CAROTID AND CORONARY DISEASE ARE PRESENT

Carotid Endarterectomy First	Coronary Artery Bypass First	Simultaneous
Transient ischemic attacks (TIA) (carotid angiogram shows stenosis >85%)	TIA with ulcer or carotid stenosis < 75%	Severe unilateral carotid artery stenosis >85% unilateral occlusion and stenosis, bilateral severe carotid stenosis
Stable angina (usually 75% or less stenosis in one or two or possibly three coronary arteries)	Three-vessel disease	
	Left main coronary artery stenosis	Left main coronary artery stenosis >75%
	Proximal left anterior descending coronary artery stenosis	Three-vessel disease
	Unstable angina	Proximal left anterior coronary artery stenosis
		Unstable angina

REFERENCES

1. Favaloro RG: Direct myocardial revascularization: A ten year journey. Myths and realities. Circulation 43:109, 1979
2. Takaro T, Hultgren HN, Lipton MJ, Detre KM: The VA cooperative randomized study of surgery for coronary arterial occlusive disease. II. Subgroup with significant left main lesions. Circulation (Suppl) 54:III-107, 1976
3. Murphy ML, Hultgren HN, Detre K et al: Treatment of chronic stable angina: A preliminary report of survival data of the randomized Veterans Administration Cooperative Study. N Engl J Med 297:620, 1977
4. The Veterans Administration Coronary Artery Bypass Surgery Cooperative Study Group: Eleven-year survival in the Veterans' Administration randomized trial of coronary bypass surgery for stable angina. N Engl J Med 311:1333, 1984
5. European Coronary Surgery Study Group: Coronary-artery bypass surgery in stable angina pectoris: Survival at two years. Lancet 1:889, 1979
6. European Coronary Surgery Study Group: Second Interim Report: Prospective randomised study of coronary artery bypass surgery in stable angina pectoris. Lancet 2:491, 1980
7. European Coronary Surgery Study Group: Prospective randomized study of coronary artery bypass surgery in stable angina pectoris: A progress report of survival. Circulation (Suppl II) 65:II-67, 1982
8. Varnauskas E, European Coronary Surgery Study Group: Survival, myocardial infarction, and employment status in a prospective randomized study of coronary bypass surgery. Circulation (Suppl V) 72:V-90, 1985
9. Coronary Artery Surgery Study Principal Investigators and Their Associates: Myocardial infarction and mortality in the Coronary Artery Surgery Study (CASS) randomized trial. N Engl J Med 310:750, 1984
10. Coronary Artery Surgery Study Principal Investigators and Their Associates: Coronary Artery Surgery Study (CASS): A randomized trial of coronary artery bypass surgery. Quality of life in patients randomly assigned to treatment groups. Circulation 68:951, 1983
11. Peduzzi P, Hultgren H, Thomsen J, Detre K: Ten-year effect of medical and surgical therapy on quality of life: Veterans Administration Cooperative Study of Coronary Artery Surgery. Am J Cardiol 59:1017, 1987
12. Killip T, Passamani E, Davis K, the Coronary Artery Surgery Study Principal Investigators and Their Associates: Coronary Artery Surgery Study (CASS): A randomized trial of coronary bypass surgery. Eight year follow-up and survival in patients with reduced ejection fraction. Circulation 72:V-102, 1985
13. Passamani E, Davis K, Gillespie MJ et al: A randomized trial of coronary artery bypass surgery. Survival of patients with a low ejection fraction. N Engl J Med 312:1665, 1985
14. Norris RM, Agnew TM, Brandt PW et al: Coronary surgery after recurrent myocardial infarction: Progress of a trial comparing surgical with nonsurgical management for asymptomatic patients with advanced coronary dis-

ease. Circulation 63:785, 1981
15. Kloster FE, Kremkau EL, Ritzmann LW et al: Coronary bypass for stable angina. A prospective randomized study. N Engl J Med 300:149, 1979
16. National Cooperative Study Group: Unstable angina pectoris: National Cooperative Study Group to compare surgical and medical therapy. In-hospital experience and initial followup results in patients with one, two and three vessel disease. Am J Cardiol 42:839, 1978
17. Luchi RJ, Scott SM, Deupree RH, Principal Investigators and Their Associates of Veterans Administration Cooperative Study No 28: Comparison of medical and surgical treatment for unstable angina pectoris. Results of a Veterans Administration cooperative study. N Engl J Med 316:977, 1987
18. Califf RM, Pryor DB, Greenfield JC Jr: Beyond randomized clinical trials: Applying clinical experience in the treatment of patients with coronary artery disease. Circulation 74:1191, 1986
19. Loop FD: CASS Continued. Circulation (Suppl II) 72:II-1, 1985
20. Kennedy JW, Kaiser GC, Fisher LD et al: Multivariate discriminant analysis of the clinical and angiographic predictors of operative mortality from the Collaborative Study in Coronary Artery Surgery (CASS). J Thorac Cardiovasc Surg 80:876, 1980
21. Kennedy JW, Kaiser GC, Fisher LD et al: Clinical and angiographic predictors of operative mortality from the Collaborative Study in Coronary Artery Surgery (CASS). Circulation 63:793, 1981
22. Douglas JS Jr, King SB, Jones EL et al: Reduced efficacy of coronary bypass surgery in women. Circulation (Suppl II) 64:II-11, 1981
23. Fisher LD, Kennedy JW, Davis KB et al: Association of sex, physical size, and operative mortality after coronary artery bypass in the Coronary Artery Surgery Study (CASS). J Thorac Cardiovasc Surg 84:334, 1982
24. Loop FD, Golding LR, Macmillan JP et al: Coronary artery surgery in women compared with men: Analyses of risks and long-term results. J Am Coll Cardiol 1:383, 1983
25. Myers WO, Davis K, Foster ED et al: Surgical survival in the Coronary Artery Surgery Study (CASS) registry. Ann Thorac Surg 40:246, 1985
26. Ringqvist I, Fisher LD, Mock M et al: Prognostic value of angiographic indices of coronary artery disease from the Coronary Artery Surgery Study (CASS). J Clin Invest 71:1854, 1983
27. Adler DS, Goldman L, O'Neil A et al: Long-term survival of more than 2,000 patients after coronary artery bypass grafting. Am J Cardiol 58:195, 1986
28. Hall RJ, Elayda MA, Gray A et al: Coronary artery bypass: Long-term follow-up of 22,284 consecutive patients. Circulation (Suppl II) 68:II-20, 1983
29. Mock MB, Ringqvist I, Fisher LD et al: Survival of medically treated patients in the Coronary Artery Surgery Study (CASS) registry. Circulation 66:562, 1982
30. Califf RM, Harrell FE Jr, Lee KL et al: The evolution of medical and surgical therapy for coronary artery disease: A 15-year perspective. N Engl J Med (in press)
31. Pryor DB, Harrell FE Jr, Rankin JS et al: The changing survival benefits of coronary revascularization over time. Circulation 76:V-13, 1987
32. Hammermeister KE, DeRouen TA, Dodge HT: Comparison of survival of medically and surgically treated coronary disease patients in Seattle Heart Watch: A nonrandomized study. Circulation (Suppl II) 65:II-53, 1982
33. Hammermeister KE, DeRouen TA, Dodge HT: Evidence from a nonrandomized study that coronary surgery prolongs survival in patients with two-vessel coronary disease. Circulation 59:430, 1979
34. Tyras DH, Kaiser GC, Barner HB et al: Left main equivalent: Results of medical and surgical therapy. Circulation (Suppl II) 64:II-7, 1981
35. Chaitman BR, Davis K, Fisher LD et al: A life table and Cox regressions analysis of patients with combined proximal left anterior descending and proximal left circumflex coronary artery disease: Non-left main equivalent lesions (CASS). Circulation 68:1163, 1983
36. Rahimtoola SH: Left main equivalence is still an unproved hypothesis but proximal left anterior descending coronary artery disease is a "high-risk" lesion. Am J Cardiol 53:1719, 1984
37. Hutter AM Jr: Is there a left main equivalent? Circulation 62:207, 1980
38. Chaitman BR, Davis KB, Kaiser GC et al: The role of coronary bypass surgery for left main equivalent coronary disease: The Coronary Artery Surgery Study Registry. Circulation (Suppl III) 74:17, 1986
39. Selden R, Neill WA, Ritzmann LW et al: Medical versus surgical therapy for acute coronary insufficiency. A randomized study. N Engl J Med 293:1329, 1975
40. McCormick JR, Schick EC Jr, McCabe CH et al: Determinants of operative mortality and long-term survival in patients with unstable angina. J Thorac Cardiovasc Surg 89:683, 1985
41. Rahimtoola SH, Nunley D, Grunkemeier G et al: Ten-year survival after coronary bypass surgery for unstable angina. N Engl J Med 308:676, 1983
42. Waters DD, Walling A, Roy D, Theroux P: Previous coronary artery bypass grafting as an adverse prognostic factor in unstable angina pectoris. Am J Cardiol 58:465, 1986
43. Kaiser GC, Davis KB, Fisher LD et al: Survival following coronary artery bypass grafting in patients with severe angina pectoris (CASS). J Thorac Cardiovasc Surg 89:513, 1985
44. Hammermeister KE, DeRouen TA, Murray JA, Dodge HT: Effect of aortocoronary saphenous vein bypass grafting on death and sudden death. Comparison of nonrandomized medically and surgically treated cohorts with comparable coronary disease and left ventricular function. Am J Cardiol 39:925, 1977
45. Holmes DR, Davis KB, Mock MB et al: The effect of medical and surgical treatment on subsequent sudden cardiac death in patients with coronary artery disease: A report from the Coronary Artery Surgery Study. Circulation 73:1254, 1986
46. Vigilante GJ, Weintraub WS, Klein LW et al: Medical and surgical survival in coronary artery disease in the 1980s. Am J Cardiol 58:926, 1986
47. Gooch JB, Garrett HE, Davis JT Jr, Richardson RL: Coronary artery bypass surgery in the septuagenarian. Texas Heart Institute Journal 10:137, 1983
48. Gersh BJ, Kronmal RA, Frye RL et al: Coronary arteriography and coronary artery bypass surgery: Morbidity and mortality in patients ages 65 or older. A report from the Coronary Artery Surgery Study. Circulation 67:483, 1983
49. Gersh BJ, Kronmal RA, Schaff HV et al: Long-term (5 year) results of coronary bypass surgery in patients 65 years old or older: A report from the Coronary Artery Surgery Study. Circulation (Suppl II) 68:II-190, 1983
50. Gersh BJ, Kronmal RA, Schaff HV et al: Comparison of coronary artery bypass surgery and medical therapy in patients 65 years of age or older. A nonrandomized study from the Coronary Artery Surgery Study (CASS) registry. N Engl J Med 313:217, 1985
51. Rahimtoola SH, Grunkemeier GL, Starr A: Ten year survival after coronary artery bypass surgery for angina in patients aged 65 years and older. Circulation 74:509, 1986
52. Foster ED: Reoperation for coronary artery disease. Circulation (Suppl V) 72:V-59, 1985
53. Foster ED, Fisher LD, Kaiser GC et al: Comparison of operative mortality and morbidity for initial and repeat coronary artery bypass grafting: The Coronary Artery Surgery Study (CASS) registry experience. Ann Thorac Surg 38:563, 1984
54. Rahimtoola SH: A perspective on the three large multicenter randomized clinical trials of coronary bypass surgery for chronic stable angina. Circulation (Suppl V) 72:V-123, 1985
55. Zubiate P, Kay JH, Dunne EF: Myocardial revascularization for patients with an ejection fraction of 0.2 or less. West J Med 140:745, 1984
56. Freeman AP, Walsh WF, Giles RW et al: Early and long-term results of coronary artery bypass grafting with severely depressed left ventricular performance. Am J Cardiol 54:749, 1984
57. Topol EJ, Weiss JL, Guzman PA et al: Immediate improvement of dysfunctional myocardial segments after coronary revascularization: Detection by intraoperative transesophageal echocardiography. J Am Coll Cardiol 4:1123, 1984
58. Kronenberg MW, Pederson RW, Harston WE et al: Left ventricular performance after coronary artery bypass surgery. Prediction of functional benefit. Ann Intern Med 99:305, 1983
59. Waters DD, Pelletier GB, Hache M et al: Myocardial infarction in patients with previous coronary artery bypass surgery. J Am Coll Cardiol 3:909, 1984
60. Crean PA, Waters DD, Bosch X et al: Angiographic findings after myocardial infarction in patients with previous bypass surgery: Explanations for smaller infarcts in this group compared with control patients. Circulation 71:693, 1985
61. DiSesa VJ, O'Neal AC, Bitran D et al: Aggressive surgical management of post-infarction angina: Results of myocardial revascularization early after transmural infarction. Texas Heart Institute Journal 12:333, 1985
62. Singh AK, Rivera R, Cooper GN Jr, Karlson KE: Early myocardial revascularization for postinfarction angina: Results and long-term follow-up. J Am Coll Cardiol 6:1121, 1985
63. Hochberg MS, Parsonnet V, Gielchinsky I et al: Timing of coronary revascularization after acute myocardial infarction. Early and late results in patients revascularized within seven weeks. J Thorac Cardiovasc Surg 88:914, 1984
64. Golding LAR, Loop FD, Hollman JL et al: Early results of emergency surgery after coronary angioplasty. Circulation (Suppl III) 74:III-26, 1986
65. Cowley MJ, Dorros G, Kelsey SF et al: Emergency coronary bypass surgery after coronary angioplasty: The National Heart, Lung and Blood Institute's Percutaneous Transluminal Coronary Angioplasty Registry experience. Am J Cardiol 53:22C, 1984
66. Killen DA, Hamaker WR, Reed WA: Coronary artery bypass following percutaneous transluminal coronary angioplasty. Ann Thorac Surg 40:133, 1985
67. Pelletier LC, Pardini A, Renkin J et al: Myocardial revascularization after failure of percutaneous transluminal coronary angioplasty. J Thorac Cardiovasc Surg 90:265, 1985
68. Weinstein GS, Levin B: The Coronary Artery Surgery Study (CASS). A critical appraisal. J Thorac Cardiovasc Surg 90:541, 1985
69. Anderson RP: Will the real CASS stand up? A review and perspective on the Coronary Artery Surgery Study. J Thorac Cardiovasc Surg 91:698, 1986
70. Kirklin JW, Blackstone EH, Rogers WJ: The plights of the invasive treatment of ischemic heart disease. J Am Coll Cardiol 5:158, 1985
71. Rahimtoola SH: Are the findings from the randomized Coronary Artery Surgery Study (CASS) of value in the management of patients soon after acute myocardial infarction? Am J Cardiol 56:179, 1985
72. Gunnar RM, Loeb HS: An alternative interpretation of the results of the Coronary Artery Surgery Study. Circulation 71:193, 1985
73. Rahimtoola SH: Some unexpected lessons from large multicenter randomized clinical trials. Circulation 72:449, 1985
74. Gunnar RM, Loeb HS: Are the CASS statisticians answering a question no clinician is asking? Am Heart J 111:1016, 1986
75. Editorial: The "overshadowed" CASS report. Clin Cardiol 7:193, 1984

76. Weiner DA, Ryan TJ, McCabe CH et al: The role of exercise testing in identifying patients with improved survival after coronary artery bypass surgery. J Am Coll Cardiol 8:741, 1986
77. Plotnick GD: Coronary artery bypass surgery to prolong life? Less anatomy/more physiology. J Am Coll Cardiol 8:749, 1986
78. Brown KA, Boucher CA, Okada RD et al: The prognostic value of serial exercise thallium-201 imaging in patients presenting for evaluation of chest pain: comparison to contrast angiography, exercise electrocardiography and clinical data (abstr). Am J Cardiol 49:967, 1982
79. Bonow RO, Kent KM, Rosing DR et al: Exercise-induced ischemia in mildly symptomatic patients with coronary artery disease and preserved left ventricular function: Identification of subgroups at risk of death during medical therapy. N Engl J Med 311:1339, 1984
80. Gohlke H, Samek L, Betz P et al: Exercise testing provides additional prognostic information in angiographically defined subgroups of patients with coronary artery disease. Circulation 68:1329, 1983
81. Kaiser GC: CABG 1984: Technical aspects of bypass surgery. Circulation (Suppl V) 72:V-46, 1985
82. Seides SF, Borer JS, Kent KM et al: Long-term anatomic fate of coronary-artery bypass grafts and functional status of patients five years after operation. N Engl J Med 298:1213, 1978
83. Campeau L, Lesperance J, Hermann J et al: Loss of the improvement of angina between 1 and 7 years after aortocoronary bypass surgery. Correlations with changes in vein grafts and in coronary arteries. Circulation (Suppl I) 60:I-1, 1979
84. Spray TL, Roberts WC: Changes in saphenous veins used as aortocoronary bypass grafts. Am Heart J 94:500, 1977
85. Palac RT, Hwang MH, Meadows WR et al: Progression of coronary artery disease in medically and surgically treated patients 5 years after randomization. Circulation (Suppl II) 64:II-17, 1981
86. Palac RT, Meadows WR, Hwang MH et al: Risk factors related to progressive narrowing in aortocoronary vein grafts studied 1 and 5 years after surgery. Circulation (Suppl I) 66:I-40, 1982
87. Campeau L, Enjalbert M, Lesperance J et al: The relation of risk factors to the development of atherosclerosis in saphenous-vein bypass grafts and the progression of disease in the native circulation. A study 10 years after aortocoronary bypass surgery. N Engl J Med 311:1329, 1984
88. Walts AE, Fishbein MC, Sustaita H, Matloff JM: Ruptured atheromatous plaques in saphenous vein coronary artery bypass grafts: A mechanism of acute, thrombotic, late graft occlusion. Circulation 65:197, 1982
89. Gould BL, Clayton PD, Jensen RL, Liddle HV: Association between early graft patency and late outcome for patients undergoing artery bypass graft surgery. Circulation 69:569, 1984
90. Cashin WL, Sanmarco ME, Nessim SA, Blankenhorn DH: Accelerated progression of atherosclerosis in coronary vessels with minimal lesions that are bypassed. N Engl J Med 311:824, 1984
91. Bourassa MG, Campeau L, Lesperance J, Grondin CM: Changes in grafts and coronary arteries after saphenous vein aortocoronary bypass surgery: Results at repeat angiography. Circulation (Suppl II) 65:II-90, 1982
92. Campeau L, Enjalberg M, Lesparance J et al: Atherosclerosis and late closure of aortocoronary saphenous vein grafts: Sequential angiographic studies at 2 weeks, 1 year, 5 to 7 years, and 10 to 12 years after surgery. Circulation (Suppl II) 68:II-1, 1983
93. Bourassa MG, Fisher LD, Campeau L et al: Long-term fate of bypass grafts: The Coronary Artery Surgery Study (CASS) and Montreal Heart Institute experiences. Circulation (Suppl V) 72:V-71, 1985
94. Gohlke H, Gohlke-Barwolf C, Sturzenhofecker P et al: Improved graft patency with anticoagulant therapy after aortocoronary bypass surgery: A prospective, randomized study. Circulation (Suppl II) 64:II-22, 1981
95. Gitler B, Gitler ES: Efficacy of antiplatelet drugs in the maintenance of aortocoronary vein bypass graft patency. Am Heart J 106:563, 1983
96. Chesebro JH, Clements IP, Fuster V et al: A platelet-inhibitor-drug trial in coronary-artery bypass operations. Benefit of perioperative dipyridamole and aspirin therapy on early postoperative vein-graft patency. N Engl J Med 307:73, 1982
97. Chesebro JH, Fuster V, Elveback LR et al: Effect of dipyridamole and aspirin on late vein-graft patency after coronary bypass operations. N Engl J Med 310:209, 1984
98. Goldman S, Copeland J, Noritz T et al: Improvement in early saphenous vein graft patency after coronary artery bypass surgery with antiplatelet therapy. Circulation 77:1324, 1988
99. Blankenhorn DH, Nissim SA, Johnson RL et al: Beneficial effects of combined colestipol-niacin therapy on coronary atherosclerosis and coronary venous bypass grafts. JAMA 257:3233, 1987
100. Passamani ER: Cholesterol reduction in coronary artery bypass patients. JAMA 257:3271, 1987
101. Bashour TT, Hanna ES, Mason DT: Myocardial revascularization with internal mammary artery bypass: An emerging treatment of choice. Am Heart J 111:143, 1986
102. Lewis MR, Dehmer GJ: Coronary bypass using the internal mammary artery. Am J Cardiol 56:480, 1985
103. Siegel W, Loop FD: Comparison of internal mammary artery and saphenous vein bypass grafts for myocardial revascularization. Exercise test and angiographic correlations. Circulation (Suppl III) 54:III-1, 1976
104. Tector AJ, Schmahl TM, Canino VR: The internal mammary artery graft: The best choice for bypass of the diseased left anterior descending coronary artery. Circulation (Suppl II) 68:II-214, 1983
105. Hanna ES, Kabbani SS, Rashour TT et al: Internal mammary coronary artery bypass surgery: Experience with 1000 cases. Texas Heart Institute Journal 10:131, 1983
106. Grondin CM, Campeau L, Lesperance J et al: Comparison of late changes in internal mammary artery and saphenous vein grafts in two consecutive series of patients 10 years after operation. Circulation (Suppl I) 70:I-208, 1984
107. Cameron A, Kemp HG, Green GE: Bypass surgery with the internal mammary artery graft: 15 year follow-up. Circulation (Suppl III) 74:III-30, 1986
108. Lytle BW, Kramer JR, Golding LR et al: Young adults with coronary atherosclerosis: 10 year results of surgical myocardial revascularization. J Am Coll Cardiol 4:445, 1984
109. Lytle BW, Cosgrove DM, Loop FD et al: Perioperative risk of bilateral internal mammary artery grafting: Analysis of 500 cases from 1971 to 1984. Circulation (Suppl III) 74:III-37, 1986
110. Lefrak EA: The internal mammary artery bypass graft: Praise versus practice. Texas Heart Institute Journal 14:139, 1987
111. Olthof H, Middlehof C, Meijne NG et al: The definition of myocardial infarction during aortocoronary bypass surgery. Am Heart J 106:631, 1983
112. Raabe DS, Morise A, Sbrabaro JA, Gundel WD: Diagnostic criteria for acute myocardial infarction in patients undergoing coronary artery bypass surgery. Circulation 62:869, 1980
113. Chaitman BR, Alderman EL, Sheffield LT et al: Use of survival analysis to determine the clinical significance of new Q waves after coronary bypass surgery. Circulation 67:302, 1983
114. Schaff HV, Gersh BJ, Fisher LD et al: Detrimental effect of perioperative myocardial infarction on late survival after coronary artery bypass. J Thorac Cardiovasc Surg 88:972, 1984
115. Namay DL, Hammermeister KE, Zia MS et al: Effect of perioperative myocardial infarction on late survival in patients undergoing coronary artery bypass surgery. Circulation 65:1066, 1982
116. Bulkley BH, Hutchins GM: Myocardial consequences of coronary artery bypass graft surgery. Circulation 56:906, 1977
117. Brindis RG, Brundage BH, Ullyot DJ et al: Graft patency in patients with coronary artery bypass operation complicated by perioperative myocardial infarction. J Am Coll Cardiol 3:55, 1984
118. Kay JH, Zubiate P, Mendez AM, Dunne EF: Myocardial revascularization and mitral repair or replacement for mitral insufficiency due to coronary artery disease. Circulation (Suppl III) 54:III-94, 1976
119. Kay PH, Nunley DL, Grunkemeier GL et al: Late results of combined mitral valve replacement and coronary bypass surgery. J Am Coll Cardiol 5:29, 1985
120. Lytle BW, Cosgrove DM, Gill CC et al: Mitral valve replacement combined with myocardial revascularization: Early and late results for 300 patients, 1970 to 1983. Circulation 71:1179, 1985
121. Richardson JV, Kouchoukos NT, Wright JO, Karp RB: Combined aortic valve replacement and myocardial revascularization: Results in 220 patients. Circulation 59:75, 1979
122. Lytle BW, Cosgrove DM, Loop FD et al: Replacement of aortic valve combined with myocardial revascularization: Determinants of early and late risk for 500 patients, 1967–1981. Circulation 68:1149, 1983
123. Mulany CJ, Elveback LR, Frye RL et al: Coronary artery disease and its management: Influence on survival in patients undergoing aortic valve replacement. J Am Coll Cardiol 10:66, 1987
124. Berkoff HA: Management of coronary artery and peripheral vascular disease combinations: A surgeon's view. Newsletter, Council on Clinical Cardiology 9(4):1, 1983
125. Berkoff HA, Levine RL: Management of the vascular patient with multisystem atherosclerosis. Progress in Cardiovascular Diseases 29:347, 1987
126. Hammermeister KE, DeRouen TA, English MT, Dodge HT: Effect of surgical versus medical therapy on return to work in patients with coronary artery disease. Am J Cardiol 44:105, 1979
127. Johnson WD, Kayser KL, Pedraza PM, Shore RT: Employment patterns in males before and after myocardial revascularization surgery. A study of 2229 consecutive male patients followed for as long as 10 years. Circulation 65:1086, 1982
128. Smith HC, Hammes LN, Gupta S et al: Employment status after coronary artery bypass surgery. Circulation (Suppl II) 65:II-120, 1982
129. Oberman A, Wayne JB, Kouchoukos NT et al: Employment status after coronary artery bypass surgery. Circulation (Suppl II) 65:II-115, 1982
130. Kornfeld DS, Heller SS, Frank KA et al: Psychological and behavioral responses after coronary artery bypass surgery. Circulation (Suppl II) 65:II-24, 1982

THE ROLE OF CARDIAC SURGERY IN THE MANAGEMENT OF ACUTE MYOCARDIAL INFARCTION

Jack M. Matloff ▪ Richard J. Gray

Coronary atherosclerosis in its various manifestations is still the leading cause of death in western society today. Mortality is often due to the occurrence of acute myocardial infarction (AMI) and its sequelae. Historically, the management of AMI has focused on medical therapy. When surgeons became involved, it was to correct mechanical complications (Table 75.1) in an attempt to directly lessen the hemodynamic burden imposed on an already impaired heart and indirectly, to optimize function of residual, noninfarcted myocardium. Primary preservation of myocardial viability by revascularization, either in the infarcted territory or in other jeopardized territories, was not a goal of such therapy.

More recently, cardiac surgeons have become increasingly involved in the dialogue concerning therapy of AMI. The two primary reasons underlying this change have been (1) a dissatisfaction with clinical outcome of classical medical therapy,[1-4] despite significant advances in monitoring and in pharmacologic therapy; and (2) an evolving change in how the morbid anatomy and pathophysiology of AMI are viewed as they affect clinical outcome and therapy thereof.

Early mortality and prognosis following AMI have been defined by a number of studies.[5,6] In the Framingham experience, sudden death and hospital (30-day) mortality for men up to age 79 years was 38%; for women it was 47%. Additionally, three-year and six-year mortalities for survivors were 26% and 38% for men and 40% and 54% for women.[7] The initial year after a first, recognized AMI carried the highest risk: 19% for males. Annual attrition (mortality) rate averaged 5.1%. Clearly, this has not been an acceptable outcome for such a prevalent illness, especially because it affects a relatively young population. This experience has been the stimulus for evolution of more aggressive therapeutic approaches.

Coinciding with this dissatisfaction with conventional medical therapy, there has been an appreciation that AMI is a pleomorphic entity, with variations in location and size as determined by specificity and dominance of the involved coronary artery and the presence or absence of collaterals contributing significantly to immediate outcome and prognosis. Further, the traditional concept of acute coronary thrombosis at the site of an atherosclerotic plaque as the pathophysiologic mechanism that results in infarction has reemerged with new therapeutic significance.[8] Finally, it has become apparent that the temporal occurrence of an AMI is not necessarily instantaneous and complete; rather myocardial infarctions can evolve. Thus, there has emerged an appreciation of the fact that there is a time interval during which the ischemic insult might be partially or completely reversible.[9-12] These considerations have also contributed to the emergence of an increasingly aggressive attitude about medical and/or surgical therapies.

As these more aggressive attitudes have evolved, it has become more difficult to separate purely medical from purely surgical treatment. In this chapter we focus on the surgical aspects of this newer, interventional therapeutic philosophy developed primarily from our clinical experience at Cedars-Sinai Medical Center, and from other experiences, which are extensively cited from the literature.

THE EVOLUTION OF SURGICAL THERAPY IN ACUTE MYOCARDIAL INFARCTION

Coronary artery bypass grafting was initially popularized by Favaloro[13] and Johnson[14] as therapy to alleviate the pain of chronic myocardial ischemia. Subsequently, it was established that proximal coronary obstructions could be effectively bypassed with predictable and acceptable rates of graft patency, relief of angina, and improved function in both ischemic segments[10] and in global ventricular function[15] as expressed by segmental wall motion and the ejection fraction. This improvement in ventricular function was more apparent in patients with acute ischemic syndromes than in those with chronic stable angina.[15,16] These reports were complemented by physiologic studies demonstrating that, where present, biochemical evidence of ischemia was reversible and that coronary reserve could be improved by successful bypass.[17] By using pacing-induced stress, it was further shown that these changes resulted in increased functional capacity as well. Lichtlen and Moccetti and co-workers, using xenon coronary blood flow studies, demonstrated that these effects resulted from increased blood flow to ischemic myocardial segments through patent bypasses.[18] Thus, it became apparent that appropriate bypass graft surgery, in addition to achieving relief of angina, could result in preservation of myocardial viability and function.

Coincident with the demonstration of these physiologic consequences of coronary bypass, debate occurred about what was appropriate therapy for unstable angina and its medically refractory subset, preinfarction angina.[19] Although disagreement often occurred because of semantic considerations, a major point of dispute involved the contrasting results reported by medical centers committed to surgical therapy for this syndrome[20] and those participating in controlled, prospective, randomized, multicenter studies.[21] In deference to their absolute

TABLE 75.1 MECHANICAL COMPLICATIONS OF ACUTE MYOCARDIAL INFARCTION

Mitral regurgitation
   Acute
   Chronic
Ventricular septal defect
Rupture of cardiac free wall
Acute ventricular aneurysm

commitment to report cumulative results, differences between individual centers were not identified, and this precluded recognition of the fact that the techniques of cardiac surgery were not being applied with equal skill and results at all participating institutions. Furthermore, since these studies involved static protocols during an extremely dynamic period in the evolution of techniques, strict adherence to these protocols often obscured rather than clarified the answers to the questions posed by these studies. This was particularly true in regard to the nonuse of specific myocardial protection with hypothermic, hyperkalemic cardioplegic agents,[22] which has probably had a more profound effect on coronary revascularization than any other single technique. Preservation of myocardial biochemical integrity has been and will remain at the core of attempts to treat AMI surgically.

Those committed to surgical therapy were able to establish that patients with acute ischemic syndromes could be successfully revascularized with excellent results, albeit with an increased incidence of perioperative myocardial infarction.[19,20] When surgical therapy was delayed in order to rule out acute infarction before surgery, as in the cooperative studies,[21] then perioperative myocardial infarction rates decreased. Thus *all* "cooling off" studies, by the simple expedient of excluding the preoperative infarctions, resulted in a decreased perioperative infarction rate. This experience helped to define the temporal dimensions of "perioperative infarction." Scrutiny of such patients has indicated that many perioperative infarctions actually occur prior to surgery; thus, in the surgery-committed experiences, patients with acute infarctions, as well as patients with unstable or preinfarction angina, were being operated. Although the operative mortality of these patients was increased significantly (4% versus 0.5% for patients with no perioperative infarction), Gray's long-term follow-up study of patients with perioperative infarctions indicated that the late course of survivors with perioperative infarctions was not statistically different from that of patients undergoing bypass surgery without perioperative myocardial infarction.[23] These experiences suggested that acute infarction, in close temporal juxtaposition to revascularization surgery, carried a different and better prognosis than one might have anticipated. The survival of these patients was also better than that of patients experiencing AMI who were treated conventionally. This historical perspective forms the basis for the evolution of reperfusion by coronary artery bypass grafting as primary surgical therapy in AMI and its complications.

MYOCARDIAL REPERFUSION TO TERMINATE EVOLVING ACUTE MYOCARDIAL INFARCTION
CORONARY BYPASS AS PRIMARY THERAPY OF ACUTE MYOCARDIAL INFARCTION

Early survival and late prognosis following myocardial infarction are significantly influenced by the amount of myocardial necrosis that occurs and its effects on left ventricular function.[1-4,24-26] Traditional medical therapy has not sought to achieve early augmentation or restoration of coronary flow to infarcted myocardium. The importance of reperfusion, initially suggested in surgical experiences,[19,20] has been underscored by experience with thrombolytic therapy. It has been suggested that the benefits of lower mortality, improved ventricular function, and freedom from recurrent ischemic events can most reliably be appreciated by individuals achieving and maintaining complete recanalization with minimum residual coronary stenosis. Aggressive application of coronary artery bypass as primary therapy for AMI is aimed at achieving these same goals, based on the presumption that myocardial necrosis is an evolving process that can be limited by early surgical revascularization.

This pioneering concept emanated from the surgical group in Spokane, Washington, beginning in 1971.[27] In a recent report of their 10-year experience with early surgery in 701 patients,[28] overall operative mortality rate was 5.2% for transmural infarction, and 3% for nontransmural infarction. With follow-up extending a maximum of 10 years, late mortality rate was 12.5% and 6.5%, respectively. While these data are encouraging, certain groups of patients had higher mortality rates. For instance, hospital mortality rate of transmural infarction patients with one-vessel disease was only 2.3%, but this rose to 4.4% and 9% for two- and three-vessel disease. Total late mortality rates with surgery for transmural infarction were 8%, 12%, and 17% for one-, two-, and three-vessel disease, respectively. The timing of surgery relative to onset of symptoms appears to affect outcome in transmural infarction. Patients operated on within six hours of symptoms had a 4% early and 8% total (early and late) mortality rate, compared to those operated on after six hours, who experienced 8% early and 21% total mortality rates.

The other large experience with urgent revascularization of infarctions is from Des Moines.[29] The most recent report of this group describes remarkably good success with 181 patients who were operated on between 1 and 36 hours of the onset of chest pain: an overall mortality rate of 4.4%. In 21 patients referred immediately after failure of intracoronary streptokinase, there were six operative deaths. However, among the remaining 160 patients operated on primarily, there were only two early deaths (1.2%). All early deaths were in patients with preoperative cardiogenic shock. Interestingly, these authors found no correlation with improvement in wall motion, based simply on time interval from onset of symptoms to reperfusion. Rather, they were able to predict wall motion improvements based on preoperative ventriculographic appearance of a trabeculated, normal-appearing endocardial surface.

In addition to relatively low hospital mortality rates, this approach benefits long-term survival as well. DeWood and co-workers[28] report an overall mortality rate of 12.5% after transmural infarction during a 10-year maximum follow-up, and Phillips and co-workers[29] report no late deaths during a maximum follow-up of 6.5 years. Impressive symptomatic benefits from this approach are reported from Alabama where, after a median follow-up of 1½ years, 97% of patients were in New York Heart Association (NYHA) Class I or II, 82% had no angina, and 6% had mild angina. None experienced reinfarction. The 1-year actuarial survival rate was 94%.[30] Although the primary claim for acute surgical therapy has been this reduction of mortality, postoperative hemodynamic and scintigraphic studies indicate significant improvements in ejection fraction,[29,31,32] stroke volume,[29] and reduced left ventricular end-diastolic pressure and volume.[29] The improved long-term results reported are as much an expression of this improved ventricular function as of successful revascularization. Most importantly, in a small group operated on within four hours, infarction size, as estimated by thallium scintigraphy, has been reported to be limited.[32]

While these results are impressive and demonstrate the feasibility of acute surgical reperfusion, they have been obtained at considerable cost of personnel and financial resources. It is apparent that time constraints are also of paramount importance, whether based upon arbitrary time units (four to six hours) or continued clinical signs of evolution. Unfortunately, it is not common that a community and its medical resources can be committed to such a therapeutic effort. In addition, these studies have been criticized as being flawed by severe patient-selection bias and by inclusion of low-risk patients with low-Killip classification status and a high frequency of single vessel disease, and for providing no basis to compare outcome in an equivalent, medically treated group.[33,34] The unoperated course of such patients will probably never be known, since it is unlikely that medical, ethical, and financial considerations will allow for a prospective randomized trial to resolve this uncertainty.

Data are rapidly being accumulated suggesting that urgent reperfusion may be the optimum therapy for AMI in the future. Whether achieved through surgical, chemical (thrombolysis), or mechanical (angioplasty) means, or by combinations of all modalities, it is clear that the result will depend on local experience with each technique, as well as on specific clinical indications. Until more objective data emerge for comparison, the choice of reperfusion versus routine conservative medical management will remain somewhat arbitrary. The published experience of the Iowa Heart Center, where all current techniques of reperfusion are available, is useful. Figure 75.1 illustrates the decision-making process that is followed once evolving myocardial infarction is diagnosed.[29] If the patient exhibits clinical signs of continuing evolution (persistent ischemic pain, emesis, diaphoresis), urgent cardiac catheterization is performed. The specific technique of reperfusion is based on catheterization data. If single-vessel disease is present, thrombolysis with streptokinase is attempted. If clot lysis does not occur or if significant residual stenosis is present, percutaneous transluminal coronary angioplasty (PTCA) is done. If these techniques fail, or if the patient has multivessel disease in addition to the infarction-related occlusion, surgical intervention is carried out immediately.

CORONARY BYPASS AFTER THROMBOLYTIC THERAPY FOR EVOLVING ACUTE MYOCARDIAL INFARCTION

The importance of acute coronary thrombosis at the site of a ruptured atheromatous plaque as the pathophysiologic mechanism underlying AMI has been noted.[8] Using intracoronary or intravenous thrombolytic agents, successful dissolution of acute coronary thrombi has been reported from many medical centers, resulting in less angina, diminished ST segment elevation, and improved ventricular function, all of which suggest preservation of myocardial viability.[35-38] The potential for success with such an approach and the relative simplicity of its application, particularly with intravenous administration, which can be performed in virtually any setting, has resulted in increasing numbers of patients being managed with this technique.

An unresolved but important issue concerns the adjunctive role of coronary bypass after thrombolytic therapy. Potential candidates for early coronary bypass would include the 10% to 40% of patients in whom initial clot dissolution cannot be achieved or those who evidence critical residual stenosis in the occluded vessel, especially where the course has been unstable after successful thrombolysis; those in whom the presence of severe obstructive disease in other vessels not totally occluded accounts for continuing or recurrent post-infarction angina; and those in whom surgically correctable mechanical complications of infarction coexist or appear. With regard to the indications for later surgical revascularization, patients with recurrent occlusion of the infarction-related vessel and those demonstrating evidence of postinfarction, recurrent angina, or evidence of myocardial ischemia should be considered for bypass. In all, between 25% and 40% of patients are candidates for post-thrombolytic surgical revascularization, either acutely or within the first few postinfarction weeks.

The potential risk of excessive postoperative hemorrhage is the major deterrent to such therapy. However, hemorrhage is not a com-

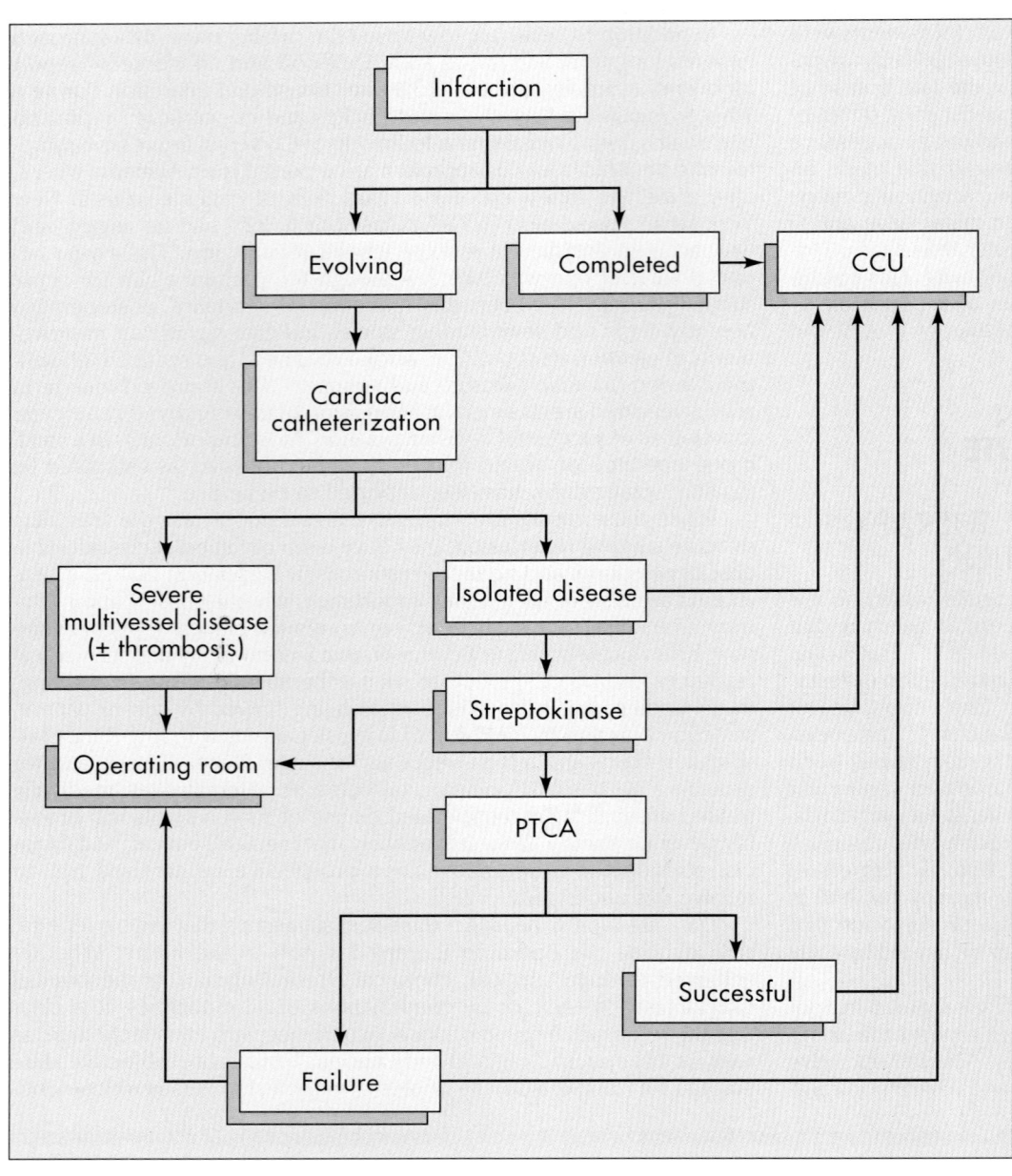

FIGURE 75.1 Schematic diagram for triage of patients. (*CCU*, coronary care unit. *PTCA*, percutaneous transluminal coronary angioplasty.) (Modified from Philips SJ: Emergency coronary artery reperfusion: A choice therapy for evolving myocardial infarction. J Thorac Cardiovasc Surg 86:679, 1983)

plication unless surgery is performed within the first four to six hours after failed thrombolysis. If the operation is performed within this time period, higher than average postoperative blood loss, need for transfusion, and reexploration for continued hemorrhage may be anticipated. Because streptokinase has a short plasma half-life, the risk of serious postoperative bleeding is more closely related to the timing of surgery than to the total dose of thrombolytic agent given.[36] Although it is not always a harbinger of the risk of clinical hemorrhage, ongoing fibrinolysis can be estimated by persistent depression of blood fibrinogen levels preoperatively.

The remaining aspects of early postoperative convalescence after such combined therapy are not remarkable. Several medical centers have reported no operative deaths[37-40] or mortality only in patients with preoperative cardiogenic shock.[35,41] These surgical results are as good as or even slightly better than those obtained when surgery is performed as the primary therapy, in spite of the potential benefit of earlier surgical intervention, especially in patients with less advanced infarction. This suggests that some measure of ischemic relief is afforded even by less than totally successful thrombolytic therapy and that such intervention may in and of itself lessen the subsequent operative risk. Longer term benefits are also apparent in that recurrent ischemic events, the appearance of angina pectoris, and intermediate term mortality are extremely uncommon.

A review of the experience at Cedars-Sinai Medical Center with 157 cases of intracoronary or intravenous streptokinase therapy indicates that 52 patients (35%) have subsequently undergone bypass surgery. Of these operated patients, half of whom had infarctions originating from left coronary occlusions, 92% have been termed "successful reperfusions." Five were operated on within six hours of reperfusion, and 47 were operated on between three days and four months (mean 2 weeks) of reperfusion. Triple-vessel or left main disease was the predominant indication for surgery in this group, although three patients, one of whom died, had single-vessel disease. Nineteen of the patients were operated on because of critical obstructions to noninfarcted myocardial segments, and most had surgery between ten and fourteen days after streptokinase therapy. Nine patients experienced recurrent postinfarction angina and were operated on within the first week after infarction. Five patients, including one with unsuccessful thrombolytic therapy who had a postinfarction ventricular septal defect, were operated on within 24 to 48 hours because of clinical instability, including ventricular tachycardia or fibrillation, congestive heart failure, and/or hypotension.

Overall, 115 vessels were grafted for an average of 3.5 distal anastomoses per patient, somewhat lower than our average of 4.3 per patient in elective cases. In 32 of 33 patients, the left anterior descending artery was involved and was bypassed. There have been two mortalities (6%), one early and one late. The early mortality was a patient with single right coronary artery disease and unsuccessful reperfusion who developed an inferior postinfarction ventricular septal defect. It was not recognized that he had also infarcted his posteromedial papillary muscle. The single late mortality was in a patient who developed constrictive pericarditis, an extremely rare complication of bypass surgery in our experience. There has been a slight increase in postoperative bleeding in these patients, which is difficult to attribute to the specific use of streptokinase owing to its short duration of action.

Although most patients had preoperative enzymatic and electrocardiographic signs of myocardial infarction, inspection of the ventricle at surgery rarely indicated transmural necrosis. This observation may suggest that urgent application of thrombolytic therapy has the potential to prevent the occurrence of a more extensive transmural myocardial infarction. Although preservation of myocardial function in the occluded territory is felt to be a potential goal of therapy, this is difficult to prove unequivocally. Accordingly, at the present time, this therapy should be considered experimental, requiring careful patient selection, adherence to the details of a specific protocol, precise management of data, and comprehensive follow-up.

As the experience from several medical centers indicates, it is feasible and relatively safe to operate in the first hours after thrombolytic therapy. Surgical revascularization early after successful or nonsuccessful thrombolytic therapy may even offer additional benefits to patients with a potential or real risk of recurrent ischemic complications. In other patients who are clinically stable and angiographically not at such risk, semielective surgery may allow for an even better operation. In this context, virtually no group reports use of internal mammary vessels when surgery is undertaken urgently. The benefits of surgery after thrombolytic therapy appear to relate to more complete reperfusion and freedom from postinfarction ischemic events, but the ultimate role of postthrombolytic coronary artery bypass remains to be defined.

REVASCULARIZATION AFTER FAILED PERCUTANEOUS TRANSLUMINAL CORONARY ANGIOPLASTY

Elective PTCA can result in acute ischemic manifestations resulting from coronary dissection, perforation, or complete thrombotic occlusion in 3% to 5% of patients treated.[42] Urgent surgical revascularization remains the treatment of choice in this clinical setting. Failure to cross the lesion or to obtain a satisfactory hemodynamic result (10%–15% of patients in most medical centers) may also be indications for surgical revascularization but usually on a less urgent basis, depending on the original indications for angioplasty.

Recently, several medical centers have begun reporting experience with angioplasty, often in conjunction with thrombolysis, in the setting of acute evolving infarction. Patients referred for urgent surgery after technical failures using this approach, as well as those referred after ischemic complications of elective angioplasty, exhibit the most severe clinical signs of acute ischemic injury. There is a high incidence of severe, unremitting chest pain, electrical instability, hypotension, and cardiac arrest.[43,44] The importance of rapid institution of cardiopulmonary bypass and reperfusion must be emphasized. The use of the intra-aortic balloon, often begun in the catheterization laboratory, is of value if it does not unduly prolong the ischemic interval, as it may reduce the extent of the evolving infarction.[43]

Although rapid surgical correction may account for only a modest increase in postoperative mortality, morbidity remains considerably higher than for elective bypass, owing to ventricular arrhythmias, hypotension, and extended perioperative myocardial infarction.[43] Obviously, these complications are more tolerable if the angioplasty and consequent surgery have been necessitated during therapy initiated for known evolving infarction. At the present time, such experience is only beginning to be accumulated.

SURGICAL REVASCULARIZATION FOR NONMECHANICAL COMPLICATIONS OF ACUTE MYOCARDIAL INFARCTION

A significant but poorly defined number of postinfarction patients experience nonmechanical complications, which have surgical implications.[45] These nonmechanical complications include (1) continuing or recurrent postinfarction angina; (2) postinfarction acute pump failure, with or without congestive heart failure and/or cardiogenic shock; (3) postinfarction ventricular arrhythmias; and (4) postinfarction complete heart block.

POSTINFARCTION ANGINA

Postinfarction anginal pain, often accompanied by electrocardiographic or hemodynamic evidence of unstable myocardial function, is the clinical expression of a pathologic substratum of continuing or threatened extension of AMI or of infarction at a distance. The persistence of ischemic symptoms beyond 6 hours should arouse suspicion and ought to be a major concern when present at 24 hours in spite of conventional medical therapy. The pathologic scenarios include extension of a subendocardial infarction to its full transmural limits, lateral extension of an established transmural myocardial infarction, or reinfarction at a distance as other significantly jeopardized myocardium experiences decreased coronary flow. Therapy must be directed at preserving ischemic but viable tissue, whether in the zone of acute infarction or adjacent to or at a distance from the AMI. This goal can best be accomplished by combined aggressive medical and surgical treatment, applied in a timely fashion to achieve minimal necrosis and maximum salvage of the ischemic zone.

In a six-month postinfarction follow-up study, infarction at a distance was found to be more common (61%) than recurrent ischemia in the infarction zone (39%). While mortality in the entire group was high (56%), it was, unfortunately, even higher (72%) among those with ischemia at a distance.[46] Although occasional patients with postinfarction angina have been identified as experiencing coronary spasm,[47,48] these data confirm that patients with postinfarction angina are not only at high risk but have a high incidence of multivessel atherosclerotic disease, potentially amenable to surgery. In the earliest reports of surgical experience with these patients, when advances in anesthesia, cardioplegia, and postoperative care had not been refined to their present state, operative mortality was as high as 20%.[49-52] While surgical mortality has been reduced more recently, largely through such nontechnical adjunctive advances, the most encouraging new information concerns the potential for excellent long-term survival (85% at five years)[53] and freedom from recurrent late infarction and severe angina.[54] The operative mortality of 1.8% has been reported even in patients operated on within 48 hours of acute infarction.[55] Thus, coronary artery bypass for postinfarction angina has major benefits over conventional therapy alone. This indication, along with acute unstable preinfarction angina, has become the primary indication for revascularization in our institution.

POSTINFARCTION ACUTE PUMP FAILURE

After AMI, congestive heart failure, whether progressing to cardiogenic shock or not, can occur in the absence of a mechanical complication. The pathologic substrate for this occurrence is simply the loss of a large volume (up to 40%) of functioning myocardium. The potential value of coronary bypass in this circumstance rests on the extent to which there is functionally impaired ischemic but viable myocardium that can regain sufficient contractility to improve global ventricular function after revascularization. Pathophysiologically, this can occur in two ways: First, hypocontractile but viable myocardium in the peri-infarction zone has been identified experimentally and may persist in the viable state for an unknown period of time.[9-12,56] Secondly, multivessel disease in patients with AMI suggests that segments remote from the zone of infarction may also be ischemic and at jeopardy. Inadequate perfusion of these segments may be due to or worsened by hypotension associated with loss of functioning myocardium, or additional myocardial ischemia may result from excessive mechanical demands occurring secondarily to sympathetic stimulation of the heart.

If congestive heart failure and/or hypotension do not respond after heart rate and/or rhythm has been stabilized or hypovolemia corrected, then hemodynamic monitoring is essential for characterization to determine subsequent medical therapy. When vasoactive drug management proves ineffective, the patient should be evaluated for intra-aortic balloon counterpulsation. Such therapy is not associated with the metabolic disadvantages of inotropic or pressor drugs and has the potential to unload the myocardium during systole and to increase blood flow to normal and jeopardized myocardial segments during diastole. This approach can stabilize the patient and allow angiography to be performed under more acceptable conditions. Unfortunately, when acute pump failure becomes established, intra-aortic balloon counterpulsation is of temporizing value only, and without eventual revascularization, weaning from the balloon may be expected in only 13% to 24% of patients.[57-61] *The temporizing value of balloon counterpulsation is therefore emphasized.* In the only available controlled trial of counterpulsation, therapy was begun 5 to 14 hours after the onset of pain, and hospital survival was similar (approximately 50%) with either medical therapy or counterpulsation therapy.[62] For best results, it is important to emphasize the need not only for rapid institution of therapy, but also for continued combined medical and balloon counterpulsation therapy.[63-65] The value of such a protocol, followed by urgent bypass, is emphasized by a recent report demonstrating hospital survival rates of 75%, when bypass was completed within 16 hours of onset of symptoms compared to only 28% survival when surgical therapy had been completed more than 18 hours after the onset of symptoms.[66] Two recent reports indicate that the prospects for hospital survival may be even brighter, with 69%[29] and 86%[53] survival rates reported in small groups of patients operated on within hours of infarction with the aid of intra-aortic balloon counterpulsation and modern surgical techniques.

The importance of the details of myocardial preservation in this setting may best be appreciated by only a 9% hospital mortality rate in a small group of cardiogenic shock patients urgently revascularized using glutamate-enriched warm blood cardioplegic induction, with meticulous attention to distribution of cardioplegia during the grafting sequence.[67] What this experience further suggests is that preservation of myocardial viability after infarction may be related more to the conditions of reperfusion than to the time factor to revascularization. If this proposition proves to be true, then we are about to embark on a new era in the treatment of AMI.

POSTINFARCTION RECURRENT VENTRICULAR ARRHYTHMIAS

During the acute phase of infarction, recurrent ventricular arrhythmias are almost never a primary indication for surgical revascularization, but these arrhythmias are often present in patients operated on for other indications. In the subacute or chronic phase of infarction, medically refractory life-threatening ventricular arrhythmia is becoming an ever-increasing indication for surgical intervention using endocardial mapping excision and/or freezing of identified arrhythmogenic foci and coronary artery bypass. The pathophysiology of these arrhythmias has traditionally been thought to be electrical instability arising from juxtaposed areas of normal, ischemic, and infarcted myocardium. While revascularization alone may have the potential to stabilize this situation, experience has indicated that unless the arrhythmia is acute, such a result is not predictable. Best results are obtained in the chronic phase, where there are large areas of scarring and even aneurysm formation. Under these circumstances, resection of the scarred endocardium and/or endocardial freezing, guided by ventricular mapping using programmed stimulation, has been reported to be effective in ablating the arrhythmia.[68-72] However, a blind technique of resection most often fails to prevent sudden arrhythmic deaths.[73,74] Despite improving results for established postinfarction scars, guidelines for the application of such techniques to the period of AMI have not been developed.

THE RESULTS OF SURGICAL THERAPY FOR NONMECHANICAL COMPLICATIONS OF ACUTE INFARCTION

At the Cedars-Sinai Medical Center, the results of myocardial revascularization in patients who were operated on for nonmechanical complications of AMI within 30 days were first reviewed in 1977.[75] Eighty-one patients (mean age 59 years) were operated on over the preceding seven-year period without benefit of specific myocardial preservation, that is, using mild-to-moderate systemic hypothermia without hypothermic, hyperkalemic cardioplegia. The location of the antecedent infarction in these patients was predominantly anterior, in contrast to elective coronary revascularization experience where remote infarctions involved the inferior wall in 67% of postinfarction cases. The temporal distribution of these operations was an almost equal division among the first 24 hours, the 2nd to 14th day, and the 3rd to 4th week. The goal of revascularization at that time was to preserve myocardial viability in other, remote ischemic areas that had not yet infarcted. There was little or no anticipation that infarction size might be reduced. Continuing or recurrent angina was the indication for surgery in 60 of these patients; in 13 patients, life-threatening ventricular arrhythmias, congestive heart failure, and/or cardiogenic shock were the primary indications for study. Following angiography, 8 patients were identified as having critical left main lesions (75% or more diameter reduction), which then became the primary indication for surgery in this group.

Of the 60 patients who were revascularized primarily because of continuing angina indicative of threatened extension, there were four perioperative deaths (6.6% mortality). Two of these deaths were due to noncardiac causes; therefore, the cardiac-related mortality was 3.3%. This initial experience with early revascularization was more encouraging than had been anticipated, and along with the advent of hypothermic hyperkalemic cardioplegia, it has resulted in our having a lower threshhold for considering surgery in such patients. There is now closer early scrutiny of postinfarction patients, and this clinical setting is becoming one of the most common indications for coronary revascularization.

Of the 21 patients who were revascularized for reasons other than angina, eight were in congestive heart failure and/or cardiogenic shock at the time of surgery; none was treated with an intra-aortic balloon, and four (19%) died. Thus, the overall hospital mortality in these 81 cases was 10% (8/81), but cardiac-related mortality was 7% (6/81).

When the mortalities were examined in relation to the timing of the surgery after AMI, mortality of patients operated on within 24 hours was 14%; this high mortality was a reflection of the more serious nature of the complication (*i.e.*, cardiogenic shock) that occurred early and required urgent surgery. From days 2 to 14 there were also four mortalities (14%); however, two of the four deaths occurred in patients who experienced a second acute infarction during this time and prior to surgery. Thus, mortality from 8 to 30 days was 5%, and no deaths occurred when surgery was undertaken from 14 to 30 days.

On late follow-up there were three additional deaths, one of which was due to recurrent ischemia. Actuarial survival was 86% at three years. These results were surprisingly good as compared to the Framingham Study,[7] in which 30-day mortality after AMI for patients up to age 79 (similar to our patients) was 38%. The long-term results also exceed those for patients in the Framingham Study, where three-year probability of survival was 74% for men and 60% for women.

To place these data in a more contemporary context, it would seem that concern about revascularizing patients within 30 days of AMI is no longer appropriate. Ventricular function is a more powerful determinant of survival, irrespective of the interval between AMI and surgery.[76] Based on the foregoing, one is encouraged to stabilize and temporize, when possible, to a time beyond one week, but if this is not possible, then surgical therapy within the first month does not carry a prohibitive mortality.

In the past several years, medical capability has advanced significantly, so that the ability to diagnose, stabilize, and temporize patients is markedly better. Major improvements in diagnosis of complications and determination of prognosis have resulted through electrocardiographic ST segment mapping, two-dimensional echocardiography, and Doppler ultrasound, noninvasive radionuclide imaging, and invasive hemodynamic monitoring. It is now apparent that the time has come when we should be capable of reducing postinfarction mortality, particularly during the high-risk period of the first 6 to 12 months. While definition of high-risk patient subsets and improved medical therapy have helped, we believe that a more profound effect on the natural history of infarction will occur from earlier application of techniques of myocardial reperfusion.

SURGICAL MANAGEMENT AFTER UNCOMPLICATED ACUTE MYOCARDIAL INFARCTION

To this point, we have focused on surgical therapy in relation to the acute event. In clinical practice at this time, such patients represent a minority of the acute infarction patients seen; the majority of survivors can be classified as being minimally symptomatic or asymptomatic. However, the diagnostic and therapeutic approach to the minimally symptomatic or asymptomatic hospital survivor of an uncomplicated myocardial infarction is extremely diverse. Cardiac death within the first year after infarction is between 10% to 20%, with the highest mortality occurring in subsets of patients with left main or multivessel disease and left ventricular ejection fraction below 50%. A recent prospective survey indicates that 40% of infarction survivors may have left main or three-vessel disease.[77] While these findings help to identify patients who could significantly benefit from elective myocardial revascularization, it is unfortunate that many such patients are not recognizable solely on the basis of symptoms and/or physical findings. Noninvasive evaluation of left ventricular function and treadmill testing have been advocated to identify, more objectively, individuals who are candidates for coronary angiography and possible angioplasty or bypass.[78]

The recently conducted Coronary Artery Surgery Study (CASS) addressed this issue by entering patients who were asymptomatic after recent infarction. Of the entire cohort of *nonrandomized* patients with three-vessel disease who were operated on, long-term survival rate was 88%, versus 63% for those treated by medical therapy.[79] In the *randomized* cohort, of those with three-vessel disease and ejection fraction below 50%, the surgical group also had long-term survival rates superior to those treated by medical therapy (84% versus 70%).[80] These data substantiated those from a previous, nonrandomized study showing improved survival with surgery, regardless of the degree of coronary involvement, in patients whose ejection fraction was between 25% and 50%.[81] Clearly then, there are good data to substantiate the recommendation that post-AMI patients with multiple-vessel disease and abnormal ventricular function be considered for revascularization, regardless of symptomatic status.

With regard to survival, quantification of the degree of viable but jeopardized myocardium is extremely important in predicting future ischemic events. In a recent *nonrandomized* retrospective comparison of medical and surgical management of patients after infarction,[82] the presence of large numbers of jeopardized myocardial segments (4 to 10) defined a group of patients with significantly improved survival rates after surgery. Jeopardized segments were defined as those ventriculographic segments exhibiting some degree of inward systolic wall motion and supplied by a coronary vessel with 70% or greater stenosis. In another *randomized* study to compare medical and surgical therapy, there was no advantage in either approach, with an enviably low annual mortality rate of 3% to 4% for both groups.[83] However, this benign outcome could have been anticipated since patients with well-preserved left ventricular function were enrolled into both groups. These two different types of studies once again confirm the importance of left ventricular function as the predominant predictor of long-term outcome in coronary disease.

If surgery is to be undertaken, its timing in relation to infarction must be considered. Although operative mortality is definitely higher in patients operated on within the first 7 to 10 days, the indications compelling early surgery, that is, acute pump failure and postinfarction angina, and the status of ventricular function are much more important determinants than timing alone. In a recently reported large series of patients, no operative deaths occurred within seven weeks of infarction when ejection fraction was greater than 50%. When ejection fraction was less than 50%, operative survival was much better if surgery could be delayed between three and four weeks after infarction (Fig. 75.2).[84] Based upon these observations, when a completely elective surgery is contemplated in patients with reduced ejection fraction, it would seem prudent to wait until three to four weeks after infarction.

From the foregoing it should be apparent that angiography and possible elective bypass definitely should be considered for the patient with early, postinfarction angina, for the asymptomatic patient with laboratory evidence of significant degrees of jeopardized myocardium, and/or for the patient with diminished left ventricular ejection fraction. Thus, the asymptomatic postinfarction patient *ought to be subjected to some form of screening process* to detect possible significant residual myocardial ischemia. At present, the treadmill test offers advantages because of its low cost and relative safety, and it should become one of the most commonly performed postinfarction studies. While treadmill testing does provide certain prognostic information when highly positive (more than 2 mm ST depression at low exercise levels, inadequate blood pressure response to exercise, and inability to complete the heart rate goal for any reason), it lacks the ability to quantitate ischemic myocardium and suffers from imperfect test sensitivity. Thallium scintigraphy and radionuclide wall motion imaging address some of these shortcomings but are much more expensive and not universally available. When available, they should probably be reserved to answer specific clinical questions, such as the confirmation of equivocal treadmill test responses.

In any event, the course and prognosis after AMI is so well defined that postinfarction patients, especially in younger age categories, should be screened and stratified to assess their candidacy for invasive therapy, which has the potential to improve their prognosis by reducing future ischemic events.

SURGICAL CORRECTION OF THE MECHANICAL COMPLICATIONS OF ACUTE MYOCARDIAL INFARCTION

The pathologic process after AMI includes a period during which macrophages clear the necrotic muscle; at this time, the process of connective tissue ingrowth is not advanced enough to give strength to the infarcted area. These simultaneous reparative processes occur from four to eight days after AMI. It is at this time that necrosis and softening of myocardium[85] and "elasticity" of the infarcted segments is maximal, and disruption of various segments of affected left ventricle may occur. Following disruption, depending on the location of the infarction, one of three mechanical complications can occur: (1) mitral regurgitation; (2) rupture of the ventricular septum; and (3) rupture of the free wall. If disruption does not occur, increased elasticity of the involved segment can result in acute left ventricular aneurysm formation. While the pathophysiologic consequences of each of these mechanical defects is different, each results in the profound hemodynamic liability, often with cardiogenic shock, that is associated with increased mortality. Historically, the grave prognosis with any form of medical therapy has been and continues to be the reason why surgical therapy is the primary consideration in the management of these complications.

MITRAL REGURGITATION AND CORONARY ARTERY DISEASE

Mitral regurgitation may coexist with coronary artery disease as separate pathologic entities or as an etiologically related entity. The prognosis in the latter situation is very different from and not as good as that for coexisting valvular and coronary disease.[86] Further comments will be limited to the treatment of mitral regurgitation etiologically related to coronary atherosclerosis.

Ischemic heart disease may be associated with mitral regurgitation in several ways (Table 75.2). Dilatation of the mitral annulus is not well documented in the acute setting but is seen more often with chronic myocardial ischemia and repeated infarction. These patients have what is essentially a chronic ischemic cardiomyopathy. Mitral regurgitation resulting from annular dilatation almost always requires correction with a ring annuloplasty or mitral valve replacement performed during the course of coronary bypass.

Papillary muscle dysfunction can occur in the presence of a normally competent mitral valve with episodic, reversible ischemia resulting in severe, transient, acute mitral regurgitation and pulmonary edema.[87] Alternately, left ventricular wall motion abnormalities can distort the spatial relationships of intrinsically normal papillary muscles and mitral leaflets within the left ventricular cavity, resulting in mitral regurgitation.[88] While papillary muscle dysfunction can occur without myocardial infarction,[87] our experience and that reported in the literature indicate that most of these patients do, in fact, have some degree of infarction of the papillary muscle and the adjacent myocardium.[89] This observation is consistent with studies that show that experimental, isolated, papillary muscle infarction without infarction of adjacent myocardium does not produce mitral regurgitation.[90] These experi-

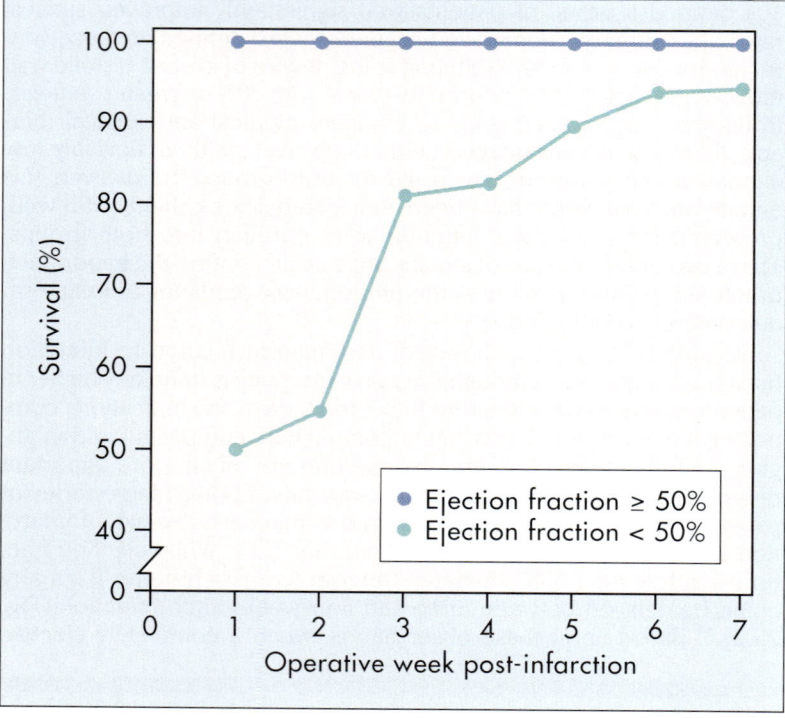

FIGURE 75.2 Survival after revascularization in 174 patients with recent myocardial infarction. The patients are divided according to their preoperative ejection fraction. Each *point* on the curve represents the cohort of patients operated upon during a particular week after myocardial infarction. (Modified from Hochberg MS, Parsonnet V, Gielchinsky I et al: Timing of coronary revascularization after acute myocardial infarction. J Thorac Cardiovasc Surg 88:914, 1984)

mental and clinical studies show that papillary muscle necrosis must be combined with a localized area of ventricular dysfunction, such as occurs in AMI, to cause regurgitation. Clinically, the existence of papillary muscle dysfunction as a mechanism of mitral regurgitation in AMI is a problematic entity since it is not always clear what the pathophysiologic mechanism is and therefore how the mitral valve should be managed. Further, mitral regurgitation during AMI may be silent and only be appreciated by specific studies.[91] Each case has to be evaluated individually, based on preoperative symptomatic status, physical findings, angiography, hemodynamics, and intraoperative observations, which most recently include Doppler color flow echocardiography. In patients operated on in relation to AMI, every attempt should be made to repair the valve by annuloplasty. However, the most significant problems have occurred in patients in whom the degree and importance of the mitral regurgitation have not been appropriately assessed or in whom appropriate correction of the mitral regurgitation was not achieved by the procedure chosen. In this respect, mitral valve replacement may result in a more predictable outcome than mitral valve repair. Coronary revascularization is always carried out as an integral part of the procedure.

While mitral regurgitation resulting from papillary muscle dysfunction in acute myocardial infarction may present a therapeutic dilemma in regard to what needs to be done and what therapy should be applied, rupture of the papillary muscle presents an equally problematic situation because of the severity of the infarction and ensuing hemodynamic instability. Papillary muscle rupture is a rare complication, estimated to be responsible for approximately 1% of all infarction deaths.[92] The posteromedial papillary muscle, which receives a single blood supply from the right coronary artery, is more commonly involved than the anterolateral papillary muscle, which receives a dual blood supply from the right and circumflex coronary arteries. It is commonly taught that papillary muscle rupture occurs most often after a first infarction where there is inadequate collateral circulation. In practice, most patients have multivessel disease, and mitral regurgitation is most often seen in the setting of a remote right or circumflex occlusion with infarction and a second acute infarction involving the reciprocal vessel. Since inferior or posterior (lateral) wall infarctions are usually not large enough to cause refractory heart failure or cardiogenic shock, papillary muscle rupture should be suspected in these cases, even in the absence of a systolic murmur.[93] Partial rupture of a papillary muscle head or rupture of the chordae to an area of papillary muscle infarction can also occur. The clinical consequences of these pathologic entities are much less severe than rupture of the entire papillary muscle; the former can be seen as a subacute and even chronic postinfarction problem, whereas the latter carries an immediate mortality of 33% and a 24-hour mortality of 50%. Unoperated, one week mortality is 80%, and only 7% are two-month survivors.[94] Papillary muscle involvement also may occur in association with a postinfarction ventricular septal defect and should always be anticipated in this setting. The diagnosis can be *suggested* by bedside insertion of a pulmonary artery flotation catheter and documentation of significant v waves in the pulmonary artery occluded tracing in the presence of a step-up in oxygen saturation at the level of the right ventricle or main pulmonary artery. However, augmented v waves can occur in the absence of mitral regurgitation, and echo Doppler evaluation is recommended.

Medical therapy should be instituted before confirming the diagnosis, since most of these patients are in cardiogenic shock. The effects of medical management may be limited, since profound systemic hypotension often precludes vasodilator therapy, while vasoconstrictor drugs that increase afterload have the potential to worsen the mitral regurgitation. Certainly when medical therapy is not effective, and perhaps in all instances, percutaneous insertion of an intra-aortic balloon is indicated. If the patient can be stabilized, catheterization and angiography can be performed in a semielective setting. While the timing of mitral valve replacement and coronary artery bypass may be dictated by the response to intra-aortic balloon pumping, it is always necessary in our experience, usually earlier than later.

The results of surgery for AMI complicated by mitral regurgitation leave much to be desired. Currently, isolated mitral valve replacement surgery, for all NYHA classes, is associated with a one-month mortality of 4%. For mitral valve replacement in patients with ischemic mitral regurgitation, triple-vessel disease (Fig. 75.3), and Class IV NYHA classification (Fig. 75.4), operative mortality is 18%. When preoperative left ventricular ejection fraction is below 35% (Fig. 75.5), early mortality is 13%, and when preoperative intra-aortic balloon pumping is necessary (Fig. 75.6), operative mortality increases to 32%. Four-year survival for triple-vessel or left main disease with ejection fraction of less than 50% is 40%, while four-year survival after use of an intra-aortic balloon pump is approximately 20%. In this experience, the use of an intra-aortic balloon pump was the most powerful predictor ($P = 0.001$) of early and late outcome.[95]

The severe pathophysiologic changes that account for this dismal outlook in treating acute mitral regurgitation after AMI are due to a variable but significant loss of left ventricular free wall, interventricular septum, and/or right ventricular free wall; an increase in end-diastolic volume and left ventricular wall tension, with resultant increases in preload and oxygen consumption; an increase in adrenergic activity, with increased heart rate reducing the ejection time and increasing afterload, both responses aggravating the degree of mitral regurgitation; and, finally, free mitral regurgitation into a normal-sized and compliant left atrium, resulting in pulmonary venous hypertension, pulmonary edema, and pulmonary hypertension. Virtually no combination of medical and/or surgical therapy is capable of correcting all elements of this downward pathophysiologic spiral. Thus the issue here is not how good or bad medical and/or surgical therapy are after the fact, but rather, how these patients can be identified before the fact in an attempt to prevent AMI with mitral regurgitation, either by appropriately performed coronary angioplasty or by bypass graft surgery.

POSTINFARCTION VENTRICULAR SEPTAL DEFECT

Postinfarction rupture of the interventricular septum is estimated to complicate from 0.5% to 2% of AMI and accounts for 5% of all postinfarction deaths.[96] Two morphologic types have been described: an inferior basal defect with dominant right coronary (or dominant circumflex posterior descending) artery occlusion and inferior septal infarction; and a midapical-to-anterior defect with left anterior descending occlusion and anteroseptal infarction. Prognostically, the former carries a higher risk of mortality, especially if the mitral valve is involved. An important factor in the pathogenesis of septal rupture is a pattern of coronary disease, where possible collateral flow to the ischemic septal zone is inhibited by significant obstructions in major reciprocal coronary arteries.[97]

Pathophysiologically, perforation of the ventricular septum exposes the unprepared, possibly infarcted right ventricle to left-sided pressures, resulting in right ventricular dysfunction. If infarcted, the

TABLE 75.2 ASSOCIATION OF ISCHEMIC HEART DISEASE AND MITRAL REGURGITATION

Papillary muscle dysfunction
  Ischemia
  Infarction
    Papillary muscle tip
    Adjacent free wall
Papillary muscle rupture
  Tip
  Head
Chordae tendineae rupture
Mitral annulus dilatation
Ischemic cardiomyopathy
Nonischemic mitral valve disease (*e.g.*, rheumatic)

right ventricle is unable to sustain the level of pulmonary blood flow needed for systemic cardiac output, resulting in cardiogenic shock.[98] In addition, the large flow across the ventricular septal defect results in an acute decrease in left ventricular forward flow, imposing a significant volume overload on a left ventricle already damaged by a recent large myocardial infarction. The septal defect cannot decrease in size during systole as the septal margins are infarcted and akinetic. Frequently, shunting continues during diastole as left ventricular end-diastolic pressures exceed those in the right ventricle.[96] The diagnosis can be made rapidly by right heart catheterization with a pulmonary artery flotation catheter and the determination of a pulmonary-to-systemic flow ratio that is usually more than 2:1 and sequential oximetry showing a blood oxygen increase at the right ventricular level.[99] Two-dimensional echocardiography, negative contrast echocardiography,[100] Doppler echocardiography,[101] and radionuclide techniques[102] can also establish the existence of a left-to-right shunt noninvasively. Although not absolutely necessary for definitive diagnosis, catheterization and angiography should be carried out to establish the pattern of coronary

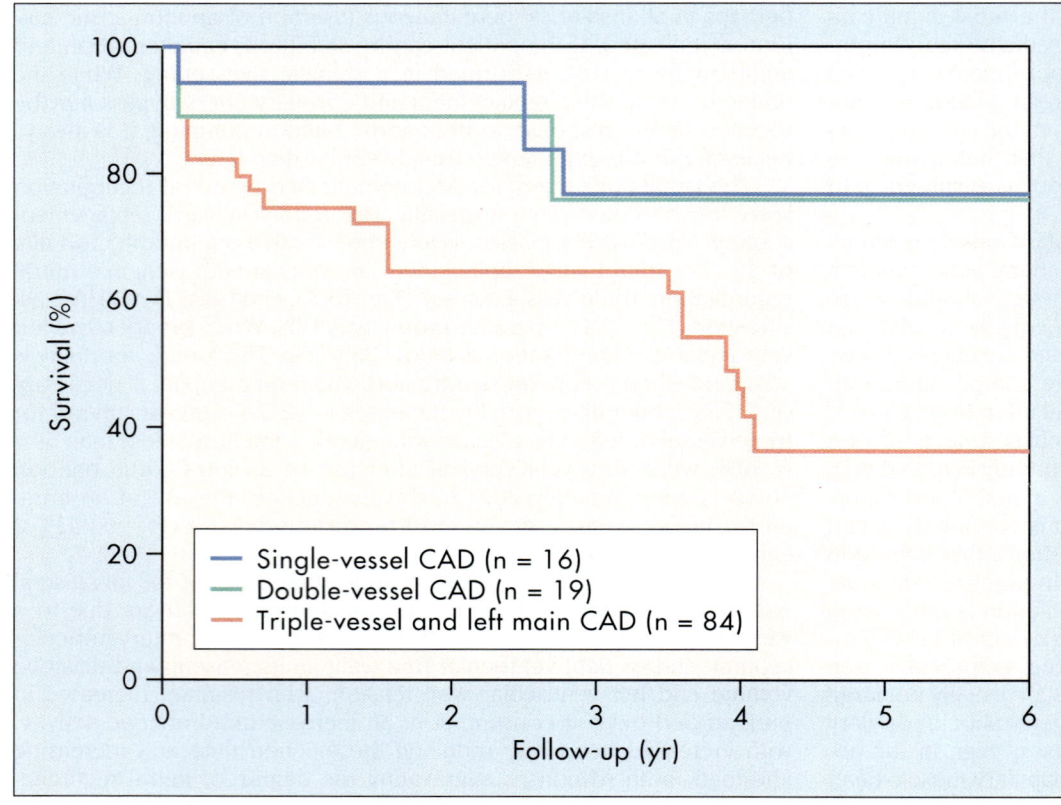

FIGURE 75.3 Survival rates by coronary artery disease (CAD) severity in patients with mitral valve replacement and coronary artery bypass grafting. Patients with triple-vessel or left main CAD had a much lower survival rate than those with single- or double-vessel CAD ($P < 0.05$). (Modified from Czer LSC, Matloff JM, Gray RJ, Chaux A: Mitral valve replacement with coronary artery disease. Duran C, Angell WW, Johnson AD, Oury JH (eds): Recent Progress in Mitral Valve Disease. London, Butterworth, 1984)

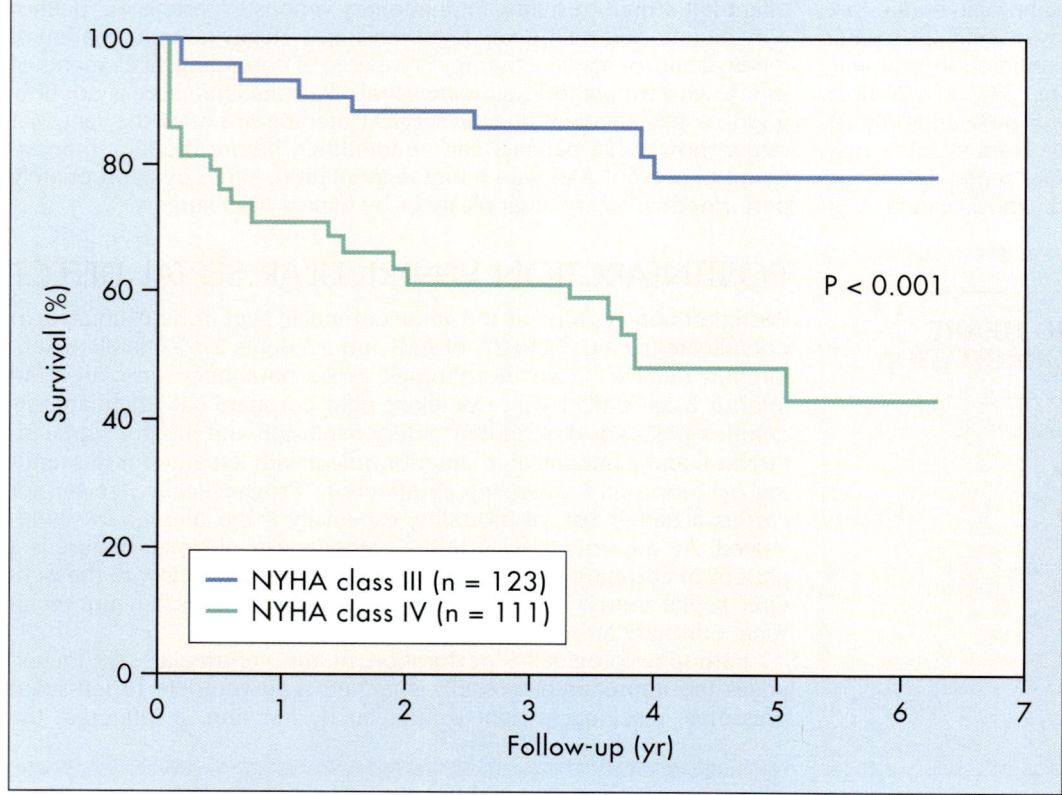

FIGURE 75.4 Survival following mitral valve replacement, stratified by preoperative NYHA class. (Modified from Czer LSC, Matloff JM, Gray RJ, Chaux A: Mitral valve replacement with coronary artery disease. Duran C, Angell WW, Johnson AD, Oury JH (eds): Recent Progress in Mitral Valve Disease. London, Butterworth, 1984)

disease and to determine whether there is coincident mitral regurgitation.

The natural history is an ominous one, with a 24-hour mortality of 24%, a one-week mortality of 46%, and a two-month mortality varying from 67% to 82%.[103,104] One-year survival rates approximate 5% to 7%. Medical management of ventricular septal rupture also has serious limitations because afterload reduction with vasodilators may be precluded by severe hypotension, and inotropic or vasoconstrictor drugs may increase myocardial oxygen consumption and increase left-to-right shunting. In the past, the presence of cardiogenic shock has largely determined outcome. Despite therapy, including surgery, patients with cardiogenic shock have experienced a 73% early mortality compared to an 18% mortality in patients with severe congestive heart failure without cardiogenic shock.[98] Notwithstanding, patients treated with optimal medical therapy experienced a 100% mortality in the series of Radford[98] and Montoya and their co-workers.[105] Immediate introduction of an intra-aortic balloon pump can decrease pulmonary capillary wedge pressure with reduction of the systemic-to-pulmonary

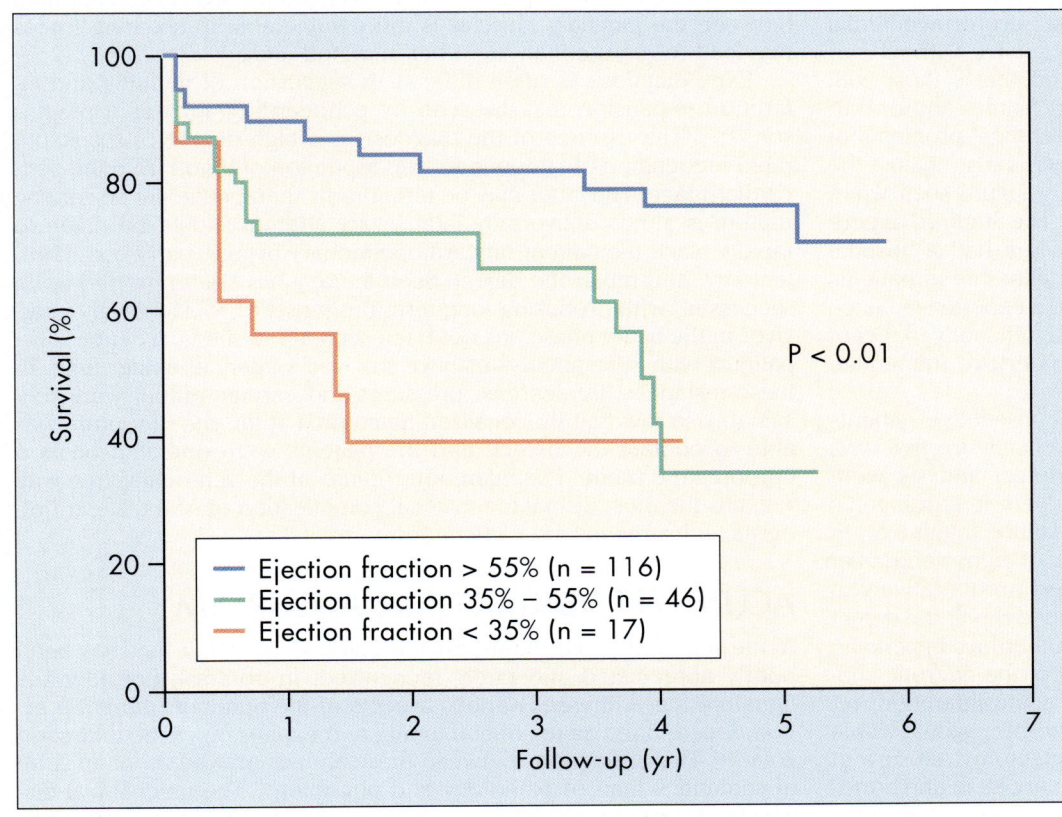

FIGURE 75.5 Effect of preoperative left ventricular ejection fraction on survival following mitral valve replacement. (Modified from Czer LSC, Matloff JM, Gray RJ, Chaux A: Mitral valve replacement with coronary artery disease. Duran C, Angell WW, Johnson AD, Oury JH (eds): Recent Progress in Mitral Valve Disease. London, Butterworth, 1984)

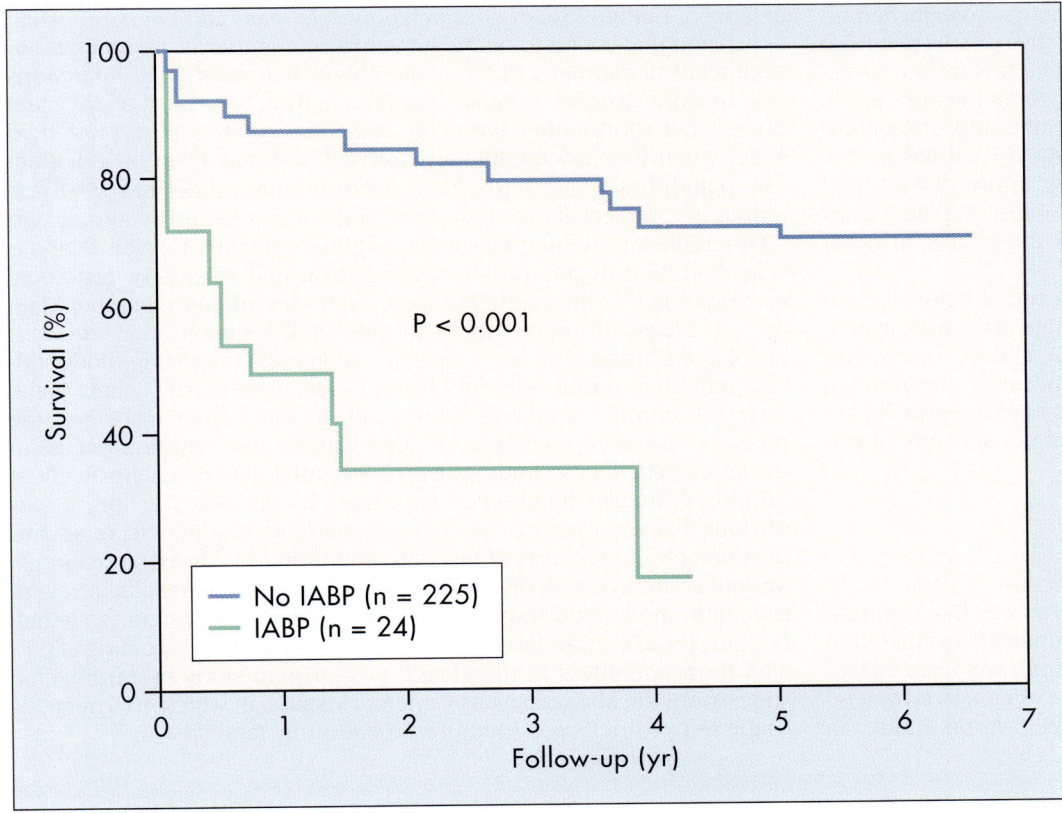

FIGURE 75.6 Survival following mitral valve replacement, stratified by use of the intra-aortic balloon pump (IABP) preoperatively or intraoperatively. (Modified from Czer LSC, Matloff JM, Gray RJ, Chaux A: Mitral valve replacement with coronary artery disease. Duran C, Angell WW, Johnson AD, Oury JH (eds): Recent Progress in Mitral Valve Disease. London, Butterworth, 1984)

flow ratio.[106] However, any period of hemodynamic stability achieved may be transient, and patients thought to be hemodynamically stable can suddenly deteriorate and die.[105]

Surgery for repair of postinfarction ventricular septal defects was initiated by Cooley,[107] and by the early 1970s, survival was improved to 32% at one year.[108] Coronary artery bypass was not a part of these operations. Mortality was prohibitive when patients were operated on within the first two weeks of the onset of the ventricular septal defect, leading to a recommendation that surgery be delayed, ideally, for three to six weeks, or until the reparative process was advanced enough so that the margins of the defect were fibrosed and more readily amenable to surgery. Unfortunately, such management selects out for surgery the best candidates, that is, those with the least severe myocardial dysfunction and, therefore, those most likely to survive without surgery. It also discriminates against those most in need, that is, those with severe biventricular dysfunction, congestive heart failure, and/or cardiogenic shock.[98] Thus one has to balance the technical problems of surgery involving nonhealing infarcted tissues, seen early, against the advanced cardiac, renal, cerebral, and pulmonary failure seen when surgery is delayed to allow some fibrosis to occur. The Stanford experience has shown that patients with end-organ failure had a hospital mortality rate of 77%, compared with a 22% mortality rate in patients without end-organ failure,[109] reconfirming Radford's experience. Since options for surgical management have improved significantly in recent years, a more current recommendation is to undertake immediate surgery.

In our recent experience, of the first eight consecutive patients operated on "early,"[110] two had been treated medically for five days after the occurrence of the ventricular septal defect and six were operated on within 18 hours. Preoperatively, six were in cardiogenic shock, five were obtunded, and two were in renal failure. In this experience, shock was related primarily to the extent of right ventricular involvement. An intra-aortic balloon was inserted preoperatively in seven. Six had anterior defects. The technique used to repair the defect involved generalized hypothermia to 23°C; hypothermic, hyperkalemic cardioplegia to 18°C; radical resection of all of the necrotic septum through a ventriculotomy at the site of the acute infarction; replacement of the septum with a patch folded over the residual viable rim of septum; left and/or right ventricular infarctectomy; closure of the residual, viable ventricular free walls to the septal patch; and aortocoronary saphenous vein bypass grafting where indicated. Six patients received an average of 2.2 grafts each. There were two hospital and no late deaths at three years follow-up. The two operative deaths occurred 36 hours and six days after surgery, respectively, the first from a supraventricular arrhythmia in a 72-year-old woman in whom the intra-aortic balloon had to be removed prematurely because of compromised circulation to her leg, and the second from continuing low cardiac output in a 56-year-old male with single right coronary artery disease and unrecognized involvement of the posteromedial mitral papillary muscle. This 75% survival compares favorably with the results of other reported cases of early surgical therapy.[105,107-109,111]

At the present time, postinfarction ventricular septal defect should constitute a surgical emergency in which immediate diagnosis, institution of medical therapy, insertion of an intra-aortic balloon pump, cardiac catheterization and angiography, and radical surgical correction of the defect with bypass of other involved vessels have the potential to improve the two-month mortality rate of 75% that occurs without surgical therapy.

POSTINFARCTION RUPTURE OF THE VENTRICULAR FREE WALL

Postinfarction rupture of the left ventricular free wall was first reported in 1647 by William Harvey.[112] Currently, cardiac rupture is estimated to complicate 1.5% to 8% of AMI and is responsible for from 5% to 24% of infarction deaths.[113] A higher incidence of rupture occurs in advanced age, in female patients, and in the presence of hypertension during the acute phase of infarction. There is an uncertain relation to chronic hypertension, the administration of anticoagulants, and level of activity. The peak incidence (54%), as with other mechanical defects, occurs from two to eight days after AMI. Severe coronary atherosclerosis, usually with total occlusion of a major vessel and no collateral circulation, is the pathologic substrate. Although 50% of transmural posterior infarctions extend into the right ventricle, rupture of the right ventricle is rare.[114] The most common site of rupture is at the junction of the infarcted and healthy tissue, the decreased tensile strength generated at this site being considered an important pathogenic factor. The greater incidence of rupture through the left lateral wall, relative to the smaller incidence of infarction in this region, suggests that this area between the papillary muscles is more vulnerable to shearing forces that lead to rupture than are other infarcted areas.[115]

Early diagnosis is often difficult. A suggestion of thinning and infarction expansion may be seen by echocardiography as a precursor.[116,117] The essence of the diagnosis is a high degree of suspicion, rapid recognition of tamponade, and aspiration of blood from the pericardial space. The latter may be temporarily therapeutic. Since cardiac rupture is almost universally fatal, every attempt should be made to rapidly place the patient on cardiopulmonary bypass, carry out infarctectomy, and repair the defect. Such therapy has been reported to be successful, with promising long-term prognosis.[118-121] However, a survivor in the acute phase has not been seen at our medical center. Five patients with false aneurysms have survived surgery at a later time. In these instances, intracardiac pressures and cardiac output were presumably so low that the localized hematoma at the site of rupture was able to contain the defect, and the patients were operated on in a chronic time frame. Postinfarction rupture of the ventricular free wall remains the most dismal mechanical complication of AMI that cardiologists and surgeons are called upon to treat.

ACUTE LEFT VENTRICULAR ANEURYSM

Acute left ventricular aneurysm formation is an entity that has been poorly appreciated and rarely recognized. In contrast, considerable literature has addressed various aspects of the entity of *infarction expansion,* defined as regional thinning and expansion of the infarction zone.[116] The distinctions between these entities may be more an issue of semantics than of pathology and physiology. The mechanical disadvantages of chronic left ventricular aneurysms have been well characterized, but the loss of contractile muscle mass and the paradoxical expansion that is said to occur with chronic aneurysms are much more significant phenomena in the acute phase. Left ventricular infarctions may be conceived as forming a continuum from their most elastic state during and shortly after the acute ischemic insult to their most rigid state, when they are completely fibrosed and may even be calcified. The pathophysiologic basis for this conceptual model has been explored in a clinical study of infarcted segments resected at surgery and characterized as to their elasticity or stiffness (length–tension relationship) and their degree of muscular necrosis and fibrosis by histologic examination.[122] Three different responses were identified and characterized, based on the acuity of the resected segment and degree of histologic fibrosis. The acute necrotic segments, consisting of identifiable infarcted muscle without fibrous tissue, were elastic, whereas the fibrosed, chronic segments were rigid. In the former instance, true paradox can occur, whereas stenting without true paradox occurs in the latter. When these findings were extrapolated to calculate an effect on left ventricular function as expressed by ejection fraction, it was obvious that aneurysms of varying sizes had different effects, related to the character or stiffness of the wall. According to this extrapolation, a muscular aneurysm involving 20% of the left ventricle results in severe reduction in ejection fraction, and 30% to 40% involvement is lethal. Further, these extrapolated data on clinical pathologic specimens parallel those identified in the classic postmortem study of cardiogenic shock from the Massachusetts General Hospital, in which 40% necrosis of the left ventricle was found to be uniformly fatal.[123]

Early during AMI, while the ischemic insult is still potentially reversible (within four to six hours), it may be that recanalization and/or revascularization have the potential to reverse some of the acute ischemic dysfunction that occurs in the distribution of the occluded major coronary artery. At present, only anecdotal clinical cases support such a surmise. Once infarction is completed, and through the eighth or ninth day when fibrosis begins to be effective, elasticity of the infarcted segment is maximal and the hemodynamic burden most severe. Infarctectomy, while theoretically attractive, has not proven to be effective, perhaps because resection of infarction extensive enough to warrant such radical therapy results in reduction of stroke volume to lethal levels. Therapy should be medical and include pharmacologic afterload reduction, inotropic agents, and, if necessary, the use of an intraaortic balloon pump. The severe hemodynamic burden should diminish as fibrosis ensues and the infarcted segment becomes a mature scar that loses its elasticity. More attention needs to be focused on this entity so that it can be better characterized and a more effective therapy developed.

CONCLUSIONS

The therapeutic dilemmas presented by complicated postinfarction patients have made it all the more apparent that a better therapeutic outcome could have been achieved *if the infarction had been prevented or contained* by more timely revascularization. Since left ventricular function is the most powerful determinant of early and late prognosis after AMI, it follows that the most effective therapy may involve immediate restoration of blood flow to the myocardium to limit the amount of myocardial damage, thereby preserving myocardial viability and function. Such a therapeutic approach has validity because AMI does not occur as an all-or-none phenomenon but is a pathophysiologic process that evolves and is potentially reversible. Recent surgical experience suggests that revascularization by coronary bypass during the first 6 hours of evolving AMI has the potential to limit the effects of acute infarction, resulting in improved early and late survival and perhaps in preservation of ventricular function as well. However, such therapy is logistically difficult to achieve. It is therefore not a generally applicable therapeutic modality. Reperfusion, by recanalizing an acutely thrombosed coronary artery with intravenous or intracoronary thrombolytic therapy or by PTCA has recently been advocated in evolving AMI. Early experience indicates that such approaches are feasible, that symptoms can be controlled, that survival may be improved, and that left ventricular viability may be preserved with maintenance of some degree of left ventricular function. Despite successful early recanalization, at least one third of patients require further therapy, either by PTCA or by early coronary bypass.

In much the same way that reciprocal considerations of medical and surgical therapy emerged from the treatment of patients with unstable angina, it would seem that a similar occurrence is on the horizon in regards to the treatment of AMI. The question should not be one of whether to use exclusively medical *or* surgical therapy, but rather, which one or combination of both best suits the case at hand. The issue is one of "when" rather than "which," since it is clear that timing is of the essence and that all infarctions are not equal and demanding of equal therapy. One should not advocate more aggressive, invasive therapies on a routine basis, but neither should they be routinely discounted.

Increasingly, cardiac surgeons are being involved in the therapy of the nonmechanical complications of AMI that include threatened extension, reinfarction, acute ventricular arrhythmias, congestive heart failure, and/or cardiogenic shock in the absence of a mechanical defect. Results of coronary bypass for these complications early after acute infarction are surprisingly good, with the possible exception of the subset with cardiogenic shock. Even there, progress has been made. At present, the existence of a postinfarction complication, whether mechanical or other, certainly constitutes an indication for study, with a decreasing threshold to recommend surgical therapy.

What is certain is that increased scrutiny and study of patients will lead to the development of newer, better therapies that will result in an improvement in presently defined outcome for AMI.

REFERENCES

1. Martin CA, Thompson PL, Armstrong BK et al: Long-term prognosis after recovery from myocardial infarction: A nine year follow-up of the Perth coronary register. Circulation 68:961–969, 1983
2. Luria MH, Knoke JD, Wachs JS et al: Survival after recovery from acute myocardial infarction. Am J Med 67:7–13, 1979
3. Weinblatt E, Goldberg JD, Ruberman W et al: Mortality after first myocardial infarction. JAMA 247:1576–1581, 1982
4. The Multicenter Postinfarction Research Group: Risk stratification and survival after myocardial infarction. N Engl J Med 309:331–336, 1983
5. Shapiro S, Weinblatt E, Frank CW et al: The HIP study of incidence and prognosis of coronary heart disease: Methodology. J Chron Dis 16:1281–1292, 1963
6. Ruberman W, Weinblatt E, Goldberg JD et al: Ventricular premature beats and mortality after myocardial infarction. N Engl J Med 297:750–757, 1977
7. Kannel WB, Sorlie P, McNamara PM: Prognosis after initial myocardial infarction: The Framingham Study. Am J Cardiol 44:53–59, 1979
8. DeWood MA, Spores J, Notske R et al: Prevalence of total coronary occlusion during the early hours of transmural myocardial infarction. N Engl J Med 303:897, 1980
9. Cox JL, McLaughlin VW, Flowers NC et al: The ischemic zone surrounding acute myocardial infarction: Its morphology as detected by dehydrogenase staining. Am Heart J 76:650, 1968
10. Maroko PR, Libby P, Ginks WR et al: Coronary artery perfusion, I. Early effects on local myocardial function and the extent of myocardial necrosis. J Clin Invest 51:2710, 1972
11. Costantino C, Corday E, Tsu-Wang L: Revascularization after 3 hours of coronary arterial occlusion: Effects on regional cardiac metabolic function and infarct size. Am J Cardiol 36:368, 1975
12. Forrester JS, Diamond GA, Chatterjee K et al: Medical therapy of acute myocardial infarction by application of hemodynamic subsets, Parts I and II. N Engl J Med 295:1356 and 1404, 1976
13. Favaloro RG: Saphenous vein autograft replacement of severe segmental coronary artery occlusion: Operative technique. Ann Thorac Surg 5:334, 1968
14. Johnson WD, Lepley D, Jr: An aggressive approach to coronary disease. J Thorac Cardiovasc Surg 59:128, 1970
15. Chatterjee K, Swan HJC, Parmley WW et al: Depression of left ventricular function due to acute myocardial ischemia and its reversal after aortocoronary saphenous vein bypass. N Engl J Med 286:1117, 1972
16. Chatterjee K, Swan HJC, Parmley WW et al: Influence of direct myocardial revascularization on left ventricular asynergy and function in patients with coronary heart disease. (With and without previous infarction). Circulation 47:276, 1973
17. Freeman MR, Gray RJ, Berman DS et al: Improvement in global and segmental left ventricular function after coronary bypass surgery. Circulation 64 (Suppl 2)II:34, 1981
18. Lichtlen P, Moccetti T, Halter J et al: Postoperative evaluation of myocardial blood flow in aorta-to-coronary artery *vein* bypass grafts using the Xenon-residue detection technique. Circulation 46:445–455, 1972
19. Bertolasi CA, Tronge JE, Riccitelli MA et al: Natural history of unstable angina with medical or surgical therapy. Chest 70:596–605, 1976
20. Sustaita H, Chatterjee K, Marty A et al: Emergency surgery in impending and complicated acute myocardial infarction. Arch Surg 105:30, 1972
21. Cooperative Unstable Angina Study Group: Unstable angina pectoris: National cooperative study to compare surgical and medical therapy, II. In-hospital experience and initial follow-up results in patients with one, two, and three vessel disease. Am J Cardiol 42:839–848, 1978
22. Kirklin JW, Conti VR, Blackstone EH: Prevention of myocardial damage during cardiac operations. N Engl J Med 301:135–141, 1979
23. Gray RJ, Matloff JM, Conklin CM et al: Perioperative myocardial infarction: Late clinical course after coronary artery bypass surgery. Circulation 66:1185, 1982
24. Caulfield JB, Leinbach R, Gold H: The relationship of myocardial infarct size and prognosis. Circulation 53:1–141, 1976
25. Braunwald E: Control of myocardial oxygen consumption. Physiologic and clinical considerations. Am J Cardiol 27:416, 1971
26. Alonso DR, Scheidt S, Post M et al: Pathophysiology of cardiogenic shock. Quantification of myocardial necrosis: Clinical, pathologic and electrocardiographic correlations. Circulation 48:588, 1973
27. Berg R Jr, Kendall RW, Duvoisin GE et al: Acute myocardial infarction. A surgical emergency. J Thorac Cardiovasc Surg 70:432–439, 1975
28. DeWood MA, Spores J, Berg R, Jr et al: Acute myocardial infarction: A decade of experience with surgical reperfusion in 701 patients. Circulation 68(II):8–16, 1983

29. Phillips SJ, Kongtahworn C, Skinner JR et al: Emergency coronary artery reperfusion: A choice therapy for evolving myocardial infartion. Results in 339 patients. J Thorac Cardiovasc Surg 86:679–688, 1983
30. Kirklin JK, Blackstone EH, Zorn GL et al: Intermediate-term results of coronary artery bypass grafting for acute myocardial infarction. Circulation 72(II):175–178, 1985
31. DeWood MA, Heit J, Spores J et al: Anterior transmural myocardial infarction: Effects of surgical coronary reperfusion on global and regional left ventricular function. J Am Coll Cardiol 1(5):1223–1234, 1983
32. Venhaecke J, Flameng W, Sergeant P et al: Emergency bypass surgery: Late effects on size of infarction and ventricular function. Circulation 72(II):179–184, 1985
33. McIntosh HD, Buccino RA: Emergency coronary artery revascularization of patients with acute myocardial infarction. You can . . . but should you? Circulation 60:247, 1979
34. Spencer FC: Emergency coronary bypass for acute infarction: An unproved clinical experiment. Circulation 68(II):17, 1983
35. Skinner JR, Phillips SJ, Zeff RH et al: Immediate coronary bypass following failed streptokinase infusion in evolving myocardial infarction. J Thorac Cardiovasc Surg 87:567–570, 1984
36. Kay P, Ahmad A, Floten S, Starr A: Emergency coronary artery bypass surgery after intracoronary thrombolysis for evolving myocardial infarction. Br Heart J 53:260–264, 1985
37. Lolley DM, Fulton R, Hamman J et al: Coronary artery surgery and direct coronary artery thrombolysis during acute myocardial infarction. Am Surg 49:296–300, 1983
38. Wilson JM, Held JS, Wright CB et al: Coronary artery bypass surgery following thrombolytic therapy for acute coronary thrombosis. Ann Thorac Surg 37(3):212–217, 1984
39. Urban PL, Cowley M, Goldberg S et al: Intracoronary thrombolysis in acute myocardial infarction: Clinical course following successful myocardial reperfusion. Am Heart J 108(4-I):873–878, 1984
40. Losman JG, Finchum RN, Nagle D et al: Myocardial surgical revascularization after streptokinase treatment for acute myocardial infarction. J Thorac Cardiovasc Surg 89:25–34, 1985
41. Walker WE, Smalling RW, Fuentes F et al: Role of coronary artery bypass surgery after intracoronary streptokinase infusion for myocardial infarction. Am Heart J 107(4):826–829, 1984
42. Gruentzig AR: Percutaneous transluminal coronary angioplasty: Six years' experience. Am Heart J 107:818, 1984
43. Murphy DA, Craver JM, Jones EL et al: Surgical management of acute myocardial ischemia following percutaneous transluminal coronary angioplasty. J Thorac Cardiovasc Surg 87:332–339, 1984
44. Roberts AR, Faro RS, Rubin MR et al: Emergency coronary artery bypass graft surgery for threatened acute myocardial infarction related to coronary artery catheterization. Ann Thorac Surg 39:116–124, 1985
45. Mundth ED, Buckley MJ, Daggett WM: Surgery for complications of acute myocardial infarction. Circulation 45:1279, 1972
46. Schuster EH, Bulkley BH: Early post-infarction angina: Ischemia at a distance and ischemia in the infarct zone. N Engl J Med 305(19):1101–1105, 1981
47. Koiwaya Y, Torii S, Takeshita A et al: Postinfarction angina caused by coronary arterial spasm. Circulation 65(2):275–280, 1982
48. Moran TJ, French WJ, Abrams HF, Criley JM: Postmyocardial infarction angina and coronary spasm. Am J Cardiol 50:197–202, 1982
49. Loop FD, Cheanvechai C, Sheldon WC: Early myocardial revascularization during acute myocardial infarction. Chest 66:478, 1974
50. Keon WJ, Bedard P, Shankar KR: Experience with emergency aortocoronary bypass grafts in the presence of acute myocardial infarction. Circulation 47 and 48(III):151, 1972
51. Levine RH, Gold HK, Leinbach RC: Safe early revascularization for continuing ischemia after acute myocardial infarction. Circulation 58(II):17, 1978
52. Wellons HA, Grossman J, Crosby IK: Early operative intervention for complications of acute myocardial infarction. J Thorac Cardiovasc Surg 73:763, 1977
53. Nunley DL, Grunkemeier GL, Teply JF et al: Coronary bypass operation following acute complicated myocardial infarction. J Thorac Cardiovasc Surg 85:485–491, 1983
54. Baumgartner WA, Borkon AM, Zibulewsky J et al: Operative intervention for postinfarction angina. Ann Thorac Surg 38(3):265–267, 1984
55. Singh AK, Rivera R, Cooper GN, Jr, Karlson KE: Early myocardial revascularization for postinfarction angina: Results and longterm follow-up. J Am Coll Cardiol 6:1121–1125, 1985
56. Braunwald E, Covell JW, Maroko PR et al: Effects of drugs and of counterpulsation on myocardial oxygen consumption: Observations on the ischemic heart. Circulation 50(Suppl 4):220, 1969
57. Scheidt S, Wilner G, Mueller H et al: Intra-aortic balloon counterpulsation in cardiogenic shock. Report of a cooperative clinical trial. N Engl J Med 288:979, 1973
58. Leinbach RC, Gold HK, Dinsmore RE: The role of angiography in cardiogenic shock. Circulation 48(III):95, 1973
59. Wajsczczuk WJ, Karakauer J, Rubenfire M: Current indications for mechanical circulatory assistance on the basis of experience with 104 patients. Am J Cardiol 33:176, 1974
60. Baron DW, O'Rourke MF: Long term results of arterial counterpulsation in acute severe cardiac failure complicating myocardial infarction. Br Heart J 38:285, 1976
61. Experiences with the intra-aortic balloon pump, No. 3. Nutley, NJ, Roche Medical Electronics, Dept. of Biomedical Research, March 1975
62. O'Rourke MF, Norris RM, Campbell TJ: Randomized controlled trial of intra-aortic balloon counterpulsation in early myocardial infarction with acute heart failure. Am J Cardiol 47:815, 1981
63. Mundth ED, Yurchak PM, Buckley NJ: Circulatory assistance and emergency direct coronary artery surgery for shock complicating acute myocardial infarction. N Engl J Med 283:1382, 1979
64. McEnany MT, Kay HR, Buckley MJ: Clinical experience with intra-aortic pump support in 728 patients. Circulation 58(I):124, 1977
65. Gay W: Cardiogenic shock: The basis for surgical therapy. In Moran JM, Michaelis LL (eds): Surgery for the Complications of Acute Myocardial Infarction, p 255. New York, Grune & Stratton, 1980
66. DeWood MA, Notski RN, Hensley GR et al: Intra-aortic balloon counterpulsation with and without reperfusion for myocardial infarction shock. Circulation 61:1105, 1980
67. Rosenkranz ER, Buckberg GD, Laks H, Mulder DG: Warm induction of cardioplegia with glutamate-enriched blood in coronary patients with cardiogenic shock who are dependent on inotropic drugs and intra-aortic balloon support. J Thorac Cardiovasc Surg 86:507–518, 1983
68. Favaloro RH, Effler DB, Groves LK: Ventricular aneurysm. Clinical experience. Ann Thorac Surg 6:227, 1968
69. Spurrell RAJ, Sowton E, Deuchar DC: Ventricular tachycardia in four patients evaluated by programmed electrical stimulation of heart and treated in two patients by surgical division of anterior radiation of left bundle branch. Br Heart J 35:1014, 1973
70. Spurrell RAJ, Yates AK, Thornburn CW: Surgical treatment of ventricular tachycardia after epicardial mapping studies. Br Heart J 37:115, 1975
71. Gallagher JJ, Oldham HN, Wallace AG: Ventricular aneurysm with ventricular tachycardia. Am J Cardiol 35:696, 1975
72. Harken AH, Josephson ME, Horowitz LN: Surgical endocardial resection for the treatment of malignant ventricular tachycardia. Ann Surg 190:456, 1979
73. Ricks WB, Winkle RA, Shumway NE: Surgical management of life-threatening ventricular arrhythmias in patients with coronary artery disease. Circulation 56:38, 1977
74. Buda AJ, Stinson EB, Harrison DC: Surgery for life-threatening ventricular tachyarrhythmias. Am J Cardiol 44:1171, 1979
75. Matloff JM, Chaux A, Sustaita H: Unstable angina. Experience with surgical therapy in the subset of patients having preinfarction angina. Cleve Clin Q 45(1): 184–188, 1978
76. Jones EL, Douglas JS, Craver JM et al: Results of coronary revascularization in patients with recent myocardial infarction. J Thorac Cardiovasc Surg 76:545, 1978
77. Betriu A, Castaner A, Sanz GA: Angiographic findings one month after myocardial infarction: A prospective study of 259 survivors. Circulation 65:1099–1105, 1982
78. Epstein SE, Palmeri ST, Patterson RE: Evaluation of patients after acute myocardial infarction. Indications for cardiac catheterization and surgical intervention. N Engl J Med 307(24):1487–1492, 1982
79. Myers WO, Davis K, Foster ED et al: Surgical survival in the Coronary Artery Surgery Study (CASS) registry. Ann Thorac Surg (in press)
80. Passamani E, Davis K, Gillespie M et al: A randomized trial of coronary artery bypass surgery: Survival of patients with a low ejection fraction. N Engl J Med 312:26, 1665–1671, 1983
81. Vleistra R, Assad-Morell J, Frye R et al: Survival predictors in coronary artery disease: Medical and surgical comparisons. Mayo Clin Proc, 52:85–90, 1977
82. Rogers WJ, Smith LR, Oberman A et al: Surgical vs nonsurgical management of patients after myocardial infarction. Circulation 62(I):67–74, 1980
83. Norris RM, Agnew TM, Brandt PWT et al: Coronary surgery after recurrent myocardial infarction: Progress of a trial comparing surgical with nonsurgical management for asymptomatic patients with advanced coronary disease. Circulation 63(4):785–792, 1981
84. Hochberg MS, Parsonnet V, Gielchinsky I et al: Timing of coronary revascularization after acute myocardial infarction: Early and late results in patients revascularized within seven weeks. J Thorac Cardiovasc Surg 88:914–921, 1984
85. Lodge-Patch I: The aging of cardiac infarcts and its influence on cardiac rupture. Br Heart J 13:37, 1951
86. Czer LSC, Gray RJ, DeRobertis M et al: Mitral valve replacement: Impact of coronary artery disease and determinants of prognosis following revascularization. Circulation 70:(Suppl I):I-198–207, 1984
87. Brody W, Criley JM: Intermittent severe mitral regurgitation. Hemodynamic studies in a patient with recurrent acute left-sided heart failure. N Engl J Med 283:673, 1970
88. De Busk RF, Harrison DC: The clinical spectrum of papillary muscle disease. N Engl J Med 281:1458, 1969
89. Shelburne JC, Rubinstein D, Gorlin R: A reappraisal of papillary muscle dysfunction: Correlative clinical and angiographic study. Am J Med 46:862, 1969
90. Mittal AK, Langston M, Jr, Cohn KE, Selzerka KW: Combined papillary

muscle and left ventricular wall dysfunction as a cause of mitral regurgitation. An experimental study. Circulation 44:174, 1971

91. Forrester JS, Diamond G, Freedman S et al: Silent mitral insufficiency in acute myocardial infarction. Circulation 44:877, 1971
92. Cederqvist L, Soderstron J: Papillary muscle rupture in myocardial infarction. A study based upon an autopsy material. Acta Med Scand 176:287, 1964
93. Radford MJ, Johnson RA, Buckley MJ et al: Survival following initial valve replacement for mitral regurgitation due to coronary artery disease. Circulation 60(Suppl I):39, 1979
94. Sanders RJ, Neubuerger KT, Ravin A: Rupture of papillary muscles: Occurrence of rupture of the posterior muscle in posterior myocardial infarction. Dis Chest 31:316, 1957
95. Czer LSC, Matloff JM, Gray RJ et al: Mitral valve replacement with coronary artery disease. Duran C, Angell WW, Johnson AD, Oury JH (eds): Recent Progress in Mitral Valve Disease, pp 304–319. Sevenoaks, England, Butterworth, 1984
96. Fox AC, Glassman E, Ison OW: Surgically remediable complications of myocardial infarction. Prog Cardiovasc Dis 21:461, 1979
97. Hutchins GM: Rupture of the interventricular septum complicating myocardial infarction. Pathological analysis of 10 patients with clinically diagnosed perforations. Am Heart J 97:165, 1979
98. Radford M, Johnson RA, Daggett WM et al: Ventricular septal rupture: A review of clinical and physiologic features and an analysis. Circulation 64:545, 1981
99. Meister SG, Helfant RH: Rapid bedside differentiation of ruptured intraventricular septum from acute mitral insufficiency. N Engl J Med 287:1024, 1972
100. Farcot JC, Boisante L, Rigaud M et al: Two-dimensional echocardiographic visualization of ventricular septal rupture after acute anterior myocardial infarction. Am J Cardiol 45:370, 1980
101. Richards KL, Hoekenga DE, Leach JK, Blaustein JC: Doppler-cardiographic diagnosis of interventricular septal rupture. Chest 76:101, 1979
102. Bedynek JL, Fenoglio JJ, McAllister HA, Jr: Rupture of the ventricular septum as a complication of myocardial infarction. Am Heart J 97:773, 1979
103. Sanders RJ, Kern WH, Blount SG: Perforation of the interventricular septum complicating infarction. Am Heart J 51:736, 1956
104. Oyamada A, Queen FB: Spontaneous rupture of the ventricular septum following acute myocardial infarction with some clinico-pathological observations on survival in five cases. Paper presented at Pan-Pacific Pathology Congress, Tripler U.S. Army Hospital, 1961
105. Montoya A, McKeever L, Scanlon P et al: Early repair of ventricular septal rupture after infarction. Am J Cardiol 45:345, 1980
106. Gold HK, Leinback RC, Sanders CA et al: Intra-aortic balloon pumping for control of recurrent myocardial ischemia. Circulation 47:1197, 1973
107. Cooley DA, Belmonte BA, Zeis LB, Schnur S: Surgical repair of ruptured interventricular septum following acute myocardial infarction. Surgery 41:930, 1957
108. Kitamura S, Mendez A, Kay JH: Ventricular septal defect following myocardial infarction. J Thorac Cardiovasc Surg 61:186, 1971
109. Iben AB, Pupello DF, Stinson EB, Shumway NE: Surgical treatment of postinfarction ventricular septal defects. Ann Thorac Surg 8:252, 1969
110. Miyamoto A, Lee M, Kass R et al: Postmyocardial infarction ventricular septal defect. J Thorac Cardiovasc Surg 86:41–46, 1983
111. Forfar JC, Irving JB, Miller HC et al: The management of ventricular septal rupture following myocardial infarction. Q J Med 49:205, 1980
112. Harvey W: Complete Works, p 127. Willis R, trans. London, Sydenham Society, 1647
113. Rasmussen S, Leth A, Kjoller E, Pedersen A: Cardiac rupture in acute myocardial infarction: A review of 72 consecutive cases. Acta Med Scand 205:11, 1979
114. Isner JM, Roberts WC: Right ventricular infarction complicating left ventricular infarction secondary to coronary heart disease. Am J Cardiol 42:885, 1978
115. Van Tassel RA, Edwards JE: Rupture of the heart complicating myocardial infarction. Analysis of 40 cases including nine examples of left ventricular false aneurysm. Chest 61:104, 1972
116. Eaton LW, Weiss JL, Bulkley BH et al: Regional cardiac dilation after acute myocardial infarction. Recognition by two-dimensional echocardiography. N Engl J Med 300:57, 1979
117. Schuster EH, Bulkley BH: Expansion of transmural myocardial infarction: A pathophysiologic factor in cardiac rupture. Circulation 60:1532, 1979
118. Cobbs BW, Hatcher CR, Robinson PH: Cardiac rupture. Three operations with two long-term survivors. JAMA 223:532, 1973
119. O'Rourke MF: Subacute heart rupture following myocardial infarction. Clinical features of a correctable condition. Lancet 2:124, 1973
120. Montegut FJ, Jr: Left ventricular rupture secondary to myocardial infarction: Report of survival with surgical repair. Ann Thorac Surg 14:75, 1972
121. Fitzgibbon GM, Hooper GD, Heggtveit HA: Successful surgical treatment of postinfarction external cardiac rupture. J Thorac Cardiovasc Surg 63:622, 1972
122. Parmley WW, Chuck L, Kivowitz C et al: *In vitro* length-tension relations of human ventricular aneurysms: The relationship of stiffness to mechanical disturbance. Am J Cardiol 32:389, 1973
123. Page DL, Caulfield JB, Kastor JA et al: Myocardial changes associated with cardiogenic shock. N Engl J Med 285:133, 1971

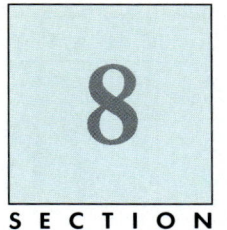

Section Editor
William W. Parmley, MD

SECTION 8

Hypertension

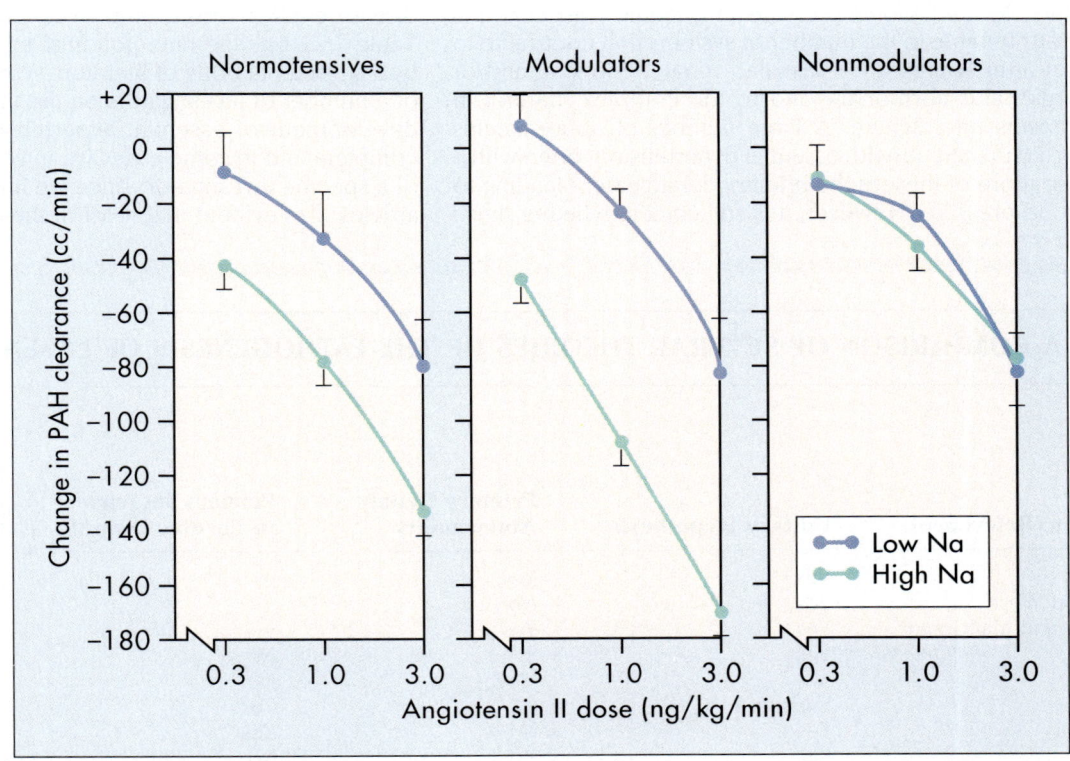

PATHOPHYSIOLOGY OF ESSENTIAL HYPERTENSION

Gordon H. Williams ▪ Norman K. Hollenberg

Undoubtedly, the major difficulty in determining the mechanism(s) responsible for the elevated blood pressure in patients with essential hypertension is attributable to the number of systems that contribute to the regulation of arterial pressure—vascular, renal, peripheral and/or central adrenergic, and hormonal—and to the complex manner in which these systems interdigitate. A large number of abnormalities have been reported in patients with essential hypertension, often with a claim that one or more of these is the primary derangement leading to the elevated blood pressure. However, it is still unclear whether these individual abnormalities are primary or secondary, reflect individual disease entities, or are simply varying expressions of a single process. Table 76.1 lists the nine potential etiologic factors that are supported by a substantial body of literature. We have also reviewed the opinions of a number of investigators on the importance of each of these in the development of essential hypertension.[1-15] The list is by no means complete and in some cases we may well have misstated the opinions of a specific investigator, since we limited our search to recent review articles. It is evident that most of these investigators still adhere to the

TABLE 76.1 A COMPARISON OF SEVERAL THEORIES OF THE PATHOGENESIS OF ESSENTIAL HYPERTENSION

Investigator (Reference)	Unitary Hypothesis	Primary Renal Abnormality	Primary Increase in Cardiac Output	Primary Arteriolar Defect	Defect in Central or Peripheral Adrenergic System
Brown et al[1]	Yes	Yes	±	No	Yes
Chalmers and West[2]	Yes	No	±	No	Yes
deWardener and MacGregor[3]	Yes	Yes	±	No	No
Doyle[4]	Yes	±	No	Yes	Yes?
Dustan[5]	No	Maybe	No	No	Yes
Folkow[6]	Variants	±	Yes	Yes	Yes
Frohlich et al[7]	Yes	No	Yes	±	Yes
Genest[8]	Yes	No	No	No	Yes
Guyton et al[9]	Yes	Yes	±	No	±
Kaplan[10]	Maybe	Yes	Yes	±	Yes
Korner[11]	±	±	Yes	Yes	Yes
Laragh[12]	No	±	No	No	±
Garay et al[13]	Yes	±	±	No	No
Safar et al[14]	Yes	Yes	±	No	No
Tobian[15]	Yes	Yes	±	Yes	Yes

Investigator (Reference)	Dysregulation of the Renin-Angiotensin System	Altered Mineralocorticoid Biosynthesis	Abnormality in Sodium Transport	Abnormal Volume Regulation	Excessive Sodium Intake
Brown et al[1]	No	No	Yes	±	Yes
Chalmers and West[2]	No	No	No	No	No
deWardener and MacGregor[3]	±	±	Yes	Yes	Yes
Doyle[4]	No	No	Yes	Yes	Yes
Dustan[5]	No	No	No	±	No
Folkow[6]	No	No	No	±	No
Frohlich et al[7]	No	No	No	No	No
Genest[8]	No	Yes	?	No	?
Guyton et al[9]	±	No	No	No	±
Kaplan[10]	Yes?	No	Yes	±	Yes
Korner[11]	No	No	±	Yes	Yes
Laragh[12]	Yes	Yes	±	Yes	Yes
Garay et al[13]	±	No	Yes	Yes	Yes
Safar et al[14]	No	No	No	Yes	Yes
Tobian[15]	No	No	±	±	Yes

"unitary derangement" hypothesis with some variations. In other words, most suspect that essential hypertension reflects a single process. A minority support the hypothesis that essential hypertension reflects several different disease processes. We support the minority position. Just as pneumonia is caused by a number of agents, even though a similar clinical picture is observed, so we believe that essential hypertension has a number of distinct causes.

In evaluating the wealth of information reported by the investigators listed in Table 76.1, we found the single etiologic factor that has received the greatest attention is the role of sodium. The potential mechanism(s) by which sodium produces an elevated blood pressure probably is better understood, particularly with the data accumulated over the past several years. Because of the space constraints imposed in writing a single chapter on this subject, we will, therefore, limit our remarks to an assessment of some of the ways sodium may be involved in the pathogenesis of essential hypertension. It is clear that sodium is not the only factor that produces an elevated blood pressure, although it may be responsible for the rise in blood pressure in the majority of the essential hypertensive population.

BACKGROUND

Sodium intake's role in the pathogenesis of essential hypertension has been assessed by a number of techniques, including the benefit of restriction of sodium intake or diuretics in treating hypertensive patients, the study of a number of animal models, and epidemiologic surveys. However, only some patients have a beneficial response to sodium restriction or diuretics, suggesting that a special sensitivity to sodium intake is not universal in the hypertensive population.[16-18] Indeed, it is uncertain whether all normotensive subjects have an equal sensitivity to sodium's pressor effects.[19] Identifying the patients with "sodium-sensitive" hypertension has, therefore, become increasingly important: success in doing so facilitates the design of specific therapy and clarifies the pathogenesis.

What is the frequency of "sodium-sensitive" hypertension? Between 50% and 60% of hypertensives respond to sodium restriction;[20] a similar percentage respond to diuretics.[21] There is also evidence to indicate that a patient who responds to a diuretic will have a similar beneficial effect from a sodium-restricted intake.[22] Finally, 50% of apparently unselected but small groups of hypertensive patients will have a pressor response to a short-term sodium load.[16,17] Thus, using a variety of techniques, most studies report that half the hypertensive population are unusually susceptible to sodium's pressor effect.

How homogeneous is the sodium-sensitive subgroup? Data from a variety of sources suggest that this subgroup is heterogeneous. For example, several secondary forms of hypertension appear to be sodium sensitive, including patients with primary aldosteronism, bilateral renal artery stenosis, and chronic renal failure sufficient to produce mild-to-moderate azotemia. Thus, each is a "volume-dependent" form of hypertension.[23] Renin-sodium profiling has been used to subclassify patients with essential hypertension and has been partially successful. Patients with "low-renin essential hypertension" have a more consistent and greater reduction in blood pressure with diuretic agents than do other subgroups of essential hypertensives.[23] However, even low-renin hypertension is unlikely to be homogeneous. In older patients or those with diabetes, the low renin levels probably reflect the vascular damage within the kidney resulting from longstanding hypertension, or in the case of diabetes, the effects of metabolic derangements.[24] In other patients with low-renin hypertension, the primary abnormality appears to be an enhanced adrenal response to angiotensin II.[25-27] Thus, in these subjects, the sodium-sensitive pressor mechanism(s) is analogous to that present in patients with primary aldosteronism. Two additional questions arise from this analysis: First, is there a common thread to the pathogenesis of hypertension in these persons? Second, do the known forms of volume-dependent hypertension account for all sodium-sensitive hypertension? There does seem to be a common thread in the pathogenesis of the known groups involving a distortion in their capacity to excrete a sodium load, whether because of renal damage, an impairment of the renal vasculature, or autonomous secretion of aldosterone. The answer to the second question is clearly no. Not only is the cumulative frequency of the secondary forms of hypertension, which may be volume dependent, too low, it is equally clear that some patients with normal-renin essential hypertension also demonstrate a special pressor sensitivity to high sodium intake.[16,17]

Several earlier hypotheses on the pathogenesis of sodium-sensitive hypertension have been discarded because of limited experimental support. These include a number of hormonal abnormalities,[28] water logging of the arterioles,[15] and a volume-dependent increase in cardiac output.[29] Recently, a more plausible hypothesis, based largely on studies in animal models, has found increasing support.[3,30-33] In this hypothesis, the elevated blood pressure does not directly result from the retained sodium but rather reflects the influence of activation of alternative mechanisms for elimination of sodium. In animal models, there has been considerable interest in the possibility that a natriuretic, ouabain-like inhibitor of sodium–potassium ATPase contributes to the pathogenesis of the hypertension. Inhibition of the usual pathways for sodium excretion, according to these hypotheses, results in the recruitment of a factor(s) that act within the kidney to promote natriuresis through inhibition of sodium–potassium ATPase.[3,30-33] Inhibition of sodium–potassium ATPase occurs in blood vessels, resulting in changes in electrolyte fluxes that enhance vascular responsiveness to normal pressor agents. Blaustein and Hamlyn hypothesized that because of the changes in sodium flux there is a parallel increase in cytosolic calcium levels, accounting for the enhanced vasoconstrictor responses.[33] Possibly in agreement with these hypotheses are several abnormalities described in some patients with essential hypertension including a circulating sodium–potassium-ATPase inhibitor, a transferable factor inhibiting cell membrane sodium transport, and abnormalities in the red blood cell sodium transport systems.[3,13,33-36] While these mechanisms may play a role in the known forms of sodium-sensitive hypertension, none of the presently available hypotheses can account for the known sodium sensitivity of some normal-renin essential hypertensives, potentially the larger subgroup. Most attempts to deal with this issue have involved a vague notion that there is a primary, intrinsic abnormality in the ability of the kidney to handle sodium.[3]

In the subsequent sections of this chapter, we will review the normal factors involved in sodium homeostasis, how derangements in these normal regulatory systems may lead to altered sodium balance, and the potential therapeutic implications of such findings.

THE RENIN-ANGIOTENSIN-ALDOSTERONE RENAL SYSTEM

Despite recent interest in a physiologic role for the renin-angiotensin system in controlling blood pressure, most of the accumulated evidence suggests that this system primarily is involved in the regulation of extracellular fluid volume, as may be appreciated by examining the evolution of the renin-angiotensin-aldosterone system. The cyclostomes and elasmobranches, the most primitive living vertebrates, have neither renin nor renal juxtaglomerular granules. However, at the next level on the evolutionary scale, the teleosts and tetrapods, renin appears.[37] The Australian lung fish has a blood pressure of only 15 mm Hg, and angiotensin is not directly pressor, suggesting that renin's role in this organism is not related to blood pressure regulation but to the control of extracellular fluid volume through an intrarenal action.[38] Aldosterone is not demonstrably present in Australian lung fish but appears to occur even later, as Berne has stated,[39] being an "invention of land living vertebrates" beginning with reptiles and amphibians.[40] Thus, the most likely interpretation of these data is that the renin-angiotensin system initially evolved as a means of controlling extracellular fluid volume, primarily by modifying renal plasma flow and thus regulating glomerular filtration rate.[41] With movement out of the sea to an increasingly more complex environment, aldosterone was drawn under the control of the renin-angiotensin system to further potentiate the ability of this system to respond appropriately to increasingly greater changes in the level of sodium intake.

As one progresses up the evolutionary scale to humans and higher vertebrates, there is no question that aldosterone plays an important role in sodium handling and that a major regulator of its secretion is the renin-angiotensin system. Controversy existed for a number of years concerning the primacy of the renin-angiotensin system in regulating adrenal responses to changes in sodium intake[42,43]; however, with documentation that the responsiveness of the adrenal to angiotensin II varies with the level of sodium intake, much of the apparent discrepant data became interpretable.[44-47]

Considerable evidence also suggests that the effect of angiotensin II on both the peripheral and renal vasculature is influenced by the level of sodium intake. For example, neither *saralasin* (a competitive antagonist to angiotensin II) nor converting enzyme inhibitors modify renal blood flow if a liberal sodium intake has been allowed. However, when sodium intake is restricted and the renin-angiotensin system activated, both classes of inhibitors induce a dose-related increase in renal blood flow with an increase in sodium excretion, suggesting that angiotensin II indeed has contributed to sodium handling by the kidney.[48,49] Similar findings have been reported for the peripheral vasculature.[50-52] These studies have led to the formulation of a hypothesis that sodium intake reciprocally influences the vascular smooth muscle and adrenal responses to angiotensin II, with sodium restriction enhancing the adrenal response and reducing the vascular response (Fig. 76.1).[45]

What factors are responsible for the change in target tissue responsiveness with changes in sodium intake? The mechanism(s) underlying these changes for the vascular smooth muscle has become increasingly clear. *In vivo* studies document that as the level of angiotensin II rises in the circulation there is a reduction in both the renal vascular and pressor responses to infused angiotensin II. These findings are similar to those observed when isolated smooth muscle strips are placed in a tissue bath, suggesting that the angiotensin II receptor is involved.[53] Data over the past several years, assessing tissue binding of radiolabeled ligands, have provided support for this conclusion. The shifts in vascular responsiveness to angiotensin II with changes in sodium intake almost certainly reflect the reciprocal relationship between its plasma level and the number of angiotensin II receptors on vascular smooth muscle (Fig. 76.2).[54,55]

What of aldosterone secretion? Here the answer is more complex and the data more controversial. Some of the controversy may be species related, but even that is uncertain. At least two possibilities exist. Either the change in sensitivity is receptor mediated, or it is secondary to a change in a postreceptor event. In the rat, an increase in the number of angiotensin II receptors on the glomerulosa cells has been reported with sodium restriction or the chronic infusion of angiotensin II.[56,57] However, binding studies using primate tissue demonstrate a reciprocal relationship between the number of binding sites on the adrenal and the circulating angiotensin II level.[58] Pharmacologic studies in both rats and humans also suggest that the circulating angiotensin II level is not the prime mediator of change in adrenal responsiveness to angiotensin II when sodium intake is modified.[59-61] For example, reducing plasma angiotensin with a converting enzyme inhibitor (enalapril) did not enhance the adrenal response to angiotensin II in normal subjects (Fig. 76.3). On the other hand, studies examining changes in enzyme activity in the glomerulosa cell with changes in sodium intake have been consistent: With sodium restriction there is an enhanced rate of conversion of corticosterone to aldosterone, with the opposite occurring with sodium loading.[59,62]

How the adrenal "knows" what the sodium intake is remains uncertain. One possibility is that there is a change in the activity of the dopaminergic system.[63,64] Dopamine levels in the adrenal increase with high sodium intake, and dopamine has been shown to inhibit aldosterone secretion specifically in response to angiotensin II. Finally, meto-

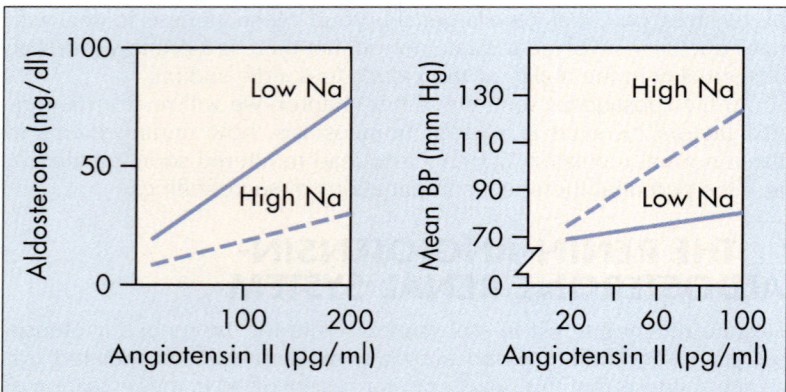

FIGURE 76.1 Sodium intake's reciprocal influence on vascular and adrenal responses to angiotensin II. With sodium restriction adrenal responses are enhanced and vascular responses are reduced. Vascular responses apply not only to blood pressure but also to renal blood flow. (Modified from Hollenberg NK, Chenitz WR, Adams DF, Williams GH: Reciprocal influence of salt intake on adrenal glomerulosa and renal vascular responses to angiotensin II in normal man. J Clin Invest 54:34, 1974)

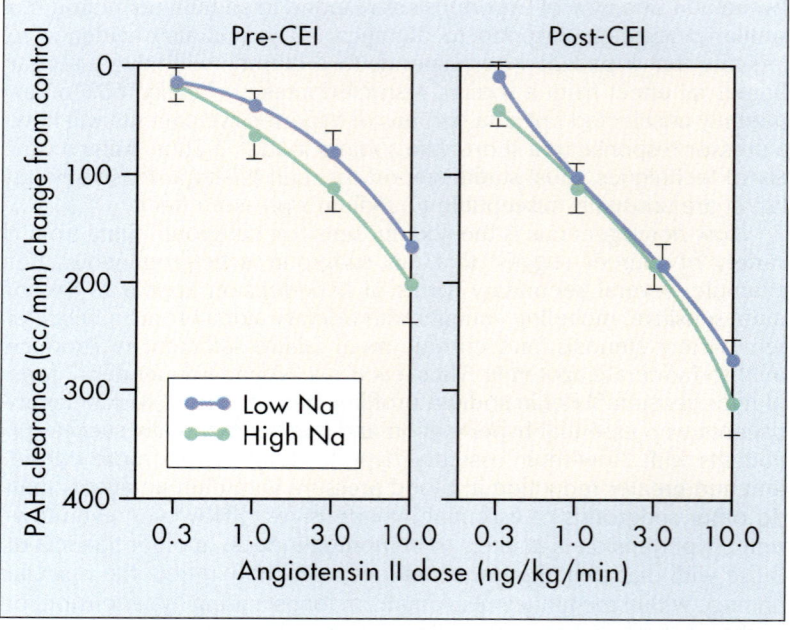

FIGURE 76.2 The effect of high sodium intake and converting enzyme inhibition (enalapril) on renal vascular responses to angiotensin II in normal controls. Sodium restriction reduces the renal vascular responses. This reduced responsiveness is completely reversed by the administration of a converting enzyme inhibitor, enalapril. Thus, the changes in renal vascular responsiveness to infused angiotensin II is secondary to the changes sodium intake produces in the circulating angiotensin II level. (Modified from Shoback DM, Williams GH, Hollenberg NK et al: Endogenous angiotensin II as determinant of sodium modulated changes in tissue responsiveness to angiotensin II in normal man. J Clin Endocrinol Metab 51:764, 1983)

clopramide, a dopamine antagonist, enhances the adrenal response to angiotensin II on a high but not a low sodium intake. Thus, dopamine may be the conveyer of the "sodium intake" information.[63,64]

ALTERED RESPONSIVENESS TO ANGIOTENSIN II IN ESSENTIAL HYPERTENSION

With the development of a clearer understanding of the normal relationship between the renal vasculature, the adrenal gland, changes in sodium intake, and responsiveness to angiotensin II, it became possible to design studies looking at potential abnormalities in this relationship in hypertensive subjects. During the 1970s several such studies were reported. In one study, for example, in normal subjects the renal blood flow increased when dietary sodium intake was changed from low to high. In some patients with essential hypertension, no change was observed.[65,66] Since one or both parents of the patients studied in this subgroup also had hypertension, it raised the intriguing possibility that the renal abnormality was inherited. In a second set of studies, some patients with essential hypertension were reported to have an alteration in the normal adrenal response to acute volume depletion (Fig. 76.4).[67] Since the response of both the renal blood supply and the adrenal to shifts in total body sodium is largely determined by angiotensin II, it was suggested that the underlying difficulty was a defect in their interaction with angiotensin II. This hypothesis was confirmed.[68] There were several other studies during this same period also reporting abnormalities in the way some patients with essential hypertension responded to sodium and/or volume changes.[26,69-71] Most did not examine in detail a potential derangement in the renal vasculature and/or the adrenal, but with accumulating evidence it appears that similar abnormalities probably were present in these patients.

Thus, a substantial body of evidence has accumulated suggesting that in some patients with normal- and/or high-renin essential hypertension, there is an apparent defect in the manner in which sensitivity of the renal vasculature and the adrenal response to angiotensin II is modified with changes in sodium intake. Since these two systems, as noted earlier, play a primary role in the response to changes in sodium intake, these abnormalities could be pathophysiologically significant.

More recent studies have extended these observations. The first series of studies defined whether the two previously described abnormalities coexist in the same patient. In one study, hypertensives younger than age 30 were examined.[72] The age restriction was used in order to minimize the likelihood that any abnormalities noted would be secondary to longstanding hypertension. Studies were performed during a high (200-mEq) and a low (10-mEq) sodium intake, followed by an additional short-term volume deficit induced by furosemide to achieve a wide span of sodium balance. Acute diuretic-induced volume depletion was used to divide the patients into two subgroups, as shown in Figure 76.4. In each patient, an aldosterone secretion rate was determined on the low-salt diet prior to administration of the diuretic and again following 24 hours of acute, diuretic-induced volume depletion. The increment in aldosterone secretion was then calculated and the individual values plotted. In normotensive subjects, the increment was always greater than 300 μg/24 hr. The hypertensive patients were divided into two subgroups—one with an increment similar to the normotensive patients and another in which there was little, if any, effect of the acute volume depletion on the aldosterone secretion rate. The response of the hypertensive patients was clearly bimodal, and each subgroup made up about half of the population. The differences in the responses were not due to differences in the response of plasma renin activity to the acute volume depletion. Renal plasma flow was then assessed on a high- and low-salt diet in the two subgroups. In those who had a normal aldosterone response to acute volume deple-

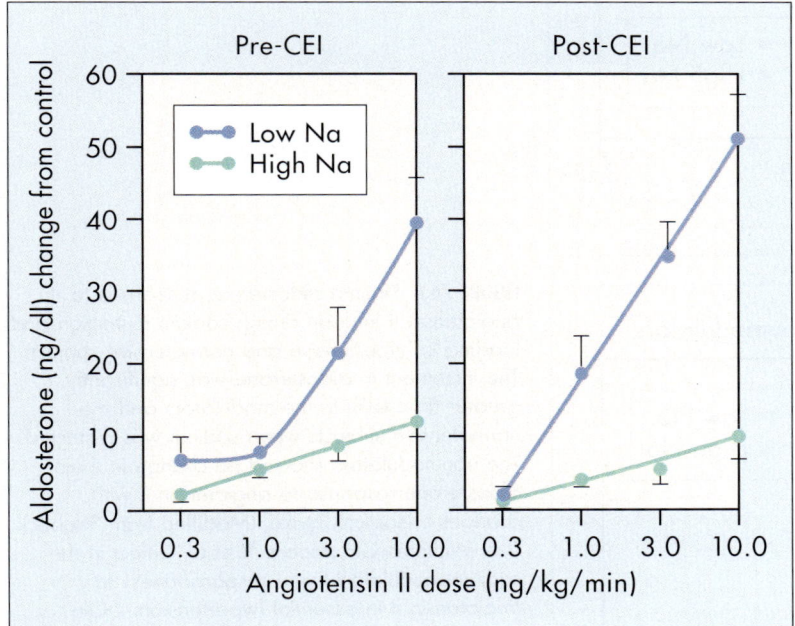

FIGURE 76.3 Modification of adrenal responses to angiotensin II by changes in sodium intake and/or converting enzyme inhibition (enalapril). The same normotensive subjects were studied on both a 10 mEq and 200 mEq sodium intake prior to and after three days of administration of enalapril, a converting enzyme inhibitor. Sodium restriction enhanced the adrenal response to angiotensin II. Since enalapril did not modify this enhanced response, the data suggest that circulating levels of angiotensin II are not the prime mediators of the change in responsiveness of the adrenal gland to angiotensin II with modification of sodium intake. (Modified from Shoback DM, Williams GH, Hollenberg NK et al: Endogenous angiotensin II as determinant of sodium modulated changes in tissue responsiveness to angiotensin II in normal man. J Clin Endocrinol Metab 51:764, 1983)

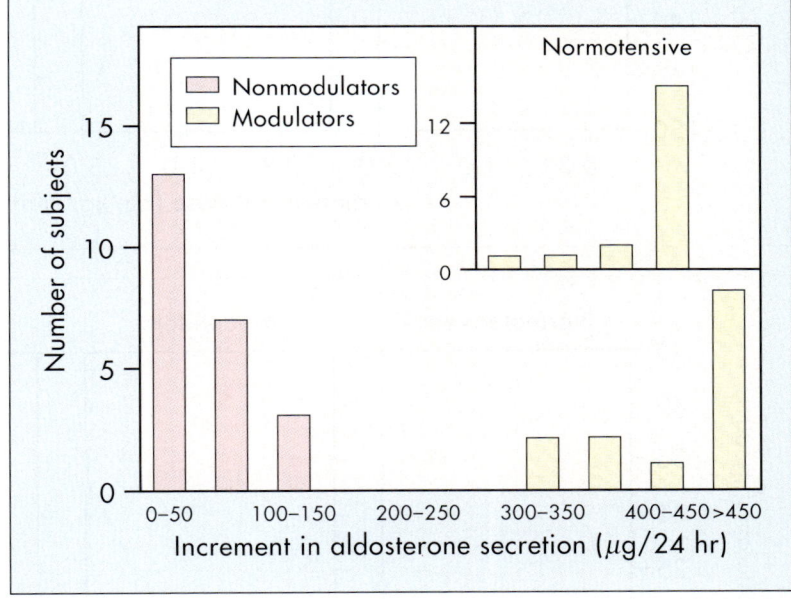

FIGURE 76.4 A histogram of the individual increments in aldosterone secretion rates induced by administration of furosemide to normal and hypertensive subjects when in balance on a low-sodium intake (10 mEq Na/100 mEq K). In all subjects, a low-salt aldosterone secretion rate was obtained, furosemide administered, and the aldosterone secretion rate repeated. The figure depicts the increment between these two secretion rates. The hypertensive subjects are divided into two groups based on their responses as compared with the normotensive controls: (1) normal responders (modulators) and (2) abnormal responders (nonmodulators). Note the distinct bimodal distribution of the responses in the hypertensives. (Modified from Williams GH, Hollenberg NK: Are non-modulating essential hypertensives a distinct subgroup? Implications for therapy. Am J Med 79(suppl 3C):3, 1985)

tion, sodium restriction appropriately reduced renal blood flow, while this maneuver had no effect on the renal blood flow in the abnormal responders. The data in this study, once again, were compatible with parallel blunting of responsiveness to angiotensin II in both systems.

This hypothesis was then directly tested.[73] Subjects in this study were divided into normal or abnormal responders based on their renal vascular response to angiotensin II. In normotensive subjects studied under similar circumstances, a decrement in para-aminohippuric acid (PAH) clearance (as an estimate of renal blood flow) of at least 120 ml/min/1.73 m^2 with the 3 ng/kg/min angiotensin II infusion rate was observed on the high sodium intake. In contrast, nearly half of the hypertensive subjects had a smaller decrement. These abnormal responders had three major characteristics distinguishing them from the normotensive subjects and the normal-responding hypertensive patients: (1) sodium intake did not modify their renal vascular response to angiotensin II (Fig. 76.5); (2) sodium intake also did not modify adrenal responses to angiotensin II (Fig. 76.6), even though the patients were not separated on the basis of their adrenal response to angiotensin II; and (3) (perhaps most important) with chronic sodium loading there was no increase in renal blood flow—a characteristic that was prominent in the normotensive subjects and the normally responding hypertensive patients (Fig. 76.7). Thus, these two avenues of investigation strongly suggest that there exists a subgroup of patients with essential hypertension who fail to modify or modulate their renal vascular and adrenal responses to angiotensin II with changes in dietary sodium intake. We have termed these patients *nonmodulators*.

Nonmodulators do not differ from other essential hypertensive patients in age, duration of hypertension, sodium and potassium balance, gender, renal function, cardiac output, and/or plasma volume. There also appear to be no clinical differences in the severity of the hyper-

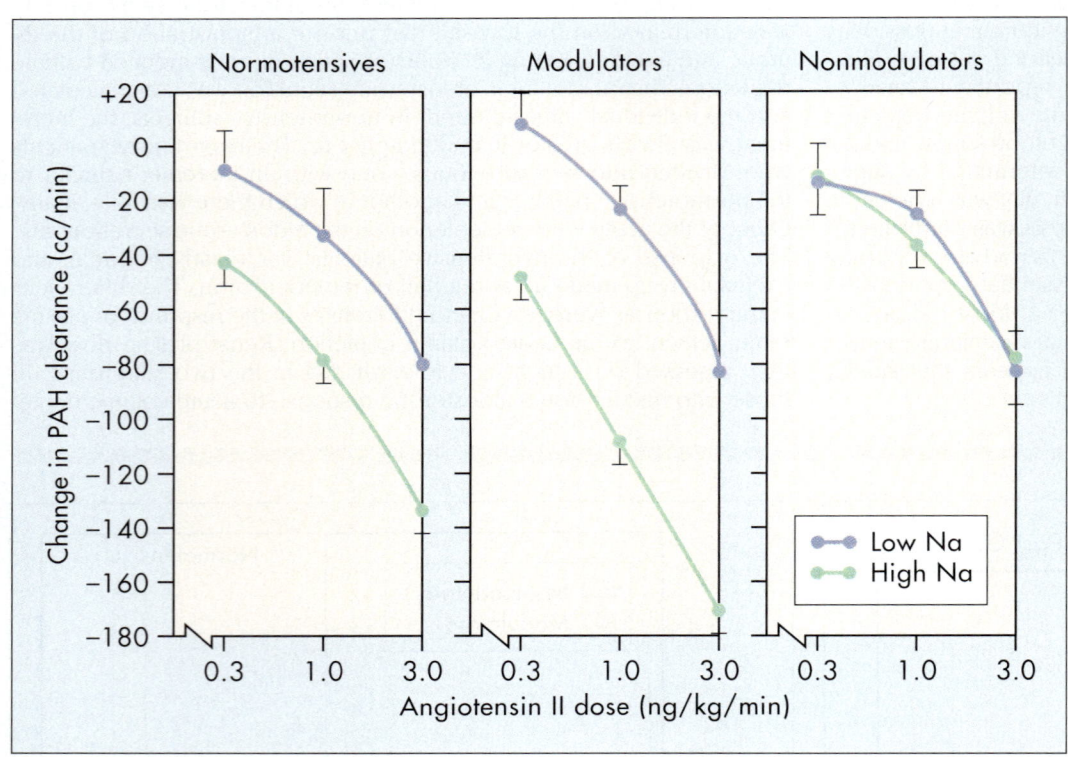

FIGURE 76.5 Changes in PAH clearance as an index of renal blood flow during angiotensin II infusion in normotensives and hypertensives. The decrement in renal blood flow during the angiotensin II infusion was significantly greater ($P < 0.01$) in the modulators (*center*; n = 8) on the high-sodium compared to the low-sodium diets, a response similar to the normotensive subjects (*left*). In contrast, in the nonmodulators (*right*), there was no significant difference in the PAH decrement during angiotensin II infusion between the low- and high-sodium diets. (Modified from Shoback DM, Williams GH, Moore TJ et al: Defect in the sodium-modulated tissue responsiveness to angiotensin II in essential hypertension. J Clin Invest 72:2115, 1983)

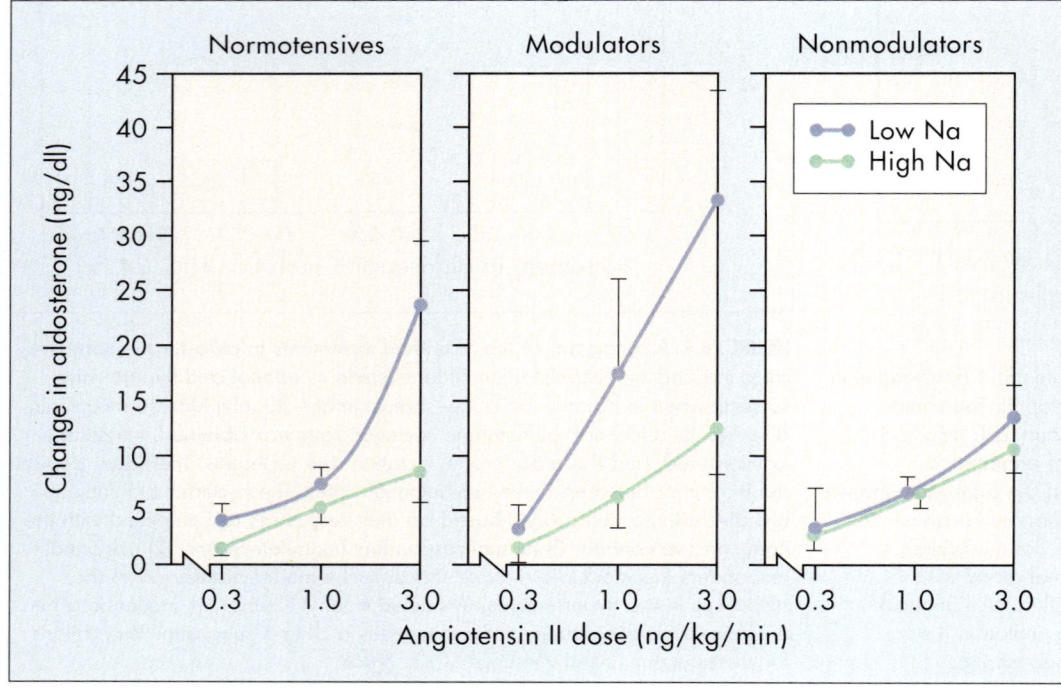

FIGURE 76.6 Plasma aldosterone responses to angiotensin II infusion during sodium restriction and loading in hypertensive and normotensive subjects. The increment in aldosterone was significantly greater ($P < 0.01$) in the modulators and the normotensive subjects when sodium was restricted. The nonmodulators showed no change in their aldosterone response to angiotensin II with changes in sodium intake. (Modified from Shoback DM, Williams GH, Moore TJ et al: Defect in the sodium-modulated tissue responsiveness to angiotensin II in essential hypertension. J Clin Invest 72:2115, 1983)

tensive process as judged by physical examination, electrocardiograms, or admission blood pressures.[65-68,72,73]

There are several additional characteristics, however, that partially distinguish the nonmodulators from other hypertensives (Table 76.2). First, as would be anticipated on the basis of the adrenal defect and the fact that the renin-angiotensin-aldosterone volume system is a closed negative feedback loop, on a sodium-restricted diet in the upright position the plasma renin activity and angiotensin II levels are higher and the plasma aldosterone levels lower in the nonmodulators than other normal- and high-renin essential hypertensive patients.[74] Second, the ability of both sodium chloride[75] and angiotensin II[76] to suppress plasma renin activity in subjects on a low-salt diet is reduced. Third, sodium/lithium countertransport in red blood cells is significantly elevated in nonmodulators compared with modulating hypertensive subjects.[77] Fourth, dopamine levels in the plasma are increased in nonmodulators, particularly on a low sodium intake, and urine dopamine excretion is fixed and does not vary with the level of sodium intake compared with what is observed in normotensive subjects and modulating hypertensive patients.[78] Finally, plasma norepinephrine levels are increased in nonmodulating patients in response to both sodium restriction and upright posture.[79]

CLASSIFICATION OF NONMODULATION

Even though there are 10 different characteristics associated with the nonmodulation phenotype (see Table 76.2), only three of them have demonstrated sufficient specificity to be useful in identifying these patients. For each of the following characteristics, there is too great an overlap between the nonmodulating and modulating hypertensive subjects: sodium/lithium countertransport in red blood cells, plasma renin activity suppression by saline or angiotensin II, plasma dopamine or norepinephrine levels, and the ratio of the increment in aldosterone to increment in renin activity in response to upright posture on a low-salt diet. The most precise way of defining "nonmodulation" is to determine the increment in aldosterone in response to a 3-ng/kg/min infusion of angiotensin II in subjects in balance on a 10-mEq sodium intake. Nearly as precise is the increment in PAH clearance (an index of renal blood flow) estimated by plasma not urine clearance techniques in a patient whose sodium intake has been changed from 10 to 200 mEq. The third technique is to assess the decrement in renal blood flow in response to a 3-ng/kg/min infusion of angiotensin II when the subject is in balance on a 200-mEq sodium intake.

Since the responses of normal subjects vary considerably with the level of sodium intake, precision in defining the level of sodium balance at the time the study is performed is of critical importance in identifying the nonmodulating patient.

HOW DOES NONMODULATION PRODUCE HYPERTENSION?

Over the past decade, it has become increasingly apparent that even in a relatively simple hypertensive model the factors responsible for the elevated blood pressure may vary under different conditions. For example, in early renal vascular hypertension resulting from unilateral renal artery stenosis, angiotensin II is certainly the prime mediator. Indeed, even in the late phases of this disease process in experimental animals, it becomes the primary mechanism if sodium intake is restricted. However, it is also apparent that other mechanisms are involved in maintaining the elevated blood pressure when these experimental animals or patients have their renin-angiotensin system suppressed by a high sodium intake.[83-85] How does this relate to the pathogenesis of essential hypertension?

Again, it is more likely to be applicable in those persons who have a derangement in their ability to handle a sodium load, as occurs in nonmodulators. In normal subjects the control of both the adrenal and the renal vasculature is dominated by angiotensin II, with changes in sodium intake reciprocally changing their responsiveness to this agent. It would, therefore, seem likely that the adrenal abnormality would be

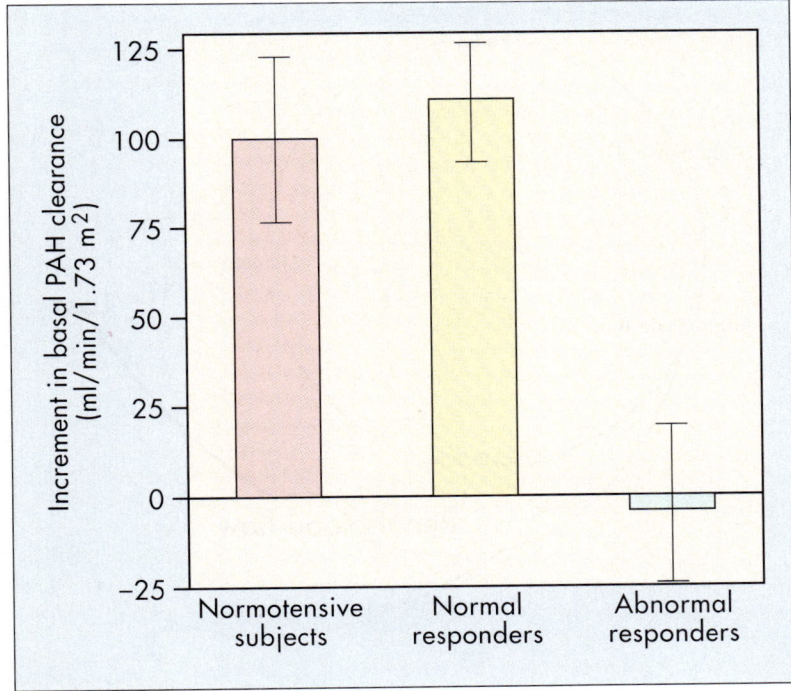

FIGURE 76.7 Effect of sodium intake on basal renal plasma flow estimated by PAH clearance (ml/min/1.73 m^2). PAH clearance was determined during a 10-mEq and a 200-mEq sodium intake. With sodium loading, PAH clearance increased significantly ($P < 0.01$, Fisher Exact Test) in normotensives and modulators (normal responders) but not in nonmodulators (abnormal responders). (Modified from Shoback DM, Williams GH, Moore TJ et al: Defect in the sodium-modulated tissue responsiveness to angiotensin II in essential hypertension. J Clin Invest 72:2115, 1983)

TABLE 76.2 CHARACTERISTICS OF THE NONMODULATING TRAIT

Trait	Corrected by Converting Enzyme Inhibitors
Decreased aldosterone response to angiotensin II on low-salt diet[73]	Yes[74]
Decreased renal blood flow response to angiotensin II on high-salt diet[73]	Yes[81]
Decreased renal blood flow response to sodium loading[73,81]	Yes[81]
Reduced sodium excretion[80]	Yes[82]
Renin suppression by angiotensin II on low-salt diet[76]	Yes[76]
Renin suppression by saline on low-salt diet[75]	No[82]
Elevated sodium/lithium countertransport in red blood cells[77]	?
Decreased increments in aldosterone divided by increments in renin in response to posture and sodium restriction[68]	?
Increased plasma dopamine levels[78]	?
Increased plasma norepinephrine levels in response to posture and salt restriction[79]	?

most evident when sodium intake is restricted, while the renal abnormality would become more evident as sodium intake increases. Thus, the expression of this abnormality is likely to be a reflection of the level of sodium intake at any given moment.

To relate these abnormalities to the elevated blood pressure, an assessment is needed of the impact of each in a situation where its function is most critical. When sodium intake is restricted in normal subjects, there is an enhancement of the adrenal response and blunting of the smooth muscle response to angiotensin II. This produces several beneficial effects: sodium retention is facilitated, the level of activation of the renin angiotensin system is less than what it would be without the enhancement of the adrenal response, and blunting of the pressor effect of the renin-angiotensin system is achieved. In nonmodulating essential hypertensive patients, the adrenal response is not enhanced. As a result, aldosterone secretion is reduced, which, as the obligatory response of this negative feedback loop, leads to an increased renin release and angiotensin II formation (Figs. 76.8 and 76.9). Thus, the sodium-restricted nonmodulator's arterial pressure will have a greater dependency on angiotensin II than the rest of the (modulating) hypertensive patients.

Several observations support this hypothesis. The nonmodulators have lower basal aldosterone and higher basal renin and/or angiotensin II levels with sodium restriction.[73,74] If the comparisons are made after the subjects are upright, the differences are accentuated.[68,86] Saralasin, a competitive antagonist of angiotensin II, reduces blood pressure in sodium-restricted, nonmodulating, high-renin essential hypertensives to a much greater degree than in other high-renin essential hypertensives.[86] This also suggests that the blood pressure of the sodium-restricted nonmodulator is more dependent on angiotensin II (Fig. 76.10).

What happens with increases in sodium intake? The renal vasculature plays a major role in producing an appropriate renal response to a sodium load by at least two mechanisms. First, glomerular filtration rate determines what sodium load is presented to the renal tubule. This rate, in part, is dependent on the renal plasma flow. Second, peritubular oncotic and hydrostatic pressure—key determinants of proximal tubular sodium reabsorption—are also regulated in part by changes in renal hemodynamics. Thus, to the degree that their renal perfusion is fixed, hemodynamic factors in these patients cannot contribute to adaptations to a high-sodium intake and require the recruitment of alternative mechanisms (see Figs. 76.8 and 76.9).[73,87] Therefore, the salt sensitivity of some normal and high-renin essential hypertensives may be an indication that they are nonmodulators.

Several findings support this hypothesis. First, the time necessary to achieve low-sodium balance is distinctly abnormal in nonmodulators. The half-time of disappearance of sodium from the urine when modulators or normotensive subjects are placed on a 10-mEq diet is approximately 24 hours. In contrast, the half-time of disappearance for the nonmodulators is nearly 50% longer (36 hours). Theoretically, this would lead to an increased sodium retention, and these persons would require longer to achieve sodium balance. There is factual support for these theoretical considerations.[80] The authors divided hypertensive patients into modulators and nonmodulators by their renal vascular response to angiotensin II. They were brought into balance on a sodium-restricted intake and then the sodium intake was increased to 200 mEq/day. Within 2 days in the modulators, sodium homeostasis

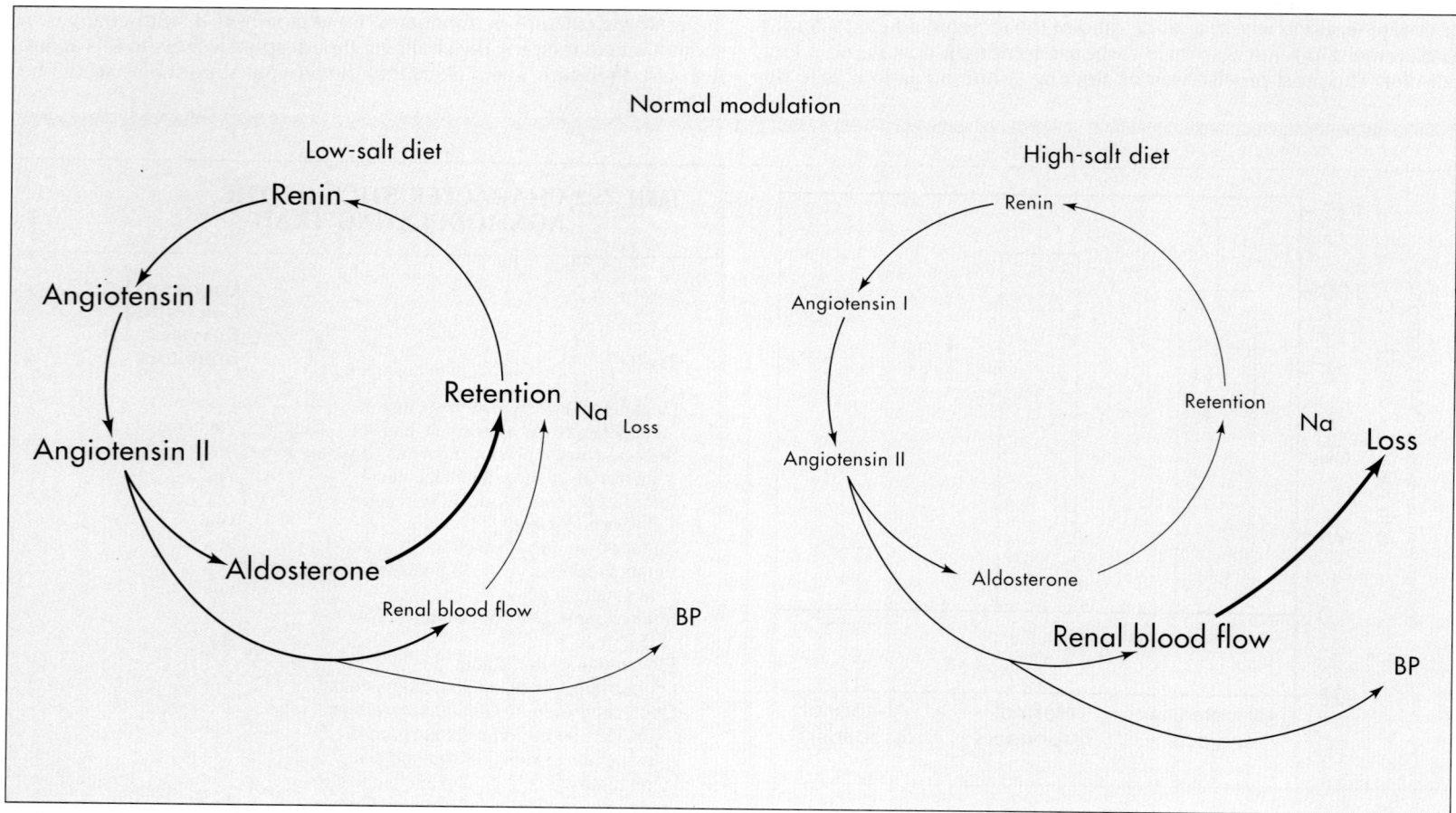

FIGURE 76.8 Schematic of the effect of changes in sodium intake on the responsiveness of the adrenal, renal vasculature, and blood pressure to angiotensin II. Note the enhanced aldosterone response to angiotensin II with sodium restriction, which modulates angiotensin II levels downward, and the increased renal blood flow on the high-salt intake, which enhances the body's ability to lose sodium. Both effects are important in preventing the rise in blood pressure with changes in sodium intake. (Modified from Williams GH, Hollenberg NK: "Sodium sensitive" essential hypertension: Emerging insights into pathogenesis and therapeutic implications. In Klahr S, Massry SG (eds): Contemporary Issues in Nephrology, 4th ed, p 303. New York, Plenum, 1985)

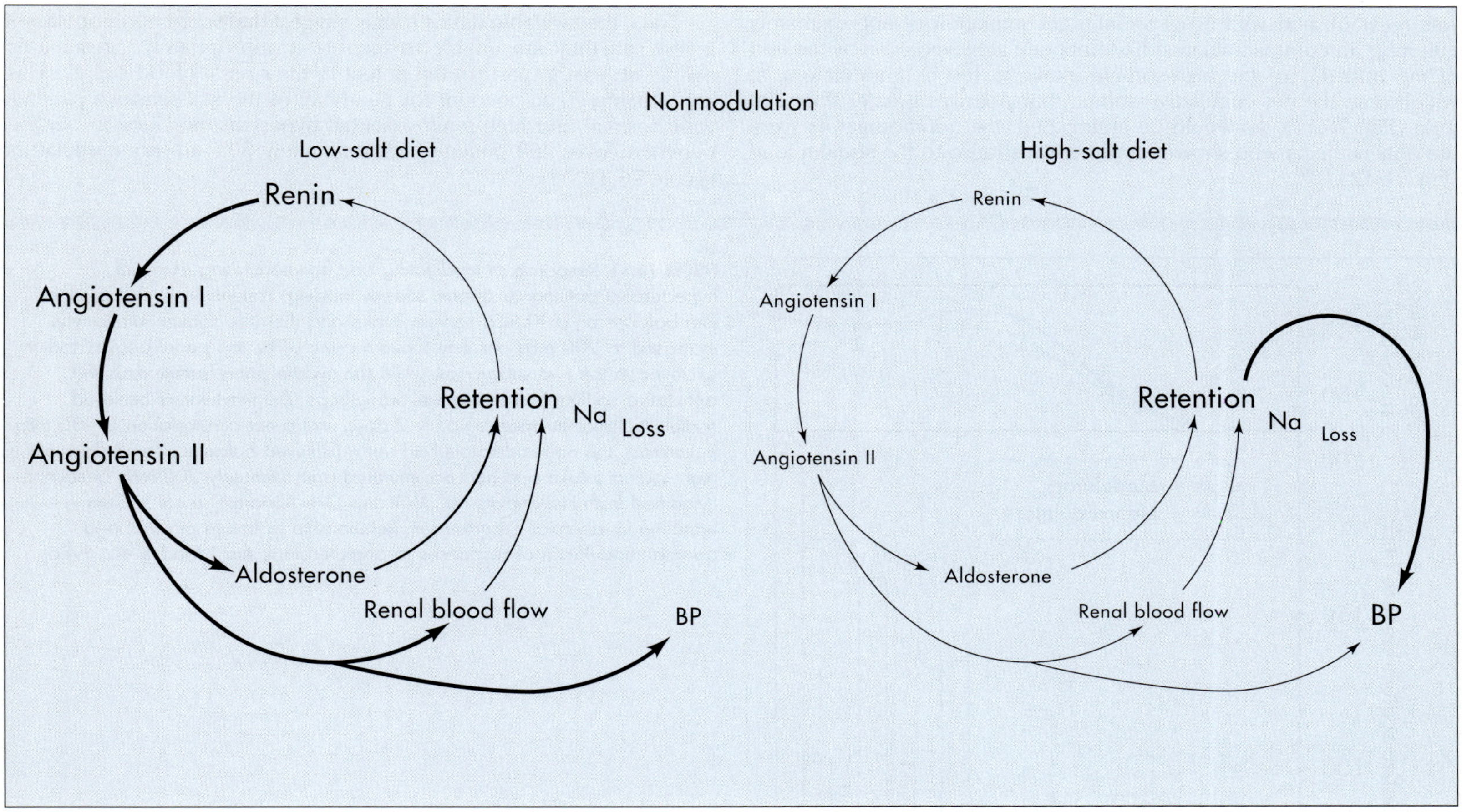

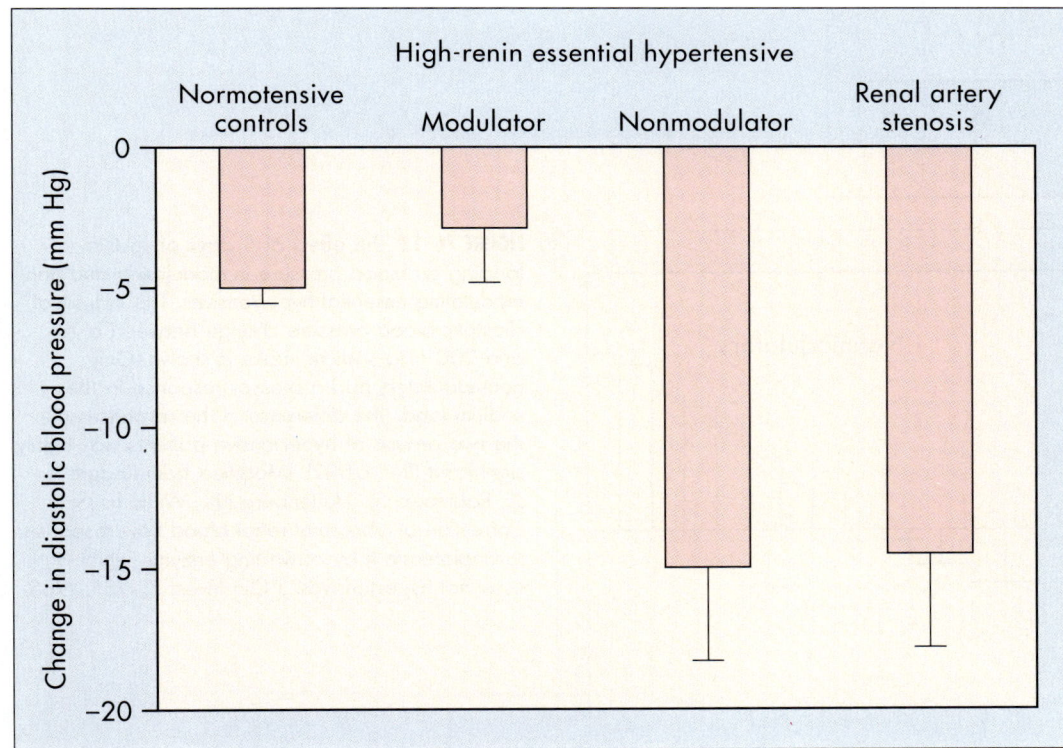

FIGURE 76.9 Schematic of consequences of nonmodulation of adrenal, renal vasculature, and pressor responses to angiotensin II with changes in sodium intake. There is a failure of the enhanced adrenal response on the low-sodium intake, resulting in an inappropriate increase in angiotensin II. The salt-loaded renal blood flow fails to increase, leading to inappropriate sodium-retentive state. Either or both conditions can result in an increased blood pressure. (Modified from Williams GH, Hollenberg NK: "Sodium sensitive" essential hypertension: Emerging insights into pathogenesis and therapeutic implications. In Klahr S, Massry SG (eds): Contemporary Issues in Nephrology, 4th ed, p 303. New York, Plenum, 1985)

FIGURE 76.10 Hypotensive response of sodium-restricted, high-renin essential hypertensive patients to saralasin, a competitive antagonist of angiotensin II. Saralasin was given in graded infusions from 0.1 to 30 μg/kg/min. The blood pressure fall was the maximum achieved during the course of the saralasin infusion. The hypertensive patients were divided into modulators (*normal ratio*) and nonmodulators (*abnormal ratio*). The depressor response to saralasin is similar in the patients with renal artery stenosis and in the nonmodulating essential hypertensives. Contrariwise, even though the renin levels were equivalently elevated in the modulating and nonmodulating essential hypertensive subgroups, the modulators had a depressor response similar to the normotensive subjects, suggesting that with sodium restriction, the blood pressure in the nonmodulators is more dependent on angiotensin II than in the modulators. (Modified from Dluhy RG, Bavli SZ, Leung FK et al: Abnormal adrenal responsiveness and angiotensin II dependency in high renin essential hypertension. J Clin Invest 64:1270, 1979)

was reestablished with a net sodium accumulation of approximately 100 mEq. In contrast, balance had not been achieved even by the end of the fifth day of the high-sodium intake in the nonmodulators, at which time the net cumulative sodium balance was greater than 200 mEq (Fig. 76.11). As would be anticipated, the nonmodulators were the only subjects who showed a pressor response to the sodium load (Fig. 76.12).[81,82]

Thus, the available data strongly suggest that when nonmodulators ingest salt they are unable to excrete it appropriately, presumably owing, at least in part, to the defect in their renal blood supply. This abnormality could account for nearly all of the salt-sensitive patients with normal- and high-renin essential hypertension, since in our experience (over 400 patients) approximately 50% are nonmodulators (Table 76.3).[88]

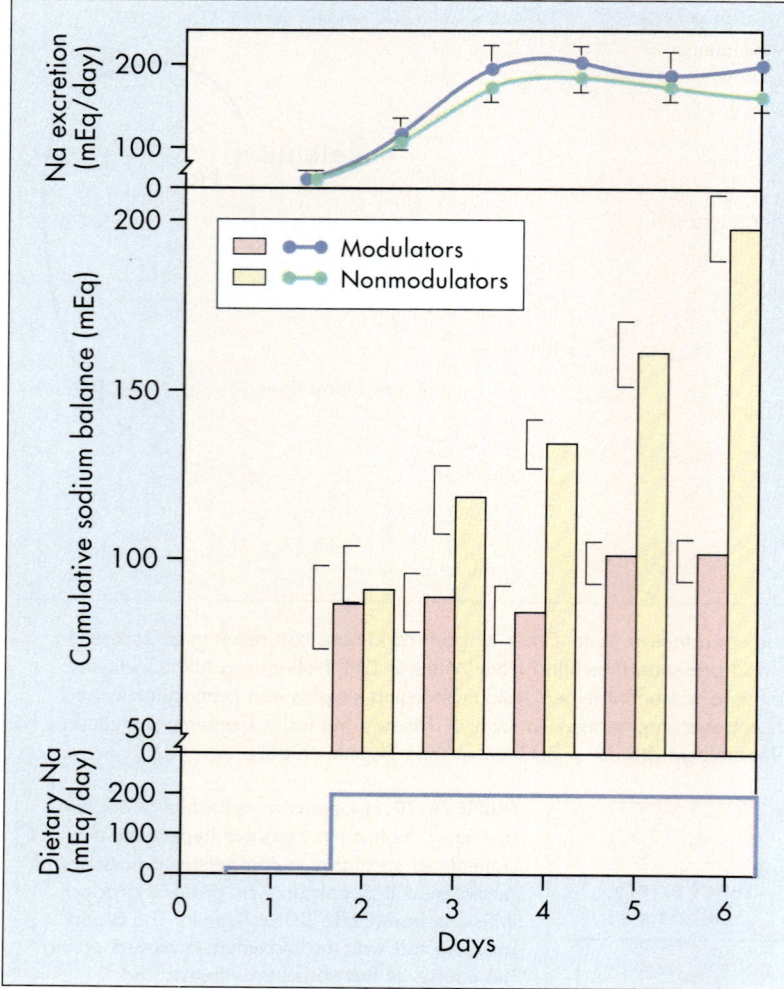

FIGURE 76.11 Response of modulating and nonmodulating essential hypertensive patients to chronic sodium loading. Patients were first brought into balance on a 10 mEq sodium intake and then the sodium intake was increased to 200 mEq per day (*bottom panel*). The top panel depicts sodium excretion in the two subgroups, while the middle panel summarizes the cumulative sodium balance in the two groups. The modulators achieved sodium balance in approximately 2 days with a net accumulation of 100 mEq. In contrast, the nonmodulators had not reachieved balance after 5 days of high-sodium intake and had accumulated approximately 200 mEq of sodium (Modified from Hollenberg NK, Williams GH: Abnormal renal sodium handling in essential hypertension: Relationship to failure of renal and adrenal modulation of responses to angiotensin II. Am J Med 81:412, 1986)

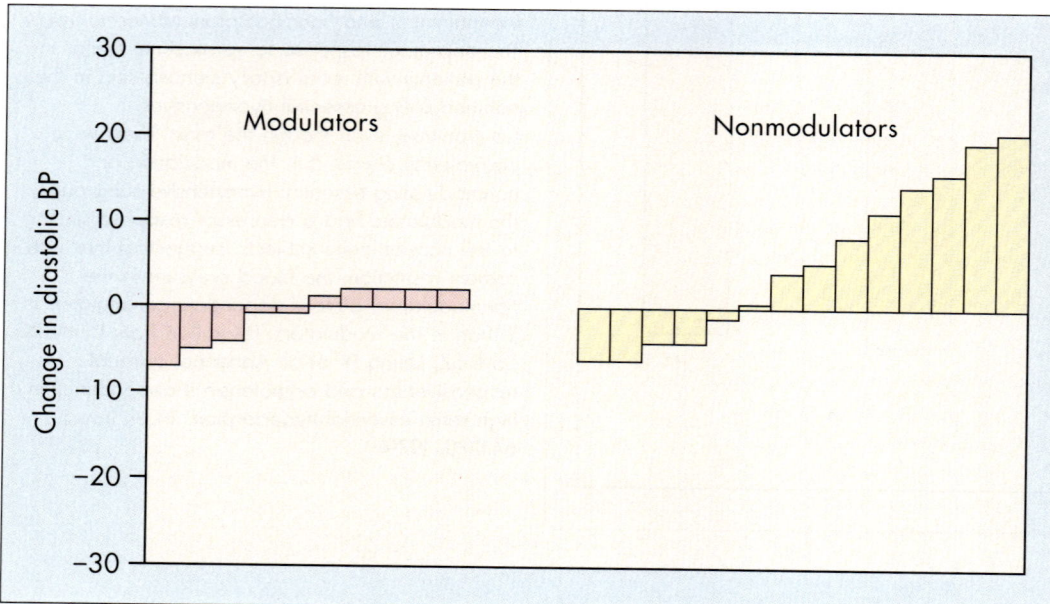

FIGURE 76.12 The effect of 5 days of sodium loading on blood pressure in modulating and non-modulating essential hypertensives. The individual diastolic blood pressure change between a 10- and 200-mEq sodium intake is shown. Only nonmodulators had a pressor response to the sodium load. The difference in the responses of the two groups of hypertensive patients was highly significant (P < 0.002). (Modified from Redgrave JE, Rabinowe SL, Hollenberg NK, Williams GH: Correction of abnormal renal blood flow response to angiotensin II by converting enzyme inhibition in essential hypertensives. J Clin Invest 75:1285, 1985)

POTENTIAL MECHANISMS UNDERLYING NONMODULATION

What could account for the absence of an effect of sodium intake on tissue responsiveness to angiotensin II? Two possibilities seem particularly appealing: differences in tissue or circulating angiotensin II levels and/or a difference in the volume status of the nonmodulating hypertensives. If the nonmodulator actually has an increase in total body sodium, one would expect, based on what occurs in normotensive subjects, a reduced adrenal responsiveness to angiotensin II. Since some studies have suggested that at least some hypertensive patients do appear to have an increase in total body sodium, this is not an unreasonable consideration.[69,70] Several lines of evidence, however, do not support this possibility. Neither the basal plasma volume nor its response to sodium restriction or loading differs among nonmodulators and other hypertensive patients.[72] Indeed, if anything, sodium restriction produces a greater fall in plasma volume among the nonmodulators, a finding that would be the opposite of what one would anticipate if the nonmodulators were volume-expanded. Second, when adrenal responsiveness to angiotensin II is assessed in normotensive patients on a high (200-mEq) and a low (10-mEq) sodium intake and then following further volume depletion with furosemide, there is a stepwise increase in the adrenal responsiveness to angiotensin II. Modulators show a similar progressive enhancement, while nonmodulators show no change with progressive volume depletion.[87] Finally, since normal subjects have an enhanced renal vascular response to angiotensin II when volume-expanded,[44,45] one would anticipate that, if volume expansion were the mechanism underlying the adrenal abnormality in nonmodulators, their renal vascular response to angiotensin II also would be enhanced. Such is not the case, thus making abnormalities in volume perception or total body sodium unlikely underlying mechanisms for nonmodulation.

An increase in the circulating angiotensin II level inappropriate for the level of sodium intake could explain the abnormal renal vascular responsiveness in the nonmodulators, accounting for both the reduced renal vascular responsiveness to infused angiotensin II on the high-sodium intake and the failure of the basal renal blood flow to increase with sodium loading. But in all of the studies cited, there were no significant differences in the circulating levels of plasma renin activity or angiotensin II in the two subgroups of hypertensive patients when sodium intake was increased. The possibility exists, however, that it is not an abnormality in circulating but intrarenal angiotensin II or in the renal angiotensin II receptor that is responsible for this apparent high angiotensin II state. Several lines of investigation support this hypothesis. First, there is the circumstantial evidence previously discussed, and secondly, there is the change in tissue responsiveness to angiotensin II after administration of converting enzyme inhibitors—pharmacologic probes that should inhibit angiotensin II generation from whatever source. Thus, the adrenal responsiveness to angiotensin II is enhanced in sodium-restricted nonmodulators but not in normotensive subjects nor modulators following converting enzyme inhibition (Fig. 76.13).[89]

Likewise, converting enzyme inhibitors modify the renal vascular responsiveness to both sodium loading and angiotensin II infusion. When hypertensive and normotensive subjects are placed on a high-sodium intake and then given a converting enzyme inhibitor for 2 days, neither modulators nor normotensive subjects show any change in the basal renal blood flow (Fig. 76.14).[81] In contrast, nonmodulators significantly increase their renal blood flow (83 ± 25 ml/min/1.73 m^2). To assess whether this renal blood flow change was a nonspecific effect of converting enzyme inhibition, rather than directly related to a reduction in angiotensin II formation, angiotensin II infusions were administered. Several studies have suggested that converting enzyme inhibitors, in addition to inhibiting angiotensin II generation, can increase the levels of vasodilators, such as bradykinins or prostaglandins.[51,52] However, bradykinins and prostaglandins blunt renal vascular responsiveness to angiotensin II. Contrariwise, if the circulating angiotensin II level is reduced prior to the addition of exogenous angiotensin II, the vascular smooth muscle responsiveness is enhanced. Nonmodulators enhance their renal vascular response to angiotensin II following con-

TABLE 76.3 FREQUENCY OF CAUSES OF SODIUM-SENSITIVE HYPERTENSION*

Cause	Frequency (%)
Primary aldosteronism	<1
Bilateral renal artery stenosis	<1
Bilateral renal parenchymal disease	3–5
Acromegaly	<1
Low-renin essential hypertension	15–25
Nonmodulating essential hypertension	35–40

* Approximately 60% of hypertensives are sodium sensitive.

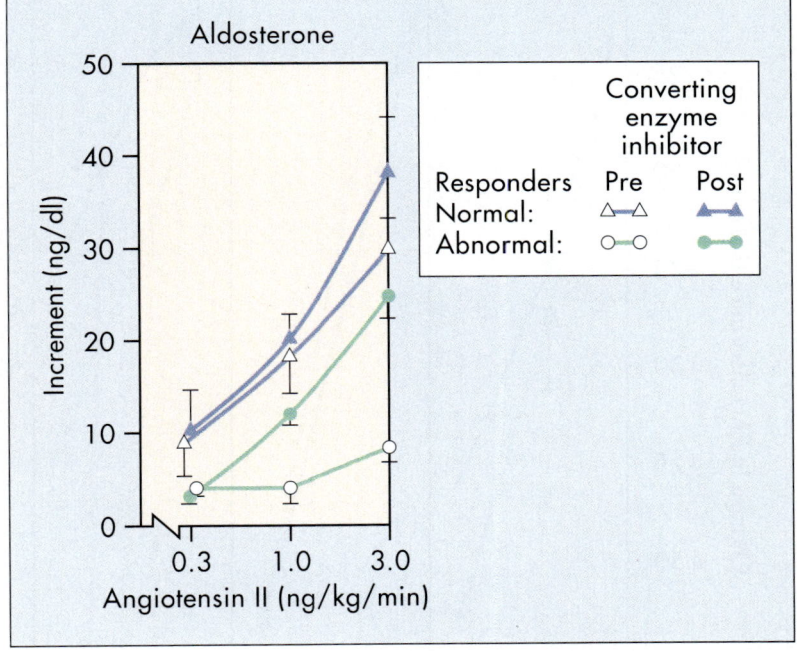

FIGURE 76.13 Effect of converting enzyme inhibition on the adrenal response to angiotensin II in hypertensive subjects. The hypertensive patients were divided into normal (modulators) and abnormal (nonmodulators) responders (mean ± SEM). Data are presented for responses both before and after the administration of a converting enzyme inhibitor (n = 31). (Modified from Taylor TT, Moore TJ, Hollenberg NK, Williams GH: Converting enzyme inhibition corrects the altered adrenal response to angiotensin II in essential hypertension. Hypertension 6:92, 1984)

verting enzyme inhibition. No significant changes in responsiveness occur in either modulators or normotensive subjects on a high sodium intake (Fig. 76.15). The enhancement in nonmodulators suggests that the increase in renal blood flow with converting enzyme inhibition indeed reflects a reduction in renal angiotensin II levels. Thus, these data would support strongly the concept that both the failure of the renal blood flow to increase with salt loading and its reduced responsiveness to angiotensin II in the high-salt state are the result of increased local concentrations of angiotensin II.

What of the other features associated with nonmodulation? Converting enzyme inhibition corrects the blunted renin suppression by angiotensin II but not by sodium chloride. The impact of converting enzyme inhibitors on the other characteristics associated with nonmodulation has not been assessed (see Table 76.2).

What does this mean to the hypertensive patient? In part, the answer becomes apparent when one examines the nonmodulator's blood pressure response to converting enzyme inhibitors when on a high-salt diet. Under these circumstances, these sodium-sensitive hypertensives should be particularly resistant to converting enzyme inhibitors, yet only the nonmodulators had a hypotensive response (Fig.

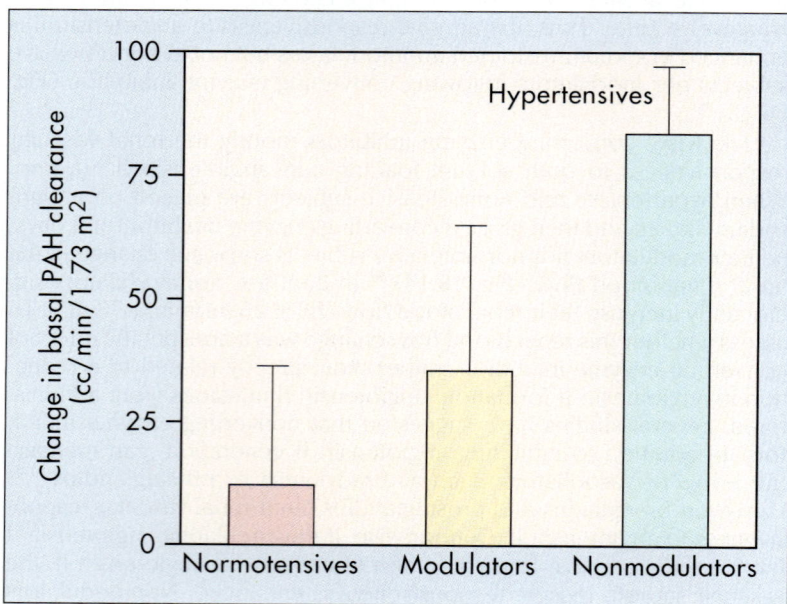

FIGURE 76.14 Renal blood flow response to a converting enzyme inhibitor (enalapril). A control renal blood flow was assessed after all subjects were in balance on a 200 mEq sodium intake. Enalapril was then administered for 48 hours and a repeat estimate of renal blood flow made. The normotensive subjects showed no significant change in renal blood flow following enalapril administration, while the nonmodulating essential hypertensives had a significant ($P < 0.01$) increase. (Modified from Redgrave JE, Rabinowe SL, Hollenberg NK, Williams GH: Correction of abnormal renal blood flow response to angiotensin II by converting enzyme inhibition in essential hypertensives. J Clin Invest 75:1285, 1985)

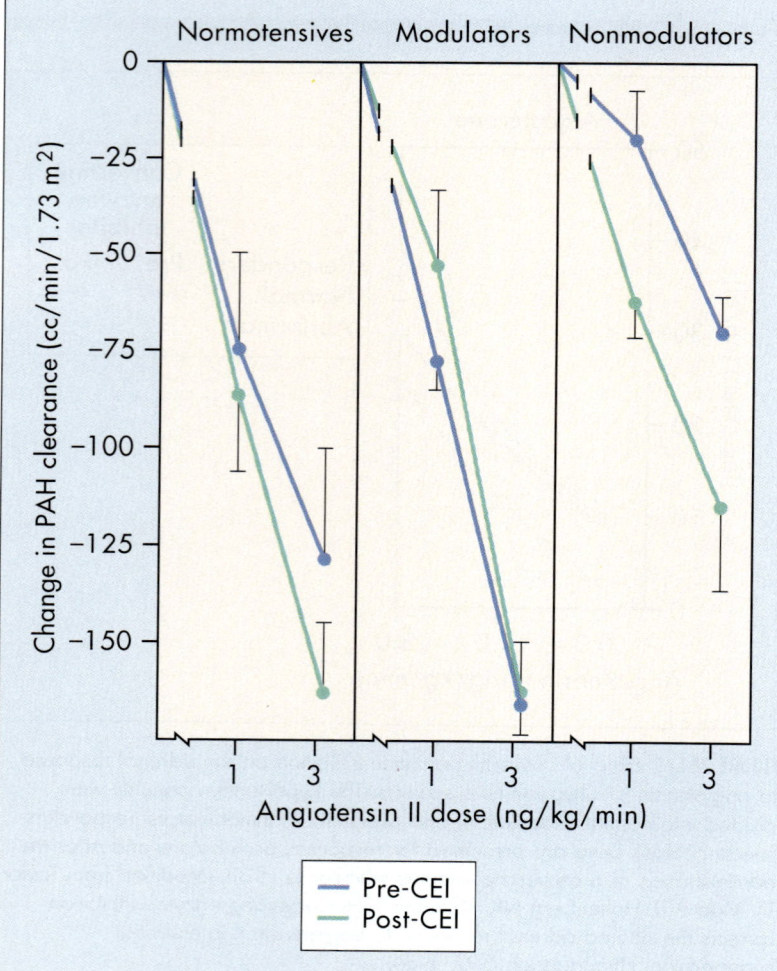

FIGURE 76.15 The effect on renal blood flow responses to angiotensin II of 2 days' administration of a converting enzyme inhibitor. Following converting enzyme inhibition (green lines), the renal blood flow response to angiotensin II was significantly enhanced ($P < 0.02$) in the nonmodulators but not in the other two groups. (Modified from Redgrave JE, Rabinowe SL, Hollenberg NK, Williams GH: Correction of abnormal renal blood flow response to angiotensin II by converting enzyme inhibition in essential hypertensives. J Clin Invest 75:1285, 1985)

76.16). Indeed, the ability of converting enzyme inhibitors to correct the underlying defects in the nonmodulators could explain a puzzling observation. Several studies have reported that approximately 50% of hypertensive patients will achieve a normal blood pressure when given a converting enzyme inhibitor, despite free access to salt. The rest require activation of the renin-angiotensin system either by salt restriction or diuretic therapy before converting enzyme inhibition is efficacious.[190] Our observations suggest that the responders to monotherapy are probably nonmodulators.

DOES NONMODULATION REFLECT A DISCRETE SUBGROUP?

What is the frequency distribution of the abnormalities that characterize nonmodulation in the essential hypertensive population? Is there really a discrete subgroup, or are the abnormalities simply part of a continuum of responsiveness, different at the extremes from that observed in the normotensive subjects? Several lines of evidence suggest that the distribution of these abnormalities is indeed bimodal in the essential hypertensive population. One of the first techniques we used to separate patients into modulators and nonmodulators was to determine their aldosterone secretory response to acute volume depletion induced by furosemide on a sodium-restricted intake, as discussed earlier (see Fig. 76.4).[67,72] The hypertensive patients divided into two distinct subgroups: In one the increment in aldosterone secretion was similar to what was observed in the normotensive subjects, while in the other little if any increase in aldosterone secretion was observed following acute volume depletion.

In 170 sodium-restricted hypertensive patients and 46 normotensive controls, the adrenal response to angiotensin II was assessed on a low sodium intake.[45,60,61,63,68,73,74,81,86,91] Again, a highly significant ($P < 0.0009$) bimodal distribution of the response of the hypertensive patients was observed. Finally, the renal plasma flow response to dietary sodium loading is also bimodal in patients with essential hypertension. Normotensive subjects have approximately a 20% increase in renal plasma flow when switched from a low to a high sodium intake. Using PAH clearance as an index of renal plasma flow, a bimodal distribution ($P < 0.01$) was observed in patients with essential hypertension (Fig. 76.17).[73,80,81,91]

HERITABILITY OF THE NONMODULATION TRAIT

Several lines of evidence suggest that the nonmodulation phenotype is not an acquired abnormality but, rather, genetically determined. First, there is a highly positive family history for hypertension in the nonmodulators.[65,66,80] Indeed, in one analysis nearly 85% of the nonmodula-

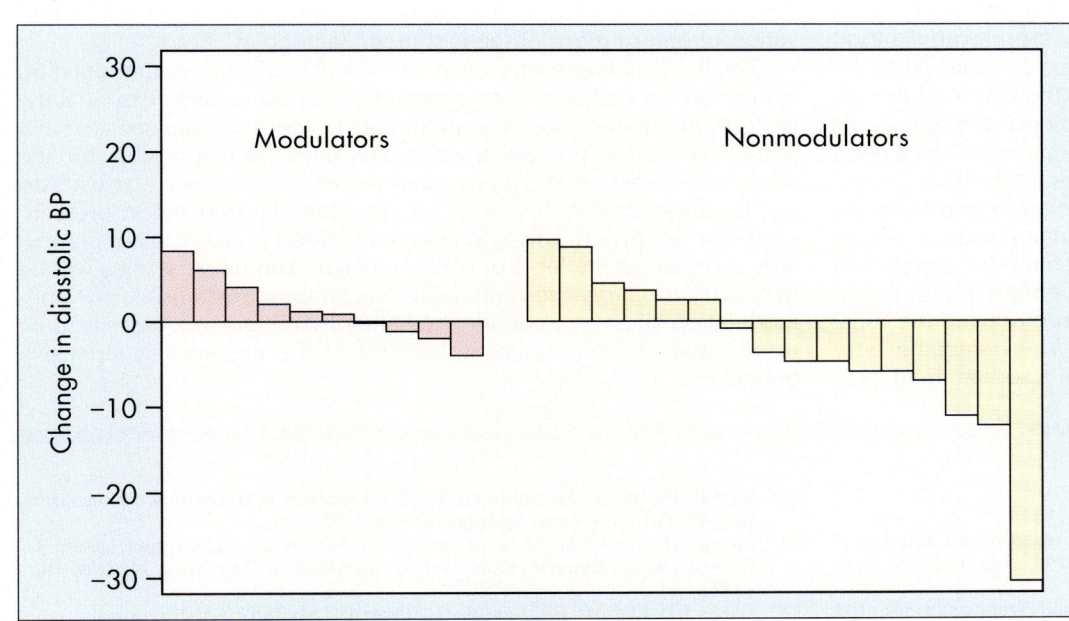

FIGURE 76.16 Individual blood pressure responses to 2 days' administration of a converting enzyme inhibitor in essential hypertensive patients on a high-sodium intake. Note that only the nonmodulators had a significant (>6 mm Hg) reduction in blood pressure after enalapril. In general, the subjects who had the greatest hypertensive response to sodium loading (shown in Fig. 76.12) also had the largest hypotensive response to converting enzyme inhibition. (Modified from Redgrave JE, Rabinowe SL, Hollenberg NK, Williams GH: Correction of abnormal renal blood flow response to angiotensin II by converting enzyme inhibition in essential hypertensives. J Clin Invest 75:1285, 1985)

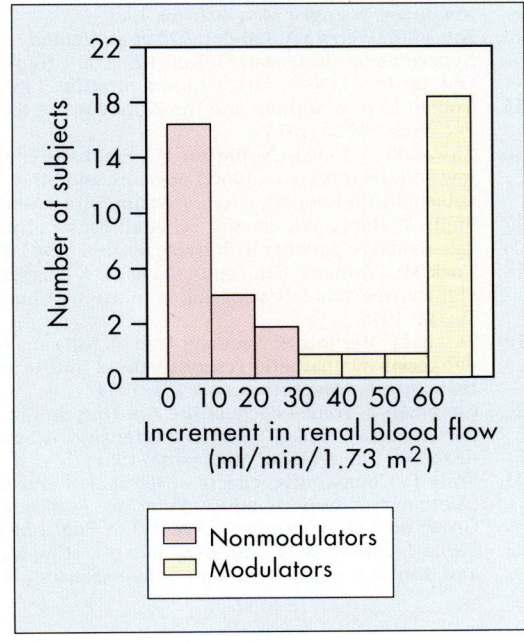

FIGURE 76.17 The effect of sodium loading on renal blood flow in 43 hypertensive subjects. Renal blood flow was estimated by PAH clearance under two sodium balance conditions: 10 mEq sodium/100 mEq potassium and 200 mEq sodium/100 mEq potassium intakes. The individual increments are shown. Normotensive subjects usually increase their renal blood flow by 15% to 20% under similar circumstances. The responses of the hypertensive patients were bimodal. In one group, the renal blood flow response was similar to that observed in normotensive subjects (modulators), and in the other, high-sodium intake had no appreciable effect on basal renal blood flow (nonmodulators). (Modified from Hollenberg NK, Williams GH: Are non-modulating patients with essential hypertension a distinct subgroup? Implications for therapy. Am J Med 79(suppl 3C):3:1985)

tors had a positive family history for hypertension, in contrast to 25% to 30% in the rest of the normal- and high-renin hypertensives. Second, the nonmodulating phenotype can be observed in normotensive subjects. In normotensive kidney donors, those with a positive family history for hypertension had a significantly lower plasma aldosterone response to a low sodium intake than did those with a negative family history, despite equivalent plasma renin activity levels, suggesting a reduced adrenal response to angiotensin II.[92] Furthermore, when normotensive subjects with a positive family history of hypertension are infused with angiotensin II, their aldosterone responses are diminished when compared with subjects with a negative family history of hypertension.[93] Finally, in families in which sibling pairs with hypertension are analyzed for the presence or absence of the nonmodulating phenotype, there is a highly significant concordance.[94] Thus, the nonmodulating phenotype is familially aggregated. Definitive proof of the inheritance of this trait will require an assessment of whether the phenotype segregates in families.

CONCLUSIONS

From the data cited in this review as well as that presented by others elsewhere (see Table 76.1), the accumulated evidence suggests that essential hypertension is not a single disease entity. It is perhaps not surprising that several factors commonly assessed in essential hypertensives appear to form a continuum. In all probability, there are a number of common homeostatic responses to the elevated blood pressure or to the mechanisms underlying the hypertension. These responses would form a continuum dependent on the extent of the underlying abnormality. For example, the actual blood pressure levels have been reported to form a continuum in most studies. Plasma renin activity in response to sodium restriction also seems to be a continuum, albeit a broader continuum than that observed in normotensive subjects. In contrast, other factors involving sodium and/or volume homeostasis are discontinuous. Indeed, they are bimodal. Nearly half of the white normal and high-renin essential hypertensive population are nonmodulators, that is, sodium intake fails to modulate the renal vascular and adrenal responses to angiotensin II. This defect, because it includes an abnormality in the renal handling of a sodium load, produces sodium-sensitive hypertension. Paradoxically, converting enzyme inhibitors, which theoretically should be relatively ineffective therapeutic agents in sodium- and/or volume-dependent hypertensives, are more effective in nonmodulators than in non-salt-sensitive essential hypertensive subjects, supporting other lines of evidence that some abnormality involving angiotensin II may underlie nonmodulation. Intriguingly, preliminary data suggest the nonmodulating trait is inherited, raising the possibility that early intervention could potentially prevent the development of hypertension.

Does this evolving theory account for all abnormalities in patients with essential hypertension? The answer is clearly no. We believe that other subgroups exist in the "modulating" hypertensive subset, who appear to be normal from the perspective of the renin-angiotensin system. Nonmodulation, however, may explain why some essential hypertensives have abnormalities in other sodium- and/or volume-regulating systems. This is based on the assumption that if the major system used by the body to adapt to varying sodium loads is defective, then secondary systems would be activated in order to restore sodium and/or volume homeostasis. Thus, it would not be surprising if nonmodulators have increased levels of a variety of natriuretic factors including ouabain-like natriuretic factors, atrial natriuretic peptide, or dopamine. While each of these would presumably facilitate sodium excretion, a price would be extracted in that tissue responsiveness to vasoconstrictors would be altered, as noted by others.[30,31,95,96] Furthermore, nonmodulators might also have abnormalities in erythrocyte sodium transport activity as a primary process or secondary to the activation of one or more of the natriuretic factors.[36,97-99]

Finally, it is important again to reemphasize that nonmodulation cannot be the pathogenic mechanism in all patients with essential hypertension, indeed, not even in all patients with sodium-sensitive hypertension. Other primary mechanisms must be responsible for the sodium sensitivity and hypertension in salt-sensitive persons who do not have the modulating defect and to the elevated blood pressure itself in those hypertensives in whom the blood pressure is not particularly sensitive to the level of sodium intake. Additional studies will be necessary to clarify the underlying mechanisms responsible for nonmodulation and also to define the pathophysiologic processes leading to elevated blood pressure in the rest of the essential hypertensive population.

REFERENCES

1. Brown JG, Lever AF, Robertson JIS et al: Blood pressure and sodium: A personal view. In Genest J et al (eds): Hypertension, 2nd ed, pp 632–645. New York, McGraw Hill, 1983
2. Chalmers JP, West MJ: The nervous system and the pathogenesis of essential hypertension. In Robertson JIS (ed): Handbook of Hypertension: Clinical Aspects of Essential Hypertension, pp 64–96. Amsterdam, Elsevier, 1983
3. de Wardener HE, MacGregor GA: The relation of a circulating sodium transport inhibitor to essential hypertension. In Kidney in Hypertension, pp 1–14. Boston, Martinus Nijhoff Publishing, 1984
4. Doyle AE: Personal views on hypertension. In Genest J et al: Hypertension, 2nd ed, pp 659–666. New York, McGraw Hill, 1983
5. Dustan HP: Personal views on the mechanisms of hypertension. In Genest J et al: Hypertension, 2nd ed, pp 667–678, New York, McGraw Hill, 1983
6. Folkow B: Personal views on the mechanisms of primary hypertension. In Genest J et al: Hypertension, 2nd ed, pp 646–658. New York, McGraw Hill, 1983
7. Frohlich ED, Musserli FH, Re RN, Dunn RG: Mechanisms controlling arterial pressure. In Pathophysiology: Altered Regulatory Mechanisms in Disease, 3rd ed, pp 75–82. Philadelphia, JB Lippincott, 1984
8. Genest J: Personal views on the mechanisms of essential hypertension. In Genest J et al: Hypertension, 2nd ed, pp 559–614. New York, McGraw Hill, 1983
9. Guyton AC, Hall JE, Lohmeier TE et al: Role of the kidney and volume control and the pathogenesis of hypertension. In Robertson JIS (ed): Handbook of Hypertension: Clinical Aspects of Essential Hypertension, pp 216–238. Amsterdam, Elsevier, 1983
10. Kaplan MM: Systemic hypertension: Mechanisms and diagnosis. In Braunwald E (ed): Heart Disease: A Textbook of Cardiovascular Medicine 2nd ed, pp 849–901. Philadelphia, WB Saunders, 1984
11. Korner PI: Does hypertension develop through long-term autoregulation? In Laragh JH, Buhler FR, Seldon DW (eds): Frontiers in Hypertension Research, pp 148–156. New York, Springer Verlag, 1981
12. Laragh JH: Personal views on the mechanisms of essential hypertension. In Genest J et al: Hypertension, 2nd ed, pp 615–631. New York, McGraw Hill, 1983
13. Garay RP, Elghozi J-L, Dagher G, Mayer P: Laboratory distinction between essential and secondary hypertension by measurement of erythrocyte cation fluxes. N Engl J Med 302:769, 1980
14. Safar ME, Weiss YA, London GM et al: Hemodynamic changes in mild early hypertension. In Onesti G, Kim KE (eds): Hypertension in the Young and Old, pp 19–27. New York, Grune & Stratton, 1981
15. Tobian L: How sodium and the kidney relate to the hypertensive arteriole. Fed Proc 33:138, 1974
16. Kawasaki T, Delea CS, Bartter FC, Smith H: The effect of high-sodium and low-sodium intakes on blood pressure and other related variables in human subjects with idiopathic hypertension. Am J Med 64:193, 1978
17. Fujita T, Henry WL, Bartter FC et al: Factors influencing blood pressure in salt-sensitive patients with hypertension. Am J Med 69:334, 1980
18. Tuck ML, Williams GH, Dluhy RG et al: A delayed suppression of the renin-aldosterone axis following saline infusion in human hypertension. Circ Res 39:711, 1976
19. Skrabal F, Herholz H, Neumayr M et al: Salt sensitivity in humans is linked to enhanced sympathetic responsiveness and to enhanced proximal tubular reabsorption. Hypertension 6:152, 1984
20. Chapman B: Some effects of the rice-fruit diet in patients with essential hypertension. In Bell ET (ed): Hypertension, A Symposium, pp 504–516. Minneapolis, University of Minnesota, 1951
21. Freis E: Comparative effects of ticrynafen and hydrochlorothiazide in the treatment of hypertension (Veterans Administration Cooperative Study Group on Antihypertensive Agents). N Engl J Med 301:293, 1979
22. Parijs J, Joossens JV, Van der Linden L et al: Moderate sodium restriction and diuretics in the treatment of hypertension. Am Heart J 85:22, 1973

23. Laragh JH: Vasoconstriction-volume analysis for understanding and treating hypertension. The use of renin and aldosterone profiles. Am J Med 55:261, 1973
24. Bell ET: Renal vascular disease in diabetes mellitus. Diabetes 2:376, 1953
25. Kisch ES, Dluhy RG, Williams GH: Enhanced aldosterone response to angiotensin II in human hypertension. Circ Res 38:502, 1976
26. Wisgerhof M, Brown RD: Increased adrenal sensitivity to angiotensin II in low-renin essential hypertension. J Clin Invest 63:1456, 1979
27. Marks AD, Marks DB, Kanefsky TM et al: Enhanced adrenal responsiveness to angiotensin II in patients with low renin essential hypertension. J Clin Endocrinol Metab 48:266, 1980
28. Porter GA: Chronology of the sodium hypothesis and hypertension. Ann Intern Med 98 (Part 2):720, 1983
29. Guyton AC, Coleman TG, Norman RA Jr et al: Overall circulatory control in hypertension. Aust NZ J Med 6:72, 1976
30. Overbeck HW, Pamnani MB, Akera T et al: Depressed function of a ouabain-sensitive sodium-potassium pump in blood vessels from renal hypertensive dogs. Circ Res 38(suppl 2):48, 1976
31. Haddy FJ, Pamnani MB, Clough DL: Humoral factors and the sodium-potassium pump in volume expanded hypertension. Life Sci 24:2105, 1979
32. Buckalew VM Jr, Gruber KA: Natriuretic hormone. In Epstein MP (ed): The Kidney in Liver Disease, 2nd ed. New York, Elsevier, 1983
33. Blaustein MP, Hamlyn JM: Role of a natriuretic factor in essential hypertension: An hypothesis. Ann Intern Med 98 (part 2):785, 1983
34. Canessa M: The polymorphism of red cell Na and K transport in essential hypertension: Findings, controversies, and perspectives. Sixth International Conference on Red Cell Metabolism. New York, Alan R Liss, Inc., 1984
35. Poston L, Sewell RB, Wilkinson SP et al: Evidence for a circulating sodium transport inhibitor in essential hypertension. Br Med J 282:847, 1981
36. Woods JW, Parker JC, Watson BS: Perturbation of sodium-lithium countertransport in red cells. N Engl J Med 308:1258, 1983
37. Sokabe H: Physiology of the renal effects of angiotensin. Kidney Int 6:263, 1974
38. Sawyer WH, Blair-West JR, Simpson PA, Sawyer MK: Renal responses of Australian lungfish to vasotoxin, angiotensin II and NaCl infusion. Am J Physiol 231:593, 1976
39. Berne HA: Hormones and endocrine glands of fishes. Science 158:455, 1967
40. Vinson GP, Whitehouse BJ, Goddard C, Sibley CP: Comparative and evolutionary aspects of aldosterone secretion and zona glomerulosa function. J Endocrinol 81:5P, 1979
41. Sokabe H, Mizogame S, Sato A: Role of renin in adaption to sea water in eruyhaline fishes. Jpn J Pharmacol 18:332, 1968
42. Boyd GW, Adamson AR, Arnold M et al: The role of angiotensin II in the control of aldosterone in man. Clin Sci 42:91, 1972
43. Steele JM Jr, Neusy AJ, Lowenstein G: The effects of des-Asp^1-angiotensin II on blood pressure, plasma aldosterone concentration, and plasma renin activity in the rabbit. Circ Res 38(suppl 2):113, 1976
44. Oelkers W, Brown JJ, Fraser R et al: Sensitization of the adrenal cortex to angiotensin II in sodium-deplete man. Circ Res 34:69, 1974
45. Hollenberg NK, Chenitz WR, Adams DF, Williams GH: Reciprocal influence of salt intake on adrenal glomerulosa and renal vascular responses to angiotensin II in normal man. J Clin Invest 54:34, 1974
46. Williams GH, Hollenberg NK, Brown C, Mersey JH: Adrenal responses to pharmacological interruption of the renin-angiotensin system in sodium restricted normal man. J Clin Endocrinol Metab 47:725, 1978
47. Swartz SL, Williams GH, Hollenberg NK et al: Primacy of the renin-angiotensin system in mediating the aldosterone response to sodium restriction. J Clin Endocrinol Metab 50:1071, 1980
48. Kibrough HM, Vaughan ED, Carey RM, Ayers CR: Effect of intrarenal angiotensin II blockade on renal function in conscious dogs. Circ Res 40:174, 1977
49. Hollenberg NK, Swartz SL, Passan DR, Williams GH: Increased glomerular filtration rate following converting enzyme inhibition in essential hypertension. N Engl J Med 301:9, 1979
50. Hollenberg NK, Williams GH, Burger B et al: Blockade and stimulation of renal, adrenal, and vascular angiotensin II receptors with 1-sar 8-ala angiotensin II in normal man. J Clin Invest 57:39, 1976
51. Williams GH, Hollenberg NK: Accentuated vascular and endocrine response to SQ 20881 in hypertension. N Engl J Med 297:184, 1977
52. Hollenberg NK, Meggs LG, Williams GH et al: Sodium intake and renal responses to captopril in normal man and in essential hypertension. Kidney 20:240, 1981
53. Strewler GJ, Hinrichs KJ, Guiod LR, Hollenberg NK: Sodium intake and vascular smooth muscle responsiveness to norepinephrine and angiotensin in the rabbit. Circ Res 31:758, 1972
54. Devynck MA, Meyer P: Angiotensin receptors in vascular tissue. Am J Med 61:758, 1976
55. Gunther S, Gimbrone MA Jr, Alexander RW: Regulation by angiotensin II of its receptors in resistance blood vessels. Nature 287:230, 1980
56. Douglas J, Catt KJ: Regulation of angiotensin II receptors in the rat adrenal cortex by dietary electrolytes. J Clin Invest 58:834, 1976
57. Aguilera G, Catt K: Regulation of aldosterone secretion by the renin-angiotensin system during sodium restriction in rats. Proc Natl Acad Sci USA 75:4057, 1978
58. Platia MP, Catt KJ, Hodgen GD, Aguilera G: Angiotensin II receptor regulation during altered sodium intake in primates. Hypertension (in press)
59. Williams GH, Hollenberg NK, Braley LM: Influence of sodium intake on vascular and adrenal angiotensin II receptors. Endocrinology 98:1343, 1976
60. Dawson-Hughes BF, Moore TJ, Dluhy RG et al: Plasma angiotensin concentration regulates vascular but not adrenal responsiveness to restriction of sodium intake in normal man. Clin Sci 61:527, 1981
61. Shoback DM, Williams GH, Hollenberg NK et al: Endogenous angiotensin II as determinant of sodium modulated changes in tissue responsiveness to angiotensin II in normal man. J Clin Endocrinol Metab 51:764, 1983
62. Haning R, Tait SAS, Tait JF: In vitro effects of ACTH, angiotensins, serotonin and potassium on steroid output and conversion of corticosterone to aldosterone by isolated adrenal cell. Endocrinology 87:1160, 1970
63. Gordon MB, Moore TJ, Dluhy RG, Williams GH: Dopaminergic modulation of aldosterone responsiveness to angiotensin II with changes in sodium intake. J Clin Endocrinol Metab 56:340, 1983
64. Carey RM, Drake CR Jr: Dopamine selectively inhibits aldosterone responses to angiotensin II in humans. Hypertension 8:399, 1986
65. Hollenberg NK, Merrill JP: Intrarenal perfusion in the young 'essential' hypertensive: A subpopulation resistant to sodium restriction. Trans Assoc Am Physicians 83:93, 1970
66. Hollenberg NK, Borucki LJ, Adams DF: The renal vasculature in early essential hypertension: Evidence for pathogenetic role. Medicine 57:167, 1978
67. Williams GH, Rose LI, Dluhy RG et al: Abnormal responsiveness of the renin-aldosterone system to acute stimulation in patients with essential hypertension. Ann Intern Med 72:317, 1970
68. Moore TJ, Williams GH, Dluhy RG et al: Altered renin-angiotensin-aldosterone relationships in normal renin essential hypertension. Circ Res 41:167, 1977
69. Tarazi RC, Frohlich ED, Dustan HP: Plasma volume in men with hypertension. New Engl J Med 278:762, 1968
70. Julius S, Pascual AV, Reilly K, London R: Abnormalities of plasma volume in borderline hypertension. Arch Intern Med 127:116, 1971
71. Streeten DHP, Schletter FE, Clift GV et al: Studies of the renin-angiotensin-aldosterone system in patients with hypertension and in normal subjects. Am J Med 46:844, 1969
72. Williams GH, Tuck ML, Sullivan JM et al: Parallel adrenal and renal abnormalities in the young patient with essential hypertension. Am J Med 72:907, 1982
73. Shoback DM, Williams GH, Moore TJ et al: Defect in the sodium-modulated tissue responsiveness to angiotensin II in essential hypertension. J Clin Invest 72:2115, 1983
74. Taylor TT, Moore TJ, Hollenberg NK, Williams GH: Converting enzyme inhibition corrects the altered adrenal response to angiotensin II in essential hypertension. Hypertension 6:92, 1984
75. Rabinowe SL, Redgrave JE, Shoback DM et al: Renin suppression by saline is blunted in non-modulating essential hypertension. Hypertension 10:404, 1987
76. Seely EW, Moore TJ, Rogacz S et al: Angiotensin-modulated renin suppression is altered in nonmodulating hypertension. Hypertension 13:31, 1989
77. Redgrave J, Canessa M, Gleason R et al: Red blood cell lithium-sodium countertransport in nonmodulating essential hypertension. Hypertension 13:721, 1989
78. Gordon MS, Steunkel CA, Conlin PR et al: The role of dopamine in non-modulating hypertension. J Clin Endocrinol Metab 69:426, 1989
79. Conlin PR, Gleason RE, Williams GH: Altered aldosterone and norepinephrine response to posture in nonmodulating hypertension. Hypertension 1990 (in press)
80. Hollenberg NK, Williams GH: Abnormal renal sodium handling in essential hypertension: Relationship to failure of renal and adrenal modulation of responses to angiotensin II. Am J Med 81:412, 1986
81. Redgrave JE, Rabinowe SL, Hollenberg NK, Williams GH: Correction of abnormal renal blood flow response to angiotensin II by converting enzyme inhibition in essential hypertensives. J Clin Invest 75:1285, 1985
82. Rystedt L, Williams GH, Hollenberg NK: The renal and endocrine response to saline infusion in essential hypertension. Hypertension 8:217, 1986
83. Brunner HR, Kirshman JD, Dealey JE, Laragh JH: Hypertension of renal origin: Evidence for two different mechanisms. Science 174:1344, 1971
84. Gavras H, Brunner HR, Vaughn ED Jr, Laragh JL: Angiotensin-sodium interaction in blood pressure maintenance of renal hypertensive and normotensive rats. Science 180:1369, 1973
85. Barger AC: Experimental renovascular hypertension. Hypertension 1:477, 1979
86. Dluhy RG, Bavli SZ, Leung RK et al: Abnormal adrenal responsiveness and angiotensin II dependency in high renin essential hypertension. J Clin Invest 64:1270, 1979
87. Gordon MB, Dluhy RG, Moore TJ, Hollenberg NK: Abnormal sodium-mediated changes in target tissue responsiveness to angiotensin II in essential hypertensives is not due to differences in total body sodium. Presented before the Endocrine Society Annual Meeting, 1982
88. Williams GH, Hollenberg NK: Abnormal adrenal and renal responsiveness to angiotensin II in essential hypertension. In Edwards CRW, Carey RM (eds): Essential Hypertension as an Endocrine Disease, pp 184–211. London, Butterworth & Co, 1985
89. Dluhy RG, Smith K, Taylor T et al: Prolonged converting enzyme inhibition in

nonmodulating hypertension. Hypertension 13:371, 1989
90. Veterans Administration Cooperative Study Group on Antihypertensive Agents. Racial differences in response to low-dose captopril are abolished by the addition of hydrochlorothiazide. Br J Clin Pharmacol 14:97S, 1982
91. Williams GH, Hollenberg NK: Are nonmodulating essential hypertensives a distinct subgroup? Implications for therapy. Am J Med 79:3, 1985
92. Blackshear JL, Garnic D, Williams GH et al: Exaggerated renal vasodilator response to calcium entry blockade in first-degree relatives of essential hypertensive subjects. Hypertension 9:384, 1987
93. Beretta-Piccoli C, Pusterla C, Stadler P, Weidmann P: Blunted aldosterone responsiveness to angiotensin II in normotensive subjects with familial predisposition to essential hypertension. J Hypertens 6:57, 1988
94. Lifton RP, Hopkins PN, Williams RR et al: Evidence for heritability of nonmodulating essential hypertension. Hypertension 13:884, 1989
95. Gruber KA, Whitaker JM, Buckalew VM Jr. Endogenous digitalis-like substance in plasma of volume-expanded dogs. Nature 287:743, 1980
96. Poston L, Sewell RB, Wilkinson SP et al: Evidence for a circulating sodium transport inhibitor in essential hypertension. Br Med J 282:847, 1981
97. Canessa M, Adragna N, Solomon HS et al: Increased sodium/lithium countertransport in red cells of patients with essential hypertension. N Engl J Med 302:772, 1980
98. Cooper R, Miller T, Trevisan M et al: Family history of hypertension and red cell cation transport in high school students. J Hypertens 1:145, 1983
99. Canessa M, Cusi D, Brugnara C, Tosteson DC: Furosemide-sensitive Na fluxes in human red cells: Equilibrium properties and net uphill extrusion. J Gen Physiol 82:28, 1983

EVALUATION AND MANAGEMENT OF THE PATIENT WITH ESSENTIAL HYPERTENSION

CHAPTER 77 VOLUME 2

Edward D. Frohlich

As recently as 1975, deaths from cardiovascular diseases accounted for over half (54%) of all deaths in the United States. Although hypertension accounted for only 2% of these deaths, it is clear that it is the major treatable risk factor underlying heart attacks and strokes that collectively account for 85% of all cardiovascular deaths.[1] Today, the death rate from cardiovascular diseases has fallen to 50% of all deaths; and this, in no small way, may be attributed to greater awareness and vigor in antihypertensive treatment programs.

The incidence rates for hypertension in the United States have increased dramatically over the past 15 years—not because of any real increase in the numbers of potential patients but because definitions have changed based on new knowledge and experience. Thus, based on National Health Survey data generated in the 1960s, there were 23 million Americans in 1970 with diastolic pressure exceeding 104 mm Hg who required medical attention. With newer data in the 1970s the estimates were increased to 35 million. The reports from the Hypertension Detection and Follow-Up Program (HDFP) permitted the conclusion that 58 million Americans had diastolic pressure greater than 89 mm Hg.[2,3] These data may provoke discussion concerning the meaning of these numbers and whether all of these patients require pharmacotherapy.[4] These questions do not detract from the facts that hypertension is a major national health problem demanding intensive and continuous medical attention; that the higher the diastolic or systolic pressure the greater the risk; and that patients whose diastolic pressure remains over 90 mm Hg are at greater risk. Whether all of these patients require pharmacologic therapy is another question yet to be resolved. Nevertheless, this supports the reason for pursuing specific nonpharmacologic treatment interventions that may be used for patients with high normal pressures (*i.e.*, diastolic pressures of 85 mm Hg through 89 mm Hg), those with mild hypertension not necessarily receiving drugs (*e.g.*, 90 mm Hg through 94 mm Hg), or even those patients receiving antihypertensive drug therapy.[5]

If one accepts these conservative generalizations, what is their justification? As indicated, no matter what the source of information (*i.e.*, Society of Actuaries, National Center for Health Statistics, the Pooling Project, the Framingham Heart Study, and so forth), the higher the systolic *or* diastolic arterial pressures, the greater the cardiovascular morbidity *and* mortality. These data and others have shown clearly that, in this country, the prevalence of hypertension increases with the age of the population as does the height of systolic and diastolic pressure (for men and women whether of the black or white race). Moreover, hypertension and its major complications are more prevalent in blacks of any age. In addition, the higher the pressure the greater the number of "all events" and deaths from cardiac disease: congestive heart failure, angina pectoris, myocardial infarction, and sudden death. While hypertension is the most powerful risk factor underlying development of heart attacks and strokes, other risk factors including cigarette smoking, obesity, diabetes mellitus, hypercholesterolemia, and hyperuricemia increase the chances for these catastrophic events.[1]

The encouraging news is that over this past decade the national health data have demonstrated a 50% reduction in death rates from stroke.[6] Reports confirm these trends and findings: the curve still descends, demonstrating reduction in morbidity and mortality for all cardiovascular diseases (especially stroke and coronary heart disease) from the 54% figure in 1975 to 50% at present. Clearly, there is no one specific factor that can account for this reduction, but improved and generally available therapy for patients with elevated arterial pressure is one of the major attributable factors. Other factors include reduced cigarette consumption, improved dietary habits, awareness of the wisdom of weight control and exercise programs, mobile and coronary care units, and new and improved cardiovascular pharmacologic agents (including the antihypertensive, antiarrhythmic, diuretic, and myocardial-preserving agents).

More than 12 years have passed since the Veterans Administration Cooperative Study Group published its dramatic and exciting findings concerning the treatment of hypertension.[7,8] These findings showed that pharmacologic treatment of hypertension results in reduced cardiovascular morbidity and mortality. In that series of studies there was a significant decrease in deaths directly related to and associated with hypertension; in terminating study events from clinical problems; in treatment failures directly attributable to hypertension (*i.e.*, pressures rose to levels demanding therapy); and in nonterminating morbid events.

This dramatic series of studies was first related to patients with diastolic pressure greater than 130 mm Hg, then to patients whose initial diastolic pressure was between 115 mm Hg and 129 mm Hg, and, finally, to patients whose initial diastolic pressure was between 90 mm Hg and 114 mm Hg. As a result, the High Blood Pressure Education Program (HBPEP) was established, receiving voluntary support from all related medical specialties, health-care professional groups, and representatives from the general public. Over the ensuing 15 years and associated with the increased enlightenment of all concerned was the significant and progressive reduction in cardiovascular mortality in the United States just described.

Unfortunately, the third VA cooperative study alluded to had too few patients whose initial diastolic blood pressure was between the levels of 90 mm Hg and 105 mm Hg, and for this reason the Joint National Committee of the HBPEP recommended that pharmacologic treatment should be pursued in all persons whose diastolic pressure exceeded 104 mm Hg.[9] At that time it was estimated that there were 23 million Americans who would derive benefit from antihypertensive therapy. The number of patients who could benefit from treatment is presently estimated to approach 60 million. This is based on a redefinition of hypertension to include patients with mild hypertension (i.e., those patients whose diastolic pressure is between 90 mm Hg and 104 mm Hg).[5]

The HDFP involved 14 major centers that screened over 187,000 Americans, resulting in the assignment of approximately 11,000 persons with essential hypertension to one of two treatment groups: The Referred Care Group received the fine medical care that is provided to patients in the community by their practicing physicians; the Stepped-Care Group received intensive medical care and follow-up by a specialized hypertension treatment team at the 14 hypertension centers.[2,3] It is important to remember that when this study was established, the community physicians were advised to treat hypertension with pharmacotherapeutic agents if diastolic pressure exceeded 104 mm Hg. Nevertheless, both groups demonstrated effective reduction in arterial pressure to levels below 90 mm Hg over the study's 5-year period. However, those patients in the Stepped-Care Group demonstrated significantly greater reduction in diastolic pressure than those in the Referred Care Group, and this reduction was associated with a significantly lesser overall and cardiovascular mortality.

The implications of the HDFP study were clear: Treatment of hypertension, mild or otherwise, with antihypertensive drugs is justified and could be expected to reduce morbidity and mortality associated with hypertension. As a result, it was determined that there were almost 60 million Americans who might benefit from treatment. This increase in numbers reflects the large number of patients with "mild essential hypertension" whose pretreatment diastolic pressure falls in the range of 90 mm Hg to 104 mm Hg.

This is not to suggest that any person with a single occasional diastolic pressure of 90 mm Hg or more should be treated. Diastolic pressure in excess of 90 mm Hg on at least three separate occasions should be documented before clinical evaluation and treatment are pursued. After that time, it is prudent to treat these patients (especially those with mild hypertension) with nonpharmacologic dietary measures to promote weight reduction, sodium restriction, reduction of alcohol intake, and cessation of cigarette consumption. However, if the desired blood pressure control is not achieved, drug treatment should be pursued. Notes of caution have been raised by important authorities because of the potential side effects of pharmacotherapy in patients with mild hypertension. These researchers have argued that patients with mild hypertension and without target organ involvement could be followed until diastolic pressure exceeds a level of 94 mm Hg; at that time pharmacotherapy could be introduced. These authorities, however, offer certain caveats and suggest that if there is evidence of target organ involvement, even with diastolic pressure between 90 mm Hg and 95 mm Hg, pharmacotherapy is a reasonable approach.

The Joint National Committee's fourth report on the detection, evaluation, and treatment of hypertension defined hypertension as a persistent diastolic pressure of 90 mm Hg or more.[5] It also indicated that normotensive persons whose diastolic pressure was 85 mm Hg through 89 mm Hg were at greater risk for later development of hypertension.

WORKUP OF THE PATIENT WITH HYPERTENSION

CLINICAL MANIFESTATIONS

In most patients with systemic hypertension there are no clinical manifestations other than the elevated pressure.[10] Therefore, unless blood pressure is measured in all patients, hypertension will remain unrecognized. Not infrequently it is reported that the most common symptoms related to hypertension are fatigue, headache, and epistaxis; however, these symptoms are among the most common complaints offered by any patient seeking medical attention. In contrast to these complaints, the most common symptoms related to the "target organs" of hypertension are decreased exercise tolerance and fatigue and nocturia as early evidence of cardiac and renal involvement, respectively. In addition, patients with mild hypertension may describe symptoms of cardiac awareness (e.g., palpitations and tachycardia) that may persist inordinately long after exertion or stress. Chest pain may occur in patients with cardiac involvement as a consequence of the increased myocardial oxygen demands associated with high pressure, left ventricular hypertrophy, or as a manifestation of coexistent coronary arterial (atherosclerotic) heart disease.

PHYSICAL FINDINGS

The small vessels of the optic fundus provide an excellent means to assess the degree of systemic vasoconstriction; this examination should be performed routinely.[10,11] The earliest stage (group I) of hypertensive vascular disease is recognized by increased arterial tortuosity and mild constriction. Coexisting arteriosclerotic changes are manifested by the discontinuity of the arterioles at arteriovenous (AV) crossings (i.e., AV nicking; group II). Appearance of exudates and hemorrhages (group III) represents accelerated hypertension, but it is with the appearance of papilledema (group IV) that diagnosis of malignant hypertension is established.

PERIPHERAL PULSES

One should always compare the femoral and brachial arterial pulsations in all patients with hypertension in a search for a delay in the propagation of the aortic pulse wave as a manifestation of coarctation of the aorta (particularly in young patients) or for evidence of atherosclerotic occlusive processes in older patients. Auscultation of the carotid arteries (for bruits) may provide signs of preventable strokes and transient ischemic attacks; and funduscopy may reveal cholesterol emboli in the retinal arterioles. Renal arterial bruits on examination of the abdomen, flanks, and back provide an important sign of renovascular hypertension. Systolic bruits are commonly detected, especially in older patients, and may not be associated with occlusive arterial disease; however, when associated with a diastolic component to the bruit there is a more significant relationship to renal arterial disease.

CARDIAC EXAMINATION

Even before cardiac structure is altered, palpation may reveal a hyperkinetic apical impulse and a faster heart rate as evidence of early functional hyperdynamic cardiac changes. But as the heart adapts structurally by hypertrophy to the increasing afterload, the increased left ventricular mass may not always be detectable by the chest roentgenogram and electrocardiogram.[10-13] The earliest clinical index of cardiac involvement in hypertension is left atrial enlargement, which may be suspected by an atrial diastolic gallop (fourth heart sound).[14,15] This auscultatory finding is highly concordant with at least two of four conventional electrocardiographic criteria of left atrial abnormality (Table

77.1). Hemodynamic[11] and echocardiographic[16] studies have demonstrated that when both the fourth heart sound and the electrocardiographic left atrial abnormality are present (even without clinical indication of left ventricular hypertrophy), there is adequate physiologic evidence of impaired left ventricular function. As ventricular hypertrophy becomes more evident by chest roentgenogram and electrocardiogram, a louder aortic component of the second heart sound is heard, the fourth heart sound is almost always present, and there is palpable sustained left ventricular lift.[17,18] Clearly the presence of a third heart sound, the ventricular diastolic gallop, connotes the presence of left ventricular failure.

LABORATORY STUDIES

It is important for the physician to discuss with the patient the appropriate preparation for laboratory tests. If possible, these should be done with the patient off *all* medications for at least 3 to 4 weeks (Table 77.2). Even a sodium-restricted diet will stimulate the adrenal cortex sufficiently to suggest the possibility of primary aldosteronism. Dietary sodium intake in excess of 100 mEq/day (2.3 g) will obviate this possibility. Oral contraceptives may not only obscure the baseline arterial pressure readings but may also alter intravascular volume, hemodynamics, and plasma renin activity. And diuretics, laxatives, and even intercurrent viral infections (causing nausea, vomiting, and diarrhea) may produce secondary hyperaldosteronism and associated hypokalemia. Antihypertensive drugs may have effects lasting for as long as four weeks, thereby providing a false concept of "baseline" pressure levels. Even the thiazide diuretics may have persistent effects for two weeks following their discontinuation. Other common medications, including sympathomimetic nose drops, nonsteroidal anti-inflammatory compounds, monoamine oxidase inhibitors, and tricyclic antidepressant drugs, as well as excessive dietary sodium intake may contribute to the high pressure reading or antagonize prescribed antihypertensive drugs.[19]

The following discussion is offered to provide for the clinician a rationale for interpretation of those laboratory studies that could be ordered in the evaluation of a patient with hypertension. Clearly, not all of these studies are necessary in the routine evaluation of a patient with hypertension; however, this discussion is offered to permit a means for understanding and evaluating a patient with hypertension who may have one or more of those diseases that frequently coexist. For the uncomplicated patient, the minimal evaluation usually includes complete blood count (without differential); determination of serum creatinine, potassium, blood sugar, uric acid, and cholesterol (with high and low density cholesterol) concentrations; and an electrocardiogram. It is clear that the fewer the number of laboratory studies the more cost effective will be the evaluation; however, using modern automated laboratory testing techniques more measurements are possible with a more comprehensive evaluation.

COMPLETE BLOOD COUNT. In addition to assessing the hematologic status of a new patient, the CBC is of broad significance. First, if anemia is present, the physician should determine whether it is a complication of the disease (*e.g.*, renal involvement), a result of therapy (*e.g.*, methyldopa-induced hemolysis), or related to an associated problem (*e.g.*, hemoglobinopathy). Conversely, an elevated hemoglobin concentration or hematocrit occurs not infrequently in hypertension. The Gäisbock syndrome is manifested by elevated arterial pressure and by "polycythemia" but without splenomegaly, leukocytosis, or thrombocytosis; and it may be explained physiologically as a "relative polycythemia" since red cell mass and erythropoietin levels are normal.[20] Therefore, the "polycythemia" of hypertension is frequently explained by a contracted plasma volume.[21-24]

BLOOD CHEMISTRIES. Several laboratory tests may be of value in evaluating the patient with hypertension (see Table 77.2). The fasting blood sugar value may be abnormal, and diabetes mellitus is a common coexistent disease. Alternately, the fasting blood sugar value may be normal, but results of a 2- or 4-hour glucose tolerance test may be abnormal. This finding should alert the clinician for other manifestations of diabetes and should suggest those patients who might develop hyperglycemia, glycosuria, or overt diabetes mellitus while receiving diuretic therapy. Therefore, it is unnecessary to order a 2- or 4-hour glucose tolerance test in all patients with hypertension. However, in those in whom diabetes mellitus is suspected (*e.g.*, patients with a family history of diabetes or who develop abnormal carbohydrate tolerance while receiving a thiazide), it may be of value. In most experts'

TABLE 77.1 CLINICAL CLASSIFICATION OF HYPERTENSIVE HEART DISEASE

Stage I
Normal-sized heart without evidence (by chest film or electrocardiogram) of cardiac enlargement

Stage II
Early left ventricular hypertrophy as detected by a fourth heart sound and two of the following ECG criteria:
P wave in lead II $\geq$ 0.3 mV and $\geq$ 0.12 sec
Bipeak interval in notched P wave $\geq$ 0.04 sec
Ratio of P wave duration to PR segment $\geq$ 1.6 (lead II)
Terminal (negative) atrial forces (in V_1) $\geq$ 0.04 sec

Stage III
Clinically evident left ventricular hypertrophy as evidenced by:
Ungerleider index $\geq$ +15% (chest film alone)
Ungerleider index $\geq$ +10% (chest film and two of the following ECG criteria):
Sum of tallest R and deepest S waves $\geq$ 4.5 mV (precordial)
LV "strain"—that is QRS and T wave vectors 180° apart
QRS frontal axis < 0°
All three ECG criteria (above)

Stage IV
Left ventricular failure

TABLE 77.2 LABORATORY STUDIES THAT *MAY* BE OF VALUE IN THE EVALUATION OF THE PATIENT WITH HYPERTENSION (SEE TEXT FOR CLINICAL JUSTIFICATIONS)

Complete Blood Count
White blood cell count (and differential)
Hemoglobin concentration
Hematocrit
Adequacy of platelets

Blood Chemistries
Sugar (fasting, 2-hr postprandial, or glucose tolerance test)
Uric acid
Cholesterol concentration (total, high-density lipoprotein and low-density lipoprotein fractions)
Renal function (serum creatinine and/or blood urea concentrations)
Serum electrolyte (Na, K, Cl, CO_2) concentrations
Calcium and phosphate concentrations
Total protein and albumin concentration
Hepatic function (alkaline phosphatase, bilirubin, serum glutamic oxaloacetic transaminase, serum glutamic pyruvic transaminase, lactic acid dehydrogenase)

Urine Studies
Urinalysis
Urine culture
24-hr collection (protein, Na, K, creatinine)

experience, for example, diabetes does not develop *de novo* in the patient with hypertension and an abnormality in carbohydrate metabolism frequently preceded the use of the diuretic.

The serum uric acid determination should also suggest which patients may develop more severe hyperuricemia or even clinical gout with diuretic therapy. My colleagues and I have reported that the higher the uric acid concentration in patients with otherwise uncomplicated essential hypertension, the lower will be the renal blood flow and the higher the renal vascular resistance.[25]

This rise in serum uric acid levels, reflecting early involvement of renal hemodynamic function in hypertension, follows the earliest echocardiographic changes of left ventricular hypertrophy.[26] Clinicians are also advised to screen their patients for hyperlipidemia.[27] The blood cholesterol determination (with high- and low-density cholesterol concentrations) is of value for detecting remediable hyperlipidemia, and the physician is cautioned to advise the patient to remain fasting from after dinner the evening before this test.[5]

The kidney is a prime target organ of hypertension, and renal functional impairment is a major complication. Therefore, it is of value to measure the serum creatinine and/or blood urea nitrogen concentrations in all patients. I usually obtain both tests; and by using the serum creatinine along with urinary creatinine excretion, it is possible to calculate the creatinine clearance (glomerular filtration rate) in those patients in whom impaired renal function is of concern. Measurement of serum electrolyte values, particularly serum potassium concentration, is valuable in excluding secondary forms of hypertension, steroidal hormone excess, and the effects of diuretic therapy. Many factors may produce hypokalemia (Table 77.3), and very few factors (other than laboratory error and red cell hemolysis) are responsible for hyperkalemia. Determination of serum calcium concentration will exclude hypercalcemia, an alteration that is associated with a high incidence of hypertension; its correction may reduce the abnormal pressure to normal levels.

Routine measurement of serum proteins and hepatic function is usually part of the automated serum chemistry determinations. Although these tests may be of little value for the patient with hypertension, they may confirm hemoconcentration (*i.e.*, plasma protein concentrations) or may provide a baseline for later possible coexisting problems (*e.g.*, myocardial infarction, hepatic diseases). Baseline hepatic function data could be of great value in evaluating intercurrent and incidental problems (*e.g.*, hepatitis, drug hepatotoxicity, or even the possible low-grade elevation of serum bilirubin with Gilbert's disease).

URINARY STUDIES. Of prime importance is the routine urinalysis to detect the glycosuria of diabetes mellitus, the impaired renal function of advancing nephrosclerosis (diminished concentratability), the alkaline urine of primary hyperaldosteronism, and the abnormal sediment in renal parenchymal disease. A 24-hour urine collection is most valuable in determining creatinine clearance as well as dietary sodium intake. If the urinary *sodium excretion* is greater than 100 mEq/24 hr (demonstrating adequate sodium intake and no dietary factor to explain aldosterone stimulation), and if the urinary excretion of potassium is less than 40 mEq/24 hr, a measured hypokalemia (<3.5 mEq/liter) is not likely to be the result of excessive adrenal cortical hormone excretion. On the other hand, if the 24-hour potassium excretion is excessive (*i.e.*, >50 mEq) in the presence of adequate sodium intake and there is no other obvious explanation for the demonstrated hypokalemia (<3.5 mEq/liter; see Table 77.3), there is a definite need to consider the possibility of hyperaldosteronism.

Further, the normal kidney should not excrete more than 200 mg to 300 mg protein daily; any amount in excess suggests either renal parenchymal disease (including nephrosclerosis) or an effect of the elevated pressure itself. However, nephrosclerosis itself will not be associated with protein excretion in excess of 400 mg to 500 mg daily. Although a severely elevated arterial pressure may be associated with massive proteinuria, it should remit with reduction of pressure to normal levels. Thus, if urinary protein excretion persists or remains in excess of 400 mg to 500 mg in 24 hours, the physician should consider other causes of renal parenchymal diseases (*e.g.*, chronic pyelonephritis, glomerulonephritis). If daily protein excretion exceeds 2 g or 3 g, the physician should conclude that chronic pyelonephritis alone is an unlikely cause; more rational diagnosis will include the various causes of nephrotic syndrome. Urine *culture* (and sensitivity) is always wise if there is a likelihood of a urinary tract infection.

CHEST ROENTGENOGRAM. Routine chest roentgenographic examination is a worthwhile baseline study for any chronic illness and is of particular value in the patient with hypertension. It permits recognition of cardiac enlargement, the stigmata of aortic coarctation, and complications of hypertension (*e.g.*, pulmonary congestion, aortic widening) and provides evidence for associated disease. The degree of cardiac enlargement is easily quantified by chest film and electrocardiogram, thus providing a means to assess changes with therapy.[12,13]

ELECTROCARDIOGRAPHY. The electrocardiogram is of particular value in determining the degree of cardiac involvement from hyper-

TABLE 77.3 FACTORS RESPONSIBLE FOR HYPOKALEMIA

Dietary Sodium Excess Associated With Diuretic Therapy

Chronic Gastrointestinal Potassium Losses
Vomiting
Diarrhea
Laxative abuse
Pyloric obstruction
Nasogastric suction
Villous adenoma
Malabsorption syndrome
Ureterosigmoidoscopy

Adrenocortical Excess
Primary aldosteronism
 (adenoma or hyperplasia)
Cushing's syndrome and disease
Other adrenal steroidal hormone excess

Drug Therapy and Food
Diuretics
Licorice
Adrenal steroids
Salicylate intoxication
Outdated tetracycline

Renal Disease (Chronic)
Potassium-wasting nephropathy
Nephrotic syndrome
Renal tubular acidosis

Secondary Hyperaldosteronism
Renal arterial disease
Cirrhosis
Congestive heart failure

Diabetes Mellitus (Acidosis)

Primary Periodic Paralysis (Hypokalemic Type)

tensive vascular disease. As indicated, left atrial abnormality is the first electrocardiographic sign of cardiac enlargement.[14,15] Although the electrocardiographic literature is replete with criteria for diagnosis of left ventricular hypertrophy, each criterion has its own false-negative and false-positive results. The McPhie criterion (the sum of the tallest R wave and deepest S wave in any of the precordial leads achieving a total voltage of 4.5 mV) has the lowest false-positive result (1.5%).[28] The criteria that we have used are detailed in Table 1 and, when used with the Ungerleider index determined from chest roentgenograms, are of great value in classifying the severity of hypertensive heart disease. These criteria have been confirmed by echocardiography and provide an excellent means to describe functional progression of hypertensive heart disease.

There is a large variety of specialized diagnostic tests available to evaluate the patient with hypertension. As a rule, none needs to be performed routinely. However, the major specialized tests are presented in Table 77.4, each with its major indications. For a more detailed discussion of these tests the reader is referred to several specialized publications dealing with them in greater detail.

ANTIHYPERTENSIVE THERAPY

With the demonstrated efficacy of antihypertensive therapy in reducing arterial pressure and reversing cardiovascular morbidity and mortality,[2–8,29] a simple, but practical, stepped-care approach was established.[9] This algorithmic approach was particularly well suited for mass population treatment programs, but recently there has been a burgeoning of new antihypertensive agents. Some of these drugs possess therapeutic mechanisms that now permit rational preselection of certain patients for specific therapy.[5,30] The discussion that follows concerns these newer agents, their role in the treatment of hypertension, and new concepts about antihypertensive therapy that permit more enlightened use of even the older agents.

CLASSIFICATION

Until recently, antihypertensive therapy was considered in three pharmacologic categories, with nonpharmacologic therapy (including discontinuance of oral contraceptives and other drugs that may elevate arterial pressure, weight control, moderation of alcohol consumption, restriction of dietary sodium intake, and cessation of cigarette consumption) not emphasized. The former three drug classes had included the diuretics as a fundamental first step, with the progressive introduction of agents from the two additional groups, the antiadrenergics and vasodilators, following in sequence.[9] In this context the antiadrenergics agents are considered to be dissociated from the vasodilators, even though both these classes of antihypertensive therapy decrease vascular smooth muscle tone and dilate arterioles. In this discussion *vasodilators* are defined as compounds that act directly on vascular smooth muscle contractile mechanisms. Nevertheless, this concept of therapy is intrinsic in the current recommendations of the Joint National Committee of the HBPEP.[5]

TABLE 77.4 SPECIALIZED STUDIES OF VALUE IN EVALUATING PATIENTS WITH HYPERTENSION*

Study	Indications
Intravenous urography	Consideration of renal parenchymal disease History of urinary tract infections, renal stones, or obstructive uropathy Persistence of hypertension after toxemia of pregnancy
Selective renal arteriography (May be preceded by digital subtraction angiography in outpatients)	Abdominal, flank, or back bruit (see text) Sudden onset of hypertension Sudden severity of known hypertension, including loss of blood pressure control on previously adequate therapy Disparity in renal lengths (by urography or scintigraphy) of ≥1 cm
Renal venous renin activities	Functional assessment of the arterial lesion(s) at the time of selective renal arteriography Possible outpatient use after digital subtraction arteriograms have demonstrated arterial disease Evaluation of progression of known renal arterial disease
Isotope renography and renal scans	Follow-up of patient with diagnosed renal arterial disease (*e.g.*, to assess reduction in renal size or to compare postoperative to preoperative studies) Postoperative assessment of the patency of renal blood supply Use in conjunction with digital subtraction arteriography Confirmation of clinical suspicion of renal arterial lesion in patient allergic to contrast material in order to obviate steroidal preparation of patient for arteriographic study
Plasma renin activity (Peripheral venous blood)	Assessment of low-renin forms of hypertension (*e.g.*, primary aldosteronism, volume-dependent hypertension) Assessment of high-renin forms of hypertension (renal arterial disease or high-renin essential hypertension) in association with pharmacologic provocative studies to aid in selection of therapeutic programs
Blood (*i.e.*, plasma) volume	Determination of volume expansion and confirmation of "pseudotolerance" to antihypertensive therapy Preoperative assessment of patient with pheochromocytoma
Hormonal studies	Catecholamines for pheochromocytoma or with clonidine suppression test Aldosterone levels for primary aldosteronism Corticosteroid levels for Cushing's disease or syndrome Thyroid function studies for hyperthyroidism or hypothyroidism Parathormone for hyperparathyroidism Growth hormone for acromegaly Insulin levels for associated diabetes mellitus

* These studies are indicated if a specific cause of hypertension is considered or if target organ involvement and other complications of the disease are suspected.

Present-day antihypertensive therapy has now been complicated further by the introduction of three new classes of agents (Table 77.5). Thus, in addition to the former groups, the β-adrenergic receptor blocking drugs were added; they are generally considered as a separate group, even though they also inhibit adrenergic function. Their mechanisms seem to operate through different means than the traditionally used antiadrenergics. A fifth group of agents that specifically inhibit the generation and effects of angiotensin II has come into important clinical use; they are considered as a separate entity. The most recent class of agents is the slow-entry calcium channel blocking drugs or calcium antagonists. These agents all dilate arterioles and reduce arterial pressure but are more heterogeneous than their classification suggests.

HEMODYNAMIC CONCEPTS

Most clinical forms of hypertension are characterized hemodynamically as being produced by a generalized increase in the tone of vascular smooth muscle.[17,18,31,32] The resulting vasoconstriction explains the increased systemic arteriolar resistance and a reduced venular capacitance. Consequently, the hemodynamic hallmark of hypertension is an increased total peripheral resistance that is more or less uniformly distributed throughout all the organ circulations.[17] The increased venular smooth muscle tone redistributes the circulating intravascular volume from the periphery to the central (i.e., cardiopulmonary) circulation and thus, early in the development of hypertension, augments venous return to the heart to increase cardiac output.[17,33] Later, in more established hypertension, the cardiac output returns toward normal and the regional or organ blood flows are normal. This reduction of cardiac output to normal reflects a contraction of intravascular (i.e., plasma) volume and a lesser return of circulating volume to the cardiopulmonary area and heart as precapillary and postcapillary resistances increase.[17,31]

Thus, as hypertensive disease progresses in severity, vascular resistance increases, raising the arterial pressure.[11,17,18,31,32] Two primary cardiovascular adaptations result from these changes: First, the heart and vessels structurally adapt to their increasing workloads, increasing cardiac (e.g., left ventricular) mass and vascular wall thickness. The second adaptive change, which has already been discussed, is the contraction of intravascular (i.e., plasma) volume in most non-volume-dependent forms of hypertension. When the heart and vessels no longer can adapt structurally and functionally, secondary hormonal substances (e.g., renin-angiotensin-aldosterone, vasopressin, catecholamines) come into play. Eventually, cardiac and circulatory failure ensue with associated expansion of effective circulating blood volume and its attendant impaired renal excretory function.[32] The sequence of these pathophysiologic changes has been demonstrated in most patients with established essential hypertension.

CLINICAL PHARMACOLOGIC CONCEPTS

The "ideal" antihypertensive agent should be one that (1) reduces vascular smooth muscle tone in order to reduce total peripheral and organ vascular resistances; (2) maintains cardiac output and organ blood flows (especially to the heart, brain, and kidneys) at normal levels; (3) does not inordinately reflexively stimulate the heart (in response to the induced hypotension) to increase its rate, contractility or ejection, and metabolism; and (4) does not expand intravascular volume in response to the reduced hydrostatic and renal perfusion pressures.

When assessing the hemodynamic effects of any antihypertensive drug, it is essential that the physician be aware that discrepancies in published reports may reflect (1) differences in the route of that drug's administration by the different investigators; (2) the dose used; (3) the time elapsed after drug administration before observations were made; (4) whether a single dose was administered or whether the patient was treated over a more extensive time; (5) the age, race, and sex of the treated subjects (recent reports emphasized the importance of these factors); (6) the severity of the hypertensive diseases; (7) previous drug therapy; and (8) whether other medications had been administered concomitantly or recently enough to alter the hemodynamic responses to the therapeutic agent in question. These points are of great significance, as are other factors, even though they may not seem to have vasoactive action. Such factors include use of tranquilizers or anesthetic agents; the time of day; time since the last meal; and ingestion of commonly used self-medications (e.g., oral contraceptives, nosedrops, steroidal compounds, and even such "non-drugs" as coffee, tea, tobacco, snuff, vitamin tablets, and laxatives).[19,34]

DIURETICS

Until recently, most authorities have considered diuretics as the first step and the mainstay of antihypertensive therapy.[5] However, with the increasing acceptance of the β-adrenergic receptor blocking drugs, with more critical evaluation of their use and value in the treatment of hypertension, with the introduction of other classes of drugs suitable for initial monotherapy of hypertension, and with recent reports from multicenter clinical trials raising some concerns about their value in patients with mild hypertension (less than 105 mm Hg), there has been a reevaluation of the general need for the diuretic as a mandatory "first step" in therapy (Table 77.6).

Question has also been raised about the "traditional" *dose* of diuretics in this country: 50 mg (but more frequently 100 mg) of hydrochlorothiazide (or equivalent doses of other thiazide congeners). This dose is clearly greater than necessary, and the Joint National Committee IV report now recommends 12.5 mg to 50 mg hydrochlorothiazide or its equivalent.[5] Another concept that has been emphasized in recent years is the concern about *hypokalemia* induced by thiazide (or congeners) therapy. In this regard, one important consideration is that excessive sodium intake will aggravate the hypokalemia induced by diuretics. Thus, the secondary aldosteronism produced by the diuretic

TABLE 77.5 CLASSES OF ANTIHYPERTENSIVE AGENTS

Diuretics
Thiazide congeners
"Loop-acting" agents
Potassium-sparing agents
    Aldosterone antagonists
    Sodium pump inhibitors

β-Adrenergic Receptor Antagonists
Cardioselective (β_1) inhibitors
Nonspecific (β_1, β_2) inhibitors
Complex molecules
    α–β-blockers
    β-blockers–vasodilators

Adrenergic Inhibitors
Centrally acting agents
Peripherally acting agents
α-Adrenergic receptor antagonists
Complex molecules (central and peripheral actions)

Direct-Acting Vasodilators
Direct vascular smooth muscle relaxing agents act primarily on arterial or smooth muscle

Renin-Angiotensin System Inhibitors
Agents that inhibit renin release from the kidney
Inhibitors of the angiotensin converting enzyme
Angiotensin II receptor antagonists
Renin inhibitors

Calcium Antagonists
Agents that inhibit calcium entry into cardiac and vascular myocytes
Agents that inhibit calcium entry into vascular myocytes

facilitates further potassium wasting from body stores as the excess dietary sodium is filtered through the kidney and is exchanged for the potassium at the level of the distal tubule. Reduced sodium intake not only facilitates the antihypertensive effectiveness of the diuretic but also reduces concern for induced secondary hypokalemia.[35]

A third concept concerning diuretics is their potential for producing *cardiac dysrhythmias* (and perhaps sudden death) resulting from the induced hypokalemia. Although still controversial, data supporting these arguments have been provided from several prospective studies that demonstrated more ectopic beats over a 24-hour period in patients receiving diuretics than in those patients who received no therapy.[36,37] These studies, however, involved small numbers of patients, but are supported in part by the as-yet incompletely explained data from the MRFIT (Multiple Risk Factor Intervention Trial).[29] In this study, the diuretic-treated mild hypertensive patients had a higher prevalence of cardiovascular (and ?sudden) death, a finding interpreted by some to suggest the possibility of hypokalemia-induced cardiac dysrhythmias. However, these special intervention–treated patients also had more "abnormal" electrocardiograms at the outset of the study than the usual care group of hypertensive patients, a condition that may have predisposed them to the dysrhythmias and possible sudden deaths. In addition, my co-workers and I reported that untreated hypertensive patients with cardiac enlargement had more ectopic ventricular beats in one day's time than patients without cardiac enlargement.[38] If we were to extrapolate these preliminary findings to patients receiving diuretic therapy, perhaps the more severe cardiac dysrhythmias (and, hence, greater potential for sudden death) may be found in patients with cardiac hypertrophy and diuretic-induced hypokalemia. Further, this factor may be aggravated by the coexistence of ischemic and obesity heart disease and emphasizes the importance of the pretreatment cardiac status.[39–41]

Following our early suggestions for tailoring the initial therapy with respect to the patient's demographic, clinical, and physiologic characteristics,[30] the Joint National Committee, in its fourth report, recommends individualization of the initial step of antihypertensive therapy.[5] In this regard, patients who may be the most suitable for diuretic therapy may be older patients, black patients, patients with volume-dependent forms of hypertension (*e.g.*, those with expanded intravascular volume, lower plasma renin activity), patients with steroid-dependent forms of hypertension, or patients who have renal parenchymal disease.

β-ADRENERGIC RECEPTOR BLOCKING DRUGS

Several therapeutic concepts have been introduced with the addition of new β-adrenergic receptor blocking drugs to the armamentarium of antihypertensive drug therapy. There are now seven β-blocking drugs available in this country. An eighth agent also possesses α-receptor inhibitory actions in its single molecule (Table 77.7).

β-Adrenergic receptors have been classified as β_1 or β_2: β_1-receptors are those located primarily on myocardial cell membranes (and in the kidney that stimulate renin release); and β_2-receptors are those found elsewhere (bronchi, gastrointestinal tract, but some in the myocardium).[42–44] Some β-blockers (*e.g.*, acebutolol, metoprolol, and atenolol) are *cardioselective;* in low pharmacologic (subantihypertensive and antianginal) doses, they selectively inhibit the β_1-receptors. However, in the doses that are used for the treatment of hypertension (or angina pectoris), they also block β_2-receptors and therefore do not confer absolute safety to the patient with asthma, history of asthma, or with chronic obstructive pulmonary disease.[44]

Although formerly considered a property of greater concern to the pharmacologist, the concept of drug *solubility* has great clinical significance. Lipid solubility relates to drug metabolism, to onset and duration of action of the agent, and to side effects. The agent that is lipid soluble has a greater avidity for tissues with greater lipid content (*e.g.*, liver and brain). Thus, when taken by mouth, the drug is absorbed through the gastrointestinal tract and passes through the portal circulation, and a greater percentage of the lipid-soluble agent will be ex-

---

TABLE 77.6 CLINICAL CONSIDERATIONS OF DIURETIC THERAPY

Dose of agent
Hypokalemia
Cardiac dysrhythmias, sudden death
Carbohydrate intolerance
Hyperuricemia
Lack of uniformity of response in all patients with hypertension
Hyperlipidemia (cholesterol, low-density lipoprotein cholesterol, triglycerides)

TABLE 77.7 β-ADRENERGIC RECEPTOR BLOCKERS AVAILABLE IN THE UNITED STATES

Generic Name	Trade Name	Pharmacologic and Clinical Features
Acebutolol	Sectral	Cardioselective; possesses intrinsic sympathomimetic activity
Atenolol	Tenormin	Cardioselective; given once daily
Metoprolol	Lopressor	Cardioselective; may be given once daily
Nadolol	Corgard	Nonselective; given once daily
Pindolol	Visken	Nonselective; possesses intrinsic sympathomimetic activity
Propranolol	Inderal	Nonselective; available longest; may be given once daily; approved for angina pectoris, migraine
Timolol	Blocadren	Nonselective; approved for glaucoma and prevention of myocardial reinfarction
Labetalol*	Normodyne; Trandate	Nonselective; α–β blockade

* Not a "pure" β-adrenergic receptor blocker

tracted and metabolized in the liver. Moreover, the lipid-soluble agent may be taken up in greater amounts in neural tissue. This concept provides explanations for the so-called first-pass phenomenon of lipid-soluble agents and for their central nervous system side effects. It also follows that patients with renal functional impairment will develop higher blood levels of water-soluble agents and patients with impaired hepatic function will have higher levels of lipid-soluble agents.

Some β-adrenergic blocking drugs not only have the ability to inhibit β-receptors, but, strangely enough, they can also stimulate adrenergic function. Those agents that have this property will produce a lesser decrease in heart rate and cardiac output than agents without *intrinsic sympathomimetic activity* (ISA).[45] As a result, these agents may have a potential role in patients with pre-existing bradycardia and low systemic blood flow states wherein β-receptor antagonists may be (at least relatively) contraindicated.

Certain agents have been said to possess *membrane stabilizing activity* (MSA) and were believed to have their antiarrhythmic effect on the basis of this property. This is no longer held to be true, although this characteristic probably confers an anesthetic effect. The only currently marketed agent not having this characteristic is timolol, making it useful in glaucoma; the ophthalmic preparation does not anesthetize the conjunctiva.

These pharmacologic concepts are vitally important in providing the clinician a base of knowledge that will permit the wise selection of a β-blocking drug for a patient for whom antihypertensive therapy with a β-blocking compound is prescribed. Moreover, it also provides a rationale for maintaining therapy with the same antihypertensive drug class should certain side effects occur or should the dose seem too great without achieving the optimal therapeutic effect. If one β-blocking drug produces side effects (*e.g.*, diarrhea, bad dreams, hallucinations), it may not be necessary to discontinue the use of this class of antihypertensive drugs to control pressure. One may only need to change to another β-blocker. Thus, if there are central nervous system side effects, the physician may prescribe a less lipid-soluble agent. For example, if one encounters complaints of cold extremities with a noncardioselective agent, the use of a cardioselective agent may be more satisfactory without need to withdraw the β-blocking therapy. Furthermore, if the patient is taking unusually high doses of one agent without achieving an optimal antihypertensive effect, better pressure control may be obtained with an alternative drug. This may be achieved with a less lipid-soluble β-blocker that may be more completely absorbed or with less of the first-pass phenomenon. In these situations the physician may transfer the therapy by simply using theoretically equivalent doses (*e.g.*, 160 mg to 480 mg propranolol to 80 mg nadolol, 100 mg atenolol, 100 mg metoprolol). Of course, if the patient reports side effects suggesting obstructive pulmonary disease, congestive heart failure, or any of the other absolute contraindications of β-blocking therapy, the drug should be discontinued.

At present the precise mechanism(s) by which arterial pressure is reduced and is controlled remains unknown and controversial. A variety of mechanisms have been postulated (Table 77.8), but none has been proved.[44] Thus, although pressure reduction was initially shown to be in direct proportion to the height of pretreatment cardiac output and heart rate, subsequent studies showed that pressure reduction could be achieved with β-blockers that do not reduce cardiac output (or agents with ISA). Others suggested that the fall in pressure was dependent on the pretreatment plasma renin activity (PRA) of the patient; however, PRA is reduced to the same extent following the immediate intravenous administration of the agent without the pressure reduction that is demonstrated with more prolonged use of the drug. A variety of other antihypertensive mechanisms has also been postulated, including several mechanisms that might produce adaptations of the circulation and its flow characteristics and modify β-receptor–mediated mechanisms in the brain or at the nerve ending. Each proposed action either has arguments against its effect or may not be achieved with other β-blockers.

It is important to recognize that, despite this frustration in providing a rational explanation for the antihypertensive action of the β-blockers, this does not preclude their clinical use. We must remember that we have made use of the diuretic agents for a longer time period and still cannot ascribe a precise action to explain why their prolonged use is associated with their effect in decreasing vascular resistance and controlling arterial pressure.

With respect to the concept of individualizing antihypertensive therapy,[5] patients who may be more amenable for therapy with β-adrenergic receptor blocking drugs include younger patients (who may have greater adrenergic activity); those patients with cardiac awareness (*e.g.*, with more rapid cardiac action or palpitations or with catecholamine-mediated ectopic cardiac beats) or with hyperdynamic circulation; patients with angina pectoris or a prior myocardial infarction; or those patients with coexisting disease that is also amenable to β-receptor blocking therapy (*e.g.*, migraine headache, mitral valve prolapse).

ANTIADRENERGICS

The α-adrenergic receptor is of at least two types pharmacologically: the peripheral α_1-receptor is located at the distal side of the synaptic cleft between the postganglionic nerve ending and the vascular smooth muscle cell; the α_2-receptor is located at the cell membrane of the postganglionic nerve ending.[46,47] When the α_1-receptor is stimulated by the natural neurohumoral agonist norepinephrine, vasoconstriction is produced. In contrast, when the α_2-receptor at the nerve ending is stimulated, further release of norepinephrine from that nerve ending is inhibited. This mechanism provides a negative feedback concept for adrenergic function at the adrenergic nerve ending.

These α_1- and α_2-receptors have been termed *postsynaptic* and *presynaptic* α-receptors, respectively. Prazosin (or trimazosin or indoramine) acts as a peripheral α_1-receptor blocker. This concept is readily understandable until one considers the role of α-receptors, centrally, in the brain. Postsynaptic α-receptors are also located on specific neurons in the brain (*e.g.*, the nucleus tractus solitarii), and when they are stimulated they behave as peripheral α_2-receptors, inhibiting adrenergic outflow from the brain center to the heart and blood vessels. This provides the mechanism of action for the centrally acting antihypertensive adrenergic inhibiting drugs (*i.e.*, methyldopa, clonidine, guanabenz, goanfacine).

VASODILATORS

The traditional pharmacologic concept of the vasodilators is that they provide direct relaxation of vascular smooth muscle. As a result, arterial pressure is reduced through a decrease in arteriolar smooth muscle tone and total peripheral resistance. With relaxation of venomotor tone, venous return to the heart may be reduced, thus diminishing

---

TABLE 77.8. POSTULATED ANTIHYPERTENSIVE MECHANISMS OF THE β-BLOCKING DRUGS

Reduced cardiac output
Readjustments of blood flow
    Preferential responses of component regional circulations
    Total body autoregulation ("reverse Guyton")
    Reduced vessel distention ("reverse Bayliss")
Readjusted baroreceptors
Altered high-pressure reflexes from the heart
Reduced plasma renin activity
Altered catecholamine biosynthesis
Inhibited presynaptic β-receptors
Central action of an active metabolite of the agent

cardiac output through a peripheral pooling of blood. Both factors—arteriolar and venular smooth muscle tone—therefore participate in controlling arterial pressure.

In response to these effects of vasodilation, reflex stimulation of the heart and vessels results, provided that the neural baroreceptor-mediated mechanisms remain intact. Most vasodilators produce predominantly arteriolar dilation, and whatever venodilation may be evoked will usually be overcome by reflex constriction. As a result of the failure of venules to dilate effectively, venous return and cardiac output fail to be reduced. The heart may also be stimulated reflexively with direct vasodilator therapy, producing an increase in its rate, contractility, and metabolism. This is why the usual vasodilator agents have not been used as a single agent or together with diuretics in most patients with intact cardiovascular reflexes; angina pectoris, myocardial infarction, further dissection of an aneurysm, or overt cardiac failure may be precipitated in the predisposed patient.

Fluid retention is another normal physiologic response following the vasodilation and hypotension induced by most vasodilators and most adrenolytic compounds. As capillary hydrostatic pressure falls, Starling's law of capillary fluid transfer comes into play and fluid moves intravascularly from extravascular sites. The result is a pre-expansion of intravascular volume, an attenuation of the previously produced hypotensive effect of the vasodilator, and a rational explanation for the so-called phenomenon of "pseudo-tolerance" to certain antihypertensive agents.[48] In addition to this effect, the reduced renal perfusion pressure permits a secondary retention of sodium and water by the kidney. The net effect of both is an expansion of blood volume, a return of pressure toward pretreatment levels, and the need for cotreatment with diuretic agents to maintain effectiveness of the antihypertensive agent.[49]

ANGIOTENSIN SYSTEM INHIBITORS

Angiotensin II, one of the most potent of the naturally occurring vasoconstrictors, is generated by the release of the enzyme renin from the kidney, which acts on its substrate, circulating angiotensin, to free the vasoinactive decapeptide angiotensin I from its protein substrate. Angiotensin I subsequently loses two peptides with its passage through the lung (in particular) through the action of the angiotensin-converting enzyme (or kininase II) and forms the vasoactive octapeptide angiotensin II. This converting enzyme not only activates the vasoconstrictor angiotensin II, but it also inactivates one of the most potent vasodilators in the body, bradykinin. (The octapeptide angiotensin II may also lose an additional peptide to form the septapeptide angiotensin III, a more specific adrenocortical agonist, which releases aldosterone.) From this cascade of biochemical events there are several potential levels of the renin–angiotensin system that can be specifically inhibited by drugs. Pharmacologic agents may inhibit the release of renin; and adrenergic inhibiting drugs as a class do just this. Other agents inhibit the angiotensin II receptor site on the vascular smooth muscle membrane. A new class of agents, synthesized from developments in molecular biology, are the renin inhibitors. These agents directly antagonize the rate-limiting enzyme of the renopressor system and have already been studied in experimental forms of hypertension. Early trials in humans are anticipated.

A number of compounds have been developed that act through inhibition of the angiotensin-converting enzyme. Three of these agents are already available (i.e., captopril, enalapril, and lisinopril). These compounds reduce arterial pressure primarily through reduced generation of angiotensin II, although it may be argued that less of the most potent naturally occurring vasodilator bradykinin is inactivated, since the angiotensin-converting enzyme (kininase II) that is inhibited is the same enzyme that inactivates bradykinin. In addition, angiotensin II gains access to the central nervous system, is also synthesized in the brain, and interacts with the naturally occurring adrenergic neurohumoral substance norepinephrine peripherally at the postsympathetic neuron. Thus, angiotensin II may stimulate adrenergic outflow from cardiovascular centers in the brain and augment adrenergic function peripherally; both functions serve to increase arterial pressure through interaction of angiotensin II with the adrenergic nervous system. Angiotensin II also promotes a release of catecholamines from the adrenal cortex. Further, angiotensin II affects renal tubular function and probably plays an important role in the local regulation of intrarenal blood flow.

Thus, lesser generation of angiotensin II through converting enzyme inhibition provides some antihypertensive action through indirect adrenergic inhibition as well as through the reduced availability of angiotensin II to stimulate angiotensin II receptors on vascular smooth muscle. And still further, because of the reduced angiotensin II, there is less stimulation of the adrenal cortex to reduce aldosterone with its resulting metabolic effects. It is vitally necessary to understand all of these actions if one is to use these effective and potent compounds clinically.

The angiotensin-converting enzyme inhibitors reduce arterial pressure through arteriolar dilation and reduced vascular resistance that is unassociated with reflex cardiac stimulation; heart rate, myocardial contractility, and cardiac output do not increase.[50-54] Associated with the pressure reduction with both agents is a significant reduction in renal vascular resistance. The decrease in renal vascular resistance is produced from efferent as well as afferent glomerular arteriolar resistance, and, as a consequence glomerular hydrostatic pressure is reduced. This creates a favorable intraglomerular hemodynamic status that should tend to retard the development of glomerulosclerosis and nephrosclerosis.[55] Experimental and clinical studies with these compounds have demonstrated regression of left ventricular mass associated with the pressure fall.

Early investigative studies with captopril were directed primarily to patients with severe hypertension whose disease was refractory to other antihypertensive therapy or who had severe renal complications of hypertensive disease (e.g., chronic renal and collagen diseases). Captopril is a compound having sulfhydryl groups, a property that may provide affinity of this drug for the basement membrane. Each of these circumstances may have added to the two major side effects that were reported initially with captopril: leukopenia and proteinuria. However, as clinical experience with this agent increased, the incidence of these two side effects has been found to diminish markedly.[56] Two other side effects associated with this drug, rash and ageusia (loss of taste), were also less common with time. A third, and more common, side effect is chronic cough. It is of particular interest that all of these side effects usually disappear with discontinuance of the medication and may not reappear if therapy is resumed. Two other side effects of these agents may be related directly to the physiologic effects of the drug. Because inhibition of angiotensin-converting enzyme will reduce angiotensin II and aldosterone while stimulating the renal release of PRA, one should anticipate the predisposition to develop hyperkalemia if potassium is prescribed with captopril therapy. The potassium elevation may be caused by dietary potassium supplementation (KI tablets, potassium in dietary salt substitutes) or by prescription of potassium-retaining agents. In addition, reports have demonstrated development of renal failure with or without associated malignant hypertension in patients with bilateral occlusive renal arterial disease or renal arterial disease in a solitary kidney.[57,58] These phenomena have been explained on the basis of the withdrawal of homeostatic intrarenal circulatory angiotensin-dependent mechanisms.

Patients who may be more responsive for initial therapy with angiotensin-converting enzyme inhibitors are those patients with more severe hypertension requiring a multiplicity of hypertensive agents; patients who have suboptimal control of pressure with other agents; patients with angiotensin-dependent forms of hypertension (e.g., essential hypertension with high plasma renin activity, renal arterial disease) and cardiac failure; and patients who have had metabolic or other side effects from prior antihypertensive treatment programs that add cost by requiring additional agents or laboratory testing or that impair quality of life.[5,30]

CALCIUM ANTAGONISTS

The slow-entry channel calcium inhibiting drugs, or the calcium antagonists, all reduce arterial pressure by reducing total peripheral resistance without associated reflex stimulation of the heart or expansion of intravascular volume. As a result, these agents do not require the additional use of an adrenergic inhibiting drug or diuretic. However, with the addition of a diuretic, a β-blocker or an angiotensin-converting enzyme inhibitor there is an augmented antihypertensive effect.

Verapamil, the first of this class of compounds, also decreases heart rate and, to some extent, myocardial contractility (the latter action is more evident under more experimental conditions than clinically). As a result, this agent was initially used as a therapeutic agent for supraventricular tachycardia. Nifedipine, a dihydropyridine derivative, does not have this cardiac action; in fact, as a result of its vasodilation and depressor action, a reflexive increase in heart rate and myocardial contractility and metabolism may occur.[59] It is not known precisely why this class of agents do not retain fluid, but among the several explanations include a natriuretic effect of these agents and some degree of postcapillary vasodilation. However, because of reflexive postcapillary constriction in some patients, an increased capillary hydrostatic pressure may result in a migration of fluid into the tissues with consequent edema unassociated with weight gain.

Some of these agents may increase renal blood flow without increasing glomerular filtration rate.[60-62] This reduction in filtration fraction, similar to that described above for the angiotensin-converting enzyme inhibitors, is related to a reduced intraglomerular hydrostatic pressure associated with efferent glomerular arteriolar dilation.[63]

Patients who may be expected to respond to calcium antagonist therapy are those who also respond well to diuretics, that is, those who are elderly or black, even though younger patients and white patients also respond well to these drugs. Patients with coronary artery disease who cannot take the β-blocking drugs or who have not responded well to these drugs are likely patients to benefit from this class of drugs. Moreover, if metabolic or other side effects complicate a successful antihypertensive treatment program, use of the calcium antagonists may obviate these problems through a rationale similar to that described for the angiotensin-converting enzyme inhibitors.

☐ MANAGEMENT OF THE PATIENT WITH ESSENTIAL HYPERTENSION

MILD HYPERTENSION

All patients with mild essential hypertension (baseline diastolic pressures from 90 mm Hg through 104 mm Hg) should be followed carefully by their attending physicians, using the following approach:[4]

1. Document that, in fact, diastolic pressure in excess of 90 mm Hg is present on three or four or more visits to the office.
2. If diastolic pressure exceeds 90 mm Hg on repeated outpatient visits, the patient might be treated for a limited period of time with nonpharmacologic therapy alone. This might include weight reduction, if indicated, or a sodium-restricted diet (less than 75 mEq to 100 mEq sodium daily). If after this limited period of time (3 to 6 months, perhaps) blood pressure still is not reduced to levels below 90 mm Hg, then consider pharmacotherapy.
3. In initiating treatment with pharmacologic agents, it is not necessary to treat all patients with essential hypertension with diuretics as a first step.
   - Diuretics may be used in all patients with mild hypertension but are perhaps most effective in those patients who are older, black, female, or volume-dependent (patients receiving oral contraceptives or other steroidal drug treatment, with history of renal infections, obesity, edema).
   - Patients may be treated with β-adrenergic receptor blocking drugs if they are young, male, and white and have symptoms of cardiac awareness (rapid heart action, palpitations, or extrasystoles).
   - Patients who are already receiving β-adrenergic blocking therapy (for angina pectoris, for example) and whose blood pressures still remain elevated might also benefit from a slow-entry channel calcium blocking drug to achieve better control of pressure.
   - Patients with intolerance to any of the foregoing agents or who may have gout, diabetes mellitus, chronic obstructive pulmonary disease, or asthma may respond well to one of the angiotensin-converting enzyme inhibitors or calcium antagonists.
   - For a more detailed rationale and explanation for selecting individualized initial therapy with angiotensin-converting enzyme inhibitors or the calcium antagonists refer to the previous discussions.[5,30]

MODERATE-TO-SEVERE ESSENTIAL HYPERTENSION

A number of recommended algorithms for therapy have been published suggesting the progressive stepwise introduction of pharmacologic agents that control arterial pressure. As previously indicated, the merit of this approach to therapy is that by adding logical selections of antihypertensive drugs lower doses of each agent may be used, thus minimizing the chance for side effects. Additionally, this approach lends itself to a reversal and slow withdrawal of one or more agents with control of pressure. However, there is little likelihood that antihypertensive therapy can or should be totally withdrawn in patients with pre-existing moderate or severe essential hypertension.

In contrast to this therapeutic approach, I have long advocated a more rational means for selecting therapy based on the clinical and physiologic characteristics of the patient. This approach would focus on the specific inhibition of disease mechanisms using knowledge of the mechanism of drug action. This is, indeed, the ideal of all clinical therapeutic challenges—a goal worthy of long-standing commitment in the field of hypertension.

In view of the foregoing discussion of the antihypertensive drugs and their respective differences with respect to clinical pharmacologic principles, the rationale for the change in recommendations by the Joint National Committee in its fourth report is clear.[5] The report now recommends the individualization of the stepped-care approach by including the use of diuretics, β-blockers, angiotensin-converting enzyme inhibitors, and the calcium antagonists for initial therapy. This is because, unlike the other adrenergic inhibitors in the direct-acting smooth muscle vasodilators, these four classes of agents do not promote an intravascular volume expansion after they reduce arterial pressure. If optimal blood pressure control is not achieved with any of these selected drugs, the clinician may elect to increase the dose of the agent chosen to full doses, change to an alternative agent (e.g., a calcium antagonist instead of the diuretic or the angiotensin-converting enzyme inhibitor instead of the β-blocker), or add a second agent (Table 77.9). If pressure is still not controlled several other options

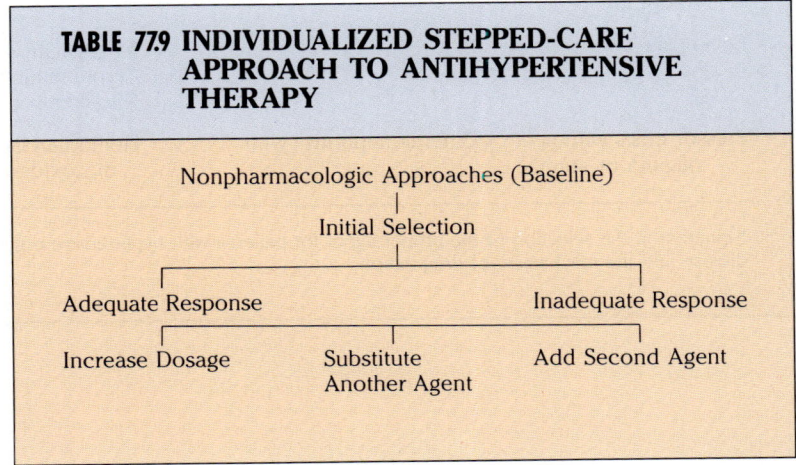

TABLE 77.9 INDIVIDUALIZED STEPPED-CARE APPROACH TO ANTIHYPERTENSIVE THERAPY

remain: (1) change to still another agent; (2) add a second agent; or (3) use high doses of either of the agents already selected.

The rationale for presenting this new option in selecting antihypertensive therapy is to provide single daily dose antihypertensive monotherapy to the maximal number of patients with essential hypertension. It is generally held that most patients with mild and moderately severe essential hypertension should respond to nonpharmacologic therapy without or with this approach of individualized stepped care.

SEVERE OR MORE RESISTANT FORMS OF ESSENTIAL HYPERTENSION

In patients with severe or more resistant forms of hypertension, therapy may have already been initiated with either of the two potential step-one agents, and a second-step agent may have also been added. If this therapeutic program includes a diuretic and a β-blocker, then a vasodilator (e.g., hydralazine, minoxidil) or a slow-entry channel calcium blocker may be added to the treatment program. With the addition of an agent that directly dilates the vascular smooth muscle to the regimen of a patient already receiving a diuretic and an adrenergic inhibitor, a fall in arterial pressure may be expected without the otherwise anticipated reflex stimulation of the heart and fluid retention. Alternatively, the physician may wish to add to the baseline treatment of a diuretic one of the angiotensin converting enzyme inhibitors. Should arterial pressure fail to respond to this more potent form of therapy, several points should be considered: the patient may not be taking the prescribed treatment for a variety of reasons (e.g., poorly explained or understood treatment program, development of side effects, and so

TABLE 77.10 TREATMENT OF HYPERTENSIVE URGENCIES OR EMERGENCIES*

Condition	Therapy	Cautions
Urgency (reduce pressure within hours or days without need for intensive-care hospitalization)	Angiotensin-converting enzyme inhibitor Slow-entry channel calcium blocking drugs Diazoxide Labetalol	Monitor serum potassium Follow renal function Check for reflex cardiac effects Watch for postural hypotension
Accelerated or malignant hypertension or	Angiotensin-converting enzyme inhibitor	See above
Acute myocardial infarction with severe hypertension	Slow-entry channel calcium blocking drugs Diuretics or Nitroprusside (IV)	When used, care should be exercised in follow-up of potassium levels
Left ventricular failure	Nitroprusside (IV) Angiotensin-converting enzyme inhibitor Diuretics	Monitor thiocyanate levels See above Monitor potassium levels
Postoperative (e.g., coronary bypass, aneurysm, hypotension)	Nitroprusside (IV) Trimethaphan camsylate	Watch for paralytic ileus
Hypertensive encephalopathy	Diazoxide (IV) Nitroprusside (IV) Trimethaphan camsylate (IV)	
Subarachnoid hemorrhage	Diazoxide (IV) Nitroprusside (IV) Trimethaphan camsylate (IV)	
Pheochromocytoma crisis	Labetalol (IV) Phentolamine (IV) with β-blocker (for cardiac arrhythmias)	Watch for fluid retention

Other cathecholamine excess syndromes
  Clonidine withdrawal
  Tyramine-containing foods and monoamine oxidase inhibitor
  Guanethidine or guanadrel and imipramine or desipramine
	Treat as pheochromocytoma crisis (or reinstitute clonidine in clonidine-withdrawal cases)	

Eclampsia	Magnesium sulfate Cryptenamine Nifedipine	May cause vomiting
Pressor crisis with acute glomerulonephritis (with oliguria or anuria)	Hemodialysis (if furosemide and diazoxide do not work)	Monitor serum potassium

* Inherent in the selection of the proper agent for patients with hypertensive urgencies or emergencies is a rational "wedding" of the underlying mechanisms of the disease and the mechanism of drug action.

forth); the patient may be retaining fluid because he is unresponsive to thiazide diuretics (*e.g.*, impaired renal function); or a secondary form of hypertension may be present (*e.g.*, development of occlusive renal arterial disease). Under these circumstances, each and all of the foregoing possibilities should be explored to the fullest with any and all of the diagnostic, therapeutic, and referral options that are available to the physician. Finally, while the treatment of hypertensive urgencies and emergencies is a more appropriate subject for a separate chapter, Table 77.10 provides a guide to therapy of the variety of conditions concerned in this grouping.

No matter what the choice of therapeutic management program, maintaining control of arterial pressure offers a brighter future with less chance of complicating disease and earlier mortality.

REFERENCES

1. Frohlich ED: Achievements in hypertension: A 25-year overview. J Am Coll Cardiol 1:225, 1983
2. Hypertension Detection and Follow-Up Program Cooperative Group: Five-year findings of the Hypertension Detection and Follow-Up Program. I. Reduction in mortality of persons with high blood pressure, including mild hypertension. JAMA 242:2562, 1979
3. Hypertension Detection and Follow-Up Program Cooperative Group: Five-year findings of the Hypertension Detection and Follow-Up Program. II. Mortality by race, sex and age. JAMA 242:2572, 1979
4. Frohlich ED: Treatment of hypertension: The case for pharmacological therapy. In Narins RG (ed): Controversies in Nephrology and Hypertension, p 93. New York, Churchill Livingstone, 1984
5. The Joint National Committee on the Detection, Evaluation, and Treatment of High Blood Pressure: The 1988 Report of the Joint National Committee on Detection, Evaluation, and Treatment of High Blood Pressure. Arch Intern Med 148:1023, 1988
6. Levy RI, Moskowitz J: Cardiovascular research: Decades of progress, a decade of promise. Science 217:121, 1982
7. Veterans Administration Cooperative Study Group on Antihypertensive Agents: Effects of treatment on morbidity in hypertension. Results in patients with diastolic blood pressure averaging 115 through 129 mm Hg. JAMA 202:1028, 1967
8. Veterans Administration Cooperative Study Group on Antihypertensive Agents: Effects of treatment on morbidity in hypertension. II. Results in patients with diastolic blood pressure averaging 90 through 114 mm Hg. JAMA 213:1143, 1970
9. Perry HM (chairman): Recommendations for a national high blood pressure program data base for effective antihypertensive therapy. Report of Task Force I. DHEW publication No (N.I.H.) 75-593. Bethesda, US Department of Health, Education and Welfare, 1973
10. Frohlich ED: Practical management of hypertension. Curr Probl Cardiol 10:1, 1985
11. Frohlich ED, Tarazi RC, Dustan HP: Clinical-physiological correlations in the development of hypertensive heart disease. Circulation 44:446, 1971
12. Ungerleider HE: Cardiac enlargement. Radiology 48:129, 1947
13. Ungerleider HE, Clark CP: Study of the transverse diameter of the heart silhouette with prediction table based on the teleroentgenogram. Am Heart J 17:92, 1939
14. Tarazi RC, Miller A, Frohlich ED, Dustan HP: Electrocardiographic changes reflecting left atrial abnormality in hypertension. Circulation 34:818, 1966
15. Tarazi RC, Frohlich ED, Dustan HP: Left atrial abnormality and ventricular pre-ejection period in hypertension. Dis Chest 55:214, 1969
16. Dunn FG, Chandraratna P, de Carvalho JGR et al: Pathophysiological assessment of hypertensive heart disease with echocardiography. Am J Cardiol 39:789, 1977
17. Frohlich ED: Haemodynamics of hypertension. In Genest J, Koiw E, Kuchel O (eds): Hypertension: Physiopathology and Treatment, p 15. New York, McGraw-Hill, 1977
18. Frohlich ED: The heart in hypertension. In Genest J, Kuchel O, Hamet P, Cantin M (eds): Hypertension: Physiopathology and Treatment, 2nd ed, p 791. New York, McGraw-Hill, 1983
19. Oren S, Grossman E, Messerli FH et al: High blood pressure: Side-effects of drugs, poisons, and food. Cardiol Clin 6(5):225, 1988
20. Gäisböck R: Die Bedeutung der Blutcruck messung fur die Praxis. Dtsch Arch Klin Med 83:363, 1905
21. Emery AC Jr, Whitcomb WH, Frohlich ED: "Stress" polycythemia and hypertension. JAMA 229:159, 1974
22. Chrysanthakopoulos SG, Frohlich ED, Adamopoulos PN et al: The pathophysiologic significance of "stress polycythemia" in essential hypertension. Am J Cardiol 37:1069, 1976
23. Kobrin I, Frohlich ED, Ventura HO et al: Stable red cell mass despite contracted plasma volume in men with essential hypertension. J Lab Clin Med 104:11, 1984
24. Tarazi RC, Frohlich ED, Dustan HP: Plasma volume in men with essential hypertension. N Engl J Med 278:762, 1968
25. Messerli FH, Frohlich ED, Dreslinski GR et al: Serum uric acid in essential hypertension: An indicator of renal vascular involvement. Ann Intern Med 93:817, 1980
26. Kobrin I, Frohlich ED, Ventura HO et al: Renal involvement follows cardiac enlargement in essential hypertension. Arch Intern Med 146:272, 1986
27. The Lipid Research Clinics Coronary Primary Prevention Trial Results. Lipid Research Clinics Program. JAMA 251:351, 1984
28. McPhie J: Left ventricular hypertrophy. Electrocardiographic diagnosis. Australas Ann Med 7:317, 1958
29. Multiple Risk Factor Intervention Trial Research Group: Multiple Risk Factor Intervention Trial. Risk factor changes and mortality results. JAMA 248:1465, 1982
30. Frohlich ED: Initial drug therapy—treatment options. In Hunt JC, Dreifus LS, Dustan HP (eds): Hypertension Update II: Pharmacotherapy and Management of Hypertension, p 22. Lyndhurst, NJ, Health Learning Systems, 1985
31. Frohlich ED: Hemodynamic factors in the pathogenesis and maintenance of hypertension. Fed Proc 41:2400, 1982
32. Frohlich ED, Messerli FH, Re RN et al: Mechanisms controlling arterial pressure. In Frohlich ED (ed): Pathophysiology: Altered Regulatory Mechanisms in Disease, 3rd ed, p 45. Philadelphia, JB Lippincott, 1984
33. Ulrych M, Frohlich ED, Dustan HP, Page IH: Cardiac output and distribution of blood volume in central and peripheral circulations in hypertensive and normotensive man. Br Heart J 31:570, 1969
34. Messerli FH, Frohlich ED: High blood pressure: A common side effect of drugs, poisons, and food. Arch Intern Med 139:682, 1979
35. Ram CVS, Garrett BN, Kaplan NM: Moderate sodium restriction and various diuretics in the treatment of hypertension. Ann Intern Med 141:1015, 1981
36. Johansson BW (ed): Electrolytes and cardiac arrhythmias. Acta Med Scand [Suppl] 647:1, 1980
37. Holland CB, Nixon JF, Kunnert L: Diuretic-induced ventricular ectopic activity. Am J Med 70:762, 1981
38. Messerli FH, Ventura HO, Elizardi DJ et al: Hypertension and sudden death: Increased ventricular ectopic activity in left ventricular hypertrophy. Am J Med 77:18, 1984
39. Frohlich ED: Diuretics in hypertension. J Hypertension (Suppl 3)5:S43, 1987
40. Frohlich ED: Potential mechanisms explaining the risk of left ventricular hypertrophy. Am J Cardiol 59:91A, 1987
41. Frohlich ED: Cardiac hypertrophy in hypertension. N Engl J Med 317:831, 1987
42. Connolly ME, Kersting F, Dollery CT: The clinical pharmacology of beta-adrenoceptor blocking drugs. Prog Cardiovasc Dis 19:203, 1976
43. Fitzgerald JD: Cardioselective beta-adrenergic blockade. Proc R Soc Med (Lond) 65:761, 1972
44. Frohlich ED: Beta-adrenergic receptor blockade in the treatment of essential hypertension. In Strauer BE (ed): The Heart in Hypertension, p 425. New York, Springer-Verlag, 1981
45. Svendsen TL, Hartling O, Trap-Jensen J et al: Adrenergic beta-receptor blockade: Haemodynamic importance of intrinsic synpathomimetic activity at rest. Clin Pharmacol Ther 29:711, 1961
46. Hausler G: Central α-adrenoceptors involved in cardiovascular regulation. J Cardiovasc Pharmacol 4:72s, 1982
47. Langer SZ, Cavero I, Massingham R: Recent developments in noradrenergic neurotransmission and its relevance to the mechanism of action of certain antihypertensive drugs. Hypertension 2:372, 1980
48. Weil JV, Chidsey CA: Plasma volume expansion resulting from interference with adrenergic function in normal man. Circulation 37:54, 1968
49. Dustan HP, Tarazi RC, Bravo EL: Dependence of arterial pressure on intravascular volume in treated hypertensive patients. N Engl J Med 286:861, 1972
50. Hollenberg NK, Meggs LG, Williams GH et al: Sodium intake and renal responses to captopril in normal man and in essential hypertension. Kidney Int 20:240, 1981
51. Frohlich ED: Newer antihypertensive drugs. In Yu PN, Goodwin JF (eds): Progress in Cardiology, p 265. Philadelphia, Lea & Febiger, 1984
52. Dunn FG, Oigman W, Ventura HO et al: Enalapril improves systemic and renal hemodynamics and regresses left ventricular mass in essential hypertension. J Am Coll Cardiol 53:105, 1984
53. Ventura HO, Frohlich ED, Messerli FH et al: Cardiovascular effects and regional blood flow distribution associated with angiotensin converting enzyme inhibition (captopril) in essential hypertension. Am J Cardiol 55:1023, 1985
54. Garavaglia GE, Messerli FH, Nunez BD et al: Immediate and short-term cardiovascular effects of a new converting enzyme inhibitor (lisinopril) in essential hypertension. Am J Cardiol 62:912, 1988

55. Hostetter TH, Rennke HG, Brenner BM: The case for intrarenal hypertension in the initiation and progression of diabetic and other glomerulopathies. Am J Med 72:375, 1982
56. Frohlich ED, Cooper RA, Lewis EJ: A review of the overall experience of captopril in hypertension. Arch Intern Med 144:1441, 1984
57. Hricik DE, Browning PJ, Kopelman R et al: Captopril-induced functional renal insufficiency in patients with bilateral renal-artery stenosis or renal-artery stenosis in a solitary kidney. N Engl J Med 308:373, 1983
58. Curtis LJ, Luke RG, Whelchel JD et al: Inhibition of angiotensin converting enzyme in renal-transplant recipients with hypertension. N Engl J Med 308:377, 1983
59. McCall D, Walsh RA, Frohlich ED et al: Calcium entry blocking drugs: Mechanisms of action, experimental studies, and clinical uses. Curr Probl Cardiol 10:7, 1985
60. Amodeo C, Ventura HO, Messerli FH et al: Immediate and short-term hemodynamic effects of diltiazem in patients with hypertension. Circulation 73:108, 1986
61. Isshiki T, Amodeo C, Messerli FH et al: Diltiazem maintains renal vasodilation without hyperfiltration in hypertension: Studies in essential hypertensive man and the spontaneously hypertensive rat. Cardiovasc Drugs Ther 1:359, 1987
62. Grossman E, Oren S, Garavaglia GE et al: Systemic and regional hemodynamic and humoral effects of nitrendipine in essential hypertension. Circulation 78:1394, 1988
63. Isshiki T, Uchino K, Kardon MB et al: Diltiazem reduces glomerular pressure in SHR: A micropuncture study. (submitted for publication)

Evaluation of Secondary Forms of Hypertension

Michael D. Cressman ▪ Ray W. Gifford, Jr

CHAPTER 78
VOLUME 2

One of the goals of the initial evaluation of the hypertensive patient is to detect a secondary cause of high blood pressure. In this chapter, secondary hypertension refers to any cause of hypertension that is not idiopathic ("primary" or "essential"). A secondary cause is present in roughly 10% of the hypertensive population and less than 50% of these cases are curable.[1] Despite this low incidence, detection of a condition other than essential hypertension (EH) may drastically alter the patient's subsequent care. Hypertension can be a manifestation of an immediately life-threatening but curable disease such as pheochromocytoma or a clue to the presence of previously undetected chronic renal disease. Surgical cure of hypertension is possible in some patients, particularly those with renovascular hypertension, primary hyperaldosteronism, and pheochromocytoma. This eliminates the expense, inconvenience, and potential adverse effects of drug therapy.

The clinical presentation and pathophysiology of the most common secondary causes of hypertension (Table 78.1) will be described in this section. An approach to the laboratory investigation and treatment options will also be discussed. Before describing specific disease entities, it is helpful to point out general features that should suggest a secondary cause of hypertension.

TABLE 78.1 SECONDARY CAUSES OF HIGH BLOOD PRESSURE

Renal
1. Renal parenchymal disease
   a. Bilateral
   b. Focal
2. Renovascular
   a. Atherosclerotic and fibrous
   b. Thromboembolic

Endocrine
1. Adrenal
   a. Pheochromocytoma
   b. Primary aldosteronism
   c. Cushing's syndrome
   d. Adrenocortical enzyme deficiencies
2. Extra-adrenal
   a. Hypothyroidism
   b. Hyperthyroidism
   c. Hyperparathyroidism
   d. Acromegaly
   e. Carcinoid syndrome
   f. Diabetes

Drug-Induced
1. Oral contraceptives
2. Alcohol
3. Corticosteroid
4. Nonsteroidal anti-inflammatory
5. Sympathomimetics
6. Sympatholytic agent withdrawal
7. Monoamine oxidase/tyramine ingestion
8. Amphetamines, cocaine, narcotics (and their withdrawal)
9. Ergotamine
10. Glycyrrhizic acid (licorice)

Neurologic
1. Increased intracranial pressure
2. Peripheral neuropathies

Post Cardiac Surgery
1. Postcoronary bypass
2. Post cardiac transplant
3. Post aortic valve replacement

CLUES TO THE PRESENCE OF A SECONDARY CAUSE

HYPERTENSION PRESENTING AT AN ATYPICAL AGE SHOULD BE SUSPECTED AS BEING SECONDARY. EH usually is detected between ages 35 and 55 years (although EH is the most common cause of adolescent hypertension). When hypertension develops abruptly in young patients or in the elderly, a search for a secondary cause is warranted, particularly if the hypertension is severe or resistant to treatment.

A POOR RESPONSE TO STANDARD TRIPLE DRUG TREATMENT SHOULD RAISE THE SUSPICION OF A SECONDARY CAUSE OF HYPERTENSION. Previously controlled hypertension that becomes resistant may also indicate the development of a secondary cause. Atherosclerotic renal artery disease frequently presents in this fashion. It should be kept in mind that many patients with secondary causes of hypertension respond well to standard drug treatment so an adequate response does not exclude the possibility that a secondary cause is present. Atypical or paradoxical responses to certain antihypertensive agents can also suggest a secondary cause. For example, the development of profound hypokalemia in a patient receiving a small dose of a thiazide diuretic should raise the suspicion of primary aldosteronism. Paradoxical hypertension has been reported after the administration of several sympatholytic agents in patients with pheochromocytoma.

THE SUDDEN APPEARANCE OF SEVERE HYPERTENSION AT ANY AGE SHOULD SUGGEST A SECONDARY CAUSE. The development of high blood pressure is gradual in most patients with EH. The massive effort to detect and treat asymptomatic hypertension in the community has undoubtedly led to a decrease in the frequency of accelerated and malignant-phase essential hypertension. Unfortunately, patients with EH in economically deprived areas still present in this fashion. However, because of the decreasing frequency of malignant hypertension due to EH, virtually all patients with this entity should be carefully evaluated for a secondary cause. In addition, the sudden appearance of severe hypertension or a sudden worsening of preexisting hypertension is suggestive even if the patient has no symptoms and does not have accelerated or malignant-phase hypertension. Correlation of the level of the blood pressure with certain clinical features can be helpful in determining the duration of the hypertension. For example, patients with severe hypertension of recent onset tend to have significant spasm in the retinal arterioles with less severe sclerotic changes (change in the light reflex or the presence of arteriovenous nicking). The absence of evidence of involvement of target organs in a patient with severe hypertension is consistent with a recent onset.

A SECONDARY CAUSE OF HYPERTENSION SHOULD BE SUSPECTED WHEN SIGNIFICANT SYMPTOMS ACCOMPANY THE HYPERTENSION. It is well known that mild to moderate essential hypertension does not, in and of itself, cause any symptoms. Symptoms in patients with EH are usually due to complications of the hypertension or the presence of an unrelated illness. In contrast, patients with pheochromocytoma generally have a variety of symptoms (*e.g.*, headache, sweating, palpitations) associated with their hypertension. Severe headaches (especially in the morning) should raise the suspicion of an intracranial mass lesion, particularly if unilateral papilledema is noted on physical examination. Muscle weakness may be a prominent feature in patients with Cushing's syndrome (particularly in patients with an ACTH-producing tumor), hypothyroidism, hyperthyroidism, peripheral neuropathies, and primary hyperaldosteronism. Polyuria and nocturia develop in patients with poorly controlled diabetes mellitus and in some patients with chronic renal failure.

A subgroup of patients with EH have symptoms of adrenergic excess (labile hypertension, palpitations, excessive sweating), suggesting the presence of diseases such as pheochromocytoma, hyperthyroidism, or other states that lead to activation of the sympathetic nervous system (SNS). These "hypernoradrenergic" patients with EH are usually young and have physical features that suggest SNS activation. These include (1) resting tachycardia, (2) systolic ejection murmurs, and/or (3) a hyperdynamic precordium. β-Blockers are quite effective in this group of patients with essential hypertension who have variably been labeled as having a "hyperkinetic circulation" or a "hyper-β-adrenergic state." It should be kept in mind that this diagnosis should only be made after conditions such as pheochromocytoma, hyperthyroidism, and other conditions subsequently described have been reasonably excluded.

RENAL HYPERTENSION

HYPERTENSION IN RENAL PARENCHYMAL DISEASE

BILATERAL RENAL PARENCHYMAL DISEASE

CLINICAL PRESENTATION. Hypertension is present at some stage in approximately 85% of patients with chronic renal failure (CRF) and is the most common non-drug-related cause of secondary hypertension.[1,2] High blood pressure can be the initial manifestation of asymptomatic chronic renal parenchymal disease. Danielson and his coworkers noted hypertension in patients with CRF even before the serum creatinine had changed significantly.[3] In their series, 35% of hypertensive patients with chronic renal parenchymal disease had serum creatinine concentrations of 1.4 mg/dl or less. Hypertension was discovered prior to or at the time of diagnosis in 50% of these patients.

Historical clues to the presence of chronic renal disease include (1) the history of previous renal disease such as "nephritis," repeated urinary tract infections, hematuria, and/or renal calculus formation; (2) polyuria and/or nocturia; (3) excessive fatigue, weakness, or anorexia; (4) the presence or history of generalized edema; or (5) the excessive use of analgesics. The patient may have been informed about an abnormal urinalysis in the past. Early in the course of CRF, there are usually no helpful physical findings to suggest the presence of renal parenchymal disease. Exceptions to this rule include the presence of palpable kidneys in patients with polycystic kidney disease or the demonstration of peripheral edema in the nephrotic syndrome. Diabetic retinopathy is virtually always present in patients with diabetic nephropathy. Cutaneous manifestations of the systemic vasculitides may be present in patients with systemic lupus erythematosus, polyarteritis nodosa, scleroderma, Henoch-Schönlein purpura, Wegener's granulomatosis, or bacterial endocarditis. Dark red papules on the lower abdomen, pubic area, buttocks, and upper thighs suggest the presence of Fabry's disease (angiokeratoma corporis diffusum).[4]

It should be kept in mind that hypertension occurs frequently in patients with acute glomerulonephritis. Hypertension can dominate the clinical picture in young patients who have a propensity to develop hypertensive encephalopathy with only moderately elevated blood pressure. Elderly patients may develop acute congestive heart failure because of the combined volume and pressure load that occur with acute renal insufficiency. The presence of significant azotemia and an abnormal urine sediment (particularly if the sediment contains red blood cell casts) points to the presence of a primary renal abnormality. However, renal insufficiency with an abnormal urinalysis can also occur in patients with accelerated or malignant-phase essential hypertension. Thus, it can be difficult to determine if hypertension produced the renal insufficiency or if a primary renal disease secondarily caused the hypertension.

PATHOPHYSIOLOGY. There are two major forms of renal parenchymal disease: glomerular diseases and tubulointerstitial diseases. In general, hypertension is more common and develops earlier in the course of chronic glomerular disease, but any type of chronic renal parenchymal disease can cause hypertension. Although the exact pathophysiology of the hypertension accompanying CRF is incompletely understood and probably varies with different etiologies of CRF, volume retention and abnormal control of the renin–angiotensin system appear to be the most important features.[2]

Brod and his co-workers found that the cardiac output and circulating blood volume were increased in approximately 33% of normotensive patients with mild renal insufficiency (glomerular filtration rate [GFR] > 50 ml/min).[5] Hypertension developed in over 90% of these patients during a 2- to 6-year period of follow-up. Volume expansion is further suggested by the presence of a natriuretic substance in the blood of patients with hypertension and chronic renal failure. The substance appears to be an ouabain-like sodium-potassium ATPase inhibitor. Volume expansion is thought to stimulate the release of this substance, which leads to natriuresis (due to inhibition of renal sodium-potassium ATPase) and vasoconstriction via a calcium-mediated enhancement of smooth muscle contraction. The importance of hypervolemia is suggested by the antihypertensive response to volume-depleting maneuvers (salt restriction, diuretic therapy, or ultrafiltration).

There is also evidence to suggest that abnormal regulation of the renin–angiotensin system contributes to the hypertension of CRF. Warren and Ferris found that saline-loaded patients with CRF did not suppress plasma renin activity (PRA) to the same degree as control subjects with normal renal function.[6] The majority of patients with CRF have PRAs less than 5 ng/ml/hr but 30% have hyperreninemia.[7] Furthermore, hypertensive patients with CRF have PRAs that are twice as high as the PRAs of normotensive patients with chronic renal failure for any given level of total exchangeable sodium. There are some patients with CRF in whom activation of the renin–angiotensin system appears to be the major mechanism of the hypertension. These patients usually have very high PRAs and do not respond to volume-depleting measures. In the past, bilateral nephrectomies were sometimes required to control the hypertension. Nephrectomies are required infrequently now that angiotensin-converting enzyme inhibitors and other potent antihypertensive medications are available.

LABORATORY INVESTIGATION. Azotemia, proteinuria, an abnormal urine sediment, and/or anemia is present in most patients with hypertension due to chronic renal parenchymal disease. The absence of any one of these laboratory abnormalities does not exclude the diagnosis. As previously stated, Danielson found that 35% of hypertensive patients with chronic renal disease had serum creatinine concentrations of 1.4 mg/dl or less.[3] It should be kept in mind that a serum creatinine that is at the upper limits of "normal" may represent a GFR which is reduced by as much as 50%. This is most likely to occur in patients with a small muscle mass (women, children, elderly patients) since the serum creatinine depends on the level of protein intake, the catabolism of muscle, and its excretion by the kidney.

Proteinuria is the cardinal laboratory manifestation of chronic renal disease. Significant proteinuria (>1.5 g/day) is noted in most patients with acute or chronic glomerulonephritis. Patients with tubulointerstitial disease also have proteinuria, but usually excrete less than 1.5 g in 24 hours. Normal patients excrete less than 150 mg in a day. Nephrotic-range (>3.0 g/24 hr) proteinuria is common in patients with idiopathic chronic glomerulonephritis and is nearly always detected by the dipstick method. However, the urine dipstick results can be "negative or trace" in patients with tubulointerstitial diseases, particularly if the urine sample is dilute. The urine dipstick is only sensitive to about 30 mg/dl of albumin. Since patients with chronic renal failure often have a renal concentrating defect, they may excrete several liters of dilute urine in a day and have negative or trace results on urine dipstick. For these reasons, it is useful to note the urine specific gravity when the degree of proteinuria is being estimated by the dipstick method. Quantitation of the daily urine protein excretion aids in the differentiation of patients with glomerular diseases from those with tubulointerstitial diseases. This differentiation requires a careful 24-hour urine collection. Specific instructions must be given to the patient to ensure adequate collection. Adequacy of the 24-hour urine specimen can be roughly estimated by measuring the creatinine (Cr) content of the specimen. Women excrete approximately 15 mg Cr/kg/day while men excrete roughly 20 mg Cr/kg/day.[8] GFR can be estimated by calculating the creatinine clearance. This requires a serum creatinine as well as the 24-hour urine creatinine. The sodium content of the urine can be measured as a general indicator of the daily sodium intake.

Patients with acute and chronic renal parenchymal diseases nearly always have some abnormality in the urinalysis if this test is carefully performed and includes a microscopic examination of the urine sediment. These abnormalities include microscopic hematuria, pyuria, crystalluria, and/or the presence of cellular casts. Patients with essential hypertension often have proteinuria but generally have a benign urine sediment. Red blood cell casts virtually always imply that glomerulonephritis is present. Patients with nephrotic-range proteinuria may have fatty casts, lipid-laden renal tubular epithelial cells ("oval fat bodies"), or lipid droplets in the urine specimen. However, these elements disintegrate in a short period of time and may not be found in a urine specimen that is not examined shortly after the patient has voided.

A normochromic, normocytic anemia occurs at a relatively early phase of chronic renal failure. Analgesic abusers frequently have a hypochromic, microcytic anemia due to the combined effects of their renal disease and gastrointestinal blood loss. Patients with polycystic kidney disease tend to have higher hematocrits at any level of renal function than patients with other forms of chronic renal parenchymal disease.

Ultrasonography is useful in patients with newly discovered chronic renal failure. A carefully performed examination will (1) virtually exclude the presence of obstructive uropathy, (2) identify patients with cystic diseases of the kidney, and (3) estimate kidney size. Its main advantage over intravenous pyelography is that the latter procedure requires the administration of potentially nephrotoxic contrast material. Computerized tomographic (CT) scanning is also helpful, but it may be difficult to visualize the renal pelvis and ureters without contrast material. Whenever possible, nephrologic consultation should be obtained when clinical and laboratory evidence suggests the presence of chronic renal disease. Renal biopsy may be required to obtain a definitive diagnosis and detect the presence of a potentially treatable renal disease. This is particularly true in patients with heavy proteinuria and normal or enlarged kidneys.

TREATMENT. This section will discuss the treatment of hypertension in patients with CRF (rather than the treatment of individual forms of CRF). As stated, hypertension develops in the vast majority of patients with CRF at some stage.[2] In addition, corticosteroid treatment of patients with certain types of glomerulonephritis and in renal transplant recipients may cause *de novo* hypertension or worsening of preexisting hypertension.

Despite the concern that renal function will deteriorate during the drug treatment of hypertension in patients with CRF, there is no good evidence that renal function deteriorates more rapidly in the long run in treated hypertensives. In fact, clinical and experimental evidence indicates that poorly controlled hypertension is a significant factor in the progression of chronic renal disease. It is true that salt restriction, diuretic therapy, and many β-blocking agents all have the potential to reduce renal blood flow or GFR. However, the effects of treatment on GFR may not persist; in fact, the serum creatinine may fall during long-term treatment. One could argue that the reduction in renal blood flow and GFR during the initial phase of antihypertensive therapy serves a protective role by favorably altering glomerular hemodynamics. If the theory of "hyperfiltration" is correct, methods to reduce renal blood flow and GFR are actually desirable in the patient with chronic renal failure.

Volume-depleting measures (salt restriction, diuretics, ultrafiltration/dialysis) are the mainstay of antihypertensive therapy in patients with hypertension due to CRF. The efficacy of the thiazide diuretics is diminished when the GFR is less than approximately 30 ml to 40 ml/min (this correlates with a serum creatinine of approximately 2.5

mg–3.5 mg/dl). Some of the newer thiazide derivatives (indapamide, metolazone) and the "loop" diuretics (bumetanide, ethacrynic acid, furosemide) are preferred in patients with more advanced renal disease. High doses of furosemide may be required in patients with severe renal insufficiency since the tubular secretion of this drug (which is required for its activity) is impaired in azotemic patients. It should be pointed out that potassium-sparing agents may cause severe hyperkalemia and should be avoided unless the patient with CRF has significant hypokalemia.

A number of options are available if volume-depleting maneuvers do not control the blood pressure. A "stepped-care" approach outlined by the Joint National Committee on Detection, Evaluation, and Treatment of High Blood Pressure can be followed in patients with CRF.[9] Although the various antiadrenergic agents (β-blockers, α_2-agonists, α_1-antagonists) have different renal hemodynamic effects, there is little evidence to document that these effects are important clinically. The dose of atenolol and nadolol should be reduced if a β-blocker is chosen as the second step in drug treatment since these agents are excreted by the kidneys and may accumulate in patients with CRF.

Converting enzyme inhibitors (captopril, enalapril) have been successfully utilized in hypertensive patients with CRF.[10] Rationale for their use is derived from the observation that an abnormal volume/pressure–renin relationship is present in these patients. Captopril has proven to be effective in patients with resistant hypertension due to CRF.[11] However, it should be kept in mind that (1) captopril and enalapril can accumulate in CRF, (2) patients with high renin levels may develop hypotension and possibly acute renal failure during the initial phase of angiotensin-converting enzyme (ACE) inhibitor treatment, and (3) captopril has been incriminated in the generation of membranous glomerulonephritis.[12] Thus, initiation of low-dose (6.25 mg–12.5 mg, two to three times daily) captopril therapy or enalapril (2.5 mg–5.0 mg once or twice daily) and vigilant observation for the toxic effects are mandatory if this agent is used in treating hypertension in the face of chronic renal failure. It is of note, however, that experimental evidence suggests that ACE inhibitors may delay progression of chronic renal insufficiency to end-stage renal failure.

Captopril is probably the drug of choice for the management of the hypertensive–renal crisis of scleroderma. This syndrome is characterized by the sudden and rapid deterioration of renal function associated with severe renin-mediated hypertension. The syndrome develops in approximately 7% of patients with scleroderma and often causes a hypertensive crisis, end-stage renal failure, and/or death.[13] Bilateral nephrectomy was formerly required to control the blood pressure but, more recently, a number of agents have been used to treat the hypertension. Control of the blood pressure has been associated with reversal of this syndrome, but treated patients may progress to end-stage renal failure despite adequate blood pressure control.[14]

"FOCAL" RENAL PARENCHYMAL DISEASE

CLINICAL PRESENTATION. Uncommonly, a unilateral disease involving all or a portion of a kidney produces hypertension. Hypertension has been noted in patients with unilateral pyelonephritis, renal cysts, renal tumors, and renal hematomas.[15–18] In addition, unilateral or bilateral urinary tract obstruction can produce hypertension.[18] A history of flank trauma, acute pyelonephritis, or a known renal cyst may come to light during the initial hypertensive evaluation. The presence of a presumed renal mass on physical examination is also suggestive. At times, an abnormal urinalysis has prompted radiographic investigation of the urinary tract. Such an investigation may bring to light the presence of a unilateral disease of the renal parenchyma. Although none of these entities is common, they should be kept in mind in patients whose hypertension appeared abruptly or is unusually severe.

PATHOPHYSIOLOGY. Several case reports have described hypertension that appeared to be "renin-dependent" in patients with (1) hypernephromas, (2) renal juxtaglomerular cell tumors, (3) unilateral ureteral obstruction, (4) solitary or multiple renal cysts, (5) unilateral pyelonephritis, or (6) unilateral or segmental hypoplasia (Ask-Upmark kidney).[15–18] In most situations, the renin dependency of these conditions has been inferred from the finding of asymmetric renin production at the time of renal venous catheterization and/or cure of the hypertension by appropriate surgery. The juxtaglomerular tumors produce renin; in most of the other situations described it is felt that ischemia due to compression of adjacent normal renal parenchyma led to the hyperreninemia and hypertension.[17]

LABORATORY INVESTIGATION. All of these forms of hypertension are very rare and laboratory confirmation may be extremely difficult. Radiographic examination of the kidneys should always be performed if examination of the bladder is unrevealing in a patient with microscopic or gross hematuria. Azotemia or significant proteinuria is infrequent since most of these entities are focal and unilateral. Intravenous pyelography and ultrasonography are both useful but neither of these procedures is universally sensitive. In addition, the presence of one of these lesions does not necessarily mean that the hypertension is related. Elevation of PRA in the peripheral venous blood or preferably in renal venous blood may suggest a relationship between the renal pathology and the hypertension. Proof of the relationship requires definitive (usually surgical) treatment.

TREATMENT. Surgical treatment is indicated in patients with renal tumors and those with ureteral obstruction (if the kidney is salvageable or the hypertension is severe). Drainage of a solitary renal cyst has resulted in amelioration of hypertension, but this is rarely required.[16] Unilateral or segmental atrophy of the kidney may also require surgery if it is felt that this will correct the hypertension. In many cases, the hypertension is mild or easily controlled with medications, and surgical therapy is not mandatory. A trial of an ACE inhibitor is reasonable if the hypertension is difficult to control or the plasma renin level is very high (particularly if the patient is not an ideal surgical candidate).

RENOVASCULAR HYPERTENSION

FIBROUS AND ATHEROSCLEROTIC RENAL ARTERY DISEASE

CLINICAL PRESENTATION. Renovascular hypertension is the most common curable cause of high blood pressure.[1] There are two major types of diseases that affect the main renal artery or its major branches. Renovascular hypertension (RVH) in young patients is usually "fibrous"; atherosclerotic disease occurs with increasing frequency in older patients (over age 50). The most frequent clues to the presence of fibrous disease of the renal arteries include (1) the abrupt onset of hypertension developing in a patient less than 35 years of age, (2) the appearance of accelerated or malignant-phase hypertension in this age group, (3) resistant hypertension, (4) the presence of vasospastic retinopathy, and (5) the detection of a systolic/diastolic bruit deep within the abdomen. Atherosclerotic renal artery disease is suggested by similar features in older patients but systolic/diastolic bruits are uncommon.

Fibrous diseases occur in both males and females but are more frequent in women. The incidence of fibrous disease is very low in black patients, and if a fibrous lesion is noted in a black hypertensive, it is particularly important to determine whether or not such a patient has renovascular disease with essential hypertension or renovascular hypertension. Takayashu's disease should be considered in Oriental patients, especially if carotid or upper extremity occlusive vascular disease is present. It should also be kept in mind that renovascular hypertension occurs in patients with von Recklinghausen's disease. Patients with atherosclerotic renal artery disease often have generalized atherosclerosis with historical evidence or physical findings suggesting cerebrovascular, coronary, or peripheral vascular disease.

The presence of a systolic/diastolic abdominal bruit is a particularly important clue to the presence of renovascular hypertension in young patients. The stethoscope should be applied with pressure to the abdomen in the epigastrium and 3 cm to 4 cm lateral to it. Systolic bruits are frequently heard in the midline, particularly in thin patients. Superficial systolic bruits generally emanate from the celiac or mesenteric arteries and are often confused with the bruit signifying the presence of renal artery disease. Systolic bruits are often heard in patients with atherosclerosis but the systolic/diastolic bruits of renal artery disease are uncommon. Radiographic investigation is generally indicated if a systolic/diastolic bruit is heard, particularly if the patient has vasospastic retinopathy and/or rapid onset of severe hypertension. In these patients, the pretest probability of renal artery disease is quite high. However, it should be pointed out that the clinical history of most patients with RVH is indistinguishable from that of patients with essential hypertension, and the absence of any of the general clues to the presence of RVH previously described does not rule out the possibility that a renal artery lesion exists.

PATHOPHYSIOLOGY. Harrison and co-workers provided a useful classification of the fibrous diseases in 1971.[19] The various fibrous lesions were characterized by radiographic and pathologic features into three major types (Table 78.2). Classification of these lesions is of more than academic interest since their natural history varies considerably. Approximately 85% of the fibrous lesions have a "beaded" appearance. Medial fibroplasia (Fig. 78.1) is the most common lesion (64%) and carries the best prognosis. The beads in medial fibroplasia represent true aneurysms, a distinction noted angiographically when the beads are larger than the lumen of the proximal main renal artery. The long-term prognosis of these lesions is good since dissection, thrombosis, or rupture of an aneurysm is uncommon. However, loss of renal mass can occur and careful monitoring of both blood pressure and renal function is required if medical treatment is chosen.

Perimedial fibroplasia occurs in approximately 20% of patients with fibrous disease and is particularly common in young women. These lesions are also beaded, but the beads appear because of areas of stenosis rather than areas of dilatation. Angiographically, the beads in perimedial fibroplasia are smaller than the diameter of the main renal artery. The potential for loss of renal mass is greater with perimedial disease than it is in patients with medial fibroplasia.

Intimal fibroplasia (Fig. 78.2), medial hyperplasia, and periarterial fibroplasia are all uncommon lesions. These uncommon lesions are not beaded and can be confused with atherosclerosis. They are usually located in the proximal or mid portion of the main renal artery and are difficult to distinguish angiographically. The age of the patient and the absence of extra-renal occlusive disease suggest that the stenosis is due to one of the fibrous lesions rather than atherosclerosis. The prognosis of the nonbeaded fibrous lesions is poor because these lesions often progress and may thrombose or dissect. Surgical treatment should be undertaken whenever possible. Atherosclerotic disease of the renal artery can have a similar appearance but the atherosclerotic lesions tend to be more proximal. These patients are usually older and have evidence of atherosclerosis in the aorta and celiac, mesenteric, or iliac vessels (Fig. 78.3). The potential of atherosclerotic renal artery disease to progress and jeopardize renal function has been adequately documented, and in some patients, elective renal revascularization may be considered to preserve renal function.

The pathophysiology of RVH depends on whether or not the stenosis is unilateral or bilateral. Unilateral RVH is the counterpart of Goldblatt's experimental two-kidney–one-clip (2K–1C) hypertension in dogs. In this model, constriction of a single renal artery leads to release of renin in the clipped kidney. Renin is a proteolytic enzyme that stimulates the formation of angiotensin I (A_I) from angiotensinogen (renin substrate), which is synthesized in the liver. The two terminal amino acids (histidyl and leucine) of A_I are cleaved by an angiotensin-converting enzyme to form the potent vasoconstrictor angiotensin II (A_{II}). Although the converting enzyme is located primarily in the lung, it is found in other capillary beds, particularly in the kidney.

The important role of the renin–angiotensin system in the pathogenesis of unilateral renovascular hypertension is suggested by the

TABLE 78.2 CLASSIFICATION OF THE FIBROUS RENAL ARTERY LESIONS

Intimal
Intimal fibroplasia (5%–10%)

Medial
1. Medial fibroplasia (60%–70%) — "beaded" lesions
2. Perimedial fibroplasia (15%–25%) — "beaded" lesions
3. Medial hyperplasia (5%–10%)
4. Medial dissection (5%–10%)

Adventitia
Periarterial fibroplasia (<1%)

(Adapted from Harrison EG, McCormack LJ: Pathologic classification of renal arterial disease in renovascular hypertension. Mayo Clin Proc 46:161, 1971)

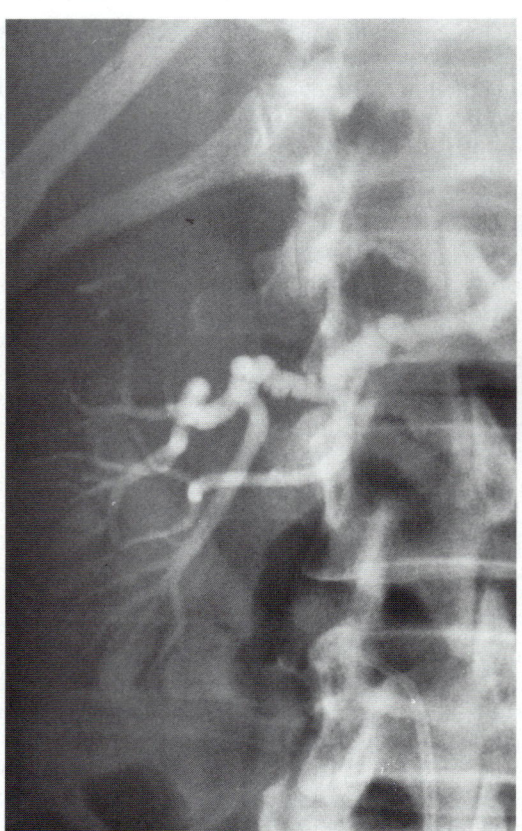

FIGURE 78.1 Medial fibroplasia is the most common fibrous lesion of the renal artery and has the most favorable prognosis.

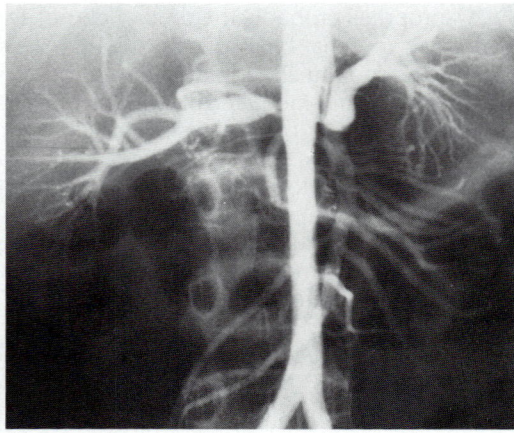

FIGURE 78.2 Intimal fibroplasia.

beneficial response to converting enzyme inhibitors (captopril, enalapril), A_{II} antagonists (saralasin), and corrective surgery. These patients generally have high peripheral PRAs and contracted or normal plasma volumes. Presumably, this occurs because of a "pressure-natriuresis" phenomenon that occurs in the unaffected kidney. The situation differs in patients with bilateral renal artery disease, when the artery to a solitary kidney is stenosed, or if renal parenchymal disease is present. In these situations volume expansion often plays a significant role in the hypertension, a finding that is suggested by a normal or suppressed peripheral PRA and an expanded blood volume.

LABORATORY INVESTIGATION. Renovascular disease is defined radiographically, but the angiographic demonstration of renovascular disease does not confirm the presence of RVH. In fact, RVH is only proven when a patient becomes normotensive after successful renal angioplasty, reconstructive arterial surgery, or nephrectomy. Nevertheless, several clinical, radiographic, and biochemical clues are useful in predicting surgical cure of the hypertension.

Several screening procedures have been advocated for the detection of renal artery disease. Unfortunately, none of these tests is specific or sensitive enough to establish the diagnosis or rule it out. Thus, a case can be made for performing formal renal arteriography as the first procedure if the clinical suspicion is high and the patient is a surgical candidate. (An example would be a young woman with acute-onset severe hypertension who has vasospastic retinopathy and a systolic/diastolic abdominal bruit.) However, there are situations when a normal rapid-sequence intravenous pyelogram (IVP), intravenous digital subtraction angiogram, or radionuclide renal flow scan can be sufficiently reassuring to postpone arteriography and attempt to control the hypertension medically while closely following renal function. The rapid-sequence IVP is a useful procedure to perform if some form of renal hypertension (RVH or hypertension due to renal parenchymal disease) is suspected on clinical grounds. A carefully performed examination allows the physician to (1) determine if the patient has one or two kidneys, (2) detect anatomical abnormalities (obstruction, cysts, tumors, segmental hypoplasia), and (3) estimate kidney size. There are several clues that suggest the presence of renal artery disease, particularly if the renal artery disease is severe and unilateral. These findings include (1) delayed appearance of contrast in the affected kidney on early (1–2 min) films, (2) discrepancy in renal size, and (3) late hyperconcentration of dye in the affected kidney.[20] These features imply that the degree of stenosis is of sufficient magnitude to impair flow while providing evidence that the kidney is functioning. An abnormal IVP is a favorable sign as a predictor for surgical cure. Nonvisualization of a kidney or visualization of a small (<10 cm) kidney generally signifies that the kidney is not salvageable. Nephrectomy may be required in this situation. However, it should be kept in mind that normal IVPs do not exclude the presence of renal artery disease. This problem was demonstrated in a young man with severe hypertension and a normal rapid-sequence IVP (Fig. 78.4). Renal arteriography (see Fig. 78.2) showed severe bilateral renal artery stenosis due to intimal fibroplasia.

The recent application of computer technology has generated a renewed interest in radionuclide methods as screening tests for renovascular disease. Nally and co-workers have shown that the initial up-

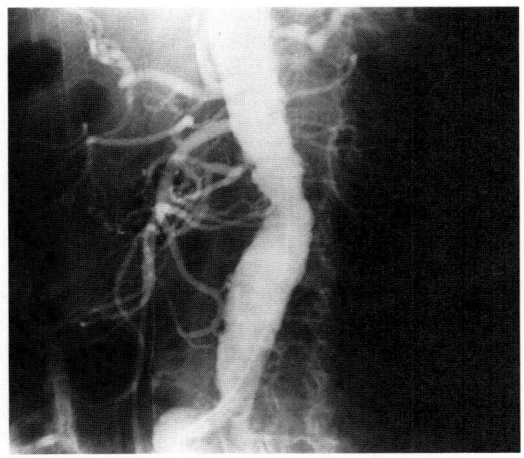

FIGURE 78.3 Renal artery stenosis in atherosclerosis is often part of a generalized process that involves the aorta and iliac, celiac, and mesenteric arteries. Atherosclerosis can progress and cause ischemic atrophy of the renal parenchyma. In this case, there is total occlusion of the left main renal artery and a nonfunctioning left kidney. There is also stenosis of the right renal artery at its origin from the aorta. Orificial involvement in atherosclerosis makes transluminal angioplasty difficult to perform. Even if the lesion can be dilated, recurrence is frequent during the course of a year.

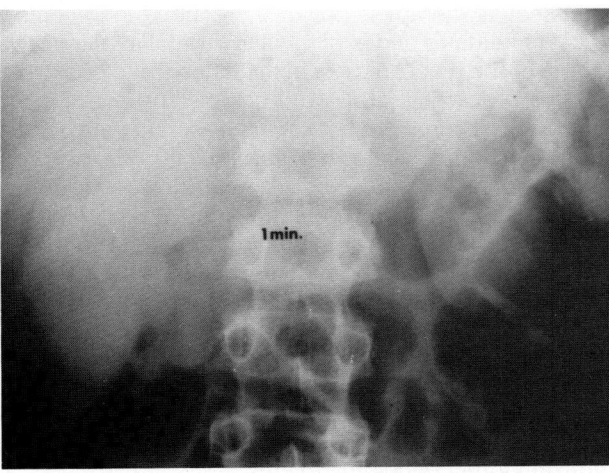 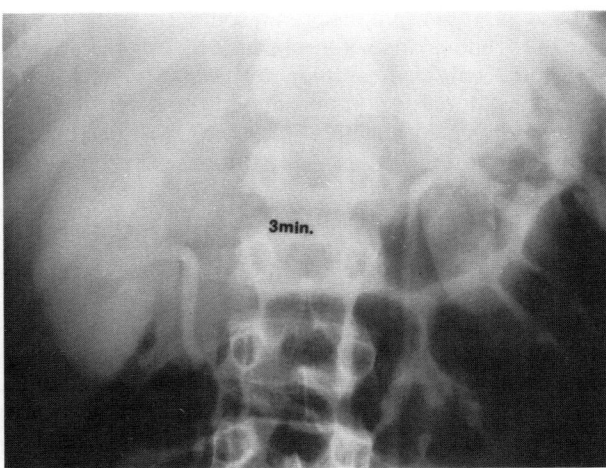

FIGURE 78.4 A normal rapid-sequence intravenous pyelogram (IVP) does not rule out renal artery disease. This young man with severe hypertension had a normal rapid-sequence IVP but underwent formal arteriography because the clinical index of suspicion for renal artery disease was high. Severe bilateral renal artery stenosis was found (see Fig. 78.2). A strong case can be made for proceeding directly to arteriography in situations like this since any of the "screening" procedures for renal artery disease have false-negative and false-positive results.

take of Tc-DTPA correlates with renal blood flow (estimated by para-aminohippurate [PAH] clearance) in dogs with 2K-1C hypertension.[21] A reasonable estimation of the contribution of each kidney to overall renal function can be made, a feature that is particularly helpful during long-term follow-up. Another important advantage of the radionuclide techniques relates to the fact that the risk of contrast-induced renal failure is eliminated. However, the radionuclide techniques lack specificity and sensitivity and are not ideal screening procedures. They are probably more helpful in serial follow-up of medically or surgically treated patients with angiographically documented renal artery disease.

Intravenous digital subtraction angiography (DSA) is probably the best noninvasive procedure currently available for the detection of renal artery disease. This is the only noninvasive method that allows for visualization of the renal arteries. Late films can be used to estimate renal size while defining the anatomy of the renal architecture and collecting systems. The major disadvantages are (1) contrast material must be used, (2) false positive and negative results occur, and (3) formal arteriography will be required before angioplasty or surgery if the test is positive or negative. Thus, conventional arteriography will be required in most cases if the DSA is positive or negative when the clinical suspicion of renal artery disease is high.

Percutaneous renal arteriography remains the "gold standard" in defining the presence of renovascular disease. In experienced hands, the incidence of groin hematoma, traumatic dissection, rupture or thrombosis of the femoral or renal artery, and contrast-induced renal failure is minimal. The latter complication is minimized (but not eliminated) by adequate hydration. Atheroemboli can also occur in patients with severe atherosclerotic disease. Since these complications do exist, renal arteriography must be reserved for patients who are surgical candidates; arteriography is rarely performed merely for diagnostic purposes (a single exception is the detection of microaneurysms in polyarteritis nodosa).

Several radiographic features suggest that a renal artery lesion has functional significance. These include the size of the involved kidney, the degree of stenosis, and the presence or absence of poststenotic dilatation. In general, obstruction of less than 65% to 75% of the renal artery does not reduce flow but the angiographic estimation of the degree of stenosis can be difficult, particularly in patients with the beaded fibrous lesions. Loss of renal parenchymal size and the presence of poststenotic dilatation are much more specific clues to the functional significance of a renal artery lesion.

Measurement of PRA from renal venous and inferior vena caval blood samples is often helpful in determining the functional significance of a renal artery lesion. This analysis is generally performed at the time of renal arteriography and requires catheterization of the femoral vein and sampling of renal venous and inferior vena caval blood. In addition to the baseline renin samples, renin secretion is stimulated acutely by giving an intravenous dose of furosemide (40 mg) or a single oral dose of captopril (25 mg). These maneuvers can unmask functional significance of an arterial lesion and increase the sensitivity of the renal vein renin studies.[22] In unilateral renal artery disease, functional significance of a lesion is suggested by a renal vein renin ratio (involved/uninvolved) of 1.5 or greater. The caval renin is obtained as an estimate of renal arterial renin and is used to determine if the uninvolved (or less involved) kidney is adding or extracting renin. This is particularly helpful in patients with bilateral disease since it allows the clinician to choose which kidney to revascularize if a surgical procedure is indicated. If both kidneys are secreting renin, surgical cure of hypertension is less likely if only one kidney is revascularized. However, the results of vein sampling must be interpreted in light of the patient's clinical history since surgical cure of hypertension occurs in patients with RVH and nonlateralizing renins. Furthermore, patients with lateralizing renins may not be cured by surgery, particularly if the hypertension is of longstanding and has been poorly controlled. In this regard, hypertension of less than 5 years' duration is probably as helpful in predicting surgical cure as the renal vein renin ratio. The chance of surgical cure falls dramatically when the hypertension has been present for longer than 5 years.[23]

Pharmacologic blockade of the renin angiotensin system with the converting enzyme inhibitor captopril or the A_{II} antagonist saralasin has been advocated as a method of screening for RVH or predicting surgical cure. It is assumed that a favorable response to one of these agents signifies A_{II}-mediated RVH and subsequent surgical cure. Unfortunately, a subgroup of patients with EH have A_{II}-mediated hypertension and respond to acute angiotensin blockade. Patients with bilateral renal artery disease may have a volume-dependent form of hypertension and not respond. Thus, these pharmacologic tests, such as the IVP, intravenous DSA, and radionuclide renal flow scan, lack both sensitivity and specificity as screening procedures. In addition, they do not necessarily provide evidence that renal angioplasty, renal revascularization, or nephrectomy in the appropriate setting will or will not cure the hypertension.

TREATMENT. Renovascular hypertension can be treated medically or surgically, or by angioplastic dilatation of the renal artery. It is extremely difficult to provide specific recommendations regarding the choice of treatment because they have not been compared in a well-controlled clinical study. The clearest indication for angioplasty or surgery is the control of drug-resistant hypertension, but revascularization should be considered in some patients in an effort to preserve renal function. The choice of therapy depends on (1) the patient's general medical condition, (2) the type and location of the lesion (or lesions), (3) the level of renal function, and (4) the expectation that angioplasty or surgery will cure the hypertension or preserve renal function. Each mode of therapy has its advantages and disadvantages and many factors need to be considered, not the least of which is the expertise of the radiologists or surgeons who perform these invasive and potentially hazardous interventions.

MEDICAL THERAPY. There is a common misconception that RVH does not respond to standard antihypertensive therapy. It is not difficult to understand why this false impression exists since resistant hypertension is a major reason to perform a careful investigation to detect renovascular disease. The degree of hypertension and the response to drug therapy are highly variable in RVH and it should not be assumed that every patient with renal artery disease will need surgery, angioplasty, or nephrectomy to control the hypertension. This is particularly true in this decade when a number of potent agents with a variety of pharmacologic properties are available to the clinician for the treatment of hypertension. The availability of orally acting converting enzyme inhibitors (captopril, enalapril) is a major advance, but these agents are not necessarily required and at times can be hazardous.

Medical therapy is obviously required in patients who are not surgical candidates and is particularly useful in patients with medial fibroplasia of the renal arteries. In the latter group of patients, renal function should be carefully followed because progressive loss of renal mass can occur, even though it occurs less frequently with this lesion than it does in patients with other forms of fibrous disease or in those with atherosclerosis. The Tc-DTPA renal flow scan combined with some index of GFR (serum creatinine, creatinine clearance, iothalamate clearance, and so on) is helpful in long-term follow-up. Surgical intervention or angioplasty may be required if the blood pressure simply cannot be controlled with antihypertensive medication or if renal function begins to deteriorate. A case can be made for following this approach in the majority of patients with renovascular disease. Exceptions include young patients with severe bilateral renal artery disease secondary to the nonbeaded renal artery lesions since spontaneous dissection or thrombosis with subsequent ischemic atrophy of the involved kidney frequently occurs.

A "stepped-care" approach to drug treatment is often effective in patients with RVH. Some physicians advocate this approach to medical therapy and reserve converting enzyme inhibitors for resistant cases.

Others favor more widespread use of converting enzyme inhibitors in patients with renal artery disease since these patients generally have angiotensin-dependent hypertension and do very well with the converting enzyme inhibitors. Converting enzyme inhibitors must be used with caution in patients with severe bilateral renal artery disease and in patients with stenosis of an artery to a solitary kidney (such as stenosis of an artery to a transplanted kidney) since renal failure can develop during the course of treatment.[24] However, bilateral renal artery disease is not an absolute contraindication to the use of converting enzyme inhibitors but careful follow-up of renal function is required in this setting. The renal insufficiency that occurs during converting enzyme inhibitor therapy may be immediate or may not develop for several weeks or a few months. It is generally reversible after discontinuation of the drug. A profound antihypertensive response to converting enzyme inhibitors occurs in some patients with RVH, particularly if pretreatment PRA is very high. For this reason, it is prudent to begin with a small dose of a converting enzyme inhibitor (6.25 mg to 12.5 mg captopril or its equivalent) and observe the patient closely.

TRANSLUMINAL ANGIOPLASTY. Percutaneous introduction of a flexible catheter with an inflatable balloon has been increasingly utilized to dilate stenosed renal arteries. The indications for percutaneous transluminal dilatation of the renal arteries have not been clearly defined but the procedure appears to be most useful in patients with the fibrous lesions.[25] Patients who have discrete fibrous dysplastic lesions with only one or two short stenotic segments seem to respond better to transluminal angioplasty than patients who have multiple areas of involvement that involve long segments of the renal artery or its branches. Transluminal dilatation of atherosclerotic renal artery disease has been less rewarding, chiefly because atherosclerotic disease tends to have a proximal location and often involves the orifice of the renal artery with its adjacent aortic wall. When the orifice is involved (see Fig. 78.3), it is difficult to dilate the lesion and recurrent stenosis is common over the course of a year, even if the lesion seems to be dilated at the time of arteriography. In patients with atherosclerotic renal artery disease not involving the orifice of the renal artery, angioplastic dilatation may be more successful. The clinician should keep in mind that perforation or rupture of the renal artery, acute renal arterial occlusion after dissection of the intima or a plaque, embolization or thrombosis at the time of dilatation, and groin hematoma can occur in patients undergoing transluminal angioplasty. Several of these conditions require emergency surgery, which can be extremely hazardous in patients who are poor surgical candidates. Surgical "standby" should always be obtained since the risk of these life-threatening complications is real. The lack of a skilled angiographer or lack of immediate access to an experienced vascular surgeon, refusal of the patient to agree to surgery in the event that complications occur, and refusal of the patient to undergo long-term hemodialysis if there is renal failure after transluminal angioplasty should all be considered as contraindications to the procedure.

For reasons previously outlined, patients with fibrous disease of the renal arteries are the best candidates for transluminal angioplasty. These patients do not generally have orificial lesions and may have lesions in intrarenal branches of the renal artery (Fig. 78.5). At times, these lesions can be dilated and spare the patient the hazards and expense of a technically very difficult surgical procedure. Transluminal angioplasty is also useful in the management of transplant renal artery stenosis, another situation that presents a difficult surgical problem. However, involvement of the orifice and adjacent iliac artery may occur in the transplant recipient, resulting in a situation analogous to atherosclerotic renal disease where orificial involvement makes angioplasty difficult and less successful. Again, the experience of the radiologists and transplant surgeons involved in the care of these patients to a large degree dictates the proper approach.

RENAL REVASCULARIZATION. Many physicians feel that surgical intervention is the treatment of choice for patients with drug-resistant renovascular hypertension and for patients who have shown a deterioration in renal function when the blood pressure has been well controlled. In properly selected patients, renal revascularization can cure or alleviate the hypertension in a high percentage of patients. This selection process requires a careful assessment of the patient's operative risk as well as a preoperative estimation of the likelihood of surgical cure. The risk assessment is particularly important in patients with atherosclerotic disease since these patients are older and have a greater incidence of significant atherosclerotic cerebrovascular and coronary artery disease. Novick and colleagues have shown that careful preoperative clinical assessment and surgical correction of signifi-

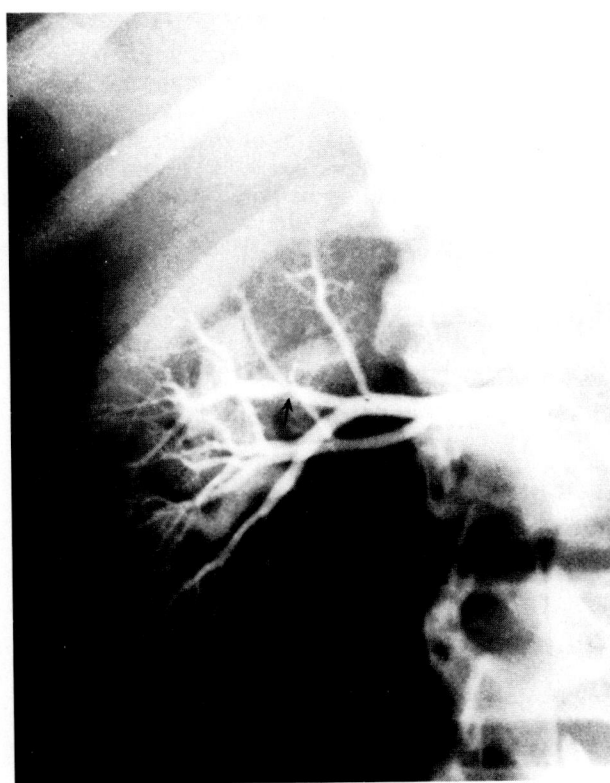

FIGURE 78.5 Intrarenal lesion. It is possible to dilate such lesions by transluminal angioplasty and spare the patient a difficult surgical procedure.

cant carotid and coronary atherosclerosis where appropriate reduces the mortality of renal revascularization to approximately 2% in patients with atherosclerotic renal artery disease.[26] In this study of 100 consecutive patients, those who had historical clues or physical findings suggesting extracranial carotid artery disease (prior stroke, transient ischemic attack, or cervical bruit) or coronary artery disease (angina pectoris, myocardial infarction, congestive heart failure, abnormal resting or exercise electrocardiogram) underwent formal cerebral or coronary arteriography. Carotid and coronary revascularization was performed prior to renal revascularization in 11% and 14% of these patients, respectively. Surgical "cure" of the hypertension occurred in 40% while 50% were improved (normotensive on medication or greater than a 15 mm Hg fall in diastolic blood pressure). The results of surgery in terms of cure of the hypertension were directly related to the extent of atherosclerosis noted preoperatively; 76% of patients with focal atherosclerosis (confined to the renal arteries) were cured. In contrast, cure of the hypertension was obtained in only 30% of patients with diffuse atherosclerosis (35% with unilateral renal artery disease, 27% with bilateral renal artery disease). Various procedures, including splenorenal bypass, hepatorenal bypass, mesenterorenal bypass, and renal autotransplantation, were performed to avoid saphenous vein bypass grafting to a severely diseased aorta. This undoubtedly contributed to the success of the surgical procedure. Twenty-two percent of the patients underwent revascularization to preserve renal function. In this subgroup, the creatinine fell in 86% of the patients, remained stable in 9%, and increased in approximately 5% of the study population.[26]

In general, patients with significant azotemia (Cr > 5 mg/dl) have severe renal parenchymal disease even if they have bilateral renal artery disease or severe stenosis of an artery to a solitary kidney. Surgical revascularization of a severely diseased kidney (poor or nonfunctioning on IVP, arteriogram, or renal flow scan with significant ischemic atrophy or nephrosclerosis noted preoperatively or intraoperatively) is not likely to result in an amelioration of hypertension or a significant preservation of renal function. In these situations, nephrectomy may be indicated if medical treatment fails to control hypertension, provided that adequate postnephrectomy renal function can reasonably be assured.

THROMBOEMBOLIC DISEASES

In situ thrombosis or embolic occlusion of the main renal artery or one of its branches can produce hypertension. Renal infarction is suggested by the presence of flank pain, hematuria, fever, elevated SGOT and/or LDH, and acute onset of hypertension, but the clinical picture is highly variable and none of these signs or symptoms is necessarily present.[27] Thrombotic occlusion can occur after trauma (including catheter-induced trauma), with atherosclerotic or fibrous disease of the renal arteries, and in patients with inflammatory diseases such as syphilis, polyarteritis nodosa, or thromboangiitis obliterans. Emboli nearly always originate from the heart (mural thrombi, valvular vegetations, tumor emboli) or the aorta. Atheroembolic renal artery disease can arise spontaneously but more often develops as a complication of catheterization of the aorta. The development of livedo reticularis or "purple toes" suggests the diagnosis, but these peripheral manifestations are not always present. Postarteriography, atheroembolic renal disease may be difficult to distinguish from contrast-induced renal failure. As a general rule, dye-induced renal failure resolves over a period of days to weeks whereas atheroembolic disease progresses, often producing end-stage renal failure over the course of weeks to months. Abdominal pain and occult gastrointestinal bleeding also suggest atheroembolic disease rather than contrast-induced renal failure.

A high index of suspicion is required for accurate diagnosis of thromboembolic renal disease since the clinical picture is highly variable and none of the classic features of renal infarction are universally present. If thromboembolic occlusion is suspected, arteriography and early surgery (within a few weeks) is indicated if the patient is a surgical candidate since restoration of renal blood flow can cure the hypertension and preserve renal function of the involved renal parenchyma. Total or segmental nephrectomy may be required if the hypertension is severe and resistant to treatment when the occlusion occurred several weeks or months before contemplated surgical intervention. A search for a cardiac source of a renal embolus by echocardiography or arteriography is warranted since recurrent emboli from a tumor, clot, or valvular vegetations can produce devastating consequences.

ENDOCRINE HYPERTENSION
ADRENAL
PHEOCHROMOCYTOMA

CLINICAL PRESENTATION. Pheochromocytoma is one of the least common but most fascinating secondary causes of hypertension. It is of utmost importance for clinicians to be aware of the varied manifestations of this neoplastic endocrinopathy since the disease is life-threatening but usually curable. Hypertension is the most consistent manifestation of pheochromocytoma although rare cases have occurred in normotensive patients. The hypertension is continuous in about 50% of the patients but marked lability of the blood pressure may be present even when the hypertension is sustained. The list of signs and symptoms that have been reported in pheochromocytoma is seemingly endless (Table 78.3), but headache, sweating, and palpitations are particularly common.[28] One of these three manifestations is present in over 90% of patients with pheochromocytoma; 70% have two of the three symptoms.

The headaches are usually pounding, severe, and frontal or occipital in location. They are discrete and short-lived rather than continuous or lingering on for days at a time. This distinguishes them from tension headaches and the headaches often described by patients with essential hypertension. Sweating is usually generalized but particularly prominent in the upper part of the body. Palpitations are usually associated

---

TABLE 78.3 CLINICAL FEATURES OF PHEOCHROMOCYTOMA

Signs and Symptoms*	Conditions Associated with Pheochromocytoma
1. Hypertension (50% sustained, 50% with normotensive intervals)	1. Neurofibromatosis
2. Headache	2. Multiple endocrine neoplasia (MEN) syndromes (types II and III)
3. Sweating	3. von Hippel–Lindau syndrome
4. Palpitations	4. Cushing's syndrome
5. Pallor	5. Acromegaly
6. Anxiety, tremulousness	6. Addison's disease
7. Nausea, abdominal discomfort	

* The paroxysmal nature and the association of the signs and symptoms in a stereotyped manner are particularly suggestive.

with tachycardia. It should be kept in mind that headache, sweating, and palpitations are all relatively frequent symptoms among patients in the general population. It is not the mere presence of these symptoms that is important; rather, it is their stereotyped order of appearance and paroxysmal and discrete nature that point to the presence of pheochromocytoma.

The paroxysms last less than an hour in approximately 80% of the patients but rarely an episode can persist for several days. Approximately 75% of the patients have one or more episodes per week, but the paroxysms can occur as often as 25 times per day or as seldom as every few months. An unexplained increase in blood pressure during the induction or maintenance of anesthesia should also suggest the diagnosis of pheochromocytoma. Pregnancy may aggravate the symptoms and increase the frequency of paroxysms. Pressure in the area of the tumor, a variety of drugs (including some sympatholytic antihypertensive medications), micturition, anxiety, and a host of other factors can precipitate a paroxysm.

A careful family history should be obtained in pheochromocytoma suspects since this entity can occur as part of a multiple endocrine neoplasia (MEN) syndrome. In MEN II (Sipple's syndrome), pheochromocytoma can be associated with medullary carcinoma of the thyroid and/or hyperparathyroidism. MEN III is characterized by the association of pheochromocytoma, medullary carcinoma of the thyroid, marfanoid habitus, multiple mucosal neuromas, thickened corneal nerves, alimentary tract ganglioneuromas, and rarely hyperparathyroidism. Bilateral pheochromocytomas are particularly common in these familial syndromes.[29] Neurofibromatosis occurs in 5% of patients with pheochromocytoma and approximately 1% of patients with neurofibromatosis have a pheochromocytoma. Some patients with von Hippel–Lindau syndrome (cerebellar hemangioblastoma and retinal angiomata), acromegaly, or Addison's disease have pheochromocytoma. Rarely, ectopic ACTH production by a pheochromocytoma can produce Cushing's syndrome (Fig. 78.6). Up to 30% of patients with pheochromocytoma have cholelithiasis for unknown reasons.

A number of clinical entities may mimic pheochromocytoma (Table 78.4). Acute anxiety attacks, hyperthyroidism, and a hyper β-adrenergic state cause the greatest diagnostic confusion. The latter condition, a variant of the hyperkinetic heart syndrome, is characterized by labile hypertension, episodic tachycardia, headache, anxiety, flushing, and occasionally diaphoresis. Plasma catecholamine levels and the urinary excretion of catecholamine metabolites are normal in this condition. The symptoms can be reproduced during an infusion of the β-agonist isoproterenol and treatment with β-adrenergic receptor blockers is usually effective. Less frequently, the menopausal syndrome, migraine headache, and acute coronary insufficiency mimic pheochromocytoma. Striking elevations of plasma catecholamines or urinary catecholamine metabolites do not occur in these conditions. In contrast, the clinical and biochemical features of pheochromocytoma can occur after the abrupt withdrawal of sympatholytic agents (clonidine, guanabenz, and occasionally methyldopa) and in patients taking monoamine oxidase inhibitors if tyramine-containing foods or beverages are ingested.

PATHOPHYSIOLOGY. Pheochromocytoma represents a neoplastic transformation of cells arising from embryologic rests of neural crest tissue. The tumors are usually located unilaterally in the adrenal medulla but may be bilateral, particularly in patients with the familial syndromes. Extra-adrenal tumors have been found at the aortic bifurcation (organ of Zuckerkandl), along the paravertebral sympathetic ganglia in the abdomen or chest, or in the wall of the urinary bladder. Other "paragangliomas" (especially of the carotid body) can produce and release catecholamines but they usually do not produce typical catecholamine excess syndromes. Tumors in association with intracranial branches of the vagus nerve (glomus jugulare tumors) generally occur along the base of the skull in the jugular foramen, in the mastoid or temporal bones, or in the middle ear.

Of the tumors, 10% metastasize or are locally invasive. "Malignancy" is determined by clinical behavior since the histologic appearance of these lesions is deceiving. The tumors are nearly always highly vascular and well encapsulated, a feature that is important diagnostically. Necrosis and fibrosis are common in large tumors. Nearly all of the tumors produce increased amounts of norepinephrine; 50% produce increased quantities of epinephrine as well. The production of large quantities of epinephrine generally implies that the tumor resides within the adrenal gland. Rarely, dopamine is the predominant catecholamine produced.

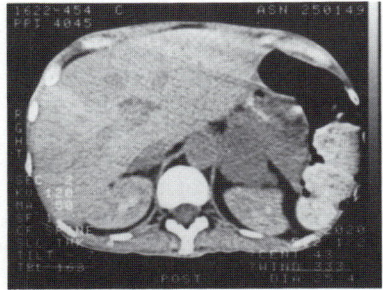
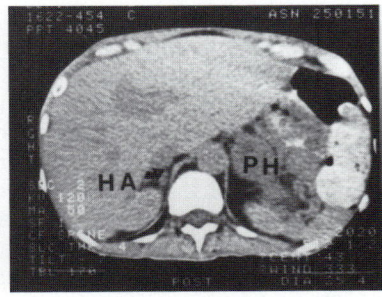
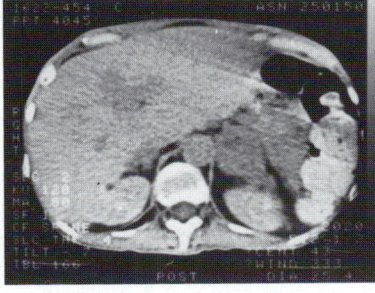
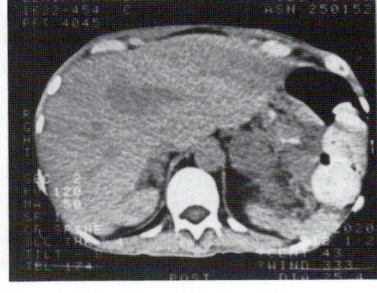

FIGURE 78.6 Pheochromocytomas (PH) are usually located in a single adrenal gland. This patient had an ACTH-producing left adrenal pheochromocytoma and hyperplasia of the right adrenal gland (HA) producing an acute Cushing's syndrome. The adrenal glands are usually located around the upper poles of the kidneys. The aorta and diaphragmatic crus are identified in this area.

TABLE 78.4 DIFFERENTIAL DIAGNOSIS OF PHEOCHROMOCYTOMA

Anxiety/tension states
Hyper-β-adrenergic circulatory state
Hyperthyroidism
Paroxysmal tachycardia
Hypovolemia
Acute coronary insufficiency
Autonomic neuropathies
Diencephalic seizure syndrome
Sympatholytic agent withdrawal
Monoamide oxidase inhibitor/tyramine interaction
Menopausal syndrome
Migraine and cluster headache
Carcinoid syndrome

Norepinephrine-mediated vasoconstriction is the major mechanism of the hypertension in pheochromocytoma. Bravo and his co-workers have presented evidence to suggest that central activation of the sympathetic nervous system is in part responsible for the hypertension of pheochromocytoma. Stored norepinephrine released from sympathetic nerve terminals during sympathetic stimulation is probably the major mechanism involved rather than vasoconstriction from the norepinephrine directly released from the tumor into the circulation.[30,31] Patients with pheochromocytomas often have a contracted blood volume due to the combined effects of vasoconstriction and "pressure-natriuresis" associated with this condition. The reduced circulating blood volume may account for the orthostatic fall in blood pressure that has sometimes been noted in patients with pheochromocytoma. In addition, the low blood volume places the patient at risk for hypotension following removal of the tumor.

LABORATORY INVESTIGATION. There are no reliable clues to pheochromocytoma obtained during the routine laboratory investigation of the hypertensive patient. However, a carefully conducted laboratory investigation is required to obtain biochemical and radiographic confirmation of pheochromocytoma whenever historical clues suggest the diagnosis. Surgical exploration should only be performed when biochemical confirmation has been obtained and radiographic localization of pheochromocytoma has been attempted. Preoperative localization is usually possible with current techniques. Rarely, exploration may be required if attempts to localize the tumor have failed and the patient has clinical and biochemical evidence of pheochromocytoma.

Laboratory confirmation depends on either demonstration of strikingly elevated plasma catecholamines in peripheral venous blood or elevation of catecholamine metabolites (particularly metanephrines) in a 24-hour urine specimen. Proper interpretation of plasma catecholamine levels requires knowledge of the conditions under which the blood samples were collected as well as the assay that a given laboratory has performed. A variety of methods have been used to measure catecholamines in the circulation. These methods include fluorometric techniques, radioimmunoassay, radioenzymatic assay, and high-pressure liquid chromatography (HPLC). The latter two procedures are probably the most reliable but are technically the most difficult to perform. Many physicians continue to rely on the excretion of urinary metanephrines to diagnose pheochromocytoma and indeed this method is quite sensitive and specific. A 24-hour urinary metanephrine of greater than 1.8 mg has a sensitivity and specificity of approximately 80% and 90%, respectively.[32] The sensitivity of urinary metanephrines is greater than the sensitivity of either urinary catecholamines or urinary vanillylmandelic acid (VMA). One of the problems in relying on urinary metanephrines relates to the difficulty in obtaining an accurate 24-hour urine collection. This is particularly problematic in children.

When carefully performed, plasma catecholamine determinations offer the most sensitive and specific method of establishing a biochemical diagnosis of pheochromocytoma. In addition to eliminating the need to collect a timed urine collection, plasma catecholamines can be measured after the acute administration of pharmacologic agents.[32] The data of Bravo and co-workers suggest that *under appropriate conditions*, a plasma catecholamine level of greater than 2000 pg/ml can be used as presumptive biochemical evidence of pheochromocytoma. If the history suggests pheochromocytoma, radiographic localization should be performed. However, it should be kept in mind that patients with a variety of acute life-threatening illnesses can have plasma catecholamine levels in this range. In addition, striking elevations in plasma catecholamines can occur after abrupt withdrawal of clonidine and in patients with the monoamine oxidase inhibitor/tyramine interaction syndrome. This is why the qualifier "under appropriate conditions" is used in interpreting the results of the total plasma catecholamine level.

There are a few patients with surgically proven pheochromocytoma who have plasma catecholamine levels of <2000 pg/ml when they are asymptomatic. If the patient is hypertensive and has a plasma catecholamine level in the 500 pg to 2000 pg/ml range, a clonidine-suppression test should be performed. Patients who do not have pheochromocytoma have a significant (usually >40%) fall in plasma catecholamine levels three hours after the oral administration of 0.3 mg of clonidine. Patients with pheochromocytoma have no significant clonidine-induced fall in plasma catecholamine levels. An occasional normotensive patient with catecholamine levels in the 500 pg to 1500 pg/ml range will benefit from a pharmacologic stimulation test. Glucagon is the most useful agent for this purpose. Pheochromocytoma is suggested by a threefold increase in plasma catecholamines to levels greater than 2000 pg/ml. Pharmacologic stimulation tests can precipitate a hypertensive crisis and intravenous phentolamine or sodium nitroprusside must be immediately available. A stimulation test should not be performed in symptomatic or severely hypertensive patients; these patients are at risk for developing a hypertensive crisis and virtually always have a diagnostic (>2000 pg/ml) elevation of plasma catecholamines if the hypertension or symptoms are due to pheochromocytoma.

Radiographic localization has been simplified since the advent of high-resolution CT. CT scanning of the abdomen and pelvis will localize pheochromocytoma in approximately 90% of cases.[33] The tumors are usually relatively large (when compared to aldosterone-producing adenomas) and located within the adrenal gland 90% of the time (see Fig. 78.6). Tumor necrosis is not uncommon, particularly if the tumor is large. The abdomen is also the most frequent site of extra-adrenal pheochromocytoma and these tumors can be visualized with the abdominal CT scan. Bladder tumors and other pelvic tumors may be found, but interpretation of the pelvic scan can be difficult. Patients who have symptoms induced by micturition should undergo cystoscopy.

The physician is faced with a difficult task if the abdominal and pelvic CT scans do not demonstrate a tumor. It is reasonable to scan the thorax and possibly the head and neck since these procedures pose no risk to the patient. Abdominal and pelvic arteriography may be required and sequential sampling of the superior and inferior vena cava for catecholamines can also aid in the localization of pheochromocytoma. These invasive procedures obviously pose a risk to the patient and are usually not required. The radioisotope ^{131}I-meta-iodobenzylguanidine (MIBG) appears promising for the localization of pheochromocytoma in selected cases.[34] The isotope accumulates in catecholamine-producing tumors and can be detected by exterior counting. It is very expensive and not generally available at present.

TREATMENT. Surgical treatment is virtually always indicated in patients with pheochromocytoma. Exceptions include patients who simply are not surgical candidates and patients with extensive metastatic disease. However, a debulking procedure may make the hypertension easier to control or alleviate symptoms and is not unreasonable in certain situations. A long midline or bilateral subcostal incision should be performed in patients with adrenal pheochromocytomas. This allows for careful examination of the contralateral adrenal gland and the entire content of the abdomen and pelvis.

The preoperative care of the patient with pheochromocytoma is controversial. Some physicians advocate preoperative α- and β-blockade in an attempt to reduce the risk of a hypertensive crisis during the induction of anesthesia or manipulation of the tumor. α-Blockade should be established (with prazosin, phenoxybenzamine, or phentolamine) before instituting β-blockers. The vasodilatation induced by α-blockers tends to expand the blood volume. Other physicians reserve preoperative adrenergic blockade for patients who are precariously ill or who have had severe hypertensive episodes. Preoperative volume expansion with whole blood or another volume-expanding solution should be performed prior to surgery particularly if preoperative α-blockade is not instituted. Sodium nitroprusside and intravenous phentolamine must be available in the operating room (this is true even in patients who have had preoperative α-blockade). Proponents of this approach argue that pretreatment with α-blockers impairs the surgeon's ability to localize unsuspected tumors by palpation and increases the incidence of postoperative hypotension.

Blood pressure should be closely monitored with an intra-arterial line throughout the procedure and in an intensive care unit postoperatively. Postoperative hypertension can be due to pain, release of stored catecholamines, volume overload, the presence of an unrecognized tumor, or inadvertent ligation of a renal artery. Hypotension suggests volume depletion, an untoward side effect of antihypertensive medication, or intra-abdominal hemorrhage.

Inoperable patients should be treated with α-blocking and possibly β-blocking drugs. Prazosin (1 mg–5 mg, three to four times daily) is probably the most useful drug. A β-blocker is added if arrhythmias develop. Oral phenoxybenzamine or phentolamine can also be used, but these nonselective α-blockers produce more side effects than prazosin does. The combined α/β-blocker labetalol would seem to be a reasonable choice on pharmacologic grounds but there is a risk of an exacerbation of the hypertension because this drug is a more potent β-blocker than α-blocker (particularly when the drug is administered orally).[35] Metastatic pheochromocytomas are generally resistant to chemotherapy and radiation therapy. However, a few patients have been successfully treated with tagged MIBG. The role of this agent in the treatment of pheochromocytoma remains to be clarified and this agent is currently investigational. In addition, new chemotherapeutic regimens are being tested and may be more effective than the regimens previously used.

PRIMARY ALDOSTERONISM

CLINICAL PRESENTATION. An investigation for primary aldosteronism is indicated for hypertensive patients who have spontaneous hypokalemia or a marked reduction in serum potassium concentration during diuretic treatment. However, a normal serum potassium (≥ 3.5 mEq/liter) does not exclude the diagnosis of primary aldosteronism.[36] The hypertension of primary aldosteronism has generally been described as being only of mild to moderate severity, but it should be kept in mind that patients with primary aldosteronism have presented with malignant hypertension. Primary aldosteronism is also a cause of resistant hypertension and should be ruled out especially if the serum potassium has been unusually low (<3.0 mEq/liter) during standard diuretic treatment (25 mg–50 mg hydrochlorothiazide or its equivalent). There are no characteristic physical findings.

It is difficult to estimate the incidence of primary aldosteronism in the hypertensive population. Detection has undoubtedly increased with advances in laboratory and radiographic techniques and the increased awareness of the varied clinical presentations of this disease. In any institution or patient population, the incidence of primary aldosteronism will be related to the vigor of the search to find this curable cause of hypertension.

PATHOPHYSIOLOGY. Primary aldosteronism is characterized by the excessive and autonomous overproduction of aldosterone by a tumor (aldosteronoma) or hyperplasia of the adrenal cortex. Aldosteronomas are virtually always unilateral while hyperplasia is almost always bilateral. Aldosterone-producing adenomas can be quite small (<1 cm), a feature that is of importance from the radiographic standpoint. For clinical purposes, the "autonomy" of aldosterone production refers to the fact that it is not under control of the renin–angiotensin system. *The continued secretion of aldosterone in the face of a saline-induced inhibition of the renin–angiotensin system promotes sodium retention and renal potassium wasting.* The laboratory investigation is designed to demonstrate this sequence of events.

LABORATORY INVESTIGATION. The biochemical evaluation of primary aldosteronism is designed to (1) determine if hypokalemia is due to renal potassium wasting, (2) assess the role of the renin–angiotensin system if hypokalemia and renal potassium wasting are present, and (3) determine if inhibition of the renin–angiotensin system by saline loading suppresses aldosterone production. In nondiuretic-treated hypertensives, it is reasonable to initiate an investigation if the serum potassium is less than 3.5 mEq/liter.[9] A firm recommendation for evaluation in diuretic-treated patients is more difficult to make and depends on the severity of the hypokalemia, the dose and type of diuretic used, and a variety of other factors including the adequacy of the patient's previous blood pressure control. An investigation is reasonable if the serum potassium is less than 3.0 mEq/liter in a patient receiving 50 mg or less of hydrochlorothiazide or its equivalent.

A carefully collected 24-hour urine specimen should be obtained if primary aldosteronism is suspected. This should be performed at least two weeks after the discontinuation of diuretics whenever possible. Renal potassium wasting, which is a hallmark of mineralocorticoid-induced hypokalemia, is present if the hypokalemic patient is excreting more than 40 mEq K^+ in a 24-hour period. If inappropriate kaliuresis is present, the role of the renin–angiotensin–aldosterone axis is assessed. This requires measurement of PRA, urine sodium excretion, and urinary aldosterone. The combination of low plasma renin (<0.5 ng/ml/hr) and increased urinary aldosterone excretion (>14 μg/24 hr) strongly suggests the diagnosis.[36] However, PRA is not universally suppressed in primary aldosteronism, particularly if the patient is consuming a low-sodium diet. In fact, as many as 36% of patients with proven primary aldosteronism have a PRA > 2.0 ng/ml/hr after a 3- to 4-day period of salt loading.

Presumptive evidence of primary aldosteronism is present when a saline-loaded patient excretes more than 14 μg of aldosterone per day. Salt loading can be accomplished in outpatients by asking the patient to add a teaspoon of table salt to each meal. After 3 to 4 days, a hemodynamically and metabolically stable patient will come into sodium balance and excrete the daily salt load. A reasonable goal of sodium loading is the maintenance of a urine sodium excretion of approximately 250 mEq/day. This corresponds to an intake of approximately 6 g of sodium (15 g of salt) per day. Laboratory evaluation for primary aldosteronism after this period of salt loading should include measurement of serum K^+, PRA, and the 24-hour urinary Na, K, Cr, and aldosterone. Patient compliance with the diet and urinary collections is the major obstacle in performing this outpatient investigation. Problems are minimized by hospitalizing the patient in an area that is familiar with metabolic investigations and giving the saline load intravenously (approximately 25 ml/kg normal saline, IV) but even then it is remarkable how difficult it can be to complete the evaluation successfully.

When a biochemical diagnosis is made, a localization procedure is required. Radiographic localization also aids in the differentiation of aldosterone-producing adenoma from adrenal hyperplasia. Computerized tomography, adrenal ultrasound, adrenal scintigraphy, and adrenal venography with adrenal vein renin sampling have all been used to differentiate aldosterone-producing adenomas from adrenal hyperplasia. CT scanning is probably the most useful procedure because it is noninvasive, generally available, useful in differentiating adenoma from hyperplasia, and fairly sensitive. Thin slices of the adrenal gland must be obtained since these tumors are often quite small (<2 cm). CT has been successful in localizing tumors as small as 1 cm. In contrast to pheochromocytoma (see Fig. 78.6) where the entire adrenal gland is enlarged and distorted, only a portion of the gland may be affected in primary aldosteronism (Fig. 78.7) and some thin sections of the adrenal gland can appear normal. Tumor necrosis and calcification are very uncommon in aldosterone-producing adenomas. Either of these findings should raise the suspicion of pheochromocytoma or an adrenal carcinoma. Tumors that are large (>5 cm) should also be viewed cautiously since large tumors are more often malignant. It should be noted that adrenal carcinomas have been identified in patients with classic biochemical features of primary aldosteronism but this is an unusual occurrence.

Aldosterone-producing adenomas account for at least 75% of all cases of primary aldosteronism. It is extremely important to make this distinction because surgical cure of hypertension is quite possible with adrenal adenomas; surgical cure is unlikely with hyperplasia.[37] Bilateral adrenalectomy for adrenal hyperplasia is contraindicated because it requires lifelong replacement of adrenal hormones. Fortunately, the two diseases have fairly distinctive radiographic features and also have some characteristic biochemical features. For example, adenomas are more likely if the hypokalemia is severe (<2.5 mEq/liter), the plasma 18-hydroxycorticosterone is >50 ng/dl, or a paradoxical postural fall in plasma aldosterone is noted.[36] It is reasonable to perform these biochemical tests if the radiographic features are confusing. In this situation, adrenal venography with bilateral adrenal vein sampling can also be helpful. This procedure is technically demanding and need not be performed if the biochemical presentation is classic and the CT scan unequivocally shows a unilateral adrenal adenoma. However, false positive CT scans are not infrequent and nonfunctioning adenomas are not rare. This is why biochemical proof and radiographic localization are mandatory before performing unilateral adrenalectomy for an aldosterone-producing adenoma.

TREATMENT. Medical therapy is required for patients with bilateral adrenal hyperplasia and is always a reasonable option for patients with an adenoma if surgery is considered to be a high-risk procedure or the patient wishes to avoid operation. There has never been a controlled trial of medical versus surgical treatment in primary aldosteronism. Most physicians choose to remove aldosterone-producing adenomas because of the fact that surgery is not particularly hazardous and the chances of curing or significantly relieving the hypertension are quite good.

Spironolactone and amiloride are the most useful agents for medical treatment since they simultaneously reduce blood pressure and renal potassium wasting. The doses of the potassium-sparing diuretics are relatively large (100 mg–200 mg/day for spironolactone, 10 mg–40 mg/day for amiloride). Painful gynecomastia is a problem when large doses of spironolactone are required. If hypertension persists during treatment, a thiazide-type diuretic can be added, provided that the serum potassium has normalized. Adequate control of the blood volume with diuretics is very successful in controlling the hypertension of primary aldosteronism.

A flank incision is used in the surgical treatment of aldosterone-producing adenomas since the disease is unilateral and has been localized preoperatively. This avoids the hazard of entering the peritoneum and reduces surgical risk. Adequate blood pressure control and potassium repletion should be accomplished preoperatively and serum potassium should be closely monitored perioperatively. Selective hypoaldosteronism frequently occurs in the early postoperative period in primary aldosteronism. The major clinical manifestation of this entity is the inability to acutely dispose of a potassium load. This is important because intravenous potassium is often given postoperatively to replenish depleted potassium stores. Life-threatening hyperkalemia can develop, particularly if the patient has been potassium repleted preoperatively. Selective hypoaldosteronism has not been a long-term postoperative problem.

CUSHING'S SYNDROME

Hypertension is a frequent manifestation of glucocorticoid excess syndromes and occurs in patients with ACTH-producing pituitary adenomas (Cushing's disease), ectopic ACTH-producing malignancies, or adrenocortical adenomas or carcinomas, and after exogenous administration of glucocorticoids.[38] Patients with hypertension due to Cushing's syndrome nearly always have typical features of glucocorticoid excess, including weakness, thin skin, obesity, easy bruising, hirsutism, impotence, purplish striae, edema, osteopenia, and mental disturbances in roughly that order of frequency. Hyperglycemia or hypokalemic metabolic alkalosis is not uncommon.

Patients with ectopic ACTH syndromes usually present with a fulminant illness characterized by rapidly progressive muscle weakness, hypokalemic alkalosis, edema, hypertension, and carbohydrate intolerance.[39] Truncal obesity and the moon facies that are common with Cushing's disease are often absent in these patients. Ectopic ACTH production is most common in patients with oat cell carcinoma of the lung but also occurs in patients with islet cell carcinoma of the pancreas, medullary carcinoma of the thyroid, thymoma, pheochromocytoma (see Fig. 78.6), ovarian tumors, and carcinoid tumors of the gut or lung. The ectopic ACTH-producing syndrome can develop years before a tumor is clinically or radiographically apparent.

The pathogenesis of hypertension in Cushing's syndrome is not entirely clear and probably depends to some extent on the etiology of the syndrome. Desoxycorticosterone and corticosterone are overproduced in some patients with Cushing's disease and in most patients with adrenal carcinoma or ectopic ACTH syndromes.[40] These mineralocorticoids are generally not overproduced in patients with unilateral adrenal adenomas. Glucocorticoids also increase pressor responsiveness to A_{II} and norepinephrine but the role of this pressor hyperresponsiveness in producing or maintaining the hypertension is uncertain.

The diagnosis of Cushing's syndrome is most frequently entertained in obese patients with hypertension, particularly if hyperglycemia has been detected. It should be kept in mind that the obesity due to Cushing's syndrome does not involve the extremities. If the diagnosis is in question, a carefully performed laboratory investigation should be undertaken. Probably the easiest screening procedure is the overnight dexamethasone suppression test. The patient is given 1 mg of dexamethasone at midnight (which should suppress glucocorticoid production) and a serum cortisol is obtained at 8 AM the following morning. Cushing's syndrome is suggested by a post-dexamethasone serum cortisol of ≥ 5 μg/dl. However, false positive tests occur in obese patients and in depressed individuals.[39] If this occurs, higher doses of dexamethasone can be given. Measurement of 24-hour urinary cortisol and the lack of a diurnal variation in serum cortisol may be helpful. Obese patients usually have a 50% fall in PM cortisol levels (compared to the morning value) and a normal 24-hour urinary free cortisol.[38]

Confirmation of Cushing's syndrome can be difficult and endocrinologic consultation is helpful, particularly in view of the importance of separating Cushing's disease from ectopic ACTH production and

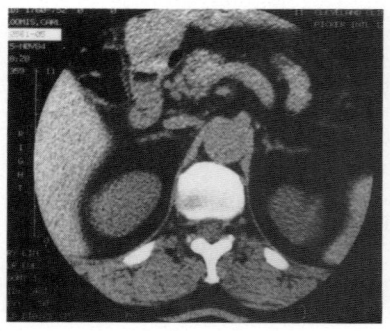 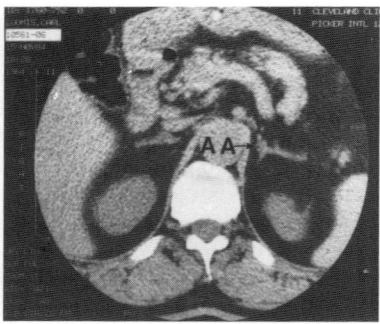 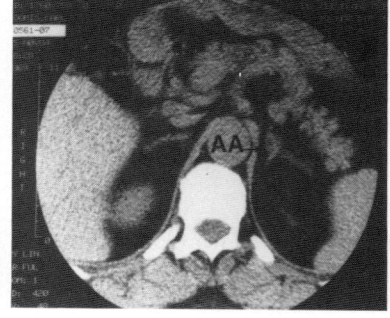 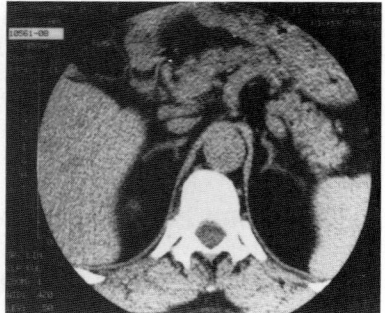

FIGURE 78.7 Aldosterone-producing adenomas (AA) are often quite small (1 cm–2 cm) and thin slices of the adrenal gland may be required to visualize them with CT. In contrast to pheochromocytoma, certain sections of the adrenal gland (the unlabeled sections) appear normal.

adrenocortical adenoma or carcinoma. The CT scan is helpful in making some of these distinctions. The treatment of adrenal adenomas and carcinomas is adrenalectomy whenever possible. Transsphenoidal hypophysectomy, pituitary irradiation, and bilateral adrenalectomy have all been used to treat patients with Cushing's disease. The latter procedure is used less frequently now because of the risks of long-term adrenal replacement. Clear recommendations for the treatment of the hypertension accompanying these glucocorticoid excess syndromes are difficult to give. Diuretics are generally used initially since volume expansion is a frequent feature of Cushing's syndrome.[38] Close attention to the serum potassium is mandatory since there is a tendency to hypokalemia. The use of a potassium-sparing diuretic with or without a thiazide diuretic is not unreasonable.

ADRENOCORTICAL ENZYME DEFICIENCIES

Deficiencies in 11-β-hydroxylase or 17 α-hydroxylase lead to impaired cortisol production and increased ACTH secretion. This stimulates deoxycorticosterone secretion, which leads to hypertension and hypokalemia. The syndromes produced by the two enzymatic defects differ in their effects on sexual characteristics. In 11-β-hydroxylase deficiency, genetic females are virilized while males have pseudo-precocious puberty. Females with 17 α-hydroxylase deficiency have hypoovarianism (primary amenorrhea, absent pubic hair, no breast development) while males are pseudohermaphrodites. There are also major differences in mineralocorticoid metabolism. Both groups of patients have hyporeninemic hypoaldosteronism and a favorable antihypertensive response to dexamethasone replacement.

Hypertension with a hypokalemic alkalosis also occurs in patients with Liddle's syndrome (a rare familial syndrome of renal tubular potassium wasting) and in the "apparent mineralocorticoid excess" syndrome. This is characterized by hyporeninemia, hypokalemic alkalosis, renal potassium wasting, subnormal production of known mineralocorticoids, a defect in peripheral cortisol metabolism, and a decrease in hypertension with spironolactone treatment.[41]

EXTRA-ADRENAL

HYPOTHYROIDISM

The incidence of diastolic hypertension appears to be increased in patients with hypothyroidism.[42] Hypothyroidism should be considered in patients who complain of excessive fatigue, weight gain, cold intolerance, dry skin, or a change in the character of their body hair. Physical features include the presence of dry skin, puffy eyelids, coarsening of the hair, thyroid enlargement, muscle weakness, and/or prolongation of relaxation of deep tendon reflexes. However, the symptoms and signs may be quite subtle and remain undetected. The patient may not have any complaints, but family members may have noted a change in personality or physical appearance.

The pathogenesis of hypertension in hypothyroidism is incompletely understood; in fact, an association between hypothyroidism and hypertension has not been universally noted. A relationship between the hypothyroidism and hypertension is suggested by the antihypertensive response to thyroid hormone replacement that has been noted in hypothyroid women with Hashimoto's thyroiditis.[42] In addition, plasma thyroxine (T_4) is reduced while thyroid-stimulating hormone (TSH) is increased in spontaneously hypertensive rats compared to their normotensive Wistar controls.[43] Coulombe and co-workers noted an increase in circulating norepinephrine (which is felt to reflect sympathetic tone) in hypothyroid patients, which suggests that sympathetic activation in response to lack of thyroid hormone could contribute to the development or maintenance of hypertension.[44]

When the history or physical examination suggests the possibility of hypothyroidism, laboratory investigation is warranted. Several screening tests have been advocated, but the serum T_4 and free thyroxine index (FTI) are probably the most useful tests. If any one of these tests suggests hypothyroidism, a TSH level should be obtained. The combination of a low T_4 or FTI and a high TSH strongly suggests the diagnosis. It should be kept in mind that the clinical presentation of thyroid disease is often atypical in the elderly patient and that hypothyroidism is not uncommon (2.3% to 7%) in an unselected population of older individuals.[45] A case could be made for "screening" elderly hypertensives for hypothyroidism since the incidence of hypertension in hypothyroidism appears to be highest in patients over age 50, and proper diagnosis using solely clinical criteria is more difficult in this age group. However, the yield of such a screening procedure is not known.

Saito and others treated 18 hypertensive women with Hashimoto's thyroiditis and hypothyroidism with thyroxine.[42] Fourteen of these patients responded by normalizing TSH, triiodothyronine (T_3), and T_4. A significant fall in blood pressure occurred in 13 of the 14 patients. The blood pressure did not change in the four patients who received inadequate thyroid replacement (manifested as a failure to normalize T_3, T_4, and TSH). Thus, a trial of thyroid replacement is reasonable in hypertensive patients with hypothyroidism. If the blood pressure does not normalize, standard antihypertensive treatment should begin. The choice of therapy depends on individual patient characteristics.

HYPERTHYROIDISM

Hyperthyroidism should be considered in patients with isolated or predominant systolic hypertension when there are symptoms and physical findings of a hyperkinetic circulation. As a general rule, hyperthyroidism elevates the systolic blood pressure while hypothyroidism elevates the diastolic blood pressure. The symptoms of hyperthyroidism may bring the diagnosis of pheochromocytoma or the hyperkinetic form of idiopathic hypertension to mind since tachycardia, palpitations, and excessive sweating occur in all of these conditions. The demonstration of lid lag, exophthalmos, thyromegaly, and/or hyperactive deep tendon reflexes lends further support to the diagnosis of hyperthyroidism. However, these features are often absent in elderly patients with "apathetic hyperthyroidism."[45] Significant diastolic hypertension in a hyperthyroid patient is more likely to be due to underlying essential hypertension or some secondary cause and the physician should not attribute the hypertension to hypothyroidism or expect treatment of the hyperthyroidism to normalize the blood pressure.

Thyroid hormone elevates cardiac output and probably causes systolic hypertension by this mechanism. The sensitivity of adrenergic receptors is felt to be increased by thyroid hormone, but this is a controversial issue. However, the observation that beta blocking agents reduce cardiac output, pulse pressure, and heart rate in hyperthyroid patients lends clinical support to this hypothesis.

The FTI and T_4 are also the best screening tests for hyperthyroidism. False negative tests occur in patients with "T_3 thyrotoxicosis" but this condition is unusual. If the diagnosis is in question, endocrinologic consultation, measurement of T_3, and evaluation of the uptake of radiolabeled iodine may all be helpful in establishing the diagnosis.

β-Blockers are probably the agents of choice for treating the hypertension that is associated with hyperthyroidism. Although these drugs do decrease some of the clinical manifestations of the hyperthyroid state, they should not be considered as definitive therapy. Hyperthyroidism can be treated medically or surgically or by using radioactive iodine; the choice of treatment varies from center to center. β-blocking drugs are particularly useful in controlling the clinical manifestations of hyperthyroidism if medical or radioactive iodine treatment is given since these modes of treatment may take several weeks to be effective in controlling the clinical manifestations of the disease.

HYPERPARATHYROIDISM

The incidence of hypertension in patients with hypercalcemia due to hyperparathyroidism (and other hypercalcemic states) also appears to be increased.[46,47] Asymptomatic hypercalcemia is noted in at least five times as many hypertensive patients as it is in normotensive controls.[47] It could be assumed that this increased incidence of hypercalcemia in hypertensive populations is a reflection of thiazide diuretic use. Thiazide diuretics cause hypocalciuria, but probably do not cause hypercalcemia. Christensson and co-workers found that 20% of their hypertensive patients with hypercalcemia were taking thiazide diuretics. Fourteen of the 20 patients underwent neck exploration; a parathyroid adenoma was found in every patient.[47] The high incidence of hyperparathyroidism in thiazide-treated patients with hypercalcemia has been noted by others and the concept that thiazide diuretics cause hypercalcemia only in patients with hyperparathyroidism is accepted by most endocrinologists.

The mechanism of the hypertension of hyperparathyroidism has not been clarified but calcium-induced renal parenchymal disease, calcium-stimulated cardiac and smooth muscle contraction, and calcium-stimulated release of vasoactive substances have all been proposed. It should be kept in mind that a significant percentage of patients with primary hyperparathyroidism are likely to have essential hypertension since these patients present at an age (usually age 40–60 years) when essential hypertension is quite common. Cure of the hypertension after parathyroid surgery provides the best evidence that a cause-and-effect relationship exists between hyperparathyroidism and hypertension. Cure of hypertension after surgery for hyperparathyroidism has been noted in several small series of patients but requires further documentation.[46,47]

ACROMEGALY

Hypertension has been noted in up to 40% of patients with acromegaly and contributes to the substantial premature cardiovascular morbidity and mortality noted in these patients.[48] Wright and co-workers reported that 50% of their acromegalic patients were dead by age 50; 90% died by age 60.[49] Carbohydrate intolerance is also present in 40% of these patients and potentiates the hypertension-related cardiovascular pathology. These growth-hormone-producing pituitary adenomas are very rare and the clinical manifestations can be quite subtle. The onset of the illness is insidious and the correct diagnosis antedates the onset of clinical manifestations by over a decade in most cases.[50]

Growth hormone has antinatriuretic effects and most patients with acromegaly have an increased total exchangeable sodium, suppressed PRA, and increased renal blood flow and glomerular filtration rate suggesting a growth-hormone-induced defect in the renal tubular handling of sodium.[51] Treatment of acromegaly by microsurgery, pituitary irradiation, or bromocriptine may not cure the hypertension even if the peripheral manifestations of the disease regress. Diuretics would seem to be a reasonable choice as the first step in drug treatment should this occur.

CARCINOID SYNDROME

A few patients with carcinoid syndrome have hypertension rather than hypotension during episodes of flushing. In addition, sustained hypertension has been noted to develop as the symptoms of carcinoid syndrome progress.[52] The clinical history at times suggests pheochromocytoma, but in the latter condition pallor occurs more frequently than flushing. If episodic flushing is a prominent symptom in a hypertensive patient, carcinoid syndrome should be evaluated by measuring 5-HIAA in a 24-hour urine specimen. Episodic flushing and hypertension are more often due to the hyper-β-adrenergic variant of essential hypertension.

DIABETES

Complications of diabetes mellitus, particularly the nephropathy and neuropathy, produce secondary forms of hypertension. Patients with hypertension due to diabetic nephropathy virtually always have a substantial amount of proteinuria, azotemia, and/or diabetic retinopathy.[53] Autonomic neuropathy can cause supine hypertension with orthostatic hypotension. These patients usually have demonstrable peripheral neuropathy or clues to suggest the presence of associated autonomic neuropathy (bladder dysfunction, diabetic gastroparesis). The incidence of hypertension appears to be higher in patients with diabetes than in the general population and the combination of glucose intolerance and high blood pressure produces an additive cardiovascular risk. A fasting venous plasma glucose is a part of the initial hypertensive evaluation for this reason.

DRUG-INDUCED

A variety of drugs can chronically increase blood pressure (see Table 78.1). Oral contraceptives have been incriminated as a major cause of reversible hypertension. The amount of progestogen, the patient's age, and the duration of oral contraceptive use directly influence the incidence of hypertension.[54] Discontinuation of oral contraceptives is reasonable if a relationship between the hypertension and the oral contraceptives is suspected and an alternative form of contraception is acceptable to the patient. The blood pressure may not return to normal for several weeks even if the oral contraceptives caused the hypertension.

An association between alcohol and hypertension has been noted in several studies; the incidence of hypertension begins to increase when three or more alcoholic beverages are consumed per day.[55] The adverse influence of alcohol is more prominent in men than in women and systolic blood pressure is generally affected more than diastolic blood pressure. There is some evidence that the hypertension is a subtle reflection of alcohol withdrawal but this hypothesis has not been rigidly tested.

Exogenous administration of glucocorticoids can induce hypertension but the incidence of high blood pressure in steroid-treated patients is substantially less than it is in patients with Cushing's disease. The nonsteroidal anti-inflammatory drugs can elevate the blood pressure in hypertensive patients and cause resistance to diuretic therapy. *De novo* hypertension secondary to the nonsteroidals does not appear to be a major problem. However, interstitial nephritis is a well-known complication of the nonsteroidals and hypertension can develop in this setting. Careful attention to the level of renal function and urinalysis is mandatory in these patients.

A number of drugs are felt to produce hypertension by stimulating the sympathetic nervous system. These include the "over-the-counter" sympathomimetics that are contained in a variety of cold remedies, withdrawal of sympatholytic agents, the monoamine oxidase inhibitor/tyramine interaction, and amphetamines, cocaine, narcotic analgesics, and withdrawal syndromes secondary to a variety of "recreational" drugs. Ergot alkaloids, which are often contained in medications to treat migraine headaches, can also produce hypertension. Finally, licorice, which contains glycyrrhizic acid, can produce hypertension and hypokalemia because of this agent's mineralocorticoid effects.

HYPERTENSION IN NEUROLOGIC DISEASES

Hypertension occurs in a variety of extracranial and intracranial neurologic diseases. Peripheral neuropathies that affect the autonomic nervous system (particularly diabetes, alcohol, heavy metal poisonings, porphyria) at times produce a syndrome mimicking pheochromocytoma. Supine hypertension with orthostatic hypotension can also occur with these peripheral neuropathies and with central lesions that affect the autonomic control of the blood pressure (idiopathic orthostatic hypotension, Shy-Drager syndrome). Inflammatory, infectious, traumatic, vascular, and neoplastic diseases of the central nervous system can produce hypertension by increasing intracranial pressure. Less frequently, invasion or compression of brain stem structures can produce severe hypertension.

HYPERTENSION AFTER CARDIAC SURGERY

POST-CORONARY-BYPASS HYPERTENSION

Systemic hypertension occurs in 30% to 60% of patients after coronary bypass surgery and places a major stress on the revascularized myocardium.[56] There is a considerable amount of evidence suggesting activation of the sympathetic nervous system as a major mechanism of this acute hypertension, which can be severe and life threatening. Unilateral stellate block has been successfully used to treat the hypertension but intravenous vasodilators are used more frequently.[57] Sodium nitroprusside and nitroglycerin given by continuous infusion are probably the drugs of choice. Fremes and co-workers recently reported a carefully controlled trial of sodium nitroprusside and nitroglycerin in post-coronary-bypass hypertension. Both drugs reduced blood pressure and increased ejection fraction, but nitroglycerin had a more favorable effect on myocardial lactate metabolism (reflected by arterial and coronary sinus lactate measurements).[56] The authors suggested that nitroglycerin should be strongly considered if there is a suspicion of myocardial ischemia because of this drug's favorable effect on myocardial metabolism.

POST-CARDIAC-TRANSPLANT HYPERTENSION

Hypertension occurs in the vast majority of stable post-cardiac-transplant patients.[58] Although the etiology of this recently described entity is currently unknown, the increased frequency of post-transplant hypertension in patients receiving cyclosporine as part of their immunosuppressive regimen raises the suspicion that the hypertension is an adverse effect of this drug. Hypertension is much less frequent in patients treated with azathioprine and prednisone, which suggests that the hypertension is not merely a manifestation of cardiac denervation.[59] Cyclosporine has significant nephrotoxic effects and a significant increase in serum creatinine concentration occurs in the post-transplant period. Indeed, Thompson and co-workers reported a mean increase in serum creatinine from 1.1 mg/dl to 2.2 mg/dl in a group of long-term survivors of cardiac transplantation.[60] This represents a 50% fall in GFR, which may well be a major mechanism for the hypertension. These patients have PRAs that are at the upper limits of "normal" but this normal PRA could be inappropriate for the level of total exchangeable sodium, a situation analogous to that described in hypertensive patients with chronic renal failure.[6] Post-cardiac-transplant hypertension is of mild to moderate severity in most cases and responds well to standard "stepped-care" antihypertensive treatment.[60]

POST-AORTIC-VALVE-REPLACEMENT HYPERTENSION

An increased incidence of hypertension has been noted in patients following aortic valve replacement, particularly in patients with aortic stenosis preoperatively. The mechanism of hypertension has not been clarified; abnormal renal function or renal emboli related to prosthesis does not appear to be the mechanism. Studies of autonomic function and hormonal profile will be required to elucidate the mechanism. Standard antihypertensive therapy usually controls hypertension in these patients.

REFERENCES

1. Gifford RW Jr: Evaluation of the hypertensive patient with emphasis on detecting curable causes. Milbank Mem Fund Q 37(2):170, 1969
2. Acosta JH: Hypertension in chronic renal disease. Kidney Int 22:702, 1982
3. Danielson H, Karnerup HJ, Olsen S, Posborg V: Arterial hypertension in chronic glomerulonephritis: An analysis of 310 cases. Clin Nephrol 19(6):284, 1983
4. Wise D, Wallace HJ, Jellinik EH: Angiokeratoma corporis diffusum: A clinical study of eight affected families. Q J Med 31:177, 1962
5. Brod J, Bahlman J, Cachovan M et al: Mechanisms for the elevation of blood pressure in human renal disease: Preliminary report. Hypertension 4(6):839, 1982
6. Warren DJ, Ferris TF: Renin secretion in renal hypertension. Lancet 1:159, 1970
7. Weidmann P, Beretta-Piccoli C, Steffen F et al: Hypertension in terminal renal failure. Kidney Int 9:294, 1976
8. Scarpioni L, Poisetti P, Ballocchi S et al: The renal handling of plasma proteins in kidney disease. Ric Clin Lab (Suppl) 8:245, 1978
9. The Joint National Committee on Detection, Evaluation, and Treatment of High Blood Pressure: The 1984 Report of the Joint National Committee on Detection, Evaluation, and Treatment of High Blood Pressure. Arch Intern Med 144:1045, 1984
10. Brunner HR, Wanters JP, McKinstry D et al: Inappropriate renin secretion unmasked by captopril in hypertension of chronic renal failure. Lancet 2:704, 1978
11. Vaughan ED, Carey RM, Ayers CR, Peach MJ: Hemodialysis resistant hypertension: Control with an orally active inhibitor of angiotensin converting enzyme. J Clin Endocrinol Metab 48(5):869, 1979
12. Frohlich ED, Cooper RA, Lewis EJ: Review of the overall experience of captopril in hypertension. Arch Intern Med 144:1441, 1984
13. Cannon P, Hassar M, Case D et al: The relation of hypertension and renal failure in scleroderma (progressive systemic sclerosis) to structural and functional abnormalities of the renal cortical circulation. Medicine 53:1, 1974
14. Brown EA, MacGregor GA, Maini RN: Failure of captopril to reverse the renal crises of scleroderma. Ann Rheum Dis 42:52, 1983
15. Delin K, Aurell M, Granerus G: Renin-dependent hypertension in patients with unilateral kidney disease not caused by renal artery stenosis. Acta Med Scand 201:345, 1977
16. Rose HJ, Pruitt AW: Hypertension, hyperreninemia and a solitary renal cyst in an adolescent. Am J Med 61:579, 1976
17. Baruch D, Corvol P, Achenc-Gelas F et al: Diagnosis and treatment of renin-secreting tumors: Report of three cases. Hypertension 6(5):760, 1984
18. Sonda LP, Konnak JW, Diskno AC: Clinical aspects of nonvascular renal causes of hypertension. Urol Radiol 3:257, 1982
19. Harrison EG, McCormack LJ: Pathologic classification of renal arterial disease in renovascular hypertension. Mayo Clin Proc 46:161, 1971
20. Bookstein JJ, Abrams HL, Buenger RE et al: Radiologic aspects of renovascular hypertension. Part 2. The role of urography in unilateral renovascular disease. JAMA 220(9):1225, 1972
21. Nally JV, Clark HS, Grecos GP et al: ^{99m}Tc-DTPA flow studies with converting enzyme inhibition in unilateral renal artery stenosis. Presented to the American Society of Nephrology, Washington, DC, 1984
22. Thibonnier M, Joseph A, Sassano P et al: Improved diagnosis of unilateral renal artery lesions after captopril administration. JAMA 251:56, 1984
23. Hughes JS, Dove HG, Gifford RW Jr, Feinstein AR: Duration of blood pressure elevation in accurately predicting surgical cure of renovascular hypertension. Am Heart J 101:408, 1981
24. Hricik DE, Browning PJ, Kopelman R et al: Captopril-induced functional renal insufficiency in patients with bilateral renal-artery stenoses or renal-artery stenosis in a solitary kidney. N Engl J Med 308(7):373, 1983
25. Levin DC: Percutaneous transluminal angioplasty of the renal arteries. JAMA 251(6):759, 1984
26. Novick AC, Straffon RA, Stewart BH, Gifford RW Jr: Diminished operative morbidity and mortality in renal revascularization. JAMA 246:749, 1981
27. Hoxie JH, Coggin CB: Renal infarction: Statistical study of two hundred fifty cases and detailed report of an unusual case. Arch Intern Med 65:587, 1940
28. Gifford RW Jr, Kvale WF, Maher FT et al: Clinical features, diagnosis and treatment of pheochromocytoma: A review of 76 cases. Mayo Clin Proc 39:281, 1964
29. Carman CT, Brashear RE: Pheochromocytoma as an inherited abnormality: Report of the tenth affected kindred and review of the literature. N Engl J Med 263:419, 1960
30. Bravo EL, Gifford RW Jr: Pheochromocytoma: Diagnosis, localization and management. N Engl J Med 311(20):1298, 1984
31. Bravo EL, Tarazi RC, Fouad FM et al: Blood pressure regulation in pheochromocytoma. Hypertension (Suppl II) 4:II-193, 1982
32. Bravo EL, Tarazi RC, Fouad FM et al: Clonidine-suppression test: A useful aid in the diagnosis of pheochromocytoma. N Engl J Med 305:623, 1981
33. Stewart BH, Straffon RA, Bravo EL, Meaney TF: A simplified, cost-effective approach to the diagnosis of pheochromocytoma. Transactions of the American Association of Genitourinary Surgery 71:101, 1979
34. Sisson JC, Frager MS, Valk TW et al: Scintigraphic localization of pheochromocytoma. N Engl J Med 305:12, 1981
35. Feck CM, Earnshaw PM: Hypertensive response to labetald in pheochromocytoma. Br Med J 281:387, 1980
36. Bravo EL, Tarazi RC, Dustan HP et al: The changing clinical spectrum of primary aldosteronism. Am J Med 74:641, 1983
37. Weinberger MJ, Grim CE, Hollifield SW et al: Primary aldosteronism: Diagnosis, localization and treatment. Ann Intern Med 90:386, 1979

38. Urbanic RC, George JM: Cushing's disease—18 years experience. Medicine 60(1):14, 1981
39. Aron DC, Tyrrell JB, Fitzgerald PA et al: Cushing's syndrome: Problems in diagnosis. Medicine 60(1):25, 1981
40. Biglieri EG, Slaton PE, Schambelan M, Kronfield SJ: Hypermineralocorticoidism. Am J Med 45:170, 1968
41. New MI, Oberfield SE, Carey R et al: A genetic defect in cortisol metabolism as the basis for the syndrome of apparent mineralocorticoid excess. In Mantero F, Biglieri EG, Edwards CRW (eds): Endocrinology of Hypertension, p 85. New York, Academic Press, 1982
42. Saito I, Ito K, Saruta T: Hypothyroidism as a cause of hypertension. Hypertension 5:112, 1983
43. Kojima A, Kubota T, Sato A et al: Abnormal thyroid function in spontaneous hypertensive rats. Endocrinology 98:1109, 1976
44. Coulombe P, Dussault JH, Walker P: Plasma catecholamine concentrations in hyperthyroidism and hypothyroidism. Metabolism 25(9):973, 1976
45. Burroughs V, Shenkman L: Thyroid function in the elderly. Am J Med Sci 283(1):8, 1982
46. Lueg MC: Hypertension and hyperparathyroidism: A five year case review. South Med J 75(11):1371, 1982
47. Christensson T, Hellstrom K, Wengle B: Hypercalcemia and primary hyperparathyroidism. Arch Intern Med 137:1138, 1977
48. Popovicci D, Buteikis A, Handoca A et al: Cardiovascular pathology in acromegaly and some effects of the 90 yttrium implant in the hypophysis. Endocrinologie 16:223, 1978
49. Wright AD, Hill DM, Lowry C, Trosen TR: Mortality in acromegaly. Q J Med 39:1, 1970
50. Davidoff LM: Studies in acromegaly. III. The anamnesis and symptomatology in 100 patients. Endocrinology 10:461, 1926
51. Falkheden T, Sjögren B: Extracellular fluid volume and renal function in pituitary insufficiency and acromegaly. Acta Endocrinol (Copenh) 46:80, 1964
52. Rosenberg EB: The carcinoid syndrome and hypertension. Arch Intern Med 121:95, 1968
53. Christlief AR: The hypertensions of diabetes. Diabetes Care 5:50, 1982
54. Royal College of General Practitioners: Oral contraception study: Effect on hypertension and benign breast disease of progestogen component in combined oral contraceptives. Lancet 1:624, 1977
55. Klatsky AL: The relationship of alcohol and the cardiovascular system. Ann Rev Nutr 2:51, 1982
56. Fremes SE, Weisel RD, Mickle AG et al: A comparison of nitroglycerin and nitroprusside: I. Treatment of postoperative hypertension. Ann Thorac Surg 39(1):53, 1985
57. Tarazi RC, Estafanous FG, Fouad FM: Unilateral stellate block in the treatment of hypertension after coronary bypass surgery. Am J Cardiol 42:1013, 1978
58. Greenberg ML, Uretsky BF, Reddy S et al: Long-term hemodynamic follow-up of cardiac transplant patients treated with cyclosporine and prednisone. Circulation 71(3):487, 1985
59. Oyer PE, Stinson EB, Jamieson SW et al: Cyclosporine in cardiac transplantation: A 2½ year followup. Transplant Proc 15:2546, 1983
60. Thompson ME, Shapiro AP, Johnsen AM et al: New onset of hypertension following cardiac transplantation: A preliminary report and analysis. Transplant Proc 15:1247, 1983

EFFECTS OF ANTIHYPERTENSIVE TREATMENT ON LEFT VENTRICULAR HYPERTROPHY AND CORONARY BLOOD FLOW

*Pierre Wicker • Fetnat M. Fouad
Robert C. Tarazi*

INTRODUCTION

Interest in the cardiac aspects of hypertension has heightened remarkably in the past few years because of a number of factors including (1) the recognition that hypertension is the most important risk factor for left ventricular (LV) hypertrophy and heart failure, (2) the better understanding and more accurate assessment of LV hypertrophy by echocardiography, and (3) the demonstration that cardiovascular structural changes can be reversed by adequate treatment. The following discussion will therefore address specifically the impact of antihypertensive treatment on LV hypertrophy and the coronary circulation, as many recent advances are renewing our understanding and possibly our clinical approach to hypertension. Moreover, LV hypertrophy was reported to be associated with impaired control of vasopressin release, possibly due to impairment of cardiopulmonary and arterial baroreceptors.[1] In addition, Grassi and colleagues[2] reported that cardiopulmonary regulation of peripheral vascular resistance is impaired in essential hypertensive patients, particularly when associated with LV hypertrophy.

Because of the association between increased heart size and the subsequent development of heart failure, and because of the observation that a shrinking cardiac silhouette heralds a concomitant improvement in cardiac status, reversal of cardiac hypertrophy has usually been viewed as a highly desirable therapeutic goal in patients with heart disease. However, this clinical impression has proven quite difficult to substantiate by more rigorous techniques. Some experimental studies raised doubts about the possibility of actual reversal of myocardial hypertrophy as opposed to only reduction in cardiac volume.[3] Further, lively controversies are still ongoing as to the beneficial or detrimental effect of hypertrophy on cardiac function.[4,5]

Recent developments in different scientific fields have led to renewed interest in this problem and opened the possibility for clinically relevant answers. Advances in echocardiography allowed noninvasive, precise, and repeatable determinations of LV wall thickness and mass in man.[6] Concomitantly, blood pressure control by medical treatment was shown experimentally to reduce actual cardiac mass in different types of hypertension.[7-9] Although earlier experimental studies had demonstrated regression of cardiac hypertrophy following cure of the causative lesion, the use of antihypertensive agents was more akin to the clinical situation in the majority of hypertensives. More important, perhaps, was the observation that all antihypertensive agents were not equipotent in that respect despite the fact that all reduced arterial pressure effectively.[7,10] Those observations prompted a reevaluation of the exact relationship between arterial pressure levels and the hypertrophic response of the heart and helped delineate a number of factors that could modulate both the development and reversal of cardiac hypertrophy.[8,10,11]

This chapter will be restricted to answer, if possible, the following questions, based mainly on clinical studies:

1. What are the evidence for and clinical features of reversibility of cardiac hypertrophy by medical treatment in man?
2. Is the reversal by antihypertensive drugs confined to a special type of agent or is it a mathematically predictable result of a reduction in arterial pressure and cardiac load, however obtained?
3. What are the implications of a reduction in cardiac mass as regards cardiac function, its impact on the coronary circulation, and its relationship if any to reversal of hypertensive vascular lesions?

REVERSIBILITY OF LV HYPERTROPHY IN MAN

The many questions raised regarding the solidity of the evidence for changes in cardiac mass with treatment have now been answered satisfactorily. The reliability and reproducibility of echocardiographic measurements and of their derived data have been demonstrated provided certain fundamental requirements are fulfilled. These include strict attention to details, sector scanner monitoring of M-mode records, double-blind readings, and use of internal checks for consistency.[6,10,12] Reproducibility of LV indices in man has been confirmed over short intervals as well as over periods of 6 to 12 months.[10,12]

The evidence first presented in man by Schlant and co-workers[13] for reversal of LV hypertrophy by antihypertensive measures has been confirmed by many investigators from different parts of the world.[10] The regression in cardiac hypertrophy achieved by blood pressure control stands in marked contrast with the difficulties experienced in obtaining regression by inotropic agents.[3,14] This contrast between the failure of digitalis and the success of antihypertensive therapy has important connotations regarding the dynamics of the hypertrophic response; clinically it underlines the major role of effective blood pressure control in the structural consequences of hypertension.

CLINICAL CORRELATES OF LV HYPERTROPHY REVERSAL

The success of antihypertensive therapy in producing regression of LV hypertrophy has raised more questions than was at first apparent. Reversal of hypertrophy did not occur in all patients treated by the same antihypertensive agents.[15-17] The factors determining this diversity of response are still not clear.

In our experience, neither age nor duration of hypertension could account for the difference in response; the question of degree of blood pressure control is more complex. This issue is separate from that of possible differences among various antihypertensive agents as regards regression of hypertrophy. It concerns the reasons for differences in response of LV mass among patients treated with the same drug. One of the main observations that emerged from large scale echocardiographic studies has been the poor correlation between LV mass and arterial pressure in treated as well as in untreated hypertensive patients.[18,19] Since those results were based mainly on office readings and because earlier studies had suggested that electrocardiogram (ECG) changes of LV hypertrophy were more closely related to home than to clinic-visit blood pressure readings,[20] the effect of treatment on regression of LV hypertrophy was reevaluated using continuous blood pressure monitoring techniques. As expected, a closer correlation was found between average diurnal blood pressure levels and variations in LV mass, but the statistical significance of these correlations should not hide their still relatively low index of determination. A typical example from Rowlands and co-workers[21] gave a correlation coefficient of 0.60 between ΔMAP and ΔLV mass, which really means that blood pressure variations could account for only 36% of the variation in LV mass. The practical implication is that attention to the evolution of LV hypertrophy during treatment could help differentiate between home and office hypertension and that factors other than blood pressure levels alone are probably involved in the reduction of LV mass by antihypertensive therapy (Table 79.1).

Many investigators have commented that reversal of hypertrophy seemed to be associated in a statistically significant way with pretreatment LV mass: the heavier the mass, the greater the reduction in LV hypertrophy by treatment.[15-17] However, much more needs to be investigated in that regard; Rowlands and co-workers[22] found that treatment with atenolol led to reduction of cardiac mass even in patients with no evident increase in LV mass or wall thickness. Further, there are many mathematical difficulties inherent in the evaluation of a correlation between the initial value of any parameter and its response to therapy.[23] Unfortunately, most published reports relating pretreatment LV mass to its change with treatment are statistically incomplete, and no final answer is available. It is obviously a matter of the greatest importance to determine whether even nonhypertrophied hearts could be made smaller by antihypertensive treatment, or whether one should expect regression only when ventricular hypertrophy has exceeded a certain degree. In that regard, another question has come forward, namely, whether the regression (or for that matter the development) of hypertrophy can occur preferentially in some parts of the left ventricle, such as in the interventricular system (IVS). Von Bibra and Richardson have reported early reduction in IVS thickness during antihypertensive therapy with little or no concomitant change in thickness of the LV posterior wall (PW). Asymptomatic septal hypertrophy has been reported in a significant number of hypertensive patients, particularly those with early or borderline hypertension[24]; this has been linked with a particular susceptibility of IVS to adrenergic stimuli or to a locally higher wall stress owing to its flatter configuration. However, an early development of septal hypertrophy does not necessarily predict an earlier regression by treatment; further, in the experience of many, the IVS/PW ratio did not change significantly during blood pressure control and reduction in LV mass.

Of obvious clinical importance is the time frame of reduction in LV mass during treatment. Folkow has demonstrated the dynamic role played by structural alterations of the cardiovascular system in the evolution of hypertension. Their hemodynamic impact is now well recognized as regards both peripheral vascular resistance and cardiac function; less well appreciated perhaps is the rapidity with which cardiovascular hypertrophy can develop or regress. The biochemical processes of hypertrophy appear within hours of imposition of an added load on the heart; demonstrable structural consequences appear in 2

TABLE 79.1 POSSIBLE FACTORS INVOLVED IN PERSISTENCE OF LV HYPERTROPHY DESPITE ANTIHYPERTENSIVE THERAPY

Blood Pressure Control
1. Duration of treatment and blood pressure control
2. Difference between office and home readings
3. Diurnal blood pressure fluctuations (stress?)

Drug-Related Factors
1. Secondary neurohumoral stimulation
2. Fluid retention and volume overload (?)
3. Direct myocardial effect of drug (?)

Patient-Related Factors
1. Age, sex, and genetic factors
2. Associated cardiac diseases (coronary arterial disease, myocardiopathy, valvular dysfunction, and so on)

weeks in experimental animals.[25] In man, definite reduction of LV mass was not usually seen, despite rapid blood pressure control, within the first 30 days of antihypertensive therapy but became evident within 8 to 12 weeks of maintained treatment (Table 79.2).[10,12] However, in some patients, changes in IVS thickness were noted in as little as 5 weeks of cessation or initiation of treatment by methyldopa or propranolol. As regards the evolution of reversal, there are no firm answers as yet. Early studies were limited in time of follow-up and left the impression that after its relatively rapid early reduction, LV mass stabilized at a new level during treatment. More recently, continued reduction in LV wall thickness was reported after even a year's therapy.[26] This could be related to the type of hemodynamic alteration induced by therapy; drugs such as metoprolol, which lead to late reductions in peripheral resistance, might be associated with much slower regression of LV hypertrophy.

REVERSIBILITY OF LV HYPERTROPHY AND TYPE OF ANTIHYPERTENSIVE THERAPY

The first studies in spontaneous hypertensive rats showed that all antihypertensive drugs were not equipotent in reversing LV hypertrophy; although methyldopa, hydralazine, and minoxidil controlled arterial pressure equally well, ventricular mass was reduced by methyldopa but actually increased by minoxidil.[7] Experience in man has similarly revealed a wide divergence in the ability of various antihypertensive drugs to induce changes in LV mass. Sympatholytics, including methyldopa and reserpine, have been definitely associated with significant regression of LV hypertrophy.[10] Addition of small doses of methyldopa to diuretics led to significant reduction of LVM with little change in blood pressure.[15] Converting enzyme inhibitors such as captopril (Fig. 79.1) and enalapril (Table 79.2) led to significant regression of hyper-

TABLE 79.2 REGRESSION OF LV HYPERTROPHY DURING ENALAPRIL THERAPY (LV MERIDIONAL WALL STRESS AND FUNCTION IN SIX PATIENTS WITH ESSENTIAL HYPERTENSION)

Variable	Control	Day 5	Month 1	Month 3
MAP (mm Hg)	134 (6.3)	110 (3.4)†	106 (2.6)†	107 (2.8)†
ESS (10^3 dynes/cm^2)	77 (9.5)	57 (5.8)*	61 (20.5)*	67 (9.0)
PSS (10^3 dynes/cm^2)	191 (22.1)	144 (4.9)	163 (27.5)	156 (13.6)
LVM (g/M^2)§	110 (4.5)	109 (2.6)	103 (6.0)	94 (5.2)†
LV% Sh	33 (3.5)	35 (2.8)	37 (5.5)	32 (2.0)
SBP/ESV (mm Hg/ml)	3.9 (0.5)	3.4 (0.5)	3.9 (0.8)	3.3 (0.6)

§ The reduction in LVM lagged behind the reduction in blood pressure; it did not appear related to changes in LV wall stress and was not associated with significant change in either cardiac performance (% Sh) or contractility (SBP/ESV).

(Average ± standard error of the mean: *$P < 0.05$ and †$P < 0.01$ vs. control by analysis of variance. MAP, mean arterial pressure; ESS, end-systolic stress; PSS, peak systolic stress; LVM, left ventricular mass; LV% Sh, left ventricular fractional shortening; SBP/ESV, ratio of systolic blood pressure to LV end-systolic volume, a load-independent index of myocardial contractility. Based on data from Fouad.)

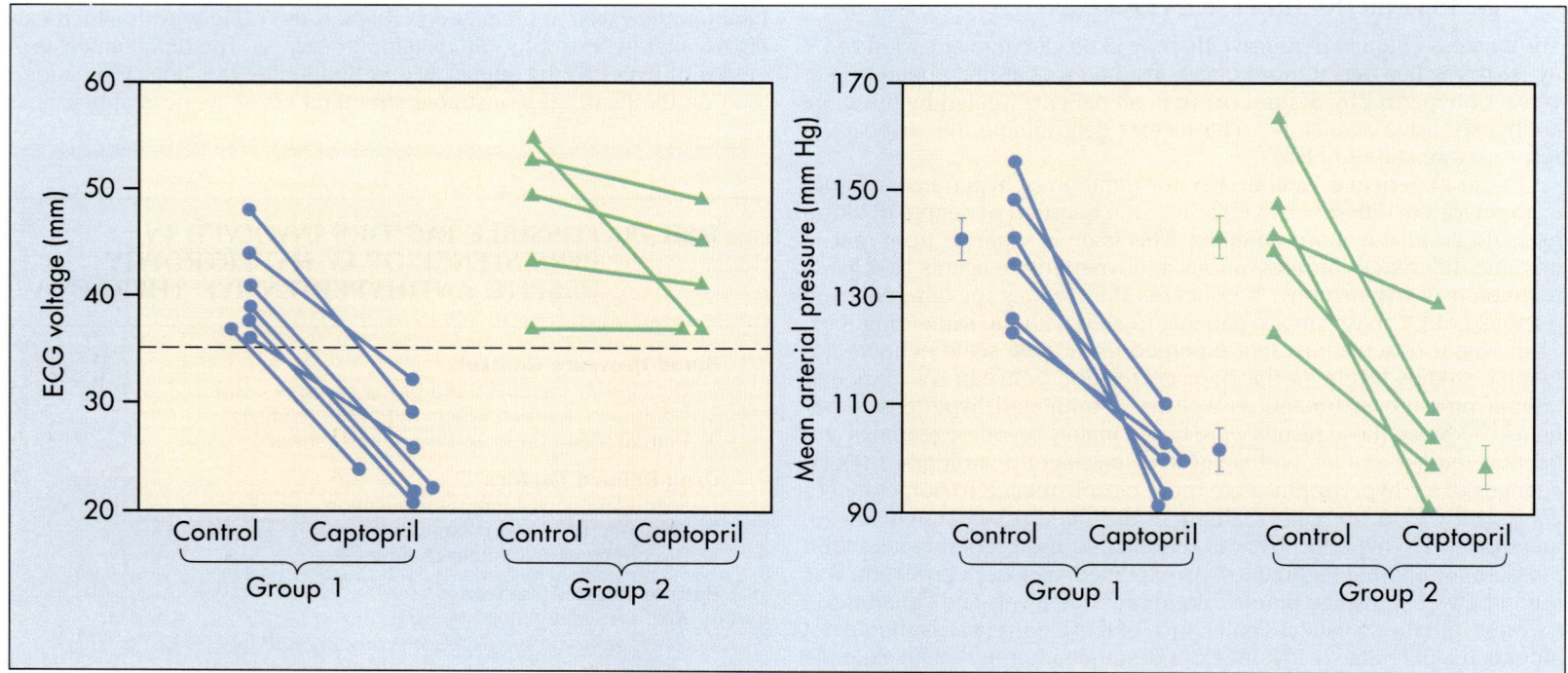

FIGURE 79.1 A. Voltage changes (S in V_1 + R in V_5) in response to captopril therapy in 12 patients with pretreatment electrocardiographic left ventricular hypertrophy (ECG-LVH). Group 1 reversal of ECG-LVH. Group 2, persistent ECG-LVH. **B.** Blood pressure response to captopril therapy in 12 patients with pretreatment ECG-LVH.

trophy; calcium entry blockers also reduced LV mass both in experimental animals and in man.[17,29-31] On the other hand, vasodilators such as hydralazine and trimazosin were not associated with regression of hypertrophy; in the exceptions reported they were used together with β-blockers.[32] Results with other antihypertensive drugs have been more disparate, an observation which might be significant *per se*. Diuretics were reported either not to reduce LV mass or to reduce it, but in a smaller proportion of patients than methyldopa.[33] Initial studies with β-blockers were controversial, but evidence is accumulating that they are indeed effective in reducing LV mass,[16,21] although Wikstrand and co-workers found that diminution in LV wall thickness occurred only after prolonged (≥8 months) therapy.[26]

In summary, the data point to some divergence in the ability of various antihypertensive drugs to induce regression of LV hypertrophy. These differences may prove to be more quantitative than qualitative; our experience with different agents and review of the literature suggest that reduction of arterial pressure and systemic resistance without reflex cardioadrenergic stimulation is probably the more important factor in inducing regression of LV hypertrophy.[12] Cardioadrenergic stimulation has been repeatedly demonstrated to produce hypertrophy in experimental animals, even in the absence of sigdifferent degrees of reflex-adrenergic stimulation by some antihypertensive agents may prevent completely or interfere partially with the regression of hypertrophy expected from relief of the pressure load alone.[27,28]

REGRESSION OF HYPERTROPHY AND CARDIAC PERFORMANCE

Analysis of the functional consequences of a reduction in LV mass depends in part on whether cardiac hypertrophy is viewed as a compensatory useful adaptation or a pathologic process. This question is usually discussed in terms of "pump performance"; a broader approach, however, is needed because the effects of hypertrophy are more pervasive and can include altered biochemical composition of the myocardium, reduced inotropic responsiveness, and disturbances in coronary blood flow.

VENTRICULAR PUMP FUNCTION

Initial studies in experimental animals suggested that the pumping action of the heart was improved with methyldopa, which reversed hypertrophy both in spontaneously hypertensive rats (SHR)[34] and renovascular hypertensive rats (RHR).[35] However, this improvement probably was due more to blood pressure reduction than to regression of hypertrophy (Fig. 79.2). Capasso and co-workers have reported that the abnormalities demonstrated in papillary muscle studies of LV hypertrophy in RHR reverted to normal with reversal of hypertrophy following nephrectomy.[36] Overall cardiac performance, however, is based on total ventricular characteristics and thus not entirely predictable from papillary muscle studies alone.

Most available studies in hypertensive patients have relied on determinations of LV ejection fraction or fractional shortening (LV% Sh); none reported a deterioration in either index at rest with reduction in LV mass.[10] However, as in the case of experimental hypertension, it is difficult to dissociate in these studies the effects of blood pressure reduction from those of regression of LV hypertrophy. Adequate assessment of the functional consequences of a reduction in ventricular mass must first take into account the effects of alterations in LV afterload on cardiac performance. This entails analysis not only of arterial pressure levels but also of changes in LV wall thickness and diameter, since LV wall stress is determined by all three indices.

Many echocardiographic studies from our group and others have revealed a close and significant correlation between LV end-systolic stress and left ventricular performance as estimated from LV% Sh. Fouad and co-workers therefore suggested that this correlation could be used to determine whether any alteration in cardiac performance concomitant with changes in LV mass during treatment was appropriate to or went beyond changes in LV wall stress. In our experience with enalapril, the relation between LV end-systolic stress and LV% Sh remained within normal ranges at the time of peak reduction in LV mass (Fig. 79.3), confirming that the regression of hypertrophy was not associated with a deterioration of ventricular pump function. More recently, reversal of myocardial hypertrophy was shown to induce im-

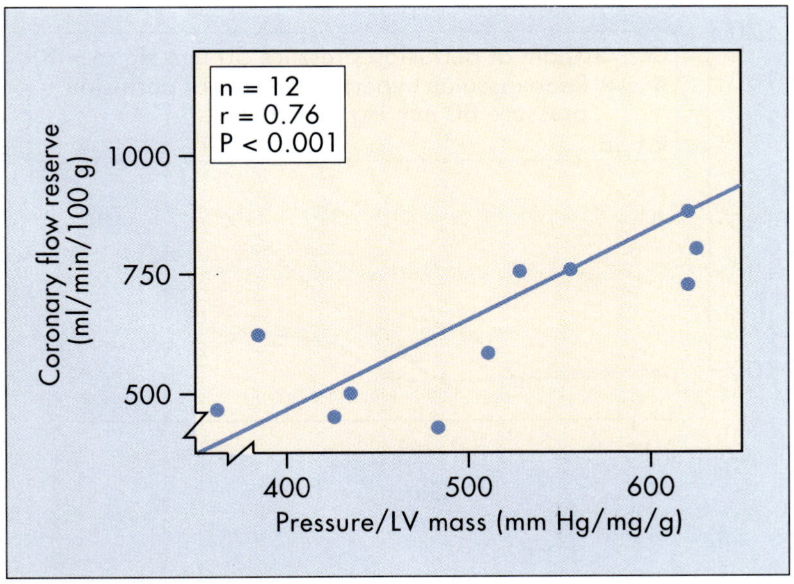

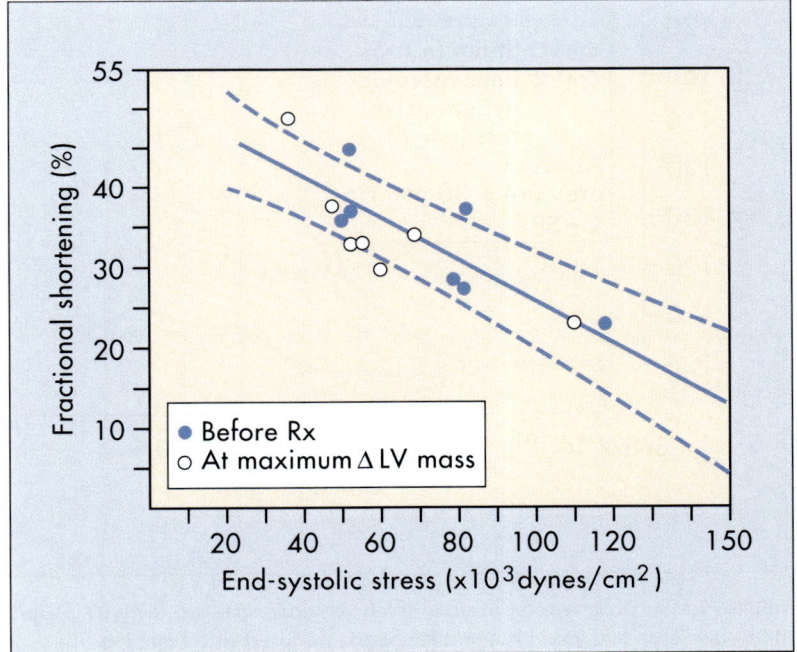

FIGURE 79.2 Coronary flow reserve is closely related to the ratio of coronary artery pressure and left ventricular mass; coronary artery pressure in hypertension is closely approximated by the aortic pressure. A reduction of pressure without a reduction in left ventricular mass would diminish coronary flow reserve, suggesting that antihypertensive treatment should aim at a balanced reduction of blood pressure and regression of LV hypertrophy. (Modified from Wicker P, Tarazi RC: Coronary blood flow in left ventricular hypertrophy: A review of experimental data. Eur Heart J 3:111, 1982)

FIGURE 79.3 Left ventricular wall stress-function with regression of left ventricular hypertrophy. Normal relation between left ventricular fractional shortening (FS%) and end-systolic stress (ESS) before treatment and at the time of maximal change in left ventricular mass (LVM) (3 to 7 months of maintenance therapy). Each point of relation between FS% and ESS at baseline (asterisks) and during treatment is located within 95% prediction limits (broken lines) of the correlation obtained in normal volunteers.

provement of LV filling pattern in hypertensive patients.[37,38] Moreover, Grassi et al.[2] have shown that regression of LV hypertrophy in hypertension is associated with improvement of cardiopulmonary reflexes "with consequent favorable effects on circulatory homeostasis."

Although this conclusion is common to most investigators, these results are as yet not complete enough to make a final decision on the value or disadvantages of a reduction in ventricular mass. More studies are needed in man of both the systolic and diastolic functions of the heart, and particularly of its ability to meet sudden overloads resulting from exercise or exacerbations or from recurrence of hypertension.

INOTROPIC RESPONSIVENESS IN LV HYPERTROPHY

The inotropic response of hypertrophied hearts to isoproterenol was repeatedly found to be reduced in hypertensive rats.[39] This reduction correlated significantly with LV weight; it was related in part to a reduction in density of β-adrenergic receptors, but other defects at various steps of the adenylate cyclase system also were shown to play possibly a more important role.[40] This impairment in inotropic responsiveness occurred with other stimuli acting through c-AMP, such as catecholamines, glucagon (Fig. 79.4) and the vasomotor intestinal peptide (VIP) as well as to α-adrenegic stimuli (Fig. 79.5). On the other hand, responses to other inotropic agents such as calcium and scillaren remained normal.[41] Interestingly, the same decline in inotropic response to β-adrenergic stimuli was described in aging hearts.[42] The clinical implications of this functional defect are slow in unfolding; to the extent that adrenergic stimulation is a "contractile reserve" helping the heart meet increased loads, the reduced response to β-adrenergic stimulation will influence the progression of hypertensive heart disease. With a reduced ability to respond by increased inotropy, the heart will depend more on the Frank-Starling mechanism to meet an

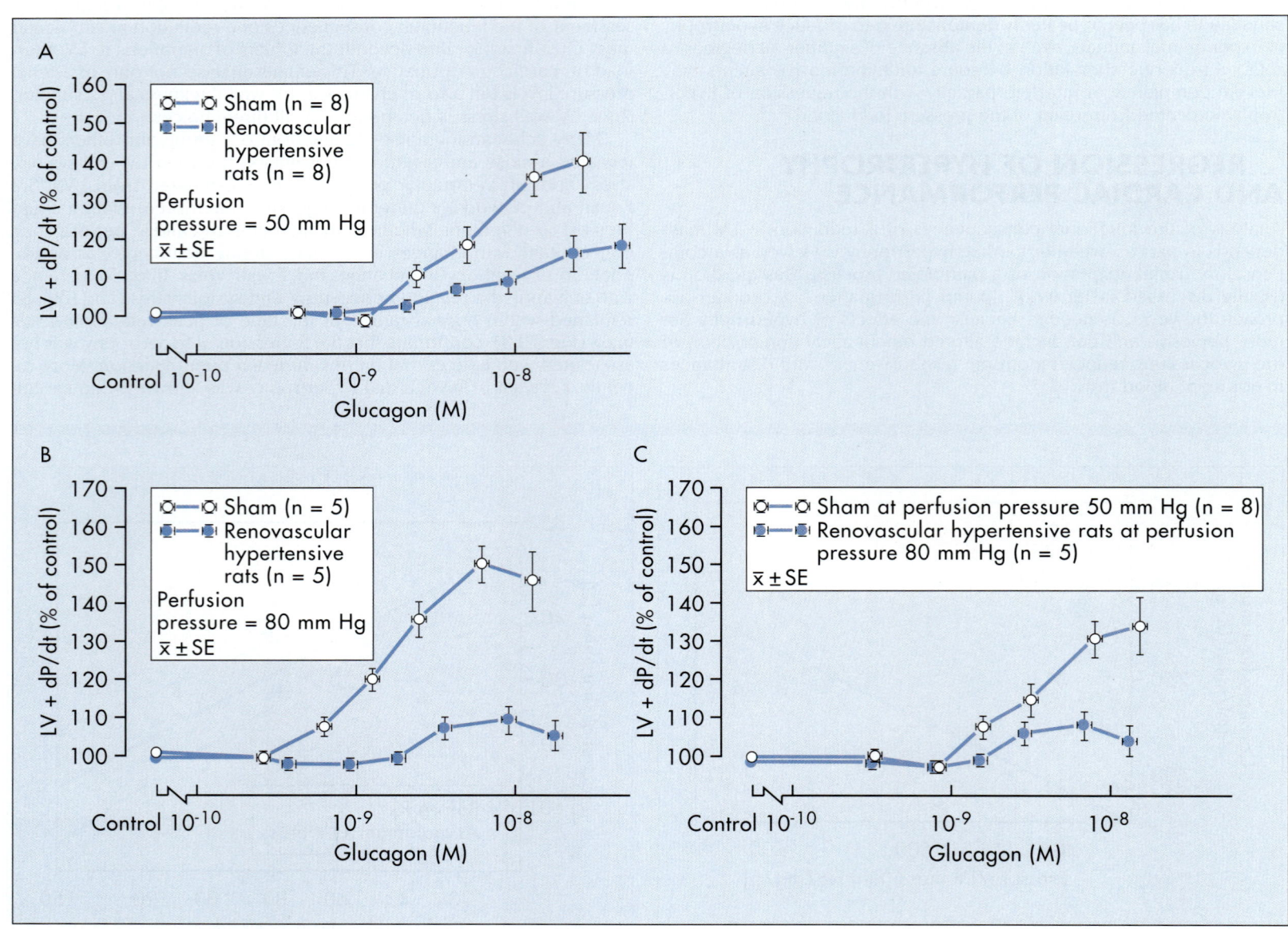

FIGURE 79.4 A. Dose-response curve of left ventricular positive dP/dt (LV + dp/dt) to glucagon infusion in isolated rat hearts perfused at 50 mm Hg. The hypertrophied hearts had a depressed curve compared with sham controls. The dose of glucagon was corrected in the individual hearts for the corresponding myocardial flow rate. **B.** Dose-response curve of LV + dP/dt to glucagon infusion in isolated rat hearts perfused at 80 mm Hg. The hypertrophied hearts had a depressed curve compared with sham controls. The dose of glucagon was corrected in the individual hearts for the corresponding myocardial flow rate. **C.** Hypertrophied hearts from RHR and normal control hearts from sham-operated rats were compared at equivalent myocardial flow rates but different perfusion pressures. Despite similar flow rates, the dose-response curve of LV + dP/dt to glucagon was depressed in the hypertrophied group.

increased load—hence the initiation of ventricular dilation and a vicious cycle of an increased load leading to further dilation and hypertrophy. Hearts in end-stage failure are practically unresponsive to adrenergic stimulation.[43] It is significant therefore that regression of LV hypertrophy by removal of the ischemic kidney or by medical control of hypertension was found to restore to near-normal the inotropic response of hypertensive hearts to isoproterenol.[44]

RELATION TO VASCULAR HYPERTROPHY

Both the heart and vessels increase in muscle mass in response to the increased pressure load imposed by hypertension; it is not clear, however, whether both follow a similar path towards regression of hypertrophy when blood pressure is reduced by treatment. Reports of reduction in wall thickness of the arterial system and particularly the resistance vessels are relatively few. A close relation was described in SHR between changes in cardiac weight with treatment and lysine incorporation in vascular walls. Regression of vascular hypertrophy, or more precisely reduction of the ratio of wall thickness to internal radius, was reported by the Goteborg group following antihypertensive treatment both in man[45] and in experimental animals.[46] The regression of vascular hypertrophy was more marked in our experience following treatment of SHR by captopril than by hydralazine. More recently, Kobayashi and co-workers[47] have shown that LV and vascular structural changes in SHR respond differently to the same therapeutic agent in the same animal; that for equal regression of vascular hypertrophy, captopril and hydrochlorothiazide had different effects on regression of LV hypertrophy; LV mass was reduced by captopril but not by hydrochlorothiazide, possibly due to differences in the pharmacodynamic effects of both drugs. Clearly more data are needed, but the impression remains that reversal of vascular hypertrophy, although possible, is more difficult to achieve unless treatment is undertaken early.

These observations are of particular importance in the case of the coronary circulation because of the disturbances in coronary reserve in hypertension and of the increased oxygen needs of the hypertrophied myocardium. The complex interrelationships between LV mass, coronary changes, and arterial pressure in hypertension and in response to therapy are discussed in the following section.

CORONARY FLOW AND REVERSAL OF LV HYPERTROPHY WITH ANTIHYPERTENSIVE DRUGS

Studies of the coronary circulation in LV hypertrophy have demonstrated various functional or structural abnormalities, such as an impaired ability of the coronary vessels to dilate or to carry an augmented flow.[48,49] Similarly, the number of capillaries per unit mass has been found to be diminished by most investigators. These findings are not of purely academic interest. Other studies indicate that these alterations have potentially adverse clinical consequences and that myocardial ischemia may ensue when myocardial oxygen needs are increased. Hypertensive patients, particularly those with LV hypertrophy, may develop symptoms suggestive of ischemia, such as angina pectoris or ST segment depression during exercise in the absence of any detectable coronary artery lesions.[50,51] Myocardial infarction is more severe in hypertensive patients or animals,[52] and the size of the infarcted area is larger in dogs with hypertensive LV hypertrophy.[53] Furthermore, these coronary circulatory abnormalities may account for the higher risk of cardiac complications or sudden death that has been observed in hypertensive patients with echocardiographic evidence of LV hypertrophy.[54] Whether reversal of LV hypertrophy with antihypertensive drugs will be associated with normalization of these coronary abnormalities and eventually improve the prognosis of these patients is a key issue in the study of coronary circulation in hypertensive LV hypertrophy.

Unfortunately, little information is available at the present time on this issue, despite its obvious clinical implications. No studies have been reported in man, mainly because of methodological limitations. Current techniques for measuring coronary blood flow in man are invasive and therefore cannot be justified ethically nor repeated easily.

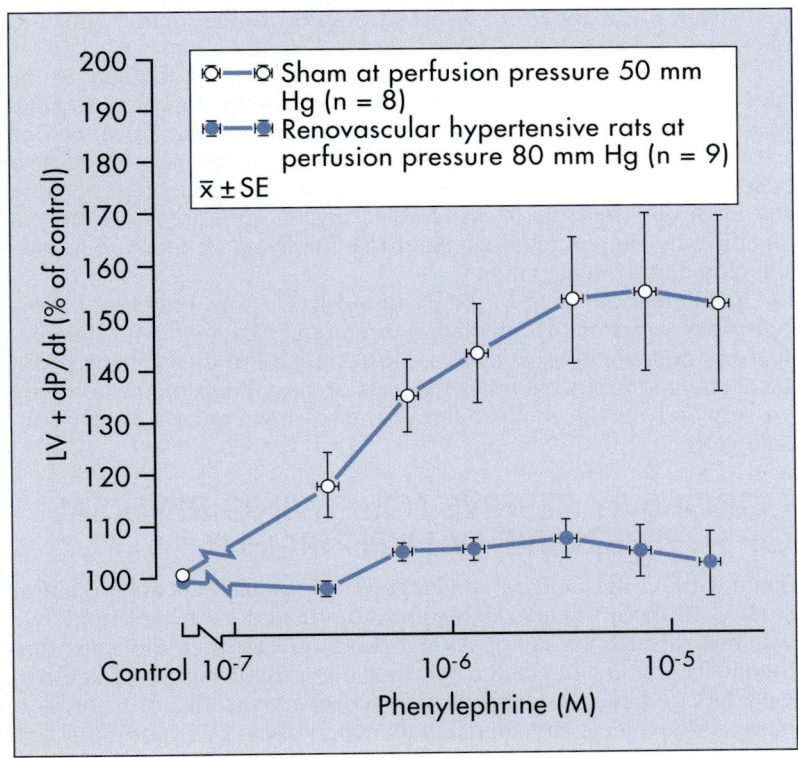

FIGURE 79.5 Inotropic response (expressed as a percentage of control value) to phenylephrine in the presence of propranolol (10^{-7} M). The different perfusion pressures used (50 mm Hg for controls and 80 mm Hg for renovascular hypertensive rats) were chosen because the myocardial flow rates under these conditions in the two groups were equal.

Only a few studies are available in animals and will be discussed in this section.

Before we proceed, however, it is necessary to review some of the definitions and concepts underlying the study of the coronary circulation. Coronary blood flow can be evaluated either at rest or in response to a coronary vasodilatory stimulus. Resting flow measurements do not provide any answer as to whether a hypertrophied ventricle is at greater risk of ischemia. By virtue of its definition, ischemia is more likely to occur when myocardial oxygen needs are increased or when coronary perfusion pressure is reduced. Thus, over the last decade, the emphasis has been shifted from studies of resting coronary blood flow to studies of the coronary circulation after various interventions in order to assess its ability to dilate and to maintain an adequate myocardial perfusion in these circumstances. The increase in coronary blood flow or the decrease in coronary resistance after maximal vasodilatory stimuli has been termed *coronary reserve* and is used as an index of the adaptive capacity of the coronary circulation.

RESTING CORONARY BLOOD FLOW DURING REVERSAL OF HYPERTENSIVE LVH

Table 79.3 summarizes the results obtained in hypertensive rats following chronic administration of a variety of antihypertensive drugs.[29,55-58] Coronary blood flow is expressed in milliliters per minute per unit mass of tissue to allow comparisons between animals with and without LV hypertrophy. The response of coronary blood flow to these different antihypertensive agents results from a complex interplay between the direct vascular effects of any particular drug and the indirect alterations in coronary resistance secondary to the changes in myocardial oxygen consumption induced by treatment. In that regard, the effects of antihypertensive treatment must be viewed along two perspectives, the immediate effects of blood pressure reduction and the long-term impact on LV mass. Similar to other conditions, resting coronary blood flow in hypertensive LV hypertrophy is closely autoregulated by myocardial oxygen demands; the latter is mainly determined by heart rate, contractility, and LV parietal stress (the force developed by the myocardial muscle fibers within the wall). LV parietal stress is directly correlated with blood pressure and ventricular size and inversely proportional to LV wall thickness. Thus, the relative magnitude of blood pressure reduction and of LV hypertrophy reversal will influence parietal stress and ultimately coronary blood flow. A precise delineation of these mechanisms would require simultaneous measurements of myocardial oxygen consumption and/or a more precise assessment of its main determinants.

However, some speculations on the potential mechanisms whereby antihypertensive drugs affect resting coronary blood flow in hypertensive LV hypertrophy can be made from presently available knowledge regarding the effects of these agents on coronary vasculature or myocardial oxygen consumption. For instance, β-blocking drugs exert little direct effect on the coronary vessels, unless resting sympathetic tone is significantly increased; the decrease in resting coronary blood flow observed with β-blockade results mainly from a reduction in heart rate and contractility.[58] On the contrary, calcium-blocking agents possess direct peripheral and coronary vasodilator properties, which probably account for most of the increase in coronary blood flow after chronic administration of nitrendipine.[29] This explanation is even more likely since nitrendipine probably reduces myocardial oxygen needs; had the autoregulatory coronary mechanism been the only one operative, coronary blood flow would have been expected to decrease. That nitrendipine will reduce myocardial oxygen needs, or at least not increase them, can be inferred from the observation that this compound decreases blood pressure more than LV mass[29] (and thus decreases parietal stress) and that it depresses myocardial contractility.

Converting enzyme inhibitors have no discernible acute direct effect on the coronary vasculature[59] unless the animal is in a sodium-depleted state.[60] Thus, the maintenance of a normal resting coronary blood flow after reversal of LV hypertrophy by captopril can be explained by the absence of any change in myocardial oxygen consumption. Heart rate was not affected by captopril in our study, and this compound possesses no known effect on cardiac contractility; moreover, blood pressure and LV mass were reduced in parallel so that parietal stress remained unchanged.

The absence of changes in coronary blood flow following hydralazine administration in rats[56] probably results from a balanced effect on myocardial oxygen needs and the coronary vasculature. However, hydralazine can elicit in some patients a marked sympathetic reflex stimulation, which can lead to both an increase in coronary blood flow and in oxygen demands. Depending on the net balance of these conflicting actions, hydralazine administration may so increase myocardial oxygen demand that angina pectoris is induced in hypertensive patients with coronary artery disease because of their limited ability to augment coronary flow.

Detailed studies of the direct coronary effects of centrally acting antiadrenergic drugs such as clonidine or methyldopa are lacking. Moreover, the few studies that are presently available have yielded conflicting results.[61] It is in fact likely that resting coronary blood flow remained unchanged after chronic treatment with these drugs because the main determinants of myocardial oxygen consumption were not significantly altered, although heart rate may tend to decrease following clonidine administration.[56]

In summary, resting coronary blood flow in hypertensive LV hypertrophy was variably affected after chronic treatment with different types of antihypertensive agents. Most if not all of these changes can be accounted for by the relative effects of these drugs on the coronary vessels and on the main determinants of myocardial oxygen consumption.

CORONARY RESERVE FOLLOWING REVERSAL OF HYPERTENSIVE LV HYPERTROPHY

Since work in this field can be judged only against the background of studies on the coronary circulation in untreated LV hypertrophy, we will first discuss the latter. A large body of evidence indicates that minimal coronary resistance per unit mass following pharmacologically induced coronary vasodilation (coronary vasodilator reserve) is elevated in patients and animals with hypertensive LV hypertrophy.[48,49] Of note is that this increase in minimal coronary resistance is a characteristic feature of pressure overload hypertrophy regardless of its

TABLE 79.3 RESTING CORONARY BLOOD FLOW IN RATS WITH HYPERTENSIVE LV HYPERTROPHY FOLLOWING CHRONIC ANTIHYPERTENSIVE TREATMENT

Author	Drug Used	Coronary Blood Flow (ml/min/100 g)
Kobayashi[29]	Nitrendipine	Increased*
Kobrin et al.[55]	Nitrendipine	
Pegram et al.[56]	Alphamethyldopa Clonidine Hydralazine	Unchanged*
Wicker et al.[57]	Captopril	
Wicker, unpublished observation	Clonidine	
Nishiyama et al.[58]	Propranolol Timolol	Decreased*

*Compared with untreated hypertensive animals

cause. Mueller and colleagues have also proposed to compute minimal coronary resistance for the *entire* LV (total minimal coronary resistance).[62] Conceptually, this parameter provides an important tool for the analysis of the respective roles of changes in LV mass and the coronary bed. Its calculation is independent of cardiac mass, and it can be viewed as an index of the total functional cross-sectional area of the coronary vasculature available for blood transport. Total minimal coronary resistance has consistently been found to be unchanged when compared with control normotensive animals; the association of these findings indicates that the size of the coronary vasculature does not keep pace with the increase in LV mass because of either functional or structural factors. An important consequence of this dissociation between mass and vasculature is that maximal coronary blood flow per unit (coronary flow reserve) will be dependent on an appropriate relationship between LV mass and coronary perfusion pressure (which is reasonably well approximated by the mean arterial blood pressure).

There are only a few reported studies of coronary reserve following reversal of hypertensive LV hypertrophy (Table 79.4).[57,63–65] In one of the first reports, we found that captopril, a converting enzyme inhibitor, decreased significantly both blood pressure and LV mass in RHR while leaving coronary flow reserve unchanged.[57] Further analysis of these data indicated that coronary flow reserve remained within normal limits because (1) *total* minimal coronary resistance remained unchanged and (2) coronary perfusion pressure and LV mass were decreased in parallel. As a consequence of this, minimal coronary resistance per unit mass (coronary vasodilator reserve), which was elevated in untreated animals, returned to near normal levels after captopril administration. Another important implication of this observation is that the only apparent effect of captopril was to reduce LV mass, while the coronary bed itself was most probably not affected by the drug. We cannot, however, exclude the possibility that captopril exerted direct effects on the coronary vessels, which were offset by directionally opposite structural or vascular changes, so that the total functional coronary cross-sectional area remained unchanged. This suggestion, however, is unlikely since very similar results were observed after treatment by nephrectomy in RHR rats in which any potential pharmacologic influence of captopril was excluded.[57]

The lack of changes in minimal total LV coronary resistance again pointed to the role of an appropriate balance between arterial pressure and LV mass in determining coronary flow reserve. Because some antihypertensive drugs have divergent effects on arterial pressure and cardiac hypertrophy, we further investigate the importance of the relationship between blood pressure and LV mass changes in two other studies in which the blood pressure to mass ratio was altered either by therapeutic manipulations or by using rat strains with different types of genetic cardiac hypertrophy with or without hypertension. Both studies confirmed that this ratio indeed played a crucial role in determining flow reserve; when pressure was low relative to LV mass, coronary flow reserve was diminished, and it was conversely increased when the blood pressure to mass ratio was high (see Fig. 79.2).[57]

These results have been confirmed recently in another study using a calcium-entry blocker. RHR and their normotensive sham-operated controls were treated with nitrendipine.[29] This agent reduced blood pressure more than LV mass *both* in normotensive and hypertensive rats. As a result, coronary flow reserve, again measured after carbochrome, was significantly reduced in normotensive treated animals and tended to decrease (although not significantly) in treated hypertensive rats as compared to their respective untreated controls.

In summary, this preliminary experience suggests that the few antihypertensive drugs evaluated so far exert beneficial effects on the coronary circulation, because the coronary resistance reserve, an index of the ability of coronary vasodilator vessels to dilate, returns toward normal levels. However, coronary flow reserve, which determines to a large extent the actual amount of blood—and thus of oxygen supply to the heart—may be impaired when the appropriate relationship between blood pressure and LV mass is altered.

POTENTIAL CLINICAL IMPLICATIONS

If confirmed in humans, these results have potentially important clinical implications for the choice of antihypertensive therapy. Antihypertensive drugs that induce reduction in blood pressure parallel to the decrease in LV mass would be preferable, as regards coronary flow reserve, to drugs that control blood pressure without affecting LV mass. In the absence of any data in man, however, these extrapolations from animal studies to clinical situations must remain speculative at the present time.

CONCLUSIONS

The manifold possible alterations in coronary circulation with reversal of hypertensive LV hypertrophy are virtually unexplored. Results from initial animal studies have already provided new and important knowledge but much remains to be learned. Obviously, these preliminary observations must be extended to clinical situations. The current development of noninvasive methods for measuring coronary blood flow in man holds promise, as these techniques will allow repeated measurements in asymptomatic hypertensive patients. Also, various experi-

TABLE 79.4 CORONARY RESERVE IN HYPERTENSIVE LEFT VENTRICULAR HYPERTROPHY: EFFECTS OF ANTIHYPERTENSIVE TREATMENT*

Author	Model	Drug	Blood Pressure	LV Mass	Coronary Vasodilator Reserve	Coronary Flow Reserve
Wicker et al.[57]	RVH/1C-2K	ACEI	↓N	↓N	↑N	↔
Tomanek et al.[63]	SHR	HZ	↓N	↔	↑N	↔
Friberg and Nordlander[64]	SHR	BB + CCB	↓N	↓	↑	—
Gosse et al.[65]	RVH/1C-2K	ACEI	↓N	↓N	↑N	↔

* All studies were performed in rats. RVH, reno-vascular hypertension; SHR, spontaneously hypertensive rats; ACEI, angiotensin-converting enzyme inhibitors; HZ, hydralazine; BB, β-blocker; CCB, calcium channel blocker; ↓ or ↑, significant decrease or increase as compared with untreated hypertensive rats with or without normalization (N); ↔, not significantly different from untreated hypertensive animals and from normotensive rats (coronary flow reserve only).

mental models of hypertension should be explored, and the effects of different classes of antihypertensive agents, alone or in combination, should be analyzed. Finally, little data are available on the transmural distribution of coronary blood flow between the superficial (*epicardial*) and inner (*endocardial*) layers after reversal of LV hypertrophy, and the ratio between endocardial and epicardial flow should be systematically assessed. Various clinical and experimental observations suggest that ischemia may occur predominantly in the endocardial layers,[66] and a determination of whether this abnormality can be effectively reversed by antihypertensive drugs would be of great interest.

REFERENCES

1. Trimarco B, De Luca N, De Simone A, et al: Impaired control of vasopressin release in hypertensive subjects with cardiac hypertrophy. Hypertension 10:595, 1987
2. Grassi G, Giannattasio C, Cleroux J, et al: Cardiopulmonary reflex before and after regression of left ventricular hypertrophy in essential hypertension. Hypertension 12:227, 1988
3. Tarazi RC: Reversal of cardiac hypertrophy: Possibility and clinical implications. In Robertson JIS, Caldwell ADS (eds): Left Ventricular Hypertrophy in Hypertension. Royal Society of Medicine International Congress and Symposium Series No. 9, p 55. London, Academic Press, and New York, Grune & Stratton, 1979
4. Grossman W: Cardiac hypertrophy: Useful adaptation or pathologic process? Am J Med 69:576, 1980
5. Meerson FZ: The myocardium in hyperfunction, hypertrophy and heart failure. Monograph 26, p 6. New York, American Heart Association, 1969
6. Devereux RB, Reichek N: Echocardiographic determination of left ventricular mass in man: Anatomic validation of the method. Circulation 55:613, 1977
7. Sen S, Tarazi RC, Khairallah PA, Bumpus FM: Cardiac hypertrophy in spontaneously hypertensive rats. Circ Res 35:775, 1974
8. Tarazi RC, Sen S, Fouad FM: Regression of myocardial hypertrophy. In Braunwald E, Mock MB, Watson J (eds): Congestive Heart Failure: Current Research and Clinical Applications, p 151. New York, Grune & Stratton, 1982
9. Sen S, Tarazi RC, Bumpus FM: Reversal of cardiac hypertrophy in renal hypertensive rats: Medical vs surgical therapy. Am J Physiol 240:H408, 1981
10. Tarazi RC, Fouad FM: Reversal of cardiac hypertrophy in humans. Hypertension 6 (Suppl) III:140, 1984
11. Frohlich ED: Left ventricular hypertrophy and the hypertensive patient. In Frishman W, Maseri A (eds) International Proceedings Journal, Cardiology, Curr Concepts Antihypertensive Ther 1(2):8, 1989
12. Fouad FM, Tarazi RC, Bravo EL: Hemodynamic and cardiac effects of enalapril. Hypertension 1 (Suppl) I:135, 1983
13. Schlant RC, Feiner JM, Heymsfield SG, Gilbert CA: Echocardiographic studies of left ventricular anatomy and function in essential hypertension. Cardiovasc Med 2:477, 1977
14. Williams JR Jr, Braunwald E: Studies on digitalis. XI. Effects of digitoxin on the development of cardiac hypertrophy in the rat subjected to aortic constriction. Am J Cardiol 16:534, 1965
15. Fouad FM, Nakashima RC, Tarazi RC, Salcedo EE: Reversal of left ventricular hypertrophy in hypertensive patients treated with methyldopa: Lack of association with blood pressure control. Am J Cardiol 49:795, 1982
16. Ibrahim MM, Madkour MA, Mossalam R: Factors influencing cardiac hypertrophy in hypertensive patients. Clin Sci 61 (Suppl) 7:105s, 1981
17. Drayer JIM, Weber MA, Gardin JM, Lipson JL: Effect of long-term antihypertensive therapy on cardiac anatomy in patients with essential hypertension. Am J Med 75 (Suppl) 3A:116, 1983
18. Hartford M, Wikstrand J, Wallentin I et al: Non-invasive signs of cardiac involvement in essential hypertension. Eur Heart J 3:75, 1982
19. Abi-Samra F, Fouad FM, Tarazi RC: Determinants of left ventricular hypertrophy and function in hypertensive patients: An echocardiographic study. Am J Med (Suppl)3A:26, 1983
20. Ibrahim MM, Tarazi RC, Dustan HP, Gifford RW, Jr: Electrocardiogram in evaluation of resistance to antihypertensive therapy. Arch Intern Med 137:1125, 1977
21. Rowlands DB, Glover DR, Ireland MA et al: Assessment of left ventricular mass and its response to antihypertensive treatment. Lancet 1:467, 1982
22. Rowlands DB, Glover DR, Stallard TJ, Littler WA. Control of blood pressure and reduction of echocardiographically assessed left ventricular mass with once-daily Timolol. Br J Clin Pharmacol 14:89, 1982
23. Williams GW, Forsythe SB, Textor SC, Tarazi RC: Analysis of relative change and initial value in biological studies. Am J Physiol 246:R122, 1984
24. Safar ME, Lehner JP, Vincent MI et al: Echocardiographic dimensions in borderline and sustained hypertension. Am J Cardiol 44:930, 1979
25. Sasayama S, Ross J, Jr, Franklin D et al: Adaptations of the left ventricle to chronic pressure overload. Circ Res 38:172, 1976
26. Trimarco B, Wikstrand J: Regression of cardiovascular structural changes by antihypertensive treatment. Hypertension 6 (Suppl)III:150, 1984
27. Fouad-Tarazi FM, Liebson PR: Echocardiographic studies of regression of left ventricular hypertrophy in hypertension. Hypertension 9(Suppl II):II-65, 1987
28. Fouad-Tarazi FM: Structural cardiac and vascular changes in hypertension: response to treatment. Curr Opinion in Cardiol 2:782, 1987
29. Kobayashi K, Tarazi RC: Effect of nitrendipine on coronary flow and ventricular hypertrophy. Hypertension 5 (Suppl)II:45, 1983
30. Motz W, Strauer BE: Regression of structural cardiovascular changes by antihypertensive therapy. Hypertension 6 (Suppl)III:133, 1984
31. Kobrin I, Frohlich ED, Ventura HO, et al: Renal involvement follows cardiac enlargement in essential hypertension. Arch Intern Med 146:272, 1986
32. Drayer JIM, Gardin JM, Weber MA, Aronow WS: Cardiac muscle mass during vasodilation therapy of hypertension. Clin Pharmacol Ther 33:727, 1983
33. Drayer JIM, Gardin JM, Weber MA, Aronow WS: Changes in cardiac anatomy and function during therapy with alphamethyldopa: An echocardiographic study. Curr Ther Res 32:856, 1982
34. Ferrario CM, Spech MM, Tarazi RC, Doi Y: Cardiac pumping ability in rats with experimental renal and genetic hypertension. Am J Cardiol 44:979, 1979
35. Kuwajima I, Kardon MB, Pegram BL et al: Regression of left ventricular hypertrophy in two-kidney, one clip Goldblatt hypertension. Hypertension 4 (Suppl)II:113, 1982
36. Capasso JM, Strobeck JE, Malhotra A et al: Contractile behavior of rat myocardium after reversal of hypertensive hypertrophy. Am J Physiol 242:H282, 1982
37. Agati L, Fedele F, Penco M, Sciomer S, Dagianti A: Left ventricular filling pattern in hypertensive patients after reversal of myocardial hypertrophy. Int J Cardiol 17:177, 1987
38. Fletcher PJ, Bailey BP, Harris PJ: Regression of hypertrophy in hypertension: effects on diastolic function. Circulation 75(Suppl II):II–297 (abstract), 1986
39. Ayobe MH, Tarazi RC: Beta-receptors and contractile reserve in left ventricular hypertrophy. Hypertension 5 (Suppl)I:192, 1983
40. Kumano K, Upsher ME, Khairallah P: Beta-adrenergic receptor response coupling in hypertrophied hearts. Hypertension 5 (Suppl)I:175, 1983
41. Fouad FM, Shimamatsu K, Said SI, Tarazi RC: Inotropic responsiveness in hypertensive left ventricular hypertrophy; impaired inotropic response to glucagon and vasoactive intestinal peptide (VIP) in renal hypertensive rats. J Cardiovasc Pharmacol 8:398, 1986
42. Rodeheffer RJ, Gerstenblith G, Becker LC et al: Exercise cardiac output is maintained with advancing age in healthy human subjects: Cardiac dilatation and increased stroke volume compensate for a diminished heart rate. Circulation 69:203, 1984
43. Bristow MR: The adrenergic nervous system in heart failure. N Engl J Med 311:850, 1984
44. Ayobe MH, Tarazi RC: Reversal of changes in myocardial beta-receptors and inotropic responsiveness with regression of cardiac hypertrophy in renal hypertensive rats (RHR). Circ Res 54:125, 1984
45. Sivertsson R: The hemodynamic importance of structural vascular changes in essential hypertension. Acta Physiol Scand 343 (Suppl)I:56, 1970
46. Lundin SA, Margareta IL, Hallback M: Regression of structural cardiovascular changes by antihypertensive therapy in spontaneously hypertensive rats. J Hypertension 2:11, 1984
47. Kobayashi H, Sano T, Tarazi RC, Fouad-Tarazi FM: Effects of antihypertensive drugs on heart and resistance vessels. Cardiovasc Res 24(2):137, 1990
48. Tomanek RJ: Response of the coronary vasculature to myocardial hypertrophy. Am J Cardiol 15:528, 1990
49. Wicker P: Coronary circulation and coronary reserve in the hypertensive heart. In Safar ME and Fouad-Tarazi FM (ed): The heart in hypertension. Dordrecht. Kluwer Academic Publishers, 253, 1989
50. Harris CN, Aronow WS, Parker DP, Kaplin MA: Treadmill stress test in left ventricular hypertrophy. Chest 63:353, 1973
51. Opherk D, Mall G, Zebe H et al: Reduction of coronary reserve: A mechanism for angina pectoris in patients with arterial hypertension and normal coronary arteries. Circulation 69:1, 1984
52. Koyanagi S, Eastham CL, Marcus ML: Effects of chronic hypertension and left ventricular hypertrophy on the incidence of sudden cardiac death following coronary occlusion in conscious dogs. Circulation 65:1192, 1982
53. Koyanagi S, Eastham CL, Harrison DG, Marcus ML: Increased size of myocardial infarction in dogs with chronic hypertension and left ventricular hypertrophy. Circ Res 50:55, 1982
54. Casale P, Devereux R, Milner M et al: Value of echocardiographic measurement of left ventricular mass in predicting cardiovascular morbid events in hypertensive men. Ann Int Med 105:173, 1986
55. Kobrin I, Sesoko S, Pegram BL, Frohlich ED: Reduced cardiac mass by nitrendipine is dissociated from systemic or regional haemodynamic changes in rats. Cardiovasc Res 18:158, 1984
56. Pegram BL, Ishise S, Frohlich ED: Effect of methyldopa, clonidine, and hydralazine on cardiac mass and haemodynamics in Wistar Kyoto and sponta-

57. Wicker P, Tarazi RC, Kobayashi K: Coronary blood flow during the development and regression of left ventricular hypertrophy in renovascular hypertensive rats. Am J Cardiol 51:1744, 1983
58. Nishiyama K, Nishiyama A, Pfeffer MA, Frohlich ED: Systemic and regional flow distribution in normotensive and spontaneously hypertensive young rats subjected to lifetime β-adrenergic receptor blockade. In Bevan JA (ed): Blood Vessels, pp 333–347. Basel, Switzerland, S. Karger, 1978
59. Noguchi K, Kato T, Ito H, Aniya Y, Sakanashi M: Effect of intracoronary captopril on coronary blood flow and regional myocardial function in dogs. Eur J Pharmacol 110:11, 1985
60. Liang C-S, Gavras H, Hood WB, Jr: Renin-angiotensin system inhibition in conscious sodium-depleted dogs. J Clin Invest 61:874, 1978
61. Tarazi RC: Hemodynamic effects of Aldomet. In Maxwell MH (ed): Aldomet (Methyldopa, MSD) In The Management of Hypertension, pp 73–81. West Point, Pennsylvania, Merck Sharp & Dohme, 1978
62. Mueller TM, Marcus ML, Kerber RE et al: Effects of renal hypertension and left ventricular hypertrophy on the coronary circulation in dogs. Circ Res 42:543, 1978
63. Tomanek RJ, Wangler RD, Bauer CA: Prevention of coronary vasodilator reserve decrement in spontaneously hypertensive rats. Hypertension 7:569, 1985
64. Friberg P, Nordlander M: Influence of long-term antihypertensive therapy on cardiac function, coronary flow and myocardial oxygen consumption in spontaneously hypertensive rats. J Hypertens 4:165, 1986
65. Gosse P, Grellet J, Bonoron S, Tariosse L, Besse P, Dallocchio M: Effets du Perindopril sur l'hypertrophie ventriculaire gauche, la reserve coronaire et les proprietes mecaniques du muscle papillaire du rat avec hypertension arterielle renovasculaire. Arch Mal Coeur 80:905, 1987
66. Hoffman JIE: Why is myocardial ischaemia so commonly subendocardial? Clin Sci 61:657, 1981

Hypertension in the Elderly

CHAPTER 80 VOLUME 2

Robert C. Tarazi

Both arterial pressure and age are continuous variables; hence, the notion of "hypertension in the elderly" can at best constitute only a relative entity, not a condition qualitatively different from increased blood pressure in the adult population. Practically, these considerations mean that there is no feature that is "unique" to hypertension in patients over age 60—in fact, this traditional threshold for "old age" is itself purely arbitrary.

Hypertension is the result of the interaction of different pressor mechanisms; these are relatively limited in number and the various types of hypertension differ from each other, not so much by the presence of any single pressor factor but rather by the way in which these factors are integrated.[1] Age affects many of these physiologic mechanisms in a graded way. There is therefore no arbitrary limit at which hypertension suddenly becomes a qualitatively different disease, but some characteristics begin gradually to assume a greater importance with advancing years, influencing both its clinical picture and response to treatment. One outstanding example is the gradual reduction in compliance of the aorta and large vessels with age; this reduction is more frequent among older patients but it certainly can occur in younger subjects[2,3] and will have the same consequences regardless of the patient's chronologic age. Its occurrence does not negate the importance of other pressor factors but will modulate their expression.

The reduced arterial distensibility with its secondary exaggeration of systolic hypertension and diminished effectiveness of baroreceptor reflexes[4] is perhaps the better known of the vascular changes that develop with age. There are others, possibly more subtle in their expression but no less important in their therapeutic consequences. These include a gradual reduction in beta-adrenergic receptors in the heart and blood vessels[5-7] and changes in liver and kidney function that can alter the excretion rate of antihypertensive agents.[8] The reduction in vascular beta-receptors would enhance the vasoconstrictor effect of alpha-adrenergic stimuli and may alter response to alpha-blocking agents; fewer cardiac beta-receptors may entail a reduction in cardiac contractile reserve.[7,9,10] A diminished excretion rate of drugs could enhance their hypotensive potential or risk from adverse side effects.

Most of these age-dependent changes can be accelerated by hypertension, whether these be reduced aortic distensibility,[11] diminution in beta-adrenergic receptors,[12] or impairment of renal function. Chronologic age therefore becomes less important than the medical history of the patient; safe and effective treatment will depend more on careful assessment of the individual than on dogmatic decisions based on arbitrary values of blood pressure and age.

THE QUESTION OF SYSTOLIC HYPERTENSION IN THE ELDERLY

Physicians have traditionally been more familiar with decisions based on diastolic blood pressure levels, both for diagnosis and treatment of hypertension. Stepped-care therapy is based entirely on the degree of diastolic pressure elevation.[13] There are many reasons for this bias, such as the assumed greater lability of systolic blood pressure and its purported dependence on cardiac action in contrast to the closer relation of diastolic pressure to peripheral arteriolar vasoconstriction[14]; both these impressions were repeatedly shown to be mistaken.[15,16] They remain, nevertheless, influential, and therefore a reflection on systolic blood pressure levels is appropriate for this chapter because of their special importance in older patients.

In fact, the discussion of hypertension in elderly patients is much too often dominated by questions about isolated systolic hypertension. Although legitimate, these questions address only part of the problem and thus sometimes distort the approach to one of the important and frequent diseases of the elderly.[8] Hypertension in patients over 60 years of age is *not* limited to isolated elevations of systolic pressure; it is just as liable to be diastolic as well as systolic or, more frequently, both. The risk of cardiovascular disease increases with elevations in either the diastolic or systolic level, often more steeply with the latter.[17,18] The epidemiologic characteristics of hypertension and its risks in the over 60 years age group have been defined in several excellent reviews.[19-21] The efficacy of treatment of diastolic hypertension in that age group was convincingly demonstrated by the Hypertension Detection and Follow-up Program (HDFP) and other studies.[8] The problems of pure systolic hypertension are, in my opinion, only partly due to the absence of definite proof of efficacy for its treatment; the clear relation between systolic pressure levels and risk from cardiovascular

---

Reprinted from Tarazi RC: Hypertension in the elderly. In Calkins E (ed): The Practice of Geriatrics. Philadelphia, WB Saunders, 1986

disease[17,18,22,23] would have tipped the decision toward treatment, were it not for the difficulties and side effects of the latter. In fact, the question raised today as regards hypertension in the elderly does not challenge its risks or the advisability of treatment as much as the safety of therapy or its practicality in that high-risk population.[24] This question is best addressed by careful consideration of the pathophysiologic mechanisms of systolic hypertension and their utilization for the choice of safe therapy.

Wiggers[25] long ago defined the relation between the diastolic pressure and distensibility of the aorta and large vessels; because this distensibility is reduced as distolic blood pressure (DBP) increases, pulse pressure (everything else being equal) increases as hypertension develops (Fig. 80.1). The implication is that added loss of elasticity of these large vessels (windkessel) will lead to an even steeper slope of the relation between systolic blood pressure (SBP) and DBP, which attains its maximum in isolated systolic hypertension due to aortic sclerosis. The practical results are that a larger drop of SBP must be expected for an equal reduction of DBP during treatment of these patients (Fig. 80.2) with a greater risk of transient but alarming side effects—hence, the need for reduced dosage of drugs and a much more gradual approach to blood pressure control.

In that respect, it is important to view the relationship of systolic to diastolic pressure levels as a continuum and *not* to subdivide hypertension into two groups only, diastolic hypertension and isolated systolic hypertension. Between these two groups there is a large number of patients who have, along with an elevated diastolic pressure, a more than expected increase in systolic pressure; this "inappropriate systolic hypertension" can be of different degrees but its implications are the same. These are the similarity in therapeutic problems in those patients with the problems encountered in isolated systolic hypertension; common to both are the marked variations in systolic pressure, the brittleness of blood pressure control, and the borderline baroreceptor adequacy.

PATHOPHYSIOLOGIC ASPECTS
CARDIAC FUNCTION AND HEMODYNAMIC PATTERNS

An increase in total peripheral resistance remains the hemodynamic hallmark of established hypertension in either young or older subjects.[26] Cardiac output can be normal for the patient's age but is more frequently reduced[3,27,28]; the combination of a small stroke volume and high pulse pressure suggests a reduced aortic distensibility (see below). There are, however, some exceptions, such as patients who present with an evident hyperkinetic circulation despite a longstanding hypertension[29]; this combination seems rare over the age of 65, but

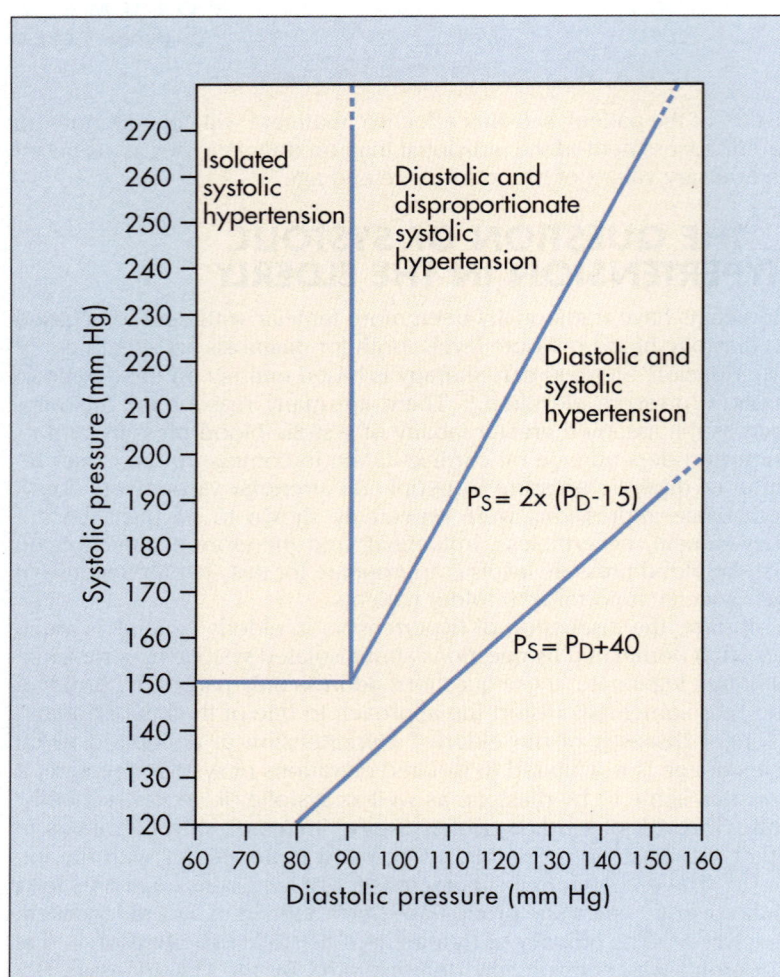

FIGURE 80.1 The relationship between diastolic (P_D) and systolic (P_S) blood pressure would have been given by the first line ($P_S = P_D + 40$) if aortic distensibility remained the same whatever the P_D level. However, since distensibility is reduced as diastolic blood pressure increases, systolic pressure rises relatively more than the diastolic, as given by the equation of the second line. Inappropriate systolic elevations for the level of diastolic pressure can cover the whole spectrum from $P_S = 2 \times (P_D - 15)$ to isolated systolic elevations. (Modified from Koch-Weser J: Am J Cardiol 32:499–510, 1973)

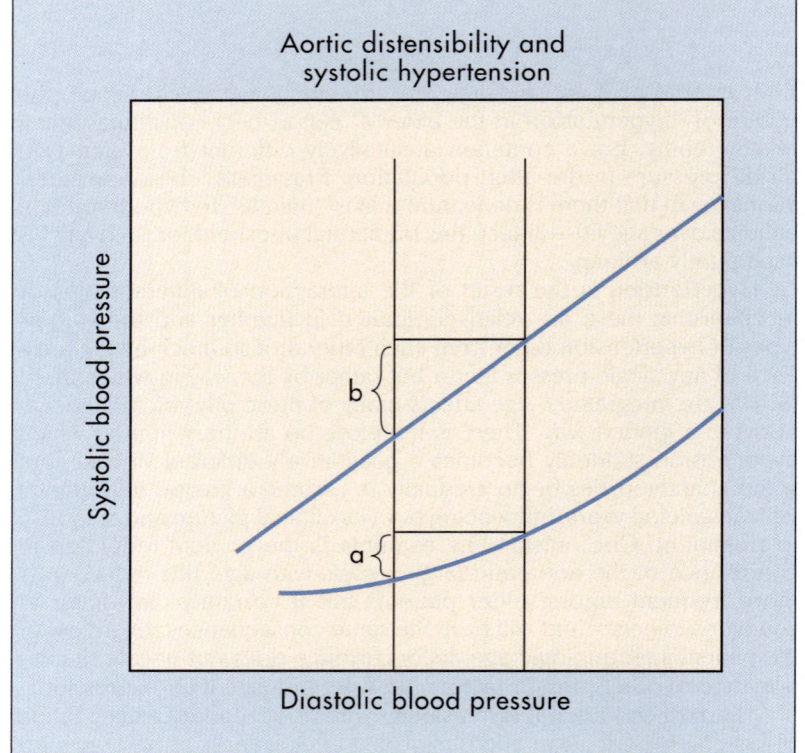

FIGURE 80.2 The steeper slope of the relation between systolic and diastolic blood pressure (see Fig. 80.1) signifies that one should expect a greater drop of systolic pressure in patients with inappropriate systolic hypertension (b > a) for the same reduction in diastolic pressure.

when present, the high cardiac output and signs of sympathetic stimulation will suggest the need for sympatholytics in therapeutic planning.

Plasma volume is frequently low in elderly hypertensives,[27,28] which helps to explain to some degree their low cardiac output. When associated with poor venous tone and static dependent edema, the low volume may contribute to their poor adjustment to upright posture.[30] Paradoxically, older patients often have a low plasma renin activity despite their low plasma volume, possibly because of reduced autonomic reflexes or of blunted end-organ responsiveness.[31] Whatever the basic mechanism (blunted baroreceptors, low renin, or contracted intravascular volume), its important practical consequences are the marked sensitivity of most elderly hypertensives to diuretics and the need to begin antihypertensive treatment with about half the adult dose.

Cardiac performance is at special risk in older hypertensive patients because of a combination of factors, including the greater incidence of coincidental coronary or arrhythmic heart disease, the reduction of cardiac output and of beta-adrenergic receptors with age and left ventricular (LV) hypertrophy,[6,7,10] and the inappropriate increase in systolic blood pressure.[32] The reduction of cardiac output with age has recently been confirmed by carefully controlled studies[7]; the results are a higher systemic resistance to blood flow and greater impedance to cardiac ejection. The reduced responsiveness to beta-adrenergic stimulation will blunt the effectiveness of cardioadrenergic drive, robbing the heart of a major supportive mechanism and reducing its contractile reserve.[9] The result is greater dependence on the Frank-Starling mechanism to meet extra-loads and a predisposition to ventricular dilation and further encroachment on cardiac reserve.

Of particular importance because of its therapeutic implications is the direct relation of systolic pressure levels to the cardiac load; it is the systolic not the diastolic pressure that is the variable used to define ventricular afterload[32] and hence the oxygen-expensive types of cardiac work. It is therefore particularly important in cases with reduced cardiac function or potential heart disease. Indications for antihypertensive therapy based exclusively on diastolic pressure levels miss the evident importance of systolic pressure for patients with inappropriate systolic hypertension or those with cardiac problems. Many studies have directly demonstrated the marked reduction in stroke volume and increase in LV end-diastolic pressure associated with even modest increases in systolic blood pressure (Table 80.1). More accurate appreciation of the impact of systolic hypertension on the heart will help explain much of the cardiac hypertrophy and diminished performance seen in older patients and offer a therapeutic possibility instead of invoking some unspecified degenerative effect of age.

When a physician is confronted with a multiplicity of causes for cardiac dysfunction, as is often the case in older patients, the more important causes in practice are those about which something can be done. Careful reduction of systolic blood pressure may help improve cardiac performance. To a purely quantitative definition of hypertension, it is appropriate to add in some cases a biologic dimension; a systolic blood pressure that depresses cardiac function is too high for that particular case and should suggest a careful consideration of antihypertensive measures.

AORTIC COMPLIANCE AND ARTERIAL DYNAMICS

Arterial compliance reflects the viscoelastic properties of the walls of the large arteries and determines the effectiveness of their role in buffering the wide fluctuations in pressure generated by the heart (windkessel effect).[25] Although there is a general tendency for arterial compliance to diminish with age and for hypertension in the elderly to be associated with aortic rigidity, there are enough exceptions to suggest that investigations are sometimes needed in problem cases.[2,3]

Many indices have been proposed to determine aortic compliance in humans[3,33-35]; some, such as the ratio of pulse pressure to stroke volume (PP/SV, mm Hg rise in pressure per ml blood ejected), can be useful as easy approximations of systemic arterial compliance (SAC).[3] Others are more precise mathematical derivations from the slope of fall in intra-arterial pressure during diastole (Fig. 80.3).[34,35] In our experience and that of others, there has been a close correlation in most older patients between PP/SV ratio and the index derived from pulse pressure tracings; many exceptions, however, were found among young subjects. The paradox is explained by the dependence of SBP on more than one factor; it depends in part on aortic distensibility but also in part on the velocity of ventricular ejection of blood. In case the

TABLE 80.1 HEMODYNAMIC EFFECTS OF INCREASED SYSTOLIC BLOOD PRESSURE*

	Control	↑Systolic Blood Pressure
Systolic pressure (mm Hg)	122 ± 6	133 ± 8†
Diastolic pressure (mm Hg)	87 ± 4	85 ± 4
LVEDP (mm Hg)	5.1 ± 0.5	6.0 ± 0.6†
Cardiac index (liters/m²)	1.71 ± 0.16	1.58 ± 0.17†
SV/EDV	0.42 ± 0.04	0.35 ± 0.04†

* Increase obtained by inserting a rigid bypass along the aorta.

† $P < 0.01$

(LVEDP = left ventricular end-diastolic pressure; SV/EDV = ejection fraction)

(Urschel C et al: Am J Physiol 214:299, 1968)

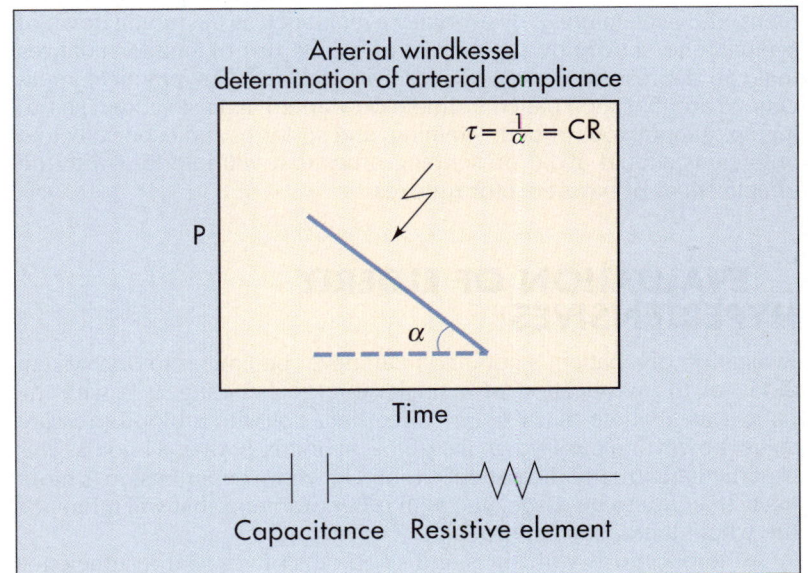

FIGURE 80.3 The fall in arterial pressure from the dicrotic notch until the beginning of the next cardiac cycle is exponential and can be likened to a simple model linking in series a capacitance (C) with a resistive element (R). Arterial compliance can therefore be calculated from the slope of the diastolic part of the pulse and from simultaneously determined total peripheral resistance. The method has been validated in humans by Simon and co-workers[34]

inappropriate elevation of SBP is related to a reduction in aortic compliance, the two indices agree, but if ventricular ejection is abnormally rapid, then SBP may be high even though arterial compliance is normal or only slightly reduced.[36]

The compliance of the arterial system is not a fixed characteristic dependent only on the biochemical and structural characteristics of its walls. The "tone" of large arteries is influenced by different neurohumoral factors, particularly sympathetic activity,[37,38] and reacts differently to various vasodilators. The work of Safar, Simon, and Levenson[39-41] has brought to light the frequent divergence between the effect of vasodilators on the small resistance vessels and their effects on the large arteries. Some, like hydralazine, lower peripheral resistance by peripheral vasodilation but reduce the diameter of the larger vessels, whereas converting enzyme inhibitors and particularly calcium entry blockers dilate both the small peripheral vessels and the large arteries.[42] As these differences are confirmed and better appreciated, they will add a new dimension to our therapeutic choice among vasodilators. Those that produce arterial as well as arteriolar dilation may prove more suitable for patients with peripheral arterial disease. This subject will be discussed further under Therapeutic Considerations, below.

BARORECEPTOR FUNCTION IN OLDER PATIENTS

One of the more significant features in circulatory homeostasis is the gradual reduction in baroreceptor sensitivity that develops with age, both in normotensive and hypertensive subjects.[4] The early clinical observations of blunted arterial pressure responses to a Valsalva maneuver in older patients were further extended and quantified by studies of the heart rate response to induced variations in systolic blood pressure; baroreceptor sensitivity was defined by the slope of the relation determined between the SBP levels and RR intervals.[43] That sensitivity was gradually reduced with advancing age, and within each decade was significantly lower in hypertensive than in normotensive subjects.[4]

The blunting of baroreceptor reflexes in older hypertensives suggests that complaints of hypotension and dizziness on standing or straining will be frequent when antihypertensive therapy is initiated in patients over 60 years old. The combined effects of age and hypertension have them living at the edge, as it were, of baroreceptor compensation. The balance can be easily tipped to inadequate postural adjustment, and even fainting, by everyday events such as the toning down of sympathetic activity by supine rest or by the use of simple sedatives that can depress baroreceptor sensitivity further.[30] The practical implications are that such patients should be warned against sudden standing up, jumping out of bed, straining, and so forth, and especially that physicians should avoid prescribing drugs that will interfere with the effectiveness of baroreceptor reflexes.

EVALUATION OF ELDERLY HYPERTENSIVES

Evaluation of a patient's condition can never be limited to one system alone or to investigation of a single abnormal finding; it is with the patient as a whole that we are concerned, not with a blood pressure value, however measured, in the office, at home, or over 24 hours. This is particularly true of the patient over 60 in whom hypertension is more likely than not to be associated with other problems that will influence the whole therapeutic approach.

Atherosclerosis with signs and symptoms of vascular insufficiency in various organs, diabetes mellitus, depression, osteoarthritis, and obstructive pulmonary disease are all common in elderly patients and each will impose its restriction on the choice of antihypertensive drug. Analgesics given over the counter may interfere with the antihypertensive effects of furosemide or of captopril; sedatives and antidepressants may impair baroreceptor reflexes and exaggerate postural hypotension. Therefore, adequate evaluation begins with a careful medical history to assess the patient's personality, his memory, and his understanding of his disease, as well as of *all* the medications he is using.

The duration of hypertension is particularly important; in the majority, hypertension dates back to their middle years and represents a classic essential hypertension.[23] Evaluation is then mostly directed to assessment of target organ damage and of concomitant atherosclerosis and other diseases, with particular attention to the heart, to the possibility of carotid or peripheral vascular disease, and to the level of renal excretory function.[23] In other patients, the increase in pressure will have developed *de novo* above the age of 55 or there has been an acute exacerbation of a stable hypertension. Under these conditions, a search for atherosclerotic renal artery stenosis is warranted.[8,44] Investigations may also be warranted for either primary or secondary aldosteronism if hypokalemia develops easily and limits therapy.[8]

BLOOD PRESSURE RECORDING

Careful, repeated measurements of blood pressure are needed in all hypertensives, young and old, in order to avoid overdiagnosis, needless anxiety, and the side effects of unnecessary treatment. Extremely wide variations in systolic blood pressure readings are common in the elderly. Multiple blood pressure measurements should therefore be obtained before deciding on treatment, at least three measurements on each of at least three office visits over a period of weeks. An alternative is to have the patients measure their own blood pressures regularly at home for a couple of weeks.

In addition, two facts must be carefully ascertained; the first is the response of arterial pressure to upright posture, and the second is the effect of arterial stiffness on auscultatory blood pressure measurements. Caird and associates,[45] reported a drop of 20 mm Hg or more in systolic pressure on standing in 24% of 494 subjects above age 64. The poor cardiovascular adjustment to posture implies the potential for more side-effects during treatment and the need to use small doses and avoid drugs that impair baroreceptor reflexes. As regards the second question, older patients frequently have a greater discrepancy between auscultatory and intra-arterial blood pressure levels than younger subjects; some with apparent severe hypertension were shown to be almost normotensive by direct intra-arterial records.[46] This "pseudohypertension" is probably related to the difficulty of compressing a stiff and possibly calcified brachial artery.

THERAPEUTIC CONSIDERATIONS

Controversies still surround the advisability and modalities of antihypertensive therapy in elderly patients.[47] The controversy will not be solved by statistics and epidemiologic studies alone; in my opinion, its persistence really reflects more a fear of complications and a reluctance to meddle with patients who have reached a great age unmolested by vascular disease. An editorial in the *Lancet*[47] expressed the situation in a most precise, elegant, and practical way; three questions summarize the physician's dilemma: (1) Is there an increased risk associated with hypertension in the elderly? (2) Is this risk reversible by therapy? (3) At what cost in iatrogenic disease might some increase in survival be purchased, and can the labor and expense of detecting and treating symptomless hypertension in this age group be justified in social and economic terms?

The answers today are quite clear for some points, still doubtful for others, and, as regards the last point, involve a value judgment rather than a scientific decision. That hypertension, whether diastolic or systolic, is associated with increased cardiovascular risk is a demonstrated fact. The favorable effects of therapy in diastolic hypertension in patients over age 60 or 65 have been proven in many trials both here[19] and abroad.[20,48] Table 80.2 is a review of the subject. There is no definite evidence that antihypertensive therapy is beneficial in elderly patients with isolated systolic hypertension, but there is no more evidence either for a harmful effect of adequate and cautious treatment.

I do not think the questions raised can be solved only by more statistical evidence. The problem is clinical, the objections stem from bedside observations, and the answer will come from a better understanding of pathophysiology applied with common sense. The *Lancet* editorial expressed this very well indeed[47]:

> Therapeutic misadventures are more likely in the elderly because of inappropriate dosage, impaired cardiovascular homoeostasis, erratic pill-taking, and polypharmacy for multiple diseases. Few would urge the conversion of a happy independent hypertensive into a depressed invalid, chair-bound or bed-bound for fear of postural hypotension, in pursuit of a theoretical prolongation of life, but such instances are grounds not so much for neglecting hypertension as for avoiding a casual approach.

This is the reason for the lengthy discussion of pathophysiology in this chapter; its reasoned application should make antihypertensive treatment safer and therefore more acceptable. There are many published discussions of antihypertensive drugs for older patients such as the excellent summary by Kirkendall and Hammond,[8] the personal opinion of Gifford,[23] and the recommendations of the National High Blood Pressure Education Committee.[44] Two basic principles are stressed by all:

1. The initial doses and subsequent increments of any antihypertensive agent selected should be quite small (half of the usual adult dose) because of the many factors that enhance their hypotensive effect in older patients. These include low plasma volume, impaired mechanisms of cardiovascular homeostasis, reduced excretion rate of some drugs, and greater sensitivity to sympatholytics and alpha-blockers because of enhanced sympathetic vasoconstrictor tone.
2. Drugs that interfere with baroreceptor reflexes should be avoided if at all possible, because of the borderline "baroreceptor compensation" of older patients.

To the extent that general rules can really be summarized in a few sentences and still be helpful, one might suggest from the preceding discussion that antihypertensive therapy in older patients could begin —if indicated—with small doses of a diuretic to which small doses of an adequate vasodilator could be added later. Hydralazine has been suggested because it does not interfere with baroreceptor reflexes and can be well tolerated; however, it could induce or worsen angina pectoris.[8] The hemodynamic pattern produced by converting enzyme inhibitors and most calcium entry blockers appears favorable; the latter can serve more than one purpose if the hypertensive patient also suffers from some form of arterial insufficiency, peripheral or coronary.

Of potential great importance is the *better understanding of vasodilators* that has been developing over the past few years. Two aspects have been added to the early concept that peripheral vasodilators are drugs that lower total peripheral resistance (TPR) by relaxing the resistance vessels: first, their effect on veins, and second, their action on the large arteries. Drugs that can be classified as vasodilators because their first hemodynamic effect is to lower TPR can be subdivided according to

1. Mode of action, whether neural, humoral, or directly on the vascular smooth muscle
2. Venodilating effect. At one end of the spectrum are those that produce marked venodilation and lower cardiac output; at the other end are those with little if any venodilating effect, which lead to marked tachycardia and increased output. Those with balanced veno-arteriolar effect will lower TPR without altering cardiac output significantly.[49]
3. Their effect on large arteries. Safar and his co-workers have pointed out in a series of impressive studies[39-42] that the effects of different vasodilators on the large (brachial) arteries differ in both time course, intensity, and, more importantly, direction from their effect on small arterioles. Thus, hydralazine dilates the resistance vessels but actually decreases the diameter of the large arteries, while converting enzyme inhibitors and calcium entry blockers dilate both the large arteries and the small resistance vessels. Nitroglycerin can dilate the brachial artery without reducing TPR.

Another approach to the choice of a vasodilator has been developed based on the patient's level of plasma renin activity. Converting enzyme inhibitors are more potent in high renin hypertension, at least acutely.[50] More relevant to our discussion is the reported marked effectiveness of calcium entry blockers in low renin conditions[51,52]; they are also particularly effective in older patients. It is not completely settled whether the enhanced effectiveness of calcium entry blockers is related to the prevalence of low renin in patients above age 60 or to the blunting of baroreceptor reflexes, which may interfere with blood pressure response to vasodilators. Nevertheless, the fact remains that treatment with calcium entry blockers might prove effective for more than one reason in older patients. It is important, however, to avoid (1) those that depress heart rate in patients with poor cardiac function or abnormal cardiac conduction, and (2) those that may overstimulate the heart in patients with angina pectoris.

TABLE 80.2 INCIDENCE OF MORBID EVENTS IN PATIENTS AGED 60 AND ABOVE AT RANDOMIZATION*

Blood Pressure Prior to Randomization (mm Hg)	Control Group			Treated Group		
	No. Randomized	Events	%	No. Randomized	Events	%
90–104	21	13	61.9	19	8	42.1
150–114	22	14	63.9	19	3	15.8
Total	43	27	62.8	38	11	28.9

* Veterans Administration Cooperative Study on Morbidity in Hypertension
(Data from Kirkendall WM, Hammond JJ: Hypertension in the elderly. Arch Intern Med 140:1155–1161, 1980)

REFERENCES

1. Tarazi RC, Gifford RW Jr: Systemic arterial pressure. In Sodeman WA Jr, Sodeman TM (eds): Pathophysiology, 6th ed, pp 198–229. Philadelphia, WB Saunders, 1979
2. Ho JK, Lin CY, Galysh FT et al: Aortic compliance: Studies on its relationship to aortic constituents in man. Arch Pathol 94:537–546, 1972
3. Tarazi RC, Magrini F, Dustan HP: The role of aortic distensibility in hypertension. In Milliez P, Safar M (eds): Recent Advances in Hypertension, pp 133–142. Reims-France, Boehringer Ingelheim, 1975
4. Gribbin B, Pickering TG, Sleight P, Peto R: Effect of age and high blood pressure on baroreflex sensitivity in man. Circ Res 29:424–431, 1971
5. Amer SM, Gomoll AW, Perhuch JL Jr et al: Aberrations of cyclic nucleotide metabolism in the hearts and vessels of hypertensive rats. Proc Natl Acad Sci USA 71:4930–4934, 1974
6. Baker SP, Potter LT: Cardiac β-adrenoceptors during normal growth of male and female rats. Br J Pharmacol 68:65–70, 1980
7. Rodeheffer RJ, Gerstenblith G, Becker LC et al: Exercise cardiac output is maintained with advancing age in healthy human subjects: Cardiac dilatation and increased stroke volume compensate for a diminished heart rate. Circulation 69:203–213, 1984
8. Kirkendall WM, Hammond JJ: Hypertension in the elderly. Arch Intern Med 140:1155–1161, 1980
9. Saragoca M, Tarazi RC: Left ventricular hypertrophy in rats with renovascular hypertension. Alterations in cardiac function and adrenergic responses. Hypertension 3(6):II-171–II-176, 1981
10. Tarazi RC: The progression from hypertrophy to heart failure. Hosp Pract 18:101–122, 1983
11. Wolinsky H: Effects of hypertension and its reversal on the thoracic aorta of male and female rats. Circ Res 28:622–637, 1971
12. Ayobe MH, Tarazi RC: Beta-receptors and contractile reserve in left ventricular hypertrophy. Hypertension 5(Suppl I):I-192–I-197, 1983
13. Joint National Committee. The 1984 Report of the Joint National Committee on Detection, Evaluation and Treatment of High Blood Pressure. Arch Intern Med 144:1045–1057, 1984
14. Fishberg AM: Hypertension and Nephritis. Philadelphia, Lea & Febiger, 1939
15. Ayman D: Essential hypertension: The diastolic blood pressure; its variability. Arch Intern Med 48:89–97, 1931
16. Berne RM, Levy MN: Cardiovascular Physiology, pp 94–108. St Louis, CV Mosby, 1981
17. Kannel WB: Role of blood pressure in cardiovascular morbidity and mortality. Prog Cardiovasc Dis 17:5–24, 1974
18. Kannell WB, Wolf PA, McGee DL et al: Systolic blood pressure, arterial rigidity and risk of stroke. JAMA 245:1225–1232, 1981
19. Five year findings of the Hypertension Detection and Follow-up Program: Part I: Reduction in mortality. Part II: Mortality by race, sex and age. Hypertension Detection and Follow-up Program Cooperative Group. JAMA 242:1562–1577, 1979
20. National Heart Foundation of Australia Study: Treatment of mild hypertension in the elderly: Report by the Management Committee. Med J Aust 2:398–402, 1981
21. Dyer AR, Stamler J, Shekelle RB et al: Hypertension in the elderly. Med Clin North Am 61:513–529, 1977
22. Colandrea MA, Friedman GD, Nichaman MZ et al: Systolic hypertension in the elderly: An epidemiologic assessment. Circulation 41:239–245, 1970
23. Gifford RW Jr: Isolated systolic hypertension in the elderly. JAMA 247:781–785, 1982
24. Jackson G, Pierscianowski TA, Mahon W, Condon JR: Inappropriate antihypertensive therapy in the elderly. Lancet 2:1317–1318, 1976
25. Wiggers CJ: Circulatory dynamics. In Physiologic Studies, Modern Medical Monograph. New York, Grune & Stratton, 1952
26. Tarazi RC: The hemodynamics of hypertension. Chapter 2, In Genest J, Kuchel O, Hamet P, Cantin M (eds): Hypertension, 2nd ed, pp 15–42. New York, McGraw-Hill, 1983
27. Adamapoulos PN, Chrysanthalkopoulis SG, Frohlich ED: Systolic hypertension: Non-homogenous disease. Am J Cardiol 36:697–701, 1975
28. Messerli FH, Sundgaard-Riise K, Ventura HO et al: Essential hypertension in the elderly: Haemodynamics, intravascular volume, plasma renin activity, and circulating catecholamine levels. Lancet 2:983–986, 1983
29. Ibrahim MM, Tarazi RC, Dustan HP et al: Hyperkinetic heart in severe hypertension: A separate clinical hemodynamic entity. Am J Cardiol 35:667–674, 1975
30. Tarazi RC, Fouad FM: Circulatory dynamics in progressive autonomic failure. In Bannister R (ed): Autonomic Failure: A Textbook of Clinical Disorders of the Autonomic Nervous System, pp 96–113. Oxford, Oxford University Press, 1983
31. Niarchos AP, Laragh JH: Hypertension in elderly. Mod Conc Cardiovasc Dis 49:43–48, 1980
32. Tarazi RC, Levy MN: Cardiac responses to increased afterload. Hypertension 4(Suppl II):II-8–II-18, 1982
33. Abboud FM, Houston JH: The effects of aging and degenerative vascular diseases on the measurement of arterial rigidity in man. J Clin Invest 40:933–939, 1981
34. Simon AC, Safar ME, Levenson JA et al: An evaluation of large arteries compliance in man. Am J Physiol 237:H550–H554, 1979
35. Randall OS, Esler MD, Bulloch GF et al: Relationship of age and blood pressure to baroreflex sensitivity and arterial compliance in man. Clin Sci Mol Med 51(Suppl 3):357s–360s, 1976
36. Tarazi RC: Hypertension in the elderly: Pathophysiological considerations and therapeutic approaches. Unpublished paper.
37. Freis ED: Hemodynamics of hypertension. Physiol Rev 40:27–54, 1960
38. Alicandri CL, Fariello R, Agabiti-Rosei E et al: Influence of the sympathetic nervous system on aortic compliance. Clin Sci Mol Med 59(Suppl 6):279s–282s, 1980
39. Simon ACh, Safar MA, Levenson GA et al: Systolic hypertension. Hemodynamic mechanism and choice of antihypertensive therapy. Am J Cardiol 44:505–511, 1979
40. Simon ACh, Safar ME, Levenson JA et al: Action of vasodilating drugs on small and large arteries of hypertensive patients. J Cardiovasc Pharmacol 5:626–631, 1983
41. Safar ME, Simon ACh, Levenson JA, Cazor JL: Hemodynamic effects of Diltiazem in hypertension. Circ Res 52(Suppl I):169–173, 1983
42. Simon AC, Levenson JA, Bouthier J, Aarek B, Safar ME: Effects of acute and chronic angiotensin converting enzyme inhibition on large arteries in human hypertension. J Cardiovasc Pharmacol 7(suppl 1):S45–S51, 1985
43. Bristow JD, Honour AJ, Pickering GW et al: Diminished baroreflex sensitivity in high blood pressure. Circulation 39:48–54, 1969
44. Statement on Hypertension in the Elderly. National High Blood Pressure Education Program, rev'd ed, pp 1–7. Bethesda, Maryland, 1980
45. Caird FI, Andrews GR, Kennedy RD: Effect of posture on blood pressure in the elderly. Br Heart J 35:527–530, 1973
46. Taguchi JT, Suwangool P: "Pipe-stem" brachial arteries. A cause of pseudohypertension. JAMA 228:733, 1974
47. Editorial: Hypertension in the elderly. Lancet 1:684–685, 1977
48. Kuramoto K, Matsushita S, Kuwajima I: The pathogenetic role and treatment of elderly hypertension. Jpn Circ J 45:833–843, 1981
49. Tarazi RC, Dustan HP, Bravo EL, Niarchos AP: Vasodilating drugs: Contrasting haemodynamic effects. Clin Sci Mol Med 51:575s–578s, 1976
50. Tarazi RC, Bravo EL, Fouad FM et al: Hemodynamic and volume changes associated with captopril. Hypertension 2:576–585, 1980
51. Buhler FR, Hulthen L, Kiowski W et al: The place of the calcium antagonist verapamil in antihypertensive therapy. J Cardiovasc Pharmacol 4:S350–S357, 1982
52. Fouad FM, Pedrinelli R, Bravo EL et al: Clinical and systemic hemodynamic effects of nitrendipine. Clin Pharmacol Ther 35:768–775, 1984

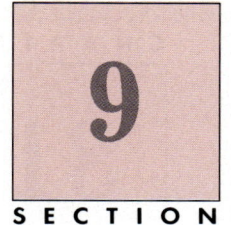

SECTION 9

Section Editor
Elliot Rapaport, MD

VALVULAR HEART DISEASE

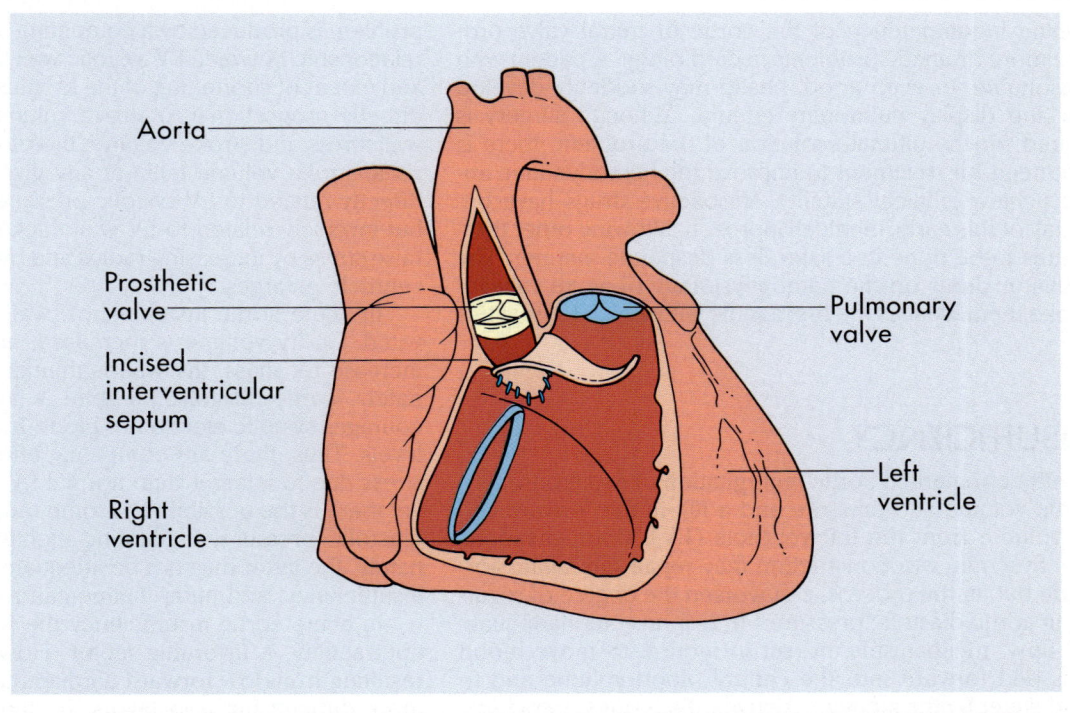

THE USE OF VASODILATOR AGENTS IN ACUTE AND CHRONIC VALVULAR REGURGITATION

Jack Kron • J. David Bristow

PATHOPHYSIOLOGY OF ACUTE VALVULAR REGURGITATION

Acutely developing incompetence of the aortic or mitral valve produces one of the more dramatic problems in cardiology. A patient who has been in reasonable, or even good, health may suddenly develop severe dyspnea and display pulmonary edema. Although surgery is frequently required for the ultimate solution of the problem, there is often immediate need for treatment to improve the hemodynamic abnormalities and achieve clinical stability. Vasoactive drugs have become the mainstay of this early, medical approach, allowing other therapeutic procedures to be done in a safer, less desperate manner. The effects of vasodilator drugs on the pathophysiology of acute valvular regurgitation make them ideal as the first agents with which to treat this disorder.

AORTIC INSUFFICIENCY

The immediate effect of marked aortic regurgitation of acute onset is a decrease in aortic volume and pressure and a fall in the forward (effective) stroke volume from the left ventricle (LV). Compensations promptly follow. Systemic vasoconstriction may repair the falling aortic blood pressure but, in the process, can worsen the degree of regurgitation by raising aortic diastolic pressure.[1] In response to inadequate systemic blood flow, mechanisms are set in motion to move blood from the venous bed forward into the central blood volume and to conserve salt and water by the kidney.[2] Tachycardia is often associated as part of a generalized increase in adrenergic tone.

Although understandable as reactions to the falling aortic blood pressure and peripheral blood flow, these compensatory responses may have adverse consequences. Peripheral vasoconstriction raises ventricular afterload and makes ejection of blood from the LV less complete. The increase in LV preload from the venous constriction and sodium and water conservation result in increased LV end-diastolic volume, given a competent right ventricle. Elevated LV diastolic, left atrial, and pulmonary capillary pressures result, with pulmonary edema as a common expression of the sequence. Premature closure of the mitral valve may occur, perhaps protecting the left atrium and pulmonary circulation somewhat.[3]

It is likely that the pericardium provides some defense against overwhelming LV dilation due to acute aortic insufficiency. In studies of cardiac and pericardial function at varied filling volumes, Holt long ago demonstrated that an increase in LV diastolic pressure produced by volume loading was associated with raised intrapericardial pressure, that is, the distending force producing LV dilation (LV cavity pressure minus pericardial pressure) was less than might have been predicted from LV diastolic pressure alone.[4] Thus, the pericardium provided some restraint to LV dilation, as shown by the positive pressure in the pericardial space. Although this mechanism may protect the structural integrity of the LV somewhat, diastolic ventricular pressure is high nonetheless.

The increase in preload allows the ventricle to take advantage of the Frank-Starling mechanism and increase its ejection volume, helping to correct the decreased forward stroke volume. From the standpoint of the mechanics of left ventricular contraction, however, a problem is produced by a competing mechanism.[5,6] There is an inverse relationship between LV systolic wall stress (afterload) and the velocity and extent of shortening of the LV muscle fibers, with shortening being directly proportional to stroke volume. The relationship between LV wall stress and stroke volume, therefore, is inverse (*i.e.*, as wall stress rises, stroke volume falls) at any given state of contractility. Stress is directly related to LV systolic pressure and the radius of the ventricle, but inversely related to LV wall thickness. Thus, acute LV dilation will raise stress by increasing radius and by decreasing wall thickness as the ventricle enlarges.

In acute aortic insufficiency, wall stress can be considerably elevated. Cavity volume is increased, and, given no opportunity yet to increase LV mass, the wall is thinner due to diastolic dilation. Fortunately, aortic diastolic pressure is sometimes subnormal, which encourages systolic ejection of blood from the LV at relatively low stress levels. Thus, there are competing effects, that is, potentially high wall stress due to a larger than normal LV with a thinner than normal wall, yet there is the possibility of some reduction in stress due to low aortic diastolic pressure, facilitating ejection from the ventricle. Unfortunately, the latter may not be adequate in the most acute form of aortic insufficiency, and pump failure can result.

In acute aortic insufficiency the LV usually starts out with normal contractility, a favorable factor. However, systemic vasoconstriction resulting from low forward cardiac output not only makes LV ejection more difficult but also favors the fundamental physiologic fault—regurgitation through the aortic valve. Thus, congestive failure, with low forward cardiac output and high LV filling pressure, can be evident despite a normal ventricle.[6] An analogous experimental preparation has shown that this can occur.[7]

If the patient survives these initial problems, additional changes occur with time. The LV mass generally increases to improve the ratio of LV radius to wall thickness, which would decrease wall stress.[6,8] Furthermore, the diastolic properties of the LV may change, allowing accommodation of a large end-diastolic volume without raised end-diastolic pressure. Given a sufficient period of time, some patients with acute aortic insufficiency can compensate sufficiently to mimic the chronic, slowly developing syndrome. This is not generally believed to be common, however.

On theoretical grounds, vasodilator therapy in aortic insufficiency should be beneficial. Decreasing the resistance to LV outflow (outflow impedance) should allow the ventricle to empty more completely, raising the total and the effective LV stroke volume. There should be less regurgitation per beat if aortic diastolic pressure is diminished. This net increase in cardiac output should attenuate those stimuli that have produced the high LV end-diastolic volume. Thus, the system could function at a lower pulmonary capillary wedge pressure and higher cardiac output. Benefits to the LV should accrue, as it operates at a smaller volume to produce a higher systemic, nonregurgitant flow. Agents with venodilating properties would also contribute to a lessening of pulmonary congestion.

MITRAL REGURGITATION

Although the general pathophysiologic principles for aortic insufficiency, above, hold for mitral regurgitation, this lesion presents additional problems. In aortic insufficiency, the filling pressures on the left side of the heart rise because LV diastolic volume is higher than normal. This is also true in mitral regurgitation, but in addition there is a direct increase in left atrial pressure produced by the retrograde pumping of blood during systole, that is, mean left atrial pressure is increased both because of an increase in LV diastolic volume *and* by the regurgitant volume entering the left atrium.[9] Furthermore, in many of the situations in which acute mitral regurgitation occurs, the LV is not normal at the onset of the valvular problem, which further compounds the hemodynamic problem. There is evidence that as mitral regurgitation leads to an increase in LV size, it further disrupts mitral valve function, and more mitral regurgitation is produced.[10] Determinants of the amount of mitral regurgitant flow during systole include the difference in pressure between the LV and the left atrium (serving as the driving force for reflux) and the size of the mitral orifice. These are the same factors, in a reverse direction, that are well recognized in determining diastolic forward blood flow in mitral stenosis. As LV volume increases, the mitral regurgitant orifice area increases, facilitating backward flow. Thus, high systemic vascular resistance will decrease LV forward ejection, will increase LV diastolic volume, and may directly worsen regurgitant flow.[10]

When the mitral valve becomes incompetent, left atrial pressure increases and forward output decreases. As in aortic insufficiency, compensatory mechanisms raise LV diastolic volume. Regurgitant blood flow into the left atrium is thus favored, as opposed to normal forward flow, by the very low resistance or impedance offered by the mitral valve and left atrium. Thus, regurgitation starts during the period that normally would be isovolumic LV systole. Early, easy ejection into the left atrium allows a lower LV wall stress than would be the case if a ventricle of equivalent size faced only aortic pressure during ejection. The LV ejection fraction is higher than would be expected for a given state of contractile depression.[11]

The pathologic process causing mitral regurgitation has an important influence on these relationships.[12] LV function may be normal in patients who rupture mitral chordae tendineae. However, mitral regurgitation due to a ruptured head of a papillary muscle is quite a different matter. These patients generally have substantial LV damage due to myocardial infarction. Severe LV dysfunction and acute mitral regurgitation can produce the lethal combination of pulmonary edema and cardiogenic shock.

Vasodilator therapy should help patients with acute mitral regurgitation. Arteriolar vasodilation should favor forward, nonregurgitant blood flow. This should reduce those stimuli that have increased the central blood volume and LV preload. Venous dilation would directly diminish venous return and LV filling, improving pulmonary congestion. Both effects should reduce LV volume and directly reduce the amount of mitral regurgitation.[10,13]

There are significant limitations to vasodilator therapy in some of these acutely ill patients. Systemic vascular resistance is relatively high in these disorders because of the need to maintain the blood pressure. Despite this, some patients with acute aortic or mitral valve regurgitation may present with low systemic pressure. In that circumstance, vasodilators must be used with great caution, since an adverse outcome with these agents can be seen in patients with low blood pressure. In desperation, they can be tried, cautiously, but other avenues may be more hopeful, such as positive inotropic drugs or prompt surgical treatment.

For the patients with hypotension and acute mitral regurgitation, consideration can be given to use of the aortic balloon pump. This not only decreases the resistance to LV outflow but also adds mechanical energy to the vascular system and will often stabilize the patient. This is a temporizing therapy, however, and a more definitive procedure must follow. The aortic balloon pump should *not* be employed in acute aortic insufficiency because of the theoretical probability of worsening regurgitant flow.

CLINICAL USE OF VASODILATORS

A number of investigators have demonstrated that afterload-reducing agents can have a salutary effect in acute or chronic severe mitral[14-17] and aortic regurgitation.[18-20] Most series have combined chronically severely ill patients with acutely ill patients, but there are a few studies that look at acute valvular regurgitation in isolation.[21]

EXPERIENCE IN SEVERE MITRAL REGURGITATION

Acute mitral regurgitation can result from a variety of causes, as listed in Table 81.1. Many of these patients will eventually require urgent surgery, but some, especially in the setting of acute myocardial infarction, will be poor surgical candidates and would benefit from medical measures.

Chatterjee and co-workers[15] studied a group of eight patients with mitral regurgitation due to dysfunction of the subvalvular apparatus, two of whom developed mitral regurgitation immediately following acute myocardial infarction. All had evidence of cardiomegaly and pulmonary venous congestion. Three of the patients had frank pulmonary edema. Pulmonary capillary wedge pressure was markedly elevated and large v waves were uniformly present. The severity of illness in these patients was further manifested by a marked reduction of forward flow and elevation of systemic vascular resistance. The infusion of sodium nitroprusside resulted in rapid improvement in hemody-

TABLE 81.1 COMMON CAUSES OF ACUTE VALVULAR REGURGITATION*

Mitral Regurgitation	Aortic Regurgitation
Papillary muscle dysfunction or rupture due to coronary artery disease	Endocarditis
Ruptured chordae tendineae due to endocarditis, Marfan's syndrome, mitral valve prolapse, rheumatic fever, trauma, or idiopathic	Dissecting aneurysm
	Marfan's syndrome
	Cusp prolapse
	Traumatic leaflet rupture
Leaflet or valvular destruction due to endocarditis	Rupture of a fenestrated leaflet
Degeneration or destruction of the mitral annulus	Rheumatic
Annular dilatation due to congestive heart failure	Following aortic valve replacement
Rheumatic damage to leaflets or fusion of commissures	
Following mitral valve repair or replacement	

* This list does not include all causes of valvular regurgitation, particularly acute exacerbations of previously stable chronic regurgitation.

namics in all patients, with LV filling pressure decreasing toward normal and with a 50% increase in cardiac output. Pulmonary capillary v waves decreased from 50 to 19 mm Hg, and systemic vascular resistance normalized. These beneficial hemodynamic effects corresponded with similar improvement in clinical status. The hemodynamic benefit in these patients was attributed primarily to reduced impedance to LV outflow (*i.e.*, resulting in reduced afterload), although the venous pooling effects of nitroprusside likely played an important role in the relief of pulmonary congestion.

Nitroprusside infusion results in similar hemodynamic improvement with mitral regurgitation that is primarily of valvular origin. A reduction in systemic vascular resistance is associated with a considerable fall in pulmonary wedge pressure and a higher (forward) cardiac output. In one report there was no increase in ejection fraction or heart rate, which the authors believed suggested that the improvement in cardiac function was not due to a reflex increase in adrenergic stimulation but mostly due to afterload reduction.[14]

Prazosin is a dual-acting vasodilator that has hemodynamic effects generally similar to nitroprusside[22,23] and that has been studied in the clinical setting of chronic severe mitral regurgitation.[17] Although none of the reported patients had acute mitral regurgitation, a degree of hemodynamic improvement similar to that of sodium nitroprusside has been demonstrated.

Unlike nitroprusside, which has arterial and venous dilating effects, hydralazine is a pure arterial dilator. Greenberg and co-workers[16] studied the effects of hydralazine in 10 patients with severe mitral regurgitation due to a variety of causes. Following 0.3 mg/kg hydralazine IV (up to 20 mg), forward stroke volume increased by 50% while calculated regurgitant stroke volume fell 33%. Pulmonary capillary wedge pressure and systemic vascular resistance fell markedly, with a decrease in v waves from 61 to 36 mm Hg. LV end-diastolic volume or pressure did not change, and this was attributed to the pure afterload-reducing effects of hydralazine.

The mechanism for hemodynamic improvement with vasodilators in patients with severe mitral regurgitation is primarily due to the afterload-reducing properties of these agents. There is one study, however, suggesting that an important effect of nitroprusside is the reduction of size of the mitral regurgitant orifice,[13] directly diminishing mitral reflux. In this study, cardiac index and stroke volume index did not change significantly, whereas left atrial pressure and LV filling pressure dropped significantly. It was therefore reported that the reduction of the regurgitation was due primarily to the venodilator effect of nitroprusside on the capacitance bed and subsequent reduction of ventricular volume.

It is likely that the effects of sodium nitroprusside are due to both reduction of preload as well as impedance to LV ejection. However, agents that are predominantly arterial dilators, such as hydralazine or nifedipine, appear to result in a similar degree of clinical improvement, exclusively by a reduction in impedance to ejection. There is no evidence that venous pooling accounts for any of the improvements seen with pure arterial dilators.

An illustrative example of the marked changes resulting from the administration of vasodilators is that of the 56-year-old man shown in Figure 81.1.

USE OF THE INTRA-AORTIC BALLOON PUMP IN MITRAL REGURGITATION

A form of afterload reduction that is infrequently used for acute mitral regurgitation is the intra-aortic balloon pump. Gold and co-workers[21] reported on the hemodynamic response to intra-aortic balloon pump placement in five patients in clinical cardiogenic shock associated with severe mitral regurgitation in the setting of acute myocardial infarction.

All patients initially had pulmonary edema, low cardiac output, and hypotension. Following placement of the intra-aortic balloon pump, these patients had an initial modest hemodynamic improvement. Following initial stabilization, however, the condition of the patients maintained on the intra-aortic balloon pump for longer than 24 hours subsequently deteriorated, and only one patient survived. Despite the poor outcome of the patients in this series, the use of the pump permitted diagnostic LV and coronary angiography to be performed safely in these critically ill patients. The augmentation of coronary blood flow and reduced impedance to LV ejection produced by the intra-aortic balloon pump may be of some use in selected patients in this setting.

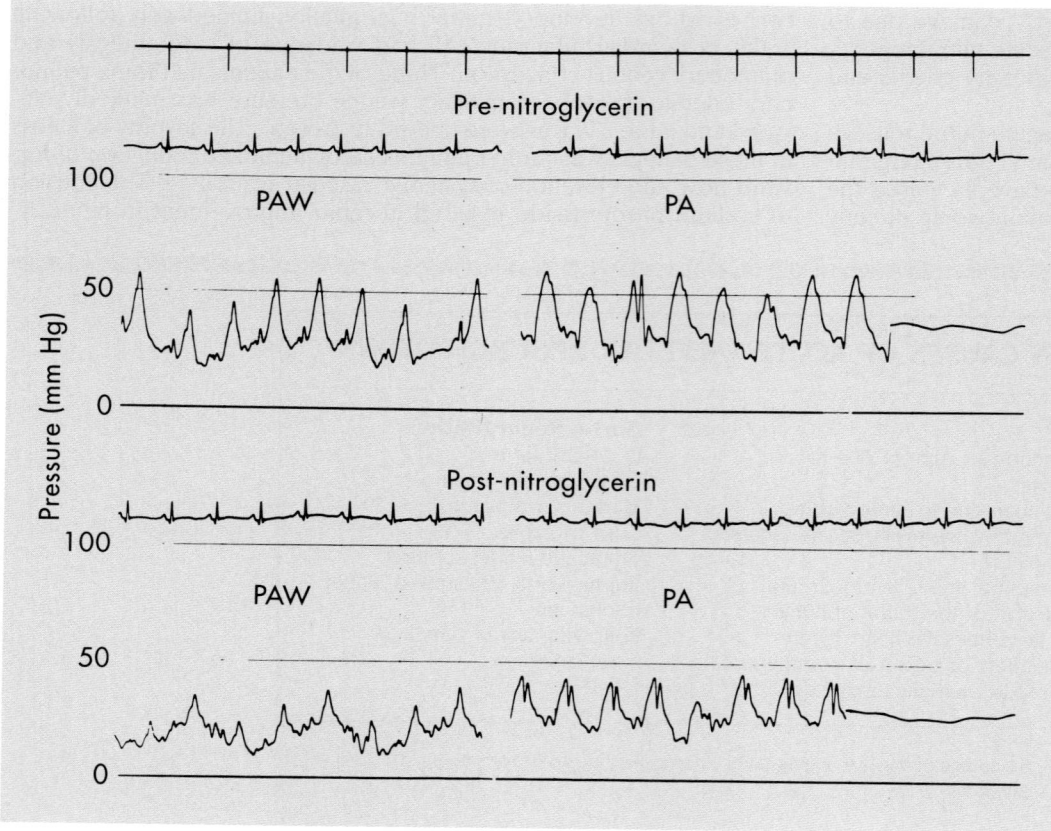

FIGURE 81.1 Example of a 56-year-old man who presented 1 year following inferior myocardial infarction with severe mitral regurgitation and congestive heart failure. On catheterization, mean pulmonary artery wedge pressure was 30 mm Hg with approximately 50-mm v waves. Following administration of 40 µg/min intravenous nitroglycerin, mean pulmonary artery wedge pressure fell to 20 mm Hg with a reduction in v waves to approximately 30 mm. Much of this benefit was probably due to venodilation and subsequent preload reduction. It should be remembered, however, as discussed in the text, that preload is an important determinant of afterload, according to the law of Laplace. Therefore, dual mechanisms may account for the hemodynamic improvement seen in this man.

USE OF AFTERLOAD REDUCTION IN ACUTE AORTIC REGURGITATION

Acute aortic regurgitation is a heterogeneous disorder, which, regardless of cause, represents an emergency.[3] The causes are manifold (see Table 81.1),[24-32] and therapy, although in most cases surgical, must also address the underlying disease process. For example, in the case of infective endocarditis, surgery may be delayed for several days while appropriate antibiotics are administered, if the patient's condition can be stabilized. In other cases, underlying medical problems may preclude immediate surgery. In such cases, a medical alternative, such as afterload reduction, may be an attractive alternative or may improve the patient's status for early operation.

The pathophysiology and hemodynamic consequences of acute aortic insufficiency have been reviewed earlier in this chapter. As noted, the major hemodynamic abnormality is an acute volume overload that results in pulmonary vascular congestion and, in some cases, low forward cardiac output and hemodynamic collapse. In animal models,[11] although myocardial fiber tension rises acutely, impedance to ejection actually falls, thus increasing stroke volume and ejection fraction somewhat. In the chronic situation, the heart will adapt by hypertrophy, thus decreasing wall stress.

Despite the decreased impedance to ejection seen acutely, there is still a relative afterload mismatch in acute aortic regurgitation,[6] which in time will result in impaired hemodynamic performance with reduction in forward stroke volume and pulmonary vascular congestion. The importance of afterload stress has been studied in aortic regurgitation. Infusion of vasoconstrictor agents was shown to increase the degree of aortic regurgitation and to worsen LV pump function.[33,34] Similarly, amyl nitrate administration has been shown to decrease the amount of regurgitant flow and hence the intensity of the murmur in patients with aortic regurgitation.[35]

Preliminary experience with sodium nitroprusside,[36] demonstrating decreased aortic compliance and reduced LV end-diastolic volume, formed a basis for subsequent trials of afterload-reducing therapy in severe aortic regurgitation. Miller and associates[18] infused sodium nitroprusside into 12 patients with documented severe aortic regurgitation. LV end-diastolic pressure decreased in all patients (23 to 11 mm Hg), with a concomitant reduction in LV end-diastolic volume. Ejection fraction increased in seven of eight patients; however, forward stroke volume only increased modestly. Interestingly, systemic vascular resistance fell markedly (1782 to 1148 dynes·sec·cm^{-5}) and regurgitant fraction decreased significantly as well. Others have demonstrated similar findings in isolated chronic severe aortic regurgitation.[37]

Hydralazine, a potent arterial dilator,[38] has been studied in isolated cases[39] that have shown sustained improvement in rest and exercise hemodynamics and a reduction of LV end-diastolic volume index. These isolated reports suggest that certain patients with significant regurgitation might be maintained long-term on afterload-reducing therapy. In subsequent studies,[40,41] Greenberg and associates confirmed the salutary effects on rest and exercise hemodynamics in severe aortic insufficiency. For the group as a whole, exercise LV filling pressure fell from 21 to 12 mm Hg following hydralazine and cardiac index increased by 31%. The major beneficial effect of hydralazine was believed to be a reduction in the amount of aortic regurgitation, due to the lowering of arterial impedance by hydralazine. In some patients it was believed that an improvement in systolic pump function performance might be playing a role as well.

Similar beneficial effects with prazosin[42] and the calcium channel blocker nifedipine[19] have been shown. In one report, sublingual administration of 20 mg nifedipine in 12 patients with isolated severe aortic insufficiency did not change LV end-diastolic pressure or ejection fraction, which favored reduction of impedance to LV ejection rather than venous pooling or altered inotropic state as the predominant mechanism.

Although most of the reported experience with vasodilators is in the setting of chronic severe aortic regurgitation rather than in the acute setting, this form of medical therapy is extremely useful in patients who are being stabilized prior to surgery. In most cases a titratable intravenous agent such as sodium nitroprusside is most appropriate; however, when surgery must be delayed for several days or weeks, an oral agent such as hydralazine or nifedipine is more appropriate.

RIGHT-SIDED VALVULAR REGURGITATION

Experience with vasodilators is limited in acute tricuspid or pulmonic regurgitation. Most often, tricuspid insufficiency is due to left-sided heart failure, producing pulmonary hypertension and right ventricular failure. Rarely, primary tricuspid valve rupture is seen with endocarditis or trauma. Pulmonic regurgitation secondary to severe pulmonary hypertension is not usually of great volume and is not, of itself, a serious problem. One special form of pulmonic valve incompetence can occur after surgical correction of tetralogy of Fallot.

Therapy for tricuspid or pulmonic regurgitation is generally directed toward the overall congestive state and left-sided heart dysfunction. Specific pulmonary vasodilators have not been consistently helpful. Thus, digitalis, diuretics, and vasodilator treatment for left-sided heart problems are more important than attempts at specific pulmonary vasodilation. Such treatment could include venodilating agents, which could decrease right-sided heart volume and decrease tricuspid regurgitation.

CHARACTERISTICS AND USE OF VASODILATOR DRUGS

Vasodilator drugs can be divided into classes that act predominantly on the venous capacitance vessels to reduce preload (such as nitroglycerin); agents that are predominant arterial dilators (afterload reducers, such as hydralazine); and agents that dilate both venous capacitance vessels and arteries (dual-acting agents such as nitroprusside and captopril) (Table 81.2).[43]

NITROPRUSSIDE

Sodium nitroprusside[44] is an iron coordination compound that is prepared by the combination of the sodium salt of ferricyanide with nitric acid. It is an unstable compound that is a powerful dilator of vascular smooth muscle, with prominent effects on both arterial and venous vessels. Its onset of action is rapid, and its duration of action is minutes; therefore, it must be administered as a continuous infusion. It is rapidly converted to cyanide and is converted in the liver to thiocyanate. Thiocyanate is excreted by the kidney and has a half-life of approximately 1 week with normal renal function. Since it is a very potent agent, it must be administered to patients with acute valvular regurgitation in an intensive care unit with arterial and pulmonary artery catheters in place.

Sodium nitroprusside is supplied in 50-mg/5-ml vials in the dihydrate form. It should be dissolved in 250 to 1000 ml of 5% dextrose in water and, because it is photosensitive, should be protected from light. Dosing is initiated at 0.25 µg/kg/min, with maximum dose recommendation of 10 µg/kg/min. The average dose is approximately 3 µg/kg/min, with adjustments to maintain blood pressure and the desired pulmonary artery wedge pressure within acceptable limits.

Such dosage adjustments can be accomplished quickly with a Swan-Ganz cathter in place, with increments of 5 µg/min every 2 to 3 minutes until cardiac output increases and pulmonary artery wedge pressure falls or until the patient becomes mildly hypotensive. Most patients will tolerate a pulmonary artery wedge pressure in the 12- to 20-mm Hg range very well. Systolic blood pressure should be maintained above 90 mm Hg, although some patients (particularly in the setting of sepsis) will perfuse their periphery and maintain urine output with a somewhat lower blood pressure. If the blood pressure is marginal, it is best to initiate therapy with an inotropic agent such as dobutamine prior to the cautious institution of sodium nitroprusside.

Thiocyanate toxicity begins to appear at levels of 5 to 10 mg/dl, with fatalities reported at levels greater than 20 mg/dl. Symptoms include nausea, fatigue, mental status changes, headache, rash, muscle twitching, seizures, and, rarely, respiratory arrest. In patients who are critically ill, it can be difficult to differentiate early symptoms of thiocyanate toxicity from those of the underlying disease. Toxicity may be predisposed by renal failure since thiocyanate is cleared by the kidney. Hydroxycobalamin may be effective in the treatment of thiocyanate toxicity.[45] If toxicity is strongly suspected, the patient should be switched to other drugs, such as a combination of nitrates and hydralazine.

HYDRALAZINE

Hydralazine is a phthalazine derivative that is a direct arteriolar dilator through an unknown mechanism. It has minimal effects on the venous capacitance vessels. It improves cardiac output by afterload reduction and has no known inotropic properties. It has been established as one of the most effective agents in the vasodilator therapy of congestive heart failure[22] and, as stated earlier, has also been useful in mitral[16] and aortic regurgitation.[20,40,41]

In the past, a starting dose of 10 mg four times daily was recommended, with gradual increase to 50 mg four times daily. However, we have found that larger doses are often necessary for the vasodilator therapy of congestive heart failure or valvular regurgitation. Therefore, we generally give an initial oral dose of 50 to 75 mg (25 mg if hypotensive or elderly). Maximal hemodynamic effects to a given dose are seen at 2 to 3 hours. If the cardiac index does not increase substantially or pulmonary wedge pressure does not fall to the 14- to 18-mm Hg range, the dose is increased in 25-mg increments until a desired endpoint is reached. If mean arterial blood pressure falls by more than 15 mm Hg or diastolic blood pressure falls below 50 mm Hg, we generally discontinue the dose, depending of course on the original level before the drug was given. Similarly, if heart rate increases by more than 15 beats per minute, we have not found further increases in dosage to be beneficial. Hydralazine can also be administered intravenously. A reasonable starting dose for valvular regurgitation is 0.3 mg/kg or 20 mg intravenously.

Hydralazine is completely orally absorbed and is metabolized in the liver where it is acetylated by N-acetyltransferase. Patients who are slow acetylators may have an augmented response to hydralazine and may be more likely to develop a lupuslike syndrome with positive antinuclear antibody test at doses greater than 200 mg daily. Side effects of hydralazine include nausea, emesis, flushing, headache, and nasal congestion. Hydralazine has also been known to precipitate myocardial ischemia and should be used cautiously in patients with severe coronary artery disease. Other rare adverse reactions include drug fever, peripheral neuropathy, rash, and blood dyscrasias.

PRAZOSIN

Prazosin is a piperazine derivative that exerts its hemodynamic effects by blocking vascular α-adrenergic receptors.[22,46] It has a dual effect on precapillary resistance and postcapillary venous capacitance vessels and therefore is both a preload and afterload reducer. There is minimal effect on the renal vasculature. Prazosin is almost completely absorbed following oral administration, and it is primarily metabolized in the liver. Its hemodynamic effects last 6 hours.

TABLE 81.2 VASODILATORS

	Site of Action	Dose and Duration	Side Effects and Precautions
IV Drugs			
Sodium nitroprusside	Arterial and venous smooth muscle (*i.e.*, afterload and preload)	0.25–10 μg/kg/min; average dose is 3 μg/kg min. Onset is immediate; ceases with cessation of drug	Use cautiously with hypotension; can alter mental status; may worsen myocardial ischemia
Phentolamine	α-Blocker with major effect on arterial smooth muscle	Start at 0.1 mg/min; increase by 0.1 mg/min every 10 minutes; most respond to 1–2 mg/min dose	May cause tachycardia or precipitate angina
Afterload Agents			
Hydralazine	Arterial smooth muscle	50–200 mg PO; duration, 6–12 hr; 0.3 mg/kg IV	Headache; gastrointestinal upset; orthostasis; lupuslike syndrome; nasal congestion
Nifedipine	Calcium blocker with major effect on arterial smooth muscle	10–40 mg q6–8h	May cause edema; hypotension
Preload-Reducing Agents			
Nitroglycerin	Major effect in venous capacitance with some arterial dilation	10–200 μg/min IV; ointment, 12.5–40 mg (1–3 inches) q3–4h; transdermal, 5–20 mg q24h	Hypotension; headache; postural symptoms
Isosorbide dinitrate		Sublingual, 2.5–15 mg q2–4h; oral, 10–40 mg q4–6h; chewable, 5–10 mg q2–3h	
Combined Agents			
Prazosin	α₁-Blocker with effects on arterial and venous capacitance	2–14 mg (lasts 6 hr)	Postural hypotension; "first-dose" effect; headache; alopecia; tachyphylaxis
Captopril	Angiotensin-converting enzyme inhibitor	Initially 6.25–25 mg; chronic, 25–100 mg q8h	Hypotension; neutropenia; proteinuria; use cautiously in chronic renal failure
Enalapril	Angiotensin-converting enzyme inhibitor	Initially 2.5–5 mg; chronic, 5–20 mg q12h	Similar to captopril

Dosing is generally recommended to start at 1 mg orally because of a "first-dose" phenomenon that has been reported in the therapy for hypertension, resulting in profound hypotension. This has not been reported in the setting of congestive heart failure. Recommended dosing in the setting of congestive heart failure has been 2 to 5 mg every 6 to 8 hours, although higher dosage may be required to overcome the tachyphylaxis commonly seen with chronic prazosin administration.[47]

Side effects, other than the first-dosing phenomenon seen with hypertension, are rare and generally do not require drug cessation. They include headaches, nausea, fluid retention, dry mouth, rash, drowsiness, urinary incontinence, and depression.

We do not recommend prazosin as a first-line drug for acute valvular regurgitation but rather a choice to consider if the patient is unable to tolerate hydralazine or nitroprusside.

NIFEDIPINE

Nifedipine[48] is a calcium antagonist that is predominantly a peripheral vasodilator with little effect on the cardiac pacemaker conduction system. It has been used for therapy for angina pectoris, hypertension, hypertrophic cardiomyopathy, Raynaud's phenomenon, pulmonary edema, and aortic insufficiency.[19] It is well absorbed orally and can be administered sublingually or orally. Its onset of action is 2 to 3 minutes sublingually and 15 to 30 minutes orally. Duration of action is 6 to 8 hours. Dosage ranges from 10 to 40 mg three to four times daily. For rapid action in the acutely ill patient we would favor sublingual administration, starting with 10 mg, with additional 10-mg increments every 30 minutes to 1 hour. The capsule can be perforated for sublingual administration in patients who are severely ill or who cannot take oral medications.

CAPTOPRIL

Captopril is an angiotensin-converting enzyme inhibitor that has been very effective in the acute and chronic management of refractory congestive heart failure.[49,50] Although its precise mechanism of action is unclear, it has been shown to have potent effects on peripheral resistance and venous tone. Therefore, it may be considered useful in situations in which a patient has had a beneficial hemodynamic response to sodium nitroprusside and requires longer-term therapy than possible by the intravenous route. In general, the acute hemodynamic response to captopril administration predicts long-term efficacy. This has been an area of controversy, however, and some patients who respond initially do not demonstrate prolonged improvement with captopril.[51] Similarly, a small percentage of patients who show little or no initial improvement with captopril do demonstrate long-term beneficial effects. There is little experience with this agent for acute valvular regurgitation. However, since it is a potent agent, with similar hemodynamic effects to those of prazosin or sodium nitroprusside, it should be considered as a possible adjunct to therapy in patients who are not immediate surgical candidates and in whom a replacement for intravenous nitroprusside must be found.

Captopril is well absorbed orally (75%). Hemodynamic effects correspond to peak levels, which are achieved in 1 to 1½ hours. Since hypotension is seen in 50% of patients following the initial dose, low initial doses are recommended to minimize symptomatic hypotension. We recommend initiating doses with 6.25 mg every 6 to 8 hours and gradually increasing to 25 mg every 6 to 8 hours. The use of hemodynamic monitoring will facilitate management of the more severely ill patient, with endpoints similar to those that we recommended with hydralazine. Most patients will not have further improvement beyond the 25-mg dose, although the occasional patient will require higher doses for clinical response. Captopril is excreted in the urine, and the dosage should be reduced in the setting of renal insufficiency.

The most common adverse effect seen with captopril is hypotension. In most cases, this will not necessitate discontinuance of the drug, but a dose reduction instead. Other adverse effects include rash (7%), which is often transient, neutropenia (0.3%), gastrointestinal disturbances (1.6%), proteinuria (1.2%), and taste alteration (3%). The incidence of neutropenia may be increased in chronic renal failure, and captopril should be used cautiously in this setting, in autoimmune disease, or with immunosuppressive therapy. Caution should also be exercised in the use of captopril in patients suspected of having intrinsic renal disease or renal arterial stenosis, since renal dysfunction may be produced or worsened.

Enalapril as an alternative is described in Chapter 18, with more information about converting enzyme inhibitors in general.

NITROGLYCERIN

Nitroglycerin predominantly acts on venous capacitance vessels and is available in oral, sublingual, topical, and intravenous forms. It also has a prominent effect on the epicardial coronary vessels. It is metabolized in the liver, and the duration of its effect depends on the form utilized, with oral forms lasting 4 to 6 hours and topical preparations up to 24 hours. Intravenous nitroglycerin is a relatively new preparation,[52] which we recommend as the first-line nitroglycerin preparation in patients who are severely compromised by pulmonary vascular congestion. Its duration of action is a few minutes, with some effects lasting up to 30 minutes.

As is the case with sodium nitroprusside, it should be administered with a Swan-Ganz catheter in place to gauge the response to therapy and to guide dosage. We recommend starting at 10 μg/min and increasing the dose in 5- to 10-μg/min increments every 5 minutes until a therapeutic endpoint is achieved. There is little benefit gained by increasing the dose beyond 200 μg/min, although doses up to 500 μg/min have been used.

Nitrates can be given orally as isosorbide dinitrate in doses of 10 to 40 mg every 6 hours; sublingually, 5 to 15 mg every 2 to 3 hours; or as a topical paste, 12.5 to 40 mg every 3 to 4 hours. In switching from nitroprusside to oral therapy, a combination of a long-acting nitrate and an afterload-reducing agent, such as hydralazine, can be very effective in selected patients.[22] Side effects are few, with hypotension and headache the most common. Methemoglobinemia is a rare complication of nitrate therapy and is characterized by cyanosis, dyspnea, headache, tachycardia, and mental status changes at very high methemoglobin levels.

PHENTOLAMINE

Phentolamine[22] is an α-adrenergic blocking agent that has prominent effects on vascular smooth muscle. It predominantly reduces afterload but also has some milder effects on the venous capacitance vessels. It is generally given intravenously, with an onset of action within 5 minutes.

It is very short acting, and hemodynamic effects are quickly reversible with cessation of the drug. The recommended starting dose is 0.1 mg/min with an increase in dosage by 0.1-mg/min increments every 10 minutes. Hemodynamic status must be monitored carefully, with attention to pulmonary artery wedge pressure, blood pressure, cardiac output, and systemic vascular resistance. Most patients respond to 1 to 2 mg/min phentolamine infusions. The predominant side effect is hypotension, and in some cases angina may be precipitated. In general, phentolamine carries little advantage over sodium nitroprusside, but it may be a useful alternative if thiocyanate toxicity is suspected. It is an expensive agent for sustained use (hours).

DOBUTAMINE AND DOPAMINE

Dopamine and dobutamine are sympathetic amines that act as β-adrenergic stimulators, with dopamine having prominent α-stimulating effects as well, particularly in larger doses.[53] Dopamine also causes mesenteric and renal vasodilatation via stimulation of dopaminergic receptors. While these agents have some β_2-peripheral vasodilatory effects, their major indication is for inotropic support. They are included in this discussion because they are often used in conjunction with vasodilators in the acutely ill, hemodynamically unstable patient. Both agents can exert similar hemodynamic effects; however, there are some notable differences.

Dopamine is a potent vasopressor whereas dobutamine has no α effect. Dopamine might be indicated in patients who are more severely hypotensive. Dobutamine tends to be less arrhythmogenic than dopamine. Additionally, dopamine has been reported to raise pulmonary artery wedge pressure in some patients, an effect not seen with dobutamine. Since increased systemic vascular resistance will increase the degree of valvular regurgitation, we generally prefer dobutamine over dopamine in the setting of acute valvular regurgitation. The usual dosage range for the two agents is similar, starting at approximately 2 $\mu g/kg/min$ with gradual titration of dose upward in 1- to 2-$\mu g/kg/min$ increments up to 15 $\mu g/kg/min$. At the higher end of the dose range dopamine has prominent vasopressor effects, similar to norepinephrine, whereas with dobutamine, tachycardia and lowering of peripheral resistance are seen, actions similar to those of isoproterenol. A reduction in myocardial oxygen consumption that may be produced by a vasodilator agent may be counteracted by increased energy demands of an inotrope.[54]

Both dobutamine and dopamine are metabolized within minutes of intravenous administration and therefore must be administered as a continuous intravenous infusion. We would reserve the use of these drugs for the patient with acute valvular regurgitation whose initial systolic blood pressure is less than 100 mm Hg and whose cardiac index is lower than 2.2 liters/min/m². Occasionally, in such a patient, starting a dobutamine infusion will permit the administration of nitroprusside, which will in turn decrease the amount of regurgitation and thus increase forward stroke volume. It should be emphasized, however, that the conditions of such patients are extremely unstable and surgery may be required quickly.

OTHER AGENTS

It is beyond the scope of this chapter to discuss in detail other agents that occasionally might be useful in the patient with acute valvular regurgitation. The loop diuretics (i.e., furosemide, ethacrynic acid, and bumetidine) are often useful in these patients and are a mainstay of therapy in patients with volume overload. They decrease preload indirectly by reducing blood volume and also by a venous pooling effect. Digitalis has little role in such acutely ill patients but can be useful in their subacute or chronic management.

Other sympathetic amines, such as isoproterenol, may be useful in certain clinical situations in which the patient does not respond to dopamine or dobutamine. Agents that are effective in the management of hypertension, such as an α-methyldopa or clonidine, will lower systemic vascular resistance and occasionally will be useful adjuncts. Nevertheless, the mainstay for acute valvular regurgitation is intravenous sodium nitroprusside, which is easily titratable and often is extremely effective.

APPROACH TO THE PATIENT WITH ACUTE VALVULAR REGURGITATION

The patient who presents with acute left-sided valvular regurgitation represents a medical emergency that in most cases eventually requires the resources of a tertiary medical center. Once recognized, the two highest priorities are medical stabilization and determination of the cause. In the setting of myocardial infarction, papillary muscle dysfunction and rupture are likely possibilities. Placement of a Swan-Ganz catheter will help confirm the diagnosis and guide subsequent management. During placement of the catheter, it is helpful to obtain right atrial, right ventricular, and pulmonary artery saturations to rule out the presence of an associated ventricular septal defect, which can at times be difficult to distinguish from papillary muscle rupture or dysfunction.

In the absence of an acute myocardial infarction, the most likely cause of acute left-sided valvular regurgitation is bacterial endocarditis. Therefore, it is mandatory to search for stigmata of endocarditis and to obtain blood cultures as part of the initial workup. A two-dimensional echocardiogram with Doppler flow study is extremely useful diagnostically. The presence of a vegetation will confirm the etiologic diagnosis as well as correctly identify the valve (or valves) involved. Doppler study will help confirm the clinical impression. Additionally, a good quality two-dimensional echocardiographic study will evaluate the status of LV function, thus facilitating further decision-making. If the patient is hemodynamically stable, close observation, with cautious diuresis if there is evidence of pulmonary vascular congestion, will suffice while appropriate diagnostic steps are taken. If there is evidence of hemodynamic instability, with evidence of high LV filling pressure, tachycardia, and borderline or low cardiac index, intravenous sodium nitroprusside is indicated. In most cases the patient can be stabilized on nitroprusside while more definitive therapy is planned. It has been the practice in our institution to take patients to the cardiac catheterization laboratory when possible, to confirm the diagnosis, evaluate LV function, rule out other valvular involvement, and define coronary anatomy, particularly in older patients. An unsuspected aortic root abscess or evidence of aortic dissection may be identified by supravalvular angiography. Alternative viewpoints have been published.[55] Following catheterization, a decision is made concerning immediate or delayed surgery or permanent nonsurgical management.

If the patient is less severely ill (i.e., mild to moderate valvular regurgitation) or if he is believed to be a very poor surgical candidate because of associated disease, poor ventricular function, or recent myocardial infarction, it may be prudent to delay surgery. In such cases, the patient should be initially stabilized on sodium nitroprusside and diuretics to attain acceptable hemodynamic variables (i.e., systolic blood pressure around 100; cardiac index > 2.2 liters/min/m²; pulmonary artery wedge pressure < 20 mm Hg). Digitalis can be instituted with a loading dose administered over a period of 24 hours. The patient may then be switched to oral or topical vasodilators. We generally start with captopril at an initial dose of 6.25 mg every 6 to 8 hours and gradually increase the dosage to 25 mg every 6 to 8 hours. Occasionally patients will benefit from doses as high as 50 mg every 6 to 8 hours. Alternatively, enalapril at an initial dose of 2.5 to 5 mg every 12 hours may be used, with a gradual increase in dosage up to 20 mg every 12 hours. If oral hydralazine is chosen, we start with an initial dose of 50 mg to 75 mg, which is increased in 25-mg increments every 3 hours until a desired hemodynamic endpoint or a dose of 200 mg is attained. If there is a high pulmonary artery wedge pressure, oral or topical nitrates are instituted concomitantly. It is important not to stop the nitroprusside precipitously, since the patient may become acutely unstable, but rather to slowly taper the nitroprusside as the oral agents are instituted. In most cases a combination of captopril or hydralazine and oral or topical nitrates will be effective. If these drugs are ineffective, other vasodilators can be used with careful hemodynamic monitoring to assess their efficacy.

PATHOPHYSIOLOGY OF CHRONIC VALVULAR REGURGITATION

The physiological principles described for the cardiac adaptation to acute valvular regurgitation similarly apply in the chronic disorder. The major difference is that time allows remodeling of the LV and an increase in its mass. Thus, the ventricle has an opportunity to enlarge, at times considerably.

There is a large LV end-diastolic volume, a large total LV stroke volume, and (with perfect adaptation) a normal forward or effective stroke volume. In either mitral or aortic regurgitation, the problem generally is similar for the LV. In aortic regurgitation, a large total stroke volume is pumped into the aorta only to have much of it, in severe cases, reflux into the LV. In mitral regurgitation, the large total stroke volume is split into a portion destined for the left atrium and the forward stroke volume for the aorta. In both cases, the LV must contract with a large diastolic volume, and this has implications concerning its mechanical properties and energetics, as described earlier. Total wall forces during systole will be high and must be compensated by an increase in muscle mass, that is, to normalize wall stress. Ultimately LV failure may occur nonetheless.

In mitral regurgitation the LV has an opportunity to begin ejection very early in systole because left atrial pressure is relatively low, in comparison with aortic pressure. Thus, a substantial proportion of the regurgitant flow into the left atrium occurs before the aortic valve opens, perhaps 50%.[56] The total LV wall stress (afterload) is lower than in aortic regurgitation, on the average.[57]

In aortic regurgitation the LV begins ejection when the aortic diastolic pressure is exceeded, in contrast to the situation in mitral regurgitation. Total force requirements, despite the low aortic diastolic pressure in this disease, can be excessive. Left ventricular mass is increased, and, at least for a time, systolic wall stress is maintained at normal level.

RATIONALE FOR VASODILATOR THERAPY

Remarkably, the LV can often sustain a very large regurgitant flow and high stroke volume for many years. The diastolic properties change, and the response to exercise is reasonably normal in many patients, in terms of meeting need for an increase in cardiac output.[58,59] Ultimately, however, the chronically dilated state of the LV leads to a decline in its systolic performance.[60] In patients not treated surgically, congestive heart failure will supervene.

Unfortunately in some patients, valve replacement after the development of LV dysfunction does not lead to improvement. One answer to forestall this problem would be surgery early in the course of the disease. This, however, exposes the patient to the risk of the operation and the continuing risks of a complication of a valve prothesis, whether mechanical or biological, before symptoms require treatment (perhaps many years).

The rationale for vasodilator therapy in chronic valvular regurgitation is to decrease the impedance to LV outflow, which should lead to decreases in regurgitant flow, in LV size, and in contractile force demands. Forward cardiac output might increase. Assuming that late LV dysfunction is related to chronic LV dilation, such changes would be desirable. The ultimate goal would be to preserve LV function so that a good surgical result could still be obtained, but later in life. There is information to support this rationale, but there are no data yet to prove that the goal can be met.

SPECIAL CASE OF MITRAL REGURGITATION

Two issues make the mitral lesion especially complex. First, the low impedance to ejection presented by the left atrium may mask the fact that LV dysfunction has developed. Thus, the ejection fraction may be preserved because, in effect, there has been afterload reduction produced by the low resistance of the mitral valve and left atrium. Such dysfunction would become manifest after valve replacement, when the ventricle must generate sufficient stress in its wall to open the aortic valve prior to onset of ejection. Thus, a fall in LV ejection fraction is not at all rare following valve replacement for chronic mitral regurgitation.

The second important factor with mitral regurgitation is related to the cause of the problem. LV dilation and dysfunction induced by disorders other than primary valve disease can result in ventricular dysfunction and thus produce mitral valve leakage. Furthermore, this may exacerbate the amount of mitral regurgitation, even in primary mitral disease. Thus, the cause of the mitral regurgitant problem is of fundamental importance in the evaluation of any patient with this valve problem. There is a spectrum that exists from intrinsic, primary valve disease (such as ruptured chordae tendineae) to primary LV dysfunction with a very low ejection fraction and secondary mitral regurgitation (such as dilated cardiomyopathy or end-stage coronary disease). The use of vasodilator agents may be appropriate at both ends of the spectrum, but the results may differ. Surgical treatment may be urgently needed in one and contraindicated in the other.

CLINICAL USE OF VASODILATORS IN CHRONIC REGURGITATION
AORTIC REGURGITATION

Several studies of the acute administration of vasodilators in chronic aortic regurgitation have been published, and the results are encouraging. LV ejection fraction remains normal, regurgitant volume falls, and forward cardiac output may increase.[19,40,41,61] Exercise hemodynamics may improve.

Long-term trials of vasodilators in chronic aortic regurgitation are few. A small randomized trial of hydralazine was conducted for 6 months (14 patients). Although calculated LV end-systolic wall stress was decreased and ejection fraction increased, changes in LV size were not found.[62]

A randomized controlled trial of hydralazine was performed in our unit in 80 patients with minimal or no symptoms who had moderate to severe aortic regurgitation.[63] LV end-diastolic volume prior to randomization averaged 166 ml/m^2. The ejection fraction was 0.65. After 2 years of hydralazine therapy, end-diastolic volume had been reduced by 30 ml/m^2 and the ejection fraction had increased slightly in the treatment group. The study demonstrated that long-term treatment with a vasodilator agent was feasible and that physiological effects could be sustained. The trial was not designed to test effects of this treatment on longevity or surgical risk, both very important issues.

Hydralazine is difficult to use because of the high incidence of side effects. Therefore, other drugs such as angiotensin-converting enzyme (ACE) inhibitors appear promising. These may be tried on a chronic basis on empiric grounds, recognizing that there are no long-term data to support their use, in terms of delaying the timing of valve replacement or preserving LV function. Nonetheless, their use would be rational in patients with severe aortic regurgitation. Vasodilator therapy may be helpful in improving symptoms in patients with severe regurgitant disease who are not candidates for valve surgery for other reasons.

MITRAL REGURGITATION

As mentioned earlier, mitral regurgitation presents at least three separate pathophysiological problems: Elevated left atrial pressure results from the direct pumping of blood from the LV retrograde; the forward cardiac output may be compromised by the regurgitant flow; and the cause of the process may have implications about LV function, which, in turn, can contribute to regurgitant flow and decreased forward output. Given these interacting factors, systemic arteriolar vasodilation and/or venodilation are desirable.

Surprisingly, little information from chronic controlled or uncontrolled trials of vasodilation is available. Intravenous nitroglycerin produced reduction of LV filling pressure, end-diastolic volume, and regurgitant volume in patients with chronic mitral regurgitation.[64] The role of nitrates in the long-term management of this disorder is problematic, given tolerance to nitrates and the fact that nitroglycerin was tested by the intravenous route.

In ten patients, intravenous hydralazine produced a marked increase in forward (nonregurgitant) stroke volume and a reduction in the amount of regurgitation. Pulmonary vascular pressure fell.[16] In another small study oral hydralazine was dramatically effective acutely, as shown by hemodynamic study. After about a year of oral therapy, clinical improvement was sustained in approximately 50% of the group.[65]

RECOMMENDATIONS FOR CHRONIC VALVULAR REGURGITATION

AORTIC REGURGITATION

There is no current justification for the use of vasodilator agents in patients with mild aortic regurgitation, given the uncertainty about beneficial effects in such a population and the potential side effects of long-term use of the available drugs. In patients with substantial enlargement of LV end-diastolic volume and signs of hemodynamically significant aortic regurgitation, however, consideration should be given to long-term use of vasodilator agents. The goals would be to attempt to decrease LV size, to preserve LV function, and, perhaps, to delay the time until valve replacement is required. It must be stated again that the latter goal is untested, although logical.

We recommend the use of an ACE inhibitor or hydralazine with the doses mentioned in Table 81.2. Although hydralazine is a logical choice, the incidence of side effects is relatively high, and it would often be our second choice. It might be the primary agent in those with renal dysfunction and those in whom there are concerns about ACE inhibitors' potential effects on the kidney. We have not employed long-term nitrate therapy in chronic aortic regurgitation.

MITRAL REGURGITATION

The decision to use chronic therapy with vasodilating agents depends on the severity of the mitral leakage and the cause of the valve dysfunction and on the status of LV performance. Equally important will be the presence of concomitant problems such as coronary disease. Given the frequency of LV dysfunction, consideration should be given to chronic use of a vasodilator in those patients with serious amounts of mitral regurgitation and/or reduced LV function. The therapeutic goals would be to maintain lower regurgitant volume and left atrial and pulmonary capillary pressures and to try to preserve LV function. Suggested dosages are listed in Table 81.2.

REFERENCES

1. Welch GH, Braunwald E, Sarnoff SJ: Hemodynamic effects of quantitatively varied experimental aortic regurgitation. Circ Res 5:546, 1957
2. Zelis R, Flaim SF: Alterations in vasomotor tone in congestive heart failure. Prog Cardiovasc Dis 24:437, 1985
3. Morganroth J, Perloff JK, Zeldis SM, Dunkman WB: Acute severe aortic regurgitation: Pathophysiology, clinical recognition and management. Ann Intern Med 87:223, 1977
4. Holt JP, Rhode EA, Kines H: Pericardial and ventricular pressure. Circ Res 8:1171, 1960
5. Wilcken DEL: Load, work and velocity of muscle shortening of the left ventricle in normal and abnormal human hearts. J Clin Invest 44:1295, 1965
6. Ross J: Afterload mismatch and preload reserve: A conceptual framework for the analysis of ventricular function. Prog Cardiovasc Dis 18:255, 1976
7. Taylor RR, Covell JW, Ross S Jr: Left ventricular function in experimental aorto-caval fistula with circulatory congestion and fluid retention. J Clin Invest 47:1333, 1968
8. Grossman W, Jones D, McLaurin LP: Wall stress and patterns of hypertrophy in the human left ventricle. J Clin Invest 56:56, 1975
9. Braunwald E: Mitral regurgitation: Physiologic, clinical and surgical considerations. N Engl J Med 281:425, 1969
10. Yoran C, Yellin EI, Becker RM et al: Dynamic aspects of acute mitral regurgitation: Effects of ventricular volume, pressure and contractility on the effective regurgitant orifice area. Circulation 60:170, 1979
11. Urschel CW, Covell JW, Sonnenblick EH et al: Myocardial mechanics in aortic and mitral valvular regurgitation: The concept of instantaneous impedance as a determinant of the performance of the intact heart. J Clin Invest 47:867, 1968
12. Kremkau EL, Gilbertson PR, Bristow JD: Acquired non-rheumatic mitral regurgitation: Clinical management with emphasis on evaluation of myocardial performance. Prog Cardiovasc Dis 15:403, 1973
13. Yoran C, Yellin E, Becker R et al: Mechanisms of reduction of mitral regurgitation with vasodilator therapy. Am J Cardiol 43:773, 1979
14. Harshaw C, Grossman W, Munro A, McLaurin L: Reduced systemic vascular resistance as therapy for severe mitral regurgitation of valvular origin. Ann Intern Med 83:312, 1975
15. Chatterjee K, Parmley WW, Swan HJC et al: Beneficial effects of vasodilator agents in severe mitral regurgitation due to dysfunction of subvalvular apparatus. Circulation 48:884, 1973
16. Greenberg BH, Massie BM, Brundage BH et al: Beneficial effects of hydralazine in severe mitral regurgitation. Circulation 58:273, 1978
17. Mehta J, Feldman RL, Nichols WW et al: Acute hemodynamic effects of oral prazosin in severe mitral regurgitation. Br Heart J 43:556, 1980
18. Miller RR, Vismara LA, DeMaria AN et al: Afterload reduction with nitroprusside in severe aortic regurgitation: Improved cardiac performance and reduced regurgitant volume. Am J Cardiol 38:564, 1976
19. Fioretti P, Bennusi B, Scardi S et al: Afterload reduction with nifedipine in aortic insufficiency. Am J Cardiol 49:1728, 1982
20. Greenberg BH, Rahimtoola SH: Usefulness of vasodilator therapy in acute and chronic valvular regurgitation. Curr Probl Cardiol 9:1, 1984
21. Gold HK, Leinbach RC, Sanders CA et al: Intraaortic balloon pumping for ventricular septal defect or mitral regurgitation complicating acute myocardial infarction. Circulation 47:1191, 1973
22. Chatterjee K: Vasodilator therapy for heart failure. In Cohn J (ed): Drug Treatment of Heart Failure, pp 151–179. New York, Yorke Medical Books, 1983
23. Miller RR, Awan A, Maxwell KS, Mason DT: Sustained reduction of cardiac impedance and preload in congestive heart failure with the antihypertensive vasodilator prazosin. N Engl J Med 297:303, 1977
24. Wigle ED, LaBrosse CJ: Sudden severe aortic insufficiency. Circulation 32:708, 1965
25. Levine RJ, Roberts WC, Morrow AG: Traumatic aortic regurgitation. Am J Cardiol 10:752, 1962
26. Marcus FI, Ronan J, Misanik LF, Ewy GA: Aortic insufficiency secondary to spontaneous rupture of a fenestrated leaflet. Am Heart J 66:675, 1963
27. O'Brien KP, Hitchcock GC, Barratt-Boyes RG, Lowe JB: Spontaneous aortic cusp rupture associated with valvular myxomatous transformation. Circulation 37:273, 1968
28. Wise JR, Cleland WP, Hallidie-Smith KA et al: Urgent aortic-valve replacement for acute aortic regurgitation due to infective endocarditis. Lancet 2:115, 1971
29. Mann T, McLaurin L, Grossman W, Craige E: Assessing the hemodynamic severity of acute aortic regurgitation due to infective endocarditis. N Engl J Med 293:108, 1975
30. Carter JB, Sethi S, Lee GB, Edwards JE: Prolapse of semilunar cusps as causes of aortic insufficiency. Circulation 43:922, 1971
31. Emanuel R, Ng RAL, Marcomichelakis J et al: Formes frustes of Marfan's syndrome presenting with severe aortic regurgitation. Br Heart J 39:190, 1977
32. Roberts WC, Morrow AG, McIntosh CL et al: Congenitally bicuspid aortic valve causing severe, pure aortic regurgitation with superimposed infective endocarditis. Am J Cardiol 47:206, 1981
33. Kloster FE, Bristow JD, Lewis RP, Griswold HE: Pharmacodynamic studies in aortic regurgitation. Am J Cardiol 19:644, 1967
34. Bolen JL, Holloway EL, Zener JC: Evaluation of left ventricular function in patients using afterload stress. Circulation 53:132, 1976
35. Delius W, Enghoff D: Studies of the peripheral and central dynamics in patients with aortic insufficiency. Circulation 42:787, 1970
36. Urschell CW, Covell JW, Sonnenblick EF et al: Effects of decreased aortic compliance on performance of the left ventricle. Am J Physiol 214:298, 1968
37. Bolen JL, Alderman EL: Hemodynamic consequences of afterload reduction in patients with chronic aortic regurgitation. Circulation 53:879, 1976
38. Koch-Weser J: Hydralazine. N Engl J Med 295:320, 1976
39. Greenberg BH, Rahimtoola SH: Long-term vasodilator therapy in aortic insufficiency. Ann Intern Med 93:440, 1980
40. Greenberg BH, DeMots H, Murphy E, Rahimtoola S: Beneficial effects of hydralazine on rest and exercise hemodynamics in patients with chronic severe aortic insufficiency. Circulation 62:49, 1980
41. Greenberg BH, DeMots H, Murphy E, Rahimtoola S: Mechanism for improved cardiac performance with arterial dilators in aortic insufficiency. Circulation 63:263, 1981
42. Mockings BE, Cope GD, Clark GM, Tallor RR: Comparison of vasodilator drug prazosin with digoxin in aortic regurgitation. Br Heart J 43:550, 1980
43. Cohn JN, Franciosa JA: Vasodilator therapy of cardiac failure. N Engl J Med 297:27, 1977
44. Palmer RF, Lasseter KC: Sodium nitroprusside. N Engl J Med 292:294, 1975
45. Cottrell JE, Casthely P, Brodie JD et al: Prevention of nitroprusside-induced cyanide toxicity with hydroxycobalamin. N Engl J Med 298:809, 1978
46. Graham RM, Pettinger WA: Prazosin. N Engl J Med 300:232, 1979
47. Awan NA, Lee G, DeMaria AN, Mason DT: Ambulatory prazosin treatment of chronic congestive heart failure: Development of late tolerance reversible by higher dosage and interrupted substitution therapy. Am Heart J 101:541, 1981
48. Singh BW, Opie LH: In Opie LH (ed): Drugs for the Heart. Orlando, FL, Grune & Stratton, 1984
49. Parmley WM: Captopril for heart failure. In Cohn JN (ed): Drug Treatment of Heart Failure. New York, Yorke Medical Books, 1983

50. Vidt DG, Bravo EL, Fetnat MF: Captopril. N Engl J Med 306:214, 1982
51. Packer M, Medina N, Yushack M, Meller J: Hemodynamic patterns of response during long-term captopril therapy for severe chronic heart failure. Circulation 68:803, 1983
52. Hill NS, Antman EM, Green LH, Alpert JS: Intravenous nitroglycerin. Chest 79:69, 1981
53. Sonnenblick EH, Frishman WH, LeJemtel TH: Dobutamine: A new synthetic cardioactive sympathetic amine. N Engl J Med 30:17, 1979
54. Hasenfuss G, Holubarsch C, Heiss W et al: Myocardial energetics in patients with dilated cardiomyopathy: Influence of nitroprusside and enoximone. Circulation 80:51, 1989
55. Hosenpud JD, Greenberg BH: The preoperative evaluation in patients with endocarditis: Is cardiac catheterization necessary? Chest 84:690, 1983
56. Eckberg DL, Gault JH, Bouchard RL et al: Mechanics of left ventricular contraction in chronic severe mitral regurgitation. Circulation 68:1252, 1973
57. Wisenbaugh T, Spann JF, Carabello BA: Differences in myocardial performance and load between patients with similar amounts of chronic aortic versus chronic mitral regurgitation. J Am Coll Cardiol 3:916, 1984
58. Lewis RP, Bristow JD, Griswold HE: Exercise hemodynamics in aortic regurgitation. Am Heart J 80:171, 1970
59. Massie BM, Kramer BL, Loge D et al: Ejection fraction response to supine exercise in asymptomatic aortic regurgitation: Relation to simultaneous hemodynamic measurements. J Am Coll Cardiol 5:847, 1985
60. Greenberg B, Massie B, Thomas D et al: Association between the exercise ejection fraction response and systolic wall stress in patients with chronic aortic insufficiency. Circulation 71:458, 1985
61. Reske SN, Heck I, Kropp J et al: Captopril-mediated decrease of aortic regurgitation. Br Heart J 54:415, 1985
62. Kleaveland JP, Reichek N, McCarthy DM et al: Effects of six-month afterload reduction therapy with hydralazine in chronic aortic regurgitation. Am J Cardiol 57:1109, 1986
63. Greenberg B, Massie B, Bristow JD et al: Long-term vasodilator therapy of chronic aortic insufficiency. Circulation 78:92, 1988
64. Elkayam U, Roth A, Kumar A et al: Hemodynamic and volumetric effects of venodilation with nitroglycerin in chronic mitral regurgitation. Am J Cardiol 60:1106, 1987
65. Greenberg BH, DeMots H, Murphy E, Rahimtoola SH: Arterial dilators in mitral regurgitation: Effects on rest and exercise hemodynamics and long-term clinical follow-up. Circulation 65:181, 1982

Chronic Valvular Insufficiency

CHAPTER 82
VOLUME 2

Hans P. Krayenbuehl • Otto M. Hess

MITRAL INSUFFICIENCY

Normal closure of the mitral valve is a complex mechanism resulting from a combination of atrial and ventricular events. Effective systolic sealing depends on proper function, size, position, and integrity of the mitral leaflets, chordae tendineae, papillary muscles, mitral valve annulus, and left ventricular and atrial walls.[1] Abnormalities of any of these structures may lead to mitral insufficiency.

ETIOLOGY

In 1972 chronic rheumatic heart disease was reported to be the most common cause of chronic mitral insufficiency.[2] A Norwegian study published in 1976[3] still found rheumatic heart disease to account for the most frequent etiology (36%) among patients with severe operative chronic mitral insufficiency. More recently, mitral valve prolapse due to myxomatous degeneration of the fibrous skeleton of the valve leaflets and chordae tendineae has become the most frequent cause of mitral insufficiency necessitating surgery (Table 82.1).[4] In underdeveloped populations rheumatic heart disease remains the largely predominant etiology of severe mitral insufficiency,[5] the age when surgery is performed being considerably lower (25 years) than in the aforementioned United States (55 years) and Swiss (52 years) surgical series.

PATHOPHYSIOLOGY

Chronic mitral insufficiency is accompanied by volume overload of the left-sided cavities. It causes enlargement of both the left ventricle and

TABLE 82.1 ETIOLOGY OF OPERATIVE MITRAL INSUFFICIENCY

	Excised Mitral Valves for Isolated Severe Chronic Mitral Insufficiency 1968–1981[4] (n = 97)	Operations for Mitral Insufficiency, 1972–1983 (Surgical Clinic A, University of Zurich) (n = 315)
Myxomatous degeneration	62%	35%
Rheumatic	3%	17%
Ischemic	30%	5%
Infective endocarditis	5%	12%
Combined with congenital defect		12%
Cardiomyopathy		5%
Reoperation		14%

atrium. Once established, mitral insufficiency tends to get hemodynamically worse with time. Because of the continuity between the left atrial endocardium and the posterior mitral leaflet the posterior cusp is pulled across its annulus so that the cusp functionally shortens as the left atrium enlarges. Thus, mitral insufficiency is augmented by atrial enlargement.[1] Mitral orifice size is also determined by the size of the left ventricular cavity because mitral annular dilatation is a common consequence of left ventricular dilatation except when there is marked rigidity of the annulus due to heavy calcification. Moreover, the lateral displacement of the papillary muscles in an enlarged left ventricular cavity results in abnormal systolic traction on the chordae tendineae, which pull the mitral leaflets laterally and downward instead of bringing them to coaptation. Hence, as with the increase of left atrial size, any increase in left ventricular volume tends to make mitral insufficiency worse. This vicious cycle has been characterized by Edwards and Burchell[6] as "mitral insufficiency begets mitral insufficiency."

Systolic backflow from the left ventricle to the left atrium causes an augmentation of the v wave in the left atrial pressure curve. The height of the v wave is variable according to the compliance of the wall of the left atrium and the pulmonary veins. Whereas in acute mitral insufficiency the v wave is greatly enhanced because the normally sized left atrium and pulmonary veins are not prepared to accommodate the regurgitant volume without a massive increase in pressure, equally severe chronic mitral regurgitation may cause only a minor increase of the v wave in the presence of a markedly dilated left atrium.[7] Accordingly, left atrial mean pressure is higher in acute cases than in most cases of chronic mitral insufficiency, and consecutive elevation of pulmonary artery pressure is more marked when severe insufficiency develops over a short period of time.

In most patients with chronic mitral insufficiency pump function of the left ventricle remains well preserved because the systolic leak into the low-pressure left atrium allows the left ventricle to empty against a reduced afterload. During ejection there is rapid unloading of the left ventricle evidenced by a marked drop of left ventricular pressure and especially of left ventricular wall stress once the respective peaks are reached in early systole. Hence, in compensated chronic mitral insufficiency the left ventricular ejection fraction is high normal. Persistence of normal peak, mean, and end-systolic wall stress in patients with already depressed myocardial contractile state allows left ventricular ejection fraction to remain in the low normal range or to be only minimally depressed.[8] Hence, favorable loading conditions may mask contractile dysfunction. It is therefore not surprising that mild to moderate degrees of reduction of preoperative ejection performance such as a systolic fractional shortening of <31% or an ejection fraction of <40% are associated with unfavorable postoperative results manifested as persistent cardiomegaly[9] or reduced survival.[10] More recent investigations, however, have raised some doubt as to whether the presence of the "low impedance" left atrium in mitral insufficiency is associated with particularly favorable systolic loading conditions of the left ventricle. In patients with depressed ejection fraction, left ventricular peak systolic, end-systolic, and mean systolic circumferential wall stress was found to be consistently increased as compared with controls.[11] Even in patients with normal ejection fraction, afterload as assessed by mean stress from aortic valve opening to aortic valve closure was increased, although end-systolic wall stress did not differ from that in controls.[11]

Acute and chronic increases of aortic pressure intensify the hemodynamic severity of mitral insufficiency (Fig. 82.1). Hence, development of arterial hypertension in mitral insufficiency may lead to rapid deterioration with the occurrence of pulmonary edema. Not only may increases of preload and afterload render mitral insufficiency more severe via an increase of ventricular size, but deterioration of myocardial contractility will accentuate mitral insufficiency because a decrease of contractile state is generally accompanied by a further increase of ventricular volume and an impairment of systolic mitral annular area reduction.

PROGNOSIS AND NATURAL HISTORY

Most patients with chronic mitral regurgitation follow a relatively benign natural course and experience few limiting symptoms until late in their illness. Dyspnea with effort and palpitations occur solely in the fourth to sixth decades. At the time of surgery, symptoms can usually be traced back ten years. When atrial fibrillation ensues, the patients become more symptomatic. Sudden massive deterioration is mostly due to chordal rupture with or without infective endocarditis. Not every chordal rupture, however, is followed by lasting clinical impairment. The patient may become relatively asymptomatic again for months or years. It is of note that in the first clinical description of mitral insufficiency, Corvisart in 1806[12] reported a 34-year-old patient in whom chordal ruptures were found at necropsy. This patient did well for 20 months after the initial episode of sudden left heart decompensation.

Five-year survival in medically treated patients with mitral insufficiency was found to be 55% after catheterization[13] and 80% after the diagnosis was established.[14] This large difference in survival is not surprising, however, because the two cohorts may not have been comparable since their etiology, age at entry into the observation period, and coronary status were unknown.

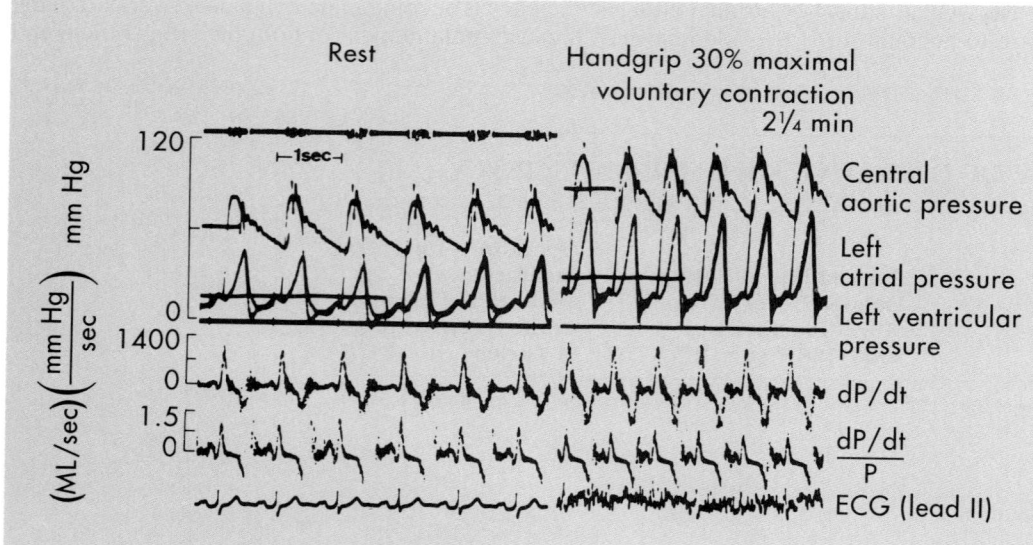

FIGURE 82.1 Effect of an acute increase in afterload by handgrip (at a strength of 30% of maximal voluntary contraction [MVC] during 2¼ minutes) on left ventricular and atrial pressures in a 65-year-old patient with severe rheumatic mitral insufficiency. During handgrip the v wave of the left atrial pressure curve increases from 40 mm Hg to 75 mm Hg, indicating a massive increase in mitral regurgitation consequent to the increase in afterload. (LAP, left atrial pressure; LVP, left ventricular pressure [micromanometry]; AoP, central aortic pressure; dP/dt, first derivative of LVP; (dP/dt)/P, instantaneous velocity of shortening of the contractile elements in muscle lengths/sec; ECG, electrocardiogram [lead II])

SYMPTOMS AND PHYSICAL EXAMINATION

SYMPTOMS
Slowly progressive dyspnea with effort is the main symptom. Patients with a massively dilated high-compliant left atrium may be limited more by fatigue than by exertional dyspnea. Palpitations may occur, mostly with the onset of atrial fibrillation. Anginal symptoms are uncommon; when they are present, an ischemic etiology of mitral insufficiency is suspected. Unlike mitral stenosis, hemoptysis is rare in mitral insufficiency.

PALPATION
The apical impulse is displaced laterally and caudally into the sixth intercostal space. In the left parasternal region a late systolic thrust may be palpable. This "precordial lift" is caused by massive systolic expansion of the left atrium anteriorly when mitral reflux is severe. The upstroke of the peripheral arterial pulse is brisk; its amplitude is small in contrast to aortic insufficiency.

AUSCULTATION
The main feature of mitral insufficiency is a holosystolic blowing, high-pitched murmur that starts immediately after a soft S_1 and continues beyond A_2. The murmur is loudest at the apex and radiates toward the axilla. Its intensity is fairly constant, even when heart rate is irregular, as in atrial fibrillation, and does not change with an ectopic beat. In patients with chordal rupture the systolic murmur is harsh and a thrill is often palpable at the apex. Expiratory wide splitting of S_2 is a typical feature of mitral insufficiency because the left ventricular ejection terminates prematurely due to low resistance to cavity emptying. In early diastole ≥ 0.12 sec after A_2, a low-frequency filling sound (S_3) is heard and may also be palpable.

In mitral valve prolapse with small reflux the regurgitant murmur is late-systolic and crescendo toward A_2. In some patients with massive mitral insufficiency the holosystolic murmur shows decreasing intensity toward A_2 because of a rapidly decreasing pressure gradient between the left ventricle and left atrium when the v wave is very high.

NONINVASIVE TESTS

ELECTROCARDIOGRAM
About two thirds of operative patients with mitral insufficiency are in atrial fibrillation. In sinus rhythm, signs of left atrial enlargement are prominent in leads I, II, V_1, V_5, and V_6 (Fig. 82.2, A and B). Left ventricular hypertrophy of moderate degree (index of Sokolow $S_{V1} + R_{V5}$ or V_6 between 3.5 mV and 5.5 mV) is present in about 50% of the patients with severe mitral insufficiency. Repolarization disturbances are often due to digitalis. Signs of right ventricular hypertrophy are rare.

RADIOLOGY
The chest roentgenogram shows enlargement of the left atrium and ventricle, which is slowly progressive over years (Fig. 82.3, A and B). When massive atrial dilatation ("giant left atrium") is present, mitral insufficiency is most likely of rheumatic origin, probably with initial inflammatory damage of the left atrial myocardium. Signs of pulmonary stasis are generally mild and contrast with the marked cardiomegaly.

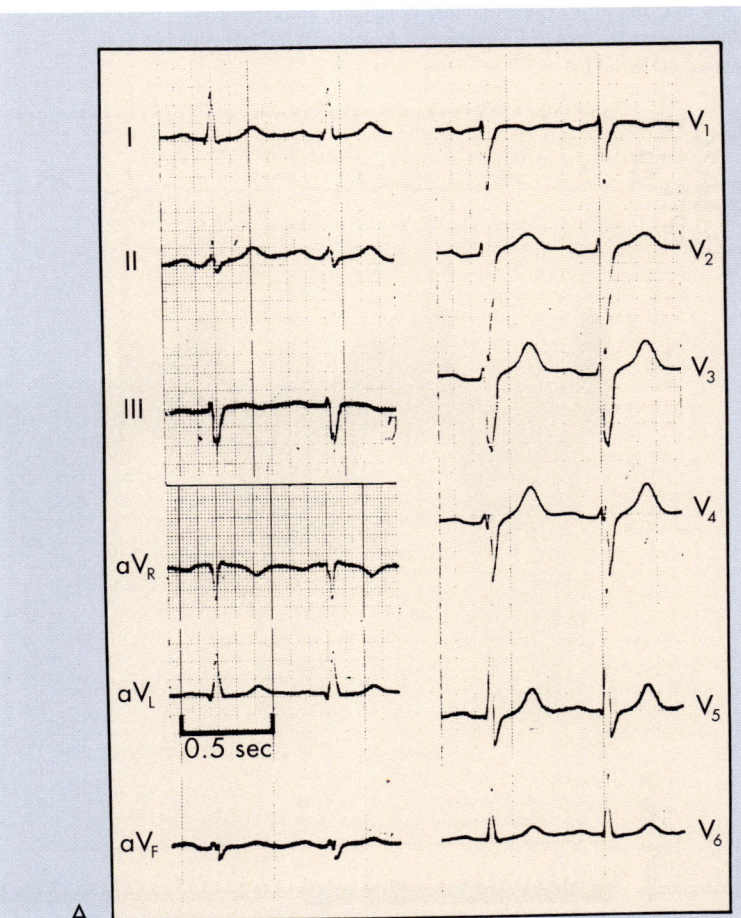
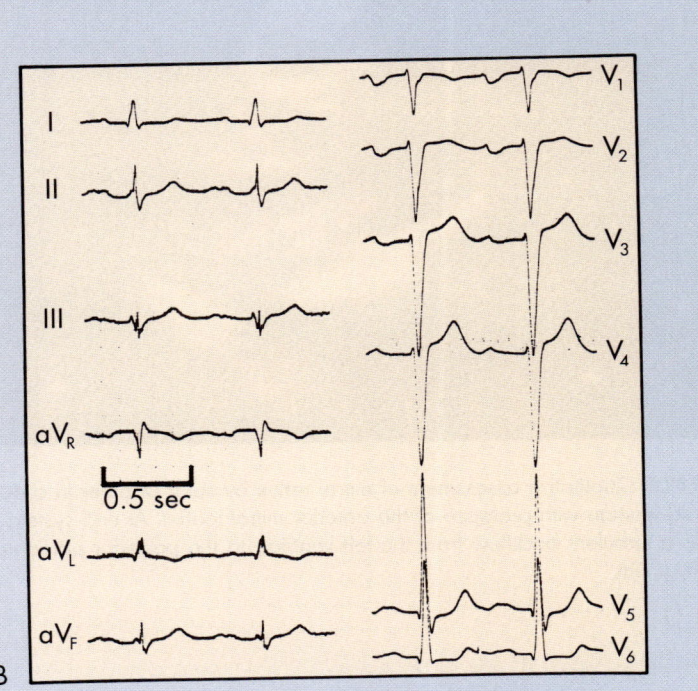

FIGURE 82.2 A. Electrocardiogram of a 56-year-old patient with moderate rheumatic mitral insufficiency. There is left ventricular hypertrophy. Sokolow index is 4.8 mV. **B.** Electrocardiogram of the same patient at age 65 (same patient as in Fig. 82.1). There is still sinus rhythm. However, signs of left atrial enlargement are prominent in leads I, II, V_1, V_5, and V_6. There is beginning left ventricular "strain." Sokolow index is now 5.1 mV.

ECHOCARDIOGRAPHY

Whereas the hemodynamic severity of mitral insufficiency cannot be assessed directly by echocardiography, the consequences of long-standing left atrial and ventricular volume overload, namely enlargement of both cavities, are reliably documented by M-mode as well as two-dimensional echocardiography. Moreover, the etiology of mitral insufficiency is usually determined because echocardiography allows the identification of mitral valve prolapse, flail leaflet with chordal rupture, vegetations, central or lateral defects of leaflet coaption in rheumatic mitral insufficiency, abnormal systolic motion of mitral leaflets in hypertrophic obstructive cardiomyopathy, and mitral annular calcification.

DOPPLER ECHOCARDIOGRAPHY

With pulsed[15] and color[16] Doppler, systolic retrograde flow on the left atrial side of the mitral valve plane is assessed with very high sensitivity and specificity (Figs. 82.4 and 82.5). Mapping of the left atrium with pulsed or color Doppler allows one to evaluate the spatial distribution

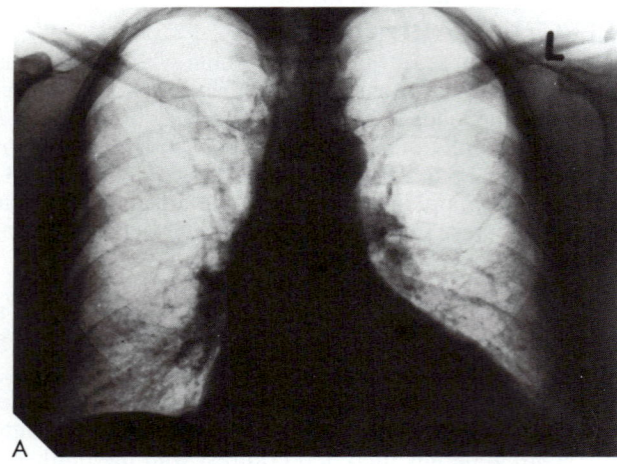
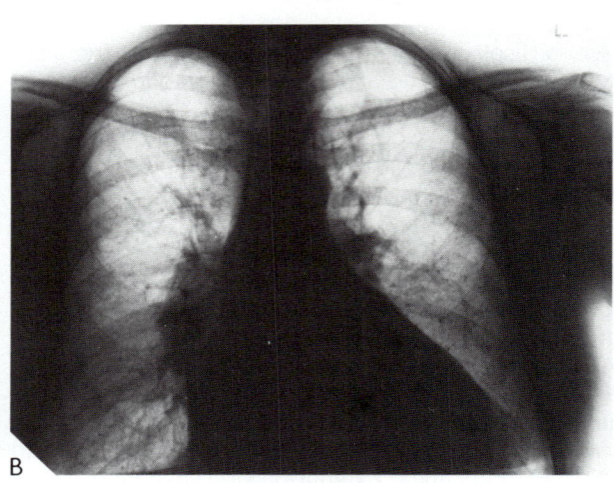

FIGURE 82.3 A. Chest roentgenogram of a 56-year-old patient with moderate rheumatic mitral insufficiency (same patient as in Fig. 82.2, A). There is slight left ventricular enlargement. (The mitral regurgitant fraction is 0.42; the left atrial v wave is 25 mm Hg) **B.** Chest roentgenogram of the same patient at age 65 (same patient in Figs. 82.1 and 82.2, B). Left ventricular enlargement is more marked than in A, the left atrium is now definitely enlarged, and there is pulmonary stasis. (Mitral regurgitant fraction, 0.52; left atrial v wave, 40 mm Hg)

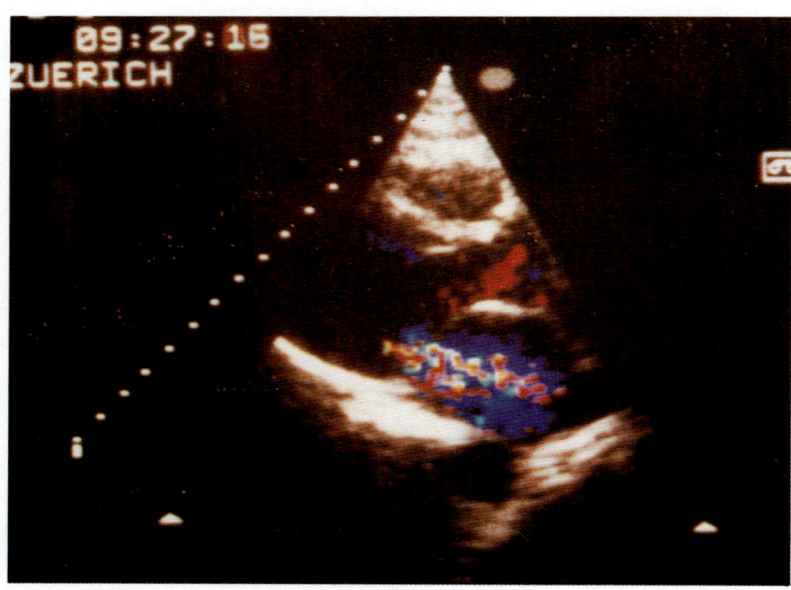

FIGURE 82.4 Qualitative assessment of mitral reflux by color Doppler in a 48-year-old woman with prolapse of the anterior mitral leaflet. At end-systole there is a turbulent backflow from the left ventricle to the posterior portion of the left atrium.

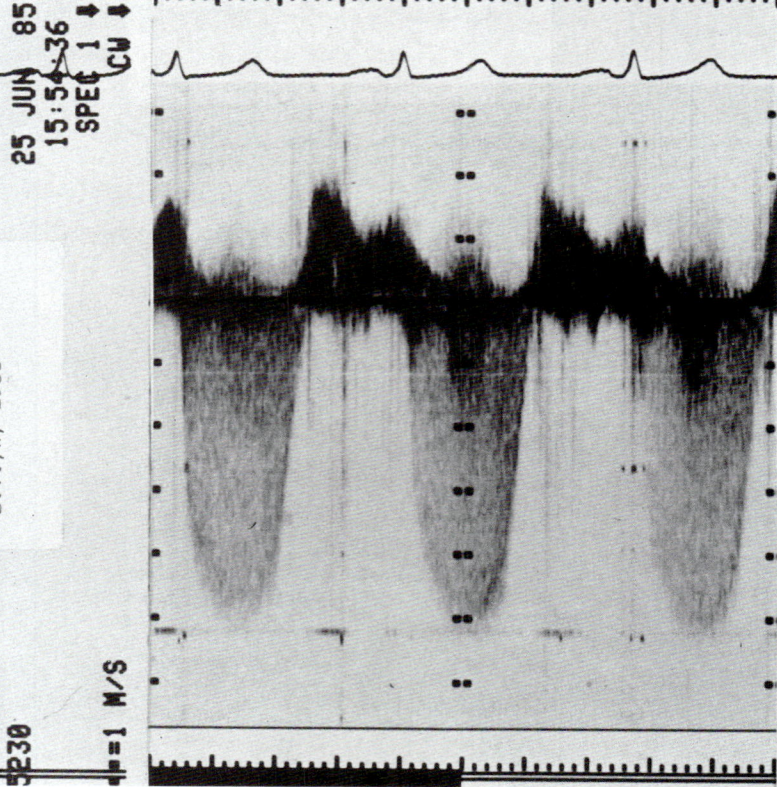

FIGURE 82.5 Qualitative assessment of mitral reflux by continuous wave Doppler in a 30-year-old woman with mild mitral insufficiency from mitral prolapse. There is a high velocity systolic backflow (peak velocity 5 m/sec) away from the transducer located at the cardiac apex. The pattern of the mitral inflow (toward the transducer) is without particularities.

of systolic mitral backflow, and hence serves as a semiquantitative measure of the hemodynamic severity of mitral insufficiency. From continuous wave Doppler spectra, accurate quantification of mitral regurgitation can be achieved based on the calculation of the systolic (left ventricular outflow tract) and diastolic (left ventricular inflow tract) time integrals of amplitude-weighted mean velocities (Fig. 82.6).[17] The quotient integral (inflow) − integral (outflow)/integral (inflow) represents the mitral regurgitation fraction. Its determination is independent of the measure of the left ventricular inflow and outflow tract area.

RADIOISOTOPE STUDIES

Gated blood pool imaging may be used for the estimation of mitral regurgitant fraction from the ratio of left ventricular minus right ventricular stroke volume/left ventricular stroke volume.[18] This approach requires the absence of any other valvular regurgitation. Moreover, the separation of the ventricular regions of interest from atrial overlap may be difficult to accomplish, especially in cases with a greatly enlarged left atrium. Thus, regurgitation as determined by radioisotope angiography provides only a rough estimate of severity of mitral regurgitation.

APEXCARDIOGRAM AND SYSTOLIC TIME INTERVALS

The apexcardiogram shows a prominent early diastolic filling wave whose peak coincides with S_3. The upstroke of the carotid pulse tracing is particularly brisk, the peak is not sustained, and the incisura occurs prematurely. In severe mitral insufficiency, left ventricular ejection time as measured from the carotid pulse tracing is consistently below 85% of normal.

PHYSICAL WORKING CAPACITY

Despite the presence of hemodynamically significant mitral insufficiency, physical working capacity remains relatively well preserved for a considerable time because reduction of peripheral resistance during dynamic exercise facilitates antegrade left ventricular emptying through the aortic valve. Physical working capacity falls with the occurrence of atrial fibrillation.

PULMONARY FUNCTION

Massive dilatation of the cardiac cavities is accompanied by reduction of vital capacity. In combined mitral valve stenosis and insufficiency, chronic pulmonary stasis is usually complicated by moderate bronchial obstruction. Maximal ventilation per minute may then be reduced. A value below 45 liters/min is considered critical when surgery is contemplated. Pulmonary compliance is diminished in longstanding pulmonary stasis but its estimation has not gained practical importance.

HEMODYNAMICS AND ANGIOCARDIOGRAPHY

The typical feature of mitral insufficiency is an augmented v wave of the left atrial and the pulmonary capillary wedge pressure (see Fig. 82.1). In severe mitral insufficiency of recent onset and pulmonary hypertension, a pulmonary arterial early diastolic v wave can occur that causes premature closure of the pulmonic valves.[19] The O_2 saturation of the blood in the peripheral portions of the pulmonary arterial tree may be slightly higher than in the central pulmonary artery because the high v wave squeezes saturated blood through the capillaries backward into the distal pulmonary arterial bed. Between the left atrial and left ventricular pressure curve there is a small gradient during the rapid filling phase because viscous forces become operative due to the high inflow rate (see Fig. 82.1). Quantitation of mitral regurgitant flow can be achieved by indicator dilution techniques with upstream and downstream sampling following indicator injection into the left ventricle, videodensitometry, or left ventricular angiocardiography.

At angiocardiography, mitral insufficiency is best visualized with left ventricular contrast dye injection in the right anterior oblique projection. Details of valve structure and motion are less well assessed than by two-dimensional echocardiography. The severity of mitral insufficiency is assessed semiquantitatively from the rate and extent of left atrial opacification. Whereas this visual evaluation is sufficient for routine purposes, the truly volumetric quantitation of mitral regurgitant flow per beat (RSVm) is carried out by subtracting the forward stroke volume (FSV, obtained by Fick or dilution cardiac output estimation) from the angiographic left ventricular total stroke volume (TSV). The mitral regurgitant fraction (fm) is represented by the ratio RSVm/TSV. A ratio of 0.3 to 0.5 corresponds to moderate mitral insufficiency; when regurgitant fraction exceeds 0.5, severe mitral insufficiency is present.

In cohorts of operative patients with mitral insufficiency, left ventricular end-diastolic volume index (EDVI) varied between 131 ml/m^2 and 148 ml/m^2,[20–23] which is roughly double the normal value. When EDVI exceeds 200 ml/m^2, left heart decompensation is the rule.[24] In most patients left ventricular ejection fraction is well preserved. An end-systolic volume index (ESVI) > 30 ml/m^2 was found to be associated with reduced left ventricular postoperative fractional shortening, and a preoperative ESVI > 60 ml/m^2 with increased risk of perioperative death from heart failure.[22] End-diastolic geometry of the left

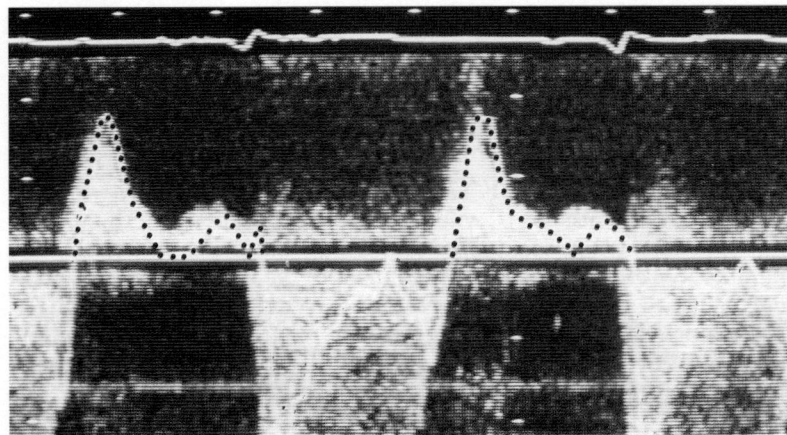
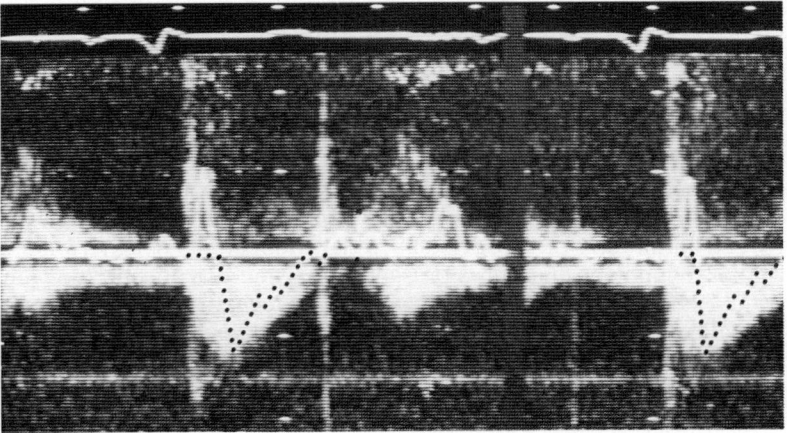

FIGURE 82.6 Amplitude-weighted mean velocities from continuous wave Doppler spectra (indicated by the dotted line) in the left ventricular inflow tract (upper panel) and in the left ventricular outflow tract (lower panel). This is a 74-year-old patient with moderate mitral insufficiency. The time integral of the amplitude-weighted mean velocity in the left ventricular inflow tract is clearly larger than that in the systolic outflow tract (corresponding to a mitral insufficiency with a mitral regurgitation fraction of 0.36).

ventricle in chronic mitral insufficiency is more spherical than normal and when left heart decompensation ensues, end-systolic left ventricular shape becomes more spherical too.[24]

DIAGNOSIS AND DIFFERENTIAL DIAGNOSIS

In most cases the diagnosis of mitral insufficiency is easily made from the pansystolic murmur at the apex with radiation to the axilla. More difficult is the diagnosis of additional mitral insufficiency in the presence of aortic stenosis with a harsh systolic murmur audible over the entire heart. In this instance, Doppler echocardiography is valid for confirmation or exclusion of mitral reflux. The differential diagnosis has to consider ventricular septal defect, hypertrophic obstructive cardiomyopathy, and tricuspid insufficiency in the presence of a greatly enlarged right ventricle.

SPECIFIC TYPES OF MITRAL INSUFFICIENCY

RHEUMATIC MITRAL INSUFFICIENCY

A pansystolic apical murmur suggestive of mitral insufficiency is heard in about 25% of the patients with acute rheumatic fever. Later, this murmur disappears in most instances because initial rheumatic damage was not such as to create a durable defect of leaflet closure. Chronic mitral insufficiency in rheumatic heart disease is the consequence of a progressive shrinkage and fibrosis of the leaflets and requires decades to become hemodynamically significant. It is unknown why rheumatic endocarditis is followed much more often by stenosis than by insufficiency of the mitral valve.

Rheumatic origin of mitral insufficiency is likely when a stenotic component is present and when reflux occurs in the mid part of the mitral orifice toward the central portion of the left atrium.[25] Failure of closure in two or more laterally located places along the valve may also cause significant reflux in rheumatic mitral valve disease.[26]

MITRAL VALVE PROLAPSE

PATHOLOGY AND PATHOPHYSIOLOGY. Typical are the ballooning, redundant cusps composed of myxomatous material. *Myxomatous degeneration*, which is associated with increased quantities of acid mucopolysaccharides in the valvular stroma, is not confined to the cusps but involves chordae tendineae and mitral annulus as well. Systolic prolapse beyond the mitral valve plane is caused by both the protrusion of the oversized billowing leaflets *per se* and the inability of the elongated thinned chordae tendineae to keep the leaflets in apposition when the cavity size is reduced during ejection.

Ischemic papillary muscle dysfunction and infarction of the ventricular wall at the base of the posterior papillary muscle can also be the cause of a prolapsing mitral leaflet.

NATURAL HISTORY AND COMPLICATIONS. Mitral valve prolapse is a benign condition with low morbidity and minimal mortality. Complications may occur, however. During a 14-year follow-up period, bacterial endocarditis, chordal rupture, and gradually progressive mitral insufficiency have been observed in 15% of patients with auscultatory signs of the mitral valve prolapse.[27] A higher rate of progression to severe mitral insufficiency has been observed in young patients with Marfan's syndrome and mitral valve prolapse.[28] The association between mitral valve prolapse and bacterial endocarditis is higher when a mitral regurgitant murmur is present than when it is absent.[27,29] Transient ischemic attacks, especially amaurosis fugax, are not uncommon in patients with mitral valve prolapse.[30] They appear to be related to cerebral embolism.

Sudden death is a rare event in patients with the mitral valve prolapse. Whether mitral valve prolapse is really the cause of death is not firmly established, although coincidence with other known heart disease has not been found at necropsy.[31]

PHYSICAL EXAMINATION. The cornerstone of the diagnosis of mitral valve prolapse is the midsystolic (nonejection) click followed by a mid- to late-systolic murmur that is crescendo toward S_2. This murmur is the correlate of late-systolic mitral reflux. Click and murmur may occur independently of each other. Sudden tensing of the chordae tendineae and leaflets at the onset of prolapse is responsible for the midsystolic click. When there is asynchronous prolapse of the individual scallops of the posterior cusp or of both the posterior and the anterior leaflets, multiple clicks may be audible. The auscultatory findings may be quite variable at consecutive examinations. Only a minority of subjects with echocardiographic mitral valve prolapse have auscultatory findings. Physical and pharmacologic interventions that lead to a reduction of left ventricular volume (sudden standing, Valsalva maneuver, amyl nitrite) result in an earlier occurrence of the click and the systolic murmur. When the murmur becomes holosystolic, the click is indistinguishable from S_1. The characteristics of the murmur may be those of a whoop or honk. Occasionally, a high-frequency early diastolic sound is heard that may be confused with an opening snap. Asthenic habitus, abnormalities of the bony thorax such as pectus excavatum, scoliosis, and straight back, T wave inversions in the inferior limb leads, premature ventricular or supraventricular beats, and atypical chest pain are all nonspecific findings not preferentially occurring in patients with mitral valve prolapse.[32]

In patients with prolapsing mitral leaflets due to *chordal rupture* the murmur at the apex is holosystolic. It contains low-frequency components and hence an apical thrill is often palpable. This murmur may radiate to the spine and to the skull ("murmur on top of the head").

ECHOCARDIOGRAPHY. In the M-mode echocardiogram the typical 90° clockwise-turned question mark sign and the U-shaped or hammock-type prolapse can be seen. False positive or false negative diagnoses may, however, be made with M-mode echocardiography. Unambiguous diagnosis or exclusion of mitral valve prolapse is best obtained by assessing mitral valve motion from the apical four-chamber view during two-dimensional echocardiography. Superior systolic displacement of the mitral leaflets with the coaption point above the annular plane is the hallmark of this diagnosis. This displacement must amount to 3 mm or more and must be present in two orthogonal apical views, because the miral annulus is nonplanar but has a "saddle-shaped" configuration.[33]

HEMODYNAMICS AND ANGIOCARDIOGRAPHY. In uncomplicated mitral valve prolapse, standard hemodynamics are within normal limits. Mitral regurgitant fraction does not exceed 0.35.[34] At left ventricular angiography, prolapse of the posterior leaflet is best visualized in the RAO projection and prolapse of the anterior leaflet in the right posterior oblique projection, with the x-ray beam in the ventrodorsal direction. Left ventricular angiographic shape and contraction are normal in the vast majority of patients. In some patients with mitral valve prolapse, however, there are left ventricular angiographic abnormalities including regional hypokinesis or akinesis and indentation of one or both papillary muscles, leading to the appearance of an "hourglass" left ventricular cavity.[35]

PAPILLARY MUSCLE DYSFUNCTION

Coronary artery disease is, with few exceptions, the cause of papillary muscle dysfunction. The posterior papillary muscle is particularly vulnerable to ischemia because, in contrast to the anterior papillary muscle, its blood supply stems solely from one (the right) coronary artery. For mitral insufficiency to occur, a severe contraction disorder of both the posterior papillary muscle and its underlying wall is necessary. Hence, chronic mitral insufficiency from papillary muscle dysfunction is mostly due to a transmural posteroinferior infarction. Enlargement of the left ventricular cavity further compromises mitral valve closure. Acute papillary muscle dysfunction with a transiently audible apical systolic regurgitant murmur can occur during an episode of severe angina pectoris.

Other conditions associated with abnormal function of one or both papillary muscles include hypertrophic obstructive cardiomyopathy, endomyocardial fibrosis, systemic neuromuscular disorders, amyloidosis, and sarcoidosis.

MITRAL INSUFFICIENCY SECONDARY TO ENLARGEMENT OF THE LEFT VENTRICULAR CAVITY

Marked enlargement of the left ventricle from any cause may lead to mitral insufficiency (see under Pathophysiology, earlier in this chapter). Its hemodynamic severity is mild. The soft apical systolic murmur is easily overlooked at routine auscultation. Following recompensation, the systolic murmur disappears simultaneously with the reduction of heart size.

MITRAL ANNULAR CALCIFICATION

Rigidity of the calcified mitral annulus interferes with systolic mitral orifice reduction and may result in mild mitral insufficiency. Mitral annular calcification is found predominantly in elderly women. From necropsy studies an incidence of 12% in females older than 70 years has been found.[36] Diabetes and hypertension appear to play an important pathogenetic role. Up to 60% of patients with angiographically or echocardiographically documented hypertrophic obstructive cardiomyopathy who were older than 55 years were reported to have calcification of the mitral annulus.[37] In dialysis patients, mitral annular calcifications can occur at an earlier age.

Mitral annular calcification is easily detected in the anteroposterior or left anterior oblique chest roentgenogram as a dense C-shaped opacity. Complications of mitral annulus calcification include conduction disturbances due to extension of the calcium deposits into the membranous septum, infection of the annulus with myocardial abscesses, and calcific embolism in rare instances. Protrusion into the inflow tract of calcific masses originating from the mitral annulus may mimic mitral stenosis, especially when the left ventricle is small and hypertrophied.

MITRAL INSUFFICIENCY IN CONGENITAL HEART DISEASE

Partial and total atrioventricular (AV) canal, corrected transposition of the great arteries, and single papillary muscle ("parachute mitral valve") are associated with mitral insufficiency. In atrial septal defect of the secundum type, mitral valve prolapse is not uncommon but mitral insufficiency, when present, is trivial. The morphologic basis of hemodynamically significant mitral insufficiency that occurs in about 4% of patients with secundum atrial septal defect consists of leaflet and chordal thickening, fibrosis, and deformity.[38]

DIASTOLIC MITRAL INSUFFICIENCY

In patients with total atrioventricular block, mitral regurgitation has been shown to occur following each atrial contraction in the diastolic interval ("atriogenic reflux").[39] In severe aortic insufficiency with mid-diastolic equilibration between aortic and left ventricular pressures at a level higher than left atrial pressure, reflux from the left ventricle to the left atrium has been documented during the second half of diastole by left atrial intracardiac phonocardiography and left ventricular cineangiography.[40] This reflux is observed when the rise of left ventricular diastolic pressure is slow at a low heart rate, whereas the more frequent premature mitral valve closure in severe aortic insufficiency is produced when the diastolic left ventricular pressure rise is steep.

MEDICAL TREATMENT

Symptomatic patients with chronic mitral insufficiency are treated with digitalis and diuretics. When dyspnea occurs for the first time or is considerably accentuated with the appearance of atrial fibrillation, conversion to sinus rhythm should be attempted in addition to the aforementioned measures. Pharmacologic conversion is best carried out with quinidine or amiodarone. In the case of failure, electrical conversion is recommended. If atrial fibrillation recurs despite adequate antiarrhythmic prophylaxis, repeated electrical conversions should not be employed. Anticoagulation prior to conversion is not necessary in mitral insufficiency because, in contrast to mitral stenosis, emboli are extremely rare. Only in cases with massive enlargement of the left atrium and low cardiac output is anticoagulation with warfarin indicated.

Because high afterload aggravates mitral insufficiency, blood pressure should be kept at a value as low as possible. Afterload reduction with hydralazine given intravenously has been shown to acutely reduce mitral regurgitant fraction and improve cardiac output,[41] and oral hydralazine given for seven weeks led to a decrease of left ventricular end-diastolic and end-systolic diameters and improved left ventricular fractional shortening.[42] Beneficial effects on symptoms lasting for at least six months were reported in 44% of patients on long-term hydralazine therapy.[43] Other afterload-reducing compounds like prazosin and angiotensin-converting enzyme inhibitors may be administered as well. Any long-term treatment with these agents requires surveillance as to development of drug tolerance.

Antibiotic endocarditis prophylaxis should be performed in all patients with chronic mitral insufficiency except in those whose mitral reflux is secondary to enlargement of the left ventricular cavity. Specific guidelines are given elsewhere in these volumes (see the Index).

SURGICAL TREATMENT

Both valve replacement and reconstructive surgery have been used in patients with mitral insufficiency.

INDICATIONS FOR SURGERY

The prerequisite is severe mitral insufficiency with a regurgitant fraction ≥ 0.50. Surgery should not be delayed until severe symptoms are present. Survival has been shown to be clearly better in patients with New York Heart Association (NYHA) class II symptoms than in those with NYHA class III to IV symptoms.[44] Many patients with slowly progressive mitral insufficiency adapt to their limited physical working capacity and report no symptoms. In these patients echocardiographic measures may guide the indications for surgery.[45] Good postoperative functional results, including regression of left ventricular end-diastolic and end-systolic size and left ventricular hypertrophy and maintenance of ejection fraction within the normal range, were observed when preoperative left ventricular end-diastolic diameter was <7 cm and end-systolic diameter was <5 cm.[46] Another study reported similar favorable postoperative results when preoperative end-systolic diameter did not exceed 2.6 cm/m^2 and fractional shortening was not smaller than 31% at the preoperative evaluation.[9]

OPERATIVE RESULTS

Surgery was shown to yield significantly better long-term survival than medical treatment in patients with mitral insufficiency and mixed mitral stenosis and insufficiency studied retrospectively.[13] The 5-year survival was 70% with surgical and 55% with medical treatment.[13] The results of mitral valve reconstruction are more favorable than those of mitral valve replacement.[47,48] Whereas 9- to 10-year survival following reconstruction was reported to be 81%[47] and 82%,[49] 8- to 10-year survival with prosthetic replacement varied between 39%[47] and 65%.[50] A similar trend was observed in other studies (Fig. 82.7). In the same cohorts late thromboembolic complications were fewer after reconstruction, the 7-year actuarial rate of patients free of thromboembolic events being 94% versus 82% after mitral valve replacement.

Following mitral valve reconstruction, an apical systolic murmur is present in >40% of the patients, signaling some degree of mitral insufficiency.[49] Recurrence of mitral insufficiency requiring reoperation occurs at a rate of 2.5% per year.[49] Mitral insufficiency of rheumatic origin[5,23] as well as that due to myxomatous degeneration[47] is amenable to reconstruction. Contraindications include extensively calcified leaflets, marked alterations of the subvalvular apparatus, and bacterial endocarditis. When mitral valve surgery is combined with aortocoronary bypass grafting, operative mortality was reported to be 10% in elective cases and 60% in emergency operations.[51] The risk of combined coronary artery bypass grafting and mitral valve replacement appears to be particularly increased with a 30-day mortality of up to 20% in patients in whom the etiology of mitral insufficiency is ischemic.[52]

Postoperative left ventricular ejection performance was generally found to be decreased compared with the preoperative data[10,21-23,46] although there are exceptions.[53,54] In most instances, reduction of ejection performance is related to a postoperative increase in afterload, although a true postoperative decrease in myocardial contractile state must also be taken into account in individual patients. The preservation of at least parts of the mitral apparatus appears to be important for postoperative left ventricular function because early postoperative ejection fraction did not decrease following valvuloplasty and valve replacement with preservation of chordae tendineae and papillary muscles in contrast to conventional mitral valve replacement.[55] The recommended indications for surgical therapy in mitral regurgitation, based on expected long-term results and their relation to preoperative left ventricular function, are summarized in Table 82.2.[56]

LONG-TERM MANAGEMENT

Patients with mechanical prostheses require lifelong anticoagulation with warfarin. After bioprosthetic mitral valve replacement, anticoagulation can be gradually discontinued after 2 to 3 months when there is sinus rhythm. When atrial fibrillation persists it appears prudent to continue anticoagulation especially in patients with large left atria. Following mitral valve reconstruction with persistent atrial fibrillation, both discontinuation after 6 weeks[47] and permanent[23] anticoagulation have been recommended. Afterload-reducing agents should be administered liberally in all patients with reduced ejection performance after mitral valve surgery.

AORTIC INSUFFICIENCY

Among patients with valvular heart disease about 10% have aortic insufficiency. Inadequate aortic valve closure results from shortening and retraction of the cusps following inflammatory damage, shrinkage of a congenitally bicuspid aortic valve, or dilatation of the aortic annulus and the ascending aorta due to connective tissue disorders or inflammation. In some patients one or more of these mechanisms may be causal. When the inflammatory or degenerative process leads to fusion of the commissures, proper opening of the valve is restricted and hence a stenotic component develops as well.

ETIOLOGY

Rheumatic heart disease is still considered the most frequent cause of chronic severe aortic insufficiency.[57] An aortic diastolic decrescendo murmur is often heard after the attack of rheumatic fever and it does not disappear, in contrast to the systolic murmur of transient rheumatic mitral insufficiency. Progressive retraction and shrinkage of a congenitally bicuspid valve may also lead to chronic aortic insufficiency. In both rheumatic heart disease and bicuspid valve, a more severe degree of aortic insufficiency develops over decades. Coexistence of coarctation and infective endocarditis aggravate aortic reflux in patients with bicuspid valves. Another congenital condition that can be associated with aortic insufficiency is the Fallot-type ventricular septal defect. In-

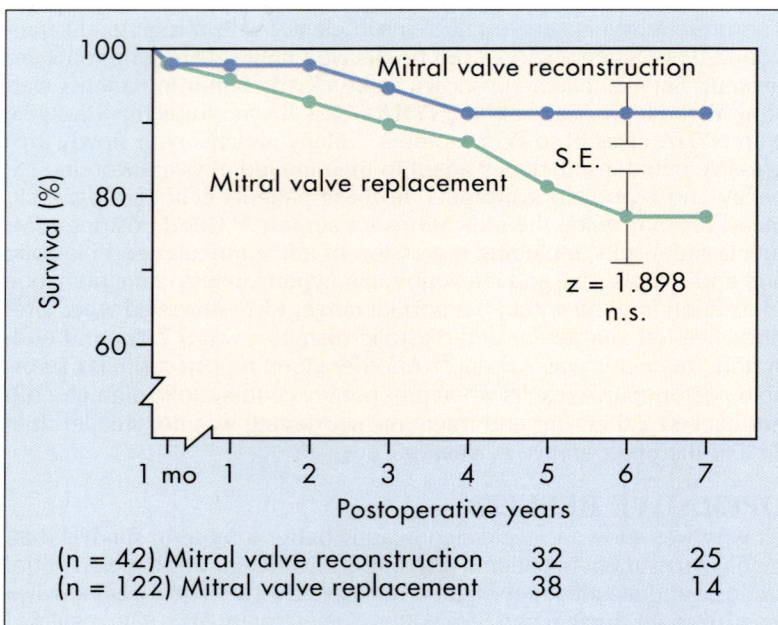

FIGURE 82.7 Actuarial survival after mitral reconstruction (n = 42) or replacement (n = 122) for mitral insufficiency, 1972 to 1982, Surgical Clinic A, University Hospital Zurich. There is a trend toward higher survival after mitral valve reconstruction than after valve replacement although statistical significance was not reached (z = 1.898). (S.E., standard error of the mean; n.s., not significant) (Modified from figure courtesy of Professor M. Rothlin)

TABLE 82.2 GUIDELINES FOR SELECTING PATIENTS WITH MITRAL REGURGITATION FOR OPERATION

1. The downhill clinical course is relatively gradual in chronic mitral regurgitation once symptoms begin, and left ventricular dysfunction may develop insidiously.
2. With significant *limiting symptoms* and severe mitral regurgitation, operation is usually indicated, provided left ventricular function is good or not severely depressed (ejection fraction <40%). Even when left ventricular function is sustained preoperatively, the ejection fraction will deteriorate to some degree after operation.
3. In patients with severe regurgitation who have *few or no symptoms*, operation should be considered to preserve left ventricular function, provided serial noninvasive studies of the left ventricle show ejection fraction <55%, fractional shortening <30%, plus either A or B:
   A. End-diastolic diameter approaching 75 mm and end-systolic diameter approaching 50 mm or 26 mm/m² body surface area (end-systolic volume approaching 60 ml/m²)
   B. Both an end-systolic diameter approaching 26 mm/m² and a radius/wall thickness ratio at end-systole × systolic pressure approaching 195 mm Hg

(Reprinted with permission from the American College of Cardiology. Ross J Jr: Afterload mismatch in aortic and mitral valve disease: Implications for surgical therapy. J Am Coll Cardiol 5:811, 1985)

sufficient support of the noncoronary aortic leaflet causes cusp prolapse and aortic reflux.

Chronic inflammations of both the proximal aorta as well as the aortic cusps can also cause chronic aortic insufficiency. These conditions include rheumatoid arthritis, ankylosing spondylitis, syphilis, and Reiter's disease. They are rare etiologies in patients who undergo aortic valve replacement.[57]

Failure of aortic valve closure may be the consequence of massive dilatation of the aortic annulus and/or the ascending aorta. Annulus dilatation is predominant in annuloaortic ectasia and in Marfan's syndrome. Dilatation of the ascending aorta is most commonly due to cystic medial necrosis with or without other signs of Marfan's syndrome. In the absence of primary involvement of the aortic annulus, aortic reflux is generally mild. It may, however, become acutely augmented with dissection of the ascending aorta. Dissection of ascending aorta without Marfan's disease may also cause aortic insufficiency. Other causes of aortic root disease that may be accompanied by aortic insufficiency are pseudoxanthoma elasticum, osteogenesis imperfecta, and Ehlers-Danlos and Hurler syndromes. Finally, aortic dilatation and insufficiency can result from longstanding arterial hypertension. Chronic severe aneurysm can also cause aortic root dilatation and hemodynamically insignificant aortic regurgitation.

Acute aortic insufficiency is most often due to infective endocarditis. The resulting severity of aortic regurgitation, however, is variable. The spectrum extends from massive backflow with rapid onset of left ventricular decompensation to mild or trivial aortic regurgitation of healed infective endocarditis. Other rare causes of aortic insufficiency are traumatic tear of the supporting structure of an aortic cusp and rupture of a congenitally fenestrated valve or a valve altered by myxomatous degeneration. Hemodynamically significant aortic regurgitation may also result from syphilis, with or without ascending aortic aneurysm.

PATHOPHYSIOLOGY

Diastolic aortic reflux represents primarily a volume overload for the left ventricle although some pressure overload may be present especially in elderly patients with increased systolic aortic pressure. The magnitude of aortic insufficiency is dependent on the diastolic aortic valve area, the diastolic gradient between aortic and left ventricular pressure, and the duration of diastole. Acute pharmacologic reduction of the peripheral resistance has been shown to be associated with a diminution of aortic reflux.[58] An increase in heart rate by right atrial pacing produced no consistent change in aortic regurgitant fraction[59] because the decrease of the duration of diastole and the increase of diastolic aortic pressure had opposite effects on the magnitude of regurgitant flow. By contrast, an increase in heart rate produced by dynamic exercise, which is associated with a decrease of peripheral resistance, leads to a decrease of aortic regurgitant fraction.[60,61] At moderately severe exercise, the decrease in regurgitant flow roughly equals the increase in forward flow. The decrease of regurgitant flow is associated with a decrease of left ventricular filling pressure provided that there is no myocardial failure.[60] Reduction of regurgitant flow, which contributes to increased forward flow and decrease of left ventricular filling pressure, explains why patients with severe aortic insufficiency may be asymptomatic and have normal physical work capacity over many years.

The increased systolic outflow into the ascending aorta and the diastolic leak into the left ventricle cause the increased pulse pressure typical of chronic aortic insufficiency. Because diastolic aortic pressure is reduced, coronary perfusion pressure is below normal. Reduced perfusion pressure and increase of myocardial O_2 requirements consequent to the increase in left ventricular muscle mass may cause an imbalance of myocardial oxygen supply/demand ratio that has been observed in some patients with aortic insufficiency during exercise.[62]

Aortic diastolic backflow leads to a sizable enlargement of the left ventricular cavity. The left ventricular wall thickness is at the upper limit of normal or slightly increased.[8,63,64] Left ventricular hypertrophy is of the eccentric type, which is thought to be achieved by a replication of sarcomeres in series. This particular "hypertrophy in length" may explain why in some patients left ventricular end-diastolic pressure is normal or minimally increased despite massive enlargement of the left ventricular cavity. To conclude from this finding that left ventricular diastolic compliance is increased, however, is misleading because instantaneous diastolic pressure–dimension and stress–strain relations were shown in most patients not to be different from normal controls.[65]

Mean systolic wall stress and peak systolic wall stress are increased in many patients with chronic aortic insufficiency.[8,66,67] There is no rapid systolic unloading as in mitral insufficiency. Hence, in aortic insufficiency the left ventricle is confronted with an elevated afterload throughout the major part of ejection. In operative patients with aortic insufficiency left ventricular end-diastolic wall stress is increased.[8,68]

A longstanding increase in preload *and* afterload in chronic aortic insufficiency finally causes myocardial dysfunction. A key point of beginning depression of left ventricular function is an increase of left ventricular end-diastolic volume disproportionate to the regurgitant stroke volume.[69] It is important to detect the beginning of myocardial depression so not to miss the optimal time for surgery.

The impact of the regurgitant jet may create left ventricular endocardial pockets that are localized mainly on the interventricular septum. The anterior mitral leaflet may show abnormal diastolic motion ("reverse doming" or "diastolic indentation") as an effect of significant aortic backflow.[70] Moreover, localized thickening of the anterior mitral leaflet may occur.

The ascending aorta dilates in chronic aortic insufficiency. This dilatation may itself intensify aortic reflux by further compromising leaflet apposition through traction on the cusps. Massive enlargement of the left ventricle leads to dilatation of the mitral annulus and, as a consequence, mitral insufficiency may ensue. In acute aortic insufficiency, massive reflux in a nonenlarged left ventricular chamber causes diastolic left ventricular pressure to rise to very high levels (Fig. 82.8). The mitral valve closes prematurely and hence prevents the

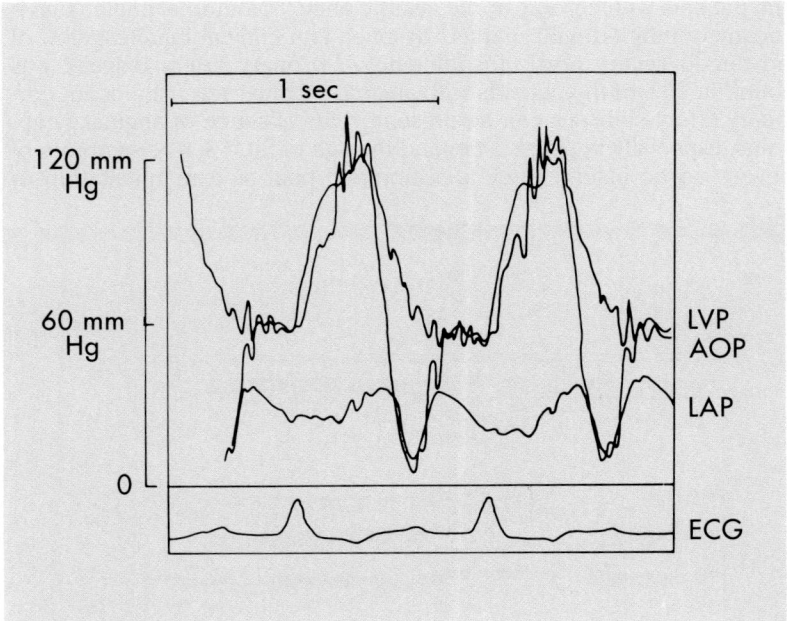

FIGURE 82.8 Severe subacute aortic insufficiency following bacterial endocarditis in a 58-year-old man. Note that 110 msec prior to the QRS, left ventricular pressure exceeds left atrial pressure leading to premature mitral valve closure (confirmed by echocardiography). Early mitral valve closure prevents the transmission of the high late diastolic left ventricular pressure to the pulmonary vascular bed. (*LVP,* left ventricular pressure; *AOP,* central aortic pressure; *LAP,* left atrial pressure; *ECG,* electrocardiogram)

transmission of the high left ventricular pressure to the pulmonary vascular bed.

NATURAL HISTORY AND PROGNOSIS

Mild aortic insufficiency is well tolerated, with a 10-year survival rate of 85% to 95%. In more severe aortic insufficiency 10-year survival rate after diagnosis is approximately 50%.[15] Younger patients diagnosed with severe aortic insufficiency in their early twenties seem to fare better. They were reported to have a 10-year survival of about 60%.[71] About 50% of patients with rheumatic aortic insufficiency followed since the end of an attack of rheumatic fever who developed moderate to marked left ventricular enlargement, ECG abnormalities including strain and hypertrophy, and diastolic blood pressure < 40 mm Hg either died or had left ventricular failure or angina within two years.[72] Congestive heart failure has an especially bad prognosis since 90% of these patients died within two years.[73] Patients in NYHA class III and IV scheduled for operation but finally not operated on for various reasons had a 5-year survival of only 37%.[74] In contrast to this grave prognosis of symptomatic patients with moderate to severe aortic insufficiency, asymptomatic patients with normal ejection performance at rest have a favorable prognosis. During a mean follow-up of 49 months none died and less than 4% per year required aortic valve replacement because symptoms of left ventricular dysfunction developed.[75] Nevertheless, even asymptomatic patients may die suddenly,[72,76] especially patients with a cardiothoracic ratio ≥ 0.60 or a left ventricular end-diastolic volume index > 200 ml/m^2.[77] The presence of ventricular premature beats was found to be associated with an overall increased mortality rate.[76]

SYMPTOMS AND PHYSICAL EXAMINATION
SYMPTOMS

Symptoms occur late in the time course of chronic aortic insufficiency. When exertional dyspnea becomes manifest, moderate to severe aortic insufficiency has been present for about 10 years. In NYHA class II patients left ventricular ejection performance is slightly to moderately depressed.[64] Palpitations and pounding sensations in the chest are frequent symptoms. Chest pain typical of angina occurs in about 20% of the patients with chronic aortic insufficiency.[78] Nocturnal angina that is mostly combined with marked dyspnea is a clinical manifestation of advanced severe aortic insufficiency. Coronary artery disease was found in 20% of the patients with angina.[79] Conversely, significant coronary artery stenoses can be present in the absence of anginal symptoms, especially in patients beyond the age of 50.[80] A rare symptom of severe aortic insufficiency is abdominal pain as a manifestation of splanchnic ischemia. In aortic root disease the patients may complain of chronic dull oppression within the chest.

INSPECTION

In chronic severe aortic insufficiency there are marked pulsations of the carotid arteries and of the aorta visible in the suprasternal region. The arterial pulsations may be transmitted to the surrounding tissues, resulting in pulse-synchronous movements of the head (Musset's sign), of the uvula (Müller's sign), and the larynx (Oliver-Cardarelli's sign). Capillary pulsations can be observed on the fingertips or the lips using slight compression with a glass slide.

PALPATION

The arterial pulse is characterized by abrupt distention and rapid fall mimicking a waterhammer (Corrigan's pulse). In the presence of a stenotic component, a bisferiens pulse is typical. In the parasternal region and in the carotid arteries a systolic thrill may be palpable. Its presence does not imply additional aortic stenosis. A diastolic thrill palpable in the upper right parasternal region is a rare finding (Fig. 82.9). It occurs with perforation or retroversion of a cusp. The apical systolic impulse is displaced laterally and caudally into the sixth intercostal space.

BLOOD PRESSURE

The pulse pressure is increased to 80 mm Hg and higher in severe chronic aortic insufficiency. This increase is due to both an increase in systolic arterial pressure and, most importantly, to a decrease in diastolic arterial pressure. Diastolic arterial pressure must be determined by the criterion of muffling of the Korotkoff sounds because they are often audible down to zero pressure. Below the age of 40, severe chronic aortic insufficiency is excluded when the diastolic arterial pressure is 70 mm Hg or higher. In elderly patients with higher systemic vascular resistance severe aortic insufficiency may be present with diastolic blood pressure ranging between 70 mm Hg and 90 mm Hg.

AUSCULTATION

A pistol shot sound is heard over the femoral arteries in moderate and severe chronic aortic insufficiency. When this early systolic sound is also present over the brachial arteries, aortic reflux is generally severe. A mild aortic stenotic component abolishes the pistol shot regardless of how severe aortic diastolic reflux is. With slight compression of the femoral artery by the stethoscope, a systolic–diastolic murmur (Duroziez's sign) may be heard. The diastolic component signals the diastolic backflow.

S_1 is soft whereas S_2 is accentuated but may become soft in severe regurgitation. In early systole there is an ejection click and in two thirds

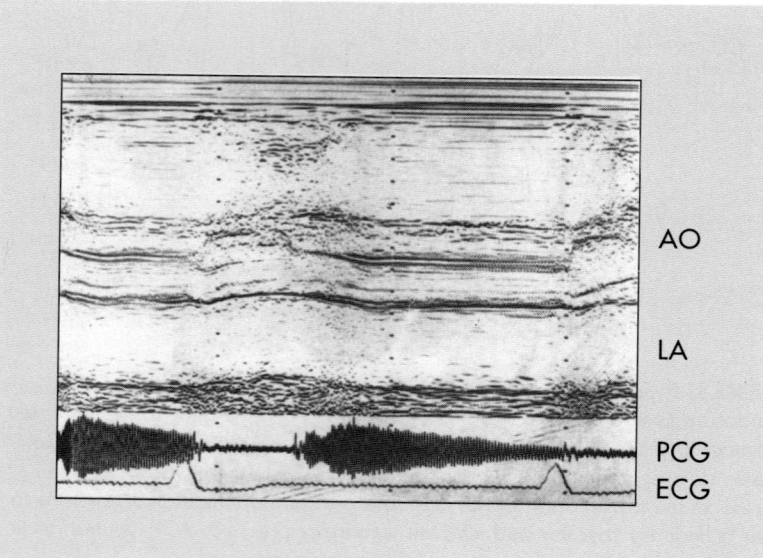

FIGURE 82.9 M-mode echocardiogram, phonocardiogram (PCG) in the second intercostal space in the right parasternal position, and lead II of the electrocardiogram (ECG) of a 72-year-old man with chronic aortic insufficiency. In the second right intercostal space a diastolic thrill was palpable. The aortic cusps show diastolic vibrations of a frequency similar to that of the diastolic murmur of the PCG. At surgery, perforations of the noncoronary and the left coronary aortic cusp were found. (AO, ascending aorta; LA, left atrium)

of patients with moderate to severe aortic insufficiency an early diastolic filling sound has been reported.[81] The S_3 gallop sound appears to be a marker of left ventricular dysfunction.

The high-pitched diastolic decrescendo murmur of chronic aortic insufficiency starts immediately after A_2. It is best heard in the parasternal region, in the second intercostal space on the right, and in the third and fourth intercostal spaces on the left with the patient in the sitting position and leaning forward. The diastolic murmur of mild aortic insufficiency extends about to mid-diastole whereas in moderate to severe aortic insufficiency it occupies all of diastole. In some patients the diastolic murmur is musical. It is known as the "seagull cry" or "dove coo" murmur.[82] A systolic ejection-type murmur is invariably present in aortic insufficiency. It is due to turbulence consequent to the increased systolic flow across the aortic valves.

In severe aortic insufficiency a diastolic rumble may be heard at the apex (Austin Flint murmur). This murmur is caused by turbulent antegrade flow across a closing mitral orifice. Partial mitral closure is produced by the rapid rise in diastolic left ventricular pressure consequent to massive aortic reflux. The Austin Flint murmur is differentiated from the diastolic rumble of organic mitral stenosis by the absence of a loud S_1 and of an opening snap. The intensity of the Austin Flint murmur is increased by vasopressors and isometric exercise.

In *acute severe aortic insufficiency* there are some particular findings with physical examination. The pulse pressure is not widened, there is tachycardia, and the aortic regurgitant murmur terminates prematurely at mid-diastole. The Austin Flint murmur is short without presystolic accentuation. S_1 is absent because the mitral valve closes in diastole. Sometimes a closure sound is produced and slight diastolic mitral regurgitation may occur, but a diastolic mitral regurgitant murmur is only detected by left atrial intracardiac phonocardiography.[40]

NONINVASIVE TESTS
ELECTROCARDIOGRAM
Patients with chronic aortic insufficiency are in sinus rhythm except far-advanced cases with secondary mitral insufficiency in whom atrial fibrillation occurs. The PR interval is prolonged in one fifth to one third of the patients. Left ventricular hypertrophy (Sokolow index ≥ 3.5 mV) may be the only ECG abnormality. When ST segment depression and T inversion are present, survival is impaired.[72] Bundle branch block and precordial QS waves are late manifestations. Twenty-four-hour electrocardiographic monitoring may reveal complex ventricular arrhythmias regardless of symptoms; the severity of arrhythmia was shown to be inversely related to left ventricular ejection fraction.[83]

RADIOLOGY
Severity and duration of aortic insufficiency determine the size of the heart. The left ventricle enlarges in a lateral and caudal direction. When the cardiothoracic ratio exceeds 0.60, the prognosis is compromised.[77] A ratio ≥ 0.64 was associated with a high rate of postoperative myocardial death and poor functional results in survivors.[84] The ascending aorta is dilated and elongated. More massive aneurysmal dilatation signals aortic root disease (annuloaortic ectasia, cystic medial necrosis) (Fig. 82.10). Aortic valvular calcifications are uncommon. In acute aortic insufficiency the heart size is little altered, but pulmonary stasis may be marked.

ECHOCARDIOGRAPHY
Of diagnostic importance is diastolic fluttering of the anterior mitral leaflet and of its chordae and eventually of an endocardial pocket of the interventricular septum. It is produced by the impact of the aortic diastolic backflow on these structures. Even mild aortic reflux is generally associated with fluttering of the anterior mitral leaflet. No fluttering is observed when the mitral leaflets are rigid as in organic mitral stenosis. Massive aortic backflow may lead to premature mitral valve closure. When the latter occurs, surgery is indicated.

Echocardiography may be helpful in defining the etiology of aortic insufficiency because it allows the detection of aortic valve vegetations, flail leaflet, and cusp retraction in aortic root disease. A prolapsing aortic leaflet may exhibit diastolic fluttering whereby the frequency of the vibrations is such as to produce a thrill and a musical murmur (see Fig. 82.9). Severe diastolic reflux in acute or subacute aortic insufficiency is eventually associated with premature opening of the aortic valve, which is caused either by the elastic recoil of the septum when the mitral valve closes prematurely, or by atrial contraction.[85]

The end-diastolic and end-systolic transverse diameters of the left ventricular cavity and systolic fractional shortening are important measures for assessing size and function of the left ventricle. Originally an end-systolic diameter > 5.5 cm and a fractional shortening $< 25\%$ were associated with poor postoperative survival.[86] More recent studies,[87,88] however, could not confirm the predictive value of these measures. The systolic fractional shortening as determined by M-mode

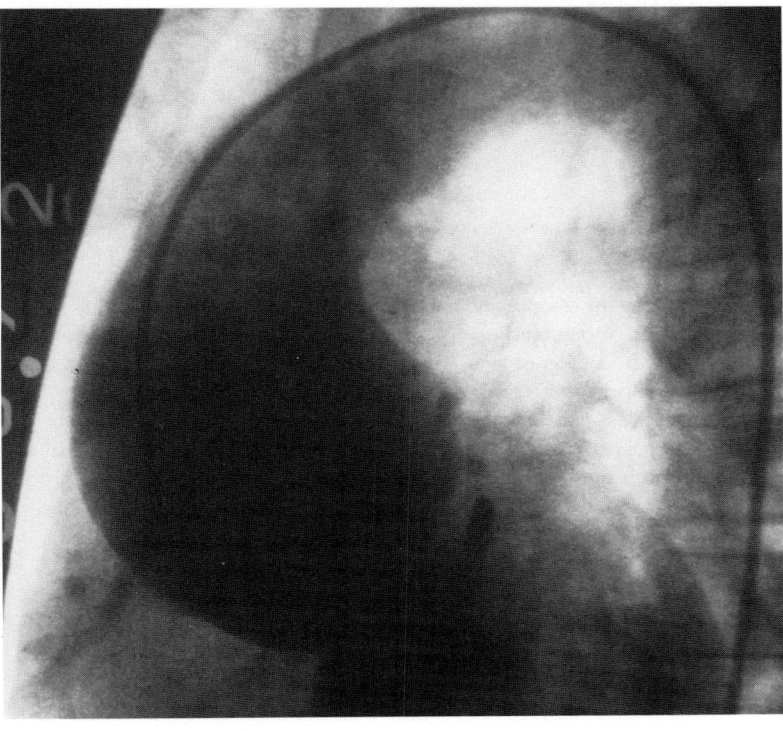

FIGURE 82.10 Massive annuloaortic ectasia in a 31-year-old man. The maximal diameter of the ascending aorta was 7.0 cm. There is regurgitation of contrast dye into the left ventricle following supra-aortic injection. Aortic regurgitant fraction from combined left ventricular volumetric measurements and cardiac output estimation by Fick amounted to 0.58. At surgery a composite graft was implanted.

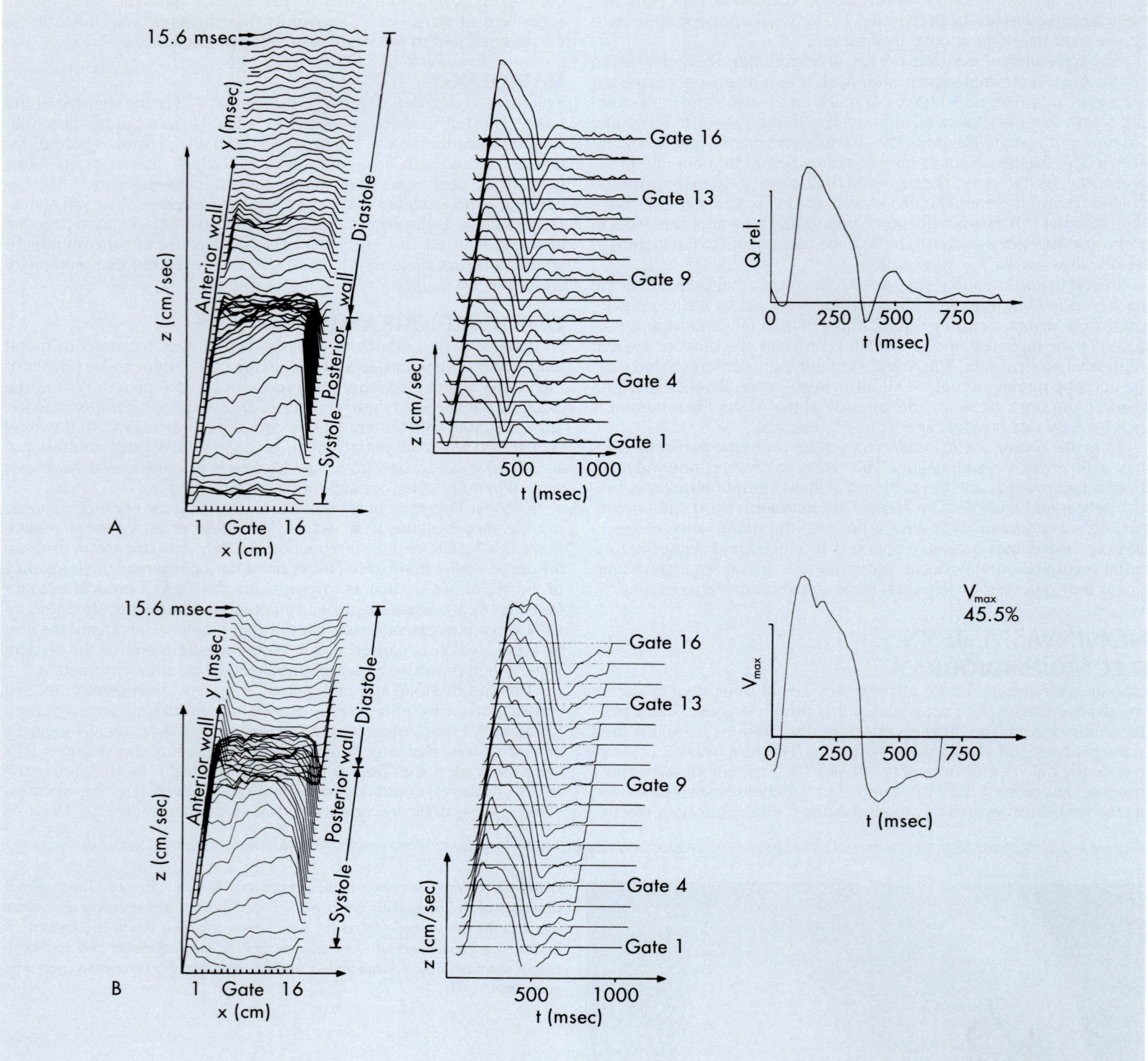

FIGURE 82.11 A. Velocity patterns in the ascending aorta of a 30-year-old normal woman obtained with a 16-gate pulsed Doppler–echo system. The plot contains the full set of velocity profiles of one cardiac cycle. The x axis corresponds to the depth divided into 16 gates, the y axis to the time within the cardiac cycle, and the z axis to the velocity. In the middle the velocity waveforms as a function of time are plotted for the 16 single-gates and to the right the weighted instantaneous mean velocity (Q rel.) is depicted. Note that there is only a short-lasting minimal backflow early in diastole. **B.** Velocity patterns in the ascending aorta of a 44-year-old woman with moderate to severe chronic aortic insufficiency. Again to the left the full set of velocity profiles of one cardiac cycle is shown. In the middle the velocity waveforms as a function of time are plotted for the 16 single-gates and to the right a composite waveform based on the instantaneous individual maximal velocities is shown. The area of the diastolic portion of the curve (backflow) amounts to 45.5% of the systolic portion. Although not identical to the hemodynamic aortic regurgitant fraction, the ratio of diastolic area/systolic area has been shown to correlate favorably with the invasively determined aortic regurgitant fraction.[94]

echocardiography overestimates left ventricular ejection performance, because shortening in the orthogonal minor axis is clearly less as documented by biplane cineventriculography.[89] Therefore, an echocardiographic value of 25% to 30% corresponds to a marked depression of ejection performance, frequently associated with left ventricular decompensation.[90]

DOPPLER ECHOCARDIOGRAPHY

Aortic insufficiency is detected reliably by examining the high left ventricular outflow tract during diastole with pulsed or color Doppler echocardiography (Figs. 82.11–82.13). Even clinically silent aortic reflux may be diagnosed correctly using this technique. Several indexes for assessing the severity of aortic insufficiency have been derived from Doppler studies and were shown to correlate well with semiquantitative angiographic measures of aortic reflux. This includes the distance from the aortic valves at which diastolic reflux is detected within the left ventricular cavity,[91] the ratio of end-diastolic amplitude of retrograde flow/maximal amplitude of systolic forward flow in the aortic arch,[92] and the regurgitant aortic valvular area explored by pulsed Doppler.[93] Figure 82.11, A and B, show the flow velocities in the ascending aorta obtained by multigated Doppler of a control subject and of a patient with chronic aortic insufficiency. The ratio of diastolic area/systolic area was shown to agree within ±15% with the aortic regurgitant fraction determined from quantitative angio-Fick studies.[94] Similarly to the estimation of mitral regurgitation fraction, aortic regurgitation fraction can be determined from continuous wave Doppler spectra based on the calculation of time integrals of amplitude-weighted mean velocities (Fig. 82.14). The aortic regurgitation fraction corresponds to the quotient systolic integral (left ventricular outflow tract) − systolic integral (right ventricular outflow tract)/systolic integral (left ventricular outflow tract).[95]

RADIOISOTOPE STUDIES

Radioisotope techniques have been used for both the quantification of aortic insufficiency[18,61] and the evaluation of ejection performance in these patients.[61,96–98] Failure of the ejection fraction to increase during dynamic exercise is considered a useful marker of early left ventricular dysfunction in asymptomatic or minimally symptomatic patients.[96,98] In contrast, a normal exercise response of ejection fraction may not necessarily be a reliable indicator of normal left ventricular function because such responses have been observed in patients with depressed ejection fraction at rest.[97] Furthermore, in the absence of depressed contractile function, ejection fraction may decrease during exercise if there is an excessive rise in arterial pressure, which increases systolic wall stress.

SYSTOLIC TIME INTERVALS

The carotid pulse tracing is characterized by a rapid upstroke and the absence of a clear-cut incisura. A double peak (bisferiens) is sometimes present, especially in patients with a component of aortic stenosis. The left ventricular ejection time is prolonged, although less than in patients with aortic stenosis.

PHYSICAL WORKING CAPACITY

Despite severe chronic aortic insufficiency, physical working capacity may be normal over many years. However, when a slight reduction of physical working capacity ensues, measures of left ventricular function are markedly depressed.[64] Moreover, in symptomatic patients a reduced exercise capacity was shown to be a predictor of unfavorable postoperative survival and compromised reversibility of left ventricular dilatation and dysfunction.[98]

PULMONARY FUNCTION

In one fifth of the patients with chronic aortic insufficiency vital capacity was found to be below 80% of normal. The reduction occurs predominantly in patients with severe aortic insufficiency and greatly enlarged left heart chambers.[60]

HEMODYNAMICS AND ANGIOCARDIOGRAPHY

Invasive evaluation of patients with clinically moderate to severe chronic aortic insufficiency is indicated when patients are symptomatic, cardiothoracic ratio exceeds 0.55, repolarization disturbances (ST segment depression, inverted T waves) are present, or echocardiographic left ventricular transverse diameter shortening is below 30%

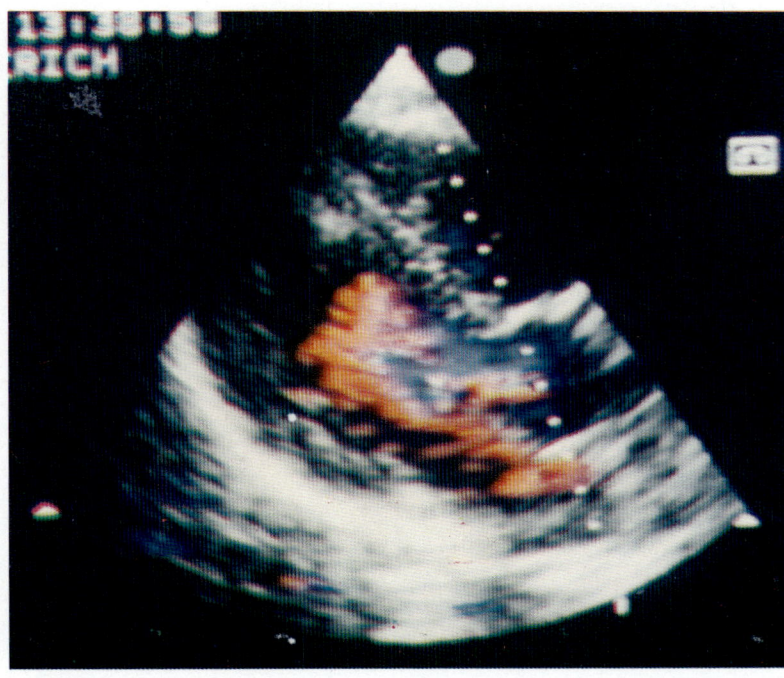

FIGURE 82.12 Qualitative assessment of diastolic aortic reflux by color Doppler in a 24-year-old man with moderately severe pure aortic insufficiency. The regurgitant flow (blue) encounters the mitral inflow (red) in the left ventricular cavity during diastole.

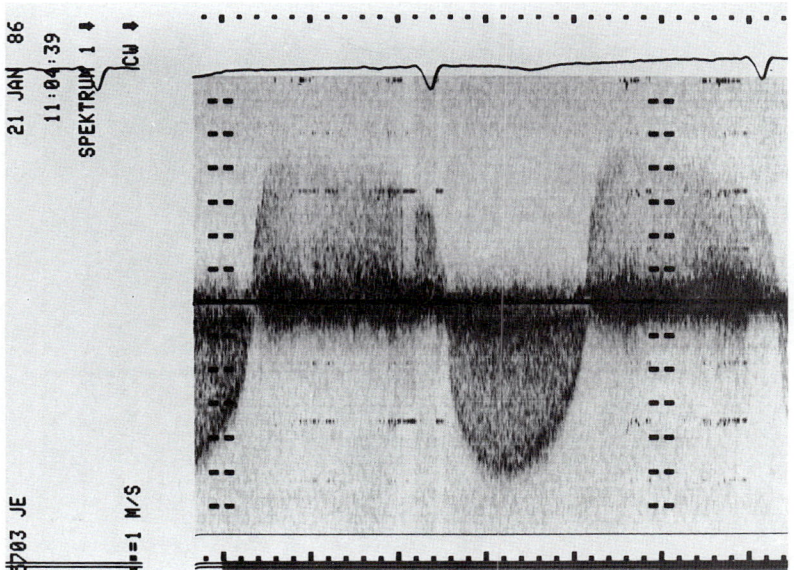

FIGURE 82.13 Qualitative assessment of diastolic aortic reflux by continuous wave Doppler in a 57-year-old woman with combined aortic valve lesion. The diastolic reflux is depicted above the zero line (diastolic flow toward the transducer located at the cardiac apex). The systolic peak velocity across the stenotic aortic valve is 5 m/sec (peak gradient = $5^2 \cdot 4 = 100$ mm Hg).

and the end-diastolic diameter exceeds 70 mm. Whether an abnormal response of ejection fraction during exercise alone, in the absence of resting left ventricular dysfunction and more marked left ventricular enlargement, justifies catheterization is a matter of debate. In general, it is probably in order to postpone catheterization, because in a well documented long-term study of patients with a normal preoperative ejection fraction at rest, it has been shown that an abnormal exercise response has no impact on the postoperative prognosis in regard to survival, resting ejection fraction, or ejection fraction response during exercise.[100]

The central aortic pressure curve shows the typically enhanced difference between peak systolic and end-diastolic pressure. Following an extrasystole, if aortic and left ventricular pressure equilibrate at end-diastole, aortic insufficiency is severe. A clearly demarcated *a* wave is absent in the left ventricular pressure curve because after atrial contraction there is no drop in left ventricular pressure due to the ongoing filling through the aortic leak. Hence, there may be difficulties in determining left ventricular end-diastolic pressure which is then measured at the peak of the R wave of the ECG.

Semiquantitative assessment of the severity of aortic insufficiency has been carried out by measuring the maximal regurgitant distance of green dye injected into the descending aorta and from visual evaluation of left ventricular opacification following injection of contrast dye into the aortic root. Quantification of aortic reflux in terms of regurgitant fraction (regurgitant volume per beat/forward volume crossing the aortic valves during systole) is achieved by indicator dilution techniques, videodensitometry, and, most commonly, by combining angiographic volumetry and cardiac output estimation with the Fick or dye dilution technique.[59] A regurgitant fraction smaller than 0.3 corresponds to mild, a fraction of 0.3 to 0.5 to moderate, and a fraction of >0.5 to severe aortic insufficiency.

In chronic aortic insufficiency left ventricular end-diastolic volume is increased twofold to threefold. In several small surgical series the average value of left ventricular end-diastolic volume index varied between 168 ml/m^2 and 218 ml/m^2 (normal, up to 120 ml/m^2).[22,64,101-104] In the same cohorts the average left ventricular ejection fraction varied between 43% and 54%, being below 50% in 4[22,64,101-104] of the 6. An ejection fraction below 50% was reported to be associated with in-creased postoperative mortality and incomplete recovery of pump function.[104,105]

The incidence of significant coronary artery disease in patients with severe aortic insufficiency is smaller than in aortic stenosis. It was reported to be 17% based on preoperative coronary arteriography in patients 36 to 72 years of age (mean, 54 years),[106] and 19% in necropsy patients 34 to 77 years of age (mean, 54 years).[107] This incidence justifies preoperative coronary arteriography in patients over 40 years of age with chronic aortic insufficiency.

DIAGNOSIS AND DIFFERENTIAL DIAGNOSIS

The high-pitched diastolic decrescendo murmur, best heard in the second right and the third left intracostal spaces, together with the increased pulse pressure and the reduced diastolic arterial pressure, is the cornerstone of the diagnosis of chronic aortic insufficiency. Patients with *acute* aortic insufficiency are generally more symptomatic; the heart rate is increased, the systolic pressure is low normal, the pulse pressure is only slightly widened, and the diastolic aortic murmur is not high-pitched and may be rather short and may not extend through the entire diastole.

The differential diagnosis has to include the following: pulmonic insufficiency secondary to chronic pulmonary hypertension (high-pitched diastolic Graham Steell murmur), rupture of an aneurysm of a sinus of Valsalva into the right ventricle or the right atrium, patent ductus arteriosus, aortopulmonary window, coronary arteriovenous fistula, and venous hum.

MEDICAL TREATMENT

Because an increase in afterload is a substantial part of the increased left ventricular burden in chronic aortic insufficiency,[8] afterload-reducing agents have an important place in medical management. In acute studies, hydralazine reduced aortic regurgitant fraction and improved left ventricular ejection fraction and exercise hemodynamics.[58,108] With oral therapy, beneficial effects, including improved left ventricular performance and reduction of left ventricular size, were documented to last for several weeks[42] or months.[109] Moreover, the

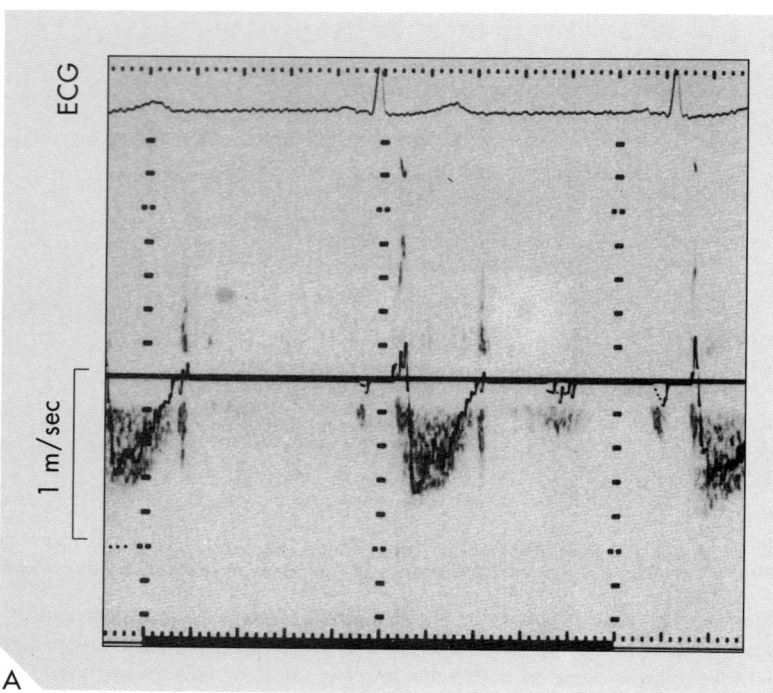 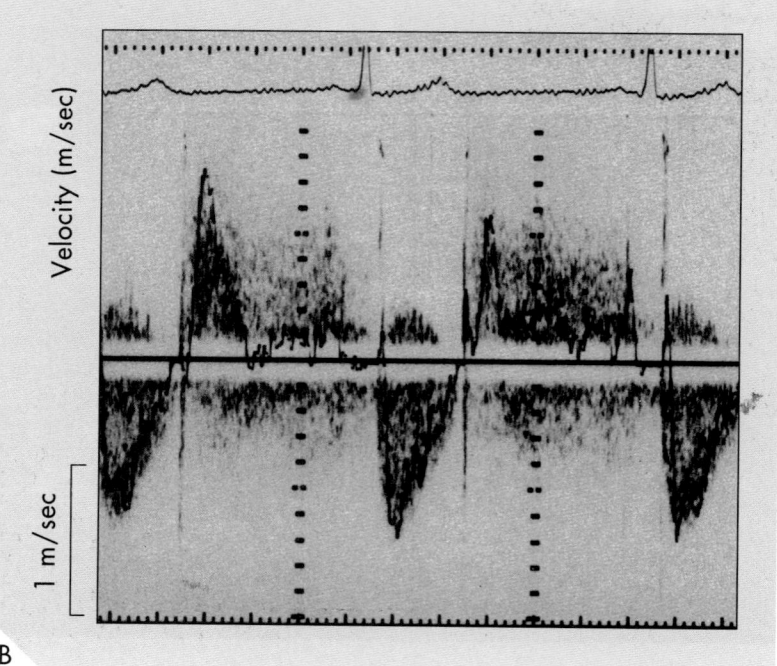

FIGURE 82.14 Quantitative assessment of aortic regurgitation from integrals of amplitude-weighted mean velocities obtained from continuous wave Doppler spectra in the right ventricular outflow tract (**A**) and the left ventricular outflow tract (**B**). The black continuous lines during systole represent the amplitude-weighted mean velocities. This is a 63-year-old man with pure aortic insufficiency (regurgitation fraction, 0.46).

need for aortic valve replacement was reduced in comparison with a placebo group.[110] Digitalis and diuretics are only indicated when there is left heart decompensation. Because bradycardia tends to increase aortic regurgitant fraction, digitalis therapy should be accompanied by vasodilators. This combined treatment is most effective for stabilizing severe decompensated patients who are awaiting surgery.

SURGICAL TREATMENT

Surgical treatment consists of aortic valve replacement with a mechanical or bioprosthetic valve. Additional aortic aneurysm may be treated by aortoplasty with net reinforcement, supracoronary graft, or composite graft with reimplantation of the coronary arteries. The latter type of surgery is particularly used when chronic aortic insufficiency is caused by annuloaortic ectasia.

INDICATION FOR SURGERY

There is no doubt that symptomatic patients should undergo aortic valve replacement without delay. Symptoms during exercise should be documented by objective stress testing. A marked reduction of physical working capacity defines a subset of patients with increased operative risk and reduced long-term survival.[99]

The attitude to adopt in asymptomatic patients with objectively proven normal physical working capacity is controversial because among these patients are some with already depressed left ventricular function. The rationale for recommending surgery is to preserve left ventricular function. The rationale for delaying operation is to expose the patient to a shorter period of being at risk of valve-related complications and to let him take the benefit of future refinements of operative technique, myocardial preservation, and prosthesis design.[111] Those who adopt the latter position indicate that valve replacement may still lead to a considerable improvement of left ventricular performance[68,104,112,113] in many patients operated on with left ventricular dysfunction. However, the bulk of the data indicate that preoperatively depressed left ventricular ejection performance,[86,105,114,115] large left ventricular end-diastolic volume,[104,116] large end-systolic volume,[22,112] and massively increased indexes of systolic wall stress[66,67] are markers of suboptimal functional response to valve replacement, as manifested by left ventricular dysfunction and congestive heart failure, or by postoperative death.[117] Hence, it appears appropriate to proceed to aortic valve replacement in asymptomatic patients when clearly abnormal left ventricular end-systolic or end-diastolic dimensions or depressed ejection performance is present. In asymptomatic patients with moderate to severe chronic aortic insufficiency having preserved left ventricular function at rest, follow-up at 6-month intervals is recommended. (An increase of left ventricular end-systolic diameter to >5 cm, of end-diastolic diameter to >7 cm, and a fall of fractional shortening below 30% appear realistic limits when aortic valve replacement should be envisaged.) The guidelines for recommendation of aortic valve replacement are summarized in Table 82.3.

OPERATIVE RESULTS

In series of aortic valve replacement published after 1979, perioperative mortality ranged between 2% and 15%, the average being 6%.[77,114,115,118-121] The 5-year survival after aortic valve replacement for aortic insufficiency varied between 63% and 86% (average 75%).[77,114,115,118,119] A comparison of two series operated between 1970 to 1974 and 1975 to 1979 shows that at similar perioperative mortality long-term survival was clearly better when surgery was performed prior to the onset of severe clinical and hemodynamic impairment as was the policy for the 1975 to 1979 period (Fig. 82.15).[77] The improved survival resulted from a massive reduction in the frequency of late postoperative death caused by heart failure.

The incidence of thromboembolic complications is similar for the

TABLE 82.3 GUIDELINES FOR SELECTING PATIENTS WITH AORTIC REGURGITATION FOR OPERATION

1. The downhill clinical course in chronic aortic regurgitation once significant symptoms occur is more gradual than in aortic stenosis, but if aortic regurgitation is severe and *limiting symptoms are present*, operation is usually indicated. Left ventricular systolic function is often normal, but even if it is moderately impaired, left ventricular size and function improve after operation.
2. In patients *without symptoms* who have normal or mildly impaired left ventricular function, careful follow-up with echocardiography is indicated, since deterioration of left ventricular function and onset of significant symptoms usually coincide.
3. Operation should be considered to prevent irreversible myocardial changes in patients in whom symptoms are *few or absent* when left ventricular dysfunction and enlargement become significant (confirmed by angiography): ejection fraction <40%, fractional shortening <25%, plus either A or B:
   A. Left ventricular end-diastolic diameter approaching 70 mm or 38 mm/m² body surface area (end-diastolic volume index approaching 200 ml/m²) and end-systolic diameter approaching 50 mm or 26 mm/m²
   B. Both end-systolic diameter approaching 26 mm/m² and a radius/wall thickness ratio at end-diastole × systolic pressure greater than 600

(Reprinted with permission from the American College of Cardiology. Ross J Jr: Afterload mismatch in aortic and mitral valve disease: Implications for surgical therapy. J Am Coll Cardiol 5:811, 1985)

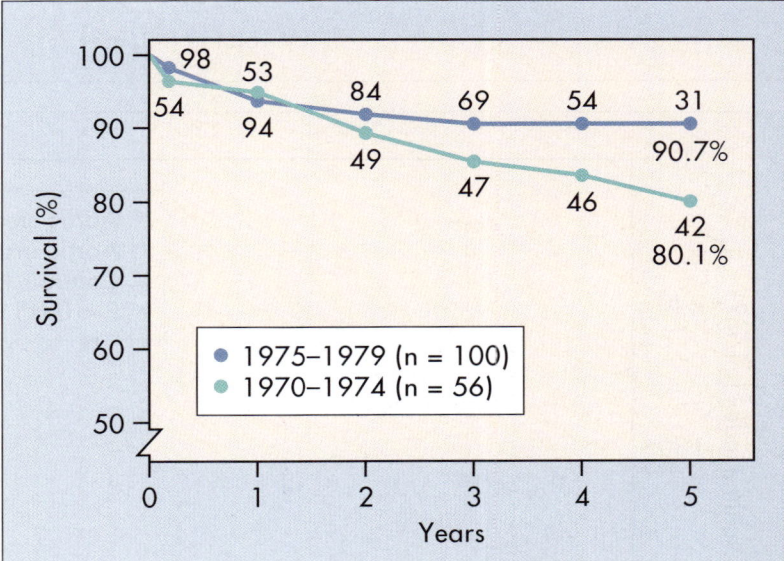

FIGURE 82.15 Survival in two groups of patients with chronic aortic insufficiency operated on from 1970 to 1974 (56 patients) and 1975 to 1979 (100 patients). The number of patients alive at the end of each period is indicated. The improvement in survival for the 1975 to 1979 period was the result of a reduction in frequency of death caused by postoperative heart failure (Modified from Turina J, Turina M, Rothlin M, Krayenbuehl HP: Improved late survival in patients with chronic aortic regurgitation by earlier operation. Circulation (Suppl) 70:I-147, 1984)

best aortic mechanical and bioprostheses.[122] It is slightly less than 2 per 100 patient-years.

When aortic valve replacement is associated with coronary revascularization, perioperative mortality is no longer significantly higher than in isolated aortic valve replacement.[121,123] Additional surgery of an ascending aortic aneurysm increases perioperative mortality (8% to 10%) if a graft (either supracoronary or composite) is implanted.[124,125] By contrast, aortoplasty in addition to aortic valve replacement is not associated with increased perioperative mortality.

Following aortic valve replacement, physical working capacity increases[64,126] and heart size decreases, although in most studies the average value of postoperative left ventricular end-diastolic volume was still above the upper limit of normal (Fig. 82.16).[127] The most marked decrease of left ventricular size occurs early, but further modest decreases in left ventricular end-diastolic diameter were documented at one year after surgery.[113] Return to an end-diastolic volume index indistinguishable from that of control subjects may require up to 85 months following valve replacement (Fig. 82.17).[128] There are, however, patients in whom left ventricular dimensions remain markedly increased despite good prosthetic valve function (Fig. 82.18).[113,116] Recovery of left ventricular ejection performance is less marked than in aortic stenosis. Four[101,102,104,129] of six angiographic studies[64,101,102,104,129,130] in which the average preoperative

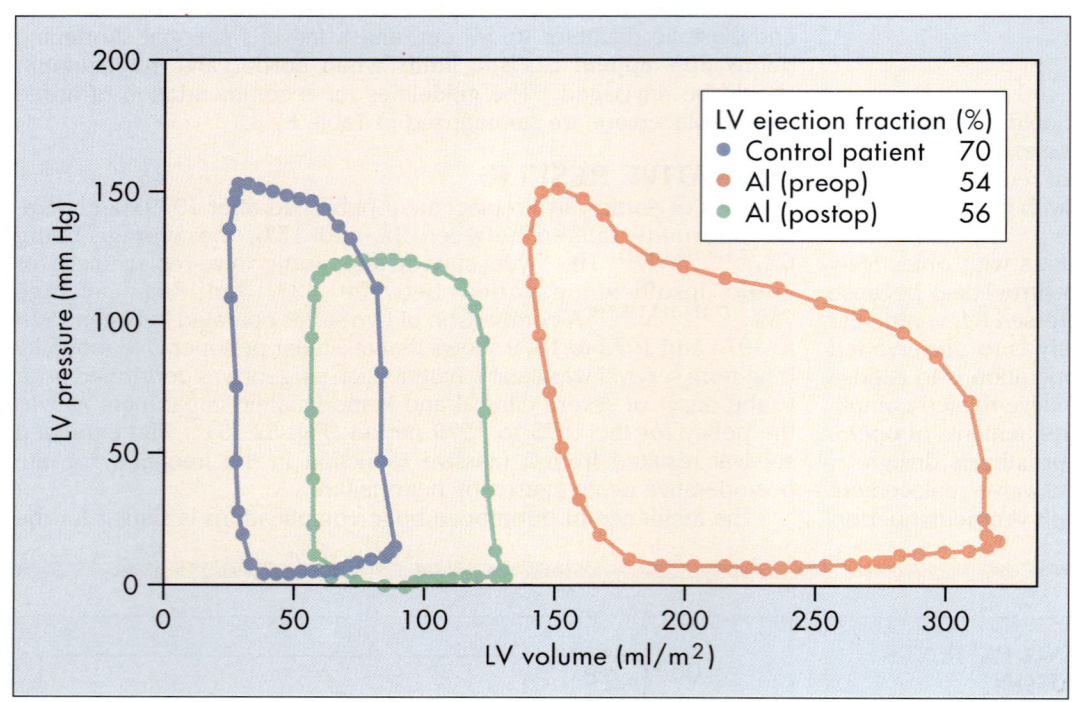

FIGURE 82.16 Left ventricular (LV) pressure–volume loops in a control patient (C) and in a 43-year-old male with severe chronic aortic insufficiency before and 25 months after successful aortic valve replacement with a Carpentier-Edwards prosthesis nr. 31. There was massive enlargement of the left ventricular cavity prior to surgery, but left ventricular ejection fraction (EF) was only minimally reduced. Aortic regurgitant fraction amounted to 0.67. Following surgery there was a substantial decrease of left ventricular volume although no normalization occurred. EF did not change.

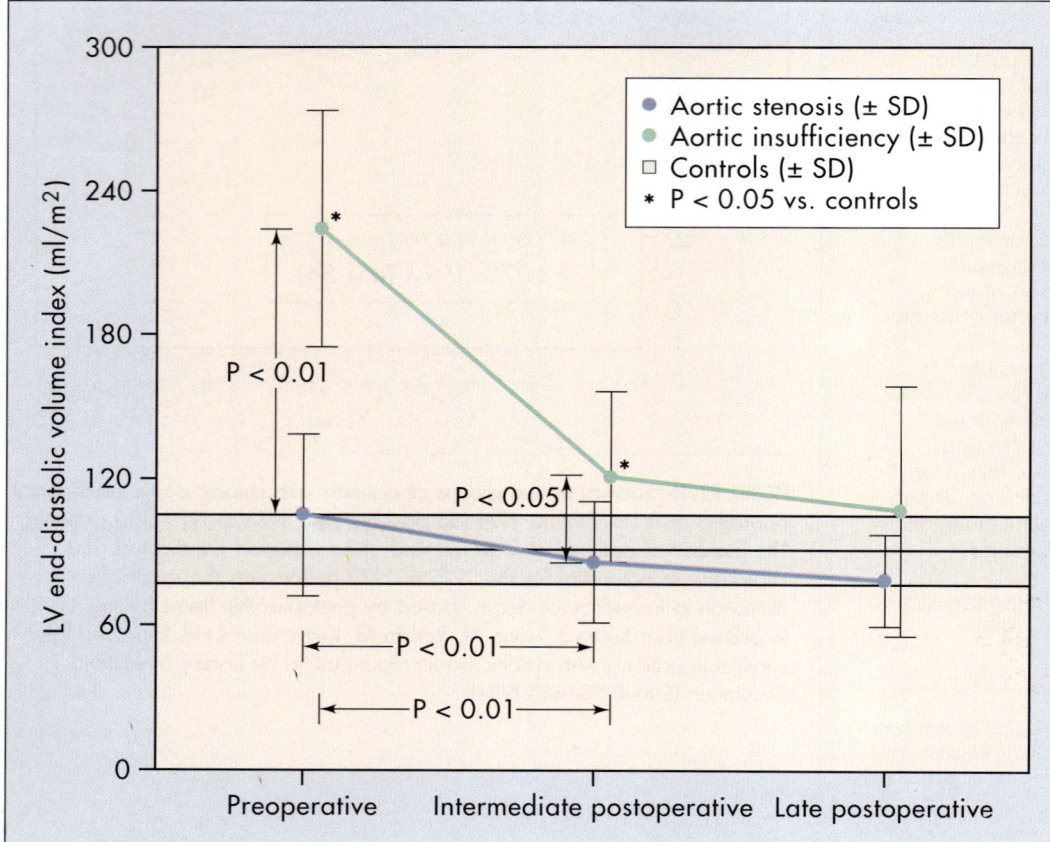

FIGURE 82.17 Left ventricular end-diastolic volume index in 11 patients with aortic stenosis and 10 patients with aortic insufficiency before, 19 and 20 months respectively (intermediate postoperative), and 108 and 85 months respectively (late postoperative) after valve replacement. The shaded area corresponds to the range found in controls (mean valve ± 1 SD). In the patients with aortic insufficiency, the left ventricular end-diastolic volume index is still significantly higher than the value in controls at the intermediate postoperative study. At 85 months postoperatively there was no difference between patients and controls. (Modified from Monrades et al., Circulation 77: 1345, 1988)

left ventricular ejection fraction was below normal reported no significant increase of ejection fraction following surgery.

LONG-TERM MANAGEMENT

Patients with mechanical prostheses require lifelong anticoagulation with warfarin whereas in patients with aortic bioprostheses anticoagulation can be gradually withdrawn after 6 to 8 weeks. During dental procedures, antibiotic prophylaxis for bacterial endocarditis is carried out. Arterial hypertension is not uncommon following aortic valve replacement and should be treated vigorously, especially when heart size is still increased. Angiotensin-converting enzyme inhibitors appear to be particularly useful because they reduce blood pressure and specifically help left ventricular muscle mass to regress. Patients with ejection performance below normal should undergo 24-hour ECG monitoring because they are at risk for complex ventricular arrhythmias.[83] It appears appropriate to treat such arrhythmias regardless of symptoms because sudden death has been reported to be the most frequent cause of late mortality in patients followed for 5 years after aortic valve replacement.[77]

PULMONIC INSUFFICIENCY

Isolated organic chronic pulmonic insufficiency is a condition that may remain undetected for a long period of time because the patients are largely asymptomatic. Because pulmonary hypertension is absent in these cases, this condition has been termed "low pressure" pulmonic insufficiency.[131] In contrast, relative or functional chronic pulmonic insufficiency is the consequence of dilatation of the valve ring in patients with longstanding pulmonary arterial hypertension. Unlike isolated organic pulmonic insufficiency the clinical manifestations of the underlying disease are generally severe and overshadow the pulmonic insufficiency, which is often an incidental auscultatory finding.[132] This is the "high pressure" type of pulmonic insufficiency,[131] which is characterized by the high-pitched diastolic Graham Steell murmur.

Chronic "low pressure" pulmonic insufficiency is due either to primary enlargement of the valve ring in massive dilatation of the main stem of the pulmonary artery (idiopathic dilatation or dilatation consequent to connective tissue disorders, such as in Marfan's syndrome) or to pulmonic valve involvement. Organic pulmonic valvular lesions resulting in chronic pulmonic insufficiency may be congenital, rheumatic,[133] due to healed bacterial endocarditis, or malignant carcinoid.[132] Pulmonic insufficiency is often found after valvotomy for pulmonic stenosis. Any chronic severe pulmonary arterial hypertension may lead to the relative "high pressure" pulmonic insufficiency. The most frequent causes are pulmonary hypertension in Eisenmenger's syndrome, primary (vascular) pulmonary hypertension, and advanced mitral valve disease.

On physical examination, patients with "low pressure" pulmonic insufficiency present with a normally sized or moderately enlarged heart. At the left parasternal area in the third and fourth intercostal space a systolic impulse is palpable. In "high pressure" pulmonic insufficiency a palpable pulmonic closure sound, a marked right ventricular parasternal heave, and signs of tricuspid insufficiency are characteristic features. At auscultation the diastolic pulmonic regurgitant murmur is fundamentally different in patients with "low" and those with "high pressure" pulmonic insufficiency. In the "low pressure" situation the diastolic murmur is low in pitch and crescendo–decrescendo in configuration. It begins with a short delay after the widely split second heart sound, the interval between P_2 and the onset of the murmur being on the order of 0.04 second. This short silent period is due to the fact that early after P_2 the pressures in the pulmonary artery and in the right ventricle are practically identical and it is only when the two pressure curves diverge (buildup of a gradient) that the murmur begins.[132] The peak intensity is reached when the pressure gradient is greatest. In "high pressure" pulmonic insufficiency the diastolic murmur (Graham Steell) is high-pitched, decrescendo in configuration and begins immediately after P_2, which is often fused with A_2. This murmur is almost identical to that of chronic aortic insufficiency. A presystolic low-frequency murmur may also be present; it is considered to be a right-sided Austin Flint murmur.

In "low pressure" pulmonic insufficiency the ECG and the echocardiogram show signs of mild to moderate right ventricular volume overload. Electrocardiographic and echocardiographic right ventricular hypertrophy, absence of an a wave and systolic notching of the posterior pulmonic cusp at echocardiography, and an abnormally short time to peak flow evaluated by pulsed Doppler[134] are all typical features of chronic pulmonary arterial hypertension and should be looked for when "high pressure" pulmonic insufficiency is suspected. An end-diastolic pressure gradient obtained by continuous wave Doppler between the pulmonary artery and the right ventricular outflow tract exceeding 12 mm Hg signals an elevated pulmonary arteriolar resistance.

Noninvasive proof of pulmonic insufficiency is probably best obtained by the combined two-dimensional echo–Doppler technique. With the sample volume in the right ventricular outflow tract, two pat-

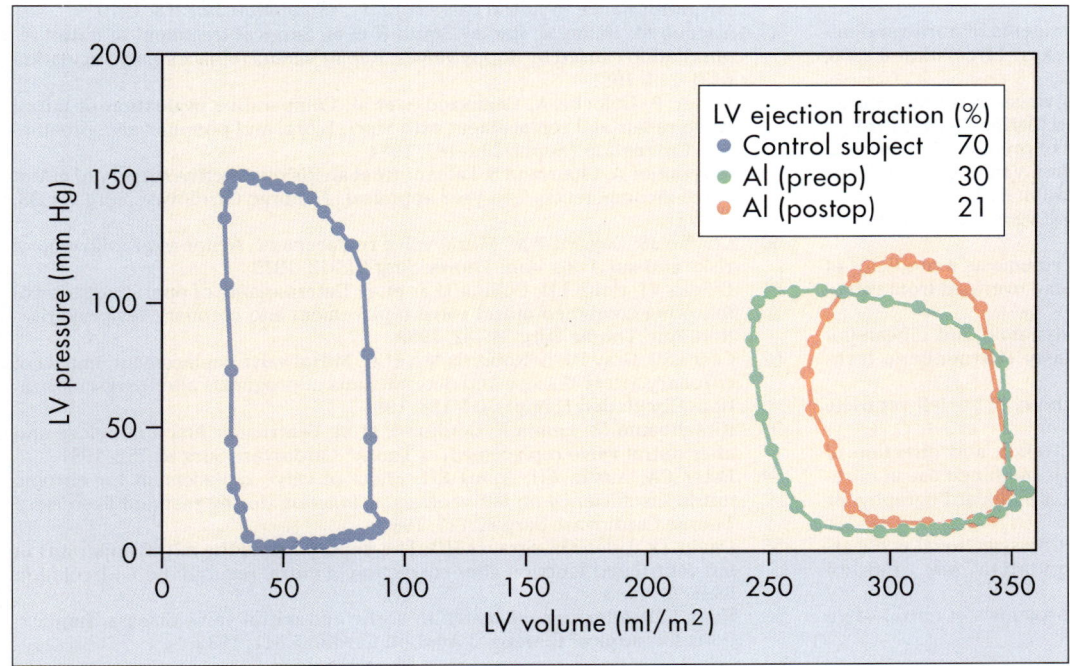

FIGURE 82.18 Left ventricular pressure–volume loops in a control subject (C) and in a 42-year-old male with chronic aortic insufficiency before and 13 months after aortic valve replacement by a Carpentier-Edwards prosthesis nr. 27. In contrast to the patient depicted in Figure 11, preoperative left ventricular ejection fraction (EF) was clearly depressed. Aortic regurgitation fraction amounted to 0.58. The functional result after aortic valve replacement was poor. Left ventricular end-diastolic volume remained massively enlarged and EF dropped to 21%. The patient died suddenly two years after valve replacement.

terns of pulmonic regurgitant Doppler signals have been described[135]: In pulmonary hypertension the maximal component of instantaneous flow velocity is sustained at about the same signal strength throughout diastole, whereas in patients with "low pressure" pulmonic insufficiency the velocity slows down gradually from early diastole to end-diastole. Invasively, pulmonic diastolic reflux can be documented by cineangiography or indicator dilution methods. The difficulty with these techniques is that they require the passage of a catheter across the pulmonic valves, which, by distorting the valves, may artificially induce pulmonic insufficiency.

Most patients with pulmonic insufficiency are managed medically. Surgery for chronic organic pulmonic insufficiency is rarely necessary. Indications include severe pulmonic reflux associated with elevated pulmonary vascular resistance and right ventricular failure.[136]

REFERENCES

1. Roberts WC, Perloff JK: Mitral valvular disease: A clinicopathologic survey of the conditions causing the mitral valve to function abnormally. Ann Intern Med 77:939, 1972
2. Selzer A, Katayama F: Mitral regurgitation: Clinical patterns, pathophysiology and natural history. Medicine 51:337, 1972
3. Amlie JP, Langmark F, Storstein O: Pure mitral regurgitation: Etiology, pathology and clinical patterns. Acta Med Scand 200:201, 1976
4. Waller BF, Morrow AG, Maron BJ et al: Etiology of clinically isolated, severe, chronic, pure mitral regurgitation: Analysis of 97 patients over 30 years of age having mitral valve replacement. Am Heart J 104:276, 1982
5. Antunes MJ, Colsen PR, Kinsley RH: Mitral valvuloplasty: A learning curve. Circulation 68:II-70, 1983
6. Edwards JE, Burchell HB: Pathologic anatomy of mitral insufficiency. Proc Mayo Clin 33:497, 1958
7. Braunwald E: Mitral regurgitation: Physiologic, clinical and surgical considerations. N Engl J Med 281:425, 1969
8. Wisenbaugh T, Spann JF, Carabello BA: Differences in myocardial performance and load between patients with similar amounts of chronic aortic versus chronic mitral regurgitation. J Am Coll Cardiol 3:916, 1984
9. Zile MR, Gaasch WH, Carroll JD, Levine HJ: Chronic mitral regurgitation: Predictive value of preoperative echocardiographic indexes of left ventricular function and wall stress. J Am Coll Cardiol 3:235, 1984
10. Phillips HR, Levine FH, Carter JE et al: Mitral valve replacement for isolated mitral regurgitation: Analysis of clinical course and late postoperative left ventricular ejection fraction. Am J Cardiol 48:647, 1981
11. Corin WJ, Monrad ES, Murakami T et al: The relationship of afterload to ejection performance in chronic mitral regurgitation. Circulation 76:59, 1987
12. Corvisart JN: Essai sur les Maladies et les Lésions Organiques du Coeur et des Gros Vaisseaux. De la Rupture Partielle du Coeur, p 256. Paris, Migneret, 1806
13. Hammermeister KE, Fisher L, Kennedy JW et al: Prediction of late survival in patients with mitral valve disease from clinical, hemodynamic, and quantitative angiographic variables. Circulation 57:341, 1978
14. Rapaport E: Natural history of aortic and mitral valve disease. Am J Cardiol 35:221, 1975
15. Pearlman AS, Scoblionko PP, Saal KA: Assessment of valvular heart disease by Doppler echocardiography. Clin Cardiol 6:573, 1983
16. Perry GJ, Nanda NC: Diagnosis and quantitation of valvular regurgitation by color Doppler flow mapping. Echocardiography 6:493, 1986
17. Jenni R, Ritter M, Eberli F et al: Quantification of mitral regurgitation with amplitude-weighted mean velocity from continuous wave Doppler spectra. Circulation 79:1294, 1989
18. Rigo P, Alderson PO, Robertson RM et al: Measurements of aortic and mitral regurgitation by gated cardiac blood pool scans. Circulation 60:306, 1979
19. Grose R, Strain J, Cohen MV: Pulmonary arterial V waves in mitral regurgitation: Clinical and experimental observations. Circulation 69:214, 1984
20. Carabello BA, Nolan SP, McGuire LB: Assessment of preoperative left ventricular function in patients with mitral regurgitation: Value of the end-systolic wall stress–end-systolic volume ratio. Circulation 64:1212, 1981
21. Huikuri HV: Effect of mitral valve replacement on left ventricular function in mitral regurgitation. Br Heart J 49:328, 1983
22. Borow KM, Green LH, Mann T et al: End-systolic volume as a predictor of postoperative left ventricular performance in volume overload from valvular regurgitation. Am J Med 68:655, 1980
23. Lessana A, Herreman F, Boffety C et al: Hemodynamic and cineangiographic study before and after mitral valvuloplasty (Carpentier's technique). Circulation (Suppl) 64:II-195, 1981
24. Vokonas PS, Gorlin R, Cohn PF et al: Dynamic geometry of the left ventricle in mitral regurgitation. Circulation 48:786, 1973
25. Miyatake K, Nimura Y, Sakakibara H et al: Localisation and direction of mitral regurgitant flow in mitral orifice studied with combined use of ultrasonic pulsed Doppler technique and two dimensional echocardiography. Br Heart J 48:449, 1982
26. Wann LS, Feigenbaum H, Weyman AE, Dillon JC: Cross-sectional echocardiographic detection of rheumatic mitral regurgitation. Am J Cardiol 41:1258, 1978
27. Mills P, Rose J, Hollingsworth J et al: Long-term prognosis of mitral-valve prolapse. N Engl J Med 297:13, 1977
28. Pyeritz RE, Wappel MA: Mitral valve dysfunction in the Marfan syndrome. Clinical and echocardiographic study of prevalence and natural history. Am J Med 74:797, 1983
29. Clemens JD, Horwitz RJ, Jaffe CC et al: A controlled evaluation of the risk of bacterial endocarditis in persons with mitral-valve prolapse. N Engl J Med 307:776, 1982
30. Barnett HJM, Boughner DR, Taylor DW et al: Further evidence relating mitral-valve prolapse to cerebral ischemic events. N Engl J Med 302:139, 1980
31. Chesler E, King RA, Edwards JE: The myxomatous mitral valve and sudden death. Circulation 67:632, 1983
32. Perloff JK, Child JS, Edwards JE: New guidelines for the clinical diagnosis of mitral valve prolapse. Am J Cardiol 57:1124, 1986
33. Levine RA, Triulzi MO, Harrigan P, Weyman AE: The relationship of mitral annular shape to the diagnosis of mitral valve prolapse. Circulation 75:756, 1987
34. Turina J, Simon R, Brunner HH et al: Linksventrikuläre Cineangiographie und Echokardiographie bei Patienten mit dem Syndrom mesosystolischer Klick–telesystolisches Geräusch. Schweiz Med Wochenschr 105:1539, 1975
35. Scampardonis G, Yang SS, Maranhao V et al: Left ventricular abnormalities in prolapsed mitral leaflet syndrome. Circulation 48:287, 1973
36. Müller F, Schneider J: Komplikationen des verkalten Anulus fibrosus mitralis des Herzens. Schweiz Med Wochenschr 110:1233, 1980
37. Kronzon I, Glassman E: Mitral ring calcification in idiopathic hypertrophic subaortic stenosis. Am J Cardiol 42:60, 1978
38. Boucher CA, Liberthson RR, Buckley MJ: Secundum atrial septal defect and significant mitral regurgitation: Incidence, management and morphologic basis. Chest 75:697, 1979
39. Rutishauser W, Wirz P, Gander M, Lüthy E: Atriogenic diastolic reflux in patients with atrioventricular block. Circulation 34:807, 1966
40. Reddy PS, Leon DF, Krishnaswami V et al: Syndrome of acute aortic regurgitation. In Physiologic Principles of Heart Sounds and Murmurs. American Heart Association Monograph 46:166, 1975
41. Greenberg BH, Massie BM, Brundage BH et al: Beneficial effects of hydralazine in severe mitral regurgitation. Circulation 58:273, 1978
42. Jensen T, Kornerup HJ, Lederballe O et al: Treatment with hydralazine in mild to moderate mitral or aortic incompetence. Eur Heart J 4:306, 1983
43. Greenberg BH, de Mots H, Murphy E, Rahimtoola SH: Arterial dilators in mitral regurgitation: Effects on rest and exercise hemodynamics and long-term clinical follow-up. Circulation 65:181, 1982
44. Salomon NW, Stinson EB, Griepp RB, Shumway NE: Surgical treatment of degenerative mitral regurgitation. Am J Cardiol 38:463, 1976
45. Peterson KL: The timing of surgical intervention in chronic mitral regurgitation. Editorial. Cathet Cardiovasc Diagn 9:433, 1983
46. Schuler G, Peterson KL, Johnson A et al: Temporal response of left ventricular performance to mitral valve surgery. Circulation 59:1218, 1979
47. Yacoub M, Halim M, Radley-Smith R et al: Surgical treatment of mitral regurgitation caused by floppy valves: Repair versus replacement. Circulation 64:II-210, 1981
48. Perier P, Deloche A, Chauvaud S et al: Comparative evaluation of mitral valve repair and replacement with Starr, Björk, and porcine valve prostheses. Circulation (Suppl) 70:I-187, 1984
49. Carpentier A, Chauvaud S, Fabiani JN et al: Reconstructive surgery of mitral valve incompetence. Ten-year appraisal. J Thorac Cardiovasc Surg 79:338, 1980
50. Chaffin JS, Daggett WM: Mitral valve replacement: A nine-year follow-up of risks and survivals. Ann Thorac Surg 27:312, 1979
51. DiSesa VJ, Cohn LH, Collins JJ Jr et al: Determinants of operative survival following combined mitral valve replacement and coronary revascularization. Ann Thorac Surg 34:482, 1982
52. Czer LSC, Gray RJ, deRobertis MA et al: Mitral valve replacement: Impact of coronary artery disease and determinants of prognosis after revascularization. Circulation (Suppl) 70:I-198, 1984
53. Kirschbaum M, Lumia F, Germon P et al: Ventricular function before and after mitral valve replacement. J Thorac Cardiovasc Surg 82:752, 1981
54. Peter CA, Austin EH, Jones RH: Effect of valve replacement for chronic mitral insufficiency on left ventricular function during rest and exercise. J Thorac Cardiovasc Surg 82:127, 1981
55. David TE, Uden DE, Strauss HD: The importance of the mitral apparatus in left ventricular function after correction of mitral regurgitation. Circulation 68:II-76, 1983
56. Ross J Jr: Afterload mismatch in aortic and mitral valve disease: Implications for surgical therapy. J Am Coll Cardiol 5:811, 1985

57. Roberts WC, Morrow AG, McIntosh CL et al: Congenitally bicuspid aortic valve causing severe, pure aortic regurgitation without superimposed infective endocarditis. Am J Cardiol 47:206, 1981
58. Greenberg BH, deMots H, Murphy E, Rahimtoola S: Mechanism for improved cardiac performance with arteriolar dilators in aortic insufficiency. Circulation 63:263, 1981
59. Judge TP, Kennedy JW, Bennett LJ et al: Quantitative hemodynamic effects of heart rate in aortic regurgitation. Circulation 44:355, 1971
60. Enghoff E: Aortic incompetence: Clinical, haemodynamic and angiocardiographic evaluation. Acta Med Scand (Suppl 538)193:3, 1972
61. Gerson MC, Engel PJ, Mantil JC et al: Effects of dynamic and isometric exercise on the radionuclide-determined regurgitant fraction in aortic insufficiency. J Am Coll Cardiol 3:98, 1984
62. Uhl GS, Boucher CA, Oliveros RA, Murgo JP: Exercise-induced myocardial oxygen supply-demand imbalance in asymptomatic or mildly symptomatic aortic regurgitation. Chest 80:686, 1981
63. Kennedy JW, Twiss RD, Blackmon JR, Dodge HT: Quantitative angiocardiography. III. Relationships of left ventricular pressure, volume, and mass in aortic valve disease. Circulation 38:838, 1968
64. Krayenbuehl HP, Turina M, Hess OM et al: Pre- and postoperative left ventricular contractile function in patients with aortic valve disease. Br Heart J 41:204, 1979
65. Hess OM, Ritter M, Schneider J et al: Diastolic stiffness and myocardial structure in aortic valve disease before and after valve replacement. Circulation 69:855, 1984
66. Kumpuris AG, Quinones MA, Waggoner AD et al: Importance of preoperative hypertrophy, wall stress and end-systolic dimension as echocardiographic predictors of normalization of left ventricular dilatation after valve replacement in chronic aortic insufficiency. Am J Cardiol 49:1091, 1982
67. Gaasch WH, Carroll JD, Levine HJ, Criscitiello MG: Chronic aortic regurgitation: Prognostic value of left ventricular end-systolic dimension and end-diastolic radius/thickness ratio. J Am Coll Cardiol 1:775, 1983
68. Krayenbuehl HP, Hess OM, Schneider J, Turina M: Physiologic or pathologic hypertrophy. Eur Heart J (Suppl A)4:29, 1983
69. Levine HJ, Gaasch WH: Ratio of regurgitant volume to end-diastolic volume: A major determinant of ventricular response to surgical correction of chronic volume overload. Am J Cardiol 52:406, 1983
70. Robertson WS, Stewart J, Armstrong WF et al: Reverse doming of the anterior mitral leaflet with severe aortic regurgitation. J Am Coll Cardiol 3:431, 1984
71. Bland EF, Wheeler EO: Severe aortic regurgitation in young people: A long-term perspective with reference to prognosis and prosthesis. N Engl J Med 256:667, 1957
72. Spagnuolo M, Kloth H, Taranta A et al: Natural history of rheumatic aortic regurgitation. Circulation 44:368, 1971
73. Massell BF, Amezcua FM, Czoniczer G: Prognosis of patients with pure or predominant aortic regurgitation in the absence of surgery. Circulation (Suppl)34:III-164, 1966
74. Haerten K, Dohn G, Dohn V et al: Natural history of patients with severe aortic valve disease under medical therapy. Z Kardiol 69:757, 1980
75. Bonow RO, Rosing DR, McIntosh CL et al: The natural history of asymptomatic patients with aortic regurgitation and normal left ventricular function. Circulation 68:509, 1983
76. Smith HJ, Neutze JM, Roche AHG et al: The natural history of rheumatic aortic regurgitation and the indications for surgery. Br Heart J 38:147, 1976
77. Turina J, Turina M, Rothlin M, Krayenbuehl HP: Improved late survival in patients with chronic aortic regurgitation by earlier operation. Circulation (Suppl)70:I-147, 1984
78. Sen S, Hahmann H, Becker D et al: Incidence and significance of angina pectoris in aortic valve disease. Z Kardiol 72:32, 1983
79. Basta LL, Raines D, Najjar S, Kioschos JM: Clinical, haemodynamic, and coronary angiographic correlates of angina pectoris in patients with severe aortic valve disease. Br Heart J 37:150, 1975
80. Miller DC, Stinson EB, Oyer PE et al: Surgical implications and results of combined aortic valve replacement and myocardial revascularization. Am J Cardiol 43:494, 1979
81. Abdulla AM, Frank MJ, Erdin RA Jr, Canedo MI: Clinical significance and hemodynamic correlates of the third heart sound gallop in aortic regurgitation. Circulation 64:464, 1981
82. Venkataraman K, Siegel R, Kim SJ, Allen JW: Musical murmurs: An echophonocardiographic study. Am J Cardiol 41:952, 1978
83. von Olshausen K, Hofmann M, Schaefer A et al: Ventricular arrhythmias before and after aortic valve replacement. Z Kardiol 72:168, 1983
84. Samuels DA, Curfman GD, Friedlich AL et al: Valve replacement for aortic regurgitation: Long-term follow-up with factors influencing the results. Circulation 60:647, 1979
85. Cohen IS, Wharton TP Jr, Neill WA: Pathophysiologic observations on premature opening of the aortic valve utilizing a technique for multiplane echocardiographic analysis. Am Heart J 97:766, 1979
86. Henry WL, Bonow RO, Borer JS et al: Observations on the optimum time for operative intervention for aortic regurgitation. I. Evaluation of the results of aortic valve replacement in symptomatic patients. Circulation 61:471, 1980
87. Turina J, Jenni R, Turina M, Krayenbuehl HP: Est-ce que l'échocardiographie est utile pour établir le pronostic à long terme après remplacement valvulaire chez des malades avec surcharge de volume du ventricule gauche? Arch Mal Coeur 73:675, 1980
88. Fioretti P, Roelandt J, Bos RJ et al: Echocardiography in chronic aortic insufficiency. Is valve replacement too late when left ventricular end-systolic dimension reaches 55 mm? Circulation 67:216, 1983
89. Johnson AD, Alpert JS, Francis GS et al: Assessment of left ventricular function in severe aortic regurgitation. Circulation 54:975, 1976
90. Rosenblatt A, Clark R, Burgess J, Cohn K: Echocardiographic assessment of the level of cardiac compensation in valvular heart disease. Circulation 54:509, 1976
91. Ciobanu M, Abbasi AS, Allen M et al: Pulsed Doppler echocardiography in the diagnosis and estimation of severity of aortic insufficiency. Am J Cardiol 49:339, 1982
92. Diebold B, Peronneau P, Blanchard D et al: Non-invasive quantification of aortic regurgitation by Doppler echocardiography. Br Heart J 49:167, 1983
93. Veyrat C, Lessana A, Abitbol G et al: New indexes for assessing aortic regurgitation with two-dimensional Doppler echocardiographic measurement of the regurgitant aortic valvular area. Circulation 68:998, 1983
94. Jenni R, Huebscher W, Casty M et al: Quantitation of aortic regurgitation by a percutaneous 128-channel digital ultrasound Doppler instrument. In Lancée CT: Echocardiology, p 241. Boston, M Nijhoff, 1979
95. Hoppeler H, Jenni R, Ritter M, Krayenbuehl HP: Quantification of aortic regurgitation with amplitude-weighted mean velocity from continuous wave Doppler spectra. J Am Coll Cardiol (in press)
96. Borer JS, Bacharach SL, Green MV et al: Exercise-induced left ventricular dysfunction in symptomatic and asymptomatic patients with aortic regurgitation: Assessment with radionuclide cineangiography. Am J Cardiol 42:351, 1978
97. Lewis SM, Riba AL, Berger HJ et al: Radionuclide angiographic exercise left ventricular performance in chronic aortic regurgitation: Relationship to resting echocardiographic ventricular dimensions and systolic wall stress index. Am Heart J 103:498, 1982
98. Huxley RL, Gaffney A, Corbett JR et al: Early detection of left ventricular dysfunction in chronic aortic regurgitation as assessed by contrast angiography, echocardiography, and rest and exercise scintigraphy. Am J Cardiol 51:1542, 1983
99. Bonow RO, Borer JS, Rosing DR et al: Preoperative exercise capacity in symptomatic patients with aortic regurgitation as a predictor of postoperative left ventricular function and long-term prognosis. Circulation 62:1280, 1980
100. Bonow RO, Picone AL, McIntosh CL et al: Survival and functional results after valve replacement for aortic regurgitation from 1976 to 1983: impact of preoperative left ventricular function. Circulation 72:1244, 1985
101. Kennedy JW, Doces J, Stewart DK: Left ventricular function before and following aortic valve replacement. Circulation 56:944, 1977
102. Pantely G, Morton M, Rahimtoola SH: Effects of successful, uncomplicated valve replacement on ventricular hypertrophy, volume, and performance in aortic stenosis and incompetence. J Thorac Cardiovasc Surg 75:383, 1978
103. Schwarz F, Flameng W, Schaper J, Hehrlein F: Correlation between myocardial structure and diastolic properties of the heart in chronic aortic valve disease: Effects of corrective surgery. Am J Cardiol 42:895, 1978
104. Clark DG, McAnulty JH, Rahimtoola SH: Valve replacement in aortic insufficiency with left ventricular dysfunction. Circulation 61:411, 1980
105. Forman R, Firth BG, Barnard MS: Prognostic significance of preoperative left ventricular ejection fraction and valve lesion in patients with aortic valve replacement. Am J Cardiol 45:1120, 1980
106. Bonow RO, Kent KM, Rosing DR et al: Aortic valve replacement without myocardial revascularization in patients with combined aortic valvular and coronary artery disease. Circulation 63:243, 1981
107. Day PJ, McManus BM, Roberts WC: Amounts of coronary arterial narrowing by atherosclerotic plaques in clinically isolated, chronic, pure aortic regurgitation: Analysis of 37 necropsy patients older than 30 years. Am J Cardiol 53:173, 1984
108. Greenberg BH, deMots H, Murphy E, Rahimtoola S: Beneficial effects of hydralazine on rest and exercise hemodynamics in patients with chronic severe aortic insufficiency. Circulation 62:49, 1980
109. Greenberg BH, Rahimtoola SH: Long-term vasodilator therapy in aortic insufficiency. Ann Intern Med 93:440, 1980
110. Greenberg B, Massic B, Bristow JD et al: Long-term vasodilator therapy of chronic aortic insufficiency. A randomized double-blinded, placebo-controlled clinical trial. Circulation 78:92, 1988
111. Hirshfeld JW Jr: Valve replacement for chronic severe aortic regurgitation: When should it be done? Int J Cardiol 3:243, 1983
112. Boucher CA, Bingham JB, Osbakken MD et al: Early changes in left ventricular size and function after correction of left ventricular volume overload. Am J Cardiol 47:991, 1981
113. Carroll JD, Gaasch WH, Zile MR, Levine HJ: Serial changes in left ventricular function after correction of chronic aortic regurgitation. Am J Cardiol 51:476, 1983
114. Greves J, Rahimtoola SH, McAnulty JH et al: Preoperative criteria predictive of late survival following valve replacement for severe aortic regurgitation. Am Heart J 101:300, 1981
115. Bonow RO, Rosing DR, Kent KM, Epstein SE: Timing of operation for chronic aortic regurgitation. Am J Cardiol 50:325, 1982

116. Donaldson RM, Florio R, Rickards AF et al: Irreversible morphological changes contributing to depressed cardiac function after surgery for chronic aortic regurgitation. Br Heart J 48:589, 1982
117. Bonow RO, Epstein SE: Is preoperative left ventricular function predictive of survival and functional results after aortic valve replacement for chronic aortic regurgitation? J Am Coll Cardiol 10:713, 1987
118. Dale J, Levang O, Enge I: Long-term results after aortic valve replacement with four different prostheses. Am Heart J 99:155, 1980
119. Macmanus Q, Grunkemeier GL, Lambert LE et al: Year of operation as a risk factor in the late results of valve replacement. J Thorac Cardiovasc Surg 80:834, 1980
120. Cohn LH, Mudge GH, Pratter F, Collins JJ Jr: Five to eight-year follow-up of patients undergoing porcine heart-valve replacement. N Engl J Med 304:258, 1981
121. Kirklin JW, Kouchoukos NT: Editorial: Aortic valve replacement without myocardial revascularization. Circulation 63:252, 1981
122. Edmunds LH: Thromboembolic complications of current cardiac valvular prostheses. Ann Thorac Surg 34:96, 1982
123. Lytle BW, Cosgrove DM, Loop FD et al: Replacement of aortic valve combined with myocardial revascularization: Determinants of early and late risk for 500 patients, 1967–1981. Circulation 68:1149, 1983
124. Egloff L, Rothlin M, Kugelmeier J et al: The ascending aortic aneurysm: Replacement or repair? Ann Thorac Surg 34:117, 1982
125. Grey DP, Ott DA, Cooley DA: Surgical treatment of aneurysm of the ascending aorta with aortic insufficiency. J Thorac Cardiovasc Surg 86:864, 1983
126. Niemelä K, Ikäheimo M, Takkunen J: Functional evaluation after aortic valve replacement. Scand J Thorac Cardiovasc Surg 17:221, 1983
127. Carroll JD, Gaasch WH: Left ventricular volume, mass, and function following surgical correction of chronic aortic regurgitation. Herz 6:131, 1981
128. Monrad ES, Hess OM, Murakami T et al: Time course of regression of left ventricular hypertrophy after aortic valve replacement. Circulation 77:1345, 1988
129. Toussaint C, Cribier A, Cazor JL et al: Hemodynamic and angiographic evaluation of aortic regurgitation 8 and 27 months after aortic valve replacement. Circulation 64:456, 1981
130. Schwarz F, Flameng W, Langebartels F et al: Impaired left ventricular function in chronic aortic valve disease: Survival and function after replacement by Björk-Shiley prosthesis. Circulation 60:48, 1979
131. De Pace NL, Nestico PF, Iskandrian AS, Morganroth J: Acute severe pulmonic valve regurgitation: Pathophysiology, diagnosis, and treatment. Am Heart J 108:567, 1984
132. Runco V, Levin HS: The spectrum of pulmonic regurgitation. In Physiologic Principles of Heart Sounds and Murmur. American Heart Association Monograph 46:175, 1975
133. Vela JE, Contreras R, Sosa FR: Rheumatic pulmonary valve disease. Am J Cardiol 23:12, 1969
134. Kitabatake A, Inoue M, Asao M et al: Noninvasive evaluation of pulmonary hypertension by a pulsed Doppler technique. Circulation 68:302, 1983
135. Miyatake K, Okamoto M, Kinoshita N et al: Pulmonary regurgitation studied with the ultrasonic pulsed Doppler technique. Circulation 65:969, 1982
136. Emery RW, Landes RG, Moller JH, Nicoloff DM: Pulmonary valve replacement with a porcine aortic heterograft. Ann Thorac Surg 27:148, 1979

MITRAL VALVE PROLAPSE

Pravin M. Shah

CHAPTER 83
VOLUME 2

HISTORICAL BACKGROUND

Barlow is credited with first drawing attention to an association between mitral valve prolapse and auscultatory findings of mid-late systolic clicks, which until then were largely interpreted as extracardiac in origin.[1] Although Reid had earlier suggested this association, the angiographic evidence of valve prolapse was provided by Barlow, hence the eponym Barlow's syndrome. A careful review of the literature reveals references to auscultatory sounds and murmurs over the cardiac apex attributed to abnormalities of the mitral valve dating back more than 100 years. However, angiographic documentation of this phenomenon was first reported by Barlow, who credits Criley with accurate interpretation of the angiograms. Criley subsequently reported a series of patients with mitral valve prolapse and correlated the timing of the systolic click with that of prolapse.[2] Shah and colleagues first reported a diagnosis of mitral valve prolapse by M-mode echocardiography.[3] This noninvasive technique, along with cardiac auscultation, was widely adopted for population surveys of mitral valve prolapse.[4-7] Kisslo and his associates reported on diagnosis by two-dimensional echocardiography utilizing parasternal views.[8] Morganroth and associates emphasized the diagnostic value of apical cross sections.[9] Ormiston and associates described an echocardiographic method of quantitating mitral annular area using multiple apical cross sections.[10] They further demonstrated enlargement of annular areas in a subset of patients with echocardiographic evidence of mitral valve prolapse independent of ventricular and atrial chamber enlargement.[11] Levine and colleagues constructed a model of mitral valve and annulus. They reasoned that the assumption of a nonplanar, saddle shaped configuration explained the common appearance of echocardiographic prolapse in otherwise normal valves using the apical cross-sections.[12] They recommended parasternal long axis views as the standard for echocardiographic diagnosis of prolapse.[13] It has been further recognized that characteristic auscultatory findings may be absent or only intermittently observed in patients with valve prolapse documented either by echocardiography or by angiocardiography. This, coupled with atypical and bizarre symptoms generally out of proportion to the cardiovascular abnormalities, has raised concern about the diagnostic role of any one technique. Considerable confusion has resulted from a lack of distinction between the occurrence of mitral valve prolapse and the existence of the mitral valve prolapse syndrome. It is therefore important to define these terms and emphasize the distinction between a functional finding and a clinical syndrome.

An additional note of historical interest is a suggestion carefully researched by Wooley, that several diagnoses in the past, such as neurocirculatory asthenia, soldier's heart, DaCosta's syndrome, and others, may have included patients who would now be recognized as having mitral valve prolapse syndrome.[14]

DEFINITIONS

The term *mitral valve prolapse* refers to a functional phenomenon in much the same way as the term *rectal prolapse* does. So defined, it is considered to be present whenever a portion of mitral valve leaflet(s) crosses the mitral annular plane posterosuperiorly into the left atrium. Any technique that permits clear delineation of the annular plane as well as separation of the left atrium from the left ventricle will provide an accurate means of diagnosis. Apical cross sections by two-dimensional echocardiography most often satisfy these requirements, and echocardiography is among the more accurate means for diagnosis. The condition of mitral valve prolapse as a functional entity may be a normal variant, since the precise relationship of coapted mitral leaflets to the annular plane is neither constant through systole nor uniform for

9.30

all normal subjects. If additional studies confirm the presence of a saddle shaped configuration of the mitral annulus as suggested by Levine and colleagues, an apparent prolapse may occur in a given plane (commonly apical four chamber view) without actual leaflet displacement above the most superior points of the mitral annulus.[12] It is suggested that their work on nonplanar configuration of the annulus be considered preliminary at present, and requiring independent confirmation as to its frequency of occurrence. Mild degrees of ventricular-valvular disproportion may develop with hypovolemia, tachycardia, or geometric distortion of the left ventricular cavity. Thus, even though mitral valve prolapse as defined functionally may be present in a variety of physiologic and pathologic states that do not primarily involve valve tissue, this should not be confused with mitral valve prolapse syndrome as defined below.

The term *mitral valve prolapse syndrome* may be used broadly to include a disorder with familial incidence, inconstant and vague symptomatology, characteristic but not always present auscultatory findings, infrequent electrocardiographic abnormality, and morphologic and functional abnormalities of the mitral valve complex generally recognized by echocardiography. Several studies in this subset of patients have identified evidence of neuroendocrine autonomic dysfunction in association with otherwise unexplained symptoms that cannot be related to valvular dysfunction. However, the only truly objective and consistent abnormalities are those related to structure and function of the mitral valve. Hence, mitral valve prolapse syndrome should be defined as morphologic (myxomatous or degenerative) changes in the valve leaflets, chordae tendineae, or annulus that result in posterosuperior displacement of the valve tissue into the left atrium. Thus defined, it may be readily distinguished from functional or anatomic prolapse with normal underlying valve structure.

It is important to stress that this disorder has been described under at least 15 different names. The more common among these are floppy mitral valve, Barlow's syndrome, billowing posterior leaflet syndrome, myxomatous degenerative valve, and mitral valve prolapse. Floppy or "myxomatous" valve is the morphologic substrate associated with and often responsible for prolapse of the valve.

In the current context of frequent attempts at surgical repair of nonrheumatic "myxomatous" floppy valves for correction of mitral regurgitation, it is vital to develop an agreement on common definitions and terminologies among internists, cardiologists, cardiac pathologists, and cardiothoracic surgeons. This would enhance communication and understanding of this frequently confused clinical entity. Surgeons and pathologists tend to see a well defined spectrum of this disorder. Similarly, cardiologists at tertiary referral centers are likely to see a symptomatic subset. There is a great need to develop a multispecialty panel of experts to recommend precise definitions of various terms commonly used in describing this clinical entity.

PATHOLOGY

In its severe forms, pathologic findings are characteristic, but in its more subtle forms, its recognition may depend on careful morphometric methods. Lucas and Edwards have proposed interchordal leaflet hooding as a major criterion of morphologic diagnosis.[15] Waller and associates suggested a morphometric approach to measure annular circumference (cm) and leaflet area (cm^2), and calculated a circumference area product (cm^3). A basis for this approach rests on characteristic leaflet redundancy and annular dilation, both of which are generally present to varying degrees.[16] Associated morphologic features include elongated chordae tendineae, fibrotic thickening of leaflet surfaces, and ventricular endocardial friction lesions.

Histologic examinations have shown an increase in the spongiosa component (the portion containing mucopolysaccharide material). This increased spongiosa has been inappropriately termed *myxoid degeneration*. More correctly, there is encroachment of the spongiosa on the fibrosa, resulting in focal disruption of the fibrosa.[15]

The posterior mitral leaflet has three well-defined scallops: medial, posterior, and lateral. Prolapse of one or more of these scallops may be observed. Although the anterior leaflet does not have any well-defined scallops, they may form with redundancy and elongation of the leaflet.

ETIOLOGY AND PREVALENCE

Familial occurrence of mitral valve prolapse has been found in both sexes in two or three generations of several families. Genetic studies suggest that the propensity for development of prolapse is inherited as an autosomal dominant trait with variable expression.[17] Expression of the prolapse gene appears to be affected by both sex and age. Women predominate in most population surveys and familial studies, and it has been suggested that echocardiographic prolapse is penetrant in 90% to 100% of women with the gene but only about 50% of the men.[18] The influence of age is somewhat complex and less well-defined. The prevalence of mitral valve prolapse is low in childhood and adolescence, but increases beyond the age of 20. Another complicating epidemiologic observation is that prevalence in women, but not in men, decreases with age.

A large recent epidemiologic study confirmed the incidence of echocardiographic mitral valve prolapse to be 5% of the total of 4,967 subjects.[19] The incidence was 3% in elderly subjects and 7% in younger ones. Females showed a progressive decline in the incidence of mitral valve prolapse: it was 17% for those in their 20s, but between 1% and 2% for those in their 70s and 80s. No such decline was noted in males. These epidemiologic observations, although interesting, should be considered only tentative, since the diagnosis of prolapse was based on M-mode echo criteria, which are not the current standards for diagnosis. Nevertheless, clinical observation of a higher frequency of males in older age groups having advanced valvular dysfunction tends to support the observation. There is also a predilection of mitral valve prolapse for certain types of body habitus. Subjects with prolapse are leaner and have narrower anteroposterior chest dimensions, longer arm spans, and a high incidence of thoracic skeletal deformities. This has led to a suggestion that a significant portion of these patients have an autosomally dominant, inherited body habitus, suggesting that mitral valve prolapse is only one component of a generalized developmental syndrome.[20]

ASSOCIATED DISEASES

There is no correlation between mitral valve prolapse and the incidence of specific cardiovascular conditions such as coronary artery disease, hypertrophic cardiomyopathy, rheumatic heart disease, or muscular dystrophy. On the other hand, prolapse is an integral feature of several distinct connective tissue diseases, including the Marfan syndrome and Ehlers-Danlos syndrome types I, III, and IV. In the family of a proband with classic type IV Ehlers-Danlos syndrome, all patients with abnormal production of type III collagen had mitral valve prolapse, while those with normal production of this collagen had no evidence of it.[21] This observation provides an etiologic link to the abnormality of a specific collagen.

CLINICAL FEATURES
SYMPTOMS

In most epidemiologic studies a large number of patients are symptom-free.[22] Others will seek medical attention for a variety of ill-defined problems that seem to have strong underlying features of anxiety neurosis. One study suggests that the incidence of these vague symptoms is no different in patients with mitral valve prolapse and in those without. Nonetheless, symptoms often thought to be associated with this disorder include the following:

1. Fatigue and lassitude.
2. Chest pain. This is generally atypical, unrelated to exertion, and often localized without a typical radiation pattern. A careful history indicates that the pain is clearly not consistent with angina pectoris.

However, in a few patients some of the features may be suggestive of angina and a diagnosis of atypical angina is often entertained.

3. Dyspnea. Patients often complain of difficulty in breathing, either on exertion or at rest. A careful history shows the sensation to be one of breath "sticking," inability to move air, feeling of a need for more oxygen, and so on, and not true dyspnea, which may accompany severe exertion.
4. Palpitations. This is a frequent symptom. It manifests as awareness of heartbeat, and frequently as localized pain and tenderness over the apical impulse. Other forms include skipped beats, a fluttering sensation, and rapid heart action.
5. Dizziness/syncope. Patients often complain of dizziness, although frank syncope is less common.
6. Agoraphobia. Some patients suffer extreme anxiety, unexplained fear, and panic. These attacks may be characterized by simultaneous anxiety and multiple cardiovascular and autonomic symptoms, including palpitations, dyspnea, chest pain, and dizziness.[23,24]

Thus, a combination of multiple, ill-defined symptoms in a patient with little objective evidence of organic cardiac disease often leads to a suspicion of underlying mitral valve prolapse. However, a number of recent epidemiologic studies have questioned this association. Thus, earlier reports of a high incidence of prolapse in panic attacks (agoraphobia) is not confirmed in more recent studies.[24] The Framingham Study of the general population examined 2,931 subjects (age range, 20 to 72 years) and concluded that cardiovascular symptoms were no more common in subjects with echocardiographic mitral valve prolapse than in those without it.[22]

Comment: There is a clear discrepancy between the clinical series in which the symptoms described above are frequently associated with mitral valve prolapse and the epidemiologic observations in the Framingham and other studies. One might question accuracy in the final diagnosis based on M-mode echocardiography as utilized in the Framingham Study,[22] which appears to have a sensitivity and specificity in the 50% to 70% range. The diagnostic criteria applied in the clinical series may be stricter. An alternative explanation lies in the selective referral of symptomatic patients who constitute the clinical series.

PHYSICAL SIGNS

The characteristic physical signs that provide important clues for the bedside diagnosis of mitral valve prolapse include the following:

1. Mid-late systolic click. A high-pitched mid-to-late systolic click heard over the apex is most commonly due to prolapse. Careful timing with selective angiocardiography and with echocardiography has shown the click to coincide with the apex of the prolapsing motion of the valve leaflet. A sudden tensing of the chordal-leaflet structure at the height of prolapse is considered to be responsible. At times, multiple clicks are present. Typically, the click or clicks may shift in timing to earlier or later portions of the systole, based on changes in left ventricular volume and geometry. Thus, maneuvers that reduce left ventricular volume result in an earlier timing of prolapse and hence of the click, and vice versa. Typically, the Valsalva maneuver is well suited to demonstrating variations in timing of the systolic click. It moves progressively earlier in systole during phases II and III, and may indeed coincide with the first heart sound. Following release of Valsalva strain during phase IV, as filling of the left ventricle increases progressively, the click moves later in systole and may fall just prior to the aortic component of the second heart sound.
2. Systolic murmur. A high-pitched, blowing, soft, systolic murmur commonly accompanies the click and is heard over the apex. It may start prior to the click, but typically follows it. In some patients a holosystolic murmur is present. A characteristic apical "whoop" or honk is also audible in some patients, especially related to body position. This is often loud, and may be heard or felt by the patient. A change in posture from sitting to supine will often eliminate the honking nature of the murmur.
3. First heart sound (S_1). Intensity of the mitral component of the first heart sound may vary, depending on the timing and type of prolapse. Tei and associates reported that early or pansystolic prolapse is generally associated with a loud S_1 over the apex, whereas mid-late systolic occurrence of prolapse is associated with normal S_1.[25] Patients with flail mitral valve secondary to rupture of chordae tendineae generally have a soft or absent S_1. This bedside clue may be helpful in characterizing the type of prolapse. The loud S_1 observed with pansystolic prolapse may merely represent coincident timing of the systolic click and S_1, whereas the attenuated S_1 in flail mitral valve is secondary to failure of leaflet coaptation at the time of valve closure.
4. Diastolic sounds. An early diastolic sound coincident with full opening of the valve leaflet may be observed in phonocardiographic recordings and may sometimes be audible. This occurs at the time of the mitral opening snap, but is generally of low intensity.
5. Jugular venous pulse and carotid arterial pulse are normal in contour.
6. Apical impulse has often shown mid-systolic retraction by apexcardiography, and may be appreciated during careful inspection and palpation of the apex beat.

BEDSIDE MANEUVERS

As pointed out earlier in this section, several bedside maneuvers may assist in providing diagnostic confirmation, especially when the auscultatory signs are not typical or prominent.

POSTURE
Assumption of upright posture, by reducing venous return and cardiac filling, results in earlier occurrence of the click and murmur, although their intensities may be softer. Opposite behavior in these physical signs is noted with squatting. As described earlier, some patients demonstrate a loud "whooping" or "honking" murmur in certain positions in a reproducible manner.

VALSALVA MANEUVER
A sustained forced expiration against a closed glottis held for 15 to 20 seconds before release results in typical changes in ventricular filling, stroke volume, blood pressure, and heart rate. An early occurrence of the click, at times coincident with S_1, and earlier initiation of the systolic murmur are noted during phases II and III, when left ventricular volume is reduced and tachycardia is present. The opposite occurs during phase IV, when left ventricular volume is increased and bradycardia is present.

AMYL NITRITE INHALATION
A decrease in arterial pressure and ensuing tachycardia are associated with reduced left ventricular volume, earlier occurrence of the click, and an earlier but softer systolic murmur.

POSTECTOPIC POTENTIATION
Following an ectopic beat, left ventricular volume increases because of the compensatory pause; thus, late occurrence of the clicks in relation to the first heart sound is expected. However, due to a marked increase in inotropy because of postectopic potentiation, the clicks occur earlier and the interval between the first heart sound and the clicks decreases. It has been suggested that in individual patients the left ventricular systolic dimension at which mitral valve prolapse occurs is relatively fixed. The first heart sound-click interval may shorten during the postectopic beat because the click dimension is reached earlier during ejection owing to a marked increase in contractility.

INTERMITTENCY OF PHYSICAL SIGNS

Characteristic auscultatory features may be intermittently present in a patient, at times without obvious explanation. The typical click and/or murmur may be absent at examination and quite evident at a subsequent time. This well known clinical finding makes the use of auscultatory signs as a "gold standard" for diagnosis somewhat unreliable. Although the presence of typical auscultatory findings strongly supports a diagnosis of mitral valve prolapse, their absence cannot be used to exclude the diagnosis. An excessive reliance on clinical findings for presence or absence of mitral valve prolapse as proposed by Perloff and associates cannot be considered accurate.[26]

PROLAPSE WITHOUT AUSCULTATORY SIGNS

It is well recognized that an obvious mitral valve prolapse, noted either by angiocardiography or echocardiography, may exist in the absence of any physical signs, even with bedside maneuvers. However, the prevalence of prolapse without auscultatory signs in population studies has not been well-defined. The Framingham Study of 2,931 subjects, which defined prolapse based on M-mode echo criteria, reported that less than 15% of patients with prolapse had a click and/or murmur heard on auscultation.[22] This question will need to be readdressed after more rigid echo criteria of diagnosis, involving both morphologic as well as functional aspects of prolapse, are widely adopted.

AUSCULTATORY SIGNS OF PROLAPSE WITHOUT ECHOCARDIOGRAPHIC CONFIRMATION

It is generally held that when typical auscultatory findings are present, it is not necessary to obtain confirmation by echocardiography, since a negative study does not exclude the clinical diagnosis. However, other less common causes of mid-late systolic clicks include interatrial septal aneurysm, intracardiac tumors, and rarely, pleuropericardial disease. In instances when auscultation is typical for prolapse but the echo is negative, it is advisable to document the presence of a typical click and murmur, in resting condition as well as with bedside maneuvers (*e.g.*, Valsalva) by phonocardiography. It is certainly possible for prolapse to be localized to a small portion of a leaflet (*e.g.*, a scallop of a posterior leaflet), which may not have been visualized by echocardiography. Such a possibility is minimized by obtaining multiple cross sections from several transducer orientations.

PATHOGENESIS OF SYMPTOMS AND SIGNS
SYMPTOMS

There is an obvious disparity between the presence or severity of symptoms, and objective evidence of the severity of heart disease. No distinct cardiac functional abnormality can readily account for such symptoms as chest pain, dyspnea, and fatigue. In uncomplicated cases of mitral valve prolapse, the cardiac chambers and their function are essentially normal, although focal asynergy of the posterobasal wall of the left ventricle has sometimes been described. The basis for chest pain has been investigated without a definite result. For instance, the severity of prolapse itself, as it may be manipulated by vasoactive drugs, it is not related to the occurrence of chest pain. Similarly, coronary vasospasm has only rarely been demonstrated as a mechanism for chest pain in these patients.[27] Rare case reports of typical anginal chest pain with reversible ST changes or with acute myocardial infarction have implicated coronary spasm.

Autonomic dysfunction has been reported in patients with mitral valve prolapse.[28-30] The various reported abnormalities of neuroendocrine and autonomic function may be summarized in this way (as suggested by Boudoulas and associates):[31]

1. Evidence of high adrenergic activity. The 24-hour urinary catecholamines were higher in symptomatic patients than in normal controls. Plasma catecholamine values at rest were higher in symptomatic patients, both in the supine and upright positions. A repeat measurement in the same patients after 6 years showed persistent elevation of plasma catecholamines.[32,33]
2. Evidence of abnormal catecholamine regulation. In patients with mitral valve prolapse syndrome, acute volume expansion with 2.5 to 3 liters of isoteric saline given intravenously over 10 hours failed to result in a decrease in plasma catecholamine values. This contrasted with the results found in normal subjects.[34]
3. Evidence of abnormal symptomatic response to adrenergic stimulation. Isoproterenol infusions reproduced symptoms including chest pain, fatigue, dyspnea, dizziness, and panic attacks only in patients with mitral valve prolapse syndrome. The increase in heart rate was significantly greater.
4. Evidence for decreased intravascular volume. Several studies have demonstrated this phenomenon. There is also an inverse relationship between plasma volume and peripheral vascular resistance on standing.[35,36]
5. Evidence for abnormal renin-aldosterone regulation. Volume depletion with intravenous furosemide resulted in a greater increase in plasma norepinephrine, a smaller increase in plasma renin activity, and a greater decrease in plasma aldosterone for mitral valve prolapse syndrome as compared with control subjects.[37]
6. Evidence for abnormal parasympathetic activity. Studies examining heart rate response to the Valsalva maneuver showed higher rates during strain period and inappropriate bradycardia during recovery, suggesting an excessive vagal tone in some patients.[29] Evidence for abnormal baroreflex modulation was a different heart rate response to phenylephrine infusion as compared with normal controls.
7. Atrial natriuretic factor. Some patients showed an increase in atrial natriuretic factor, associated with a lower blood volume. A second group had normal values. The meaning of these differences is not known.

While these studies stress abnormal autonomic and neuroendocrine function, the basic mechanisms involved and their precise correlations with symptoms remain to be investigated.[38]

SIGNS

The underlying mechanisms of physical signs are more clearly defined and can be related to the timing and occurrence of valve prolapse. Thus, the systolic click coincides with the apex of leaflet prolapse, and multiple clicks may represent different scallops of the valve prolapsing at slightly different times. The systolic murmur is one of mitral regurgitation.

Up to 40% of patients with mitral valve prolapse may also demonstrate tricuspid valve prolapse, and the physical findings may be indistinguishable other than a more defined localization of click(s)/murmur along the lower left sternal edge. If clicks are heard along the lower right sternal edge, associated tricuspid valve prolapse is likely to be present. Occasionally, tricuspid valve prolapse may occur as an isolated finding. Therefore, a careful evaluation of the tricuspid valve should also be undertaken by echo in patients with typical auscultatory findings indicative of valve prolapse but without abnormalities of the mitral valve.

LABORATORY DIAGNOSIS
ROUTINE 12-LEAD ELECTROCARDIOGRAM

Approximately 10% to 15% of patients with mitral valve prolapse demonstrate abnormal ST and T wave changes in the inferior and lateral leads. The basis for this abnormality is not understood. A combination of ECG changes along with auscultatory findings is referred to as an "auscultatory-echocardiographic" subset of the mitral valve prolapse syndrome. Supraventricular and/or ventricular dysrhythmias may be observed on routine ECG.

CHEST X-RAY FILM

The cardiac silhouette is most often normal, although narrowed anteroposterior dimensions, pectus excavatum, loss of dorsal spine curvature ("straight back"), and varying degrees of kyphoscoliosis may be observed. Thoracic skeletal abnormalities occur in approximately 60% to 70% of patients, although they are often not pronounced.

ECHOCARDIOGRAPHIC DIAGNOSIS
M-MODE ECHOCARDIOGRAPHY

Although M-mode parameters for mitral prolapse were developed prior to the advent of two-dimensional echocardiography,[3-7] the limitations of M-mode include uncertain or "blind" beam direction and lack of spatial display with a limited window. Nonetheless, the following criteria on M-mode echocardiography may complement the two-dimensional echocardiographic diagnosis:

1. Mid-late systolic buckling. A sharp mid-late systolic posterior displacement is a highly characteristic finding, but it is observed in less than 40% of cases with known mitral valve prolapse. Thus, although this finding is highly specific, its sensitivity is relatively low.
2. Holosystolic posterior displacement or hammocking. This feature, although often present in patients with mitral valve prolapse, is nonspecific. In an effort to improve its diagnostic accuracy, it has been suggested that only when posterior displacement exceeds 2 mm should a diagnosis of prolapse be made. This arbitrary figure is subject to a number of vagaries and, although helpful, is not always reliable.
3. Thickened mitral leaflet with normal or increased excursion. This too is a nonspecific finding consisting of multilayered mitral valve echoes, suggesting thickening of the leaflet(s), and normal or exaggerated opening amplitude.
4. Early systolic prolapse. This consists of posterior displacement of the valve leaflet immediately after the closure point.
5. Flail mitral valve syndrome. This syndrome features (1) holosystolic posterior displacement of a mitral leaflet, (2) abnormal anterior diastolic opening motion of the posterior mitral leaflet, (3) coarse chaotic diastolic flutter of a mitral valve leaflet, (4) systolic fluttering of a leaflet, and (5) appearance of valve echo in the left atrium during systole. These findings are very useful, and when two or more are present, they are diagnostic of the flail mitral valve syndrome.

TWO-DIMENSIONAL ECHOCARDIOGRAPHY

As a result of better spatial orientation and ease of determining the mitral annular plane, two-dimensional echo has become the standard by which the diagnosis of functional mitral valve prolapse is made. In some patients, the main limitation of the method is a technical inadequacy in obtaining the multiple anatomic cross sections needed to image all major segments of both valve leaflets. All cross sections providing a separation between the left ventricle and the left atrium and a view of the mitral annular plane may be used to diagnose prolapse. In all views, the point of coaptation of the leaflets is an important observation. In mitral valve prolapse, the tip coaptation is preserved, although it may be displaced superiorly, and the body of a leaflet protrudes or billows into the left atrium. In contrast, the flail mitral valve syndrome is associated with failure of tip coaptation in at least one cross-sectional view that best highlights the flail portion of the leaflet.

The more important two-dimensional characteristics of primary mitral valve prolapse include the following:

1. Functional prolapse of a localized portion of one or both leaflets may be observed. This is seen as a systolic displacement of the prolapsing segment of the valve into the left atrium posterosuperior to the mitral annular plane. The two-dimensional cross section that permits its visualization would depend on the segment of the leaflet involved in prolapse. The parasternal or apical long axis view transects the medial aspect of the anterior leaflet and the middle scallop of the posterior leaflet. Prolapse of these components would be best diagnosed using the long axis views. The apical four chamber view visualizes the medial aspect of the anterior leaflet and the lateral scallop of the posterior leaflet. The apical two chamber view permits visualization of the lateral aspect of the anterior leaflet and the medial scallop of the posterior leaflet. Thus, the two dimensional view with the most diagnostic information will depend on the segment or segments of the leaflet involved. Two cautionary notes are important. First, the body of the anterior leaflet may appear to prolapse in the apical four chamber in some normal subjects. It is not clear if this represents nonplanar mitral annulus. However, even in this view, posterosuperior displacement of the coaptation point or of the posterior leaflet is never a normal finding. Second, the apical two chamber view is a posteriorly oriented cross section. Since the entire heart moves anteriorly during systole, this cross section may transect the leaflets in diastole and the posterior annulus in systole. This may give an erroneous suggestion of prolapse, since the annulus is normally curved posteriorly. Nevertheless, it must be emphasized that all available two-dimensional views should be utilized in order to diagnose functional mitral valve prolapse, which may be a focal abnormality. A recent suggestion[12] that only long axis views be used to make the diagnosis is inappropriate, since a distinct prolapse of the lateral scallop of the posterior leaflet may easily be missed. Evidence presented to support the contention that apical views are not useful is simply too feeble.[13]
2. Thickened mitral valve leaflets with redundant tissue on one or both. These are generally subjective visual assessments, although comparisons with a structure such as the posterior aortic wall may compensate for differences in gain settings. The thickening may also be focal and has been examined in multiple views.
3. Dilation of the mitral annulus. This is best evaluated by using apical views to reconstruct the annulus and measure its circumference and area.[10,11,39]
4. Coexistence of prolapse of other cardiac valves. The commonest association is with tricuspid valve prolapse, which is best seen in the views from the right ventricular apex with visualization of the right ventricle, the right atrium, and the tricuspid annular plane. Idiopathic prolapse of the aortic valve cusp is less common, and may be seen in the parasternal or the apical long axis views. Redundancy and prolapse of the pulmonary valve may occasionally be present.

Flail mitral valve is diagnosed using the following two-dimensional echo criteria:

1. Absence of leaflet coaptation at the tips or free margins may be noted in one or more apical or parasternal cross sections, depending on the size of the flail leaflet.
2. Sudden whipping motion of a leaflet from the left ventricle to the left atrium may be observed when a large portion of a leaflet is flailing.
3. Prolapse of a leaflet or a portion of one into the left atrium, beginning in presystole after the end of the P wave and continuing into ventricular systole. A frame-by-frame evaluation showing presystolic prolapse is characteristic of a flail leaflet and is generally not observed in the other forms of mitral valve prolapse. Flail mitral valve is most often indicative of ruptured chordae tendineae, leaving unsupported leaflet time. Similar but less pronounced echocar-

diographic appearances may be observed in the case of elongated chordae without rupture.

DOPPLER ECHOCARDIOGRAPHY

Pulsed Doppler technique provides additional evidence of valve regurgitation. The sample volume is located in the mitral apparatus or immediately proximal to the mitral valve in the left atrium. A late systolic flow velocity turbulence has been reported, indicative of mitral regurgitation. Furthermore, the abnormal velocity signal is observed even in the absence of a systolic murmur. Color flow imaging permits visualization of a mitral regurgitation flow jet, which is often eccentric in mitral valve prolapse. The severity of regurgitation may be judged from the area of the regurgitation jet. Trivial short-lived regurgitation is not uncommon in a normal valve. Mild or moderate degrees of regurgitation, especially when late systolic or eccentric, are nearly always pathologic and frequently associated with mitral valve prolapse syndrome even in the absence of a murmur.

WHEN DOES PROLAPSE VISUALIZED ON ECHOCARDIOGRAPHY CONSTITUTE A PATHOLOGIC SYNDROME OF MITRAL VALVE PROLAPSE?

As stated in the section on definitions, echocardiographic evidence of mitral valve prolapse may represent a nonpathologic functional state resulting from changes in left ventricular geometry and size. What then is the significance of echocardiographic mitral valve prolapse? When should an echocardiographic diagnosis of "definite," "probable," or "cannot exclude mitral valve prolapse" be made?[40] Given present knowledge, which is admittedly in a state of evolution, the following guidelines may be useful in the clinical setting:

1. Definite mitral valve prolapse syndrome with clinical-pathologic significance may be diagnosed when two or more of the following echocardiographic signs are present:
   a. Leaflet prolapse into the left atrium.
   b. Thickened, redundant valve leaflets.
   c. Dilated mitral annulus.
   d. Associated tricuspid valve prolapse with dilation of the tricuspid annulus.
   e. Associated aortic valve prolapse.
   The emphasis in making a diagnosis of definite mitral valve prolapse is on the combination of functional as well as structural changes. This subset of patients generally exhibits the typical physical signs.
2. Probable mitral valve prolapse may be diagnosed when the following is present: Functional prolapse on two-dimensional echocardiography with clinical signs to support the diagnosis but without structural changes (i.e., thickened leaflets or dilated annulus).
3. Possible (consistent with but not diagnostic of) mitral valve prolapse may be diagnosed when the following are noted:
   a. Mild hammocking on M-mode or borderline for functional prolapse by two-dimensional echocardiography with or without questionable leaflet thickening and no supporting clinical signs.
   b. Suggestive physical findings without any functional or structural abnormalities on echocardiography.

A diagnosis of possible mitral valve prolapse should be viewed as a likely normal variant and may not constitute the basis for pathology, unless longitudinal follow-up provides more diagnostic clues.

TREADMILL EXERCISE TESTING

Since one of the presenting complaints of mitral valve prolapse is chest pain, these patients may undergo diagnostic treadmill stress testing for suspected myocardial ischemia. One of the characteristic clues is an inappropriate heart rate response, suddenly increasing during an early stage of exercise. Some patients demonstrate orthostatic tachycardia with assumption of the upright posture. Abnormal repolarization changes (i.e., ST–T abnormalities) may be observed in some patients with prolapse.[41] Since coronary artery disease may coexist in older patients, coronary angiography may be required to document the presence or absence of coronary arterial occlusions. Therefore, while a negative test may be helpful for excluding significant symptomatic coronary artery disease, a positive test has little validity.

THALLIUM STRESS TEST

Some patients with a positive treadmill stress test may undergo thallium stress testing for further diagnostic evaluation.[42] Once again, a negative test may be helpful; however, a falsely positive thallium stress test has been reported.

AMBULATORY ELECTROCARDIOGRAPHIC MONITORING

Ambulatory ECG monitoring is usually undertaken either for symptomatic patients (i.e., having palpitations, dizziness, syncope) or those showing an abnormal resting ECG with or without arrhythmia in the routine tracing. Patients in hazardous occupations, such as airline pilots, should also receive Holter monitoring.

COMPLICATIONS

The complications of mitral valve prolapse include progressive mitral regurgitation and heart failure, chordal rupture with flail mitral valve, sudden death, infective endocarditis, and systemic embolism.

Although the incidence of these complications appears to be low, and the subset of patients susceptible to a given complication is not accurately defined, the serious nature of many of them cannot be ignored.

PROGRESSIVE MITRAL REGURGITATION AND HEART FAILURE

In affluent parts of the world where the incidence of rheumatic fever has been sharply reduced, mitral valve prolapse syndrome is a common cause of mitral regurgitation.[43] The mechanisms for a progressive increase in mitral regurgitation in the absence of chordal rupture include (1) increasing degrees of prolapse resulting from more extensive leaflet degeneration and redundancy and/or elongation of chordae tendineae, and (2) progressive dilation of the mitral annulus, which in the initial stages is primary (i.e., unrelated to the size of the left ventricle and/or left atrium). In later stages, secondary annular dilation is superadded from increased mitral regurgitation and chamber enlargement.

The incidence of progressive mitral regurgitation in a population of patients with mitral valve prolapse is not known. It generally reaches the symptomatic stage beyond the fifth decade. For reasons still not understood, it appears that males are more prone to develop this complication. This is in striking contrast to the greater prevalence of prolapse among females in the second and third decades. Increased physical exertion, higher systemic arterial blood pressure, or some as yet unknown factor(s) may be responsible for this disparity.

Presenting symptoms are often those of pulmonary congestion with effort, dyspnea, orthopnea, and paroxysmal nocturnal dyspnea. The physical signs are those of severe mitral regurgitation with left ventricular enlargement, a holosystolic mitral regurgitation murmur, and S_3 gallop with or without mid-diastolic flow murmur. In many patients, the first heart sound (S_1) over the apex is accentuated and is associated with early systolic or pansystolic prolapse.

Progressive pulmonary hypertension, right heart chamber dilation, and chronic congestive heart failure are late developments. Ideally, surgical correction should be undertaken prior to this stage of advancement.

FLAIL MITRAL VALVE SYNDROME

Rupture of the chordae tendineae, which results in flail mitral valve syndrome, is most often secondary to the degenerative mitral valve prolapse syndrome, although other causes include infective endocarditis and blunt chest trauma. The chordal rupture in patients with mitral valve prolapse is commonly spontaneous. Rupture of primary chords attached to or near the free margins of the leaflets results in increased mitral regurgitation. Severity of regurgitation is related to the extent of unsupported leaflet tissue, based on size and number of ruptured chordae. The degree of annular dilation and of leaflet redundancy is variable.

Presenting symptoms are similar to those described above, although acute onset may be heralded by rupture of a chord, resulting in prolapse of a large volume of unsupported valve tissue. More usual is a subacute course with symptoms progressing over weeks, or a more chronic course. The physical signs are as described above in more chronic cases, except for an attenuated or absent S_1. The signs of acute mitral regurgitation are rather characteristic, and consist of a short early systolic murmur, prominent S_4, early signs of pulmonary hypertension, and right ventricular decompensation. In more acute cases, the cardiac chambers are only slightly dilated.

Management of the flail mitral valve syndrome is surgical, although timing of surgery may be guided by severity and progression of symptoms and of left ventricular function.

CARDIAC DYSRHYTHMIAS

Early reports emphasized a high incidence of ventricular and supraventricular arrhythmias in patients with mitral valve prolapse.[44] In some cases these arrhythmias were serious enough to be life-threatening, and sudden death has generally been associated with malignant ventricular dysrhythmias.[45] Early ambulatory ECG monitoring studies revealed a 50% to 80% incidence of premature ventricular contractions (PVCs), and complex or frequent PVCs were noted in 30% to 50% of patients. Ventricular arrhythmias are typically reduced in frequency at night and exaggerated following exercise. Incidence of sustained or nonsustained ventricular tachycardia in patients seen at tertiary referral centers has varied between 10% and 25%. Brief spontaneous episodes of ventricular fibrillation may occur and "torsade de pointes" has been reported. Mechanisms of ventricular dysrhythmias have not been clarified. Focal cardiomyopathy has been offered as an explanation. Vectorcardiographic evidence that the majority of PVCs originate in the posterobasal left ventricular myocardium may lend support to this theory.[46] The dysrhythmias have not correlated with prolapse of one or both leaflets; however, severity of mitral leaflet thickening as judged by echocardiogram has correlated with a higher incidence of arrhythmias. Prolongation of QT interval has also been implicated. Additionally, there is a high incidence of repolarization abnormalities in the resting electrocardiogram.

Supraventricular arrhythmias are also common in patients with mitral valve prolapse. Paroxysmal supraventricular tachycardia is probably the most common sustained tachyrhythmia seen in patients with the mitral valve prolapse syndrome.[47] Electrophysiologic studies have implicated atrioventricular nodal reentry as the mechanism in some, and a high incidence of bypass tracts precipitating the tachycardia has been reported. Although earlier reports emphasized a preponderance of left-sided accessory pathways in cases of mitral valve prolapse, a recent study found no pattern of association with the location of the accessory pathway.[48]

Metabolic studies by Boudoulas and associates have examined the neuroendocrine system and have correlated diurnal variations of urinary catecholamines with variations of PVC frequency. Similarly, an increase in plasma catecholamines after exercise was also substantially greater in association with an increase in PVC frequency.[49] A study utilizing induced psychological stress (anxiety) demonstrated increased frequency of ventricular dysrhythmias resulting from the intervention. This lends further support to a role of the autonomic nervous system.[50]

A study of programmed ventricular stimulation with three extrastimuli in 36 patients with mitral valve prolapse reported that in those with transient cerebral symptoms and documented nonsustained ventricular tachycardia or PVCs, ventricular tachycardia or fibrillation is inducible in 65%.[51] The clinical relevance or applicability of this finding is unclear.

Conduction abnormalities have also been reported, and associated with mitral valve prolapse.[52] Sinus node dysfunction and varying grades of atrioventricular block as well as bundle branch block may be noted. Electrophysiologic studies have revealed abnormal sinus node function, prolongation of atrioventricular interval, and intra-hisian block as well as functional bundle branch block.

Although some of the earlier studies used comparisons with age-matched and sex-matched controls, results were compromised by selection bias.[53] The Framingham Study using M-mode echocardiographic mitral valve prolapse screened 2,840 patients by 1-hour ambulatory ECG monitoring, and an age-stratified sample of 179 subjects by 24-hour ambulatory ECG monitoring.[54] Dysrhythmias occurred with similar frequency on resting 12-lead, exercise, and 1-hour ambulatory ECGs whether prolapse was present or not. However, 24-hour monitoring revealed a higher incidence of ventricular and supraventricular arrhythmias in those with prolapse. Another study matched symptomatic patients who had mitral valve prolapse with a group of control subjects who were also highly symptomatic. This study demonstrated that populations of highly symptomatic patients, regardless of the presence or absence of prolapse, have a high prevalence of arrhythmias. Despite this report questioning a special predilection of prolapse for ventricular dysrhythmias, clinical experience would suggest that a high-risk subset of patients (i.e., highly symptomatic, severe prolapse with valve thickening, abnormal resting ECG) should be carefully monitored and appropriately managed.

SUDDEN DEATH

A number of reports as well as much clinical experience indicate that sudden death may occur in persons with mitral valve prolapse as the only pathologic cardiac finding.[55] In most such instances serious recurrent ventricular dysrhythmias had been previously observed.[56] In some cases, complete atrioventricular block or sinoatrial arrest was an underlying factor. A role for antiarrhythmic agents in preventing sudden death remains to be established.

INFECTIVE ENDOCARDITIS

Occurrence of infective endocarditis in patients with mitral valve prolapse has been recognized, although it is not certain if this represents a coincidental association or is indicative of an increased risk due to valvular pathology.[57] A controlled study confirmed a higher risk of endocarditis associated with mitral valve prolapse. It has been suggested that persons with prolapse are five to eight times more likely to have infective endocarditis than normal persons.[57] Although clinical reports have demonstrated occurrence of endocarditis irrespective of the presence or absence of an associated murmur, a murmur of mitral regurgitation is thought to provide additional risk. It also appears that thickened redundant valves and severe prolapse are more frequently associated with infection.[58]

It has been recommended that prophylaxis for infective endocarditis be instituted only for patients with a heart murmur. This seems somewhat illogical, since patients with clicks alone are known to have suffered from endocarditis, and murmurs may be intermittent. I subscribe to the view that patients who fulfill stringent criteria for diagnosis based on both structural and functional evidence of mitral valve prolapse should receive prophylaxis against endocarditis, irrespective of the physical findings.

SYSTEMIC EMBOLISM

A large body of clinical evidence implicates mitral valve prolapse as a cause of transient ischemic attacks (TIA) or stroke, especially in younger patients.[59] The neurologic literature is replete with association of TIA, stroke, and mitral valve prolapse. Patients are also reported to develop retinal emboli. A study of 141 patients over 45 years of age (mean, 64.7 years) and 40 patients under 45 (mean, 33.9) showed the incidence of valve prolapse in the older group to be 5% to 7%, and in younger patients to be 40%.[59] Some patients also had other potential causes for cerebral ischemia, suggesting that detection of prolapse does not confirm an etiologic role, and other causes should be looked for. A precise mechanism for systemic embolism has not been defined, although platelet aggregates over a redundant and thickened valve may provide an explanation. A study of patients with prolapse has reported increased platelet coagulant activity, and those with thromboembolism also demonstrated an increased proportion of circulating platelet aggregates.[60] This appears to support a potential role for platelets in the assumed association of thromboembolism and mitral valve prolapse.

NATURAL HISTORY

It is difficult to define with accuracy the natural history of so common and varied a disorder as mitral valve prolapse. Most long-term follow-up studies originate from tertiary referral centers and have to a large extent included retrospective data analysis. Whereas this approach defines the complications that may develop during the lifetime of a patient with this disorder, current evidence points to a specific subset of patients being more at risk for some of these complications, as discussed earlier.

Most long-term follow-up studies demonstrate that the vast majority of patients remain stable and without progression of mitral regurgitation.[61] Incidence of infective endocarditis appears to be low and may be largely preventable. Progression of mitral regurgitation appears to develop more frequently in older men with redundant, thickened valves and often with associated chordal rupture. Sudden death is a rare complication and almost always involves malignant ventricular dysrhythmias.[62] Patients with an abnormal resting ECG appear to be at increased risk. Systemic embolism is also a rare complication; younger patients (<45 years) with thickened redundant valve leaflets appear to be at greater risk.

MANAGEMENT

Mitral valve prolapse is generally a benign condition with a low incidence of complications. However, some of these may be quite devastating, and a physician often faces a real dilemma as to the wisdom of informing a patient of the presence of this condition, and educating him or her as to the possibility of serious complications. The basic principles of management are patient education and reassurance, management of symptoms, prevention of complications, and treatment of complications.

PATIENT EDUCATION AND REASSURANCE

This is a most important therapeutic intervention, once a diagnosis of definite or highly probably mitral valve prolapse is established. It is especially necessary in symptomatic patients who suffer from high-level anxiety. It is generally advisable to educate even the asymptomatic patient in whom the condition is discovered accidentally. Lack of a careful explanation may be misinterpreted as indicating a more serious prognosis. Most patients are reassured by detailed communication as to the nature of the condition, its frequency, its generally benign course, and its rare but often preventable complications.

SYMPTOMATIC TREATMENT

Since many of the symptoms have no well-defined organic basis, there is little reason to use cardioactive drugs for chest pain, palpitations, dizziness, and so on. Beta-blocking agents have been used and can produce relief of a variety of vague symptoms, including anxiety attacks. In more persistent cases, use of tranquilizers may be indicated. However, it is much more important to listen to patients' symptoms and give reinforcing assurance of the excellent long-term prognosis for the disorder.

In occasional patients, where coronary artery spasm can be documented, treatment with calcium channel blockers or with nitrates may be indicated. Similarly, specific treatment aimed toward arrhythmias or hypotension may relieve associated symptoms.

PREVENTION OF COMPLICATIONS

Even though they are infrequent, complications do tend to have serious consequences, and a prophylactic approach is advisable.

INFECTIVE ENDOCARDITIS

It is controversial whether all patients in whom a diagnosis of mitral valve prolapse is made by clinical and/or echocardiographic criteria should receive prophylaxis against endocarditis. Clemens and Ransohoff have estimated the early risk of endocarditis for a person with prolapse to be approximately 5 per 100,000. This low risk, despite increased overall risk compared with the normal person, can be explained by the high prevalence of prolapse in the general population and the relative rarity of endocarditis (1.1 cases per 100,000 per year).[63] It has been suggested that routine prophylaxis with *parenteral penicillin* is not only cost-ineffective, but may actually cause a net loss of life. This is because the risk of endocarditis after dental procedures would be outweighed by the risk of anaphylaxis. Thus, for routine prophylaxis, oral antibiotics are recommended.

Groups at increased risk for infective endocarditis include patients with thickened redundant valve leaflets by echocardiography, patients with associated systolic murmurs, and patients with frequent bacteremia (*e.g.*, drug addicts).

Those with only a systolic click and structurally normal appearing valve leaflets on echocardiogram and a mild degree of prolapse should not, according to some authors, receive routine prophylaxis. However, such patients may demonstrate an intermittent systolic murmur, and the degree of prolapse and valve thickness may alter with time. I recommend the use of routine prophylaxis against endocarditis with all patents in whom a definite or highly probable diagnosis of prolapse is made, based on considerations given under Laboratory Diagnosis earlier in this chapter.

SUDDEN DEATH

The most frequent underlying cause of sudden death is cardiac dysrhythmias. Hence, prevention consists of proper recognition and effective treatment of arrhythmias. Since mitral valve prolapse is such a common condition, it would not appear practical to carry out ambulatory ECG monitoring on all patients with this diagnosis. The following guidelines are offered as a practical approach for undertaking 24-hour Holter monitoring:

1. Presence of cardiac arrhythmias on routine 12-lead ECG.
2. Presence of repolarization abnormalities (ST and T changes) on 12-lead ECG.
3. Symptomatic patients with palpitations, dizziness, or syncope.

4. Prolonged QT interval or pre-excitation syndrome on ECG.
5. Special work-related categories (*e.g.*, pilots).

Although class I antiarrhythmics (*i.e.*, quinidine, procainamide) are commonly used, their effectiveness and safety are not established. In many patients, propranolol appears to be effective. Similarly, phenytoin sodium has been used with some success. In more recalcitrant cases with malignant forms of ventricular dysrhythmia, it would be appropriate to use more potent drugs such as amiodarone, despite a risk of side effects. In some patients, use of mechanical devices such as an implanted defibrillator may have to be considered.

Occasional success in reducing life-threatening ventricular dysrhythmias has been reported following replacement of the mitral valve. However, this radical form of therapy is generally not indicated for arrhythmias, and should be reserved for patients with severe mitral regurgitation and hemodynamic compromise.

SYSTEMIC EMBOLISM

It has been proposed that patients with a history of systemic embolism should receive antiplatelet agents to prevent recurrence. Although this approach is a reasonable one, no definite evidence of efficacy exists at present. The use of anticoagulants may be reserved for patients with embolism in vital areas of the body.

CONGESTIVE HEART FAILURE

Since this complication may develop either from a progressive increase in mitral regurgitation or a rupture of chordae tendineae, no adequate prophylactic measure is known.

TREATMENT OF COMPLICATIONS
INFECTIVE ENDOCARDITIS

Specific antibiotic therapy is guided by the infecting organism. Indications for mitral valve surgery are based on evidence of hemodynamic compromise and on recurrent systemic emboli with echocardiographic evidence of vegetative lesions.

ARRHYTHMIAS

Specific therapy is directed to the type and complexity of the arrhythmias. Some patients with potentially serious ventricular arrhythmias are unresponsive to commonly used antiarrhythmic agents. It may be necessary to resort to such potent drugs as amiodarone.

PROGRESSIVE MITRAL REGURGITATION WITH CONGESTIVE HEART FAILURE

Symptomatic patients with hemodynamic compromise should be considered for mitral valve reconstructive surgery. This has been successful in a large portion of such patients, and it is clearly a more desirable choice than valve replacement. Reconstructive surgery is particularly appropriate for patients who have posterior leaflet prolapse with annular dilation. Localized anterior leaflet pathology with valvular redundancy may be amenable to wedge resection. Similarly, elongated chordae tendineae may be shortened, and in some instances repair of a torn chorda is feasible. Mitral valve replacement is generally required for more extensive disruption of the valve, and for predominant involvement of the anterior mitral leaflet.

Acute chordal rupture with severe mitral regurgitation may initially be managed with vasodilator therapy. Following stabilization of the patient, valve surgery may be considered.

REFERENCES

1. Barlow JB, Bosman CK, Pocock WA et al: Late systolic murmur and nonejection (mid-late) systolic clicks. Br Heart J 30:203, 1968
2. Criley JM, Lewis KB, Humphries JO et al: Prolapse of the mitral valve: Clinical and cineangiocardiographic findings. Br Heart J 28:488, 1966
3. Shah PM, Gramiak R: Echocardiographic recognition of mitral valve prolapse (abstr). Circulation (Suppl 3) 42:45, 1970
4. Kerber RE, Isaeff PM, Hancock EW: Echocardiographic patterns in patients with the syndrome of systolic click and late systolic murmur. N Engl J Med 284:691, 1971
5. Dillon JC, Haine CL, Chang S et al: Use of echocardiography in patients with prolapsed mitral valve. Circulation 43:503, 1971
6. Popp RL, Brown OR, Silverman JF et al: Echocardiographic abnormalities in the mitral valve prolapse syndrome. Circulation 49:428, 1974
7. DeMaria AD, King JF, Bogren JG et al: The variable spectrum of echocardiographic manifestations of the mitral valve prolapse syndrome. Circulation 50:33, 1974
8. Kisslo J, von Ramm OT, Thurstone FL: Cardiac imaging using a phased-array ultrasound system. II: Clinical technique and application. Circulation 53:262, 1976
9. Morganroth J, Mardelli TJ, Naito M et al: Apical cross sectional echocardiography: Standard for the diagnosis of idiopathic mitral valve prolapse syndrome. Chest 79(1):23, 1981
10. Ormiston JA, Shah PM, Tei C, Wong M: Size and motion of the mitral valve annulus in man. I: A two-dimensional echocardiographic method and findings in normal subjects. Circulation 64:113, 1981
11. Ormiston JA, Shah PM, Tei C, Wong M: Size and motion of the mitral valve annulus in man. II: Abnormalities in mitral valve prolapse. Circulation 65:713, 1982
12. Levine RA, Triulzi MO, Harrigan P, Weyman AE: The relationship of mitral annular shape to the diagnosis of mitral valve prolapse. Circulation 75:756, 1987
13. Levine RA, Stathogiannis E, Newell JB, Harrigan P, Weyman AE: Reconsideration of echocardiographic standards for mitral valve prolapse: Lack of association between leaflet displacement isolated to the apical four chamber view and independent echocardiographic evidence of abnormality. J Am Coll Cardiol 11:1010, 1988
14. Wooley CF: Where are the diseases of yesteryear? DaCosta's syndrome, soldier's heart, the effort syndrome, neurocirculatory asthenia—and the mitral valve prolapse syndrome. Circulation 53:749, 1976
15. Lucas RV Jr, Edwards JE: The floppy mitral valve. Curr Probl Cardiol 7:1, 1982
16. Waller BF, Morrow AG, Maron BJ et al: Etiology of clinically isolated, severe, chronic, pure, mitral regurgitation: Analysis of 97 patients over 30 years of age having mitral valve replacement. Am Heart J 104:288, 1982
17. Devereux RB, Brown T, Kramer-Fix R, Sachs I: Inheritance of mitral valve prolapse: Effect of age and sex on gene expression. Ann Intern Med 97:826, 1982
18. Strahn NV, Murphy EA, Fortuin NJ et al: Inheritance of the mitral valve prolapse syndrome: Discussion of a three-dimensional penetrance model. Am J Med 74:967, 1983
19. Savage DD, Garrison RJ, Devereux RB et al: Mitral valve prolapse in the general population. 1. Epidemiologic features: The Framingham Study. Am Heart J 106:571, 1983
20. Schute JE, Gaffney FA, Blend L, Blomquist CG: Distinctive anthropometric characteristics of women with mitral valve prolapse. Am J Med 71:533, 1981
21. Jaffe AS, Geltman EM, Rodey GE, Utto J: Mitral valve prolapse: A consistent manifestation of Type IV Ehlers-Danlos syndrome: The pathogenic role of the abnormal production of Type III collagen. Circulation 64:121, 1981
22. Savage DD, Devereux RB, Garrison RJ et al: Mitral valve prolapse in the general population. 2. Clinical features: The Framingham Study. Am Heart J 106:577, 1983
23. Venkatesh A, Pauls DL, Crowe R et al: Mitral valve prolapse in anxiety neurosis (panic disorder). Am Heart J 100:302, 1980
24. Mavissakalin M, Salerni R, Thompson ME, Michelsen L: Mitral valve prolapse and agoraphobia. Am J Psychiatry 140:1612, 1983
25. Tei C, Shah PM, Cherian G et al: The correlates of abnormal first heart sound in mitral valve prolapse syndromes. N Engl J Med 307:334, 1982
26. Perloff JK, Child JS, Edwards JE: New guidelines for the clinical diagnosis of mitral valve prolapse. Am J Cardiol 57:1124, 1986
27. Mautner RK, Katz GE, Held BJ, Phillips JH: Coronary artery spasm: A mechanism for chest pain in selected patients with the mitral valve prolapse syndrome. Chest 79:499, 1981
28. Gaffney FA, Bastian BC, Lane LB et al: Abnormal cardiovascular regulation in the mitral valve prolapse syndrome. Am J Cardiol 52:316, 1983
29. Coghlan HC, Phares P, Cowley M et al: Dysautonomia in mitral valve prolapse. Am J Med 67:236, 1979
30. Gaffney FA, Karlsson ES, Campbell W et al: Autonomic dysfunction in women with mitral valve prolapse syndrome. Circulation 59:894, 1979
31. Boudoulas H, Kolibash AJ, Baker P, King BD, Wooley CF: Mitral valve prolapse and the mitral valve prolapse syndrome: A diagnostic classification and pathogenesis of symptoms. Am Heart J 118:796, 1989
32. Boudoulas H, Reynolds JC, Mazzaferri E, Wooley CF. Metabolic studies in mitral valve prolapse syndrome. Circulation 61:1200, 1980
33. Boudoulas H, Reynolds JC, Mazzaferri E, Wooley CF: Mitral valve prolapse syndrome: The effect of adrenergic stimulation. J Am Coll Cardiol 2:638, 1983
34. Rogers JM, Boudoulas H, Malarkey WB, Wooley CF: Mitral valve prolapse:

Disordered catecholamine regulations with intravascular volume maneuvers (Abstr). Circulation (Supp 3)68, 1983

35. Fontana ME, Wooley CF, Leighton RF, Lewis RP: Postural changes in left ventricular and mitral valvular dynamics in the systolic click-late systolic murmur syndrome. Circulation 51:167, 1975
36. Gaffney AF, Lane LB, Pettinger W, Blomquist GC: Effects of long-term clonidine administration on the hemodynamic and neuroendocrine postural responses of patients with dysautonomia. Chest 83:436, 1983
37. Rogers JM, Boudoulas H, Wooley CF: Abnormal reninaldosterone response to volume depletion in mitral valve prolapse. (Abstr) Circulation (Suppl 2)336, 1984
38. Pasternac A, Latour JG, Leger-Gauthier C, Lambert M, Cantin M, de Champlain J: Stability of hyperadrenergic state, atrial natriuretic factor, and platelet abnormalities in mitral valve prolapse syndrome. In: Boudoulas H, Wooley CF (eds): The Mitral Valve Prolapse and the Mitral Valve Prolapse syndrome, pp 455–63. Mount Kisco, NY: Futura, 1988
39. Vijayaraghavan G, Boltwood CM, Tei C et al: Simplified echocardiographic measurement of the mitral annulus. Am Heart J (in press)
40. Shah PM: Update of mitral valve prolapse syndrome: When is echo prolapse a pathological prolapse? Echocardiography: A review of cardiovascular ultrasound 1(1):87, 1984
41. Gardin JM, Isner JM, Ronan JA, Fox SA: Pseudoischemic "false positive" ST segment changes induced by hyperventilation in patients with mitral valve prolapse. Am J Cardiol 45:952, 1980
42. Gaffney FA, Wohl AJ, Blomquist CG et al: Thallium-201 myocardial perfusion studies in patients with the mitral valve prolapse syndrome. Am J Med 64:21, 1978
43. Tresch DD, Doyle TP, Boncheck LI et al: Mitral valve prolapse requiring surgery: Clinical and pathologic study. Am J Med 78:245, 1985
44. Winkle RA, Lopes MG, Popp RL, Hancock EW: Life threatening arrhythmias in mitral valve prolapse syndrome. Am J Med 60:961, 1976
45. Wei JY, Bulkley BH, Schaeffer AH et al: Mitral valve prolapse syndrome and recurrent ventricular tachyarrhythmias: A malignant variant refractory to conventional drug therapy. Ann Intern Med 86:6, 1978
46. Lichstein E: Site of origin of ventricular premature beats in patients with mitral valve prolapse. Am Heart J 100:450, 1980
47. Josephson ME, Horowitz LN, Kastor JA: Paroxysmal supraventricular tachycardia in patients with mitral valve prolapse. Circulation 57:111, 1977
48. Drake CE, Hodsden JE, Sridharan MR, Flowers NC: Evaluation of the association of mitral valve prolapse in patients with Wolff-Parkinson-White type ECG and its relationship to the ventricular activation pattern. Am Heart J 109:83, 1985
49. Boudoulas H, Reynolds J, Mazzaferri E, Wooley CF: Metabolic studies in mitral valve prolapse syndrome: A neuroendocrine cardiovascular process. Circulation 61:1200, 1980
50. Combs RL, Shah PM, Klorman RS, Klorman R: Effects of induced psychological stress on click and rhythm in mitral valve prolapse. Am Heart J 99:714, 1980
51. Morady F, Shen E, Bhandari A et al: Programmed ventricular stimulation in mitral valve prolapse: Analysis of 30 patients. Am J Cardiol 53:135, 1984
52. Ware JA, Magro SA, Luck JC et al: Conduction system abnormalities in symptomatic mitral valve prolapse: An electrophysiologic analysis of 60 patients. Am J Cardiol 53:1075, 1984
53. Kramer HM, Kligfield P, Devereux RB et al: Arrhythmias in mitral valve prolapse: Effect of selection bias. Arch Intern Med 144:2360, 1984
54. Savage DD, Levy D, Garrison RJ et al: Mitral valve prolapse in the general population: Three dysrrhythmias: The Framingham Study. Am Heart J 106:582, 1983
55. Pocock WA, Bosman CK, Chester E et al: Sudden death in primary mitral valve prolapse. Am Heart J 107:398, 1984
56. Bharati S, Granston AS, Lichson PR et al: The conduction system in mitral valve prolapse syndrome with sudden death. Am Heart J 104:667, 1981
57. Corrigall D, Bolen J, Hancock EW, Popp RL: Mitral Valve prolapse and infective endocarditis. Am J Med 53:215, 1977
58. Clemens JD, Horwitz RI, Jaffee CC et al: A controlled evaluation of the risk of bacterial endocarditis in persons with mitral valve prolapse. N Engl J Med 307:776, 1982
59. Barnett HJM, Bongliner DR, Taylor W et al: Further evidence relating mitral valve prolapse to cerebral ischemic events. N Engl J Med 302:139, 1980
60. Steele P, Weiley H, Rainwater J et al: Platelet survival time and thromboembolism in patients with mitral valve prolapse. Circulation 60:43, 1979
61. Bisset GS, Schwartz DC, Meyer RA et al: Clinical spectrum and long-term follow up of isolated mitral valve prolapse in 119 children. Circulation 52:423, 1980
62. Oakley CM: Mitral valve prolapse: Harbinger of death or variant of normal: Br Med J 288:1853, 1984
63. Clemens JD, Ransohoff DF: A quantitative assessment of predental antibiotic prophylaxis of patients with mitral valve prolapse. J Chronic Dis 37:531, 1984

> # VALVULAR HEART DISEASE: PROSTHETIC VALVE REPLACEMENT

L. Henry Edmunds, Jr
V. Paul Addonizio, Jr ▪ Nicholas A. Tepe

The ideal prosthetic heart valve does not exist. Modern prosthetic valves are still plagued by an operative mortality and morbidity and by problems of thromboembolism, anticoagulant-related bleeding, infective endocarditis, durability, hemolysis, and noise. No prosthetic valve has all of these problems, but none matches the performance of the normal cardiac valve. Nevertheless, approximately 80,000 prosthetic heart valves were implanted worldwide in 1984, and approximately half of these were placed in Americans. Prosthetic valves offer symptomatic patients an attractive alternative to the restricted activity, progressive morbidity, and eventual mortality due to malfunction of one or more cardiac valves. This chapter reviews the current status of prosthetic heart valves.

A wide variety of pathologic processes including congenital malformations and disorders, infections, ischemia, inflammatory diseases, and degenerative changes afflict cardiac valves. Rheumatic fever, once the dominant cause of valvular heart disease, is now only one of many causes of valve dysfunction. Although causes of valve disease are important, hemodynamic consequences produce symptoms. With rare exception, activity-limiting symptoms are prerequisite for implantation of a prosthetic valve.

The decision to replace a cardiac valve is made when symptoms, quality of life, and prognosis, predicted by natural history data, are less attractive than the morbidity and mortality associated with a prosthetic valve. This is an important concept, for as the mortality and morbidity of prosthetic valves approach zero, operation can be prescribed earlier and before ventricular morphology and contractility are injured by a period of valvular dysfunction. Even with current valve prostheses, the majority of late cardiac deaths are due to cardiac causes, which are not related to prosthetic valve function. Arrhythmias and heart failure are, in part, consequences of myocardial fibrosis initiated by the pathologic process, or are the result of adaptive changes caused by valve dysfunction (*e.g.*, ventricular fibrillation). Earlier operation may reduce the incidence of these late non-valve-related cardiac deaths, but cannot be prescribed until operative and late morbidity and mortality approach that of the normal valve.

HISTORY

As early as 1902, Sir Lander Brunton suggested an operation for relief of mitral stenosis, the details of which were determined in laboratory animals and humans.[1] Brunton's suggestions, however, met with a storm of criticism occasioned by the then popular belief that the problem in patients with mitral stenosis occurred from weakened myocardium rather than a deformed valve. In 1923, following renewed interest in developing a surgical attack on the stenotic mitral valve, a "cardio-valvulotome" was inserted through the apex of the left ventricle to relieve severe stenosis in an 11-year-old girl. The operation was technically a success, but the underlying disease process progressed relentlessly. Indeed, although Henry Souttar realized in 1925 that digital dilatation of the mitral valve could be performed safely through the left atrial appendage,[2] when results of mitral surgery were reviewed in 1929, only 2 of 10 patients remained as survivors.[3] Then, in the 1940s, Dr. Dwight Harken and Dr. Charles Bailey independently performed successful "mitral commissurotomies."[4,5]

The surgical attack on the stenotic pulmonic valve began in 1947 when T. Halveo Sellors[6] incised the leaflets of a stenotic pulmonary valve through the main pulmonary artery. Following this pioneering effort, Lord Brock performed several successful valvotomies through the right ventricular apex using a newly developed valvulotome.[7]

Solution of the surgical problems associated with aortic valve surgery required development of the heart–lung machine. In the 1940s Charles Hufnagel began to construct an aortic valve prosthesis. Finally, after approximately 10 years of research, Hufnagel inserted a mechanical plastic ball valve in the descending thoracic aorta of a patient with aortic regurgitation in 1952.[8]

In 1953, open heart surgery became feasible when Gibbon performed the first cardiac procedure using a pump oxygenator. Meanwhile, numerous advances in the design of mechanical valves were introduced after Hufnagel's pioneering efforts. In 1960, Harken successfully replaced an aortic valve,[9] and Starr inserted a mitral valve prosthesis.[10] The success of the Starr-Edwards prosthesis ushered in the modern era of valve replacement surgery. Preserved heterograft valves were introduced in 1965.[11,12]

INDICATIONS FOR VALVE REPLACEMENT

Prosthetic valves are prescribed for ongoing symptoms or life-threatening complications. The natural history of cardiac valve disease is well established but includes the coincident development of ventricular dysfunction, which is due in part to the hemodynamic burden imposed by the diseased valve.[13] To some extent, ventricular dysfunction may progress independently of symptoms so that irreversible ventricular damage develops before valve replacement surgery is recommended. Since irreversible ventricular dysfunction increases late mortality and morbidity, optimal timing of operation must consider ventricular contractility and dynamics as well as symptoms and weigh these considerations against the total morbidity and mortality of a prosthetic valve.

AORTIC STENOSIS

The onset of symptoms in aortic stenosis is associated with a markedly decreased life expectancy. The average life expectancy for patients with aortic stenosis and angina or syncope is 3 years, and for patients with aortic stenosis and congestive heart failure only 1.5 years.[14] In addition, a significant portion of patients who have tight aortic stenosis (valve area < 0.5 cm^2/m^2) have sudden death as their first symptom. Criteria for defining this asymptomatic patient group have not yet been developed. Although dependent on cardiac output, most cardiologists consider a resting valvular gradient of 50 mm Hg an indication for operation. Therefore, the indications for valve replacement in patients with aortic stenosis are

1. Aortic stenosis associated with angina, syncope, or congestive heart failure

2. Peak systolic gradients ≥ 50 mm Hg
3. Valve area ≤ 0.7 cm²/m²

MITRAL STENOSIS

Patients with mitral stenosis usually have a 10- to 20-year asymptomatic latent period and a subtle onset of symptoms. However, once symptoms become significant, life expectancy is shortened. Five-year survival in patients with mitral stenosis who are New York Heart Association (NYHA) class III is 62% and NYHA class IV is 15%.[15] The usual causes of death are pulmonary edema, pulmonary hypertension with right ventricular failure, systemic embolization, pulmonary emboli, and infective endocarditis. Of patients with mitral stenosis 20% will develop emboli and 25% of those develop recurrent emboli.[16] The indications for mitral valve replacement in patients with mitral stenosis are

1. NYHA class III or IV
2. Valve area of 1.0 cm² or less
3. Systemic emboli

Active rheumatic pancarditis and cerebral embolization both require delay in surgery. Elevations in pulmonary artery pressure do not contraindicate surgery, and patients with pulmonary artery pressure > 120 mm Hg systolic should not be denied mitral valve replacement.

AORTIC REGURGITATION

Chronic aortic regurgitation in itself carries a reasonable prognosis with a 5-year survival of 75% and a 10-year survival of 50%.[17] However, once a patient becomes symptomatic, irreversible left ventricular damage has often already occurred and the prognosis worsens to a life expectancy of 5 years for aortic regurgitation and angina, and 2 years for aortic regurgitation and congestive heart failure.[18] At this point, there is usually irreversible fibrosis of the left ventricle with distention of the remaining myocardial fibers. For aortic regurgitation in an asymptomatic patient, the goal is to time surgery just prior to the development of left ventricular dysfunction.[19]

Several noninvasive methods have been used to detect the onset of irreversible left ventricular dysfunction in asymptomatic patients with aortic regurgitation. Unfortunately, cardiomegaly by chest x-ray and electrocardiographic voltage criteria correlate poorly with the degree of aortic regurgitation and fail to predict symptomatic status.[20] Early ventricular dysfunction can be reversed,[21-23] but if operation is delayed, operative mortality and morbidity greatly increase, and there may be little or no improvement in left ventricular function and long-term survival.[22,24,25] Ultrasound may help identify asymptomatic, high-risk patients. Clark[25] found a 94% 5-year survival in patients with preoperative ejection fractions over 45% versus a 33% 5-year survival in patients with lower ejection fractions. Henry[26] found that a left ventricular end-systolic minor axis diameter > 55 mm or a percent fractional dimension shortening of < 25% correlated with operative death or severe postoperative heart failure. At present, there are no universally accepted criteria for valve replacement in asymptomatic patients with aortic regurgitation.

Acute aortic regurgitation secondary to bacterial endocarditis or aortic dissection requires immediate aortic valve replacement because of an unacceptably high mortality rate when this condition is treated medically.

Morgan[27] has summarized the indications for valve replacement for aortic regurgitation as follows:

1. NYHA class III or IV
2. NYHA class II with
   a. Left ventricular systolic minor axis 5.5 cm or greater
   b. A 3+ or 4+ aortic regurgitation with ejection fraction ≤ 50%
3. Increasing ventricular volumes or decreasing ejection fraction
4. Any *acute* aortic regurgitation

MITRAL REGURGITATION

Mitral regurgitation is similar to aortic regurgitation in that the lesion can be tolerated well for many years, but that severe symptoms may herald the onset of irreversible left ventricular dysfunction. Survival in 70 selected patients with mitral regurgitation was 80% at 5 years and 60% at 10 years.[13] However, despite these apparently optimistic data, patients with mitral regurgitation should have mitral valve replacement prior to onset of severe symptoms.[28]

Left ventricular dimensions can be obtained by echocardiogram and ejection fraction and regurgitant fraction can be approximated by radionuclear angiogram. Morgan[27] summarizes the indications for valve replacement for mitral regurgitation as follows:

1. NYHA class III or IV
2. NYHA class II with
   a. Left ventricular diastolic minor axis 5 cm or greater
   b. Regurgitant fraction 40% or greater
   c. A 4+ mitral regurgitation with ejection fraction 60% or less
3. Increasing ventricular volumes or regurgitant fraction
4. Acute severe mitral regurgitation

TRICUSPID STENOSIS AND REGURGITATION

Isolated tricuspid valve disease is rare; most often, tricuspid disease occurs in association with mitral valve disease. Tricuspid insufficiency is more common than stenosis and usually develops in association with pulmonary hypertension secondary to mitral stenosis or regurgitation. Rheumatic fever, endocarditis, and trauma are often causes of tricuspid insufficiency; tricuspid stenosis is nearly always rheumatic.

Tricuspid valves are usually repaired rather than replaced. Valvuloplasty techniques are often successful in opening stenotic valves and in reducing the dilated annulus of regurgitant valves. The decision to replace the valve is made at operation usually on the basis of destroyed or infected leaflets.

OPERATION AND EARLY POSTOPERATIVE MANAGEMENT

Once the decision for cardiac valve replacement has been made and accepted, the patient is prepared for operation. Preparation will be minimal if the patient's hemodynamic condition is unstable or unsatisfactory, and in these patients, expeditious transfer to the operating room is wise. In extreme situations, operation may be started in an unconscious or lethargic patient simultaneously with endotracheal intubation and anesthesia. The immediate goal is to initiate cardiopulmonary bypass as rapidly as possible to maintain adequate perfusion of essential organs.

For elective operations the patient deserves both psychological and medical preparation. Although others may contribute, the senior operating surgeon should explain to the patient and close relatives the indications for operation, alternatives to operation, what exactly is planned, and the expected result. Both benefits and risks should be explained, and all questions should be truthfully answered. Others may provide detailed supplementary material and obtain signatures on "informed consent" forms. However, the interview with the senior operating surgeon is essential to obtain the patient's trust and to strengthen his confidence.

The patient must be fully evaluated medically. Both the type and severity of associated diseases of other organs and organ systems should be catalogued. Routinely all patients have an electrocardiogram, chest roentgenogram, and laboratory tests to determine hemoglobin, white and platelet counts, blood type, serum electrolytes, BUN, creatinine, sugar, total protein, prothrombin time, and partial thromboplastin time. Pulmonary function tests, liver chemistries, bleeding time, fibrinogen concentration, and other special studies are dictated by historical and physical findings. Note is made of medications, allergies, and special problems. Carious teeth should be removed before operation (with antibiotic coverage). Arrhythmias should be controlled and cardiac function optimized to the extent possible with medical measures. If possible, the patient should receive respiratory therapy training preoperatively.

The anesthesiologist usually visits the patient before operation and describes the planned anesthesia and the induction experience. The anesthesiologist thoroughly reviews the patient's hospital chart and notes the presence of associated diseases, allergies, and medications. Premedication orders for the anesthetic are written by the anesthesiologist.

The surgeon specifies when medications are to be stopped, the number of units of blood to be cross-matched, whether or not fresh-frozen plasma or platelet transfusions are likely to be required, and the doses and type of preoperative antibiotics. Usually a broad-spectrum antibiotic, such as cephalothin or vancomycin (for patients allergic to penicillin), is given in the operating room just before induction of anesthesia. Body hair over planned and possible incisions is removed before transfer to the operating room. A depilatory is preferred to shaving.

In the operating room, electrocardiographic leads and monitoring catheters in the radial artery and internal jugular vein (Swan-Ganz catheter) are placed with local anesthesia, and sedation is provided by premedication. After induction of anesthesia, an endotracheal tube is passed and secured. Nasopharyngeal and rectal temperature probes, an esophageal stethoscope, a Foley catheter, and the grounding pad for an electrocautery are placed after induction of anesthesia. The electrocardiogram (usually two leads), temperatures, and arterial, central venous, and pulmonary arterial pressures are monitored continuously.

The midline sternotomy incision is the most common approach for operations on the cardiac valves.[29] All four valves can be easily exposed through this incision. Satisfactory exposure of the mitral valve may be obtained via a right or left thoracotomy. The tricuspid valve can be seen through a right thoracotomy. A transverse incision across the sternum and into both the left and right chest may be used to expose the aortic valve and great vessels as well as other valves.[30] For most patients, including those who require reoperation, a midline sternotomy incision is made. In exceptional circumstances, other incisions and special cannulation techniques for the heart-lung machine may be used.[30]

After exposure of the heart and administration of intravenous heparin (3 mg/kg), the ascending aorta just upstream to the innominate artery is cannulated. Optionally, a femoral artery may be cannulated, and this is routinely done by some surgeons prior to thoracotomy in patients who have had previous cardiac operations. For isolated aortic valve replacement, one large catheter may be placed in the right atrium to capture most of the venous return to the heart. For operations on the mitral, tricuspid, or pulmonary valves, both the inferior and superior vena cavae are cannulated via the right atrium. Double venous cannulation is often used for combination operations on the coronary arteries and aortic valve. Tourniquets are placed around both cannulated cavae during bypass to prevent blood reaching the right atrium when the tricuspid or pulmonary valve is exposed.

After cardiopulmonary bypass is started, the patient is usually cooled to 26°C to 28°C (nasopharyngeal temperature). With the heart decompressed, the aorta is clamped and the heart is arrested with cold cardioplegic solution injected into the aortic root.[31] In patients with aortic insufficiency, the aorta is incised and cardioplegic solution is injected directly into the right and left coronary ostia. Simultaneously, the heart is bathed in cold (1°C-4°C) saline solution to achieve arrest. Cardioplegic solution and external cold saline are renewed approximately every 20 minutes to maintain myocardial protection. Either blood or crystalloid cardioplegic solution can be used.

The aortic and mitral valves are most commonly replaced. Replacement of the pulmonary valve is almost exclusively limited to reconstructive operations of the right ventricular outflow tract in patients with congenital cardiac disease. Tricuspid valve replacement is uncommon and represents about 1% to 2% of prosthetic valve operations.[32] Approximately 12% to 15% of patients who require valve prostheses have multiple valve replacements.[33-36] In patients who require simultaneous coronary bypass grafts, distal vein or artery graft anastomoses are usually made before valves are replaced to avoid annular suture line stresses when the heart is manipulated.

The aortic valve is exposed by an oblique incision in the aortic root placed 1 cm to 1.5 cm downstream from the right coronary orifice. The incision is carried into the noncoronary sinus to adequately reveal the valve and valve annulus. Exposure is facilitated by placing a catheter into the left ventricle via the left atrial–right superior pulmonary venous junction or left ventricular apex to aspirate left ventricular blood.[30]

The diseased valve is completely excised. Calcium attached to the annulus, adjacent to the aortic wall, anterior leaflet of the mitral valve, and ventricular septum, is carefully removed so that the tissues and structure of the left ventricular outflow tract are not destroyed. Debridement must be thorough to achieve the maximum annular diameter and to permit healing between the annulus and prosthesis. Occasional patients with endocarditis may have annular abscesses or fistulas that require closure and reconstruction of the annulus and left ventricular outflow tract before the prosthesis is inserted.

After preparation, the annulus is sized. The prosthetic valve can be inserted using interrupted single or mattress sutures or a continuous suture. Small Teflon felt pledgets may be used above or below the annulus to buttress mattress sutures. The valve annulus must be snugly opposed to the valve sewing ring around the circumference to prevent paravalvular leak. Valve function must not be compromised by adjacent tissue. While the patient is rewarmed, the aortic incision is closed with a double suture line.

Small aortic annuli can be incised and patched to accommodate a larger prosthesis. Incisions and patches in either the left coronary or noncoronary sinuses add 1 cm to 2 cm to the annular circumference.[30] An incision into the right coronary sinus (medial to the right coronary ostium) into both the ventricular septum and right ventricular outflow tract permits almost unlimited enlargement of the aortic annulus but requires prosthetic patching of the ventricular septum, right ventricle, and aorta (Fig. 84.1).[37] The aortic valve and ascending aorta may be replaced with a composite valved conduit sutured to the aortic annulus and distal ascending aorta. In this operation, both coronary ostia and any coronary bypass grafts are directly sutured to the conduit downstream to the prosthetic valve.[38]

The mitral valve may be exposed three different ways. Usually the left atrium is incised posterior to the interatrial septum. The incision is carried posterior to the inferior vena cava and superiorly into the right superior pulmonary vein–left atrial junction to expose the valve. Alternatively, a superior left atrial incision, made by retracting the aorta medially and the superior vena cava laterally, or an incision in the interatrial septum via a right atriotomy may be used. An enlarged left atrium improves exposure when the atrial septal approach is used. When both aortic and mitral valves are replaced, the mitral valve is replaced first.

In recent years, more aggressive and innovative attempts to reconstruct the mitral valve have become popular.[39] However, when the valve must be replaced, it is excised so that a 1-mm to 2-mm rim of leaflet tissue is left attached to the annulus. Chordae are completely excised, but the papillary muscles are preserved. If a bioprosthetic mitral valve is used, chordal attachments may be preserved by excising only the midportion of the anterior leaflet.[40] Calcium is meticulously debrided, but this must be done very carefully if large amounts of calcium are deposited in the mural annulus of elderly patients. In such patients calcium may actually extend through to the epicardial surface near the circumflex coronary artery. Once the valve is excised and the annulus is prepared, the proper sized prosthesis is sutured in place with pledgeted interrupted mattress sutures, single interrupted sutures, or two or three continuous sutures. To prevent annular tissue from interfering with closure of mechanical valves, pledgeted mattress sutures should be placed so that the pledget is on the atrial surface of the annulus. A Foley catheter is temporarily placed through the prosthetic valve to decompress the left ventricle and to facilitate removal of air until cardiopulmonary bypass is discontinued. The left atrium is closed with a single or double running suture around the catheter but is not tied closed until all air is evacuated from the left heart.

No good techniques are available to enlarge the mitral annulus, but this is seldom necessary in adults and older children. In patients with large left ventricular aneurysms, the mitral valve can be excised and replaced through the ventriculotomy.

Tourniquets around both cannulated cavae and an aortic clamp produce a dry operative field when the right atrium is opened to expose the tricuspid valve or mitral valve via an incision in the interatrial septum. In most patients the tricuspid valve can be reconstructed using valvuloplastic procedures and techniques to reduce the circumference of the tricuspid annulus.[41] When the valve must be excised and replaced, all chordae are removed, but papillary muscles are not cut. Calcium seldom, if ever, involves the tricuspid annulus, but thick fibrous tissue can involve the valve annulus, leaflets, and chordae. Along the septal leaflet near the conduction system, anchoring sutures for the prosthesis are passed through the annulus and a rim of leaflet to avoid injury to the bundle of His. Many surgeons prefer bioprosthetic valves for tricuspid valve replacement.

The pulmonary valve is rarely excised and replaced. More often, a bioprosthesis is used within a conduit to bypass or replace the right ventricular outflow tract and main pulmonary artery. Although bioprostheses calcify and deteriorate with time in the pulmonary circuit,[42] mechanical prostheses are poorly tolerated (thrombosis, emboli) and are rarely used. If the tricuspid valve is competent and pulmonary vascular resistance is not increased, most patients do well without a pulmonary valve if obstruction to flow from the right ventricle to the lungs is completely relieved.

After insertion of valves and closure of cardiac chambers, all air must be evacuated from the heart before the aortic clamp is released. Furthermore, ventricular distention must be assiduously avoided until the ventricles resume reliable contractions. Temporary atrial and ventricular pacing wires are placed to facilitate management of cardiac rhythm postoperatively. Direct measurement of left atrial pressure via a small polyethylene catheter in the left atrium is optional.

Cardiopulmonary bypass is stopped after the patient is rewarmed to a nasopharyngeal temperature of 37°C and a rectal temperature of 33°C or more, and after spontaneous or paced ventricular contractions at the rate of 70 to 90 beats per minute are established. Pulmonary ventilation is started and abnormalities in serum electrolytes and blood gases are corrected before bypass stops. The aorta is usually vented for possible air as the patient is weaned from the heart–lung machine. The surgeon must carefully observe cardiac performance and contractility and closely monitor ventricular filling pressures, arterial pressure, and cardiac rhythm and rate during this critical period. Thermodilution cardiac output measurements are frequently helpful. Intravenous calcium, epinephrine, an infusion of other catecholamines, and/or vasodilator drugs may be helpful. In exceptional cases the use of the intra-aortic balloon pump, inserted via the femoral artery or less commonly via a polyfluorotetraethylene (PFTE) graft sutured to the ascending aorta, may be required.[43] Venous cannulas are not removed until an adequate and stable circulation is established. After venous cannulas are removed, protamine is given to neutralize heparin, and wound hemostasis is secured. Much of the blood within the bypass system is returned to the patient during the immediate post-bypass period; the remainder of the perfusate and blood aspirated from the surgical field is washed and concentrated, and eventually returned to the patient as packed cells.

POSTOPERATIVE CARE

After placement of prosthetic cardiac valves, patients are monitored and nursed in a surgical intensive care unit.[44] Electronic monitoring, constant surveillance, and correction of abnormalities before crises occur are fundamental to a successful outcome.

The electrocardiogram, arterial blood pressure, central venous pressure, and left atrial or pulmonary arterial pressure are continuously monitored. Chest tube drainage, urine volume, and rectal temperature are monitored at least every hour. Thermodilution cardiac output, arterial blood P_{O_2}, P_{CO_2}, and pH, and blood hematocrit, potassium, and calcium are measured from time to time. Arterial blood gases are usually obtained whenever ventilator settings are changed. A mixed venous P_{O_2} is periodically obtained in patients who have low cardiac output. Serum electrolytes, creatinine, urea nitrogen, total protein, glucose, prothrombin time, partial thromboplastin time, and white cell and platelet counts are measured the morning after operation and thereafter as needed. In some patients, measurements of myocardial enzymes and liver function tests are also made. A chest film (portable anteroposterior) and 12-lead electrocardiogram are obtained shortly after the patient arrives in the intensive care unit and at least once daily while the patient is in the unit. The type and amount of all fluids given

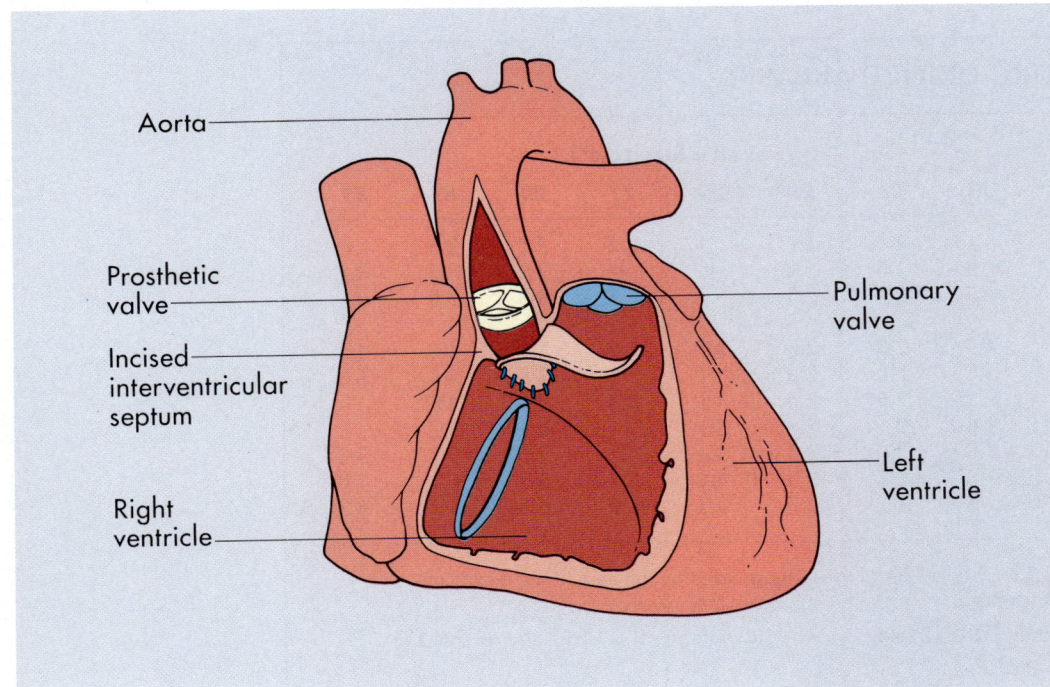

FIGURE 84.1 Diagram of a method to enlarge a small aortic annulus to accommodate a larger prosthesis. The aortotomy is extended across the annulus medial to the right coronary ostium into both the outflow tract of the right ventricle and also into the ventricular septum. The prosthesis is sewn to the aortic annulus and to an elliptical patch sewn to the incision in the ventricular septum. This patch is continued cephalad to close the aortotomy. A second patch is used to close the right ventricular outflow tract and necessarily this patch must be sewn to the first at the aorta. (Modified from Konno S, Imai Y, Iida Y et al: A new method for prosthetic valve replacement in congenital aortic stenosis associated with hypoplasia of the aortic valve ring. J Thorac Cardiovasc Surg 70:909, 1975)

to or removed from the patient are measured and recorded hourly. The patient is weighed daily.

The goal of postoperative care is to maintain a satisfactory cardiac output (>2.2 liters/m^2/min) and satisfactory function of all organ systems while the heart recovers from operative trauma, cardioplegia, and the new dynamics produced by the prosthetic valve. Cardiac output, a product of heart rate and stroke volume, is closely monitored and managed. Arrhythmias are promptly recognized and treated; atrial, ventricular, or sequential pacing using temporary pacing wires is commonly used. Stroke volume is manipulated by monitoring right or left ventricular filling pressures, myocardial contractility, and right and left ventricular afterload. In adult patients usually left ventricular performance is more precarious early after operation than is right ventricular function. Therefore, pulmonary end-diastolic pressure (or left atrial pressure) and systemic vascular resistance are managed by fluids and vasodilator drugs to improve cardiac output. Myocardial contractility is manipulated by avoiding drugs which decrease contractility and by using catecholamines, calcium, and digoxin to increase contractility. Occasional patients will require intra-aortic balloon pumping to reduce afterload and to increase coronary blood flow[43]; rare patients may require left or biventricular mechanical assistance using extracorporeal circulatory assist technology.[45]

Most patients are mechanically ventilated after valve replacement until fully awake from anesthesia and until central circulatory dynamics are both stable and clearly adequate. The endotracheal tube is removed when the patient is able to maintain adequate blood ventilation as confirmed by measurement of arterial blood gases. Other measures are directed toward preventing common postoperative respiratory complications: pneumothorax, atelectasis, pneumonia, pleural effusion, and aspiration.

Excessive bleeding after prosthetic valve operations is not uncommon and may be due to failure of blood to clot or to open vessels or leaking sutures lines. Additional protamine, fresh-frozen plasma, platelet transfusions, and increased end-expiratory airway pressure are some nonsurgical means to control postoperative bleeding. Reexploration is indicated if blood losses exceed 10 ml/kg/hr during the first hour after operation and 5 ml/kg/hr any hour thereafter. Pericardial tamponade, if recognized and untreated, can cause low cardiac output and death.

Patients with prosthetic valves may develop any complication associated with open cardiac surgery in the first few days or weeks after operation. In addition to those mentioned above, acute transmural or subendocardial myocardial infarction, cerebral embolus or hemorrhage, renal failure, infection, and hepatitis are important possible complications. In patients who require anticoagulation, either intravenous heparin or coumadin, or both, is started shortly after the chest tubes used to drain the operative field are removed.

AVAILABLE PROSTHETIC VALVES

Ideally, prosthetic valves should achieve the same performance as undiseased natural valves. Unfortunately, the interaction between a natural valve and adjacent structures[46,47] and the inability of prosthetic valves to grow in children ensure the inferiority of prosthetic valves. Nevertheless, achievable criteria that define desirable characteristics of prosthetic valves can be established. These criteria include minimal opening impedance; minimal closing backflow; minimal leak when closed; availability in a wide range of sizes; low profile; lack of noise; structural strength and durability; nonthrombogenicity; minimal injury to red cells; minimal activation of platelets, white cells, and coagulation proteins; and resistance to infection.

The effective cross-sectional orifice area (EOA) of the opened valve *in vivo* is calculated using a modified hydraulic formula.[48,49]

$$\text{Aortic valve area (cm}^2\text{)} = \frac{F}{44.5}\sqrt{\Delta P}$$

$$\text{Mitral valve area (cm}^2\text{)} = \frac{F}{38.0}\sqrt{\Delta P}$$

where F equals flow across the orifice in milliliters per second, ΔP equals the mean pressure difference, and the numbers represent empirical constants that adjust for turbulence and other dynamic factors.[48] Flow must be adjusted for the duration of systole or diastole by dividing the measured cardiac output (milliliters per minute) by heart rate times systolic ejection time (sec) or diastolic filling time (sec). The formula estimates valve orifice area and is not accurate in the presence of regurgitation because regurgitant flow cannot be quantitated.

The effective orifice area (EOA) for normal adult aortic valves ranges between 2.6 cm^2 and 3.5 cm^2 and for normal mitral valves 4 cm^2 to 6 cm^2. Because of the necessity of a sewing ring, all prosthetic valves have smaller geometric orifice areas and EOAs than normal valves (Table 84.1). Furthermore, because of turbulence and other factors, all prosthetic valves produce more impedance to opening than

TABLE 84.1 GEOMETRIC ORIFICE AREAS *

Valve	Valve Size (cm^2)							
	19	21	23	25	27	29	31	33
Starr-Edwards		1.4	1.7	†	2.2	2.6	2.9	
Sutter	1.2	1.6	1.8	†	†	2.9	3.6	4.1
Bjork-Shiley (standard)	1.5	2.0	2.5	3.1	3.8	4.6	4.6	4.6
Bjork-Shiley (convexo-concave)	1.5	2.0	2.5	3.1	3.8	4.6	4.6	4.6
Omniscience	1.5	2.0	2.5	3.1	3.8	3.8	4.5	5.3
Medtronic-Hall		2.0	2.5	3.1	3.8	4.5	4.5	
St. Jude	1.6	2.1	2.6	3.1	3.7	4.4	5.2	
Hancock	1.5	2.0	2.5	3.8	4.2	4.9	5.7	5.5
Carpentier-Edwards	1.8	2.7	3.5	4.4	4.7	5.3	6.1	7.0
Ionescu-Shiley	1.8	2.1	2.7	3.3	4.0	4.5	5.3	6.2

* For mechanical valves, actual areas are smaller than those listed by the area of the occluding mechanism when the valve is open.

† Size not available: #24 Sutter 2.1; #26 Sutter 2.4; #24 Starr-Edwards 1.8; #26 Starr-Edwards 1.9.

do undiseased normal valves. The amounts of impedance and backflow vary with valve design and size as well as with heart rate and cardiac output. Effective orifice areas *in vivo* are generally smaller than geometric orifice areas because of anatomical and dynamic factors.

Prosthetic cardiac valves are currently divided into two classes: mechanical and bioprosthetic. Mechanical valves include all valves that do not contain any biologic tissue. These valves are manufactured from metals, plastics, and textiles that are carefully selected for durability, biocompatibility, and fabrication qualities. Components of mechanical valves can be made or machined to close tolerances, and representative valves can be intensively tested *in vitro* for manufacturing defects, structural fatigue, and wear. The wide range of biocompatible materials, defined as materials that are not antigenic and that do not react with host chemicals and enzymes, permit the design and construction of very durable mechanical prostheses.

Bioprosthesis is the term used to describe prosthetic valves that contain animal tissue. These manufactured valves are not strictly biocompatible, as defined above, and cannot be extensively tested *in vitro* for wear and structural fatigue. Moreover, individual valves of the same size and design may vary subtly since the animal tissue is handsewn to metal or plastic frames and textile sewing rings. Quality control largely depends on careful inspection during manufacture. The animal tissue is not living, is not antigenic, and is chemically treated before it is sewn to the frame. Durability of these valves is less certain than that of mechanical valves because the animal tissue may react *in vivo* with host chemicals and enzymes, and because the distribution of stresses on the flexing animal components may vary from valve to valve.[50]

Currently available mechanical valves may be subdivided into three basic designs: ball, tilting disc and bileaflet (Fig. 84.2). Ball valves are represented by the Starr-Edwards valve (American Bentley, Santa Ana, California) and the Sutter valve (formerly Smeloff-Cutter valve, Sutter Biomedical Inc., San Diego, California). In the Starr-Edwards valve, a barium-impregnated, silicone rubber ball moves within an outflow metal cage formed by three (aortic) or four (mitral) struts joined at the apex. During closure the ball rests against a metal seating ring, which is 0.88 the diameter of the ball. The Sutter valve has both inflow and outflow cages formed by metal struts, which are not joined, and the diameters of the ball and seating ring are identical.

Current ball valves are quiet and have a very low incidence of mechanical failure (*e.g.*, ball variance or escape). Because of the central ball, blood flows circumferentially through the valve orifice.[51] The design produces partial obstruction to flow at three levels: the seating ring; the space between the seating ring and the opened ball; and the space between the opened ball and aortic or ventricular wall. In patients with a narrow proximal aorta, the proximity of the cage and aortic wall may increase turbulence, peak flow velocity, and the pressure gradient across the valve, particularly during exercise. Furthermore, the high profile of the valve cage may complicate closure of the aortotomy. In patients with pure mitral stenosis and normal sized left ventricles, the cage may abut against the ventricular wall or partially obstruct the left ventricular outflow tract. Resting diastolic pressure gradients across smaller sized mitral ball valve prostheses are generally higher than those with other types of prostheses.[52–54] Backflow across ball valves is significantly less than with other mechanical prostheses.[55]

Tilting disc valves use a flat or convexo-concave disc to occlude

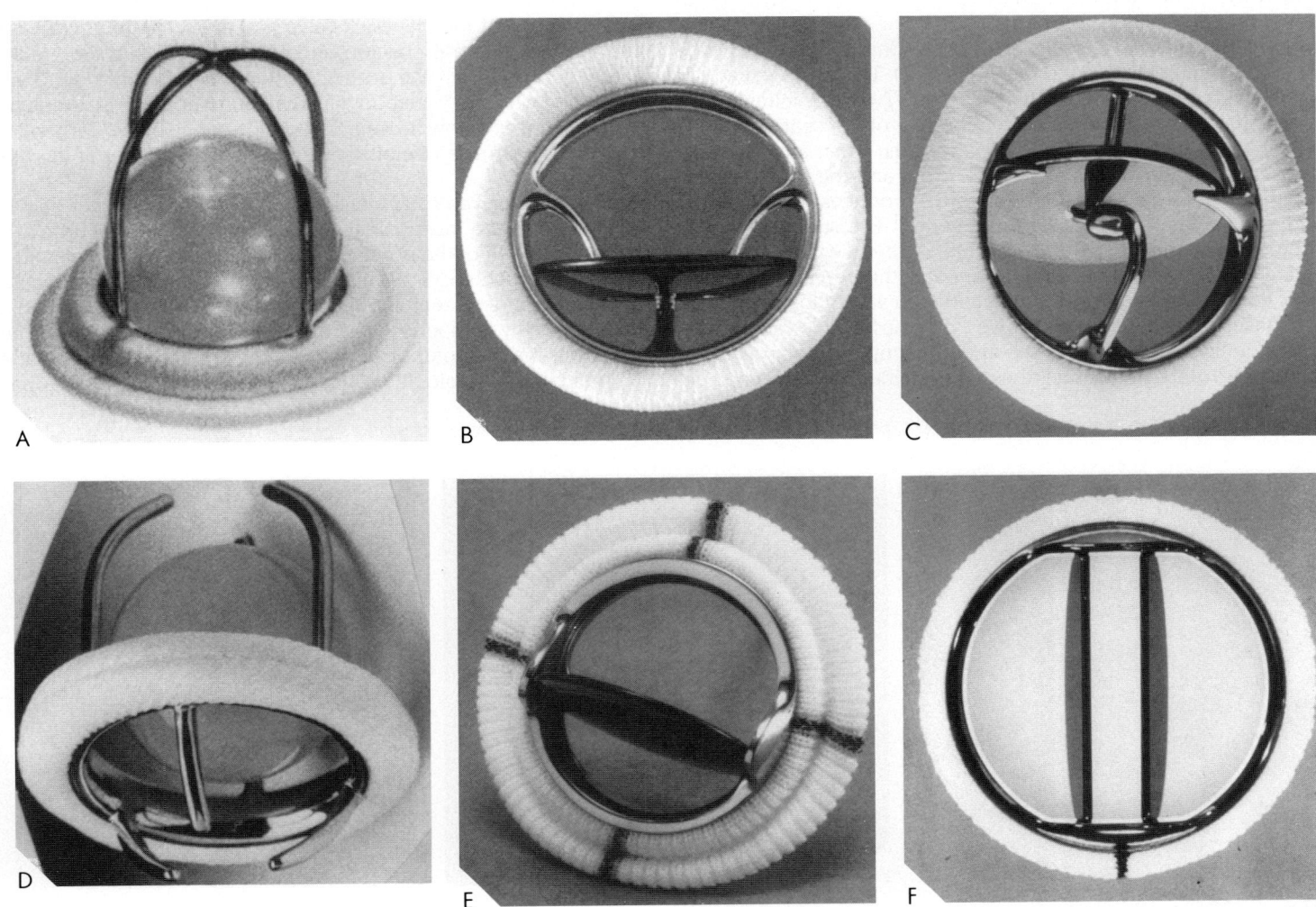

FIGURE 84.2 Mechanical valvular prostheses currently available in the United States. (A) Starr-Edwards ball valve; (B) Bjork-Shiley convexo-concave tilting disk; (C) Medtronic-Hall tilting disk; (D) Sutter ball; (E) Omniscience tilting disk; and (F) St. Jude bileaflet valve.

the valve orifice. When open, the disc tilts to an angle of 60° to 75° with the plane of the seating ring. Although materials and designs differ, the mechanism by which the moving disc is trapped largely distinguishes the three designs that are currently available (see Fig. 84.2). In all tilting disc valves the pivot point occurs along a minor chord of the disc; this produces a major and minor orifice for blood passing through the seating ring. The functional cross-sectional area of the opened valve is reduced by the obliquity of the tilted disc and the struts or protrusions of the disc-trapping mechanism.

Tilting disc valves usually close with a click, which may be audible in thin patients. In recent years, the valve-trapping mechanism and metal seating ring are machined out of one piece of metal to avoid welds. Welded struts of the Bjork-Shiley convexo-concave valve have fractured in numerous patients, usually with fatal results.[56] Failure of strut welds of earlier standard Bjork-Shiley valves and/or rupture of the disc are rare.[56] Mechanical failure of other tilting disc valves and of the new unwelded Bjork-Shiley convexo-concave valve are also uncommon.[57]

Tilting disc valves produce more central flow than ball valves, but generally more turbulence.[58] The height (profile) of the valve is low, which obviates problems of aortotomy closure and left ventricular outflow tract obstruction. Tilting disc valves can be rotated by the surgeon after insertion to partially direct flow through the major orifice and to ensure free motion of the disc. Pressure differences across tilting disc valves are slightly lower than differences across comparable ball valves.[52,58,59] On the other hand, backflow across tilting disc valves is approximately twice that observed with ball valves at comparable heart rates and flows.[55,60] *In vitro*, at high simulated heart rate (140 strokes/min) and low flow, backflow is approximately 30% of forward flow.[55] Protrusion of the valve-trapping mechanism and the necessity of a minor valve orifice tend to increase the incidence of valve thrombosis in patients with tilting disc valves.

Only one bileaflet valve is available in the United States (St. Jude Medical Inc., St. Paul, Minnesota) (see Fig. 84.2). This valve is made of graphite that is coated with pyrolytic carbon. Two hemicircular flat leaflets are attached to the inner circumference of the seating ring by butterfly hinges, which allow the leaflets to open to an angle of 85°. When closed the leaflet edges meet each other and the inner edge of the seating ring at an angle of 23°. This valve produces nearly central flow and only a small amount of turbulence.[61] Pressure differences across the valve are as low as or lower than differences across similar sized tilting disc valves.[59] Backflow, defined as the percentage of forward flow that passes backward during and after valve closure, is similar to that observed with tilting disc valves.[55,60] The St. Jude valve closes with a distinct click, is difficult to see at fluoroscopy or on x-ray films, and cannot be rotated after insertion. The incidence of mechanical failure is extremely low; leaflet fractures or escape have not been reported except when excessive force has been used during insertion of the valve.

BIOLOGIC TISSUE VALVES

Homograft valves were first used in 1962 and proved to be virtually free of thromboembolic complications.[62] Use of homograft valves, unfortunately, has been limited by difficulties in procurement and uncertainties concerning long-term durability.[63] Not surprisingly, homograft valves are currently employed only in a few centers worldwide. Use of glutaraldehyde to permit preservation of *heterograft* valves, however, was first employed by Carpentier,[12] and this technique permitted the development of the current generation of bioprostheses.

There are three commercially available bioprostheses: the Hancock valve, the Carpentier-Edwards valve, and the Ionescu-Shiley valve (Fig. 84.3). While all these use glutaraldehyde to stabilize tissues, substantial differences exist in the composition of the stabilizing solutions. Furthermore, the Ionescu valve is fashioned from bovine pericardium, whereas both the Hancock and Carpentier valves are derived from porcine valvular tissue. The Hancock valve features a cloth-covered sewing ring and cloth-covered stents composed of polypropylene. Likewise, the Carpentier valve features a cloth-covered sewing ring and cloth-covered stents. In the Carpentier valve, the stents are composed of Elgiloy, an alloy of steel, and the base is consequently flexible. Theoretically, the Ionescu valve, which is fashioned from bovine pericardium, should be free of the natural variation which would characterize harvested valves. This, however, has never been proven to be of clinical importance. The frame of the Ionescu valve is also cloth-covered, but composed of titanium.

The hemodynamic performance of bioprostheses is not ideal.[64-66] Early editions of the Hancock valve had mean diastolic gradients of 6 mm Hg in the mitral position and average peak systolic gradients of nearly 20 mm Hg in the aortic position. With the introduction of the "modified orifice,"[67] hemodynamics improved but remain of concern with valve sizes below 23 mm. The performance of the Carpentier valve with thinner struts and cloth covering is similar to that of the modified Hancock.

The Ionescu valve has a calculated area actually larger than that for comparably sized mechanical valves (see Table 84.1). Further, lacking the muscle shelf of the porcine valves, improved hemodynamic performance is expected.[68,69] While this is true in the aortic position,[70] a significant gradient remains in the mitral position.[68,69] Nevertheless, the valve probably is superior in its hydraulic performance to the Hancock valve, but may be inferior to the new "supra-annular" Carpentier.[65]

In summary, biologic valves differ in source, manner of preserva-

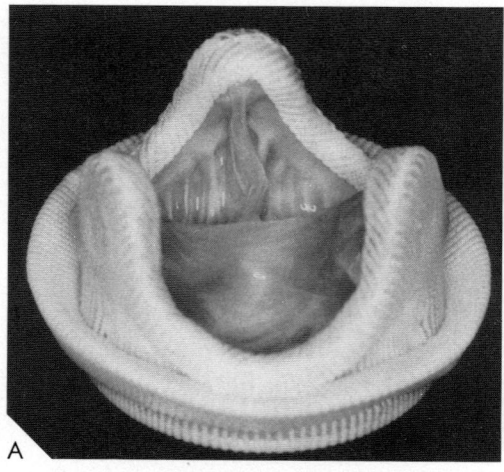
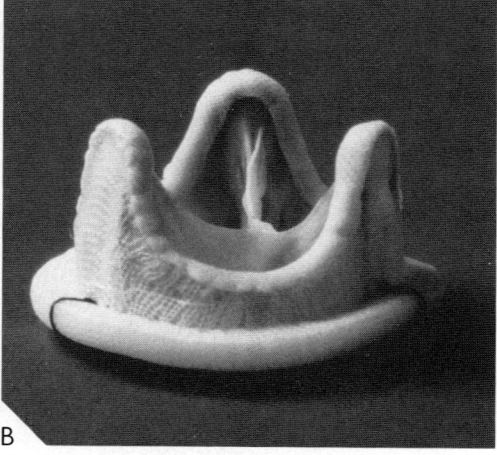
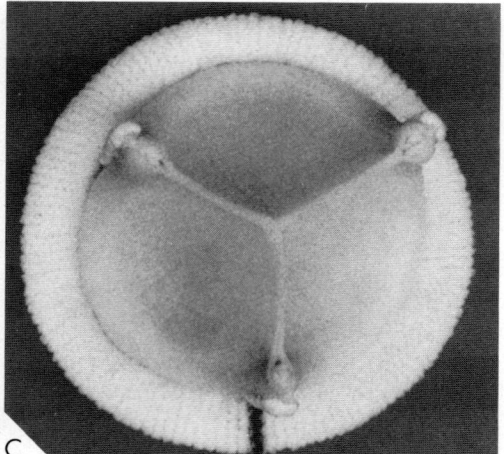

FIGURE 84.3 Bioprosthetic valves currently available in the United States. (A) Hancock porcine heterograft; (B) Carpentier-Edwards porcine heterograft; (C) Ionescu-Shiley bovine pericardial bioprosthesis.

tion, and hydraulic performance. In small sizes (e.g., <23 for the aortic position), none provide the low systolic pressure gradients of the better mechanical valves, but all have minimal backflow.[55,60] An important advantage of bioprosthetic valves is freedom from anticoagulation. The thromboembolic complication rate for bioprosthetic valves *without* anticoagulation is roughly equal to that for mechanical valves with anticoagulation. On the other hand, durability is uncertain so that life expectancy of the valve may be less than that of the recipient.

COMPLICATIONS OF PROSTHETIC VALVES

Of the long-term adverse consequences of valve replacement, three are particularly devastating and account for the majority of significant complications of prosthetic valves. These three are prosthetic valve endocarditis, equally common for mechanical and biologic valves; thromboembolism, which is more frequently associated with mechanical valves; and valve degeneration, which occurs with tissue valves. Each will be considered in detail separately.

PROSTHETIC VALVE ENDOCARDITIS

Prosthetic valve endocarditis (PVE) is one of the most serious complications of cardiac surgery. Most centers report an overall incidence of 2% to 4%.[71] Interestingly, this incidence has declined from the 12% reported in 1966.[72] This decline is probably multifactorial, with prophylactic antibiotics, improved technique, and better material all contributing. By convention, prosthetic valve endocarditis has been classified as early, if appearing within 60 days of surgery, and late, if appearing beyond that point.[73] The incidence of each is about equal, with the caveat that the incidence of late PVE will vary with length of follow-up.

The prosthesis in the aortic position may be more prone to infection than one in the mitral position.[74] However, no definite pattern of infection occurs when double prosthetic valves are present.[75,76] Currently, there does not appear to be significant differences in infectability between mechanical and biologic valves,[71] and the incidence of PVE following replacement of an infected native valve is only 4%.[77]

The most commonly isolated species is *Staphylococcus*, which accounts for approximately 50% of early PVE. Indeed, it accounts for more than 30% of late PVE as well.[75] Of staphylococcal species, *Staphylococcus epidermidis* is the most common and, unfortunately, this organism is demonstrating increasing evidence of methicillin resistance.[78] *Sreptococcus viridans* remains as a common isolate during late PVE, accounting for approximately 30% of cases.[77] There is no relationship between any organism and valve type. An important rule of thumb, however, is that the further from surgery a patient is, the more likely it will be that the microbiology will resemble that of native valve endocarditis.

The hallmark of PVE is the valve ring abscess, which makes surgical extirpation of the infection particularly difficult. There is a lower incidence of valve ring abscess with biologic valves, which has led some to believe that infections involving biologic valves are easier to eradicate.[78]

The clinical manifestations of PVE can be subtle, particularly early after operation.[79] Fever is the most common manifestation, occurring in 97% of patients with new or changing murmurs (56%) and petechiae (26%–38%) following in frequency. As with the microbiology, the farther from surgery the patient is in his course, the more likely it will be that the manifestations will resemble native valve endocarditis. Clearly, the presentation of early and late PVE is often dramatically different. Early PVE is often confused with other problems (e.g., fever from atelectasis or postpericardiotomy syndrome) that often accompany open cardiac surgery. Petechiae and splenomegaly occur uncommonly. Interestingly, for both early and late PVE, the incidence of emboli from an infected valve varies widely.[74,80]

The laboratory is often unhelpful in making a diagnosis of PVE. Although anemia is present in 74% of patients, leukocytosis and hematuria occur in only 50%. An elevated sedimentation rate and positive rheumatoid factor are even less commonly observed. Furthermore, routine x-ray films and special studies including echocardiography and cardiac catheterization are rarely specific and, consequently, not very helpful.[81-84] Blood cultures are the cornerstone of the diagnosis of PVE and are positive in over 90% of cases.[73,85] Culture-negative PVE is exceedingly uncommon. However, noncardiac sources of positive blood cultures must always be considered in surgical patients.[86] When blood cultures are positive, an aggressive approach to recognized extracardiac sources of infection is mandatory since seeding of a prosthesis from an extracardiac source is associated with a 100% mortality.[87]

The therapy for PVE is similar to that for native valve endocarditis. Once the diagnosis is confirmed by positive blood cultures (or sooner if the clinical suspicion is strong), aggressive antibiotics are indicated with multiple bactericidal agents employed intravenously for a minimum of six to eight weeks. As with native valve endocarditis, surgical intervention is indicated for any signs of hemodynamic deterioration, ongoing sepsis, embolization, and certain particularly invasive or resistant organisms.[71,78,79,88]

The extremely high mortality of PVE with medical management alone has prompted consideration of early operative intervention.[89] However, the decision to reoperate on a patient for PVE soon after valve replacement can be extremely difficult. Objective criteria for the decision have been suggested,[88] but because delay is associated with high mortality, early intervention is usually preferred. Overall mortality for early PVE is in the range of 75% and, for late PVE, approximately 45%.[74]

In summary, PVE has a much higher mortality than native valve endocarditis and differs from native valve endocarditis in pathogenesis and clinical expression. A high index of suspicion is required to prompt appropriate diagnosis and therapy, which should be aggressive and involve both medical and surgical approaches.

THROMBOEMBOLIC COMPLICATIONS

Thromboembolic complications continue to threaten recipients of prosthetic heart valves and this threat delays referral for native valve replacement. One associates thromboembolism largely with mechanical valves even though recipients of biologic valves are also at significant risk.

It is exceedingly uncommon for recipients of mechanical valves to be maintained without some form of antithrombotic therapy. Unfortunately, no single agent has emerged as the ideal form of antithrombosis. The mainstay of acute anticoagulation is heparin, a "polydisperse" molecule with a molecular weight of approximately 6,000 to 14,000. Heparin is extremely effective as an anticoagulant, with only 0.01 unit per milliliter of plasma needed to prolong the thrombin time.[90] Yet, heparin can be a very potent procoagulant and even induce a 1.5- to 2-fold potentiation of platelet activation.[91] Clearly, to the extent that platelet activation participates in the thrombotic potential of mechanical valves, heparin represents a poor choice of antithrombotic agent.

Warfarin interferes with the synthesis of all vitamin K-dependent coagulant factors, including II, VII, IX, and X, and remains the mainstay of anticoagulation for chronic use. However, warfarin also inhibits synthesis of protein C, a naturally occurring anticoagulant. Slow onset of therapeutic concentrations and two weeks for all clotting times to reflect a sensitivity to a variety of commonly prescribed drugs are disadvantages of warfarin.[92]

Conventional antiplatelet therapy with aspirin and dipyrimadole is an appealing adjunct to warfarin anticoagulation but, in the setting of valve replacement, remains promising but unproven.[93-96] Reductions in thromboembolic complications have been reported[95] but are usually associated with an increase in bleeding complications.[97] Platelet inhibitors without coumadin have been used in a few patients with mitral bioprostheses.[98,99] Most patients with aortic bioprostheses are not anticoagulated.

Thromboembolism remains a major complication of prosthetic cardiac valves. Most emboli are undetected and most detected emboli (80%–90%) are cerebral. Since the brain receives only 14% of the cardiac output, it follows that most emboli are undetected.[100] Variations in thoroughness of follow-up and in definitions of an embolic event also obscure the true incidence of thromboemboli and weaken comparisons between reports. Approximately 10% to 15%[101,102] of thromboembolic events are fatal and approximately half of cerebral emboli produce a permanent defect.[102]

Bleeding episodes must also be factored into the equation of valve-related thromboembolic complications. Most would accept a fatal complication rate of 0.15 instance per 100 patient-years (pt-yrs) and 0.5 to 6.3 instances of nonfatal but serious complications.[103] As with embolic episodes, bleeding problems are probably underreported. Approximately 15% of serious bleeding episodes, defined as those requiring transfusion or hospitalization or those that cause a residual neurologic defect, are fatal.[100,103] Unfortunately, the incidence of bleeding complications, which average 3% to 4%/year, remains as long as the prosthetic heart valve patient is anticoagulated.

All patients with mechanical valves require permanent anticoagulation, usually with warfarin. Although spot checks show that up to 40% of patients are not anticoagulated,[100] omission of anticoagulants increases the incidence of thromboembolism by about 6-fold in patients with mechanical valves.[33,100,104] Some investigators have also found that atrial fibrillation, atrial clot at operation, large left atrium, and history of emboli increase the incidence of emboli[100]; however, others have not.[102] Some reports also indicate that the risk of thromboembolism is greatest during the first 3 to 6 months after operation,[35,105] but others do not.[28,101,106–108]

DEGENERATION OF BIOPROSTHETIC VALVES

The major drawback of bioprosthetic valves is uncertain durability and the possible need to replace the valve during the patient's lifetime. Fortunately, degeneration of bioprosthetic valves is usually slow; thus, catastrophic emergencies, which happen with thrombosis of mechanical valves, do not occur.[27,109–112] When new symptoms or murmurs appear, cardiac ultrasound may be diagnostic of bioprosthetic degeneration.[113,114]

Several factors increase the risk of late bioprosthetic valve degeneration and most of these involve calcium and phosphorus metabolism.[115] Young age (<25 years),[116] chronic renal failure, pregnancy, and high-calcium diets increase the likelihood of bioprosthetic valve degeneration. Location of the prosthesis (aortic, mitral, tricuspid), type (porcine heterograft or bovine pericardium), supplier, shelf-life, size, and year of implantation do not affect the incidence.[110,111,117–119]

Degenerated bioprosthetic valves develop cusp tears and perforations, flail or immobile leaflets, and deposits of thrombus, fibrous tissue, or calcium (Fig. 84.4). Approximately 90% of sterile, degenerated valves have abnormal valve calcification, which is of two types.[120] One is an extrinsic deposit and is related to calcification of surface thrombi and vegetations. The other type is intrinsic calcification of the valve leaflet and involves dystrophic calcium deposits within the spongiosa itself.[113,120–122] This latter pattern of calcification causes leaflet stiffness, weakness, perforation, and failure and is related to cell membrane damage.[113] Fibrous overgrowth, collagen degeneration, and fibrous thickening of leaflets are non-calcium-related causes of bioprosthetic valve failure.

The histologic structure of normal porcine valves may relate to the development of valve calcification. The normal porcine valve has an inferior inflow surface, a middle layer called the spongiosa, and a superior outflow surface. The inflow and outflow surfaces are normally covered with endothelium overlying a basement membrane. The spongiosa consists of a combination of loose and dense connective tissue.[123] In preparing a bioprosthetic valve, the normal porcine valve is treated with glutaraldehyde, which increases collagen cross-links. Examination of these prepared porcine valves shows that the endothelium is stripped off the inflow and outflow surfaces, and that proteoglycans and glycoaminoglycans are removed from their spaces within the collagen network of the spongiosa.[120,121,123,124] This change exposes the collagen network directly to the bloodstream and opens areas within the network to blood components and plasma proteins.[124] In valves implanted for less than 2 months, Ferrans found infiltration of plasma proteins and penetration of erythrocytes into surface crevices, formation of a thin fibrin surface layer, and deposition of macrophages, giant cells, and platelets.[124] Valves examined after 2 months of implantation showed progressive disruption of collagen, erosion of the valve surface, formation of platelet aggregates, and accumulation of lipids. In this way, the inert bioprosthesis interacts with blood to accumulate the cells and cell components involved with dystrophic calcification. In addition to infiltrating cells and cell components, the collagen interface itself may initiate the calcification process.[115,121]

The relationship of the immune system, valve preparation, and tissue stress to the development of valve calcification has also been studied. Although there is some evidence of circulating antibodies to components of the valve,[125] there is little evidence that immunity is involved in the calcification process.[111,120,126,127] Residual glutaraldehyde from inadequate rinsing may accelerate the calcification process,[115] but probably does not initiate it. Similarly, areas of maximum stress correspond to areas of maximal calcium and degeneration.[128,129]

Currently, efforts to inhibit bioprosthetic valve calcification involve modification of gluteraldehyde cross-linking,[130] use of detergents and

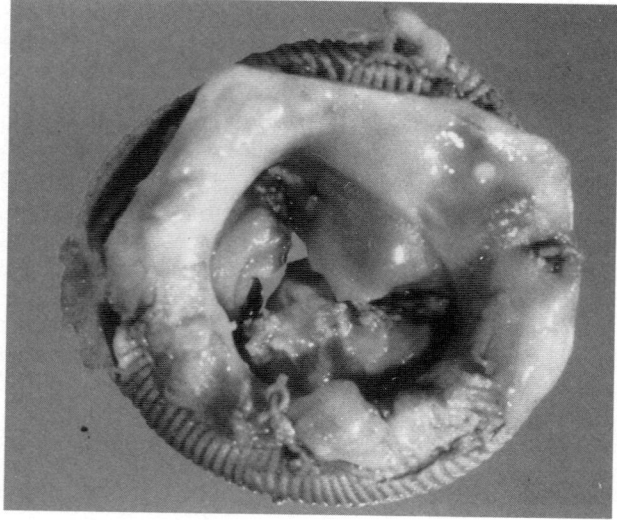

FIGURE 84.4 Undersurface of a degenerated mitral bioprosthetic valve removed at operation. One leaflet was torn and others were immobile because of dystrophic calcification.

surfactants,[122] the use of diphosphonates to sterically block propagation of hydroxyapatite crystals,[131] and changes in valve design to reduce areas of stress.[120]

RESULTS

Operative mortality is defined as death within 30 days of operation or death before hospital discharge. The advent of cold potassium cardioplegia,[31] improved management of postoperative cardiac output, and a host of other evolutionary changes has steadily reduced the risk of operation. Other factors such as advanced age, advanced cardiac decompensation, and multiple organ systems dysfunction have partially offset reductions in operative mortality and encouraged cardiologists and surgeons to offer operation to essentially all patients with symptomatic valvular dysfunction.

In consecutive series, overall operative mortality for aortic valve replacement ranges between 3% and 12%.[33-36,104-108,118,132-136] Factors that increase risk include advanced age,[137] advanced New York Heart Association classification,[132,134,137] aortic regurgitation,[132,137] atrial fibrillation,[137] prosthetic endocarditis,[138,139] renal dysfunction,[137] emergency operation,[139] previous operation,[139] and the addition of coronary artery bypass grafts.[140]

Replacement of the mitral valve in consecutive series generally has an operative mortality that is 1 to 3 percentage points higher than the aortic mortality.[33,35,36,104,107,108,134-136] Factors associated with an increased operative mortality for mitral valve replacement include advanced age,[141,142] advanced New York Heart Association functional class,[143] prosthetic valve infection,[138] liver dysfunction, ascites, ischemic mitral valve disease,[107] mitral insufficiency, associated coronary artery revascularization,[136,144] renal dysfunction, bar calcification of the mitral annulus, reoperation,[143] and emergency operation.[143] Age over 70 years[141,142] or ischemic mitral insufficiency increases operative mortality to 20% to 25%.[107,145] Operative mortality in patients with acute myocardial infarction, mitral insufficiency, and cardiogenic shock is approximately 50%.[146] Pulmonary hypertension (unless suprasystemic)[147] and tricuspid valve insufficiency are not associated with an increased operative mortality.

Operative mortality for replacement of both aortic and mitral valves varies widely between zero[104,107,148] and 28%,[136] with a median around 12%.[36,108,134] Factors that influence operative mortality in these patients are similar to those for single valve replacement. The introduction of cold potassium cardioplegia was particularly influential in reducing operative mortality in patients who require double valve replacement.[148]

Inadequate cardiac contractility is the most common cause of operative mortality and morbidity. Other causes include stroke due to hemorrhage; thrombus or air; uncontrolled bleeding; recurrent arrhythmias; heart block; acute myocardial infarction; pulmonary embolus; sepsis; valve disruption; rupture of a suture line, bypass graft, or posterior left ventricular wall[149]; renal or pulmonary dysfunction; mesenteric ischemia; and valve malfunction due to thrombosis, suture, or tissue interference.[150] Problems with the prosthetic valve, including sepsis, account for 20% to 30% of operative deaths.[101] Early valve thrombosis is peculiar to mechanical valves; iatrogenic tears are a complication of tissue valves.[150]

Type of valve (mechanical or tissue), design, and construction have a greater influence on late morbidity and mortality than on hospital mortality. Because late results have been comparatively unfavorable, many prosthetic valves implanted in the past are no longer used. Structural wear or fracture, tissue ingrowth, or a high incidence of valve thrombosis and thromboembolism have retired the Braunwald-Cutter,[151] Beall,[152] Cross-Jones, Kay-Shiley,[153] Lillehei-Kaster,[154] Harken, DeBakey, Wada-Cutter,[155] Magovern-Cromie,[156] Cape Town (UCT),[157] fascia lata, dura mater, and aortic allograft valves.[158] Only the Starr-Edwards bare strut and Sutter (Smeloff-Cutter) ball valves survive from the earlier era. Cloth-covered struts were abandoned when a higher incidence of valve thrombosis and tissue interference was recognized.[159]

SURVIVAL

Although the mortality rate for patients with prosthetic heart valves exceeds that of the age-matched general population, most series indicate that 75% to 85% of operative survivors live an additional 5 years (see Table 84.2). At 10 years actuarial curves indicate that 47% to 72%[106,160,161] of hospital survivors are still alive. The location of the prosthesis (aortic or mitral, or both) does not appear to influence survival (Table 84.2). Age,[162] preoperative functional classification,[35,132] the presence of coronary artery disease, and the development of valve-related complications adversely affect survival. Patients who have simultaneous replacement of aortic, mitral, and tricuspid valves have cumulative survival rates of 55% at 5 years and 40% at 10 years.[163]

Congestive heart failure, coronary disease, and arrhythmia are the most common causes of late death[160,164] after prosthetic valve replacement and account for 28%[162] to 47%[107,132] of all late deaths. The incidence of these non-valve-related cardiac deaths is strongly associated with the preoperative functional status of the patient and the presence of associated coronary artery disease.[35,132,135] Sudden, unexpected, and usually unexplained late deaths cause an additional 15% to 25% of all late deaths.[33,134,160,162] These deaths are presumably due to an unrecognized arrhythmia or stroke and invariably occur outside the hospital without postmortem examination. Consequently, a small coronary or

TABLE 84.2 FIVE-YEAR ACTUARIAL SURVIVAL BY VALVE*

Valve	Aortic	Mitral	Multiple
Starr-Edwards (bare-strut)	66,†[106] 77,[176] 78,[175] 80[105]	71,[101] 76,[105] 77,[176] 78,†[160] 79[175]	
Smeloff-Cutter	69,[177] 77,[178] 80[161]	74[178]	
Bjork-Shiley (standard)	73,†[135] 83,[105] 84,†[33] 86[28]	69,[28] 78,[105] 85,†[33]	75,[28] 80,†[33]
Omniscience	82[165]	80[165]	
Medtronic-Hall	81[168]	75[168]	81[168]
St. Jude	91[104]	90[104]	95[104]
Porcine	68,†[35] 78,[111] 83,†[36] 87[134]	73,†[35] 77,†[36] 80,[111] 83†[134]	72,†[35] 80,†[36] 81†[134]
Ionescu-Shiley	80,[136] 88[133]	72[136]	

*Numbers indicate 5-year actuarial survival for the series indicated by the superscript reference number. Except when indicated by a dagger, survival rates do *not* include operative mortality.

cerebral embolus cannot be excluded. Overall, non-valve-related and sudden cardiac deaths account for roughly 40% to 60% of all late deaths in patients with prosthetic heart valves.

Thromboembolism, anticoagulant-related hemorrhage, prosthetic endocarditis, reoperation, and mechanical dysfunction of the prosthesis are fatal complications that are directly related to the prosthesis.[101] These valve-related deaths cause 12% to 34% of late deaths.[34,36,101,104,106,108,134,164] The incidence is higher in patients with prosthetic mitral valves[36,101] than in patients with aortic prostheses.[36,101] Although there is great variability between reports in the incidence of valve-related late deaths, the incidence appears higher in patients with the Bjork-Shiley prosthesis as compared to ball valve or bioprosthesis.[34,36,101,106,134,135,164] There are insufficient data regarding other tilting disk valves and bileaflet valves.

FUNCTIONAL IMPROVEMENT

The majority of hospital survivors are symptomatically improved after valve replacement operations, but functional improvement bears little relationship to the type of prosthesis used. After aortic valve replacement, 74%[105,135] to 92%[104,107] of patients improve at least one NYHA class within the first year and 53%[105] to 99%[34,104] achieve class I or II status. At 5 and 10 years, approximately 85% to 90% of surviving patients remain in NYHA class I or II.[135] After isolated mitral valve replacement, 80%[105] to 95%[104] improve at least one NYHA class within the first year and 70%[104] to 99%[34,105] reach class I or II status. At 5 and 10 years, 85% to 90% of surviving patients remain in class I or II status. After replacement of both aortic and mitral valves, most patients improve at least one functional class and approximately 90% are in class I or II.[104] At 5 years, the majority of surviving patients remain in class I or II.[34,35]

VALVE-RELATED MORBIDITY

Thromboembolism, anticoagulation-related bleeding, endocarditis, paravalvular leak, reoperation, and mechanical failure of the prostheses are the major causes of valve-related morbidity. Other infrequent causes of valve failure are hemolysis, tissue ingrowth (Fig. 84.5), and progressive obstruction due to "stent creep" of porcine heterograft valves. The reported incidence of all valve-related morbidity varies between reports, and perhaps between valves, although this cannot be clearly documented. The total incidence of valve-related morbidity ranges between 2.5% and 8.5%[101] (episodes per 100 pt-yrs), with a median of about 5%.

The incidence of thromboembolism varies between valve types and between valve locations. Overall, the incidence of thromboembolism from aortic prostheses ranges between 0.5% and 3.0%/pt-yr. Although the majority of patients with bioprosthetic valves do not receive anticoagulants,[36,134,136] the incidence of thromboemboli is the same as or less than the incidence in anticoagulated patients with mechanical valves.[33,34,101,107,135] When warfarin anticoagulation is used, serious bleeding, defined as that which requires transfusion or hospitalization, or which causes stroke or death, occurs at a constant rate of 3% to 4% for the remainder of the patient's life. Omission of anticoagulants without an increase in embolization or valve thrombosis is the major advantage of bioprosthetic aortic valves as compared to mechanical prostheses. If thromboembolic and bleeding complications are added, the combined incidence for bioprosthetic aortic valves is approximately 2 episodes/100 pt-yrs versus 4 or 5 for mechanical aortic valves.[97,103]

The incidence of thromboembolism of mitral prostheses varies between 2.5% and 4.0%/pt-yr and does not differ appreciably between bioprosthetic and mechanical prostheses. Because of atrial fibrillation or other concerns, approximately half of patients with bioprosthetic mitral valves are anticoagulated.[35,108] For mechanical and bioprosthetic mitral valves, the combined incidence of thromboembolism and serious bleeding ranges between 4% and 8%/pt-yr. The combined incidence for bioprosthetic mitral valves tends to be lower at 1.5% to 4%/pt-yr. Patients who cannot tolerate long-term anticoagulation should have bioprosthetic mitral valves since anticoagulants can be omitted with little or no increase in the incidence of thromboembolism.[94,98,99]

The incidence of thromboembolic complications in patients with multiple prosthetic valves ranges between 2%[28,33,34,165] and 5%/pt-yr.[36,108,134,136] When added to the incidence of anticoagulated bleeding, the combined incidence is similar to that observed in patients with mechanical mitral prostheses.

Valve thrombosis is a major complication of Bjork-Shiley[28,33,34,105,132] (standard model) and Omniscience valves,[165,166] but occurs rarely in patients with ball valves,[101,106,160] bileaflet valves,[104,107] and bioprostheses.[35,36,136] The reported incidence for Bjork-Shiley standard valves ranges between 0.2% and 1.3% and is even higher in patients with both aortic and mitral Bjork prostheses.[28,34] Preliminary data suggest that the incidence of valve thrombosis is less with the convexo-concave Bjork valve[28,167] and with the Medtronic-Hall valve.[168] There is little evidence that anticoagulation for 3 to 6 months after operation reduces the incidence of thromboembolic complications of aortic bioprostheses.

Prosthetic endocarditis is a major complication of prosthetic valves and one that usually requires reoperation. The overall incidence of endocarditis ranges between 0.1%[132] and 3.9%/pt-yr,[136] but most investigators report a 0.5% to 1.5%/pt-yr incidence. The incidence may be slightly higher in patients with double prosthetic valves[35,108] and in patients with single aortic as compared to single mitral valves.[74] *Staphylococcus,* particularly *S. epidermidis,* streptococci (beta-hemolytic and *S. viridans*), and enterococci are the most common organisms; gram-negative organisms and fungi cause less than 20% of cases.[138,169] Reoperation for early postoperative prosthetic endocarditis has a 60% to 75% mortality rate[139,169]; for late endocarditis, operative mortality is 20%[169] to 60%.[170] Emergency operation and severe congestive heart failure are factors that increase reoperative mortality.[138,169]

Paravalvular leak has an incidence of 0.2%[134] to 3.3%/pt-yr,[166] which averages about 1%/pt-yr. Causes include endocarditis as well as sterile detachments due to sutures pulling out or breaking. Paravalvular leak increases hemolysis and reoperation may be required because of anemia, infection, or heart failure.

Mechanical failure of mechanical prosthetic valves is uncommon. In recent years there are no instances of mechanical failure of ball

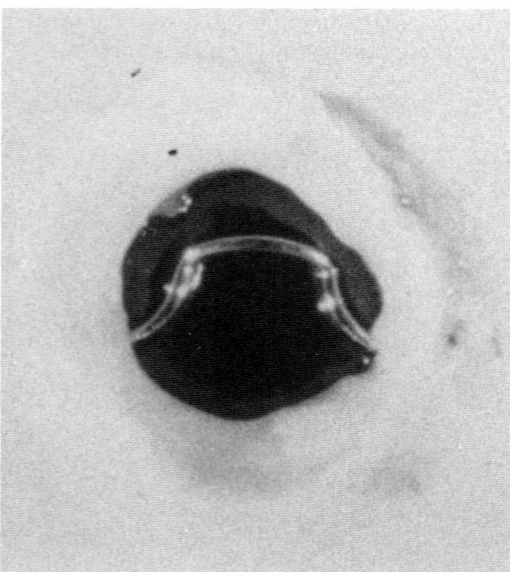

FIGURE 84.5 Excised size 19 standard Bjork-Shiley aortic prosthesis that shows concentric tissue overgrowth. This tissue impaired movement of the disk and reduced the effective orifice area of the valve.

valves. Reported instances of leaflet dislodgement or fracture of bileaflet valves are rare.[171] Strut fractures have occurred with welded convexo-concave Bjork-Shiley valves, and these valves have been recalled.[56] Strut fractures have not been observed in tilting disk valves that have been machined from one piece of metal.[57,168]

Occasionally, tissue ingrowth has narrowed the effective orifice of ball and tilting disk valves or interfered with closure of tilting disk valves (Fig. 84.5). This problem was more common in cloth-covered ball valves and requires reoperation if valve function is compromised.

The durability of bioprosthetic valves has been a major concern since these valves were introduced. Fresh or preserved homograft valves generally fail 1 to 3 years after operation and consequently were abandoned. In adults over 25 years of age, bioprosthetic valves have a failure rate between 0.1%[36] and 1.7%/pt-yr; however, this rate may increase beyond 8 to 10 years after operation.[111,172] Five years after implantation, 97% of aortic porcine heterografts and 96% of mitral heterografts remain mechanically sound[111,140]; however, by 10 years, only 71% of prostheses in each position are satisfactory.[111,172] The results with bovine pericardial valves are generally similar.[136,173] In children, aortic and mitral bioprosthetic valves develop calcium deposits, thrombi, and tears in 60% of patients by 5 years. At the present time, bioprosthetic valves are contraindicated in patients under 20 years except in right ventricular outflow tract conduits.[116] "Stent creep" wherein the prosthetic commissures bend inward to reduce the effective valve orifice is an uncommon complication.[174]

The incidence of reoperation does not vary significantly between valve locations and ranges between 0.1%[132] and 5.2%/pt-yr,[136] with an average of approximately 1%/pt-yr. Indications for reoperation include endocarditis, valve thrombosis, paravalvular leak, mechanical failure, recurrent emboli, and hemolysis. Operative mortality averages approximately 10%,[143] but increases substantially for emergencies[170] and in patients with endocarditis.[169]

REFERENCES

1. Brunton L: Preliminary note on the possibility of treating mitral stenosis by surgical methods. Lancet 1:352, 1902
2. Souttar HS: The surgical correction of mitral stenosis. Br Med J 2:603, 1925
3. Cutler EC, Beck CS: The present status of the surgical procedures in chronic valvular disease of the heart. Arch Surg 18:403, 1929
4. Bailey CP: The surgical treatment of mitral stenosis (mitral commissurotomy). Dis Chest 15:377, 1949
5. Harken DE, Ellis LB, Ware PF et al: The surgical treatment of mitral stenosis. N Engl J Med 239:801, 1948
6. Sellors TH: Surgery of pulmonary stenosis: A case in which the pulmonary valve was successfully divided. Lancet 1:988, 1948
7. Brock RC: Pulmonary valvulotomy for the relief of congenital pulmonary stenosis: Report of three cases. Br Med J 1:1121, 1948
8. Hufnagel CA: The use of rigid and flexible plastic prostheses for arterial replacement. Surgery 37:165, 1955
9. Harken DE, Sorof HS, Taylor WJ et al: Partial and complete prosthesis in aortic insufficiency. J Thorac Cardiovasc Surg 40:744, 1960
10. Starr A, Edwards ML: Mitral replacement: Clinical experience with a ball valve prosthesis. Ann Surg 154:726, 1961
11. Binet JP, Carpentier A, Langlois J et al: Implantation de valves heterogenes dans le traitement de cardiopathies aortiques. C R Acad Sc Paris 261:5733, 1965
12. Carpentier A, Lemaigre G, Robert L et al: Biological factors affecting long-term results of valvular heterografts. J Thorac Cardiovasc Surg 58:467, 1969
13. Rapaport E: Natural history of aortic and mitral valve disease. Am J Cardiol 35:221, 1975
14. Frank S, Johnson A, Ross J: Natural history of valvular aortic stenosis. Br Heart J 35:41, 1973
15. Oleson KH: Natural history of 271 patients with mitral stenosis under medical treatment. Br Heart J 24:349, 1962
16. Akins CW, Kirklin JK, Block DC et al: Preoperative evaluation of subvalvular fibrosis in mitral stenosis: A predictive factor in conservative versus replacement surgical therapy. Circulation (Suppl I) 60:I-71, 1979
17. Heglin R, Scheu H, Rothlin M et al: Aortic insufficiency. Circulation (Suppl V) 34:V-77, 1968
18. O'Rourke RA, Crawford MM: Timing of valve replacement in patients with chronic aortic regurgitation. Circulation 61:493, 1980
19. Rahimtoola SH: Valve replacement should not be performed in all asymptomatic patients with severe aortic incompetence. J Thorac Cardiovasc Surg 79:163, 1980
20. Goldschlager N, Pfeifer J, Cohn K et al: The natural history of aortic regurgitation: A clinical and hemodynamic study. Am J Med 54:577, 1973
21. Kennedy JW, Doces J, Stewart DK: Left ventricular function before and following aortic valve replacement. Circulation 56:944, 1977
22. Pantely G, Morton M, Rahimtoola SH: Effects of successful uncomplicated valve replacement on ventricular hypertrophy, volume, and performance in aortic stenosis and in aortic incompetence. J Thorac Cardiovasc Surg 75:383, 1978
23. Gaash WH, Andrias WC, Levine HJ: Chronic aortic regurgitation: The effect of aortic valve replacement on left ventricular volume, mass, and function. Circulation 58:825, 1978
24. Borow K, Green LH, Mann T et al: End-diastolic volume as a predictor of postoperative left ventricular function in volume overload from valvular regurgitation. Circulation (Suppl III) 56:III-40, 1977
25. Clark DG, McAnulty JH, Rahimtoola SH: Results of valve replacement in aortic incompetence with left ventricular dysfunction. Circulation 61:411, 1980
26. Henry WL, Bonow RO, Borer JS et al: Observations on the optimum time for operative intervention for aortic regurgitation. I. Evaluation of the results of aortic valve replacement in symptomatic patients. Circulation 61:471, 1980
27. Morgan RJ, Davis JT, Fraker TD: Current status of valve prostheses. Surg Clin North Am 65:699, 1985
28. Bjork VO, Henze A: Ten years' experience with the Bjork-Shiley tilting disc valve. J Thorac Cardiovasc Surg 78:331, 1979
29. Waldhausen JA, Pierce WS (eds): Johnson's Surgery of the Chest, 5th ed, p 56. Chicago, Year Book Medical Publishers, 1985
30. Cooley DA: Techniques in Cardiac Surgery. Philadelphia, WB Saunders, 1984
31. Gay WA, Ebert PA: Functional, metabolic and morphologic effects of potassium-induced cardioplegia. Surgery 74:284, 1973
32. Kirklin JW, Pacifico AD: Surgery for acquired valvular heart disease. N Engl J Med 288:133, 1973
33. Daenen W, Nevelsteen A, Van Cauwelaert P et al: Nine years experience with the Bjork-Shiley prosthetic valve: Early and late results of 932 valve replacements. Ann Thorac Surg 35:651, 1983
34. Karp RB, Cyrus RJ, Blackstone EH et al: The Bjork-Shiley valve. J Thorac Cardiovasc Surg 81:602, 1981
35. Oyer PE, Stinson EB, Reitz BA et al: Long-term evaluation of the porcine xenograft bioprosthesis. J Thorac Cardiovasc Surg 78:343, 1979
36. Zussa C, Ottino G, DiSumma M et al: Porcine cardiac bioprostheses: Evaluation of long-term results in 990 patients. Ann Thorac Surg 39:243, 1985
37. Konno S, Imai Y, Iida Y et al: A new method for prosthetic valve replacement in congenital aortic stenosis associated with hypoplasia of the aortic valve ring. J Thorac Cardiovasc Surg 70:909, 1975
38. Bentall HA, DeBono A: A technique for complete replacement of the ascending aorta. Thorax 23:338, 1968
39. Carpentier A: Cardiac valve surgery—the "French" connection. J Thorac Cardiovasc Surg 86:323, 1983
40. David TE, Uden DE, Strauss HD: The importance of the mitral apparatus in left ventricular function after correction of mitral regurgitation. Circulation (Suppl II) 68:II-76, 1982
41. Carpentier A, DeLoche A, Hanania G et al: Surgical management of acquired tricuspid valve disease. J Thorac Cardiovasc Surg 71:53, 1976
42. Agarwal KC, Edwards WD, Feldt RH et al: Clinical pathological correlates of obstructed right-sided porcine-valve extracardiac conduits. J Thorac Cardiovasc Surg 81:591, 1981
43. Macoviak JA, Stephenson LW, Edmunds LH Jr et al: The intra-aortic balloon pump: An analysis of 5 years experience. Ann Thorac Surg 29:451, 1989
44. Edmunds LH Jr: Cardiac surgery. In Dudrick S (ed): Manual of Preoperative and Postoperative Care, p 382–411. American College of Surgeons. Philadelphia, WB Saunders, 1982
45. Rose DM, Laschinger J, Grossi E et al: Experimental and clinical results with a simplified left heart assist device for treatment of profound left ventricular dysfunction. World J Surg 9:11, 1985
46. Padula RT, Cowan GSM Jr, Camishon RC: Photographic analysis of the active and passive components of cardiac valvular action. J Thorac Cardiovasc Surg 56:790, 1968
47. Thubrikar M, Bosher LP, Nolan SP: The mechanism of opening of the aortic valve. J Thorac Cardiovasc Surg 77:863, 1979
48. Cohen MV, Gorlin R: Modified orifice equation for the calculation of mitral valve area. Am Heart J 84:839, 1972
49. Gorlin R, Gorlin E: Hydraulic formula for calculation of area of stenotic mitral valve, other valves and central circulatory shunts. Am Heart J 41:1, 1951
50. Thubrikar M, Piepgrass WC, Deck JD et al: Stresses of natural versus prosthetic aortic valve leaflets in vivo. Ann Thorac Surg 30:230, 1980
51. Yoganathan AP, Corcoran WH: In vitro velocity measurements in the vicinity of aortic prostheses. J Biomech 12:135, 1979
52. Glancy DL, O'Brien KP, Reis RL et al: Hemodynamic studies in patients with 2M and 3M Starr-Edwards prostheses: Evidence of obstruction to left atrial

emptying. Circulation (Suppl I) 39:113, 1969

53. Gottwik M, Fentrop T, Kobel K et al: Hemodynamic properties of St. Jude Medical and Bjork-Shiley valvular prostheses in mitral position in the pulse duplicator. Thorac Cardiovasc Surg 29:307, 1981
54. Smeloff EA, Huntley AC, Davey TB et al: Comparative study of prosthetic heart valves. J Thorac Cardiovasc Surg 52:841, 1966
55. Dellsperger KC, Wieting DW, Baehr DA et al: Regurgitation of prosthetic heart valves: Dependence on heart rate and cardiac output. Am J Cardiol 51:321, 1983
56. Bjork VO: Metallurgic and design development and response to mechanical dysfunction of Bjork-Shiley heart valves. Scand J Thorac Cardiovasc Surg 19:1, 1985
57. Bjork VO, Lindblom D, Henze A: The monostrut strength. Scand J Thorac Cardiovasc Surg 19:13, 1985
58. Yoganathan AP, Stevenson DM, Williams FP et al: In vitro fluid dynamic characteristics of the Medtronics-Hall pivoting disc heart valve prosthesis. Scand J Thorac Cardiovasc Surg 16:235, 1982
59. Yoganathan AP, Reamer HH, Corcoran WH et al: The Bjork-Shiley aortic prosthesis: Flow characteristics of the present model vs the convexo-concave model. Scand J Thorac Cardiovasc Surg 14:1, 1980
60. Steenhoven A, vanVerlaan CWJ, Veenstra PC et al: An in-vivo cinematographic analysis of the behavior of the aortic valve. Am J Physiol 240:H286, 1981
61. Yoganathan AP, Chaux A, Gray RJ et al: Flow characteristics of the St. Jude prosthetic valve: An in vitro and in vivo study. Artif Intern Organs 6:288, 1982
62. Barratt-Boyes G: Cardiac surgery in the antipodes. J Thorac Cardiovasc Surg 78:804, 1979
63. Stinson EB, Griepp RB, Shumway NE: Long-term results of isolated aortic and mitral valve replacement with fresh aortic allografts. In Davila JC (ed): Second Henry Ford Symposium on Cardiac Surgery. New York, Appleton-Century-Crofts, 1977
64. Lurie AJ, Miller RR, Maxwell K et al: Postoperative hemodynamic assessment of the glutaraldehyde-preserved porcine heterograft in the aortic and mitral positions. Circulation (Suppl 2) 53,54:II–148, 1976
65. Carpentier A, Dubost C, Lane E et al: Continuing improvements in valvular bioprostheses. J Thorac Cardiovasc Surg 83:27, 1982
66. Stinson EB, Griepp RB, Oyer PE et al: Long-term experience with porcine aortic valve xenografts. J Thorac Cardiovasc Surg 73:54, 1977
67. Levine FH, Buckley MJ, Austen WG: Hemodynamic evaluation of Hancock modified orifice aortic position bioprostheses. Circulation (Suppl 3) 55,56:III–28, 1971
68. Ionescu MI, Tandon AP, Mary DA et al: Heart valve replacement with the Ionescu-Shiley pericardial xenograft. J Thorac Cardiovasc Surg 73:31, 1977
69. Tandon AA, Sengupta SM, Lukacs L et al: Long-term clinical and hemodynamic evaluation of Ionescu-Shiley prostheses in the mitral position. J Thorac Cardiovasc Surg 76:763, 1978
70. Revuelta T, Garcia-Rinaldi R, Johnston RM et al: The Ionescu-Shiley valve: A solution for the small aortic root. J Thorac Cardiovasc Surg 88:234, 1984
71. Baumgartner WA, Miller CD, Reitz BA et al: Surgical treatment of prosthetic valve endocarditis. Ann Thorac Surg 35:87, 1983
72. Geraci JE, Dale AJD, McGoon DC et al: Bacterial endocarditis and endarteritis following cardiac operations. Wis Med J 62:302, 1963
73. Dismukes WE: Prosthetic valve endocarditis: Factors influencing outcome and recommendations for therapy. In Bisno A (ed): Treatment of Endocarditis, p 167. New York, Grune & Stratton, 1981
74. Gnann JW Jr, Cobbs CG: Infections of prosthetic valves and intravascular devices. In Mandell GI (ed): Principles and Practice of Infectious Disease, p 530. New York, John Wiley & Sons, 1985
75. Dougherty SH, Simmons RL: Infections in implanted prosthetic devices: Prosthetic valve endocarditis. Curr Probl Surg 19:269, 1982
76. Masur H, Johnson WD Jr: Prosthetic valve endocarditis. J Thoracic Cardiovasc Surg 80:31, 1980
77. Jones EL, Schwarzmann SW, Check WA et al: Complications from cardiac prostheses: Infection, thrombosis and emboli associated with intracardiac prostheses. In Sabiston DC, Spencer FC (eds): Surgery of the Chest, p 1253. Philadelphia, WB Saunders, 1983
78. Magilligan DJ, Quinn EL, Davila JC: Bacteremia, endocarditis and the Hancock valve. Ann Thorac Surg 24:508, 1977
79. Wilson WR, Jaumin PM, Danielson GK et al: Prosthetic valve endocarditis. Ann Intern Med 82:751, 1975
80. Watanakunakorn C: Prosthetic valve endocarditis: A review. Prog Cardiovasc Dis 22:181, 1979
81. Stinson EB, Castellino RA, Shumway NE: Radiologic signs in endocarditis following prosthetic valve replacement. J Thorac Cardiovasc Surg 55:554, 1968
82. Miller HC, Gibson DG, Stephens JD: Role of echocardiography and phonocardiography in diagnosis of mitral paraprosthetic regurgitation with Starr-Edward prostheses. Br Heart J 35:1217, 1973
83. Nagata S, Park Y-D, Nagae K et al: Echocardiographic features of bioprosthetic valve endocarditis. Br Heart J 51:263, 1984
84. Welton DE, Young JB, Raizner AE et al: Value and safety of cardiac catheterization during active infective endocarditis. Am J Cardiol 44:1306, 1979
85. Washington JA: The role of the microbiology laboratory in the diagnosis and antimicrobial treatment of infective endocarditis. Mayo Clin Proc 57:22, 1982
86. Weinstein L: Infected prosthetic valves: A diagnostic and therapeutic dilemma. N Engl J Med 286:1108, 1972
87. Sande MA, Johnson WD Jr, Hook EW et al: Sustained bacteremia in patients with prosthetic cardiac valves. N Engl J Med 286:1067, 1972
88. Gnann JW, Dismukes WE: Prosthetic valve endocarditis: An overview. Herz 8:320, 1983
89. Raychaudhury T, Cameron EWJ, Walbaum PR: Surgical management of prosthetic valve endocarditis. J Thorac Cardiovasc Surg 86:112, 1983
90. Rosenberg RD: Heparin antithrombin system. In Colman RW et al (eds): Hemostasis and Thrombosis, p 738. Philadelphia, JB Lippincott, 1982
91. Ellison N, Edmunds LH Jr, Colman RW: Platelet aggregation following heparin and protamine administration. Anesthesiology 48:65, 1978
92. Gallop PM, Liam TB, Haukochka PV: Carboxylated calcium-binding proteins and vitamin K. N Engl J Med 302:1460, 1980
93. Hetzer R, Gerbode F, Keith WJ et al: Thrombotic complications after valve replacement with porcine heterografts. World J Surg 3:505, 1979
94. Altman R, Boullon F, Rouvier J et al: Aspirin and prophylaxis of thromboembolic complications in patients with substitute heart valves. J Thorac Cardiovasc Surg 72:127, 1976
95. Chesebro JH, Fuster V, Pumphrey CW et al: Combined warfarin-platelet inhibitor antithrombotic therapy in prosthetic heart valve replacement. Circulation (Suppl 4) 64:76, 1981
96. Sullivan JM, Harken DE, Gorlin R: Pharmacologic control of thrombotic complications of cardiac-valve replacement. N Engl J Med 284:1391, 1971
97. Douglas PS, Hirshfeld JW Jr, Edie RN et al: Clinical comparison of St. Jude and porcine aortic valve prostheses. Circulation (Suppl II) 72:II–135, 1985
98. Hill JD, Szarnicki RJ, Avery GJ II et al: Risk-benefit analysis of warfarin therapy in Hancock mitral valve replacement. J Thorac Cardiovasc Surg 83:718, 1982
99. Nunez L, Aguado MG, Larria JL et al: Prevention of thromboembolism using aspirin after mitral valve replacement with porcine valve prosthesis. Ann Thorac Surg 37:84, 1984
100. Edmunds LH Jr: Thromboembolic complications of current cardiac valvular prostheses. Ann Thorac Surg 34:96, 1982
101. Miller DC, Oyer PE, Stinson EB et al: 10-15 year reassessment of the performance characteristics of the Starr-Edwards Model 6120 mitral valve prosthesis. J Thorac Cardiovasc Surg 85:1, 1983
102. Fuster V, Pumphrey CW, McGoon MD et al: Systemic thromboembolism in mitral and aortic Starr-Edwards prostheses: A 10-12 year follow-up. Circulation 66:I-157, 1982
103. Addonizio VP Jr, Edmunds LH Jr: Thromboembolic complications of prosthetic valves. Cardiology Clinics 3:431, 1985
104. Baudet EM, Oca CC, Roques XF et al: A five and one-half year experience with the St. Jude Medical cardiac valve prosthesis. Early and late results of 737 valve replacements in 671 patients. J Thorac Cardiovasc Surg 90:137, 1985
105. Murphy DA, Levine FH, Buckley MJ et al: Mechanical valve: A comparative analysis of the Starr-Edwards and Bjork-Shiley prostheses. J Thorac Cardiovasc Surg 86:746, 1983
106. Miller DC, Oyer PE, Mitchell RS et al: Performance characteristics of the Starr-Edwards Model 1260 aortic valve prosthesis beyond 10 years. J Thorac Cardiovasc Surg 88:193, 1984
107. Chaux A, Czer LS, Matloff JM et al: The St. Jude Medical bileaflet valve prosthesis. A five year experience. J Thorac Cardiovasc Surg 88:706, 1984
108. Janusz MT, Jamieson WRE, Allen P et al: Experience with the Carpentier-Edwards porcine valve prosthesis in 700 patients. Ann Thorac Surg 34:625, 1982
109. Cohn LM, Mudge GH, Pratter F et al: Five to eight-year follow-up of patients undergoing porcine heart valve replacement. N Engl J Med 304:258, 1981
110. Craver JM, Jones EL, McKeown P et al: Porcine cardiac xenograft valves: Analysis of survival, valve failure, and explanation. Ann Thorac Surg 34:16, 1982
111. Magilligan DJ, Lewis JW, Tilley B et al: The porcine bioprosthetic valve 12 years later. J Thorac Cardiovasc Surg 89:499, 1985
112. Rossiter SJ, Miller DC, Stinson EB et al: Aortic and mitral prosthetic valve reoperation: Early and late results. Arch Surg 114:1279, 1979
113. Alam M, Lakier JB, Pickard SD et al: Echocardiographic evaluation of porcine bioprosthetic valves: Experience with 309 normal and 59 dysfunctioning valves. Am J Cardiol 52:309, 1983
114. Lentz DJ, Pollock EM, Olsen DB et al: Prevention of intrinsic calcification in porcine and bovine xenograft materials. Trans Am Soc Artif Intern Organs 28:494, 1982
115. Dunn JM, Marmon LM: Mechanisms of calcification of tissue valves. Cardiology Clinics 3:385, 1985
116. Dunn JM: Porcine valve durability in children. Ann Thorac Surg 32:357, 1981
117. Gallo I, Ruiz B, Duran CG et al: 5–8 year follow-up of patients with the Hancock cardiac bioprosthesis. J Thorac Cardiovasc Surg 86:897, 1983
118. Ott DA, Cooley DA, Reul GJ et al: Ionescu-Shiley bovine pericardial bioprosthesis. Cardiology Clinics 3:343, 1985
119. Ionescu MI, Smith DR, Hasan SS et al: Clinical durability of the pericardial xenograft valves. Ten years' experience with mitral replacement. Ann

Thorac Surg 34:265, 1982
120. Schoen FJ, Levy RJ: Bioprosthetic heart valve failure: Pathology and pathogenesis. Cardiology Clinics 2:717, 1984
121. Ferrans VJ, Boyce SW, Billingham ME et al: Calcific deposits in porcine bioprostheses: Structure and pathogenesis. Am J Cardiol 46:721, 1980
122. Levy RJ, Zenker JA, Bernhard WF: Porcine bioprosthetic valve calcification in bovine LV-aorta shunt. Studies of the deposition of Vitamin K-dependent proteins. Ann Thorac Surg 36:187, 1983
123. Riddle JM, Stein PD, Magilligan DJ: A morphologic review of the porcine bioprosthetic heart valve. Henry Ford Hosp Med J 30:139, 1982
124. Ferrans VJ, Spray TL, Billingham ME et al: Structural changes in glutaraldehyde treated porcine heterografts used as substitute cardiac valves. Transmission and scanning electron microscopic observations in 12 patients. Am J Cardiol 41:1159, 1978
125. Heinzerling RM, Stein PD, Riddle JM et al: Immunologic involvement in porcine bioprosthetic valve degeneration: Preliminary studies. Henry Ford Hosp Med J 30:146, 1982
126. Levy RJ, Schoen FJ, Levy JT et al: Biologic determinants of dystrophic calcification and osteocalcin deposition in glutaraldehyde-preserved porcine aortic valve leaflets implanted subcutaneously in rats. Am J Pathol 113:143, 1983
127. Levy RJ, Schoen FJ, Howard SL: Mechanism of calcification of porcine bioprosthetic aortic valve cusps. Role of t-lymphocytes. Am J Cardiol 52:629, 1983
128. Fishbein MC, Levy RJ, Ferrans VJ et al: Calcification of cardiac valve bioprostheses. J Thorac Cardiovasc Surg 83:602, 1982
129. Thubrikar MJ, Deck JD, Aouad J et al: Role of mechanical stress in calcification of aortic bioprosthetic valves. J Thorac Cardiovasc Surg 86:115, 1983
130. Gallop DM, Paz MA: Post translational protein modification with special attention to collagen and elastin. Physiol Res 55:418, 1975
131. Fleish M: Diphosphonates, history and mechanism of action. Metastic Bone Disease Related Research 4-5:279, 1981
132. Cohn LH, Allred EN, DiSessa VJ et al: Early and late risk of aortic valve replacement. J Thorac Cardiovasc Surg 88:695, 1984
133. Gonzalez-Lavin L, Chi S, Blair TC et al: Five-year experience with the Ionescu-Shiley bovine pericardial valve in the aortic position. Ann Thorac Surg 36:270, 1983
134. Pelletier LC, Chaitman BR, Baillot R et al: Clinical and hemodynamic results with the Carpentier-Edwards porcine valve prosthesis. Ann Thorac Surg 34:612, 1982
135. Cheung D, Flemma RJ, Mullen DC et al: Ten year follow-up in aortic replacement using the Bjork Shiley prosthesis. Ann Thorac Surg 32:138, 1981
136. Brais MP, Bedard JP, Goldstein W et al: Ionescu-Shiley pericardial xenografts: Follow-up of up to six years. Ann Thorac Surg 39:105, 1985
137. Scott WC, Miller DC, Haverich A et al: Determinants of operative mortality for patients undergoing aortic valve replacement. J Thorac Cardiovasc Surg 89:400, 1985
138. Rossiter SJ, Stinson EB, Oyer PE et al: Prosthetic valve endocarditis. J Thorac Cardiovasc Surg 76:795, 1978
139. Wideman FE, Blackstone EH, Kirklin JW et al: Hospital mortality of re-replacement of the aortic valve. Incremental risk factors. J Thorac Cardiovasc Surg 82:692, 1981
140. Craver JM, Goldstein J, Jones EL et al: Clinical hemodynamic and operative descriptors affecting outcome of aortic valve replacement in elderly versus young patients. Ann Surg 199:733, 1984
141. Stephenson LW, MacVaugh H III, Edmunds LH Jr: Surgery using cardiopulmonary bypass in the elderly. Circulation 58:250, 1978
142. Salomon NW, Stinson EB, Griepp RB et al: Patient-related risk factors as predictors of results following isolated mitral valve replacement. Ann Thorac Surg 24:519, 1977
143. Husebye DG, Pluth JR, Piehler JM et al: Reoperation on prosthetic heart valves. An analysis of risk factors in 552 patients. J Thorac Cardiovasc Surg 86:543, 1983
144. Lytle BW, Cosgrove DM, Gill CC et al: Mitral valve replacement combined with myocardial revascularization: Early and late results for 300 patients, 1970–1983. Circulation 71:1179, 1985
145. Rostad H, Hall KV, Froysaker T: Mitral insufficiency following myocardial infarction. Scand J Thorac Cardiovasc Surg 13:277, 1979
146. Tepe NA, Edmunds LH Jr: Operation for acute post-infarction mitral insufficiency and cardiogenic shock. J Thorac Cardiovasc Surg 89:525, 1985
147. Manners JM, Monro JL, Ross JK: Pulmonary hypertension and mitral valve disease: 56 surgical patients reviewed. Thorax 32:691, 1977
148. Stephenson LW, Edie RN, Harken AH et al: Combined aortic and mitral valve replacement: Changes in practice and prognosis. Circulation 69:640, 1984
149. Dark JH, Bain WH: Rupture of posterior wall of left ventricle after mitral valve replacement. Thorax 39:905, 1984
150. Roberts WC: Complications of cardiac valve replacement: Characteristic abnormalities of prostheses pertaining to any or specific site. Am Heart J 103:113, 1982
151. Blackstone EH, Kirklin JW, Pluth JR et al: The performance of the Braunwald-Cutter aortic prosthetic valve. Ann Thorac Surg 23:302, 1977
152. Silver MD, Wilson GJ: The pathology of wear in the Beall Model 104 heart valve prosthesis. Circulation 56:617, 1977
153. Wellons HA Jr, Strauch RS, Nolan SP et al: Isolated mitral valve replacement with a Kay-Shiley disc valve. Actuarial analysis of the long-term results. J Thorac Cardiovasc Surg 70:862, 1975
154. Mitha AS, Matisonn RE, LaRoux BT et al: Clinical experience with the Lillehei-Kaster cardiac valve prosthesis. J Thorac Cardiovasc Surg 72:401, 1976
155. Schaeffer JW, Marks SD, Wolf PS et al: Systemic embolization of the disk occluder of the Wada-Cutter prosthetic valve. A late complication. Chest 71:44, 1977
156. Scott SM, Sethi GK, Flye MW et al: The sutureless aortic valve prosthesis: Experience with and technical considerations for replacement of the early model. Ann Surg 184:174, 1976
157. Ellis FH Jr, Healy RW, Alexander S: Mitral valve replacement with the modified University of Cape Town (UCT) prosthesis: Clinical and hemodynamic results. Ann Thorac Surg 23:26, 1977
158. Stinson EB, Griepp RP, Bieber CP et al: Aortic valve allograft for mitral valve replacement. Surgery 77:861, 1975
159. Stein DW, Selden R, Starr A: Thrombotic phenomena with non-anticoagulated, composite-strut aortic prostheses. J Thorac Cardiovasc Surg 71:680, 1976
160. Sola A, Schoevaerdts JC, Jaumin P et al: Review of 387 isolated mitral valve replacements by the Model 6120 Starr-Edwards prosthesis. J Thorac Cardiovasc Surg 84:744, 1982
161. Starr DS, Lawrie GM, Howell JF et al: Clinical experience with a Smeloff-Cutter prosthesis: One to 12 year follow-up. Ann Thorac Surg 30:448, 1980
162. Barnhorst DA, Oxman AJ, Connolly DC et al: Long-term follow-up of isolated replacement of the aortic or mitral valve with the Starr-Edwards prosthesis. Am J Cardiol 35:228, 1975
163. Gersh BJ, Schaff HV, Vatterott PJ et al: Results of triple valve replacement in 91 patients: Perioperative mortality and long-term follow-up. Circulation 72:130, 1985
164. Marshall WG Jr, Kouchoukos NT, Karp RB et al: Late results after mitral valve replacement with the Bjork-Shiley and porcine prostheses. J Thorac Cardiovasc Surg 85:902, 1983
165. De Wall R, Pelletier LC, Panabianco A et al: 5-year clinical experience with Omniscience cardiac valve. Ann Thorac Surg 38:275, 1984
166. Fananapazir L, Clarke DB, Dark JF et al: Results of valve replacement with the Omniscience prosthesis. J Thorac Cardiovasc Surg 86:621, 1983
167. Marshall WG Jr, Kouchoukos NT, Pollock SB et al: Early results of valve replacement with a Bjork-Shiley convexoconcave prosthesis. Ann Thorac Surg 37:398, 1984
168. Nitter-Hauge S, Semb B, Abdelnoor M et al: A five year experience with the Medtronic-Hall disk valve prosthesis. Circulation (Suppl II) 68:II-169, 1983
169. Richardson JV, Karp RB, Kirklin JW et al: Treatment of infective endocarditis: A 10-year comparative analysis. Circulation 58:589, 1978
170. Bosch X, Pomar JL, Pelletier LC: Early and late prognosis after reoperation for prosthetic valve replacement. J Thorac Cardiovasc Surg 88:567, 1984
171. Odell JA, Durandt J, Shama DM et al: Spontaneous embolization of a St. Jude prosthetic mitral valve leaflet. Ann Thorac Surg 39:569, 1985
172. Mitchell RS, Miller DC, Stinson EB et al: Perspective on the porcine xenograft valve. Cardiology Clinics 3:371, 1985
173. Gabbay S, Bortolotti U, Wasserman F et al: Long-term follow-up of the Ionescu-Shiley mitral pericardial xenograft. J Thorac Cardiovasc Surg 88:758, 1984
174. Schoen FJ, Schulman LJ, Cohn LH: Quantitative anatomic analysis of "stent creep" of explanted Hancock standard porcine bioprostheses used for cardiac valve replacement. Am J Cardiol 56:110, 1985
175. MacManus Q, Grunkemeier GL, Lambert LE et al: Non-cloth-covered caged-ball prostheses. J Thorac Cardiovasc Surg 76:788, 1978
176. Macmanus Q, Grunkemeier GL, Lambert LE et al: Year of operation as a risk factor and the late results of valve replacement. J Thorac Cardiovasc Surg 80:834, 1980
177. Lee SJK, Barr C, Callaghan JC et al: Long-term survival after aortic valve replacement using the Smeloff-Cutter prosthesis. Circulation 52:1132, 1975
178. McHenry MM, Smeloff EA, Matlof HJ et al: Long-term survival after single aortic or mitral valve replacement with the present model of Smeloff-Cutter valves. J Thorac Cardiovasc Surg 75:709, 1978

CATHETER BALLOON VALVULOPLASTY

James P. Srebro • Thomas A. Ports

In the past decade there has been significant expansion in the role of the cardiac catheterization laboratory. Whereas their original mission was to obtain relevant hemodynamic and angiographic data for diagnostic purposes, cardiac catheterization laboratories in most large hospitals now provide a range of interventional therapeutic procedures. These include percutaneous transluminal coronary angioplasty, closure of atrial septal defects and patent ductus arteriosus by catheter techniques, acute thrombolytic therapy, and, most recently, catheter balloon valvuloplasty. A chronology of interventional procedures using balloon catheters is shown in Table 85.1.

Balloon dilatation of stenotic valves has been performed on all four valves of the heart. Table 85.2 lists the normal valve areas and those associated with significant and severe hemodynamic impairment. This chapter reviews the available data on these procedures, summarizes the technical aspects, and provides perspective with regard to standard surgical approaches. In many cases, surgery still represents the "gold standard" of care. It should be emphasized that most forms of valvuloplasty are still experimental and that much of the available data must be viewed as tentative. With the exception of pulmonic stenosis, these procedures should be performed routinely only in patients in whom other accepted forms of therapy are not possible. Further, patients should be made aware of the experimental nature of the procedure and entered into an approved protocol. Only after substantial cumulative clinical experience will the final role of balloon dilatation of heart valves be known.

PULMONARY VALVULOPLASTY
PULMONIC VALVULAR STENOSIS

Stenosis of the pulmonic valve generally occurs as a congenital anomaly. It may occur as a single entity or in association with complex congenital heart disease. Isolated pulmonary valve stenosis was observed in 7.5% of 10,624 children with congenital heart disease over a 20-year observation period in a leading university hospital.[1] Pulmonary stenosis may also be seen in association with other complex congenital malformations such as tetralogy of Fallot, double-outlet right ventricle, single ventricle, and hypoplastic right ventricle.

There are two pathologically different and morphologically distinguishable forms of pulmonic stenosis. One results from inadequate commissural separation during the embryologic development and the other is caused by dysplasia of the pulmonic valve. The most common variety is commissural fusion in which the valve leaflets become rigid and thickened with age. As a general rule, the diagnosis is made by hemodynamic measurements and a characteristic appearance on ventriculography. During systole, the fused leaflets appear to form a conical or dome-shaped funnel and produce an obvious jet of contrast (Fig. 85.1). The less common form of congenital pulmonic stenosis is dysplasia of the pulmonary valve. It is recognized by replacement of the delicate leaflets by multiple pedunculated or sessile nodules arising from the valve annulus. The dysplastic pulmonary valve may occur in the setting of Noonan's syndrome or the syndrome of polyvalvular dysplasia. The obstruction of the pulmonic valve may be complicated by subvalvar infundibular hypertrophy or an underdeveloped pulmonic annulus.

Acquired pulmonic stenosis is extremely rare. It has been described with advanced rheumatic valvular disease and is invariably associated with stenosis of other cardiac valves. There have been only a few reported cases of balloon valvuloplasty in acquired pulmonic stenosis.

The conventional and conservative approach to pulmonic stenosis dictates surgical correction when the right ventricular pressure approaches or exceeds systemic pressure. Early surgical procedures employed rigid instruments and a closed technique. The introduction of cardiopulmonary bypass allowed pulmonary valvulotomy to be performed under direct vision, and excellent long-term results have been obtained. Consequently, surgery has been the treatment of choice since the mid-1960s. Surgical visualization of the abnormal anatomy and outflow tract also allows for concomitant infundibulectomy or enlargement of the pulmonic annulus if required at the time of surgery.

HISTORY OF PULMONARY BALLOON VALVULOPLASTY

The first therapeutic, nonsurgical procedure to relieve valvular pulmonic stenosis was performed by Semb and associates in 1979.[2] In a Rashkind-like maneuver, a balloon inflated with carbon dioxide was withdrawn across a stenotic pulmonic valve, with encouraging hemodynamic improvement. The first report of balloon valvuloplasty as we understand the procedure today was published by Kan and colleagues in 1982.[3] Shortly thereafter, Pepine and associates extended the technique to an adult.[4] In 1983, Lababidi and Wu published the first series of patients.[5] In their group of 18 patients, the majority of whom were children, they documented significant acute reductions in transvalvular gradient and right ventricular pressures. Later that year, Kan and coworkers published follow-up data from Johns Hopkins Hospital on 20 patients in whom they had performed pulmonic valvuloplasty.[6] Again, the vast majority of these patients were infants and children; however, one adult was included. They include long-term follow-up with repeat catheterization an average of 7 months after the procedure. They corroborated the observations of earlier investigators with excellent acute hemodynamic improvement and documented sustained beneficial effect. Rocchini and associates also documented the safety and efficacy of pulmonic valvuloplasty by comparing rest and exercise hemodynamics before and after the procedure.[7] Since that first case of a successful dilatation of a stenotic pulmonary valve in an 8-year-old child, there have been multiple case reports including refinements and modifications of the procedure and several relatively large series. These are summarized in Table 85.3. There is clear evidence that the procedure is useful in acutely relieving pulmonic valvular obstruction and that these beneficial effects persist over several years. Percutaneous balloon valvuloplasty has become the treatment of choice for most patients with congenital pulmonic stenosis.

PHYSIOLOGIC AND ANATOMICAL EFFECTS

There have been several reports that expand our understanding of the physiology of pulmonic stenosis, right ventricular pressure overload, and acute obstruction of the outflow tract. These include a study by Shuck and colleagues, in which the role of right-to-left shunting

TABLE 85.1 CHRONOLOGY OF INTERVENTIONAL VASCULAR DILATATION PROCEDURES WITH BALLOON CATHETERS

Procedure	Year First Performed
Peripheral arteries	1964
Renal arteries	1977
Coronary arteries	1977
Pulmonic valve	1979
Aortic valve (children)	1982
Coarctation of aorta	1983
Pulmonary veins	1984
Mitral valve	1984
Aortic valve (adults)	1986
Subaortic membrane	1986
Porcine tricuspid valve	1986
Tricuspid valve	1987

TABLE 85.2 NORMAL VALVE AREAS AND THOSE ASSOCIATED WITH HEMODYNAMIC IMPAIRMENT

Valve	Normal Area (cm^2)	Hemodynamic Impairment Significant	Severe
Pulmonic*	2–3	<0.8	<0.5
Tricuspid*	5–10	<1.5	<1.5
Aortic	2.6–3.5	<0.8	<0.5
Mitral	4–6	1.5–2.5	1.0–1.5

* Because of the rarity of pulmonic and tricuspid stenosis, there is not a clear consensus on accepted normal valve areas. The grading of the severity of pulmonic stenosis varies with authors. Rather than emphasizing valve areas, ratio of the peak right ventricular (RV) pressure to the peak systemic arterial (SA) pressure is used: RV/SA <0.5, mild; RV/SA 0.5 to 0.75 moderate; RV/SA >0.75, severe.

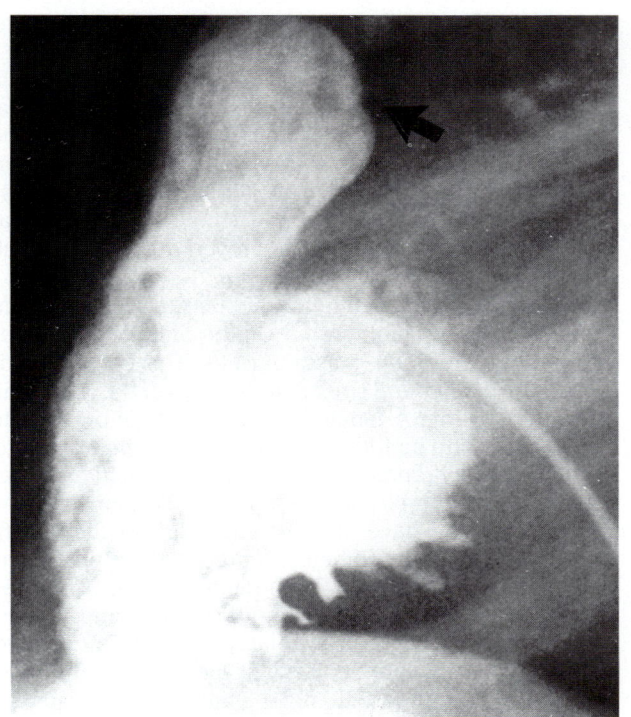

FIGURE 85.1 Cineradiograph demonstrating pulmonic stenosis. This left lateral projection of a right ventriculogram demonstrates the doming pulmonic valve frequently seen in congenital pulmonic stenosis. Note the absence of infundibular hypertrophy.

TABLE 85.3 REPORTED SERIES OF PULMONIC VALVULOPLASTY

Investigator	Year	Number of Patients	Age (yr)	Gradient (mm Hg) Predilatation	Postdilatation	Follow-Up
Lababidi and Wu[5]	1983	19	0.9–19.0	81	23	Acute
Kan et al.[6]	1984	20	0.02–14, 22, 56	68	23	Acute + 2–12 mo
Rocchini et al.[7]	1984	7	1.5–9.9	90	49	Acute, exercise 4–5 mo
Khalilullah et al.[11]	1985	3	17–28	115	59	Acute
Kveselis et al.[12]	1985	19	0.5–18	78	38	Acute + 1 yr
Ali-Khan et al.[14]	1986	32	0.5–12	99	23	Acute + 6 mo
Yeager et al.[15]	1986	10	0.8–12	72	30	Acute
Rao et al.[13]	1987	22	0.3–2.0	93	44	Acute + 6–28 mo

through a patent foramen ovale was documented.[8] By measuring changes in exercise hemodynamics before and after the procedure, they documented improvements in dynamic stress indices. Ben-Shachar and co-workers reported a case in which infundibular obstruction became manifest acutely after balloon valvuloplasty.[9] This patient required surgical correction shortly after the valvuloplasty. Visualization of the previously dilated valve intraoperatively provided the first insight into the mechanism of dilatation in balloon valvuloplasty. In this case there were two tears in the valve leaflets extending to the annulus. These were closely adjacent to the commissures but did not split the commissures themselves. The pulmonary artery and right ventricular outflow tract were undamaged, but a small (2 mm × 3 mm) subendocardial hemorrhage was noted beneath a pulmonic valve cusp.

Tynan and associates successfully used the procedure in a 6-day-old neonate.[10] A small series of young adults was reported by Khalilullah and co-workers.[11] Kveselis and colleagues similarly reported a series of 19 children, with hemodynamic follow-up at 1 year in 7 patients.[12] Again, significant and sustained reductions in the right ventricular systolic pressure and outflow tract gradient were documented. In most patients the calculated pulmonic valve area increased at the end of 1 year, presumably demonstrating normal growth of the great vessels and valvular apparatus. They further looked at regression of electrocardiographic evidence of right ventricular hypertrophy and found that the height of the R wave in lead V_1 decreased significantly over the follow-up period. The surface electrocardiographic results were corroborated by vectorcardiographic reductions in the maximal right spatial voltage with clockwise loop. Their study also incorporated an echo-Doppler estimation of the right ventricular outflow tract gradient and documented the utility of this noninvasive technique in following these patients.

There have been technical modifications and refinements in the technique, including ways to reasonably estimate the balloon size, period of inflation, and maximal inflation pressure. Rao studied the relationship between the size of the balloon and the degree of relief from pulmonary stenosis.[13] In this study, 26 valvuloplasties were performed and followed over a period of 6 months to 28 months (mean, 12 months). Immediately after the valvuloplasty there was no significant difference in residual gradients (44 mm Hg vs. 43 mm Hg). In those with a balloon-to-pulmonary annulus ratio greater than 1 (mean, 1.32), there was a significant reduction in the residual pulmonic gradient (18 mm Hg vs. 80 mm Hg) at follow-up catheterization. This study suggests that although the immediate results of pulmonic valvuloplasty are significant, a large balloon-to-annulus ratio produces a more sustained result. In other words, the restenosis rate is less when an aggressive dilatation is performed. The authors conclude that balloons larger than the pulmonary annulus should be used. Ali-Khan and co-workers published a relatively large series of patients who had undergone pulmonary valvuloplasty.[14] In their series, two patients required a double-balloon technique to dilate the stenotic valve adequately as judged by residual gradient. This may further support the need to dilate the valve adequately even if two balloons are required. Yeager and associates found similar results.[15]

PATIENT SELECTION

Ideal patients for pulmonary valvuloplasty are those with documented or suspected commissural fusion without significant infundibular hypertrophy. Those with dysplastic valves fall into an intermediate category where individual judgment is required. Those with true anular hypoplasia and moderate or severe infundibular hypertrophy are poor candidates for pulmonary valvuloplasty. In these patients, surgical correction is appropriate. It is not uncommon that patients who have significant valvular pulmonary stenosis will also have some degree of infundibular hypertrophy, which may contribute to the outflow gradient by dynamic obstruction. One would postulate that if the primary process were obstruction of the valve and this were relieved, the hypertrophy would regress. This hypothesis has not been adequately studied but appears to occur in at least some patients. Infundibular "spasm" has also been postulated to explain unusually high gradients immediately following the procedure. This phenomenon may be observed by a high residual gradient using the central lumen of the balloon-dilatation catheter, which resolves over a short period of time. Recrossing the valve with a catheter that is more flexible and soft may alleviate this potential problem.

PROCEDURE

If pulmonic stenosis is highly likely based on the clinical history, physical examination, and echocardiographic and Doppler data, it is reasonable to perform pulmonic valvuloplasty at diagnostic catheterization if the diagnosis is confirmed by catheterization. Most centers perform the procedure with mild sedation and local anesthesia; however, some have administered general anesthesia.

The usual approach involves cannulation of the femoral vein and a femoral artery by the Seldinger technique. Baseline hemodynamic data are obtained, including measurement of cardiac output by the thermodilution method or Fick principle. Biplane right ventriculography is ideal for visualizing the right ventricle, outflow tract, pulmonary valve, and proximal pulmonary arteries. The size of the pulmonic annulus should be estimated by echocardiogram and corroborated by the angiographic data. An arterial sheath is used for blood pressure monitoring and left heart catheterization if indicated.

A variety of techniques may be used to cross the stenotic pulmonary valve. These include the use of balloon-tip flotation catheters, tip-deflecting catheters, and guide wire techniques. If the stenotic valve is particularly difficult to cross with the diagnostic catheters, an exchange wire may be used. This allows repeated access to the stenotic segment if multiple dilatations or balloon catheters are to be used. Anticoagulation is generally employed during the valvuloplasty if there are no contraindications.

The valvuloplasty catheter most commonly used and the only one commercially available in the United States is produced by Mansfield Scientific, Watertown, Massachusetts. This catheter is the only one approved by the Federal Drug Administration for pulmonary valvuloplasty as of this writing. A family of balloon-dilatation catheters is shown in Figure 85.2. The balloon catheters have a shaft diameter ranging from 5 French to 14 French, with balloons varying in diameter from 5 mm to 30 mm when completely inflated. The balloons vary in length from 2 cm to 6 cm and have metallic end markers that are fluoroscopically visible. The balloon catheter is prepared by purging repeatedly with carbon dioxide and filling with dilute contrast. A more dilute contrast solution is preferable (3 to 1 or 4 to 1) to minimize the viscosity. In our laboratory, the size of the inflated balloon is checked with a sterile architectural template because it is not unusual for inflated balloons to be 1 mm to 2 mm less than the stated diameter at the recommended inflation pressures. Most operators will select a balloon identical to or slightly larger than the estimated annulus size. There have been reports of dilatation up to 120% to 150% of the measured diameter without untoward effects, and at least one study suggests restenosis is less common with a balloon-to-annulus ratio greater than 1.[13] Balloon diameters and corresponding cross-sectional areas for commonly used balloons are shown in Table 85.4. The balloon catheters generally require 4 to 6 atmospheres (50 psi–90 psi) of inflation pressure, which may be measured by manometer. Occasionally the balloons may rupture, typically by a longitudinal tear. In carefully prepared balloons, there are no complications related to balloon rupture.

Because of the relatively large size of the balloon compared to the intraluminal shaft and the viscosity of the dilute contrast, the inflation and deflation times are relatively long. Generally, it requires 5 to 10 seconds to inflate the balloon completely and 5 to 10 seconds to deflate it rapidly by aspiration.

The length of the balloon is chosen with two opposing principles in mind. Larger and longer balloons require more time to inflate, making it difficult to prevent intracavitary and intraluminal rocking, which may traumatize these structures. Similarly, they require more time to deflate and may be problematic in the setting of significant hemodynamic compromise. Longer balloons necessarily straighten the segment over which they are inflated and may unnecessarily distort the normal anatomy. On the other hand, the shorter balloons are more difficult to maintain in proper position during inflation and are more easily expelled by the contractile force of hypertrophic ventricle as they begin to occlude the orifice. Consequently, it may be impossible to deliver the maximal transaxial pressure to the area of interest, even on multiple attempts. The operator must choose the length of the balloon based on the individual patient and personal experience.

The prepared valvuloplasty balloon catheter is introduced over the guide wire. The venous sheath may be removed and the valvuloplasty balloon catheter inserted directly over the guide wire after enlargement and dilatation of the access site. The balloon catheter is advanced under fluoroscopic control to the stenotic valve. Once the balloon catheter is in position, the balloon is rapidly inflated by hand injection of dilute contrast. An area of narrowing generally becomes obvious as the balloon is inflated. This is referred to as a *waist*. The dilating valve usually resists but eventually is overcome by the transaxial pressure transmitted by the expanding diameter of the balloon. The amount of time required to inflate the balloon and the amount of time the balloon is left inflated are generally determined by the operator and the size of the balloon-dilatation catheter. Relatively short inflation times with the minimum amount of pressure required to alleviate the waist would seem to be the least traumatic way to achieve the desired result. Some feel that relatively longer inflation times are required. There is no clear consensus nor are there convincing data to support either position. As the balloon is inflated, it is common to see the right ventricular pressure rise above systemic pressure. Systemic pressure generally falls because of reduced left ventricular preload. It has been clearly documented that during this period, a previously closed foramen ovale may open with right-to-left shunting.[8] This may be well tolerated but raises the possibility of paradoxical embolus and creation of sustained right-to-left shunt. These problems seem more theoretical than real based on the available data.

After the first balloon dilatation is performed, time is allowed for the rhythm and hemodynamic disturbances to stabilize. The procedure is repeated until the desired result is obtained. The accepted end point is an appropriately-sized balloon inflating without difficulty and without a discernible waist. Repeat hemodynamic measurements are made across the stenotic segment either by employing a separate catheter in the right ventricle and the distal lumen of the balloon catheter in the pulmonary artery or by a pullback procedure. An impressive reduction in the gradient and right ventricular pressure is generally expected.

In some cases, especially in adults, a two-balloon technique must be used. Care must be taken to avoid wrapping of the guide wires and balloon-dilatation catheters. When both catheters are in proper position, the two balloons are inflated simultaneously and repeat hemodynamics are recorded. A sequence of cineradiographs is shown in Figure 85.3, illustrating some elements of pulmonary valvuloplasty.

COMPLICATIONS

Few complications and no deaths have been reported with pulmonary valvuloplasty. The procedure may not give the desired beneficial results, especially if the pulmonic valve is dysplastic. The stenosis may recur and require surgical intervention. Development or worsening of pulmonary insufficiency may occur, but this does not appear to cause problems following pulmonary valvuloplasty.[16] Complications are similar to those of right heart catheterization including bleeding, infection, embolus, local vascular problems, cardiac tamponade, and arrhythmias. Loss of consciousness with convulsions, thrombosis of the inferior vena cava, and occlusion of the femoral and common iliac veins have been observed.[12] The development of a transient or persistent intracardiac shunt related to the opening of a foramen ovale has been described.[8] It may be hazardous to perform valvuloplasty in patients with a critically obstructed valve where the deflated balloon catheter may completely obstruct the orifice during positioning. Lababidi's group recently experienced a rupture of the papillary muscle of the tricuspid valve when an extra-long balloon was used.[17]

MECHANISM OF DILATATION

The exact mechanism by which the opening of the stenotic segment occurs is a matter of controversy. Kan and associates suggested that the procedure produces rupture of valvular tissue.[3,6] Lababidi and Wu reported the gross anatomical findings in a patient with tetralogy of Fallot who underwent surgical repair 1 day after pulmonic valvulo-

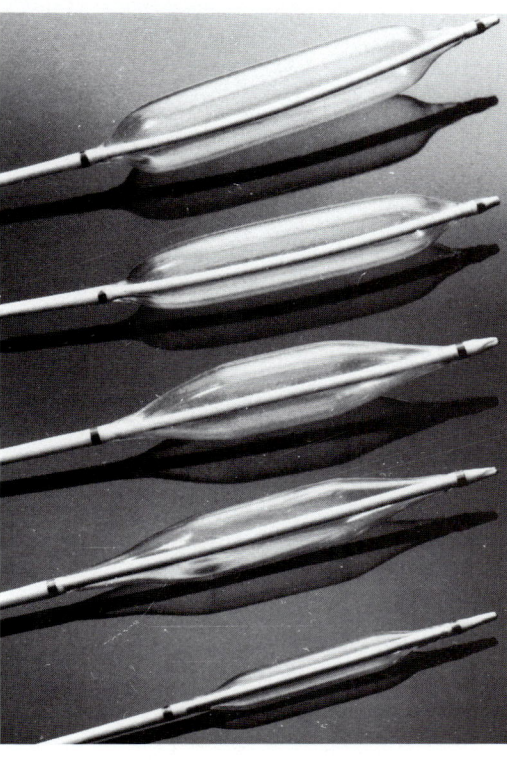

FIGURE 85.2 Valvuloplasty balloon-dilatation catheters. A family of balloon-dilatation catheters is available from several manufacturers. The catheters depicted here are manufactured by Mansfield Scientific and range in size from 8 mm to 25 mm and 3 cm to 5 cm in length. All accommodate a 0.038 guide wire. (By permission of Mansfield Scientific)

TABLE 85.4 BALLOON DIAMETER AND CORRESPONDING CROSS-SECTIONAL AREA

Balloon Diameter (mm)	Cross-sectional Area (cm²)
5	0.19
10	0.78
15	1.76
18	2.54
20	3.14
22	3.80
25	4.90

plasty.[5] The pulmonic valve was found to be bicuspid with a tear alongside the anterior valve raphe, suggesting that the mechanism of dilatation involved tearing of the valvular tissue.

RESULTS OF PULMONARY BALLOON VALVULOPLASTY

There have been seven published series of patients who have undergone percutaneous balloon valvuloplasty since the procedure was first performed in 1982 (see Table 85.3). The first series, by Lababidi and Wu, included the results of 19 patients who had undergone pulmonic valvuloplasty.[5] All patients had isolated pulmonic stenosis with no associated cardiac anomalies. There was no comment on the etiology of the pulmonic stenosis. Their technique used relatively high pressure (up to 120 psi) with relatively long inflation times (10 seconds). There was no significant change in cardiac output, but each patient had an improved transvalvular gradient. On the average, the gradient dropped from 80 mm Hg to 20 mm Hg. Similarly, the right ventricular peak systolic pressure decreased dramatically. There were no significant complications. This was an acute study and did not provide information on long-term follow-up. The authors felt that success in increasing the diameter of the valve was related to the high balloon pressure used. They later reviewed their long-term experience with this technique both in pulmonic and aortic stenosis[18] and found similar results.

Kan and associates published the first case report and later presented their data on an additional 20 patients in 1984.[6] This study had the advantage of providing relatively long-term follow-up on about half the patients. Their study again documented a dramatic decrease in the peak systolic pressure gradient across the pulmonic valve and right ventricular pressures. They did not experience any complications. They found sustained beneficial results 2 to 12 months after the procedure. They dilated one patient with a dysplastic pulmonary valve and achieved a modest, acute reduction in right ventricular pressure (from 78% to 54% of systemic pressure). However, follow-up catheterization showed that the right ventricular pressure had increased (to 71% of the systemic pressure), suggesting that the dilated segment returned to its prior conformation or that restenosis had occurred. The patient underwent a repeat balloon valvuloplasty with similar results acutely and chronically. These observations parallel the experience of the surgical valvulotomy–debridement procedure in dysplastic pulmonary valves. Consequently, valve resection or replacement is recommended for these patients.

Rocchini and co-workers reported on 7 patients who underwent pulmonary valvuloplasty.[7] Their data included both resting and exercise hemodynamics. They documented acute hemodynamic improvements with follow-up data at 3 months. Each patient sustained clinical and hemodynamic benefit over this period of time. Other investigators have found similar acute and follow-up results. Long-term follow-up over several years will be necessary before the final role of pulmonic valvuloplasty is known. In most cases it is the initial method of choice for treatment of congenital valvular pulmonic stenosis.

In addition to these data, there is an accumulating body of evidence in the privately funded pediatric registry on valvuloplasty, angioplasty, and congenital anomalies (VACA). Although there have been no published results to date, review of the preliminary data is consistent with acute and chronic hemodynamic improvement with few complications.[19]

SURGICAL RESULTS

The surgical treatment of pulmonary valve stenosis carries a low risk and leads to long-term excellent results. Surgery has the disadvantage of requiring more prolonged hospitalization, the risks attendant with major surgery and general anesthesia, and a higher likelihood of exposure to blood products. For most patients, the surgical scar is cosmetically unappealing. Percutaneous pulmonary valvuloplasty has the advantage of being a less invasive technique that does not require prolonged hospitalization or general anesthesia, does not usually require blood products, and does not leave a significant scar.

PULMONARY ARTERY STENOSIS AND VENOUS CHANNELS

Although not specifically related to pulmonic valvuloplasty, a few studies have been performed that deal with balloon dilatation of hypoplastic and stenotic pulmonary arteries in humans. In 1981, Lock and associates reported a study of experimental pulmonary artery stenosis in 27 newborn lambs.[20] These animals underwent left thoracotomy and

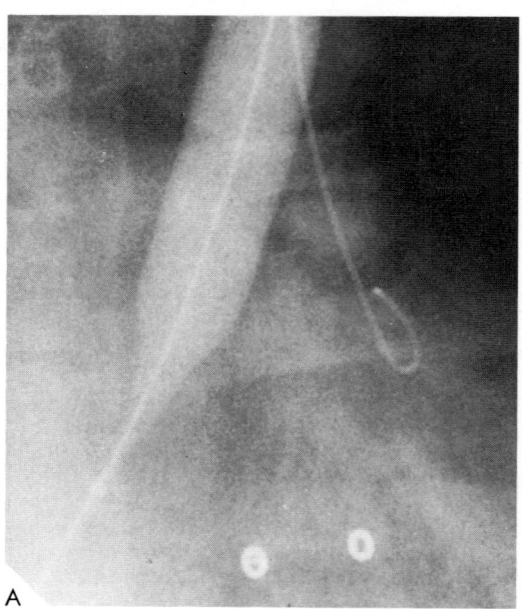
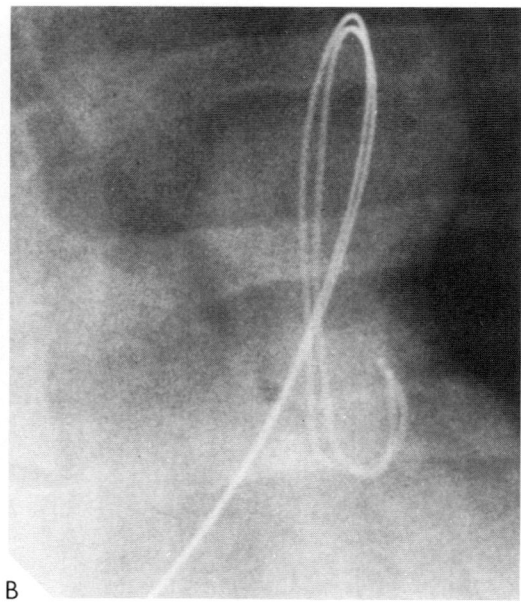
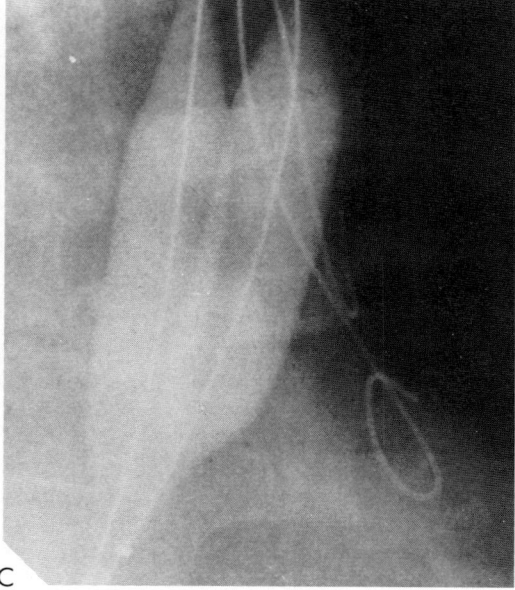

FIGURE 85.3 Sequence of cineradiographs of pulmonary valvuloplasty. **A.** Anteroposterior projection of inflated balloon-dilatation catheter across the pulmonic valve. The guide wire terminates in the left pulmonary artery. Radiopaque markers are used to size the annulus. **B.** A single balloon pulmonary valvuloplasty proved inadequate in this adult patient. A second guide wire was positioned in preparation for a double balloon valvuloplasty. **C.** The balloons are aligned and inflated simultaneously to perform a double balloon valvuloplasty. Each of the balloons is 5 cm in length. One is 20 mm while the other is 18 mm in diameter.

creation of bilateral branch pulmonary artery stenosis by partial ligation. Interrupted sutures were placed around the right pulmonary artery. Of the 27 lambs, 15 developed right ventricular dilatation and a low cardiac output syndrome and died during surgery or in the next 4 days; 2 died over the next 4 weeks, and 9 were long-term survivors. Thirteen arteries underwent dilatation by a modified balloon-dilatation catheter. Flows were measured using radioactive microspheres, and hemodynamic data were obtained by repeat catheterization. Sixteen weeks after dilatation, the average gradient remained below 10 mm Hg despite considerable growth in the animals. Late pathologic data showed multiple inner tears in the intima in recently dilated cases but complete intimal healing at 2 months. No significant morbidity was attributed to the dilation.

Based on these findings, Lock and co-workers undertook a study of balloon angioplasty in 7 children with stenosis or hypoplasia of both the right and left pulmonary arteries. They were unsuccessful for technical reasons in 2 patients. In the remaining 5 children, balloon dilatation of the affected arteries was successful as measured by a significant fall in right ventricular pressure, the gradient across the stenotic segment, and the percentage of pulmonary blood flow by quantitative perfusion scintigraphy. No morbidity was observed. Follow-up angiograms in 3 of 5 patients at 2 to 12 months documented persistence of the anatomical and physiological improvement.

A more ambitious series by Lock's group involved balloon dilatation of congenital or operative narrowings of venous channels.[21] This was a heterogeneous group of patients who had complex congenital heart disease or previous reparative procedures. The venous channel most often dilated was the common pulmonary vein, but there were also examples of dilatation of the right and left lower pulmonary veins and the superior and inferior limbs of baffles created during Mustard procedures. Complications included tearing and hemorrhage of the vein, acute hemoptysis, and bradycardia. The majority of patients died within several months or had no demonstrable improvement. The most successful results were obtained in those patients who had undergone previous Mustard procedures and required dilatation of the baffle. In these 4 patients there was resolution of edema and hepatic congestion at 6 months. One patient required tricuspid valve replacement as a separate and unrelated procedure.

These studies have provided useful information on the effects of balloon dilatation on pulmonary vessels. Although not specifically related to dilatation of the valve or valve annulus, there may be pathologic correlates. The studies in humans are anecdotal and should be performed only in centers with special interest and experience. It appears that they are appropriate only for selected critically ill patients who are not surgical candidates. The likelihood of long-term clinical benefit is low.

TRICUSPID VALVULOPLASTY

Tricuspid stenosis is a rare form of valvular heart disease. In native valves the only known etiology is related to rheumatic fever. It is usually seen in combination with stenotic disease of the aortic or mitral valves.

A case of tricuspid catheter valvuloplasty was reported by Al-Zaibag, Ribeiro, and Al-Kasab in 1987 using a two-balloon technique.[22] Their patient was a 45-year-old man with a history of rheumatic fever who had right heart failure and a mean gradient of 6.3 mm Hg. The tricuspid valve area was calculated to be $0.9\ cm^2$. Immediately following the two-balloon procedure, the mean gradient was 2.1 mm Hg. The patient underwent repeat cardiac catheterization 5 months after the procedure and was found to have a mean gradient of 1.7 mm Hg, indicating a sustained beneficial effect.

Another case report by Feit and co-workers illustrated the feasibility of dilating a porcine bioprosthesis.[23] Their patient required valve replacement for endocarditis and received a No. 31 Hancock heterograft. After 10 years the patient developed right heart failure and on catheterization was found to have a tricuspid mean diastolic gradient of 22 mm Hg. The prevalvuloplasty valve area was calculated to be $0.69\ cm^2$. After a single 20-mm balloon was inflated across the valve, the gradient dropped to 15 mm Hg, corresponding to a valve area of $1.22\ cm^2$. At 1 month the patient had increased exercise tolerance and decreased peripheral edema.

These two cases illustrate the utility of catheter-balloon valvuloplasty for patients with tricuspid stenosis, as it pertains to both the native and bioprosthetic valves. It needs to be emphasized that at this point the experience is only anecdotal.

AORTIC VALVULOPLASTY
ETIOLOGY

The four major causes of aortic stenosis are (1) congenital aortic stenosis, which may include congenital commissural fusion alone or in association with unicuspid or bicuspid aortic valves; (2) postinflammatory (rheumatic) aortic stenosis; (3) senile calcific aortic stenosis; and (4) aortic stenosis after infective endocarditis. Many cases of severe congenital aortic stenosis are treated with balloon valvuloplasty by pediatric cardiologists, and there are a number of studies demonstrating the efficacy of this technique in the pediatric population.

The primary forms of aortic stenosis of interest to the adult cardiologist are senile calcific aortic stenosis, rheumatic aortic stenosis, and bicuspid aortic valve. When the valve is heavily calcified and deformed, it may be difficult to discern the number of aortic leaflets. It is important not to miss an unrecognized bicuspid calcific aortic valve because effects of valvuloplasty are less predictable. Complications including restenosis and regurgitation may be higher with calcified bicuspid valves. Consequently, aortic valve replacement is recommended if the patient is a surgical candidate. A rare form of aortic stenosis is a late result of infective endocarditis. To date, valvuloplasty has not been reported in such cases.

Isolated rheumatic aortic stenosis is also rarely seen in industrialized nations but is the major etiology in many underdeveloped countries. The inflammatory process initiates reaction at the free edges of the cusps, which may involve thrombotic deposits, and eventually leads to commissural fusion.[24,25] Fusion usually affects all three commissures equally but rarely involves only one commissure, giving rise to an acquired bicuspid valve. Because the primary pathological process at this stage of the disease is commissural fusion, balloon valvuloplasty may have significant beneficial acute and long-term effects. Calcification is commonly found in patients over 40 years of age and may limit the long-term effectiveness of the procedure. However, aortic balloon valvuloplasty becomes especially attractive when viewed in the context of limited health care resources, which in many cases, precludes the surgical option.

THE NATURAL HISTORY OF AORTIC STENOSIS

This topic is covered in detail elsewhere in these volumes. A number of classic studies demonstrate that once the symptoms of aortic stenosis become manifest, there is a predictable and well-understood progression of disease. The natural history of patients who are candidates for aortic balloon valvuloplasty was recently reviewed by O'Keefe and associates at the Mayo Clinic.[26] The actuarial survival at 1, 2, and 3 years was 57%, 37%, and 25%, respectively, compared to 93%, 85%, and 77%, for age- and sex-matched controls. Patients may develop secondary congestive heart failure, angina pectoris, or syncope with exertion. These symptoms suggest advanced disease and generally warrant further evaluation by noninvasive or invasive means.

In advanced calcific aortic stenosis, the pathology relates primarily to heavy calcification of the leaflets, which prevents opening by the available contractile force. In advanced cases, both the increasing stiffness of the valve and reduction of the valve-opening force contribute to the reduction of effective orifice area. This concept has its correlates in clinical practice and in the catheterization laboratory. It is often difficult to evaluate whether the primary problem is the stenotic valve, which may have a relatively small gradient, or the depressed ejection fraction and low cardiac output. A series of patients with critical stenosis and low cardiac output was reviewed by Wyman and associates at Beth Israel Hospital.[27] They found a marked improvement in radionuclide left ventricular ejection fraction at 4 months (39% immediately post-valvuloplasty and 58% at 4 months).

It is generally accepted that once a patient becomes symptomatic and moderate to severe aortic stenosis is documented, the patient should undergo aortic valve replacement. The matter of timing surgery requires an assessment of the severity of symptoms and surgical risk, including the age of the patient and concurrent medical problems. Many patients are surgical candidates for aortic valve replacement either alone or in combination with coronary artery bypass grafting. Generally it is advisable to perform cardiac catheterization to document the severity of the hemodynamic impairment, assess left ventricular function, and evaluate coronary artery disease. Coronary angiography is especially important in patients with angina pectoris. There are occasional patients in whom it may be possible to proceed directly to surgery based on the clinical history, physical examination, and data obtained by echo-Doppler techniques.

SURGICAL EXPERIENCE

Open and closed debridement valvulotomy is not a new technique among cardiothoracic surgeons. A number of studies in the early days of cardiovascular surgery considered this approach to aortic stenosis, but because of the generally poor long-term results and the concurrent development of acceptable replacement valves in the mid 1960s, the operation fell into rather profound disfavor. The three most recent, relatively large surgical series will be reviewed as they may provide a model for catheter balloon valvuloplasty.

In 1967, Barratt-Boyes and co-workers reported their experience at Green Lane Hospital, New Zealand, from 1959 through 1964.[28] They had 61 patients with isolated aortic stenosis, 31 of whom had bicuspid aortic valves. All patients had moderate to severe calcification on fluoroscopy and ranged in age from 19 to 71 years. They found that 13 of these original 61 patients died during the procedure or in the early postoperative period. Of the 48 who were discharged, 10 experienced late deaths, which were not well documented as to their etiology but were felt to be cardiovascular in nature. The remaining 38 patients were the subject of the long-term follow-up study. Their review showed that 29 of these 38 underwent recatheterization from 27 to 70 months after their debridement valvulotomy. The mean gradient in these patients was 74 mm Hg (12 mm Hg–155 mm Hg). One patient had severe aortic regurgitation. At the time of publication, 8 had undergone aortic valve replacement and the remaining 21 were symptomatic but had not undergone surgery, presumably because of stable clinical course or refusal. There were 9 patients of the original group of 38 who did not undergo recatheterization; 5 had undergone aortic valve replacement on clinical grounds and the remaining 4 refused further evaluation. Figure 85.4 outlines the clinical course of these patients. These results, although quite poor when compared to aortic valve replacement in terms of morbidity and mortality, do suggest that a majority of patients (38) survived more than 2 years following the procedure. In patients who may not be candidates for surgery and who may be markedly debilitated with their disease, these results may be viewed as encouraging.

In 1973, Hill reported the experience from Guys Hospital, London, from 1962 to 1965.[29] They likewise performed debridement valvulotomy for calcific aortic stenosis and had a 100% follow-up over 10 years. The mean age of their patient population was 50.2 years at the time of operation. In this series of 16 patients, 3 died during the procedure or in the early postoperative period. There were 4 late deaths, which occurred primarily due to cardiac failure, within several months of the procedure. Nine patients (56%) had a 7- to 10-year survival. Two patients required aortic valve replacement due to restenosis. One patient developed angina pectoris but was controlled medically. Six patients remained asymptomatic over the 7- to 10-year period. This led the authors to conclude that there was a 33% restenosis rate among patients who survived.

Another series by Rees and associates looked at the long-term follow-up of valvuloplasty in aortic stenosis at Cornell University Medical Center from 1956 through 1969.[30] In their series of 40 patients, 21 were felt to have congenital bicuspid aortic stenosis and 19 were rheumatic in origin. In this series, there were 5 early deaths, 10 late deaths with a mean period of palliation of 2.1 years, and a mean survival of 2.7 years. Over the next 5 years, 19 patients underwent reoperation. A variety of procedures were performed on these patients, including aortic valve replacement (15), aortic valve replacement and mitral valve replacement in combination (2), aortic valve replacement and mitral valvuloplasty in combination (1), and repeat valvuloplasty (1). In this subgroup of 19 patients, 6 experienced early death prior to discharge from the hospital, 7 experienced late death, and 6 remained asymptomatic at the end of their second procedure. Of the original group of 40 patients who had not experienced early or late mortality or reoperation, 6 patients remained asymptomatic from 3 to 10 years after the procedure.

All of these surgical studies of debridement valvulotomy are quite discouraging when compared to the morbidity, mortality, and long-term results of aortic valve replacement, especially in patients who are at low risk for anticoagulation and who can receive a mechanical prosthesis. The important point to make is that the majority of patients who undergo percutaneous aortic valvuloplasty should be considered high risk for surgery. In this group, the natural history of their disease puts these patients at substantial risk for short-term morbidity and mortality. Additionally, there are no studies of the risk of valve replacement in the very elderly patient (>85 years of age), but it is generally felt to be substantially higher than that of younger patients. Consequently, for selected groups of patients, percutaneous valvuloplasty may be the only therapeutic option.

HISTORY OF AORTIC BALLOON VALVULOPLASTY

The first clearly described aortic valvuloplasty using a balloon technique was performed in 1982 by Lababidi on an 8-year-old boy.[31] In a manner similar to that described previously for pulmonary valvuloplasty, a 14-mm balloon catheter was advanced across the stenotic valve and inflated. Progressively increasing pressures were used to a maximum of 120 psi for 5 seconds. The only complication was sinus bradycardia and transient hypotension. A dramatic drop (85 mm Hg to 28 mm Hg) in the systolic aortic valve gradient was noted. There was no evidence of aortic insufficiency after the procedure. Lababidi's group postulated at that time that the primary role of the procedure would be to allow younger children to grow to an age when surgical repair would be done at less risk. This initial success led them to perform the procedure in an additional group of 23 patients, which they reported in 1984.[32] These patients were 2 to 17 years of age and were all felt to have congenital aortic stenosis. The mean gradient fell from 113 mm Hg to 32 mm Hg, and peak systolic pressure decreased from 149 mm Hg to 121 mm Hg. Mild aortic regurgitation was noted in 10 patients. Over a 9-month follow-up period, 2 patients required open aortic commissurotomy using cardiopulmonary bypass, which provided an opportunity to observe valves that had undergone balloon valvuloplasty. In both instances, bicuspid valves were found. There were small tears measuring 1 mm to 4 mm near the ends of the aortic commissures. Six patients had repeat cardiac catheterizations, which showed very little increase in the peak systolic gradient (35 ± 25 mm Hg vs. 38 ± 32 mm Hg). The remaining patients were felt to be doing well clinically. The authors felt that the short-term results were encouraging but long-term benefits were speculative. Although they only had two opportunities to observe the effects of valvuloplasty, it was their impression that the mechanism of improvement in the stenotic valve was related to stretching of the valve leaflets and minor tearing of the aortic commissures.

Rickards and Somerville performed aortic valvuloplasty on a 10-year-old boy with severe aortic stenosis, pulmonary hypertension, and patent ductus arteriosus.[33] After the procedure, the patient improved dramatically with a decrease of the peak systolic gradient from 92 mm Hg to 10 mm Hg with trace aortic regurgitation noted on Doppler examination.

Attention was drawn to the utility of this technique in adult patients with acquired aortic stenosis by Cribier and co-workers in January, 1986.[34] They presented preliminary results in 3 patients with severe calcific aortic stenosis. These initial patients were offered valvuloplasty because they were not surgical candidates for various reasons. In each patient, the transvalvular gradient fell significantly and the aortic valve area, as calculated by the Gorlin formula, increased roughly by a factor of 2. There was no worsening of aortic regurgitation and no significant complications. Clinical follow-up showed sustained benefit at 3 to 5 months. Culling's group performed the procedure in a 65-year-old woman and found that over 2 weeks, her initial clinical improvement deteriorated.[35] A second valvuloplasty was performed using a larger balloon and a prolonged benefit was obtained. They were the first to employ a brachial approach and noted no local vascular complications.

McKay and colleagues studied the effect of balloon inflation on patients who were to undergo aortic valve replacement surgically and in a group of acute postmortem specimens.[36] They performed three evaluations: (1) postmortem valvuloplasty in which the baseline and post–balloon inflation specimens were grossly inspected; (2) intraoperative valvuloplasty in which the stenotic valve was dilated under direct vision while on cardiopulmonary bypass but before explantation; and (3) percutaneous valvuloplasty in 2 patients at the time of diagnostic catheterization. Both of these patients were elderly (93 and 86 years of age) and refused surgical intervention. Their results showed that in a total of 10 patients who had undergone postmortem and intraoperative valvuloplasty, the majority were felt to have senile calcific aortic stenosis. Of these 10, 7 had extensive nodular calcification of the valve leaflets. McKay's group observed no evidence of tearing of the valve cusps, liberation of calcific or other valvular debris, or disruption of the valve annulus. They felt that the cusps were less rigid after the procedure. Only in half of the patients studied was there commissural separation or leaflet fracture. Two patients who had percutaneous valvuloplasty experienced improved acute hemodynamics and clinical course. They found marked improvement in the left ventricular ejection fraction at 6 weeks in one patient but lack of successful palliation of angina in the second patient who also had severe coronary artery disease. Their observations have been challenged by Robicsek and Harbold, who performed valvuloplasties on 16 intraoperative patients. They found no significant increase in the aortic valve area.[37]

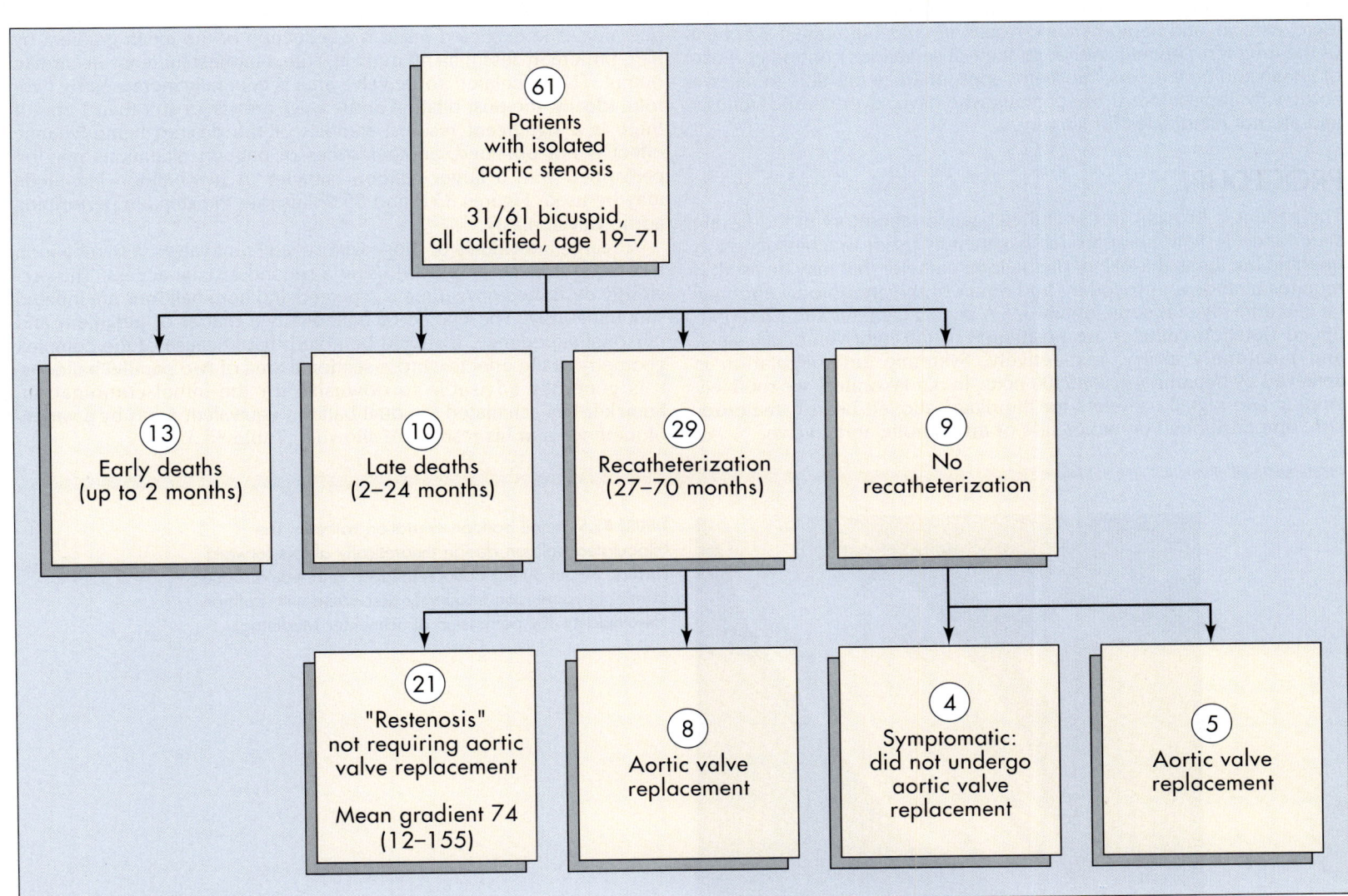

FIGURE 85.4 Debridement valvulotomy for aortic stenosis (Green Lane Hospital, New Zealand 1959–1964). This study by Barratt-Boyes and associates at Green Lane Hospital, New Zealand, shows their results with surgical debridement valvulotomy from 1959 to 1964. These results are poor compared to aortic valve replacement (AVR). Note that 21/61 (33%) had "restenosis" but did not require valve replacement up to 155 months (13 years) following the procedure. (Modified from Hurley PJ, Lowe JB, Barratt-Boyes BG: Debridement-valvuloplasty for aortic stenosis in adults: A follow-up of 76 patients. Thorax 22: 314, 1967)

Meier reported a successful aortic valvuloplasty in a 12-year-old boy using a trefoil balloon catheter.[38] It was postulated that the trilobulated balloon configuration would allow sufficient blood flow through the interstices of the three smaller balloons when fully inflated. As it is currently manufactured, it requires a 17-French sheath. The acute results using this design were essentially identical to those cases previously studied. The trefoil catheter is shown in Figure 85.5.

Walls, Lababidi, and others reported a series of pediatric patients who had undergone aortic valvuloplasty.[16] They experienced a drop in the systolic gradient from 125 mm Hg to 35 mm Hg while maintaining similar cardiac outputs. They provided follow-up data averaging 7 months after the procedure. In each case, sustained hemodynamic benefit was documented.

PATIENT SELECTION

Because the primary pathologic process of most adult patients with aortic stenosis in the United States is calcific and fibronodular in nature, balloon dilatation may be expected to provide little benefit over a long period of time. In a study of 16 patients undergoing aortic valve replacement, Robicsek and Harbold meticulously studied the geometric effects of balloon dilatation.[37] They found that the majority of patients (63%) had no apparent change in the orifice area after dilatation with two 15-mm balloons. Minimal improvements were seen in 25%, and only 12% had moderate improvements. They concede that the visual appearance of the orifice area may not correlate with the physiologic, clinical, and hemodynamic results *in vivo,* but remain skeptical of the long-term benefit. Although their observations contradict those of Safian and co-workers,[39] it seems appropriate at this time to reserve aortic valvuloplasty for those patients who have severe aortic stenosis and are not candidates for surgery.

PROCEDURE

The patient is brought to the catheterization laboratory in the fasting state, and the femoral approach is generally used. Brachial access is possible but limits the size of the balloon catheter that may be used. It requires a cutdown procedure and repair of the arteriotomy and may be less attractive for some operators. A pacing catheter and a balloon-tipped flotation catheter are positioned in the right ventricular apex and pulmonary artery, respectively. Systemic anticoagulation is achieved by heparin, usually 5000 units. In our laboratory we routinely employ two pigtail catheters for the diagnostic left heart catheterization, one positioned on either side of the stenotic aortic valve.

A guide wire technique is generally used across the valve. After the hemodynamic assessment is performed, a 0.038 heavy-duty exchange wire with a double bend is positioned in the left ventricle. The pigtail catheter is removed with the guide wire left in place. The diagnostic 7 or 8 arterial sheath is removed and the access site is enlarged using a 10-French dilator. If desired, a 12- or 14-French sheath is inserted over the guide wire. Some of the sheaths useful in valvuloplasty are shown in Figure 85.6. A previously prepared balloon valvuloplasty catheter is advanced over the guide wire and positioned across the aortic valve. The balloon catheter is initially inflated to approximately 4 to 5 atmospheres (50 psi–60 psi). It is not uncommon for the balloon catheter to rock back and forth or be expelled from the left ventricle. The balloon catheter is quite stiff due to its size, and it is possible to lacerate or perforate the left ventricle with the catheter or guide wire. This motion should be minimized by stabilizing the catheter as much as possible during balloon inflation.

It is frequently possible to observe a waist as the balloon is inflated and transaxial pressure is transmitted to the stenotic valve. Proper positioning of the balloon for aortic valvuloplasty is shown in Figure 85.7. Hypotension and arrhythmias are frequently noted as aortic outflow is completely obstructed. As a general rule, these resolve with balloon deflation. Occasional patients will experience syncope or near-syncope and shortness of breath.

The procedure is repeated until the balloon can be fully inflated across the valve without a noticeable waist. Measurement of the gradient is repeated as is the cardiac output to calculate aortic valve orifice area. The expected result is a reduction of the mean gradient by half, preferably less than 40 mm Hg, with a modest increase in cardiac output. The calculated aortic valve area is generally increased by twofold. Ideally, the post-dilation aortic valve area is greater than 1 cm^2. If there is a significant residual stenosis or the desired hemodynamic effect is not obtained, another series of balloon dilatations may be performed with a larger balloon catheter. A two-balloon technique may be used. Figures 85.8 and 85.9 illustrate the steps in performing aortic valvuloplasty.

In large individuals or those with recalcitrant valves, a two-balloon technique may be employed using a second arterial access. The previously described procedure is repeated and both balloons are inflated simultaneously. The choice of balloons is a matter of judgment and personal experience. It should be noted that because of the complex geometry of the effective cross-sectional area of two parallel balloons, it is generally advisable to downsize for the initial combination. Smucker has calculated the dual balloon equivalent areas by a variety of methods and his results are shown in Table 85.5.

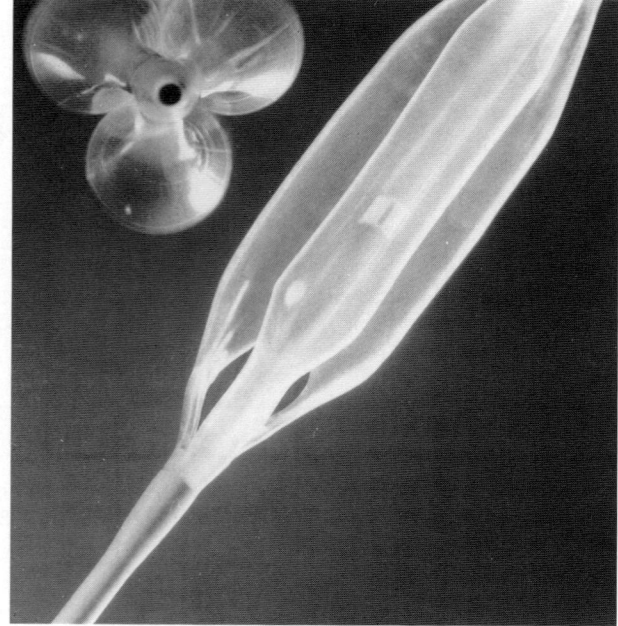

FIGURE 85.5 Trefoil balloon-dilatation catheter. The trilobulated balloon design theoretically allows forward cardiac output during balloon inflation and would reduce transient hypotension frequently associated with balloon valvuloplasty. (By permission of Schneider Medintag)

At the end of the procedure, all catheters and guide wires are removed and hemostasis is achieved by manual compression. In our laboratory, a sheath is not generally used for the balloon valvuloplasty *per se*, but may be used to occlude the arterial puncture site while the anticoagulant effect of heparin dissipates as the patient is being transported to the CCU. It is generally advisable to monitor patients closely for the first 24 to 48 hours after the procedure.

MECHANISM OF DILATATION

In contrast to the underlying disease process of congenital valve stenosis, advanced acquired aortic stenosis is characterized by calcific deposits. In a study of intraoperative and postmortem aortic valvuloplasty in elderly patients, Safian and associates found that valve orifice dimensions and leaflet mobility increased in all patients.[39] The mechanism of successful dilatation included fracture of calcified nodules, separation of fused commissures, and grossly inapparent microfractures. There was leaflet avulsion in 1 of 39 patients studied, which was related to an oversized balloon. There was no evidence of valve ring disruption, midleaflet tears, or liberation of calcific debris. Their findings seem to be consistent with the clinical experience. Their observations on improvements in orifice area and pliability are a matter of controversy.[37]

RESULTS OF AORTIC VALVULOPLASTY

Cribier has the largest single experience with aortic balloon angioplasty to date. His most recent review included 218 patients whose mean age was 73 years (range, 30–90 years). The majority (44%) of patients were between 71 and 80 years of age, with 25% being older than 80 years. Aortic valvuloplasty was performed because the patients were judged "high risk" for surgery (60%), refused to consider surgery

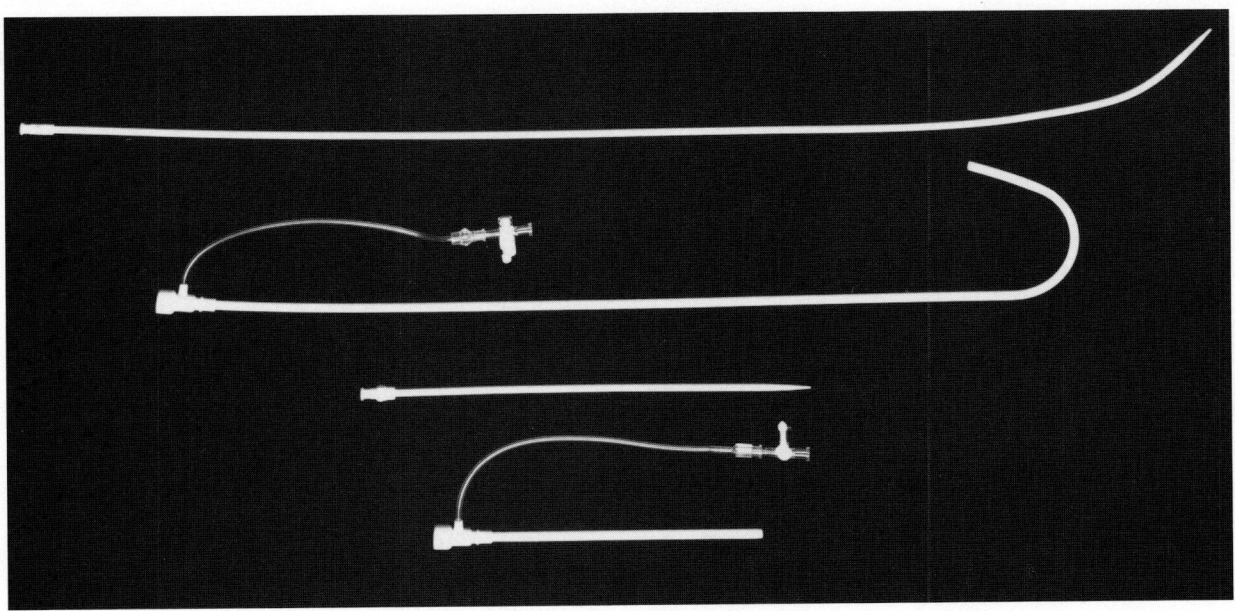

FIGURE 85.6 Sheaths used in performing valvuloplasty. From top to bottom, dilator used with Brockenbrough needle in performing atrial punctures in mitral valvuloplasty; a Mullins sheath; 10-French dilator used to dilate access site; 12-French sheath with backflow adaptor that may be used in the arterial or venous system. Similar sheaths are available in sizes ranging to 17 French.

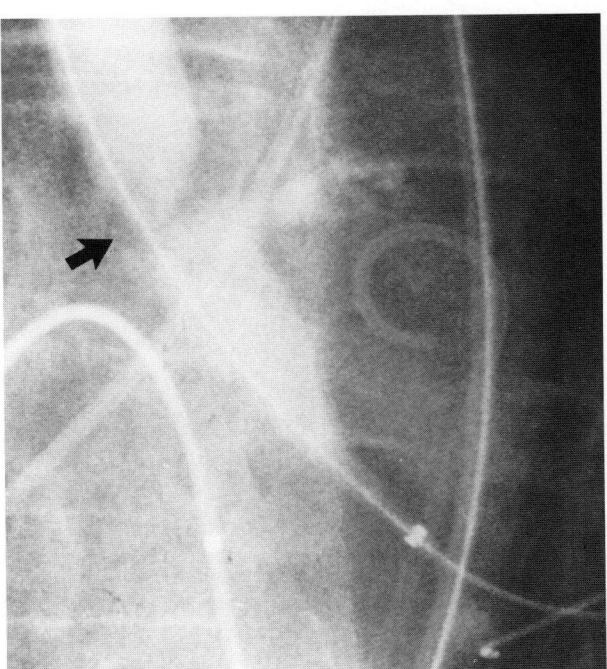

FIGURE 85.7 Waist observed during aortic balloon valvuloplasty. Magnified anteroposterior view of aortic balloon valvuloplasty demonstrating a waist as the balloon is inflated. Calcification can be seen in the aortic annulus. A pigtail catheter is seen in the descending aorta and a bipolar pacing catheter is positioned in the right ventricular apex.

(14%), or expressed a strong personal preference. Their technique employed an 18-mm balloon-dilatation catheter in most cases (67%). In 54 (25%) patients a larger balloon was required and in 16 (8%) a smaller one was used. After balloon dilatation, the mean gradient fell from 72 mm Hg to 29 mm Hg, with no significant change in cardiac output. The calculated aortic valve area increased from 0.5 cm^2 to 0.93 cm^2. The acute hemodynamic effects were somewhat less impressive in patients who were older than 80 years of age. Prior to valvuloplasty, 26% of all patients had New York Heart Association (NYHA) Class III or IV angina pectoris and 74% had Class III or IV congestive heart failure. Afterwards, the functional class improved to NYHA Class I or II for 85% of patients with angina and for 97% of patients with heart failure.

At 5-month follow-up, data were available on 148 (68%) patients. Of these, 24 (16%) were known to have died, 7 within the first month after the procedure. Their mean age was 77 years, and the post-dilatation aortic valve area averaged 0.7 cm^2. Recatheterization was per-

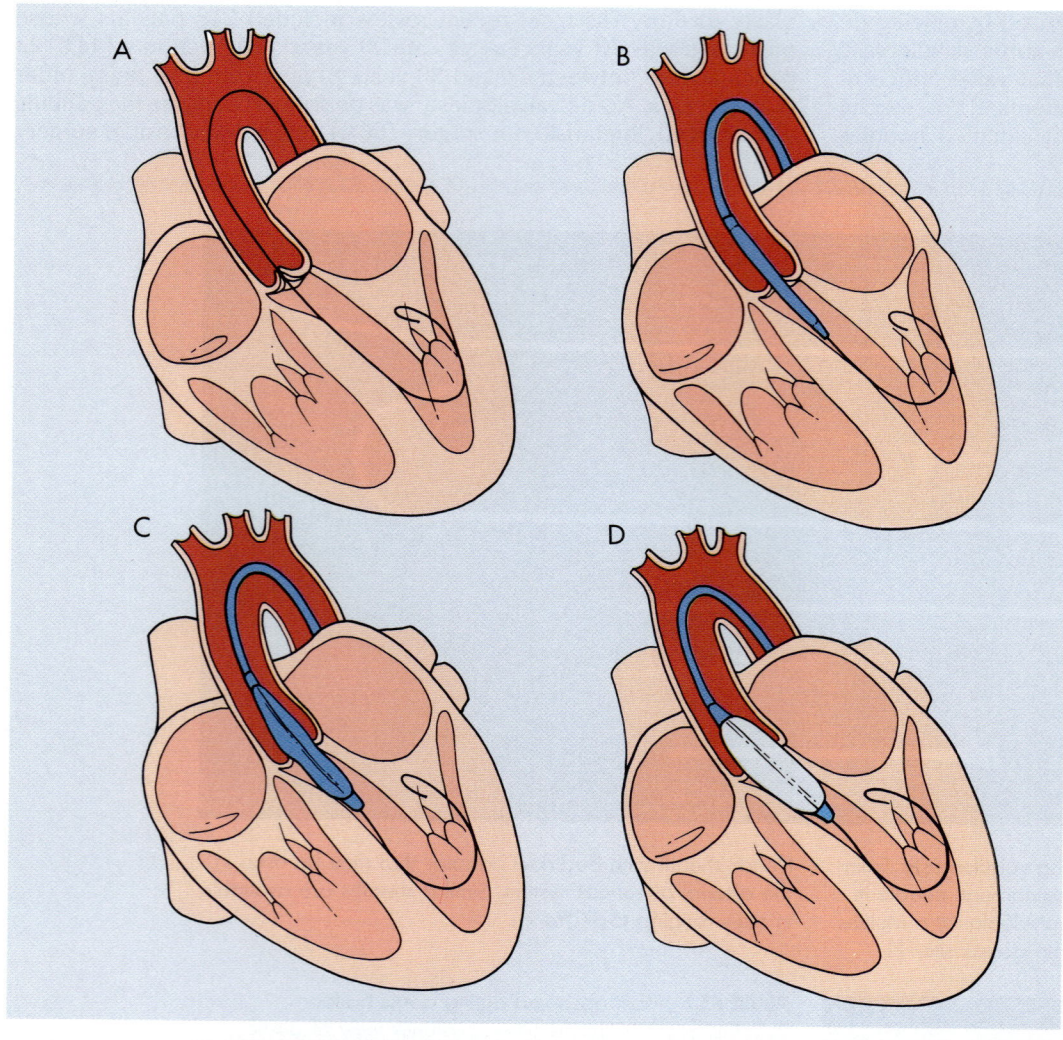

FIGURE 85.8 Technique of aortic valvuloplasty by the femoral approach. **A.** The double-bend guide wire across the stenotic aortic valve. **B.** The deflated balloon-dilatation catheter in position across the aortic valve. **C.** The balloon-dilatation catheter as it is filled with contrast. A noticeable "waist" is seen as the balloon is inflated across the stenotic aortic valve. **D.** The balloon-dilatation catheter when completely filled. The aortic orifice is dilated to the size of the balloon-dilatation catheter.

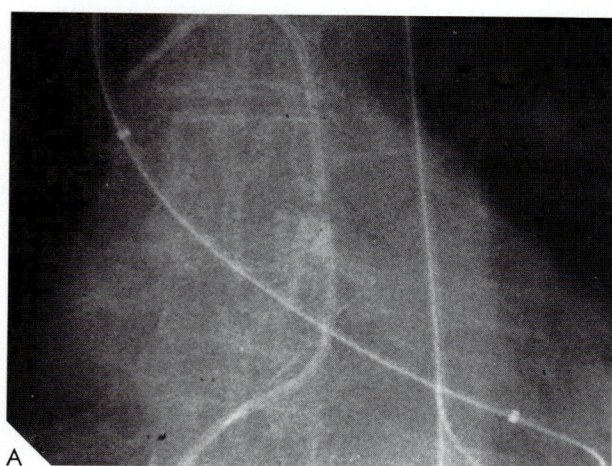
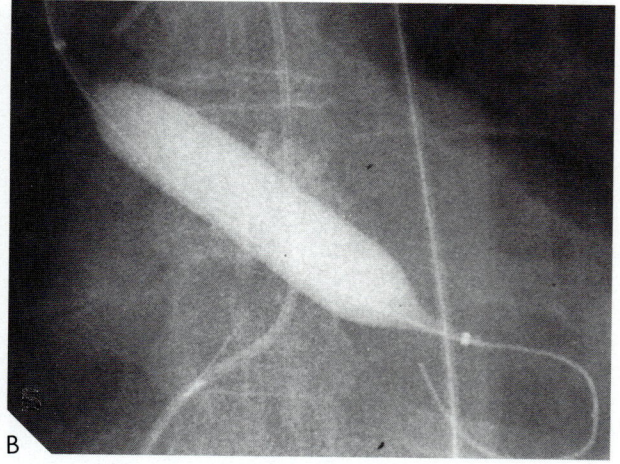

FIGURE 85.9 Anteroposterior cineradiographs of aortic valvuloplasty. **A.** The guide wire and balloon-dilatation catheter in place across a calcified and stenotic aortic valve. **B.** The balloon is inflated at 4 atmospheres (60 psi) of pressure. A pace-port Swan-Ganz catheter is shown in the pulmonary artery with the pacing wire in the right ventricular outflow tract.

formed on 45 patients. By defining restenosis as a 50% loss in the valve area initially gained by the procedure, they documented a 33% restenosis rate. Of the patients who were restudied, 50% had a reduction in the post-valvuloplasty valve area but not greater than the 50% used in their definitions. Only 17% had maintained the previously achieved hemodynamic result.

A number of centers are performing valvuloplasties in the United States. Most are relatively low volume; however, several have performed rather large studies. The Harvard experience (McKay and Block) is similar to that of Cribier. In 100 patients at the Beth Israel Hospital, McKay and associates were able to demonstrate significant improvement in the acute hemodynamic profile. Their patients averaged 76 years of age (35–93 years). Three quarters had symptoms of congestive heart failure. After valvuloplasty, the mean gradient decreased from 55 mm Hg to 30 mm Hg, with a concomitant increase in cardiac output from 4.6 liters to 4.9 liters/min. The calculated aortic valve area increased from 0.6 cm^2 to 1 cm^2. In their laboratory, they report a 97% primary success rate with a 30% restenosis rate by Doppler at 8-month follow-up. There were no deaths during the procedure, but 5 deaths occurred prior to discharge. An additional 16 patients died within the follow-up period.

The results at the Massachusetts General Hospital are somewhat less encouraging. In reviewing the data on 118 aortic valvuloplasties, the mean age of the patients was 79 years (52–93 years). The aortic valve area increased from 0.5 cm^2 to 0.9 cm^2. Follow-up data were available on 30 patients (25%), 10 (8%) of whom underwent repeat catheterization. All 10 had gradients and valve areas similar to those obtained prior to the initial balloon dilatation. Eight underwent repeat valvuloplasties. Of the 30, 13 (43%) died, and 1 had valve replacement surgery. Only 6 of the 30 (20%) had a sustained benefit. It is unclear why these patients did less well than those reported by other investigators. It could be related to the small number of patients on whom follow-up data were available, differences in technique (choice of balloon size, antegrade vs. retrograde approach), the criteria for repeat catheterization in the follow-up group, or other factors.

A study comparing the results of antegrade versus retrograde percutaneous balloon valvuloplasty was performed by Block and Palacios.[40] In a demographically similar series of patients, they documented similar hemodynamic results without any local vascular complications. The incidence of other complications was unchanged. Their study demonstrated the feasibility of the antegrade approach, which may be the only alternative in patients who also have severe peripheral vascular disease. The obvious drawback is the need for transseptal technique and the complications associated with it. In the future, it may be possible to improve the safety of atrial puncture by echocardiographic visualization of the Brockenbrough needle fitted with a transponder tip.[41] The results of these series and the University of California-San Francisco experience are shown in Table 85.6.

COMPLICATIONS

Although reported serious complications of aortic balloon valvuloplasty are relatively infrequent, a variety of acute and chronic complications have been observed. Estimated rates from pooled data are shown in Table 85.7.

The most common complication associated with aortic balloon valvuloplasty is local vascular events related to the size of the balloon-dilatation catheters used. These include laceration of the femoral artery, persistent bleeding and hematoma formation, blood transfusion, loss of distal pulse, and peripheral embolus. Although bleeding at the insertion site is generally controlled by applying local pressure, relatively long periods of compression may be required to achieve complete hemostasis. Protamine may be given to reverse the heparin effect if necessary. Frequent groin checks are imperative in the first 12 hours after the procedure.

Hemodynamic alterations during balloon placement and inflation are common, expected, and occasionally of major significance. Transient hypotension with syncope occurs relatively frequently (10% to 20%). It is surprising that more patients do not become severely hypotensive as the balloon is inflated across the stenotic valve and outflow is obstructed. Left ventricular perforation can occur as the guide wire and balloon catheter rock in and out of the ventricle during inflation. Cardiac tamponade may result from chamber perforation or, rarely, rupture of the aorta below the pericardial reflection.[42] As a general rule, aortic insufficiency is not a major problem post-valvuloplasty, especially if none was present before the procedure and left ventricular function was not severely depressed. In up to 5% of cases, however, patients will develop or experience worsened aortic insufficiency related to the procedure.

Embolic phenomena are another major complication of balloon valvuloplasty. Embolic cerebrovascular accident (CVA) occurs in up to 3% of patients and peripheral emboli are seen approximately 1% of the time. In an autopsy and intraoperative series reported by Safian and co-workers, there was no liberation of calcific debris.[39] It is unclear whether these emboli are caused by fragmentation of valvular material, atheroma within the central arterial circulation that are disturbed by catheter manipulations, or thrombi forming on the catheter and guide wires themselves. In a comprehensive evaluation of the risk of systemic embolization after balloon valvuloplasty, Davidson and associates found embolization to be an uncommon event even when vigorously sought with head computed tomography (CT), serial neurologic examinations, ocular fundoscopic examination, and myocardial enzymes.[43] In 24 patients studied, they had one subclinical event.

Arrhythmias are commonly seen during the procedure. Almost all patients will experience frequent ectopic beats and nonsustained runs of ventricular tachycardia. High-grade, malignant arrhythmias are less common, but occasionally cardioversion may be required. Bradyar-

TABLE 85.5 DUAL-BALLOON AREA EQUIVALENTS *

		\multicolumn{7}{c}{Balloon #1 Diameter (mm)}						
		10	12	15	18	20	23	25
	10	15.1	16.6	19	21.5	23.2	25.7	27.4
	12	16.6	18.1	20.4	22.8	24.5	27	28.6
Balloon #2	15	19	20.4	22.6	24.9	26.5	28.9	30.6
Diameter	18	21.5	22.8	24.9	27.1	28.7	31	32.6
(mm)	20	23.2	24.5	26.5	27.7	30.2	32.5	34
	23	25.7	27	28.9	31	32.5	34.7	36.2
	25	27.4	28.6	30.6	32.6	34	36.2	37.7

* Computed by M. L. Smucker, M.D. Used by permission.

TABLE 85.6 RESULTS OF STUDIES OF AORTIC VALVULOPLASTY

Study	Number of Patients	Mean Age (yr)	Age Range (yr)	Pre-Valvuloplasty					Balloon Size (mm)	Post-Valvuloplasty				
				Mean Gradient (mm Hg)	Cardiac Output (liters)	Aortic Valve Area (cm²)	Angina Class III–IV	Congestive Heart Failure Class III–IV		Mean Gradient (mm Hg)	Cardiac Output (liters)	Aortic Valve Area (cm²)	Angina Class III–IV	Congestive Heart Failure Class III–IV
French Registry	635	75		77	2.6	0.47		Mean EF 52%	<15 (12%) >15 (88%)	36	2.7	0.8		Mean EF 56%
Cribier (included in French Registry)	218	73	30–93	72	2.8	0.5	26%	74% Mean EF 49%	18 (67%) >18 (25%) <18 (08%)	29	2.8	0.93	4%	28% Mean EF 51%
Block (Massachusetts General Hospital)	118 25 A 30 R	79 79 79	52–93	59 A 63 R	3.6 A 3.5 R	0.5 0.5 A 0.4 R		100% A 96% R	15–20 15–20	29 A 35 R	3.6 A 3.5 R	0.9 0.8 A 0.7 R		
McKay (Beth Israel Hospital)	100	76	35–93	55	4.6	0.6		75%		30	4.9	1.0		
UCSF (very elderly)	23	92	85–100	68	3.9	0.47	25%	85%	20 (86%) >20 (14%)	29	4.3	0.94	10%	15%
Totals	876	79		66	3.6	0.51				32	3.8	0.91		

(Data presented at the Conference on New Directions in Interventional Cardiology, Santa Barbara, CA, October 23–25, 1987)

(EF, ejection fraction; A, antegrade; R, retrograde; UCSF, University of California Hospitals, San Francisco)

TABLE 85.7 ACUTE AND CHRONIC COMPLICATIONS ASSOCIATED WITH AORTIC BALLOON VALVULOPLASTY (POOLED DATA)

Complication	Estimated Rate
Arrhythmia	
Transient left bundle branch block	10%–20%
Advanced atrioventricular block	1%–2%
Embolic	
Cerebrovascular accident	1%–3%
Peripheral	<1%
Hemodynamic	
Syncope during procedure	10%–20%
Left ventricular perforations	2%
Cardiac tamponade	1%–3%
Worsened aortic insufficiency	1%–5%
Mortality	
During procedure	1%
Early (prior to discharge)	4%–7%
Late (after discharge, 8–12 mo)	16%–25%*
Restenosis	
(Defined as 50% reductions in post-valvuloplasty aortic valve area, 8–12 mo)	33%–50%*
Vascular	
Hematoma	10%–15%
Transfusion	25%

*Incomplete follow-up in most reported series

rhythmia may be seen after balloon inflation and may be unresponsive to atropine, suggesting mechanisms other than those mediated by the vagus nerve. The most commonly reported arrhythmic complications are transient left bundle branch block and advanced atrioventricular block. For these reasons, a temporary pacing catheter is recommended during the procedure and may be necessary in the recovery period (24–48 hours) if the abnormalities persist. To date, heart block requiring permanent pacing has not been reported following balloon valvuloplasty.

Mortality during the procedure is estimated to be 1%. A larger number of patients will die prior to discharge (4%–7%). The exact cause of death is not always clear but may be related to failed balloon valvuloplasty, low-output syndromes, or myocardial infarction. Rarely, other complications, such as CVA or hemorrhage, may contribute to the patients demise. Long-term mortality data are often incomplete, but mortality approaches 25% at one year.

The most significant chronic complication of aortic balloon valvuloplasty is restenosis. The best available "long-term" results are discussed in the previous section. Although the follow-up is incomplete in most series, the restenosis rate varies from 33% to 100%, depending on the definition. Realistically, restenosis is likely to occur in patients with calcific aortic stenosis as pliability diminishes following the procedure. Long-term follow-up data on a large series of patients are required before any definitive statement can be made.

SIMULTANEOUS PROCEDURES

Percutaneous transluminal coronary angioplasty (PTCA) may be performed either before or after dilatation of the aortic valve. In performing the PTCA first, one may protect against ischemia caused by the hypotension frequently observed during valvuloplasty. This may also permit the use of the same arterial sheath. In this case, the PTCA is performed first and afterward the sheath is removed and the site is dilated to accommodate the valvuloplasty balloon catheter. After dilation of the valve, the catheter is removed and a smaller sheath (typically 10–12 French) is inserted to aid in hemostasis during the recovery period.[44] Some investigators have done the procedure in reverse, with the intent of addressing the primary (*i.e.*, aortic stenosis) pathophysiologic problem first. There have been relatively few simultaneous procedures, but there does not appear to be a significant increase in morbidity and mortality.

There have been a few cases of combined aortic and mitral valvuloplasty in patients with advanced multivalvular heart disease.[45] Because of the need for a transseptal approach to the mitral valve in most centers, an antegrade approach to the aortic valve is possible when a combined procedure is planned. In the few cases to date, there does not appear to be extraordinary risk.

MITRAL VALVULOPLASTY
HISTORY

The mitral valve is anatomically the most inaccessible valve of the heart. It is interesting therefore that percutaneous balloon valvuloplasty for severe mitral stenosis was performed in adults more than two years before the technique was applied to the relatively more accessible aortic valve. Transvenous mitral commissurotomy by a balloon catheter was first performed by Inoue and associates in 1984.[45] Their approach was to use a transseptal technique to introduce a guide wire into the left atrium and then into the left ventricle. A "pillow-shaped" balloon catheter made of nylon micromesh was then positioned across the mitral valve. In their series of 6 patients, ranging in age from 32 to 62 years of age, successful mitral valvuloplasty was performed in 5 patients with significant hemodynamic improvement. The average mitral valve gradient was reduced from 14.0 mm Hg to 6.4 mm Hg. A single-balloon technique was employed with balloons ranging in size from 22 mm to 26 mm. All 5 patients demonstrated sustained clinical improvement from 2 to 16 months after the procedure. The hemodynamic improvements were associated with increased excursion of the mitral valve leaflets on two-dimensional echocardiography.

A second study by Lock and co-workers looked at the value of performing percutaneous catheter commissurotomy in 8 young children and adults with rheumatic mitral stenosis.[46] A similar technique was performed using a standard 25-mm valvuloplasty catheter. There was an immediate decrease in the gradient across the stenotic valve with a concomitant increase in cardiac output. The mitral valve area was approximately doubled. Minimal mitral regurgitation was observed in only 1 of 8 patients. These early results suggested that this was an effective and safe treatment modality for patients with rheumatic mitral stenosis.

A different technique was employed by Babic's group in treating a 60-year-old patient with severe mitral stenosis and refractory congestive heart failure.[47,48] They used a "Kurry intravascular retriever catheter" with a snare guide wire in an effort to avoid creation of the relatively large atrial septal defect necessary for the advancement of the balloon-dilatation catheter. A two-wire technique was used such that a wire with an end loop was advanced through the Brockenbrough needle into the left atrium. In the left ventricle it was snared with the J guide wire and retrieved through the femoral artery. The balloon-dilatation catheter could then be advanced in a retrograde fashion across the aortic and mitral valves by placing traction on the transvenous wire. Their initial case report was followed by two additional patients who had undergone mitral valvuloplasty using the same technique. In these patients the mitral valve gradient was reduced from 17 mm Hg to 8.6 mm Hg. The authors felt that the advantages of this approach were the technical ease of the procedure, that both ends of the guide wire were under manual control and allowed better fixation of the balloon catheter across the valve, and that larger balloon catheters could be used. They postulated balloon rupture and embolization would be less likely and that there would be less danger of creating a large iatrogenic atrial septal defect.

Kveselis and associates reported three cases in children and adolescents who were felt to have congenital and rheumatic mitral stenosis.[49] Their hemodynamic findings were typical of severe mitral stenosis. After valvuloplasty the patients had marked reduction in the transmitral gradient. Kveselis' group characterized the effects of valvuloplasty by two-dimensional echo and Doppler studies. They found an increase in the pressure half-time and a modest improvement in mitral valve orifice area. In 1 of the 3 patients they were unsuccessful in advancing the balloon catheter, and 2 months later the patient was noted to have a left atrial thrombus. It was uncertain as to whether the thrombus was related to the procedure, low-output state, polycythemia, or a combination of factors.

Al-Zaibag and associates published the first case report using a two-balloon technique.[50] Two balloons were required in 7 of 9 patients with severe mitral stenosis in order to achieve satisfactory hemodynamic results. In their study, the mitral valve area increased from 0.7 cm^2 to 1.4 cm^2. The initial findings were confirmed 6 weeks after the procedure by repeat catheterization and by echocardiographic measurement of the mitral valve. They published a follow-up series of 9 patients in whom double-balloon procedures had been performed. In 7 of 9 patients with severe mitral stenosis, the transmitral end-diastolic gradient fell significantly. The cardiac output was not affected. The net result was dramatic improvement in the calculated mitral valve area. The beneficial effects were sustained over 6 weeks when the patients were restudied. Al-Zaibag's group felt that their first two patients developed restenosis because of the small balloons used (12 mm). Consequently, they planned to use larger balloons in future cases. It was their feeling that commissural splitting was the mechanism of dilatation based on two other cases performed under direct vision.

A case report by McKay and associates illustrates the utility of this technique in an elderly patient with calcific rheumatic mitral stenosis.[51] They reported two complications of the procedure: mitral regurgitation and shunt. Specifically, after single-balloon mitral valvuloplasty, they noted an increase in the mitral regurgitation from 1+ to 2+. They also

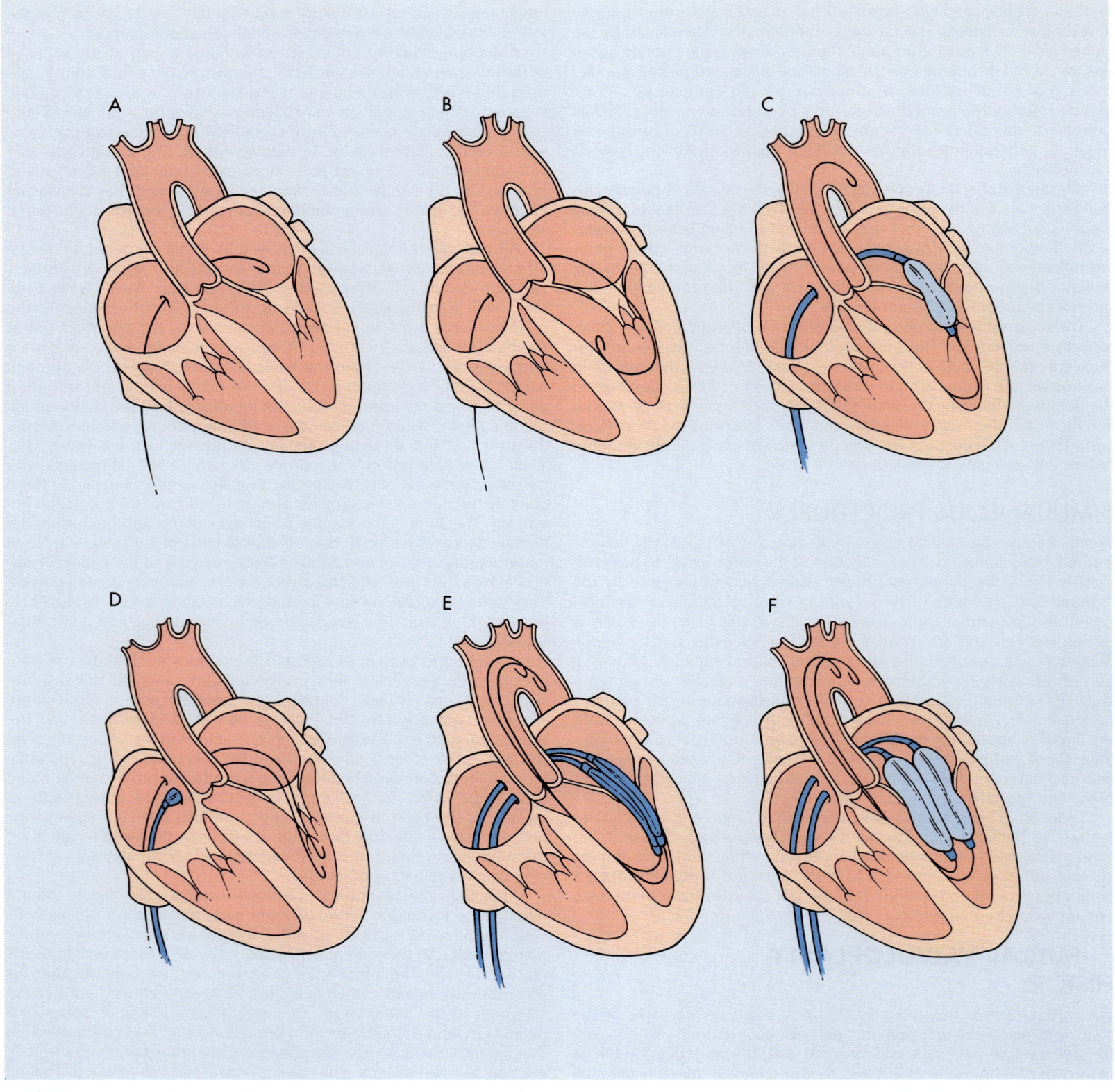

FIGURE 85.10 Technique of double-balloon mitral valvuloplasty. **A.** The position of the guide wire in the left atrium after left atrial puncture using the Brockenbrough needle. **B.** The position of the guide wire as it is advanced into the left ventricle across the stenotic mitral valve. **C.** Partial inflation of a single-balloon catheter across the stenotic mitral valve when a single-balloon valvuloplasty is to be performed. Notice that the guide wire may be advanced into the aorta in an antegrade fashion to provide greater stabilization. **D.** Dilatation of the atrial septum using an Olbert catheter in anticipation of performing a two-balloon mitral valvuloplasty. **E.** The two valvuloplasty catheters across the stenotic mitral valve. **F.** The appearance of the two simultaneously inflated balloons as the two-balloon valvuloplasty is being performed.

found a pulmonary-to-systemic shunt of 1.8 after the procedure. Another difficulty of atrial septal defect associated with mitral stenosis is that it can interfere with the hemodynamic assessment of the mitral stenosis, making the post-valvuloplasty determinations difficult to interpret.

PROCEDURE

Right heart catheterization is usually performed and a temporary pacing wire is positioned in the right ventricular apex. Simultaneous pulmonary capillary wedge and left ventricular pressures are recorded and calculation of the mitral valve area is performed using Fick or thermodilution cardiac outputs. In anticipation of performing the left atrial puncture using the Brockenbrough needle, a pulmonary angiogram with levophase visualization of the left atrium is often helpful. Additionally, a pigtail catheter may be positioned in one of the sinuses of Valsalva to make the anatomical relationship of these structures as clear as possible. Some of the aspects of the procedure are illustrated in Figures 85.10 and 85.11.

In the standard technique, a transseptal sheath is preloaded with a Brockenbrough needle and introducer. The assembled system is advanced under fluoroscopic control and positioned below the limbus of the atrial septum. Proper positioning of the Brockenbrough needle should be confirmed by anteroposterior and lateral fluoroscopy. If proper position is confirmed, the atrial septum is punctured and a saturation specimen is obtained. If the oxygen saturation is identical to the arterial specimen and a left atrial pressure waveform is obtained, the dilator and sheath are advanced into the left atrium. Once this has been accomplished, the needle and dilator may be removed and a balloon-tipped Berman-type catheter can be advanced into the left atrium and manipulated across the mitral valve and into the left ventricle. Systemic anticoagulation is then achieved by heparin. Some authors advocate anticoagulation with warfarin for at least 3 weeks prior to the procedure to reduce the risk of atrial or ventricular thrombus or embolization. If atrial thrombus is detected, the procedure is contraindicated. A specially prepared 0.038 J-tipped double-curved guide wire is then advanced into the left ventricle through the balloon-tipped catheter. The Berman catheter is carefully withdrawn while the guide wire is left in place.

It is necessary to dilate the intra-atrial septum to allow the passage of the valvuloplasty catheter(s). This can be performed with an Olbert dilatation catheter or a standard peripheral angioplasty catheter. Typically, we dilate to #15 French (8 mm). The septal-dilatation catheter is removed and the balloon-dilatation catheter is advanced over the guide wire and manipulated across the mitral valve. Because of the possibility of balloon rupture, it is prudent to purge the balloon with carbon dioxide prior to flushing and filling with dilute (3:1 or 4:1) contrast. If a single-balloon mitral valvuloplasty is to be performed, the balloon is inflated under fluoroscopic control until completely filled. It is not uncommon to observe a waist as the balloon is being inflated.

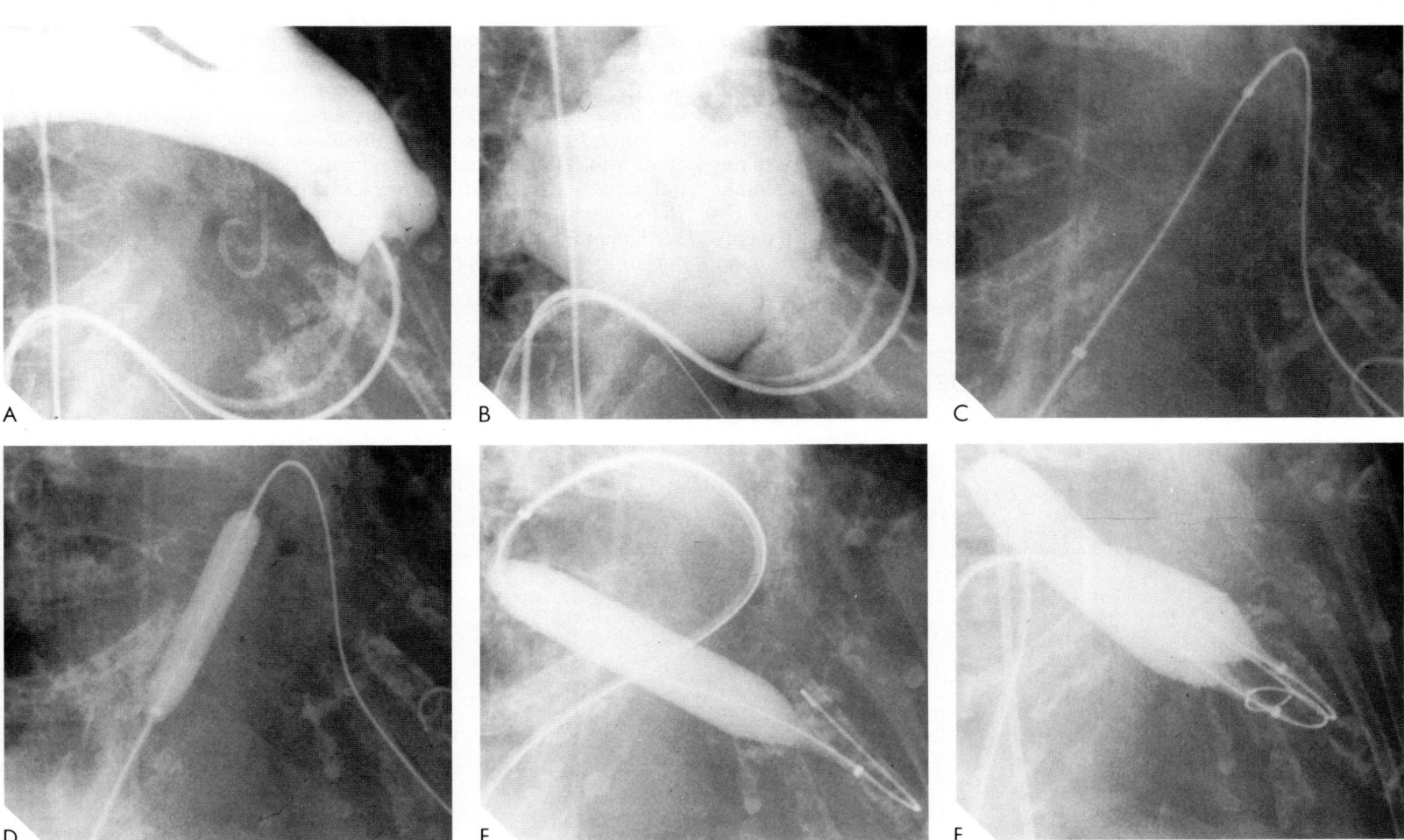

FIGURE 85.11 Anteroposterior cineradiographs of mitral valvuloplasty. **A.** A pulmonary angiogram, which may be performed at the beginning of the procedure to make clear the relationship of the left atrium and aortic root. Note the location of the pigtail catheter in the non-coronary cusp. **B.** Levophase left atrial filling and ventriculogram. **C.** The guide wire across the atrial septum with an Olbert catheter in place. Note the end markers of the balloon catheter. **D.** The atrial septum is dilated as the Olbert catheter is inflated. The end of the double J guide wire is in the left ventricle. **E.** A single-balloon mitral valvuloplasty as the balloon-dilatation catheter is fully inflated. **F.** A double-balloon mitral valvuloplasty is shown with two balloon-dilatation catheters being simultaneously inflated across the stenotic mitral valve.

Repeat hemodynamics can be performed using the tip of the balloon-dilatation catheter if desired.

In cases where a two-balloon technique is to be employed, the entire procedure using the Brockenbrough needle, dilator, sheath, and the Olbert catheter is repeated utilizing a second atrial septal site. Alternatively, some have employed a two-lumen angiographic catheter to advance a second guide wire through the original atrial septal puncture. Conceivably this could make it more difficult to manipulate the catheter across the mitral valve and may tear the septum but would lower the risk associated with a second atrial puncture. In a two-balloon technique, it is important to align the balloon catheters and to inflate them as simultaneously as possible.

It is not uncommon during balloon inflations to experience hypotension and ventricular ectopy. Generally these problems resolve as the balloon is deflated. After the procedure, repeat hemodynamic measurements are made and a left ventriculogram is performed to assess mitral insufficiency. One should check right-sided saturation data at the end of the procedure to evaluate the significance of the left-to-right shunt. As a general rule we do not use sheaths for the balloon-dilatation catheters and hemostasis must be achieved by manual compression once the catheters are removed. Being venous punctures, there is less risk of local vascular complications than in retrograde aortic balloon valvuloplasty, but frequent groin checks and CCU monitoring for the first 24 hours are recommended.

MECHANISM OF DILATATION

Because of the preponderance of rheumatic heart disease among patients with severe mitral stenosis, the underlying pathology is thought to be that of thickening and fusion of the commissures. Consequently, the dilatation procedure is envisioned to split the fused commissures and permit the leaflets to open more completely during diastole. Because of the low transvalvular pressure gradient even in severe mitral stenosis and the lack of significant contractile force of the left atrium, adequate dilatation is imperative. Reid and co-workers recently reported their echocardiographic and Doppler findings in 12 patients who had undergone double-balloon mitral valvuloplasty.[52] They found that gains in the diastolic mitral valve area occurred along the commissures and were related to a widening of the bicommissural angles. The procedure was less effective when the mitral valve was heavily calcified and when the leaflets were rigid. Although mitral regurgitation developed or worsened after balloon dilatation in as many as a third of patients, it was usually not clinically significant. There was a poor correlation between the Doppler estimate of the mitral valve area and that obtained at cardiac catheterization after balloon valvuloplasty. They postulated that this may be due to undetected shunts or inherent problems with the Doppler pressure half-time method. The long-term results will have to be compared with the established surgical approaches to rheumatic mitral stenosis, open and closed commissurotomy. It is hoped that the balloon dilatation procedure will compare favorably with the long-term excellent results of surgery.

RESULTS OF MITRAL VALVULOPLASTY

The acute effects of mitral valvuloplasty are well documented. From the available hemodynamic and clinical data, it appears that the gradient may be reduced by half and the calculated mitral valve area doubled. A summary of the studies published to date is found in Table 85.8.

The largest database on mitral valvuloplasty is the French Registry. Their preliminary data was recently reviewed.[53] As of September, 1987, 156 patients were enrolled and 133 were successfully dilated, yielding a primary success rate of 85%. Unlike most patients undergoing aortic valvuloplasty, the majority of patients (113, 85%) undergoing mitral valvuloplasty were considered good surgical candidates. The mean age was 40 years (13–70 years) and the vast majority of patients (120, 90%) were symptomatic with heart failure. Chronic atrial fibrillation was present in 43 (32%). Previous surgical commissurotomy had been performed in 38 (29%). The physicians participating in the registry employed a double-balloon technique in 108 (81%) patients and a trefoil balloon in 25 (19%). They found that the mean gradient fell from 16 mm Hg to 6 mm Hg and that the cardiac index rose from 2.7 liters to 2.9 liters/min/m². The calculated mitral valve area increased from 1 cm² to 2 cm². Only 18 (13.5%) had a post-procedure mitral valve area

TABLE 85.8 RESULTS OF STUDIES OF MITRAL VALVULOPLASTY

Study	Number of Patients	Mean Age (yr)	Age Range (yr)	Pre-Valvuloplasty MV Gradient (mm Hg)	Pre-Valvuloplasty MV Flow (liters)	Pre-Valvuloplasty MV Area (cm²)	Balloon Diameter (mm)	Post-Valvuloplasty MV Gradient (mm Hg)	Post-Valvuloplasty MV Flow (liters)	Post-Valvuloplasty MV Area (cm²)	Notes
Inoue et al.[45]	6		30–62	14	NR	NR	1 each—22.5, 23, 23, 24, 26	6	NR	NR	"Pillow-shaped" balloon
Lock et al.[46]	8	15	9–23	21	3.8 (I)	0.7	1–18; 2–20; 5–25	10.1	4.9 (I)	1.3	
Al-Zaibag et al.[50]	9	25	16–23	13	2.6 (I)	0.7	2–12 ×2; 7–15 ×2	1.9	3.0 (I)	2.0	Double balloon
McKay et al.[55]	12	43	25–70	16	4.4 (O)	1.0	2–15 ×2; 7–15, 18; 3–18 ×2	5	5.5 (O)	2.4	Double balloon
Palacios et al.[54]	35	49	13–87	18	3.9 (O)	0.8	1–15; 2–20; 17–25; 4–15 ×2; 2–18 ×2; 2–15, 18; 6–15, 18	7	4.6 (O)	1.7	Double balloon
McKay et al.[57]	18	49	23–75	15	4.3 (O)	0.9	25 or 18 ×2	9	5.1 (O)	1.6	Double balloon
Totals	88	36 + 15		16.5		0.83		4.5		1.8	

(MV = mitral valve; NR = not reported; (I) = cardiac index; (O) = cardiac output)

of less than 1.5 cm². Their most common complication was syncope or presyncope (see Table 85.9 for details).

Palacios and associates recently reported their experience with 35 patients who underwent mitral balloon valvuloplasty.[54] Their patients were primarily female (83%) and had a mean age of 49 years (13–87 years). They found that there was a significant decrease in the mitral gradient (18 mm Hg to 7 mm Hg) and a significant increase in the cardiac output (3.9 liters to 4.6 liters/min) and mitral valve area (0.8 cm² to 1.7 cm²) after balloon dilatation. They used a variety of balloons ranging from 15 mm to 25 mm in diameter. Some patients (40%) underwent a double-balloon procedure. They found that improvements in the mitral valve area correlated best with the balloon size index (effective balloon-dilating diameter per square meter of body surface area). Improvement did not correlate with the degree of mitral regurgitation, age, prior mitral commissurotomy, or degree of mitral calcification. They did not report follow-up data, but felt that the encouraging short-term results were likely to persist based on correlates to surgical commissurotomy.

McKay, Kawanishi, and Rahimtoola reported a series of 12 patients who had undergone double-balloon mitral valvuloplasty.[55] They found that the mitral valve gradient decreased in all patients (16 mm Hg to 5 mm Hg). The cardiac output increased from 4.4 liters to 5.5 liters/min with a concomitant increase in the mitral valve area (1.0 cm² to 2.4 cm²). They documented small left-to-right shunts related to the transseptal approach but did not observe increased mitral regurgitation. In 11 of 12 patients the functional class improved prior to discharge. They did not present follow-up data in their initial report, but recently restudied 16 patients who underwent double-balloon mitral valvuloplasty. They found that at 3 months there were persistent improvements in the mitral valve area, rest and exercise hemodynamics, and exercise performance.[56]

McKay and associates reported their study of 18 patients who had undergone mitral balloon valvuloplasty and 5 postmortem valvuloplasties.[57] They found the expected decrease in transmitral gradient (15 mm Hg to 9 mm Hg), pulmonary artery pressure, and pulmonary artery wedge pressure. There was an increase in cardiac output (4.3 liters to 5.1 liters/min) and mitral valve area (0.9 cm² to 1.6 cm²). They also demonstrated an increase in the left ventricular peak filling rate by serial radionuclide ventriculography. Echocardiographically, they also observed improvement in the mitral valve excursion, mitral E to F slope, and left atrial diameter. All patients improved clinically prior to discharge. They concluded that there was acute and significant improvement in valvular function after valvuloplasty and that successful dilatation was characterized by commissural separation and fracture of nodular calcium.

All of these studies corroborate the general clinical observations that the stenotic embarrassment of the mitral valve is lessened by the balloon-dilatation procedure. It follows from the surgical experience with open and closed commissurotomy that the acute results should persist for several years. There is relatively little long-term follow-up data available in the literature. Although the initial results are encouraging, and there is reason to be optimistic, the final assessment of this modality must remain for the future.

COMPLICATIONS

The potential complications of performing mitral valvuloplasty relate primarily to those associated with performing the left atrial puncture and manipulating a large catheter across the mitral valve. The most common complication of mitral valvuloplasty using a transseptal technique is residual intra-atrial shunt, which may be detected in as many as a third of patients. Transient arrhythmias, including left bundle branch block, nonsustained ventricular tachycardia, and atrial fibrillation, are also seen in approximately as many cases. Vasovagal episodes, left atrial perforation, cardiac tamponade, cerebrovascular accidents, mitral annulus rupture, and severe mitral regurgitation have all been reported. Mitral valvuloplasty does not cause significant mitral regurgitation in most cases. However, if mitral regurgitation is present prior to the balloon valvuloplasty, worsening of the mitral regurgitation

TABLE 85.9 COMPLICATIONS OF MITRAL VALVULOPLASTY AND THEIR ESTIMATED RATES

	French Registry	Block (Massachusetts General Hospital, Boston)	McKay (Beth Israel Hospital, Boston)	Al-Zaibag (Saudi Arabia)	McKay (USC, Los Angeles)
Number of patients	133	80	61	60	40
Arrhythmia					
Advanced atrioventricular block		1%			
Vagal		1%			2%
Embolic—CVA	1%	3%	3%		0%
Hemodynamic					
Syncope or presyncope	16%				
Hemopericardium/pericardial tamponade	8%	2%	2%	3%	0
Worsened mitral regurgitation	"Occasional"	50%			33%
Intra-atrial shunt (Qp/Qs >1:1.5)	10%	8%	21%	0* (two-puncture technique)	10%
Mortality					
During procedure		2%	2%		2%
Early		1%	2%		
Vascular	0				0

(From personal communication and data presented at the Conference on New Directions in Interventional Cardiology, Santa Barbara, CA, October 23–25, 1987)

* Follow-up at 1 yr by catheterization in 30 (50%) patients

is frequently observed. Patients with greater than 2+ mitral regurgitation are not good candidates for valvuloplasty. The complications of mitral valvuloplasty and their estimated rates from pooled data are shown in Table 85.9.

REMAINING QUESTIONS

Percutaneous balloon valvuloplasty of the mitral valve appears to be a useful technique in relieving the hemodynamic problems associated with severe mitral stenosis. It holds more promise for long-term benefit than aortic valvuloplasty in adults because the primary pathologic process associated with rheumatic mitral stenosis is commissural fusion. Clearly, balloon valvuloplasty can rupture leaflet adhesions and occasionally tear the valvular tissue. If the leaflets are supple enough to remain mobile and competent, the procedure will have appeal, especially in underdeveloped nations where access to cardiothoracic surgery is limited.

Questions that will have to be answered with increasing experience are the restenosis rate and factors that may influence it, the progression and significance of mitral regurgitation, and the likelihood of various potential complications. Issues relating to patient selection will necessarily follow and the final role of mitral balloon valvuloplasty will become clear. It is highly likely that equipment advances will make the procedure more technically appealing in the future, and concerns relating to operator training, experience, and certification will have to be addressed.

REFERENCES

1. Nadas AS, Flyer DC: Pediatric Cardiology. Philadelphia, WB Saunders, 1978
2. Semb BKH, Tjonneland S, Stake G, Aabyholm G: Balloon valvuloplasty of congenital pulmonary valve stenosis with tricuspid valve insufficiency. Cardiovasc Radiology 2:239, 1979
3. Kan JS, White RI, Mitchell SE, Gardner TJ: Percutaneous balloon valvuloplasty: A new method for treating congenital pulmonary-valve stenosis. N Engl J Med 307(9):540, 1982
4. Pepine CJ, Gessner IH, Feldman RL: Percutaneous balloon valvuloplasty for pulmonic valve stenosis in the adult. Am J Cardiol 50:1442, 1982
5. Lababidi Z, Wu JR: Percutaneous balloon pulmonary valvuloplasty. Am J Cardiol 52:560, 1983
6. Kan JS, White RI, Mitchell SE et al: Percutaneous transluminal balloon valvuloplasty for pulmonary valve stenosis. Circulation 69(3):554, 1984
7. Rocchini AP, Kveselis DA, Crowley D et al: Percutaneous balloon valvuloplasty for treatment of congenital pulmonary valvular stenosis in children. J Am Coll Cardiol 3(4):1005, 1984
8. Shuck JW, McCormick DJ, Cohen IS et al: Percutaneous balloon valvuloplasty of the pulmonary valve: Role of right to left shunting through a patent foramen ovale. J Am Coll Cardiol 4(1):132, 1984
9. Ben-Shachar G, Cohen MH, Sivakoff MC et al: Development of infundibular obstruction after percutaneous pulmonary balloon valvuloplasty. J Am Coll Cardiol 5:754, 1985
10. Tynan M, Jones O, Joseph MC et al: Relief of pulmonary valve stenosis in first week of life by percutaneous balloon valvuloplasty. Lancet: 273, 1984
11. Khalilullah M, Bahl VK, Choudary A et al: Pulmonary balloon valvuloplasty for the non-surgical management of valvular pulmonary stenosis. Indian Heart J 37:150, 1985
12. Kveselis DA, Rocchini AP, Snider R et al: Results of balloon valvuloplasty in the treatment of congenital valvar pulmonary stenosis in children. Am J Cardiol 56:527, 1985
13. Rao PS: Influence of balloon size on short term and long term results of balloon pulmonary valvuloplasty. Texas Heart Institute Journal 14:57, 1987
14. Ali-Khan MA, Al-Yousef S, Mullins CE: Percutaneous transluminal balloon pulmonary valvuloplasty for the relief of pulmonary valve stenosis with special reference to double-balloon technique. Am Heart J 112(1):158, 1986
15. Yeager SB, Neal WA, Balian AA, Gustafson RA: Percutaneous balloon pulmonary valvuloplasty. W Va Med J 82:169, 1986
16. Miller G: Balloon valvuloplasty and angioplasty in congenital heart disease. Br Heart J 53:520, 1985
17. Attia I, Weinhaus L, Walls J, Lababidi Z: Rupture of tricuspid valve papillary muscle during balloon pulmonary valvuloplasty. Am Heart J 114:(5):1233, 1987
18. Walls JT, Lababidi Z, Curtis J, Silver D: Assessment of percutaneous balloon pulmonary and aortic valvuloplasty. J Thorac Cardiovasc Surg 88:352, 1984
19. Stanger P, University of California-San Francisco Hospital, Department of Pediatric Cardiology: Personal communication, October 6, 1987
20. Lock JE, Castaneda-Zuniga WR, Fuhrman BP, Bass JL: Balloon dilatation angioplasty of hypoplastic and stenotic pulmonary arteries. Circulation 67(5):962, 1983
21. Lock JE, Bass JL, Casteneda-Zuniga W et al: Dilatation angioplasty of congenital or operative narrowings of venous channels. Circulation 70(3):457, 1984
22. Al-Zaibag M, Ribeiro P, Al-Kasab S: Percutaneous balloon valvotomy in tricuspid stenosis. Br Heart J 57:51, 1987
23. Feit F, Stecy PJ, Nachamie MS: Percutaneous balloon valvuloplasty for stenosis of a porcine bioprosthesis in the tricuspid valve position. Am J Cardiol 58:636, 1986
24. Stein PD, Sabbah HN, Pitha JV: Continuing disease process of calcific aortic stenosis: Role of microthrombi and turbulent flow. Am J Cardiol 39:159, 1977
25. Tweedy PS: The pathogenesis of valvular thickening in rheumatic heart disease. Br Heart J 18:173, 1956
26. O'Keefe JH, Vlietstra RE, Bailey KR, Holmes DR: Natural history of candidates for balloon aortic valvuloplasty. Mayo Clin Proc 62:986, 1987
27. Wyman RM, Berman AD, Safian RD et al: Balloon aortic valvuloplasty in patients with critical aortic stenosis and low gradient (abstr). Circulation (Suppl IV) 56:IV-75, 1987
28. Hurley PJ, Lowe JB, Barratt-Boyes BG: Debridement-valvuloplasty for aortic stenosis in adults: A follow up of 76 patients. Thorax 22:314, 1967
29. Hill DG: Long-term results of debridement valvotomy for calcific aortic stenosis. J Thorac Cardiovasc Surg 65(5):708, 1973
30. Rees JR, Holswade GR, Lillehei CW, Glenn F: Aortic valvuloplasty for stenosis in adults: Late results. J Thorac Cardiovasc Surg 67(3):390, 1974
31. Lababidi Z: Aortic balloon valvuloplasty. Am Heart J 10:751, 1983
32. Lababidi Z, Jiunn-Ren W, Walls JT: Percutaneous balloon aortic valvuloplasty: Results in 23 patients. Am J Cardiol 53:194, 1984
33. Rickards AF, Somerville J: Successful balloon aortic valvotomy in a child with a pulmonary hypertensive duct and aortic valve stenosis. Br Heart J 56:185, 1986
34. Cribier A, Saoudi N, Berland J et al: Percutaneous transluminal valvuloplasty of acquired aortic stenosis in elderly patients: An alternative to valve replacement? Lancet 63, 1986
35. Culling W, Papouchado M, Jones J Vann: Percutaneous transluminal valvuloplasty. Lancet 909, 1986
36. McKay RG, Safian RD, Lock JE et al: Balloon dilatation of calcific aortic stenosis in elderly patients: Postmortem, intraoperative and percutaneous valvuloplasty studies. Circulation 74(1):119, 1986
37. Robicsek F, Harbold N: Limited value of balloon dilatation in calcific aortic stenosis in adults: Direct observations during open heart surgery. Am J Cardiol 60:857, 1987
38. Meier B, Friedli B, Oberhanssli I: Trefoil balloon for aortic valvuloplasty. Br Heart J 56:292, 1986
39. Safian RD, Mandell VS, Thurer RE et al: Postmortem and intra-operative balloon valvuloplasty in elderly patients: Mechanisms of successful dilatation. J Am Coll Cardiol 9(3):655, 1987
40. Block PC, Palacios IF: Comparison of hemodynamic results of anterograde versus retrograde percutaneous balloon aortic valvuloplasty. Am J Cardiol 60:659, 1987
41. Landzberg J, Franklin J, Langberg J et al: Echo guided transponder catheter placement in the right atrium. Circulation (Suppl II) 76(4):IV-192, 1987
42. Lembo NJ, King SB, Roubin GS et al: Fatal aortic rupture during percutaneous balloon valvuloplasty for valvular aortic stenosis. Am J Cardiol 60:733, 1987
43. Davidson CJ, Skelton TN, Kisslo KB et al: A comprehensive evaluation of the risk of systemic embolization after percutaneous balloon valvuloplasty (abstr). Circulation (Suppl IV) 76:IV-188, 1987
44. Ports TA, Srebro JP, Manubens SM et al: Simultaneous percutaneous aortic valvuloplasty and coronary artery angioplasty in an elderly patient. Am Heart J 115:672, 1988
45. Inoue K, Owaki T, Nakamura T et al: Clinical application of transvenous mitral commissurotomy by a new balloon catheter. J Thorac Cardiovasc Surg 87:394, 1984
46. Lock J, Khalilullah M, Shrivastava S et al: Percutaneous catheter commissurotomy in rheumatic mitral stenosis. N Engl J Med 313:1515, 1985
47. Babic U, Sreten MV, Grujicic M: Percutaneous transarterial balloon valvuloplasty for end-stage mitral valve stenosis. Scand J Thorac Cardiovasc Surg 20:189, 1986
48. Babic UU, Pejcic P, Djurisic Z et al: Percutaneous transarterial balloon valvuloplasty for mitral stenosis. Am J Cardiol 57:1101, 1986
49. Kveselis DA, Rocchini AP, Beekman R et al: Balloon angioplasty for congenital and rheumatic mitral stenosis. Am J Cardiol 57:348, 1986
50. Al-Zaibag M, Al-Kasab S, Ribeiro A, Al-Fagih MR: Percutaneous double-balloon mitral valvotomy for rheumatic mitral stenosis. Lancet 757, 1986
51. McKay RG, Lock JE, Keane JF et al: Percutaneous mitral valvuloplasty in an adult patient with calcific rheumatic mitral stenosis. J Am Coll Cardiol 7:1410, 1986
52. Reid CL, McKay CR, Chandaratna PAN et al: Mechanisms of increase in mitral valve area and influence of anatomic features in double-balloon, catheter balloon valvuloplasty in adults with rheumatic mitral stenosis: A Doppler and two-dimensional echocardiographic study. Circulation 76(3):628, 1987

53. Data presented at the Conference on New Directions in Interventional Cardiology, Santa Barbara, CA, October 23–25, 1987
54. Palacios I, Block P, Brandi S et al: Percutaneous balloon valvulotomy for patients with severe mitral stenosis. Circulation 75(4):778, 1987
55. McKay CR, Kawanishi T, Rahimtoola SH: Catheter balloon valvuloplasty of the mitral valve in adults using a double balloon technique. JAMA 257(13):1753, 1987
56. McKay C, Kawanishi D, Kotlewski A et al: Long-term improvement in rest and exercise hemodynamics and in treadmill performance. Circulation (Suppl IV) 76:IV-77, 1987
57. McKay R, Lock J, Safian R et al: Balloon dilatation of mitral stenosis in adult patients: Post-mortem and percutaneous valvuloplasty studies. J Am Coll Cardiol 9(4):723, 1987

Infective Endocarditis

Gabriel Gregoratos

CHAPTER 86
VOLUME 2

Infective endocarditis is a microbial infection of the cardiac valves, the endocardium adjacent to a congenital or acquired cardiac defect, or the endothelium of a vascular malformation or an arteriovenous fistula. It may be caused by a large variety of microorganisms and the infection may pursue either a prolonged or a fulminant course. In the preantibiotic era, endocarditis was uniformly fatal.

The microbiologic, clinical, and therapeutic features of infective endocarditis have changed dramatically during the past three decades.[1] Patients with "classic" manifestations such as fever, splenomegaly, "changing murmurs," signs of peripheral embolization, and multiple positive blood cultures have become distinctly unusual. Weinstein and Rubin have suggested that if physicians were to rely on these classic diagnostic criteria, they would fail to suspect the diagnosis of infective endocarditis in as many of 90% of patients presenting today with this disease process.[2] Factors responsible for the changing pattern of this disease include the decreasing incidence of rheumatic and syphilitic heart disease, the longer survival of patients with rheumatic and congenital heart disease, the increasing use of antimicrobial agents, the general increase in the life expectancy of the population, and advances in medicine, such as cardiac surgery, intravenous hyperalimentation, and the widespread use of indwelling central venous catheters, as well as the progressively increasing numbers of habitual intravenous narcotic drug users.

Originally, endocarditis was classified primarily as acute or subacute depending on the duration of the disease and the infecting microorganism. Patients dying in less than 8 weeks from the onset of the disease were classified as having the acute form and those surviving 8 weeks or longer were said to have the subacute form.[3] Today, with modern medical therapy, survival of 60% to 80% of all patients can be expected and the distinction blurs. Similarly, patients with endocarditis due to *Staphylococcus aureus, Neisseria gonorrhoeae, Neisseria meningitidis, Hemophilus influenzae,* or *Streptococcus pyogenes* were considered to have the acute form of the disease because of the invasiveness of the infecting microorganism. Patients with endocarditis due to *Streptococcus viridans* or *Staphylococcus epidermidis,* less invasive organisms, were considered to have subacute disease. This is an important clinical differentiation since the duration of the disease, the nature and frequency of complications, and the final outcome in the two groups of patients differ greatly. However, it has recently become evident that the clinical course in many instances bears no relationship to the invading organism. Patients with acute disease have been converted to the subacute form by appropriate therapy whereas patients with subacute endocarditis have been known to suddenly develop acute life-threatening complications such as valve perforation with consequent fulminant heart failure. For these reasons, Lerner and Weinstein have suggested that the modifiers *acute* and *subacute* be abolished.[4]

GENERAL CONSIDERATIONS

INCIDENCE

The incidence of infective endocarditis is difficult to ascertain precisely. Variable diagnostic criteria and the inclusion or exclusion of culture-negative patients account in part for this difficulty. In one study, infective endocarditis was listed as the admitting diagnosis in 0.16 to 5.4 patients per thousand hospital admissions from data obtained from 10 different hospitals in the United States.[5] Some institutions have reported a decrease in the incidence of infective endocarditis since the introduction of antimicrobial agents in clinical practice, whereas others have noted no change in the incidence of the disease over a 30-year period[6] and other investigators have reported a definite increase in the frequency of endocarditis over the past 25 years.[4] The increasing number of predisposing factors and the recent increase in the population subgroups at risk (see below) tend to support the contention that the true incidence of endocarditis is rising.

Notwithstanding the conflicting evidence concerning the incidence of endocarditis, there is general agreement regarding a change in the age distribution of this disease during the past 30 years. Whereas in the preantibiotic era endocarditis was seen primarily in young adults, it now affects mainly elderly individuals, with the mean age of affected persons reported to be between 55 and 57 years and with 55% of cases occurring in individuals over the age of 60 years.[7] Endocarditis continues to be an uncommon disease in the first decade of life, and when it occurs in infants under the age of 2 years, it is usually of the acute variety with involvement of normal cardiac valves. Children with congenital cardiac abnormalities are at particular risk for the development of endocarditis and in some instances the increased susceptibility to infection persists despite surgical correction of the defect.[8] Men predominate in practically all reported series. Male-to-female ratios have ranged from 2:1 to as high as 9:1 in the older age groups.[4,5] Endocarditis tends to involve women at an earlier age than men, but it is uncommon during pregnancy.[9]

PREDISPOSING CONDITIONS

Infective endocarditis develops most commonly in patients with preexisting cardiac disease. In a recently reported retrospective study, 72% of patients with endocarditis had evidence of preexisting structural cardiac abnormalities.[10] Congenital cardiac defects were encountered as frequently as rheumatic heart disease in this series (26% versus 27%) presumably because of the decreasing incidence of rheumatic valvular heart disease and the classification of isolated valvular aortic stenosis as probably congenital in origin. Isolated valvular aortic stenosis was the congenital defect most often associated with endocarditis, followed in frequency by ventricular septal defect, tetralogy of

Fallot, idiopathic hypertrophic subaortic stenosis, and atrial septal defect (uncommon).

In patients with valvular disease, the mitral valve is involved most often, followed by aortic valve endocarditis and combined mitral and aortic valve infection.[5] Until recently, tricuspid valve endocarditis was reported uncommonly, with a mean incidence of 2% in reported series. Endocarditis involving both sides of the heart was also uncommon, with a mean reported incidence of 1%. At variance with the above are the more recent studies such as the University of Washington series in which the aortic valve was the most frequently infected, followed in order by the mitral valve, multivalvular involvement, tricuspid valve, and other sites of infection.[10]

Several other cardiac and vascular structural abnormalities predispose to the development of infective endocarditis. Infection of atheromatous deposits of the aortic cusps and of a calcified mitral valve annulus have been reported.[11,12] Infection of a "prolapsing" mitral valve is being identified with increasing frequency.[13] Although on an individual basis this valvular lesion does not carry a high risk for infective endocarditis, it is a significant problem because of the high incidence of mitral valve prolapse, reported to occur in 6% to 10% of the population at large.[14,15] A prior episode of infective endocarditis also increases the susceptibility of the individual to new infection presumably because of residual valvular or endocardial abnormalities. Cardiac surgery, especially the introduction of prosthetic valves and other prosthetic material, constitutes a major risk factor for the development of the disease and is discussed in more detail later in this chapter. Similarly, the large group of endocarditis cases associated with parenteral narcotic drug use is covered later in this chapter under Special Considerations. Other, relatively unusual, predisposing factors include myocardial infarction, ventricular aneurysm[16] with the presence of a thrombus that may become infected, infection of an atrial myxoma,[17] and infective endocarditis in patients with peritoneovenous (LeVeen) shunts or arteriovenous shunts or fistulas for the purpose of hemodialysis. These predisposing factors are listed in order of their relative risk in Table 86.1.

ETIOLOGY: INFECTIVE MICROORGANISMS

Infective endocarditis is caused by numerous diverse species of bacteria, fungi, and other microorganisms. To a great extent, however, this diversity is the result of sporadic infections with unusual organisms when, in fact, the majority of cases are caused by the various streptococcal and staphylococcal species. The frequent involvement of these gram-positive cocci in infective endocarditis is probably the result of their inherent ability to adhere to platelet–fibrin thrombi and damaged or even normal valvular endocardium.[18,19]

Although the various streptococcal species are still the most common causative organisms,[5] a striking decline in the incidence of streptococcal endocarditis has been seen in the past three decades.[2] Whereas in the preantibiotic era *Streptococcus viridans* was responsible for approximately 90% of the subacute and 70% of all cases of endocarditis, currently this organism is thought to be responsible for only 35% to 50% of all cases[2] and in more recent studies has been surpassed by the staphylococci as the most common causative microorganism.[10] In part, this is due to other streptococcal species replacing *S. viridans*. Both microaerophilic and anaerobic streptococci are now seen more commonly, emphasizing the need for concomitant anaerobic and aerobic blood cultures in order to isolate the responsible organism. *Streptococcus bovis* is responsible for approximately 50% of cases caused by group D streptococci.[20] It is seen especially in association with cancer of the colon, ulcerative colitis, and Crohn's disease of the bowel.[21,22] The various enterococcal species have been causing infective endocarditis with increasing frequency and are currently thought to be responsible for approximately 10% of all cases.[2,5,10] Enterococcal infections have been reported primarily in women of childbearing age and elderly men.[23] Whereas most cases of *S. viridans* or *S. bovis* endocarditis fall in the category of subacute or indolent disease, enterococci are approximately equally responsible for acute and subacute disease.

Staphylococcus aureus is the most common microorganism producing *acute* endocarditis. In recent reported series from large urban institutions, this organism was responsible for 30% to 34% of endocarditis cases and, in at least one series, was the most frequently isolated agent.[10] *S. aureus* has been shown to be responsible for more than 50% of the acute, rapidly progressive forms of infective endocarditis[4] and in approximately one half of these cases the organism involved previously normal cardiac valves. *S. aureus* is the most common causative organism in intravenous drug users.[24] In the early antibiotic era (up to 1967) it was also the most common infective organism in endocarditis complicating open heart surgery. More recently it has been found to be responsible for only 14% of post open heart surgery endocarditis cases, probably because of the widespread use of antibiotic prophylaxis with penicillinase-resistant penicillins or cephalosporins during the perioperative period.[5]

The coagulase-negative *Staphylococcus epidermidis* has been reported to be responsible for up to 13% of cases of infective endocarditis. The importance of this microorganism lies in the fact that it is the most common pathogen in endocarditis complicating open heart surgery despite the usual extensive use of perioperative antibiotic prophylaxis. *S. epidermidis* has been responsible for both "early" (27%) and "late" (23%) prosthetic valve infections.[25]

Several other microorganisms may be responsible for infections of the endocardium. Pneumococcal endocarditis has declined in frequency from approximately 15% in the preantibiotic era to less than 5% since the introduction of penicillin,[5] and when seen today it frequently coexists with pneumococcal meningitis.[2] Gonococcal endocarditis has

---

TABLE 86.1 RELATIVE RISK OF VARIOUS PREDISPOSING CONDITIONS FOR INFECTIVE ENDOCARDITIS

High Risk	Intermediate Risk	Low/Negligible Risk
Prosthetic valves	Mitral valve prolapse	Degenerative heart disease
Aortic valve disease	Mitral stenosis	Atrial septal defect
Mitral regurgitation	Tricuspid valve disease	Luetic aortitis
Patent ductus arteriosus	Hypertrophic obstructive cardiomyopathy	Transvenous pacemakers
Arteriovenous fistula	Calcific aortic sclerosis	Surgically corrected congenital lesions (no prosthesis)
Ventricular septal defect	Tetralogy of Fallot	
Coarctation of the aorta	Indwelling right heart and pulmonary artery catheters	Aortocoronary bypass surgery
Indwelling right heart catheters (hyperalimentation)	Nonvalvular intracardiac prosthesis	Cardiac pacemakers
Previous infective endocarditis		
Marfan's syndrome		

(Adapted from Dascomb HE: The current status of prophylaxis against infective endocarditis. J La State Med Soc 132:91, 1980)

declined from 5% to 10% of all cases in the preantibiotic era to an occasional sporadic case. A double daily temperature elevation and a relatively high incidence of involvement of the right side of the heart have been reported as characteristic of gonococcal endocarditis in approximately 50% of patients.[2] Many other gram-negative microorganisms may also be responsible for occasional infections of the endocardium. Overall, gram-negative endocarditis remains uncommon except as a complication of open heart surgery and in drug addicts.[2,5] The various *Hemophilus* species were the most common organisms isolated in a recent series of 56 patients with gram-negative infective endocarditis,[26] although among addicts other gram-negative organisms predominate.[27] Numerous other microorganisms, including *Erysipelothrix, Listeria monocytogenes, Serratia marcescens,* various *Salmonella* species, *Coxiella burnetii, Chlamydia psittaci,* and clostridia have been reported as responsible for sporadic cases.

Endocarditis due to yeasts and fungi is an unusual occurrence in the general population in the absence of predisposing factors. Infections due to various species of *Candida, Aspergillus,* and *Histoplasma* form the bulk of fungal endocarditis cases. The common predisposing factors include prolonged antibiotic or corticosteroid administration, preexisting bacterial infective endocarditis, diabetes mellitus, prolonged intravenous glucose infusions, polyethylene catheter embolization, open heart surgery, immunosuppressed status, and narcotic intravenous drug abuse.[5] Total parenteral hyperalimentation and indwelling intravenous catheters are particularly common predisposing factors to *Candida* infection.

The incidence of "culture-negative" endocarditis has declined from 10% in the early antibiotic era to approximately 3%.[1] This decline is probably related to improved microbiologic techniques that allow the isolation of anaerobic and other fastidious organisms as well as the recognition of nonbacterial agents that were formerly difficult to isolate from blood.

Polymicrobial endocarditis is distinctly uncommon. When seen, these infections occur in patients following open heart surgery or in intravenous drug users. In a recent series, *Pseudomonas aeruginosa, Streptococcus faecalis,* and *Staphylococcus aureus* were the most common organisms involved. Clinically, polymicrobial endocarditis has been reported to be indistinguishable from single-organism disease, except that mixed infections carry a high mortality rate (over 30%) and over half of the patients require surgery to control the infection or to repair cardiac defects resulting from the infection. It appears that prognosis in these cases depends more on the species involved rather than on the number of microorganisms isolated.[28] The incidence of responsible infective agents in different forms of endocarditis is listed in Table 86.2.

PATHOGENESIS AND PATHOLOGY
SOURCE OF INFECTION

Invasion of the bloodstream by microorganisms is the initial essential element in the development of endocarditis. Most often, the bacteremia (or fungemia) that initiates the infection is transient and arises from the oropharynx, genitourinary or gastrointestinal mucosa, lungs, or skin. Okell and Elliott first studied the incidence of transient streptococcal bacteremia following dental extractions in 1935 and documented a 61% rate in their 138 patients.[29] Subsequent studies have documented the incidence of transient bacteremia associated with dental manipulations to vary from 18% to 85%.[30] The organisms that inhabit the oropharynx are most commonly streptococci of the alpha type and occasionally enterococci. The bacteremia rarely persists for more than 15 to 20 minutes because of the existence of efficient clearing mechanisms for microorganisms that enter the bloodstream. Since few species of microorganisms can actually multiply in the circulation, the level of bacteremia rapidly declines after a limited period of invasion. Clearance of microorganisms depends on the combined function of fixed macrophages and circulating leukocytes. The presence of large arteriovenous fistulas that bypass the splanchnic and hepatic vascular beds results in a more prolonged bacteremia and has been observed to cause spontaneous infective endocarditis in the experimental animal.[31]

Dental procedures (other than extractions) that have been found to be associated with transient bacteremia include vigorous brushing of teeth, periodontal operations, cleaning and scaling of teeth, dental prophylaxis, use of unwaxed dental floss, and the use of oral irrigation devices (*e.g.*, Water-Pik).[30] Spontaneous transient bacteremia has been documented in normal individuals.[32] It may be related to minor focal infections and has been reported to occur in as many as 11% of patients with periodontitis, 8% of patients with periapical abscesses, and 9% of patients prior to tonsillectomy.[29,33]

Invasion of the circulation by microorganisms also occurs commonly following trauma or manipulation of mucous membranes colonized by either indigenous or pathogenic organisms. Bacteremia has been documented to occur in 30% of patients following tonsillectomy, 16% of patients following nasotracheal intubation, 15% of patients following rigid bronchoscopy, 10% of patients after upper gastrointestinal

TABLE 86.2 MICROORGANISMS RESPONSIBLE FOR INFECTIVE ENDOCARDITIS

Organism	% Incidence
Native Valves	
Streptococcus viridans	30–40
Enterococci	5–15
Other streptococci	15–20
Staphylococcus aureus	10–30
Staphylococcus epidermidis	1–3
Gram-negative bacilli	2–10
Fungi (*Candida, Aspergillus, Histoplasma*)	2–4
Diphtheroids	2–4
Miscellaneous*	2–5
Culture-negative	5–10
In Narcotic Addicts	
Streptococci	
Enterococci	8–10
Nonenterococcal	10–15
Staphylococcus aureus	50–60
Staphylococcus epidermidis	2–5
Gram-negative bacilli	4–8
Fungi	4–5
Diphtheroids	1–2
Miscellaneous	<1
Culture-negative	5–8
Prosthetic Valves	
Streptococcus viridans	5–20
Enterococci	5–10
Other streptococci	1–5
Staphylococcus aureus	15–20
Staphylococcus epidermidis	20–30
Gram-negative bacilli	10–20
Fungi	5–15
Diphtheroids	5–10
Miscellaneous	0–2
Culture-negative	<5

(Adapted from Karchner AW: Infective endocarditis in the 1980's: Clinical features and management. Baylor College of Medicine Cardiology Series 7(3):6, 1984; Reisberg BE: Infective endocarditis in the narcotic addict. Prog Cardiovasc Dis 22:193, 1979; and Sande MA: Infective endocarditis. In Stein JH (ed): Internal Medicine, p 537. Boston, Little, Brown & Co, 1983)

* Miscellaneous microorganisms are gonocarti, pneumococci, meningococci, *Listeria, Hemophilus,* rickettsiae, *Chlamydia,* cell-wall defective bacteria, *Eikenella,* clostridia.

endoscopy, 10% of patients undergoing sigmoidoscopy, 11% of patients undergoing barium enema examination, and between 11% (sterile urine) and 58% (infected urine) of patients undergoing a variety of urologic maneuvers.[30] In general, the incidence of transient bacteremia following uncomplicated vaginal delivery and various gynecologic procedures has been low. However, in a recent study approximately 85% of patients undergoing suction abortion were found to have transient bacteremia and in some instances microorganisms were found in the circulation following simple bimanual pelvic examination.[34] History of a previous procedure associated with transient bacteremia can be elicited in only half of patients with infective endocarditis. Patients with *Staphylococcus aureus* endocarditis are more likely to have a demonstrable source of infection (68%) than patients with streptococcal disease (42%). Similarly, patients with the subacute form of the disease are less likely to have an apparent source of infection than are patients with acute endocarditis.[4] The important predisposing factors are summarized in Table 86.3.

CARDIAC PATHOLOGY

Once microorganisms gain access to the circulation, several factors combine to promote their deposition on damaged or normal endothelium. It appears likely that endocarditis develops following implantation of a microorganism on a preexisting sterile thrombotic vegetation present at a point of structural endocardial abnormality.[35]

The localization of infective vegetations depends on hemodynamic factors as well as structural changes. It has been shown experimentally that bacteria are often deposited in areas of high blood flow velocity with decreased lateral pressure.[36] Consequently, vegetations develop more frequently on insufficient rather than stenotic valves and then on the low pressure side of the regurgitant valve (*i.e.*, on the atrial side of the mitral valve in mitral regurgitation and the ventricular aspect of the aortic valve in aortic regurgitation) (Fig. 86.1). In ventricular septal defects with a small orifice and high left-to-right shunt velocity, the vegetations usually are located on the right side of the interventricular septum at the circumference of the defect. Similarly, in coarctation of the aorta the lesions are found on the rim of the stenotic area distal to the narrowing, and in patent ductus arteriosus with left-to-right shunt, vegetations are seen most often on the pulmonary artery end of the ductus. Endocarditis involves the left side of the heart much more frequently than the right, although the rise in drug abuse has caused an increase in tricuspid valve disease.

Histologically, vegetations consist of an amorphous mass of fibrin, platelets, leukocytes, and red blood cell debris along with bacterial colonies. In general, fibrin and few leukocytes predominate near the surface of the vegetation whereas deeper toward the base of the vegetation the leukocytes become more numerous and masses of stainable bacteria are often present. The inflammatory cells consist chiefly of mononuclear cells, lymphocytes, and histiocytes. Very few polymorphonuclear cells are present. Giant cells containing phagocytized bacteria are also seen. The valve leaflet underlying the vegetation most often is the site of a destructive process that can be either localized or extend to both surfaces of the leaflet (Fig. 86.2). Early healing is a prominent feature (especially with antibiotic therapy) and the lesion contains numerous capillaries and fibroblasts. This destructive process may cause an aneurysm of the leaflet or frank perforation and extensive loss of valvular tissue with consequent grave hemodynamic aberrations.

Mitral valve vegetations may extend along the chordae tendineae toward the papillary muscles, causing their rupture. Aortic valve endocarditis is often complicated by the development of ring abscess. This is especially true with aggressive infective organisms such as *Staphylococcus aureus*. These abscesses may become large and burrow into the interventricular septum where they may disrupt the conduction system or may rupture into the pericardial space causing cardiac tamponade and death.[37] Ring abscesses are seen primarily with infections of the aortic valve and are rare in tricuspid or mitral valve endocarditis, presumably because of the different anatomical structure of the aortic valve annulus, which predisposes to extension of the infection.

Vegetations may also extend downstream along the jet of a regurgitant or shunt lesion. Thus, in cases of ventricular septal defect endocarditis, vegetations may be found on the right ventricular wall opposite the defect, the site of the jet impact. When endocarditis involves a mitral regurgitant lesion, vegetations may be found on the wall of the left atrium in the area termed MacCallum's patch where the regurgitant jet strikes the atrial wall and produces endocardial thickening. Similarly, vegetations may localize on the chordae tendineae of the anterior mitral leaflet as a result of aortic valve endocarditis, with the aortic regurgitant stream being responsible for chordal and endocardial abnormalities that allow bacterial implantation.

More distant cardiovascular lesions result from embolization of vegetation fragments containing viable microorganisms. Mycotic aneurysms of the anterior ascending aortic wall have been described and coronary embolization may result in the development of myocardial abscesses and myocardial fibrosis. A vasculitis involving small myocardial arteries and arterioles has been reported to complicate infective endocarditis and to persist despite successful treatment of the infection.[38]

TABLE 86.3 THE IMPORTANT INVASIVE PREDISPOSING FACTORS TO BACTERIAL ENDOCARDITIS

Dental procedures
Oral and upper respiratory tract surgery
Certain gastrointestinal procedures
Genitourinary surgery
Cardiac surgery
Certain trauma
Alimentation catheters in the right heart
Pressure monitoring catheters
Intravenous drug use

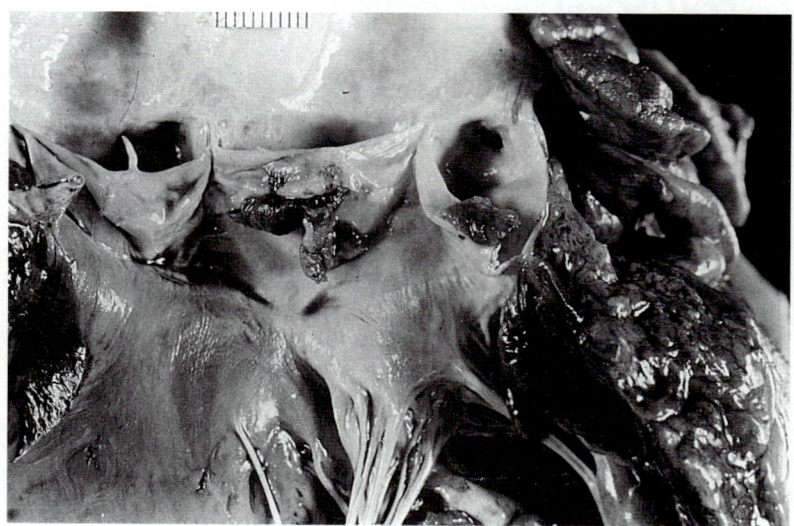

FIGURE 86.1 Polypoid vegetations due to *Staphylococcus aureus* on the ventricular aspect of aortic valve cusps. (Courtesy of Colin M. Bloor, M.D., Department of Pathology, University of California, San Diego)

EXTRACARDIAC PATHOLOGY

Systemic embolism is a common finding in infective endocarditis, having been reported to occur in over 50% of necropsied cases.[39,40] Practically any tissue or organ may be involved, but the most common sites of embolic complications are the kidneys, skin, mucous membranes, spleen, eyes, and central nervous system. Immunologic factors also play an important role in the development of extracardiac lesions and there is increasing evidence that in fact many of the so-called embolic phenomena actually represent "immune-complex" depositions in small systemic arteries.[41] The extracardiac manifestations of infective endocarditis are discussed in more detail in the following section. Pulmonary embolic complications are almost always seen in the setting of right-sided valvular endocarditis. When the infective organism is *Staphylococcus aureus*, multiple pulmonary abscesses are a frequent result of pulmonary embolization.

CLINICAL MANIFESTATIONS

The symptoms and signs of infective endocarditis are the result of four distinct pathophysiologic mechanisms: (1) infection of the valve and other cardiac structures; (2) metastatic infection; (3) remote embolization and its sequelae; and (4) the production of abnormal immunoglobulins and circulating immune complexes and their deposition in various organs. All these mechanisms are not operative at the same time in any one patient and their relative importance varies considerably in the acute and subacute forms of the disease.[42] Although the distinction between acute and subacute endocarditis is not absolute, from the clinical standpoint it is useful to think in terms of these two categories.

PRESENTING SYMPTOMS

Patients with *subacute* infective endocarditis usually present with nonspecific constitutional symptoms of insidious onset, especially malaise, fatigability, fever, and weight loss. The presence of fever and nonspecific constitutional complaints in a patient with preexisting valvular or congenital cardiac defects should immediately raise the suspicion of infective endocarditis. Occasionally patients will present with minimal temperature elevations and totally nonspecific symptoms such as myalgias, arthralgias, or back pain. Similarly, an occasional patient will present with an extracardiac catastrophe such as a stroke and the true diagnosis may be missed. It is noteworthy that patients presenting with primarily central nervous system symptoms (stroke, delirium, and coma) had a significantly higher mortality rate in at least one series.[10] In some series the frequency of musculoskeletal symptoms has been reported to be as high as 44%.[43,44]

The presentation of *acute* infective endocarditis is more dramatic with the abrupt onset of a toxic illness with "spiking" fevers and rigors. Most of the episodes of acute endocarditis are caused by *Staphylococcus aureus*, an invasive microorganism, with resultant rapid valvular tissue disruption and a high incidence of peripheral embolic events when the organism involves left-sided valves. With right-sided staphylococcal endocarditis, initially pulmonary symptoms will predominate, frequently as a result of pulmonary embolization and microabscess formation. Pneumonia and septic pulmonary embolism are said to occur in 70% to 100% of patients with tricuspid valve endocarditis.[24]

PHYSICAL FINDINGS

Classically, a heart murmur has been the *sine qua non* for the diagnosis of infective endocarditis. It is now recognized that as many as 15% of patients may have no detectable murmurs at the time of the initial examination.[2,4,45] Cardiac murmurs may appear first during therapy or not until sometime after the therapy has been completed or may fail to develop altogether. Cardiac murmurs may not be detected in the early stages of the disease in approximately one third of patients with acute endocarditis involving the left side. Similarly, up to two thirds of patients with acute tricuspid valve endocarditis may have no detectable murmur initially.[2,4] It should be noted, however, that the vast majority of patients with infective endocarditis will eventually develop a cardiac murmur during the course of their illness.

Although the literature on endocarditis is full of references to "changing murmurs" as part of the clinical picture, this concept needs to be reexamined and "change" defined. Numerous factors other than valve destruction are responsible for changes in the characteristics of a cardiac murmur. For example, alterations in cardiac output, body temperature, or hematocrit may produce impressive changes in the intensity and quality of a cardiac murmur completely independent of changes in valvular integrity. On the other hand, when after careful, regular examinations a patient develops a *new* organic regurgitant murmur in a setting of acute sepsis this is virtually diagnostic of infective endocarditis. Real changes in intensity and quality of cardiac murmurs are more likely to occur in the acute disease where the highly

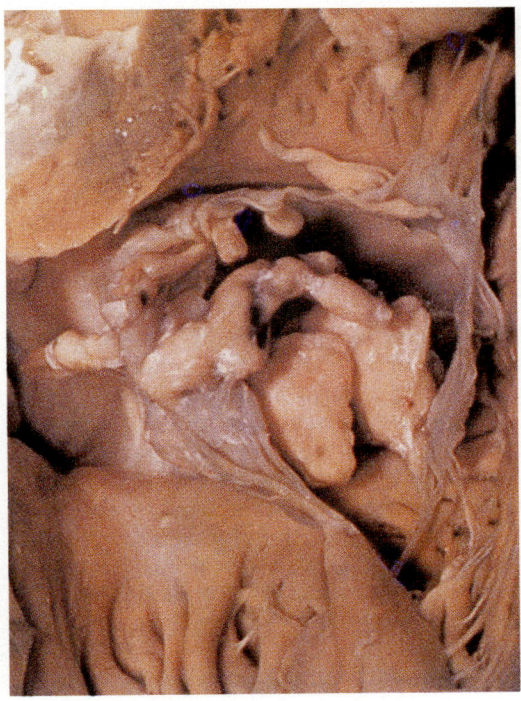
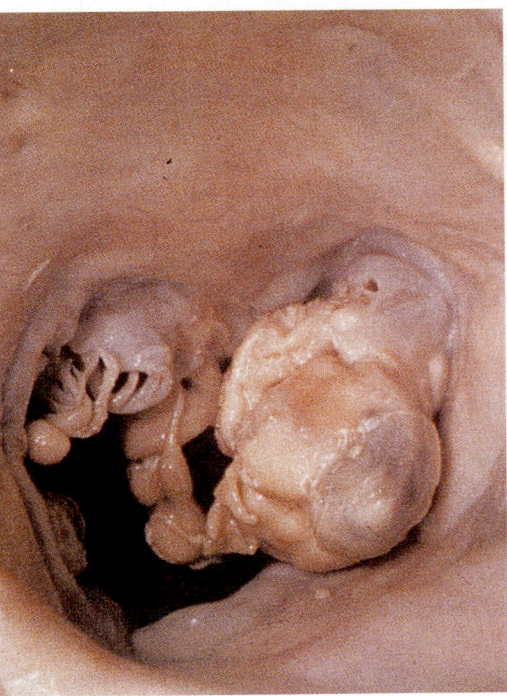

FIGURE 86.2 Unusually large vegetation due to *Streptococcus viridans*. The bulk of the vegetation is on the atrial side of the mitral leaflets (*right panel*) but also extends to involve the ventricular aspect of the valve (*left panel*). Note the leaflet destruction. Chordal rupture has occurred with consequent prolapse of portion of the leaflets at the posteromedial commissure.

destructive valvular lesions cause rapidly progressive hemodynamic alterations and, therefore, changes in the intensity and quality of the cardiac murmur.[42]

The frequency of clinical findings in 125 episodes of infective endocarditis is summarized in Table 86.4. Although fever is the most frequent initial clinical manifestation, it is not invariably present. This is particularly true in elderly patients and in patients who have been previously partially treated with antibiotic agents. Similarly, in the presence of massive intracerebral or subarachnoid hemorrhage due to embolism or a ruptured mycotic aneurysm, severe congestive heart failure, or uremia, the temperature may be normal or subnormal. A characteristic clinical pattern of recurring episodes of remission and relapse of a febrile illness in response to repeated short courses of antibiotic therapy should alert the physician to the possibility of infective endocarditis.[2]

CUTANEOUS MANIFESTATIONS

The most common cutaneous manifestations are petechiae, which are seen in 20% to 40% of cases, a remarkable reduction by more than one half from the 85% incidence in the preantibiotic era.[2,4] Furthermore, the presence of petechiae has lost much of its specificity. A considerable number of patients undergoing cardiac surgery under cardiopulmonary bypass develop subconjunctival and subungual "splinter" hemorrhages due to lipid microembolism,[46] a potentially false positive sign. However, the development of "splinter" hemorrhages or petechiae while a patient is under observation and in the absence of trauma is clinically significant and suggests the presence of endocarditis in the setting of a febrile illness.

Osler's nodes and Janeway's lesions have long been considered to be hallmarks of infective endocarditis, but their incidence has decreased markedly in the past 25 years. Osler's nodes are *tender*, subcutaneous, purplish erythematous papules that develop in the pulp of the distal fingers. They may occasionally necrotize and ulcerate. Janeway's lesions are larger, erythematous, *nontender*, nodular lesions that may develop on the palms or soles. They are usually nontender and do not necrotize. Both Osler's nodes and Janeway's lesions are distinctly uncommon today, occurring perhaps in less than 10% of cases of subacute infective endocarditis, and are even rarer in the more fulminant acute disease. Pathologically, both lesions are described as showing a vasculitis with inflammation and central necrosis.[45] Cultures taken from Osler's nodes have been generally found to be sterile and most investigators have concluded that these lesions represent a hypersensitivity angiitis.[2,41,47] However, in a recent study the causative organisms were isolated from aspirates of Osler's nodes, thereby supporting Osler's original belief that the skin lesions that bear his name were "in all probability caused by minute emboli."[48]

Clubbing of the fingers is a rare clinical manifestation today. Although formerly it was seen in almost all patients with subacute infective endocarditis, clubbing is now found in only 10% to 20% of cases, probably because of the marked reduction in the number of chronic or subacute cases of the disease and their prompt treatment with antibiotic agents.[2,4]

OCULAR MANIFESTATIONS

The eyes are occasionally involved in patients with endocarditis, especially the subacute type. In addition to the subconjunctival petechiae mentioned above, small hemorrhages may be seen in the sclera and the retina where they appear to be circular or flame-shaped. The so-called Roth spot has the appearance of a flame-shaped hemorrhage with a pale center and occasionally takes the form of a "cotton wool" exudate. Far from being specific for infective endocarditis, Roth spots are also seen in a variety of hematologic diseases, including severe anemia, leukemia, scurvy, and collagen vascular diseases. Retinal lesions are distinctly uncommon today, occurring in fewer than 5% of patients with infective endocarditis.

COMPLICATIONS
CONGESTIVE HEART FAILURE

The most common and probably the most serious complication of infective endocarditis is the development of congestive heart failure despite adequate treatment of the infectious process. Congestive heart failure develops most often as a result of severe acute aortic regurgitation resulting from perforation or destruction of aortic valve cusps. In a recently reported series of 125 patients, the prevalence of this complication was 67%.[10] In the same series, heart failure of recent onset carried a higher risk of death (59%) compared to preexisting or aggravated congestive heart failure, which carried a mortality of 39%. Severe mitral regurgitation and combined mitral and aortic regurgitation are responsible for one third of the cases of severe heart failure associated with infective endocarditis.[49] Patients with multivalvular involvement have the poorest prognosis, with a 97% mortality recorded in the series reported by Pelletier and Petersdorf.[10] The extremely high mortality rates that have been recorded in patients with congestive heart failure in this disease have stimulated interest in the aggressive surgical approach to repair or replace incompetent valves even in the face of active infection (see below).

EXTRAVALVULAR CARDIAC COMPLICATIONS

Many other cardiac complications, besides valvular disruption, contribute to the morbidity and mortality of infective endocarditis. These include myocardial infarction and myocardial abscess formation secondary to coronary embolization of fragmented vegetations, sudden death caused by occlusion of a coronary ostium by valvular vegetations,[50,51] extension of the infection through the myocardium resulting in the formation of fistulas, aneurysms, and perforations, as well as the development of interventricular septal fistulas and atrioventricular block. Purulent pericarditis, with or without cardiac tamponade, may result from rupture of an aortic ring abscess into the pericardium.[2,42]

The aortic annulus is particularly susceptible to involvement in cases of endocarditis, especially when the infective organism is aggressive (*e.g., Staphylococcus aureus*). As a result, the development of annular destruction and formation of annular abscesses are much more common in aortic than in mitral valve endocarditis. In a postmortem study of patients who died of native endocarditis, Arnett and Roberts found annular involvement with abscess formation in 41% of aortic and only 6% of mitral infections.[37]

TABLE 86.4 INCIDENCE OF CLINICAL FINDINGS IN INFECTIVE ENDOCARDITIS

Symptoms	%	Signs	%
Fever	84	Heart murmur	89
Chills	41	Fever	77
Weakness	38	Embolic events	50
Dyspnea	36	Skin manifestations	50
Sweats	24	Splenomegaly	28
Anorexia, weight loss	24	Septic complications	19
Malaise	24	Mycotic aneurysms	18
Cough	24	Glomerulonephritis	15
Skin lesions	21	Digital clubbing	12
Stroke	18	Retinal lesions	9
Nausea, vomiting	17		
Chest pain	16		

(Adapted from Pelletier LL Jr, Petersdorf RG: Infective endocarditis: A review of 125 cases from the University of Washington hospitals, 1963–72. Medicine 56:287, 1977)

Aortic ring abscesses frequently progress and cause other structural complications: perivalvular leaks, ventricular septal defects, atrioventricular block, "aneurysms" of the sinuses of Valsalva, and fistulous communications between the aortic root and other cardiac chambers have all been reported as consequences of aortic valve endocarditis.[52] Occasionally, such aneurysms of the sinuses of Valsalva may reach gigantic proportions (Fig. 86.3). Ring abscesses may burrow into the interventricular septum or may involve a coronary artery (Fig. 86.4). Precise delineation of these extravalvular complications of endocarditis by modern imaging techniques (see below) is crucial, if surgical therapy is to be undertaken.

SYSTEMIC AND PULMONARY EMBOLISM

After congestive heart failure, systemic arterial emboli are the most frequent complication of infective endocarditis. The incidence of major embolic phenomena is thought to be between 15% and 35% in all cases of endocarditis today,[2] although in some recently reported series embolic complications occurred in 50% of the patients.[10] The most common sites involved are the coronary arteries, kidneys, and spleen. Splenic emboli are rarely detected during life but have been reported at necropsy to be present in as many as 44% of cases of endocarditis. Splenic abscess may develop as a consequence of septic embolism and has been reported to carry a high mortality if not treated promptly with splenectomy.[53] Splenic rupture is an unusual sequela of embolism and infarction of the spleen[54] and may be the first manifestation of infective endocarditis or may occur while the disease appears to be under control. Hemorrhage into a splenic infarct may cause a large subcapsular hematoma and massive splenomegaly.[55] Most often, major systemic embolic events result from infections that produce large, mobile vegetations, such as those caused by *Hemophilus parainfluenzae*, other slow-growing, fastidious, gram-negative bacilli, nutritionally variant *Streptococcus viridans,* and fungi, especially *Aspergillus*.[2,56] Embolic occlusion of a *large* artery is unusual in infective endocarditis and when it occurs should suggest a fungal etiology. Late embolic events are rather common and do not necessarily imply inadequate anti-infective therapy.[2,4]

Pneumonia and septic pulmonary embolism develop in 60% to 100% of patients with tricuspid valve endocarditis.[24] Cough, sputum production, hemoptysis, pleuritic chest pain, and dyspnea are the most common presenting symptoms. The chest roentgenogram demonstrates nodular and segmental multiple infiltrates that frequently appear sequentially in different parts of the lung parenchyma with a predilection for the lower lobes.[24] Cavitation of the pulmonary infiltrates with development of pulmonary abscesses, empyema, and pleural effusions are common sequelae of septic pulmonary embolism. Occasionally systemic embolism occurs in isolated tricuspid valve endocarditis, probably originating from septic thrombi formed in the pulmonary veins.

MYCOTIC ANEURYSMS

Mycotic aneurysms are another major complication. They develop either as a response to embolic occlusion of the vasa vasorum or because of direct bacterial invasion of the arterial wall. They occur most frequently in the sinuses of Valsalva[10] but have also been reported in cerebral and pulmonary arteries, the celiac axis, ligated ductus arteriosus, and at the sites of atherosclerotic disease in the aorta and its major branches.[2] They are seen most frequently when the infective organisms are relatively noninvasive and are less common when the infective microorganism is *Staphylococcus aureus*.[2]

NEUROLOGIC COMPLICATIONS

Several different neuropsychiatric syndromes occur in approximately 10% to 50% of patients with infective endocarditis. The most common syndromes encountered are listed in Table 86.5. Major stroke is uncommon but occasionally may be the presenting manifestation. Therefore, the clinical adage "in hemiplegia in young adults (or children) always think of subacute bacterial endocarditis" is as useful now as

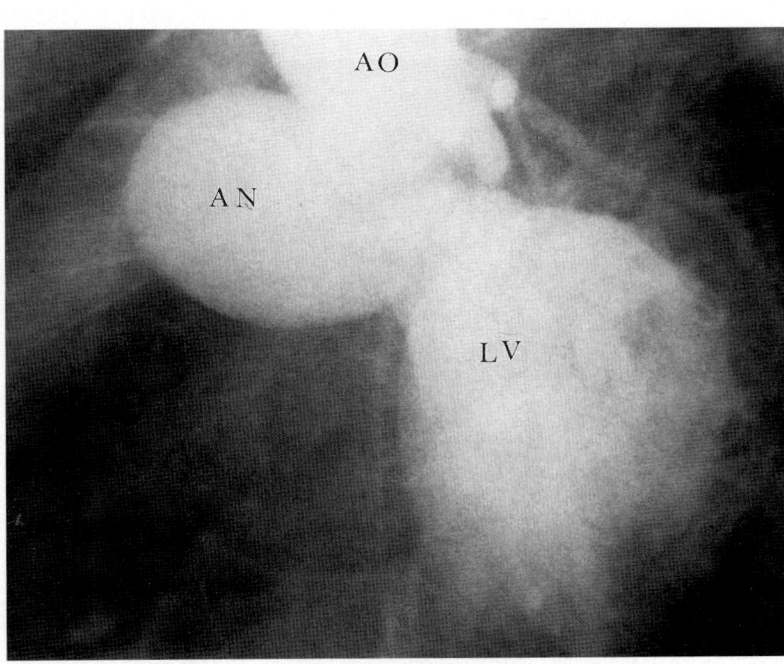

FIGURE 86.3 Aneurysm of the right coronary sinus following an incompletely treated case of *Streptococcus viridans* aortic valve endocarditis. Single frame from cineangiogram of an aortic root (AO) injection in the left anterior oblique projection: Severe aortic regurgitation is present with dense opacification of the left ventricle (LV); the aneurysm of the right coronary sinus (AN) measures 5.5 cm in its largest diameter and impinges on the right ventricular outflow tract and right atrium.

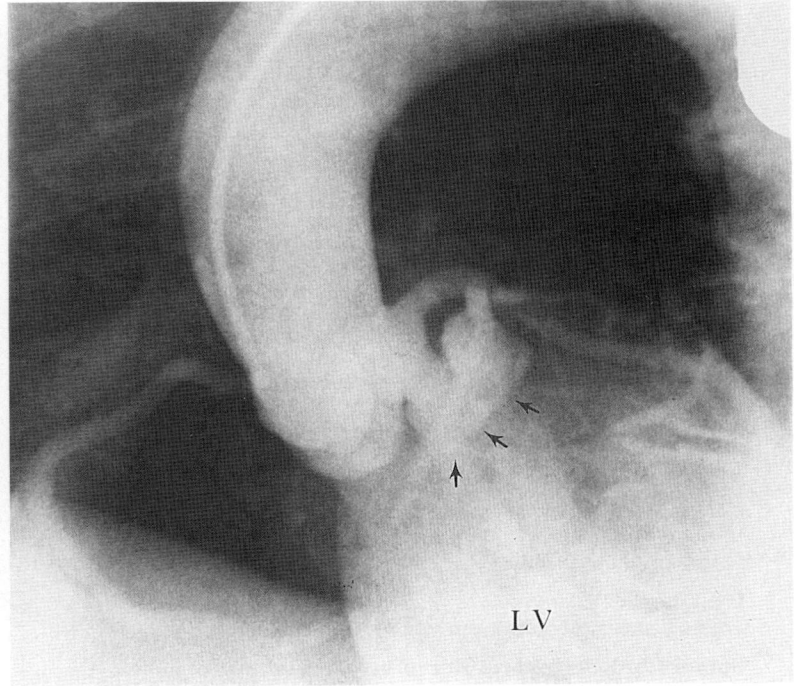

FIGURE 86.4 Single frame from aortic root cineangiogram in the left anterior oblique projection: Aortic ring abscess (arrows) originating from the area of the left coronary sinus is seen to extend posteriorly and superiorly just below the left main coronary artery and its bifurcation. Severe aortic regurgitation is present with dense opacification of the left ventricle (LV).

when originally enunciated in 1924.[57] Mycotic aneurysms of the cerebral arteries are said to occur in 2% to 10% of patients with infective endocarditis.[2] Patients are usually asymptomatic until the aneurysm ruptures, but the development of a mycotic aneurysm may be accompanied by symptoms due to concomitant cerebral ischemia, meningoencephalitis, increased intracranial pressure, or cranial nerve palsies.[58] Asymptomatic cerebrospinal fluid pleocytosis may be present in patients with mycotic cerebral aneurysms and does not imply active central nervous system infection. Cerebral mycotic aneurysms may rupture as late as one to two years following bacteriologic cure.[58]

RENAL COMPLICATIONS

Renal involvement is common in patients with both acute and subacute infective endocarditis and the kidneys are second only to the spleen in frequency of embolization.[4,59] Although renal infarction is not commonly recognized during life, it has been found in 56% of patients with infective endocarditis coming to necropsy (Fig. 86.5); renal infarcts have seldom been related to serious disturbances of renal function.[4] Most episodes of renal embolization are asymptomatic, but others may cause clinical manifestations of variable severity, including flank pain, gross or microscopic hematuria, and proteinuria.

Acute and chronic proliferative glomerulonephritis associated with infective endocarditis is due to immune-mediated injury. Depositions of IgG, IgM, and complement in a granular, nodular, or lumpy bumpy pattern in the glomerular basement membrane suggest an immune injury as the cause of the glomerulonephritis.[60] The presence of circulating immune complexes and the reduction of serum complement levels further support the notion that immune complex deposition and complement consumption injury are responsible for this complication. In contrast to embolic renal infarcts, glomerulonephritis may cause azotemia and progress to renal failure. Renal function will most often return to normal once effective antibiotic therapy has been started. Recovery of renal function usually continues for weeks or months after all other laboratory and clinical evidence of active infection has subsided. Occasionally, patients may be left with significant residual renal dysfunction.

HEMATOLOGIC COMPLICATIONS

A normochromic, normocytic anemia is seen frequently (up to 70% of cases) in infective endocarditis. The syndrome of fever, anemia, petechiae, and splenomegaly should always raise the possibility of infective endocarditis in the mind of the clinician and does not necessarily imply a primary hematologic disorder. A thrombotic thrombocytopenic purpura-like (TTP) syndrome has been recently reported as the presenting feature in some patients with infective endocarditis.[61] Serum complement levels were found to be low in this condition and high levels of circulating immune complexes were detected with return to normal as the TTP syndrome subsided after the institution of specific antimicrobial therapy.

SPECIAL CONSIDERATIONS
ENDOCARDITIS IN NARCOTIC DRUG ABUSERS

The increasing use of illicit narcotic agents and especially intravenous heroin is responsible for important changes in the frequency and clinical manifestations of infective endocarditis. Cherubin and co-workers reported the incidence of endocarditis in an addict population of approximately 50,000 individuals to be 1.4 per 10,000 per year.[62] This incidence is thirty times higher than in the general population and four times higher than the incidence of endocarditis in young adults with chronic rheumatic heart disease. Pelletier and Petersdorf reported that 15% of their patients were parenteral drug addicts.[10] The most common infective microorganism in this subgroup is *Staphylococcus aureus*, reported to be responsible for 50% to 60% of all cases.[10,24,63,64] This organism usually produces acute endocarditis, with high fever, systemic toxicity, pulmonary infiltrates, and minimal or absent cardiac murmurs despite extensive valvular destruction. *S. aureus* and *S. epidermidis* are the commonly reported organisms in mainline heroin addicts. Endocarditis in morphine or opium addicts is due to a variety of microorganisms, including enterococci, *Pseudomonas aeruginosa*, *Enterobacter aerogenes*, *Escherichia coli*, and candida. Infection by multiple microorganisms has been reported in parenteral drug users.[65]

Infective endocarditis in narcotic addicts most often involves the

TABLE 86.5 NEUROPSYCHIATRIC SYNDROMES IN INFECTIVE ENDOCARDITIS

Toxic Symptoms
Headache, decreased concentration, lethargy, insomnia, vertigo, irritability

Psychiatric Symptoms
Confusion, disorientation, psychosis, hallucinations, emotional lability, personality/behavior changes

Stroke
Hemiplegia, hemiparesis, diplegia, paraplegia, aphasia, coma, stiff neck

Meningoencephalitis
Acute brain syndrome

Cranial Nerve Involvement
Visual disturbances, ocular palsy, facial palsy, pupillary inequality, sensory impairment

Dyskinesia
Tremor, ataxia, parkinsonism, chorea, convulsions, myoclonus

Spinal Cord/Peripheral Nerve Involvement
Girdle pain, weakness, myalgias, mononeuritis, peripheral neuropathy

(Adapted from Ziment I: Nervous system complications in bacterial endocarditis. Am J Med 47:593, 1969)

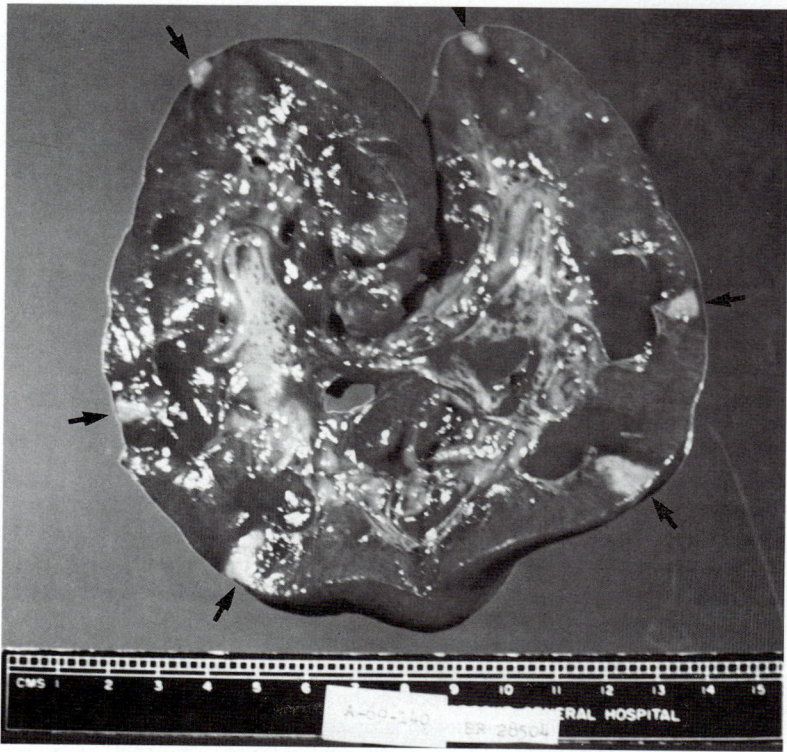

FIGURE 86.5 Multiple cortical renal infarcts (*arrows*) from a case of streptococcal endocarditis of the aortic valve. This patient had mild microscopic hematuria.

tricuspid,[63,64] frequently the aortic, and occasionally the pulmonic valve. Valves on both sides of the heart may be affected in some cases.[2] In the series of Pelletier and Petersdorf the mortality of addicts with left-sided endocarditis was 80%.[10] In addition to the variant and polymicrobial nature of this disease in addicts, a major problem is the propensity of some of these individuals to reinfect themselves by continuing to "mainline" during therapy even in the hospital.

PROSTHETIC VALVE ENDOCARDITIS

Infection of valvular prostheses is a particularly serious and sometimes malignant form of endocarditis. It is customary to distinguish early-onset prosthetic valve endocarditis (within two months after surgery) and late-onset endocarditis developing more than two months postoperatively.[10,62,65-67] There are important clinical and bacteriologic differences between early-onset and late-onset endocarditis that make this distinction useful to the clinician. Prosthetic valve endocarditis occurring within two months of surgery carries a high mortality rate of between 63% and 88%[10,67,68] whereas late-onset endocarditis has a considerably lower mortality rate of between 25% and 45%.[65] The microbiology of early and late prosthetic valve endocarditis is also characteristically different. Early-onset endocarditis is usually caused by microorganisms resistant to the antibiotic agents administered prophylactically at the time of the operation (*Staphylococcus epidermidis*, *Staphylococcus aureus*, and gram-negative bacilli). In late-onset endocarditis the most frequently isolated microorganisms have been the streptococci, especially *Streptococcus viridans* species, *Staphylococcus epidermidis*, gram-negative bacilli, and *Staphylococcus aureus*, in that order.[10,66,68]

The major consequences of prosthetic valve endocarditis relate to the development of valvular dysfunction. Detachment of the prosthesis causing severe regurgitation has been reported to occur in up to 80% of patients with an infected prosthetic aortic valve, but only in approximately 30% of patients with an infected mitral valve prosthesis.[67] Conversely, obstruction of the valve by vegetations and thrombus is reported to occur mainly in infections of mitral valve prostheses (71%) and only in 7% of infected prosthetic aortic valves. Common complications of prosthetic aortic valve endocarditis include the development of high-grade atrioventricular conduction abnormalities and, in at least one series, the universal development of annular infection and ring abscesses.[67] In other series, the incidence of ring abscesses in prosthetic aortic valve endocarditis has been much less, having been reported in only 50% of patients.[66] Other complications include a relatively high incidence of embolic events and the development of ventricular or aortic aneurysms.[2]

Although mortality in prosthetic valve endocarditis is high, most studies suggest that early, aggressive therapy with bactericidal antimicrobial agents and early surgical replacement of the infected prosthesis provide the best chance of effective therapy.[66] Early reports on infective endocarditis involving porcine heterografts (Hancock valve) suggest that this valve may be resistant to early postoperative bacteremias and is probably easier to sterilize than rigid prostheses and more durable than other tissue valves in the face of endocarditis.[69]

The development of prosthetic valve dysfunction, manifested by a new regurgitant murmur, decreased intensity of opening and closing valve sounds, and abnormal "rocking" of the valve on fluoroscopic examination, is strong evidence for endocarditis in a patient in whom this diagnosis is suspected.[45]

HEMODIALYSIS AND INFECTIVE ENDOCARDITIS

As mentioned previously, experimentally produced arteriovenous fistulas in dogs predispose to the spontaneous development of infective endocarditis.[31] More recently it has become evident that arteriovenous shunts or fistulas created in patients for the purpose of hemodialysis also predispose to the development of infective endocarditis in humans.[70] Clinical experience indicates that endocarditis occurs in these patients only in the presence of endarteritis of the arteriovenous fistula. When the shunt is infected, the resultant bacteremia together with the hemodynamic stress imposed on the cardiac valves by the high-output state of renal failure and hemodialysis are responsible for the development of endocarditis. If bacteremia is documented in such patients, immediate surgical removal of the arteriovenous shunt has been recommended since it may be impossible to sterilize the blood otherwise.[71] It has been reported that the presence of peritoneovenous (Le Veen) shunts for the control of intractable ascites also poses an increased risk for the development of right-sided infective endocarditis.[72]

MITRAL VALVE PROLAPSE AND INFECTIVE ENDOCARDITIS

Mitral valve prolapse is the predisposing lesion in many patients with infective endocarditis. In the series of Corrigall and co-workers, mitral valve prolapse was present in one third of 25 consecutive patients with mitral regurgitation and infective endocarditis.[15] In a more recent report, mitral valve prolapse was the most common predisposing factor.[14] Although the risk of endocarditis for the individual patient with mitral valve prolapse is low, the importance of this lesion as a predisposing factor is due to its high prevalence; as many as 6% to 10% of the population may have various degrees of the mitral valve prolapse syndrome.[73] Therefore the possibility exists that large numbers of patients with mitral valve prolapse are at risk. With increasing awareness and recognition of the syndrome, the question of antibiotic chemoprophylaxis becomes particularly important. Although the efficacy of prophylactic therapy has not been absolutely documented, it appears prudent and reasonable to administer antibiotics during periods of potential bacteremia to those patients with evidence of mitral valve prolapse and a murmur of valvular regurgitation.

NOSOCOMIAL ENDOCARDITIS

The incidence of hospital-acquired infections has progressively increased as medical technology, including invasive vascular procedures, has expanded. Nosocomial infective endocarditis is a rare occurrence but one of great importance because of its high mortality rate and because it is potentially preventable. In a recent series, 13% of all cases of infective endocarditis treated in that particular institution were considered to be nosocomial in origin.[74] Several procedures have been identified as potential risks for the development of nosocomial endocarditis. These include urinary bladder catheterization and cystoscopy, central or peripheral venous indwelling catheter insertion, flow-directed pulmonary artery bedside catheterization, and cardiac output determinations by the thermodilution technique.[74-77] Review of recently reported cases suggests that the development of hospital-acquired endocarditis following vascular or genitourinary invasive procedures is related to improper technique, failure to administer prophylactic antibiotics during the procedure to patients with known preexisting cardiac abnormalities, leaving intravascular catheters *in situ* for prolonged periods of time, and performance of cardiac output determinations with contaminated injectate solutions. It has been shown by several autopsy studies that indwelling intravascular catheters in the right side of the heart produce traumatic, initially sterile, endocardial lesions which then become infected during an episode of transient bacteremia.

LABORATORY DIAGNOSIS
MICROBIOLOGIC STUDIES

Isolation of the infective microorganism is required for the definitive diagnosis of infective endocarditis. Furthermore, isolation of the infectious agent is important for determination of specific appropriate antimicrobial therapy. Blood cultures must be obtained before the initiation of antimicrobial treatment. An important question to be considered is how many blood cultures are usually sufficient when the diagnosis of infective endocarditis is considered before beginning antimicrobial therapy. Although it has been demonstrated that intravascular infections usually produce continuous bacteremia,[78] other studies have suggested that the bacteremia associated with infective endocarditis is qualitatively continuous, but quantitatively discontinuous,[79] that is, that organisms are always present but that their numbers vary considerably. It is therefore possible for many blood specimens to be drawn and no positive cultures to be obtained.[80] On the other hand, in well-conducted studies where three sets of blood cultures were obtained within 24 hours in patients with bacteremia, the yield was 80% in the first set of cultures, 89% in the second set, and 99% in the third set.[81] It is therefore generally agreed that three sets of blood cultures obtained within 24 hours are usually sufficient, provided the patient had not received antimicrobial therapy within two weeks.[82]

In the past, the incidence of persistently negative blood cultures in infective endocarditis was reported to be 12% to 25%.[4] The usual causes of culture-negative infective endocarditis are (1) administration of antibiotics before blood cultures are drawn; (2) poor bacteriologic techniques with reference to microorganisms with special growth requirements (e.g., anaerobic bacteria, nutritionally deficient streptococci, L forms); and (3) nonbacterial causes of endocarditis. With improvement in microbiologic techniques, the incidence of culture-negative endocarditis has declined and its most common cause remains the administration of antibiotic agents prior to the drawing of the blood specimens. It must be emphasized that blood must be inoculated into both aerobic and anaerobic media in view of the recent increase of anaerobic and microaerophilic organisms causing infective endocarditis.[83] Duration of blood culture incubation has varied, but a minimum of two weeks is recommended in order to maximize the yield of this procedure.[81,82] Blood specimens are best obtained from a peripheral vein because of its accessibility. Arterial blood cultures offer no distinct advantage over venous blood. On occasion, bone marrow cultures will be positive in the face of negative peripheral venous blood cultures.[84] Cultures of blood obtained downstream, distal, or close to the suspected valve involved also do not appear to provide any additional advantage.

OTHER LABORATORY STUDIES

The erythrocyte sedimentation rate is elevated in up to 90% of cases of infective endocarditis, but this is a nonspecific finding. However, a normal sedimentation rate becomes an important negative finding when the diagnosis of infective endocarditis is considered. A normochromic normocytic anemia may occur in up to 70% of cases and the white blood cell count may be elevated or normal. Rheumatoid factor is present in the serum of one third to one half of patients with infective endocarditis[85] and the titer decreases with appropriate antimicrobial therapy. The presence of phagocytic reticuloendothelial cells in a peripheral blood smear and teichoic acid antibodies have on occasion been of help in diagnosing infective endocarditis in patients with negative blood cultures. Intraleukocytic bacteria may be demonstrated in concentrates of venous blood in approximately 50% of patients and therefore this finding may also help confirm the diagnosis in patients with negative blood cultures.[86]

Patients with endocarditis demonstrate no specific abnormalities on the electrocardiogram. However, the electrocardiogram may be helpful in detecting and following complications such as the development of pericarditis or atrioventricular conduction abnormalities. Similarly, the electrocardiogram may be helpful in ascertaining the presence of preexisting hemodynamically significant valvular abnormalities.

ROENTGENOGRAPHY AND RADIONUCLIDE STUDIES

The chest roentgenogram does not demonstrate specific abnormalities in infective endocarditis. It is, however, a most useful technique in evaluating the complications of the disease, especially the development of congestive heart failure.[87] Many patients with acute left heart failure demonstrate inconspicuous cardiac enlargement. In these patients interstitial pulmonary edema is the most impressive finding and can be detected easily by chest radiography. In right-sided endocarditis, especially due to *Staphylococcus aureus*, the characteristic roentgenographic findings are those of septic pulmonary emboli manifested as multiple peripheral, pleural-based, frequently cavitating densities. A specific sign of septic pulmonary embolism, the target lesion, has been recently described.[88] Fluoroscopy and cinefluorography may be helpful in identifying prosthetic valve dysfunction. Excessive motion of the prosthetic valve ring implies partial detachment from the valve annulus. Incomplete excursion of radiopaque prosthetic valve elements suggests invasion of the prosthesis by thrombus or vegetations.[87] It is of course necessary for the physician performing the examination to be familiar with the normal appearance and motion of the prosthetic valve in order that abnormalities may be appreciated.

Recently, radionuclide studies have been applied to the diagnosis of infective endocarditis. It has been reported that gallium-67 citrate will concentrate in portions of the myocardium and endocardium involved in the infectious process. Of 11 patients with the clinical diagnosis of infective endocarditis, 7 demonstrated positive scans 3 to 8 days following the injection of the radioisotopic tracer.[89] The disadvantages of this test include insufficient resolution, the length of time required for localization of the radionuclide, and a 40% incidence of false negative results presumably due to the small mass of involved tissue.[90] Although technetium pyrophosphate scan has been reported to demonstrate the vegetations in experimental endocarditis, the clinical application of this technique has not been established.

ECHOCARDIOGRAPHY

Since the original report of Dillon and associates in 1973 regarding the utility of echocardiography in the detection of valvular vegetations,[91] this technique has assumed progressively greater importance in the diagnosis, management, and follow-up of infective endocarditis. It is now generally agreed that two-dimensional (cross-sectional) echocardiography is superior to M-mode techniques in evaluating patients with infective endocarditis.[92-99] The advantages of two-dimensional echocardiography include (1) increased sensitivity in diagnosing the presence of valvular vegetations; (2) improved visualization of extravalvular extension of the infection (e.g., perivalvular abscesses)[98]; (3) greatly improved visualization of the tricuspid and pulmonic valves[94] as well as the right ventricle; and (4) more accurate measurement of vegetation size. Notwithstanding the above, M-mode echocardiography is a useful complementary technique that offers advantages over two-dimensional echocardiography particularly in the area of precise chamber dimension measurements and functional evaluation of regurgitant lesions.

IDENTIFICATION OF VALVULAR VEGETATIONS

Vegetations appear on M-mode echocardiography as characteristically fuzzy echoes in the region of the affected valve. Improper gain settings of the echocardiography may produce artifacts that may be falsely interpreted as vegetations. On two-dimensional presentation, vegetations appear as echo-dense, sessile, or pedunculated masses of variable dimensions that appear to be attached to the valve leaflet involved (Fig. 86.6). Frequently aortic valve vegetations prolapse in the left ventricular outflow tract, mitral valve vegetations are seen to cross the plane of the mitral valve annulus with each cardiac cycle, and tricuspid valve vegetations are seen to prolapse deep in the right ventricular cavity. Current information suggests that two-dimensional echocardiography can detect valvular vegetations in more than 50% of patients with infective endocarditis and in some series this rate is 80%.[93] The sensitivity of M-mode echocardiography alone is considerably less, perhaps 30% to 40% of all patients with endocarditis.[99] The dimensions of vegetations influence the detection rate. Although calcified lesions as small as 1 mm can be detected, there is general agreement that the vegetation must measure at least 2 mm to 3 mm to be reliably visualized on echocardiographic studies.[100] The size of visualized vegetations has important prognostic information. Despite considerable disagreement in published studies, my experience and that of others suggest that large vegetations (greater than 10 mm) are associated with a higher incidence of congestive heart failure, systemic embolization, and valvular surgery.[101,102] Fungal endocarditis has been classically described as causing large vegetations. Recent studies, however, suggest that large vegetations are produced by the same infective organisms as smaller vegetations[101] and therefore the presence of a large vegetation cannot be considered diagnostic of fungal endocarditis.

CONFIRMATION OF DIAGNOSIS

Patients with tricuspid or pulmonic valve endocarditis frequently present with fever and pulmonary symptoms but with a paucity of cardiac findings. The murmurs associated with tricuspid and pulmonic regurgitation may be atypical or totally absent on initial presentation.[103] The identification of a tricuspid or pulmonic valve vegetation in a septic patient therefore provides valuable information and confirms the diagnosis. Similarly, patients with acute severe aortic regurgitation may present without the usual peripheral findings (i.e., wide pulse pressure). In this setting, the documentation of fluttering of the anterior mitral valve leaflet on M-mode echocardiography will strongly suggest the presence of aortic regurgitation that might otherwise have been missed.

FUNCTIONAL ASSESSMENT OF VALVULAR REGURGITATION

Early mitral valve closure has been described as an indicator of acute severe aortic regurgitation. In at least one study, all patients with mitral valve closure preceding the onset of the QRS complex due to acute aortic regurgitation secondary to endocarditis required surgical replacement of the infected valve because of hemodynamic deterioration.[104]

IDENTIFICATION OF THE EXTRAVALVULAR INFECTION

Extension of the infectious process beyond the confines of the involved valve may occur in up to 30% of patients, especially when the aortic valve is infected. The presence of this complication is known to be associated with a higher mortality and a more fulminant course. The identification, therefore, of perivalvular abscesses is important from both the prognostic and management standpoint. Two-dimensional echocardiography has been recently shown to be a useful technique in identifying this complication.[98] Although the sensitivity of this technique has not been studied, experience suggests that to date it is the best technique available, possibly better than selective angiography. The proposed criteria for diagnosing an aortic perivalvular abscess are (1) rocking of the prosthetic valve ring; (2) the presence of sinus of Valsalva aneurysm; (3) anterior or posterior aortic root thickness of 10 mm or greater; and (4) the presence of a perivalvular density in association with an interventricular septal thickness of 14 mm or greater. In addition to identifying perivalvular abscesses, two-dimensional echocardiography has been found to be useful in following the stability of such lesions over a prolonged period of time[95] and in identifying more remote extravalvular complications (e.g., mycotic aortic aneurysms and satellite vegetations).[105,106]

More recently, transesophageal two-dimensional and Doppler echocardiography has been found to extend the sensitivity of ultrasound studies in detecting abnormalities of the aortic root. Most studies reported to date deal with the value of this technique in detecting aortic dissection,[107] with intraoperative monitoring of left ventricular function, and with adequacy of repair of complex congenital cardiac defects.[108] In our hands, however, transesophageal echocardiography has proven to be an invaluable tool in assessing the presence of aortic annular abscesses (Fig. 86.7), fistulous tracts, septal excavations, and perivalvular leaks. The success of this technique has been such that we consider transesophageal echocardiography the preferred method of imaging the aortic root and aortic annulus in cases of aortic valve endocarditis.

EVALUATION OF BIOPROSTHETIC VALVES

Bioprosthetic cardiac valves are subject to dysfunction because of primary tissue failure, dehiscence of the valve ring, development of thrombus, or involvement by an infectious process. Two-dimensional echocardiography has been helpful in identifying bioprosthetic valve dysfunction.[97] Findings of valve dysfunction include (1) a discordant motion of the valve ring; (2) increased size of the bioprosthetic leaflet image (seen in 62% of cases due to endocarditis); and (3) prolapse of leaflet echoes either below the level of the bioprosthetic sewing ring or antegradely beyond the level of the stents, implying leaflet tear. Unfortunately, the echocardiographic appearance of bioprosthetic valve dysfunction often does not distinguish primary leaflet degeneration from infection.

CARDIAC CATHETERIZATION AND ANGIOCARDIOGRAPHY

Cardiac catheterization and selective angiocardiography are studies that are frequently employed to define precisely the anatomical abnormalities and hemodynamic aberrations in patients with infective endocarditis and congestive heart failure severe enough for surgery to be considered. These invasive procedures have been of greatest value in multivalvular left heart lesions or when myocardial, pericardial, or pulmonary disease coexists and when it is necessary to delineate associated extravalvular infection accurately.[109] Cineangiography is probably the most useful diagnostic procedure. In one study, among patients

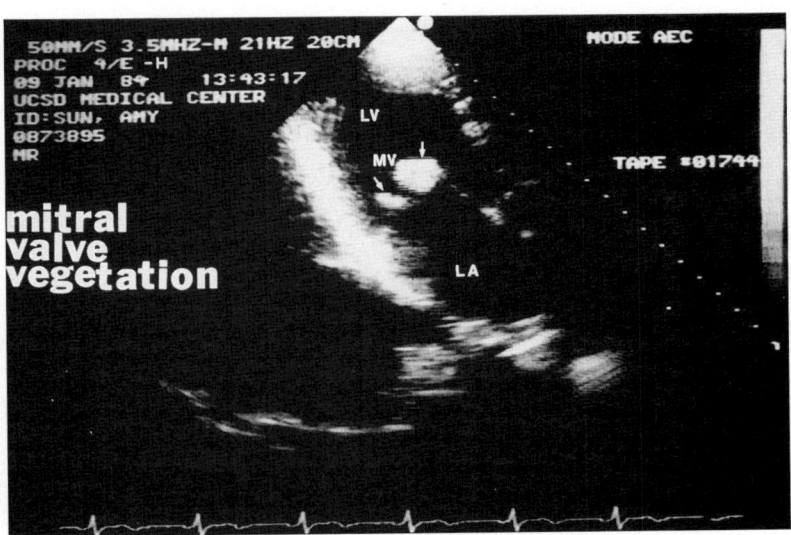

FIGURE 86.6 Two-dimensional echocardiographic (parasternal long axis view) presentation of large streptococcal vegetations involving both mitral leaflets (arrows). Despite the size of the vegetations, this patient has followed a chronic course and remains compensated three years after the episode of endocarditis. (From the Echocardiography Laboratory, University of California, San Diego; courtesy of K. L. Peterson, M.D., and Ms. Nancy Dalton)

in whom valvular involvement was uncertain, cineangiography correctly identified each occurrence of significant valvular insufficiency.[109] Supravalvular aortic root angiography can help identify such extravalvular lesions as aneurysmal erosions of the aortic root, sinus of Valsalva aneurysms, and fistulous tracts through the interventricular septum. Mills and co-workers reported that angiography failed to identify 50% of the aortic root abnormalities subsequently discovered at surgery[109]; however, in a later study Hosenpud and Greenberg demonstrated angiography to have 83% sensitivity and 100% specificity in evaluating myocardial invasion (abscess formation).[110] It is generally agreed that patients with isolated, clear-cut mitral regurgitation probably do not require invasive diagnostic procedures, although an occasional unsuspected mitral valve annular abscess may be discovered by this type of a study when clinical and echocardiographic examinations are unrevealing (Fig. 86.8).

In general, the risk of cardiac catheterization and angiocardiography in patients with active endocarditis is acceptably low and does not differ significantly from the risk of comparably ill patients without intravascular infection.[111] The usual risks quoted include aggravation of severe congestive heart failure related to the administration of contrast media and systemic embolization due to fragmentation of friable vegetations dislodged by the catheter manipulation. The first of these risks

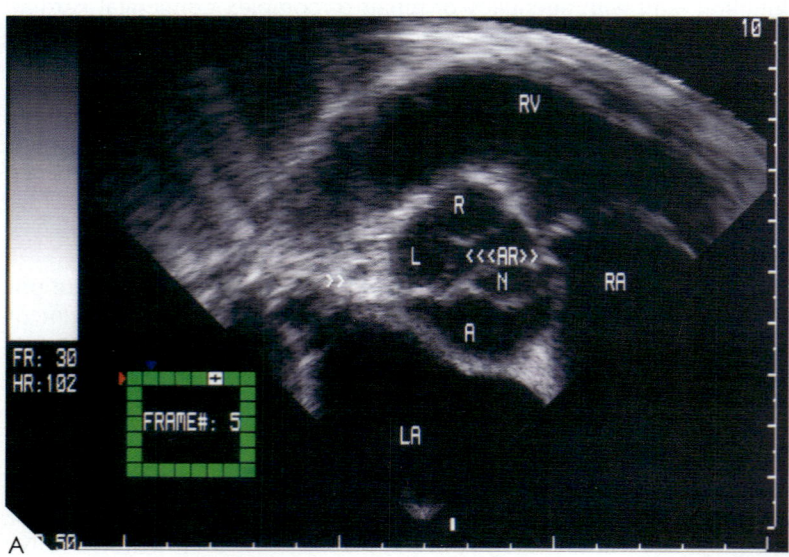

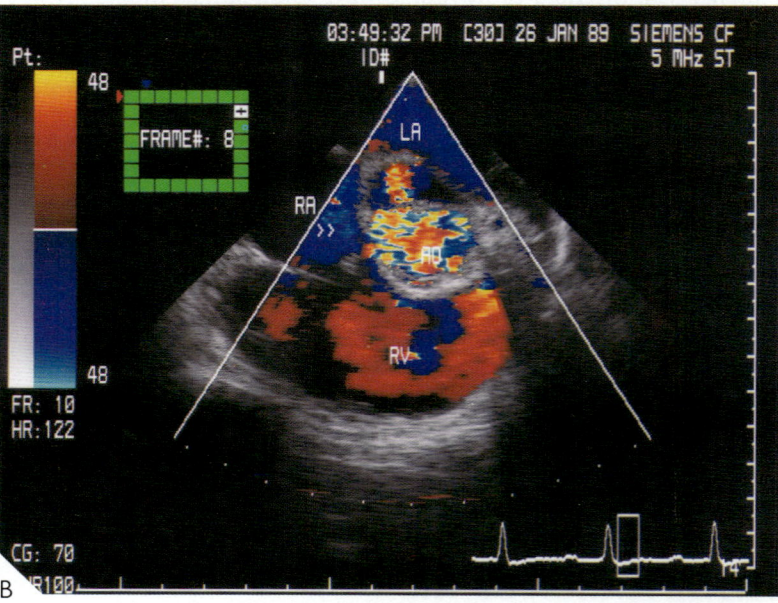

FIGURE 86.7 Two still frames of two-dimensional and color-flow Doppler transesophageal echocardiographic study from a patient with aortic valve endocarditis and annular involvement. (**A**) Echolucent space labeled A is seen posterior to the left (L) and noncoronary (N) sinuses of Valsalva. This abscess/aneurysm distorts the cusps and prevents coaptation thereby producing regurgitation (area marked AR). Other structures identified: right coronary sinus (R), right atrium (RA), left atrium (LA), right ventricle (RV). (**B,** inverted image) With the addition of color-flow Doppler the area of communication between the aortic lumen (AO) and the abscess is visualized; a high-velocity jet (mosaic) is seen to originate from the junction of the left and noncoronary sinuses and extend into the abscess/aneurysm center. (From the Echocardiography Laboratory, University of California, Davis Medical Center. Courtesy of Dr. William Bommer)

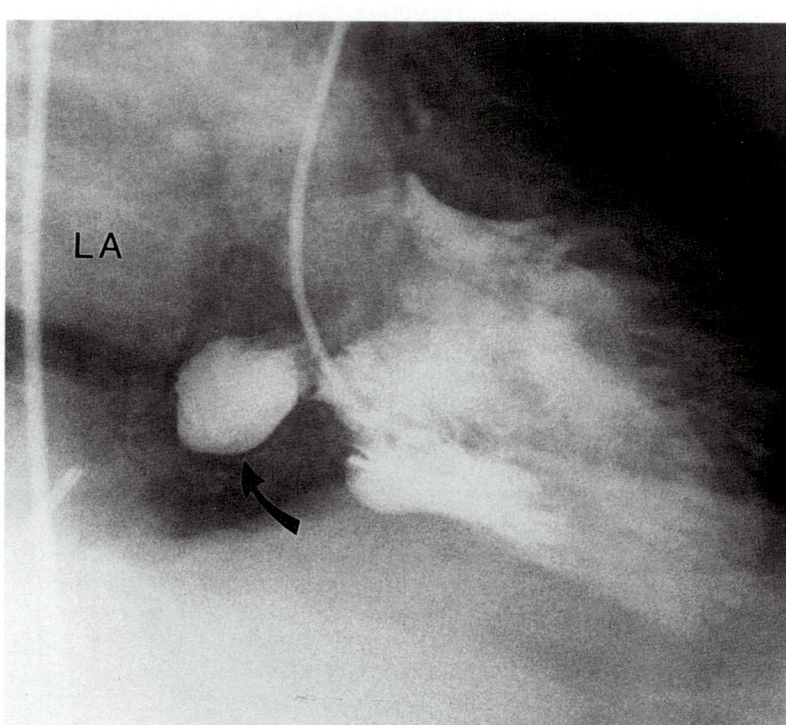

FIGURE 86.8 End-diastolic frame of a selective left ventricular cineangiogram from a patient with hypertrophic cardiomyopathy and *Streptococcus bovis* endocarditis of the mitral valve. The left atrium (LA) is opacified due to mitral regurgitation. The globular density (*curved arrow*) represents opacification of an annular abscess. This was confirmed at surgery and had not been detected by echocardiography.

can be minimized by keeping the volume of contrast media administered low and by being prepared to support the failing circulation in a standard fashion. The risk of embolization appears to be low and can be further minimized by not passing the catheter across an infected valve. In fact, crossing of an infected tricuspid valve with a balloon flotation catheter for a right heart catheterization has not been associated with recognizable episodes of pulmonary embolism in over 20 cases studied by the author.

Right heart catheterization has been employed to confirm and quantitate the degree of heart failure through measurement of pulmonary artery wedge pressure and cardiac output. In general, it appears that this may not be a valid reason for performing a right heart catheterization since clinical and echocardiographic studies can diagnose congestive heart failure with high sensitivity and specificity.[110] Additionally, cardiac catheterization has been used to help localize the infectious involvement of a valve that may be producing minimal or no physical findings. Intracardiac phonocardiography and indicator dilution studies have been used to good advantage, and, according to some investigators, quantitative cultures of blood samples taken from sites proximal and distal to the tricuspid and pulmonic valve at the time of catheterization may be of value in localizing the infection.[112,113] False localization of the site of infective endocarditis by this technique has been reported and was probably due to the presence of intermittent rather than continuous bacteremia.[114]

Current medical practice is to perform preoperative catheterization and angiography in the patient with infective endocarditis when the accuracy of the clinical and noninvasive assessment is in question. This position is supported by the potentially disastrous consequences of referring a patient to cardiac surgery with an erroneous or incomplete diagnosis.

TREATMENT
GENERAL PRINCIPLES

In considering the therapy of infective endocarditis, it is important to classify cases into two groups: (1) patients with uncomplicated streptococcal endocarditis and (2) patients with complicated disease. Patients should be placed in the *uncomplicated* group if their infection is caused by *Streptococcus viridans*, *Streptococcus bovis*, or *Streptococcus faecalis*, all organisms relatively sensitive to penicillin. In addition, there should be no evidence of hemodynamically significant valvular disease. Generally, prognosis in this group is good with 90% to 97% bacteriologic cure with four weeks of therapy. Organisms do not become resistant during therapy, and treatment regimens have been standardized for years and have been well tested and accepted. Disc diffusion studies are usually adequate to guide the clinician as to therapy, and elaborate serum bactericidal tests are not usually required. On the other hand, patients should be classified in the *complicated* group if the causative organism is a staphylococcus, a fungus, or a gram-negative bacterium, or when one is dealing with "culture-negative" endocarditis. Additionally, patients with intracardiac prostheses, those allergic to indicated antibiotics, narcotic users, and pregnant women should be placed in the complicated group because of the frequently poor outcome. Finally, all patients with heart failure, renal failure, distal embolization, mycotic aneurysm, intracerebral abscess, or aortic annular involvement also should be classified in the complicated group. The prognosis of the complicated group is uncertain, with only 20% to 80% bacteriologic cure having been reported in various series.[2,4,5,10,45,115] The organisms commonly involved in this group may become resistant during therapy, and therapeutic regimens are not well standardized. Special microbiologic techniques and special sensitivity studies are often necessary as a guide to therapy, and prolonged periods of treatment may be required. Cardiovascular surgery support is often necessary to achieve cure and/or treat complications. It is therefore evident that whereas patients with uncomplicated infective endocarditis can be effectively treated in almost any well-staffed facility with an adequate microbiologic laboratory, patients with complicated disease are best treated in a tertiary referral center where sophisticated microbiologic and surgical consultative services are available.

Several general principles must be kept in mind when treating patients with infective endocarditis. (1) Early establishment of microbiologic diagnosis is crucial along with early and accurate assessment of the susceptibility of the isolated organism to various antibiotic agents. (2) The early institution of empiric antimicrobial therapy is necessary in patients with acute fulminant infective endocarditis. In this setting, antimicrobial therapy should be instituted immediately after three sets of blood cultures have been obtained at 10- to 15-minute intervals. The selection of an empiric regimen is discussed below. (3) Early consultation with a cardiac surgeon is desirable for patients with aortic valve endocarditis or patients with a valvular prosthesis even though initially they may not be hemodynamically compromised. (4) Within 48 hours after initiation of antibiotic therapy, repeat blood cultures should be obtained to assess the efficacy of treatment. Persistently positive blood cultures despite appropriate antimicrobial chemotherapy may indicate the presence of extravalvular infection, erroneous sensitivity studies, or errors in the administration and dosage of the antimicrobial agent. (5) Daily physical examinations should be performed without failure since subtle changes may precede abrupt hemodynamic catastrophes. (6) Current practice indicates that antimicrobial chemotherapy should be administered parenterally in a hospital setting, since absorption of orally administered antibiotics may be unpredictable and compliance always in question. Exceptions to this rule have been reported and are discussed below. (7) Patients should be examined in search for the portal of entry. Especially the oral cavity should be carefully investigated and patients should have dental x-ray studies and a consultation with an oral surgeon so that necessary dental work can be performed while the patient is receiving therapy for endocarditis. Patients with infective endocarditis caused by *Streptococcus bovis* should undergo sigmoidoscopy and barium enema examination of the colon during the course of therapy. The specific antimicrobial regimens currently recommended for treatment of the more common forms of endocarditis are listed in Table 86.6.

TABLE 86.6 SUGGESTED ANTIBIOTIC THERAPY REGIMENS FOR INFECTIVE ENDOCARDITIS IN ADULTS

Streptococcus viridans* and *Streptococcus bovis
1. Aqueous penicillin G, 10–20 million units/day IV in divided doses q4h for 4 weeks
2. Aqueous penicillin G as above plus streptomycin, 0.5 g IM q12h for initial 2 weeks
3. Procaine penicillin G, 1.2 million units IM q6h for 4 weeks plus streptomycin as above

Enterococci
1. Aqueous penicillin G, 20–40 million units/day IV in divided doses, or ampicillin, 12 g/day IV, plus streptomycin, 0.5 g IM q12h, or gentamicin 1 mg/kg IV q8h for 4–6 weeks
2. Vancomycin, 0.5 g q6h IV (for patients allergic to penicillin) plus streptomycin or gentamicin as above for 4–6 weeks

Staphylococcus aureus
1. If penicillin-sensitive, aqueous penicillin G, 20 million units IV in divided doses q4h for 4–6 weeks
2. If penicillin-resistant, nafcillin or oxacillin, 1.5 to 2.0 g IV q4h for 6 weeks
3. If methicillin-resistant, vancomycin, 0.5 g q6h IV for 6 weeks

Staphylococcus epidermidis
1. Methicillin-susceptible, same as *S. aureus*, 2, above
2. Methicillin-resistant, vancomycin, 0.5 g q6h IV, plus rifampin, 300 mg PO q8h for 6 weeks

STREPTOCOCCAL ENDOCARDITIS

Streptococcus viridans and *Streptococcus bovis* are organisms that are usually highly sensitive to penicillin as evidenced by a zone of inhibition of 30 mm or more surrounding a 10-μg penicillin disc or a minimum inhibitory concentration (MIC) of less than 0.1 unit. Despite this high degree of penicillin sensitivity, streptomycin or gentamicin are frequently added to the regimen because of experimental evidence showing that the combination of penicillin and an aminoglycoside antibiotic is synergistic against penicillin-sensitive organisms both *in vitro* and *in vivo*.[116] The various antibiotic regimens recommended for this disease are noted in Table 86.6. Gray states that for naturally occurring endocarditis due to *S. viridans* sensitive to penicillin, oral amoxicillin and probenecid constitute the regimen of choice and case reports supporting this assertion have recently appeared in the literature.[117,118] However, until more information is gained, parenteral therapy for a minimal period of two weeks followed by oral therapy for an additional two weeks is indicated.

ENTEROCOCCAL ENDOCARDITIS

Streptococcus faecalis organisms generally demonstrate "intermediate sensitivity" to penicillin by disc testing. The combination of penicillin and streptomycin is most effective in treating this organism because of its demonstrated synergism. It is generally agreed that aqueous penicillin should be given in doses of 20 million units daily intravenously combined with streptomycin, 0.5 g to 1.0 g, intramuscularly twice daily for a minimum period of four weeks. In some cases, a 6-week course of therapy may be necessary. If the organism is relatively resistant to streptomycin, gentamicin or tobramycin should be used. Ampicillin may be substituted for penicillin in this regimen because enterococci are more sensitive *in vitro* to this agent than to penicillin. However, ampicillin alone cannot be relied on to cure *S. faecalis* endocarditis and therefore an aminoglycoside agent should still be used. Despite the *in vitro* observations, the results of therapy have been equally good with both regimens and currently there is no evidence to recommend ampicillin over penicillin.[115,116]

STAPHYLOCOCCAL ENDOCARDITIS

Patients with disease due to *Staphylococcus aureus* are often acutely ill and clearly fall in the complicated group. The antibiotic agents of choice are the penicillinase-resistant penicillins (methicillin, nafcillin, or oxacillin). Despite differences of *in vitro* activity, protein binding, and other pharmacodynamics, all three agents listed above have proven to be equally effective in the treatment of staphylococcal endocarditis in both the experimental animal and in clinical practice.[119] Nafcillin and oxacillin are preferred because of the occasional development of interstitial nephritis with methicillin therapy. Treatment should be continued for a minimum of four weeks, and in many instances six weeks will be required. Relapses may occur and must be retreated. The development of a relapse in staphylococcal endocarditis should strongly suggest the presence of myocardial abscesses or other extravalvular extension of infection. Vancomycin is the agent of second choice and can be used both in patients allergic to penicillin and in those with semisynthetic penicillin-resistant staphylococcal infections.[116] Both cephalosporins and clindamycin also have been used successfully to treat staphylococcal endocarditis in selected cases.

CULTURE-NEGATIVE INFECTIVE ENDOCARDITIS

In the usual patient with infective endocarditis and negative blood cultures, it is common practice to direct initial therapy against *Streptococcus faecalis* and use regimens as outlined above. Exceptions to this general rule include narcotic addicts, the postoperative cardiosurgical patient, and patients with an acute fulminant septic course. In these three situations, a regimen consisting of an aminoglycoside antibiotic and a semisynthetic penicillin must be used until the microorganism is positively identified.[45]

PROSTHETIC VALVE ENDOCARDITIS

The difficulties inherent in treating infections of foreign body implants are well recognized.[69] Treatment of prosthetic valve endocarditis, irrespective of the infective organism, is prolonged and requires large doses of antimicrobial agents frequently in combination regimens and a combined "team approach" to include specialists in infectious disease, cardiology, nephrology, and cardiovascular surgery. Available data suggest that early aggressive bactericidal antimicrobial therapy alone or in combination with early surgery can successfully cure a substantial number of patients.[69] Surgical removal of the prosthesis may be necessary in cases where the infective organism is a fungus, when the infection relapses despite adequate antimicrobial therapy, or if there is major embolization or evidence of prosthetic valve malfunction.[25]

ALLERGY TO PENICILLIN

Patients with documented allergy to penicillin present a difficult therapeutic problem because the alternative agents are generally less effective than the penicillin–aminoglycoside combinations commonly used. History of penicillin allergy, however, is often unsubstantiated and the so-called allergy is either insignificant or nonexistent. Skin testing should be undertaken and should definite penicillin allergy exist, the clinician has the choice of either desensitizing the patient (a minimally risky procedure) or preferably substituting another effective antimicrobial agent. The concurrent administration of corticosteroids to suppress the hypersensitivity reaction in allergic patients cannot be recommended.

FUNGAL ENDOCARDITIS

Amphotericin B has been demonstrated to be an effective agent in the treatment of infections caused by several varieties of yeasts and fungi. However, there has been a high incidence of primary drug failures in treating native and prosthetic valve endocarditis with amphotericin B alone.[120] Current concepts suggest the need for surgical removal of the infected valve and continuation of amphotericin B chemotherapy for a period of 6 to 8 weeks. Valve resection without prosthetic replacement has been recommended for fungal tricuspid endocarditis but has not gained widespread acceptance due to the frequently intolerable hemodynamic burden it places on the right heart.[121] Amphotericin B can be administered in accordance to one of several different regimens. Administration is usually begun at a level of 0.25 mg/kg on day one and then the dosage is increased by 0.25 mg/kg each day until a dose of 1 mg/kg to 1.5 mg/kg a day is achieved. In order to minimize the venous sclerosing and other unpleasant drug side effects, an alternate-day regimen has been recommended with the individual daily dose not to exceed 90 mg.[122] Two new antifungal agents have been recently made available: 5-flucytosine and ketoconazole. The exact role that these agents will play in the therapy of fungal endocarditis remains to be determined.

SURGICAL MANAGEMENT

Congestive heart failure due to the development of acute aortic regurgitation continues to be the leading cause of death from infective endocarditis.[2,104] Patients developing pulmonary edema during the active phase of left-sided endocarditis have a particularly poor prognosis on medical therapy alone; the mortality associated with this complication has been reported to range from 50% to 80%.[123,124] For these reasons, early operative treatment with replacement of the incompetent valve has been advocated and extensively studied during the past ten years.[104,125-130] Gratifying reductions in mortality have been documented ranging from 8% to 28% when valve replacement was undertaken during the active phase of the infection[129,130] and as low as 0% for valve replacement during the inactive phase of endocarditis.[130]

Pulmonic and tricuspid valve resection without valve replacement has been advocated and utilized in cases of right-sided endocarditis caused by organisms relatively resistant to antimicrobial chemotherapy. *Pseudomonas aeruginosa* and fungi were the common organisms isolated in these cases.[121] It has been reported that an otherwise normally functioning right ventricle tolerates the presence of tricuspid or pulmonic insufficiency well.[131] However, late right ventricular failure occurs and current thinking suggests that maintaining tricuspid valve competence by insertion of a prosthesis is hemodynamically preferable.[128]

Other indications for early surgery in infective endocarditis include recurrent embolization, uncontrolled sepsis despite adequate antimicrobial chemotherapy, fungal infection, the development of extravalvular complications (conduction defects or pericarditis), and the development of prosthetic valve dysfunction. DiNubile has recently reviewed in detail the role of surgery and has proposed major and minor criteria for early surgical intervention.[132] He suggests that the presence of one major criterion mandates early surgical intervention whereas the presence of two or three minor criteria necessitates serious consideration of operative therapy. Table 86.7 lists a slightly modified version of these recommendations.

PREVENTION

Prophylactic antimicrobial therapy is commonly prescribed for the prevention of infective endocarditis in susceptible patients.[30] The rationale for this practice rests on numerous studies that have documented the occurrence of transient bacteremia after a variety of procedures including dental treatments and surgical procedures or instrumentations involving mucosal surfaces or contaminated tissue.[30] Furthermore, recent studies have confirmed the fact that pretreatment of patients with antimicrobial drugs markedly reduces the incidence and extent of postprocedure bacteremia.[133] It has therefore become accepted medical practice to administer antibiotic chemoprophylaxis to susceptible patients (see Table 86.1) for procedures with the potential for developing transient bacteremia (Table 86.8).

Although the effectiveness of antibiotic prophylaxis for endocarditis has not been absolutely documented,[134] the American Heart Association has proposed specific recommendations and antimicrobial chemotherapeutic regimens.[135] A summary of the current recommendations of the American Heart Association is listed in Tables 86.9 and 86.10.

Recent evidence suggests that the risk of developing infective endocarditis from transient bacteremia is low especially in such conditions as mitral valve prolapse.[136] Apparent failures of prophylactic regimens have been reported[14] and serious problems exist with patient compliance to recommended antibiotic regimens despite meticulous instructions.[137] The above notwithstanding, the potential complications and sequelae of infective endocarditis are of such gravity that vigorous adherence to the current American Heart Association recommendations is strongly advised.

CLINICAL IMPLICATIONS

Infective endocarditis is a potentially lethal disease that affects primarily patients with preexisting structural cardiac defects and, today, intravenous drug abusers. Transient bacteremia is the initiating event and the disease may be prevented by adequate antimicrobial prophylaxis.

The disease takes the form of either an acute fulminant sepsis or a more chronic/subacute process. In general (but not always), the infective microorganism is responsible for the acuteness of the disease. Thus, streptococcal infections tend to pursue a slow, indolent course whereas infections with more pathogenic organisms such as *Staphylococcus aureus* tend to pursue a more fulminant course. Subacute endocarditis frequently presents with nonspecific symptoms such as low-grade fever, headache, and nonspecific musculoskeletal complaints. Acute endocarditis often presents with rigors and high fever. Infective disease must be seriously considered in all patients with *S.*

TABLE 86.7 CRITERIA FOR SURGERY IN INFECTIVE ENDOCARDITIS

Major Criteria
Congestive heart failure, progressive or unresponsive to "simple" measures
Recurrent systemic emboli
Persistent bacteremia despite adequate antibiotic therapy
Fungal etiology
Extravalvular infection (atrioventricular block, purulent pericarditis)
Prosthetic valve dehiscence or obstruction
Recurrence of infection despite adequate therapy

Minor Criteria
Congestive heart failure, resolved with medical therapy
Single systemic embolic event
Large aortic or mitral vegetations on echocardiography
Premature mitral valve closure in acute aortic insufficiency
Flail valvular leaflet(s)
Prosthetic valve infection due to organisms other than highly penicillin-sensitive streptococci
Tricuspid endocarditis due to gram-negative bacilli
Persistent fever without other identifiable cause
New regurgitation in an aortic prosthesis
Lack of appropriate cell wall antibiotics

(Adapted from DiNubile MJ: Surgery in active endocarditis. Ann Intern Med 96:950, 1982)

TABLE 86.8 PROCEDURES REQUIRING PROPHYLACTIC ANTIBIOTICS

All dental procedures likely to induce gingival bleeding (not simple adjustment of orthodontic appliances or shedding of deciduous teeth)
Tonsillectomy and/or adenoidectomy
Surgical procedures or biopsy involving respiratory mucosa
Bronchoscopy, especially with a rigid bronchoscope*
Incision and drainage of infected tissue
Certain genitourinary and gastrointestinal procedures

(Shulman ST, Amren DP, Bisno AL et al: Prevention of bacterial endocarditis: A statement for health professionals by the Committee on Rheumatic Fever and Infective Endocarditis of the Council on Cardiovascular Disease in the young. Circulation 70:1123A, 1984. Reproduced with permission. © Prevention of Bacterial Endocarditis. American Heart Association)

* The risk with flexible bronchoscopy is low, but the necessity for prophylaxis is not yet defined.

aureus bacteremia even if signs of valvular involvement are absent. Rapid destruction of valve leaflets and extension of the infection beyond the confines of the valve involved are the hallmarks of acute endocarditis caused by *S. aureus*. Numerous other microorganisms can cause infections of the endocardium and endothelium, including yeasts and fungi as well as gram-negative bacilli. In general, disease due to the less common microorganisms is seen in narcotic drug addicts and in patients who are immunosuppressed or have had recent open heart surgery.

The clinical findings of endocarditis depend on the extent of cardiovascular tissue involvement. From 20% to 40% of patients with this disease will have evidence of cutaneous embolic events and hematuria due to either renal embolization or immune complex glomerulonephritis. The development of a pericardial friction rub or a new atrioventricular conduction abnormality in a patient with aortic valve infection strongly suggests the presence of an aortic ring abscess with extension of the infection in the interventricular septum or partial rupture into the pericardial sac. Patients with prosthetic valves are particularly prone to develop major complications from endocarditis. Infection of an aortic valve prosthesis is associated with a high incidence of annular abscesses and valve dehiscence whereas infection of a mitral valve prosthesis is frequently complicated by valve obstruction due to a combination of vegetations and thrombus.

The diagnosis of endocarditis, once the disease is suspected, depends on the isolation of the infective microorganism from the blood. At least three blood cultures should be obtained before the onset of antibiotic chemotherapy. Both aerobic and anaerobic cultures are required since the incidence of anaerobic and microaerophilic streptococci is increasing. Patients who are acutely ill and who are suspected of harboring *S. aureus* should be treated as soon as blood cultures have been obtained before cultural identification of the organism has been accomplished. Elevation of the erythrocyte sedimentation rate can be expected in about 90% of patients with infective endocarditis and, although a nonspecific finding, is useful in making the diagnosis. Echocardiography (especially two-dimensional) is an important adjunct in diagnosing endocarditis by visualizing valvular vegetations in as many as 80% of patients with this disease. In addition, echocardiography is most useful in assessing the functional significance of acute aortic regurgitation (early mitral valve closure) and in diagnosing extension of the infection beyond the confines of the involved valve.

TABLE 86.9 PROPHYLACTIC ANTIBIOTIC REGIMENS FOR DENTAL AND RESPIRATORY TRACT PROCEDURES

Standard Regimen	
For dental procedures that cause gingival bleeding, and oral/respiratory tract surgery	Penicillin V 2.0 g orally one hour before, then 1.0 g six hours later. For patients unable to take oral medications, 2 million units of aqueous penicillin G IV or IM 30–60 minutes before a procedure and 1 million units six hours later may be substituted
Special Regimens	
Parenteral regimen for use when maximal protection desired (*e.g.*, for patients with prosthetic valves)	Ampicillin 1.0 g–2.0 g IM or IV plus gentamicin 1.5 mg/kg IM or IV, one-half hour before procedure, followed by 1.0 g oral penicillin V six hours later. Alternatively, the parenteral regimen may be repeated once eight hours later
Oral regimen for penicillin-allergic patients	Erythromycin 1.0 g orally one hour before, then 500 mg six hours later
Parenteral regimen for penicillin-allergic patients	Vancomycin 1.0 g IV slowly over one hour, starting one hour before. No repeat dose is necessary

Note: Pediatric doses: ampicillin 50 mg/kg per dose; erythromycin 20 mg/kg for first dose, then 10 mg/kg; gentamicin 2.0 mg/kg per dose; penicillin V full adult dose if greater than 60 lb (27 kg), one-half adult dose if less than 60 lb (27 kg); aqueous penicillin G 50,000 units/kg (25,000 units/kg for follow-up); vancomycin 20 mg/kg per dose. The intervals between doses are the same as for adults. Total doses should not exceed adult doses.

(Shulman ST, Amren DP, Bisno AL et al: Prevention of bacterial endocarditis: A statement for health professionals by the Committee on Rheumatic Fever and Infective Endocarditis of the Council on Cardiovascular Disease in the young. Circulation 70:1123A, 1984. Reproduced with permission. © Prevention of Bacterial Endocarditis. American Heart Association)

TABLE 86.10 PROPHYLACTIC ANTIBIOTIC REGIMENS FOR GASTROINTESTINAL AND GENITOURINARY PROCEDURES

Standard Regimen	
For genitourinary/gastrointestinal tract procedures listed in the text	Ampicillin 2.0 g IM or IV plus gentamicin 1.5 mg/kg IM or IV, given one-half to one hour before procedure. One follow-up dose may be given eight hours later
Special Regimens	
Oral regimen for minor or repetitive procedures in low-risk patients	Amoxicillin 3.0 g orally one hour before procedure and 1.5 g six hours later
Penicillin-allergic patients	Vancomycin 1.0 g IV slowly over one hour, plus gentamicin 1.5 mg/kg IM or IV given one hour before procedure. May be repeated once 8–12 hours later

Note: Pediatric doses: ampicillin 50 mg/kg per dose; gentamicin 2.0 mg/kg per dose; amoxicillin 50 mg/kg per dose; vancomycin 20 mg/kg per dose. The intervals between doses are the same as for adults. Total doses should not exceed adult doses.

(Shulman ST, Amren DP, Bisno AL et al: Prevention of bacterial endocarditis: A statement for health professionals by the Committee on Rheumatic Fever and Infective Endocarditis of the Council on Cardiovascular Disease in the young. Circulation 70:1123A, 1984. Reproduced with permission. © Prevention of Bacterial Endocarditis. American Heart Association)

Therapy will depend on the infective microorganism. In general, penicillin-sensitive streptococcal endocarditis should be treated with parenteral penicillin, 10 to 20 million units daily for a minimum of four weeks. Enterococcal endocarditis is treated with a minimum of 20 million units penicillin daily combined with either streptomycin or gentamicin for a period of four to six weeks. *S. aureus* endocarditis is most often treated with a semisynthetic penicillin (nafcillin or oxacillin) in doses of 12 g daily for a period of four to six weeks. Treatment regimens of other organisms will depend on their sensitivity to the antibiotic agents.

Early surgery with valve replacement is currently advocated for cases of infective endocarditis with associated severe heart failure, recurrent embolization, persistent bacteremia despite adequate therapy, and for those cases with evidence of extravalvular extension of the infection. Patients with prosthetic valve endocarditis and those with fungal infections will almost always require removal of the infected valve.

The prognosis of infective endocarditis has improved over the past three decades. Bacteriologic cure may be expected in up to 90% of patients with streptococcal endocarditis of a native valve without the requirement for surgery. Staphylococcal endocarditis cure rates vary from 40% to 80% with combined antibiotic and surgical therapy. Patients with multivalvular involvement and especially intravenous drug abusers have the worst prognosis.

REFERENCES

1. Brandenburg RO, Giuliani ER, Wilson WR, Geraci JE: Infective endocarditis: A 25 year overview of diagnosis and therapy. J Am Coll Cardiol 1:280, 1983
2. Weinstein L, Rubin RH: Infective endocarditis—1973. Prog Cardiovasc Dis 16:239, 1973
3. White PD: Heart Disease, 4th ed. New York, MacMillan, 1956
4. Lerner PI, Weinstein L: Infective endocarditis in the antibiotic era. N Engl J Med 274:199, 259, 323, 388, 1966
5. Watanakunakorn C: Changing epidemiology and newer aspects of infective endocarditis. Adv Intern Med 22:21, 1977
6. Cherubin CE, Neu HC: Infective endocarditis at the Presbyterian Hospital in New York City from 1938–1967. Am J Med 51:83, 1971
7. Cantrell M, Yoshikawa TT: Infective endocarditis in the aging patient. Gerontology 30:316, 1984
8. McNamara DG, Latson LA: Long-term followup of patients with malformations for which definitive surgical repair has been available for 25 years or more. Am J Cardiol 50:560, 1982
9. Payne DG, Fishburne JI Jr, Rufty AJ, Johnston FR: Bacterial endocarditis in pregnancy. Obstet Gynecol 60:247, 1982
10. Pelletier LL Jr, Petersdorf RG: Infective endocarditis: A review of 125 cases from the University of Washington hospitals 1963–72. Medicine 56:287, 1977
11. Korn D, DeSanctis RW, Sell S: Massive calcification of the mitral annulus: A clinicopathologic study of fourteen cases. N Engl J Med 267:900, 1962
12. Watanakunakorn C: Staphylococcus aureus endocarditis on the calcified mitral annulus fibrosus. Am J Med Sci 266:219, 1973
13. Clemens JD, Horwitz RI, Jaffe CJ et al: A controlled evaluation of the risk of bacterial endocarditis in persons with mitral valve prolapse. N Engl J Med 307:776, 1982
14. Durack DT, Kaplan EL, Bisno AL: Apparent failures of endocarditis prophylaxis: Analysis of 52 cases submitted to a national registry. JAMA 250:2318, 1983
15. Corrigall D, Bolen J, Hancock EW, Popp RL: Mitral valve prolapse and infective endocarditis. Am J Med 63:215, 1977
16. Venezio FR, Thompson JE, Sullivan H et al: Infection of a ventricular aneurysm and cardiac mural thrombus. Survival after surgical resection. Am J Med 77:551, 1984
17. Graham HV, von Hartitzch B, Medina JR: Infected atrial myxoma. Am J Cardiol 38:658, 1976
18. Gould K, Ramirez-Ronda CH, Holmes RK, Sanford JP: Adherence of bacteria to heart valves in vitro. J Clin Invest 56:1364, 1975
19. Scheld WM, Valone JA, Sande MA: Bacterial adherence in the pathogenesis of endocarditis. Interaction of bacterial dextran, platelets and fibrin. J Clin Invest 61:1394, 1978
20. Mollering RC Jr, Watson BK, Kunz LJ: Endocarditis due to group D streptococci. Comparison of disease caused by Streptococcus bovis with that produced by enterococci. Am J Med 57:239, 1974
21. Keusch GT: Opportunistic infections in colon carcinoma. Am J Clin Nutr 27:1481, 1974
22. Klein RS, Recco RA, Catalano MT et al: Association of Streptococcus bovis with carcinoma of the colon. N Engl J Med 297:800, 1977
23. Koenig MG, Kaye D: Enterococcal endocarditis. Report of 19 cases with long-term followup data. N Engl J Med 264:257, 1961
24. Reisberg BE: Infective endocarditis in the narcotic addict. Prog Cardiovasc Dis 22:193, 1979
25. Watanakunakorn C: Prosthetic valve infective endocarditis. Prog Cardiovasc Dis 22:181, 1979
26. Geraci JE, Wilson WR: Endocarditis due to gram negative bacteria. Mayo Clin Proc 57:145, 1982
27. Cohen PS, Maguire JH, Weinstein L: Infective endocarditis caused by gram negative bacteria: A review of the literature, 1945–1977. Prog Cardiovasc Dis 22:205, 1980
28. Saravolatz LD, Burch KH, Quinn EL et al: Polymicrobial infective endocarditis: An increasing clinical entity. Am Heart J 95:163, 1978
29. Okell CC, Elliot SD: Bacteremia and oral sepsis with special reference to the etiology of subacute bacterial endocarditis. Lancet 2:869, 1935
30. Everett ED, Hirschman JV: Transient bacteremia and endocarditis: A review. Medicine 56:61, 1977
31. Lillehei CW, Bobb JRR, Visscher MB: The occurrence of endocarditis with valvular deformities in dogs with arteriovenous fistulas. Proc Soc Exp Biol Med 75:9, 1950
32. Hockett RN, Beers RL, Loesche WL: Low-level bacteremia in humans. American Society of Microbiology, Annual Meeting (Abstracts), M6, 1972
33. Elliott SD: Bacteremia and oral sepsis. Proc R Soc Med 32:747, 1939
34. Ritro R, Monroe P, Andreole VT: Transient bacteremia due to suction abortion. Implications for SBE prophylaxis. Yale J Biol Med 50:471, 1977
35. Angrist AA, Oka M, Nakao K: Vegetative endocarditis. In Sommers S (ed): Pathology Annual, pp 155–212. New York, Appleton-Century-Crofts, 1967
36. Rodbard S: Blood velocity and endocarditis. Circulation 27:18, 1963
37. Arnett EW, Roberts WC: Valve ring abscess in active infective endocarditis: Frequency, location and clues to clinical diagnosis from the study of 95 necropsy patients. Circulation 54:140, 1977
38. Shanes JG, Lyons MF, Saffitz J et al: Persistent endomyocardial biopsy-proven vasculitis following cure of endocarditis. Am Heart J 108:614, 1984
39. Buchbinder NA, Roberts WC: Left sided valvular active infective endocarditis: A study of 45 necropsy patients. Am J Med 53:20, 1972
40. Wilson LM: Pathology of fatal bacterial endocarditis before and since the introduction of antibiotics. Ann Intern Med 58:84, 1963
41. Cream JJ, Turk JL: A review of the evidence for immunocomplex deposition as a cause of skin disease in man. Clin Allergy 1:235, 1971
42. Weinstein L, Schlessinger JJ: Pathoanatomic, pathophysiologic and clinical correlations in endocarditis. N Engl J Med 291:832, 1122, 1974
43. Churchill MA Jr, Geraci JE, Hunder GG: Musculoskeletal manifestations of bacterial endocarditis. Ann Intern Med 87:754, 1977
44. Meyers OL, Commerford PJ: Musculoskeletal manifestations of bacterial endocarditis. Ann Rheum Dis 36:517, 1977
45. Kaye D: Changes in the spectrum, diagnosis and management of bacterial and fungal endocarditis. Med Clin North Am 57:941, 1973
46. Kilpatrick ZM, Greenberg PA, Sanford JP: Splinter hemorrhages—their clinical significance. Arch Intern Med 115:730, 1965
47. Farrior JB III, Silverman ME: A consideration of the differences between a Janeway's lesion and an Osler's node in infectious endocarditis. Chest 70:239, 1974
48. Alpert JS, Krous HF, Dalen JE et al: Pathogenesis of Osler's nodes. Ann Intern Med 85:471, 1976
49. Robinson MJ, Ruedy J: Sequelae of bacterial endocarditis. Am J Med 32:922, 1962
50. Greenberg BH, Hoffman P, Schiller NB et al: Sudden death in infective endocarditis. Chest 71:794, 1977
51. Pfeiffer JF, Lipton MJ, Oury JH et al: Acute coronary embolism complicating bacterial endocarditis: Operative treatment. Am J Med 37:920, 1974
52. Schaff HV, Danielson GK: Annular destruction. In Magilligan DJ Jr, Quinn EL (eds): Endocarditis: Medical and surgical management. New York, Marcel Dekker, 1986
53. Johnson JD, Raff MJ, Barnwell PA, Chun CH: Splenic abscess complicating infectious endocarditis. Arch Intern Med 143:906, 1983
54. Vergne R, Selland B, Gobel FL, Hall WH: Rupture of the spleen in infective endocarditis. Arch Intern Med 135:1265, 1975
55. Gregoratos G, Karliner JS: Infective endocarditis: Diagnosis and management. Med Clin North Am 63:173, 1979
56. Wilson WR, Giuliani ER, Danielson GK, Geraci JE: Management of complications of infective endocarditis. Mayo Clin Proc 57:162, 1982
57. Jones HR Jr, Siebert RG, Geraci JE: Neurologic manifestations of bacterial endocarditis. Ann Intern Med 71:21, 1969
58. Ziment I: Nervous system complications in bacterial endocarditis. Am J Med 47:593, 1969
59. Baehr G: Renal complications of endocarditis. Trans Assoc Am Physicians 46:87, 1931
60. Gutman RA, Striker GE, Guilliland BC, Cutler RE: The immune complex glomerulonephritis of bacterial endocarditis. Medicine 51:1, 1972
61. Bayer AS, Theofilopoulos AN, Eisenberg R et al: Thrombotic thrombocytopenic purpura-like syndrome associated with infective endocarditis. JAMA 238:408, 1977

62. Cherubin CE, Baden M, Kavaler F et al: Infective endocarditis in narcotic addicts. Ann Intern Med 69:11091, 1968
63. Banks T, Fletcher R, Ali N: Infective endocarditis in heroin addicts. Am J Med 55:444, 1973
64. Menda KB, Gorbach SL: Favorable experience with bacterial endocarditis in heroin addicts. Ann Intern Med 78:25, 1973
65. Child JA, Darrell JH, Rhys Davies N, Davis-Dawson L: Mixed infective endocarditis in a heroin addict. J Med Microbiol 2:293, 1969
66. Anderson DJ, Bulkley BH, Hutchins GM: A clinicopathologic study of prosthetic valve endocarditis in 22 patients: Morphologic basis for diagnosis and therapy. Am Heart J 94:325, 1977
67. Arnett EN, Roberts WC: Prosthetic valve endocarditis. Am J Cardiol 38:281, 1976
68. Wilson WR, Jaumin PM, Danielson GK et al: Prosthetic valve endocarditis. Ann Intern Med 82:751, 1975
69. Magilligan DJ Jr, Quinn EL, Davila JC: Bacteremia, endocarditis and the Hancock valve. Ann Thorac Surg 24:508, 1977
70. King LH Jr, Bradley KP, Shires DL Jr et al: Bacterial endocarditis in chronic hemodialysis patients: A complication more common than previously suspected. Surgery 69:554, 1971
71. Cross AS, Steigbigel RT: Infective endocarditis and access site infections in patients on hemodialysis. Medicine 55:456, 1976
72. Valla D, Pariente E, Degott C et al: Right-sided endocarditis complicating peritoneovenous shunting for ascites. Arch Intern Med 143:1801, 1983
73. Procacci PM, Savran SV, Schreiter SL, Bryson AL: Prevalence of clinical mitral valve prolapse in 1,169 young women. N Engl J Med 294:1086, 1976
74. Friedland G, von Reyn CF, Levy B et al: Nosocomial endocarditis. Infect Control 5:284, 1984
75. Rowley KM, Clubb KS, Smith GJW, Cabin HS: Right-sided endocarditis as a consequence of flow-directed pulmonary artery catheterization. N Engl J Med 311:1152, 1984
76. Tsao MMP, Katz D: Central venous catheter-induced endocarditis. Rev Infect Dis 6:783, 1984
77. Stiles GM, Singh L, Imazaki G, Stiles QR: Thermodilution cardiac output studies as a cause of prosthetic valve bacterial endocarditis. J Thorac Cardiovasc Surg 88:1035, 1984
78. Bennett IL Jr, Beeson PB: Bacteremia: A consideration of some experimental and clinical aspects. Yale J Biol Med 26:241, 1954
79. Beeson PB, Bramnon ES, Warren JV: Observations on the sites of removal of bacteria from the blood in patients with bacterial endocarditis. J Exp Med 8:9, 1945
80. Griffith GC, Levinson DC: Subacute bacterial endocarditis: A report on 57 patients treated with massive doses of penicillin. Calif Med 71:403, 1949
81. Washington JA: Blood cultures, principles and techniques. Mayo Clin Proc 50:91, 1975
82. Washington JA: The role of the microbiology laboratory in the diagnosis and antimicrobial treatment of infective endocarditis. Mayo Clin Proc 57:22, 1982
83. Cannady PB Jr, Sanford JP: Negative blood cultures in infective endocarditis: A review. South Med J 69:1420, 1976
84. Mallen MS, Hube EL, Brenes M: Comparative study of blood cultures made from artery, vein and bone marrow in patients with subacute bacterial endocarditis. Am Heart J 33:692, 1947
85. Gleckman R: Culture negative endocarditis: Confirming the diagnosis. Am Heart J 94:125, 1977
86. Powers DL, Mandell GL: Intraleukocytic bacteria in endocarditis patients. JAMA 227:312, 1974
87. Ellis K, Jaffe C, Malm JR, Bowman FO Jr: Infective endocarditis—roentgenographic considerations. Radiol Clin North Am 11:415, 1973
88. Zelefsky MN, Lutzker LG: The target sign: A new radiologic sign of septic pulmonary emboli. Am J Roentgenol 129:453, 1977
89. Wiseman J, Rouleau J, Rigo P et al: Gallium-67 imaging for the detection of bacterial endocarditis. Radiology 110:135, 1976
90. Miller MH, Casey JI: Infective endocarditis: New diagnostic techniques. Am Heart J 96:123, 1978
91. Dillon JC, Feigenbaum H, Konecke LL et al: Echocardiographic manifestations of valvular vegetations. Am Heart J 86:698, 1973
92. Mintz GS, Kotler MN, Segal BL, Parry WR: Comparison of two-dimensional and M-mode echocardiography in the evaluation of patients with endocarditis. Am J Cardiol 43:738, 1979
93. Martin RP, Meltzer RS, Chia BL et al: Clinical utility of two-dimensional echocardiography in infective endocarditis. Am J Cardiol 46:379, 1980
94. Nakamura K, Satomi G, Sakai T et al: Clinical and echocardiographic features of pulmonary valve endocarditis. Circulation 67:198, 1983
95. Burger AJ, Messineo FC, Schulman P, Geller D: Mycotic aneurysm of the sinus of Valsalva due to Eikinella corrodens bacterial endocarditis. Cardiology 71:220, 1984
96. Cassling RS, Rogler WC, McManus BM: Isolated pulmonic valve endocarditis: A diagnostic elusive entity. Am Heart J 109:558, 1985
97. Effron MC, Popp RL: Two-dimensional echocardiographic assessment of bioprosthetic valve dysfunction and infective endocarditis. J Am Coll Cardiol 2:597, 1983
98. Ellis SG, Goldstein J, Popp RL: Detection of endocarditis-associated perivalvular abscesses by two-dimensional echocardiography. J Am Coll Cardiol 5:647, 1985
99. Wann LS, Hallam CC, Dillon JC et al: Comparison of M-mode and cross-sectional echocardiography in infective endocarditis. Circulation 60:728, 1979
100. Gilbert BW, Haney RS, Crawford F et al: Two-dimensional echocardiographic assessment of vegetative endocarditis. Circulation 55:346, 1977
101. Wong D, Chandraratna AN, Wishnow RM et al: Clinical implications of large vegetation in infectious endocarditis. Arch Intern Med 143:1874, 1983
102. O'Brien JT, Geiser EA: Infective endocarditis and echocardiography. Am Heart J 108:386, 1984
103. Panidis IP, Kotler MN, Mintz GS et al: Right heart endocarditis: Clinical and echocardiographic features. Am Heart J 107:759, 1984
104. Mann T, McLaurin L, Grossman W, Craige E: Assessing the hemodynamic severity of acute aortic regurgitation due to infective endocarditis. N Engl J Med 293:108, 1975
105. Kisslo J, Guadalajara JF, Stewart JA, Stack RS: Echocardiography in infective endocarditis. Herz 8:271, 1983
106. Nguyen NX, Kessler KM, Bilsker MS, Myerburg RJ: Echocardiographic demonstration of satellite lesions in aortic valvular endocarditis. Am J Cardiol 55:1433, 1985
107. Mohr-Kahaly S, Erbel R, Renolet H et al: Ambulatory followup of aortic dissection by transesophageal two-dimensional and color-coded Doppler echocardiography. Circulation 80:24, 1989
108. Cyran SE, Kimball TR, Meyer RA et al: Efficacy of intraoperative transesophageal echocardiography in children with congenital heart disease. Am J Cardiol 63:594, 1989
109. Mills J, Abott J, Utley JR, Ryan C: Role of cardiac catheterization in infective endocarditis. Chest 72:576, 1977
110. Hosenpud JD, Greenberg BH: The preoperative evaluation in patients with endocarditis. Is cardiac catheterization necessary? Chest 84:690, 1984
111. Cheitlin MD, Mills J: Infective endocarditis. Is cardiac catheterization usually needed before cardiac surgery? Chest 86:4, 1984
112. Peterson KL: Infective endocarditis: Role of newer diagnostic techniques. Chest 72:553, 1977
113. Pazin J, Peterson KL, Griff FW et al: Determination of site of infection in endocarditis. Ann Intern Med 82:746, 1975
114. Bennish M, Weinstein RA, Kabins SA, Jain MC: False localization of site of endocarditis by cardiac catheterization with quantitative cultures. Am J Clin Pathol 83:130, 1985
115. Durack DT: Practical therapy of infective endocarditis. Pract Cardiol 3:79, 1977
116. Sande MA, Scheld WM: Combination antibiotic therapy of bacterial endocarditis. Ann Intern Med 92:390, 1980
117. Gray IR: Management of infective endocarditis. J R Coll Physicians Lond 15:173, 1981
118. Guntheroth WG, Cammarano AA, Kirby WMM: Home treatment of infective endocarditis with oral amoxicillin. Am J Cardiol 55:1231, 1985
119. Egert J, Carrizosa J, Karfe D, Kobasa WD: Comparison of methicillin, nafcillin and oxacillin in therapy of Staphylococcus aureus endocarditis in rabbits. J Lab Clin Med 89:1262, 1977
120. Kay JH, Bernstein S, Tsuji HK et al: Surgical treatment of Candida endocarditis. JAMA 203:621, 1968
121. Arbulu A, Thomas NW, Wilson RF: Valvulectomy without prosthetic replacement. J Thorac Cardiovasc Surg 64:103, 1972
122. Bindschadler DD, Bennett JE: A pharmacologic guide to the clinical use of amphotericin B. J Infect Dis 120:427, 1969
123. Richardson JV, Karp RB, Kirklin JW, Dismukes WE: Treatment of infective endocarditis: A 10 year comparative analysis. Circulation 58:589, 1978
124. Parrott JCW, Hill JD, Kerth WJ, Gerbode F: The surgical management of bacterial endocarditis: A review. Ann Surg 183:289, 1976
125. Jung JY, Saab SB, Almond CH: The case for early surgical treatment of left sided primary infective endocarditis. J Thorac Cardiovasc Surg 70:509, 1975
126. Okies JE, Bradshaw MW, Williams TW: Valve replacement in bacterial endocarditis. Chest 63:898, 1973
127. Perry LS, Tresch DD, Brooks HL et al: Operative approach to endocarditis. Am Heart J 108:561, 1984
128. Silverman NA, Levitsky S, Mammana R: Acute endocarditis in addicts: Surgical treatment for multiple valve infection. J Am Coll Cardiol 4:680, 1984
129. Kay PH, Oldershaw PJ, Dawkins K et al: The results of surgery for active endocarditis of the native aortic valve. J Cardiovasc Surg 25:321, 1984
130. Nelson RJ, Harley DP, French WJ, Bayer AS: Favorable 10 year experience with valve procedures for active infective endocarditis. J Thorac Cardiovasc Surg 87:493, 1984
131. Black S, O'Rourke RA, Karliner JS: Role of surgery in the treatment of primary infective endocarditis. Am J Med 56:357, 1974
132. DiNubile MJ: Surgery in active endocarditis. Ann Intern Med 96:950, 1982
133. Batch AL, Shaffer C, Hammer MC et al: Bacteremia following dental cleaning in patients with and without penicillin prophylaxis. Am Heart J 104:1335, 1982
134. Ramphal R, Shands JW Jr: The therapy for infective endocarditis. Cardiovasc Clin 14:285, 1984
135. Shulman ST, Amren DP, Bisno AL et al: Prevention of bacterial endocarditis: A statement for health professionals by the Committee on Rheumatic Fever and Infective Endocarditis of the Council on Cardiovascular Disease in the Young. Circulation 70:1123A, 1984
136. Bor DH, Himmelstein DV: Endocarditis prophylaxis for patients with mitral valve prolapse: A quantitative analysis. Am J Med 76:711, 1984

137. Bertel O, Braun H-P, Gradel E: Non-compliance with the AHA recommendations for antibiotic prophylaxis of bacterial endocarditis in patients with valvular heart disease. Circulation 68(Suppl III):205, 1983

GENERAL REFERENCES

Durack DT: Current issues in prevention of infective endocarditis. Am J Med (Suppl 6B)78:149, 1985

Gnann JW, Dismukes WE: Prosthetic valve endocarditis: An overview. Herz 8:320, 1983

Karchmer AW: Infective endocarditis in the 1980's: Clinical features and management. Baylor College of Medicine Cardiology Series 7(3):6, 1984

Neugarten J, Baldwin DS: Glomerulonephritis in bacterial endocarditis. Am J Med 77:297, 1984

Reisberg BE: Infective endocarditis in the narcotic addict. Prog Cardiovasc Dis 22:181, 1979

Symposium on Infective Endocarditis. Mayo Clin Proc 57:3(Pt 1);57:81(Pt 2);57:145(Pt 3), 1982

TRICUSPID VALVE DISEASE

Gordon A. Ewy

CHAPTER 87 VOLUME 2

Tricuspid valve disease is a commonly seen clinical entity resulting from malformation or malfunction of any of a number of interrelated structures referred to as the tricuspid valve "complex." When tricuspid valve disease is severe, the diagnosis is obvious. However, subtle presentations are much more common. Noninvasive and/or invasive techniques may be required to confirm the diagnosis or to quantify the severity of the defect. Since tricuspid valve disease rarely presents as an isolated finding, its presence should stimulate a search for one of the multiple etiologies.

ANATOMY

The anatomy of the tricuspid valve is complicated and somewhat variable. The tricuspid valve complex is composed of several structures whose integrated function is essential for tricuspid valve competence.[1-3] These structures, the leaflets, chordae, papillary muscles, annulus, and the right atrial and right ventricular myocardium, must all be anatomically and physiologically sound.

The normal tricuspid leaflets are delicate, translucent structures that have a scalloped appearance when closed (Fig. 87.1, *left*). The scalloped appearance is due to a variety of chordal attachments. The name of the valve is derived from the presence of three leaflets: anterior, septal, and posterior. The anterior leaflet is the largest, the septal leaflet the smallest. The posterior leaflet is intermediate in size and is characterized by the presence of from one to three clefts. The clefts in the posterior leaflet can be quite prominent, creating the illusion of multiple tricuspid valve leaflets. The free edges of the three leaflets are longer than the circumference of the annulus, thereby providing complete and unobstructed opening as the leaflets drop curtain-like into the right ventricle during diastole (Fig. 87.1, *right*).

When the right heart is opened through the acute margin (Fig. 87.2), the three largest fan-shaped chordae identify the three commissures. Two of the three large fan-shaped chordae arise from the papillary muscles. The anterior papillary muscle supplies fan-shaped chordae to the anterior and posterior leaflets identifying the anteroposterior commissure. The medial papillary muscle supplies fan-shaped chordae to the posterior and septal leaflets and identifies the posteroseptal commissure. The large fan-shaped chordae to the anterior and the septal leaflets arise from the septal wall (Fig. 87.2).

An average of 25 chordae tendineae attach to the tricuspid valve leaflets.[2] In contrast to mitral chordae, the chordae tendineae to the tricuspid leaflets are quite variable; Silver and co-workers have identified five separate types.[1] Identification of each type of chorda is probably not important, although from an anatomical and functional point of view, some types are of interest. In addition to the large fan-shaped chordae that identify the commissures, there are small fan-shaped chordae to the clefts of the posterior leaflet of the tricuspid valve (Fig. 87.2). Two interesting types of chordae not seen in the mitral apparatus include the "free edge chordae" that are long and attach to the free edge of the leaflets and the "deep chordae" that are short and attach to the basal portion of each leaflet.[1-3] Of greatest interest are the short chordae that arise directly from the muscle of the septum and posterior wall and attach to the septal leaflet (Fig. 87.3). This configuration limits the mobility of the septal leaflet and may predispose the tricuspid valve to incompetence.[3] As illustrated in Figure 87.3, the fixed septal leaflet allows for little compensation should the free wall of the right ventricle dilate.

The circumference of the tricuspid valve annulus is 11 cm to 12 cm.[2,3] The tricuspid valve leaflets attach to the annulus at different levels. The highest part of the tricuspid valve's attachment occurs at the anteroseptal commissure, which is located near the membranous interventricular septum (see Fig. 87.2). As will be emphasized below, the tricuspid annulus plays an important role in tricuspid valve competence. In addition, the atrial and ventricular myocardium and perhaps the sequence of electrical activation are all important for normal function of the tricuspid valve complex.[3]

Like the mitral valve, the tricuspid valve leaflets consist of three layers: the fibrosa on the ventricular surface, the atrialis on the atrial surface, and the thicker spongiosis layer sandwiched between the atrialis and the fibrosa.

PHYSIOLOGY OF NORMAL TRICUSPID APPARATUS

The pressure generated by right ventricular contraction produces the force that closes the tricuspid valve. The right ventricular–right atrial pressure crossover precedes tricuspid valve closure by an average of 50 msec.[4] Abrupt deceleration of the valve apparatus contributes to the tricuspid component of the first heart sound. In normal subjects with two major components to the first sound, the first component coincides with mitral closure and the second with tricuspid closure.[5,6] The tricuspid component of the first sound is nearly synchronous with the mitral component in normal subjects with a single first heart sound.[5,6] In situations where the mitral and tricuspid closures are grossly asynchronous, each valve closure has an associated sound.[5,6] The tricuspid component is soft when right ventricular contractility is decreased or with a prolonged electrocardiographic PR interval, and is accentuated with a forceful right ventricular contraction or a short electrocardiographic PR interval.

The motion of the tricuspid annulus was studied with biplane videoangiograms in normal, intact, anesthetized dogs. Two to six weeks earlier, beads had been placed on the tricuspid ring during cardiopulmonary bypass.[7] With this technique, Tsakiris and associates found that there was a rhythmic reduction of the tricuspid annular area by an average of 29%. Approximately two thirds of the total ring narrowing was associated with atrial systole.[7]

More recently, the human tricuspid valve leaflets and their annular attachments were studied in detail by two-dimensional echocardiography.[8] The size of the human tricuspid annulus was also observed to change dramatically.[8] Figure 87.4 shows the change in tricuspid annular area in a normal subject.[8] Maximal size occurred just prior to atrial systole. The major reduction in area occurred with atrial systole and the minimal size was reached in mid-systole. In normal subjects the annular circumference measured 12 ± 1 cm prior to atrial contraction and narrowed to 10 ± 1 cm in mid-systole, a 19% reduction in circumference. The annular area was reduced by 33%.[8] These findings suggest that one of the functions of atrial contraction is the reduction in size of the tricuspid valve orifice prior to the onset of systole. With atrial fibrillation, the loss or modification of this sphincter-like motion, especially with annular dilatation, may contribute to tricuspid valvular regurgitation.

ACQUIRED TRICUSPID VALVE DISEASE
FUNCTIONAL TRICUSPID REGURGITATION

The most common abnormality of the tricuspid valve is functional tricuspid regurgitation. Even in patients with rheumatic heart disease, functional tricuspid regurgitation is common.[9] It is generally accepted that functional tricuspid regurgitation results from annular dilatation secondary to right ventricular failure, and right heart failure is most often secondary to left heart failure. Compared to normal, the annular circumference of patients with tricuspid regurgitation (TR) is larger (normal 12 ± 1 cm versus TR 14 ± 1 cm) and the percent circumfer-

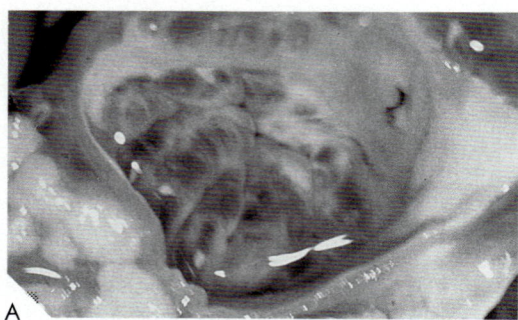
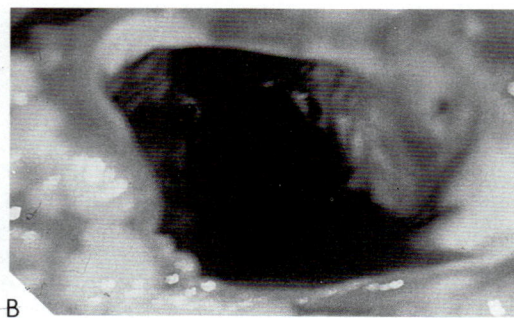

FIGURE 87.1 Tricuspid valve viewed from the atrium. **A.** Systole. **B.** Diastole.

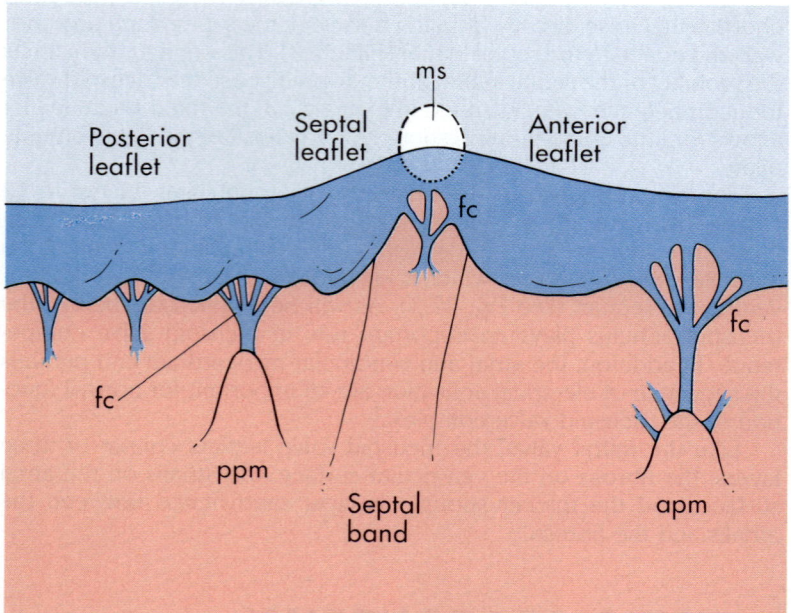

FIGURE 87.2 Diagrammatic representation of the tricuspid valve as viewed following incision through the acute margin of the right heart. The posterior, septal, and anterior leaflets are identified. The anterior papillary muscle identifies the anteroposterior commissure. The fan-shaped chordae (fc), membranous septum (ms), anterior papillary muscle (apm), and posterior papillary muscle (ppm) are labeled. Small fan-shaped chordae identify clefts in the posterior leaflet.

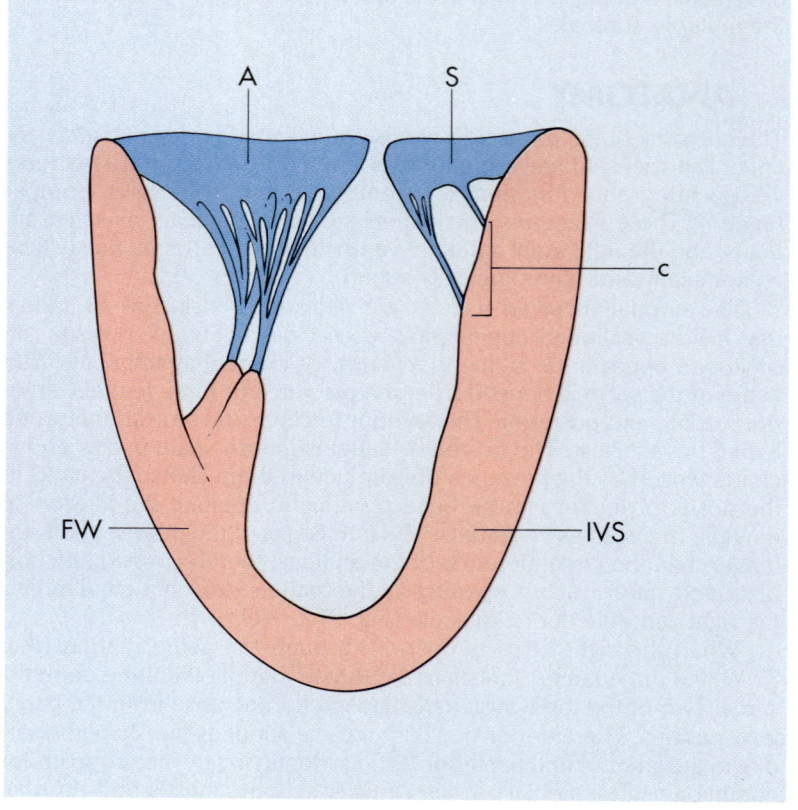

FIGURE 87.3 Schematic of the right ventricular free wall (FW) and intraventricular septum (IVS) with chordal attachments to the anterior (A) and septal (S) leaflets. Many of the chordae tendineae (c) to the septal leaflet arise directly from the muscle of the septum or posterior wall. (Modified from Silver MD, Lam JH, Ranganathan N et al: Morphology of human tricuspid valve. Circulation 44:333, 1971.)

ential reduction from pre-systole to mid-systole is less (normal 19% versus TR 10%).[8] Because the percent reduction of the annulus is less, the minimum systolic tricuspid annular area is markedly larger in patients with functional tricuspid regurgitation than that of normal subjects—almost twice normal (normal 7.6 ± 1.4 cm^2 versus TR 13 ± 1.4 cm^2).[8] The normal maximal diameter of the tricuspid valve is about 21 mm/m^2. The critical diameter is estimated to be 27 mm/m^2, since above this size, functional tricuspid regurgitation is common.[9]

A continued pressure load of the right ventricle from birth usually results in right ventricular hypertrophy with a relatively competent tricuspid valve until heart failure occurs. In contrast, increased afterload applied to the thin-walled right ventricle of an adult is more likely to result in dilatation and right ventricular failure. It is generally agreed that the thin-walled right ventricle handles a volume overload better than a pressure overload.

RHEUMATIC TRICUSPID VALVE DISEASE

Rheumatic tricuspid valve stenosis is the result of chronic scarring and fibrosis of the tricuspid valve leaflets with commissural fusion (Fig. 87.5). There is associated fibrosis, thickening, and fusion of the chordae tendineae.[10-12] The resultant limitation of leaflet mobility and reduction in tricuspid orifice size may obstruct right ventricular filling. Fibrosis and distortion of leaflet architecture may result in tricuspid regurgitation.

Rheumatic heart disease, and therefore rheumatic involvement of the tricuspid valve, is rare in the Western world but still occurs in areas where rheumatic fever is rampant. Dr. Paul Wood postulated that rheumatic involvement of the heart was a pancarditis, involving all parts of the heart.[12] He reasoned that mitral valve disease was the most important long-term sequela since the mitral valve is subject to the greatest pressure, normally having to withstand a systolic pressure of about 120 mm Hg during acute rheumatic pancarditis and thereafter. The aortic valve has to withstand a pressure of 80 mm Hg in diastole. The tricuspid valve has a systolic pressure stress of only 15 to 25 mm Hg. Following this line of reasoning, Dr. Wood postulated that rheumatic involvement of the aortic valve was always associated with rheumatic mitral valve disease and that rheumatic tricuspid disease was always associated with rheumatic involvement of the aortic and mitral valves.[12]

This postulate proved to be relatively sound. Approximately 15% to 30% of all patients with rheumatic valvular heart disease have evidence at necropsy of rheumatic involvement of the tricuspid valve.[13,14] Clinically recognized tricuspid stenosis occurs in approximately 5% of patients with rheumatic heart disease. Rheumatic tricuspid valve disease virtually never occurs in the absence of rheumatic involvement of the mitral valve.[15-19] The natural history of rheumatic tricuspid valve lesions is dictated by the severity of the associated mitral and/or aortic valve lesion.[20]

The diagnosis of rheumatic tricuspid stenosis is often difficult, yet important, since residual tricuspid stenosis may preclude clinical improvement despite successful surgical correction of mitral or mitral and aortic valvular lesions.[11,15] The low cardiac output imposed by associated severe mitral stenosis may result in such low flow across the stenotic tricuspid valve that many of the classical bedside and hemodynamic features of tricuspid stenosis are absent. Often it is only after repair of other valvular lesions that the resultant increased tricuspid valve flow allows the clinical diagnosis.

Significant tricuspid regurgitation is relatively common in patients with chronic rheumatic heart disease. In a recent series of such patients undergoing diagnostic cardiac catheterization, one third (35 of 99) had angiographic evidence of tricuspid regurgitation.[21]

RIGHT VENTRICULAR INFARCTION

Right ventricular infarction, a condition that occurs almost exclusively with transmural infarction of the left ventricular inferior wall, may result in tricuspid regurgitation.[22,23] With right ventricular infarction, tricuspid regurgitation is probably the result of infarction and dysfunction of the papillary muscle complex including its free wall attachments. The dysfunction may be transient, with normal hemodynamics following recovery.[24] Rupture of a right ventricular papillary muscle following acute myocardial infarction is rare.[25]

ENDOCARDITIS

Right-sided endocarditis involves the tricuspid valve in 95% of cases and frequently develops on a previously normal valve.[26] Intravenous

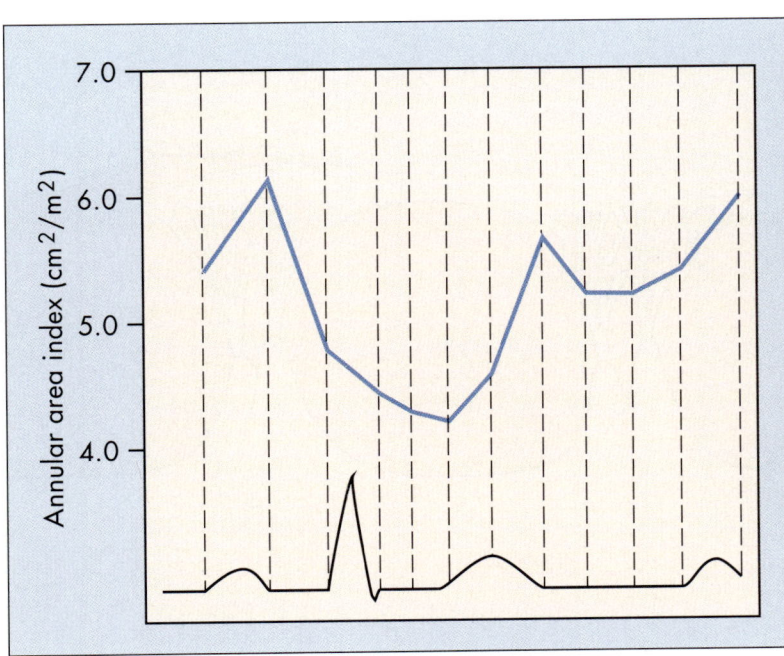

FIGURE 87.4 The changes in tricuspid annular area indices during the cardiac cycle in a normal subject. (Modified from Tei C, Pilgrim JP, Shah PM et al: The tricuspid valve annulus: Study of size and motion in normal subjects and in patients with tricuspid regurgitation. Circulation 66:665, 1982)

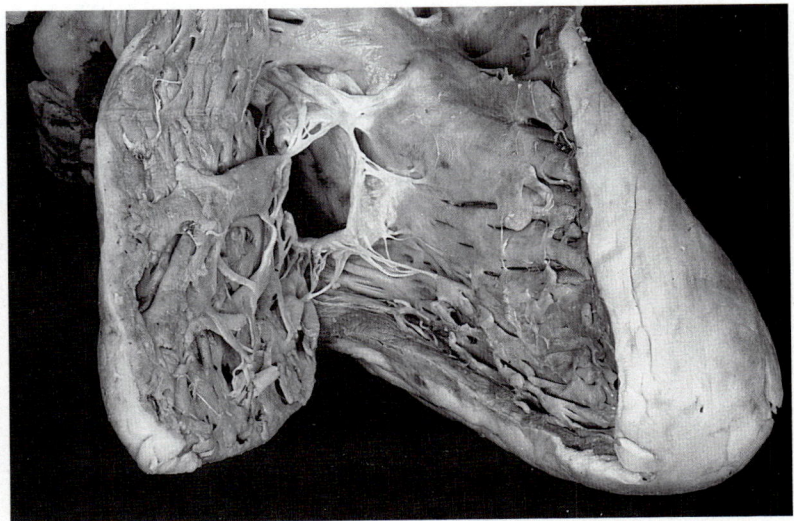

FIGURE 87.5 Rheumatic involvement of the tricuspid valve as viewed from the right ventricle. (Courtesy of Dr. Jesse Edwards)

drug abusers are especially prone to develop right-sided endocarditis. Reports from medical examiners emphasize the frequency of aortic and mitral valve involvement from acute bacterial endocarditis. Reports from large city hospitals, however, emphasize the frequency of tricuspid valve involvement. This apparent dicrepancy may be due to the fact that endocarditis of the tricuspid valve does not always result in acute severe hemodynamic embarrassment and rapid deterioration. It is now apparent that infective endocarditis in drug abusers involves the tricuspid valve alone in about 40% of cases.[27]

Patients with infective endocarditis are often acutely ill with fever, chills, rigors, and pulmonary symptoms. The pulmonary symptoms include cough, hemoptysis, pleuritic chest pain, and dyspnea.[28] Chest roentgenograms are extremely helpful in the diagnosis since they show abnormal findings in 70% of patients at initial presentation. Multiple bilateral infiltrates may be noted as a result of septic emboli from the tricuspid valve.[29] The characteristic murmur of tricuspid regurgitation is present in only one third of patients at the time of initial presentation.[29]

TRAUMATIC INJURY

Penetrating and nonpenetrating trauma can result in tricuspid regurgitation from rupture of the leaflets, chordae tendineae, or papillary muscle.[30,31] These abnormalities are illustrated in Figure 87.6. Rarely, traumatic tricuspid insufficiency leads to right atrial enlargement, elevation of mean right atrial pressure, and acquired cyanosis from right to left shunting via a patent foramen ovale.[32]

TRICUSPID VALVE PROLAPSE

Isolated tricuspid valve prolapse is rare, as there have been fewer than 50 reported patients in the English literature.[33] In contrast, the combination of tricuspid and mitral valve prolapse is relatively common. The prevalence of concomitant tricuspid valve prolapse in patients with mitral valve prolapse varies widely among reported series, but the combined prevalence of the nine largest series averages 37%.[33-37] Since prolapse of the mitral valve is relatively common, affecting almost 6% of the population, tricuspid valve prolapse may be present in 2% to 3% of the population. Patients with combined mitral and tricuspid valve prolapse tend to be older and more symptomatic than patients with isolated mitral valve disease.[34] Women predominate by a 2:1 ratio in isolated mitral valve prolapse and by a 3:1 ratio in combined atrioventricular prolapse.[34]

The clinical features, symptoms, and signs are similar to those of mitral valve prolapse. These include chest pain, dyspnea, palpitations, nonejection systolic clicks, and late systolic murmurs. The identification of tricuspid valve disease is sometimes possible by auscultation. The click is reportedly more prominent at the lower left sternal border. With inspiration, the click occurs later in systole and may merge with the second heart sound. Occasionally the click is heard along the lower right sternal border. The systolic murmur is also more prominent at the lower left sternal border. With inspiration, the murmur may increase in intensity and be shorter in duration. Thus, auscultatory changes are thought to be secondary to increased right ventricular volume with inspiration.[34,37]

Skeletal abnormalities including the straight back syndrome, scoliosis, and pectus excavatum may be more common in patients with bivalvular involvement.[37]

The spectrum of primary tricuspid prolapse is wide, varying from trivial abnormalities of the leaflets or chordae, or both, to severe redundancy of the valvular tissue and marked elongation of the supporting chordae.[33,38-41] The distinguishing pathologic feature of primary tricuspid valve disease is excessive myxomatous tissue in the middle, or spongiosis, layer of the valve leaflet. Edwards and associates have observed an association between pulmonary emphysema and mitral and tricuspid valve prolapse (Fig. 87.7). In such patients, myxomatous changes in the tricuspid valve are more commonly present and to a greater degree than similar changes in the mitral valve.[42] Edwards and co-workers postulate that these observations may indicate a common factor of connective tissue weakness in the lungs and cardiac valves: "In the lungs this weakness is manifested by emphysema; in the valves by the 'floppy state'. Given the pulmonary and right ventricular hypertension that accompany emphysema, the tricuspid valve with intrinsically weak connective tissue is challenged, with the resultant prolapsed state becoming evident."[42] Figure 87.8 is a striking example of tricuspid valve involvement in a patient with emphysema and associated mitral valve prolapse.

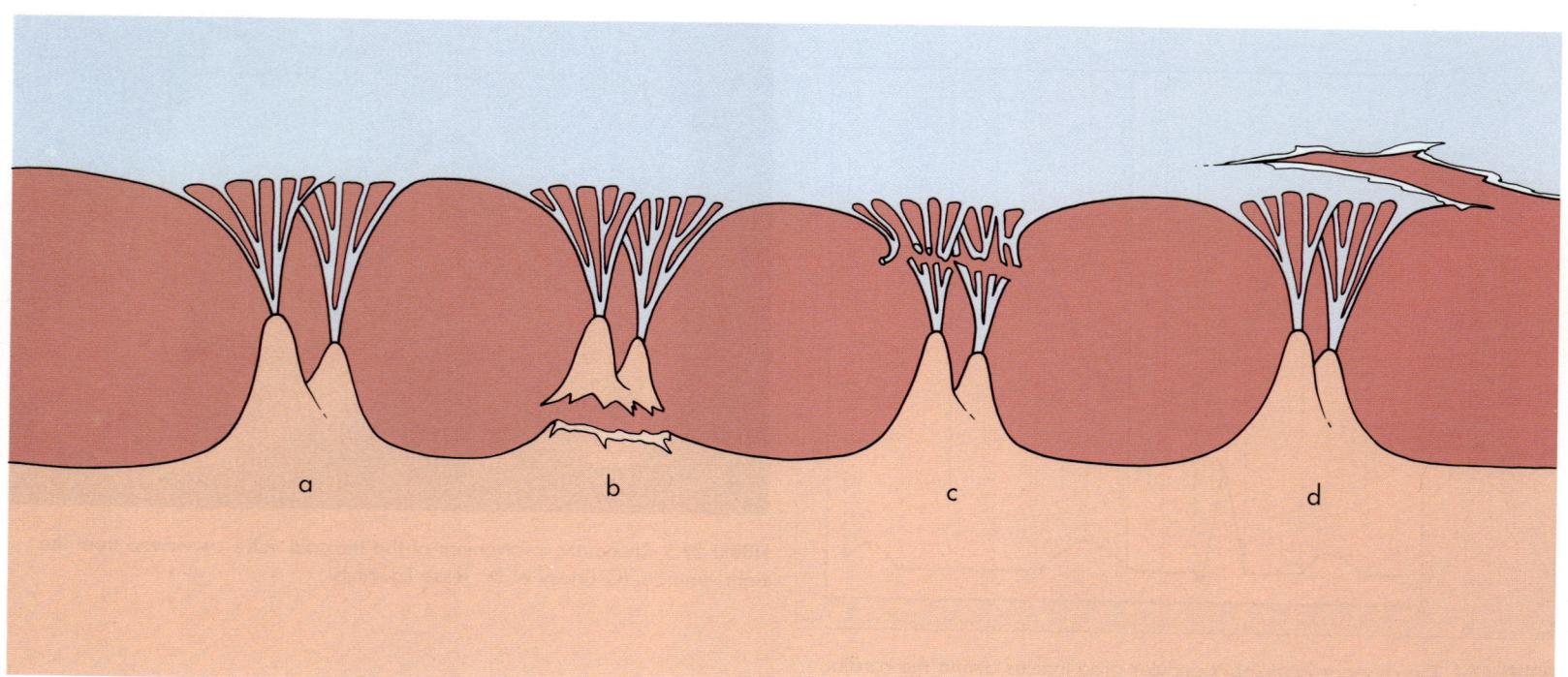

FIGURE 87.6 Schematic representation of the types of lesions that result in traumatic tricuspid regurgitation: (a) normal, (b) traumatic rupture of papillary muscle, (c) traumatic rupture of chordae tendineae, and (d) rupture of tricuspid leaflet. (Modified from figure courtesy of Dr. Jesse Edwards)

CARCINOID SYNDROME HEART DISEASE

Carcinoid syndrome is a relatively rare cause of acquired cardiac disease. Patients with the carcinoid heart disease almost always have tricuspid valve involvement.[43-45] Cardiac involvement usually occurs in patients who have hepatic metastases from ileocecal tumors.[44,45] However, cardiac involvement has also been documented in carcinoid tumors of ovarian and bronchial origin without hepatic metastases.[46,47] Although the primary tumors and their metastases tend to have the histological appearance of malignancy, they often follow an indolent course. Therefore, cardiac failure accounts for significant morbidity and mortality in this syndrome.[43,45]

The tricuspid and pulmonic valves are the most common sites of cardiac involvement. Tricuspid regurgitation is the most common clinical abnormality. The pulmonic valve, if involved, is generally stenotic. Tricuspid stenosis with or without tricuspid regurgitation also occurs.

Although the clinical features of tricuspid regurgitation resemble those of other etiologies, the two-dimensional echocardiographic features are relatively characteristic. The tricuspid leaflets are thickened and appear similar to those seen with rheumatic tricuspid stenosis, but the mitral valve is normal, indicating that the right-sided valvular lesions are not due to rheumatic heart disease.[48-51] The right atrium is enlarged. The most severely involved valves are virtually immobile with a fixed orifice, resulting in both stenosis and regurgitation.[48] In less severely involved valves the leaflets appear stiff and straightened, moving in a boardlike fashion with diminished total excursion.[50] In some there is coaptation of the nodular thickened lesions at the beginning of systole. The leaflets are increasingly pulled apart as right ventricular systole proceeds, due to traction on the leaflets by the thickened chordae tendineae.[48] This finding is thought to account for the particularly severe tricuspid regurgitation that is seen in some patients with carcinoid heart disease.[48] Occasionally, the leaflets and the right ventricular papillary muscles appear more highly reflective of ultrasound than normal, suggesting endocardial coating by carcinoid-related fibrous plaque.[49] Doming of the tricuspid valve has been described in patients with tricuspid stenosis. The M-mode echocardiogram is often not sensitive enough to completely define the tricuspid valve.[51,52] Yet, in an adult, the abnormal tricuspid valve (Fig. 87.9) and a normal mitral valve should bring to mind the possibility of carcinoid involvement.[53]

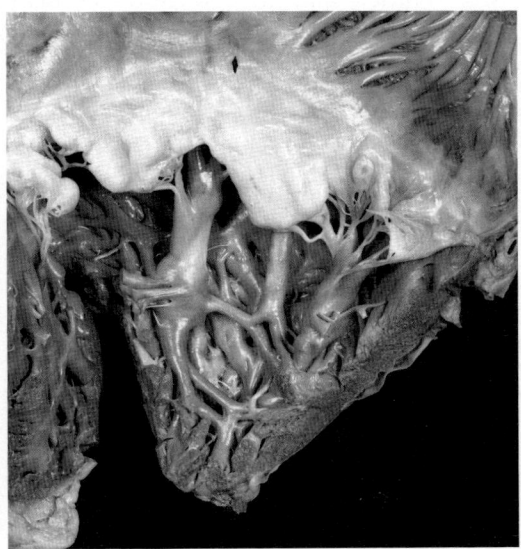

FIGURE 87.7 Tricuspid valve prolapse with thickening and redundancy of the tricuspid leaflets in a patient with pulmonary emphysema. (Courtesy of Dr. Jesse Edwards)

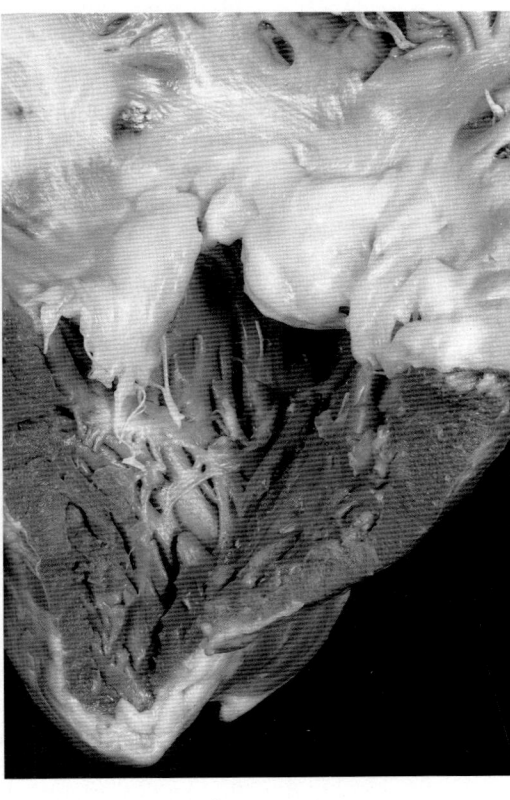

FIGURE 87.8 Enlarged and thickened tricuspid valve. Right ventricular hypertrophy is present secondary to emphysema. (Courtesy of Dr. Jesse Edwards)

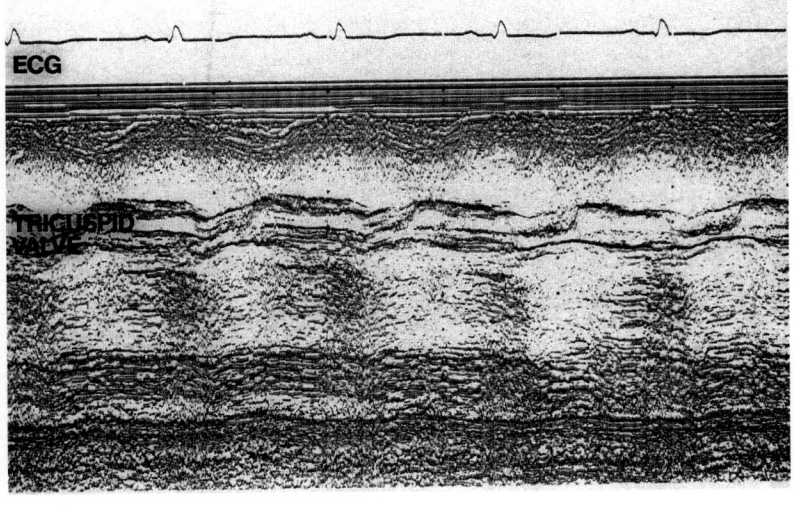

FIGURE 87.9 M-mode echocardiographic appearance of the tricuspid valve of a patient with the carcinoid syndrome.

There have been several reports of tricuspid valve replacement with prosthetic valves in patients with the carcinoid syndrome, but there is no consensus on which type of prosthetic valve is preferable.

MYXOMAS

Right atrial myxomas can produce tricuspid stenosis or tricuspid regurgitation, or both. It is easy to imagine how a large myxoma could produce apparent tricuspid stenosis. Tricuspid regurgitation can occur if the myxoma is calcified. In these patients the myxoma swings in and out of the tricuspid valve orifice, grating and destroying the tricuspid leaflets with the rough calcified areas on its surface.

Atrial myxomas are the most common primary cardiac tumor and right atrial myxomas account for approximately 25% of cardiac intracavitary myxomas.[54–56] This diagnosis should be considered in any patient who has clinical findings of tricuspid valve disease in the absence of aortic and mitral disease. Systemic symptoms of fever, anorexia, and weight loss, as well as changing auscultatory findings, suggest either tumor, progressive vasculitis, or endocarditis. The diagnosis of right atrial myxoma can be made with a high degree of accuracy by two-dimensional echocardiography.[57] In the rare case of right atrial tumor calcification, the diagnosis can be made by chest roentgenogram or fluoroscopy.

RARE CAUSES OF ACQUIRED TRICUSPID VALVE DISEASE

There are a variety of rare causes of tricuspid valve disease that include fibroelastosis,[58] endocardial fibrosis,[59] systemic lupus erythematosus,[60] metastatic tumors,[61,62] scleroderma,[63] hyperthyroidism,[64] catheter- or pacemaker-induced thrombus,[65] catheter or pacemaker entanglements,[66–68] and diseases of the pericardium.[69–71]

CONGENITAL ABNORMALITIES
EBSTEIN'S ANOMALY

Ebstein's malformation is one of the most common congenital abnormalities of the tricuspid valve in adults, provided that tricuspid valve prolapse is classified as an acquired condition.

Ebstein's anomaly consists of downward displacement of fused, malformed portions of tricuspid valvular tissue into the right ventricular cavity.[72,73] The leaflets are attached in part to the tricuspid annulus and in part to the right ventricular wall below the annulus.[72,73] In general, the large anterior leaflet is least affected or is enlarged. The posterior leaflet may be rudimentary or entirely absent.[74] In some patients, tricuspid valve tissue forms a large curtain across the right ventricular cavity.[75] The right ventricle may be thin and the right ventricular portion that is above the abnormal insertion of the tricuspid valve is said to be "atrialized." The right atrium is enlarged. The majority of patients have either an incompetent or patent foramen ovale or an ostium secundum atrial septal defect.[74]

The hemodynamic alterations of Ebstein's anomaly are related to the malformed tricuspid valve and the dysfunction of the right ventricle.[76] All gradations of severity exist,[73,76] and thus this abnormality may be compatible with a relatively long and active life.[77] When symptoms appear, dyspnea, fatigue, and weakness are most common.[76] Palpitations are usually due to atrial dysrhythmias. Death is due to congestive heart failure, hypoxia, and dysrhythmias.[76,77] Cyanosis occurs in 50% to 80% of patients. Perloff emphasizes the chronologic sequence of cyanosis as a useful diagnostic feature of the history. Neonatal cyanosis may regress or disappear and then return at a later date. He states, "The functionally inadequate right ventricle copes poorly with the high pulmonary vascular resistance in the newborn. The right atrial pressure rises and a right to left shunt develops through an interatrial communication. When the pulmonary pressure drops to normal, the burden on the right heart is relieved; the right atrial pressure declines, the right to left shunt diminishes or disappears and with it the cyanosis. As time goes on, cyanosis may reappear since the inadequate right ventricle, burdened by tricuspid regurgitation, ultimately fails again. Right ventricular end-diastolic pressure rises together with right atrial pressure and a right to left shunt is re-established."[76] The degree of cyanosis does not always coincide with the patient's symptoms.[77,78] In fact, a history of relatively good effort tolerance despite cyanosis favors the diagnosis of Ebstein's anomaly.[76]

The jugular venous pulse may be normal in spite of tricuspid incompetence because of the commodious right atrium. On auscultation, the first heart sound is widely split due to the delay in closure of the tricuspid valve. The smaller and poorly contracting right ventricle and the increased excursion of the large anterior leaflet results in a delayed tricuspid component of the first heart sound.[79] This early systolic sound is prominent and is due to the large sail-like tricuspid valve reaching the limits of its systolic excursion. Referred to as the "sail sound," this may be the most specific auscultatory finding in Ebstein's anomaly.[79] The second heart sound splitting is variable. Systolic murmurs are also quite variable; they may be totally absent or quite prominent. They are best heard along the lower left sternal border. The murmur of tricuspid regurgitation is not necessarily pansystolic because this lesion is present in the absence of pulmonary hypertension. In the absence of pulmonary hypertension, the end-systolic pressure difference between the right ventricle and the v wave of the right atrium is small, and flow is decreased in late systole. In Ebstein's anomaly the murmur of tricuspid regurgitation does not necessarily increase with inspiration. This may be due to the inability of the small right ventricle to increase its stroke volume.[76] Third and fourth heart sounds are common. These sounds may summate due to tachycardia or prolonged electrocardiographic PR interval, or both. Early diastolic sounds have been described and are attributed to the "opening snap" of the large anterior tricuspid leaflet or to the rapid filling of a small nondistensible right ventricle. The cadence created by the first heart sound (mitral valve closure), the early systolic sound (tricuspid valve closure), the second heart sound, and the early diastolic sound has been likened to the chugging of a steam locomotive.[76]

The electrocardiogram is usually abnormal in the adult with Ebstein's anomaly. The P waves may be prominent and the PR interval prolonged. Preexcitation (Wolff-Parkinson-White) has been described in as many as 20% to 25% of patients with Ebstein's anomaly, and, as would be anticipated, the atrioventricular bypass tracts are usually located on the right.[76] Although paroxysmal supraventricular tachycardia occurs from reentry over the bypass tract, other atrial dysrhythmias, such as atrial flutter and fibrillation, are also common because of the enlarged right atrium.[76]

The echocardiographic features of Ebstein's anomalies are characteristic. The M-mode recording shows an increased excursion of the tricuspid valve when the echo beam traverses the large anterior leaflet. The most characteristic feature is delayed closure (50 msec or more) of the tricuspid valve when compared with that of the mitral valve.[76] In the apical four-chamber view of the two-dimensional echocardiogram, the right ventricular displacement of the leaflet and right atrial enlargement can be visualized.[76] The diagnosis can be confirmed at cardiac catheterization by using a catheter that has an electrode near the lumen used for recording pressures. In the right atrium, atrial pressure and an intra-atrial electrocardiogram are recorded, but the atrialized portion of the right ventricle generates an *intracavitary right ventricular electrogram* while registering an *atrial* pressure pulse. As the catheter tip is advanced across the tricuspid valve, a right ventricular pressure tracing and an intracavitary right ventricular electrogram are recorded.[76]

RARE CAUSES OF CONGENITAL TRICUSPID VALVE DISEASE

Rare causes of congenital tricuspid valve disease include congenital tricuspid atresia and stenosis.[80–83] Tricuspid stenosis is usually associated with an underdeveloped right ventricle. Congenital clefts of the tricuspid valve can be seen as part of the endocardial cushion defects. A straddling tricuspid valve can be part of maldevelopment of the ventricles (single ventricle). The tricuspid valve is the left-sided atrioventricular valve in l-transposition (congenital corrected transposition). In this situation, Ebstein's anomaly is frequent.[76] Tricuspid regurgitation has been reported from Ehlers-Danlos syndrome.[84]

DIAGNOSIS OF TRICUSPID REGURGITATION
CLINICAL FINDINGS

Gross tricuspid regurgitation can be diagnosed at the patient's bedside. Lateral head bobbing, large regurgitant *cv* waves in the jugular veins, and lateral chest wall motion are characteristic. Subtle presentations are much more common. Attention must be focused on minor alterations of the jugular venous pulse and trivial changes in the frequency or intensity of precordial murmurs with respiration if less severe degrees of tricuspid regurgitation are to be appreciated at the bedside.

Normal jugular venous pulsation consists of a presystolic *a* wave, a systolic *x* descent, a late systolic *v* wave, and a diastolic *y* descent (Fig. 87.10, *top*). In normal patients with a slow heart rate, an *h* wave follows the *y* descent and ends with the onset of the next *a* wave. A *c* wave may interrupt the early portion of the *x* descent (Fig. 87.10). In right atrial tracings the *c* wave occurs with the bulging of the tricuspid valve into the right atrium at the onset of systole. The larger *c* waves that are at times present in the neck of some patients are due to impulses transmitted from forceful carotid pulsations. The *v* wave is the result of continued passive filling of the right atrium during ventricular systole.[85] Moderate to severe leakage of the tricuspid valve results in a systolic wave that begins with a *c* wave and peaks at the time of the normal *v* wave (Fig. 87.10, *bottom*). These regurgitant waves are called *cv* waves or *s* waves. Small *cv* waves may do little more than obliterate the *x* descent. As the *cv* waves become larger, they are easier to recognize as a systolic venous pulse that wells up from the base of the neck. The *cv* wave should not be confused with the Cannon wave. Cannon *a* waves result from atrial contractions against a closed tricuspid valve such as occurs with junctional rhythms, advanced degrees of heart block, premature ventricular contractions, or with atrioventricular dissociation. Compared to the slow-rising regurgitant *cv* wave, the Cannon *a* wave has a quicker rate of rise and is nonsustained. These features cause the Cannon *a* wave to have a more flipping quality. Regurgitant *cv* waves must also be differentiated from large *c* waves transmitted from forceful carotid pulsations. This differential is easily made if the examining physician applies light pressure with the lateral aspect of his or her hand to the base of the neck just above the clavicle. This maneuver obstructs the internal jugular vein and obliterates regurgitant *cv* waves, but has no effect on carotid pulsations.[84]

It is difficult to quantitate the degree of tricuspid regurgitation.[86,87] The height of the regurgitant *cv* wave is determined by right atrial size and venous compliance as well as by the amount of regurgitation. A large right atrium might absorb a considerable amount of tricuspid regurgitation without altering the venous pulse. Likewise, trivial tricuspid regurgitation may not alter the venous wave form even in patients with a normal-sized right atrium.[86,87]

Significant tricuspid regurgitation may result in palpable hepatic pulsations. The method I have found most helpful in feeling hepatic pulsation is to make a fist and place the knuckles and the back side of the metacarpals in the rib interspaces over the liver. Firm pressure facilitates the sensing of rhythmic systolic outward motion of the chest wall. This technique appears to be more sensitive than trying to feel hepatic pulsations below the rib cage with the palmar surface of the fingers. Lesser degrees of tricuspid regurgitation may not produce liver pulsations and must be diagnosed by careful inspection of the jugular venous pulsations, or by use of noninvasive techniques.

The classic auscultatory finding of tricuspid regurgitation is a systolic murmur best heard over the lower sternal area that increases with inspiration (Fig. 87.11). Although the murmur of tricuspid regurgitation is most often heard over the fourth and fifth left intercostal spaces, it may be loudest over the lower right sternal border or over the xiphoid.[88] With right ventricular dilatation, the murmur may extend across the entire precordium, mimicking murmurs of ventricular septal defect, obstructive cardiomyopathy, or mitral regurgitation.

The murmur of tricuspid regurgitation is classically holosystolic, but it can be late systolic or early systolic in timing. At times, holosystolic murmurs of tricuspid regurgitation may be recorded by intracardiac (right atrial) phonocardiography when no or only a mid-systolic murmur can be recorded on the precordium. Rios and associates have emphasized that early systolic murmurs are a feature of tricuspid regurgitation *without* elevated right ventricular systolic pressures.[89] In this situation, regurgitant flow is thought to decrease in the latter part of systole as the right atrial *v* wave and the right ventricular systolic pressures tend to equilibrate.[89] The intensity and the frequency of the murmur are variable. The intensity of the murmur is not helpful in determining the severity of tricuspid regurgitation. Gross tricuspid regurgitation can be present with little or no murmur. Loud "musical," "honking," or "whooping" murmurs may result from trivial tricuspid regurgitation.[33,38-41] This type of musical murmur is most frequently reported in patients with tricuspid valve prolapse.[33,38-41]

The murmurs resulting from tricuspid and mitral valve regurgitation

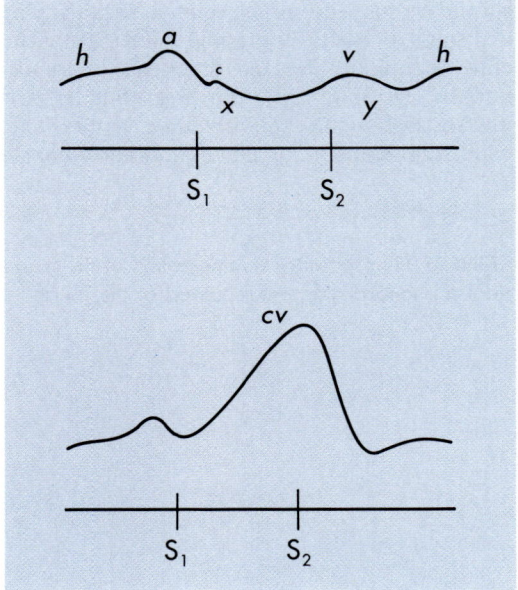

FIGURE 87.10 (Top) Normal jugular venous pulse illustrating the *a* and *v* waves and the *x* and *y* descents. The *c* wave follows the *a* wave and interrupts the *x* descent. The *h* wave is also shown. First heart sound is labeled S_1 and the second heart sound is labeled S_2. (Bottom) Schematic representation of a cv wave of tricuspid regurgitation. Note the relationship of the cv wave to S_1 and second heart sound (S_2). A small presystolic *a* wave is shown but is not labeled.

may be similar in character and have overlapping auscultatory areas. Therefore, emphasis has been placed on inspiratory augmentation of the intensity of tricuspid valve murmurs. Since 1946, when Rivero-Carvallo described this inspiratory increase, this sign has been considered the most important auscultatory feature of tricuspid regurgitation.[90] The absence of Carvallo's sign has been referred to as "silent" regurgitation.[91] The inspiratory increase in the intensity of the murmur is thought to be due to increased venous return. The intensity of the murmur can be augmented by applying manual pressure below the liver either before or during inspiration. Occasionally, the murmur may appear only during inspiration while applying manual abdominal pressure.[92] Gooch and associates refer to the technique of applying abdominal pressure during inspiration as the "augmented Carvallo sign."[92] The increase in murmur intensity is most marked during early inspiration, but the increased intensity is lost if inspiration is held.[88] In the presence of right heart failure, right heart output cannot be further increased by inspiration. Thus, the Carvallo sign may be absent in patients with tricuspid regurgitation and right heart failure only to appear after therapy. Occasionally, the murmur of tricuspid regurgitation will appear with the onset of atrial fibrillation and disappear with the return to normal sinus rhythm.[88]

Rios and associates described the auscultatory features of acute tricuspid regurgitation as a short, decrescendo murmur heard over the tricuspid area associated with a right-sided fourth heard sound.[89] The decrescendo configuration of the murmur is associated with end-systolic equalization of right ventricular and right atrial pressures.[89] Thus, the auscultatory findings in acute tricuspid regurgitation are similar to those found in acute mitral regurgitation.

ELECTROCARDIOGRAM AND CHEST ROENTGENOGRAM

The electrocardiogram may provide evidence of right atrial enlargement with increased voltage and rightward shift of the P-wave vector. The chest roentgenogram often shows rightward displacement of the right heart border (which is formed by the right atrium). The maximal distance of the right heart border of the heart from the midline exceeds the normal value of 4 cm.

ECHOCARDIOGRAPHY

Echocardiography is used to identify not only the etiology but also the pathologic consequence of tricuspid regurgitation. Echocardiography can be helpful in identifying specific causes of tricuspid regurgitation. Tricuspid valve prolapse, chordal rupture, endocarditis, rheumatic involvement, carcinoid syndrome, and myxomas, all have relatively specific two-dimensional echocardiographic appearances.[93,94] Echocardiography has also identified the indirect signs of tricuspid regurgitation (i.e., indicators of right ventricular volume overload). On motion-mode echocardiograms there is an increase in the diameter of the right ventricular chamber or paradoxical septal motion, or both. These findings, obviously, are not specific for tricuspid regurgitation since there are other causes of right ventricular volume overload. Similar abnormalities are also seen with two-dimensional echocardiography. In addition, dilatation of the tricuspid annulus and reduced systolic shortening of annular size have also been identified by two-dimensional echocardiography.[8]

Contrast echocardiography can detect tricuspid regurgitation. When a bolus of saline or indocyanine green is injected into a peripheral vein, microcavitation can be visualized in the right heart chambers.[95] In tricuspid regurgitation there is systolic microcavitation in the inferior vena cava. Three distinct patterns of contrast appearance in the inferior vena cava have been observed. "V wave synchronous" patterns are seen in patients with tricuspid regurgitation; "a wave synchronous" and "random" patterns are seen in patients without tricuspid regurgitation. The movement of microcavitation back and forth across the tricuspid valve has also been reported.

DOPPLER FLOW STUDIES

The addition of Doppler flow studies to the basic or anatomical echocardiographic imaging modalities has enhanced the physician's ability to diagnose abnormalities of the tricuspid valve. By analyzing the returning echoes for a change or shift in the returning sound wave frequency (the Doppler principle), the velocity of blood movement can be estimated.[96] Continuous-wave and single-point Doppler techniques are available.[96–99] Color flow imaging, a technique that provides a real-time two-dimensional image of blood flow superimposed on a real-time two-dimensional anatomical image, results in images that resemble regurgitant flows or stenotic flow jets seen on x-ray cineangiography. The images are color coded to display the direction and relative velocities of the blood flow.

Tricuspid regurgitation results in reverse or disturbed flow in the right atrial chamber (Figs. 87.12 and 87.13) and at times in the inferior vena cava or hepatic veins.[97–99] Severe tricuspid regurgitation is readily documented by single-point or range-gated pulsed Doppler (Figs. 87.12 and 87.13). However, normal individuals may demonstrate a small systolic flow disturbance in the right atrium. Thus, the sensitivity and specificity of this technique for the diagnosis of mild tricuspid regurgitation are unknown. As the severity of the regurgitation increases, the depth of penetration and the duration and extent of retrograde flow in the right atrium increase. In severe tricuspid regurgitation the disturbed flow can be detected at the roof of the right atrium. Using this criterion alone, a jet lesion can result in an overestimation of the degree of tricuspid regurgitation.

SUMMARY OF NONINVASIVE TECHNIQUES

Moderate tricuspid regurgitation can be diagnosed by radionuclide techniques. Some quantitative assessment of the severity of isolated tricuspid regurgitation is feasible by estimating regurgitant index. If the regurgitant index is less than 15, significant tricuspid regurgitation should be suspected. The relative sensitivity and specificity of the physical signs, echocardiographic microcavitation technique, and radionuclide techniques for the diagnosis of tricuspid regurgitation are unknown. Doppler echocardiography is very sensitive, and better methods of quantification will be forthcoming. In all probability, clinically significant tricuspid regurgitation can be diagnosed at the bed-

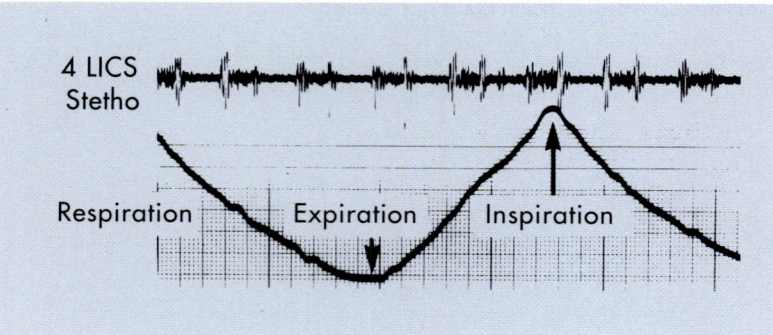

FIGURE 87.11 Inspiratory augmentation of the murmur of tricuspid insufficiency from a phonocardiogram recorded at the fourth left intercostal space (4LICS).

side. Although insensitive, the presence of *cv* waves in the jugular venous pulse, associated with an inspiratory increase in the intensity of a lower left sternal border murmur, is relatively specific.

HEMODYNAMICS AND ANGIOGRAPHY

Careful analysis of the right atrial pressure contour obtained during cardiac catheterization can provide information diagnostic of tricuspid regurgitation. Normally, the phasic and mean right atrial pressures decrease with inspiration with little change in the wave form. In contrast, patients with mild tricuspid regurgitation may have augmented *v* waves (and thus *y* descents) with inspiration. With more than trivial regurgitation, the *v* waves may be increased during all phases of respiration and become more prominent than the *a* wave. With severe regurgitation, the right atrial pressure pattern becomes "ventricularized"; that is, the contour of the right atrial pressure is similar, but of lower amplitude, than the contour of the right ventricular pressure. This pattern has been recorded in one third of patients with severe tricuspid regurgitation.[100]

Although angiographic techniques are sensitive methods for detecting mitral and aortic regurgitation, the angiographic diagnosis of tricuspid regurgitation was originally less well accepted since the catheter had to traverse the tricuspid valve. However, with the development of preshaped catheters and optimal techniques, right ventricular angiography has been shown to be a reliable way to evaluate the tricuspid valve. If the catheter traverses the valve perpendicular to the plane of the tricuspid annulus and no premature ventricular contractions are induced during the injection, the presence or absence of regurgitation can be determined with a high degree of accuracy.[100] The degree of tricuspid regurgitation has been arbitrarily graded as follows: 1+, minimal systolic regurgitant jet with rapid clearing; 2+, regurgitant jet with partial opacification of the right atrium; 3+, dense opacification of the entire right atrium; and 4+, dense opacification of the entire right atrium with vena caval reflux.[100] Figure 87.14 shows three right ventricular angiograms with no regurgitation, 2+ tricuspid regurgita-

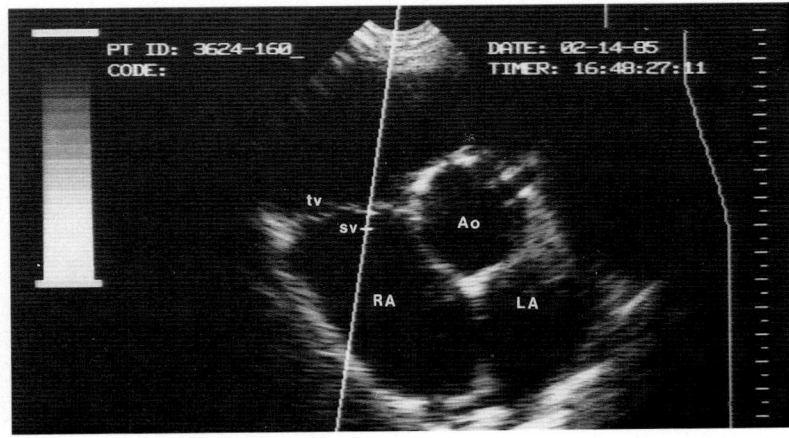
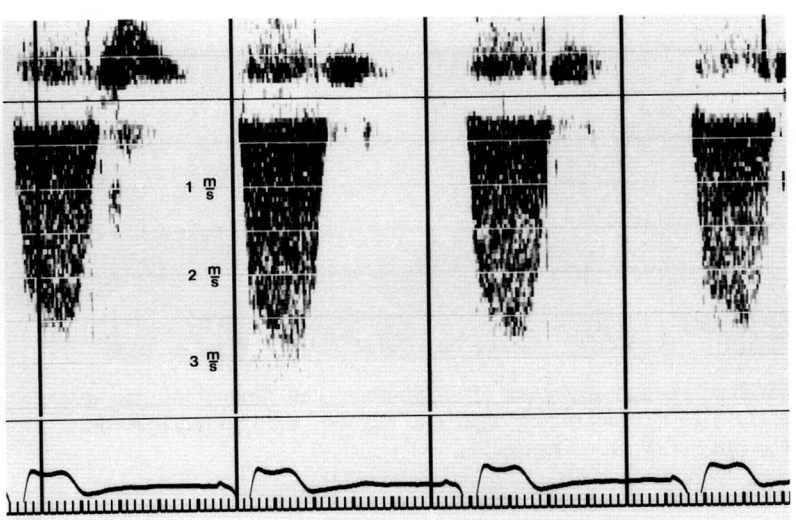

FIGURE 87.12 (*Left*) Parasternal short axis, two-dimensional echocardiogram with Doppler sample volume (*SV*) positioned proximal to the tricuspid valve (*TV*). Other structures visualized are the aorta (*Ao*), right atrium (*RA*), and left atrium (*LA*). (*Right*) Doppler flow velocity profile showing peak systolic regurgitant flow of about 2.5 m/sec, obtained from the sample volume shown above. (Courtesy of Dr. Keith Comess)

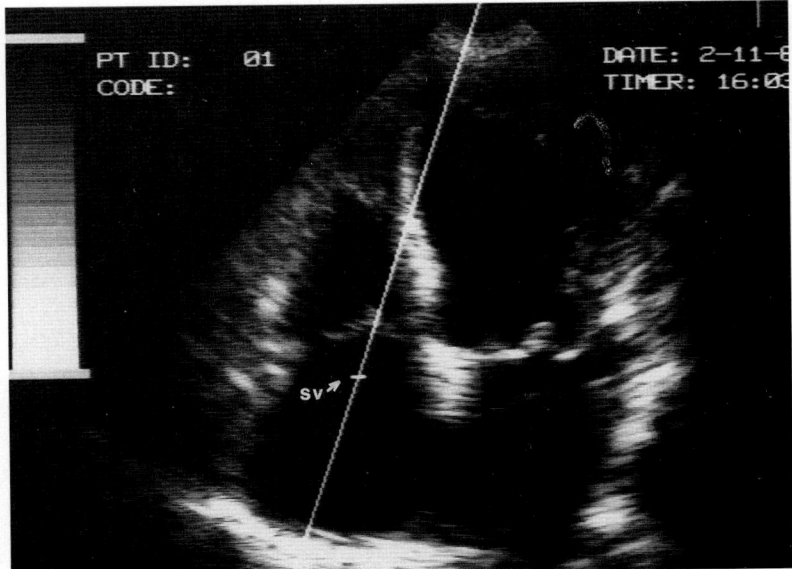
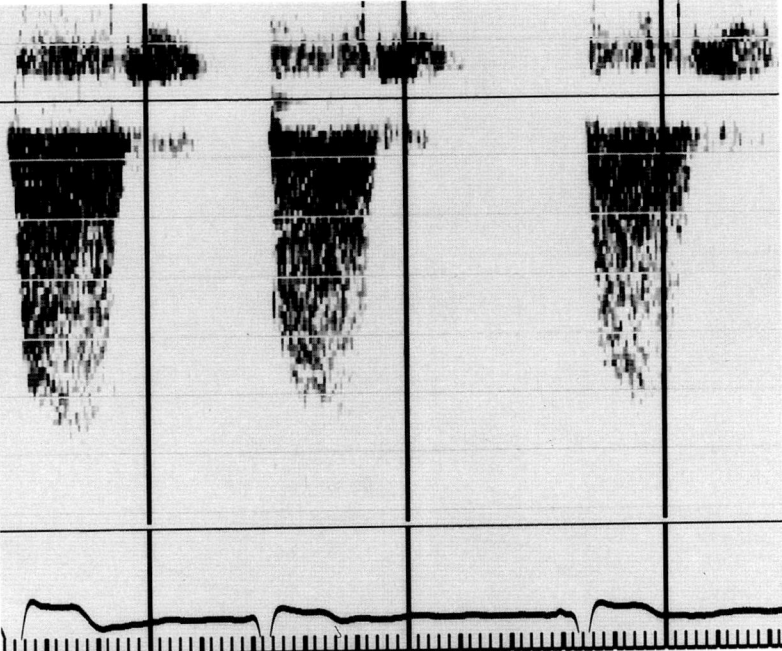

FIGURE 87.13 (*Left*) Two-dimensional echocardiographic apical four-chamber view with Doppler sample volume (*SV*) positioned in the right atrium proximal to the tricuspid valve. (*Right*) Doppler flow velocity profile showing peak systolic regurgitant flow. (Courtesy of Dr. Keith Comess)

tion, and 4+ tricuspid regurgitation.[98] Others classify tricuspid regurgitation as mild, moderate, or severe as follows: *mild*, partial, nonhomogenous opacification of the right atrium, including constant early or mid-systolic regurgitation; *moderate*, almost complete and homogenous filling of the right atrium; and *severe*, immediate filling of the whole right atrium and both caval veins.[100]

Intracardiac phonocardiography is another method of diagnosing tricuspid regurgitation (Fig. 87.15). The appearance of a marked increase in intensity of a systolic murmur when a microtip catheter is withdrawn from the right ventricle to the right atrium is diagnostic. However, intracardiac phonocardiography cannot be used to quantitate the degree of regurgitation.

DIAGNOSIS OF TRICUSPID STENOSIS
CLINICAL FINDINGS

Tricuspid stenosis should be suspected in all patients with rheumatic valvular heart disease, but especially in those with elevated venous pressure, fatigue, and fluid retention.[15] At the bedside, the diagnosis of tricuspid stenosis is made by observing the jugular venous wave form and by auscultation. Stenosis of the tricuspid valve results in an increase in the height of the *a* wave of the jugular venous pulse (Fig. 87.16). In the setting of rheumatic mitral stenosis, the presence of a giant *a* wave in the jugular venous pulse is almost pathognomonic of tricuspid stenosis. In other settings a large *a* wave is not diagnostic of tricuspid stenosis since a more common cause is decreased right ventricular compliance. In addition, advanced tricuspid stenosis often results in right atrial enlargement and atrial fibrillation. With the onset of atrial fibrillation the *a* wave disappears. Since tricuspid stenosis limits the rapidity with which the right atrium empties, a more specific venous abnormality is the slow *y* descent and the absence of the *y* trough (Fig. 87.17).

When the patient is in sinus rhythm, a crescendo–decrescendo presystolic murmur is the most important auscultatory sign of tricuspid stenosis. In contrast to the presystolic murmur of mitral stenosis which is crescendo, increasing in intensity until truncated by a loud first heart sound, the "atrial systolic" murmur of tricuspid stenosis has a distinct

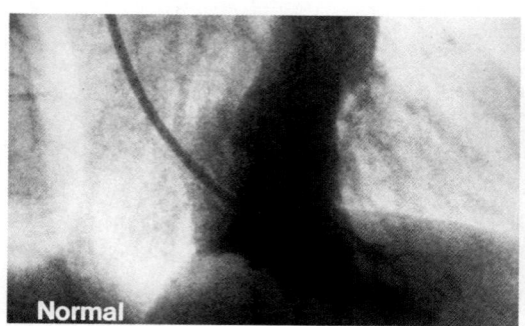 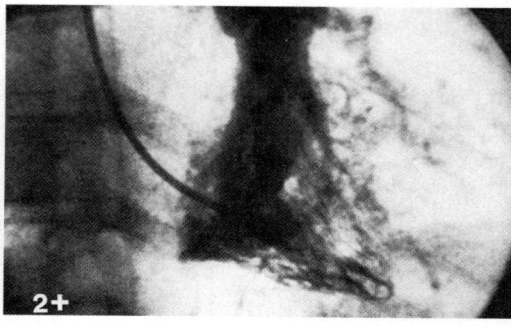 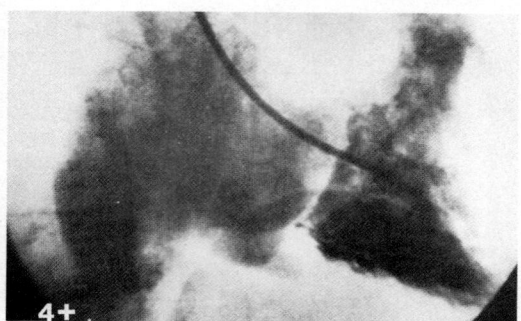

FIGURE 87.14 Right ventricular cineangiograms. (*Left*) Normal tricuspid valve; (*middle*) 2+ tricuspid regurgitation; and (*right*) 4+ tricuspid regurgitation. (Courtesy of Dr. Alan Gooch)

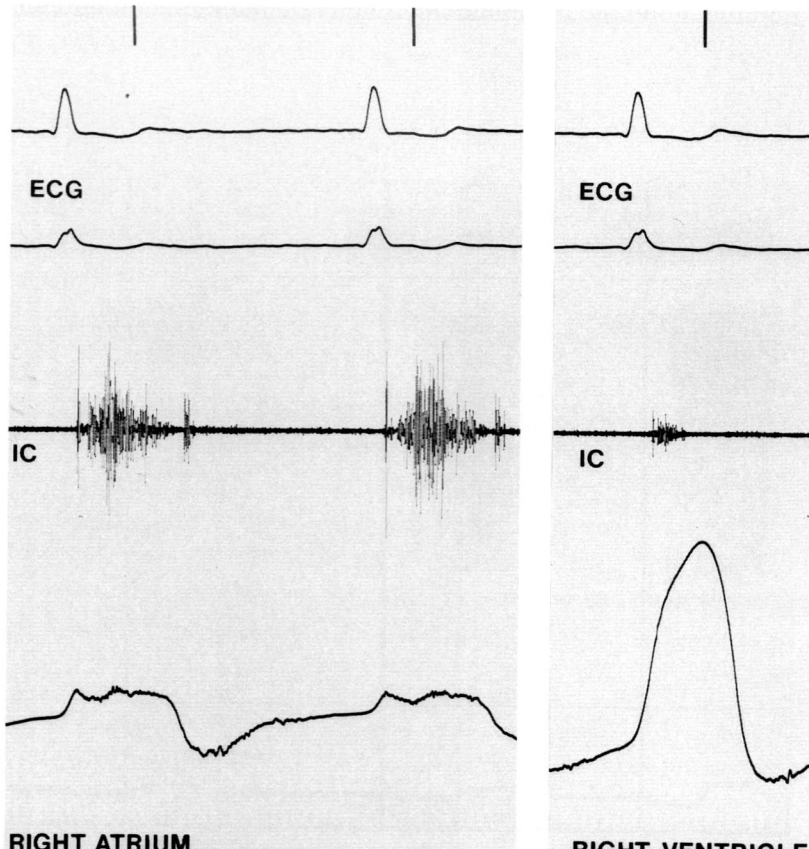

FIGURE 87.15 Intracardiac phonocardiogram (*IC*) revealing prominent murmur in right atrium that is not present in the right ventricle.

crescendo–decrescendo configuration that ends before right ventricular systole (Fig. 87.18). This murmur parallels the right ventricular–right atrial diastolic pressure gradient at the time of the atrial *a* wave.[101] The separation of the presystolic murmur of tricuspid stenosis and the first heart sound is made more distinct by the presence of first-degree heart block, a not uncommon finding in this clinical setting.

The low-frequency diastolic rumble of tricuspid stenosis is best heard along the lower left sternal border. A mid-diastolic murmur is most common in patients with atrial fibrillation. Classically, this rumble increases with inspiration (Fig. 87.19). In general, the configuration of the diastolic murmur (as well as the atrial presystolic murmur) parallels the pressure gradient envelope. A low-frequency early diastolic murmur is likewise not diagnostic of tricuspid stenosis, since similar murmurs can be produced by increased flow across a normal tricuspid valve, as seen in patients with a large shunt from an atrial septal defect. The opening snap of tricuspid stenosis is not a helpful diagnostic sign since it is rarely appreciated at the bedside. Occasionally, the tricuspid opening snap can be recorded (Fig. 87.18).

ELECTROCARDIOGRAM AND CHEST ROENTGENOGRAM

The electrocardiographic findings in patients with tricuspid stenosis include evidence of right atrial or biatrial enlargement or conduction abnormalities in the absence of electrocardiographic evidence of right ventricular hypertrophy.[15,102] First-degree heart block and atrial fibrillation are also common. The chest roentgenogram is seldom characteristic but is reported to show a prominent right heart border with a relatively inconspicuous pulmonary artery.[15,102]

ECHOCARDIOGRAPHY

Although rheumatic involvement of the tricuspid valve can be detected with the M-mode technique, two-dimensional echocardiography is more sensitive and specific. The normal tricuspid valve leaflets are seen on two-dimensional echocardiography as two thin, freely moving structures.[94] In the parasternal long axis views, the imaging plane tran-

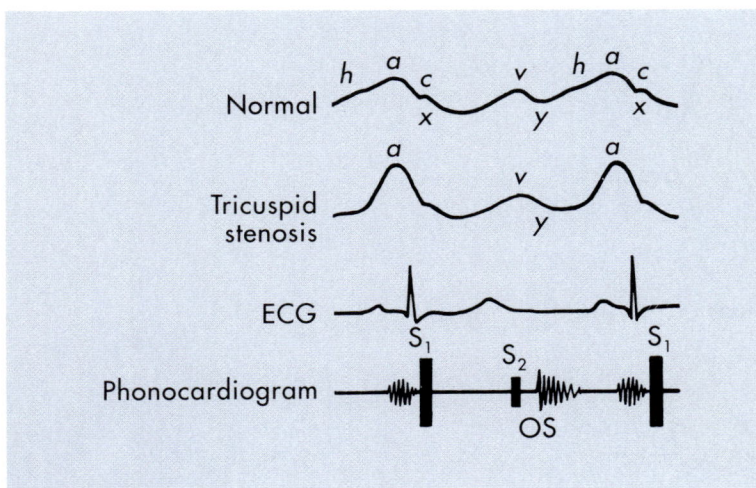

FIGURE 87.16 Comparison of the normal jugular venous pulse with that seen in patients with tricuspid stenosis (see text). The auscultatory findings of tricuspid stenosis are demonstrated on the phonocardiogram illustrated below the electrocardiogram (ECG).

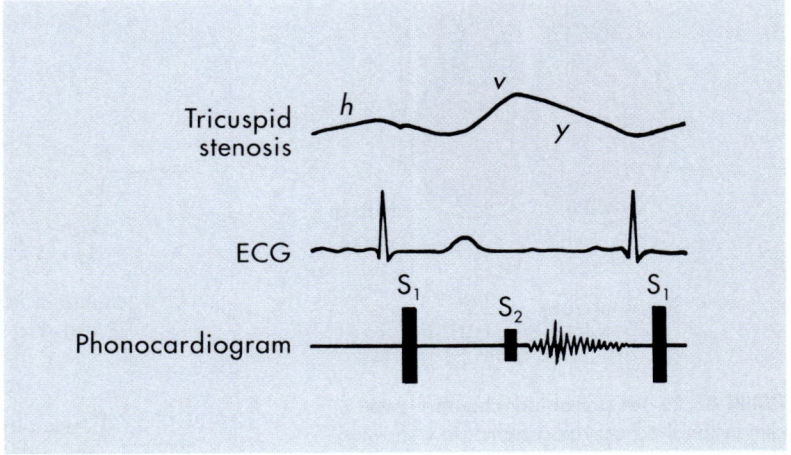

FIGURE 87.17 Illustration of the jugular venous pulse, electrocardiogram, and phonocardiogram in a patient with tricuspid stenosis and atrial fibrillation.

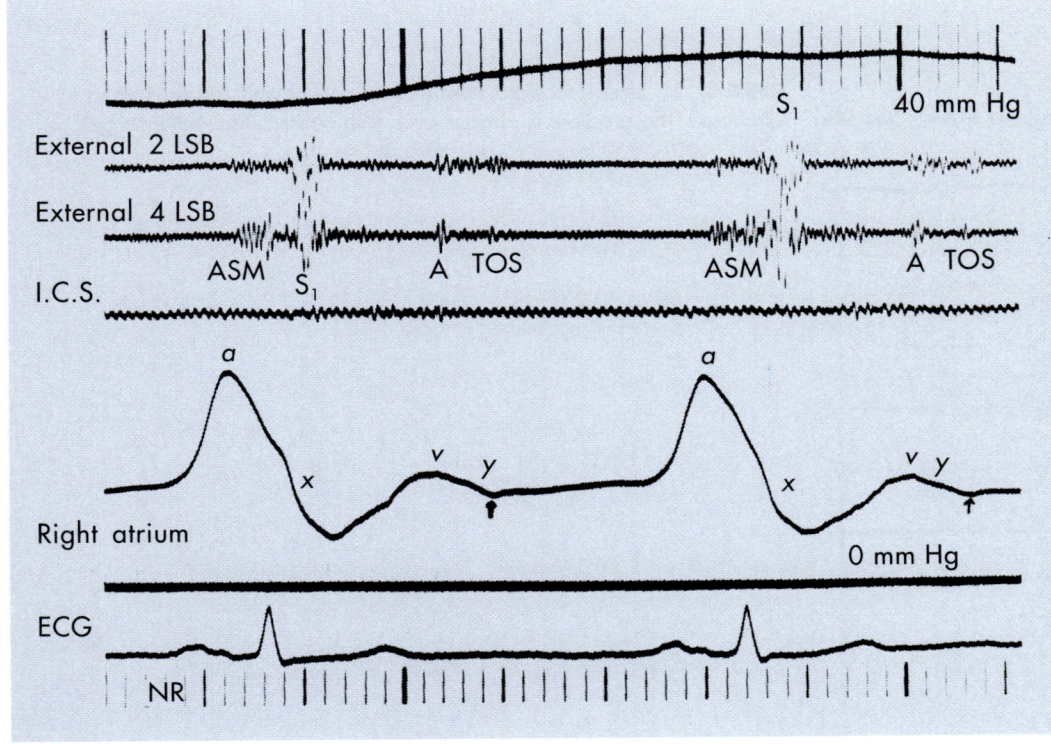

FIGURE 87.18 Right atrial pressure pulse of tricuspid stenosis as recorded with a manometer catheter. (Top to bottom) Respirometer recording (downward deflection indicates inspiration); external (Ext) phonocardiogram at second left intercostal space, left sternal border (LSB); external phonocardiogram at fourth left intercostal space, left sternal border; intercardiac sound (I.C.S.) recording, right atrium; right atrial pressure pulse; electrocardiogram (EKG). (A, aortic component, S_2; ASM, atrial systolic murmur; S_1, first heart sound; TOS, tricuspid opening snap; arrows indicate time of tricuspid opening snap in relation to pressure pulse.) Scale is 0 to 40 mm Hg; recording speed is 100 mm/sec; time lines are 40 m/sec. (Wooley CF, Fontana ME, Kilman JW, Ryan JM: Tricuspid stenosis: Atrial systolic murmur, tricuspid opening snap, and right atrial pressure pulse. Am J Med 78:375, 1985)

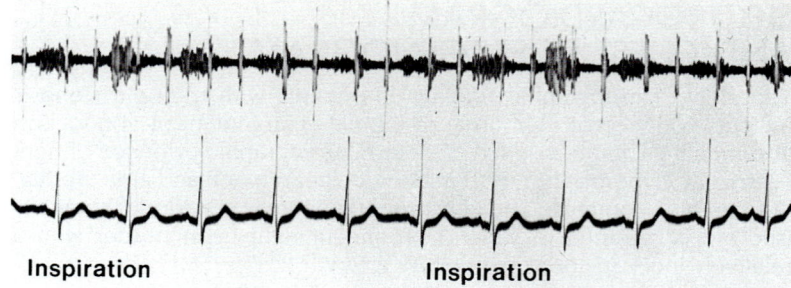

Inspiration   Inspiration

FIGURE 87.19 Murmur of tricuspid stenosis from a prosthetic porcine valve in the tricuspid position. Note the inspiratory increase in the diastolic murmur.

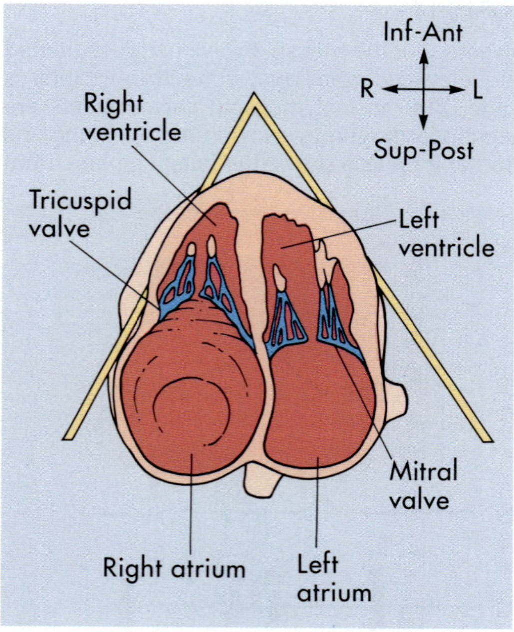

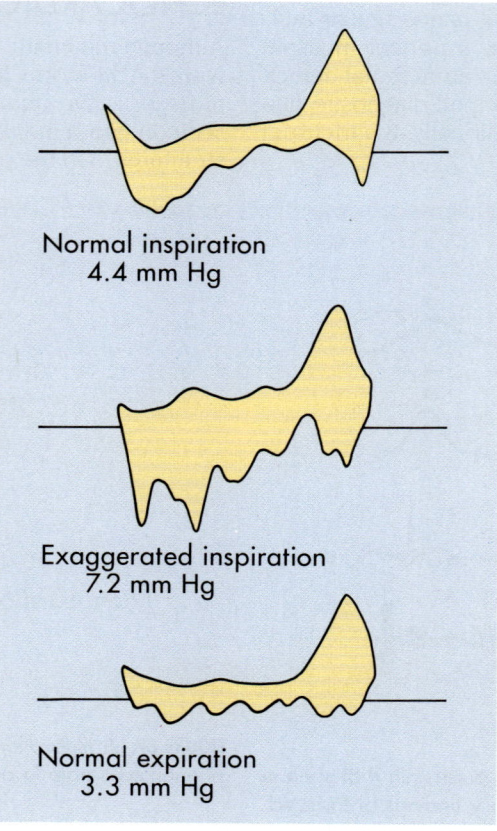

FIGURE 87.20 An apical four-chamber two-dimensional echocardiographic view showing doming of the tricuspid valve in diastole with thickening and doming of the anterior and septal tricuspid leaflets, chordal thickening, and fibrosis of the subvalvular inflow portion of the tricuspid valve. There is right atrial enlargement and bulging of the atrial septum toward the left. (Modified from Sahn DJ, Anderson F: An Atlas for Echocardiographers: Two Dimensional Anatomy of the Heart. New York, John Wiley & Sons, 1982)

FIGURE 87.21 Tricuspid valve pressure gradient. Right atrial pressures change very little with normal or exaggerated inspiration. The gradient increase with inspiration is related to a fall in right ventricular diastolic pressure. (Modified from Wooley CF, Fontana ME, Kilman JW, Ryan JM: Tricuspid stenosis: Atrial systolic murmur, tricuspid opening snap, and right atrial pressure pulse. Am J Med 78:375, 1985)

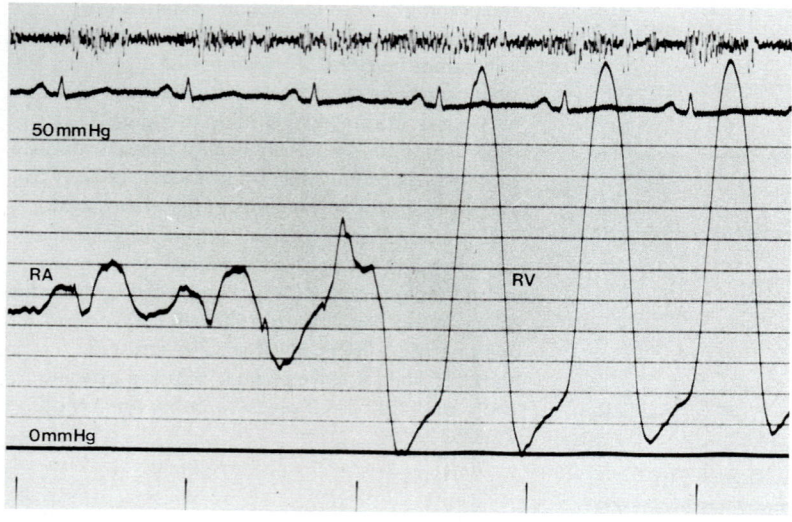

FIGURE 87.22 Severe tricuspid stenosis in a patient with carcinoid heart syndrome. The gradient is obvious even with nonsimultaneous tracings.

sects the anterior and posterior cusps of the tricuspid valve. In the apical and subcostal four-chamber views, the imaging plane transects the anterior and septal leaflets. These leaflets are seen to coapt in systole and to open freely during diastole. Reduced motion and incomplete opening of the valves occurs in any state causing decreased right ventricular inflow.

Two-dimensional echocardiography has been found to have a high predictive accuracy for the diagnosis of tricuspid stenosis when the following echocardiographic criteria are used: (1) evidence of rheumatic involvement of the mitral valve; (2) diastolic doming of the anterior tricuspid leaflet (*i.e.,* restriction of leaflet tip motion with greater mobility of the body of the leaflet); (3) reduced excursion of the septal or posterior leaflet, or both; and (4) a reduction in the tricuspid orifice diameter relative to the annular diameter recorded in the same scan plane.[94] Thickening and reduced motion of the posterior or septal tricuspid leaflets, or both, with normal anterior leaflet motion may be present with rheumatic involvement but are not considered to represent valvular stenosis.[93,94] The two-dimensional echocardiographic appearance of tricuspid stenosis is illustrated in Figure 87.20.

HEMODYNAMICS

The hemodynamic diagnosis of tricuspid stenosis often depends on the accurate measurement of a small pressure gradient (Fig. 87.21). Precise simultaneous pressure recordings from the right atrium and right ventricle are required.[3] Pressure recordings obtained during withdrawal of the catheter tip from the right ventricle to the right atrium are inadequate except in patients with severe tricuspid stenosis (Fig. 87.22). The "pullback" recording technique is limited because (1) atrial fibrillation makes it difficult to superimpose atrial and ventricular pressure curves; (2) tricuspid regurgitation, which frequently accompanies rheumatic tricuspid stenosis, elevates mean right atrial pressure and can create the appearance of a diastolic gradient; and (3) small diastolic gradients, which are typical of tricuspid stenosis, are often overloaded if the "pullback" technique is used.[102,103] Since simultaneous right atrial and right ventricular pressure tracings are not obtained on a routine basis, the diagnosis of tricuspid stenosis is frequently overlooked unless this lesion is suspected from the bedside or noninvasive precatheterization evaluation prior to catheterization, and the study is designed to specifically determine the presence or absence of tricuspid stenosis.[3] Even when simultaneous recording techniques are used, low flow across a stenotic tricuspid valve may result in deceivingly small gradients. Exercise or other methods of increasing the cardiac output may be required for hemodynamic diagnosis.

MANAGEMENT

The management of tricuspid valve disease is determined by the etiology of the condition and its severity. In the majority of patients with functional tricuspid regurgitation, therapy is initially directed at the contributing abnormality. This approach may require treatment of left heart failure, correction of mitral valve disease, thrombolytic therapy of massive pulmonary emboli, or chronic oxygen therapy in patients with cor pulmonale secondary to chronic lung disease and arterial oxygen desaturation. Specific therapy may be necessary: antibiotics and/or surgery for endocarditis, and surgery for myxomas, tricuspid stenosis, traumatic rupture of major chordae or heads of the papillary muscle, and so on.[104,105]

Since the most common cause of functional tricuspid regurgitation is right heart failure, early therapy of failure is of prime importance. Once severe tricuspid regurgitation is present, diuretics must be used with discretion. Because a large *cv* wave elevates the mean venous pressure, the physician is tempted to use increasing doses or combinations of diuretics in an effort to lower the venous pressure. Since the *cv* waves are systolic in timing, the true right ventricular end-diastolic or filling pressure is the pressure at the trough of the venous wave just before its onset. The top of the venous wave is produced by right ventricular systolic pressure. Excessive diuresis may result in an excessively decreased right ventricular filling pressure, decreased cardiac output, and increased fatigue.

Surgery is generally reserved for patients with advanced valvular disease.[106–108] It was thought that the tricuspid valve was not necessary for survival since total excision was performed in some patients with endocarditis.[109] However, it is now evident that complete removal of the tricuspid valve without replacement eventually results in congestive heart failure.[110] Surgical management may require annuloplasty or replacement with a prosthetic valve. Tricuspid annuloplasty should be considered because of its simplicity, safety, and effectiveness. Although tricuspid regurgitation may lessen and disappear in many patients simply as a result of correction of the left-sided valvular disease, this response is not predictable. In patients with severe tricuspid malfunction, valve replacement may be necessary. The mortality of tricuspid valve replacement is high when associated with replacement of the aortic and/or mitral valve.[106] On the other hand, unrecognized and uncorrected rheumatic tricuspid stenosis can have a deleterious effect on the results of surgery for aortic and mitral valve disease.[111,112]

CONCLUSIONS

An appreciation of tricuspid valve disease adds significantly to the physician's clinical acumen. Tricuspid valve disease may be an incidental finding or its presence may provide a clue to otherwise unexplained cardiovascular signs or symptoms. Tricuspid regurgitation is the most commonly seen lesion, and when present is most often functional. However, acquired and congenital defects must be excluded. Tricuspid stenosis is seen much less frequently but must be considered in patients with rheumatic heart disease who have involvement of both the mitral and aortic valves, especially if there is failure to improve after corrective surgery.

The clinical diagnosis of severe tricuspid valve disease, particularly tricuspid regurgitation, is usually not difficult. However, clinical signs of mild to moderate disease may be quite subtle and noninvasive techniques such as echo-Doppler or invasive techniques such as right ventricular angiography may be necessary for confirmation or quantification. However, slight tricuspid regurgitation can be detected by Doppler in many normals.

Management of tricuspid valve disease is based on the etiology and severity of the disease and is frequently directed at the contributing abnormality. Surgical therapy is usually reserved for patients with advanced valvular disease.

REFERENCES

1. Silver MD, Lam JH, Ranganathan N et al: Morphology of human tricuspid valve. Circulation 43:333, 1971
2. Wooley CF: Rediscovery of the tricuspid valve. Curr Probl Cardiol 6:8, 1981
3. Wooley CF: The Spectrum of Tricuspid Regurgitation. Dallas, American Heart Association, Monograph #46, 1975
4. Mills PG, Chamusco RF, Moos S et al: Echophonocardiographic studies of the contribution of the atrioventricular valves to the first heart sound. Circulation 54:944, 1976
5. Waider W, Craige E: First heart sound and ejection sounds: Echocardiographic and phonocardiographic correlations with valvular events. Am J Cardiol 35:346, 1975
6. Leatham A, Leech G: Observations on relation between heart sounds and valve movements by simultaneous echo and phonocardiography (abstr). Br Heart J 37:557, 1975
7. Tsakiris AG, Mair DD, Seki S et al: Motion of the tricuspid valve annulus in anesthetized intact dogs. Circ Res 36:43, 1975
8. Tei C, Pilgrim JP, Shah PM et al: The tricuspid valve annulus: Study of size and motion in normal subjects and in patients with tricuspid regurgitation. Circulation 66:665, 1982
9. Ubango J, Figueroa A, Ochoteco A et al: Analysis of the amount of tricuspid valve annular dilatation required to produce functional tricuspid regurgitation. Am J Cardiol 52:155, 1983
10. Hollman A: The anatomical appearance in rheumatic tricuspid valve disease. Br Heart J 19:211, 1957

11. Yu PN, Harken DE, Lovejoy FW Jr et al: Clinical and hemodynamic studies of tricuspid stenosis. Circulation 13:680, 1956
12. Wood P: Chronic rheumatic heart disease. In Wood P (ed): Diseases of the Heart and Circulation, 3rd ed, pp 690–699. Philadelphia, JB Lippincott, 1968
13. Chopra P, Tandon HD: Pathology of chronic rheumatic heart disease with particular reference to tricuspid valve involvement. Acta Cardiol 32:423, 1977
14. Edwards WD, Peterson K, Edwards JE: Active valvulitis associated with chronic rheumatic valvular disease and active myocarditis. Circulation 57:181, 1978
15. Gibson R, Wood P: The diagnosis of tricuspid stenosis. Br Heart J 17:552, 1955
16. Goodwin JF, Rab SM, Sinha AK et al: Rheumatic tricuspid stenosis. Br Med J 2:1383, 1957
17. Kitchin A, Turner R: Diagnosis and treatment of tricuspid stenosis. Br Heart J 26:354, 1964
18. Guyer DE, Gillam LD, Foale RA: Comparison of the echocardiographic and hemodynamic diagnosis of rheumatic tricuspid stenosis. J Am Coll Cardiol 3:1135, 1984
19. Daniels SJ, Mintz GS, Kotler MN: Rheumatic tricuspid valve disease: Two dimensional echocardiographic, hemodynamic, and angiographic correlations. Am J Cardiol 51:492, 1983
20. Gutner RN: Trivalvular rheumatic stenosis: Documentation of disease progression by serial cardiac catheterization. Am J Med Sci 280:185, 1980
21. Ubago JL, Figueroa A, Colman T et al: Right ventriculography as a valid method for the diagnosis of tricuspid insufficiency. Cathet Cardiovasc Diagn 7:433, 1981
22. McAllister RG, Friesinger GC, Sinclair-Smith BC: Tricuspid regurgitation following inferior myocardial infarction. Arch Intern Med 136:96, 1976
23. Zone DD, Botti RE: Right ventricular infarction with tricuspid insufficiency and chronic right heart failure. Am J Cardiol 37:445, 1976
24. Bracchetti D, Capucci A: Right ventricular infarction with tricuspid insufficiency. Case report. Am J Cardiol 39:133, 1977
25. Eisenberg S, Suyemato J: Rupture of a papillary muscle of the tricuspid valve following acute myocardial infarction. Circulation 30:588, 1964
26. Roberts WC: Characteristics and consequences of infective endocarditis (active or healed or both) learned from morphologic studies. In Rahimtoola SH (ed): Infective Endocarditis. New York, Grune & Stratton, 1978
27. Stimmel B, Dack S: Infective endocarditis in narcotic addicts. In Rahimtoola SH (ed): Infective Endocarditis. New York, Grune & Stratton, 1978
28. Reid CL, Chandraratua PAN, Rahimtoola SH: Infective endocarditis: Improved diagnosis and treatment. In O'Rourke RH: Current Problems in Cardiology. Chicago, Year Book Medical Publishers, 1985
29. Chambers HF, Koreniowski OM, Sande MA: National Collaborative Endocarditis Study Group. Staphylococcus aureus endocarditis: Clinical manifestation in addicts and non-addicts. Medicine 63:170, 1983
30. Watanabe T, Katsume H, Matsukubo H et al: Ruptured chordae tendineae of the tricuspid valve due to nonpenetrating trauma. Chest 80:751, 1981
31. Naccarelli GV, Haisty WK, Kahl FR: Left ventricular to right atrial defect and tricuspid insufficiency secondary to nonpenetrating cardiac trauma. J Trauma 20:887, 1980
32. Bardy GH, Talano JV, Meyers S, Lesch M: Acquired cyanotic heart disease secondary to traumatic tricuspid regurgitation. Am J Cardiol 44:1401, 1979
33. Weinreich DJ, Burke JF, Bharati S, Lev M: Isolated prolapse of the tricuspid valve. J Am Coll Cardiol 6:475, 1985
34. Mardelli TJ, Morganroth J, Chen CC et al: Tricuspid valve prolapse diagnosed by cross-sectional echocardiography. Chest 79:201, 1979
35. Ogawa S, Hayashi J, Sasaki H et al: Evaluation of combined valvular prolapse syndrome by two-dimensional echocardiography. Circulation 65:174, 1982
36. Morganroth J, Jones RH, Chen CC et al: Two-dimensional echocardiography in mitral, aortic and tricuspid valve prolapse: The clinical problem, cardiac nuclear imaging considerations and proposed standard for diagnosis. Am J Cardiol 46:1164, 1980
37. Maranhao V, Gooch AS, Yang SS et al: Prolapse of the tricuspid leaflets in the systolic murmur-click syndrome. Cathet Cardiovasc Diagn 1:81, 1980
38. Bashour T, Lindsay J Jr: Midsystolic clicks originating from tricuspid valve structures: A sequela of heroin-induced endocarditis. Chest 67:620, 1975
39. Sasse L, Froelich CR: Echocardiographic tricuspid prolapse and non-ejection systolic click. Chest 73:869, 1978
40. Doi YL, Sugiura T, Bishop RL et al: High-speed echophonocardiographic detection of tricuspid valve prolapse in mitral valve prolapse with discrepancy in onset of systolic murmur. Am Heart J 103:301, 1982
41. Tei C, Shah PM, Tanaka H: Phonographic-echographic documentation of systolic honk in tricuspid prolapse. Am Heart J 103:294, 1982
42. Shrivastava S, Guthrie R, Edwards JE: Prolapse of the mitral valve. Modern Concepts of Cardiovascular Disease 46:57, 1977
43. Thorson A, Biorck G, Bjorkman G et al: Malignant carcinoid of the small intestine with metastases to the liver, valvular disease of the right side of the heart (pulmonary stenosis and tricuspid regurgitation without septal defects), peripheral vasomotor symptoms, bronchoconstriction, and an unusual type of cyanosis. A clinical and pathological syndrome. Am Heart J 47:795, 1954
44. Roberts WC, Sjoerdsma A: The cardiac disease associated with the carcinoid syndrome (carcinoid heart disease). Am J Med 36:5, 1964
45. Trell E, Ransing A, Ripa J et al: Carcinoid heart disease: Clinicopathologic findings and follow-up in 11 cases. Am J Med 54:433, 1973
46. Sworn MJ, Edlin GP, McGill DAF et al: Tricuspid valve replacement in carcinoid syndrome due to ovarian primary. Br Med J 280:85, 1980
47. Erhlichman RT: Carcinoid tumor. Johns Hopkins Med J 145:170, 1979
48. Davies MK, Lowry PJ, Littler WA: Cross sectional echocardiographic feature in carcinoid heart disease: A mechanism for tricuspid regurgitation in this syndrome. Br Heart J 51:355, 1984
49. Howard RJ, Drobac M, Rider WD et al: Carcinoid heart disease: Diagnosis by two-dimensional echocardiography. Circulation 66:1059, 1982
50. Baker BJ, McNee VD, Scovil JA et al: Tricuspid insufficiency in carcinoid heart disease: An echocardiographic description. Am Heart J 101:107, 1981
51. Callahan JA, Wrobleski EM, Reeder GS et al: Echocardiographic features of carcinoid heart disease. Am J Cardiol 50:762, 1982
52. Forman MB, Byrd BF III, Oates JA et al: Two-dimensional echocardiography in the diagnosis of carcinoid heart disease. Am Heart J 107:492, 1984
53. Okada RD, Ewy GA, Copeland JG: Echocardiography and surgery in tricuspid and pulmonary valve stenosis due to carcinoid syndrome. Cardiovasc Med 4:871, 1979
54. Zitnik RS, Giuliani ER: Clinical recognition of atrial myxoma. Am Heart J 80:689, 1970
55. Bulkley BH, Hutchins GM: Atrial myxomas: A fifty year review. Am Heart J 97:639, 1979
56. McAllister HA: Primary tumors and cysts of the heart and pericardium. Curr Probl Cardiol 4:1, 1979
57. Giuliani ER, Nasser FN: Two-dimensional echocardiography in acquired heart disease—Part I. Curr Probl Cardiol 5:1, 1981
58. Dennis JL, Hansen AE, Corpening TN: Endocardial fibroelastosis. Pediatrics 12:130, 1953
59. Davies JNP, Ball JD: The pathology of endomyocardial fibrosis in Uganda. Br Heart J 17:337, 1955
60. Gibson R, Wood P: The diagnosis of tricuspid stenosis. Br Heart J 17:552, 1955
61. Thomas JH, Panoussopoulos DG, Jewell WR et al: Tricuspid stenosis secondary to metastatic melanoma. Cancer 39:1732, 1977
62. DeCock KM, Gikonyo DK, Lucas SB et al: Metastatic tumour of right atrium mimicking constrictive pericarditis and tricuspid stenosis. Br Med J 285:1314, 1982
63. Sackner MA, Heinz ER, Steinberg AJ: The heart in scleroderma. Am J Cardiol 17:542, 1966
64. Dougherty MJ, Craige E: Apathetic hyperthyroidism presenting as tricuspid regurgitation. Chest 63:767, 1973
65. Zager J, Berberich SN, Eslava R et al: Dynamic tricuspid valve insufficiency produced by a right ventricular thrombus from a pacemaker. Chest 74:455, 1978
66. Greco MA, Senesh JD, Aleksic S et al: Tricuspid stenosis secondary to entanglement of ventriculoatrial catheter in the valve leaflets. Surg Neurol 18:34, 1982
67. Lee ME, Chaux A: Unusual complications of endocardial pacing. J Thorac Cardiovasc Surg 80:934, 1980
68. Gibson TC, Davidson RC, DeSilvey DL: Presumptive tricuspid valve malfunction induced by a pacemaker lead: A case report and review of the literature. Pace 3:88, 1980
69. Beaver WL, Dillon JC, Jolly W: Pseudo-tricuspid stenosis: A rare entity. Chest 71:772, 1977
70. Cintron GB, Snow JA, Fletcher RD et al: Pericarditis mimicking tricuspid valvular disease. Chest 71:770, 1977
71. Wray TM, Prochaska J, Fisher RD et al: Traumatic pericardial hematoma simulating tricuspid valve obstruction. Johns Hopkins Med J 137:147, 1975
72. Ebstein W: On a very rare case of insufficiency of the tricuspid valve caused by severe congenital malformation of the same. Arch Anat Physiol Wissensch Med Leipz 238, 1866. Translated by Schiebler GL, Gravenstein JS, Van Mierop LHS. Am J Cardiol 22:867, 1968
73. Vacca JB, Bussman DW, Mudd JG: Ebstein's anomaly: Complete review of 108 cases. Am J Cardiol 2:210, 1958
74. Edwards JE: Pathologic features of Ebstein's malformation of the tricuspid valve. Proc Staff Meet Mayo Clinic 28:89, 1953
75. Goodwin JF, Wynn A, Steiner RE: Ebstein's anomaly of the tricuspid valve. Am Heart J 45:144, 1953
76. Perloff JK: Ebstein's anomaly of the tricuspid valve. In Perloff JK: The Clinical Recognition of Congenital Heart Disease, 2nd ed. Philadelphia, WB Saunders, 1978
77. Genton E, Blount SG Jr: The spectrum of Ebstein's anomaly. Am Heart J 73:395, 1967
78. Kumar AE, Flyer DC, Miettinsen OS et al: Ebstein's anomaly: Clinical profile and natural history. Am J Cardiol 28:84, 1971
79. Fontana ME, Wooley CF: Sail sound in Ebstein's anomaly of the tricuspid valve. Circulation 46:155, 1972
80. Mehl SJ, Kaltman AJ, Kronzon I et al: Combined tricuspid and pulmonic stenosis: Clinical, echocardiographic, hemodynamic, surgical, and pathological features. J Thorac Cardiovasc Surg 74:55, 1977
81. Cox JN, de Seigneux R, Bolens M et al: Tricuspid atresia, hypoplastic right ventricle, intact ventricular septum and congenital absence of the pulmonary valve. Helv Paediatr Acta 30:389, 1975
82. Greenwood RD: Ossification of the right auriculoventricular opening of the

83. Oeconomos NS, Camilaris DH, Petritis J et al: Congenital tricuspid valvular stenosis. J Cardiovasc Surg 16:100, 1975
84. Leier CV, Call TD, Fulkerson PK et al: The spectrum of cardiac defects in the Ehlers-Danlos syndrome, types I and III. Ann Intern Med 92:171, 1980
85. Ewy GA: Venous and arterial pulsations. In Horwitz LD, Groves BM: Signs and Symptoms in Cardiology, p 132. Philadelphia, JB Lippincott, 1985
86. Cairus KB, Kloster FE, Bristow JD et al: Problems in the hemodynamic diagnosis of tricuspid insufficiency. Am Heart J 75:173, 1968
87. Hansing CE, Rowe GG: Tricuspid insufficiency: A study of hemodynamics and pathogenesis. Circulation 45:793, 1972
88. Levine SA, Harvey WP: Clinical Auscultation of the Heart, p 339. Philadelphia, WB Saunders, 1959
89. Rios JC, Massumi RA, Breesmen WT et al: Auscultatory features of acute tricuspid regurgitation. Am J Cardiol 23:4, 1969
90. Rivero-Carvallo M: Signo para el diagnostico de las insuficiencias tricuspideas. Arch Inst Cardiol Mex 16:531, 1946
91. Muller O, Schillingford J: Tricuspid incompetence. Br Heart J 16:195, 1954
92. Gooch AS, Maranhao V, Scampardonis G et al: Prolapse of both mitral and tricuspid leaflets in systolic murmur-click syndrome. N Engl J Med 287:1218, 1972
93. Feigenbaum H: Echocardiography, 3rd ed, p 284. Philadelphia, Lea & Febiger, 1981
94. Nanna M, Chandraratna PA, Reid C et al: Value of two-dimensional echocardiography in detecting tricuspid stenosis. Circulation 67:221, 1983
95. Seward JB, Tajik AJ, Hagler DJ et al: Peripheral venous contrast echocardiography. Am J Cardiol 39:202, 1977
96. Hatle L: Doppler Ultrasound in Cardiology: Physical Principles of Clinical Applications, 2nd ed. Philadelphia, Lea & Febiger, 1985
97. Pearlman AS, Stevenson JC: Doppler echocardiography: Applications, limitation, and future directions. Am J Cardiol 46:1256, 1980
98. Miyatake K, Okamoto M: Evaluation of tricuspid regurgitation by pulsed Doppler and two dimensional echocardiography. Circulation 66:777, 1982
99. Diebold B, Touati R, Blanchard D et al: Quantitative assessment of tricuspid regurgitation using pulsed doppler echocardiography. Br Heart J 50:443, 1983
100. Cha SD, Gooch A: Diagnosis of tricuspid regurgitation. Arch Intern Med 143:1763, 1983
101. Wooley CF, Fontana ME, Kilman JW, Ryan JM: Tricuspid stenosis: Atrial systolic murmur, tricuspid opening snap and right atrial pressure pulse. Am J Med 78:375, 1985
102. Perloff JK, Harvey WP: Clinical recognition of tricuspid stenosis. Circulation 22:346, 1960
103. Sanders CA, Harthorne JW, DeSanctis RW et al: Tricuspid stenosis: A difficult diagnosis in the presence of atrial fibrillation. Circulation 33:26, 1966
104. Brandenburg RO, McGoon DC, Campeau L et al: Traumatic rupture of the chordae tendineae of the tricuspid valve: Successful repair twenty-four years later. Am J Cardiol 18:911, 1966
105. Tachovsky TJ, Giuliani ER, Ellis FH Jr: Prosthetic valve replacement for traumatic tricuspid insufficiency: Report of a case originally diagnosed as Ebstein's malformation. Am J Cardiol 26:196, 1970
106. Kochoukos NT, Stephenson LW: Indications for and results of tricuspid valve replacement. Adv Cardiol 17:199, 1976
107. Sanfelippo PM, Giuliani ER, Danielson GK et al: Tricuspid valve prosthetic replacement: Early and late results with the Starr-Edwards prosthesis. J Thorac Cardiovasc Surg 71:441, 1976
108. Breyer RH, McClenathan JH, Michaelis LL et al: Tricuspid regurgitation: A comparison of non-operative management, tricuspid annuloplasty, and tricuspid valve replacement. J Thorac Cardiovasc Surg 72:867, 1976
109. Arbulu A, Thoms NW, Wilson RF: Valvulectomy without prosthetic replacement: A lifesaving operation for tricuspid pseudomonas endocarditis. J Thorac Cardiovasc Surg 64:103, 1972
110. Robin E, Belamaric J, Thoms NW et al: Consequences to total tricuspid valvulectomy without prosthetic replacement in treatment of pseudomonas endocarditis. J Thorac Cardiovasc Surg 68:461, 1974
111. Sheikhzadeh A, Tarbiat S, Paydar D, Shakibi J: Rheumatic tricuspid stenosis: A clinical overview. Acta Cardiol 33:431, 1978
112. Watson H, Lowe K: Severe tricuspid stenosis revealed after aortic valvotomy. Br Heart J 24:241, 1962

Aortic Stenosis

Robert C. Schlant

ETIOLOGY

Aortic stenosis[1-6] is one of the more frequent forms of isolated valvular heart disease. Valvular aortic stenosis is the most common fatal cardiac valve lesion except for mitral regurgitation secondary to myocardial or coronary artery disease. Aortic stenosis frequently occurs as a mixed lesion, with some degree of aortic regurgitation. In postinflammatory aortic stenosis due to rheumatic fever, involvement of the mitral valve is often clinically apparent and is virtually always detected at autopsy.

Aortic stenosis may occur either on a congenital or an acquired basis.[7-11] Congenital aortic stenosis may be either supravalvular, valvular, or subvalvular. *Supravalvular aortic stenosis,* which occurs just above the aortic valve in the ascending aorta and only rarely in adults,[12] is the least frequent of the three types. It may be classified into the following types: (1) a focal hourglass construction, (2) a fibromuscular narrowing, and (3) a generalized hypoplasia of the ascending aorta. Supravalvular aortic stenosis sometimes occurs in association with multiple stenoses or coarctations of major branches of the pulmonary artery or with mental retardation and a characteristic facies (*Williams syndrome*). *Subvalvular aortic stenosis,* which can also occur in adult patients,[13] may be classified into the following three types: a membranous diaphragm, a fibromuscular narrowing or tunnel deformity, and muscular subaortic hypertrophy. Discrete subaortic stenosis (DSS) is usually associated with aortic regurgitation that is caused by damage to the leaflets of the aortic valve produced by the jet of blood through the subaortic obstruction. In contrast to valvular aortic stenosis, an ejection click is not heard in supravalvular or subvalvular aortic stenosis. Supravalvular and subvalvular congenital aortic stenoses are discussed elsewhere in these volumes, as is left ventricular outflow tract obstruction as part of hypertrophic obstructive cardiomyopathy (see the Index for specific chapters).

Congenital valvular aortic stenosis is usually produced by either unicuspid (or unicommissural) or bicuspid aortic valves. In contrast to congenital pulmonic stenosis, the valve is very rarely acommissural with a dome type of deformity. Congenitally acommissural aortic valves usually produce severe stenosis very early in life. A congenitally bicuspid aortic valve occurs much more frequently than a unicuspid valve, but the latter is responsible for a significant number of infants with severe obstruction. Rare instances have been encountered in adult life. Very rarely, congenital aortic stenosis is produced by a congenital tricuspid aortic valve, usually with unequal valve leaflets.

A *bicuspid aortic valve* is the most common type of congenital heart disease encountered in adults except for mitral valve prolapse.[14] In some studies it has been found to occur in 1% to 2% of infants and three to four times more frequently in males than in females. In adults in the United States a congenital bicuspid aortic valve is today the most frequent etiology of calcific aortic stenosis. It is also the most frequent cause of congenital aortic regurgitation. Although the majority of bicuspid valves do not produce significant hemodynamic obstruction in infancy or childhood, in some infants the commissures are fused at birth or in early childhood and produce severe obstruction. Thus, congenital bicuspid aortic valve disease is a very important cause of severe aortic stenosis in infancy, childhood, and adolescence. In most patients, however, the bicuspid valve produces a murmur and ejection click but does not produce significant obstruction to left ventricular emptying for 40 to 50 years, over which time the increased hemodynamic stresses on the slightly unequal valve leaflets slowly and progressively result in calcific aortic stenosis (Fig. 88.1). A bicuspid valve is always highly susceptible to infective endocarditis.

Acquired valvular aortic stenosis is usually the result of one of the following: fibrosis and dystrophic calcification of a congenitally unicommissural or bicuspid aortic valve; rheumatic fever and perhaps other inflammatory conditions of a normal tricuspid aortic valve; or "wear and tear" degenerative changes in a normal tricuspid valve. Very rare causes include familial hypercholesterolemia, rheumatoid heart disease, systemic lupus erythematosus,[15] and methylsergide (Sansert) therapy. It has been postulated, but not well proven, that viral or rickettsial valvulitis might also produce chronic aortic valve stenosis.[16] Severe familial hypercholesterolemia can produce aortic stenosis due to supravalvular stenosis due to xanthomata.[17] Similar nodules may also occur in the aortic leaflets and in the sinuses of Valsalva, where they can produce obstruction of the coronary ostia. Severe atherosclerosis of the epicardial coronary arteries is also very frequent. Rheumatoid aortic disease is produced by rheumatoid nodules in the leaflets of the aortic valve and the proximal aorta. Very rarely, aortic stenosis can be produced by massive vegetations from infective endocarditis or ochronosis.[18,19]

Rheumatic aortic stenosis, which according to some series occurs somewhat more frequently in males, is thought to be associated virtually always with gross or microscopic involvement of the mitral valve, although this involvement may not be apparent clinically or echocardiographically (Fig. 88.2). One of the hallmarks of the postinflammatory, or rheumatic, type of aortic stenosis is fusion of the valve commissures, a feature that is usually not significant in the "wear and tear" aortic stenosis of the elderly. Cuspid vascularization and fibrosis, with or without significant calcification, is also usually present. The myocardium may also show Aschoff nodules and perivascular fibrosis. At times, the latter may contribute significantly to myocardial dysfunction in patients with chronic rheumatic heart disease. Gross or microscopic evidence of involvement of the mitral valve is virtually always found in patients with rheumatic valve disease.[20]

After the age of 65 to 70 years, the most frequent cause of aortic stenosis in the United States is referred to by several names, including "wear and tear," progressive sclerosis and calcification of the elderly, or *Mönckeberg's* aortic stenosis of a tricuspid aortic valve.[21-23] This condition can at times be found in patients in their 50s; it may be more frequent in individuals with valve leaflets of slightly unequal size, systemic hypertension, elevated serum cholesterol, or Paget's disease of bone. It is quite possible that this condition might develop in all individuals if they were to live long enough. In most instances there is marked fibrosis and calcification of the aortic valve; sometimes, lipid-laden cells are also present (Fig. 88.3). Significant commissural fusion is characteristically not present. The calcification of the aortic valve may extend into the aortic annulus and may occur together with mitral annular calcification, which may be associated with mitral regurgitation, and with calcification in the atrioventricular node, bundle of His, or left bundle branch, which may be associated with varying degrees and types of heart block. Electrophysiologic studies in patients with aortic stenosis have shown that prolongation of the HV time > 50 msec is relatively frequent.[24] The incidence of degenerative aortic stenosis appears to be approximately equal in males and females, in contrast to congenitally unicommissural and bicuspid valves or even postinflammatory aortic stenosis, which are usually found more frequently in males. It is probable that this type of degenerative, or "wear and tear," calcification of the aortic valve leaflets, aortic annulus, and ascending aorta is related to the many unknown factors responsible for aging. Of interest, calcific aortic stenosis is a frequent cause of death in conditions associated with premature aging such as progeria and Werner's syndrome.

PATHOPHYSIOLOGY

The basic hemodynamic feature of aortic stenosis is an obstruction to left ventricular ejection that usually develops over a number of years. In general, the valve orifice must be decreased to considerably less than one third of normal size before any significant hemodynamic obstruction is produced. In response to the increased impedance to left ventricular ejection, the left ventricle develops progressive *concentric hypertrophy*, in which the thickness of the individual myocardial cells markedly increases from 10 μ to 15 μ to 50 μ to 70 μ and which produces an increase in the thickness of the left ventricular free wall and ventricular septum. In contrast, the internal diameter of the left ventricular chamber at end-diastole does not increase but may actually decrease. As the severity of aortic stenosis progressively increases over a number of years, one or more of the following must occur to maintain the same cardiac output: the pressure difference across the valve during systole may increase; the rate of flow may decrease; or the duration of systolic ejection may lengthen. Most patients with aortic stenosis develop both an increased pressure difference across the valve and a prolongation of left ventricular systole; interestingly, many patients maintain a normal cardiac output at rest until very late in the course of the disease. On the other hand, patients with moderate to severe aortic stenosis are usually not able to increase their cardiac output significantly during exercise.[25-27] Some patients with aortic stenosis develop asymmetric septal hypertrophy, apparently as an adaptive mechanism.[28]

The left ventricle in severe aortic stenosis (<0.75 cm²) may generate systolic pressures of 240 mm Hg and, for brief periods, up to 300 to 320 mm Hg. The calculated wall tension or stress, which is increased by increased systolic pressure in the ventricular cavity and by any increased diameter of the left ventricle, is decreased by increased thickness of the ventricular wall. Thus, the calculated left ventricular wall stress may often be maintained at normal or near-normal values by the marked concentric hypertrophy.[29] On the other hand, the calculated wall tension may be abnormally increased in patients with aortic stenosis who have systolic failure and left ventricular dilatation.

In most patients the obstruction to left ventricular ejection becomes critical only when the valve area is reduced from the normal adult valve area of 2.6 cm² to 3.5 cm² to about 0.5 cm² to 0.75 cm². In infants and children who have a normal cardiac output, the stenosis is usually considered severe when there is a valve area less than 0.5 cm²/m² or a peak systolic pressure difference of 80 mm Hg or more between the left ventricle and aorta. The stenosis is considered moderate in infants and children with a valve area between 0.5 cm² and 0.8 cm²/m² or a peak pressure difference between 50 mm Hg and 79 mm

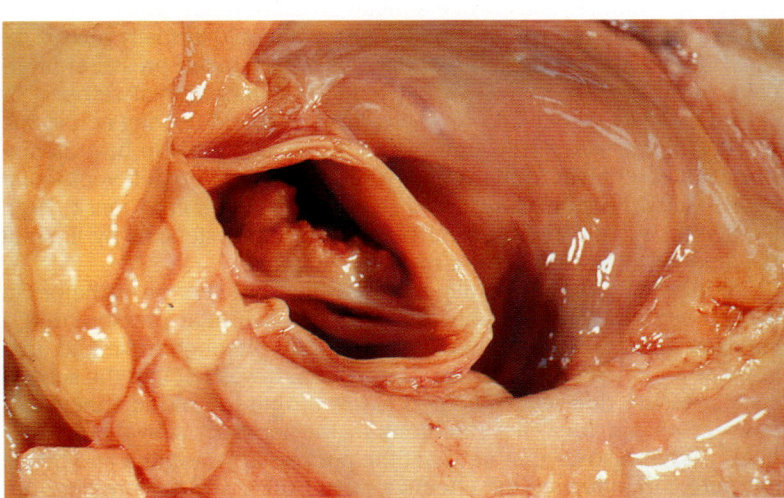

FIGURE 88.1 Bicuspid aortic valve of an 80-year-old man with moderately severe aortic stenosis and coronary artery disease who died of acute myocardial infarction while awaiting cardiac surgery.

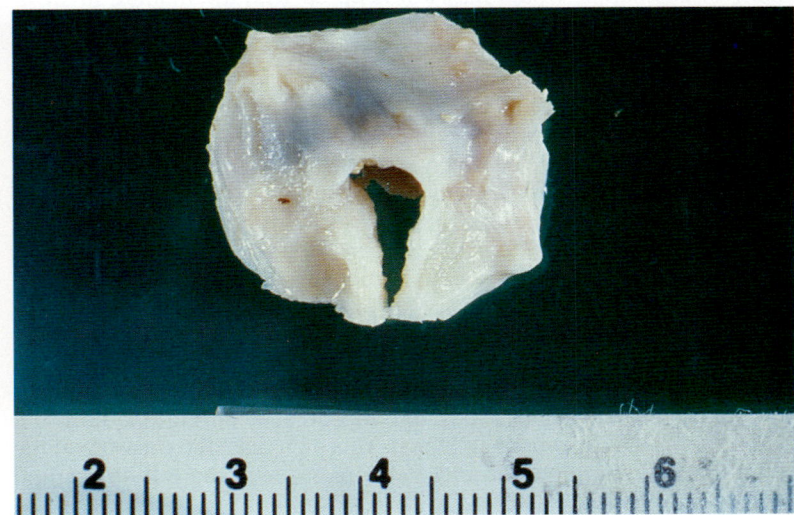

FIGURE 88.2 Aortic valve removed at surgery from a 48-year-old woman with rheumatic combined aortic and mitral stenosis. Note the characteristic fusion of the commissures.

FIGURE 88.3 Aortic valve of a 73-year-old man with severe calcific aortic stenosis (Mönckeberg's stenosis). There is some fusion of one commissure.

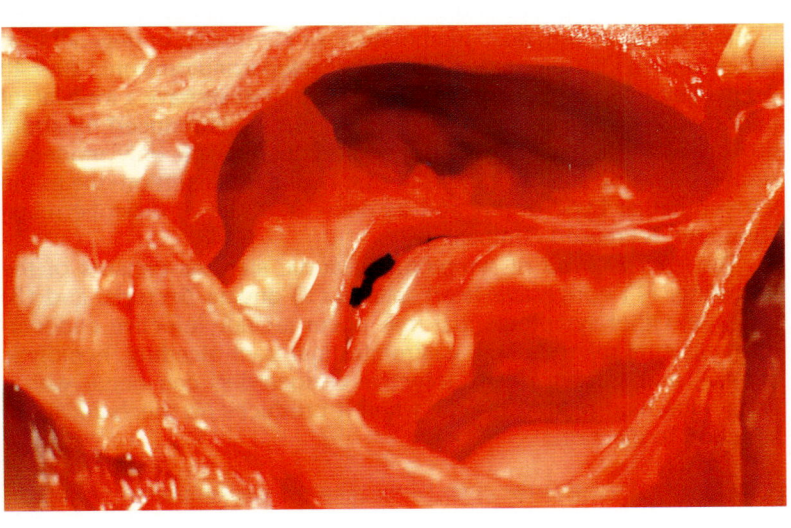

Hg, whereas the stenosis is considered to be mild if the area is 0.9 cm^2/m^2 or greater or the peak pressure difference is less than 50 mm Hg. In the presence of aortic regurgitation, which requires an even larger forward flow of blood with each systole, or of significant coronary artery disease, which may limit coronary blood flow, lesser degrees of stenosis may be hemodynamically significant.

The marked left ventricular hypertrophy that develops in response to significant aortic stenosis may be able to maintain a normal cardiac output at rest with normal or relatively normal indices of *ventricular systolic function*, although ultimately these usually become abnormal.[2] On the other hand, the marked hypertrophy is associated relatively early with varying degrees of abnormalities of *ventricular diastolic function*, including decreased left ventricular compliance, decreased rate of ventricular relaxation, and an elevated end-diastolic pressure.[8] Initially, the elevation of end-diastolic pressure is probably due only to myocardial hypertrophy, but subsequently there is added left ventricular diastolic myocardial dysfunction. Increased myocardial fibrosis is also present in the late stages. The decreased rate of isovolumic relaxation also contributes to the limited capacity of the ventricle to respond with increased cardiac output during tachycardia or exercise.[25-27]

Myocardial ischemia is especially likely to occur in the left ventricular subendocardium, which has been described as the Achilles' heel of the heart. The left ventricular endocardium normally shortens more than the epicardium and has a greater oxygen consumption and a lower tissue oxygen tension. In patients with marked concentric hypertrophy, perfusion of the endocardium may be compromised by a number of mechanisms, including the following: the increased mass and thickness of the left ventricular wall; the vasculature growth, especially of capillaries, which may not keep up with the marked myocardial hypertrophy; the increased diffusion distance from myocardial capillaries to the center of the hypertrophied myocardial cells; the lengthening of systole, which shortens diastole, during which most coronary flow to the left ventricle occurs, and which increases the systolic tension–time product; the elevated diastolic pressure in the cavity of the left ventricle, which impedes coronary flow into the subendocardium; the high intramyocardial pressure, which throttles coronary flow during systole and impedes flow during diastole; and the relatively low aortic diastolic pressure in the aorta to perfuse the coronary arteries. Patients with severe aortic stenosis can develop myocardial infarction without significant coronary artery disease.

Some patients with severe aortic stenosis develop symptoms of exertional dyspnea or even pulmonary edema and congestion due to the high diastolic pressures that are necessary to fill the hypertrophied left ventricle. Initially, this may only be present during exertion, but subsequently it is also present at rest. This high diastolic pressure in the left ventricle is reflected in elevated pressures in the left atrium and pulmonary capillaries and in the clinical symptoms of dyspnea on exertion. Some patients may have significant *diastolic dysfunction* while maintaining a normal left ventricular systolic function and cardiac output, with a normal or even increased left ventricular ejection fraction. Such patients may subsequently develop left ventricular *systolic dysfunction* with a decrease in cardiac output, stroke volume, ejection fraction, rate of ejection, and other indices of systolic function.[30] The end-systolic volume may also increase somewhat, at which time some patients develop modest left ventricular dilatation and increased end-diastolic volume, which are associated with even greater elevation of left ventricular diastolic pressure and left atrial pressure.[31] Both the decrease in systolic function and the increase in end-systolic volume of the ventricle decrease the potential contribution of *diastolic suction*, from both elastic recoil and active relaxation of the myocardium, to filling of the ventricle on the next beat. At this stage, the systolic wall tension may be increased significantly.

Whenever the left ventricle is markedly hypertrophied, the relative importance of atrial contraction to ventricular filling is increased. This final presystolic "atrial kick" produced by the "booster pump" function of the left atrium may momentarily elevate the left-ventricular end-diastolic pressure to 20 mm Hg to 35 mm Hg, even when there is no other evidence of left ventricular systolic or diastolic failure and when the mean left atrial pressure is not sufficiently elevated to produce pulmonary congestion or dyspnea. Since the left atrial pressure is elevated only for a brief period, pulmonary edema is not produced even though the left atrial *a* wave may be 30 mm Hg to 35 mm Hg. When such patients develop atrial failure due to atrial fibrillation, however, there may be signs of acute pulmonary edema together with marked elevation of the left ventricular diastolic and left atrial pressures.

Very rarely, aortic valve disease may result in such marked hypertrophy of the ventricle that the hypertrophy of the ventricular septum produces an obstruction to the ejection of blood from the right ventricle into the pulmonary artery and a pressure difference between right ventricular and pulmonary artery systolic pressures. This syndrome is referred to as the *Bernheim phenomenon*. The opposite condition, in which an obstruction to ejection from the left ventricle is produced by marked hypertrophy of the upper ventricular septum that occurs in conditions that produce right ventricular hypertrophy, has been referred to as the *reversed Bernheim phenomenon*. Both conditions are very rare.

The basic relationship between pressure and flow across a critically narrowed orifice requires that if the flow is doubled, the pressure difference across the orifice is increased fourfold. Because of this fundamental hydraulic principle (expressed in the Gorlin and Gorlin formula, discussed elsewhere in these volumes), it is important in evaluating patients with aortic stenosis to calculate the *aortic valve area* by measuring the mean pressure difference across the valve during systole, the total volume of forward flow across the valve, and the duration of systole per minute. Thus, while a mean pressure difference of 100 mm Hg in a patient with isolated aortic stenosis would virtually always be associated with severe stenosis, patients with a mean pressure difference of 30 mm Hg may have either mild or insignificant stenosis or severe stenosis, depending on the volume of blood flowing across the valve. Patients with aortic stenosis are especially likely to have diminished left ventricular forward flow when there is severe left ventricular systolic failure or coexisting mitral stenosis. The latter can "mask" both the symptoms and the physical findings of aortic stenosis by limiting the amount of blood entering the left ventricle.[32]

Studies employing laterally mounted micrometers on catheters in the left ventricle have demonstrated large subvalvular pressure differences in patients with isolated aortic stenosis although none had anatomical evidence of subvalvular obstruction. It was felt that the subvalvular pressure differences helped to overcome the blood's inertia to convective and local accelerations in the tapering subvalvular flow field.[33] It has also been noted that the peripheral resistance and blood pressure can influence the effective valve orifice and the pressure difference across a stenotic aortic valve.[25,34]

SYMPTOMS

Individuals with severe congenital aortic stenosis may have symptoms in infancy, childhood, or adolescence, but most patients with bicuspid aortic stenosis or with postinflammatory, or rheumatic, or degenerative (Mönckeberg's) aortic stenosis do not develop symptoms until after 40 years of age. Most adult patients with aortic stenosis have a long latent period with no symptoms until the valve orifice is reduced by about 60% to 75%. On the other hand, some patients with only moderate stenosis develop slightly increased dyspnea during exertion due to the left ventricular hypertrophy and its decreased rate of diastolic relaxation and decreased compliance.

The *classic triad* of symptoms in aortic stenosis consists of the following: (1) congestive heart failure, (2) angina pectoris, and (3) syncope. Other symptoms that may occur include infective endocarditis, cerebral microemboli, gastrointestinal tract bleeding, hemolytic anemia, and sudden death. Infective endocarditis can occur with a congenital bicuspid valve even when it produces no mechanical obstruction to ejection.

As noted above, some patients with aortic stenosis may have dyspnea on exertion and other symptoms of left ventricular *diastolic dysfunction* that are usually associated with the clinical syndrome of congestive heart failure, at a time when the systolic function of their left ventricle is normal or near normal. Other symptoms of diastolic dysfunction may include orthopnea, paroxysmal nocturnal dyspnea, and, occasionally, systemic edema. Later, the left ventricular *systolic function* may also decline.

Angina pectoris can occur in severe aortic stenosis in the absence of coronary artery disease.[35] It is produced by the imbalance between the supply and demand of oxygen to the massively hypertrophied myocardium.[36-38] For the reasons noted above, the left ventricular subendocardium is especially susceptible to ischemia in aortic stenosis. Patients with severe aortic stenosis often have a limited *coronary reserve*, that is, a limited ability to increase coronary blood flow under conditions of increased demand. Patients with aortic stenosis and angina pectoris may also frequently have significant coronary artery disease, particularly older patients.[39] Prior to aortic valve surgery, patients who are over the age of 35 or who have coronary risk factors[40] should have cardiac catheterization and coronary arteriography to determine the status of their coronary arteries even if there are no complaints of angina pectoris.

Syncope or near syncope usually occurs with exertion but may occur at rest. It may be produced by the following several mechanisms: an inability during exertion to increase or maintain cardiac output in association with metabolic vasodilatation of the systemic arterioles; reflex peripheral vasodilatation originating from baroreceptors in the walls of the left ventricle[41]; ventricular tachycardia or even fibrillation; atrial tachycardia, fibrillation, or flutter; or transient heart block. Sudden death is probably due to a ventricular tachyarrhythmia initiated by one of the same mechanisms; it occurs in about 15% to 20% of patients with severe aortic stenosis and may be the first symptom of the disease in about 3% to 5% of patients. It is more likely to occur in patients with pulmonary hypertension.[42]

The development of atrial fibrillation, which eliminates the atrial booster pump filling of the left ventricle, is often associated with a marked worsening of symptoms of pulmonary congestion or even syncope. In many such patients prompt electrical cardioversion is appropriate and even life saving.

In general, the onset of any of the "classic triad" of symptoms (failure, angina, or syncope) is ominous. Different clinical series have indicated varying mean survival times of 2 to 5 years after the onset of any of these three symptoms.[1,43-45] In general, definite congestive heart failure has the most ominous prognosis. The clinical picture of chronic "right heart failure" with distended jugular veins, enlarged liver, ascites, and marked peripheral edema occurs but is unusual in patients with isolated aortic stenosis.[42] When such findings occur in a patient with aortic stenosis, a coexisting cause of the symptoms and signs of clinical right heart failure should be sought.

COMPLICATIONS

Infective endocarditis can occur on any deformed valve. It is the major source of difficulty in most patients with congenitally bicuspid aortic valves before the valves become stenotic. A small percentage of patients with a congenital bicuspid aortic valve may also have *coarctation of the aorta*, which can cause cerebral vascular hemorrhage. *Gastrointestinal tract bleeding due to angiodysplasia* may occur in patients with severe aortic stenosis. It is particularly likely to occur in the ascending colon and may require hemicolectomy although it often subsides following replacement of the aortic valve.[46,47] *Aortic regurgitation* can occur in all forms of valvular aortic stenosis and especially in congenital subvalvular aortic stenosis. Any regurgitant volume increases the total volume of blood flowing forward across the valve during systole and may cause the systolic pressure difference across the valve to increase markedly. *Atrial fibrillation* removes the "atrial kick" or booster pump, which provides the final, brief filling of the left ventricle and the final, end-diastolic sarcomere stretch. When this is lost with the onset of atrial fibrillation, the patient may develop acute heart failure with pulmonary congestion, diminished cardiac output, and even hypotension. Emergency electrical cardioversion may be life saving. *Mitral annular calcification* and *calcification of the atrioventricular node* may occur, particularly in patients with Mönckeberg's aortic stenosis, and may produce mitral regurgitation (or, very rarely, mitral stenosis) and varying degrees of heart block. *Aortic dissection* occurs as a rare complication of aortic stenosis, perhaps related to the impact of the jet on the aortic wall. *Hemolytic anemia*, which is produced by trauma to red blood cells passing through the stenotic valve orifice, can occasionally occur but is usually mild.

PHYSICAL FINDINGS

Most patients with aortic stenosis have normal growth and development. Infants and children with significant aortic stenosis usually have a loud spindle-shaped mid-systolic murmur at the base, oftentimes with a palpable systolic thrill. The systolic murmur is often well heard over the entire precordium and at the apex, where the murmur tends to have the same configuration but a higher pitch than in the second right interspace or further downstream over the carotids. In about 5% of patients the systolic murmur is loudest at the apex; usually this is found in patients with an increase in chest anterior–posterior diameter from chronic lung disease. There may be a blowing, decrescendo diastolic murmur of aortic regurgitation. This is usually loudest along the mid-left sternal border but may be loudest at the apex or in the second right interspace. Occasionally, it may be heard only at the apex. In patients with severe stenosis, there may be evidence of pulmonary congestion. Infants and children with a bicuspid aortic valve without significant stenosis usually have only a relatively mild, grade 1 to grade 3 mid-systolic murmur loudest at the base or along the left sternal border, and an "opening" or "ejection" click, which is often heard loudest at the apex. The findings of congenital aortic stenosis in infants and children are discussed further elsewhere in these volumes (see the Index).

The characteristic arterial pulse in patients with significant aortic stenosis is of low amplitude, with a slow rate of rise and a prominent anacrotic shoulder on the ascending limb, and a low, rounded, delayed peak. Often a systolic thrill is readily felt over the carotid arteries. The *parvus et tardus* pulse is best appreciated in the carotid arteries. Most adult patients below the age of approximately 65 years will have a *parvus et tardus* (small and late peaking) pulse if the aortic stenosis is significant; however, some will have it with only mild stenosis. On the other hand, in some patients who are above the age of approximately 65 and who have aortic stenosis due to "degenerative" or Mönckeberg's sclerosis of a tricuspid aortic valve, the arterial pulse may not be significantly altered from normal due to the decreased elasticity and distensibility of the aorta and great vessels. Infants or young children with severe aortic stenosis may also have a carotid arterial pulse that is not remarkable. Thus, the characteristic *parvus et tardus* pulse may not be found in the very young or the very old. An *anacrotic* shoulder on the ascending limb of the carotid pulse is occasionally palpable, especially in patients with severe aortic stenosis. *Pulsus alternans* is occasionally encountered in patients with severe aortic stenosis and is due to an alternation in the contractility of the ventricle. This may be associated with an alternating strength not only of the arterial pulse but also of the loudness of the systolic murmur (*auscultatory alternans*).

In most patients the jugular venous pressure is within normal limits although a significant number of patients will have an increased prominence of the *a* wave. This is probably related to the increased vigor of right atrial contraction secondary to left ventricular and ventricular septal hypertrophy, which decrease the compliance of the right ventricle. In the small percentage (5%–10%) of patients with severe aortic stenosis who develop marked pulmonary hypertension and right ventricular hypertension,[42] the jugular venous pulse and pulse waves may be markedly increased; however, this is much less commonly encountered in aortic stenosis than in mitral valve disease.

The apex impulse in most patients with aortic stenosis is not displaced or is only minimally displaced. On the other hand, there is often a palpable *a* wave, which corresponds to the audible S_4 sound, together with a sustained, forceful systolic impulse produced by the impact of the hypertrophied left ventricle against the chest wall. In a relatively small percentage of patients with aortic stenosis who develop both severe diastolic and systolic left ventricular failure, there may be moderate left ventricular dilatation with displacement of the apex impulse laterally and inferiorly. In these patients a loud third heart sound is frequently present, and the systolic murmur occasionally becomes less loud. In most patients with aortic stenosis there is no parasternal impulse of right ventricular hypertrophy although this may be present in the approximately 5% of patients with aortic stenosis who have disproportionate or severe pulmonary hypertension.

The characteristic murmur of aortic stenosis is a loud, harsh, midsystolic crescendo–decrescendo or spindle-shaped murmur maximal in the first or second right intercostal space or along the left sternal border that radiates to the carotid arteries, especially on the right.[48] There is often a palpable systolic thrill in the second right interspace, which may radiate to the carotid arteries, especially on the right side. In approximately 10% of patients the systolic murmur is louder at the apex, particularly in older patients or in patients with emphysema or an increased anteroposterior chest diameter. The pitch of the murmur characteristically is higher at the apex than along the left sternal border but is lower pitched downstream over the carotid arteries. In some elderly patients the systolic murmur at the apex is described as having a "cooing dove" character. Patients with degenerative (Mönckeberg's) aortic stenosis may have calcification of the mitral annulus and a distinct holosytolic murmur of mitral regurgitation at the apex. Most patients with aortic stenosis have a regular rhythm, and the presence of many premature complexes or a nodal rhythm or especially atrial fibrillation is likely to precipitate severe and acute heart failure with pulmonary congestion and edema. An ejection sound is heard, usually at the apex, in most patients with a bicuspid aortic valve only as long as at least one valve leaflet is mobile and not restricted in motion by fibrosis and calcification. A fourth heart sound is present in most patients with severe aortic stenosis but may be present with minimal or mild stenosis. A third heart sound usually indicates significant left ventricular dysfunction, which is often both diastolic and systolic. In general, however, neither a third or a fourth heart sound is highly specific or sensitive for severe aortic stenosis in patients over the age of 40.

Some clues to the severity of the stenosis may be gained from auscultation. Thus, the finding of two distinct components of the second heart sound is, in general, evidence against there being significant aortic stenosis, since A_2, the aortic component of the second heart sound, is not audible in about 90% of patients with severe aortic stenosis. In patients with mild or moderate degrees of aortic stenosis, however, there may be paradoxic splitting of the second heart sound, with P_2 occurring prior to A_2, which is delayed due to the prolongation of left ventricular ejection. As the degree of aortic stenosis becomes more severe, the peaking of the loudness of the systolic murmur occurs later during systole.[49] In addition, the systemic arterial pulse pressure tends to become narrow with more severe degrees of aortic stenosis. In general, severe systemic hypertension is not frequently encountered in younger patients with significant aortic stenosis although systolic blood pressures of 160 mm Hg to 200 mm Hg can sometimes be found in older patients with aortic stenosis.[50] In patients who have both aortic stenosis and aortic regurgitation, the finding of *pulsus bisferiens* on palpitation of the carotid arteries implies that the aortic regurgitation is at least moderately severe and that regurgitation is usually the predominant lesion.

ELECTROCARDIOGRAM

The electrocardiogram classically shows normal sinus rhythm with left ventricular hypertrophy (LVH) with increased voltage and secondary ST-T wave changes. There is usually evidence of left atrial enlargement. A perfectly normal electrocardiogram is rare in adult patients with severe aortic stenosis, but voltage criteria for LVH may not be present in a small percentage, occasionally due to associated chronic lung disease. The electrical axis is usually not markedly leftward. In some patients there is poor progression of the R wave or a QS pattern in the right precordial leads that can mimic the findings of old anterior myocardial infarction. In general, the electrocardiographic (or vectorcardiographic) evidence of left ventricular hypertrophy correlates with severity of stenosis better in infants and children than in adults although there is some correlation between the 12-lead QRS amplitude and the peak systolic pressure difference across the aortic valve.[51] In patients who have severe aortic stenosis there may be occasional premature ventricular complexes. Ventricular arrhythmias have been documented on 24-hour recordings of electrocardiograms in a significant percentage of patients with aortic stenosis.[52,53] The severity of arrhythmias appears to be related more with the performance of the left ventricle than with the systolic pressure difference across the valve. Patients who have aortic stenosis of the elderly may also have calcium that extends into the atrioventricular node, producing varying degrees of heart block. Electrophysiologic studies have indicated that a significant number of patients with significant aortic stenosis have latent conduction abnormalities.[24] Mitchell and co-workers[1] reported that atrioventricular block or bundle branch block occurred in 26% of 455 patients with aortic stenosis.

CHEST ROENTGENOGRAM

In most patients with critical aortic stenosis the transverse diameter of the heart is not significantly increased although there may be some increased convexity of the left border of the left ventricle (Fig. 88.4). Prominence of the ascending aorta due to poststenotic dilatation is usually present. When the left ventricle markedly "fails," it may dilate modestly, and the left ventricular chamber may be enlarged. This is a relatively late finding in isolated aortic stenosis and implies significant left ventricular dysfunction. A very useful roentgenographic finding is the presence of calcium in the aortic valve. In most adult patients with aortic stenosis there is a fairly good correlation between the amount of calcium and the severity of stenosis.[54] The calcium can be seen on a frontal or especially on a lateral or left anterior oblique chest film; however, it is much better appreciated and quantified by cinefluoroscopy.[55] In adults, the absence of significant calcium by cinefluoroscopy is strong evidence against the presence of severe aortic stenosis. In some patients who have aortic stenosis of the elderly, calcium may also be noted in the aortic annulus, the wall of the aorta, and the mitral annulus. The lung fields usually are within normal limits unless patients have severe elevation of the left ventricular diastolic pressure, which may be reflected in some increased prominence of the venous flow in the upper lobes of the chest film, Kerley B lines, or even interstitial pulmonary edema. In the small percentage of patients with aortic stenosis who develop severe pulmonary hypertension, the main pulmonary artery and right ventricle are prominent.

ECHOCARDIOGRAM

Echocardiography is extremely useful in evaluating patients for aortic stenosis. This is particularly so if one is able to demonstrate the absence of calcium and a rapid, wide opening of the aortic valve. On the other hand, the finding of markedly thickened or calcified aortic valve leaflets may occur in the absence of severe or moderate stenosis.[56] In adults, echocardiographic evidence of minimal calcification of the aortic leaflets or of normal or nearly normal motion of the valve leaflets is strong evidence against the presence of severe stenosis. The finding of aortic valve systolic flutter on M-mode echocardiography is also strong evidence against significant aortic stenosis, but the absence of aortic valve systolic flutter does not permit one to predict reliably the severity of aortic stenosis. Most patients with moderate or severe aortic stenosis have concentric hypertrophy and many have a wide ascending aorta, ascribed to poststenotic dilatation. The use of combined two-dimensional echocardiography and Doppler echocardiography (Fig. 88.5) frequently is useful in the evaluation of patients with aortic stenosis and may provide a fairly accurate index of the severity of the stenosis.[57-65]

Echocardiography is useful in the diagnosis of a bicuspid aortic valve, either by demonstrating an abnormal eccentric position of the closed aortic valve leaflets in the aorta during diastole on M-mode recording or by direct two-dimensional imaging of the two leaflets. Echocardiography is also very useful in the evaluation of left ventricular function. Unfortunately, some older patients, particularly those with severe emphysema, may not have technically satisfactory echocardiograms, and cardiac catheterization may be necessary to rule out severe aortic stenosis. Echocardiography during or immediately following exercise is also useful in following systolic and diastolic function of the left ventricle and may be of particular value in patients with evidence of aortic stenosis but minimal or no symptoms.[66]

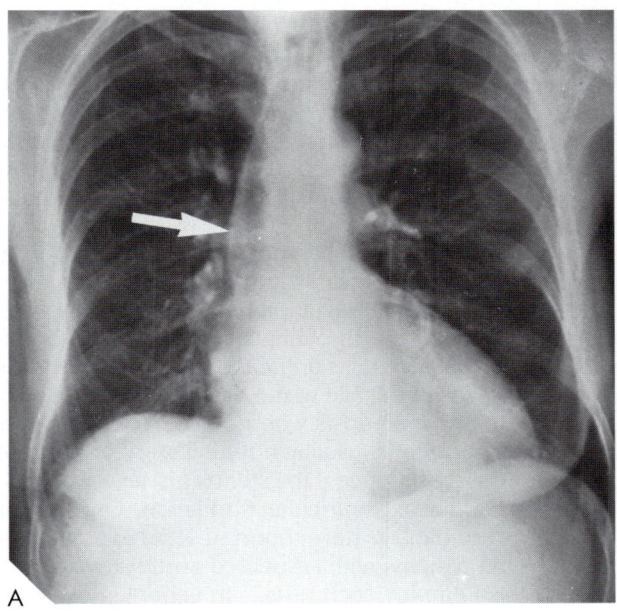
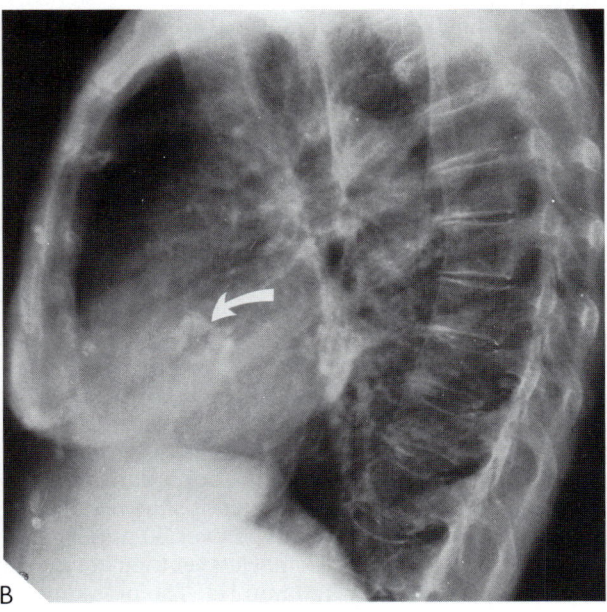

FIGURE 88.4 A. Posteroanterior roentgenogram of a patient with calcific aortic stenosis. There is slight prominence of the left cardiac border in the region of the left ventricle and slight prominence of the ascending aorta from poststenotic dilatation (*arrow*). **B.** Lateral film showing extensive calcium in the area of the aortic valve (*arrow*).

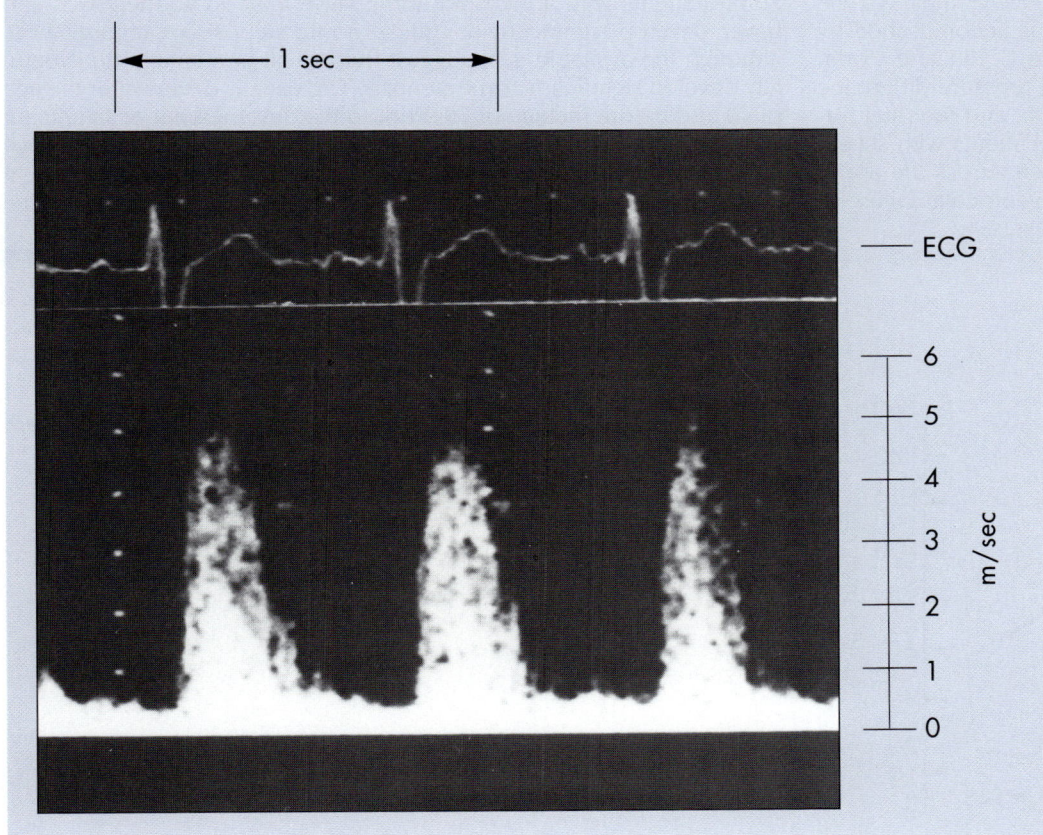

FIGURE 88.5 Doppler echocardiogram from the suprasternal notch of a 70-year-old woman with aortic stenosis. The mean peak aortic flow velocity is 4.5 m/sec, which results in an estimated pressure difference between the left ventricle and the aorta of 81 mm Hg ($P = 4V^2$). At cardiac catheterization, the patient's peak-to-peak pressure difference was 78 mm Hg and the mean difference was 63 mm Hg. The calculated valve area was 0.5 cm². (*P*, pressure; *V*, velocity)

PHONOCARDIOGRAPHY AND PULSE RECORDINGS

Recordings of the arterial pulse and phonocardiography were formerly used routinely in the evaluation of the severity of aortic stenosis. At present they are less widely used and are thought to be less specific and less sensitive than other diagnostic techniques in the hands of most physicians. In skilled hands, however, the techniques can be very useful both for screening purposes and for serial follow-up studies. Except in the very young or old, a normal systolic upstroke time is strong evidence against the presence of severe critical aortic stenosis. On the other hand, a prolonged upstroke time and prolonged left ventricular ejection can be present in both severe and mild stenosis. A systolic murmur that peaks later in systole is compatible with severe stenosis although this finding has only limited diagnostic value. Occasionally, phonocardiography can detect the presence of both the aortic and the pulmonic second heart sounds, a finding that is moderately strong evidence against critical stenosis, when this cannot be determined by auscultation. It may also detect the presence of an ejection click of the aortic valve, a finding that usually implies that there is not heavy calcification of all valve leaflets; phonocardiography may also document paradoxic splitting of the two components of the sound heart sound.

CARDIAC CATHETERIZATION

The basic defect in aortic stenosis is an abnormal pressure difference between the chamber of the left ventricle and the aorta during systole (Fig. 88.6). In most patients with critical aortic stenosis the mean pressure difference across the valve in systole will be over 50 mm Hg and sometimes more than 100 mm Hg. The maximal left ventricular systolic pressure encountered is approximately 320 mm Hg. The pressure difference across any critical orifice or obstruction is related to the square of the blood flow across the obstruction. Thus, if the blood flow across a critical obstruction doubles, the pressure difference will increase fourfold if the duration of flow remains the same. Accordingly, in the evaluation of patients with aortic stenosis, it is necessary to make sure that severe stenosis is not present despite a relatively small systolic pressure difference across the aortic valve. This is accomplished by calculation of the aortic valve orifice area by the Gorlin and Gorlin formula, which takes into account both the mean pressure difference across the valve, the duration of systole per minute, and the total forward blood flow across the valve during systole. Patients with severe aortic stenosis may have a low pressure difference across the aortic valve due to a diminished stroke volume from left ventricular failure or from concomitant mitral stenosis, which limits inflow into the left ventricle.[32]

The diastolic pressure in the left ventricle is characteristically elevated, both in early and mid-diastole and after the *a* wave. Oftentimes, the final, end-diastolic pressure is elevated to 18 mm Hg to 35 mm Hg even when the systolic function and ejection fraction of the ventricle are well preserved. In most patients with aortic stenosis the cardiac output is well preserved until late in the course of the disease. Occasionally it is even slightly increased, despite the severe outflow tract obstruction. In contrast, studies of ventricular filling have indicated that the relaxation and filling characteristics of the left ventricle are diminished relatively early. This may be due to the marked hypertrophy as well as to fibrosis or even ischemia. These changes are best appreciated during the early period of isovolumic relaxation. In patients who have severe aortic stenosis the cardiac output usually does not increase significantly during exercise although the diastolic pressure in the left ventricle and the pulmonary capillary pressure may increase significantly.[25-27,30] The systemic blood pressure occasionally falls during exercise, possibly related to baroreceptor reflexes originating in the walls of the left ventricle.[41]

Coronary arteriography should be performed in all patients who have coronary risk factors[40] or who are over the age of 35 and who undergo cardiac catheterization for aortic stenosis, whether or not they have angina pectoris. In patients with stenosis who have angina pectoris the prevalence of significant coronary artery disease increases progressively with the age of the patient.[39] It may also occur in patients with severe aortic stenosis who do not have angina pectoris.

Exercise testing is usually not necessary or appropriate in patients with aortic stenosis since if the stenosis is severe, it may induce ventricular tachycardia or ventricular fibrillation. On the other hand, some pediatric cardiologists have reported serial exercise tests to be of value in following patients with suspected aortic stenosis. Some adult cardiologists also employ such tests.[67] In general, however, it is not necessary and is potentially hazardous, particularly when performed by those without special skills in such testing.

NATURAL HISTORY AND PROGNOSIS

Some patients with a bicuspid aortic valve may go all their lives and never develop significant or critical aortic stenosis or regurgitation, although the available data suggest that a high percentage do eventually develop significant aortic stenosis. This usually occurs after the age of 40 and before the age of 70. Prior to the development of significant obstruction, the main risk to the patient is the development of infective endocarditis. In patients who develop rheumatic aortic stenosis, it usually is at least 10 years after the attack of rheumatic fever before the

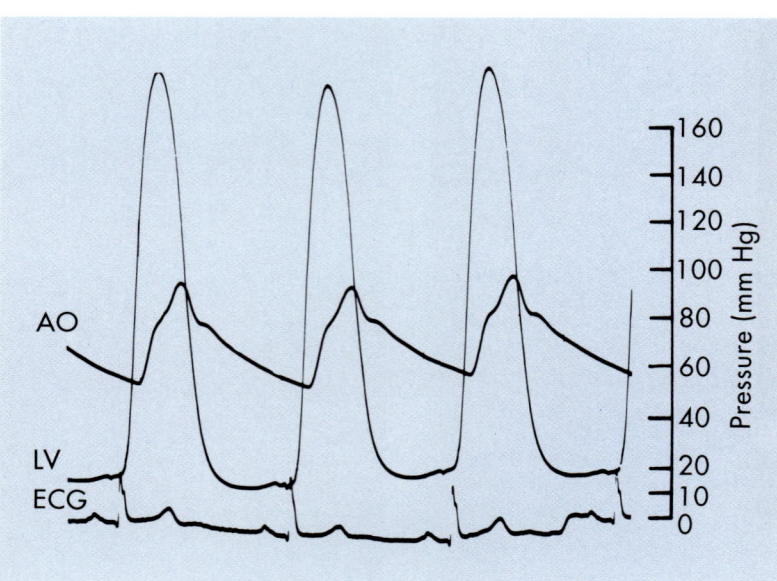

FIGURE 88.6 Simultaneous recordings of aortic pressure (AO), left ventricular pressure (LV), and electrocardiogram (ECG) in a 36-year-old woman with rheumatic aortic stenosis and mitral stenosis. There was a peak-to-peak pressure difference between the LV and AO of 88 mm Hg. The calculated aortic valve area was 0.8 cm^2, and the calculated mitral valve area was 1.3 cm^2.

stenosis becomes critical or significant. There is a moderate variation in the rate of progression of rheumatic aortic valve disease, however, and some patients progress rapidly while others progress slowly over many decades. The author and others[68–70] have noted that some patients with degenerative or aortic stenosis of the elderly may progress rapidly over a few years from little or no obstruction to very significant obstruction. Similar observations have been made in children.[71,72] Thus, it is necessary periodically to reevaluate such patients even if they have had cardiac catheterization and documentation of a low-pressure difference between the left ventricle and the aorta. In general, after the appearance of any of the classic triad of symptoms of aortic stenosis (failure, angina pectoris, or syncope), the 3-year mortality is about 40%, the 5-year mortality is 50%, and the 10-year mortality is 80%.[44] Approximately 15% to 20% of patients die suddenly, and in this group, about 3% to 5% have had no preceding symptoms.

MANAGEMENT

The major medical treatment of patients with bicuspid aortic valve or with noncritical aortic stenosis (rheumatic, degenerative, lupus, or atherosclerotic aortic stenosis) is to prevent infective endocarditis by appropriate antibiotic prophylaxis prior to dental work or surgery of any type during which bacteremia might occur. Patients with rheumatic aortic stenosis should receive daily prophylaxis against recurrent streptococcal infection with either oral sulfadiazine or penicillin. In these patients it is reasonable to continue this therapy for life.

In general, it is probably wise to counsel children with bicuspid aortic valves or with rheumatic fever involving the aortic valve not to participate in sports or activities that require extreme exertion, since this may extremely rarely be associated with sudden death in patients who have developed significant aortic stenosis. In addition, it is psychologically difficult for a young person to become very proficient in a sport only to have to give up this sport for health reasons during middle age. If atrial fibrillation occurs in a patient with significant aortic stenosis, it may precipitate acute left ventricular failure. This may require electrical cardioversion and/or the use of digoxin or other antiarrhythmic agents.

Once the onset of any of the classic triad (congestive heart failure, angina, or syncope) occurs, cardiac catheterization and surgery should be done promptly in most patients. This is particularly true in patients who have evidence of pulmonary hypertension. Some patients develop acute heart failure with the onset of atrial fibrillation or flutter; often, these patients can be significantly improved by electrical cardioversion. Digitalis is appropriate for heart failure and may cause some improvement, particularly if the symptoms are primarily related to systolic dysfunction of the ventricle. Prazosin, hydralazine, or intravenous sodium nitroprusside can occasionally cause an improvement in patients with heart failure due to aortic stenosis.[73,74] These drugs must be given very cautiously, however, because they can cause an excessive decrease in venous return and can markedly decrease cardiac output and arterial pressure unless their use is monitored very carefully. It is seldom appropriate to delay surgery significantly in order to treat the patient with digoxin or vasodilators.

Cardiac catheterization should be performed in most patients prior to valve surgery; however, in a few patients it may not be possible to catheterize the left ventricle from the aorta, and surgery can be appropriate in such patients without catheterization of the left ventricle to measure the pressure difference across the aortic valve and the left ventricular pressures and to evaluate left ventricular performance. Coronary arteriography should be performed whenever possible, particularly in patients with coronary risk factors[40] or in patients over the age of 35 years.

Valve replacement is indicated in patients with isolated valvular aortic stenosis that produces any of the classic triad of symptoms and who at catheterization have either a valve area of 0.75 cm^2 or less or a peak to peak pressure difference between the left ventricle and the aorta of 75 mm Hg or more with a normal cardiac output. The management of patients who are proven to have severe aortic stenosis but who deny symptoms must be individualized. In some patients it is appropriate to recommend surgery, whereas in other patients there is less risk in waiting for the development of symptoms.

In infants and children, surgery is generally indicated in patients with either a calculated aortic valve area of $0.5 \text{ cm}^2/\text{m}^2$ or less or a peak-to-peak pressure difference between the left ventricle and aorta of 75 mm Hg or more. If the infant or child is symptomatic or has cardiomegaly or S-T wave changes on the electrocardiogram, surgery may be appropriate with a peak pressure difference in children of 40 mm Hg or more. Surgery is usually offered to patients with subvalvular aortic stenosis that produces a pressure difference of 30 mm Hg or more in order to prevent progressive deformity of the aortic valve.

Catheter balloon valvuloplasty (CBV) of the aortic valve can be used as a palliative procedure in older patients who are not candidates for aortic valve replacement.[75–78] CBV appears to produce fractures of calcific nodules and, less frequently, grossly inapparent microfractures or separation of fused commissures. In general, CBV produces only a modest increase in valve area, but this may be sufficient to produce a significant improvement in symptomatology and left ventricular function. Unfortunately, the results of CBV are often temporary, and many patients have a recurrence of severe stenosis by 6 to 12 months. In selected cases, CBV can be useful as a palliative procedure before major noncardiac operations or invasive procedures, or as a bridge to valve replacement in a patient with severe aortic stenosis, at times with cardiogenic shock.[79–81] CBV has also been used in selected infants, children, and young adults with congenital aortic stenosis.

Patients who have angina pectoris and who have severe coronary artery disease demonstrated by coronary arteriography should usually undergo simultaneous coronary artery bypass graft surgery. Patients with subvalvular or supravalvular aortic stenosis are surgically treated by excision of the obstruction. Patients with supravalvular stenosis may also require enlargement of the aorta.[82]

The presence of severe left ventricular systolic and diastolic dysfunction or failure is not a contraindication to valve replacement, although the presence of such dysfunction or failure increases operative morbidity and mortality. Many patients may have a significant improvement in systolic and diastolic ventricular function after relief of the outflow tract obstruction.[83–86]

The overall average operative mortality for isolated aortic valve replacement is about 3% to 6%, but it is higher for patients who are in New York Heart Association functional class IV. It is somewhat higher for patients over 70 years of age and for patients requiring concurrent mitral valve replacement or coronary artery surgery.[87,88]

The life expectancy after isolated aortic valve replacement is generally good, with about 80% of patients alive at 5 years and 60% at 10 years.[89,90] The incidence of arterial thromboembolism in patients on chronic anticoagulant therapy with warfarin after aortic valve replacement is approximately 2% to 3% per year if the control is good but the incidence is several times more frequent if the therapy is less adequate. Bleeding complications, such as significant gastrointestinal, genitourinary, or intracranial bleeding, are less frequent, usually approximately 1% to 2% per year. The use of a bioprosthesis in the aortic position avoids the necessity of anticoagulation in most patients, but the pressure difference across these valves may be greater than across ball valve or disc valves of comparable size. Although the long-term durability of xenograft valves is uncertain, the results to date after 10 years of use are cautiously encouraging. Unfortunately, in children and patients under the age of 30 to 35 years, these valves undergo relatively rapid fibrosis and calcification.

Patients who undergo surgical replacement with a prosthetic aortic valve should be carefully followed for the development of the following complications: perioperative myocardial infarction; postpericardiotomy syndrome; postperfusion syndrome; periprosthetic leak with aortic regurgitation; "ball variance" due to swelling or change in shape of a caged ball; persistence of left ventricular dysfunction; interference with movement of a leaflet, disc, or ball by thrombus or by fibrosis and calcification of a porcine xenograft; hemolytic anemia from damage to erythrocytes; arterial emboli from thrombus on the prosthetic valve; infective endocarditis; and myocardial ischemia or infarction from progression of coronary artery disease. After valvular surgery and before discharge from the hospital, patients should have a chest roentgenogram, electrocardiogram, echocardiogram, and phonocardiogram. Serial echocardiography is useful in following patients with prosthetic valves, particularly heterografts. Serial cinefluoroscopy and phonocardiography are also useful, especially in patients with synthetic (disc or ball) prosthetic valves, and may detect dysfunction before it is clinically manifest.

REFERENCES

1. Mitchell AM, Sackett CH, Hunzicker WJ, Levine SA: The clinical features of aortic stenosis. Am Heart J 48:684, 1954
2. Dexter L, Harken DE, Cobb LA Jr et al: Aortic stenosis. Arch Intern Med 101:254, 1958
3. Wood P: Aortic stenosis. Am J Cardiol 1:553, 1958
4. Hancock EW, Fleming PR: Aortic stenosis. Q J Med 29:209, 1960
5. Selzer A: Changing aspects of the natural history of aortic stenosis. N Engl J Med 317:91, 1987
6. Lombardo JT, Selzer A: Valvular aortic stenosis: A clinical and hemodynamic profile of patients. Ann Int Med 106:292, 1987
7. Edwards JE: Pathology of left ventricular outflow tract obstruction. Circulation 31:586, 1965
8. Roberts WC: The structure of the aortic valve in clinically isolated aortic stenosis: An autopsy study of 162 patients over 15 years of age. Circulation 42:91, 1970
9. Schlant RC: Calcific aortic stenosis. Am J Cardiol 27:581, 1971
10. Roberts WC: Aortic valve stenosis and the congenitally malformed aortic valve. In Roberts WC (ed): Congenital Heart Disease in Adults, pp 416–426. Philadelphia, FA Davis, 1979
11. Subramanian R, Olson LJ, Edwards WD: Surgical pathology of pure aortic stenosis: A study of 374 cases. Mayo Clin Proc 59:683, 1984
12. Pansegrau DG, Kioshos JM, Durnin RE, Kroetz FW: Supravalvular aortic stenosis in adults. Am J Cardiol 31:635, 1973
13. Sung CS, Price EC, Cooley DA: Discrete subaortic stenosis in adults. Am J Cardiol 42:283, 1978
14. Roberts WC: The congenitally bicuspid aortic valve: A study of 85 autopsy cases. Am J Cardiol 26:72, 1970
15. Lerman BB, Thomas LC, Abrams GD, Pitt B: Aortic stenosis associated with systemic lupus erythematosus. Am J Med 72:707, 1982
16. Chandy KG, John TJ, Cherian G: Coxsackieviruses and chronic valvular heart disease. Am Heart J 100:578, 1980
17. Beppu S, Minura Y, Sakakibara H et al: Supravalvular aortic stenosis and coronary ostial stenosis in familial hypercholesterolemia: Two-dimensional echocardiographic assessment. Circulation 67:878, 1983
18. Roberts WE, Ewy GA, Glancy DL, Marcus FL: Valvular stenosis produced by active infective endocarditis. Circulation 36:449, 1977
19. Gould L, Reddy CVR, Depalma D: Cardiac manifestations of ochronosis. J Thorac Cardiovasc Surg 72:788, 1976
20. Roberts WC: Anatomically isolated aortic valvular disease. The case against its being of rheumatic etiology. Am J Med 49:151, 1970
21. Mönckeberg JG: Der normale histologische Bau und die Sklerose der Aortenklappen. Virchow Arch [A] 176:471, 1904
22. Roberts WC, Perloff JK, Constantino T: Severe valvular aortic stenosis in patients over 65 years of age: A clinicopathologic study. Am J Cardiol 27:497, 1971
23. Pomerance A: Isolated aortic stenosis. In Pomerance A, Davies MJ (eds): The Pathology of the Heart, pp 327–342. London, Blackwell Scientific Publications, 1975
24. Rasmussen K, Thomsen PEB, Bagger JP: HV interval in calcific aortic stenosis. Relation to left ventricular function and effect of valve replacement. Br Heart J 52:82, 1984
25. Anderson FL, Tsagaris TJ, Tikoff G et al: Hemodynamic effects of exercise in patients with aortic stenosis. Am J Med 46:872, 1969
26. Bache RJ, Wang Y, Jorgensen CR: Hemodynamic effects of exercise in isolated valvular aortic stenosis. Circulation 44:1003, 1971
27. Oldershaw PJ, Dawkins KD, Ward DE, Gibson DG: Diastolic mechanisms of impaired exercise tolerance in aortic valve disease. Br Heart J 49:568, 1983
28. Hess OM, Schneider J, Turina M et al: Asymmetric septal hypertrophy in patients with aortic stenosis: An adaptive mechanism or a coexistence of hypertrophic cardiomyopathy? J Am Coll Cardiol 1:783, 1983
29. Levine HJ, McIntyre KM, Lipana JG, Bing OH: Force-velocity relations in failing and nonfailing hearts of subjects with aortic stenosis. Am J Med Sci 259:79, 1970
30. Schlant RC, Nutter DO: Heart failure in valvular heart disease. Medicine 50:421, 1971
31. Spann JF, Bove AA, Natarajan G, Kreulen T: Ventricular performance, pump function and compensatory mechanisms in patients with aortic stenosis. Circulation 62:576, 1980
32. Zitnik RS, Piemme TE, Messer RJ et al: The masking of aortic stenosis by mitral stenosis. Am Heart J 69:22, 1965
33. Bird JJ, Murgo JP, Pasipoalarides A: Fluid dynamics of aortic stenosis: Subvalvular gradients without subvalvular obstruction. Circulation 66:835, 1982
34. Silove ED, Vogel JHK, Grover RF: The pressure gradient in ventricular outflow obstruction: Influence of peripheral resistance. Cardiovasc Res 2:234, 1968
35. Bertrand ME, Lablanche JM, Tilmant PY et al: Coronary sinus blood flow at rest and during isometric exercise in patients with aortic valve disease: Mechanism of angina pectoris in presence of normal coronary arteries. Am J Cardiol 47:199, 1981
36. Kennedy JW, Twiss RD, Blackmon JR, Dodge HT: Quantitative angiocardiography: III. Relationships of left ventricular pressure, volume, and mass in aortic valve disease. Circulation 38:838, 1968
37. Buckberg G, Edber L, Herman M, Gorlin R: Ischemia in aortic stenosis: Hemodynamic prediction. Am J Cardiol 35:778, 1975
38. Johnson LI, Sciacca RR, Ellis K et al: Reduced left ventricular myocardial blood flow per unit mass in aortic stenosis. Circulation 57:582, 1978
39. Hancock EW: Aortic stenosis, angina pectoris, and coronary artery disease. Am Heart J 93:382, 1977
40. Ramsdale DR, Faragher EB, Bennett DH et al: Preoperative prediction of significant coronary artery disease in patients with valvular heart disease. Br Med J 284:223, 1982
41. Mark AL: The Bezold-Jarisch reflex revisited: Clinical implications of inhibitory reflexes originating in the heart. J Am Coll Cardiol 1:90, 1983
42. McHenry MM, Rice J, Matloff HJ, Flamm MD: Pulmonary hypertension and sudden death in aortic stenosis. Br Heart J 41:463, 1979
43. Ross J Jr, Braunwald E: Aortic stenosis. Circulation (Suppl V)38:61, 1968
44. Frank S, Johnson A, Ross J Jr: Natural history of valvular aortic stenosis. Br Heart J 35:41, 1973
45. Rapaport E: Natural history of aortic and mitral valve disease. Am J Cardiol 35:221, 1971
46. Love JW: The syndrome of calcific aortic stenosis and gastrointestinal bleeding: Resolution following aortic valve replacement. J Thorac Cardiovasc Surg 83:779, 1982
47. Shbeeb I, Prager E, Love J: The aortic valve-colonic axis. Dis Colon Rectum 27:38, 1984
48. Perloff JK: Clinical recognition of aortic stenosis: The physical signs and differential diagnosis of the various forms of obstruction to left ventricular outflow. Prog Cardiovasc Dis 10:323, 1968
49. Nakamura T, Hultgren HN, Shettigar UR, Fowles RE: Noninvasive evaluation of the severity of aortic stenosis in adult patients. Am Heart J 107:959, 1984
50. Ikram H, Marshall DE, Moore SM, Bones PJ: Hypertension in valvular aortic stenosis. NZ Med J 89:204, 1979
51. Siegel RJ, Roberts WC: Electrocardiographic observations in severe aortic valve stenosis: Correlative necropsy study to clinical, hemodynamic, and ECG variables demonstrating relation of 12-lead QRS amplitude to peak systolic transaortic pressure gradient. Am Heart J 103:210, 1982
52. Olshausen KV, Schwarz F, Apfelbach J et al: Determinants of the incidence and severity of ventricular arrhythmias in aortic valve disease. Am J Cardiol 51:1103, 1983
53. Kostis JB, Tupper B, Moreyra AE et al: Aortic valve replacement in patients with aortic stenosis. Effect on cardiac arrhythmias. Chest 85:211, 1984
54. Glancy DL, Freed TA, O'Brien KP, Epstein SE: Calcium in the aortic valve: Roentgenologic and hemodynamic correlations in 148 patients. Ann Intern Med 71:245, 1969
55. Dancy M, Leech G, Leatham A: Comparison of cinefluoroscopy and M mode echocardiography for detecting aortic valve calcification: Correlation with severity of stenosis of non-rheumatic aetiology. Br Heart J 51:416, 1984
56. DeMaria AN, Bommer W, Joye J et al: Value and limitations of cross-sectional echocardiography of the aortic valve in the diagnosis and quantification of valvular aortic stenosis. Circulation 62:304, 1980
57. Richards KL: Doppler echocardiographic diagnosis and quantification of valvular heart disease. Curr Probl Cardiol 10(2):2, 1985
58. Carrie PJ, Seward JB, Reeder GS et al: Continuous-wave Doppler echocardiographic assessment of severity of calcific aortic stenosis: A simultaneous Doppler-catheter correlative study in 100 adult patients. Circulation 71:1162, 1985
59. Smith MD, Dawson PL, Elion JL et al: Systematic correlation of continuous-wave Doppler and hemodynamic measurements in patients with aortic stenosis. Am Heart J 111:245, 1986
60. Yeager M, Yock PG, Popp RL: Comparison of Doppler-derived pressure gradient to that determined at cardiac catheterization in adults with aortic valve stenosis: Implications for management. Am J Cardiol 57:644, 1986
61. Zoghki WA, Farmer KL, Soto JG et al: Accurate noninvasive quantification of stenotic aortic valve area by Doppler echocardiography. Circulation 73:452, 1986
62. Richards KL, Cannon SR, Miller JF et al: Calculation of aortic valve area by

Doppler echocardiography: A direct application of the continuity equation. Circulation 73:964, 1986
63. Otto CM, Pearlman AS, Comess KA et al: Determination of the stenotic aortic valve area in adults using Doppler echocardiography. J Am Coll Cardiol 7:509, 1986
64. Oh JK, Taliercio CP, Holmes DR Jr: Prediction of the severity of aortic stenosis by Doppler aortic valve area determination: Prospective Doppler-catheterization correlation in 100 patients. J Am Coll Cardiol 11:1227, 1988
65. Otto CM, Pearlman AS, Gardner CL: Hemodynamic progression of aortic stenosis in adults assessed by Doppler echocardiography. J Am Coll Cardiol 13:545, 1989
66. Dancy M, Leech G, Leatham A: Changes in echocardiographic left ventricular minor axis dimensions during exercise in patients with aortic stenosis. Br Heart J 52:446, 1984
67. Areskos NH: Exercise testing in the evaluation of patients with valvular aortic stenosis. Clin Physiol 4:201, 1984
68. Cheitlin MD, Gertz EW, Brundage BH et al: Rate of progression of severity of valvular aortic stenosis in the adult. Am Heart J 98:689, 1979
69. Wagner S, Selzer A: Patterns of progression of aortic stenosis: A longitudinal hemodynamic study. Circulation 65:709, 1982
70. Nestico PF, DePace NL, Kimbiris D et al: Progression of isolated aortic stenosis: Analysis of 29 patients having more than one cardiac catheterization. Am J Cardiol 52:1054, 1983
71. Friedman WF, Modlinger J, Morgan JR: Serial hemodynamic observations in asymptomatic children with valvar aortic stenosis. Circulation 43:91, 1971
72. El-Said G, Galioto FM, Mullins CE et al: Natural hemodynamic history of congenital aortic stenosis in childhood. Am J Cardiol 30:6, 1972
73. Greenberg BH, Massie BM: Beneficial effects of afterload reduction in patients with congestive heart failure and moderate aortic stenosis. Circulation 61:212, 1980
74. Awan NA, DeMaria AN, Miller RR et al: Beneficial effects of nitroprusside administration on left ventricular dysfunction and myocardial ischemia in severe aortic stenosis. Am Heart J 101:386, 1981
75. Safian RD, Berman AD, Diver DJ, et al: Balloon aortic valvuloplasty in 170 consecutive patients. N Engl J Med 319:125, 1988
76. Holmes DR Jr, Nishimura RA, Reeder GS et al: Clinical follow-up after percutaneous aortic balloon valvuloplasty. Arch Int Med 149:1405, 1989
77. Sherman W, Hersham R, Lazza C et al: Balloon valvuloplasty in adult aortic stenosis: Determinants of clinical outcome. Ann Int Med 110:421, 1989
78. Nishimura RA, Homes DR Jr, Reeder GS: Percutaneous balloon valvuloplasty. Mayo Clinic Proc 65:198, 1990
79. Roth RB, Palacios IF, Block PC: Percutaneous aortic balloon valvuloplasty: Its role in the management of patients with aortic stenosis requiring major noncardiac surgery. J Am Coll Cardiol 13:1039, 1989
80. Hayes SN, Homes DR Jr, Nishimura RA, Reeder GS: Palliative percutaneous aortic balloon valvuloplasty before noncardiac operations and invasive procedures. Mayo Clin Proc 64:753, 1989
81. Berland J, Cribier A, Savin T et al: Percutaneous balloon valvuloplasty in patients with severe aortic stenosis and low ejection fraction. Circulation 79:1189, 1989
82. Flaker G, Teske D, Kilman J et al: Supravalvular aortic stenosis: A 20-year clinical perspective and experience with patch aortoplasty. Am J Cardiol 51:256, 1983
83. Ross J Jr, Morrow AG, Mason DT, Braunwald E: Left ventricular function following replacement of the aortic valve. Hemodynamic responses to muscular exercise. Circulation 33:507, 1966
84. Borer JS, Bacharach SL, Green MV et al: Left ventricular function in aortic stenosis: Response to exercise and effects of operation. Am J Cardiol 41:382, 1978
85. Smith N, McAnulty JH, Rahimtoola SH: Severe aortic stenosis with impaired left ventricular function and clinical heart failure: Results of valve replacement. Circulation 58:255, 1978
86. Thompson R, Yacoub M, Ahmed M et al: Influence of preoperative left ventricular function on results of homograft replacement of the aortic valve for aortic stenosis. Am J Cardiol 43:929, 1979
87. Jamieson WR, Dooner J, Munro I et al: Cardiac valve replacement in the elderly: A review of 320 consecutive cases. Circulation 64(Suppl II):177, 1981
88. Arom KV, Nicoloff DM, Lindsay WG et al: Should valve replacement and related procedures be performed in elderly patients? Ann Thorac Surg 38:466, 1984
89. Cohn LH: The long-term results of aortic valve replacement. Chest 85:387, 1984
90. Miller DC, Oyer PE, Mitchell RS et al: Performance characteristics of the Starr-Edwards Model 1260 aortic valve prosthesis beyond ten years. J Thorac Cardiovasc Surg 88:193, 1984

MITRAL STENOSIS

Elliot Rapaport

The past four decades have witnessed a startling decline in the prevalence of mitral stenosis. This has occurred in large measure because of the introduction of penicillin and its use in acute streptococcal infections resulting in a remarkable fall in the incidence of rheumatic fever. Coupled with the introduction of effective surgical techniques for relieving mitral valve stenosis by Harken[1] and Bailey[2] in the late 1940s and, subsequently, the introduction of open heart mitral valvuloplasty and prosthetic valve replacement, we no longer witness on a daily basis the terminally bedridden patient with mitral facies, cardiac cachexia, and congestive heart failure suffering the end-stages of mitral stenosis. Despite the striking decline in the prevalence of mitral stenosis, it still remains an important clinical problem, not only in Third World countries where the occurrence of rheumatic fever is often in epidemic proportions, but also in the industrialized world where rheumatic fever is still endemic.

☐ PATHOLOGY

The normal mitral valve ring has a circumference of approximately 10 cm.[3] The greatest diameter of the orifice extends from the anterolateral to the posteromedial commissure. The commissures do not extend to the valve ring; there is approximately 0.5 cm to 1 cm of commissural tissue between the edge of the two cusps and the valve ring. Thus, the approximate area of a normal mitral valve orifice is 5 cm^2 to 6 cm^2. The valve is bicuspid, with the anterior cusp roughly twice the size of the posterior cusp.

Approximately 60% of patients with relatively pure mitral stenosis will recall a history suggestive of prior acute rheumatic fever. In contrast, patients with multivalvular disease will have a prior history in over 90% of cases. Approximately half of the patients who admit to a prior history of rheumatic fever will have had only one recognizable earlier episode. One in eight of these will have had chorea alone as their clinical manifestation. Although this is a relatively small incidence, children who present with chorea alone usually develop mitral stenosis as their manifestation of rheumatic heart disease. The average latent period following the initial episode of rheumatic fever, in those countries where rheumatic fever occurs sporadically, is approximately 20 years. In their classic 20-year report on 1000 patients followed since childhood in Boston, Bland and Jones found that nearly two thirds of those in whom mitral stenosis ultimately developed had no clinical evidence of mitral stenosis 10 years after the original episode of rheumatic fever.[4] Thus, most patients are in their late 20s or early 30s when they first develop symptoms. An average further lapse of 7 years is seen from the onset of symptoms to the time in which the patient is significantly disabled as a result of mitral stenosis. In countries where rheumatic fever occurs in epidemic proportions, the latent period is distinctly shorter and patients may present in their teens with significant mitral stenosis. The average age at the time of mitral commissurotomy in over 3700 consecutive patients in Vellore, India, was 27 years.[5]

Rheumatic fever produces varying degrees of commissural fusion. In one patient, there may be only a small amount causing a fish-mouth type of stenosis; in another, there may be marked fusion resulting in a small buttonhole valve. Thickening and calcification of the cusps may also contribute to the degree of stenosis through resultant immobility. Finally, chordal thickening and fusion may restrict valve leaflet movement contributing to the reduction in orifice area. Chordal fibrosis, calcification, and fusion with shortening may also create subvalvular stenosis, which at times may be even more significant than the orifice stenosis itself.

The left atrium characteristically enlarges as the mitral valve orifice narrows and left atrial pressure rises. The enlargement is generally less pronounced than is seen in rheumatic mitral insufficiency. Left atrial thrombi, particularly within the left atrial appendage, frequently occur. Biopsy samples of atrial appendices show an approximate 50% incidence of Aschoff lesions. These are more likely to be seen in biopsies from younger patients than from older ones.[6] Although this suggests a continuing active rheumatic state, the correlation of positive Aschoff bodies in atrial biopsies with evidences of "smoldering" rheumatic carditis has not borne out clinically, and the finding has no real clinical relevance.

Longstanding hemodynamically significant mitral stenosis is generally associated with marked structural changes in the pulmonary circulation. The smaller branches of the pulmonary artery, the so-called pulmonary arterioles, will demonstrate marked hypertrophy of the muscular layer together with intimal proliferation and some fibrosis. Additionally, some of the larger branches of the pulmonary arteries may show not only similar intimal and medial changes but also branches of the pulmonary artery with thrombosis *in situ*. The major branches of the pulmonary artery will be dilated, reflecting the presence of pulmonary hypertension. Within the pulmonary parenchyma, there will be thickening of the basement membrane of the capillaries together with interstitial edema and fibrosis, as well as hemosiderin deposition in cases with repeated hemoptysis. Although these parenchymal changes may contribute to a lowering of arterial Po_2, they may also beneficially assist in resisting the increased capillary hydrostatic pressure and thus help to prevent pulmonary edema formation. Areas of the lung may also show evidences of prior pulmonary infarction, reflecting either local thrombosis with infarction or the results of thromboemboli arising from right atrial or deep venous thrombi.

Right ventricular hypertrophy results when pulmonary arterial pressure climbs out of proportion to the passive rise from pulmonary venous hypertension due to the large increase in pulmonary arteriolar resistance. Eventually when right ventricular failure ensues, right ventricular and right atrial dilatation is also seen.

☐ PATHOPHYSIOLOGIC BASIS OF SIGNS AND SYMPTOMS

The symptoms of rheumatic heart disease with mitral stenosis are the pathophysiologic consequences of a significantly obstructed orifice. Scarring of the mitral valve in itself produces no symptoms. During the years that the orifice is gradually narrowing from a normal 5 cm^2 or 6 cm^2 to 2 cm^2, the patient will usually be asymptomatic. Rarely, symptoms in the adult at this stage may be present, reflecting chronic smoldering rheumatic activity in the absence of significant mitral valve obstruction. This may give rise to a patient, usually in the older age group, who has auscultatory findings of mitral stenosis and atrial fibrillation. The patient has no hemodynamically significant obstruction at the mitral valve but shows evidence of impaired left ventricular function manifested clinically by pulmonary congestive symptoms and a low cardiac output.

Although symptoms due to left ventricular failure are rare, laboratory evidence of impaired left ventricular function in pure mitral stenosis is seen much more commonly.[7] This may be noted during a resting examination, but sometimes it becomes apparent only under situations where left ventricular outflow impedance is increased. Various explanations have been put forward to explain left ventricular dysfunction in mitral stenosis, including segmental wall motion abnormalities, particularly posterobasal hypokinesis due to myocardial scarring; subvalvular fibrosis; the direct effects of reduced left ventricular filling; active myocardial changes reflecting smoldering carditis; and septal dysfunction and bulging into the left ventricular cavity resulting from increased right ventricular volumes and pressures. Reduced coronary blood flow due to a decrease in cardiac output, with or without associated coronary artery atherosclerosis or coronary embolic disease, may also play a role in some patients. Despite these abnormalities in left ventricular function that can be detected by echocardiography, radionuclide angiography, or contrast ventriculography, a reduced cardiac output in mitral stenosis normally does not result from left ventricular dysfunction, but rather from a high pulmonary vascular resistance. A reduced left ventricular ejection fraction when seen probably reflects the presence of some increase in afterload in the face of a reduced preload rather than intrinsic muscle dysfunction, since the ratio of end-systolic stress to end-systolic volume of the left ventricle, a sensitive index of contractility thought to be independent of preload, remains normal in patients with mitral stenosis.[8]

PULMONARY CAPILLARY HYPERTENSION

When the mitral valve area falls below 2 cm^2, patients who are asymptomatic at rest may begin to exhibit symptoms during heavy exercise while left ventricular diastolic pressure remains basically the same. The shortened diastolic filling period resulting from the tachycardia consequent to exercise, together with the ensuing slight increase in stroke output, requires a diastolic pressure gradient to supply the necessary kinetic energy to accelerate the stroke output across the stenotic mitral valve orifice. This results in transient elevations of left atrial pressure and, therefore, passive pulmonary venous and capillary hypertension during heavy exercise while left ventricular diastolic pressure remains essentially the same. The corresponding increase in pulmonary blood volume with its associated increase in lung stiffness and work of breathing results in dyspnea on exertion. As soon as exercise ceases, left atrial, pulmonary venous, and pulmonary capillary pressures will rapidly return to normal and the patient is again asymptomatic. Therefore, dyspnea on exertion is the most common presenting symptom in patients with mitral stenosis.

As progressive scarring of the mitral orifice continues and the mitral valve orifice area eventually falls below 1.5 cm^2, the patient is likely to become symptomatic with ordinary exertion. Patients now may note dyspnea on mild to moderate exertion; however, it is not until the mitral valve orifice falls to under 1.2 cm^2 that most of the cardiorespiratory complaints associated with pulmonary congestion are commonly observed. The patient may note not only dyspnea on mild exertion but also a nocturnal cough, orthopnea, hemoptysis, and paroxysmal nocturnal dyspnea. At this stage, a normal cardiac output is usually observed. However, it is maintained at the expense of a significant diastolic pressure gradient across the mitral valve orifice, which results in pulmonary capillary and left atrial pressures that are elevated at rest while left ventricular diastolic pressure remains normal (Fig. 89.1). This gradient is sensitive to mitral valve flow, and in accordance with the Gorlin formula will vary roughly with the square of changes in flow.[9] Thus, a two-fold increase in mitral valve flow produces a fourfold increase in the pressure gradient across the mitral valve. Relatively little exercise is now accompanied by significant immediate further rises in left atrial and pulmonary capillary pressures to levels of 30 to 40 mm Hg, which can only be tolerated for short periods of time before requiring the patient to cease such activity.

The pulse contour of the pulmonary capillary pressure will also be altered in the presence of significant mitral stenosis. *A* waves will be absent if atrial fibrillation is present. The *v* wave is comparatively small in relation to the overall pressure pulse. Particularly noteworthy will be the relatively slow *y* descent after opening of the mitral valve.

PULMONARY VASCULAR DISEASE

Left atrial and pulmonary capillary pressures cannot rise at rest chronically to levels significantly greater than 25 to 30 mm Hg and still be consistent with survival. Beyond these levels capillary hydrostatic pressure exceeds plasma oncotic pressure. Unopposed by significant interstitial pressure, this would rapidly produce sufficient transudation of plasma into the interstitial and intra-alveolar spaces as to exceed the capacity of the pulmonary lymphatics to handle. The only alternative remaining to ensure that pulmonary capillary pressure remains below pulmonary edema levels is for the diastolic mitral valve flow to decrease when mitral valve area begins to fall below approximately 1 cm^2. The mechanism responsible for this reduction in cardiac output appears to be the development of increased pulmonary vascular tone in the smaller branches of the pulmonary circulation (so-called pulmonary vascular disease). This appears to be a vasoconstrictive response since it is usually reversible after successful mitral valve surgery that results in a return of left atrial and pulmonary venous pressures toward normal.[10,11] It appears to be initiated by chronic elevations in left atrial and pulmonary venous pressures; for example, it can be seen in patients with congenital cor triatriatum biventricularis where similar elevations in the proximal left atrial chamber and pulmonary venous pressures occur. It has also been observed in rare cases of granulomatous disease in the lung, sparing the left atrium but wrapping around the pulmonary veins such as to produce obstruction and resultant pulmonary venous hypertension in the absence of left atrial hypertension.

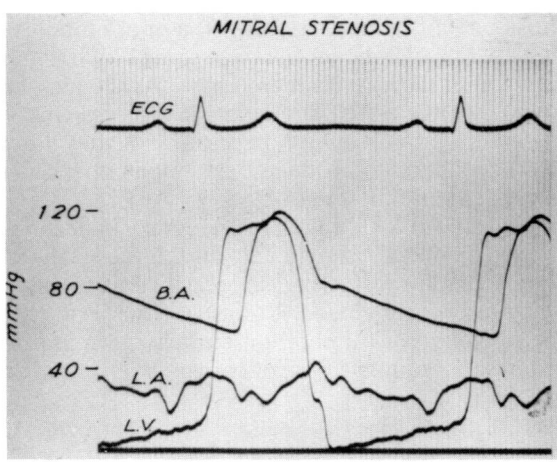

FIGURE 89.1 Simultaneous recording of brachial arterial, left atrial, and left ventricular pressure in a patient with mitral stenosis. The demonstration of a diastolic pressure gradient between left atrium and left ventricle is the *sine qua non* for the diagnosis of hemodynamically significant mitral stenosis. Left atrial mean pressure is approximately 30 mm Hg. Note the slow *y* descent to the left atrial pressure pulse following opening of the mitral valve.

This apparent reflex pulmonary vasoconstriction does not appear to be under the control of the autonomic nervous system since it is unaffected by sympathectomy.

Pulmonary arteriolar vasoconstriction not only causes cardiac output to fall, thus allowing left atrial pressure to remain below pulmonary edema levels, but also results in pulmonary arterial hypertension out of proportion to the rise in pulmonary capillary pressure. Pulmonary arterial pressures may eventually climb as high as systemic pressures, or even higher, and over time will lead to right ventricular hypertrophy, subsequent right ventricular dilatation, and congestive heart failure. Patients increasingly note easy fatigability and tiredness, reflecting the chronically reduced cardiac output as well as a marked decrease in exercise tolerance. When congestive heart failure ensues, all of the symptoms and signs normally associated with heart failure (as described elsewhere in these volumes) become apparent. The presence of congestive heart failure carries a poor prognosis, with approximately half the patients dying in the subsequent year after failure ensues.

The progression of pulmonary vascular disease with resultant severe pulmonary arterial hypertension and eventual cardiac failure varies strikingly in individual patients. One may see a child or a young adult who within a matter of but one or two years can go from auscultatory but hemodynamically insignificant mitral stenosis to tight mitral stenosis and severe pulmonary vascular disease. At the other extreme, a patient may have auscultatory evidence of mitral stenosis for decades without demonstrating significant hemodynamic abnormalities. In general, however, more rapid progression of hemodynamic abnormalities is more frequently seen in those parts of the world where rheumatic fever and rheumatic heart disease are epidemic, compared to those areas where cases occur sporadically.

Although pulmonary vascular disease develops as a result of chronic pulmonary capillary and left atrial hypertension, patients frequently develop severe pulmonary vascular disease without having had prior significant orthopnea or paroxysmal nocturnal dyspnea. In his classic description of the clinical features of mitral stenosis, Paul Wood observed that 78% of patients with severe pulmonary vascular disease had never experienced orthopnea or paroxysmal cardiac dyspnea,[12] suggesting that when extremely high pulmonary vascular resistance develops in patients with mitral stenosis, it may occur in some patients relatively early in the course of the disease. However, it has been my experience that pulmonary vascular disease will not be seen in the absence of some chronic elevation in left atrial pressure and, therefore, with a valve area that will calculate to something under 1.2 cm^2 and usually under 1.0 cm^2. High pulmonary vascular resistance in patients with mitral stenosis inevitably implies tight mitral stenosis in the absence of other coexisting valve problems or chronic obstructive pulmonary disease.

Early in the understanding of pulmonary vascular disease it was thought that such enormous elevations in pulmonary arterial pressure might reflect not only the pathophysiologic consequences of increased pulmonary vascular resistance secondary to mitral stenosis, but also the development of relatively silent pulmonary thromboembolic episodes that would result in a fixed form of pulmonary vascular disease that would be irreversible after successful mitral valve surgery. Attempts were made to define patients whose pulmonary vascular disease was primarily neurogenic from those in whom it might be predominantly anatomical by the use of hemodynamic measurements following administration of 100% oxygen, acetylcholine, hexamethonium, and other vasodilator agents. The responses were seen to be extremely variable and an inconsistent relationship was observed between the hemodynamic studies with these agents and the subsequent surgical outcome. In general, it can be said that the most dramatic falls in pulmonary vascular resistance after surgery are seen in patients with the most severe degrees of pulmonary vascular disease. Severe pulmonary hypertension should never be considered a contraindication to mitral stenosis surgery. On the contrary, it is a prime indication of the need for surgery. One can rest assured that successful mitral valve surgery will almost always result in dramatic falls in pulmonary vascular resistance if tight mitral stenosis is present and has been successfully attacked surgically.

ATRIAL FIBRILLATION

At times patients with relatively mild to moderate mitral stenosis may manifest their first symptoms of mitral stenosis with the onset of paroxysmal atrial fibrillation. Early in the natural history of mitral stenosis the patient is usually in normal sinus rhythm. However, on occasion atrial fibrillation may occur paroxysmally prior to the development of surgically significant mitral stenosis. When this happens, the patient usually presents with a fast, irregular heart rate. The shortened diastolic filling period associated with the fast ventricular response may also result in the development of a diastolic pressure gradient similar to that seen with severe exercise, producing sudden elevations in left atrial, pulmonary venous, and pulmonary capillary pressures to pulmonary edema levels. The result will be the sudden appearance of shortness of breath and at times even clinical acute pulmonary edema. However, after slowing of the ventricular response with acute digitalis administration or β-adrenergic receptor blockade, any acute cardiorespiratory symptoms will disappear. As advanced narrowing of the orifice occurs and the patient develops chronic left atrial hypertension, established atrial fibrillation is the most common rhythm observed. Nevertheless, a significant number of patients, particularly those who develop pulmonary vascular disease, will still exhibit normal sinus rhythm even after congestive heart failure develops.

Once chronic atrial fibrillation is present in patients with pure mitral stenosis, it signifies tight mitral stenosis. There are two minor exceptions to this generally useful diagnostic truism. The first is the presence of atrial fibrillation in the very young. Atrial fibrillation in the child or adult under the age of 20 should suggest active rheumatic carditis, and coexistent mitral stenosis may not be the cause of the patient's symptomatology. Care should be exercised in assuming that symptoms under this circumstance reflect obstruction at the mitral valve rather than the consequences of active rheumatic carditis. The other exception is the occasional elderly patient with auscultatory evidence of mitral stenosis and the presence of atrial fibrillation. Some of these patients may be significantly symptomatic, presenting with a low cardiac output in the absence of pulmonary vascular disease. Such a combination should suggest the possibility that the enlarged heart, low output state, and atrial fibrillation are due more to left ventricular dysfunction, either from smoldering rheumatic carditis, progressive mitral insufficiency, or coexisting coronary disease than to the presence of significant mitral valve obstruction.

Approximately 10% to 15% of patients with mitral stenosis will have one or more systemic emboli in the course of the disease related to the presence of thrombi in the left atrium. Of these embolic episodes, 90% will occur while the patient is in atrial fibrillation; it is quite uncommon to see a systemic embolus develop when normal sinus rhythm is present in the preoperative patient. Unfortunately, of those who embolize, approximately 75% will have a cerebral embolus.[12] It is of interest that examination of the left atrium at the time of surgery will not distinguish those patients who have suffered a prior embolus since approximately 20% to 25% of patients will have some clot in the left atrium regardless of whether they have suffered a prior systemic embolus. The relatively low incidence of left atrial clots in patients who have suffered a prior systemic embolus may reflect the fact that the entire thrombus has been dislodged to produce the embolic phenomena, leaving the atrial cavity temporarily free of clot.

Chronic atrial fibrillation is generally not seen until mitral stenosis is hemodynamically significant. Furthermore, the development of embolic episode following successful mitral valve commissurotomy, whether open or closed, is unusual. Thus, one of the best measures for the prevention of a cerebral embolus in mitral stenosis is successful mitral valve surgery. This, of course, does not necessarily hold if mitral valve replacement is required and a prosthesis is implanted. Thromboembolic complications occur in the years following surgery even with bioprosthetic valves. Routine anticoagulation is commonly performed, even in patients with bioprosthetic valves if left atrial enlargement is present or chronic atrial fibrillation persists postoperatively.

HEMOPTYSIS

Hemoptysis is common in patients with mitral stenosis and may reflect a variety of different pathophysiologic mechanisms. Pink, frothy sputum may accompany pulmonary congestion due to pulmonary edema. Other patients may cough up minor amounts of dark red blood because of pulmonary infarction from pulmonary emboli arising either from the right atrium secondary to atrial fibrillation or from the deep venous system of the extremities or pelvis. Still others may show dark blood mixed with discolored sputum, reflecting the propensity of patients with mitral stenosis to develop chronic bronchitis. Finally, patients with mitral stenosis may cough up relatively large amounts of bright red blood. This results from the presence of bronchial vein varices developing as a result of chronic bronchial vein and pulmonary venous hypertension. These bronchial varices, which wrap around terminal bronchioles, may rupture, with the coughing up of bright red blood, which can at times be alarming in volume. Hemoptysis of significant amounts of bright red blood implies by itself the presence of tight mitral stenosis since bronchial varicosities do not develop unless there has been longstanding, resting pulmonary venous hypertension. This in turn must mean that there is surgically significant obstruction at the mitral valve.

CONGESTIVE HEART FAILURE

Congestive heart failure in mitral stenosis normally reflects the end stage of the disease. In pure mitral stenosis, congestive heart failure implies extremely tight mitral stenosis, since it is not seen in the absence of pulmonary vascular disease with secondary marked pulmonary artery hypertension. When the mitral valve area is reduced to approximately 1.0 cm^2, left atrial, pulmonary venous, and pulmonary capillary pressures sit close to pulmonary edema levels. Pulmonary artery pressure will be passively raised to a corresponding level. This degree of pulmonary arterial hypertension is insufficient to produce significant right ventricular hypertrophy such as to be detectable on the standard electrocardiogram, and this degree of stroke work is well maintained by the right ventricle. Consequently, right ventricular dilatation and eventual failure do not occur. On the other hand, as the mitral valve area falls below 1.0 cm^2 and pulmonary arterial pressure climbs out of proportion to the pulmonary capillary pressure as the pulmonary arteriolar resistance increases, the right ventricle now must contract against a severe outflow impedance. The ventricle will undergo pronounced hypertrophy; evidence of pulmonary hypertension is apparent on physical and laboratory examination, including a marked parasternal heave from right ventricular overactivity, a snapping pulmonic component of the second sound, marked main pulmonary artery segment dilatation on chest x-ray film with abrupt tapering of the major branches of the pulmonary artery, and right ventricular hypertrophy on the electrocardiogram. As long as the right ventricle remains competent, mean right atrial and central venous pressures will remain in the normal range, although giant *a* waves may be detected in the central venous pulse. The patient will note a marked increase in easy fatigability and tiredness as well as a reduced exertional tolerance reflecting the severe pulmonary vascular disease. At times a relatively localized, left upper sternal, high-pitched decrescendo diastolic murmur of pulmonic insufficiency will be audible. Eventually the right ventricle is unable to tolerate the high systemic pressures in the pulmonary artery, and right ventricular dilatation and failure will ensue. The syndrome of congestive heart failure then dominates the clinical picture, with clinical signs and symptoms typical of heart failure. Once cardiac congestive heart failure appears, approximately 50% of patients will expire in the ensuing one to two years.

PHYSICAL EXAMINATION AND LABORATORY EXAMINATION

GENERAL APPEARANCE

Patients with mitral stenosis who have developed pulmonary vascular disease will have skin changes reflecting the chronic low-output state. Peripheral cyanosis involving the lips, fingers, toes, and mucous membranes is common as skin and mucous membrane blood flow falls. Part of the cyanosis in some patients may be central in origin, arising from the increase in alveolar–arterial PO_2 gradient consequent to thickening of capillary basement membranes, interstitial fibrosis from chronic pulmonary capillary hypertension, and/or an increase in pulmonary interstitial fluid. A characteristic facial appearance described as "mitral facies" refers to skin changes from the low-output state that are particularly prominent over the malar areas of the face. Prominent skin capillaries with an associated cyanotic hue give a characteristic appearance, suggesting that the mitral patient is suffering from pulmonary hypertension.

ARTERIAL PRESSURE AND PERIPHERAL PULSE

The arterial pressure is likely to be normal in patients with mitral stenosis. If pulmonary vascular disease has caused a reduction in cardiac output, there is usually an increase in systemic vascular resistance that ensures maintenance of a normal arterial pressure in the presence of a reduced cardiac output. In these cases the peripheral pulse is likely to be small as the stroke output is reduced. In approximately half of the patients, the pulse will be irregular due to the presence of atrial fibrillation.

PRECORDIAL EXAMINATION

The apical impulse is usually in the normal location. It is characteristically tapping in quality, nonsustained and relatively brief. However, a significant parasternal lift is frequently observed in the third and fourth interspaces along the left sternal border. If limited to early in systole, it may reflect relatively mild degrees of pulmonary hypertension resulting in a moderate increase in right ventricular stroke work. However, a prolonged systolic outward movement along the parasternal border is generally felt when moderate or severe pulmonary hypertension is present.

The first heart sound at the apex is characteristically increased in intensity and snapping in character. This is a reflection not only of the fibrocalcific changes in the valve leaflets themselves but also, more importantly, to their position at the onset of ventricular systole. Normally the mitral valve leaflets have floated back to an approximately halfway closed position at the onset of ventricular systole[13]; therefore, their closure occurs in response to a relatively low rate of left ventricular systolic pressure change with respect to time (dP/dt). In mitral stenosis with elevation in left atrial pressure, the valve leaflets are held apart during the early development of isovolumic systole since left atrial pressure still exceeds that present in the left ventricle. Closure will occur later as left ventricular contraction causes left ventricular systolic pressure to exceed left atrial pressure during early systole. The left ventricle is at this point changing its systolic pressure rapidly with respect to time (high dP/dt). This will result in an abrupt arrest of the valve leaflets by the chordae with the production of a loud, snapping first sound.

The opening snap of the mitral valve, which is normally not heard in the absence of mitral stenosis, may be thought of as analogous in origin to a snapping first heart sound. With the onset of ventricular relaxation and a fall in left ventricular diastolic pressure below that existing in the left atrium, the funnel- or cone-shaped mitral valve descends into the ventricular cavity as it opens, only to be abruptly arrested by the commissural fusion. Clinically, the presence of an opening snap suggests continued mobility of the leaflets and subvalvular apparatus. When significant mitral valve calcification is present and there is decreased distensibility of the leaflets and rigidity of the valve apparatus, the opening snap may disappear; thus, the presence of an opening snap is a hopeful sign increasing the likelihood that the valve anatomy will permit open mitral commissurotomy to be successfully undertaken in lieu of prosthetic valve replacement. Additionally, the interval between the second sound and the opening snap of the mitral valve is a measure of the severity of mitral stenosis when pure mitral stenosis is present. With the onset of ventricular relaxation, the time from closure of the aortic valve to the opening of the mitral valve will be shorter if left atrial pressure is elevated than if it is normal. Tight mitral stenosis is usually reflected in a A_2-OS interval in the neighborhood of 0.05 to 0.06 second. In contrast, relatively mild mitral stenosis with resting left atrial pressures that are normal or only minimally elevated will result in a A_2-OS interval closer to 0.10 to 0.12 second. An apical S3 is never present in pure severe mitral stenosis; however, if congestive heart failure is present, a right ventricular S_3 may be present at the lower left sternal border.

Immediately following the opening snap of the mitral valve, one may hear the classic apical diastolic rumble of mitral stenosis. The murmur is characteristically low-pitched, well localized to the apical area, and best heard with the patient lying in the left lateral recumbent position with the bell of the stethoscope lightly placed against the apex. Early in the development of mitral stenosis, the murmur may be short in duration, dying out in early or mid-diastole. As mitral stenosis progresses and a gradient is present throughout diastole, the murmur may extend in duration, encompassing all of diastole with presystolic accentuation associated with atrial systole leading into the snapping first sound. Although duration of the mitral diastolic rumble reflects severity, intensity does not. Loud apical diastolic murmurs with thrills may be heard in relatively mild mitral stenosis. Furthermore, as pulmonary vascular disease develops, there may be significant changes in the character and intensity of the apical diastolic murmur. The resultant right ventricular hypertrophy causes the right ventricle to occupy more of the anterior portion of the precordium, and the mitral valve rotates correspondingly into a more posterior location and further from the chest wall. This, together with the reduction in stroke output associated with the increase in pulmonary vascular resistance, may result in a marked diminution in the intensity of the mitral diastolic rumble. In some patients the murmur may become totally inaudible despite tight mitral stenosis.

Another cause for the apical diastolic rumble of mitral stenosis to be short and terminate before the first heart sound is the presence of atrial fibrillation. In this circumstance one may lose the presystolic accentuation that normally results from atrial systole. As a consequence, the apical diastolic rumble will be present with an irregular duration depending on the diastolic filling period of that beat, with the murmur dying out before the snapping first heart sound.

At times, there may be a differential diagnostic problem in distinguishing aortic insufficiency producing a concomitant apical diastolic rumble (the so-called Austin Flint murmur) from combined rheumatic aortic insufficiency and mitral stenosis. Echocardiographic studies reveal that the anterior mitral valve leaflet classically flutters in the presence of aortic insufficiency. This fluttering suggests that eddies are forming within the apex of the ventricle, and these have been suggested as a cause of the low-pitched apical diastolic rumble; however, a more likely explanation for the apical diastolic rumble that may be seen in free aortic insufficiency has been elucidated by echocardiographic studies that reveal that the mitral valve closes prematurely in severe aortic insufficiency. This premature closure in the presence of continuing atrioventricular flow produces a functional obstruction at the mitral valve resulting in a diastolic rumble in the absence of organic mitral stenosis. Echocardiography has made this diagnostic problem academic, since it permits one to establish the presence or absence of concomitant rheumatic mitral valve disease in patients with free aortic insufficiency who have an apical diastolic rumble as well.

It is important to appreciate that severe pulmonary hypertension may lead to functional tricuspid insufficiency even if organic tricuspid valve disease is absent. Such patients may have a loud pansystolic murmur located at the apex as the right ventricle hypertrophies and comes to occupy the apical area. This may lead to an erroneous interpretation of dominant mitral insufficiency in a patient with mitral stenosis when, in fact, pure, tight mitral stenosis may be present, with the apical systolic murmur reflecting tricuspid rather than mitral insufficiency.

CHEST X-RAY EXAMINATION

Gross cardiomegaly is normally not seen in patients with pure mitral stenosis. Overall size is usually either normal or only mildly increased from left atrial enlargement unless right ventricular dilation and congestive failure have occurred. Left atrial enlargement can be recognized by elevation of the left main stem bronchus, displacement of the esophagus posteriorly particularly evident with a barium swallow, a prominent left atrial appendage, or, on occasion, a double density in the posteroanterior projection overlying the superior aspect of the right atrium. The pulmonary artery segment in the posteroanterior projection is usually quite prominent. Depending on the presence or absence of severe pulmonary vascular disease, there may be disproportionate enlargement of the main branches of the pulmonary artery with sudden tapering of these vessels and relative avascularity of the peripheral lung fields. In the absence of severe pulmonary vascular disease, however, the findings of pulmonary venous hypertension will be seen with typical upper lobe revascularization and prominent pulmonary venous hilar markings. Kerley B lines may be seen extending up from the costophrenic angles if pulmonary congestion is present. Although calcification of the mitral valve can be seen on the plain chest x-ray film, it is usually better identified when present by cardiac fluoroscopy, cineangiography, or echocardiography. Figure 89.2 illustrates the chest x-ray film in a patient with pure mitral stenosis. The left main stem bronchus is elevated and the pulmonary vascular markings are increased with some upper lobe redistribution.

ELECTROCARDIOGRAM

The electrocardiogram may display certain distinctive features in the presence of mitral stenosis. The P wave may have the so-called P mitrale appearance characterized by an increased duration with notching best seen in extremity leads I and II. Its appearance in V_1 may be even more distinctive with a prominent negative or a prominent negative component to a bifid P wave, which has increased voltage and is widened. P mitrale is more likely to be seen in the presence of hemodynamically significant mitral stenosis as left atrial pressure increases and left atrial hypertrophy develops.

The degree of right ventricular hypertrophy will depend on the pulmonary vascular resistance. When severe pulmonary vascular disease with marked pulmonary hypertension is present, the characteristic electrocardiographic appearance of right ventricular hypertrophy is seen; however, even when milder increases of pulmonary hypertension are present, there will be a suggestion of early right ventricular hypertrophy in the electrocardiogram. This is recognized by a rather nondescript QRS complex in V_1 with marked diminution in the amplitude of the S wave, together with some vertical shift in the frontal plane leads of the electrocardiogram. Left ventricular hypertrophy should never be seen in the electrocardiogram of a patient with pure mitral stenosis. Its presence indicates either associated aortic valve disease, mitral incompetence, or systemic hypertension.

ECHOCARDIOGRAPHY AND DOPPLER ULTRASOUND

The M-mode echocardiogram readily permits identification of rheumatic mitral valve disease. Characteristically, the valve is thickened with anterior motion of the posterior leaflet, a decreased E to F slope, and an absent or markedly diminished *a* wave. However, M-mode echocardiography does not lend itself to assessing the severity of mitral stenosis.

Continuous-wave Doppler ultrasonic recordings have proven highly useful in quantifying mitral stenosis. Figure 89.3 reveals a recording from the left atrium and ventricle in the patient whose x-ray film is shown in Figure 89.2. The velocity of blood flow permits estimation of the pressure gradient across the mitral valve using the Bernoulli theorem relating the conversion of pressure energy to kinetic energy. In this example, peak velocity as shown in Figure 89.3 is 2.4 m/sec. Since $P_2 - P_1 = 4V^2$, the peak diastolic gradient was approximately $4(2.4)^2$ or 23 mm Hg. This gradient, although useful, is dependent on the existing cardiac output.

Hatle and co-workers[14] have introduced an approach based on the time required for the Doppler-measured maximal velocity to fall by one half. This method permits an estimation of the actual mitral valve area. Figure 89.4 illustrates the calculation of mitral valve area by the P½ method using the recording in Figure 89.3. Peak velocity at the onset of diastole in this patient has a value of 2.4 m/sec. Pressure half-time is calculated by measuring the time required for the peak velocity to fall to one half of the maximum. One-half the maximum velocity can be readily calculated by dividing the maximal velocity by the square root of 2. In Figure 89.3, this results in a value of 1.7 m/sec. The time for the maximal velocity to fall from 2.4 to 1.7 in this case was 310 msec. Mitral valve area is then estimated by dividing the empirical constant value of 220 by 310 msec. For this beat a value of approximately 0.7 cm² was obtained. The values from a series of beats were averaged and equaled 0.8 cm², signifying tight mitral stenosis in this patient. Actual mitral valve area by the Gorlin formula at cardiac catheterization was 0.9 cm².

Mitral valve area can also be estimated using two-dimensional echocardiography. Most present-day two-dimensional echo machines

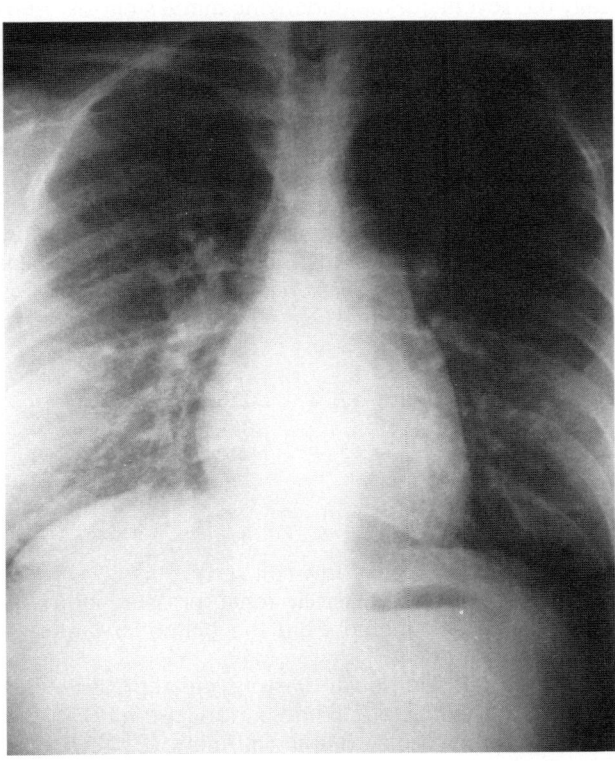

FIGURE 89.2 Chest x-ray film in a 22-year-old woman with tight mitral stenosis. There is increased pulmonary vascular markings with some redistribution to the upper lobes. The pulmonary artery segment and left atrial appendage are prominent, and the left main stem bronchus is elevated.

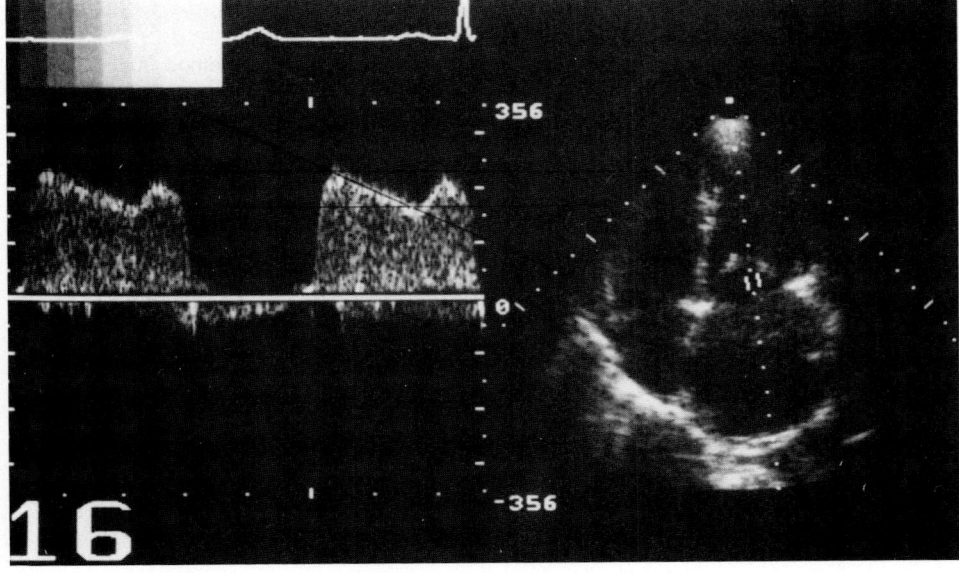

FIGURE 89.3 Continuous-wave Doppler recording of disturbed diastolic flow being recorded from a sampling site just above the mitral valve.

permit one to make freeze-frame images. When such freeze-frame images of the mitral valve orifice area are recorded in diastole using the short axis view, the mitral valve orifice area can be traced on the video screen with a light-pen system that permits direct estimation of the area of the orifice. Good correlations have been obtained with both Doppler ultrasonic and two-dimensional echo methods of estimating the mitral valve area.[15] In patients with mitral stenosis in whom the valve area has been estimated at cardiac catheterization using the Gorlin formula, however, comparisons after mitral valve commissurotomy have shown the Doppler pressure half-time to be superior to area estimation from two-dimensional echocardiography in determining residual mitral valve area.[15]

An additional benefit from Doppler interrogation of the patient with mitral stenosis is an evaluation of the status of the other cardiac valves as well as evaluation of any coexisting mitral insufficiency.

DIAGNOSIS

The diagnosis of mitral stenosis is generally evident after taking a history and performing a physical examination. Patients usually present with a history of one or more cardiorespiratory complaints such as dyspnea on exertion, orthopnea, paroxysmal nocturnal dyspnea, hemoptysis, and nocturnal cough, as well as easy tiredness or fatigability and decreased exercise tolerance. Patients may also present with signs and symptoms of congestive heart failure if the condition has progressed to critically tight mitral stenosis with the subsequent development of pulmonary hypertension. Physical examination reveals either normal sinus rhythm or atrial fibrillation, a parasternal lift, a snapping first sound, an opening snap of the mitral valve followed by an apical diastolic rumble with or without presystolic accentuation, and accentuation of the pulmonic component of the second sound. The electrocardiogram and chest x-ray film will mirror the pathophysiologic stage of the patient. The electrocardiogram may vary from normal to one with characteristic P wave changes and right ventricular hypertrophy. Similarly, the chest x-ray film may show only mild left atrial enlargement or may show the findings of pulmonary venous hypertension, frank pulmonary edema, or severe pulmonary vascular disease. M-mode echocardiography confirms rheumatic mitral valve disease with the demonstration of a decrease in the E–F slope, anterior movement of the posterior leaflet, and thickening and/or calcification of the mitral valve leaflets. In addition, the rare case of left atrial myxoma, which may clinically masquerade as mitral stenosis, can be readily identified either by M-mode or two-dimensional echocardiography.

The major question generally is not one of establishing the presence of mitral stenosis but in determining whether the natural history of the disease has reached the point where surgical intervention is justified. Although certain clinical clues will provide ready evidence of tight mitral stenosis, noninvasive laboratory procedures today permit a ready measurement of the severity of mitral stenosis. In particular, Doppler ultrasound interrogation of the mitral valve and two-dimensional echocardiography estimation of the area of the stenotic orifice provide accurate methods for assessing the severity of mitral stenosis. Under these circumstances, the necessity for cardiac catheterization in the preoperative evaluation of the patient has lessened. It is reasonable to send the patient to surgery for mitral stenosis when the patient is clearly symptomatic with cardiorespiratory complaints, the clinical picture is clear-cut, and Doppler and echocardiographic examinations confirm tight mitral stenosis (valve area ≤ 1.2 cm^2). In such patients, catheterization is necessary only if one has to evaluate the status of the coronary circulation. Thus, older-age patients should probably have coronary arteriography performed before open heart surgery for mitral stenosis to determine whether concomitant bypass surgery is advisable. Additionally, cardiac catheterization to evaluate the severity of mitral stenosis is desirable whenever there is a dichotomy between the clinical and the laboratory estimates of severity. Relatively asymptomatic patients with noninvasive estimates of severe mitral stenosis or patients unduly symptomatic with cardiorespiratory complaints who seemingly have relatively little stenosis after noninvasive evaluation are prime candidates for hemodynamic evaluation to establish unequivocally the severity of the underlying mitral stenosis. Hemodynamic evaluations, including contrast ventriculography and/or ascending aortography, are also desirable in the patient with mitral stenosis who has other valvular disease as well.

Hemodynamic evaluation requires measurement of the gradient across the mitral valve together with a concomitant determination of cardiac output. Under these circumstances, one may calculate the approximate mitral valve area using the formula of Gorlin and Gorlin with the constant modified when one is directly recording left ventricular diastolic pressure rather than assuming the normal mean value of 5 mm Hg.[16] The formula is

$$\text{MVA} = \frac{\text{CO/DFP}}{38\sqrt{\text{LA}_{dm} - \text{LV}_{dm}}}$$

where

CO/DFP = mitral valve flow (ml/sec)
LA$_{dm}$ = left atrial diastolic mean pressure either recorded directly or estimated from the pulmonary artery wedge pressure (mm Hg)
LV$_{dm}$ = left ventricular diastolic mean pressure (mm Hg)
DFP = the diastolic filling period (sec/min)
CO = the cardiac output (ml/min)

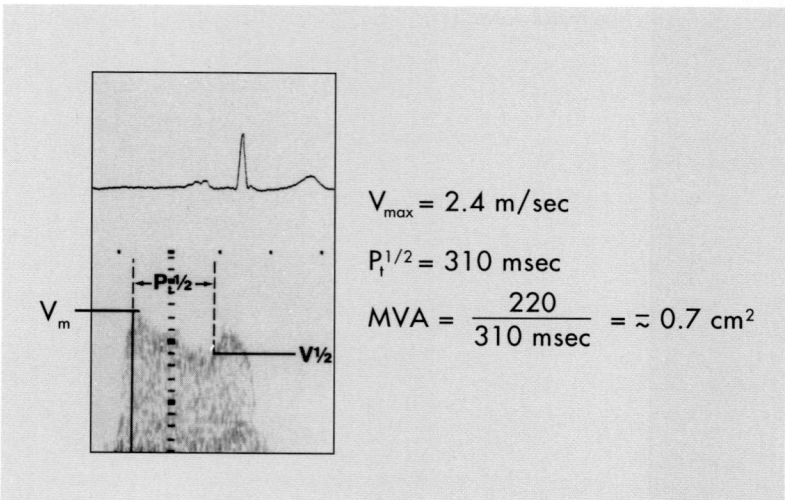

FIGURE 89.4 Calculation of mitral valve area by the P½ method from the same patient as illustrated in Figure 89.3 (see text).

The pulmonary artery wedge pressure obtained from a wedged end-hole catheter or distal to a balloon-inflated right heart catheter may be substituted for left atrial pressure in the above equation (Fig. 89.5). It should be noted that the Gorlin formula for calculation of mitral valve area loses its validity in the presence of significant mitral insufficiency. Cardiac output is no longer appropriate for the calculation of mitral valve flow since mitral valve flow represents the sum of the cardiac output plus the mitral regurgitant flow. Calculation of the mitral valve area under these circumstances will result in an overestimation of the severity of the mitral stenosis. A valve area less than that which anatomically is present in proportion to the ratio of the cardiac output to the sum of the regurgitant flow plus cardiac output will be calculated. In other words, if the regurgitant flow is equal to the cardiac output the calculated valve area will be half that which is actually present. The primary benefit of calculating the mitral valve area by the Gorlin formula is the requirement that the pressure gradient across the mitral valve area will be measured at the same time that mitral flow is being measured. The pressure gradient across a stenotic valve orifice varies as the square of changes in flow. Therefore, a 40% increase in cardiac output from factors such as anxiety on the catheterization table may cause the pressure gradient to double from that which would have otherwise been present (square root of 2 = 1.4). It is therefore mandatory to calculate the mitral valve area by determining the cardiac output simultaneously with the pressure gradient. It is also important to minimize the error inherent in calculating the mitral valve area from the Gorlin formula if the pressure gradient is very small. When a small resting gradient is present, mitral valve area should be calculated during steady-state exercise when the gradient will be increased as mitral valve flow is increased with exercise.

SURGERY

The development of closed mitral valve commissurotomy or valvuloplasty, almost simultaneously by Bailey in Philadelphia and Harken in Boston, resurrected the surgical approach to relieving mitral stenosis that lay fallow following the disastrous experiences of Cutler, Levine, and Beck during the 1920s.[17] It became readily apparent that closed commissurotomy could significantly enlarge the mitral valve orifice without producing significant additional mitral insufficiency when properly performed, thus restoring left atrial pressure from pulmonary edema levels back toward normal. With the drop in left atrial pressure, it also became obvious that patients with severe degrees of pulmonary vascular disease would reverse their pulmonary artery hypertension, with pulmonary arterial pressures dropping far out of proportion to the drop in left atrial pressure in the days and weeks following successful commissurotomy. Seemingly hopeless class IV cardiac patients could be restored to functional class I or II patients. The open valvuloplasty subsequently developed in the 1950s has become a far more popular operation today in the United States, although in many countries where the volume of mitral stenosis surgery is enormous, closed commissurotomy is still successfully performed in many patients. During the 1960s prosthetic valves became available, and many patients with combined mitral insufficiency and stenotic or calcified and distorted valve orifices unsuitable for valvuloplasty are now managed successfully with prosthetic valve replacement. The results of prosthetic valve surgery for mitral stenosis are detailed elsewhere in these volumes.

In general, a significant postoperative decrease in the intensity of the apical mitral diastolic murmur will be observed if the patient has had a good clinical response. Failure of the murmur to decrease or the development of a loud apical systolic murmur is generally a poor prognostic sign following mitral valvuloplasty and correlates with a poor postoperative result.[18] When a high-pitched, localized, diastolic murmur of pulmonic insufficiency is heard in association with mitral stenosis, it usually reflects secondary pulmonary vascular disease with marked pulmonary hypertension. Successful surgery will frequently result in disappearance of this murmur as the pulmonary hypertension reverses.

Regardless of the severity of pulmonary vascular disease, successful surgical correction of the obstruction at the mitral valve will result in a significant return of pulmonary vascular resistance toward the normal. This will not take place within the first one to two hours after valvotomy or valve replacement but takes days to occur.[19] Pulmonary arterial pressure, which has been elevated out of proportion to the rise in left atrial, pulmonary venous, and pulmonary capillary pressures, now falls out of proportion to the fall in left atrial, pulmonary venous, and pulmonary capillary pressures. Usually pulmonary arterial pressure will fall to the upper limits of normal or sometimes it will remain mildly elevated. Generally some degree of residual pulmonary vascular disease persists in that relatively mild exercise will cause an abnormal rise in pulmonary arterial pressure that is not seen normally. This regression of pulmonary vascular disease and resultant pulmonary hypertension after mitral valve surgery is also seen in children who have successful mitral valve surgery for mitral stenosis.

Patients who have undergone successful open mitral commissurotomy or valve replacement who were in atrial fibrillation at the time of surgery should have direct cardioversion attempted after surgery. Approximately half of these patients can be discharged from the hospital in normal sinus rhythm. The actuarial maintenance rate of patients discharged from the hospital in sinus rhythm is 50% seven years after surgery. Among patients who maintain sinus rhythm late postoperatively, approximately one third have had atrial fibrillation for more than one year preoperatively. A number of these patients have significantly enlarged left atria. Thus, essentially all patients should have an attempt at restoration of sinus rhythm after successful mitral valve surgery regardless of the duration of prior atrial fibrillation or heart size on chest x-ray film. If atrial fibrillation recurs relatively early after hospital discharge, another attempt at restoring sinus rhythm should be done, and the patient should then be placed on maintenance quinidine; however, if atrial fibrillation recurs again despite quinidine, the quinidine should be stopped and the patient should be placed on digitalis to control the ventricular response and anticoagulated if prior anticoagulation is not already being carried out because of the insertion of a mitral valve prosthesis.

The risk of death following mitral valve surgery primarily involves those patients who have either associated advanced coronary artery disease or severe pulmonary vascular disease complicating their mitral stenosis. Coexistent, frequently clinically silent, coronary artery dis-

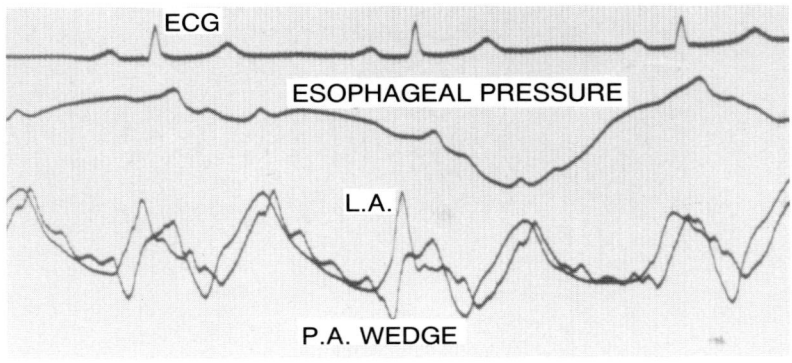

FIGURE 89.5 Esophageal pressure from a balloon catheter and left atrial and pulmonary artery wedge pressures are recorded simultaneously during a transthoracic left heart catheterization. Esophageal pressure falls during inspiration. Note the close comparability of the left atrial and pulmonary artery wedge tracings with the wedge pressure temporally lagging the pressure pulse changes in the left atrium.

ease is commonly found in patients over the age of 40 with mitral stenosis. In a series of 96 consecutive patients over age 40 with severe mitral stenosis, 28% had angiographically significant coronary artery disease.[20] Older patients with hemodynamically significant mitral stenosis should have coronary arteriography performed at the time of cardiac catheterization. If obstructive coronary vascular disease is demonstrated and the lesions are amenable to bypass surgery, it is advisable to perform this surgery at the time of mitral valve surgery.

BALLOON VALVULOPLASTY

The recent surge of interest in percutaneous transluminal coronary angioplasty has led to attempts at balloon dilatation of both congenital and adult forms of mitral stenosis.[21-24] Early results in children and young adults have suggested that this may be a safe and effective treatment in selected patients. Currently it is clearly a clinical experimental approach and is not recommended for routine use.

REFERENCES

1. Harken DE, Ellis LB, Ware PF, Norman LR: The surgical treatment of mitral stenosis. N Engl J Med 239:801, 1948
2. Bailey CP: The surgical treatment of mitral stenosis (mitral commissurotomy). Dis Chest 15:377, 1949
3. Rusted IE, Scheifley CH, Edwards JE: Studies of the mitral valve. I. Anatomic features of the normal mitral valve and associated structures. Circulation 6:825, 1952
4. Bland EF, Jones TD: Rheumatic fever and rheumatic heart disease. A twenty year report on 1000 patients followed since childhood. Circulation 4:836, 1951
5. John S, Bashi VV, Jairaj PS et al: Closed mitral valvotomy: Early results and long-term follow-up of 3724 consecutive patients. Circulation 68:891, 1983
6. McNeely WF, Ellis LB, Harken DE: Rheumatic "activity" as judged by the presence of Aschoff bodies in auricular appendages of patients with mitral stenosis. II. Clinical aspects. Circulation 8:337, 1953
7. Colle JP, Rahal S, Ohayon J et al: Global left ventricular function and regional wall motion in pure mitral stenosis. Clin Cardiol 7:573, 1984
8. Toutouzas P: Left ventricular function in mitral valve disease. Herz 9:297, 1984
9. Gorlin R, Gorlin SG: Hydraulic formula for calculation of the area of the stenotic mitral valve, other cardiac valves, and central circulatory shunts. I. Am Heart J 41:1, 1951
10. Aryanpur I, Paydar M, Shakibi JG et al: Regression of pulmonary hypertension after mitral valve surgery in children. Chest 71:354, 1977
11. Dexter L, McDonald L, Rabinowitz M et al: Medical aspects of patients undergoing surgery for mitral stenosis. Circulation 9:758, 1954
12. Wood P: An appreciation of mitral stenosis. Part I. Clinical features. Br Med J 1:1051, 1954
13. Criley JM, Chambers RD, Friedman NJ: Departures from the expected auscultatory events in mitral stenosis. In Likoff W (ed): Valvular Heart Disease, p 191. Philadelphia, FA Davis, 1973
14. Hatle L, Angelsen B, Tromsdal A: Noninvasive assessment of atrioventricular pressure half-time by Doppler ultrasound. Circulation 60:1096, 1979
15. Smith MD, Handshoe R, Handshoe S et al: Comparative accuracy of two-dimensional echocardiography and Doppler pressure half-time methods in assessing severity of mitral stenosis in patients with and without prior commissurotomy. Circulation 73:100, 1986
16. Rapaport E: Calculation of valve areas. Eur Heart J 6(Suppl C):21, 1985
17. Cutler EC, Levine SA, Beck CS: The surgical treatment of mitral stenosis: Experimental and clinical studies. Arch Surg 9:689, 1924
18. Spiegl RJ, Long JB, Dexter L: Clinical observations in patients undergoing finger fracture mitral valvuloplasty. I. Auscultatory changes. Am J Med 12:626, 1952
19. Richman HG, Long JB, Rapaport E: Central circulatory changes accompanying mitral commissurotomy. Circulation 22:563, 1960
20. Mattina CJ, Green SJ, Tortolani AJ et al: Frequency of angiographically significant coronary arterial narrowing in mitral stenosis. Am J Cardiol 57:802, 1986
21. Al Zaibag M, Ribeiro PA, Al Kasab S, Al Fagih MR: Percutaneous double-balloon mitral valvotomy for rheumatic mitral-valve stenosis. Lancet 1:757, 1986
22. Lock JE, Khalilullah M, Shrivastava S et al: Percutaneous catheter commissurotomy in rheumatic mitral stenosis. N Engl J Med 313:1515, 1985
23. Kveselis DA, Rocchini AP, Beekman R et al: Balloon angioplasty for congenital and rheumatic mitral stenosis. Am J Cardiol 57:348, 1986
24. Inoue K, Owaki T, Nakamura T et al: Clinical application of transvenous mitral commissurotomy by a new balloon catheter. J Thorac Cardiovasc Surg 87:394, 1984

SECTION 10

Section Editor
Melvin D. Cheitlin, MD

Myocardial, Pericardial, and Endocardial Diseases

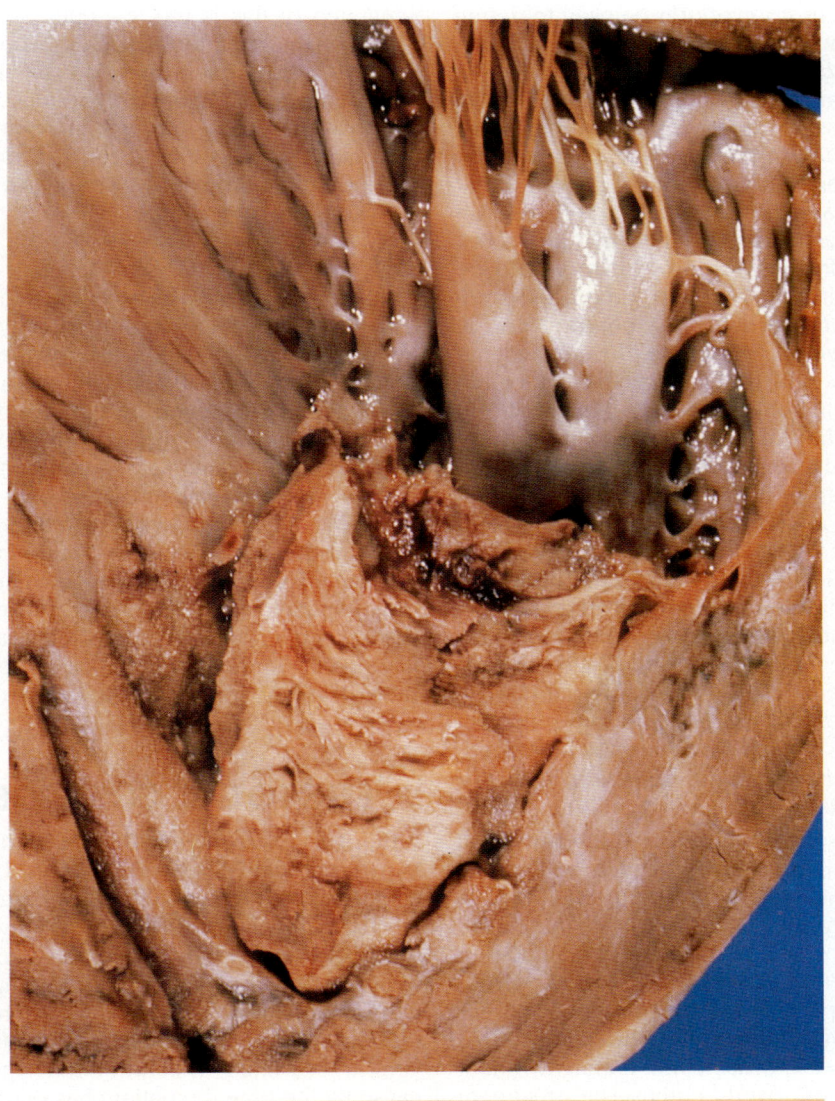

Dilated Cardiomyopathy

Ralph Shabetai

DEFINITION AND CLASSIFICATION

The English translation of the term *cardiomyopathy* is abnormality of heart muscle. It took several years for the various authorities to agree on the word, and agreement has still not been reached on its proper use and exact definitions. The terms *myocardosis* and *myocardiopathy* have fallen for the most part into disuse but may still be encountered. The term *primary myocardial disease* was popular until different authors began to use *primary* in different senses, some using it interchangeably with *idiopathic* and others using it to describe either idiopathic or secondary myocardial disease when the principal, or primary, manifestation was myocardial. *Idiopathic cardiomyopathy* then became the preferred term for disease of the myocardium of unknown etiology. This decision seemed to resolve the matter until the World Health Organization proposed that *cardiomyopathy* be used to define disease of unknown etiology of the myocardium, thus rendering inclusion of the qualifying term *idiopathic* redundant. The World Health Organization thus recommended that the use of the term *cardiomyopathy* be limited to myocardial disease of unknown etiology and that what used to be called *secondary myocardial disease,* or *secondary cardiomyopathy,* now be called *specific heart muscle disease.*[1] What may seem to the reader a quibble assumes importance, because according to the World Health Organization scheme, *myocarditis,* a disease frequently indistinguishable from cardiomyopathy, would be classified as a specific myocardial disease, and furthermore the commonly used *ischemic cardiomyopathy*[2] would be a contradiction in terms. Nevertheless, the term *ischemic cardiomyopathy* has become well established, partly because no one has suggested a better but equally short alternative. Apart from the objections raised by the World Health Organization task force on the definition and classification of cardiomyopathies, *ischemic cardiomyopathy* can be a misleading term since the patients alleged to suffer from it may or may not have sustained myocardial infarction, which may or may not have been overt, and may or may not have evidence of ongoing ischemia. Several investigators have failed to find significant differences in the prognosis and treatment of heart failure regardless of whether the original cause was cardiomyopathy or ischemic heart disease[3] and therefore have pressed for the continuing use of the term *ischemic cardiomyopathy.* I use the term *cardiomyopathy* to mean idiopathic myocardial disease and recommend that in place of *ischemic cardiomyopathy,* more descriptive terms applicable to specific clinical syndromes be employed. These would include *ischemic left ventricular dysfunction, ischemic left ventricular failure,* and *ischemic heart failure.*

When a functional classification of the cardiomyopathies was first proposed,[4] the major types were congestive, hypertrophic, and restrictive. The clinical hallmark of congestive cardiomyopathy was congestive heart failure of unknown etiology and its pathologic stigmata were passive congestion of the lungs and systemic viscera and dilatation of the cardiac chambers. The introduction of powerful diuretics, which, when necessary, can be used in especially potent combinations, has made congestive heart failure a relatively uncommon disorder, so that there may be severe myocardial disease or ischemic damage without clinically apparent *congestion.* Indeed, overly enthusiastic treatment may result in dehydration in the face of severe cardiac dysfunction. For this reason, the term *dilated cardiomyopathy,* emphasizing the principal pathologic abnormality, has been substituted for *congestive cardiomyopathy.* Even this change does not satisfy all cases, because in some instances of cardiomyopathy, and in some cases of left ventricular dysfunction secondary to past or present hypertension, the left ventricle may not be dilated but is abnormally stiff, causing diastolic, but not systolic, dysfunction.[5]

There is no doubt that from the time of the original descriptions of dilated or congestive cardiomyopathy until quite recently, investigators had in mind systolic pump failure of the left or both ventricles. Dilated cardiomyopathy must now be fitted into a classification of the cardiomyopathies that includes cardiomyopathy other than classic restrictive cardiomyopathy that is manifest principally by diastolic dysfunction. Before leaving the topic of classification, I should emphasize that classification of disease is an attempt by medical scientists to simplify the complexities of nature, which, while it may work some of the time, is bound to break down on occasion. Perhaps the most lamentable consequence of this is the tendency to use the terms *heart failure* and *cardiomyopathy* interchangeably, a practice that can only add further confusion and should therefore be strongly discouraged. Since heart failure may be an important manifestation of dilated cardiomyopathy, the two have many features in common, but congestive failure may also result from volume overload, pressure overload, metabolic and nutritional abnormalities, hypertension, and coronary artery disease.

MYOCARDITIS

Although myocarditis is discussed in detail elsewhere in these volumes, aspects relevant to cardiomyopathy are summarized here. Classic myocarditis is an acute, usually viral inflammation of the myocardium following a generalized viral infection and manifest by acute heart failure often accompanied by significant arrhythmia. At other times, the preceding prodromal illness is muted or absent and proof of preceding viral infection is lacking. The patient then presents with acute, or relatively acute, heart failure of unknown etiology,[6] which is also the most common presentation of idiopathic dilated cardiomyopathy. The differential diagnosis between dilated cardiomyopathy and myocarditis, and the possible connections between preceding myocarditis and cardiomyopathy, will be discussed subsequently. Here it suffices to note that short of endomyocardial biopsy, and perhaps even after this examination has been performed, it is not always possible to distinguish between myocarditis and dilated cardiomyopathy.

ETIOLOGIC CONSIDERATIONS

Although, by definition, dilated cardiomyopathy is a disease of unknown etiology, consideration must be given to factors that may precipitate or play a role in the development of this disorder.

The frequency with which the myocardium is invaded by virus in the acute stage of viral infection is unknown. However, it has been hypothesized that a common, perhaps the most common, cause of cardiomyopathy is a preceding viral infection. An accepted concept is that cardiomyopathy is the autoimmune manifestation of preceding viral myocarditis.[7] This attractive hypothesis is difficult to prove[8] because by the time the patient has cardiomyopathy the virus had disappeared from the myocardium. Furthermore, although it is known that the heart is susceptible to infection by a variety of viruses, especially coxsackieviruses and echoviruses, in the vast majority of patients, even those studied close to the clinical onset of dilated cardiomyopathy, viral studies are often uninformative. This also is true to a lesser extent for the onset of myocarditis.

The myocardial injury that precedes cardiomyopathy is not necessarily viral but may be secondary to exposure to a variety of other living organisms or to metabolic or environmental toxins.

Reduced suppressor T-cell function and excess T-helper cell activity have been observed in idiopathic dilated cardiomyopathy.[9,10] The future holds hope that the pathogenesis of cardiomyopathy and its relation to myocarditis will become clearer as a result of scanning magnetic resonance imaging studies, positron emission tomography, histochemical studies of biopsy material, and studies of the status of β- and α-adrenergic receptors.

ALCOHOL

The literature bears adequate testimony to an association between excessive consumption of alcohol and the subsequent development of dilated cardiomyopathy.[11] Administration of alcohol to experimental animals, normal human subjects, and patients with heart failure produces transient impairment of cardiac function, tachycardia, and arrhythmia. In experimental animals, corresponding morphologic changes have been observed. However, there is as yet no satisfactory animal model of alcohol-induced chronic dilated cardiomyopathy.[12] Furthermore, overt dilated cardiomyopathy is an uncommon complication of chronic alcoholism and a relationship between alcoholic liver dysfunction and cardiomyopathy cannot be established.[13] If anything, there tends to be an inverse relationship.

There are no specific histologic or ultrastructural criteria that separate cardiomyopathy in the alcoholic from idiopathic dilated cardiomyopathy. On the other hand, withdrawal of alcohol may sometimes be associated with dramatic improvement of cardiomyopathy. Thus, it may be that alcohol is not so much a cause of cardiomyopathy as an aggravating factor working through unknown mechanisms. One possibility is that in some cases, alcoholic myocarditis rather than viral myocarditis represents the myocardial injury triggering the autoimmune response that results in dilated cardiomyopathy.

PERIPARTUM CARDIOMYOPATHY

The view applied to alcoholic cardiomyopathy may apply to this entity. Once more, there is no doubt that there may be a significant association between the peripartum condition and the totally unexpected appearance of dilated cardiomyopathy.[14] Furthermore, the condition may remit, only to reappear in association with a subsequent pregnancy. As in alcoholic patients, there is no morphologic criterion to separate peripartum from idiopathic cardiomyopathy. Perhaps a metabolic alteration associated with pregnancy is the cause of the initial myocardial injury. This is a particularly distressing variant of cardiomyopathy, since it frequently afflicts otherwise healthy young women.

A rigorous search for heart disease of other etiology unmasked by pregnancy should be made. One distinguishing feature is that peripartum cardiomyopathy usually becomes manifest late in the last trimester or more commonly in the puerperium, whereas other heart disease becomes evident earlier and nearer the time of maximal hemodynamic burden.[15]

TOXIC CARDIOMYOPATHY

In this age of concern regarding environmental toxins and their safe disposal, it is especially prescient to recognize the possible role of toxins as triggers of cardiomyopathy. The best-known example, and one that may serve as a model for innumerable as yet undescribed toxins, is cobalt.[16] In two locations, one in the United States and the other in Canada, there was a sudden increase in the number of patients reporting to hospitals with dilated cardiomyopathy. The increase was so dramatic that an epidemic of viral myocarditis was suspected. However, subsequent inquiries revealed that the patients all drank beer to which the manufacturers had added cobalt so that the beverage would retain a large frothy head when poured into a glass or tankard. It is possible that other toxins and excesses or deficiencies of trace elements may act in a similar manner.

FAMILIAL CARDIOMYOPATHY

That asymmetric hypertrophic cardiomyopathy may be inherited as an autosomal dominant trait is well known. Much less commonly, dilated cardiomyopathy may also be familial. This familial dilated cardiomyopathy is distinct from cardiomyopathies associated with muscular and neuromuscular disorders. The prognosis tends to be poor and the response to cardiac transplantation satisfactory. The illness is manifest in young persons.

DIABETES

It has not been easy for clinicians to pinpoint diabetic cardiomyopathy as a specific entity. Although experimental or hereditary diabetes in animals can induce heart failure, the problem in clinical medicine is more complex because of the association between diabetes and premature coronary atherosclerosis and a suspected association between diabetes and disease of the small coronary branches and microvascular circulation. The decreased force of ventricular contraction observed in experimental diabetes[17] and its correction by antidiabetic treatment have been related to the activity of calcium-dependent myosin adenosine triphosphatase.

HYPERTENSION

The usual response to systolic overload is concentric hypertrophy, but myocardial fibrosis and dilatation supervene in a proportion of patients with hypertension, with the hypertrophy then becoming eccentric. The pathologist examining the heart of such a patient at autopsy cannot distinguish between dilated cardiomyopathy and hypertensive heart disease if the examination is confined to the heart and the history of hypertension is not revealed. The clinician must depend on a history of hypertension and other stigmata of hypertensive disease.

OBESITY

Obesity may cause circulatory congestion secondary to increased blood pressure and volume or true cardiac failure with severe eccentric hypertrophy.[18]

INADEQUATE MYOCARDIAL PROTECTION DURING CARDIOPULMONARY BYPASS

A number of patients are seen for the first time for heart failure some weeks or months following coronary artery bypass operation. Whether they have ischemic left ventricular dysfunction, perhaps related to previous or intraoperative myocardial infarction, or whether the myocardium was irreversibly damaged during the bypass operation is often difficult to tell. However, the syndrome occurs sufficiently frequently in the absence of evidence of heart failure before the operation, or myocardial infarction during operation, to suggest that intraoperative myocardial injury is a significant cause of heart failure. Distinction from postoperative constrictive pericarditis may be difficult because the computed tomographic scan in such cases may not show a thick pericardium. The role for endomyocardial biopsy is not yet clear.

PATHOLOGY

By definition, significant coronary atherosclerosis, intrinsic valve disease, congenital malformation, or other specific cardiac disease is absent. The heart is hypertrophied, often weighing between 500 g and 700 g and sometimes up to 1 kg. Because of the dilatation, the ventricular walls are not abnormally thick and may be even thinner than normal in spite of the hypertrophy. Where there has been preceding hypertension, wall thickness may be slightly greater than in other cases, so that the myocardial volume-to-mass ratio is improved, and this may have a favorable effect on prognosis, because of relatively reduced left ventricular wall stress and afterload.

The left ventricle is severely dilated, assuming a more spherical configuration and an abnormally smooth endocardial surface due to stretching of the trabeculae (Fig. 90.1). There is often dilatation of the right ventricle and of the atria as well. The cardiac valves are free from calcification, but the orifices of the atrioventricular valves may be considerably enlarged secondary to dilatation and stretching of their rings. In a proportion of cases, a mural thrombus, commonly in the left ventricle, is found. The pericardium should be normal in appearance, but there may be pericardial transudate.

On microscopic section, the myocytes are seen to be hypertrophied and their nuclei appear bizarre. In addition, fibrosis, varying from minimal and scattered, through more dense and focal, to extensive in amount and distribution, may be found.

ENDOMYOCARDIAL BIOPSY

Increasingly, the opportunity to study the endomyocardium during life is presented to the pathologist because of the desire to distinguish early in the course of disease between myocarditis and cardiomyopathy. Until recently, criteria for the diagnosis of myocarditis have not been agreed on, a deficiency that must be addressed before the results of endomyocardial biopsy can be used to distinguish between cardiomyopathy and myocarditis. A few round cells may be observed in the endomyocardial biopsy specimens of patients with dilated cardiomyopathy.[19] In myocarditis these cells are considerably more numerous; five or more per high power field have been suggested. The cells should be distinguishable as T lymphocytes and should be associated with myocyte necrosis.[20] As in cardiomyopathy, variable fibrosis may be present in addition.

OTHER ORGANS

The pathologic findings in the lungs and systemic organs are those of passive congestion. In addition, evidence of hypoxic injury, embolism, or thrombosis *in situ* may be found.

FUNCTIONAL DERANGEMENTS

The diagnosis of dilated cardiomyopathy is based on the demonstration of dilated ventricular cavities, with depressed systolic function (Table 90.1). Although the left ventricle is almost always involved, concomitant functional impairment of the right ventricle is more frequently observed in idiopathic dilated cardiomyopathy than in ischemic heart disease. Reduction of both contractile and pump function occurs. The ratio of the left ventricular end-systolic stress and volume, an index of contractile function, is significantly lower than in normal controls.

Left ventricular ejection fraction is the most commonly used index of systolic pump failure in patients with dilated cardiomyopathy. While ventricular ejection fraction is highly dependent on afterload, and therefore cannot be construed as a pure index of ventricular performance, in clinical practice depression of left ventricular ejection fraction is by far the most useful way to assess impairment of the systolic function of the left ventricle. Ejection fraction can be applied in this way, because, in the absence of severe aortic stenosis or hypertension, changes in ejection fraction mediated by afterload are an order of magnitude less than those caused by the cardiomyopathic process itself. In most series, the ejection fraction of the left ventricle averages 25%, with severe cases having an even lower ejection fraction. In milder cases, left ventricular ejection fraction may be in the range of 40% to 50%. In that minority of patients with relatively well preserved left ventricular function, the nearly normal ejection fraction fails to increase, and may even decrease during the performance of muscular exercise. When the ejection fraction is severely depressed, the signal-

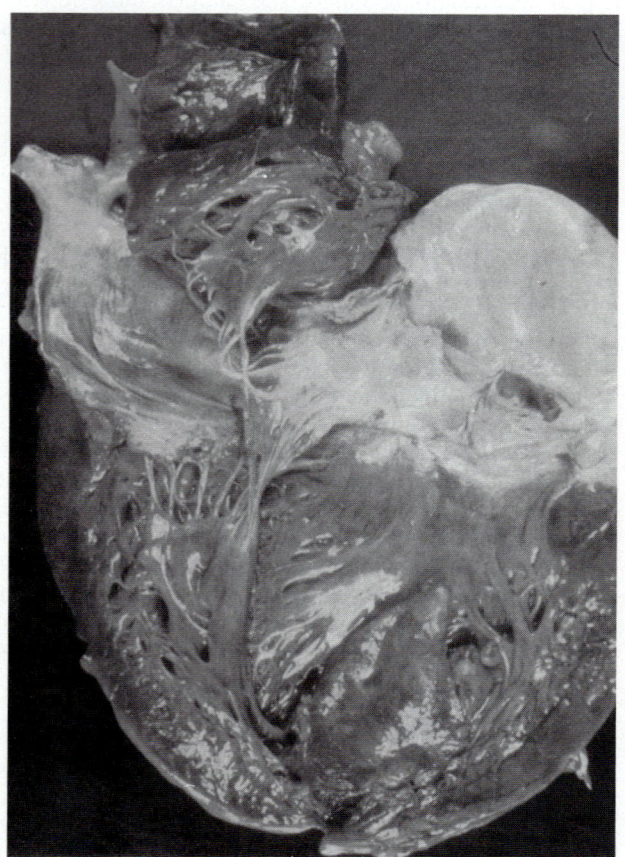

FIGURE 90.1 Heart showing the postmortem features of cardiomyopathy. The left ventricle is dilated, is unduly spherical and smooth, and contains a mural thrombus.

TABLE 90.1 FUNCTIONAL ABNORMALITIES IN DILATED CARDIOMYOPATHY

Parameter	Dilated Cardiomyopathy
Left ventricular volume	
End-diastolic	Increased
End-systolic	Increased
Left ventricular mass	Increased
Volume/mass ratio	Increased
Systolic function	
Ejection fraction	Decreased
Normalized ejection rate	Decreased
Myocardial fiber shortening	Decreased
Wall stress	Increased
End-diastolic function	
Pressure/volume	Decreased
Wall stress/volume	Decreased
Diastolic function	
Chamber stiffness	Decreased or normal
Myocardial stiffness	Increased or normal
Negative dp/dt	Decreased
Tau	Prolonged

to-noise ratio deteriorates significantly, and therefore the computed value becomes less accurate. Severe arrhythmia impedes signal averaging and thus also impairs the reliability of the result. It is important for the clinician to bear these limitations in mind, especially when using serial ejection fractions to determine whether a given patient's condition is improving or deteriorating. Clinicians should insist on having the data run in list mode for patients with atrial fibrillation or other chaotic rhythms. Left ventricular ejection fraction for a given severity of dilated cardiomyopathy, as in other diseases of the heart, tends to be higher when there is severe mitral regurgitation; usually, however, even then the ejection fraction in badly affected cases seldom exceeds 35%.

By definition, left ventricular end-diastolic volume is increased. The principal cause of this increase is the cardiomyopathy itself, but further increases, which are to some extent reversible, relate to functional mitral regurgitation and increased blood volume. In most cases, left ventricular end-diastolic volume stabilizes for a relatively long time after treatment has been initiated and a maintenance regimen has been implemented. Increase in the left ventricular end-systolic dimension is a more direct marker of impaired contractile function of the left ventricle.

Left ventricular segmental wall motion abnormalities are common in dilated cardiomyopathy, even in the absence of coronary artery disease. Analysis of regional ejection fraction may reveal areas of akinesis, dyskinesis, and hypokinesis in patients both with and without coronary artery disease. Analysis of ventriculographic patterns demonstrates that in some patients the left ventricle not only is dilated but also assumes a more rounded shape and shows uniformly poor motion (generalized hypokinesis). In other patients, localized abnormalities of contraction are also seen. These abnormal zones of contraction are similar to those that occur in patients with coronary artery disease. Thus, the presence of asynergy in dilated cardiomyopathy does not automatically establish the presence of coronary artery disease.

Depressed myocardial function can be demonstrated in animal models of cardiomyopathy as well as in patients with this disease. In the former, a reduction in the maximum velocity of unloaded shortening, V_{max}, of the papillary muscle has been observed. The force and the rate of force development in the heart muscle of Syrian hamsters with hereditary cardiomyopathy are less than normal. In patients with dilated cardiomyopathy, endocardial fiber-shortening velocity (VCF) is less than normal and there is a downward shift of the force–velocity relation, indicating depressed myocardial function. The isovolumic indices of contractility, peak dp/dt, V_{pm}, and V_{max}, are also depressed. The end-systolic pressure–volume or wall stress–volume relation provides a reliable index of contractile function in the intact heart. In patients with dilated cardiomyopathy, end-systolic volume increases markedly and increased wall thickness usually does not occur. The end-systolic pressure–volume or wall stress–volume relation therefore shifts downward and to the right, indicating reduced contractile function.

The total left ventricular mass increases; however, due to excessive cavity dilatation, the ratio of left ventricular volume to mass increases considerably and, consequently, wall stress is greatly increased. This is in contrast to hypertrophic cardiomyopathy, which is characterized by a decrease of this ratio.

Information available is inadequate to explain the variability of the changes in ventricular function that may be found in dilated cardiomyopathy. Some hemodynamic studies have indicated decreased peak rate of fall of left ventricular pressure during isovolumetric relaxation (peak negative dp/dt), prolongation of the rate constant of this pressure decline (tau), and decreased rate of early diastolic circumferential lengthening, indicating impaired relaxation. Chamber stiffness derived from the pressure–volume relationship may be increased or remain normal, but myocardial stiffness derived from the left ventricular stress–strain relationship is normal, or even increased.

In patients in whom chamber as well as myocardial compliance decreases, the symptoms are to a considerable extent caused by increased left ventricular diastolic pressure with consequent pulmonary congestion. In some patients with heart failure, usually of hypertensive or ischemic etiology, diastolic function is severely impaired but systolic function as manifest by the left ventricular ejection fraction and the cardiac output remains normal. By definition, such cases should not be included in the category of dilated cardiomyopathy. However, in some patients with dilated cardiomyopathy and depressed systolic function, diastolic dysfunction is a prominent feature.

INITIAL PRESENTATION

When patients first seek medical attention the disease is often far advanced. There may be a history of preceding fever, joint pains, and other features of a "flu"-like illness occurring some weeks before the first cardiac symptoms. A few patients will have had myopericarditis with the attendant pericardial pain, pericardial friction rub, and diffuse ST segment elevation, and perhaps PR segment depression on the electrocardiogram. Most patients have three principal symptoms, any one of which may be the chief complaint. These are fatigue, weight gain, and the various manifestations of dyspnea.

Retrospectively, many of the patients are able to recollect exertional dyspnea but many do not report it until there has been an episode of paroxysmal nocturnal dyspnea or until they begin to suffer orthopnea. The abnormal gain in weight is often impressive, frequently amounting to 20 or more pounds. Many of the patients recognize that they are retaining fluid. Complaints of swelling of the legs or ankles, increased abdominal girth, and pain or tenderness of the right upper quadrant of the abdomen are common.

Severe dyspnea accompanied by cough, especially with lying down or during exertion, is commonly the predominant early symptom, leading all too often to the incorrect diagnosis of pneumonia and a futile attempt at treatment with antibiotics. Many patients being evaluated by a cardiologist give this history.

SYMPTOMS IN THE PATIENT WITH ESTABLISHED DILATED CARDIOMYOPATHY

Following initial diuresis and the institution of conventional treatment for heart failure, a number of the patients become symptomless. In others there is persistence of dyspnea and generalized fatigue that particularly affects the legs, representing reduced cardiac output or inadequate response of cardiac output to the demands of exercise. Only a third of the patients complain of palpitation even though ambulatory electrocardiographic monitoring shows that severe arrhythmias are almost universal in dilated cardiomyopathy.[21]

A number of patients, including some in whom ischemic heart disease has been ruled out by coronary arteriography, complain of chest pain. The pain may be a persistent ache in the region of the cardiac apex, which is a type of pain commonly associated with massive cardiomegaly. In others, the pain may stimulate angina pectoris. It is difficult in this population to document myocardial ischemia because the electrocardiogram often displays abnormalities that would invalidate ST segment changes occurring during exercise and by definition the coronary arteriogram is normal. Nevertheless, it is probable that chest pain in a portion of these patients represents myocardial ischemia, a number of studies having demonstrated impaired coronary reserve in dilated cardiomyopathy.[22] Several factors may account for angina in dilated cardiomyopathy. These patients have a large thin-walled left ventricle in which wall stress is greatly increased and therefore impaired coronary reserve may not be well tolerated. With exertion, the demand for myocardial oxygen consumption is further increased because of increased wall tension and increased heart rate; furthermore, coronary vascular resistance is increased because of the raised sympathetic tone and the high levels of circulating catecholamines.

DYSPNEA

In many patients distressing attacks of paroxysmal nocturnal dyspnea or pulmonary edema, orthopnea requiring the use of three or more pillows, and severe exertional dyspnea can be ameliorated by treatment. In a minority, however, the symptoms are resistant to treatment. This lack of response is most common in patients with severely increased ventricular diastolic pressure and pulmonary hypertension. More often, exertional dyspnea is the major abnormality of breathing reported by the well-treated patient.

The concept that exertional dyspnea in chronic heart failure is directly related to increased pulmonary venous pressure has been extrapolated from studies of acute heart failure in which this relationship holds true. In chronic heart failure there is no relation between dyspnea and left atrial pressure at rest or even during exercise.[23] As yet, the pathophysiology of dyspnea in heart failure is unknown. In addition to pulmonary venous hypertension, metabolic acidosis, and other metabolic adaptations, tachypnea caused by stimulation of juxtacapillary receptors when the lungs are abnormally stiff contributes to exertional dyspnea.

FATIGUE

Depending on the stage and severity of cardiomyopathy, the arteriovenous oxygen difference may be widened to between 5.5 and 11 vol% and the cardiac output at rest may be significantly reduced. In less severely affected or particularly well-compensated cases, these parameters are normal at rest, but during exercise the arteriovenous oxygen difference becomes abnormally wide while cardiac output and oxygen consumption rise inadequately. On this basis, fatigue either at rest or with attempts to exercise is a frequent complaint. Peripheral factors also contribute to fatigue. The enormous increase in blood flow to working muscles when normal persons exercise is severely restricted in patients with heart failure. Consequently, muscle metabolism is strikingly different from normal. Lactic acid accumulates early in the course of exercise, owing in part to the greater use of anaerobic metabolism. Abnormalities of skeletal muscle and of the peripheral circulation independent of abnormalities of cardiac output have been demonstrated in patients with dilated cardiomyopathy.[24] These patients also complain that their legs give out on walking or attempting hills and stairs. In assessing this complaint, the clinician must distinguish it from intermittent claudication secondary to occlusive disease of the arteries of the lower extremities.

OTHER CLINICAL FEATURES
SLEEP DISORDERS

A commonly associated complaint, but one without a well-understood pathophysiologic basis, is insomnia in the absence of orthopnea, nocturnal dyspnea, or other symptoms that keep the patient awake. Insomnia may be secondary to diminished activity and increased sleep during the day or to sleep disorders of cardiac rate and rhythm,[25] which I often encounter in patients with heart failure. In some patients, sleep is disturbed by orthopnea, attacks of paroxysmal nocturnal dyspnea, anxiety, nightmares, and the action of diuretics.

DIZZINESS AND SYNCOPE

Less common than the previously discussed symptoms are complaints of lightheadedness, fainting attacks, and blurred vision, which are manifestations of decreased cerebral blood flow, the most common cause in this setting being hypotension. These features occur either because of an intrinsic lack of left ventricular contractile power or because of the action of vasodilators, the hypotensive effect of which may be enhanced by diuretic-induced hypovolemia. In a smaller proportion of the patients, these complaints are secondary to arrhythmia; furthermore, it should not be forgotten that when one is dealing with older patients who have cardiomyopathy there may be transient cerebral ischemic attacks secondary to occlusive cerebrovascular disease. In addition, in a small minority, cerebral embolization from a mural thrombus may be responsible.

NONSPECIFIC SYMPTOMS

Patients may complain of pleuritic pain in association with pulmonary infarction. Oliguria and hemoptysis may occur. Many patients have severe symptoms of anxiety and numerous psychosomatic complaints. There may also be a variety of symptoms secondary to administration of drugs to treat heart failure or arrhythmia.

Investigators have turned increasingly to the use of questionnaires to assess the quality of life of patients with cardiomyopathy and their impression of the impact of this disorder on their health and well-being. Analysis of patient responses indicates that in addition to the well-known conventional symptoms of heart failure, many patients complain of depression, anxiety, feelings of inadequacy, undue awareness of the heart and heart beat, forgetfulness, and inability to function satisfactorily at work or in society.

A useful way to keep track of symptoms and their progression, or their response to treatment, is by means of the visual analogue scale. A printed question is followed by a long horizontal line marked at one end with a phrase such as "not at all" and at the other with a phrase indicating that the complaint is maximal. The patient is asked to mark the line at a point that represents the best answer on this scale.

IMPOTENCE

The vast majority of men with advanced heart failure secondary to dilated cardiomyopathy are impotent. Many do not complain of this spontaneously, but its presence is readily acknowledged in response to the direct question. To what extent it is due to the hemodynamic disturbances of heart failure, to the action of drugs that the patient may be receiving, or to psychosomatic factors has not been discerned.

CLINICAL EXAMINATION

There is a wide spectrum of clinical findings depending on the stage and development of cardiomyopathy.

Commonly, the patient when first seen has obvious dyspnea. The pulse rate is rapid; the usual rhythm is sinus tachycardia, but occasionally it is atrial fibrillation. Sympathetic overdrive often generates mild hypertension with disproportionate elevation of the diastolic pressure, giving a narrow pulse pressure. Tachycardia and hypertension are other manifestations of sympathetic overdrive. Pulsus alternans is found in a small minority of severe cases but may persist for months or years and is not therefore as grave a prognostic sign as was previously thought.

The jugular venous pulse is elevated. When the heart is very dilated, tricuspid regurgitation ensues, creating a dominant systolic wave and y descent of the venous pulse. When the cardiac apex is palpable, it is usually displaced inferiorly and laterally. A left ventricular heave, and less commonly a right ventricular heave, may be found. Systolic thrills are unusual.

The most prominent and diagnostically useful finding on cardiac auscultation is a loud third heart sound. This is best appreciated with the bell of the stethoscope placed lightly but accurately over the cardiac apex with the patient in the left lateral position. In some patients there may also be a right ventricular third heart sound. When the heart rate is rapid, it is not always possible to distinguish between a third heart sound and a fourth heart sound. A fourth heart sound is audible in some patients but has much less diagnostic importance than the third heart sound. Functional regurgitation of the mitral and tricuspid valves may give rise to corresponding systolic murmurs. Irregularities of the heart owing to extrasystoles are frequently appreciated.

When the patient is seen before treatment has begun, there may well be crepitations in the lung fields and often dullness to percussion and diminished breath sounds owing to pleural effusion. Varying degrees of pitting edema, abdominal distention, ascites, and enlargement of the liver may be found.

When patients are seen after treatment has been established and are being followed in the office, the clinical findings are modified. In the vast majority of cases, pulmonary crepitations are either greatly diminished or abolished. Diuretics remove evidence of peripheral edema in all but the most stubborn cases. The heart rate is slower, and the blood pressure is lower.

Depending on the severity of heart failure and the presence or absence of tricuspid regurgitation, the venous pressure may return to normal or show less elevation than at the initial presentation. By far the most useful physical findings to follow on a serial basis are the third heart sound, the jugular venous pressure, and the patient's weight. In peripartum cardiomyopathy, dyspnea, edema, weight gain, raised venous pressure, and a third heart sound may be difficult to evaluate since they may occur in late pregnancy without heart disease or as evidence of toxemia.[26] In dilated cardiomyopathy with fully compensated heart failure, the clinical examination may be normal. In elderly patients an ejection systolic murmur unrelated to cardiomyopathy and probably caused by mild aortic stenosis is not uncommon.

CHEST ROENTGENOGRAM

Severe or well-advanced dilated cardiomyopathy is characterized by cardiac enlargement, the cardiothoracic ratio typically being about 55% or more. This degree of cardiomegaly is often present when the patient first seeks medical attention. Occasionally massive cardiomegaly is encountered, but in other instances the cardiothoracic ratio is normal or nearly so. Isolated dilatation of the left ventricle seldom increases the cardiothoracic ratio, roentgenographic cardiac enlargement being evidence of multichamber dilatation.[27] The chest roentgenogram often displays evidence of left atrial enlargement, but the left atrial appendage is less prominent than in rheumatic mitral disease. In the lateral projection, selective enlargement of the left ventricle betrayed by posterior displacement of its posterior wall is a common finding. Slight encroachment of the anterior clear space on the lateral projection of the chest roentgenogram may be caused by either an enlarged left ventricle pushing the heart forward or by true enlargement of the right ventricle. Severe encroachment of the anterior clear space, especially from the middle third upward, usually implies right ventricular dilatation.

Before treatment is initiated, pleural effusion that may be bilateral, evidence of pulmonary venous congestion and signs of interstitial and sometimes alveolar edema may be seen. In stabilized patients receiving chronic treatment, pleural effusions are much less common; redistribution of blood flow in the lungs often is the sole remaining evidence of pulmonary congestion, and even this sign may disappear. Kerley B lines are common in the acute phase and usually disappear with treatment but may persist in chronic cases even when severe dyspnea is absent. Calcification of cardiac valves characteristically is absent; its presence, especially in the leaflets, raising great doubts as to the accuracy of the diagnosis. Significant calcification of the pericardium should likewise be absent. Calcification of the coronary arteries may be found in patients with heart failure secondary to ischemic heart disease, and it has been suggested that fluoroscopic detection of coronary calcification is a reasonable means of distinguishing between idiopathic cardiomyopathy and ischemic heart failure,[28] although differentiation by this means is far from perfect. Dilation of the azygous vein may be recognized as prominence of the superior portion of the right border of the heart in patients with greatly elevated systemic venous pressure.

The chest roentgenogram performed serially is an excellent means of following the course of dilated cardiomyopathy. Dramatic decrease in heart size occurs in a small but significant proportion of cases (Fig. 90.2). This change may indicate a good prognosis and perhaps recovery from myocarditis, but in some cases cardiomegaly recurs after some years, heralding relapse. Striking reduction in heart size may be observed when some patients with dilated cardiomyopathy abstain from alcohol. Less dramatic fluctuations of cardiomegaly are useful in following this disease and for adjusting treatment.

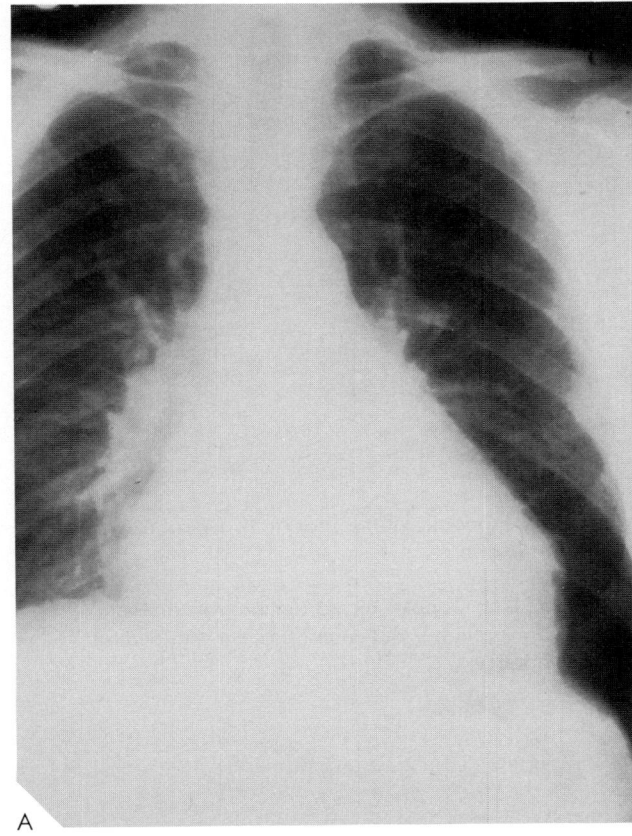
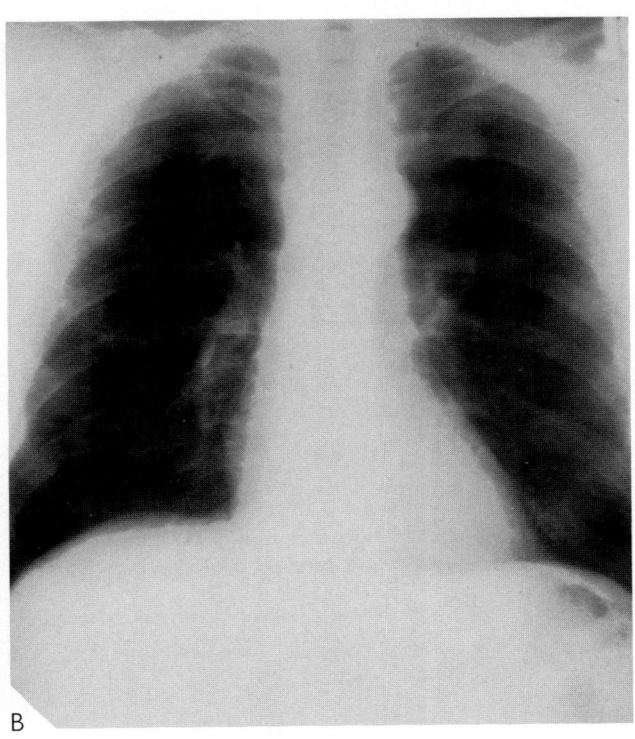

FIGURE 90.2 A. Chest roentgenogram of a patient admitted to the hospital for unexplained heart failure of unknown cause. **B.** Improvement occurred following conventional treatment. No immunosuppressive treatment was administered.

ELECTROCARDIOGRAM

The electrocardiogram is almost always abnormal. The most common abnormalities are left ventricular hypertrophy, usually with T-wave inversions, left bundle branch block, and complex ventricular extrasystoles. A number of other electrocardiographic abnormalities may be seen. As in most patients with severe heart failure, there is frequently disproportionately low QRS voltage in the frontal plane and increased voltage in the horizontal plane.[29] Atrial fibrillation is reported in up to 10% of patients. A wide-notched P wave in lead II and a broad posterior P vector in V_1 (P mitrale) is common, and left anterior hemiblock, right bundle branch block, and first-degree atrioventricular block may be present. In some cases the abnormality comprises nonspecific ST- and T-wave changes, which, especially in patients receiving digitalis and diuretics, are difficult to evaluate.

AMBULATORY ELECTROCARDIOGRAPHIC MONITORING

Long-term monitoring shows a high incidence of ventricular extrasystoles, which are frequently complex.[30] Runs of ventricular tachycardia are common. Less common, but by no means infrequent, are atrial extrasystoles and supraventricular tachycardia.

INVASIVE ELECTROPHYSIOLOGIC STUDIES

The high prevalence of arrhythmia has opened the question of the role for electrophysiologic investigation, particularly programmed stimulation, in dilated cardiomyopathy. Unfortunately, results to date have been conflicting; some reports claim that the studies lead to long-term effective pharmacologic treatment,[31] but others report a low incidence of inducing sustained monomorphic tachycardia and minimal benefit from the studies.[21] These studies should be reserved for patients with symptomatic arrhythmia, patients in whom arrhythmia appears to exert a detrimental hemodynamic effect, and patients who are not at the end stage of the disease (unless awaiting cardiac transplantation). Before embarking on electrophysiologic studies, electrolyte imbalance, drug interactions, and catecholamine excess must be addressed.

ECHOCARDIOGRAM

The echocardiographic features of dilated cardiomyopathy are highly characteristic (Fig. 90.3), although it is usually not possible by this means to distinguish between idiopathic cardiomyopathy and ischemic left ventricular failure or dysfunction. M-mode echocardiography shows that the left ventricular end-diastolic dimension is greatly increased, in severe cases up to 7 cm or 8 cm (Fig. 90.3, A). Both the septum and the posterior wall show diminished motion and wall thickening. Mitral valve opening is diminished, and the E to F slope of mitral valve closure may be slow when the left ventricular diastolic pressure is elevated; a B bump may interrupt the slope in such cases. Diminished opening of the mitral valve within a large ventricular cavity (Fig. 90.3, B) makes a highly characteristic echocardiographic picture, and the resulting separation of the E point of mitral valve opening from the posterior endocardial surface of the interventricular septum is characteristic of severe dysfunction of the left ventricle.[32] By M-mode echocardiography the motion of the aorta is seen to be diminished, and as a reflection of reduced stroke volume the aortic valve may not open to its full extent even though the cusps are not thickened. The M-mode echocardiogram frequently documents enlargement of the left atrium. Echocardiographic evidence of pericardial effusion is uncommon in cardiomyopathy.

TWO-DIMENSIONAL REAL-TIME ECHOCARDIOGRAPHY

The technique of two-dimensional real-time echocardiography confirms enlargement and hypocontractility of the left ventricle. Although cardiomyopathy is a global disease of the myocardium, particularly as it affects the left ventricle, there may be regional variations in the degree of hypokinesis, with better function sometimes being found at the base of the left ventricle.[33] Depending on the stage and severity of cardiomyopathy, the two-dimensional study may or may not show enlargement and hypocontractility of the right ventricle. When there is associated tricuspid regurgitation, motion of the interventricular septum becomes paradoxic. Enlargement of the right atrium, undetectable by M-mode echocardiography, may be seen clearly by two-dimen-

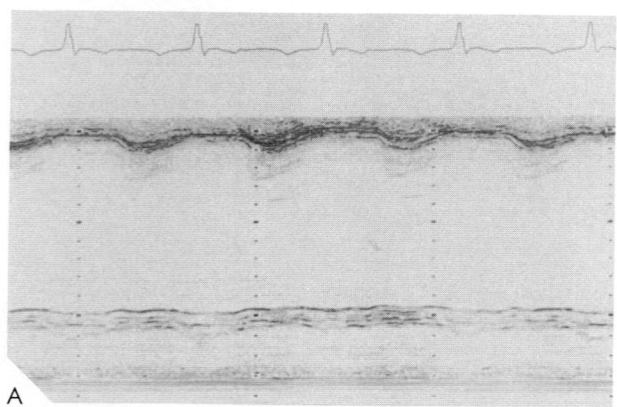
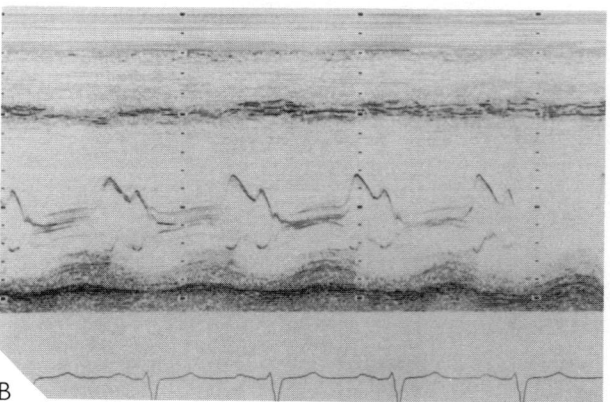

FIGURE 90.3 M-mode echocardiogram of patient with severe dilated cardiomyopathy. **A.** Marked dilatation and hypokinesis, especially of the septum. **B.** Typical appearance of the mitral valve.

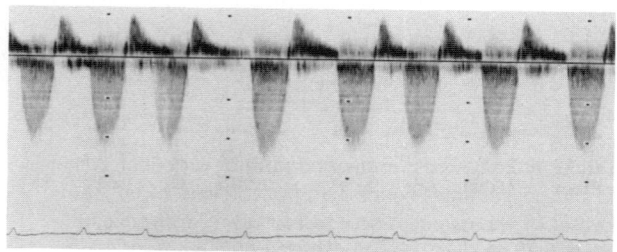

FIGURE 90.4 Echo-Doppler record demonstrating severe secondary mitral regurgitation in a patient with dilated cardiomyopathy.

sional echocardiography when present. The two-dimensional study is particularly helpful in the search for mural thrombi, and this should be done with maximal care.

VOLUME-TO-MASS RATIO OF THE LEFT VENTRICLE

With good resolution, reliable measurements of the diastolic dimensions, area and wall thickness of the left ventricle can be obtained by echocardiography. From these it is possible to estimate the volume of the ventricle and the mass of its myocardium. These calculations show that the volume-to-mass ratio is usually too high; ventricular dilatation, which increases wall stress, is not accompanied by sufficient hypertrophy to return wall stress to normal. When the increased wall stress, or afterload, is not met by preload reserve (i.e., the ability of the ventricle to dilate further and increase stroke volume), the mismatch precipitates clinically overt congestive heart failure.

ECHO-DOPPLER STUDIES

Echo-Doppler techniques frequently demonstrate mitral and tricuspid regurgitation in patients with dilated cardiomyopathy (Fig. 90.4). Regurgitation as documented by this technique may be present when the lesions are difficult to detect or evaluate clinically and when the clinician is not certain whether one or both of the atrioventricular valves is incompetent. Echo-Doppler[34] or radionuclide[35] techniques are also useful in following stroke volume and both systolic and diastolic cardiac function. Peak filling rate and time to peak filling of the left ventricle may be slow and prolonged in cases without severe mitral regurgitation.[36]

LABORATORY EXAMINATION

When the patient is first seen, the clinical laboratory is employed to help distinguish between specific myocardial diseases and cardiomyopathy. Sound clinical judgment mandates that laboratory tests be ordered in a discretionary fashion. There are simply too many systemic disorders that may affect the myocardium to allow for indiscriminate screening against all of them. This consideration is becoming increasingly important in any case because of the emphasis on containment of costs for medical diagnosis and treatment. Pointers may come from the results of routine laboratory studies and from such simple screening tests as the erythrocyte sedimentation rate. The history, family history, or clinical examination may give clues to systemic disorders. These clues should then be followed by ordering the appropriate laboratory tests. Specific heart muscle disorders are discussed elsewhere in this volume. In the vast majority, clinical manifestations are not confined to the heart and the diagnosis can be made on clinical grounds and confirmed in the laboratory. Rarely, diseases such as amyloidosis may affect the heart predominantly or exclusively. The diagnosis may then be suspected on echocardiographic findings and be detected by endomyocardial biopsy. The results of routine laboratory tests often help to identify aggravating factors such as anemia, infection, or thyroid dysfunction.

Routine laboratory screening is also of value in assessing the severity, following the course, and formulating prognosis in dilated cardiomyopathy. Depressed plasma sodium concentrations connote advanced disease, a poor prognosis,[37] and frequently the need to modify the diuretic regimen and fluid intake. Frequent monitoring of plasma potassium and magnesium concentrations, blood urea nitrogen value, and creatinine value help to guide therapy and provide prognostic information. Uric acid concentration may be increased by diuretics and should be monitored. In patients with a major component of right-sided heart failure, liver function tests and urinalysis should be performed periodically.

The plasma level of norepinephrine is increased particularly in the more advanced cases, and counterbalancing increases in atrial natriuretic factor and prostaglandin E are found, but routine monitoring of the concentrations of these substances in the plasma has not yet found its way into clinical practice.

RADIONUCLIDE STUDIES

Reduced left ventricular ejection fraction is a hallmark of dilated cardiomyopathy. The first-pass technique has the advantage that an individual cardiac chamber is imaged serially at a time when radioactivity is not present in the other cardiac chambers, and it permits estimation of transit time within the circulation. Unfortunately, the combination of low cardiac output, pulmonary congestion, and dilated cardiac chambers results in poorer temporal separation. Equilibrium-gated techniques are therefore commonly used in evaluation. With these, greater reliance must be placed on the associated computer in assigning regions of interest. The left ventricular ejection fraction is greatly reduced, often to values in the region of 20%, and this value increases little if at all during exercise. The right ventricular ejection fraction commonly is depressed. A subjective impression of cardiac chamber enlargement is gained by radionuclide ejection fraction studies, and abnormalities or regional wall motion can be documented with reasonable precision.

ECHOCARDIOGRAPHY OR RADIONUCLIDE STUDY?

In most cases it is not necessary to evaluate the patient with both echocardiography and scintigraphy. Steadily improving resolution of two-dimensional echocardiograms, the increasing availability of software to determine the volume, the filling and emptying characteristics, and the regional behavior of the ventricles, together with echo-Doppler techniques have been responsible for a shift in emphasis from radionuclide studies that require the intravenous injection of a radiopharmaceutical to echocardiography, which is truly noninvasive. However, some patients cannot be satisfactorily imaged by echocardiography and radionuclide studies are preferred unless esophageal echocardiography is available. Changes in cardiac performance during or immediately after exercise are more easily assessed in the radionuclide than in the echocardiographic laboratory, but exercise echocardiography is being developed and in some laboratories actively applied. Except in research centers, it is seldom necessary to perform both examinations except when the results of one are not concordant with the clinical evaluation.

CARDIAC CATHETERIZATION
INDICATIONS

Cardiac catheterization and angiography provide the information necessary for assessing the severity of myocardial damage and the compensatory adaptations that may have taken place. This assessment is based primarily on measurement of left ventricular end-diastolic volume and ejection fraction, cardiac output, pulmonary arterial pressure, and left ventricular end-diastolic pressure. Observation of the heart rate and calculation of the systemic and pulmonary vascular resistances help in this assessment. The degree of mitral and tricuspid regurgitation can be quantified, and right ventricular function can be assessed using techniques similar to those applied to the left ventricle. In milder cases it may be necessary to repeat a number of these measurements during stress (commonly exercise). In severe cases cardiac reserve can be estimated by repeating measurements after beneficial interventions such as the administration of a vasodilator or inotropic agent or by observing cardiac performance in postextrasystolic beats.

The main reason for carrying out invasive studies on patients with dilated cardiomyopathy is to obtain a coronary arteriogram so as to make a definitive distinction between cardiomyopathy and ischemic heart disease. Without coronary arteriography, it may be impossible to distinguish between these two disease entities, particularly when there is no history or electrocardiographic evidence of myocardial infarction. Since not all patients with ischemic heart disease have angina and some patients with cardiomyopathy have chest pain that is difficult or impossible to distinguish from angina, proof of dilated cardiomyopathy must rest on a coronary arteriogram of good quality. Since by definition coronary artery disease is absent in cardiomyopathy, the coronary arteriogram should not disclose any occlusion exceeding 50% in any major coronary arterial branch. On occasion the clinician will encounter patients with both cardiomyopathy and coronary artery disease, but in the absence of acceptable criteria for the diagnosis of coincident idiopathic and ischemic myocardial disease the diagnosis cannot be established with certainty.

When patients are to be included in a research study of idiopathic cardiomyopathy, cardiac catheterization should be carried out whenever possible before the study is begun to avoid the hazard of accidentally including a patient who in reality has ischemic heart disease. In the more common clinical circumstance the decision regarding cardiac catheterization rests mainly on the judgment of the individual physician taking care of the patient. When a patient has no evidence of ongoing ischemia but has severe congestive failure or left ventricular dysfunction manifest by cardiomegaly, a reduced ejection fraction, a third heart sound, raised jugular venous pressure, and pulmonary congestion, the treatment is the same regardless of etiology. The physician may thus elect to treat the patient without performing coronary arteriography.

In some cases, chest pain, electrocardiographic abnormalities, the results of treadmill testing, or regional wall motion abnormalities lead to the suspicion of ischemic heart disease, which in spite of a degree of cardiac failure or left ventricular dysfunction might respond to myocardial revascularization or resection of a left ventricular aneurysm. In such cases cardiac catheterization and coronary arteriography are fully justified.

HEMODYNAMICS

Cardiac output should be measured, preferably employing the Fick method in addition to any indicator dilution technique that may be used. When the catheter is passed in the right side of the heart, special attention should be paid to the size of the right atrium and to the waveform and level of right atrial pressure. Frequently, when there is right-sided heart failure prominent x and y descents are seen; respiratory variation is absent, or right atrial pressure increases during inspiration. The waveform may also reveal the prominent v wave of tricuspid regurgitation, although considerable tricuspid regurgitation may be present without generating a large systolic wave when the right atrium is enlarged and compliant. In such cases a steep and rapidly inscribed y descent is commonly recorded.

RIGHT VENTRICULAR PRESSURE

In patients with mild hemodynamic impairment, the right ventricular pressure at rest is normal. More commonly, there is a degree of elevation of the right ventricular systolic pressure, which on occasion may be severe and in the worst cases approaches systemic level. The right ventricular diastolic pressure and right atrial pressure are elevated when biventricular failure is present, in the worst cases to levels around 20 mm Hg. When the right ventricle is more hypertrophied than dilated, a prominent a wave is recorded. Even when respiratory variation of right atrial pressure is absent or reversed, right ventricular systolic pressure falls during inspiration. The pulmonary arterial systolic pressure is the same as the right ventricular systolic pressure, and the pulmonary arterial diastolic pressure is similar to the left ventricular end-diastolic pressure unless there is a significant component of increased pulmonary vascular resistance. The pulmonary wedge pressure is characteristically elevated to a level dependent on the severity of left ventricular dysfunction. Mitral regurgitation may generate a substantial systolic wave of pulmonary venous pressure. The left ventricular diastolic pressure is elevated in all but the mildest or best-compensated cases.

Characteristically, systemic vascular resistance is increased, mostly as a result of reduced cardiac output. Pulmonary vascular resistance is also elevated in a significant number of cases.

In a mild or particularly well-compensated case, the hemodynamics are normal when the patient is studied at rest, although in the vast majority of such cases the left ventricular ejection fraction is severely reduced. To bring out latent hemodynamic deficiency, an intervention that stresses the heart is carried out; in the cardiac catheterization laboratory the most appropriate means is supine bicycle ergometry. Often the simple act of raising the lower extremities and placing the feet on the ergometer pedals is enough to elevate normal left ventricular diastolic and pulmonary wedge pressures abnormally.

Several abnormalities become apparent as the patient performs exercise. The left ventricular diastolic and pulmonary wedge pressures, instead of remaining unchanged or falling slightly, increase, often dramatically. Most of the patients cannot exercise as long or as much as normal subjects of their age. The increase in cardiac output and oxygen consumption with exercise is greatly blunted with corresponding abnormal widening of the arteriovenous oxygen difference. If exercise is impractical, for instance when cardiac catheterization is performed through the femoral vessels, another stress may be employed. In contrast to ischemic heart disease, pacing is not particularly informative in patients with cardiomyopathy, but the response of left ventricular diastolic pressure and stroke volume or stroke work to increased afterload is highly informative. For this purpose angiotensin infusion is perhaps the optimal technique.

What may be expected from treatment in the acute stage of the illness can be judged by measuring the increase in cardiac output and the fall in left ventricular end-diastolic pressure, systemic vascular resistance, and pulmonary vascular resistance in response to intravenously administered vasodilators or positive inotropic drugs. Unfortunately, the outcome of such studies is of little or no value in predicting response to long-term treatment with the same or comparable drugs given by mouth.[38] Nevertheless, new drugs for the treatment of heart failure are frequently evaluated by administering them to patients during the course of hemodynamic studies.

Even when right ventricular diastolic pressure is substantially elevated, it is almost always considerably lower than left ventricular diastolic pressure, but when right ventricular dilatation has been relatively acute, the two diastolic pressures may be equal, especially during inspiration.[39] This phenomenon may give the mistaken impression of constrictive pericarditis, but when the clinical picture is taken into account, this particular source of confusion seldom arises.

In the majority of cases left ventriculography proves and quantifies the left ventricular dilatation. There is generalized hypokinesis, but this is often less severe at the cardiac base.[40] Mitral regurgitation can frequently be demonstrated, and this may be severe even in the absence of organic mitral valve disease. Right ventriculography shows comparable but usually less severe reduction of right ventricular ejection fraction, and tricuspid regurgitation of varying severity may be present. The left and right ventriculograms may disclose previously unsuspected mural thrombosis. In patients with left ventricular dysfunction secondary to ischemic heart disease, left ventricular aneurysm may be demonstrated, but would not be expected in dilated cardiomyopathy.

In addition to revealing hitherto unsuspected coronary artery disease, on occasion cardiac catheterization turns up a major congenital malformation, an element of valvular heart disease, or a pericardial abnormality that had been missed on clinical examination and laboratory investigation. In such instances, the diagnosis of idiopathic cardiomyopathy must be abandoned. Digital angiography is particularly useful because it permits assessment of global and regional function of both ventricles after a single intravenous injection of contrast medium.

ENDOMYOCARDIAL BIOPSY

Endomyocardial biopsy, as discussed earlier in this chapter, is increasingly carried out during cardiac catheterization for dilated cardiomyopathy. This procedure is most safely accomplished using the Stanford technique from the internal jugular vein to biopsy the right side of the interventricular septum.[41] Physicians experienced in the technique of puncturing the internal jugular vein between the two heads of the sternocleidomastoid muscle fairly rapidly acquire the needed skills to obtain the specimens safely. Some physicians working in cardiac catheterization laboratories lack experience in accessing the right side of the heart by the internal jugular vein. Furthermore, in laboratories in which the vast majority of hemodynamic studies are performed via the femoral vessels, many physicians prefer to obtain biopsy specimens without the need for additional cannulation at the neck. Endomyocardial biopsies from the right side of the interventricular septum can be obtained using a bioptome passed into the right ventricle via a long sheath inserted over a guide wire and pigtail catheter from the femoral vein.[42] A similar technique can be used to biopsy the left side of the septum via the femoral artery.[42] Bioptomes used for these techniques are longer and more flexible than the Stanford bioptomes, and torque control is less precise. The jaws of bioptomes introduced from the groin are somewhat smaller than those of the Stanford bioptome; biopsy specimens are therefore on the average, somewhat smaller.

The hazards of inadvertently puncturing the carotid artery with a large-bore needle or catheter introducer while performing this procedure are minimal when carried out by a well-trained physician. Biopsies should not be taken until it has been ascertained beyond doubt that the jaws of the bioptome have contacted the interventricular septum. After the bioptome has been passed through the tricuspid valve, its position in the right ventricle should be confirmed by inducing ventricular extrasystoles and by fluoroscopy in the right anterior and left anterior oblique projections. If the bioptome is inadvertently advanced into the coronary sinus where biopsy would inevitably lead to cardiac tamponade, its posterior position is readily apparent from the left anterior oblique projection. Transfer of the specimens from the bioptome to containers must be accomplished as atraumatically as possible; small hypodermic needles are generally used for this purpose. Several specimens should be obtained to reduce sampling errors and at a minimum several samples should be placed in formalin for histologic examination. In many centers, specimens are also placed in glutaraldehyde for examination under the electron microscope. Additional specimens can be frozen at $-70°C$ for subsequent special staining and immunochemical and receptor studies.

The two principal reasons for undertaking endomyocardial biopsy in cases of dilated cardiomyopathy are to rule out myocarditis and to detect a specific myocardial disease masquerading as idiopathic cardiomyopathy. The latter has a comparatively small yield in patients who have undergone clinical and extensive laboratory investigation, including in all cases echo-Doppler studies and in many cases cardiac catheterization. The yield is somewhat higher in patients referred to highly specialized national centers where selection skews the pathology toward the more obscure and uncommon diseases. Although the incidence of myocarditis in patients with unexplained heart failure reported in the literature varies from 5% to 63%,[43-47] vastly increasing experience suggests that the true figure is around 10% or less. My colleagues and I reviewed the experience in our institution[48] and found that of 90 biopsies performed for recent unexplained heart failure (60% less than 4 months) histologic proof of myocarditis was obtained in only 4.4%. Thus, the yield derived from the two most important indications for endomyocardial biopsy myocarditis and suspected dilated cardiomyopathy is small. Furthermore, whether immunosuppressive treatment is superior to conventional treatment remains entirely unknown, although the question is the subject of intense clinical investigation.

The future role of endomyocardial biopsy in dilated cardiomyopathy will rely heavily on the answer to the question of how myocarditis should be treated, because if identical treatment proves appropriate for both dilated cardiomyopathy and myocarditis, the most frequent indication for endomyocardial biopsy in patients with dilated cardiomyopathy will have been removed. On the other hand, endomyocardial biopsy will become part of the standard initial workup of patients with dilated cardiomyopathy, if it is proved that immunosuppression is clearly superior to conventional treatment of heart failure due to myocarditis, especially if endomyocardial biopsy continues to be the optimal diagnostic procedure for differentiating between myocarditis and cardiomyopathy. Until these questions relating to the diagnosis and treatment of myocarditis have been answered, endomyocardial biopsy for dilated cardiomyopathy should be restricted to large cardiac centers with extensive experience in endomyocardial biopsy.

Endomyocardial biopsy slides should be read by pathologists specifically trained and experienced in this task. It is not always possible to distinguish dilated cardiomyopathy from ischemic left ventricular failure; therefore, except in patients under 30 years of age, proposed endomyocardial biopsy should be preceded by coronary arteriography, and if severe occlusive lesions are identified the procedure need not be done. By far the safest technique, and one with the advantage that it has been performed the most frequently, is that employing the Stanford bioptome via the right internal jugular vein. There appears to be no diagnostic advantage in performing the slightly more hazardous left ventricular endomyocardial biopsy.

Unfortunately, the findings in dilated cardiomyopathy are remarkably nonspecific, correlate poorly with ventricular function, and, in most studies, have not been found to provide useful prognostic information. The principal changes are hypertrophy of the myocytes, enlargement and bizarre appearance of the nuclei, thickening of the endocardium, and fibrosis and are indistinguishable from those of heart failure secondary to valvular heart disease. Contraction bands seen under light and electron microscopy are fixation artifacts, unrelated to contraction bands found in experimental myocardial ischemia.

ASSESSMENT OF FUNCTIONAL STATUS

Assessment of the functional status of patients with cardiomyopathy has proved to be surprisingly difficult. Patients are often classified according to the New York Heart Association scheme, but this is highly subjective and serves only as a rough nonparametric guide for statistical purposes. Attempts have been made to improve on it by using a semiquantitative assessment of cardiac symptoms. Most often, the patient's ability to perform a number of common household or occupational tasks is assessed.[27] This technique is superior to the New York Association classification but is still somewhat subjective and far from perfect. Nevertheless, it gives the physician a better understanding of the patient's limitations and where to emphasize treatment. Furthermore, a detailed score based on a large number of symptoms and daily activities is superior for following the course of patients with cardiomyopathy than a scheme recognizing only four classes.

Over the past 2 decades there has been a tendency to limit assessment of the functional status of patients to objective criteria such as the left ventricular ejection fraction, performance on a treadmill, or serial hemodynamic studies. Although such criteria are important to medical scientists, and may prove important in prognosis, they sometimes have surprisingly little bearing on the well-being of the patient. There has been a refreshing rekindling of interest in symptoms and how they adversely influence the life of the patient and family. The "quality of life instrument" is becoming an increasingly popular means of assessing heart failure in patients with cardiomyopathy.[49]

Treadmill exercise can be a valuable means of assessing functional capacity. By and large, there is a fairly good correlation between symptoms and the duration of treadmill exercise. The Bruce protocol has little application here, but patients with dilated cardiomyopathy can follow more gentle protocols such as the Naughton or the Balke Ware. Attention should be paid not only to the duration of exercise but also to the heart rate and blood pressure response, the development of arrhythmia during or after exercise, and the limiting factor, which may be breathlessness or leg fatigue. If the treadmill stages are short, dyspnea is the limiting factor, whereas treadmill protocols that employ long stages are limited by fatigue, even though the pulmonary wedge pressure achieved is the same for both rapid and slow exercise protocols.[50] If the patient truly has dilated cardiomyopathy, angina pectoris ought not to be the symptom that limits exercise. In research centers oxygen consumption is measured during the performance of treadmill exercise tests,[51] as it is a more objective measurement than the duration of exercise, which can be altered by a number of subjective reactions on the part of the patient or those supervising the test. Some investigators use the anaerobic threshold but the technique is difficult and subject to important limitations.

Of considerable interest and great practical importance is the lack of correlation between ventricular function and exercise capacity whether judged by New York Heart Association classification, assessment of symptoms, performance on the treadmill, or measurement of oxygen consumption.[52] It is common to encounter patients with cardiomyopathy who deny symptoms, can exercise for 15 to 20 minutes on the treadmill, and achieve relatively high levels of oxygen consumption whose left ventricular ejection fraction is 20% or less and whose left ventricular dimensions are greatly enlarged. This discrepancy can to some extent be explained by the adaptive mechanisms that ensue when the heart fails.[53] These include maintenance of cardiac output by tachycardia and of stroke volume by ventricular enlargement. Less well understood are redistribution of cardiac output and adaptations in the systemic and pulmonary vascular beds. Functional status compares somewhat better with right ventricular function than left.[54]

PROGNOSIS

In general the prognosis is poor once a patient presents with congestive heart failure, the chances of surviving beyond 5 years being slim. There are considerable variations within this overall pattern; the course may be rapid and virulent, or a patient may live well beyond 5 years after the diagnosis is made, but in most series 5-year mortality exceeds 50%.

VENTRICULAR FUNCTION

Most investigators agree that prognosis can be related to the degree of impairment of left ventricular function, particularly the ejection fraction,[55] but a minority have reported lack of correlation[56] and this is true for our series. It is difficult to provide the prognosis in months or years for an individual patient even when left ventricular performance is greatly impaired, especially when the clinical condition is stable. The true end stage of dilated cardiomyopathy can often be recognized by a progressive increase in symptoms and refractoriness to treatment. This development is frequently rapid, occurring over a matter of weeks or a few months, but preceded by a period of years during which ventricular function, although grossly abnormal, is stable and little progression in symptoms occurs. This feature of the clinical course of cardiomyopathy adversely affects selection for cardiac transplantation.

Numerous processes may lead to the final picture that we recognize as dilated cardiomyopathy; furthermore, that picture has many variants. Dysfunction and failure may be confined to the left ventricle or be bilateral, and there are variations in the degree of dilatation and hypertrophy. Radiographically, the heart may appear enormous or only slightly enlarged and the range of morphologic, conduction, and rhythm abnormalities of the electrocardiogram is wide. This diversity has led to a number of attempts to identify features or combinations of features that predict prognosis. The findings on endomyocardial biopsy vary from virtually normal to extensive fibrosis, and the extent of myolysis, myofibrillar hypertrophy, and nuclear abnormalities is extremely variable.

In one study of 69 patients, the mortality rate at 1 year was 35% and the most powerful predictors were intraventricular conduction delay, ventricular arrhythmias, and right atrial pressure.[57] There was no relation between prognosis and the findings on endomyocardial biopsy. The latter finding is in agreement with another study of 68 patients, which showed strong correlation between survival and left ventricular ejection fraction, but not with a quantitative assessment of morphologic abnormality as seen in endomyocardial biopsy.[58] However, others[59] have found a strong correlation between prognosis and myocardial volume fraction, defined as the ratio of myocytes to all other elements found by morphometric measurement of biopsy specimens. The role of quantitation of myocardial biopsies in the assessment of cardiomyopathy thus remains unsettled. Opinion varies about whether a component of alcoholism in the etiology favorably or adversely affects prognosis, although there is general agreement that when some of these patients abstain from alcohol significant improvement results.[60] Hemodynamic abnormalities such as high left ventricular diastolic pressure and low cardiac output, especially when associated with increased pulmonary vascular resistance, are associated with poorer prognosis.

ARRHYTHMIA

Among the various factors that may affect prognosis arrhythmia is of particular interest, because here there is at least the possibility of favorably influencing prognosis with treatment. Unfortunately, in this arena, too, opinions are divided.[61] This is because there is a strong association between the magnitude of left ventricular dysfunction and the severity of arrhythmia. This association makes it difficult to determine to what extent ventricular arrhythmia, an almost universal finding in severe cardiomyopathy, is an independent risk factor for death. In a study of 74 patients with dilated cardiomyopathy, the combination of ejection fraction below 40% and frequent episodes of ventricular tachycardia or couplets prognosticated high risk for sudden death.[62] This finding differed from that of an earlier study of 35 patients in whom ventricular tachycardia was believed not to predict prognosis.[63] In either case the strong association between ventricular tachycardia and an advanced stage of cardiomyopathy militates against the importance of ventricular tachycardia in prognosis, even if it is a separately identifiable risk factor.

PLASMA CATECHOLAMINE LEVEL

Dilated cardiomyopathy that has progressed to the stage of overt heart failure is associated with a high concentration of circulating norepinephrine. The sympathetic nervous system and renin–angiotensin–aldosterone system are activated and vasopressin release is augmented. The resulting vasospasm increases afterload, a burden that is poorly tolerated by the cardiomyopathic ventricle. Norepinephrine may also play a role in the genesis of arrhythmia in such patients. It is therefore not surprising that high plasma levels of this catecholamine are associated with poor prognosis.[64]

CLINICAL COURSE

From what has been said about prognosis, it appears that the clinical course is usually one of deterioration, sometimes slower and sometimes faster, but on the average occurring over a course of 3 to 7 years, during which progressive deterioration in exercise tolerance occurs and the heart size increases. Patients become increasingly refractory to diuretics, which leads to escalating dose requirements and in turn to progressive electrolyte imbalance and further increase in plasma catecholamine levels. The most common mode of death is sudden, occurring in patients with advanced symptoms and evidence of severe ventricular dysfunction. Less common but highly important are sudden death in patients who are subjectively well and in whom ventricular dysfunction is less severe and sudden death due to a major thromboembolic accident. As the disease progresses azotemia aggravated by diuretic treatment makes its appearance. The majority of patients cease to be employed within a year of diagnosis. This is one of several factors, including impotence, longer and more frequent hospital admissions, and side-effects of drug treatment, leading to depression, a degree of which is common in patients with well-established dilated cardiomyopathy.

It is fortunate that the most useful means of following the clinical course are simple. They include symptoms, weight, jugular venous pressure, arterial blood pressure, heart rate, especially when sinus rhythm is present, and prominence of the third heart sound. Somewhat less important are the intensity of the murmurs of mitral and tricuspid regurgitation, crepitations in the lung fields, and peripheral edema. When clinical signs deteriorate, the physician must distinguish between the occurrence of some exacerbating factor and progression of the disease. Serial changes in echocardiographic dimensions and in the ejection fraction are not especially useful in following the clinical course of dilated cardiomyopathy, because for a prolonged period the changes are small, falling within the range of error of the measurements, and when significant changes do occur deterioration is readily apparent without resort to laboratory investigation.

Some patients recover; in others the course is prolonged over 10 years to 20 years; and in yet others the course is short and virulent.

DIAGNOSIS

The diagnosis of dilated cardiomyopathy is partly one of exclusion but partly one of recognition of a characteristic clinical picture. The diagnosis cannot be made with acceptable certainty in the presence of heart disease of other etiology. Diagnosis may thus seem at first a daunting task, but the rapid appearance of heart failure with significant fluid retention evident to both patient and physician in a patient with no previous evidence of heart disease and no other systemic disorder is so characteristic that one can often make a strong presumptive diagnosis at the time of an initial visit, especially if an electrocardiogram and chest roentgenogram are included. To confirm the diagnosis, other nosologic entities and specific diseases of myocardium including myocarditis must be excluded.

DIFFERENTIAL DIAGNOSIS
RHEUMATIC HEART DISEASE

Cardiac failure, cardiomegaly, and especially enlargement of the left atrium and the murmurs of mitral and or tricuspid regurgitation may mislead the unwary to the misdiagnosis of rheumatic heart disease. However, since these are murmurs of functional not organic valve incompetence, they tend to decrease following successful treatment. This behavior is in contrast to the murmurs of organic mitral and tricuspid regurgitation, which become louder with increasing cardiac compensation. Care should be taken not to mistake a third heart sound for the opening snap of mitral stenosis. Also, the third heart sound of dilated cardiomyopathy may be long enough to be confused with a short mitral diastolic rumbling murmur. Atrial fibrillation is considerably more common in rheumatic than in idiopathic heart disease (10% in our series). Correct differentiation can almost always be made by clinical examination, but on occasion the clinician relies on the echocardiogram to rule out mitral stenosis.

CORONARY ARTERY DISEASE

The entities that have been described under the somewhat misleading term *ischemic cardiomyopathy* have been discussed in preceding sections. In the majority of patients with coronary artery disease, this diagnosis can be suspected from a history of angina or previous myocardial infarction and electrocardiographic evidence of ischemia or myocardial infarction. However, angina pectoris does not exclude the possibility of dilated cardiomyopathy. Furthermore, it is only the unwise or the inexperienced physician who takes the patient's word that he has had a heart attack as evidence of previous myocardial infarction. To diagnose dilated cardiomyopathy with absolute certainty requires coronary arteriography, although this degree of certainty is often not required in clinical practice.

MYOCARDITIS

Myocarditis is discussed under etiology and classification and under endomyocardial biopsy.

SYSTEMIC MYOCARDIAL DISEASES

Involvement of the myocardium in such systemic disorders as neoplasia, pathologic infiltrates, collagen vascular disorders, metabolic abnormalities, and neuromuscular diseases can usually be identified from the history and physical examination and confirmed by appropriate laboratory tests. On rare occasions hemodynamic investigation and endomyocardial biopsy are used to establish the diagnosis, but more often when these procedures are carried out it is for confirmation or to obtain a tissue diagnosis rather than for primary diagnosis.

CONGENITAL MALFORMATIONS

The congenital malformations most likely to be confused with dilated cardiomyopathy are those in which the heart is enlarged and in which murmurs are not necessarily prominent. Good examples are atrial septal defect and Ebstein's anomaly. The large, volume-loaded heart of atrial septal defect is easily confused with that of dilatation because of intrinsic myocardial disease (Fig. 90.5). The widely split second heart sound can be confused with a third heart sound, and right bundle branch block is consistent with dilated cardiomyopathy. The pulmonary ejection murmur may not be recognized for what it is, and in some cases the murmur of tricuspid regurgitation is audible. Finally, pulmonary hyperemia may be mistaken for pulmonary vascular congestion.

Ebstein's anomaly is frequently characterized by a large globular heart (and clear lung fields), which can simulate dilated cardiomyopathy with tricuspid regurgitation (Fig. 90.6). The murmur is often scratchy and superficial. Finally, third and fourth heart sounds are common in Ebstein's anomaly.

Endocardial fibroelastosis has many of the same features as dilated cardiomyopathy but usually occurs in childhood and should be considered a separate entity, although each may occur in members of the same family.

PERICARDIAL EFFUSION

When the unexpected discovery of a large heart is made by chest roentgenography, dilated cardiomyopathy and pericardial effusion enter into the differential diagnosis. When the pericardial effusion is complicated by cardiac tamponade, the venous pressure is increased and the roentgenographic picture is that of generalized cardiomegaly with relatively clear lung fields. These findings simulate dilated cardiomyopathy, because in this disorder, too, the venous pressure is increased, and when there is tricuspid regurgitation, the lung fields may be relatively clear, even when the transverse diameter of the heart is appreciably increased. However, when the diagnosis is not made on clinical grounds, as it almost always can be, the issue is rapidly settled by echocardiography, which in the case of pericardial effusion demonstrates the effusion and underlying normal function and size of the cardiac chambers.

CONSTRICTIVE PERICARDITIS

The manifestations of constrictive pericarditis are difficult to distinguish from those of dilated cardiomyopathy with congestive heart failure. In both conditions the jugular venous pressure is high, edema is common, an additional heart sound occurs early in diastole, and atrial fibrillation may supervene. Dyspnea and pulmonary congestion are common to both. Often in chronic constrictive pericarditis the heart shadow seen by chest roentgenography is enlarged. A systolic murmur is audible in a number of patients with constrictive pericarditis, and in both heart failure and constrictive pericarditis the jugular venous pressure may show a prominent v wave and precipitous y descent. Constrictive pericarditis, although much less common than congestive heart failure, must always be considered in evaluation of what appears to be right-sided heart failure. If constrictive pericarditis is the correct diagnosis, increased pericardial thickness, a restrictive pattern of ventricular filling, and preserved systolic function can be demonstrated by appropriate imaging and hemodynamic techniques.

COR PULMONALE

The initial presentation of dilated cardiomyopathy is frequently with massive weight gain, edema, ascites, and pleural effusion. These same findings are common manifestations of severe decompensated cor pulmonale. In the latter, the results of pulmonary function and blood gas studies together with a history of severe respiratory symptoms should establish the correct diagnosis. Of greater practical importance is the occurrence of dilated cardiomyopathy in patients who have a degree of chronic obstructive airway disease but who do not have cor pulmonale. Here there is often evidence of significant airway obstruction, but apart from a large a wave, the jugular venous pressure is normal and right ventricular hypertrophy is absent. In the patient with dilated cardiomyopathy and moderately severe obstructive airway disease without cor pulmonale, the critical issue is to correctly apportion dyspnea and edema to heart or lung disease. In some cases, this assignment can be very difficult without the aid of laboratory testing, which should show severe impairment of left ventricular function. Selective right ventricular hypertrophy or dysfunction shown by radionucleotide angiography would point more to a pulmonary origin of symptoms. However, rarely the physician may encounter right ventricular dysplasia[65] in which the right ventricle is greatly dilated and hypocontractile but the left ventricle is spared. Ventricular dysrhythmia is an important complication of this uncommon form of dilated cardiomyopathy.

When the issue cannot be resolved by clinical and noninvasive means, hemodynamic studies may be helpful, particularly measurement at rest and during exercise of minute ventilation, oxygen consumption, cardiac output, and pulmonary wedge or left ventricular diastolic pressure.

HYPERTENSIVE HEART DISEASE

The cardiac manifestations of hypertensive heart disease may be indistinguishable from those of dilated cardiomyopathy. The clinician must therefore rely on a history of hypertension and evidence of other manifestations of hypertensive disease. Although hypertensive heart failure may take the form of a dilated hypokinetic left ventricle, on occasion systolic function is well preserved, the major abnormality being decreased left ventricular diastolic compliance.[66]

TREATMENT

The treatment of heart failure, including the use of various drugs, and the treatment of myocarditis are discussed elsewhere in these volumes. The following discussion is limited to aspects that deal specifically with cardiomyopathy.

Only rarely does the physician have the opportunity to treat dilated cardiomyopathy at an early stage. Prolonged bed rest, perhaps up to a year,[67] has long since been abandoned. Most physicians continue to administer digitalis on a long-term basis to patients with established dilated cardiomyopathy, although its efficacy in the treatment of chronic heart failure has been seriously questioned.[68]

The loop diuretic is the agent that has had the most profound effect on the manifestations and clinical course of dilated cardiomyopathy. It is to this class of agents that we owe the change in name from congestive to dilated cardiomyopathy. The clinical course of dilated cardiomyopathy is often characterized by progressive increase in the requirement for diuretics so that it is not uncommon to find patients receiving from 160 mg to over 300 mg/day of furosemide or the equivalent dose of bumetanide. One cannot overemphasize the importance of salt restriction in this setting. Potassium-sparing diuretics may be used in conjunction with furosemide and similar drugs, but it is essential to carefully monitor plasma levels of sodium, chloride, blood urea nitrogen, creatinine, and potassium, especially in patients receiving captopril or other inhibitors of angiotensin converting enzyme. Decreased weight and lowered venous pressure are often bought only at the price of higher blood urea nitrogen and creatinine levels. In refrac-

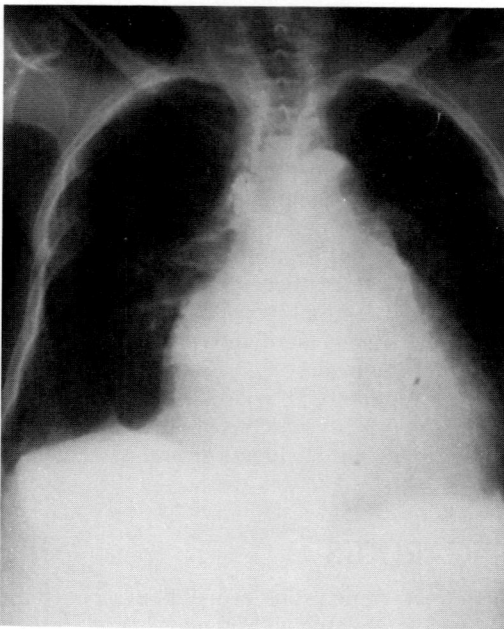

FIGURE 90.5 Chest roentgenogram of patient with dilated cardiomyopathy. The appearance suggests atrial septal defect.

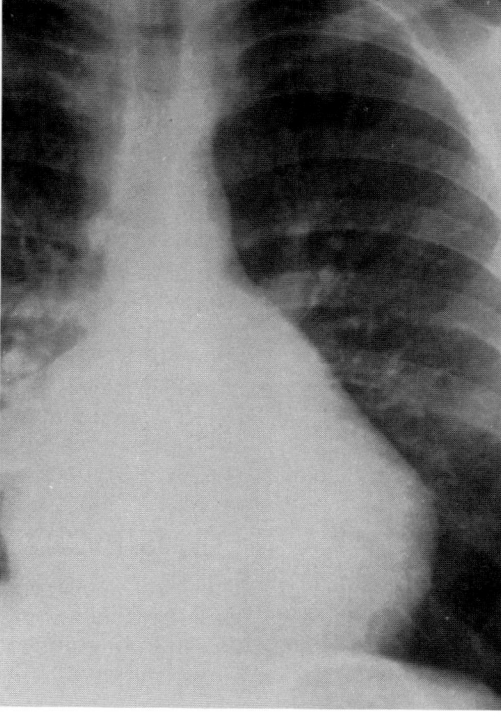

FIGURE 90.6 Chest roentgenogram of a 12-year-old patient referred for treatment of Ebstein's anomaly. Investigation ruled out this malformation but proved cardiomyopathy. Several years earlier the child's mother had been diagnosed as having Ebstein's anomaly, but she and the patient's siblings had familial dilated cardiomyopathy.

tory cases the combination of a large dose of furosemide and a small dose of metolazone may be tried, but this potent combination may lead to symptomatic nitrogen retention and hypovolemia. At one extreme it is essential that the physician not strive for some theoretic construct of the patient's dry weight and on the other not insist on normal concentration of blood urea nitrogen and creatinine. The best compromise is struck by balancing symptoms, the state of hydration, and the degree of congestion to achieve maximum comfort.

Perhaps the most controversial issue in the treatment of dilated cardiomyopathy is the place or lack of it of antiarrhythmic agents. High-grade ventricular arrhythmia is an almost universal occurrence in cardiomyopathy and becomes worse with increasing ventricular dysfunction. Supraventricular arrhythmias are also common. When serious arrhythmia occurs in patients in whom the 1-year prognosis appears favorable, symptoms are not too disabling, and ventricular function is relatively well preserved, every effort should be made to control ventricular arrhythmia, even though proof is lacking that this prevents sudden death. Likewise, symptoms, particularly lightheadedness and syncope, and aggravation of cardiac failure by arrhythmia mandate a serious effort to treat. On the other hand, even though sudden death is common in cardiomyopathy, considerable restraint in attempting to prevent arrhythmia in patients with late or end-stage cardiomyopathy is in order because arrhythmia is the mechanism but not the primary cause of sudden death and may not be preventable by antiarrhythmic drugs. At that stage of the disease, patients have a variety of symptoms and are taking large quantities of inotropic agents, potassium supplements, vasodilators, and diuretics. In such circumstances, it is usually unwise to add other drugs that require multiple dosing and have negative inotropic effects and a variety of cardiac and noncardiac toxic effects. It should also be recalled that these drugs, especially in the presence of electrolyte imbalance, may precipitate the very arrhythmias they are designed to prevent. Theoretically, amiodarone, which has less negative inotropic action than conventional antiarrhythmics, should be the agent of choice, but its severe toxic profile is a major limiting factor. When amiodarone treatment is resorted to, the dose should be kept as low as possible (*e.g.*, 200 mg 5 days per week).

VASODILATORS

Vasodilator treatment is playing an increasing role in the management of heart failure. Intensive research sponsored by the pharmaceutical industry on a large variety of vasodilators having different modes and sites of action has resulted in an extensive literature that need not be detailed in this chapter. However, investigation of vasodilators for the treatment of heart failure is best carried out in patients with myocardial disease but without obstructive valve disease, ongoing ischemia, serious congenital malformations, or cor pulmonale; in other words, the ideal subjects are those with idiopathic dilated cardiomyopathy or so-called ischemic cardiomyopathy. There is thus a large accumulated experience of the effects of vasodilators on dilated cardiomyopathy.

When vasodilators are administered early in the course of flagrant cardiac failure, a dramatic increase in cardiac output and fall in pulmonary wedge pressure can usually be demonstrated. Attempts to verify the continuing effects of these drugs over the ensuing months and years rely principally on serial exercise testing. Many investigators have tried to use echocardiographic and radionuclide indexes of cardiac performance, but the expected changes are too small to be measured meaningfully in individual patients, and indeed it has proved difficult to establish that these drugs continue to benefit the patient over the long term. Other investigators have observed cardiac output, arterial blood pressure, and pulmonary wedge pressure before administering a vasodilator, early after the institution of vasodilator treatment and again some weeks or months later, after which the effects of withdrawal of the vasodilator have also been studied. To date, although a large number of vasodilators are available, only captopril has met the Food and Drug Administration's criteria for safety and efficacy in the treatment of chronic heart failure.

While striking improvement of hemodynamics can be demonstrated with purely arteriolar vasodilators such as hydralazine, venodilators have a more pronounced effect on symptoms and exercise capacity because they reduce ventricular preload. Mixed arteriolar and venodilation can be accomplished by combinations of hydralazine and isosorbide or the administration of mixed vasodilators such as prazosin or captopril. It should be reemphasized that there is a poor correlation between the acute hemodynamic effects of vasodilators and the long-term results. Combined treatment with hydralazine and isosorbide appears to effect a small but statistically significant improvement in survival.[69]

Vasodilators are still sometimes used to treat only refractory heart failure; indeed some of the pharmaceutical houses have required until recently that patients selected for investigation be resistant to treatment with digitalis and diuretics. Administering large doses of digitalis in chronic heart failure is unwise, and excessive reliance on diuretics induces metabolic derangement and may precipitate arrhythmia. Thus, particularly when there is evidence of increased systemic vascular resistance, vasodilators, especially captopril, can be introduced early, and their administration to patients who are not receiving digitalis and who do not require extraordinary doses of a diuretic is rational and appropriate. It may well be that treatment should begin early in the course of the disease with a combination of doses of digoxin, an angiotensin-converting enzyme inhibitor, and a diuretic to obtain maximal benefit with the least incidence of unwanted drug effects.

POSITIVE INOTROPIC AGENTS

In dilated cardiomyopathy, unlike ischemic heart disease, valvular heart disease, and congenital malformations of the heart, there is no role short of cardiac transplantation for surgical treatment. Almost total reliance is therefore placed on pharmacologic treatment. Digitalis is a relatively weak inotropic agent, possibly may not be effective in the long term, and is highly toxic; therefore safer, purer, and stronger inotropic agents are being sought. Success in the treatment of acute heart failure with positive inotropic agents, most of which must be administered intravenously, has stimulated a search for agents that can be administered orally and remain effective for several years. Amrinone was the first and most promising of a new generation of non-glycoside-positive inotropic agents unrelated to the catecholamines. Its introduction was greeted with virtually uncritical enthusiasm, its combination of positive inotropic and vasodilating effects being considered particularly salutary. This enthusiasm, however, has been quickly tempered by the results of long-term studies that show it is not effective in long-term management of heart failure, certainly not in the doses that can be administered before serious side-effects occur,[70] and that in reality it may be nothing more than yet another vasodilator.[71] Intravenous amrinone may be used in the emergency treatment of exacerbations of dilated cardiomyopathy when cardiac failure is severe, with extreme reduction of cardiac output and elevation of pulmonary wedge pressure, but is no longer available for chronic treatment. Milrinone, a newer analogue, is under clinical trial and has been given to a considerable number of patients with dilated cardiomyopathy. In a recent trial,[72] it was shown that milrinone is not superior to digitalis in improving the exercise tolerance of patients with heart failure, making it unlikely that milrinone will displace digotin as a primary drug for heart failure. It is still not known whether it is beneficial, ineffective, or even harmful to chronically administer powerful positive inotropic agents to patients with dilated cardiomyopathy.[73] A number of other positive inotropic agents are also being investigated, principally in patients with dilated cardiomyopathy or ischemic heart failure.

An ingenious approach to treatment is represented by xamoterol, a partial β_1-agonist. The rationale of its use is that when the patient is at rest and sympathetic tone is low, the drug acts as an agonist and is inotropic but during exercise or other conditions of heightened sympathetic tone it acts as an antagonist, thus preventing excessive tachycardia. The role of drugs of this class in the treatment of dilated cardiomyopathy has not yet been worked out.

β-ADRENERGIC BLOCKING AGENTS

Since chronic stimulation of the failing heart muscle with positive inotropic agents may not be possible, or even desirable, much of the treatment of dilated cardiomyopathy is aimed at correcting overcompensation of congestive heart failure. Nowhere is this principle more apparent than in the administration of diuretics. Vasoconstriction triggered by cardiac dilatation and low cardiac output may also be excessive and explain the beneficial effects of reducing arteriolar vascular resistance. Likewise, vasoconstriction, tachycardia, and other manifestations of dilated cardiomyopathy may be explained by overshoot of the response of the sympathetic nervous system; thus it is being proposed that treatment with cardioselective β-adrenergic blocking agents such as metoprolol should decrease symptoms and improve exercise capacity and cardiac performance[74] and even survival.[75] The seeming paradox of treating decompensated dilated cardiomyopathy with an agent that has negative inotropic action may in part be explained by its up-regulation effect on the abnormally down-regulated myocardial β-adrenergic receptors, which characterizes at least a subset of patients with dilated cardiomyopathy.[76] Initiation of this form of treatment is usually best done with the patient in a monitored hospital bed, starting cautiously with small doses of a cardioselective agent such as metoprolol, 5 mg twice a day by mouth. The dosage is slowly increased to the conventional 50 mg twice daily over the ensuing months but must remain lower if the higher dosages are not well tolerated. Although the proper place for treatment of dilated cardiomyopathy with β-adrenergic blocking agents remains to be settled, clinicians will follow with interest the good results that have been reported so far.

REFERENCES

1. Report of the WHO/IFSC task force on the definition and classification of the cardiomyopathies. Br Heart J 44:672, 1980
2. Burch GE, Giles TD, Colcolough HL: Ischemic cardiomyopathy. Am Heart J 79:291, 1970
3. Franciosa JA, Wilen M, Ziesche S et al: Survival in men with severe chronic left ventricular failure due to either coronary heart disease or idiopathic dilated cardiomyopathy. J Am Coll Cardiol 51:831, 1983
4. Goodwin JF, Hollman GH, Gordon H et al: Clinical aspects of cardiomyopathy. Br Med J 1:69, 1961
5. Topol EJ, Traill TA, Fortuin NJ: Hypertensive hypertrophic cardiomyopathy of the elderly. N Engl J Med 312:277, 1985
6. Dec GW Jr, Palacios IF, Fallon JT et al: Active myocarditis in the spectrum of acute dilated cardiomyopathies. N Engl J Med 312:885, 1985
7. Goodwin JF: The frontiers of cardiomyopathy. Br Heart J 48:1, 1982
8. Lie JT: Myocarditis and endomyocardial biopsy in unexplained heart failure. Ann Intern Med 109:525, 1988
9. Eckstein R, Mempel W, Bolte HD: Reduced suppressor cell activity in congestive cardiomyopathy and myocarditis. Circulation 65:1224, 1982
10. Sanderson JE, Koech D, Iha D et al: T-lymphocyte subsets in idiopathic dilated cardiomyopathy. Am J Cardiol 55:755, 1985
11. Ahmed SS, Howard M, Hove W et al: Cardiac function in alcoholics with cirrhosis. Absence of overt cardiomyopathy—myth or fact? J Am Coll Cardiol 3:696, 1984
12. Regan TJ: Alcoholic cardiomyopathy. Prog Cardiovasc Dis 27:141, 1984
13. Regan TJ, Levinson GE, Olderwurtal HA et al: Ventricular function in non cardiac with alcoholic fatty liver: Role of alcohol in the production of cardiomyopathy. J Clin Invest 48:397, 1969
14. Demakis JG, Rahimtoola SH: Peripartum cardiomyopathy. Circulation 44:964, 1971
15. Homans DC: Peripartum cardiomyopathy. N Engl J Med 312:1432, 1985
16. Alexander CS: Cobalt-beer cardiomyopathy. Am J Med 53:395, 1972
17. Fein FS, Strobeck JE, Malhorta A et al: Reversibility of diabetic cardiomyopathy with insulin in rats. Circ Res 49:1251, 1981
18. Alexander JK: The cardiomyopathy of obesity. Prog Cardiovasc Dis 27:325, 1985
19. Zee-Cheng CS, Tsai CC, Palmer DC et al: High incidence of myocarditis by endomyocardial biopsy in patients with idiopathic congestive cardiomyopathy. J Am Coll Cardiol 3:63, 1984
20. Aretz HT, Billingham ME, Edwards WD et al: Myocarditis: Histopathologic definition and classification. Am J Cardiovasc Pathol 1:3, 1987
21. Poll DS, Marchlinski FE, Buxton AE et al: Sustained ventricular tachycardia in patients with idiopathic dilated cardiomyopathy: Electrophysiologic testing and lack of response to antiarrhythmic therapy. Circulation 7:451, 1984
22. Opherk D, Schwartz F, Mall G et al: Coronary dilatory capacity in idiopathic dilated cardiomyopathy: Analysis of 15 patients. Circulation 51:1657, 1983
23. Poole-Wilson PA: Causes of symptoms in chronic congestive heart failure and implications of treatment. Am J Cardiol 62:31A, 1988
24. Wiener DH, Maris J, Chance B et al: Detection of skeletal muscle hypoperfusion during exercise using phosphorus-31 nuclear magnetic resonance spectroscopy. J Am Coll Cardiol 12:353, 1986
25. Guilleminault C, Connoly SJ, Winkle RA: Cardiac arrhythmia and conduction disturbance during sleep in 400 patients with sleep apnea syndrome. Am J Cardiol 52:490, 1983
26. Julian DG, Szekely P: Peripartum cardiomyopathy. Prog Cardiovasc Dis 27:223, 1985
27. Engler RL, Ray R, Higgins CB: Clinical assessment and followup of patients with chronic congestive cardiomyopathy. Am J Cardiol 49:1832, 1982
28. Johnson AD, Laiken SL, Shabetai R: Non-invasive diagnosis of ischemic cardiomyopathy by fluoroscopic detection of coronary artery calcification. Am Heart J 96:521, 1978
29. Goldberger AL, Dresselhaus T, Bhargava V: Dilated cardiomyopathy: Utility of the transverse: Frontal plane QRS voltage ratio. J Electrocardiol 18:35, 1980
30. Meinertz, Hofman T, Kasper W: Significance of ventricular arrhythmia in idiopathic dilated cardiomyopathy. Am J Cardiol 53:902, 1985
31. Stamato NJ, O'Connell JB, Murdock DK et al: The response of patients with complex ventricular arrhythmias secondary to dilated cardiomyopathy to programmed electrical stimulation. Am Heart J 112:505, 1986
32. Lew W, Henning G, Schelbert H: Assessment of mitral valve E point–septal separation as an index of left ventricular performance in patients with acute and previous myocardial infarction. Am J Cardiol 41:836, 1978
33. Greenberg JM, Murphy JH, Okada AD et al: Value and limitations of radionuclide angiography in determining the cause of reduced left ventricular ejection fraction: Comparison of idiopathic DCM and coronary artery disease. Am J Cardiol 55:541, 1985
34. Gardin JM, Iseri LT, Elkayan U et al: Evaluation of dilated cardiomyopathy by pulsed Doppler echocardiography. Am Heart J 106:1057, 1983
35. Bryhn M: Abnormal left ventricular filling in patients with sustained myocardial relaxation: Assessment of diastolic parameters using radionuclide angiography and echocardiography. Clin Cardiol 7:639, 1984
36. Takenaka K, Dabestani A, Gardin J et al: Pulsed Doppler echocardiographic study of left ventricular filling in dilated cardiomyopathy. Am J Cardiol 58:143, 1986
37. Lee WH, Packer M: Prognostic importance of serum sodium concentration and its modification by converting enzyme inhibition in patients with severe chronic heart failure. Circulation 73:257, 1986
38. Franciosa JA, Konkman WB, Leddy CL: Hemodynamic effects of vasodilators and long-term response in heart failure. J Am Coll Cardiol 3:1521, 1984
39. Boltwood CM Jr, Shah PM: The pericardium in health and disease. Curr Probl Cardiol 9(5):10, 1984
40. Goodwin JF, Roberts WC, Wenger NK: Cardiomyopathy. In Hurst JW (ed): The Heart, p 1307. New York: McGraw-Hill, 1982
41. Caves PK, Stinson EB, Billingham ME et al: Percutaneous transvenous endomyocardial biopsy in human heart recipients: Experience with a new technique. Ann Thorac Surg 16:325, 1973
42. Brooksby IAB, Swanton RH, Jenkins BS et al: Long sheath technique for introduction of catheter tip manometer or endomyocardial bioptome into the right or left ventricle. Br Heart J 36:908, 1974
43. Fowles RE, Mason JW: Role of cardiac biopsy in the diagnosis and management of cardiac disease. Prog Cardiovasc Dis 27:153, 1984
44. Fenoglio JJ Jr, Ursell PC, Kellog CF et al: Diagnosis and classification of myocarditis by endomyocardial biopsy. N Engl J Med 308:12, 1983
45. Daly K, Richardson PJ, Olsen EGJ et al: Acute myocarditis: Role of histological and virological examination in the diagnosis and assessment of immunosuppressive treatment. Br Heart J 51:30, 1984
46. Mason J: Endomyocardial biopsy: The balance of success and failure. Circulation 71:185, 1985
47. Strain JE, Grose RM, Factor SM et al: Results of endomyocardial biopsy in patients with spontaneous ventricular tachycardia but without apparent structural heart disease. Circulation 68:1171, 1983
48. Chow LC, Dittrich HC, Shabetai R: Endomyocardial biopsy in patients with unexplained congestive heart failure. Ann Intern Med 109:535, 1988
49. Wenger NK, Mattson ME, Furberg CD: Assessment of quality of life in clinical trials of cardiovascular therapies. Am J Cardiol 54:908, 1984
50. Lipkin DP, Canepa-Anson R, Stephens MR et al: Factors determining symptoms in heart failure: Comparison of fast and slow exercise tests. Br Heart J 55:439, 1986
51. Matsumura N, Nishuimah KS: Determination of anaerobic threshold for as-

52. Franciosa JA, Park M, Levine TB: Lack of correlation between exercise capacity and indexes of left ventricular performance in heart failure. Am J Cardiol 47:33, 1981
53. Litchfield RL, Kerber RE, Benge W et al: Normal exercise capacity in patients with severe left ventricular dysfunction: Compensatory mechanisms. Circulation 66:129, 1982
54. Baker BJ, Wilen MM, Boyd CM et al: Relation of right ventricular ejection fraction to exercise capacity in chronic left ventricular failure. Am J Cardiol 54:596, 1984
55. Cohn JN, Rector TS: Prognosis of congestive heart failure and predictors of mortality. Am J Cardiol 62:25A, 1988
56. Wilson JR, Schwarz S, St. John Sutton M et al: Prognosis in severe heart failure. Relation to hemodynamic measurements and ventricular ectopic activity. J Am Coll Cardiol 2:403, 1983
57. Unverferth DV, Magorien RD, Moeschberger ML et al: Factors influencing the one year mortality of dilated cardiomyopathy. Am J Cardiol 54:147, 1984
58. Schwartz F, Mall G, Horst Z et al: Determinants of survival in patients with congestive cardiomyopathy: Quantitative morphologic findings and left ventricular hemodynamics. Circulation 70:923, 1984
59. Figula HR, Rahlf G, Nieger M et al: Spontaneous hemodynamic improvement of stabilization and associated biopsy findings in patients with congestive cardiomyopathy. Circulation 71:1095, 1985
60. Goodwin JF: Overview and classification of the cardiomyopathies. In Shaver JA (ed): Cardiomyopathies, Clinical Presentation, Differential Diagnosis and Management. Philadelphia, F.A. Davis, 1988
61. Wilson JR: Use of antiarrhythmic drugs in patients with heart failure: Clinical efficacy, hemodynamic results and relation to survival. Circulation (suppl IV):IV-64, 1987
62. Meinertz T, Hofmann T, Kasper W: Significance of ventricular arrhythmias in idiopathic dilated cardiomyopathy. Am J Cardiol 53:902, 1984
63. Huang SK, Messer JV, Dewes P: Significance of ventricular tachycardia in idiopathic dilated cardiomyopathy: Observations in 35 patients. Am J Cardiol 51:507, 1983
64. Cohn JN, Levine TB, Olivari MT et al: Plasma norepinephrine as a guide to prognosis in patients with congestive heart failure. N Engl J Med 311:819, 1984
65. Marcus FI, Fontaine GH, Guiraudon G et al: Right ventricular dysplasia: A report of 24 adult cases. Circulation 65:384, 1982
66. Soufer R, Wohlgelernter D, Vita NA et al: Intact systolic left ventricular function in clinical congestive heart failure. Am J Cardiol 55:1032, 1985
67. Burch GE, Walsh JJ, Ferrans VJ et al: Prolonged bed rest in the treatment of the dilated heart. Circulation 32:852, 1965
68. Mulrow CD, Feussner JR, Valez R et al: Reevaluation of digitalis efficacy. Ann Intern Med 101:113, 1984
69. Cohn JN, Archibald DG, Ziesche S et al: Effect of vasodilator therapy on mortality in congestive heart failure: Results of a Veterans Administration co-operative study. N Engl J Med 314:1547, 1986
70. Dibianco R, Shabetai R, Silverman BD: Oral amrinone for the treatment of chronic congestive heart failure: Results of a multicenter randomized double-blind and placebo controlled withdrawal study. J Am Coll Cardiol 4:855, 1984
71. Wilmshurst PT, Thompson DS, Jenkins BS et al: The hemodynamic effects of intravenous amrinone in patients with impaired left ventricular function. Br Heart J 49:77, 1983
72. DiBianco R, Shabetai R, Kostuk W: A comparison of oral milrinone, digohn and their combination in the treatment of patients with chronic heart failure. N Engl J Med 320:677, 1989
73. Packer M, Medina M, Yushak M: Hemodynamic and clinical limitations of long-term inotropic therapy with amrinone in patients with severe chronic heart failure. Circulation 70:1038, 1984
74. Waagstein F, Hjalmarson A, Swederg K et al: Beta-blockers in dilated cardiomyopathy: They work. Eur Heart J 4(suppl A):173, 1983
75. Swedberg K, Waagstein F, Hjalmarson A et al: Prolongation of survival in congestive cardiomyopathy by beta receptor blockade. Lancet 1:1347, 1979
76. Fowler MB, Bristow MR, Laser JA et al: Beta blocker therapy in severe heart failure: Improvement related to beta adrenergic receptor up regulation? Circulation 70(suppl II):II–112, 1984

HYPERTROPHIC CARDIOMYOPATHY

E. Douglas Wigle

Although pathologic descriptions of hypertrophic cardiomyopathy (HCM) were reported in the mid-nineteenth century, it remained for the virtually simultaneous reports of Brock in 1957 and Teare in 1958 to draw modern attention to this entity.[1,2] In the ensuing quarter of a century, a remarkable fascination for the various features of this condition has developed and has intrigued many investigators involved in the cardiovascular sciences. As a result of the intense interest, great strides have been made in our understanding of this entity, but many basic questions remained unanswered and/or debated. Thus, what is the cause and significance of myocardial fiber disarray? Do the systolic pressure gradients indicate hemodynamically significant obstruction? What determines the rate of relaxation and the diastolic filling characteristics of these hypertrophied ventricles? Which patients are at risk of atrial and ventricular arrhythmias and why? What constitutes optimal therapy for the different clinical and pathophysiologic manifestations of HCM? What factors determine prognosis? These are but a few of the important questions that have been debated over the years and must be answered if patient management is to be scientifically based and optimal.

HCM was basically a clinical and hemodynamic entity in the early 1960's and most cases were recognized because of symptoms of angina, dyspnea, and/or syncope, occurring in patients with an apical systolic murmur and an intraventricular pressure gradient. Thus, the systolic abnormalities held the focus of attention at that time, although, from the very beginning, it was clearly recognized that abnormal diastolic function was important,[3,4] and indeed could be the dominant pathophysiologic abnormality.[4] The use of various pharmacologic agents to manipulate the severity of the intraventricular pressure gradient and to elucidate its mechanism was popular in the 1960's.[5,6] In the 1970's the introduction of first one- and then two-dimensional echocardiography focused attention on the causes of ventricular septal hypertrophy[7] and the significance of systolic anterior motion of the anterior[8] (or posterior[9]) mitral leaflet. More recently a number of studies have reported on the extent of hypertrophy that may be encountered in HCM.[10,11] The correlation of echocardiographic and hemodynamic parameters has further elucidated the pathophysiologic features in both systole and diastole.[12-14] Nuclear cardiologic studies have been particularly helpful in clarifying the abnormalities of systolic and diastolic function and the effect of drug interventions thereon.[15,16] Studies using Doppler techniques and velocity flow measurements have focused attention on the systolic ejection profiles in the different hemodynamic subgroups of HCM,[17,18] while indicator dilution and Doppler techniques have elucidated the relation of the mitral regurgitation to the presence of the outflow tract obstruction and the occurrence of systolic anterior motion of the mitral leaflets.[11] Clearly, the technological explosion that has occurred in cardiology in the past 25 years has expedited our understanding and appreciation of HCM in all of its many aspects. At the same time, no other cardiologic entity has had an equivalent constellation of pathophysiologic abnormalities suitable for investigation by the currently available investigative techniques of cardiology. It is as though HCM and modern cardiologic technology were "meant for each other." Undoubtedly, nuclear magnetic resonance

TABLE 91.1 TYPES OF HYPERTROPHIC CARDIOMYOPATHY

	Approximate Incidence* (%)
Left Ventricular Involvement	
Asymmetrical hypertrophy	
Ventricular septal hypertrophy	90
Midventricular hypertrophy	1
Apical hypertrophy	3
Posteroseptal and/or lateral wall hypertrophy	1
Symmetrical (concentric) hypertrophy	5
Right Ventricular Involvement	

* At the Toronto General Hospital. The incidence of the different types of hypertrophic cardiomyopathy varies considerably among different centers.

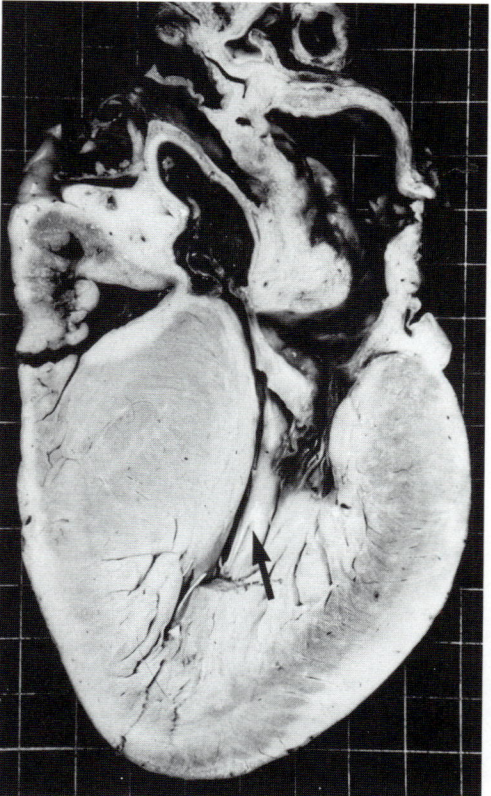

FIGURE 91.1 Longitudinal section of the heart of a 32-year-old woman with hypertrophic obstructive cardiomyopathy who died suddenly while on propranolol therapy. Hemodynamic investigation had confirmed the presence of muscular subaortic stenosis as well as mitral regurgitation that was partially due to an abnormal mitral valve (insertion of anomalous papillary muscle (arrow) onto the ventricular surface of a fibrotic anterior mitral leaflet). Note asymmetrical hypertrophy with grossly thickened ventricular septum and a narrowed outflow tract between the upper septum and anterior mitral leaflet. (Reprinted, by permission, from Silver MD (ed): Cardiovascular Pathology, p 499. New York, Churchill Livingstone, 1983. Original specimen courtesy of Dr. L. Horlick, Saskatoon, Saskatchewan)

imaging, positron emission tomography, and other developing techniques will also contribute to the further elucidation of the still-unresolved problems of HCM in the years to come.

DEFINITION

HCM may be defined as ventricular hypertrophy without identifiable cause that is usually, but not always, associated with microscopic evidence of myocardial fiber disarray.[11] Although the left ventricle is the predominant site of involvement, right ventricular involvement may occur in apparent isolation or in association with left-sided involvement. Table 91.1 lists the presently known varieties of HCM and their approximate incidence.

OCCURRENCE AND MODE OF INHERITANCE

HCM is believed to occur in both sporadic and familial forms. By history, about two thirds of cases appear to be sporadic and one third familial, and the condition appears to affect males twice as often as females. Autosomal dominance has generally been accepted as the mode of inheritance. A recent study of 70 family pedigrees indicated that HCM was genetically transmitted in 55% and occurred sporadically in 44%.[19] No single mode of inheritance was typical, suggesting that HCM may not be a single etiologically distinct disease entity. However, autosomal dominant transmission was most common, being evident in 76% of family pedigrees. It is of note that different types of HCM (Table 91.1) may occur in the same pedigree, and a history of sudden death may be very common in some families but not in others. The degree of penetrance may vary considerably between families. Several groups of authors have suggested that there is both association and linkage between the HLA complex and HCM, but others have not been able to confirm this.

PATHOLOGY

In his original description of the pathology of asymmetrical hypertrophy of the heart, Teare described nine patients, all of whom at postmortem examination were reported to have ventricular septal hypertrophy (Fig. 91.1).[2] In five of the nine cases, the hypertrophy extended into the anterolateral wall of the left ventricle. As a result of subsequent pathologic and two-dimensional echocardiographic observations, it has been recognized that the extent of septal hypertrophy may vary tremendously between patients and that HCM may infrequently present as concentric, apical, midventricular, or rarer forms of cardiac hypertrophy (Table 91.1, Fig. 91.2). Since HCM is due to ventricular (asymmetrical) septal hypertrophy in 90% of cases in the author's experience (Table 91.1), in this discussion the term HCM is equated with this form of asymmetrical hypertrophy, unless otherwise specified (such as when apical, midventricular, or concentric hypertrophy is discussed).

Microscopically, Teare noticed short, plump, hypertrophic myocardial fibers in apparent disarray, interspersed with loose intercellular connective tissue in the involved areas of the myocardium (Fig. 91.3).[2] This loosely arranged connective tissue appears at times to undergo transformation to dense fibrous tissue, a change that would have obvious implications regarding both systolic and diastolic function of the left ventricle. The extent, distribution, and indeed the very significance of myocardial fiber disarray have at times been hotly debated. Earlier reports suggested that disarray was a relatively sensitive and specific marker for HCM, but subsequently it has been shown that myocardial fiber disarray may occur in certain well-defined locations in developing and normal hearts, as well as in other forms of heart disease. Present evidence would suggest that there is usually, but not always, a quantitative difference between the extent of myocardial fiber disarray that is seen in HCM and that encountered in normals or in other forms of heart disease. Thus, patients with HCM usually have extensive myocardial fiber disarray (although 5% have none), whereas the degree of myocardial fiber disarray in other conditions (with the possible exception of aortic and pulmonary atresia) is not only limited, but is usually restricted to certain sites in the myocardium such as the junction of the free wall with the ventricular septum, at the left ventricular apex, and in the subaortic area.[20,21]

The cause and significance of myocardial fiber disarray is unknown. Goodwin has championed the view that an abnormality of catecholamine metabolism may account for some of the pathophysiologic abnormalities of HCM.[22] Perloff has reviewed this subject extensively and has suggested that a supersensitivity to catecholamines may result in a failure of regression of fetal myocardial fiber disarray and septal hypertrophy.[23] It has been suggested that myocardial fiber disarray causes isometric contraction and leads to myocardial hypertrophy.[23] Workers from Johns Hopkins University have, however, suggested the opposite, that is, that isometric contraction causes myocardial fiber disarray and thence hypertrophy.[21] These investigators have suggested that the myocardial fiber disarray seen in aortic or pulmonary atresia or in the septum in HCM is the result of isometric contraction.[21] These differences of opinion are unresolved.

Some authors have suggested that myocardial fiber disarray may be genetically determined, in which case the observation that there is an alteration of the nonhistone nuclear proteins that affect gene expression in myocardial tissue removed at the time of surgery may be of importance.[24] Similar changes in these proteins have been reported in the genetically determined hamster cardiomyopathy. A primary calcium overload of the myocardial cells in HCM has also been postulated. Myocardial fiber disarray may play a role in the observed incoordination of systolic and diastolic function, in the impaired relaxation in diastole, and in the genesis of ventricular arrhythmias that are so characteristic of HCM. The precise significance of myocardial fiber disarray is, however, unknown at this time.

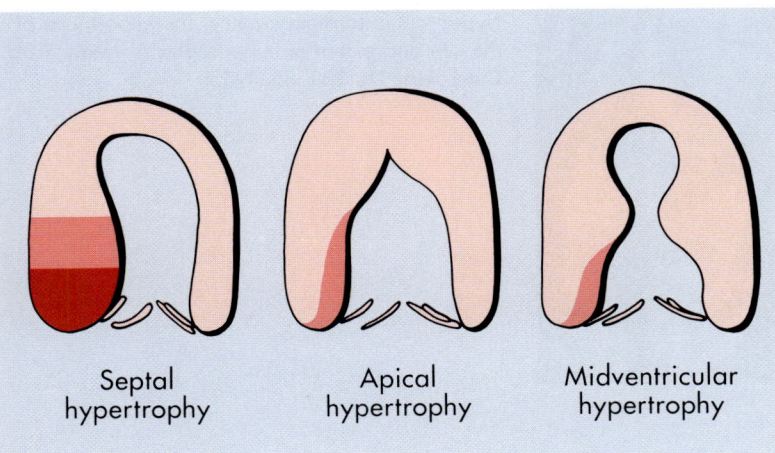

FIGURE 91.2 Diagrammatic representation of three common varieties of asymmetrical hypertrophy of left ventricle as they would be seen in the apical four chamber view of a two-dimensional echocardiogram. Septal hypertrophy may involve only the basal one third of the septum (subaortic area) or it may involve the basal two thirds of the septum (down to papillary muscles) or the hypertrophy may extend from base to apex, involving the whole septum. In apical hypertrophy the principal involvement is in the apical one third of the ventricle and there may be considerable asymmetry in this area. The apical hypertrophy may extend up the septum toward the base in which case obstruction to outflow may occur. In midventricular hypertrophy the maximal thickening occurs at the level of the papillary muscles. Basal septal hypertrophy may also occur in this variety of hypertrophic cardiomyopathy and thus give rise to muscular subaortic stenosis, as well as midventricular obstruction (see Tables 91.1 and 91.3 and Fig. 914). (Modified from Wigle ED, Sasson Z, Henderson M, et al: Hypertrophic cardiomyopathy: The importance of the site and extent of hypertrophy. A review. Prog Cardiovasc Dis 28:1, 1985)

Just as myocardial fiber disarray is not specific for HCM, neither is a disproportionately thickened ventricular septum.[7] Disproportionate septal thickening has been recognized in fetal and neonatal hearts, in athletes, and in many forms of congenital and acquired heart disease. The *de novo* development of HCM has been reported following aortic valve replacement surgery.[25] In most but not all of these instances of septal hypertrophy, there is a developmental, pathologic, or hemodynamic reason for its development. Systolic overload of the left ventricle because of aortic valve stenosis or systemic hypertension is probably the commonest cause of disproportionate septal thickening other than HCM itself.

DISTRIBUTION OF HYPERTROPHY BY ECHOCARDIOGRAPHY

As indicated, two-dimensional echocardiography has contributed significantly to our knowledge of the pathologic anatomy of HCM (Table 91.1, Figs. 91.2, 91.4).[11] This technique has been particularly useful in the recognition of the different varieties of the HCM spectrum including the site and extent of hypertrophy in the different types (Table 91.1, Figs. 91.2, 91.4). Figure 91.2 indicates diagrammatically the apical four-chamber, two-dimensional echocardiographic appearance of three varieties of HCM—septal, apical, and midventricular hypertrophy. Figures 91.2 and 91.4 indicate the variable extent of ventricular (asymmetrical) septal hypertrophy that was encountered in a study of 100 cases of this entity, as defined by one-dimensional echocardiographic criteria (ventricular septum $\geq$ 15 mm, septal-posterior wall ratio $\geq$ 1.5:1).[11] Figure 91.4 indicates that in 25% of cases the septal hypertrophy was localized to the basal septum (subaortic area); in approximately 25% of cases the septal hypertrophy extended down to the papillary muscles (basal two thirds of the septum); and in approximately 50% of cases, the hypertrophy involved the whole septum from base to apex.[11] Anterolateral wall extension of the hypertrophy was not seen with localized subaortic hypertrophy, whereas it was seen in 91% of cases when the whole septum was hypertrophied (Fig. 91.4). These studies indicate that the extent of hypertrophy is extremely variable in HCM with predominantly septal involvement. This is an important observation in that there is now evidence to suggest that the extent of hypertrophy is an important determinant of many of the manifestations of this disorder.[11]

HEMODYNAMIC CLASSIFICATION

HCM may be classified into hemodynamic subgroups according to the presence or absence of obstruction to left ventricular outflow (Table 91.2). In this respect, the terms *muscular subaortic stenosis* and *resting obstruction* are synonymous with the terms *idiopathic hypertrophic subaortic stenosis* (IHSS) and *hypertrophic obstructive cardiomyopathy* (HOCM).

A patient with resting obstruction consistently has a pressure gradient across the left ventricular outflow tract at rest that is caused by mitral leaflet-septal contact. Labile obstruction is the situation in which the left ventricular outflow tract pressure gradient appears to come and go for no apparent reason, and in our experience is relatively rare. In some patients this lability may be explained by changing afterload or contractility; in other patients, however, the lability may be more apparent than real and be due to inadvertent movement of a retrograde catheter from a high- to a low-pressure area in the left ventricle. In latent obstruction there is no pressure gradient at rest, but one appears with suitable provocation such as amyl nitrite inhalation, isoproterenol infusion, or in the postextrasystolic beat. In nonobstructive HCM there is no pressure gradient across the left ventricular outflow tract at rest or on provocation. In midventricular obstruction, the pressure gradient occurs at the level of the papillary muscles and is due to muscular occlusion at the midventricular level (Fig. 91.2).[11] This form of obstruction is not due to mitral leaflet-septal contact. Although this hemodynamic classification does not take into account the diastolic properties of the left ventricle, it has both clinical and therapeutic implications based on the presence or absence of obstruction to left ventricular outflow and the concomitant mitral regurgitation.

CORRELATION BETWEEN THE EXTENT OF HYPERTROPHY AND THE HEMODYNAMIC SUBGROUPS

The variable extent of septal and anterolateral wall hypertrophy in HCM has been described, and the different hemodynamic subgroups defined, elsewhere. It is important now to indicate the extent of hypertrophy that is encountered in the different hemodynamic subgroups of HCM. Table 91.3 indicates that latent obstruction is associated with

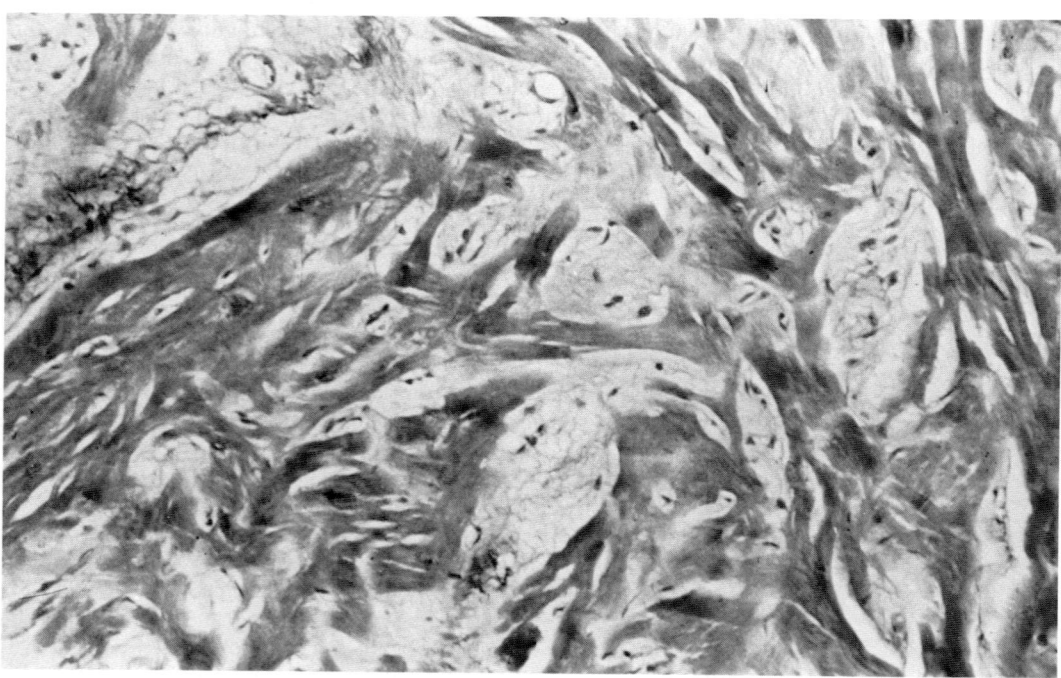

FIGURE 91.3 Microscopic section taken from the ventricular septum of a 28-year-old patient with hypertrophic cardiomyopathy who died suddenly while jogging. The section shows a typical area of myocardial fiber disarray with the fibers running in various directions. The nuclei are large and hyperchromatic. Note the extensive amount of loose intercellular connective tissue (Original magnification $\times$ 100) (Reprinted, with permission, from Wigle ED, Sasson Z, Henderson M, et al: Hypertrophic cardiomyopathy: The importance of the site and extent of hypertrophy. A review. Prog Cardiovasc Dis 28:1–83, 1985)

localized subaortic hypertrophy, involving the basal one third of the septum, in 53% of instances. In 35% of cases of latent obstruction, the hypertrophy extends down to the papillary muscles, involving the basal two thirds of the ventricular septum. Thus, in 88% of cases of the latent form of subaortic obstruction, the hypertrophy involves the basal one third to two thirds of the septum. The whole length of the septum is involved in only 12% of latent cases.[11]

Precisely the opposite situation prevails in resting obstruction in which 72% of patients have involvement of the entire length of the ventricular septum and only 8% have the localized subaortic form of hypertrophy (Table 91.3).[11] The extent of the hypertrophy in nonobstructive HCM is similar to, but somewhat less than, that seen in resting obstruction (Table 91.3). These differences in the extent of hypertrophy in the different hemodynamic subgroups of HCM become even more dramatic when it is recalled that full-length septal hypertrophy is associated with hypertrophy extending into the anterolateral wall in 91% of instances, whereas localized subaortic hypertrophy is not associated with this extension (Fig. 91.4). These truly dramatic differences in the extent of hypertrophy in the three major hemodynamic subgroups of HCM go a long way toward explaining the different clinical manifestations and courses of these patients. Thus, patients with latent obstruction and localized subaortic hypertrophy have normal left ventricular diastolic filling characteristics, a low incidence of atrial and ventricular arrhythmias, and a good prognosis. Patients with resting obstruction and nonobstructive HCM, with more extensive hypertrophy, have problems with poor relaxation and low compliance in diastole, a higher incidence of atrial and ventricular arrhythmias, and a poorer prognosis.[11] Latent obstruction has often been thought of as being somewhere between nonobstructive HCM and resting obstruction, which it is in terms of left ventricular outflow tract obstruction. In terms of the extent of hypertrophy, however, most patients with latent obstruction are very much at the mild end of the HCM spectrum, whereas those with resting obstruction are at the severe end of the spectrum, with the nonobstructive HCM patients being somewhere between.[11]

MECHANISM OF THE OBSTRUCTIVE SUBAORTIC PRESSURE GRADIENT AND MITRAL REGURGITATION IN MUSCULAR SUBAORTIC STENOSIS

MECHANISM OF MITRAL LEAFLET SYSTOLIC ANTERIOR MOTION

My concept of the mechanism for the outflow tract obstruction and mitral regurgitation in HCM is depicted in Figure 91.5.[6,11]

In muscular subaortic stenosis, the outflow tract is narrowed by ventricular septal hypertrophy. As a result, early systolic ejection is rapid (and unobstructed) and the ejection path passes closer to the mitral leaflets than is normal. Systolic anterior motion of the anterior (or posterior) mitral leaflets results from a Venturi effect on these leaflets caused by the rapid early ejection.[6] The obstruction to outflow results from subsequent mitral leaflet–septal contact. The mitral regurgitation is caused by the mitral leaflets being out of their normally closed position during systole (Fig. 91.5).

Evidence supporting the concept that a Venturi effect or similar hydrodynamic mechanism is the cause of systolic anterior motion of the mitral leaflets is as follows:

1. HCM patients with outflow tract obstruction have thicker septa and narrower outflow tracts than do patients without obstruction, setting the stage for a Venturi effect to be operative.[26,27]

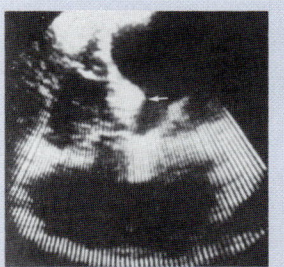
A. Localized (Subaortic)

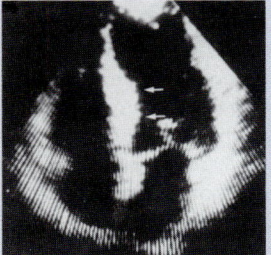
B. To Papillary Muscles

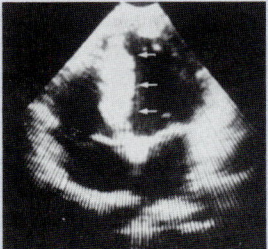
C. To Apex

FIGURE 91.4 Apical four-chamber two-dimensional echocardiographic views of the variable extent of septal hypertrophy that may be encountered in hypertrophic cardiomyopathy. The horizontal arrows point to the extent of hypertrophy in each instance. Septal hypertrophy may involve (**A**) the basal one third of the septum (localized subaortic hypertrophy) in 25% of cases, or (**B**) the basal two thirds of the septum (extending down to the papillary muscles) in 25% of cases, or (**C**) the whole septum from base to apex in approximately 50% of cases. Anterolateral wall extension of the hypertrophy was not seen with localized subaortic hypertrophy (**A**) but was seen in 35% of cases when the hypertrophy involved the basal two thirds of the septum (**B**) and in 91% of cases when the whole septum was hypertrophied (**C**). (Reprinted, with permission, from Wigle ED, Sasson Z, Henderson M, et al: Hypertrophic cardiomyopathy: The importance of the site and extent of hypertrophy. A review. Prog Cardiovasc Dis 28:1–83, 1985)

TABLE 91.2 HEMODYNAMIC CLASSIFICATION OF HYPERTROPHIC CARDIOMYOPATHY

Resting obstruction	Midventricular obstruction
Labile obstruction	Nonobstructive hypertrophic
Latent obstruction	cardiomyopathy

TABLE 91.3 EXTENT OF VENTRICULAR SEPTAL HYPERTROPHY RELATED TO THE HEMODYNAMIC SUBGROUPS IN 100 CASES OF HYPERTROPHIC CARDIOMYOPATHY*

Hemodynamic Subgroup	Number of Cases	Extent of Septal Hypertrophy (%)	
Latent obstruction	34	Basal 1/3	18 53
		Basal 2/3	12 35
		Whole septum	4 12
Nonobstructive Hypertrophic Cardiomyopathy	27	Basal 1/3	4 14
		Basal 2/3	7 26
		Whole septum	16 59
Resting obstruction	39	Basal 1/3	3 8
		Basal 2/3	8 20
		Whole septum	28 72

* The presence of ventricular septal hypertrophy was determined by one-dimensional echocardiographic criteria (see text). The extent of septal hypertrophy was determined by two-dimensional echocardiography. Hemodynamic subgrouping was carried out by means of combined transseptal and retrograde left heart catheterization.

2. Using a modeled left ventricle to reproduce the situation in muscular subaortic stenosis, Bellhouse and Bellhouse demonstrated that when the ejection jet was rapid and close enough to the mitral leaflets, the latter demonstrated systolic anterior motion.[28]
3. Ventriculomyectomy operation, by thinning the septum and widening the outflow tract, reduces the ejection velocity and displaces the path of ejection away from the mitral leaflets, thus reducing the Venturi forces on these leaflets and abolishing systolic anterior motion, the obstruction to outflow, and the mitral regurgitation. A laterally placed myectomy incision results in the abolition of systolic anterior motion laterally where the outflow tract has been widened, but not medially, where the outflow tract remains narrowed.[11]
4. A Venturi mechanism can also explain systolic anterior motion associated with concentric left ventricular hypertrophy, abnormally long mitral leaflets, mitral annular calcification, or tissue mitral valve prostheses, as well as hyperkinetic ventricles.[11]
5. Any known maneuver that can affect the pressure gradient in muscular subaortic stenosis can be explained by the Venturi mechanism causing systolic anterior motion of the mitral leaflets.[11] Preload, afterload, and contractility affect the stroke volume of normal persons and also affect the degree of systolic anterior motion and the pressure gradient magnitude in muscular subaortic stenosis. Diminished afterload or increased contractility would increase the early ejection velocity, which in turn would increase the Venturi forces on the anterior mitral leaflet and thus increase systolic anterior motion, the pressure gradient, and the mitral regurgitation (Fig. 91.6). Increased afterload or diminished contractility would reduce early systolic velocity and the Venturi forces on the anterior mitral leaflet, and consequently would reduce or abolish systolic anterior motion, the pressure gradient, and the mitral regurgitation (Fig. 91.6). Preload could affect these events by increasing or decreasing the anatomical size of the left ventricular outflow tract. The intensification of mitral systolic anterior motion, the pressure gradient, and mitral regurgitation in the postextrasystolic beat can be explained by the increased contractility (postextrasystolic potentiation) and decreased afterload (lower aortic diastolic pressure after the long pause) predominating over the increased preload (which would tend to lessen mitral systolic anterior motion).[11]

As a result of the above considerations, Venturi forces acting on the mitral leaflets would appear to be the most plausible explanation for the phenomenon of systolic anterior motion of these leaflets in muscular subaortic stenosis. It is not known whether maintenance of mitral leaflet-septal contact is due to continued Venturi effect on the mitral leaflets, or to hydrodynamic factors. The fact that mitral leaflet-septal contact ceases at approximately 75% of the systolic ejection period could be due to late systolic reduction in ejection velocity (reducing the Venturi forces) or to decreasing left ventricular systolic pressure.[11,13]

A number of other mechanisms to explain systolic anterior motion of the mitral leaflets have been suggested; these include papillary muscle contraction tethering the leaflets against the septum, as well as the leaflets being pushed anteriorly by posterior wall hyperkinesis, or the phenomenon of cavity obliteration.[29] If any of these contraction mechanisms were responsible for systolic anterior motion and mitral leaflet-septal contact, then leaflet-septal contact should be present until the end of contraction, that is, until end systole. Echocardiographic observations, however, indicate that mitral leaflet-septal contact ceases well before end systole (Fig. 91.7), rendering these mechanisms unlikely if not untenable. In addition, systolic anterior motion bears no relation to inward movement of the posterior wall of the left ventricle.[13]

EVIDENCE THAT MITRAL LEAFLET-SEPTAL CONTACT CAUSES THE PRESSURE GRADIENT AND MITRAL REGURGITATION

1. Patients with resting obstruction have severe systolic anterior motion of the mitral leaflet(s) in which mitral leaflet-septal contact exists for greater than 30% of echocardiographic systole. Patients with latent or no obstruction have no, mild, or at most, moderate systolic anterior motion.[8,26,27]
2. Simultaneous hemodynamic and echocardiographic studies indicate that the onset of the pressure gradient (defined as the peak of the aortic percussion wave) occurs virtually simultaneously with the onset of mitral leaflet-septal contact (Fig. 91.7).[13] Furthermore, the time of onset and duration of mitral leaflet-septal contact determines the magnitude of the pressure gradient.[11,14] Thus, large pressure gradients are associated with early and prolonged mitral leaflet-septal contact, whereas small pressure gradients are associated with late and brief mitral leaflet-septal contact. No pressure gradient develops if mitral leaflet-septal contact occurs after 55% of left ventricular ejection time.[11]
3. Abolition of systolic anterior motion and mitral leaflet-septal contact pharmacologically or surgically results in abolition of the pressure gradient and mitral regurgitation (Fig. 91.6).[11]
4. Provocation of systolic anterior motion and mitral leaflet-septal contact pharmacologically or in the postextrasystolic beat results in

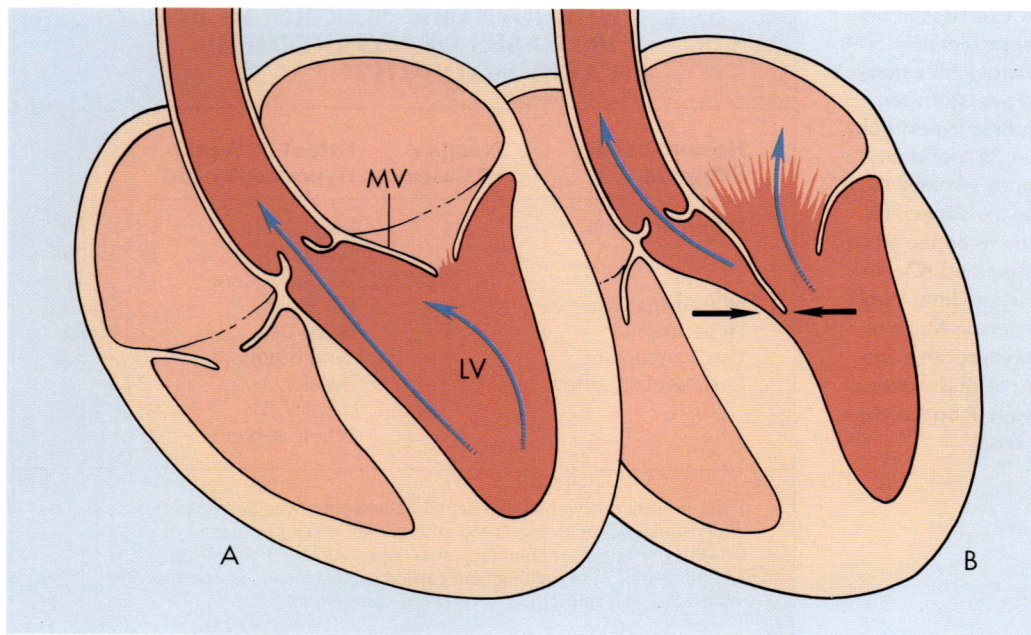

FIGURE 91.5 Proposed mechanism of systolic anterior motion of the anterior mitral leaflet in muscular subaortic stenosis. **A.** In normals blood is ejected from the left ventricle in a relatively direct path into the aorta through a wide open outflow tract. **B.** In muscular subaortic stenosis the ventricular septum is thickened (*left horizontal arrow*) resulting in a narrowed outflow tract. Because of this narrowing, the ejection of blood from the ventricle occurs at a high velocity and the ejection path is closer to the anterior mitral leaflet than is normal. As a result, the anterior leaflet is drawn into the outflow tract toward the septum, by Venturi effect (*right horizontal arrow*). Mitral leaflet—septal contact results in obstruction to left ventricular outflow. Mitral regurgitation (*upper right oblique arrow*) results from the anterior mitral leaflet being out of its normal systolic position (see text). (*LV*, left ventricle; *MV*, mitral valve.) (Adapted from Wigle ED, Sasson Z, Henderson M, et al: Hypertrophic cardiomyopathy: The importance of the site and extent of hypertrophy. A review. Prog Cardiovasc Dis 28:1–83, 1985)

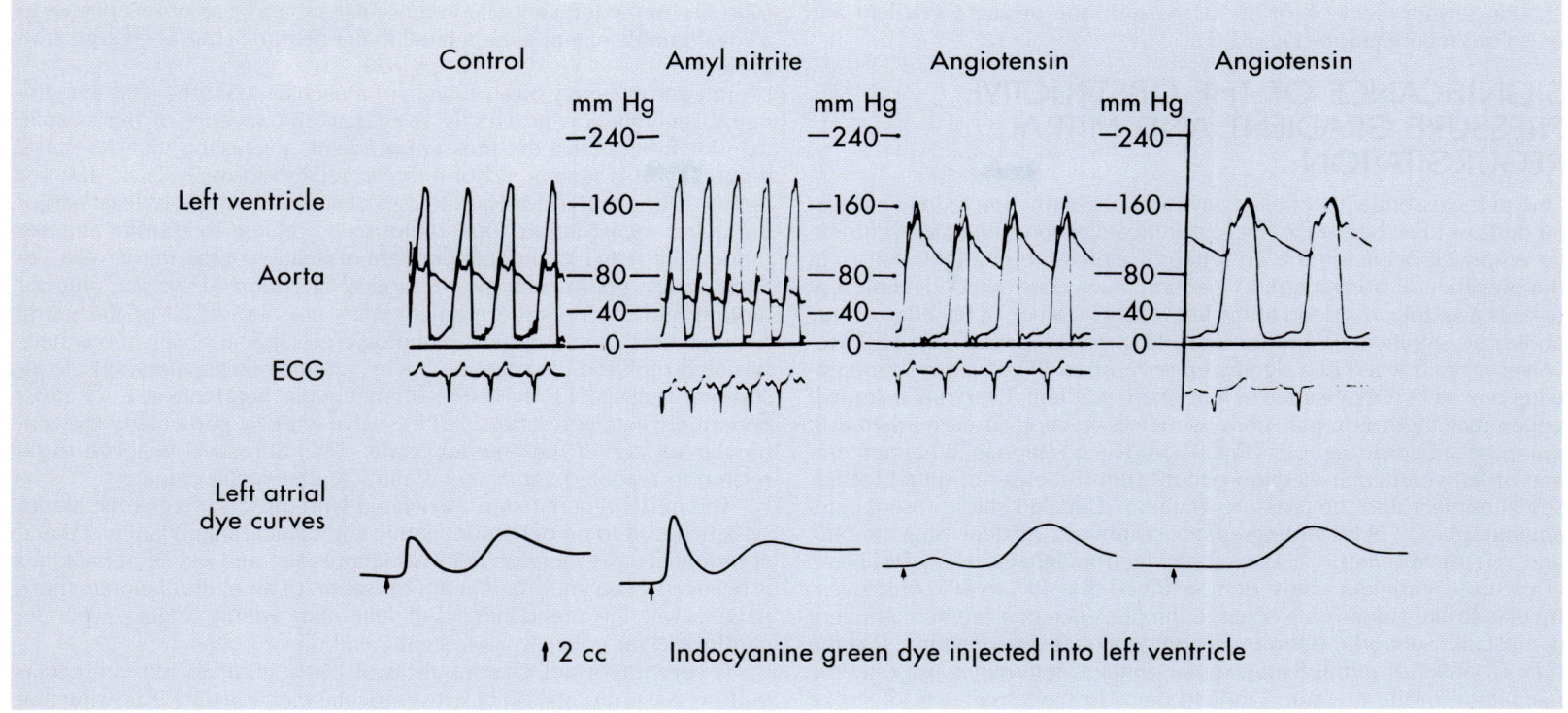

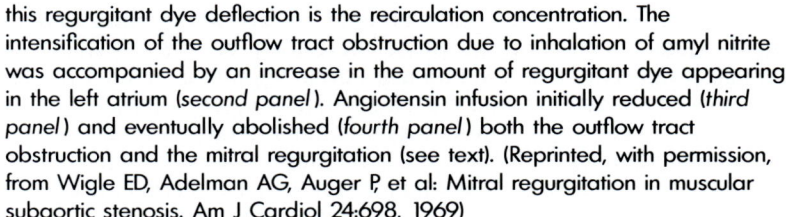

FIGURE 91.6 Simultaneous left ventricular and aortic pressure recordings (*top*) and left atrial dye dilution curves (*bottom*) inscribed from left to right, after left ventricular injection of 2 ml indocyanine green dye in a patient with muscular subaortic stenosis, in control conditions (*first panel*) after amyl nitrite inhalation (*second panel*), and during angiotensin infusion (*third and fourth panels*). The amount of dye leaking back into the left atrium is indicated by the upward deflection of the dye curve that occurs immediately to the right of the arrow, which indicates the time of left ventricular injection of the dye. To the right of this regurgitant dye deflection is the recirculation concentration. The intensification of the outflow tract obstruction due to inhalation of amyl nitrite was accompanied by an increase in the amount of regurgitant dye appearing in the left atrium (*second panel*). Angiotensin infusion initially reduced (*third panel*) and eventually abolished (*fourth panel*) both the outflow tract obstruction and the mitral regurgitation (see text). (Reprinted, with permission, from Wigle ED, Adelman AG, Auger P, et al: Mitral regurgitation in muscular subaortic stenosis. Am J Cardiol 24:698, 1969)

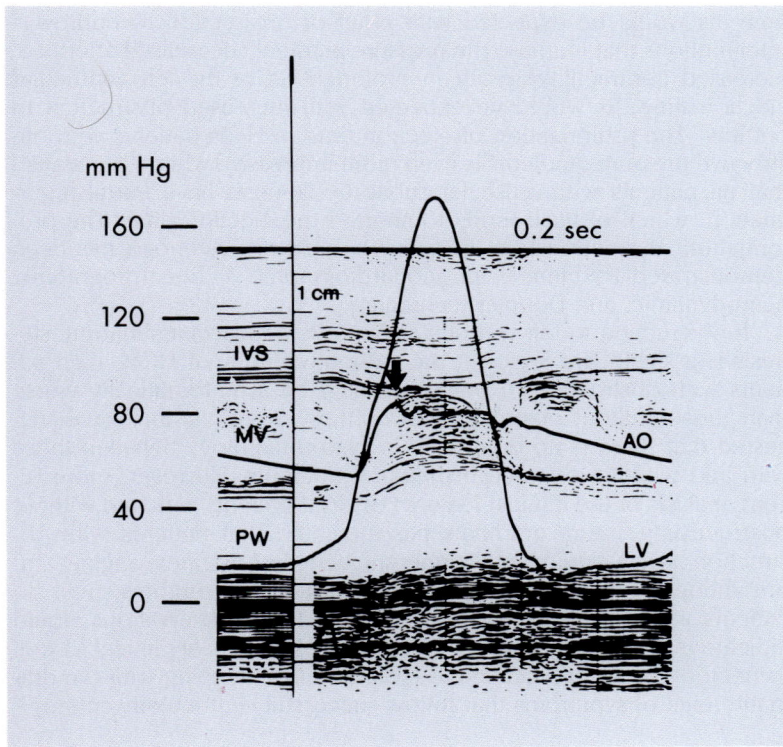

FIGURE 91.7 Simultaneous hemodynamic and one-dimensional echocardiographic recordings in a patient with muscular subaortic stenosis (gradient 86 mm Hg). The arrow indicates the onset of mitral leaflet-septal contact and the onset of the pressure gradient (defined as the peak of aortic percussion wave), which are virtually simultaneous. The small pressure gradient that exists between the left ventricle and aorta prior to the aortic percussion wave (*arrow*) is believed due to an impulse gradient and the anterior mitral leaflet approaching the septum. Following mitral leaflet-septal contact the large obstructive pressure gradient develops. Note how early in systole the mitral leaflet-septal contact and the pressure gradient occur in patients with severe outflow tract obstruction. (IVS, interventricular septum; MV, mitral valve; PW, posterior wall; AO, central aortic pressure; LV, left ventricular pressure.) (From Pollick C, Morgan CD, Gilbert BW, et al: Muscular subaortic stenosis: The temporal relationship between systolic anterior motion of the anterior mitral leaflet and pressure gradient. Circulation 66:1087, 1982. By permission of the American Heart Association, Inc.)

the development of, or an increase in, the pressure gradient and mitral regurgitation (Fig. 91.6).

SIGNIFICANCE OF THE OBSTRUCTIVE PRESSURE GRADIENT AND MITRAL REGURGITATION

One of the essential features of any form of obstruction to left ventricular outflow must be the fact that a significant proportion of left ventricular emptying occurs in the presence of a pressure gradient, that is, in the presence of obstruction to ejection. Such obstructed ejection represents a systolic overload to the left ventricle. Much of the controversy about the significance of the subaortic pressure gradient in HCM revolves around whether a significant proportion of left ventricular emptying occurs in the presence of a pressure gradient. Everyone acknowledges that there is rapid, nonobstructed ejection in early systole in muscular subaortic stenosis (Fig. 91.5). The question is, What percentage of left ventricular ejection occurs after the onset of mitral leaflet-septal contact and the pressure gradient? Detailed studies using cineangiographic,[11] echocardiographic, combined nuclear angiographic and micromanometric,[30] as well as electromagnetic[31] and Doppler[18] aortic flow techniques have demonstrated that 40% to 80% of left ventricular stroke volume is ejected in the presence of a pressure gradient in muscular subaortic stenosis. Recent work has demonstrated that the time of onset of mitral leaflet-septal contact determines not only the magnitude of the pressure gradient but also the percentage of stroke volume that is ejected against the obstruction and the degree of prolongation of left ventricular ejection time.[11] Thus, when mitral leaflet-septal contact occurs early in systole, there is a large pressure gradient, a large proportion of left ventricular stroke volume is ejected in the presence of obstruction, and the left ventricular ejection time is greatly prolonged. When mitral leaflet-septal contact occurs later in systole, the pressure gradient is smaller, the percentage of stroke volume that is obstructed is dramatically less, and left ventricular ejection time is only mildly prolonged.[11,14] The fact that a significant percentage of left ventricular ejection occurs in the presence of a pressure gradient in muscular subaortic stenosis is crucial to the understanding of the hemodynamic significance of these pressure gradients in HCM.

Mitral regurgitation has been recognized to be a potentially important part of the pathophysiology of muscular subaortic stenosis from the time of early indicator dilution and angiographic studies of this condition.[32] Both indicator dilution and Doppler studies have indicated the invariable occurrence of mitral regurgitation in the presence of mitral leaflet-septal contact and a pressure gradient.[6,11,32] These studies have indicated there is usually, but not always, a direct relationship between the magnitude of systolic anterior motion, the pressure gradient, and the mitral regurgitation in any given case, supporting the view that the mitral regurgitation is related to the degree of systolic anterior motion.[11] Pharmacologic or surgical amelioration or abolition of systolic anterior motion of the mitral leaflets usually results in amelioration or abolition of the pressure gradient and the mitral regurgitation. HCM patients with latent or no obstruction with lesser degrees of, or no, systolic anterior motion tend to have little or no mitral regurgitation.[11]

Cineangiography has contributed to an understanding of the relationship between systolic anterior motion, the pressure gradient, and the mitral regurgitation. The sequence of events as viewed in the left anterior oblique, left ventricular cineangiogram is essentially eject/obstruct/leak.[11] Thus, early systole is characterized by rapid early ejection into the aorta during which time systolic anterior motion of the anterior leaflet commences. The end of this phase is marked by the development of a radiolucent line in the left ventricular outflow tract, signifying the onset of mitral leaflet-septal contact. Aortic valve partial closure also occurs at this time. Although a small amount of mitral regurgitation may be noted in early systole during the development of systolic anterior motion, the major portion of mitral regurgitation is noted in the last half of systole after mitral leaflet-septal contact. The end-systolic size of the left ventricle in muscular subaortic stenosis appears to a considerable extent to be related to the degree of mitral regurgitation present.[11]

In approximately 80% of cases of muscular subaortic stenosisi, the mitral regurgitation is directly related to the severity of the systolic anterior motion and the pressure gradient, suggesting that the mitral regurgitation is mainly, if not entirely, related to the systolic anterior motion of the mitral leaflets.[11] In 20% of cases, however, at least part of the mitral regurgitation appears not to be related to systolic anterior motion but rather to independent abnormalities of the mitral valve. In these cases, pharmacologic or surgical abolition of systolic anterior motion and the pressure gradient does not abolish all of the mitral regurgitation. In such cases, pathologic or surgical observations have revealed ruptured chordae tendineae, anomalous papillary muscle insertions (Fig. 91.1), evidence of rheumatic heart disease, or most commonly extensive fibrosis of the valve leaflets, particularly the ventricular surface of the anterior leaflet. This fibrosis is believed to be related to repeated and forceful mitral leaflet-septal contact.[11]

The mitral regurgitation associated with muscular subaortic stenosis is believed to be of hemodynamic and clinical significance in that it contributes to an increase in left atrial pressure and size, and the latter is believed to be important in the causation of atrial fibrillation in these patients with the attendant risks of pulmonary edema, angina, syncope, cardiovascular collapse, or systemic emboli.

A very important characteristic of obstruction to left ventricular outflow is a prolongation of left ventricular ejection time. Knowing that a significant proportion of left ventricular emptying occurs in the presence of a pressure gradient and hence obstruction to outflow, one is not surprised that left ventricular ejection time is prolonged in muscular subaortic stenosis in direct relation to the magnitude of the pressure gradient.[33] Indeed, the time of onset of mitral leaflet-septal contact determines both the magnitude of the pressure gradient and the degree of prolongation of left ventricular ejection time, as well as the percentage of stroke volume that is obstructed.[11,14] Interventions that decrease the pressure gradient (increased afterload, decreased contractility, successful surgery) also decrease left ventricular ejection time, as would be expected with relief of obstruction to outflow.[33] Interventions that increase the pressure gradient (decreased afterload, increased contractility) result in prolongation of the left ventricular ejection time, as would be expected with increased obstruction to outflow. The prolongation of ejection time in HCM patients with obstructive pressure gradients is even more impressive when it is recalled that all patients with muscular subaortic stenosis have mitral regurgitation, which of itself tends to shorten the ejection time. The prolongation of ejection time in muscular subaortic stenosis has been demonstrated by clinical, phonocardiographic, echocardiographic, hemodynamic, and Doppler techniques.

If obstruction to left ventricular outflow in muscular subaortic stenosis is a significant factor in the pathophysiology of HCM, then patients with obstruction to outflow should be symptomatically worse than those without obstruction to outflow. Some authors have suggested that there is no difference in symptomatology between those with and without obstructive pressure gradients. However, more recent analysis of the clinical features of HCM patients with and without obstructive pressure gradients has indicated that patients with obstruction have a significantly higher incidence of dyspnea, angina, and presyncope-syncope, as well as more disabling symptoms, than do patients without obstruction to outflow.[11] These observations would indicate that obstruction to left ventricular outflow is of clinical as well as hemodynamic significance in HCM and is in keeping with the dramatic relief of symptoms that follow successful ventriculomyectomy.

THE NONOBSTRUCTIVE VIEWPOINT

Before the discussion of the nonobstructive viewpoint in HCM is presented, it is important to be aware of the four different types of intraventricular pressure differences that may be encountered in these patients (Table 91.4). The impulse gradient,[17] due to rapid early systolic ejection, and the pressure gradient due to midventricular obstruction (at the level of the papillary muscles) can easily be distinguished from the outflow tract pressure gradient encountered in muscular subaortic stenosis (Table 91.4). Of greater importance is to distinguish between an intraventricular pressure difference due to catheter entrapment as the result of cavity obliteration from the obstructive pressure gradient seen in muscular subaortic stenosis. This can readily be done by means of transseptal left-heart catheterization and utilization of the left ventricular inflow tract pressure concept (Fig. 91.8) and the many ancillary methods that have been described.[34] As indicated in Table 91.4, there are many clinical, echocardiographic, cineangiographic, as well as hemodynamic differences that may help differentiate an obstructive pressure gradient in muscular subaortic stenosis from an intraventricular pressure difference due to cavity obliteration. All studies reported from this center on the hemodynamics of muscular subaortic stenosis have utilized the inflow tract pressure concept, and ancillary measures, to ensure that the pressure gradients have been obstructive in nature.[34]

Criley,[29] Goodwin,[22] and Murgo,[17] and their associates have been prominent in espousing the nonobstructive viewpoint in HCM, but for different reasons. Criley and Siegel believe that the intraventricular pressure differences in HCM are related to cavity obliteration and not to obstruction to outflow or to entrapment of the catheter recording the elevated ventricular pressure in an area of cavity obliteration.[29] These authors suggest that pressure differences are created between rapidly and slowly emptying regions of the ventricle, but do not provide a scientific basis for this claim. They have suggested that mitral leaflet systolic anterior motion and aortic valve notching are caused by posterior wall hyperkinesis or cavity obliteration, but these suggestions appear to be untenable.[11,13] It is my belief that the intraventricular pressure differences in Criley's studies are either due to catheter entrapment in obliterated areas of the myocardium as he himself originally suggested, or are true obstructive pressure gradients, and methods have been described to distinguish between these two types of intraventricular pressure difference (Table 91.4, Fig. 91.8). Of importance is that many patients with muscular subaortic stenosis do not demonstrate abnormally high ejection fractions.[11] In such cases it would be rather difficult to ascribe the pressure gradient to cavity obliteration when in fact there is none! It is important to realize that cavity obliteration is not a disease entity, but rather a nonspecific manifestation of left ventricular hypertrophy, and is often but not invariably present in HCM. The degree of cavity obliteration in any form of left ventricular hypertrophy is related to the degree of hypertrophy, left ventricular systolic function, and to the degree of obstruction to left ventricular outflow and the presence or absence of mitral regurgitation.[11] Goodwin[22] speaks of cavity elimination rather than cavity obliteration, but this viewpoint appears to be rather similar to that of Criley and associates.

Murgo and associates do not believe there is a hemodynamically significant obstruction to left ventricular outflow in muscular subaortic stenosis, in that internally recorded aortic velocity flow profiles are similar in HCM patients with and without pressure gradients.[17] Recent reanalysis of this work, however, indicates that the onset of outflow obstruction during systole in muscular subaortic stenosis does in fact significantly alter the aortic ejection flow profile, in that both the flow time and ejection time become prolonged when compared to those in

TABLE 91.4 DIFFERENTIATION OF INTRAVENTRICULAR PRESSURE DIFFERENCES THAT MAY BE ENCOUNTERED IN HYPERTROPHIC CARDIOMYOPATHY

	Muscular Subaortic Stenosis	Cavity Obliteration	Impulse Gradient	Midventricular Obstruction
Hemodynamics				
Elevated LV inflow pressure	+	−	+	−
Entrapment criteria*	−	+	−	−
Time of peak systolic gradient	Late	Late	Early	Late
Spike-and-dome aortic pressure	+	−	−	−
Spike-and-dome aortic flow	+	−	−	−
LV ejection time	Increased	Normal (or short)	Normal (or short)	?
Cineangiography				
Mitral-septal contact (radiolucent line)	+	−	−	−
LV end-systolic volume	Variable	Small	Normal	Base small apex large
Mitral regurgitation	++	±	−	−
LV cavity obliteration	± Late if +	+ Early	−	−
Echocardiography: 1D				
Severe SAM	+	−	−	−
Left atrial enlargement	+	−	−	±
Aortic valve notch	+	−	−	−
Echocardiography: 2D				
Mitral leaflet–septal contact	+	−	−	−
Clinical				
Apical murmur	3–4/6	0–2/6	±	?
Reversed split S$_2$	+	−	−	−

* See text. (LV, Left ventricle; SAM, systolic anterior motion of mitral leaflet; 1D and 2D, one- and two-dimensional echocardiography; S$_2$, second heart sound)

patients without obstruction to outflow.[11] In addition, ascending aortic velocity flow profiles measured by Doppler echocardiography,[18] electromagnetic flow meters,[31] or pressure differential techniques reveal distinct differences between HCM patients with and without pressure gradients. Those with pressure gradients demonstrate a sharp deceleration of aortic flow in early systole, virtually coincident with mitral leaflet-septal contact, and may demonstrate additional late systolic flow giving rise to a spike-and-dome flow profile. HCM patients without pressure gradients have velocity flow profiles that resemble those seen in normals. For detailed analysis of both the obstructive and nonobstructive viewpoints, the reader is referred to a recent review.[11]

DIASTOLIC FILLING

From the time of earliest reports of HCM it was clearly recognized that there were abnormalities of diastolic filling of these hypertrophied ventricles,[3,4] even though more attention was paid to the systolic abnormalities at that time. The elevated ventricular end-diastolic and atrial pressures were attributed to a decrease in ventricular compliance.[3,4] Subsequently it has been suggested that we should speak of chamber stiffness (dp/dv) rather than chamber compliance (dv/dp),[35] and our knowledge and understanding of the relaxation process has improved dramatically, largely as the result of the basic work of Brutsaert and co-workers.[36,37] There is reason to believe that the extent of hypertrophy in HCM profoundly affects both chamber stiffness and the relaxation process.[11] The manner in which these factors affect diastolic filling in HCM has recently been described in some detail and will be summarized here because of the important therapeutic implications of understanding diastolic filling in this disorder (Tables 91.5 and 91.6, Figs. 91.9–91.11).[11]

CHAMBER STIFFNESS

Chamber stiffness is directly related to myocardial mass and myocardial stiffness and inversely related to ventricular volume (Table 91.5). In HCM, all three factors that affect chamber stiffness are altered such that chamber stiffness would be increased, in that myocardial mass and stiffness are increased and ventricular volume is decreased. The volume/mass effects are believed to be more important than the myocardial stiffness effect in accounting for the increased chamber stiffness in HCM.[35]

RELAXATION

Relaxation is under the control of three basic factors: load, inactivation, and nonuniformity of load and inactivation in space and time (Table 91.5).[36,37] Thus, "relaxation is governed by the continuous interplay of the sensitivity of the contractile system to the prevailing relaxation load, dissipating activation (inactivation), and to the temporal and regional (spatial) nonuniform distribution of load and inactivation."[36,37]

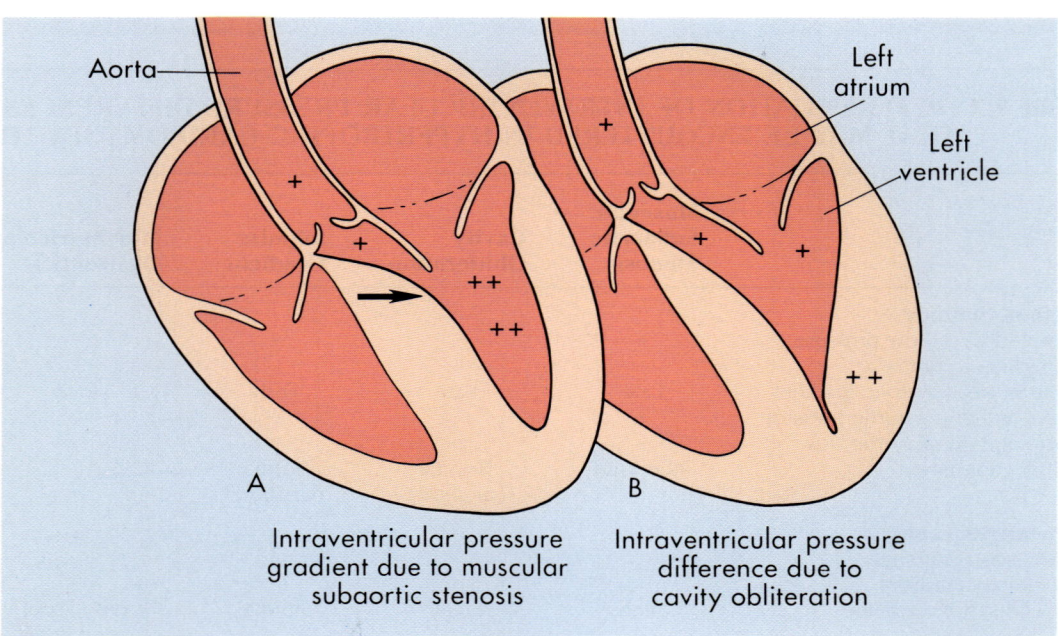

FIGURE 91.8 The left ventricular inflow tract pressure concept. **A.** In muscular subaortic stenosis, because the obstruction to left ventricular outflow (arrow) is caused by anterior mitral leaflet—ventricular septal apposition, the intraventricular pressure distal to the stenosis (and proximal to the aortic valve) is low (+), whereas all ventricular pressures proximal to the stenosis, including the one just inside the mitral valve (the inflow tract pressure) are elevated (++). **B.** When an intraventricular pressure difference is recorded, due to catheter entrapment by the myocardium as the result of cavity obliteration, the elevated ventricular pressure is recorded only in the area of cavity obliteration (++). The intraventricular systolic pressure in all other areas of the left ventricular cavity, including that in the inflow tract, just inside the mitral valve, is low (+) and equal to the aortic systolic pressure. Note that in cavity obliteration, there is an intraventricular pressure difference between the apex and the inflow tract and also the outflow tract. In muscular subaortic stenosis, there is no intraventricular pressure difference between the apex and the inflow tract as they are both elevated above the outflow tract pressure. The three areas of the left ventricle represented by the +'s in each of these diagrams are, from above downward, the outflow tract just below the aortic valve (subaortic region), the inflow tract just inside the mitral valve, and the left ventricular apex. (Modified from Wigle ED, Sasson Z, Henderson M, et al: Hypertrophic cardiomyopathy: The importance of the site and extent of hypertrophy. A review. Prog Cardiovasc Dis 28:1–83, 1985)

LOADS THAT AFFECT RELAXATION

There are five loads that may affect diastolic relaxation in man (Table 91.5, Fig. 91.9).[36,37] An increase in one—the contraction load—impedes relaxation, whereas an increase in any of the four relaxation loads enhances relaxation.

CONTRACTION LOAD. Isolated muscle contraction loading in the first half of systole results in a prolongation of contraction (ejection) and a delay in the onset of relaxation, as well as slower relaxation.[36,37] I have suggested that the early onset of outflow tract obstruction in systole in muscular subaortic stenosis may be considered a human counterpart to isolated muscle contraction load clamping, that is, in both situations a load applied in the first half of systole prolongs left ventricular contraction (ejection), thereby delaying the onset of relaxation as well as slowing the rate of relaxation (Table 91.5, Fig. 91.9).[11] Surgical relief of muscular subaortic stenosis (the contraction load) results in a shortened ejection (contraction) time with a lowering of left ventricular end-diastolic pressure (? improved relaxation). This is the only load that delays or impairs left ventricular relaxation and has obvious importance in cases of HCM with obstruction to left ventricular outflow.[11]

RELAXATION LOADS. The remaining four loads that affect the left ventricle during relaxation (relaxation loading) together explain the almost explosive character of the rapid filling phase of diastole.[36,37] These loads normally prevail over inactivation in controlling relaxation, yet they are inactivation dependent, that is, their effect is dependent on active calcium reuptake by the sarcoplasmic reticulum, with resultant lowering of myoplasmic calcium, which in turn permits disengagement of the force-generating sites (actin-myosin cross bridges). High myoplasmic calcium levels (calcium overload, ischemia, caffeine) cause relaxation to become load-independent.[36,37]

LATE SYSTOLIC LOAD. In contrast to contraction loading in the first half of systole, a load applied in the last half of systole results in the early onset of relaxation.[36,37] It does not appear that this type of relaxation loading is of any importance in HCM.

END-SYSTOLIC DEFORMATION LOAD (RESTORING FORCES). Internal and external restoring forces are generated during systolic shortening and deformation and are stored as potential energy for release during diastole, principally during the period of isovolumic relaxation (Fig. 91.9).[36,37] There is reason to believe that these forces may be increased in HCM and may account for the exaggerated changes in shape during the isovolumic relaxation period[12] as well as the occurrence of normal left ventricular diastolic pressures in the presence of massive hypertrophy. They are unlikely, however, to have a dominant effect since relaxation is usually impaired in HCM and these restoring forces (load) act to improve relaxation.[11]

CORONARY FILLING LOAD. The degree of filling of the coronary vascular tree during isovolumic relaxation represents a third load that may augment diastolic relaxation by applying an intramural load to the already relaxing myocardium (Table 91.5, Fig. 91.9).[36,37] The degree to which this "coronary kick" could be blunted in HCM is considerable. Thus, coronary perfusion pressure would be variably reduced by a low

---

TABLE 91.5 FACTORS AFFECTING LEFT VENTRICULAR DIASTOLIC FILLING IN HYPERTROPHIC CARDIOMYOPATHY

$$\text{Chamber Stiffness} \propto \frac{\text{Myocardial Mass} \cdot \text{Myocardial Stiffness}}{\text{Ventricular Volume}}$$

Relaxation
Loads
  Contraction load
    Subaortic stenosis
  Relaxation loads
    Late systolic loading
    End-systolic deformation (restoring forces)
    Coronary filling
    Ventricular filling
Inactivation
Nonuniformity of load and inactivation in space and time

Pericardial Constraint and Ventricular Interaction

Effect of Extent of Hypertrophy on Chamber Stiffness, Relaxation, and Pericardial Constraint/Ventricular Interaction

---

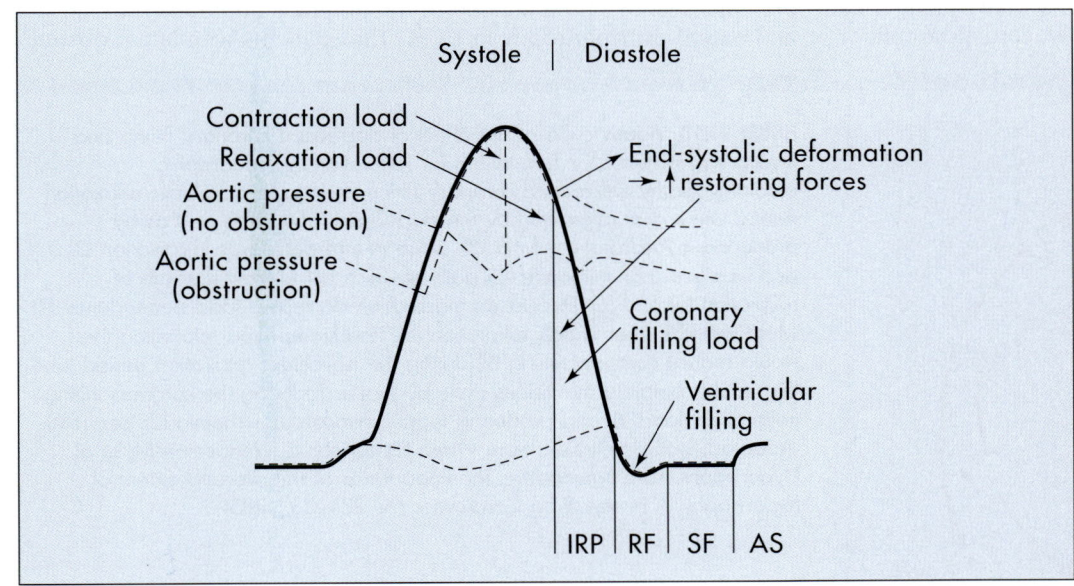

FIGURE 91.9 Diagram of left atrial, ventricular, and aortic pressures (with and without obstruction to outflow) together with the various loads that may affect diastolic relaxation in hypertrophic cardiomyopathy. A contraction load (the obstruction) applied in the first half of systole would delay the onset and slow the rate of relaxation. A load applied in the last half of systole could cause the early onset of relaxation. Exaggerated end-systolic deformation due to the extensive hypertrophy could generate increased restoring forces that would be released principally during the isovolumic relaxation period (IRP) and could account for the excessive shape changes that occur during this period. The coronary filling load (during IRP) and ventricular filling load (during RF) are reduced in hypertrophic cardiomyopathy as a result of the extent of hypertrophy and other factors (see text). (SF, slow filling period; RF, rapid filling period; AS, atrial systolic filling.) (Adapted, with permission, from Wigle ED, Sasson Z, Henderson M, et al: Hypertrophic cardiomyopathy: The importance of the site and extent of hypertrophy. A review. Prog Cardiovasc Dis 28:1–83, 1985)

aortic diastolic pressure and a high left ventricular end-diastolic pressure. Intramyocardial blood flow could be reduced by small vessel disease, by the decreased capillary-fiber ratio of hypertrophy, by septal perforator artery compression, and by decreased vasodilator capacity. The hypertrophy itself would lessen the impact of the coronary filling load. Decreased myocardial relaxation from any cause would of itself reduce coronary filling during the isovolumic relaxation period, particularly in areas of the myocardium in which systolic compression of the coronary arteries occurred. Consideration of all of these factors leads to the conclusion that the coronary filling load applied to the myocardium during isovolumic relaxation is reduced in HCM.

VENTRICULAR FILLING LOAD. The fourth relaxation load on the left ventricle is due to ventricular filling after mitral valve opening and is determined by the Laplace relationship ($T = P \times r/2h$) (Table 91.5, Fig. 91.9).[36,37] In normals, although the filling pressure (P) is low, the rapid decrease in wall thickness (h) and increase in left ventricular radius (r) result in an increased tension (T) or load on the left ventricular wall and ensure rapid diastolic filling. In HCM, however, wall thickness is increased, the rate of thinning of the wall is reduced, and the radius is reduced, all of which would decrease the wall tension or load that would aid relaxation during rapid ventricular filling.[36,37] Counteracting these effects to some extent would be the elevated left atrial filling pressure (P) which would increase the load on the left ventricular wall during rapid filling. An elevated ventricular filling pressure would partially compensate for, but not overcome, the effects of increased wall thickness and diminished radius which act to diminish the hemodynamic load during rapid filling in HCM.[11] The reduced ventricular and coronary filling loads in HCM would both act to impair diastolic relaxation.

INACTIVATION

Inactivation is the second major factor affecting relaxation of the left ventricle. With unchanging loads on the left ventricle, the rate of inactivation of the contractile process is a principal determinant of the rate of relaxation. Factors known to retard inactivation and hence relaxation are ischemia, calcium overload, caffeine, and the absence of an active sarcoplasmic reticulum.[36,37] All of these factors impair relaxation by elevating myoplasmic calcium and slowing the rate of deactivation of the force-generating sites. A number of authors have suggested that there may be a primary calcium overload in HCM. Myocardial ischemia, due to the same factors that reduced the coronary filling load, would decrease inactivation as well as cause myocardial nonuniformity, both factors acting to impair relaxation. Thus, a vicious cycle is set up in which diminished coronary filling causes ischemia and impaired inactivation and relaxation, which in turn further impedes coronary filling, leading to further ischemia, and so on (Fig. 91.10).[11]

Not only does reduced inactivation impair relaxation directly, but it also leads to a diminution of load dependency.[36,37] This double-edged sword effect of reduced inactivation may have particularly deleterious consequences in HCM patients in whom the principal relaxation loads are already diminished.

NONUNIFORMITY OF LOAD AND INACTIVATION IN SPACE AND TIME

Physiologic nonuniformity is believed to be present in the normal heart and is increased to a pathologic degree in hypertrophy, particularly in HCM, as a result of the asymmetrical hypertrophy, myocardial fiber disarray, and interstitial fibrosis, as well as by nonuniform myocardial ischemia and asynchrony of contraction and relaxation.[16] In light of these factors, it is believed that nonuniformity is one of the principal causes of impaired relaxation in HCM.

In summary, the impaired relaxation that is so characteristic of HCM can be attributed to an increased contraction load, in those with obstruction to outflow, as well as to a reduction in the principal relaxation loads, impairment of inactivation with its associated diminished load dependency, and to a pathologic degree of nonuniformity. Thus, all factors that are involved in the triple control of relaxation are altered in HCM in a manner that impairs relaxation.

PERICARDIAL CONSTRAINT AND VENTRICULAR INTERACTION

Pericardial constraint and ventricular interaction are believed to be important in a number of clinical situations. It has been suggested that the degree of pericardial constraint may be important in HCM in the presence of atrial fibrillation or following surgery, depending on how completely the pericardium is sutured. It is also possible that the degree of ventricular interaction is limited in HCM by the extent of the septal hypertrophy. The role played by these factors in determining the diastolic filling characteristics in HCM is unknown.[11]

EXTENT OF HYPERTROPHY

Previous sections have alluded to the potential importance of the site and extent of hypertrophy in HCM. Thus patients with latent obstruc-

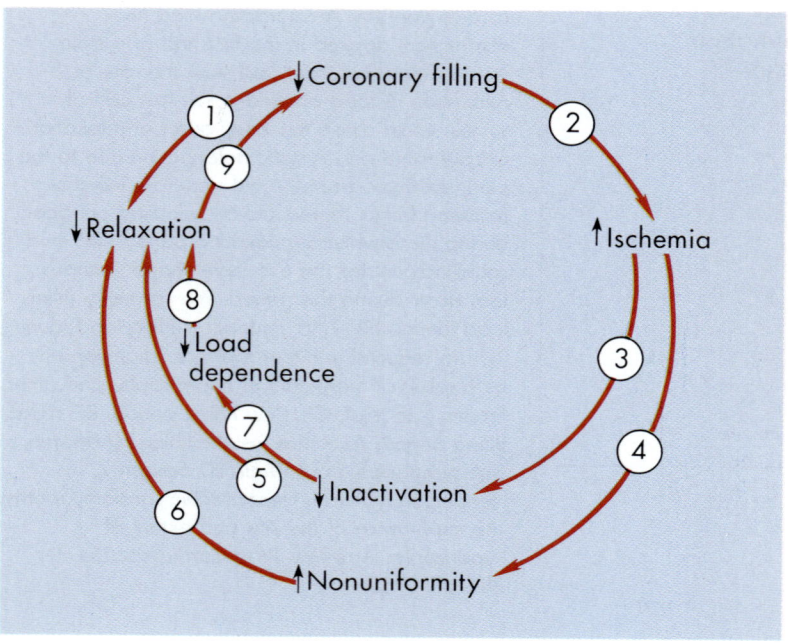

FIGURE 91.10 Vicious cycle of the effect of decreased coronary filling and myocardial ischemia on left ventricular relaxation in hypertrophic cardiomyopathy. Decreased coronary filling during the isovolumic relaxation period will impair relaxation by the decreased load (1) as well as by producing myocardial ischemia (2), which in turn decreases inactivation (3), and increases nonuniformity (4), both of which act to slow the rate of relaxation (5) and (6). Decreased inactivation decreases load dependency (7) which would further impair relaxation (8). Finally, impaired relaxation itself would reduce coronary filling (9) during the isovolumic relaxation period, and this would complete the vicious cycle by further reducing the coronary filling (relaxation) load (1), and producing further myocardial ischemia (2) (see text). (Adapted, with permission, from Wigle ED, Sasson Z, Henderson M, et al: Hypertrophic cardiomyopathy: The importance of the site and extent of hypertrophy. A review. Prog Cardiovasc Dis 28:1–83, 1985)

tion usually have a limited extent of hypertrophy, normal left ventricular filling pressures, and a good prognosis, whereas patients with resting obstruction usually have extensive hypertrophy, high filling pressures, and a poor prognosis. Figure 91.11 delineates the means by which the extent of hypertrophy in HCM profoundly affects the factors that control chamber stiffness and the rate of relaxation, which are the principal determinants of ventricular diastolic filling.[11] The extent of hypertrophy will determine the increase in myocardial mass, the decrease in chamber volume and the increase in myocardial stiffness (due to fibrosis), all of these factors acting to increase left ventricular chamber stiffness (decrease compliance). Extensive hypertrophy at the base of the septum results in a contraction load (subaortic stenosis) which would slow relaxation, as would the diminished hemodynamic relaxation loads (during coronary and rapid ventricular filling). The extent of hypertrophy and myocardial fiber disarray would further impair relaxation by decreased inactivation (due to primary or ischemic myoplasmic calcium overload) and by increased nonuniformity. Decreased inactivation would diminish the sensitivity of the relaxation process to the already reduced relaxation loads, impairing relaxation by yet another mechanism.

It is also possible that extensive hypertrophy may lead to exaggerated end-systolic deformation and the generation of increased restoring forces for release during the isovolumic relaxation period. If this were true, it might explain the exaggerated changes in shape that occur during this period in hypertrophic cardiomyopathy. There is no information available about whether the extent of hypertrophy may affect the degree of pericardial constraint or ventricular interaction.

CLINICAL MEASURES OF ABNORMAL DIASTOLIC RELAXATION

There are a number of clinically measurable indices of left ventricular relaxation in HCM that have been derived from echophonocardiographic,[12] angiographic, micromanometric, and nuclear angiographic techniques.[15,16,38] Table 91.6 indicates the relaxation load(s) that are applicable, together with the indices of relaxation that are measurable, for each time period of diastole. It is important to emphasize that impaired relaxation not only affects the indices measured during isovolumic relaxation and rapid filling, but also the duration of the slow filling period and the volume of atrial systolic filling. Thus, slow relaxation prolongs the duration and decreases the volume of rapid filling, while shortening the slow filling period and increasing the volume of atrial systolic filling. Calcium blocking agents may reverse these abnormalities by improving relaxation.

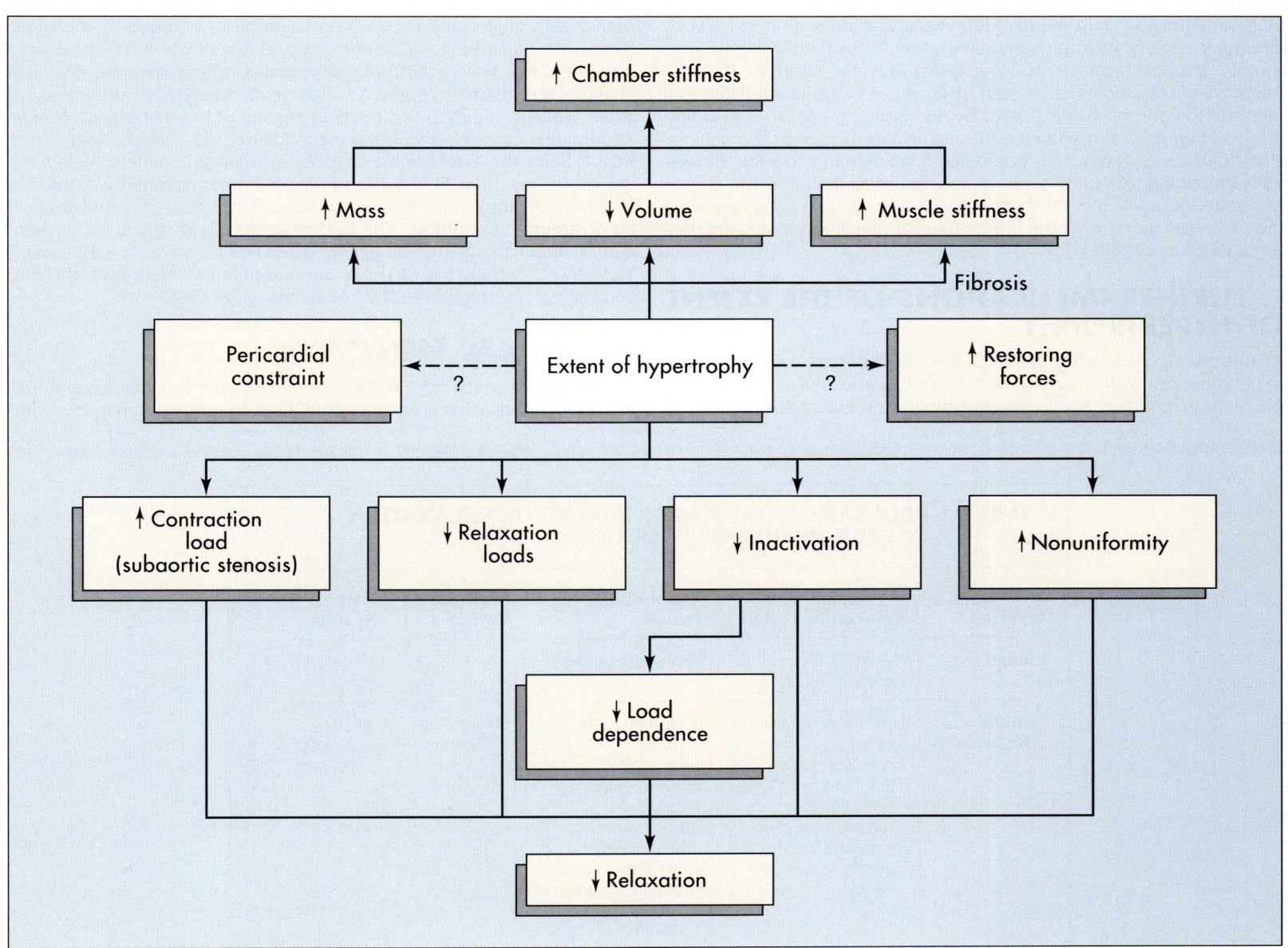

FIGURE 91.11 The effect of the extent of hypertrophy on left ventricular diastolic filling in hypertrophic cardiomyopathy. (Modified from Wigle ED, Sasson Z, Henderson M, et al: Hypertrophic cardiomyopathy: The importance of the site and extent of hypertrophy. A review. Prog Cardiovasc Dis 28:1–83, 1985)

During the isovolumic relaxation period, impairment of relaxation in HCM has been documented by prolongation of the isovolumic relaxation time[12] and the relaxation time index[12] as well as by prolongation of the time constant of isovolumic pressure decline.[38,39] Peak negative dp/dt is reduced and this effect may be reflected in the left ventricular pressure wave form.[39] Exaggerated changes in shape of the left ventricle have been reported during this period in HCM[12] and could possibly be related to increased restoring forces.[11]

During the rapid filling period, impaired left ventricular relaxation is reflected by a reduced peak filling rate, a prolonged time-to-peak filling rate,[38] by diminished posterior wall thinning and minor diameter lengthening, and by a reduced rapid filling volume together with prolongation of rapid filling.[15] In a few cases, left ventricular diastolic filling pressure has declined during rapid filling, an observation that could be explained only by a prolonged period of relaxation.[38,39] When rapid filling is decreased in volume and increased in duration due to impaired relaxation, the slow filling phase may be abbreviated and the volume of atrial systolic filling increased to compensate for the reduced filling during the rapid filling phase.[15] These clinical measurements of left ventricular relaxation indicate that all phases of diastole may be affected by impairment of the relaxation process.

It is important to note that the calcium antagonist drugs, verapamil, nifedipine, and diltiazem, have been reported to improve left ventricular relaxation as reflected in a return toward normal of these various clinically measurable indices of relaxation in HCM.[11,12,15,16,38,39] Calcium antagonists could improve left ventricular relaxation in HCM by altering the loads, by improving inactivation, or by decreasing nonuniformity. By their negative inotropic effect they can decrease the contraction load (the obstruction) and by coronary vasodilatation they can increase the coronary filling load. By decreasing the level of myoplasmic calcium they can enhance the inactivation process and help restore load dependency, thus improving relaxation in two ways. Finally, calcium antagonists have been demonstrated to decrease the degree of nonuniformity.[16] It is for these reasons that calcium antagonists are the preferred therapy for the impairment of relaxation that is encountered in patients with HCM.

FURTHER IMPLICATIONS OF THE EXTENT OF HYPERTROPHY

As described in preceding sections, the extent of hypertrophy appears to be important with regard to the presence or absence of outflow tract obstruction in systole and to the severity of ventricular filling abnormalities in diastole. It also appears that the extent of hypertrophy is an important determinant of the presence or absence of septal perforator artery compression, ECG evidence of left ventricular hypertrophy, and the occurrence of atrial and/or ventricular arrhythmias.

SEPTAL PERFORATOR ARTERY COMPRESSION

Although septal perforator artery compression has been observed in other forms of left ventricular hypertrophy, it appears to be most prevalent in HCM, in which its presence has been demonstrated to correlate with the extent of hypertrophy and the occurrence of angina.[11] Since the extent of hypertrophy is greatest in patients with resting obstruction, septal perforator compression is encountered significantly more frequently in this hemodynamic subgroup than in patients with latent or no obstruction to outflow. The potential for septal perforator artery compression to cause myocardial ischemia is enhanced by the diminished coronary filling load and the impaired relaxation in HCM, both of which appear to be affected by the extent of hypertrophy.[11]

ELECTROCARDIOGRAM

Pathologic Q waves in the inferior and left lateral precordial ECG leads together with tall R waves in the right precordial leads in HCM have been interpreted by some to indicate left-to-right depolarization of the hypertrophied septum. The fact that the development of right bundle branch block increases and a left septal incision decreases or abolishes these abnormalities would tend to support this viewpoint.[40] The development of free wall hypertrophy also results in the diminution of these changes and the development of left ventricular hypertrophy and/or strain. Recent studies indicate that the extent of hypertrophy in HCM is significantly correlated with the presence of LVH and/or strain in the ECG.[11] Since the extent of hypertrophy is greatest in patients with resting obstruction, the ECG in these patients demonstrates LVH and/or strain significantly more frequently than in HCM patients with latent or no obstruction to outflow. The ECG of patients with apical HCM often demonstrates the giant T negativity syndrome (T waves ≥ -10 mm in V_4 to V_6).[41,42] Thus, the ECG has the potential to reflect both the site and the extent of hypertrophy in patients with HCM.

VENTRICULAR TACHYCARDIA

A number of studies have drawn attention to the fact that asymptomatic ventricular tachycardia is encountered frequently in patients with

TABLE 91.6 RELAXATION LOADS AND INDICES OF RELAXATION IN EACH PERIOD OF DIASTOLE*

Diastolic Period	Isovolumic Relaxation Period	Rapid Filling Period	Slow Filling Period	Atrial Systole
Load	Restoring forces Coronary filling	Ventricular filling	—	—
Indices of Relaxation	Isovolumic relaxation time Relaxation time index Time constant (T) of isovolumic pressure decline Peak negative dp/dt Geometric changes LV pressure waveform	Peak filling rate (PFR) Time to PFR Posterior wall thinning Minor diameter lengthening Rapid filling volume Rapid filling duration LV pressure waveform	Slow filling duration	Atrial systolic volume

* Adapted with permission from reference 11.

HCM, and that the incidence of sudden death is eight times higher in those with this arrhythmia than in those without.[43,44] Some have described ventricular tachycardia as a marker for the risk of sudden death in HCM.[43,44]

Studies from this center have indicated that the occurrence of ventricular tachycardia on 72-hour ambulatory rhythm monitoring is significantly correlated with the extent of hypertrophy determined by two-dimensional echocardiography.[11] As with other phenomena related to the extent of hypertrophy, ventricular tachycardia was significantly more common in patients with resting obstruction than in the other hemodynamic subgroups. Since the ECG reflects the extent of hypertrophy in HCM, the risk of the occurrence of ventricular tachycardia in these patients can be assessed by the presence or absence of left ventricular hypertrophy and/or strain or pathologic Q waves.[11] All patients with these ECG changes and/or two-dimensional echocardiographic evidence of extensive hypertrophy should undergo extended ambulatory rhythm monitoring.

ATRIAL FIBRILLATION

Atrial fibrillation in HCM is encountered most frequently in patients with extensive hypertrophy, resting obstruction, and left atrial enlargement. The latter is highly correlated with the presence of resting obstruction and is believed related to the presence of impaired diastolic filling and mitral regurgitation.[11,27] When atrial fibrillation occurs in HCM patients without obstruction to outflow, it is usually associated with extensive hypertrophy and left atrial enlargement.

These studies indicate that the occurrence of arrhythmias in hypertrophic cardiomyopathy is significantly correlated with the extent of hypertrophy determined by echocardiography and reflected in the ECG. Since ventricular tachycardia selects out a population of patients at risk of sudden death, it would appear that the extent of hypertrophy should be considered a significant prognostic factor.[11] This would be consistent with the fact that the extent of hypertrophy also appears to be an important determinant of the systolic and diastolic abnormalities in HCM.

VARIATIONS ON THE HYPERTROPHIC THEME

RIGHT VENTRICULAR INVOLVEMENT

Right ventricular involvement in HCM is common, but the manifestations of this involvement are usually much less evident than those on the left side of the heart. Occasional cases have been described, however, in which right-sided involvement has been the dominant presenting feature. Obstruction to right ventricular outflow may occur in the outflow tract as a result of hypertrophy of the crista supraventricularis and its septal and parietal bands, or at midright ventricular level, where at times the hypertrophied septum bulges into the right ventricular cavity to such an extent that the cavity is virtually occluded. Right ventricular outflow obstruction in HCM is reflected by a systolic ejection murmur in the pulmonary area, whereas when the obstruction is more proximal in the right ventricle, the murmur may be maximal in the third or fourth left intercostal space. In studying pressure gradients on the right side of the heart in HCM, one must take care to avoid catheter entrapment in areas of cavity obliteration, particularly at the right ventricular apex. I have found the initial inflow tract pressure concept to be as valid on the right side of the heart as on the left in distinguishing between obstruction and an entrapment intraventricular pressure difference.[11]

Abnormalities of right ventricular diastolic filling are present clinically and hemodynamically in a significant percentage of patients with HCM. These are evident hemodynamically by elevation and an inspiratory rise, rather than a fall, in right ventricular end-diastolic pressure and the right atrial A wave, and clinically by an inspiratory rise in jugular venous A wave and a right atrial gallop sound.[4] It is probable that right ventricular chamber stiffness is increased and relaxation impaired to account for these abnormalities of right ventricular diastolic filling.

RESTRICTIVE DIASTOLIC FILLING DEFECT

Although impaired relaxation and increased chamber stiffness combine to account for the altered diastolic filling characteristics of most patients with HCM, a few patients manifest only increased chamber stiffness with the result that they demonstrate abnormalities compatible with a restrictive cardiomyopathy.[11] Thus, they have prominent third and fourth heart sounds and a dip-and-plateau configuration to the ventricular diastolic pressure wave form in both left and right ventricles. These patients have supranormal rapid diastolic filling but very little atrial systolic filling, in contrast to patients with impaired relaxation, who demonstrate impaired rapid filling and enhanced atrial systolic filling. Myocardial fibrosis is the likely cause of this restrictive diastolic filling defect. Although these patients are relatively rare, it is important to recognize them in that calcium antagonists would be of little benefit and could be harmful.

APICAL HYPERTROPHIC CARDIOMYOPATHY

Japanese authors first reported this variant of HCM in the late 1970's, drawing attention to the fact that the apical hypertrophy caused a spade-shaped left ventricle at end diastole in the left ventricular angiogram and also the echocardiogram.[41,42] Apical cavity obliteration was noted in systole. These patients, when they have severe apical hypertrophy, will manifest the giant T negativity syndrome in the ECG (T waves ≥ -10 mm in V_4 to V_6). With lesser degrees of apical hypertrophy the T wave negativity may be less dramatic. Apical HCM is a variant of nonobstructive HCM and hence apical systolic murmurs are unimpressive. In some patients, however, there is coexisting septal or concentric hypertrophy that can result in outflow obstruction.[11] Pathologic specimens demonstrate myocardial fiber disarray, and apical HCM can occur in families in whom other members have predominantly septal or concentric hypertrophy. Apical HCM should essentially be managed as any other patient with nonobstructive HCM (*vide infra*).

MIDVENTRICULAR OBSTRUCTION

Midventricular obstruction is a very rare manifestation of HCM (Table 91.1) and is usually recognized at left ventricular cineangiography,[45] although it can be detected by two-dimensional echocardiography or nuclear angiography.[11] The condition is characterized by midventricular occlusion or cavity obliteration at the level of the papillary muscles with an apical and basal left ventricular chamber being evident at end-systole. It must be distinguished from typical muscular subaortic stenosis (Table 91.4), as well as from end-systolic papillary muscle approximation without obstruction. In a number of cases of midventricular obstruction, apical myocardial infarction with aneurysm formation has been evident and was reflected in the apical ECG leads by ST segment elevation.[11] In these cases it is not known whether the midventricular obstruction resulted from apical infarction in patients with nonobstructive HCM and cavity obliteration, or whether midventricular obstruction with a high left ventricular apical pressure resulted in infarction and apical aneurysm formation.[11] Indeed, there is some question whether the midventricular obstruction in these cases with apical infarction truly is an obstruction, or whether we should refer to it as midventricular obliteration or occlusion with apical aneurysm formation. Very little blood leaves the apical chamber in systole, as evidenced by the low ejection fraction of this chamber and the absence of a clinically significant murmur in some cases. Surgery has rarely been performed for this variant of HCM.

PATIENT RECOGNITION, INVESTIGATION, AND MANAGEMENT

The following is a discussion of patient recognition, investigation, and management based upon which of the major hemodynamic subgroups the patient belongs to—resting obstruction (muscular subaortic stenosis), latent obstruction, or nonobstructive HCM. Table 91.7 lists these three major hemodynamic subgroups together with the most important (but not all) features noted on clinical examination and on noninvasive and invasive investigation.

PATIENT RECOGNITION

Certain signs reflect the obstruction to left ventricular outflow and concomitant mitral regurgitation, and thus are found only in patients with resting obstruction. These patients usually have a grade 3 to 4 out of 6 apical systolic murmur, a diastolic inflow murmur (reflecting the mitral regurgitation), a single or paradoxically split second heart sound, rarely a mitral leaflet-septal contact sound, a double systolic apex beat (left ventricular impulse before and after the onset of obstruction), a triple apex beat (palpable left atrial gallop sound plus a double systolic apex beat), as well as a fast rising, sharp cutoff arterial pulse that may rarely be felt as a spike-and-dome configuration.[11] All of the noninvasive and invasive investigations (Table 91.7) reflect the mechanism of obstruction and its consequences (Fig. 91.5). Patients with latent or no obstruction have none of the clinical or investigative signs of obstruction to outflow at rest, although these may be provoked in patients with latent obstruction.

Signs of impaired left ventricular filling (third and fourth heart sounds) and right ventricular involvement are encountered most frequently in patients with resting obstruction who usually have the most extensive hypertrophy. Thus, patients with resting obstruction may manifest the total clinical picture of HCM, *i.e.*, evidence of biventricular inflow and outflow tract obstruction.[4] These patients are also significantly more symptomatic than those with latent or no obstruction. Congestive heart failure is unusual in HCM in sinus rhythm, but is the rule with the onset of atrial fibrillation, which usually worsens all symptoms.

PATIENT INVESTIGATION

All patients suspected of having HCM should undergo a careful history and physical examination together with an ECG, chest film, and one- and two-dimensional echocardiographic examination. The aim of this diagnostic workup is to establish the diagnosis and the hemodynamic subgroup by clinical and/or echocardiographic means, to measure the extent of hypertrophy by two-dimensional echocardiography, and to assess the need for ambulatory rhythm monitoring. Doppler echocardiography is useful in estimating the outflow tract gradient and the degree of mitral regurgitation, and in assessing left ventricular relaxation by estimating the volume of rapid ventricular filling versus that which occurs during atrial systole. Nuclear angiography is best suited to assess left ventricular relaxation parameters as well as to assess left ventricular systolic function. Hemodynamic and angiographic investigations should be reserved (1) for preoperative assessment, (2) to establish definitively the hemodynamic subgroup when this is in doubt after noninvasive investigation, or (3) to test acutely the effect of various pharmacologic agents on the degree of outflow tract obstruction and/or impairment of relaxation. All patients with extensive hypertrophy, resting obstruction, a history of presyncope-syncope, palpitations, or sudden death in the family should have extended ambulatory rhythm monitoring (72 hours).

PATIENT MANAGEMENT

Three manifestations of HCM are amenable to medical and/or surgical therapy: (1) the obstruction to left ventricular outflow in systole; (2) impaired relaxation in diastole; and (3) atrial and ventricular arrhythmias. An approach to the management of HCM by hemodynamic subgroup is outlined in Table 91.8.

TABLE 91.7 MAJOR HEMODYNAMIC SUBGROUPS OF HYPERTROPHIC CARDIOMYOPATHY

Hemodynamic Subgroup	Hemodynamics	Echocardiography	Doppler	Nuclear Angiogram	Clinical Signs
Resting obstruction	Pressure gradient at rest	Severe SAM, LAE, and AVN Thickest septum Extensive hypertrophy	Subaortic gradient Mitral regurgitation	Increased EF* Impaired relaxation	Signs of obstruction and mitral regurgitation 3–4/6 apical M Mitral diastolic M Reversed split S_2 ML–SC sound Double systolic apex Triple apex Jerky or bifid arterial pulse
Latent obstruction	Provocable pressure gradient	Mild-moderate SAM LAE and AVN rare Hypertrophy usually restricted to basal 1/3 or 2/3 of septum	Provocable subaortic gradient Provocable miral regurgitation	Increased EF* Relaxation usually normal	1–2/6 apical M No signs of obstruction
Nonobstructive HCM	No pressure gradient	Mild or no SAM LAE rare No AVN Moderately extensive hypertrophy	No gradient No significant mitral regurgitation	Increased EF* Impaired relaxation	0–1/6 apical M No signs of obstruction

* Ejection fraction may occasionally be reduced.

SAM, Systolic anterior motion of anterior (or posterior) mitral leaflet(s); LAE, left atrial enlargement; AVN, aortic valve notch, EF, ejection fraction; M, murmur; S_2, second heart sound; ML–SC, mitral leaflet-septal contact.

RESTING OBSTRUCTION

By virtue of the extent of hypertrophy, these patients often manifest impairment of relaxation, atrial and/or ventricular arrhythmias, as well as obstruction to left ventricular outflow. Medical management of the obstruction to outflow involves the administration of a negative inotropic agent to decrease the velocity of the early (unobstructed) ejection (Fig. 91.5) and thereby lessen the Venturi forces on the mitral leaflets with a resultant decrease in mitral systolic anterior motion and amelioration or abolition of the obstruction to outflow and mitral regurgitation (Table 91.8).

β-Adrenergic blocking agents, calcium antagonists, and the antiarrhythmic agent disopyramide have been used for this purpose. β-Adrenergic blocking agents have been used for some 20 years in patients with resting obstruction, and the reported results have been variable. Administration of these drugs does not significantly affect the degree of resting obstruction (although they block provocation of it) nor do they appear to influence the incidence of atrial and/or ventricular arrhythmias or sudden death. Using doses of propranolol (160 mg to 240 mg/day) sufficient to cause a resting heart rate of 60, with a blunted heart rate response to exercise, I found these agents to be of greatest value in patients with mild outflow obstruction and mild symptoms. Patients with more significant obstruction to outflow either did not benefit or did so temporarily. In follow-up studies, a significant number of these patients died or required surgery. Larger doses of propranolol were not well tolerated in that they resulted in increased fatigue and/or presyncope. This experience suggested that β-adrenergic blocking drugs did not represent effective therapy for patients with significant obstruction to outflow. Other authors, however, have reported symptomatic benefit with high-dose propranolol therapy.

Calcium antagonists have been used in the treatment of both the obstructive and nonobstructive varieties of HCM for some 10 to 15 years.[46,47] Although verapamil (240 mg to 480 mg/day in divided doses) has been utilized most extensively, benefits have also been attributed to nifedipine and diltiazem. The negative inotropic effect of these drugs should decrease the obstruction to left ventricular outflow while their vasodilator properties have the potential to worsen it. Verapamil usually results in a significant decrease in the magnitude of the pressure gradient, but unpredictably, in some cases, the gradient may be dangerously intensified. Left ventricular relaxation may be improved by decreasing the obstruction to outflow (the contraction load),[11] by decreasing the degree of nonuniformity,[16] by lowering myoplasmic calcium, and/or by increasing the coronary filling load. In spite of this multitude of actions, left ventricular relaxation is not improved in a significant number of patients on verapamil therapy. In patients with resting obstruction and elevated filling pressures, there is approximately a 10% chance of causing left heart failure, and some of these patients go on to cardiogenic shock and death.[47] This sequence may be attributable to the vasodilatation-induced intensification of the obstruction, while the negative inotropic effect could impair systolic function, as well as relaxation. For these reasons I have infrequently used verapamil in patients with resting obstruction and have never used nifedipine, because of its potent vasodilator properties. Others, however, claim significant symptomatic benefit in these patients, while at the same time adding a note of caution about their use.[47] Common sense dictates that if verapamil is to be used in patients with resting obstruction and elevated filling pressures, great care must be taken in its administration, and the patient should be carefully observed thereafter for indications of adverse effects. Although acute intravenous verapamil therapy usually decreases the outflow gradient in the majority of patients with resting obstruction, provokable gradient usually remains unchanged. Furthermore, following oral maintenance therapy, even resting gradient may not change, although symptomatic improvement may result in many patients.[48] It has been suggested that the major mechanism for symptomatic improvement with chronic verapamil therapy is improvement in diastolic function.

It needs to be emphasized that nifedipine, because of its potential vasodilating property, may be detrimental in patients with HCM with resting left ventricular outflow obstruction. It has been reported to increase filling pressures without demonstrating any beneficial effects on outflow gradient and diastolic function.[49]

The antiarrhythmic and negative inotropic agent disopyramide has been demonstrated to abolish mitral systolic anterior motion, the pressure gradient, and mitral regurgitation; to decrease the ejection time and improve cardiac output; and to result in symptomatic improvement in some 40 patients given this form of negative inotropic therapy.[11,50] As with other negative inotropic agents used to decrease or abolish the pressure gradient in patients with resting obstruction, the effect of disopyramide can be tested acutely in the heart catheterization laboratory by administering 100 mg to 150 mg intravenously in divided doses over 10 to 15 minutes. Alternatively, the effect of this drug can be ascertained after oral administration by assessing the loudness of the apical systolic murmur, the severity of mitral systolic anterior motion on echocardiography, or the outflow tract pressure gradient by Doppler techniques. The usual starting dose is 100 mg qid, the daily dose is increased by 50 mg qid until on the third day the patient is taking 200 mg qid. The ECG is checked for QT interval prolongation and inquiry made about the anticholinergic side-effects (dry mouth, difficulty in micturition, constipation, blurred vision). These can be treated with long-acting pyridostigmine (160 mg bid) or, alternatively, the dose of disopyramide can be reduced to alleviate the side-effects. A number of patients with mild-to-moderate obstruction appear to have long-term benefit, but patients with more significant

TABLE 91.8 TREATMENT OF HYPERTROPHIC CARDIOMYOPATHY BY HEMODYNAMIC SUBGROUP

Hemodynamic Subgroup	Aim of Therapy	Medical Therapy		Surgery	
		Preferred	*Alternative*	*Preferred*	*Alternative*
Resting obstruction	Relief of obstruction to LV outflow (which will also improve relaxation[11])	Disopyramide*	Calcium antagonists† β-adrenergic blocking drugs	Ventriculomyectomy	Mitral valve replacement (only under special circumstances; see text)
Latent obstruction	Prevent provocation of obstruction	β-adrenergic blocking drugs	?Calcium antagonists† ?Disopyramide*	Ventriculomyectomy (rarely)	Mitral valve replacement (only under special circumstances; see text)
Nonobstructive HCM	Improve LV relaxation	Calcium antagonists	β-adrenergic blocking agents	N/A	N/A

* Disopyramide will lessen or abolish resting obstruction and thereby improve relaxation.[11]
† Calcium antagonists (particularly nifedipine, but also verapamil) by their vasodilator action could worsen or provoke obstruction to outflow.

obstruction do not appear to sustain the improvement and subsequently require surgery. The advantages of disopyramide appear to be the lack of significant adverse reactions other than the anticholinergic side-effects and its inherent antiarrhythmic action.

There is the potential for using a combination of negative inotropic agents in HCM patients with resting obstruction. Both β-adrenergic blocking agents and disopyramide as well as β-adrenergic blocking agents and calcium antagonists have been used in this way Such combinations, particularly if used in addition to antiarrhythmic agents, have the potential for further impairing left ventricular function and causing heart failure. Double or triple negative inotropic therapy should be used only in unusual circumstances and only if the patient is not a surgical candidate.

When patients with resting obstruction have significant symptoms in spite of adequate medical therapy, when they are intolerant of their medical therapy, and/or when they are dissatisfied with their disease-imposed physical limitations, ventriculomyectomy should be recommended. This form of surgery is believed to be successful because of the ventricular septal thinning and the widened outflow tract, which result in the abolition of mitral systolic anterior motion, the obstruction to outflow, and the mitral regurgitation. Figure 91.12 indicates the means by which ventriculomyectomy is believed to be successful.

Numerous reports have documented the short- and long-term symptomatic and hemodynamic benefits of this surgery, which can be carried out at a risk of 5% or less in centers that have experience with the procedure.[51-54] Annual mortality of all patients with HCM is estimated at 3% to 4%, and that of patients with resting obstruction may be higher. Following surgery, the annual mortality (including surgical mortality) is 2.6% to 3.5%, while the postoperative annual mortality is 1.5% to 1.8%.[53,54] In my experience, after having followed some 120 patients through ventriculomyectomy, the symptomatic and hemodynamic benefits of this procedure far exceed those obtained with any current form of medical therapy. Following completely successful surgery, patients have no obstruction to outflow, no mitral regurgitation, no symptoms, and none of the physical signs of obstruction or mitral regurgitation. Even when surgery is not completely successful, the patients are more easily managed with medical therapy postoperatively. This form of surgery has very definite benefits to patients who have been troubled with recurrent or chronic atrial fibrillation preoperatively. Successful surgery will result in a decrease in left atrial size and restoration of normal sinus rhythm in patients under 40 to 45 years of age,[55] while older patients—although left atrial enlargement and atrial fibrillation will remain postoperatively—are much better able to tolerate this arrhythmia in the absence of the outflow obstruction and mitral regurgitation. Before surgery it is pointed out to all patients that the operation is directed at abolishing the obstruction to outflow and does not affect the underlying cardiomyopathy. Postoperatively these patients are still prone to ventricular arrhythmias but appear to tolerate them better.

I continue to favor ventriculomyectomy for relief of the outflow tract obstruction and mitral regurgitation when the latter can be demonstrated to be related to mitral systolic anterior motion and the pressure gradient (Fig. 91.6). Previously, the relationship of the mitral regurgitation to systolic anterior motion and the pressure gradient had to be ascertained by invasive studies (Fig. 91.6).[32] Today, this relationship can be determined noninvasively by the use of echocardiography and Doppler techniques during pharmacologic intervention.[11] In cases where there is moderate-to-severe mitral regurgitation that is independent of mitral systolic anterior motion and the pressure gradient, consideration should be given to replacing the mitral valve with or without a myectomy. Cooley has favored mitral valve replacement as the surgery of choice in patients with resting obstruction in that it removes the offending mitral leaflets.[56] However, mitral valve replacement would unnecessarily subject these patients to all the attendant risks of prosthetic valves in the short and the long term. A particular risk for mitral prostheses in patients with HCM is the danger of the prosthesis impinging on the ventricular myocardium because of the small ventricular volume. If a tissue prosthesis was used, there would be a greater risk of systolic anterior motion of the prosthetic leaflet closest to the outflow tract.

LATENT OBSTRUCTION

The vast majority of patients with latent obstruction to outflow have only a limited extent of hypertrophy (Table 91.3), and therefore are not usually troubled with problems of impaired relaxation or significant arrhythmias. However, the limited degree of septal hypertrophy is located in the subaortic area and these patients therefore have the potential for developing outflow obstruction with suitable provocation. For some 20 years now I have managed these patients with β-adrenergic blocking agents to prevent provocation of the obstruction by adrenergic stimuli (Table 91.8). This form of therapy in some 70 patients has resulted in significant symptomatic benefit, and surgery has rarely been advised for these patients. No patient with latent obstruction and a limited extent of hypertrophy has died as a result of heart disease.[11]

Disopyramide or calcium-blocking agents represent alternative forms of therapy for patients with latent obstruction (Table 91.8). I have rarely reverted to these forms of therapy because disopyramide has the disadvantage of impairing relaxation, while the vasodilator action of the calcium antagonists (particularly nifedipine) has the unwanted potential of provoking obstruction to outflow.[11]

NONOBSTRUCTIVE HYPERTROPHIC CARDIOMYOPATHY

The calcium antagonists (verapamil, nifedipine, and diltiazem) represent the preferred line of therapy for HCM patients without obstruction to outflow. Left ventricular relaxation is improved by a lowering of myoplasmic calcium, by a decrease in the asynchrony of contraction and relaxation,[16] and by an increase in the coronary filling load,[11] while left ventricular systolic function could be improved by the afterload-reducing characteristics of these drugs. However, the negative inotropic effect of these drugs would depress left ventricular systolic function; both verapamil and nifedipine have caused heart failure in nonobstructive HCM with impaired systolic function.[11] In spite of this potential danger, the use of these agents is the therapy of choice in symptomatic patients with nonobstructive HCM. All three agents have been demonstrated to improve the indices of left ventricular relaxation and to result in symptomatic improvement. Verapamil has been used most extensively for this purpose in doses varying between 240 mg and 480 mg/day in divided doses.[46,47] Nifedipine in doses of 40 mg to 80 mg/day has resulted in symptomatic improvement in 50% of patients, but a significant percentage complained of flushing, dizziness, headache, and postural hypotension which limited the usefulness of the drug. Long-acting forms of nifedipine may circumvent these problems. Diltiazem has also been reported to have beneficial effects. I use verapamil in preference to nifedipine to improve relaxation in these patients, but only because of the frequency of side-effects with the latter.

MANAGEMENT OF ARRHYTHMIAS

Both atrial and ventricular arrhythmias are a significantly greater problem in HCM patients with resting obstruction than in those with latent or no obstruction. Atrial fibrillation in HCM is almost invariably associated with left atrial enlargement,[55] which is the rule with resting obstruction (due to the concomitant mitral regurgitation) and is rare in the other hemodynamic subgroups.[27]

Atrial arrhythmias in HCM result in dramatic hemodynamic and clinical deterioration as a result of loss of atrial transport function, and everything possible must be done to restore sinus rhythm. As previously indicated, recurrent or established atrial fibrillation in patients with resting obstruction is an indication for surgical intervention. Patients with chronic or recurrent atrial fibrillation require long-term anticoagulant therapy because of the risk of systemic emboli.

First-line drug therapy for atrial arrhythmias in HCM consists of the use of quinidine, procainamide, and disopyramide. Although some authors favor amiodarone, I reserve its use for older patients and those who do not respond to type 1 antiarrhythmic agents or to surgical

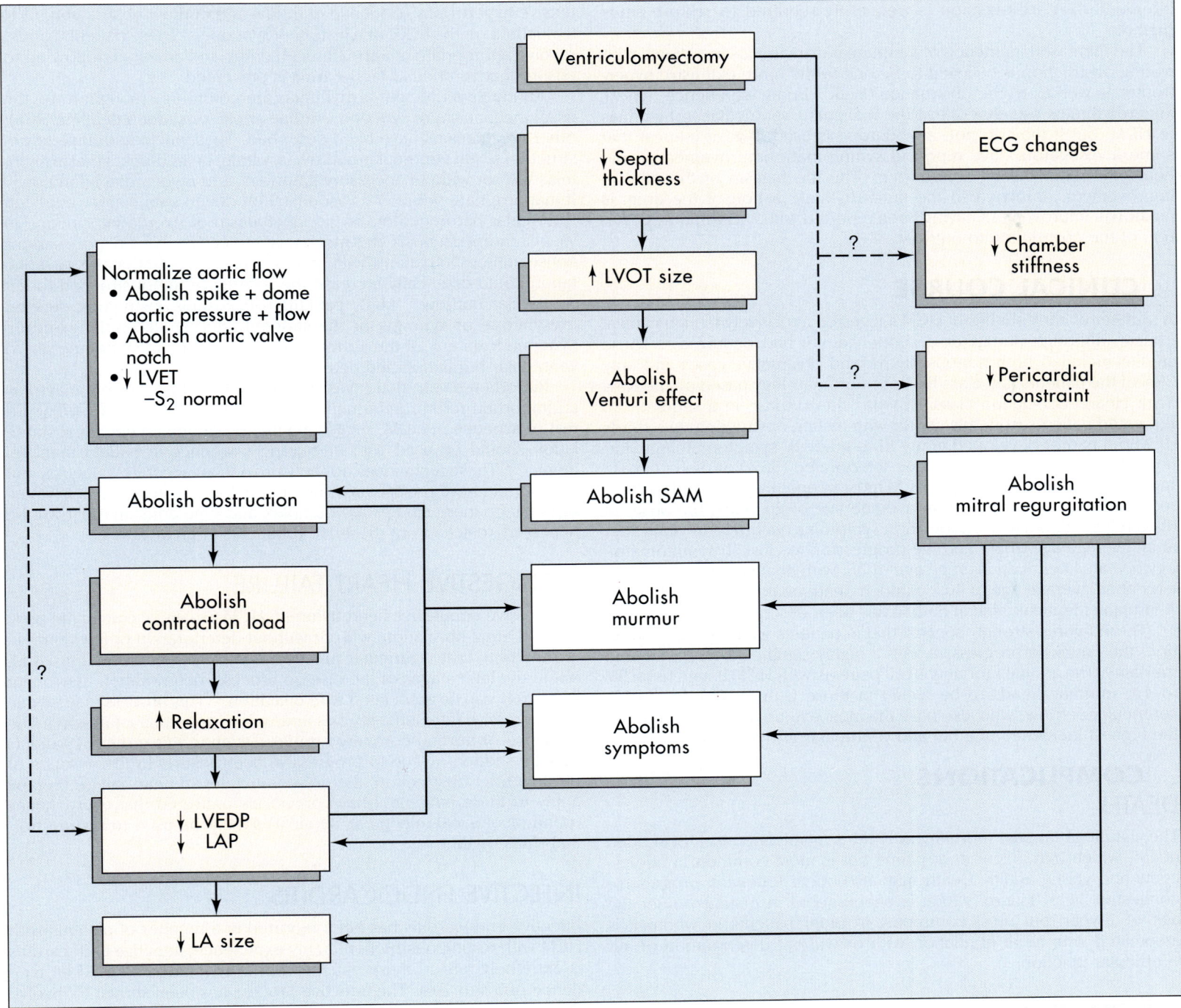

FIGURE 91.12 Diagram indicating the proposed mechanism(s) by which ventriculomyectomy affects the hemodynamic and clinical findings in HCM patients with resting obstruction (muscular subaortic stenosis). By decreasing septal thickness, ventriculomyectomy increases the size of the left ventricular outflow tract (LVOT) and results in the early systolic ejection path being displaced away from the mitral leaflets, thus reducing or abolishing the Venturi forces on these leaflets. This results in the abolition of the mitral leaflet systolic anterior motion (SAM) as a result of which the obstruction to outflow and mitral regurgitation is abolished. The abolition of the obstruction normalizes aortic flow as a result of which the spike-and-dome aortic flow and pressure profiles and aortic valve notch are abolished. Left ventricular ejection time (LVET) is no longer prolonged, and splitting of the second heart sound (S_2) becomes normal. Abolition of the obstruction abolishes the early systolic contraction load on the left ventricle which results in improved LV relaxation and a reduction in LV end-diastolic (LVEDP) and left atrial pressures (LAP). Abolition of the obstruction together with the lowering of LVEDP should also improve relaxation by increasing the hemodynamic coronary filling load that is applied to the relaxing myocardium. Abolition of mitral regurgitation would also decrease LVEDP and LAP as well as LA size, thus rendering the patient less vulnerable to atrial arrhythmias. Abolition of the apical systolic murmur results from abolition of obstruction and mitral regurgitation, while these latter two factors plus the lowering of LVEDP and LAP result in a lessening or abolition of the patient's symptoms. It is not known whether a decrease in chamber stiffness or in the degree of pericardial constraint could also favor symptomatic benefit following ventriculomyectomy. There is evidence that surgically induced ventricular conduction defects do not explain the beneficial effects of this surgery. (Modified from Wigle ED, Sasson Z, Henderson M, et al: Hypertrophic cardiomyopathy: The importance of the site and extent of hypertrophy. A review. Prog Cardiovasc Dis 28:1–83, 1985)

intervention. Cardioversion is frequently required to restore sinus rhythm.

The increased incidence of ventricular arrhythmias in patients with resting obstruction is believed to be due to the more extensive hypertrophy as well as to the obstruction itself.[11] In my experience, type 1 antiarrhythmics usually control the malignant ventricular arrhythmias in HCM, but if they do not, amiodarone is used. It is of interest that some investigators have reported symptomatic improvement in patients with HCM taking amiodarone. The mechanism of this clinical improvement, unrelated to the antiarrhythmic action of the drug, is unknown, improvement having been reported with and without alleviation of the obstruction to outflow.

CLINICAL COURSE

A number of early studies of HCM suggested a relatively benign clinical course, although unexpected sudden death had occurred.[57] These studies included both nonobstructive and obstructive cases and only 25% of the patients had class III–IV symptomatology based on the New York Heart Association classification.[57] In contrast, in a series of 26 untreated patients from this center with resting obstruction, two thirds of whom had or developed grade III to grade IV symptomatology during a 4-year follow-up, 66% either deteriorated (55%) or died (11%).[58] In an adult patient population, HCM most frequently presented with the recognition of a murmur at an average age of 20 years; the onset of class II New York Heart Association symptoms occurred 10 years later at an average age of 30; and the progression to class III symptomatology 5 years later at an average age of 35, with death occurring 5 years later at an average age of 40.[58] Sudden death could occur at any time. A virtually identical clinical course has been described by others.

These figures strongly suggest that in patients with resting obstruction, the course is progressive with a highly significant morbidity and mortality. The annual mortality of all patients with HCM is said to be 3% to 4%; mortality tends to be higher in those with obstruction to left ventricular outflow, who also have the most extensive hypertrophy and the highest incidence of atrial and ventricular arrhythmias.

COMPLICATIONS

DEATH

The significant annual mortality in HCM is mainly the result of sudden death, which may occur at any time but is most common in adolescents and young adults. Death may also occur following progressive congestive heart failure, which is encountered in patients under the age of 1 year, but most commonly in older patients in whom it is associated with atrial fibrillation with or without deterioration of left ventricular function.

SUDDEN DEATH

Risk factors for sudden death are young age, history of syncope, symptomatic status, a family history of malignant HCM and sudden death, and the occurrence of asymptomatic ventricular tachycardia on ambulatory rhythm monitoring.[43,44,58,59] The risk of sudden death is eight times as great in patients with asymptomatic ventricular tachycardia on ambulatory rhythm monitoring as it is in patients without this arrhythmia.[43-44] This arrhythmia is found most frequently in patients with extensive hypertrophy, evidence of inflow and outflow obstruction, LVH +/− strain on the ECG, or a history of syncope.[11] These patients should receive appropriate antiarrhythmia therapy and adequate follow-up to ensure that ventricular tachycardia is prevented.

Although ventricular arrhythmias are commonly thought to be the usual mechanism of syncope, cardiac arrest, or sudden death in HCM, other mechanisms have been described. These include complete obstruction to left ventricular outflow, asystole, heart block, atrial arrhythmias with or without accessory pathways, and myocardial infarction.[59] If inappropriate peripheral vasodilatation due to stimulation of the left ventricular baroreceptors is the mechanism of exertional syncope in valvular aortic stenosis, this mechanism would have even more serious consequences in patients with resting obstruction, in that the vasodilatation could drastically increase the severity of the obstruction to left ventricular outflow.[11] Many patients with resting obstruction develop presyncope or syncope or die suddenly during strenuous exertion. Syncope from any of the above causes could ultimately deteriorate to ventricular fibrillation and death.

Reports indicate that invasive electrophysiologic testing may play an important role in determining the exact mechanism of cardiac arrest or syncope in HCM, suggesting that programmed electrical stimulation should be used with increasing frequency in patient management.[59,60] These techniques not only provide an accurate diagnosis, but also permit more precise tailoring of drug therapy than previously possible. Since these studies are complex and time consuming, it will be necessary to select out those HCM patients at greatest risk.

CONGESTIVE HEART FAILURE

Progressive congestive heart failure in HCM usually occurs in the presence of atrial fibrillation, with or without deterioration of left ventricular function. Left ventricular function is usually supranormal in HCM, but in the later stages of the disease process, deterioration may occur and rarely can be associated with dilatation.[61] This process may be due to progressive interstitial fibrosis and/or to myocardial infarction in the presence of normal coronary arteries. Death in this group of patients may be sudden or due to progressive heart failure. In the absence of outflow tract obstruction, the usual principles of heart failure therapy apply to these patients. I have previously indicated that every means (pharmacological, electrical, surgical) should be used to restore normal sinus rhythm.

INFECTIVE ENDOCARDITIS

Infective endocarditis has been reported in a number of patients with HCM with resting obstruction. In my experience, infective endocarditis is extremely rare in these patients, but others have reported an incidence of 5% to 10%. The infective process has been shown to involve the mitral and aortic valves or both in any given case, and has resulted in aortic regurgitation, or increased mitral regurgitation. The management of infective endocarditis in HCM should not differ significantly from that associated with other types of heart disease. If surgical intervention is required, it is important to determine preoperatively which valve(s) are involved. I am unaware of infective endocarditis occurring in patients with either latent obstruction or nonobstructive HCM. Thus, antibiotic prophylaxis is advised only in patients with resting obstruction.

REFERENCES

1. Brock RC: Functional obstruction of the left ventricle. Guys Hosp Rep 106:221, 1957
2. Teare RD: Asymmetrical hypertrophy of the heart in young adults. Br Heart J 20:1, 1958
3. Braunwald E, Morrow AG, Cornell WP, et al: Idiopathic hypertrophic subaortic stenosis. Am J Med 29:924, 1960
4. Wigle ED, Heimbecker RO, Gunton RW: Idiopathic ventricular septal hypertrophy causing muscular subaortic stenosis. Circulation 26:325, 1962
5. Braunwald E, Lambrew C, Rockoff S, et al: Idiopathic hypertrophic subaortic stenosis: I. Description of the disease based upon an analysis of 64 patients. Circulation 29 and 30 (suppl 4):3, 1964
6. Wigle ED, Adelman AG, Silver MD: Pathophysiological consideration in muscular subaortic stenosis, in Wolstenholme GEW, O'Connor M (eds): Hypertrophic Obstructive Cardiomyopathy, p. 63. Ciba Foundation Study Group, No. 47, London, Churchill, 1971
7. Larter W, Allen H, Sahn D, et al.: The asymmetrically hypertrophied septum. Further differentiation of its causes. Circulation 53:19, 1976
8. Shah P, Gramiak R, Kramer D: Ultrasound localization of left ventricular outflow obstruction in hypertrophic obstructive cardiomyopathy. Circulation 40:3, 1969
9. Maron BJ, Harding AM, Spirito P, et al: Systolic anterior motion of the posterior mitral leaflet: A previously unrecognized cause of dynamic subaortic obstruction in patients with hypertrophic cardiomyopathy. Circulation 68:282, 1983

10. Maron BJ, Gottdiener JS, Epstein SE: Patterns and significance of distribution of left ventricular hypertrophy in hypertrophic cardiomyopathy. Am J Cardiol 48:418, 1981
11. Wigle ED, Sasson Z, Henderson M, et al: Hypertrophic cardiomyopathy. The importance of the site and the extent of hypertrophy. A review. Prog Cardiovasc Dis 28:1, 1985
12. Hanrath P, Mathey DG, Siegert R, et al: Left ventricular relaxation and filling pattern in different forms of left ventricular hypertrophy. An echocardiographic study. Am J Cardiol 45:15, 1980
13. Pollick C, Morgan CD, Gilbert BW, et al: Muscular subaortic stenosis: The temporal relationship between systolic anterior motion of the anterior mitral leaflet and pressure gradient. Circulation 66:1087, 1982
14. Pollick C, Rakowski H, Wigle ED: Muscular subaortic stenosis: The quantitative relationship between systolic anterior motion and the pressure gradient. Circulation 69:43, 1984
15. Bonow RO, Frederick RM, Bacharach SL, et al: Atrial systole and left ventricular filling in hypertrophic cardiomyopathy: Effect of verapamil. Am J Cardiol 51:1386, 1983
16. Bonow R, Vitale D, Bacharach S, et al: Regional left ventricular asynchrony and impaired global left ventricular diastolic filling in hypertrophic cardiomyopathy: effect of verapamil (abstr). Circulation 70(suppl 2):303, 1984
17. Murgo JP, Alter BR, Dorethy JF, et al: Dynamics of left ventricular ejection in obstructive and nonobstructive hypertrophic cardiomyopathy. J Clin Invest 66:1369, 1980
18. Maron BJ, Gottdiener JS, Arce J, et al: Dynamic subaortic obstruction in hypertrophic cardiomyopathy: Analysis by pulsed Doppler echocardiography. J Am Coll Cardiol 6:1, 1985
19. Maron BJ, Nichols PF, Pickle LW, et al: Patterns of inheritance in hypertrophic cardiomyopathy: Assessment by M-mode and two-dimensional echocardiography. Am J Cardiol 53:1087, 1984
20. Maron BJ, Roberts WC: Hypertrophic cardiomyopathy and cardiac muscle cell disorganization revisited: Relation between the two and significance. Am Heart J 102:95, 1981
21. Bulkley BH, Weisfeldt ML, Hutchins GM: Isometric cardiac contraction: A possible cause of the disorganized myocardial pattern of idiopathic hypertrophic subaortic stenosis. N Engl J Med 296:135, 1977
22. Goodwin JF: The frontiers of cardiomyopathy. Br Heart J 48:1, 1982
23. Perloff JK: Pathogenesis of hypertrophic cardiomyopathy: Hypotheses and speculations. Am Heart J 101:219, 1981
24. Liew CC, Sole MJ, Silver MD, et al: Electrophoretic profiles of nonhistone nuclear proteins of human hearts with muscular subaortic stenosis. Circ Res 46:513, 1980
25. Thompson R, Ahmed M, Pridie R, et al: Hypertrophic cardiomyopathy after aortic valve replacement. Am J Cardiol 45:33, 1980
26. Henry WL, Clark CE, Griffith JM, et al: Mechanism of left ventricular outflow obstruction in patients with obstructive asymmetric septal hypertrophy (idiopathic hypertrophic subaortic stenosis). Am J Cardiol 35:337, 1975
27. Gilbert BW, Pollick C, Adelman AG, et al: Hypertrophic cardiomyopathy: Subclassification by M mode echocardiography. Am J Cardiol 45:861, 1980
28. Bellhouse BJ, Bellhouse FH: The fluid mechanics of subaortic stenosis in a model left ventricle. University of Oxford, Department of Engineering Science, Report No. 1032/72, 1972
29. Criley JM, Siegel RJ: A non-obstructive view of hypertrophic cardiomyopathy, in Goodwin JF (ed). Heart Disease, p. 157. Lancaster, MTP Press Ltd.
30. Bonow RO, Ostrow DR, Rosing RO, et al: Dynamic pressure-volume alterations during left ventricular ejection in hypertrophic cardiomyopathy: Evidence for true obstruction to left ventricular outflow (abstr). Circulation 70 (suppl 2):17, 1984
31. Ross J Jr, Braunwald E, Gault JH, et al: Mechanism of the intraventricular pressure gradient in idiopathic hypertrophic subaortic stenosis. Circulation 34:558, 1966
32. Wigle ED, Adelman AG, Auger P, et al: Mitral regurgitation in muscular subaortic stenosis. Am J Cardiol 24:698, 1969
33. Wigle ED, Auger P, Marquis Y: Muscular subaortic stenosis: The direct relation between the intraventricular pressure difference and left ventricular ejection time. Circulation 36:36, 1967
34. Wigle ED, Marquis Y, Auger P: Muscular subaortic stenosis. Initial left ventricular inflow tract pressure in the assessment of intraventricular pressure differences in man. Circulation 35:1100, 1967
35. Gaasch WH, Levine HJ, Quinones MA, et al: Left ventricular compliance: Mechanisms and clinical implications. Am J Cardiol 38:645, 1976
36. Brutsaert DL, Housmans PR, Goethals MA: Dual control of relaxation. Its role in the ventricular function in the mammalian heart. Circ Res 47:637, 1980
37. Brutsaert DL, Rademakers FE, Sys SU: Triple control of relaxation: Implications in cardiac disease. Circulation 69:190, 1984
38. Bonow RO, Ostrow HG, Rosing DR, et al: Effects of verapamil on left ventricular systolic and diastolic function in patients with hypertrophic cardiomyopathy: Pressure-volume analysis with a nonimaging scintillation probe. Circulation 68:1062, 1983
39. Lorell BH, Paulus WJ, Grossman W: Modification of abnormal left ventricular diastolic properties by nifedipine in patients with hypertrophic cardiomyopathy. Circulation 65:499, 1982
40. Wigle ED, Baron R: The electrocardiogram in muscular subaortic stenosis: The effect of a left septal incision and right bundle branch block. Circulation 34:585, 1965
41. Sakamoto T, Tei C, Murayama M, et al: Giant negative T wave inversion as a manifestation of asymmetric apical hypertrophy (AAH) of the left ventricle. Echocardiographic and ultrasonocardiotomographic study. Jpn Heart J 17:611, 1976
42. Yamaguchi H, Ishimura T, Nishiyama S, et al: Hypertrophic nonobstructive cardiomyopathy with giant negative T waves (apical hypertrophy): Ventriculographic and echocardiographic features in 30 patients. Am J Cardiol 44:401, 1979
43. Maron BJ, Savage DD, Wolfson JK, et al: Prognostic significance of 24 hour ambulatory electrocardiographic monitoring in patients with hypertrophic cardiomyopathy: A prospective study. Am J Cardiol 48:252, 1981
44. McKenna WJ, England D, Doi YL, et al: Arrhythmia in hypertrophic cardiomyopathy. I: Influence on prognosis. Br Heart J 46:168, 1981
45. Falicov RE, Resnekov L, Bharati S, et al: Midventricular obstruction: A variant of obstructive cardiomyopathy. Am J Cardiol 37:432, 1976
46. Kaltenbach M, Hopf R, Kober G, et al: Treatment of hypertrophic obstructive cardiomyopathy with verapamil. Br Heart J 42:35, 1979
47. Epstein SE, Rosing DR: Verapamil: Its potential for causing serious complications in patients with hypertrophic cardiomyopathy. Circulation 64:437, 1981
48. Chatterjee K, Raff G, Anderson D, Parmley WW: Hypertrophic cardiomyopathy—therapy with slow channel inhibiting agents. Prog Cardiovasc Dis 25:193, 1982
49. Betocchi SB, Cannon RL III, Watson RM et al: Effects of sublingual nifedipine on hemodynamics of systolic and diastolic function in patients with hypertrophic cardiomyopathy. Circulation 72:1001, 1985
50. Pollick C: Muscular subaortic stenosis. Hemodynamic and clinical improvement after disopyramide. New Engl J Med 307:997, 1982
51. Morrow AG, Brockenbrough EC: Surgical treatment of idiopathic hypertrophic subaortic stenosis: Technic and hemodynamic results of subaortic ventriculomyotomy. Ann Surg 154:181, 1961
52. Wigle ED, Chrysohou A, Bigelow W: Results of ventriculomyotomy in muscular subaortic stenosis. Am J Cardiol 11:572, 1963
53. Maron BJ, Epstein SE, Morrow AG: Symptomatic status and prognosis of patients after operation for hypertrophic obstructive cardiomyopathy: Efficacy of ventricular septal myotomy and myectomy. Eur Heart J 4 (suppl F):175, 1983
54. Beahrs MM, Tajik AJ, Seward JB, et al: Hypertrophic obstructive cardiomyopathy: 10–21 year follow-up after partial septal myectomy. Am J Cardiol 51:1160, 1983
55. Watson DC, Henry WL, Epstein SE, et al: Effects of operation on left atrial size and the occurrence of atrial fibrillation in patients with hypertrophic subaortic stenosis. Circulation 55:178, 1977
56. Cooley DA, Leachman RD, Sukasch DC: Diffuse muscular subaortic stenosis: Surgical treatment. Am J Cardiol 31:1, 1973
57. Frank S, Braunwald E: Idiopathic hypertrophic subaortic stenosis. Clinical analysis of 126 patients with emphasis on the natural history. Circulation 37:759, 1968
58. Adelman AG, Wigle ED, Ranganathan N, et al: The clinical course in muscular subaortic stenosis: A retrospective and prospective study of 60 hemodynamically proved cases. Ann Int Med 77:515, 1972
59. Lever HM, Schiavone WA, Gill CC: Sudden death in hypertrophic cardiomyopathy. Cleve Clin Q 51:65, 1984
60. Kowey PR, Eisenberg R, Engel TR: Sustained arrhythmias in hypertrophic obstructive cardiomyopathy. New Engl J Med 310:1566, 1984
61. Oakley CM: Hypertrophic obstructive cardiomyopathy: Patterns of progression, in Wolstenholme GEW and O'Connor M (eds): CIBA Foundation Study Group 37, p 9. London, J&A Churchill, 1971

Diseases of the Pericardium

David H. Spodick

SYNOPSIS OF PERICARDIAL ANATOMY

The pericardium is an anatomically specialized organ, its structure designed to subserve its surprisingly complex physiology.[1] The two major components of the pericardium are its mesothelial sac (serosa), a cell monolayer covering the heart and juxtacardiac great vessels and, in humans, the pulmonary veins, and continuing over the inner aspect of its other major component, the fibrosa, which clasps the serosa externally and continues up over the arch of the aorta where it blends with the deep cervical fascia.[2] The fibrosa is attached to the central tendon of the diaphragm and loosely anchored by ligaments to the manubrium and xiphoid. The monocellular serosa covering the heart surface is the visceral pericardium ("epicardium"). The rest of the serosa together with the fibrosa which it lines internally form the parietal pericardium ("pericardium"). The pericardium encloses the terminal portions of the vena cava and pulmonary veins in the shape of an inverted "U" behind the left atrium, enclosing a recess, the oblique sinus. Between the atria and superior vena cava behind, and the ascending aorta and pulmonary artery in front, there is another pericardial space, the transverse sinus.[2]

Ultrastructural details of the serosal cells show microvilli that presumably bear friction and facilitate fluid and ion exchange (Fig. 92.1). Oblique during diastole, they become relatively perpendicular in systole. Despite a basal lamina, the mesothelium detaches at a touch. The cells tend to interdigitate and overlap—a design permitting changes in surface configuration while maintaining mechanical stability. Actin filaments within the cells appear to be involved in shape changes, while cytoskeletal filaments provide structural support.[1]

The fibrosa consists of fibrocollagenous tissue that is very wavy in youth and straightens with aging, interspersed with elastic fibers that become less densely distributed with aging. The fibrous tissue is further specialized into bundles (fascicles) that seem to be purposefully organized and are thickest over the thinner parts of the myocardium. Their orientation seems determined by mechanical factors, particularly extrapericardial traction forces (*e.g.*, respiratory movements) and internal pressures. For example, parallel, almost ligamentous, prolongations over the aortic arch may buttress it against the thrust of systole.[2]

The internal thoracic arteries supply the superior, lateral, and inferior pericardium, while aortic twigs ramify posteriorly. Bronchial arteries supply some blood. Lymph drains to the anterior and posterior mediastinal nodes from corresponding aspects of the parietal pericardium. There are usually one or two lymph nodes within the fibrosa, near the mouth of the inferior vena cava. The visceral pericardium drains to tracheal and bronchial nodes via the superficial plexus of cardiac lymphatics. The phrenic nerves supply most of the pericardium; some posterior innervation derives from the esophageal plexus of the vagi.

PERICARDIAL PHYSIOLOGY: FUNCTION OF THE NORMAL PERICARDIUM

Clinical and experimental observations yield a concept of the role of the healthy pericardium as outlined in Table 92.1.[1] Because the heart adapts to congenital and surgical absence of the pericardium it is obviously not needed to sustain life; with a normal heart and chest, the pericardium appears to have little influence on cardiac pressures, dimensions, or chamber interactions. Yet under a variety of physiologic and pathologic challenges, the mechanical effect of the parietal pericardium and metabolic activity of both pericardial layers exert both subtle and profound influences on cardiac function and symptom provocation. Thus, the pericardium has mechanical, membranous, and ligamentous roles. Each derives from the structure of the pericardium and its components.

Mechanical functions mainly relate to the relative stiffness of the parietal pericardium, the effects of a chamber filled with fluid at slightly subatmospheric pressure, and incompletely understood circulatory "feedback" regulation via pericardial neuro- and mechanoreceptors.[1] Both the pressure-volume curve of the intact pericardium and the stress-strain curve of excised pericardial tissue show initial distensibility with rapid resistance on increasing stretch.[3] Each curve thus has a J shape, that is, an initial slow rise of pressure as volume increases (and of stress as strain increases) followed by an "elbow" and a sharp, almost vertical rise. In intact pericardium, pressure changes with early increase of pericardial fluid are small due to the pericardial reserve volume provided by the normal slight slackness of the membrane and the oblique and transverse sinuses within it, as well as straightening of the wavy collagen bundles and stretching of the elastin fibers. (At necropsy the pericardium is distended by 100 ml to 200 ml of fluid, but during life smaller amounts may have detectable effects.) The steep rise in pressure with further increase of pericardial contents applies to an acute change; patients with extremely enlarged hearts have *normal pericardial fluid pressure* (equal to and varying with pleural pressure during respiration: −5 mm Hg to +5 mm Hg). Chronic slow increase in pericardial size is accommodated by gradual stretch and subsequent pericardial hypertrophy (increased weight and surface area).

The parietal pericardium provides a relatively inelastic cardiac envelope that appears to limit acute cardiac dilation, notably acute ventriculoatrial regurgitation. Normal ventricular compliance (volume-elasticity relation) is maintained, chamber compliance being less with the pericardium intact than with it open or absent. Moreover, output responses to venous inflow loads and heart rate fluctuations are maintained better with the pericardium intact. The pericardial hydrostatic system—pericardium plus the normal 15 ml to 50 ml of pericardial fluid—distributes hydrostatic forces over the epicardial surfaces, favoring equality of transmural end-diastolic pressure throughout the ventricles and therefore uniform stretch of muscle fibers (*i.e.*, preload), permitting the Starling mechanism to operate uniformly at all intraventricular pressures.[1] The pericardium also constantly compensates for changes in gravitational and inertial forces, distributing them evenly around the heart, and provides a mutually restrictive chamber favoring balanced output from both ventricles integrated over several cardiac cycles. Ventricular interaction also depends partly on the relative stiffness of the pericardium, explaining reduced ventricular compliance when there is increased pressure in the opposite ventricle. Moreover, either ventricle generates greater isovolumic pressure from any diastolic volume with the pericardium intact. It is assumed that the presence of the parietal pericardium maintains a functionally optimal cardiac shape.

Pericardial pressure curves resemble a mirror image of the pressure in the adjacent cardiac chamber, particularly on the right. With normal cavitary pressures, *pericardial* transmural pressure is zero because pericardial pressure is approximately equal to and varies with pleural pressure at the same hydrostatic level. Pericardial pressure affects *myocardial* transmural pressure by the following relation: transmural pressure equals cavitary pressure minus adjacent intrapericardial pressure. Because myocardial transmural pressure is the actual chamber distending (*i.e.*, true filling) pressure, the normally negative pericardial pressure ensures a distending pressure greater than cavitary pressure.[3] Moreover, because of the closed pericardial chamber at slightly subatmospheric pressure, the level of transmural cardiac pressures will be low relative to even large increases in "filling pressures" referred to atmospheric pressures (*i.e.*, atrial pressure). Because of more negative pericardial pressure when the ventricles shrink during ejection, pericardial pressure changes aid atrial filling.

Pericardial mechanical function (perhaps also membranous function) includes incompletely understood "feedback" cardiocirculatory regulation by pericardial servomechanisms. These utilize neuroreceptors that signal by means of the vagus nerves to lower heart rate and blood pressure, and mechanoreceptors that lower blood pressure and contract the spleen.

Membranous functions of the pericardium result from its physical presence and are partly inferential. Thus, the pericardium seems to reduce friction due to heart movements, to be a barrier to inflammation from contiguous structures, and to buttress thinner parts of the

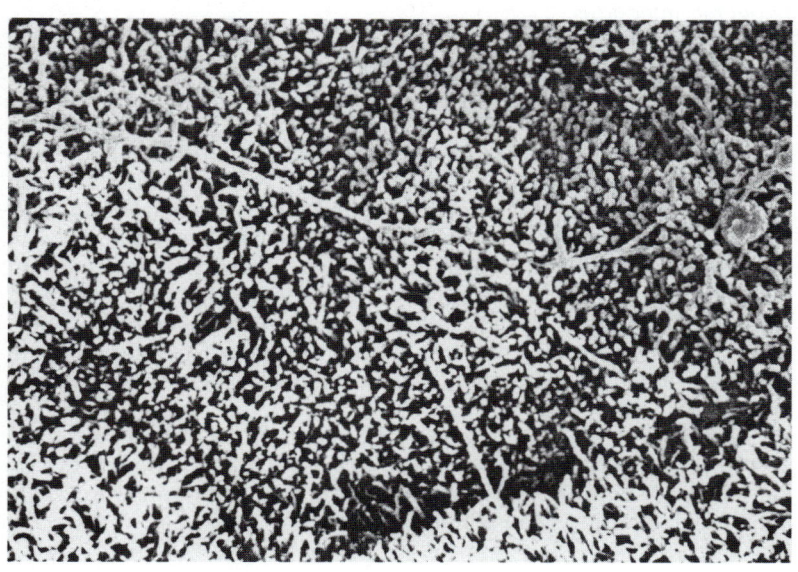

FIGURE 92.1 Electron photomicrograph of pericardial mesothelium showing microvilli (original magnification × 2600). (Courtesy Jerome Jacobs, Ph.D.)

TABLE 92.1 PHYSIOLOGY OF THE NORMAL PERICARDIUM

Mechanical Function: Promotion of Cardiac Efficiency, Especially During Hemodynamic Overloads

I. Relatively inelastic cardiac envelope
  A. Limitation of excessive acute dilation
  B. Protection against excessive ventriculoatrial regurgitation
  C. Maintenance of normal ventricular compliance (*volume-elasticity relation*)
  D. Defense of the integrity of the Starling curve: *Starling mechanism operates uniformly at all intraventricular pressures because of presence of pericardium:*
    1. Maintains ventricular function curves
    2. Limits effects of increased left ventricular end-diastolic pressure
    3. Supports output responses to
      (a) Venous inflow loads and atrioventricular valve regurgitation (especially acute)
      (b) Rate fluctuations
    4. Hydrostatic system (pericardium plus pericardial fluid) distributes hydrostatic forces over epicardial surfaces
      (a) Favors equality of *transmural* end-diastolic pressure throughout ventricle, therefore uniform stretch of muscle fibers (preload)
      (b) Constantly compensates for changes in gravitational and inertial forces, distributing them evenly around the heart
  E. Ventricular interaction: relative pericardial stiffness
    1. Reduces ventricular compliance with increased pressure in the opposite ventricle (*e.g.*, limits right ventricular stroke work during increased impedance to left ventricular outflow)
    2. Provides a mutually restrictive chamber favoring balanced output from right and left ventricles integrated over several cardiac cycles
    3. Permits either ventricle to generate greater isovolumic pressure from any volume
  F. Maintenance of functionally optimal cardiac shape
II. Provision of closed chamber with slightly subatmospheric pressure in which:
  A. The level of *transmural* cardiac pressures will be low, relative to even large increases in "filling pressures" referred to atmospheric pressures
  B. Pressure changes aid atrial filling through more negative pericardial pressure during ventricular ejection
III. "Feedback" cardiocirculatory regulation via pericardial servomechanisms
  A. Neuroreceptors (via vagus): lower heart rate and blood pressure
  B. Mechanoreceptors: lower blood pressure and contract spleen
IV. ?? Limitation of hypertrophy associated with chronic exercise

Membranous Function

I. Reduction of external friction due to heart movements
II. Barrier to inflammation from contiguous structures
III. Buttressing of thinner portions of the myocardium
  A. Atria
  B. Right ventricle

IV. Defensive immunologic constituents in pericardial fluid
V. Fibrinolytic activity in mesothelial lining
VI. Prostacyclin release into pericardial sac

Ligamentous Function: Limitation of Undue Cardiac Displacement

myocardium, like the atria and right ventricle (RV). Complement components and other immunologic constituents have been found in pericardial fluid. Prostacyclin and prostacyclin synthetase are released into the pericardial sac continually and may influence its function and affect underlying coronary vessels. The mesothelial lining has fibrinolytic activity, which opposes intrapericardial blood clotting and adhesions.

The ligamentous function of the pericardium limits cardiac displacement through the superior, inferior, lateral, and anterior attachment by ligaments to adjacent structures.

NORMAL RESPIRATORY EFFECTS

Pericardial pressure both approximates and varies with pleural pressure. Initially, inspiratory reduction of pleural pressure normally reduces pericardial, right atrial (RA), RV, pulmonary wedge, and systemic arterial pressure very slightly. Pericardial pressure, however, decreases somewhat more than atrial pressure so that RA and other central transmural (i.e., distending) pressures increase, augmenting right heart filling and consequently right ventricular preload. Although pulmonary arterial flow velocity increases with inspiration, both aortic transmural pressure and aortic flow decrease while systemic venous return is increasing. Inspiratory "pooling" of the increased RV output in the lungs tends to reduce left heart filling. Inspiration also increases LV transmural pressure, slightly increasing LV "afterload" and contributing, with underfilling, to reduce LV output. Thus, changes in right heart pressures and output vary inversely, and changes in LV output and arterial blood pressure vary directly, with changes in pericardial (and pleural) pressure.

NORMAL PERICARDIAL FLUID

The pericardium in health contains 15 ml to 50 ml of serous fluid, which appears to be an ultrafiltrate of plasma, possibly with some overflow of myocardial interstitial fluid. The electrolyte concentrations are as predicted for a plasma ultrafiltrate while the protein concentration is lower than in plasma (but with a relatively higher albumin ratio, owing to albumin's lower molecular weight and ease of transmembrane transport). This yields an osmolarity consistent with an ultrafiltrate (therefore less than plasma). Small amounts of complement (C_3, C_4, CH50), other immune factors, myocardial cellular enzymes, and prostacyclin and related compounds are continually released into the pericardial fluid.

DISEASES OF THE PERICARDIUM

Table 92.2 makes it clear that every category of disease can involve the pericardium. By far the most frequently encountered clinically is acute pericarditis, although many cases may be clinically silent, including some with relatively small pericardial effusions ("clinically dry" pericarditis).

INFLAMMATION OF THE PERICARDIUM
PATHOGENESIS[2]

Inflammatory agents involve the pericardium through contiguity, the bloodstream, lymphatic spread, or by traumatic irritation. Contiguous inflammation spreads from lungs, pleura, mediastinal lymph nodes, myocardium, aorta, esophagus, or diaphragm (and liver). Myocarditis, aortitis, and especially myocardial infarction may injure the visceral pericardium, while most acute pericarditis involves the superficial myocardium to some extent (myopericarditis). Hematogenous inflammation arises from septicemia, immunopathic, and hypersensitivity states, "circulating toxins," noncontiguous neoplasms, and metabolic abnormalities. Lymphangeal involvement occurs from noncontiguous malignancies and, rarely, nonpenetrating esophagitis. Pericarditis also arises from direct or indirect trauma. Wounds and penetrating esophageal ulcers directly attack the pericardium. Indirect injury follows nonpenetrating chest trauma or therapeutic irradiation.

PATHOLOGY

Inflammation, diffuse or local, provokes a fibrinous pericardial exudate with or without serous effusion. The extent of the inflammatory reaction varies but is more or less characteristic for a given etiology, for example, the frequently intense inflammation in bacterial pericarditis. The normal pericardium is transparent and glistening because of its thinness and the regularity of its cellular arrangement, while the inflamed sac is usually dull, opaque, and sometimes "sandy." The mesothelium is usually lost and there is edema with capillary engorgement and proliferation. Cellular infiltration is best seen in the subepicardial connective and fatty tissue. Leukocytes are especially prominent in pyogenic infections.

PERICARDIAL SCARRING: ADHESIONS AND FIBROSIS

The plastic fibrinous exudate of acute pericarditis tends to form temporary adhesions but it is either reabsorbed or becomes a matrix for later fibrous, fibrogranulomatous, or sometimes calcified scars. (Neoplastic tissue can also cause adhesions.) These are usually clinically and physiologically unimportant, but can go on to circulatory impairment (cardiac constriction) and, if very thick, to roentgenographic changes. Table 92.3 classifies pericardial adhesions and fibrosis, from which functional significances can be inferred. Recurrent pericarditis and persistent inflammation may add new fibrinous exudate and cellular infiltrations.

All forms of pericarditis can cause adhesions and fibrosis. However, more severe inflammation and more severe trauma destructive of the serosa, especially with bleeding, have greater potential for both pericardial adhesions and ultimate constriction.

PERICARDIAL EFFUSION
PATHOPHYSIOLOGY

Pericardial effusion appears when fluid is produced too fast to be reabsorbed. The size of inflammatory, traumatic, and malignant effusions is increased by serosal cell damage, compression of veins and lymphatics (limiting reabsorption), and the oncotic effects of the proteinaceous exudate and molecular breakdown of any blood components. In general pericardial effusion has four consequences: (1) slow production of clinically insignificant amounts of fluid; (2) demonstrable fluid without symptoms or signs; (3) smaller or larger effusion, compressing the heart but checked by compensatory mechanisms; (4) cardiac tamponade.

Effusion fluid may be serous, suppurative, hemorrhagic, or mixed (serosanguineous). True effusion (exudate) almost always contains large amounts of fibrin and a significant protein content, while hydropericardium (noninflammatory transudate) has much less protein and no fibrin or blood. Hydropericardium usually occurs during sodium and water retention, as in cardiac failure, and should be distinguished from true (inflammatory or irritative) pericardial effusion. Hemorrhagic exudates occur in almost any type of pericarditis, but especially with severe infections and malignancies. They should be distinguished from hemopericardium, which follows hemorrhage into the sac, as with rupture of myocardial infarct or aortic aneurysm, wounds, or excessive anticoagulation. Suppurative effusions are mainly due to pyogenic bacteria and contain cellular debris and large numbers of leukocytes. In a given case, pericardial fluid may remain serous, suppurative, or hemorrhagic or may be transiently of one kind or another. In adults, pneumopericardium occurs almost exclusively with either hemopericardium or some other type of effusion and follows wounds and fistulas to adjacent air-containing organs. Introduction of air during paracentesis produces iatrogenic pneumopericardium. Infections by gas-producing organisms simulate pneumopericardium.

Noncompressing pericardial effusions range from very small (well under 100 ml) to several liters. Keys to their noncompressing status are the rate of fluid accumulation and the biomechanical characteristics of the pericardium. As long as the fluid does not accumulate faster than the rate at which the pericardium yields, there will be no significant increase in intrapericardial pressure. The threshold at which an effusion begins to be significantly compressive, therefore, is a function of the individual case. Recently, however, it has been shown that in patients who have small to large, hemodynamically inactive effusions, respiration markedly affects the systolic time intervals (STI) as compared to control patients with dry pericarditis whose respiratory STI vary normally.[4]

CLINICAL MANIFESTATIONS

Noncompressing pericardial effusions and hydropericardium will be asymptomatic unless they are large enough to compress adjacent organs, as in occasional patients who develop dysphagia, cough, dyspnea, hoarseness, hiccups, abdominal fullness, and nausea. Reliable physical findings may be absent. With massive effusions, the heart sounds may be distant and there may be a Ewart-Pins-Bamberger sign: percussion dullness and tubular breath sounds between the angle of the left (occasionally right) scapula and spine.[2]

LABORATORY DATA

Roentgenography showing enlargement of the cardiopericardial silhouette usually requires well over 200 ml of fluid, leaving it for echocardiography to identify smaller and confirm larger amounts of fluid. Chest films cannot distinguish between pericardial effusion and cardiac enlargement, with many effusions simulating cardiomegaly. Yet, a triangular or waterbottle "heart" outline, without the normal arcuate contours, especially in the presence of clear lung fields, strongly suggests pericardial effusion (Fig. 92.2). A well-penetrated lateral chest film may show pericardial fat lines (Fig. 92.3). Cardioangiography and various scanning techniques that show an abnormally wide "dead" space between the heart and the liver and lungs also strongly suggest pericardial effusion. Electrocardiography is not helpful in identifying an effusion although it may show signs of a related pericarditis, or electric alternation.

Echocardiography (Table 92.4) is the standard for identifying and following the course of pericardial effusions since it is highly reliable, although perhaps somewhat less so than the finer tissue identifying techniques, such as computed tomography (CT) and nuclear magnetic resonance imaging (MRI). Small, moderate, and large effusions can be recognized, but nonuniform distribution precludes fine quantitation. Fluid first appears as systolic separation of epicardium and posterior pericardium, progressing to add diastolic separation. Moderate-sized effusions constantly separate epicardial and pericardial echoes with the pericardial echo flat or moving only slightly. Unless there are anterior pericardial adhesions, fluid also appears anteriorly in moderate to large effusions. Only very large effusions penetrate behind the mitral annulus and lower left atrium, that is, into the pericardial oblique sinus. Especially with M-mode echoes, diagnostic problems—false-positives—arise from left pleural effusions (common in pericardial disease[1]), epicardial fat, tumor tissue and intrapericardial cysts, adhesions, and

---

TABLE 92.2 DISEASES OF THE PERICARDIUM*

I. Acute and subacute inflammatory pericardial disease
  A. Acute pericarditis and myopericarditis
    1. Noneffusive
    2. Effusive
      (a) Without cardiac compression
      (b) With tamponade of the heart
    3. Pneumohydropericardium
  B. Recurrent acute pericarditis
  C. "Subacute pericarditis"
  D. Pericardial fat necrosis
II. Noninflammatory excess pericardial contents
  A. Hydropericardium
  B. Hemopericardium
    1. Traumatic
    2. In association with pathologic bleeding
      (a) Hemorrhagic states
      (b) Rupture of contiguous organs
  C. Chylopericardium
  D. Pneumopericardium
  E. Intrapericardial herniation of other organs
III. Chronic and constrictive pericardial disease
  A. Granulomatous
  B. Pericardial scarring
    1. Pericardial fibrosis/adhesions
    2. Pericardial calcification/ossification
    3. Inflammatory cysts and diverticula
  C. Chronic pericardial effusion
  D. Amyloidosis of pericardium
IV. Congenital pericardial abnormalities
  A. Congenital pericardial abnormalities
    1. Partial
      (a) Incidental
      (b) With herniation of portions of the heart
    2. Total
  B. Congenital cysts of the pericardium

* (Categorical; see also Table 7)

TABLE 92.3 PERICARDIAL ADHESIONS AND FIBROSIS

Anatomical
I. Pericardial thickening without adhesions
  A. Visceral
  B. Parietal
  C. Visceral and parietal
II. Internal pericardial adhesions
  A. Obliterative
    1. Complete
    2. Incomplete
  B. Focal
    1. "Milk spots"
    2. Individual strands, bridges, and bands
    3. Inflammatory pseudocysts and diverticula
III. External pericardial adhesions
IV. Perivascular pericardial adhesions
V. Combined adhesions (two or more of the preceding)

Clinical
I. Clinically and hemodynamically silent
II. Producing clinical signs without dynamic significance
III. Dynamically significant
  A. Constriction of the heart and/or
  B. Constriction of one or more great vessels
IV. With other findings (sometimes etiologically related)
  A. Endocardial (esp. valvular) lesions
  B. Mediastinal lesions
  C. Lesions of other serosae
  D. Pericardial calcification/ossification
V. Combinations of the preceding

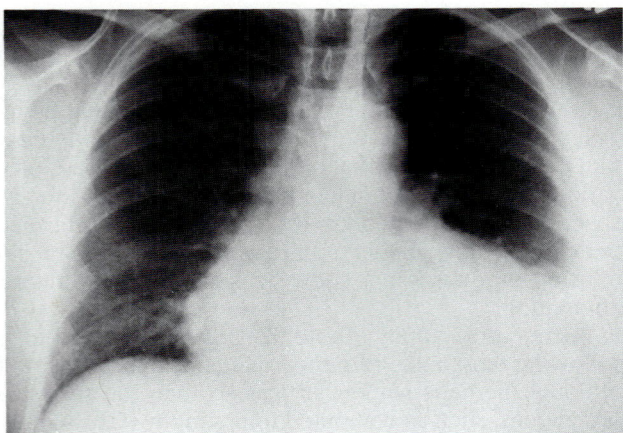

FIGURE 92.2 Anteroposterior chest film of patient with pericardial effusion showing unilateral (left) pleural effusion. Left pleural effusion (if there is a pleural effusion) is the rule in uncomplicated pericardial disease (with or without pericardial effusion).

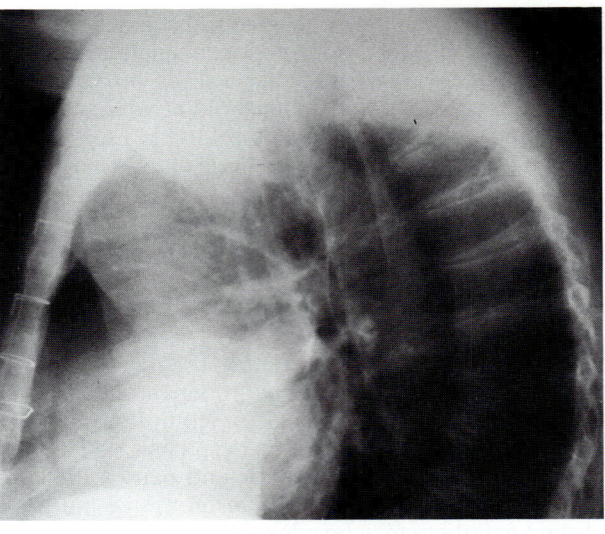

FIGURE 92.3 Lateral chest film of patient with postoperative pericardial effusion showing a pericardial fat line, an almost vertical clear streak parallel to the sternum behind the lower two metal sutures.

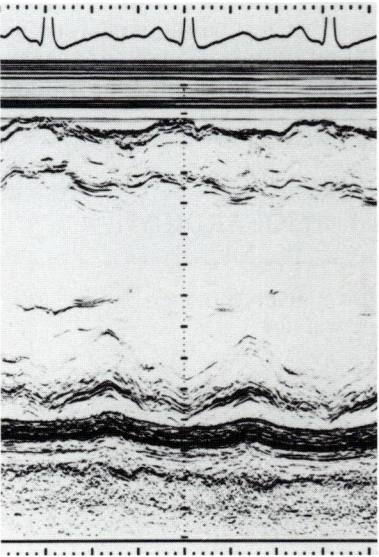

FIGURE 92.4 Pericardial effusion (with pericardial thickening). M-mode echocardiogram showing anterior and mostly posterior fluid, probably a small to moderate-sized effusion. Fluid separates the thickened parietal pericardium from the visceral pericardium in both systole and diastole. Parietal pericardium shows two zones: the more posterior is narrow and solid black, probably the parietal pericardium. Over it is a layer of thickening that could be either fibrosis (chronic) or fibrin (acute).

TABLE 92.4 ECHOCARDIOGRAM AND DOPPLER FLOW IN PERICARDIAL EFFUSION AND CARDIAC TAMPONADE (VARYING SENSITIVITES AND SPECIFICITIES)

I. Pericardial effusion
  A. Echo-free space—posterior to LV (small-to-moderate effusion)
     Posterior and anterior (moderate-to-large effusion)
     Behind left atrium (large-to-very large effusion)
  B. Decreased movement of posterior pericardium-lung interface
  C. RV pulsations brisk (with anterior fluid)
  D. "Swinging heart" (large effusions)
     Periodicity 1:1 or 2:1
     RV and LV walls move synchronously
     Mitral/tricuspid pseudoprolapse
     Alternating mitral E-F slope and aortic opening excursion
II. Cardiac tamponade: Changes of effusion plus
  A. RV compression
       RV diameters decreased, especially outflow tract
       Early diastolic collapse of RV
  B. RA free wall indentation (collapse) during late diastole or isovolumic contraction
  C. LA free wall indentation (cases with fluid behind LA)
  D. LV free wall paradoxic motion
  E. SVC and IVC congestion (unless volume depletion)
  F. Inspiratory effects (with pulsus paradoxus)
     RV expands
     IV septum shifts to left
     LV compressed
     Mitral D-E amplitude decreased
       E-F slope decreased or rounded
       Open time* decreased
     Aortic valve* opening decreased; premature closure
     Echographic stroke volume decreased
  G. Notch in RV epicardium during isovolumic contraction
  H. Course oscillations of LV posterior wall
III. Doppler studies
  A. Generally reduced flows/stroke volume
  B. Inspiratory augmentation of right-sided and decrease of left-sided flows

*Often difficult to define during pericardial effusion; mitral valve may open only with atrial systole during inspiration. (IV, interventricular; IVC, inferior vena cava; LA, left atrium; LV, left ventricle; RA, right atrium; RV, right ventricle; SVC, superior vena cava; 2D, two dimensional)

certain structures visualized posteriorly: enlarged left atrium, descending aorta, coronary sinus, foramen of Bochdalek hernia. Foramen of Morgagni hernia may produce an echo-free space anteriorly. LV pseudoaneurysms produce spaces anteriorly or posteriorly. With very large effusions there may be exaggerated cardiac motion, particularly rotational "swinging," sometimes associated with mitral and tricuspid pseudoprolapse and with false systolic anterior motion of the atrioventricular valves. Table 92.4 summarizes the echocardiographic and Doppler flow findings in pericardial effusion and cardiac tamponade (Figs. 92.4 and 92.5). Although M-mode usually suffices, cross-sectional echocardiography is superior in ruling out the above effusion mimics. Pleural effusions and tumors may extend behind the left atrium (LA), but do not permit visualization of left atrial contractions as do pericardial effusions behind that structure (Figs. 92.4 and 92.5). Copious epicardial fat (situated mainly anteriorly, but frequently also posteriorly) can exactly simulate effusions, requiring CT scans for diagnosis. Finally, a strictly anterior echo-free space should not be accepted as indicating effusion, except when there is reason to expect posterior adhesions, for example, postoperatively and with a rapidly constricting process.

Echocardiography is the standard imaging tool for diagnosing pericardial effusion because it is convenient, is nearly always adequate, and costs much less than other modalities, specifically computed tomography and magnetic resonance imaging. The latter procedures, when gated, give much better definition of most structures. In the case of computed tomography this can be striking when there is a good layer of epicardial fat (Fig. 92.6). Magnetic resonance imaging (Fig. 92.7) is especially good in complicated cases because it is the best method (when gated) for diagnosing pericardial thickening and identifying loculated pericardial effusions. In the latter case echocardiography may be sufficient, but magnetic resonance imaging permits broader views; since blood gives a higher intensity signal then serous or hydrous fluids, it can also distinguish between uncomplicated pericardial effusion and hematoma. Magnetic resonance imaging can also

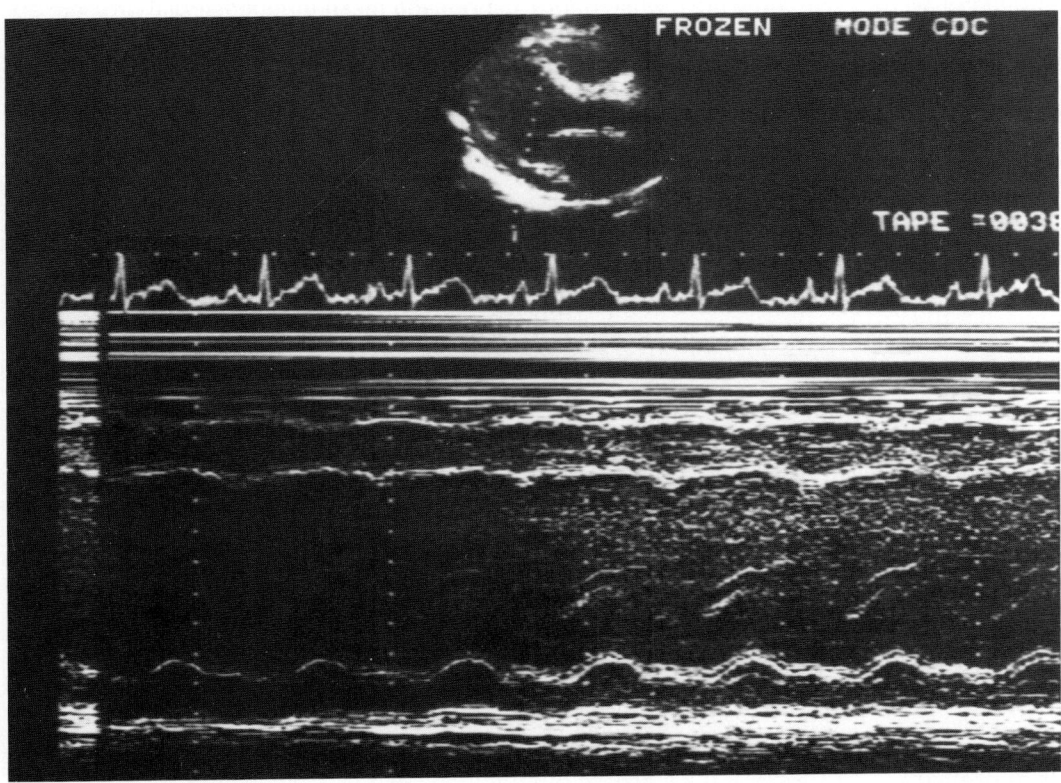

FIGURE 92.5 Pericardial effusion. Combined two-dimensional and M-mode echocardiogram. The M-mode record, obtained as a "cut" from anterior to posterior, indicated by the cursor (*dotted line in 2-D tracing*). Both recordings show anterior and posterior pericardial fluid, probably a moderate-sized effusion. The M-mode tracing has been damped (*left half*) to show attenuation of other cardiac structures and retention of the posterior cardiopericardial junction.

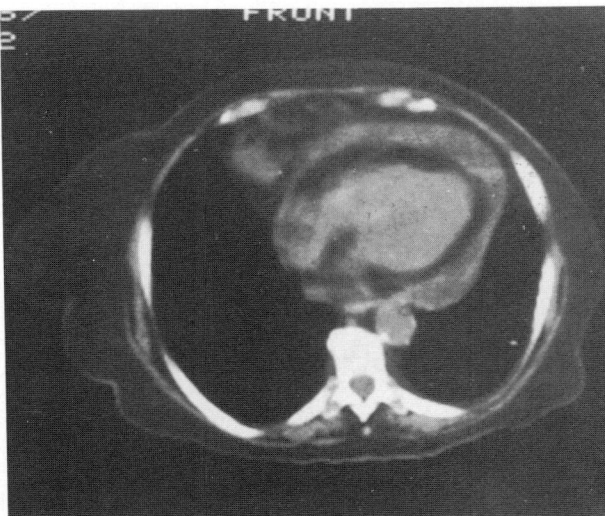

FIGURE 92.6 Computed tomogram showing pericardial effusion separated from the heart image by an unusually thick epicardial fat layer. (Black zone is fat.)

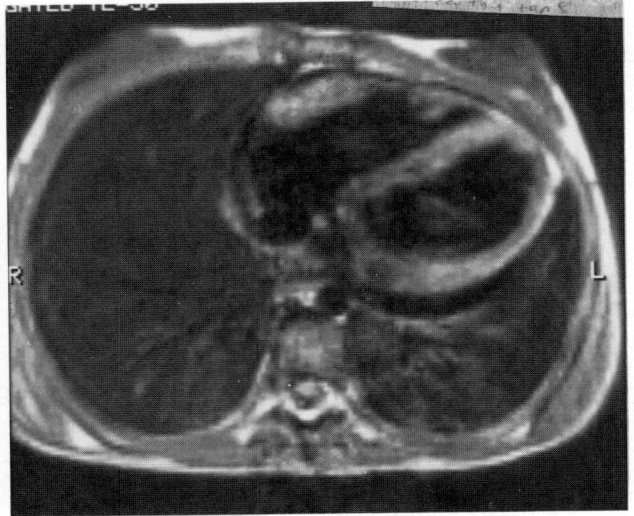

FIGURE 92.7 Magnetic resonance image (gated) showing pericardial effusion (dark zone, wider posteriorly). (Courtesy of Charles B. Higgins, M.D.)

discriminate inflammatory from fibrous tissue and thus can reflect the acuteness or chronicity of a process. Finally, gated magnetic resonance imaging is excellent for defining intracardiac and paracardiac masses. It can demonstrate cystic tumors, particularly when there is necrosis within the tumor, which on echocardiography can simulate a loculated pericardial effusion.

MANAGEMENT

Asymptomatic pericardial effusions need not be treated unless there is a need for fluid or tissue for diagnosis, including identifying any systemic disease that could be etiologic or a primary cause of the pericardial lesion.

▢ DECOMPENSATED PERICARDIAL EFFUSION: ACUTE CARDIAC TAMPONADE
PATHOPHYSIOLOGY

Cardiac tamponade is defined as "the decompensated phase of cardiac compression resulting from an unchecked increase in intrapericardial pressure."[2] "Cardiac tamponade" may also be used to describe *any* degree of cardiac compression. Since even rather small, clinically innocent effusions are not entirely without physiologic effects,[4] cardiac tamponade represents a pathophysiologic continuum—one that is prone to more or less sudden breakdown of compensation due to progressive increase in pericardial contents (Fig. 92.8). Here, the first definition of "tamponade" is used to emphasize the dramatically altered physiologic, clinical, and therapeutic characteristics of the acute decompensated phase.

Two key factors produce cardiac compression by pericardial contents: the rate of fluid accumulation and the ability of the parietal pericardium to stretch. With rapid fluid accumulation the limit of stretch is quickly attained, due to the pericardium's J-shaped pressure-volume curve. Decompensated cardiac tamponade tends to be a "last straw" phenomenon, the last small aliquot of fluid putting the chamber on the steep portion of its pressure-volume curve. Although the heart as a whole is compressed, the primary point of attack is on the thinner right heart,[1,2] especially the right atrium.[5]

Normally, intrapericardial pressure is lower than right atrial pressure (so that right atrial transmural pressure is higher than its cavitary pressure), while during tamponade mean intrapericardial pressure approximates mean atrial pressure (particularly in inspiration); cardiac filling is maintained only by a parallel rise in systemic venous pressure,

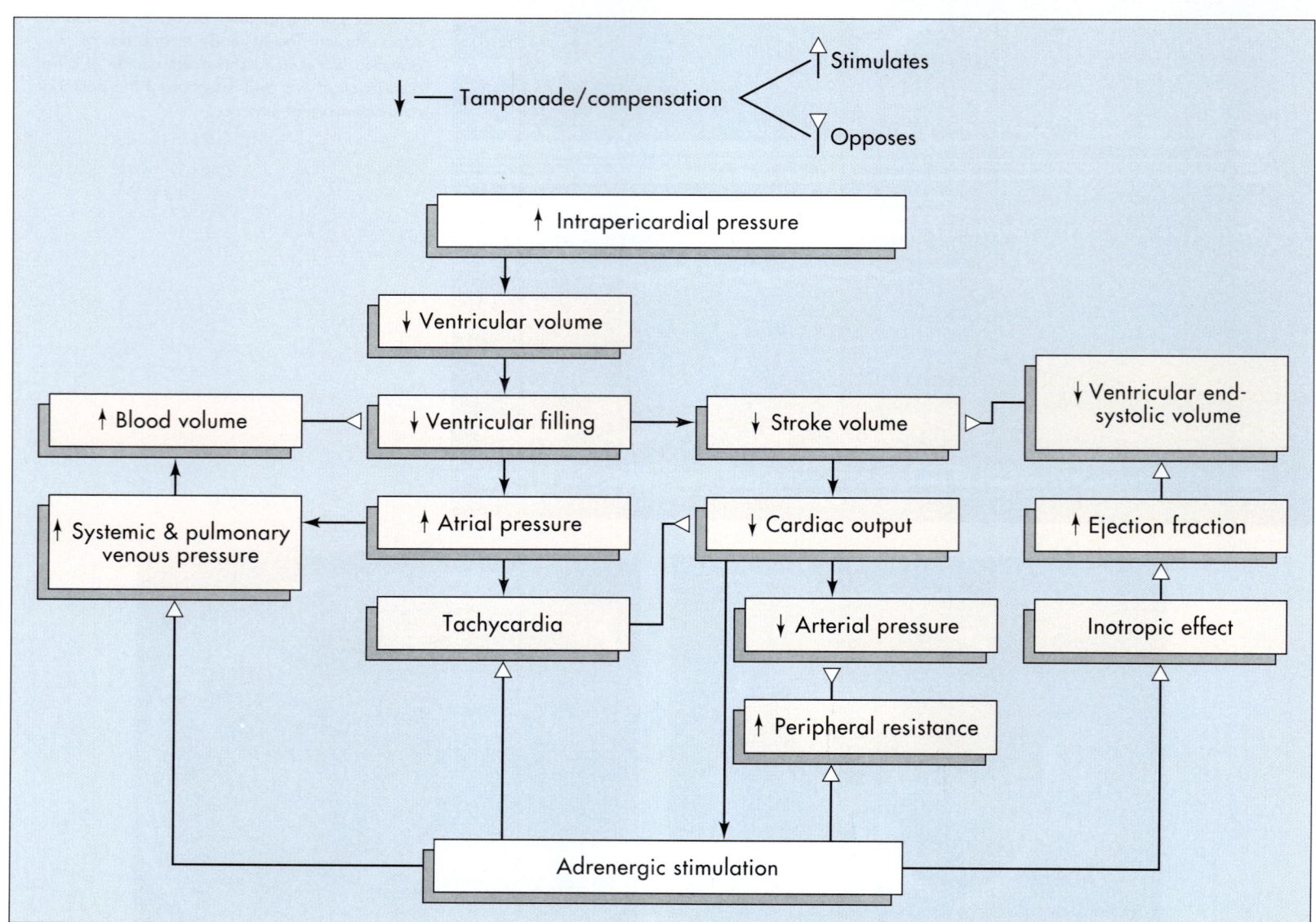

FIGURE 92.8 Cardiac tamponade: Physiology. Schema of the effects of increased intrapericardial pressure and the far-reaching set of compensatory responses. Plain arrows indicate tamponade effects. Open-headed arrows represent compensatory responses. Those with a pointed head indicate stimulation of a response while the flat-headed arrows represent opposition to an effect. (Spodick DH: The normal and diseased pericardium: Current concepts of pericardial physiology, diagnosis and treatment. J Am Coll Cardiol 1:240–251, 1983. Adapted with permission from the American College of Cardiology)

due to sodium and fluid retention and reflex venoconstriction. (Since right atrial mean (RAM) pressure approximates intrapericardial pressure, left ventricular diastolic transmural pressure can be estimated by subtracting RAM pressure from pulmonary wedge pressure.)[1]

Diastolic pressures in both ventricles and the pulmonary artery all equilibrate with mean RA and wedge pressures, at approximately intrapericardial pressure—the cardinal hemodynamic finding of uncomplicated cardiac tamponade. *Equilibrate* means pressures within a few mm Hg of each other, the differences being least, nil, or reversed during inspiration. (Equisensitive catheters show that equilibration is not absolute and there is *inspiratory tracking*, that is, pressure equilibration is nearer perfect in inspiration.) Ascending intrapericardial pressure reduces—and, during inspiration, eventually annihilates—mean cardiac *transmural pressures*, which are the distending, that is, true filling, pressures. Indeed, temporary reversal of the transmural gradient causes RV collapse early in diastole and RA collapse in late diastole (Table 92.4). Though the RA collapse may precede arterial hypotension, it indicates a 20% to 25% decrease in cardiac output. Filling may occur only during differential pressure fluctuations. For example, the atria fill only during ventricular ejection. Ventricular ejection corresponds to the *x* descent of atrial pressure curves. The *y* descent, corresponding to rapid ventricular filling, is amputated in tamponade. The jugular venous pulse faithfully reflects this characteristic. In severe tamponade, the ventricles may fill only when atrial systole propels blood into them. Ventricular pressure curves show an immediate and steady diastolic rise from the low point following atrioventricular valve opening. Fluid-filled catheters with poor resonance characteristics may falsely suggest a "dip and plateau" as seen in pericardial constriction.

COMPENSATORY RESPONSES

Salt and fluid retention are part of a widespread compensatory response with a major adrenergic component, primarily stimulated by decreased cardiac output. The dynamic events of tamponade and compensation[1] are schematized in Figure 92.8. Tachycardia helps to increase minute cardiac output for the diminished stroke output; increased peripheral resistance opposes hypotension; inotropic effects of adrenergic stimulation minimize ventricular end-systolic volume and improve ejection fraction (normal-to-high in tamponade). The equilibrated end-diastolic and mean pressures usually range between 15 mm Hg and 30 mm Hg. Systolic arterial pressure varies from normal down to "shocky" levels (70 mm Hg to 80 mm Hg), except in some hypertensive individuals who may experience florid tamponade at 140 mm Hg or higher. Diastolic arterial pressure is usually normal, but is occasionally as high as 100 mm Hg.

Although tachycardia is the rule, the usual level tends to be modest, that is, between 100 and 120 beats/min; occasional patients, notably uremics, have lower heart rates; others, particularly anemic and wounded bleeding patients, may have higher heart rates. In hemorrhaging patients (whether into the pericardium or elsewhere), compensatory mechanisms may be preempted by blood loss and shock so that venous pressure cannot be adequately utilized to maintain right heart filling. In general, all compensatory mechanisms are less efficient with hypovolemia. Finally, coronary artery flow is reduced by tamponade and may become abnormally retrograde in some branches.[1]

ATYPICAL TAMPONADE

In volume-depleted patients, *low pressure tamponade*[6] may occur at mean atrial and diastolic pressures as low as 6 mm Hg. There may be no systemic hypotension and few symptoms. Right-sided pressures are slightly raised with abnormal pulse contours, and it may be necessary to expand the blood volume to elicit diagnostic pulse waves (occult cardiac tamponade).[7] *Right-sided cardiac tamponade*, with right-sided diastolic pressures exceeding left, occurs with a low compliance LV, or when fluid is loculated over the right side of the heart (*e.g.*, after cardiac surgery).

PULSUS PARADOXUS
PATHOPHYSIOLOGY

Systolic arterial pressure normally drops during inspiration (arbitrarily, by up to 10 mm Hg). Pulsus paradoxus represents exaggeration of the phenomenon (Fig. 92.9). Although common in obstructive airway disease and occasional in hemorrhagic shock, RV infarction, pulmonary embolism, and restrictive cardiomyopathy, pulsus paradoxus is characteristic of uncomplicated cardiac tamponade and occurs very occasionally in constrictive pericarditis. (Most cases of constriction with significant "pulsus" probably have residual pericardial fluid or pulmonary disease.)

Pulsus paradoxus in cardiac tamponade is a phenomenon of multiple simultaneous and sequential mechanisms (Fig. 92.10).[1] Although normal respiratory pressure changes are sharper for the right side of the heart, in tamponade with pulsus paradoxus, aortic flow and pressure fluctuations are similar to those in the pulmonary artery, though opposite in phase. This is due to the increased effect on ventricular interaction of a filled pericardium.

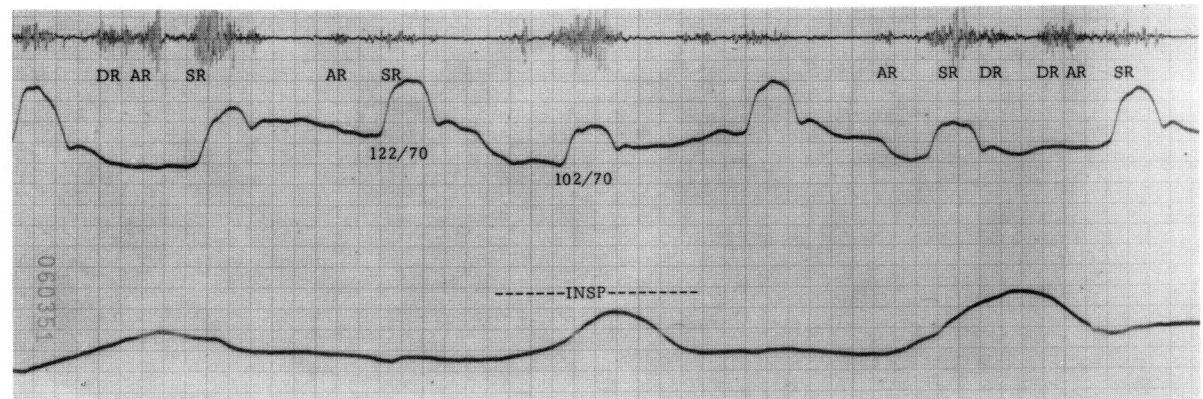

FIGURE 92.9 Pulsus paradoxus (noninvasive study). Phonocardiogram, carotid displacement pulse, respiratory thermistor trace (top to bottom). The phonocardiogram shows a three-component pericardial rub. The rub increases with inspiration and decreases markedly with expiration, sometimes losing components, depending on the time in the respiratory cycle. The carotid pulse diminishes with inspiration. Brachial arterial pressures, listed under the carotid pulse, show a 20 mm Hg fall in systolic pressure and no change in diastolic pressure. Since the respiratory rate is approximately half the heart rate, the pulsus paradoxus here is fortuitously also a "pulsus alternans." (*DR*, diastolic rub; *AR*, atrial (presystolic) rub; *SR*, systolic rub)

The appearance of pulsus paradoxus signifies a very large reduction in ventricular volume, dramatically seen in two-dimensional echocardiograms (Fig. 92.11). The fall in inspiratory systolic pressure relative to the pulse pressure is generally related to the degree of cardiac compression. Yet, because of interpatient differences, numerical quantitation is best for following a given patient.

Intrapericardial and pleural pressures normally vary equally during breathing, but in tamponade the pericardial pressure during inspiration decreases less than pleural pressure, and increases rapidly as the right side of the heart fills. Directional respiratory changes in flow and filling are normal, and the percent increase in right-sided heart filling is greater than normal, while absolute cardiac filling is less than normal. Inspiratory increase in right ventricular size (filling) has two effects: it (1) further raises pericardial pressure and (2) causes the interventricular septum to bulge to the left (Fig. 92.12), raising LV pressure; this further decreases LV transmural pressure and LV chamber compliance. Septal bulging additionally resists, and decreased transmural pressure further reduces, LV filling so that the LV operates on a steeper Starling curve during inspiration. The ensuing inspiratory decrease in arterial flow and pressure reflects decreased LV stroke output. Two other factors augment the difference between inspiratory and expiratory measurements: (1) transmission of inspiratory negative pleural pressure to the aorta and systemic arteries (increasing their transmural pressures) and (2) time for the inspiratorily increased RV output to cross the lungs and appear on the left (partly a function of heart rate). Moreover, the lungs may act to an unknown degree as a capacitor, "pooling" the RV output during inspiration, thus reducing or even reversing the pulmonary artery-left atrial gradient, which reduces left heart inflow (Fig. 92.10). Finally, aortic flow has been observed to decrease within one beat of the onset of inspiration so that other (left-sided) factors must add to this effect. Systolic time intervals reflect the LV preload and stroke volume reduction respectively by a greater than normal inspiratory increase in the LV pre-ejection period and decrease in ejection time index.[1]

ABSENCE OF PULSUS PARADOXUS

Pulsus paradoxus during tamponade requires respiratory changes alternately favoring right- and left-sided heart filling against a common pericardial stiffness. If LV diastolic pressures exceed RV and pericardial pressures as in *marked LV hypertrophy* or severe *left-sided heart failure* (common in uremia), pericardial pressure equilibrates only with right-sided heart pressures, because both are determined by the pericardial compliance.[8] In *atrial septal defect*, increased respiratory venous return is balanced by shunting to the left atrium. *Severe aortic regurgitation* produces sufficient regurgitant filling to damp respiratory fluctuations. With *extreme hypotension*, as in shock and severe tamponade, respiratory pressure change may be unmeasurable.

DIAGNOSIS OF CARDIAC TAMPONADE

Cardiac tamponade is a continuum, not "all or none."[8] Thus, without a severe acute change in the patient's condition (*e.g.*, intrapericardial hemorrhage—"surgical" tamponade), its onset may be rather subtle ("medical" tamponade). In general, tamponade must be suspected in anyone known to have pericardial disease or recent chest trauma and an enlarged (though occasionally normal) cardiopericardial silhouette, in the absence of marked dyspnea and pulmonary engorgement ("clear lungs"). Patients may have exertional dyspnea, rarely orthopnea. Air hunger may be conspicuous with severe tamponade; oliguria due to reduced renal function is common. Occasional patients lose consciousness or have seizures.

In this setting, suspicion should be raised by elevated venous pressure, sometimes with hepatomegaly. Falling systolic blood pressure

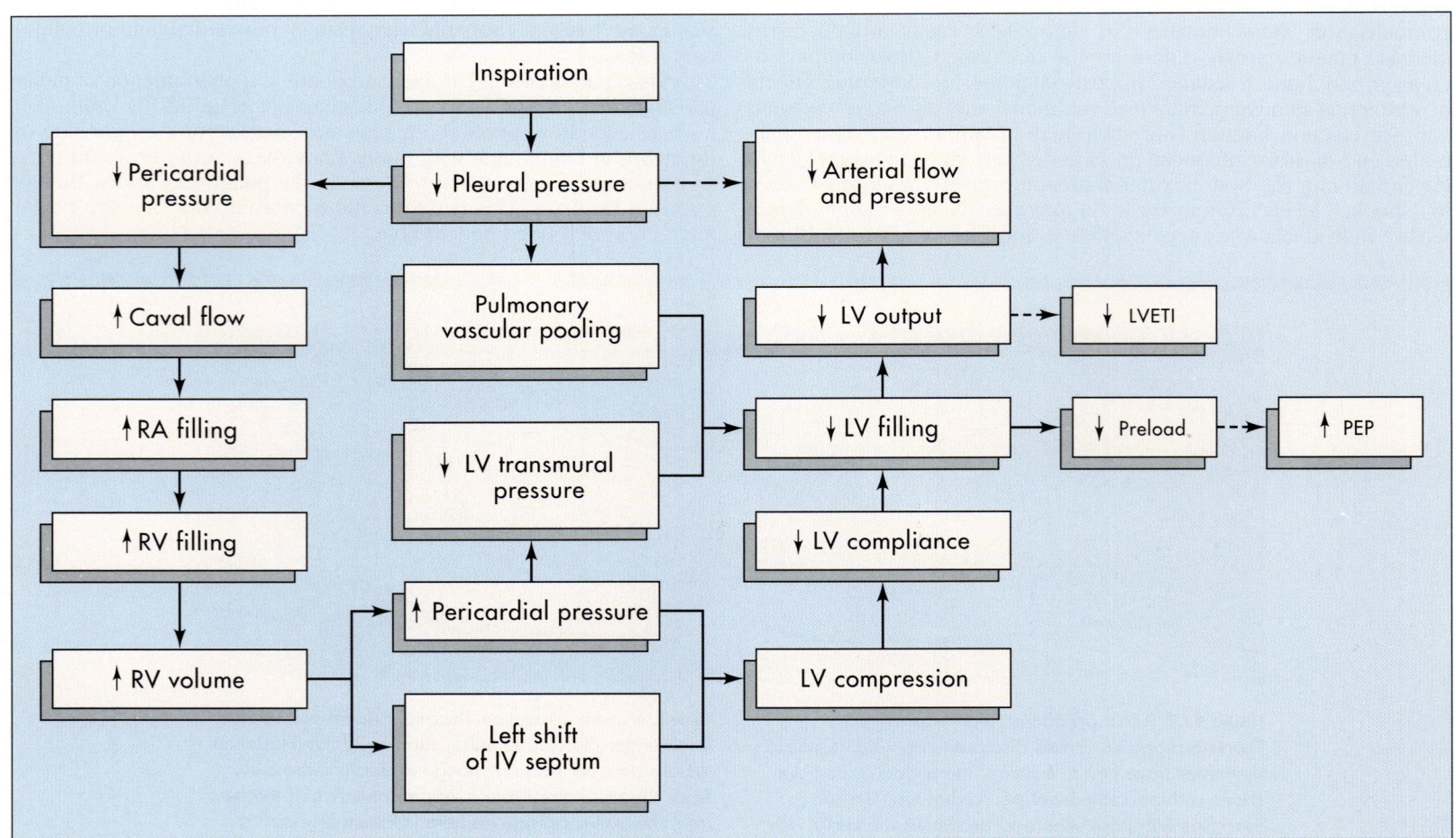

FIGURE 92.10 Pulsus paradoxus. Schema of physiology (see text). In smaller print at the right of the figure are listed changes as reflected by systolic time intervals that change reciprocally with respiration. (*LVETI*, LV ejection time index; *PEP*, preejection period)

and ultimate pulsus paradoxus strongly indicate tamponade. Changes in the degree of "pulsus" (inspiratory systolic pressure drop) roughly parallel the degree of cardiac compression in a given patient. Heart sounds may or may not be faint. Fluoroscopy may or may not show diminished cardiac pulsations. The electrocardiogram (ECG) may be virtually normal, or show changes of acute pericarditis or low voltage, but QRS electric alternation (Fig. 92.13), and particularly the rare P-QRS alternans, is quasipathognomonic of tamponade in the appropriate setting. In addition to the echo signs of effusion [Table 92.4 (I)] diagnosis is greatly aided by the echo-Doppler studies listed in Table 92.4 (II and III): The RV is compressed. RA, and occasionally LA, free wall collapse during late diastole and the ensuing isovolumic contraction period is strong evidence of cardiac compression, as is early RV diastolic collapse (correlating with absent atrial and jugular y descent). The inspiratory effects listed in Table 92.4 (II E) are also frequently present, particularly with pulsus paradoxus, but some or all can be missing. With tamponade, the whole "squeezed" heart is often easily seen within the effusion and, in the absence of heart disease, shows reduced chamber sizes with excellent systolic function (up to 90% ejection fraction). Doppler studies document reduced flows, reduced stroke volumes, and inspiratory increase of right-sided and decrease of left-sided flows that parallel pulsus paradoxus. Inspiratory decrease in left ventricular filling is particularly marked (and occurs to a greater than normal degree in nontamponading effusions[4]). Indeed, in severe

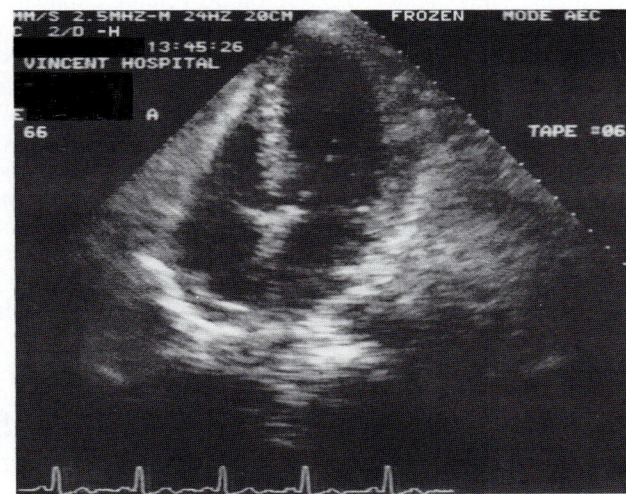

FIGURE 92.11 Cardiac tamponade. Two-dimensional echocardiogram, apical four-chamber view in early diastole. Fluid is seen posteriorly, laterally, apically, and along the right ventricular border. There is diastolic collapse of the right ventricle and slight invagination of the right atrium.

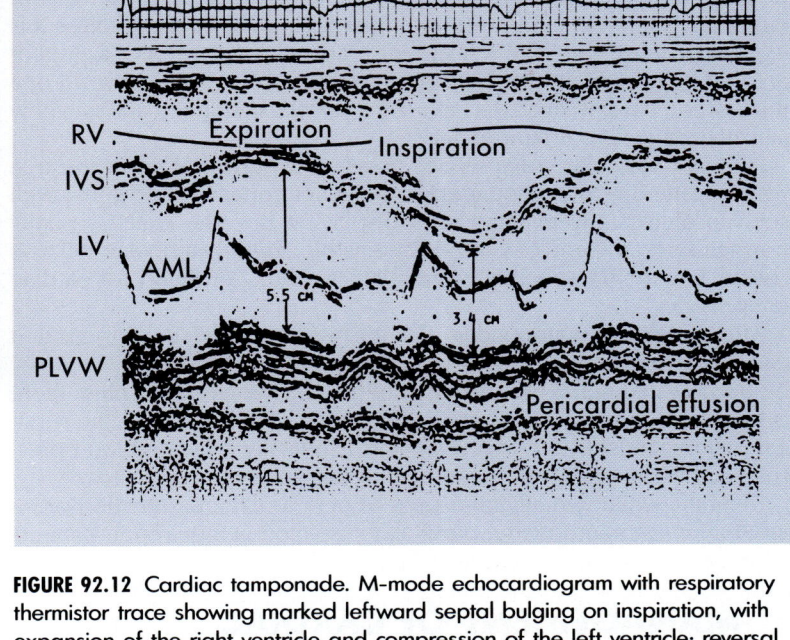

FIGURE 92.12 Cardiac tamponade. M-mode echocardiogram with respiratory thermistor trace showing marked leftward septal bulging on inspiration, with expansion of the right ventricle and compression of the left ventricle; reversal on expiration. Pericardial effusion is mainly posterior. In this case, the mitral anterior leaflet slope does not reflect changing chamber compliance or filling. The ECG (top) shows first beat normal, next three paced. (RV, right ventricle; IVS, interventricular septum; LV, left ventricle; PLVW, posterior left ventricular wall; AML, anterior mitral leaflet)

FIGURE 92.13 Electric alternation and cardiac swinging during tamponade. **Inset.** Clinical ECG showing more marked alternation in a precordial lead (less apparent in ECG of echocardiogram because of small complexes). Right ventricular anterior wall (top of echocardiogram) shows marked swinging toward and away from the chest wall artifact. Intracardiac structures move with this. Anterior mitral leaflet shows both pseudosystolic anterior motion and pseudoprolapse. Posterior echo is left atrial. Pericardial fluid reveals typical atrial contractions and, because fluid extends behind the left atrium (in the oblique sinus), indicates a very large effusion.

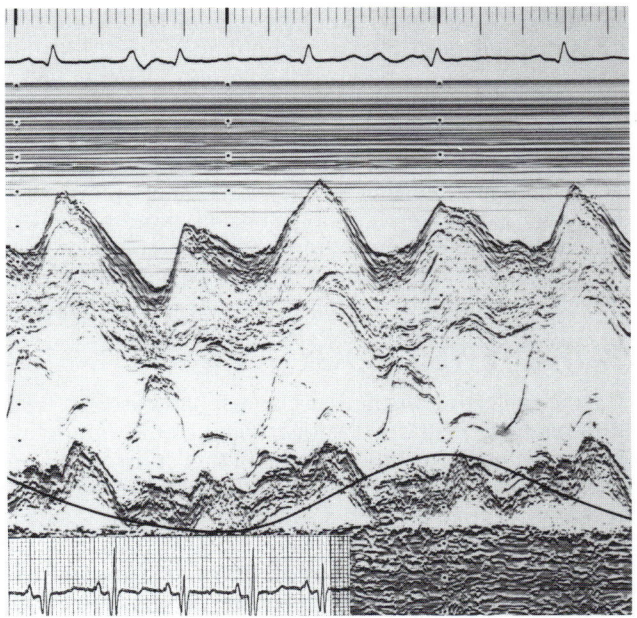

tamponade there may be no rapid filling period of the left ventricle during inspiration, with the mitral valve staying closed in early diastole and opening to permit filling only during atrial systole.

Because they also appear in incipient tamponade, as well as advanced tamponade, recognition of chamber collapses (Fig. 92.11 and Table 92.4 [II A, B, C, and D]) has great importance. Left atrial and biatrial collapse are much less frequent than right atrial and right ventricular collapse, whereas left ventricular collapse has only been seen with adjacent loculated effusion (note: loculated effusions may be associated with diastolic collapse of any chamber). Right atrial collapse has a 90% to 100% sensitivity and a somewhat lower specificity for cardiac tamponade. It occurs immediately following atrial systole (i.e., in late ventricular diastole or isovolumic contraction), and the atrial wall remains invaginated to a variable degree during early ventricular systole but disappears by the end of ventricular systole. It often has a reverse "L" configuration, best seen in either the apical or subcostal four-chamber and the parasternal short axis views. D'Cruz has quantified this phenomenon: the greatest normal reduction in echo area of either atrium is less than 16%. In tamponade, atrial collapse raises this to 20% or more, and the left atrium tends to collapse over a greater area than the right atrium. Duration of right atrial collapse beyond one third of the cardiac cycle has almost a perfect specificity and is highly sensitive as a sign of tamponade.

Right ventricular collapse occurs as an inward motion of the free wall in early diastole, appearing as a distinct concavity or "dent" well seen in almost any imaging view displaying the free wall. It usually normalizes by the end of ventricular diastole. Right ventricular collapse has an 80% to 90% specificity and a 90% to 100% sensitivity for cardiac tamponade.

In "surgical" tamponade—patients with rapidly decompensated cardiac compression—many signs may be absent due to very low blood flows. Minimal pericardial contents may be present unless there is hemorrhage into a preexisting effusion. Postoperative cardiac surgical patients must be observed for this, especially if falling blood pressure and hematocrit follow removal of temporary pacing wires.

Finally, while virtually all causes of pericardial inflammation or injury can cause tamponade, particular suspicion is required in patients with the most common causes (Table 92.5).

MANAGEMENT OF CARDIAC TAMPONADE

Tamponade is usually a first order emergency and removal of pericardial fluid by paracentesis or surgical drainage is mandatory. Needle paracentesis may suffice, but a pericardial catheter should be introduced for continued drainage and to avoid cardiac trauma. The optimal site for paracentesis is best determined by, and the procedure monitored by, 2-D echocardiography (cross-sectional echocardiography), which shows about half of all effusions to be closest to the subxiphoid approach. Except in an emergency, paracentesis probably should be avoided if there is less than 5 mm echo depth of anterior effusion. Because there is no universally accepted approach route, the technique[2] should be learned from an experienced mentor.

Subxiphoid surgical drainage, which is extrapleural and extraperitoneal, can be done under local or general anesthesia; it is effective and permits digital and endoscopic[9] exploration of the pericardium as well as biopsy and creation of a pleuropericardial window. (Care is required to avoid pneumothorax.) Although their effectiveness is controversial, medical therapies may be employed while waiting for drainage. They include oxygen, blood volume expansion with intravenous fluids, and stroke volume increase with inotropic agents that increase ejection fraction, particularly norepinephrine (which also supports systemic resistance) or dopamine. Afterload reducing agents may be useful in patients with adequate blood pressure. Thoracotomy with pericardial resection is necessary under certain circumstances: (1) most cases of severe suppurative pericarditis (particularly in children), (2) recurrence of cardiac tamponade after partial (subxiphoid) resection, (3) recurrence of malignant pericardial effusion, and (4) tamponade in dialysed uremics that is unresponsive to increased dialysis and local treatment. Before induction of anesthesia, cardiac compression should be relieved. Any anticoagulant or anti-inotropic treatment should be discontinued.

CONSTRICTIVE PERICARDIAL DISEASE
PATHOGENESIS

Constrictive pericarditis follows a clinically evident or silent episode of acute pericarditis that heals (cicatrizes) so as to restrict diastolic filling. Corticosteroid treatment in the acute phase does not prevent constriction. Traditionally this has been a chronic condition. Perhaps because the major etiologic factors have changed and because of earlier diagnosis, most cases now seen in developed countries are either subacute or even acute. Arbitrarily,[10] subacute constriction appears 3 to 12 months after an episode of pericarditis and acute constriction occurs within 3 months of an acute attack, for example, resolution of a tamponading effusion after which the cardiopericardial size is stable but the venous and central pressures increase.[10] Occasionally, a clotted hemopericardium causes rather acute constriction or effusive-constrictive pericarditis. Usually, postinflammatory scarring unites the parietal and visceral pericardia over all or most cardiac surfaces. Occasionally, loculated and bandlike scarring occurs in one or more locations, while rarely, either the parietal or visceral pericardium alone constricts, or both fibrose without adhesions.[10] In the usual chronic case constriction is by nonspecific fibrous tissue with few, if any, inflammatory cells, and with microscopic to gross calcium deposits. Depending on etiology, granulomas and giant cells may be present. (Etiology can be almost any kind of acute pericarditis, except, perhaps, acute rheumatic fever.) Subacute and acute phases show mixtures of leukocytes in lighter, less collagenized, more nucleated fibrous tissue. Rarely, localized constriction produces conditions indistinguishable from obstruction of valves, the aorta or pulmonary artery (resembling valvular stenosis), or a cardiac chamber (resembling heart failure).[10]

PATHOPHYSIOLOGY

Classic uniform constriction clamps the heart in a tightening vise that progressively restricts diastolic filling of the ventricles and atria. The ventricles begin to fill normally, but as constriction progresses this is sharply cut off at an earlier and earlier time, giving their pressure curves an early diastolic dip with a sharp transition to a plateau ("square root" sign) permitting no further filling (Fig. 92.14). This differs from tamponade, which restricts diastole from the onset of filling. During the dip, early diastolic filling is extremely rapid due to the concomitant rise

TABLE 92.5 COMMON ETIOLOGIES OF CARDIAC TAMPONADE

Neoplasia
Idiopathic (usually viral) pericarditis
Nonviral infection
    Tuberculous
    Suppurative
Intrapericardial hemorrhage with or without pericarditis
    Wounds, including surgery
        Chest
        Heart
        Pericardium
        Blind pericardiocentesis
    Dissecting aortic hematoma
    Anticoagulant therapy
Postpericardiotomy syndrome
Uremia
Mediastinal and juxtamediastinal radiation therapy
Vasculitis-connective tissue disease group

in atrial (and consequently venous) pressures. This summates with two related processes after the atrioventricular valves open: diastolic suction and the "rubber bulb" effect.[10] The latter is due to springing back of the tensed pericardium after its deformation during systole. Systolic pressure in the RV and pulmonary artery usually is moderately raised (30 mm Hg to 45 mm Hg), with RV end-diastolic at least one third of RV systolic pressure.

As in tamponade, mean diastolic pressures in all chambers tend to equilibrate. Unlike tamponade, atrial and venous wave forms are exaggerations of the normal, with a deep y descent and a variable x descent yielding M or W curve shapes (Fig. 92.15). Blood flow in the systemic veins accelerates phasically toward the heart much as it does normally, that is, both during ventricular ejection (x descent) and following atrioventricular valve opening (y descent), mainly the latter. Moreover, pericardial cavity obliteration by the thick "peel" around the heart insulates atria and ventricles from intrathoracic pressure changes, so that inspiration produces little or no decrease in RA pressure. Resistance to venous inflow is thus continuous and the systemic venous pressure tends to increase with inspiration. The neck veins, being extrathoracic, may visibly swell in inspiration—Kussmaul's sign. For similar reasons, pulsus paradoxus, which depends on increased inspiratory filling of the right side of the heart, is usually absent unless there is some fluid remaining in the pericardial cavity (effusive-constrictive pericarditis) or local constriction of the left side of the heart. Similarly, Kussmaul's sign cannot occur in acute cardiac tamponade, unless the tamponading fluid overlies an epicardial constriction, since respiratory dynamics are qualitatively normal.

Reduction of filling and consequently stroke volume evokes tachycardia which, since it tends to amputate the mid- to end-diastolic filling plateau, does not of itself reduce filling by much. Systolic function is usually normal except in patients who had had a large element of myocardial involvement with their pericardial inflammations and others who, due to chronicity, have myocardial "disuse" atrophy. Thus, features like ejection fraction, velocity of circumferential shortening, and systolic time intervals are usually normal and distinguish this condition from myocardial failure and restrictive cardiomyopathy, both of which can pose diagnostic problems. Eventually 70% to 80% of ventricular filling occurs within the first 20% to 30% of diastole, also distinguishing constrictive pericarditis from most cases of nonpericardial diastolic restriction, in which this is accomplished by about mid-

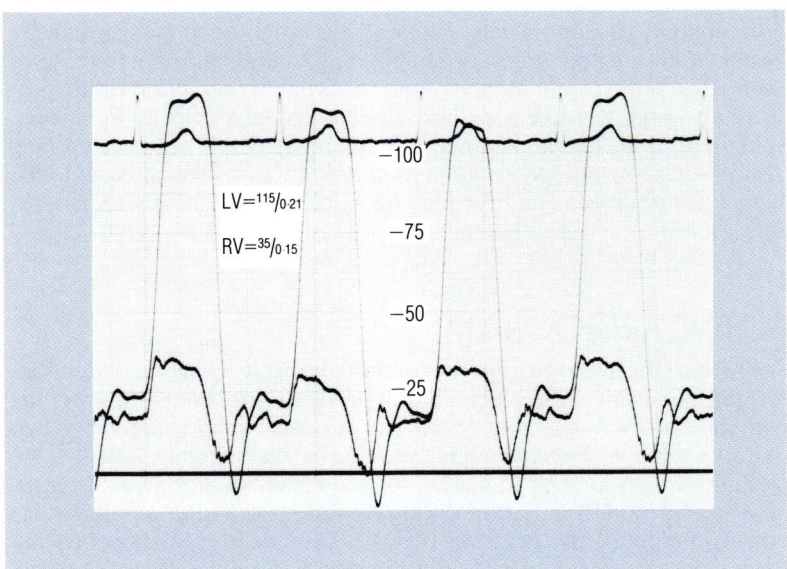

FIGURE 92.14 Constrictive pericarditis. Ventricular hemodynamics. Left and right ventricular pressure curves (fluid-filled catheters) showing diastolic plateau with near equilibration of mid- to end-diastolic pressures and the "square root" sign (see text).

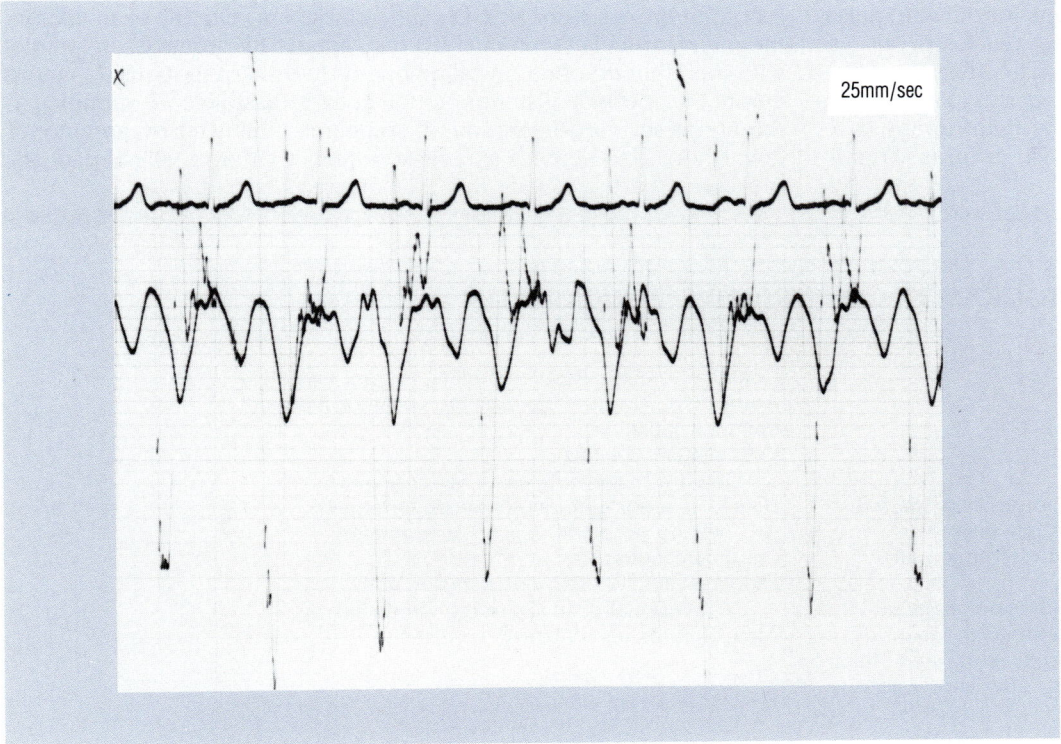

FIGURE 92.15 Constrictive pericarditis. Right atrial pressure curve showing deep x and larger y trough (also recordable from a jugular venous pulse).

diastole. (This is not reliable for diagnosis.) The systemic response resembles that of congestive heart failure with renal sodium and fluid retention that maintains the elevated venous pressure supporting cardiac filling.

CLINICAL PHYSIOLOGY OF CONSTRICTION

Echocardiography, radiologic and nuclear imaging techniques, and angiocardiography show normal to greatly decreased ventricular diastolic volume. The coronary arteries are within rather than at the edges of the cardiopericardial silhouette. The superior and inferior venae cavae and hepatic veins are dilated and the RA outer border tends to be straight. Frame-by-frame analysis of cross-sectional echocardiograms or angiograms shows very rapid early diastolic filling with abrupt ("kneelike") transition to quite slow filling, the transition point corresponding to the nadir of the atrial y descent and the beginning of the ventricular pressure plateau (Figs. 92.14 and 92.15). The hepatic veins do not collapse in inspiration.

SYMPTOMS

Early in classic generalized constriction, and often for most of its course, symptoms are closely related to the degree of systemic venous congestion and fluid retention. There is visible venous distention, edema, ascites (sometimes without edema), and abdominal discomfort due to splanchnic engorgement. Although frank pulmonary edema is rare, elevation of central venous pressures produces cough, exertional fatigue, and dyspnea and occasionally orthopnea. These are accentuated by frequent, often bilateral, pleural effusions and fixation of diaphragmatic excursion by marked ascites.

PHYSICAL EXAMINATION

The earliest sign may be pedal edema or jugular and systemic venous distention. Some patients develop anasarca, often with chronic muscle wasting of the chest and extremities. Some have peripheral cyanosis and pallor. Behavior of the distended veins contrasts to that in myocardial failure: If the patient has walked to the physician and rested on a chair, the level of jugular venous distention tends to remain high, whereas in cardiac failure it frequently falls with upright rest. Prominent y and x descents are recognized if viewed as collapses from a high standing level. (In constriction one should not look for outward pulsations.) Arrhythmia, very rapid heart rates, and obese necks will obscure these findings. Kussmaul's sign may be present. The arterial pulse is usually unremarkable and, as indicated earlier, pulsus paradoxus is uncommon in the absence of residual pericardial fluid. In any case, inspiratory fall in arterial pressure in pure constriction is virtually always under 10 mm Hg and very rarely exceeds 14 mm Hg. In some of the latter, pulmonary rather than pericardial disease is responsible.

Chronic cases are also likely to have atrial fibrillation with an irregularly irregular pulse. Subacute and acute forms of constriction nearly always have sinus tachycardia. The first and second heart sounds tend to be soft, mirroring the hemodynamic impairment, with the second sound having either a fixed split or, in cases with some degree of pulsus paradoxus, an unusual inspiratory splitting (requiring phonocardiography) due to abrupt early registration of the aortic component (brief decrease in LV ejection time due to decreased stroke volume in inspiration). The cardinal auscultatory sign of cardiac constriction is the abnormal early diastolic sound (EDS). The EDS occurs at the abrupt transition from rapid to slow diastolic filling, approximately at the nadir of the jugular y (Fig. 92.15). It is earlier than most other third sounds (S_3) in that it occurs between 60 (usually 100) and 120 milliseconds after A_2. When its intensity and frequency exceed that of most low-pitched S_3 gallops, it justifies the term *pericardial knock* and it is easily palpated. Indeed, it may be mistaken for the first heart sound, so that timing with other events (*e.g.*, jugular pulsations) is useful. In occasional patients, a mid-diastolic rumble, similar to that in mitral or tricuspid valve stenosis, is heard at the apex or along the lower left sternal edge; the mechanism appears to be due to localized constriction, respectively, at the right (or left) A-V ring.

Palpation usually reveals a sharp precordial thrust (which can be mistaken for the apex beat) corresponding to the abnormal third heart sound and often terminating a paradoxic systolic retraction of the precordium (well seen on apexcardiograms).[10] Occasionally, in chronic constriction, these events are visible. Otherwise, the precordium may be rather quiet, though sometimes the pulmonic second sound (P_2) seems accentuated. The liver may be palpable, particularly in patients with ascites.

ECHOCARDIOGRAM

Pericardial thickening is the rule, although this is always a difficult interpretation, since it is very gain-dependent and thickening occurs without constriction (Table 92.6). The pericardium may appear as two or more parallel lines, though this, too, is nonspecific. Usually, the posterior LV endocardium has flat to no diastolic motion with displacement of no more than 1 mm during diastole (even after atrial systole) corresponding to the pressure plateau. The aortic root shows abrupt early diastolic posterior motion corresponding to the atrial y descent. (Restricted ventricular filling curves are seen on frame-by-frame analysis of the cross-sectional, 2-D echocardiogram.) On 2-D examination, the interventricular septum (IVS) may appear to "bounce" in systole, with the M-mode often revealing one or two sharp motions: (1) more abrupt than normal posterior motion in early diastole corresponding to the abnormal third heart sound, sometimes followed by an anterior "overshoot" (sometimes in reverse sequence) in over 90% of patients;

TABLE 92.6 ECHOCARDIOGRAM IN CONSTRICTIVE PERICARDITIS*

Pericardial thickening
Interventricular septum
    Paradoxic systolic motion
        Anterior (type A)
        Flat (type B)
    Accentuated posterior motion in early diastole
    Abrupt anterior motion in early diastole
    Abrupt posterior, then anterior, motion after atrial systole
    Septal "bounce" (cross-sectional echograms)
Gradual to absent diastolic ventricular expansion:
    LV posterior wall approximately equidistant from chest wall in early and late diastole

Quantitative echo: Restricted filling in early diastole
Aortic root: Abrupt early diastolic posterior motion
Pulmonic valve
    Premature opening
    Marked respiratory fluctuations of a wave
Dilated superior and inferior venae cavae and hepatic veins with restricted respiratory fluctuations
Esophageal echo: RA wall excursion and dimensional change markedly reduced
Atria: Both or one enlarged

(2) rapid posterior followed by anterior motion following atrial systole in one third of patients in sinus rhythm; these are of unknown specificity. On 2-D examination the right ventricle and atria may be enlarged but are usually normal. IVS systolic motion may be "paradoxic" of type A (anterior) or type B (flat). Superior and inferior venae cavae and hepatic veins are dilated. The pulmonic valve may open prematurely due to high RV end-diastolic pressure and its *a* wave depth may vary remarkably with respiration.[1] *Esophageal echocardiography* shows markedly reduced RA wall excursion and dimensional change, indicating impaired reservoir and pump function. Magnetic resonance imaging and cardiac computed tomography may provide comparable diagnostic features.

CLINICAL LABORATORY RESULTS

Some degree of anemia (normocytic) may be found depending on chronicity. Patients with liver engorgement or cardiac "cirrhosis" may have findings consistent with hepatic failure. High systemic venous pressure is sometimes associated with protein-losing enteropathy or with nephrotic syndrome and proteinuria (particularly in children, in whom it can be the presenting manifestation of constriction). Either or both of these, like hepatic failure, produce hypoalbuminemia. The ascitic fluid tends to be an exudate, at least in early stages of hepatic congestion. Later, a mixed picture with lower specific gravity and a lower concentration of protein may be found.

CHEST FILM

The cardiopericardial silhouette is normal or modestly enlarged, the latter due to extreme thickening of the pericardium, residual pericardial fluid, or both. In approximately one third of patients, and best in lateral views, pericardial calcification is seen—a nonspecific finding that must be distinguished from other cardiac and coronary calcification. Most patients show pleural effusion and many, a dilated superior vena cava. *Unequal constriction* of the LV or RV or constricting bands in the AV groove may cause mitral or tricuspid obstruction with left and/or right atrial enlargement, best seen in the oblique views.

ELECTROCARDIOGRAPHIC CHANGES

Electrocardiographic changes are nonspecific (Fig. 92.16); sometimes the ECG is virtually normal. T waves may be generally flat or inverted. Many patients with chronic constriction and sinus rhythm have intra-atrial block (notched P) resembling P mitrale. The P wave axis may be vertical or left deviated from the normal +40° to 60°. Occasional localized or unequal constriction can give ECG findings of "upstream" chamber overload. Some patients have localized T wave inversions, particularly in II, III, and a VF, although these tend to be subacute cases.

OTHER FORMS OF CONSTRICTION

Effusive-constrictive pericarditis is characteristic of subacute and acute constriction. Here, either the parietal or visceral pericardium is mainly involved, with entrapment, sometimes in locules, of a layer of pericardial fluid under pressure. Mixed clinical pictures result, depending upon whether there is greater tamponade or constriction. Some present as tamponade and show a constrictive pattern only after fluid is removed. An abnormal third heart sound may or may not be present, but will often appear after removal of the fluid. The *x* descent is dominant if there is a prominent element of tamponade. Others present as constriction with a significant pulsus paradoxus and both *x* and *y* venous troughs. CT scanning is ideal to confirm the diagnosis, but usually echocardiography suffices.

Elastic constriction occurs with little or no fluid, the constricting pericardium being relatively yielding so that a third heart sound may be absent, but a fourth heart sound is heard. This may occur in early subacute constriction or, less commonly, with constricting neoplasms, without either fluid or constrictive fibrosis.

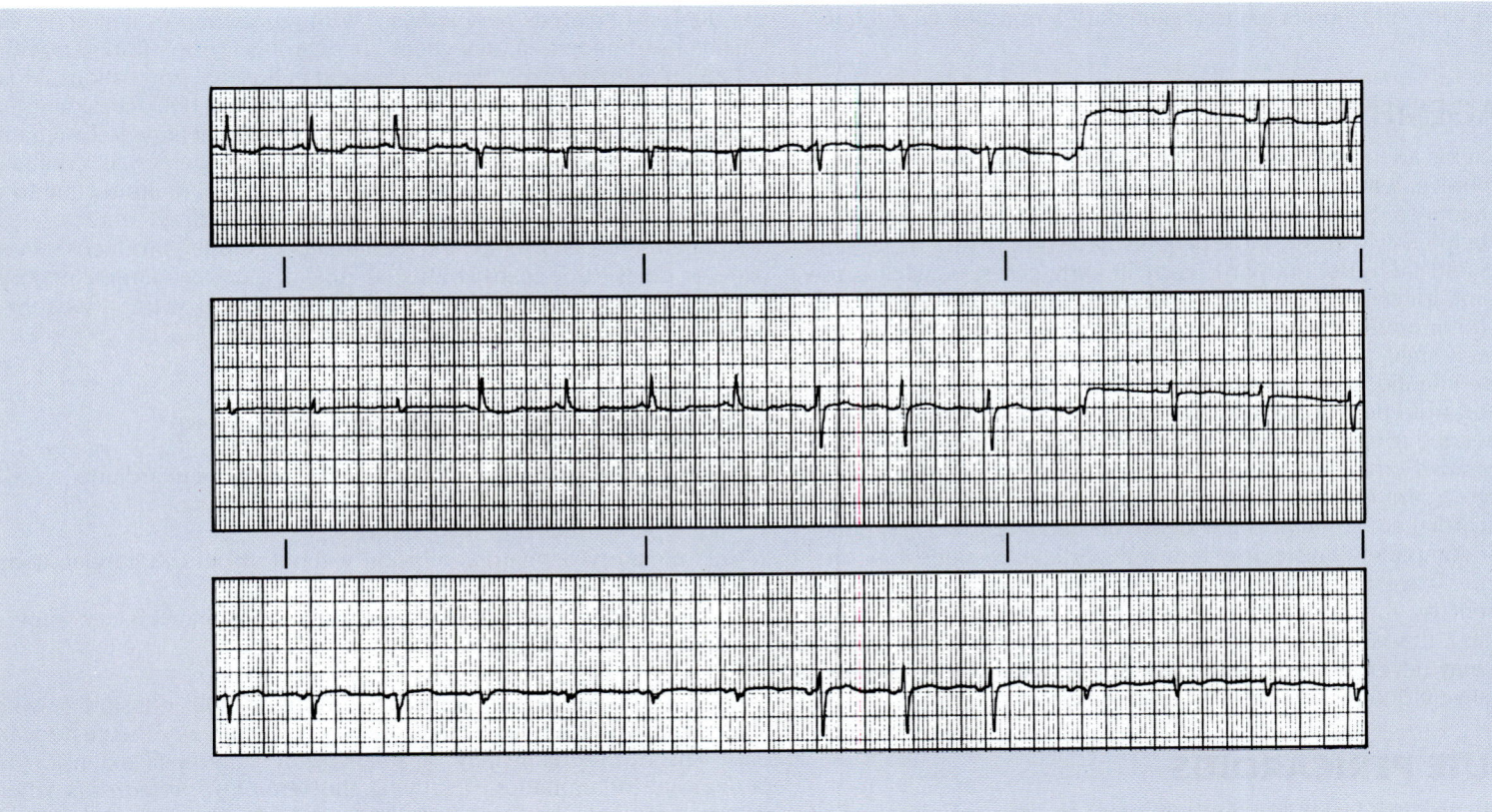

FIGURE 92.16 Constrictive pericarditis. ECG. Reduced voltage and nonspecific T wave abnormalities. The P wave axis (−20°) is left of its "normal" range.

LATENT (OCCULT) CONSTRICTION

Rarely, latent constriction[10] with normal central hemodynamics can be exposed by rapid infusion of up to 1 liter of warm saline to provoke an RV dip and plateau, accentuated RA y collapse and right- and left-sided diastolic pressure equilibration.[7] (Normal individuals have little or no rise in pressures and patients with most cardiac abnormalities do not equilibrate.) Latent constriction should be suspected in patients who have mild dyspnea, fatigue, and persistent or recurrent chest pain and who may have a history of pericarditis. ECG, chest films, and clinical laboratory findings are not helpful. Echocardiograms may show some pericardial fluid and suggestions of diastolic restriction. Pericardiectomy restores the normal response to volume expansion.

DIAGNOSIS OF CLASSIC CONSTRICTIVE PERICARDITIS

Patients with systemic venous congestion and edema or ascites must be distinguished from those with myocardial and valve failure, venous obstructive syndromes, nephrotic syndrome, Laënnec's cirrhosis, and abdominal malignancy. Suggestive but nonspecific data include history of acute pericarditis or any disorder listed in Table 92.2; an abnormal early diastolic sound (particularly if very early, very loud, and palpable); and, usually, absence of murmurs. Chest films may show pericardial calcification, the echocardiogram may show the findings described in Table 92.6, and the ECG may show changes—all individually nonspecific. In the absence of complicating cardiac disease, systolic function is exceptionally good for the dramatic systemic findings. Systolic time intervals are within normal limits.[1] Since surgical treatment is definitive, cardiac catheterization is necessary to confirm restrictive dynamics, rule out valve disease, and assess the coronary arteries. In some cases pericardial biopsy may be needed. When there is a strong possibility of primary myocardial disease, endomyocardial biopsy may decisively rule it in (but not out). As of yet, there is no absolute preoperative differentiation from restrictive cardiomyopathies. In superior vena cava syndrome, the distended neck veins and visible collaterals are nonpulsatile. In cirrhosis, the cardiac findings and elevated pressures are absent. CT demonstrates thick pericardium (which may be enhanced with intravenous contrast material), a nonspecific but helpful finding.

MANAGEMENT

A few patients adequately compensate for their constriction when it is not progressive, leaving them with only mild systemic congestion and its consequences. Here, diuretics and low salt diet suffice (digitalis is not very helpful). However, most patients have progressive symptoms and signs and the question, particularly in early cases, is, what is the optimal time for definitive therapy—pericardiectomy? In patients who have not deteriorated due to chronicity, well-developed technique and an extremely small perioperative mortality favor early operation. Those with active infections should be treated before surgery to sterilize and limit spread from pericardial lesions. Digitalis or antiarrhythmic agents may be needed for arrhythmias. Postoperative improvement is related to preoperative circulatory status, liver and kidney integrity, and, to some degree, the extensiveness of the operation. In occasional patients epicardial constriction is too dense and adherent or even penetrating for completely satisfactory removal, particularly since the coronary arteries have to be spared. Patients with extensive myocardial involvement by the pericardial inflammation (previous or ongoing myocarditis), fibrosis, and calcification, as well as myocardial "disuse atrophy" may never recover completely and occasionally go downhill postoperatively due to intractable cardiac dilation.

ACUTE PERICARDITIS

Acute pericarditis is by far the most important and most common of all pericardial disorders. The relative frequency of pericardial scarring at autopsy indicates that many cases are subclinical or missed. For example, rheumatoid arthritis produces pericardial adhesions and fibrosis in 40% to 50% of patients at necropsy, while relatively few patients have clinical manifestations. Yet, because of the large numbers of patients with rheumatoid arthritis, millions must have had subclinical rheumatoid pericarditis.

ETIOLOGIES

The enormous range of etiologies of acute pericarditis (Table 92.7) makes it apparent that conditions in every branch of medicine and surgery affect the pericardium. While a purist might have to consider the whole list for any new case of pericarditis, in most patients cause is never demonstrated (idiopathic pericarditis). On the other hand, viral pericarditis and most cases of acute pericarditis of unknown etiology produce approximately the same syndrome, so most cases of idiopathic acute pericarditis are ascribable to viral infection. Moreover, the idiopathic pericarditis syndrome can be considered the epitome of acute pericarditis in that it frequently produces all of the characteristic manifestations: pain, typical (Stage I) ECG changes, and a pericardial rub. Effusion, usually without tamponade, is common and occasionally constrictive pericarditis ensues. The next category, pericarditis due to living agents, fundamentally applies to any organism that can reach the pericardium. In the modern era, this applies mostly to a large number of viruses, notably the coxsackie group. Bacterial pericarditis still occurs despite the great reduction in suppurative infections, while tuberculosis is greatly diminished in more advanced countries. One of the largest generators of acute pericarditis and its consequences is the vasculitis-connective tissue disease group. (Here, rheumatoid pericarditis may be the most common but it is rarely of clinical significance.) The worst pericarditis in this group appears in systemic lupus erythematosus. Another important group is immunopathic pericarditis including "hypersensitivity" states, in which the pericardium can be the shock organ for drug reactions and for sensitization to antimyocardial antibodies. Diseases of contiguous structures, mainly myocardial infarction, but also the other conditions listed in Table 92.7, involve the pericardium frequently. Among disorders of metabolism two kinds of acute pericarditis are frequent in renal failure: uremic pericarditis and the stubborn "dialysis pericarditis." With the great prevalence of various types of neoplasia, malignant "pericarditis" (often fibrinous without an inflammatory reaction) is frequent in hospital populations. Most is secondary (by metastasis or direct extension), but occasionally a mesothelioma or other tumor arises from pericardial tissues. Traumatic pericarditis includes direct pericardial trauma in accidental, criminal, or surgical wounds and the rare "foreign body" pericarditis due to a juxtapericardial foreign body (e.g., shrapnel); indirect trauma (e.g., nonpenetrating chest injury and radiation pericarditis) produces immediate or delayed pericardial effects. Finally, there is a large category, pericarditis of uncertain origin and in association with various syndromes; its enormous range is indicated in Table 92.7 (IX).

THE SCOPE OF ACUTE PERICARDITIS

In general, there are three acute disorders of the pericardium:

1. Acute pericarditis and myopericarditis.
2. Inflammatory pericardial effusion without significant cardiac compression.
3. Acute cardiac tamponade—pericardial effusion with decompensated cardiac compression.

The most common is acute pericarditis without effusion or with clinically insignificant amounts of fluid—"*clinically dry*" acute pericarditis. The myocardium may be involved by superficial extension of pericardial inflammation, justifying the term *myopericarditis* when myocardial involvement is clinically apparent or dominates the picture. This is more common in children and in some viral episodes in adults.

CLINICALLY DRY (NONEFFUSIVE) PERICARDITIS

The most common clinical presentation of acute pericarditis is that of an inflammatory (fibrinous) lesion.

SYMPTOMS. Although patients may have no pain or only vague precordial distress, the cardinal symptom of acute pericarditis is central chest pain, usually pleuritic, very sharp and persistent and exacerbated by body movements, notably breathing. It may migrate to one side of the chest, radiate in any anginal distribution, or remain precordial. Onset may be gradual but surprisingly often is sudden, may interrupt sleep, and can be precipitated by effort. Like angina, pericardial pain is frequently less on sitting up, though this is not a dependable sign. It is relatively common for pericardial pain to be simultaneously perceived

TABLE 92.7 ETIOLOGY OF ACUTE PERICARDITIS AND MYOPERICARDITIS

I. Idiopathic (Syndrome)
II. Living Agents
   A. Bacterial
      1. Suppurative: any organism
      2. Tuberculous
   B. Viral
      1. Coxsackie
      2. Influenza
      3. Other
   C. Mycotic (fungus)
   D. Rickettsial
   E. Parasitic
   F. Spirochetal
   G. *Spirillum* infection
   H. *Mycoplasma pneumoniae*
   I. Infectious mononucleosis
   J. *Leptospira*
   K. *Listeria*
   L. Lymphogranuloma venereum
   M. Psittacosis (chlamydiaceae)
   N. AIDS (probably viral; HIV; other)
   O. Other (many)
III. Vasculitis–Connective Tissue Disease Group
   A. Rheumatoid arthritis
   B. Systemic lupus erythematosus (SLE); drug-induced SLE
   C. Scleroderma
   D. Sjögren's syndrome
   E. Whipple's disease
   F. Mixed connective tissue disease (MCTD)
   G. Reiter's syndrome
   H. Ankylosing spondylitis
   I. Inflammatory bowel disease
   J. Serum sickness
   K. Wegener's granulomatosis
   L. Vasculitis
   M. Polymyositis (dermatomyositis)
   N. Behçet's syndrome
   O. Familial Mediterranean fever
   P. Dermatomyositis
   Q. Panmesenchymal reaction of steroid hormone withdrawal
   R. Polyarteritis
   S. Thrombohemolytic thrombocytopenic purpura
   T. Other
IV. Immunopathies and "Hypersensitivity" States
   A. Drug reactions
   B. Serum sickness
   C. Allergic granulomatosis
   D. Giant urticaria
   E. Other sensitivity reactions (see V-A, 2 and 3)
V. Diseases of Contiguous Structures
   A. Myocardial infarction
      1. Acute myocardial infarction
      2. Postmyocardial infarction syndrome
      3. Postpericardiotomy syndrome
      4. Ventricular aneurysm
   B. Dissecting aortic aneurysm
   C. Pleural and pulmonary diseases
      1. Pneumonia
      2. Pulmonary embolism
      3. Pleuritis

VI. Disorders of Metabolism
   A. Renal failure
      1. Uremic (chronic/acute renal failure)
      2. "Dialysis" pericarditis
   B. Myxedema
   C. Cholesterol pericarditis
   D. Gout
VII. Neoplasms
   A. Secondary (metastatic, hematogenous, or by direct extension): Carcinoma, sarcoma, lymphoma, leukemia, other
   B. Primary: Mesothelioma, sarcoma, fibroma, lipoma
VIII. Trauma
   A. Direct
      1. Pericardial perforation
         (a) Penetrating chest injury
         (b) Esophageal perforation
         (c) Gastric perforation
      2. Cardiac injury
         (a) Cardiac surgery (see also V-A, 3)
         (b) During catheterization
            (1) Pacemaker insertion
            (2) Diagnostic
      3. "Foreign body" pericarditis
   B. Indirect
      1. Radiation pericarditis
      2. Nonpenetrating chest injury
IX. Uncertain Origin or In Association With Various Syndromes
   A. Postmyocardial and pericardial injury syndromes (? immune disorders)
   B. Inflammatory bowel disease
      1. Colitis (ulcerative, granulomatous)
      2. Segmental enteritis
   C. Löffler's syndrome
   D. Thalassemia (and other anemias)
   E. "Specific" drug reaction (psicofuranine, minoxidil, ? others)
   F. Pancreatitis
   G. Sarcoidosis
   H. Fat embolism
   I. Bile fistula (to pericardium)
   J. Wissler's syndrome
   K. "P.I.E." syndrome
   L. Stevens-Johnson syndrome
   M. Gaucher's disease
   N. Diaphragmatic hernia
   O. Atrial septal defect
   P. Giant cell aortitis
   Q. Takayasu's syndrome
   R. Mucocutaneous lymph node syndrome
   S. Fabry's disease
   T. Kawasaki's disease
   U. Degos' disease
   V. Other

in the trapezius ridge, usually on the left, but sometimes bilaterally or on the right, and this can occur without any chest pain. Trapezius ridge pain is almost pathognomonic for acute pericarditis.

Though there may be tachypnea with shallow, splinted breathing due to increased pain during inspiration, pericarditis does not cause true dyspnea. Yet, true dyspnea may accompany or precede the pericardial attack if there is also a pulmonary, bronchial, pleural, or cardiac disorder. More often there is a history of recent or concomitant upper respiratory infection. Painful swallowing (*odynophagia*) is rare but may be the only symptom. Patients with mild pericarditis, particularly with coxsackie infection, may have skeletal muscle pains, suggesting a generalized myositis.

Fever in acute infectious pericarditis varies according to etiology, but is usually between 100°F and 102°F (37.0°C to 38.8°C). Some patients have considerable anorexia and some are markedly anxious.

SIGNS. The cardinal sign of acute pericarditis is the pericardial rub (friction sound).[11] This auscultatory phenomenon is considered to arise from friction between inflamed pericardial surfaces. Yet, rubs are common with very large pericardial effusions. While some rubs are faint, many are unmistakable due to their tendency to be superficial and because they have peculiar shuffling, creaking, scratching, or grating qualities. Rubs are nearly always loudest at the left mid- to low-sternal border,[11] possibly because here the heart (specifically the RV free wall) is closest to the chest wall. This is also where intense rubs may be palpable, sometimes producing thrills not unlike the murmur of ventricular septal defect.[11] Rubs must be sought diligently from the very first suspicion of pericardial disease because they tend to wax and wane and even change location over short time periods and with changes in body position.[2] Some pericardial rubs are heard only with the patient in the knee-chest position.

In over 50% of cases rubs have three components,[11] each distinguishable by careful auscultation, even at rather rapid heart rates (Fig. 92.17). A fully developed rub is composed of the presystolic atrial rub, preceding the first heart sound; a systolic component, the ventricular systolic rub, between the first and second sounds and coincident with the peak of the carotid pulse; and the early diastolic rub, following the second heart sound (usually the faintest; its absence accounts for most two-component rubs during sinus rhythm). The loudest component is usually the ventricular systolic rub, occasionally the atrial rub. In the absence of atrial systole (*e.g.*, atrial fibrillation) there will be no atrial component. When three components are distinguishable, similar sounding murmurs are ruled out. While the classic description of pericardial rubs as "to and fro" thus is usually wrong, such rubs occur in 30% to 40% of cases.[11] Moreover, at rapid heart rates and with first degree atrioventricular block, the atrial and early diastolic components run together (summation rub)[11]; taken with the systolic rub, this often gives a "to and fro" effect, though sometimes each diastolic component is distinguishable as a change in quality during atrial systole. Many other rubs seem genuinely "to and fro" due to the weakness or absence of the early diastolic rub. Approximately 20% of patients have only a monophasic rub (even with frequent auscultation), nearly always the ventricular systolic rub. Finally, pleuropericarditis produces a pleuropericardial rub, with a persistent cardiac component and an intermittent, usually rougher, pleural component that may mask the pericardial rub unless respiration is suspended.

LABORATORY DATA. Unless there is significant accompanying myocarditis or heart disease, true cardiomegaly does not occur in association with pericarditis. As with percussion (an undependable index), more than 250 ml of pericardial fluid is also needed to detectably enlarge the roentgenologic cardiac outline. The etiologic agent or any primary illness will dictate the variations in white blood cell count and sedimentation rate. Moderate leukocytosis is the rule, but leukopenia and even leukemoid reactions may occur. The variability of any accompanying myocarditis makes the results of cardiac enzyme studies vary widely from normal to small increases. Occasionally a major increase (*e.g.*, CPK-MB up to 130 units) is appreciated, and is consistent with considerable myocardial involvement, otherwise evident by definite ST-T abnormalities.

ELECTROCARDIOGRAM.[12] ECG changes in acute pericarditis occur as typical (including typical variants) and atypical (including no change). A typical or typical variant ECG (Fig. 92.18) is virtually diagnostic, in particular Stage I of four sequential stages.

Stage I, characteristic of pericarditis, shows new J-point elevations, nearly always with concave ST elevations above the TP baseline, recorded in all leads except aV_R and occasionally V_1 (rarely also V_2) (Fig. 92.18). In aV_R the ST is always depressed or isoelectric.

TYPICAL VARIANTS. In hearts with a vertical ($> +60°$) QRS axis, ST in aV_L can be isoelectric or slightly depressed; if QRS voltage in lead I is algebraically zero or negative, ST in lead I can be isoelectric. With a horizontal axis ($< +30°$) ST in lead III can be isoelectric or slightly depressed. If QRS voltage in aV_F is algebraically zero or negative, ST in aV_F can be isoelectric. Atypical ECGs include all those that never develop any of the above Stage I combinations.[13]

In Stage II, all ST segments (*i.e.*, J-points) return to baseline nearly "in phase" with each other, with little change in the T wave itself until later. PR segments may be depressed, except elevated in aV_R.[16] In the transition from Stage II to Stage III, the T waves progressively flatten and invert in the leads that had ST elevations. Thereafter, the Stage III ECG shows widespread T inversions, indistinguishable from that of diffuse myocardial injury or myocarditis (indeed, it reflects involvement of the subepicardial myocardium). In Stage IV, T waves eventually assume their original directions and amplitude. This ECG evolution

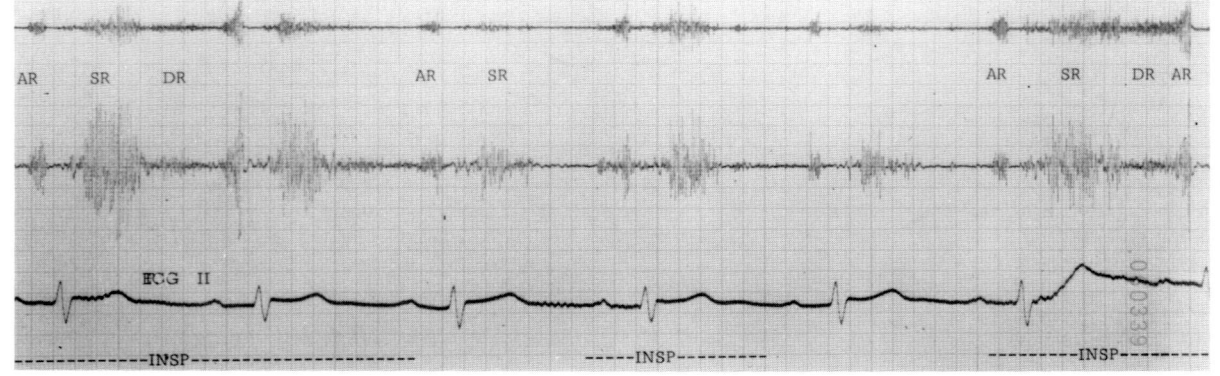

FIGURE 92.17 Acute pericarditis. Pericardial friction. Phonocardiogram and ECG; inspiration indicated by signal. The tripartite pericardial rub is shown increasing with inspiration and decreasing with expiration in a patient who also had a pericardial effusion and tamponade. Full three-part rubs are seen near peak inspiration at both ends of the trace and in the middle cycle. Other rub components wax and wane depending on the respiratory phase. (*AR*, atrial rub; *SR*, ventricular systolic rub; *DR*, diastolic rub)

may occur in days to weeks. Usually transition from Stage III to Stage IV is relatively slow while Stage II may evolve rapidly. Some patients have permanent T wave abnormalities in some or all leads.

Variants of the ECG sequence include nonresolution from Stage III to Stage IV and nonappearance of Stage III. The latter—return to normal after Stage I—is quite common, especially in mild attacks. Depending on the frequency of monitoring, one or another stage can be missed, though a daily ECG may register all stages. The rule, however, is that as long as a typical Stage I or a typical variant is recorded at some time, the ECG is virtually diagnostic of acute pericarditis.

Atypical ECGs (no Stage I)[13] occur in over 40% of cases of mixed etiology and can be perplexing, especially when only a few leads are affected. The latter suggests local rather than general injury, and therefore myocardial infarction or atypical (Prinzmetal) angina—by definition, "local" disorders. But unlike infarction, "reciprocal" ST deviations in such tracings are rare. The ECG may also be preempted by another disease which has already caused important changes.

PR SEGMENT DEVIATIONS.[12] PR segment depressions, below the TP baseline, appearing in most leads (with elevation always occurring in lead aV_R) are almost as common as J-ST elevations.[12] This sign thus has great sensitivity but unknown specificity. Moreover, it may be the only ECG abnormality and is commonly misread, due to optical illusion, as "ST segment elevation."

ELECTRICAL BASIS OF ECG ABNORMALITIES

Typical ECG changes in acute pericarditis result from inflammation of the subepicardial myocardial "shell" (essentially myopericarditis).[2,12] Because of superficiality, this inflammation does not produce QRS deformities, and preexisting S waves are usually not obliterated when the ST segments are displaced. Since the entire subepicardial zone is involved, the changes in so-called "epicardial" lead recordings develop in phase with each other; if one plots the net ST vector it is usually directed to the left and inferiorly, that is, toward the apex, usually between $+30°$ and $+60°$ (Fig. 92.19).[12]

On the ECG the apparent stage I J-ST displacement is a systolic event. Yet, direct current-coupled instruments (impractical for clinical use) reveal that J-ST displacement arises from incomplete polarization of the injured zone and can occur in systole or diastole or both (Fig. 92.19).[2,12]

SYSTOLIC INJURY CURRENT

During depolarization, the activation wave responsible for the QRS advances normally to the epicardium (Fig. 92.19). The superficial myocarditis probably alters phase 2 of the transmembrane action potential (TMP) and causes decreased intensity and duration of activity in the subepicardial muscle, which remains partly polarized. This causes a potential difference between it and the completely depolarized remainder of the myocardium in systole, expressed as an ST segment shift. The injured myocardium appears to repolarize early since it never completely depolarizes (Fig. 92.19).

DIASTOLIC INJURY CURRENT

The injured layer remains partly depolarized during diastole (probably due to loss of resting TMP). The rest of the myocardium is again completely polarized, causing a potential difference between the two zones and resulting in a diastolic injury current opposite in direction to the systolic injury current and causing a shift in electrical diastole—the TQ interval (Fig. 92.19). Since this interval corresponds to the ECG baseline (TP interval) and cannot be detected by the clinical ECG, the shift appears as a J-ST displacement in the opposite direction. Thus, the ST displacements of the Stage I ECG are the net result of either the systolic or diastolic injury current, or both. Because the duration of activation in the injured area tends to be shortened during Stage I, the QT_c interval tends to diminish.

In Stage II the ST segment becomes isoelectric because the electrical potential difference between the injured shell of myocardium and the rest of the myocardium is minimized or eliminated. In Stage III

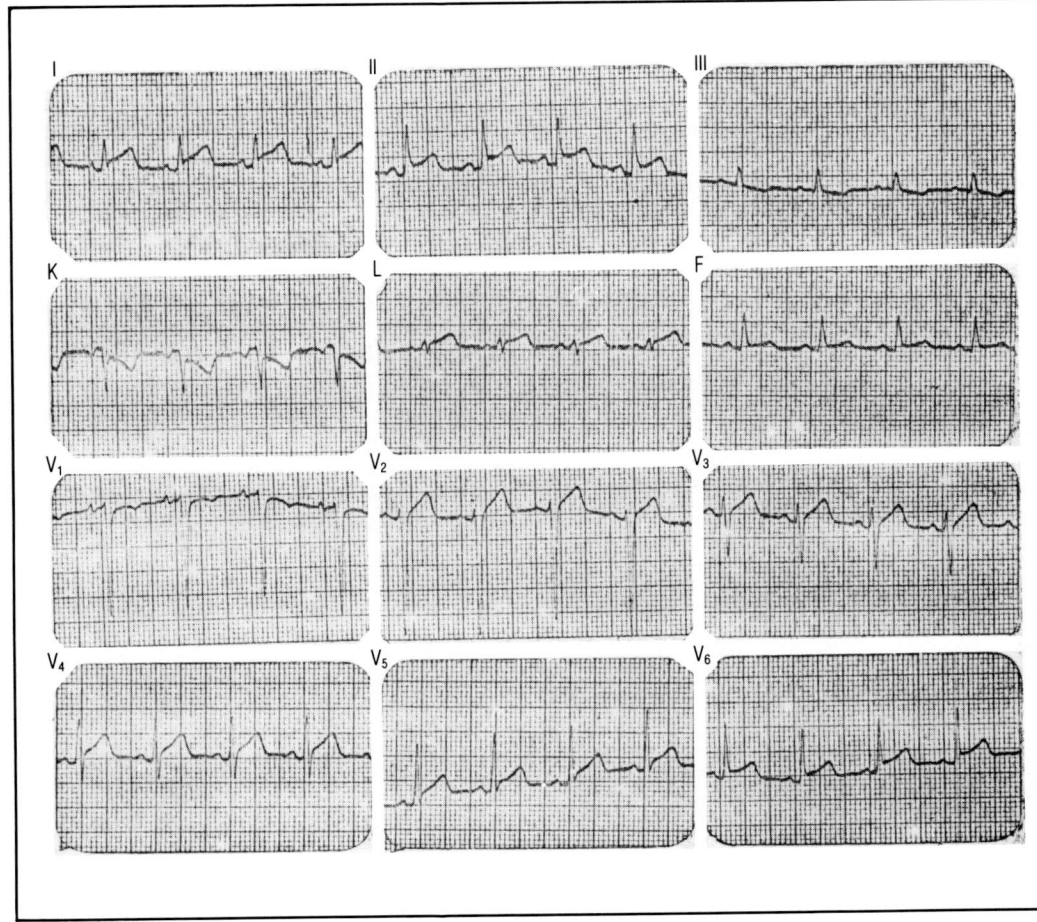

FIGURE 92.18 Acute pericarditis. Typical (stage I) ECG. J point (ST junction) elevations in all leads excepting lead III and depressions (not "reciprocal") in leads aV_R and V_1. PR segment depressions in leads I, II, aV_L, aV_F, and V_2–V_6. Note: the TP interval is the ECG baseline. Deviations of J-ST and of PR are to opposite sides of that baseline.

the mean direction of myocardial repolarization is now approximately opposite to normal so that T wave inversion occurs mainly in leads that had shown ST elevation. Thus, the T vector is now reversed, but not perfectly (180°), because during repolarization electric activity is less homogeneous.[12] Activity is now abnormally prolonged in the injured zone and the QT_c tends to increase. In Stage IV the T waves become normally oriented due to subsiding inflammation. The duration of activity in the subepicardial layer approaches normal, with gradual normalization of the QT_c and the T vector.

During typical evolution, ECG abnormalities usually occur almost simultaneously and in the same direction in most limb and precordial leads that record "epicardial" patterns, with corresponding oppositely directed changes only in aV_R and other so-called cavity leads, notably V_1 and occasionally V_2. In most cases of acute pericarditis with typical ECGs, the anatomical distribution of myocardial injury is general, so that there are no "reciprocal" elevations and depressions of ST segments in "regional" lead groups,[12] as in acute myocardial infarction. (Note: virtually every atypical case with restricted ST-T changes also will fail to show "reciprocal" changes,[13] resembling a pattern common in atypical [Prinzmetal] angina.)

PR SEGMENTS

Unlike the ventricles, subepicardial myocarditis over the thin-walled atria cannot be very superficial. The atrial T-wave (T_A) shifts to an early position, becoming visible in the PR segment (between the P and Q waves).[12] Since the atria do not have an electrical "gradient" corresponding to the "ventricular gradient," the normal orientation of the atrial T wave, opposite to the P wave, is preserved. This is seen as a PR shift opposite in direction to the P waves. Most P wave vectors are between +40° and +60°, so that the PR segment vector is approximately 180° opposite at −120° to −150°.[12]

RATE AND RHYTHM ABNORMALITIES

The heart rate in acute pericarditis is usually rapid but can be surprisingly slow, particularly in uremic patients. Many patients, particularly younger people, have rates between 90 and 120 beats/min when the inflammation is most intense. Rhythm abnormalities are often declared to be associated with pericarditis. This is not the case. All formally investigated, nonanecdotal evidence indicates no such association unless the patient has coexistent heart disease, including very severe myocarditis, or during cardiac tamponade (equivalent to heart disease).[14] Although the sinus node is approximately 1 mm deep to the pericardium, careful anatomic studies show that inflammatory cells do not invade the node proper. This does not exclude pericarditis as having some facilitating role, but the patient must have an arrhythmogenic cardiac disorder. Nevertheless, acute pericarditis *per se* does not appear to be a cause of arrhythmias.[14]

PERICARDIAL EFFUSION

Fluid surrounding the heart may alter transmission of electric signals so as to reduce QRS and T voltages (Fig. 92.20). Massive effusions reduce P wave voltage. Some voltage reduction may be related to hemodynamic impairment. Finally, a left pleural effusion (relatively common in pericardial disease)[1] can reduce voltage independently, as may any general tendency to fluid retention. Cardiac tamponade may reduce voltage both from the nonspecific fluid effect and from compressing effects producing cardiac angulation, reduction and distortion of coronary flow, and restriction of filling. Potassium leaking from bloody pericardial contents can produce ST-T changes.

Electric alternation[2] occurs in perhaps 20% to 25% of cases of tamponade and, although it often indicates serious tamponade, may be persistent or intermittent (Fig. 92.13).[15] It is definitely related to a variable but individually critical heart rate, often near 100 beats/min. The exact rate probably is related to some ratio or harmonic relation between the heart's frequency and its "pendular moment"—its tendency to freely oscillate when pericardial fluid relieves it from external restraint. Electric alternation can occur in massive effusions without obvious cardiac compression, but nearly always indicates tamponade. Oscillation usually has a 2:1 periodicity, reflecting the "swinging heart" seen on echocardiography (Fig. 92.13). Electric alternation implies a single pacemaker with an alternating direction (vector) of activation (QRS) in every other beat. T wave alternation may also be seen but is more difficult to discern because of the slow inscription and lower amplitude of the T wave. When (rarely) P waves also alternate—*simultaneous alternation*—the result is pathognomonic for cardiac tamponade. Because QRS and QRS-T alternans occur in few other conditions, tamponade should always be suspected. Removal of a quite small aliquot of fluid usually abolishes alternation, indicating there may be a hemodynamic as well as an oscillatory anatomical contribution to it. Electrical alternans is sometimes associated with auscultatory alternans, and, rarely, with pulsus alterans (Fig. 92.9).

"EARLY REPOLARIZATION"

An ECG pattern almost indistinguishable from the J-ST deviations of Stage I acute pericarditis[1,16] is found relatively frequently, particularly in young males who are often neurotic or even psychotic. Chest pain in such individuals may produce a clinical mimic of acute pericarditis.

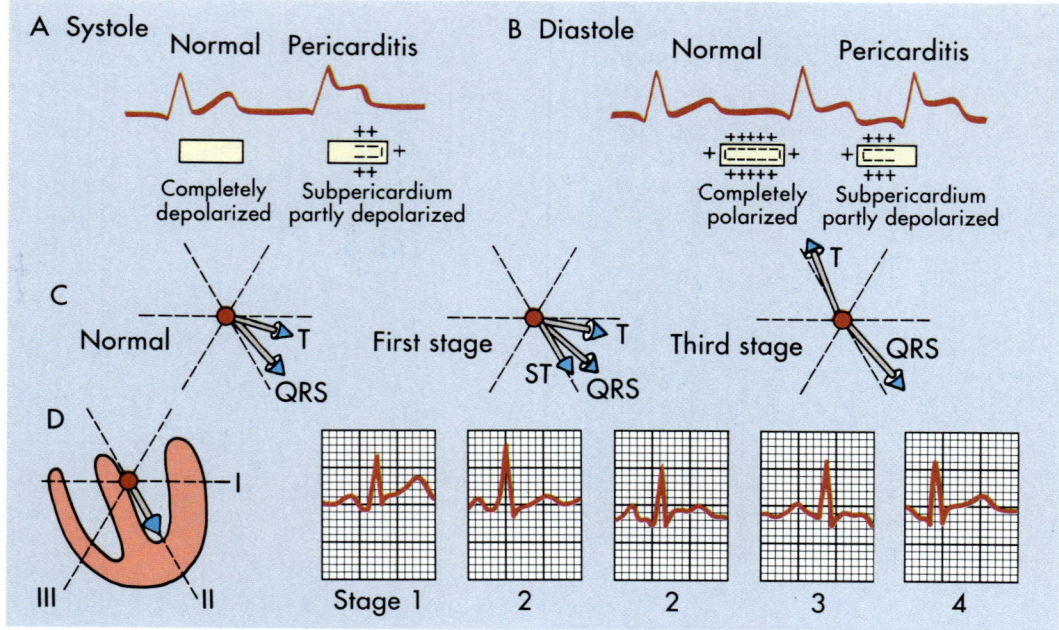

FIGURE 92.19 Acute pericarditis. Electrical basis of ECG changes (see text). **A.** Systolic J-ST displacement. **B.** Diastolic J-ST "displacement" due to depression of TP interval. **C.** Spatial representation of QRS, ST, and T vectors. **D.** Net ST vector, usual orientation: inferiorly, anteriorly, and leftward. Bottom trace shows representative complexes from stages I, II, III, and IV of ECG evolution of acute pericarditis (see text).

There are certain points permitting ECG differentiation, the most important being "early repolarization" as the patient's permanent ECG.

Patients with early repolarization (unless they also have pericarditis) will not have a rub or fever of pericardial origin. Usually the J-ST elevations follow a slurred QRS downstroke, just above and including the J point and best seen in precordial leads with tall R and T waves. PR segment deviations are uncommon and never as marked or widespread as they often are in acute pericarditis.[16] One differential point is the ratio of the height of the J point to the peak of the T wave in lead V_6, using the PR segment as a baseline. A J height exceeding 25% of that of the T wave apex makes pericarditis more likely. Although this sign reflects the tendencies to relatively lower T waves in pericarditis and T wave peaking in early repolarization,[16] it is of unknown sensitivity and specificity and probably useful only late in Stage I. Exercise testing is undependable because it appears to induce comparable changes (ST return to baseline) in both.

TREATMENT OF ACUTE PERICARDITIS: GENERAL CONSIDERATIONS

Treatment of acute pericarditis is directed toward suppression of symptoms and destruction of etiologic agents. Relief of tamponade has been discussed.

SYMPTOMATIC THERAPY

Management of symptoms should be commensurate with the patient's distress. Often, 300 mg to 600 mg of aspirin every 4 to 6 hours will control both pain and fever. Codeine (rarely, more powerful opiates) may be added and is particularly useful for coughing. While the patient is awaiting analgesia, severe pain may respond to an icebag placed on the precordium, if tolerated (note: not for ischemic patients). Nonsteroidal anti-inflammatory agents (NSAIDs) other than aspirin act more rapidly, particularly ibuprofen, 300 mg to 600 mg every 6 hours. Ibuprofen produces fewer side-effects than aspirin. Any NSAID, in fact, may be tried with attention to contraindications and side-effects. When large nontamponading effusions cause significant thoracic or abdominal distress, a palliative pericardiocentesis may be performed. Tranquilizers may be needed for anxious patients, notably those with heart disease (related or unrelated). Finally, corticosteroids should be avoided unless pericarditis is part of a syndrome for which such treatment is necessary, or when all other means of controlling symptoms have failed, and then at minimal effective doses. This is because growing numbers of individuals with recurrent pericarditis are "hooked" on a corticosteroid and must repeatedly take the agent or cannot discontinue it without experiencing disabling discomfort.

DESTRUCTION OF ETIOLOGIC AGENTS

When pericarditis is a part of a generalized disorder for which there is specific or suppressive therapy, the appropriate systemic treatment is indicated. Thus, for uremic pericarditis, intense hemo- or peritoneal dialysis is required. Bacteria and parasites should be attacked with appropriate agents, administered systemically. Most antibiotics tested produce effective levels in pericardial fluid. Intrapericardial instillation of antibiotic agents may provoke adhesions. On the other hand, malignant involvement of the pericardium has been treated successfully with antineoplastic agents both systemically and intrapericardially.

SPECIFIC FORMS OF ACUTE PERICARDITIS

Most forms of acute pericarditis manifest some or all of the general picture described. Therefore, symptoms, signs, ECG, and other laboratory findings will not be individually detailed, except when their presence or absence is conspicuous for the particular kind of acute pericarditis.

VIRAL PERICARDITIS

Most cases of acute pericarditis of unknown origin (idiopathic pericarditis; nonspecific pericarditis; "acute benign pericarditis") are of viral origin or at least completely duplicate syndromes due to identified viruses. A large number of viruses have been found in association with pericarditis. The most common are coxsackie B and A, enteroviruses, and adenovirus. Others include influenza, hepatitis, infectious mononucleosis (Epstein-Barr virus), mumps, varicella, and poliomyelitis. Pericarditis is relatively common during enteroviral epidemics. Viral pericarditides (particularly coxsackie) frequently include varying elements of myocarditis–*myopericarditis*.

Pericarditis usually appears in the course of, or 1 to 3 weeks following, a systemic infection, particularly one that includes the upper respiratory or gastrointestinal tract. It is thus usually too late to find proof of viral origin. (Indeed, even the pericardial fluid, an ultrafiltrate of blood, may merely reflect viremia, and biopsies are not often warranted.) Many patients with viral pericarditis have a cough; from 25% to 50% of them have pulmonary infiltrates and pleural effusions.

Viral pericarditis or idiopathic pericarditis syndrome is remarkably

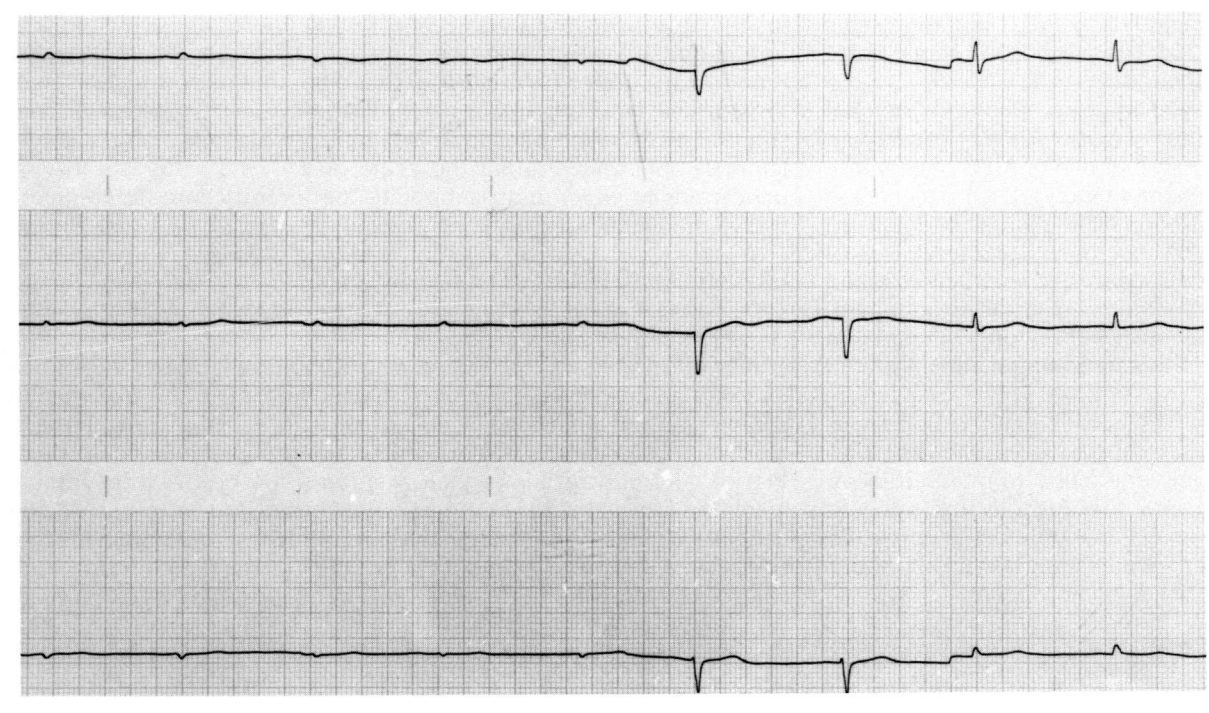

FIGURE 92.20 Pericardial involvement in myxedema. ECG. Very low voltage, nonspecific T wave abnormality and bradycardia.

more common in men than in women, with a sex ratio of 3 or 4 to 1. It should be suspected in basically healthy male patients who have had a prodromal respiratory or gastrointestinal illness. Other etiologies must always be considered, since viruses will probably not be recoverable or may not be definitively associated with the pericarditis. Even the customary fourfold rise in neutralizing antibody titers over the first 3 weeks after onset is only supporting evidence for a viral diagnosis, but is helpful when other feared conditions do not seem present. In women the latter applies particularly to systemic lupus erythematosus (SLE). Otherwise, trauma, other infections of the pericardium, or a dominant myocarditis (particularly in children) must be differentiated. In older patients, less likely to have viral infections, a different set of disorders must also be differentiated: neoplasia, myocardial infarction, tuberculosis, and vasculitis.

Clinically, this syndrome is the epitome of acute pericarditis in that all or nearly all characteristic manifestations are likely to be present. The acute illness lasts from a few days to 2 or 3 months, but averages 2 weeks. Recurrences (often a single relapse) must be anticipated in 15% to 25% of cases. These usually are shorter and milder than the initial episode. However, multiple attacks may occur for many years and some patients become dependent on therapy, particularly corticosteroid agents—which may, in fact, have a role in inducing recurrent and unremitting pericarditis.

The vast majority of cases are self-limited, but complications in addition to unresolved inflammation may occur (hence the discarded name, "acute benign pericarditis"). These include continuing myocarditis (rarely leading to cardiomyopathy), pericardial effusion with or without tamponade, and constrictive pericarditis either shortly after an attack (usually with tamponade) or developing over months to many years.

General rules of treatment are as described and apply until effective and safe antiviral agents become available. In any case, patients should be followed for at least several months to detect complications.

SUPPURATIVE PERICARDITIS

Among infectious pericarditides, pyogenic bacterial infection remains the most serious and often the most severe. (Very severe viral pericarditis is much less common. Fungal, protozoal, and acute tuberculous pericarditis can be severe, but these forms are quite uncommon in most developed countries.) Lower incidence and easy control of bacterial infections, except in compromised hosts, has contributed to a lower prevalence of suppurative pericarditis. Thus, it is more likely in patients with contiguous infection and abscesses, such as after thoracic surgery, during bacterial endocarditis, or in bacteremia. During infective endocarditis, a pericardial effusion may be sterile, but a suppurative effusion, a pericardial rub, or pericarditis by ECG often represents penetration of myocardium or valve ring (usually aortic), septic coronary embolus, or ruptured mycotic aneurysm.

"New" patient categories are particularly susceptible to bacterial and fungal pericarditis, specifically after extensive surgery or with impaired immune systems of unknown cause or due to AIDS or immunosuppressive treatment (*e.g.*, cancer chemotherapy). Such patients are usually hospitalized and may have nosocomial infections, often due to resistant organisms and gram-negative bacteria. Leading causes of suppurative pericarditis include *Staphylococcus, Pneumococcus,* and *Neisseria* (particularly *Neisseria meningitidis*—with or without meningitis). *Hemophilus influenzae* is particularly common in children, in whom any bacterial pericarditis is apt to cause tamponade and rapid constriction.

Although bacterial infections may be clinically silent, especially in patients with severe systemic diseases, they are more often dramatic, particularly in younger individuals. Only one fourth to one third have chest pain, but nearly all have fever and considerable toxicity, with chills and night sweats; dyspnea and cough are common. Tachycardia is nearly always present, but a rub is detected in only about half. About the same proportion develop overt cardiac compression.

LABORATORY DATA

Leukocytosis with a marked left shift is characteristic, although often absent with debilitation and a compromised immune system. Blood culture may reveal the organism, but it is better to culture pericardial fluid. If there are signs of hemodynamically important cardiac compression, the material can be obtained at full thoracotomy. The pericardial fluid is an exudate, usually turbid, with many polymorphonuclear leukocytes, and with high lactate dehydrogenase and low glucose levels.

In the absence of a pericardial rub or Stage I ECG (which actually occur frequently), suspicion of pericardial involvement in septic patients calls for an echocardiogram, since this condition nearly always has copious exudate and sometimes a quite large effusion.

SPECIFIC THERAPY

Mortality in purulent pericarditis has been reduced from almost 100% to well under 50% by surgical drainage alone. Antibiotics have further cut the toll. Yet, this remains a dangerous disease and, particularly in compromised hosts, together with general sepsis still can be fatal if not rapidly controlled. This is difficult to achieve early in patients without pain, other localizing signs, or laboratory data. Unless there is rapid and complete remission, the treatment is drainage—preferably surgical, when the diagnosis is uncertain—as soon and as complete as possible, and large doses of effective antibiotics. Because of the danger of constriction, complete pericardiectomy should be considered at the time of drainage.

TUBERCULOUS PERICARDITIS

Despite the drop in serious clinical tuberculosis in advanced countries, tuberculous pericarditis remains a very popular "rule out." In the United States it is practically confined to occasional elderly persons and immigrants from countries where tuberculosis remains common. Yet, because we have effective therapy for what can be a very destructive process, the usually fruitless diagnostic effort is worthwhile.

Difficult to manage *atypical mycobacteria* (e.g. *M. avium*) must be anticipated in immunocompromised (notably AIDS) patients.

PATHOGENESIS[2]

Tuberculous infection reaches the pericardium hematogenously from remote foci or miliary seeding or by direct involvement from tuberculous mediastinal lymph nodes. Occasionally, pericarditis is the first overt manifestation (clinically primary tuberculous pericarditis). The exudate in early lesions contains mainly polymorphonuclear leukocytes; later, lymphocytes or monocytes predominate. Granulomas may be found in the parietal and visceral pericardia, and if they caseate, tuberculous myocarditis may ensue, but the most common complication is constrictive pericarditis—greatly reduced by chemotherapy. Rare cases produce cholesterol pericarditis. One reason why tuberculosis of the pericardium can be so destructive, with subsequent constriction, may be the frequency of antiheart (antimyosin and antimyolemmal) antibodies during the acute phase. This contrasts to viral pericarditis in which both antibodies and constriction are comparatively infrequent.

CLINICAL CHARACTERISTICS

Tuberculous pericarditis can present in several ways: typical, painful, acute pericarditis with minimal to large amounts of pericardial fluid; silent pericardial effusion; tamponade without other acute symptoms except, perhaps, fever; subacute constriction; pericardial calcification without hemodynamic consequences; or fever of unknown origin. Most often, the clinical onset of tuberculous pericarditis contrasts to that of viral pericarditis in that symptoms can be the least striking manifestation and the acute phase may be missed in up to half the patients. Without advanced tuberculosis elsewhere, or tamponade, patients can appear well, even with very large tuberculous effusions. With cardiac compression, a frequent chief complaint is dyspnea on minimal exertion, sometimes with edema. Younger patients and those with milder disease may have a more painful, acute onset.

Effusion is the rule, generally large to massive, and sometimes loculated by adhesions. Some liquid often persists even with severe constriction. The fluid almost invariably contains old and new blood, at least during the initial tap, which may also reveal large numbers of white cells, particularly lymphocytes. The peripheral white blood cell count is usually normal, occasionally increased. Tuberculin tests are almost always positive (if negative, the patient should be checked for the presence of anergy), but tuberculin testing is not of specific diagnostic help.

Tuberculous pericarditis is difficult to diagnose, since definitive findings include tubercle bacilli in the pericardial fluid or pericardial biopsy. Extrapericardial tuberculosis only makes the diagnosis presumptive so that both fluid and biopsy material should be smeared for the presence of acid-fast bacilli, appropriately cultured, and injected into guinea pigs. Chronicity makes it increasingly difficult to obtain organisms, and the histology becomes increasingly nonspecific. Indeed, a negative biopsy does not rule out tuberculous pericarditis.

Tuberculous pericarditis should be listed with diagnoses of "pyrexia of unknown origin," particularly when there is enlargement of the cardiopericardial silhouette in a patient who has had tuberculous exposure or is in a high-risk group for tuberculosis, or has tuberculosis in another organ. Any very large effusion, especially in patients with relatively few symptoms, should raise suspicion of tuberculosis, since this is a "treatable" disease and inadequate treatment can lead to serious consequences.

Three factors seem to be associated with poor prognosis: (1) ease of bacteriologic proof, (2) age over 50 years, and (3) gradual, relatively painless development. Yet, the high mortality before specific antituberculous therapy became available has been drastically reduced and even patients with active disease can be safely operated on under antibiotic cover.

SPECIFIC THERAPY

The treatment of tuberculous pericarditis is that of any active or potentially active form of tuberculosis, preferably with triple drug therapy (*e.g.*, rifampin, isoniazid, and ethambutol) and long-term vigilance regarding complications. When pericardial involvement appears during therapy of extracardiac tuberculosis, additional antituberculosis agents may be added. Any tendency to tamponade or constriction while the patient is under appropriate therapy should be dealt with surgically.

FUNGUS AND RELATED DISEASE

Fungi affect the pericardium either through sufficient natural exposure or in immunocompromised hosts. The more common "natural" fungal infections include histoplasmosis and coccidioidomycosis. Occurring both naturally and in compromised hosts are candidiasis, blastomycosis, aspergillosis and, intermediate between fungi and bacteria, nocardiosis and actinomycosis.

HISTOPLASMOSIS

The great prevalence of subclinical histoplasmosis in endemic areas, like parts of the Midwest, makes pericardial involvement in the systemic disease unsurprising. *Histoplasma* pericarditis may present as effusion with or without tamponade, constriction, or asymptomatic pericardial calcification. An acute pericarditis syndrome is rare, pericardial involvement usually being discovered during *Histoplasma* pneumonia or dissemination with severe multiple organ involvement producing constitutional symptoms and signs, including anemia and leukopenia. *Histoplasma* endocarditis and myocarditis may accompany.

COCCIDIOIDOMYCOSIS

Common in endemic areas such as the San Joaquin Valley, coccidioidomycosis also occurs in immunocompromised hosts. In them, as in naturally occurring severe coccidioidomycosis, the generalized illness usually dominates the picture. Clinically recognized pericarditis can develop as a typical acute pericarditis syndrome, pericardial effusion with or without tamponade, or constrictive pericarditis.

OTHER FUNGI

Infections arising from *Candida*, *Blastomyces*, *Aspergillus*, and the semifungi, *Actinomycetes* and *Nocardia*, usually occur after surgery, in the context of immunocompromised patients and debilitating disease (particularly in the elderly). In recognized disease with any of these organisms, even without manifest pericardial involvement, suspicion of pericarditis warrants careful auscultation and echocardiography or other imaging procedure.

DIAGNOSIS

History of exposure to particular organisms in endemic areas always suggests an etiology for generalized or local disease. Serum and skin tests, where applicable, will identify exposure to the organism, but definitive diagnosis by biopsy may be desirable when there is an important differential diagnosis, that is, conditions that resemble fungal pericarditis, like tuberculosis, brucellosis, sarcoidosis, and Hodgkin's disease. However, organisms must be identified since, as in tuberculous pericarditis, granulomatous responses are common to a number of inflammations.

TREATMENT

In addition to the general management of acute pericarditis, cardiac tamponade, and constriction, specific agents are available for treating some fungal infections. Amphotericin B (with appropriate vigilance toward side-effects) is effective against several.

PARASITIC DISEASE

In keeping with the rule for all etiologic living agents, any parasite that can reach the pericardium can attack it, producing acute or chronic disease and constrictive pericarditis, due to the extreme irritation caused by parasites and their products. Apart from its occurrence in certain immigrants, parasitic pericarditis is mainly a disease of countries with endemic parasitoses, notably dracunculosis, cysticercosis, echinococcosis, and filariasis. Amebic pericarditis is common in endemic areas and has been found in the United States. Almost always, amebae acutely involve the pericardium by perforation from a hepatic amebic abscess; occasionally the lung and pleura are involved before rupture into the pericardium. The acute illness usually resembles suppurative pericarditis, although serous pericardial effusions occur with unruptured liver abscesses and some patients may develop sterile tamponade. Even after pericardial perforation, fluid may be negative for the presence of amebae, and biopsy will be necessary. Toxoplasmosis may produce acute pericarditis with characteristic humoral antibody titers but is more often found as an "innocent" lesion at autopsy, along with *Toxoplasma* myocarditis. Echinococcosis rarely involves the pericardium and mainly occurs in sheep-raising areas like Greece and Uruguay. Eosinophilic leukocytosis is characteristic.

PERICARDITIS IN THE VASCULITIS-CONNECTIVE TISSUE DISEASE GROUP

Although this disease category overlaps the next (immunopathies and "hypersensitivity" states), many members resemble each other clinically.

ACUTE RHEUMATIC FEVER (ARF)

Rheumatic fever is disappearing in more advanced countries, though prevalent and severe in much of the Third World. Nearly all patients dying of ARF have microscopic pericarditis, and about 70% have gross pericarditis.[2] Similarly, most patients with chronic rheumatic valve disease in the absence of active carditis often have pericardial thickening or adhesions or even obliteration of the pericardial sac.[10] In contrast, pericarditis is clinically diagnosable in only 5% to 10% of ARF patients, but always accompanies severe cardiac involvement.

CLINICAL CHARACTERISTICS. Acute rheumatic pericarditis is most frequent in children and adolescents. Unlike the situation in most forms of pericarditis, there is no male preponderance. Occasionally, pericarditis is the first sign of ARF so that for any child with pericarditis without demonstrable sepsis, ARF should be ruled out. Usually, however, symptoms and signs appear in the first week after fever and arthritis, with chest pain (often quite severe), secondary temperature rise, and disproportionate tachypnea. Any dyspnea is probably due to myocarditis and myocardial failure. Classically, an intense rub is detectable for several days. Pericardial effusion is the rule, but tamponade is rare and must be distinguished from heart failure. The pericardial fluid is usually clear amber with many shreds of fibrin.

LABORATORY DATA. As a result of ARF, the usual acute phase reactants are abnormal. The antistreptolysin-0 titer is high in up to 90% of patients with ARF, and with pericarditis is usually 400 or more. Typical Stage I ECG changes are uncommon. PR interval prolongation, probably a nonspecific streptococcemic effect, is common but is even more frequent without pericarditis.

DIAGNOSIS. It is important to rule out other members of the vasculitis group, juvenile rheumatoid arthritis, childhood exanthemata, and the occasional case of idiopathic (presumably viral) pericarditis that presents with arthralgias. Without definite signs of rheumatic carditis, ARF pericarditis is diagnosed on circumstantial evidence, including (1) fever and arthritis preceding pericarditis (usually); (2) comparative youth (most patients); (3) serologic evidence of beta hemolytic streptococcal infection; (4) absence of evidence of SLE.

PROGNOSIS. Pericarditis always indicates active rheumatic carditis with a relatively poor prognosis, especially in young children. There is no conclusive proof that it ever leads to constriction, despite the sometimes exuberant adhesions provoked.

TREATMENT. Pain and fever can be controlled with aspirin, which will also attack the rheumatic process. Treatment of myocardial failure, penicillin, and rest complete the usual approach. There is no proof that corticosteroid therapy is superior to aspirin or other nonsteroidal anti-inflammatory agents.

SYSTEMIC LUPUS ERYTHEMATOSUS (SLE)

Clinical pericarditis occurs in about half the patients with SLE; autopsy prevalence reaches almost 90%. Pericarditis may be dry or effusive, sometimes as part of a SLE polyserositis. Renal failure may add uremic pericarditis. Drug-induced SLE also causes pericarditis, but this clears with discontinuation of the drug. Occasional patients have cardiac tamponade with fluid that is serous to grossly hemorrhagic, containing immunoglobulins, increased protein, low glucose levels, and leukocyte counts under $10,000/ml^3$, mostly polymorphonuclear, and typical LE cells. Acute pericarditis can be the first overt manifestation of SLE and may be diagnosed as idiopathic pericarditis. Thus, women with idiopathic pericarditis syndrome should be tested for SLE. Both spontaneous and drug-induced SLE rarely lead to constriction. Treatment is the same as for the systemic disease.

RHEUMATOID ARTHRITIS

While rheumatoid arthritis is an uncommon cause of clinical pericarditis, at necropsy about half the patients have pericardial adhesions[10]— evidence of the great frequency of subclinical pericarditis. Indeed, on rheumatology services casual auscultation discloses rubs in patients with no chest complaints who are admitted because of their arthritis. Rheumatoid nodules of the pericardium, microscopically indistinguishable from subcutaneous nodules, are rare, but may even be seen on x-ray films. Rheumatoid arthritis pericarditis occurs in juvenile as well as adult rheumatoid arthritis, rarely as typical acute pericarditis or tamponade, more often as subacute and chronic constriction. Effusion fluid is a serous or hemorrhagic exudate containing IgG, often with low complement and positive latex-fixation titers and quite high leukocyte counts, some of the cells having cytoplasmic inclusion bodies. There is nothing distinctive about the clinical features of the ECG, and the possibility of other types of pericarditis in a patient with rheumatoid arthritis must always be considered. Only symptomatic pericarditis need be treated.

SCLERODERMA

Like rheumatoid arthritis, scleroderma involves the pericardium at necropsy in about half the patients, clinically, in fewer, usually as silent pericardial effusions. Some are transudates due to frequent myocardial failure (often a restrictive cardiomyopathy) or renal failure. Typical acute pericarditis can occur, identified by a pericardial rub, since the ECG usually is nonspecific. Occasional patients develop cardiac tamponade; chronic pericardial effusion (transudate or exudate) is more frequent. Exudative effusions have high protein levels but relatively low cell counts, and no immune complexes or autoantibodies. Constriction is rare though restrictive cardiomyopathy in patients with noncompressing pericardial fibrosis or calcification can mimic it so closely as to require thoracotomy for differential diagnosis.

OTHER CONNECTIVE TISSUE DISORDERS

Dermatomyositis, Sjögren's syndrome, Reiter's syndrome, Felty's syndrome, and mixed connective tissue disease are occasionally complicated by pericarditis that may be difficult to differentiate from intercurrent infectious pericarditis. Lesions may be noted postmortem in polyarteritis. Occasional patients with severe ankylosing spondylitis have clinical acute pericarditis with a definite rub, usually in the presence of aortic or cardiac involvement. Fibrous obliteration of the pericardium with nodular and granulomatous lesions at autopsy is more common.

PERICARDITIS IN IMMUNOPATHIES AND "HYPERSENSITIVITY" STATES

Pericarditis occasionally occurs in many of these conditions. There is considerable pathogenetic overlap with other categories (Table 92.7). For example, the sterile pericardial effusions that may occur with extracardiac amebic abscesses or in patients convalescing from meningococcal infection (who also have other immunopathic manifestations, like arthritis, ophthalmitis, and pleuritis). Similarly, the postmyocardial infarction and other postcardiac injury syndromes and some drug-associated pericarditis probably have an immunopathic basis.

More obvious "hypersensitivity" states include allergic reactions, serum sickness, allergic granulomatosis, and even bronchial asthma. Indeed, pathogenesis of ARF as a manifestation of β-hemolytic streptococcal "sensitivity" is a case in point. Other disorders, possibly of autoimmune origin, include Behcet's syndrome, Henoch-Schönlein purpura, Kawasaki's disease and some cases of polyarteritis with hepatitis-B antigen, inflammatory bowel disease, and temporal arteritis.

PERICARDITIS IN DISEASES OF CONTIGUOUS STRUCTURES

ACUTE MYOCARDIAL INFARCTION ("EPISTENOCARDIAC PERICARDITIS")

Pericarditis is found at autopsy in approximately 40% of patients dying of acute myocardial infarction. The pericardial inflammation is nearly always localized over the infarct, though fibrinous exudate may spread throughout the pericardium.[2,17] Although it does not affect the patient's in-hospital prognosis adversely, acute pericarditis is found only with anatomically transmural infarcts. (The discovery of a pericardial rub is thus the only noninvasive method to identify transmural infarcts since the ECG cannot do this reliably.[17]) Small pericardial effusions are not uncommon although they may be confused with hydropericardium associated with fluid retention. Tamponade is rare, as is hemorrhagic effusion, in the absence of anticoagulant therapy or cardiac rupture.

CLINICAL CHARACTERISTICS AND DIAGNOSIS. In only 6% to 20% of acute infarctions is pericarditis clinically detected, because a typical Stage I ECG is extremely rare, and because rubs may be faint or evanescent.[17] Most often the physician is alerted to the possibility of pericarditis by pleuritic central chest pain. Since this could also be due to pleuropulmonary complications, it is only with pain in one or both trapezius ridges that, in the absence of a rub, the diagnosis can be made with some confidence. There may be a secondary temperature rise and the pain is nearly always interpreted by the patient as different from (and sometimes worse than) that at the onset of infarction. The first 4 days after admission account for almost all cases of diagnosed infarct pericarditis. Most rubs are detected during this period, especially on the second day.[17] It is moot whether late rubs are related to the postmyocardial infarction (Dressler's) syndrome unless there are also other manifestations. Spread of the exudate throughout the pericardial sac accounts for rubs being heard equally well with anterior and posterior infarcts.[17] As in most cases of pericarditis, they are usually loudest at or restricted to the left mid- to low-sternal edge.[11]

DIFFERENTIAL DIAGNOSIS. Usually the rubs' quality is unmistakable, but when they have a single systolic component they can be confused with a new murmur of mitral or tricuspid regurgitation or septal rupture. Unlike the pain of increased ischemia, pericarditic pain does not respond to nitrates. Moreover, new ischemic pain is likely to be accompanied by new "local" ECG changes. The occasional case of tamponade may need differentiation from heart failure, which is often fairly easy because of the common presence of a third heart sound with failure and its suppression by tamponade. With RV infarction there may also be hypotension, jugular venous distention, and a Kussmaul sign—all common to constrictive pericarditis. Indeed, distention of the infarcted RV appears to tighten the basically normal pericardium, producing steep atrial and jugular y descents and a "square root" sign in the RV pulse, both helping to rule out tamponade. Imaging studies should show RV involvement and usually absence of significant pericardial fluid.

TREATMENT. Though pain of infarction pericarditis can be so mild that no treatment is needed, most patients will wish to be treated. The mainstay is aspirin or another nonsteroidal anti-inflammatory agent, with a corticosteroid only as a last resort.

DISSECTING AORTIC HEMATOMA

Intrapericardial rupture is common in dissecting aortic aneurysm. True pericardial irritation can result when blood leaks beneath the epicardium or constricts the coronary ostia to produce infarction-related pericarditis.[2] Whatever the mechanisms, pericardial rubs are not rare with dissections, and the ECG may resemble that of pericarditis. With intrapericardial rupture there is usually shock with catastrophic tamponade and often electromechanical dissociation. Slower dissections may be recognized by back or abdominal pain, aortic widening, aortic regurgitation, and markedly discrepant pulses.

PULMONARY EMBOLISM

Infarction of lung segments immediately adjacent to the heart may be heralded by central pleuritic pain and a pleuropericardial or even a strictly pericardial rub that may be the first sign of pulmonary embolism. In such patients, with only external pericardial irritation, the pulmonary embolism is the main problem. (Embolized patients recovering from cardiac surgery may also have surgical pericarditis.)

ESOPHAGEAL DISEASES

Inflammation, ulcers, malignancies, and perforating foreign bodies of the esophagus have caused pericarditis either by direct involvement or by retrograde lymphatic spread. Indeed, ECG changes in the presence of esophageal disease merit investigation for pericardial involvement.

POSTMYOCARDIAL AND PERICARDIAL INJURY SYNDROMES

Pericarditis has been associated with injury of the heart and pericardium in the presence of antiheart antibodies. While antipericardial antibodies have not yet been identified, the usual presentation of these syndromes is pericarditic rather than myocarditic (although the latter must be assumed when there are ECG changes). These pericarditic syndromes are probably immunopathic because of their common features: (1) a latent period; (2) recurrences; (3) response to corticosteroids; (4) sterile cultures; and (5) fever with pulmonary infiltration and pleuritis.

POSTMYOCARDIAL INFARCTION SYNDROME (PMIS)

Originally described by Dressler, PMIS, characterized by pericarditis, pleuritis, fever, and frequent pneumonitis, follows a myocardial infarction by a week to several months. Most patients have not had typical acute infarct-associated pericarditis. Unlike that form, the inflammatory lesion in PMIS should be diffuse rather than localized—probably the reason why the majority produce rubs and some pericardial effusion. In very early first attacks, absence of pleuritis and pneumonitis may make distinction from infarct pericarditis difficult, while these features are characteristic of many relapses. The pain is usually more severe than that of infarct pericarditis and may be both angina-like and pleuritic. There may be a pleural rub and the chest film often shows pleural effusion and transient pulmonary infiltrates as well as some enlargement of the cardiac silhouette. Half of the patients have ECG changes suggesting, but not always diagnostic of, pericarditis.

DIAGNOSTIC CONSIDERATIONS. PMIS should be suspected in patients with an unusual duration of fever after infarction and new pleuropericardial pain. Pulmonary embolism and congestive heart failure should be ruled out. Tamponade is relatively common while late constriction is rare.

TREATMENT. Anticoagulant therapy should be withdrawn and the patient hospitalized unless he has only minor discomfort. Nonsteroidal anti-inflammatory agents will usually suffice; corticosteroid therapy should be a last resort.

POSTPERICARDIOTOMY SYNDROME (PPS) AND RELATED SYNDROMES

Following cardiac surgery, self-limited traumatic pericarditis is "routine." Another form may follow that is related to pericarditis after other cardiac injury, for example, direct or indirect chest trauma, catheter perforation, and epicardial pacemaker implantation. The PPS is more common in younger patients, particularly children (over age 2) with complex congenital heart disease, a contributing factor being the extent of surgery and consequent pericardial manipulation. Antiheart antibodies (nonspecific for cardiac trauma or injury of any kind) are pathogenetic in the presence of viral infection.[18] There is a strong resemblance to the PMIS in that pleuritis and pleural effusion are common, though in PPS they may be due to surgical pleural injury.

CLINICAL CHARACTERISTICS. The immediate postoperative course may be satisfactory with or without significant "surgical" pericarditis. From 1 week to 6 months postoperatively, but usually between the second and fourth weeks, the patient develops pleuritic pain, usually with low-grade fever, and occasional dyspnea, arthralgia, and cough (sometimes with hemoptysis). A new pericardial rub is common, and often a pleural rub. Up to one half the patients will have pericardial effusions by echocardiography, and a few will develop tamponade with or without the other acute findings.

TREATMENT. The usual agents for pericarditis should be used to treat pain and fever. With tamponade, postoperative pericardial changes and adhesions warrant a surgical approach rather than needle paracentesis.

TRAUMATIC PERICARDITIS
DIRECT TRAUMA

The pericardium cannot escape injury in cardiac wounds, so that the majority of such patients rapidly develop shock as well as cardiac tamponade, often complicated by injuries to coronary vessels, the cardiac conducting system, and other chest and abdominal organs. In some patients bleeding is slow and cardiac compression delayed. Signs and symptoms of pericarditis may appear within the first 24 hours, and suppurative pericarditis ensues when the wounding agent is contaminated by bacteria (e.g., knife wounds or anterior perforation of the esophagus by swallowed bones). If there is pericardial inflammation, typical ECG Stage I changes usually occur after the first day and may persist for days to weeks, followed by long-lasting T wave inversion. However, conduction defects and secondary T wave abnormalities, with or without abnormal Q waves, may confound the interpretation. The very rapidity of tamponade in most cases makes it more difficult to diagnose, because of shock due to blood loss and vasoconstriction from the outset—not characteristic of inflammatory tamponade. Unless there is slow intrapericardial bleeding, there is no time for compensatory transfer of fluid to the venous system. Thus, though the neck veins might pulsate, they need not be distended. The usual treatment for tamponade may be applied, but there is growing evidence that in anything but trivial wounds, immediate surgical drainage is best. Larger pericardial lacerations also warrant earlier surgery since the heart can herniate through the pericardial defect with compression of coronary arteries and other structures. If the injury at first seems slight, close observation may disclose no need for immediate intervention, but emergency surgery should be anticipated.

NONPENETRATING INJURY

Crush injuries of the chest (e.g., steering wheel trauma), blast injuries, and objects striking the chest can contuse the heart and pericardium, producing a range of findings from clinically dry pericarditis to a small effusion with rapid recovery. Sufficient injury to coronary vessels or the myocardium may produce hemorrhagic pericarditis followed by insidious or rapid tamponade. Occasional patients develop pneumopericardium. All patients with any kind of traumatic pericarditis should be followed to detect late constriction.

RADIATION PERICARDITIS

High-voltage radiation therapy for mediastinal lymphomas, Hodgkin's disease, or carcinoma of the lung or breast can produce severe pericardial injury, although modern techniques have drastically reduced this. The range of damage includes acute clinically dry pericarditis, noncompressing effusion, cardiac tamponade, and subacute and chronic constrictive pericarditis. Moreover, while clinically dry pericarditis occurs during treatment or within a few weeks thereafter, constriction may appear up to years later. The treated neoplasms are also capable of causing tamponade and effusive-constrictive pericarditis, making it difficult to decide whether the pericardial disorder is due to radiation, to malignancy, or to both. The picture may be further complicated by radiation injury of any of the cardiac structures. Clinically dry pericarditis should be managed like any other type. Patients showing the slightest evidence of pericardial involvement must be followed indefinitely to detect late tamponade or constriction.

PERICARDITIS IN DISORDERS OF METABOLISM
RENAL FAILURE (UREMIC PERICARDITIS)

Acute pericarditis may complicate acute or, more often, chronic renal failure (CRF). With acute renal failure, blood urea nitrogen (BUN) averages well over 100 mg/dl and with chronic renal failure over 60 mg/dl (usually over 100 mg/dl). Yet, serum constituents like creatinine and urea when placed in the pericardial cavity do not provoke pericarditis,[2] and the pathogenesis of this condition remains unknown. Most patients have sterile fluid although secondary bacterial or viral infection may occur. (Hepatitis virus is common in dialysis units.) Before the antibiotic era, pneumococcal infection, often with pericarditis, was fairly frequent in uremic patients. In CRF, pericarditis usually appears shortly before or after the start of dialysis, which successfully treats most of these patients (as does transplantation). In patients who die there is usually a sterile acute fibrinous, hemorrhagic or serofibrinous exudate, unless infective pericarditis is superimposed. Though the pericardium may contain abundant inflammatory cells, these usually do not involve the myocardium significantly despite destruction of the mesothelium, gross hemorrhage, and frequent tamponade. Pericardial destruction is often sufficient to cause adhesions and, with prolonged survival, uremic constriction, usually the subacute effusive-constrictive type, is appearing more frequently.

Many patients are asymptomatic although up to one half have chest pain (sometimes quite severe) or precordial distress. In severely uremic patients with stupor, symptoms may be difficult to elicit. A rub is usually detected, often loud, and palpable at the left lower sternal edge. Cardiac tamponade may be precipitated by serous fluid accumulation or by either intrapericardial hemorrhage or volume depletion during dialysis decompensating an existing effusion. In many uremic patients, LV hypertrophy or failure buffers or suppresses some signs of tamponade, particularly pulsus paradoxus. Typical Stage I ECGs are rare in uremic pericarditis, probably due to failure of the inflammation to sufficiently involve the subepicardial myocardium. With uremia, a Stage I ECG, therefore, implies infection. Tamponade may appear as unexplained hypotension during or between dialyses. Thus uremic patients must be monitored to determine cardiac size and to visualize the pericardium by echocardiography, if there is any suggestion of circulatory embarrassment.

Very large or compressing effusions should first be treated with intense dialysis, avoiding excessive volume depletion. Nonsteroidal anti-inflammatory drugs such as ibuprofen or sulindac can be given. Any sign of resistance to treatment calls for careful drainage under atropine premedication. Although appropriate clinical trials are lacking, pericardial instillation of a nonabsorbable corticosteroid like triamcinolone appears to be effective. Alternatively, the pericardial sac may be drained for a day or two by catheter, with or without subsequent intrapericardial medication.

DIALYSIS PERICARDITIS

Successful hemodialysis has resulted in the emergence (usually after a period of pericarditis-free dialysis) of a new form of pericarditis, dialysis pericarditis, which is distinguished from ordinary uremic pericarditis because it fails to resolve with aggressive dialysis. Patients may or may not have had previous uremic pericarditis, and can have normal BUN levels. The cause is not known, although "middle molecules" may play a role, since pericarditis occurs much less frequently with peritoneal dialysis than with hemodialysis. Treatment is the same as for uremic pericarditis, except that resistance to treatment and tamponade will call for surgical removal of the pericardium, or, in sicker patients, subxiphoid surgical drainage and a pericardial "window" into the left pleural space.

MYXEDEMA

Although myxedematous pericardial disease is only rarely accompanied by inflammation, it responds readily to thyroid hormone treatment; and it seems logical to include myxedema with the metabolic pericardial disorders. Myxedema produces large pericardial effusions, occasionally with tamponade requiring drainage. The fluid is usually clear with high protein and cholesterol levels and very few blood cells. The lowest ECG voltage is seen with myxedema effusions (probably due also to myocardial involvement), along with nonspecific T wave changes and conspicuous bradycardia (Fig. 92.20).

CHOLESTEROL ("GOLD PAINT") PERICARDITIS

"Gold paint pericarditis" is named for the yellowish to golden, often spangled, fluid that may contain cholesterol crystals. Pericardial tissue shows cholesterol plaques and clefts, often with crystals that probably provoke the concomitant subacute or chronic inflammation. In many cases the etiology is unknown, but cholesterol pericarditis can follow antecedent hemopericardium of any etiology, myxedema, RA, tuberculosis, or other granulomatous pericarditides. Large effusions are the rule with slowly developing tamponade in a few cases; constriction is rare. Either complication indicates pericardiectomy.

OTHER CONDITIONS

Pericarditis has been reported during gout, addisonian crisis, and diabetic ketoacidosis, although no clear dependence on the systemic disease has been established. In ketoacidosis, an ECG mimicking the Stage I ECG of acute pericarditis has been found both with and without other markers of pericardial involvement.

NEOPLASTIC PERICARDIAL DISEASE

Primary tumors of the pericardium are rare, the most important being mesothelioma; even scarcer are sarcoma and benign tumors including lipoma, fibroma, hemangioma, hamartoma, and teratoma. Secondary tumors often associated with simultaneous cardiac involvement include solid tumor (including pleural mesothelioma) metastases, lymphomas, and leukemia and occur in up to 10% of patients with malignancies. Bronchogenic and mammary carcinomas are the most important lesions, although metastasis from a variety of tumors has been reported. Hodgkin's disease is the most important of the lymphomas.

CLINICAL CHARACTERISTICS

Neoplasia can cause both clinically dry and effusive pericardial disease. Abundant effusion is the rule, particularly in patients with hypoalbuminemia, although suppurative pericarditis may occur. While an abundant fibrinous reaction occurs, there may be little or no inflammation. Pericardial adhesions are frequent. Subacute and even chronic constriction may develop from neoplastic tissue and fibrinous adhesions. Most metastatic tumors confined to the heart are clinically silent. Although less so for tumors involving the pericardium, the majority are asymptomatic and found by accident or at autopsy. A common presentation is a large pericardial effusion, often first manifest as cardiac tamponade. Indeed, pericardial involvement may develop before evidence of the primary lesion. On the other hand, tamponade may not be diagnosed because cancer patients can have hypotension, tachycardia, and dyspnea from other causes. Signs and symptoms of pericarditis, dry or wet, in a patient known to have malignant disease, must be considered strong evidence of metastases. Electric alternation is probably most often seen with malignant effusions. The ECG is usually nonspecific.

Constrictive syndromes can occur from pure tumor encasement of the heart, sometimes as an elastic constriction with an S_4 but not an S_3 and mimicking a pericardial effusion on the M-mode echo. Effusive-constrictive or classic fibrotic constrictive pericarditis also occur.

DIAGNOSIS

Malignant disease must always be considered in evaluating cardiac tamponade of unknown etiology, particularly with large and especially bloody effusions that tend to reaccumulate rapidly. Enlargement of the cardiopericardial silhouette necessitates differentiation from myocardial disease, which can be difficult in patients treated with antineoplastic agents that induce cardiomyopathy (often with hydropericardium). Occasional cases mimic acute idiopathic pericarditis. Indeed, intercurrent infection should always be considered since many patients with malignancies are immunocompromised. If there is also a superior vena cava syndrome, neck vein pulsations will be absent and the face, neck, and arms may be edematous. Whether serous or hemorrhagic, pericardial fluid should be examined to detect malignant cells by appropriate stains. There is a better yield of "positives" with solid tumor metastases (though these must be distinguished from damaged mesothelial cells). Lactate dehydrogenase activity in the fluid tends to be far above the patient's serum level, but this is nonspecific. Biopsy may be necessary, particularly open biopsy through a subxiphoid approach to obtain a large tissue sample.

TREATMENT

Treatment, including systemic and intrapericardial chemotherapy and local radiation, is keyed to the cytology of any malignant lesion. Drainage of effusions is followed by instillation of antineoplastic agents. (Bleomycin can be used to cause effusion-suppressing adhesions.) A direct surgical attack is needed for any constricting lesion.

CHYLOPERICARDIUM

Chylopericardium is a rare disorder producing large amounts of milky intrapericardial chyle containing cholesterol, fat, triglycerides, and protein. Cardiac compression is uncommon and because chyle is bactericidal, the inflammation is unlikely to be infected. The condition may be idiopathic (primary chylopericardium) or related to a tumor, particularly lymphangiomatous hamartoma of the mediastinum or to an abnormal communication between pericardium and thoracic duct, which may follow neoplastic obstruction or ductal damage during thoracic surgery. Lymphangiography shows lymph leakage into the pericardium. When no communication is visible, Sudan III dye taken orally usually appears in the pericardial fluid. While the more common chylous peritoneal and pleural effusions tend not to cause adhesions, chylopericardium may inflame the pericardium and produce scarring. If the condition cannot be controlled by diet utilizing medium-chain triglycerides, definitive treatment (not always successful) is ligation of the thoracic duct low in the right side of the chest and resection of any tumor tissue. Pericardial resection may be required.

DRUG-ASSOCIATED PERICARDIAL DISEASE

A number of medicinal substances, including antineoplastic agents, occasionally provoke pericardial effusion and rarely lead to tamponade or constriction. Some occur as a "sensitivity" phenomenon, sometimes with eosinophilia; others, particularly procainamide and hydralazine, as drug-induced lupus erythematosus. If discontinuing the offending agent does not produce remission, treatment is as for any form of pericardial inflammation, effusion, or constriction. Minoxidil therapy can be associated with large pericardial effusions, but the cause-and-effect relation is not definite.

CHRONIC PERICARDIAL EFFUSION

Long-standing pericardial effusions, usually idiopathic, may be discovered by accident during investigation of an enlarged cardiopericardial silhouette or during cardiac echo studies. Some have a probable etiology, notably tuberculosis, but even most of these have lost specific markers. Some chronic effusions are in the pluricausal group also causing cholesterol pericarditis. Treatment is directed at the pericardial contents if there is any sign of cardiac compression or unpleasant symptoms due to the size of these sometimes massive effusions. Asymptomatic effusions unassociated with known disease may pose a difficult decision. Since most chronic effusions remain indefinitely stable, and in an occasional case constriction follows drainage, a conservative approach, that is, observation, may be justified. Yet this decision must be individualized, including consideration of the patient's psychological response to knowledge of the condition. Surgical pericardiectomy is, of course, definitive.

INFLAMMATORY CYSTS AND DIVERTICULA

Inflammation of the pericardium may leave areas of encapsulated exudate and effusion, usually cystic (pericardial pseudocyst) and only rarely with an opening into the general pericardial cavity (pericardial diverticulum).[10] These tend to be innocent and only rarely contribute to the differential diagnosis of distortion of the cardiopericardial silhouette. Hydatid cysts, sometimes calcified, occur in sheep-raising areas due to echinococcosis. However, they may rupture, producing an acute pericardial syndrome.[10]

CONGENITAL DEFECTS OF THE PERICARDIUM

Total absence of the pericardium is extremely rare and produces no recognizable problems. Congenital defects are usually left-sided, sometimes occurring with other congenital anomalies.[19] This partial absence may be silent but can entrap the left atrium, its appendage, or other cardiac structures, or compress coronary vessels. LA entrapment has been associated with sudden death. More often, nonspecific symptoms like chest pain, dizziness, and palpitations bring attention to a distorted cardiopericardial silhouette.[10] There may be no objective findings, but ECGs often show incomplete right bundle branch block, often with right axis deviation and large single-peaked P waves in leads V_1 to III; some combinations suggest RV hypertrophy. The apex impulse may be hypokinetic and shifted to the left along with a palpable or even visible pulmonary artery pulsation, correlating with chest films showing leftward cardiac displacement, usually with a bulge (pulmonary artery) at the upper left border. More lung than usual may be seen between heart and diaphragm. Echocardiograms may show "RV volume overload," with paradoxic systolic septal motion due to cardiac displacement and exaggerated rotation. Two-dimensional recordings may demonstrate locally abnormal LV contour and an incomplete pericardial echo. Angiography also confirms the location of the heart while CT scans document absence of the left pericardium. Air injected into the pleural space (usually left) may be seen on the side opposite the defect. The most important diagnostic problem is differentiation from more common conditions: atrial septal defect, idiopathic PA dilation, hypertrophic cardiomyopathy, ventricular aneurysm, and mitral valve disease. Management of left-sided partial absence (and the even scarcer right-sided partial absence) is surgical.

CONGENITAL PERICARDIAL CYSTS

Usually detected as a protuberance from a border of the cardiac silhouette, congenital cysts can be discovered at any time of life, most often by accident. Most are small projections at the right costophrenic angle. However, size and shape vary widely with some being as large as or larger than the heart itself. Rarely, they occur within the pericardial cavity, mimicking pericardial effusion. Cysts are lined by mesothelium and contain clear watery liquid that may contain hyaluronic acid.[2] There are usually no symptoms. Imaging techniques differentiate them from solid tumor or aneurysm (particularly important at the left heart border). No treatment is required even if the cyst wall calcifies.

PERICARDIAL FAT NECROSIS

An obscure, rare lesion, associated with chest pain that can be unremitting, is pericardial fat necrosis, diagnosable by biopsy. Of unknown origin, necrosis affects the epicardial fat, particularly in patients with a large fat pad.[2] Chest films may suggest haziness of the fat pad outline, although this is not a reliable sign.

REFERENCES

1. Spodick DH: The normal and diseased pericardium: Current concepts of pericardial physiology, diagnosis and treatment. J Am Coll Cardiol 1:240, 1983
2. Spodick DH: Acute Pericarditis. New York, Grune & Stratton, 1959
3. Shabetai R: The pericardium: An essay on some recent developments. Am J Cardiol 42:1036, 1978
4. Spodick DH, Paladino D, Flessas AP: Respiratory effects on systolic time intervals during pericardial effusion. Am J Cardiol 51:1033, 1983
5. Fowler NO, Gabel M: The hemodynamic effect of cardiac tamponade: Mainly the result of atrial, not ventricular compression. Circulation 71:154, 1985
6. Antman EM, Cargill V, Grossman W: Low-pressure cardiac tamponade. Ann Intern Med 91:403, 1979
7. Bush CA, Stang JM, Wooley CF, et al: Occult constrictive pericardial disease. Circulation 56:924, 1977
8. Reddy PS, Curtiss EI, O'Toole JD, et al: Cardiac tamponade; Observations in man. Circulation 58:265, 1978
9. Cabrera R, Leon-Galindo J, Maldonado O et al: Cardiovascular disease in Colombia. In Hurst JW: Clinical Essays on the Heart, vol 5, pp 390-50. New York, McGraw-Hill, 1985
10. Spodick DH: Chronic and Constrictive Pericarditis. New York, Grune & Stratton, 1964
11. Spodick DH: The pericardial rub: A prospective, multiple observer investigation of pericardial friction in 100 patients. Am J Cardiol 35:357, 1975
12. Spodick DH: Diagnostic electrocardiographic sequences in acute pericarditis: Significance of PR segment and PR vector changes. Circulation 48:575, 1973
13. Bruce MA, Spodick DH: Atypical electrocardiogram in acute pericarditis: Characteristics and prevalence. J Electrocardiol 13:61, 1980
14. Spodick DH: Frequency of arrhythmias in acute pericarditis determined by Holter monitoring. Am J Cardiol 53:842-845, 1984
15. Spodick DH: Electrocardiographic changes in acute pericarditis. In Fowler NO (ed): The Pericardium in Health and Disease, pp 79-96. Mt. Kisco, NY, Futura, 1985
16. Spodick DH: Differential characteristics of the electrocardiogram in early repolarization and acute pericarditis. N Engl J Med 295:523, 1976
17. Krainin FM, Flessas AP, Spodick DH: Infarction-associated pericarditis: Rarity of diagnostic electrocardiogram. N Engl J Med 3111:1211, 1984
18. Engle MA, Gay WA Jr, Zabriskie JB, et al: The postpericardiotomy syndrome: 25 years experience. J Cardiovasc Med 9:321, 1984
19. Nasser WK: Congenital diseases of the pericardium. In Spodick DH (ed): Pericardial Diseases, pp 271-286. Philadelphia, FA Davis, 1976

GENERAL REFERENCES

Fowler NO: The Pericardium in Health and Disease. Mt. Kisco, NY, Futura, 1985
Reddy PS, Leon DF, Shaver JA (eds): Pericardial Disease. New York, Raven Press, 1982
Shabetai R: The Pericardium. New York, Grune & Stratton, 1981
Spodick DH (ed): Pericardial Diseases. Philadelphia, FA Davis, 1976

Noninfective Endocardial Disease

Edwin L. Alderman

NONINFECTIVE THROMBOTIC ENDOCARDITIS

Since the 1920s pathologists have observed in postmortem examinations valvular vegetations that did not show an inflammatory reaction consistent with bacterial endocarditis and were noted in clinical settings that were inconsistent with bacterial, rheumatic, or syphilitic infection. The patients typically were debilitated and cachectic, and commonly had chronic progressive diseases, prominently malignancy. Libman in 1923[1] substituted the term *noninfective thrombotic endocarditis* for a variety of earlier descriptors, including terminal endocarditis, marantic endocarditis, endocarditis simplex, and degenerative verrucal endocarditis. Although the original pathologic view was that these valvular lesions were a terminal event in patients with wasting diseases and were unassociated with clinical manifestations, there has been increasing awareness that systemic thromboembolism can occur as a result of this relatively silent form of endocarditis. In a series of postmortem examinations in patients with noninfective thrombotic endocarditis, MacDonald and Robbins[2] noted that 27% had evidence of arterial thromboses, half of which were in cerebral vessels. Fifty-four percent of these patients had either cancer or congestive heart failure. In addition to neurologic manifestations, emboli to the spleen, kidneys, coronary arteries, bowel, and lower extremities have, in this and other reports, led to clinical events resulting in recognition of an endocarditic process.[2,3] Pathologic series have pointed out that the aortic and mitral valves are involved in near-equal proportions with an additional 10% of occurrences involving right-sided valves. More recent reports have shown that right heart valvular noninfective endocarditic lesions may occur in association with chronically in-dwelling pulmonary artery pressure monitoring catheters. An autopsy study of 36 patients with chronic right heart catheters revealed aseptic valvular vegetations in 8% to 11% of patients, almost exclusively located on the pulmonic valve.[4] Postmortem examination of noncatheterized patients suggests a much lower prevalence of 0.4% of aseptic valvular vegetation, 90% of which involve left-sided valves.[2]

Clinical and pathologic observations suggest that a combination of minor valve surface abnormalities, mucin-producing malignancy, and coagulopathy with predisposition to sterile platelet and fibrin deposition together promote vegetation formation.

PATHOLOGY

Microscopically, the vegetations are composed of a fibrin matrix which, along with trapped platelets, is tightly adherent to an intact leaflet surface (Fig. 93.1). The valve itself typically shows degenerative changes, sometimes the result of prior rheumatic inflammation but often an age-related thickening with a ground-glass histologic appearance. The valve is generally free of leukocytes and lacks the active inflammation and direct extension of vegetation into valve tissue commonly seen with infective endocarditis. The adherence of platelets and development of a fibrin matrix on the surface of valve leaflets may in part reflect age-related changes in valve structure, residue of prior rheumatic or infective episodes, or deposition of immune complexes elicited by ongoing malignant processes.[5] Further development of platelet fibrin thrombus may continue as a sterile process or may form a nidus for retention of circulating bacteria as a stage in the development of bacterial endocarditis.

The association of noninfective thrombotic endocarditis (sometimes referred to as nonbacterial thrombotic endocarditis) with malignancy, with thrombophlebitis, and with disseminated intravascular coagulopathy has been noted with increasing frequency. In most pathologic series, neoplastic disorders (usually metastatic), commonly adenocarcinoma of the pancreas and lung, hematologic, and lymphoreticular neoplasms account for nearly half of reported cases.[6] Among chronic non-neoplastic disorders, cardiac and hepatic failure predominate.

CLINICAL FEATURES

Clinically, arterial embolization is the most prominent and usually initial manifestation of noninfective thrombotic endocarditis. Cerebral embolism was noted in one third and involvement of other organs in two thirds of the autopsy series reported by Biller and colleagues.[6] Twenty-one percent of patients had distinct coagulation abnormalities,

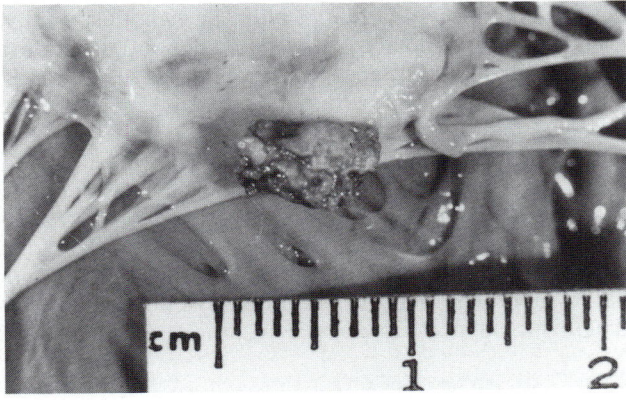

FIGURE 93.1 The mitral anterior leaflet in an 18-year-old who died of Hodgkin's disease exhibits a large vegetation adherent to the surface of this minimally fibrotic leaflet. (Courtesy Margaret Billingham, MD, Department of Pathology, Stanford University Medical Center)

with 10% having disseminated intravascular coagulopathy. Clinically, the occurrence of thrombophlebitis or cerebral or systemic emboli should raise a high level of suspicion of a silent noninfective endocarditic process. The hallmarks of disseminated intravascular coagulopathy include depressed circulating fibrinogen, thrombotic episodes, and elevated circulating fibrin split products.

Physical examination often reveals a soft systolic murmur, but rarely causes the changing murmurs or valvular incompetence that typically results from active bacterial endocarditis. Two-dimensional echocardiography has increased the sensitivity of detection of vegetations; however, it may not consistently detect valvular excrescences below 2 mm in diameter. Transesophageal echocardiography may be superior to transthoracic echocardiography for the detection of small atrioventricular valvular vegetations. Cardiac hemodynamic dysfunction is uncommon unless pre-existing myocardial or valvular disease is present. Coronary emboli may occur with resultant infarction although in elderly debilitated patients, coronary disease may be responsible. If coronary arteriography is performed weeks or months later, the offending coronary artery may be normal in appearance, despite clear ventriculographic evidence of prior infarction.

Recognition of noninfective endocardial disease is based primarily on arterial embolization, typically in the absence of fever, prominent or changing murmurs, and microembolic phenomena that are typically associated with infective endocarditis. Premortem recognition of the syndrome has been relatively uncommon. When cerebral embolic episodes occur, the decision to prescribe anticlotting therapy may be difficult. Prior experience in patients with bacterial endocarditis suggests an increased likelihood of hemorrhagic cerebral infarction when anticoagulants are given.[5] However, the experience of Rogers et al.[7] suggests that intravenous heparin is beneficial if cerebral angiography and tomographic imaging confirm the presence of multiple cerebral lesions without evidence of bacterial infection or atherosclerotic vascular etiology. Heparin therapy was not complicated by intracranial hemorrhage detectable by cerebral tomographic imaging, although autopsy evidence of hemorrhagic infarction was found in half the patients.

ENDOMYOCARDIAL FIBROSIS

Endomyocardial fibrosis is an indolent disease primarily confined to the rain forest belts of Africa, Asia, and South America in which progressive, severe endocardial scarring affects the inflow tract of right, left, or both ventricles, resulting in valvular regurgitation and severe congestive heart failure. The presence of eosinophilia, although common in patients living in the tropics, and the pathologic similarities with the end-stages of eosinophilic endomyocardial disease (Löffler's endocarditis) have suggested the possibility of a common pathophysiology secondary to eosinophilic tissue injury.

EPIDEMIOLOGY

Endomyocardial fibrosis was first reported by Bedford and Konstam[8] in 1946 in West African soldiers serving in the Middle East during World War II. Multiple subsequent reports by Davies (1954) and others have documented its occurrence, primarily in the tropical rain forest belts of Africa, Asia, and South America. Endomyocardial fibrosis is uncommon in the desert and savannah ecological zones of northern and southern Africa, but much more frequently found in the hot and humid coastal areas with tropical forest vegetation. There is some concentration of endomyocardial fibrosis in specific ethnic groups in Nigeria and Uganda, with a particular predominance in lower socioeconomic classes. There does not appear to be sufficient geographic overlap with malarial zones to suggest any etiologic association. Cases have been described in Brazil, Venezuela, and Columbia.[9] The occurrence of endomyocardial fibrosis in Europeans working in tropical zones has also been reported.

PATHOLOGY

The end-stages of endocardial fibrosis are characterized by marked fibrosis of the endocardium, often several millimeters in thickness, involving the right ventricle in 11%, the left ventricle in 38%, and both ventricles in 51% of patients.[10] Right ventricular endocardial fibrosis leads to progressive obliteration of the apex with shortening of the tricuspid cords and resultant tricuspid regurgitation. Left ventricular fibrosis leads to extensions of thick endocardium into the region beneath the mitral valve leaflets, into the apex, and into the outflow tract. Involvement of mitral valve leaflets, chordae tendineae, and papillary muscles is common. Thrombus formation with systemic embolization is not uncommon and, on occasion, an embolic event is the presenting manifestation of the disease.

Microscopically, thick and deep layers of loosely arranged collagen tissue, although primarily localized to the endocardium, may extend strands into the underlying myocardium. Although eosinophilia with resultant myocarditis and vasculitis has been implicated in the pathogenesis of endocardial fibrosis, the fibrotic endocardium which is the initial presentation of most tropical cases does not exhibit any tissue eosinophilia, and the arteries show only nonspecific intimal thickening. The wider use of endomyocardial biopsy techniques, coupled with greater availability of echographic diagnosis of the earlier stages of endocardial fibrosis, may permit a better understanding of the earlier stages and pathogenesis of this disease.

CLINICAL FEATURES

Endomyocardial fibrosis makes its appearance in tropical countries as an advanced restrictive cardiomyopathy, typically with manifestations of right heart failure predominating. Ascites, hepatomegaly, peripheral edema, and a chronic indolent course characterize endomyocardial fibrosis. Patients have variable degrees of left heart restriction and mitral regurgitation, which is manifested as exertional dyspnea, cough, and occasional hemoptysis. Generalized symptoms of fatigue, lassitude, and abdominal discomfort are prominent. Thromboembolism and onset of atrial fibrillation, with associated hemodynamic decompensation, may also be presenting manifestations. Table 93.1 summarizes the major clinical features of endocardial fibrosis as it presents in tropical countries, compared with temperate climates. In temperate climates, endomyocardial fibrosis generally is the late result of an active carditis associated with systemic manifestations, whereas in the tropics the initial presentation is in the late fibrotic restrictive cardiomyopathic stage.[11]

Physical examination reveals prominent hepatomegaly, ascites, peripheral edema, and pulmonary congestion. Systolic murmurs consistent with mitral or tricuspid regurgitation are often auscultated, along with a prominent gallop sound. A positive Kussmaul sign may be present. Restrictive hemodynamics result in a characteristic venous pressure pulse that is markedly elevated, with an early diastolic dip followed by a plateau with prominent a and v waves and deep x and y descents. Nonspecific electrocardiographic changes are observed, with atrial fibrillation occurring in later stages. Painless pericardial effusion is frequently present, resulting from right heart failure, and usually does not cause tamponade of the ventricular chambers. Cardiac size on chest radiographs typically is modestly enlarged; however, considerable variability is observed, dependent upon the amount of valvular regurgitation and endocardial restriction. Occasionally a left ventricular thrombus becomes calcified, producing a linear stripe on chest radiographs.

Echocardiography has been increasingly useful in identifying apical obliteration of one or both ventricles by a mass of endocardial fibrotic tissue.[12] The apical four-chamber echographic position is optimally suited for demonstration of apical obliteration. Restricted wall motion, particularly in areas of increased endomyocardial echo reflectance, and evidence of tricuspid or mitral valve thickening provide additional diagnostic support. In general, ventricular dimensions remain at the upper limits of normal, with left and right atrial size dependent upon the extent of atrioventricular (AV) valve regurgitation. Echocardiographic techniques are particularly helpful in identifying the earlier stages of endomyocardial fibrosis. Pericardial constriction exhibits similar restrictive hemodynamics to that of endomyocardial fibrosis; however, absence of pericardial thickening, prominence of endocardial reflectance, and AV valve involvement all suggest an endocardial disease process.

PATHOPHYSIOLOGY

Because the endocardial fibrosis found in temperate climates is pathologically indistinguishable from that observed in tropical regions, an etiologic common denominator has been sought.[11] The intense eosinophilia and carditis observed as a precursor of endocardial fibrosis in temperate climates has not ordinarily been detectable in tropical zones. In the tropics, patients with endomyocardial fibrosis commonly have eosinophilia, but not distinguishable from cohorts of control subjects living in the same areas, reflecting the fact that parasitic infections are common in these tropical regions. There is the possibility of abnormal immunologic responses to parasites in some subjects due to repeated and prolonged exposure during growth and development, possibly accentuated by individual, racial, economic, and nutritional factors. A subclinical early stage of endomyocardial fibrosis is currently being sought using echographic and endomyocardial biopsy techniques.

TREATMENT

Medical therapy comprises management of severe, unremitting, but indolent, right-sided failure. Vigorous diuresis and occasional drainage of symptomatic ascites is standard. In 1971, Charles Dubost[13] performed the first endocardiectomy, which consists of decorticating the fibrosed endocardium in a manner similar to resection of constricting densely fibrotic pericardium. The operation may include resection of the fibrotic endocardial layer in the right ventricle, left ventricle, or both, depending upon the predominant location of the restrictive process. The mitral or tricuspid valves may be subject to replacement or repair depending upon the extent of involvement of the papillary muscles and chordae. Metras and co-workers,[14] in a review of their experience with 55 patients, emphasize conservation of a thin rim of fibrosis near the conduction tissue with successful avoidance of complete heart block. The authors believed their results were enhanced by creation of a cleavage plane between fibrosis and myocardium, carrying out the dissection from apex toward annulus through a transatrial approach. They also favored mitral reconstruction over replacement in this younger group of patients. Although the operative mortality was 16%, the clinical and hemodynamic results were favorable, particularly for those with predominant left ventricular restriction.

In a report of 108 patients from Brazil followed for two years,[15] survival was influenced by the extent of biventricular involvement, New York Heart Association functional class, intensity of right ventricular fibrosis, and presence of tricuspid and mitral regurgitation. Fifty NYHA Class 3/4 patients treated surgically had a 68.5% 40-month survival, compared to 49.2% survival among medically treated patients. Tricuspid regurgitation was twice as common in patients selected for surgery as in medically treated patients. The extent to which recurrent fibrosis develops is not known; however, it has not yet emerged in a few long-term cases as a problem. In clinically advanced situations, a direct surgical approach to endomyocardial fibrosis may be the only therapy with substantial long-term benefit.

EOSINOPHILIC ENDOMYOCARDIAL DISEASE (LÖFFLER'S ENDOCARDITIS)

A rapid progressive endocardial disease occurring in temperate climates was described in 1936 by Löffler, who associated prominent eosinophilia, active carditis, and multiorgan involvement.[16] Pathologic specimens showed an eosinophilic myocarditis, a tendency toward endocardial thrombosis, and clinical manifestations of thromboembolism and acute heart failure. This combination may be referred to as an early necrotic stage of the disease (Table 93.2). Later fibrotic stages of the disease show marked endocardial scarring and thickening, pathologically identical to cases of chronic endocardial fibrosis observed in tropical climates. Examination of a large series of pathologic specimens of patients in temperate and tropical locations suggests that both endomyocardial fibrosis and eosinophilic endomyocardial disease may be part of a spectrum of heart disease in which eosinophilic damage plays an important pathophysiologic role.

PATHOLOGY

Löffler, in his original report of two patients with prominent eosinophilia, documented 3-mm endocardial thickening that was macroscopically visible.[16] Histologic examination showed layers of loosely arranged fibrous tissue comprising a thickened endocardium which, on its surface, had superimposed layers of fibrin. These findings are typical of the late fibrotic stage of the disease reported in 16 patients by Brockington and Olsen.[11] This stage, reached on average 24.5 months following symptom onset, is pathologically indistinguishable from en-

TABLE 93.1 COMPARISON OF ENDOMYOCARDIAL FIBROSIS (EMF) IN TEMPERATE AND TROPICAL REGIONS

Temperate Regions	Tropical Regions
EMF is late stage of earlier carditis	EMF is initial clinical presentation
Systemic manifestations and active carditis common	Early necrotic stage not recognized; presents as restrictive myopathy with ascites and periorbital edema
Marked eosinophilia common (hypereosinophilic syndrome, etc.)	Moderate variable eosinophilia (nonspecific parasitic infections)
Male predominance	Equal sex incidence
Ages 20–40	Ages 8–30
Usually biventricular with mitral regurgitation	Greater predominance of RV involvement
Embolic episodes common	Emboli rarely may be presenting symptom
Rapid progressive clinical course	Indolent clinical course

(Modified from Davies J, Spry CJF, Vijayaraghavan G et al: A comparison of the clinical and cardiological features of endomyocardial disease in temperate and tropical regions. Postgrad Med J 59:179, 1983)

domyocardial fibrosis. An acute necrotic stage, reached on average 5 weeks following onset of illness, is characterized by an intense eosinophilic myocarditis frequently limited to the inner layers of the myocardium (Fig. 93.2). During this stage of the disease, a periarteritis is identifiable with surrounding intense eosinophilic infiltrates. Degranulated eosinophils are found in both the endocardium and the myocardium, and may be freely circulating. An overlapping thrombotic stage (Table 93.2) is characterized by development of varying degrees of thrombosis within intramyocardial vessels as well as thrombus formations layering on the endocardial surface resulting in progressive thickening. This stage is reached on average ten months following onset of illness; often there are small thrombi and fibrinoid material layered on the endocardial surface, and there is associated vulnerability to embolization. The inflammatory stages of the disease merge gradually into later phases of fibrosis and fibrin deposition, with progressive endocardial thickening, involvement of the AV valves, apical obliteration, and restrictive hemodynamic alterations.

CLINICAL MANIFESTATIONS

Table 93.2 summarizes the initial clinical presentation of eosinophilic endomyocardial disease in relation to the pathologic stage of the disease. The intense eosinophilia associated with myocarditis may have multiple etiologies. In one retrospective series of 90 patients, the origin was idiopathic in 48%, reactive (periarteritis, asthma, parasitic infection, Hodgkin's disease, carcinoma, drug hypersensitivity) in 28%, and the result of eosinophilic leukemia in 24%.[17] In the past, the idiopathic hypereosinophilic syndrome was attributed to an eosinophilic leukemia; however, it has been recognized in follow-up that these patients have prolonged survivals with persisting high eosinophil counts in a range between 10,000 and 50,000/mm^3. The diagnosis of the idiopathic hypereosinophilic syndrome requires a peripheral blood eosinophilia of greater than 1.5×10^9/L of six months or longer duration; absence of allergic, parasitic, malignant or other known causes of secondary eosinophilia; and evidence of organ dysfunction. Neurologic and cutaneous manifestations are commonly encountered. Cardiac dysfunction occurred in 56% of one series of patients with idiopathic hypereosinophilia and was manifest as pump dysfunction atrioventricular valvular regurgitation and arterial emboli.[18]

Eosinophilic endomyocardial disease commonly presents as a systemic disorder during the acute necrotic or thrombotic phase.[19-21] The illness may be manifest as thromboembolic episodes affecting the brain, peripheral blood vessels, visceral organs, or eye. Systemic manifestations include fever, anorexia, pulmonary and gastroenterologic symptoms, possibly reflecting diffuse vasculitis. Some cases are detected primarily because of the prominent eosinophilia, and these patients are subsequently noted to have developed carditis or evidence of progressive cardiac restriction. In the later fibrotic stages of the disease, most patients present with established right- or left-sided heart failure with manifestations of exertional dyspnea, ascites, and peripheral edema. The intensity of the eosinophilic endomyocarditis typically leads to bilateral involvement. Mitral and/or tricuspid regurgitation are common features, along with hemodynamics of a restrictive cardiomyopathy. The clinical features of the late fibrotic stage of eosinophilic endomyocardial disease are very similar to those of endomyocardial fibrosis as listed in Table 93.1.

DIAGNOSIS

Myocardial biopsy during the early stage of the disease can be quite helpful in documenting acute necrosis, along with eosinophilic infiltrate. This procedure is of most value in patients who have prominent numbers of degranulated circulating eosinophils. The biventricular nature of the carditis permits right ventricular biopsy techniques to achieve a high yield of positive findings while minimizing the risk of thromboembolic complications from left-sided biopsy. In the later fibrotic stages of the disease, endomyocardial biopsy may become technically more difficult, yielding only collagen and fibrin material for examination.

Cardiac catheterization when carried out in the later fibrotic stages of the disease yields elevated right and left ventricular filling pressures of a dip-and-plateau configuration consistent with restrictive hemodynamics. Equilibration of diastolic pressures in both chambers may mimic pericardial constrictive disease. Variable degrees of tricuspid and mitral regurgitation may be present. Angiography typically shows well-retained systolic contractions in areas of unaffected ventricular wall (typically the outflow tract), whereas apical obliteration and immobility of the inflow area are consistent with both location and severity of the endocardial fibrosis.

TREATMENT

During the acute carditic phases of eosinophilic endomyocardial disease, steroids and immunosuppressive drugs have yielded impressive resolution of acute myocarditis and associated heart failure within sev-

TABLE 93.2 INITIAL CLINICAL PRESENTATION AND STAGES OF EOSINOPHILIC ENDOMYOCARDIAL DISEASE

Necrotic Stage (Early Stage)
Hypereosinophilia with systemic illness (20%–30%)
  Fever, sweating
  Lymphadenopathy, splenomegaly
Acute carditis (20%–50%)
  Anorexia, weight loss, cough, pulmonary infiltrates, skin and retinal lesions
  AV valve regurgitation
  Biventricular failure

Thrombotic Stage
Thrombotic emboli (10%–20%)
  Cerebral, splenic, renal, and coronary infarction
  Splinter hemorrhages

Fibrotic Stage (Late Stage)
Restrictive myopathy (10%)
  AV valvular regurgitation
  Right- and left-sided congestive heart failure

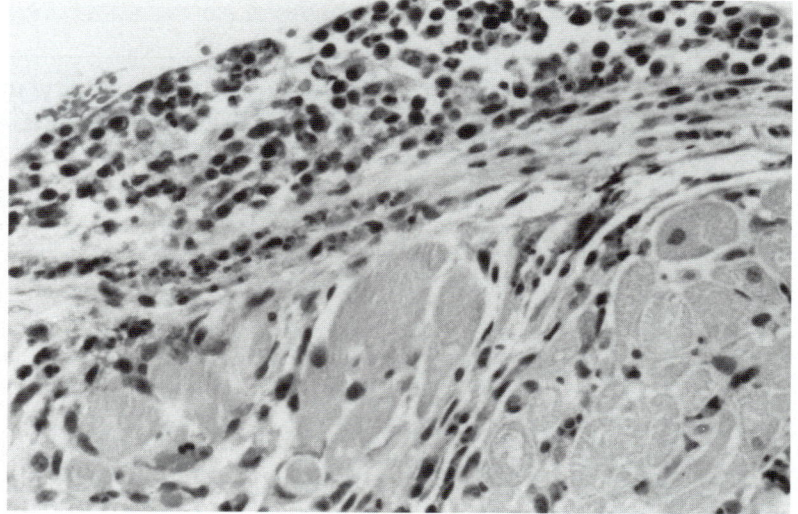

FIGURE 93.2 The endocardial surface of the left ventricle exhibits thickening and a prominent eosinophilic infiltrate in a patient who died of progressive ventricular failure (H & E stain; original magnification × 300). (Courtesy Margaret Billingham, MD, Department of Pathology, Stanford University Medical Center)

eral weeks of initiation of treatment. Disappearance of tissue eosinophils and substantial reductions in numbers of circulating eosinophils result from steroid therapy. Occasional patients develop mitral regurgitation of a severity which in and of itself dominates the clinical picture. Mitral valve replacement in this setting has led to substantial benefit in these selected patients. Endocardiectomy has been performed in those patients with advanced chronic endocardial fibrosis.[22] The procedure is assisted by the fact that in the earlier stages of the disease, fibrous septae may not have extended significantly into the adjacent myocardium, permitting a relatively clean plane of cleavage for surgical excision. Substantial clinical benefit has resulted from this procedure, although AV block has been a common complication.

PATHOPHYSIOLOGY

Substantial evidence has accumulated that documents the cardiotoxicity of eosinophils.[17] The intensity and timing of the active carditis is closely related to the severity of the circulating eosinophilia. It has been speculated that those patients, particularly in the tropics, who present with later fibrotic stages of endomyocardial disease may either have had transient earlier bouts of moderate eosinophilia with spontaneous resolution, or may have had only moderate levels of eosinophilia leading to a low-grade endomyocarditis with gradual progressive fibrosis.

There is substantial evidence that the basic proteins contained within the eosinophil granule can cause myocardial cell injury. This has been demonstrated in tissue cultures when incubated with extracts of eosinophil basic proteins or when incubated with intact blood eosinophils.[23] Metabolic studies of eosinophils suggest that the basic proteins contained within the granules have a dose-dependent cytotoxic effect with inhibition of multiple enzyme systems.[24] The development of monoclonal antibodies specific for the secreted forms of eosinophilic protein permits staining of myocardial and vascular tissue in order to localize these proteins and relate their presence to the various stages of the disease. These secreted eosinophil granule proteins are readily identified in the subendocardial and vascular tissues and in the endocardial thrombus during the acute necrotic and thrombotic stages, but much less evident in the myocardium and in the later fibrotic stage of disease.[25] However, the precise mechanism for selectivity of the endomyocardium is not understood. Similarly, it is unclear why tropical endomyocardial disease occurs only in sporadic selected individuals with moderate eosinophilia. The presence of circulating degranulated blood eosinophils in large numbers or elevated blood levels of the basic proteins normally found in eosinophil granules, and the presence of eosinophils within myocardial tissue, are relatively reliable correlates of active acute necrotic cardiac disease.[26] In individual cases, the intensity of eosinophilic infiltrates and the presence of degranulation have correlated with the extent of active carditis and disease progression and with subsequent regression of disease.

REFERENCES

1. Libman E: Characterization of various forms of endocarditis. JAMA 80:813, 1923
2. MacDonald RA, Robbins SL: The significance of non-bacterial thrombotic endocarditis: An autopsy and clinical study of 78 cases. Ann Intern Med 46:255, 1957
3. Chino F, Kodama A, Otake M: Non-bacterial thrombotic endocarditis in a Japanese autopsy sample. Am Heart J 90:190, 1975
4. Lange HW, Galliani CA, Edwards JE: Local complications associated with indwelling Swan-Ganz catheters: Autopsy study of 36 cases. Am J Cardiol 52:1108, 1983
5. Schwartzman RJ, Hill JB: Neurologic complications of disseminated intravascular coagulation. Neurology 32:791, 1982
6. Biller J, Challa VR, Toole JF et al: Non-bacterial thrombotic endocarditis. A neurologic perspective of clinical pathologic correlations of 99 patients. Arch Neurol 39:95, 1982
7. Rogers LR, Cho ES, Kempin S et al. Cerebral infarction from nonbacterial thrombotic endocarditis. Clinical and pathological study including the effects of anticoagulation. Am J Med 83:746, 1987
8. Bedford DE, Konstam GLS: Heart failure of unknown aetiology in Africans. Br Heart J 8:236, 1946
9. Hutt SR: Epidemiology aspects of endomyocardial fibrosis. Postgrad Med J 59:142, 1983
10. Shaper AG, Hutt MSR, Coles RM: Necropsy studies of endomyocardial fibrosis and rheumatic heart disease in Uganda. Br Heart J 30:391, 1968
11. Brockington IF, Olsen EGJ: Löffler's endocarditis and Davies' endomyocardial fibrosis. Am Heart J 85:308, 1973
12. Acquatella H, Schiller NB, Puigbo JJ et al: Value of two-dimensional echocardiography in endomyocardial disease with or without eosinophilia. A clinical and pathologic study. Circulation 67:1219, 1983
13. Dubost C, Maurice P, Gerbaux A et al: The surgical treatment of constrictive fibrous endocarditis. Ann Surg 184:303, 1976
14. Metras D, Coulibaly A, Ouattara K: The surgical treatment of endomyocardial fibrosis: Results in 55 patients. Circulation 72 (suppl II):274, 1985
15. Barretto ACP, Lux PL, Oliveira S et al: Determinants of survival in endomyocardial fibrosis. Circulation 80(Suppl I):I-177, 1989
16. Löffler W: Endocarditis parietalis fibroplastica mit Blueteosinophilie. Ein eigenartiges Krankheitsbild. Schweiz Med Wochenschr 18:817, 1936
17. Olsen EGJ, Spry CJF: Relation between eosinophilia and endomyocardial disease. Prog Cardiovasc Dis 27:241, 1985
18. Fauci AS, Harley JB, Roberts WC et al: The idiopathic hypereosinophilic syndrome: Clinical, pathophysiologic and therapeutic considerations. Ann Intern Med 97:78, 1982
19. Davies J, Spry CJF, Sapsford R et al: Cardiovascular features of eleven patients with eosinophilic endomyocardial disease. Quart J Med 52:23, 1983
20. Parillo JE, Borer JS, Henry WC et al: The cardiovascular manifestations of the hypereosinophilic syndrome. Prospective study of 26 patients, with review of the literature. Am J Med 67:572, 1979
21. Spry CJF, Davies J, Tai P-C et al: Clinical features of fifteen patients with the hypereosinophilic syndrome. Quart J Med 52:1, 1983
22. Davies J, Sapsford R, Brooksby I et al: Successful surgical treatment of two patients with eosinophilic endomyocardial disease. Br Heart J 46:438, 1981
23. Spry CJF, Poh-Chun T, Davies J: The cardiotoxicity of eosinophils. Postgrad Med J 59:147, 1983
24. Gleich GJ, Frigas E, Loegering DA et al: Cytotoxic properties of eosinophil major basic protein. J Immunol 123:2925, 1979
25. Tai PC, Spry CJF, Olsen EGJ et al: Deposits of eosinophilic granule proteins in cardiac tissues of patients with eosinophilic endomyocardial disease. Lancet 1:643, 1987
26. Wassom DL, Loegering DA, Solley GO et al: Elevated levels of the eosinophil granule major basic protein in patients with eosinophilia. J Clin Invest 67:651, 1981

PULMONARY HEART DISEASE INCLUDING PULMONARY EMBOLISM

John A. Paraskos

Pulmonary heart disease (cor pulmonale) may be defined as an alteration in the function or structure of the right ventricle that is caused by an alteration in the structure or function of the lungs or their vasculature. This definition specifically excludes right ventricular dysfunction caused by elevation in left atrial pressure or by large left-to-right shunts.[1] The hemodynamic abnormality common to all forms of pulmonary heart disease is an elevation in the impedance to right ventricular emptying caused by a wide variety of respiratory, pulmonary parenchymal, or pulmonary vascular problems.

If a sufficient rise in pulmonary arterial impedance occurs suddenly in a previously normal subject, the right ventricle fails abruptly and is unable to sustain more than a modestly elevated pulmonary artery pressure. This is the clinical presentation of most cases of massive pulmonary embolism and may also be seen with any acute overwhelming respiratory disease.

If the elevation in pulmonary arterial impedance rises sufficiently slowly so that the right ventricle can accommodate and hypertrophy, the pulmonary artery pressure will be significantly elevated. Pulmonary hypertension is common to all forms of chronic pulmonary heart disease and its severity reflects the extent of increased pulmonary arterial impedance. Indeed, it is useful to consider this form of heart disease as hypertensive disease of the right side of the circulation. This description remains valid despite evidence that in pulmonary heart disease the left ventricle is affected to some extent by a generalized disorder of the myocardium.[2,3] Just as an understanding of the dynamics of systemic pressure, resistance, and cardiac output is essential to any discussion of hypertensive left ventricular disease, so is knowledge of pulmonary vascular hemodynamics central to an understanding of pulmonary heart disease.

The incidence of chronic pulmonary heart disease has been variably estimated at 7% to 10% of all heart disease in the United States. Of the 30,000 people who die of chronic obstructive lung disease in the United States annually, most have had significant right ventricular dysfunction. In some locales where air pollution is high, cigarette smoking prominent, or occupational exposure common, as in industrial areas of the United Kingdom or mining areas of Appalachia, pulmonary heart disease may account for as much as 25% of all heart disease. The incidence of acute pulmonary heart disease is more difficult to estimate. However, one of the most common causes of acute pulmonary heart disease is pulmonary thromboembolism. Pulmonary embolism is recognized to be one of the commonest lung disorders in general hospitals; it has been estimated that as many as 15% of all hospital admissions may be complicated by pulmonary embolism, with a total incidence of 630,000 cases annually in the United States. The annual mortality in the United States may exceed 200,000. In 67,000 cases, the event presents as sudden cardiac death with survival of less than 1 hour.[4] Of the patients who survive longer than 1 hour, most of those who succumb do so without the correct diagnosis or appropriate therapy.

PATHOPHYSIOLOGY

The basic pathophysiologic mechanisms that provoke right ventricular alterations in pulmonary heart disease are quite similar to those that provoke left ventricular alterations in systemic hypertension. The most important mechanism is the increased impedance to right ventricular emptying. The increase in impedance causes an elevated afterload or increase in "pressure work." The simplest and most available measure of this pressure work is the systolic pulmonary artery pressure. Another mechanism often operative in patients with pulmonary disease is an increase in cardiac output provoked by hypoxemia. This increase may lead to a significant volume overload affecting both ventricles.

These two mechanisms, if operative over a long enough period, are expected to lead to compensatory hypertrophy of the right ventricle (and, to a smaller extent, of the left ventricle). While initially this hypertrophy is beneficial in sustaining the circulation, eventually increased ventricular stiffness, myocardial ischemia, and muscle failure develop. Additional complicating factors such as hypoxemia, acidosis, fluid and sodium retention, and other electrolyte abnormalities may affect ventricular contractility, compliance, and "preload."

Ultrastructural and biochemical abnormalities develop along with the hypertrophy and dilatation of the ventricles. Depletion of catecholamines and high-energy phosphates is common to all forms of dilated cardiomyopathy. Experimentally, these abnormalities have been observed in both ventricles of animals with "right" ventricular failure provoked by binding the pulmonary artery.[5]

PULMONARY HEMODYNAMICS

The pressure within the pulmonary artery (P_{PA}) varies directly with the pressure within the pulmonary veins (P_{PV}), and the cardiac output ($\dot{Q}$), as well as with the forces opposing flow across the pulmonary vascular bed (*i.e.*, the pulmonary vascular resistance, PVR). The mean pulmonary artery pressure is related to these other variables according to the formula

$$P_{PA} = \dot{Q} \times PVR + P_{PV}$$

The normal mean pressure in the pulmonary artery at rest is rarely greater than 15 mm Hg. Mean pressures greater than 20 mm Hg are considered high. The systolic pressure is normally 30 mm Hg or less. The normal pulmonary artery diastolic pressure is 10 mm Hg or less (barely higher than the pulmonary venous or left atrial pressures). An elevation of the P_{PA} into the abnormal range may be caused by a rise in $\dot{Q}$, PVR, or P_{PV}.

The normal pulmonary vasculature is a highly distensible low-resistance vascular bed. Normally, large increases in cardiac output occur during exercise with minimal increases in pulmonary arterial pressure. As the pulmonary blood flow rises, the pulmonary resistance drops because the effective radius of the pulmonary vasculature is augmented by distention of patent vessels and by opening or recruitment of closed microvessels.

Another factor which influences the pulmonary vascular resistance is the minimum pressure necessary to keep a significant number of vascular pathways open. This "critical opening pressure" must also be considered in calculating the forces that oppose pulmonary blood flow. In the normal lung, this critical opening pressure is low. In pathologic states, however, it may be significantly increased and affect the calculation of pulmonary vascular resistance.[6]

Vasomotion with active dilatation or constriction of muscular arterial walls also affects the pressure-flow relationship. β-Adrenergic drive during exercise lowers the vascular resistance by causing pulmonary vascular dilatation. In the normal individual, the P_{PA} does not rise significantly until the pulmonary blood flow ($\dot{Q}$) exceeds 2.5 times that of the basal state.

Poiseuille's law states that the pressure (P) within a rigid tube is inversely related to the internal radius (r) and is directly related to the rate of flow ($\dot{Q}$), the length of the tube (L), and the viscosity of the fluid (μ):

$$\Delta P = \frac{8 \cdot \mu \cdot L \cdot \dot{Q}}{\pi r^4}$$

Changes in vessel length are obviously rarely a factor. Clinically, however, the pulmonary blood flow, the internal cross-sectional radius of the vessels, and blood viscosity all contribute to the pressure within the vessel. Note that the most potent variable is the vessel radius.

Another factor that obviously affects pulmonary arterial pressure is the intrathoracic pressure. This is often neglected but is especially important when measuring intrathoracic vascular pressures in a patient who is being mechanically ventilated, especially with continuous positive-pressure ventilation. Also, in patients with chronic obstructive lung disease, the elevated intrathoracic pressures undoubtedly contribute to the level of pulmonary hypertension. Table 94.1 lists the pathophysiologic mechanisms that lead to pulmonary hypertension and gives a partial list of clinical states in which the mechanisms are operative.

At this point we will discuss each of the major mechanisms and each mechanism's potential impact in various diseases.

PULMONARY BLOOD FLOW

The "hyperkinetic" pulmonary hypertension of large left-to-right shunts is caused largely by the torrential pulmonary blood flow. In contrast, the increases in pulmonary blood flow imposed by hypoxemia are relatively small. Nevertheless, in many disease states the compliance of the pulmonary vasculature is markedly lowered so that even modest increases in cardiac output can be expected to elevate the pulmonary artery pressure significantly. Associated conditions such as anemia, fever, stress, and exercise will further augment the cardiac output and the pulmonary hypertension.

Direct communication between systemic arteries and pulmonary arteries will cause intrapulmonary left-to-right shunts. In severe bronchiectasis, enlarged bronchial and intercostal arteries may directly connect with branches of the pulmonary arteries and veins, bringing about a considerable increase in pulmonary blood flow and thereby contributing to pulmonary hypertension.[7]

VISCOSITY

Chronic respiratory diseases that result in poor tissue oxygenation cause an increase in erythropoietin secretion and an expansion of the red cell mass. The hematocrit will rise substantially, but if there is a concomitant increase in plasma volume this rise will be blunted. The rise in red cell mass initially helps local oxygen delivery to the tissues. However, as the hematocrit exceeds 55%, a rise in blood viscosity occurs, which can contribute to pulmonary hypertension. The detrimental effect of increasing viscosity on the cardiac output and systemic oxygen transport may actually negate any improvement in local tissue oxygen delivery once the hematocrit exceeds 60%. Regional blood flow may be affected, especially in the cerebral circulation, so that muscle fatigue, headaches, and confusion are common.

RADIUS OF PULMONARY ARTERIAL BED

Decreases in the total cross-sectional radius of the pulmonary arterial bed cause an exponential rise in the pulmonary artery pressure. This diminution in overall radius may be brought about in three ways: obliteration or loss of functional pulmonary vessels, diffuse anatomical narrowing of pulmonary vessels, or pulmonary vasoconstriction.

Loss of pulmonary vessels must exceed 60% of the total pulmonary vasculature before the resting pulmonary artery pressure will rise. Excision of a lung or an equivalent degree of embolic occlusion is, therefore, unlikely to provoke pulmonary hypertension unless other pathogenetic factors coexist. In the otherwise normal individual, the vascular resistance of the remaining lung can drop to accommodate the increased blood flow and maintain the cardiac output. Obviously, the patient's capacity to further augment cardiac output without significant rises in pulmonary artery pressure will be curtailed. Recurrent pulmonary thromboembolism can lead to chronic pulmonary hypertension if there is inadequate time for clot lysis or recanalization. Tumor and parasites may also cause recurrent embolism, while fat, bone marrow, air, gas, and amniotic fluid embolisms are more likely to be acute and self-limited. Schistosomiasis and filariasis are known to cause pulmonary hypertension. The filariae of *Wuchereria bancrofti* are thought to be sequestered in the pulmonary vasculature at night. The eggs of *Schistosoma mansoni* and *Schistosoma haematobium* embolize the pulmonary circulation and cause a granulomatous arteriolitis. These egg microemboli from the portal circulation are made possible by portal-systemic venous collaterals in the diseased liver.

Pulmonary fibrosis from sarcoidosis, scleroderma, the Hamman-Rich syndrome, and from drugs such as bleomycin and amiodarone may also cause pulmonary hypertension. In scleroderma, pulmonary hypertension is particularly associated with the CREST syndrome (calcinosis cutis, Raynaud's phenomenon, esophageal disease, sclerodactyly, and telangiectases). While obliteration of pulmonary vessels occurs with a wide variety of diseases producing fibrosis, inflammation, infiltration, and so forth, emphysema is by far the most common chronic pulmonary process that results in such vascular loss.

Compressive diseases of the thorax such as kyphoscoliosis, severe pectus excavatum, and pleural scarring may cause severe pulmonary hypertension with less than 50% apparent vascular loss. It is likely in

TABLE 94.1 MECHANISMS AND CAUSES OF PULMONARY HYPERTENSION

Mechanisms	Clinical Causes
Increased pulmonary blood flow	Left-to-right shunts Increased cardiac output Bronchiectasis
Increased blood viscosity	Polycythemia
Decreased radius of pulmonary arterial bed	
Loss of vessels	Pneumonectomy Embolism
Luminal narrowing	
Anatomical	Emphysema Embolism Chronic hypoxia Thoracic deformity Vasculitis Neoplasm Fibrosis Inflammation Infiltration
Vasoconstrictive	Hypoxia Acidosis Toxins Primary pulmonary hypertension
Increased pulmonary venous pressure	Left atrial hypertension Venous thrombosis Mediastinitis Veno-occlusive disease
Increased intrathoracic pressure	Chronic obstructive pulmonary disease

these situations that the compliance of the apparently spared vessels is also significantly affected. An alternative suggestion is that a humoral vasoconstrictive agent is produced by the compressed lung in a manner analogous to that of a compressed kidney.[8]

In many circumstances, loss of patent vessels and luminal narrowing may be reversible, for example, by lysis or fragmentation of emboli, by resolution of inflammation, and by reversal of infiltration. It should also be remembered that transient increases in the intra-alveolar or interstitial pressure may cause a reversible collapse of portions of the pulmonary capillary bed.

Diffuse and widespread *anatomical or structural narrowing* of vessels is usually caused by intimal proliferation, arterial smooth muscle hypertrophy (as in chronic hypoxia), eccentric intimal fibrosis and web formation (thromboemboli), and plexiform lesions (primary pulmonary hypertension). Such diffuse vascular obliteration is largely irreversible. These intimal and medial arterial changes are the basis for the Heath and Edwards histologic grading of pulmonary hypertension.[9] In infants with pulmonary hypertension associated with congenital shunts, there may be an absolute reduction in the number of peripheral pulmonary arteries. This reduction in vessels is likely to be caused by inadequate growth of the vascular bed rather than by obliterative changes alone.[10]

Pulmonary vasoconstriction results in a potentially reversible narrowing of the vascular lumen. Clinically, the most important stimulus to vasoconstriction is alveolar hypoxia. Although the mechanism is not clear, it is hypothesized that the synthesis or release of a vasodilator peptide, such as prostaglandin, may be dependent on the alveolar P_{O_2}.[11] When the P_{O_2} drops below 60 mm Hg, pulmonary artery pressure rises significantly with considerable variability among individuals and among species. Those individuals with greater sensitivity to lowered alveolar P_{O_2} are most likely to develop high-altitude pulmonary hypertension and pulmonary edema. Yaks and cameloid species, such as llamas, alpacas, and vicuñas, are highly resistant to high-altitude sickness, whereas cows quickly develop pulmonary hypertension, right ventricular failure, and dependent edema (*i.e.,* "brisket disease"). Indeed, cows may be bred to have greater or lesser proclivity to hypoxic pulmonary edema.

At usual altitudes, hypoventilation is the commonest mechanism producing alveolar hypoxia. *General hypoventilation* exists if all alveoli are inadequately ventilated in a diffuse pattern. Such hypoventilation occurs in patients with decreased central ventilatory drive (Ondine's curse), upper airway obstruction (sleep apnea, morbid obesity, epiglottitis, foreign body obstruction), and mechanical restriction to ventilation (morbid obesity, muscular dystrophies, pleural scarring, kyphoscoliosis, ankylosing spondylitis). Early in the course of these diseases, hypercapnia may coexist with arterial hypoxemia.

Most respiratory diseases lead to spotty rather than general hypoventilation. In these situations, the areas with alveolar hypoxia are large enough to produce an overall *"net" hypoventilation,* even when total ventilation is excessive. In these cases, at the outset, the arterial hypoxemia is associated with a normal or even depressed P_{CO_2}. Chronic obstructive pulmonary disease (COPD) is the commonest cause of net hypoventilation. Among patients with COPD, those with chronic bronchitis and severe bronchospasm have the greatest inequality in ventilation and perfusion. The maldistribution of inspired air contributes to the net hypoventilation, with more severe hypoxemia and earlier development of pulmonary hypertension.

Genetic predisposition to lung disease and to pulmonary hypertension may be caused by variable sensitivity to alveolar hypoxia, as has been suggested in the animal models of high-altitude disease. This has not been proven, however. Among genetic disorders causing severe lung disease is cystic fibrosis, which results in severe lung disease as a result of abnormal exocrine gland secretions within the airways.[12] Deficiency in α_1-protease inhibitor has been associated with the premature development of emphysema and appears to be determined by autosomal codominant alleles at a single locus. Other genetic diseases of connective tissue (Marfan's, generalized elastosis, Ehlers-Danlos syndrome) and several inherited immunologic abnormalities have also been associated with high familial aggregations of chronic obstructive pulmonary disease.[13] Since only 10% of heavy smokers develop severe chronic lung disease, it has been hypothesized that other genetic determinants of bronchitis and emphysema are involved in a complex multifactorial pattern of inheritance.[14] Clear evidence for this is still lacking, however.[13]

Acidosis (whether respiratory or metabolic) potentiates the vasoconstrictive effect of hypoxia. It is likely that the associated intracellular hypokalemia lowers the threshold for vascular smooth muscle contraction. In most clinical situations, the reversal of hypoxia and acidosis is the most valuable tool for lowering pulmonary artery pressure.

Rarely, specific vasoactive toxins may be implicated in the production of pulmonary vascular constriction. From 1966 to 1968 in Austria, Germany, and Switzerland, there was a rapidly progressive form of pulmonary hypertension associated with the use of aminorex fumarate, an anorectic agent.[15] The drug has not caused pulmonary hypertension in experimental animals, however. Pulmonary hypertension has also been linked with fenfluramine, an anorectic agent that is still available.[16] The toxic oil syndrome is a multisystem disorder that first appeared in 1981 as an epidemic in central and northeastern Spain. It is a non-necrotizing, nongranulomatous, obliterative vasculitis involving vessels of every size and type. It often presents with noncardiac pulmonary edema and acute respiratory distress syndrome. A significant number of patients develop mild to moderate pulmonary hypertension of a benign course.[17] This disease has been associated with the consumption of an as yet unidentified toxin in denatured rapeseed oil. In rats, the ingestion of pyrrolizidine alkaloids causes pulmonary hypertension.[18] These substances are found in the plants *Senecio jacobaea* and *Crotalaria spectabilis*. Leguminous plants of these and related species are not infrequently used in third world countries for making "bush tea." While these toxins are thought to cause hepatic veno-occlusive disease in humans, only rarely have they been implicated in producing pulmonary hypertension.[19]

Prostaglandin $F_{2\alpha}$ and angiotensin II are the most potent pulmonary vasoactive peptides. Their role in the production of human disease, however, has not been demonstrated.

PULMONARY VENOUS PRESSURE

Elevations in left atrial pressure are the most frequent cause of pulmonary hypertension and right ventricular failure. In accordance with our definition, these cases do not represent instances of pulmonary heart disease.

Widespread veno-occlusive disease is expected in most generalized obliterative processes of the pulmonary vasculature. Much less commonly, abnormalities may develop primarily in the pulmonary veins themselves. *In situ* thrombosis (as in sickle cell anemia) or sclerosing mediastinitis (as with the use of methesergide) may cause pulmonary hypertension. A veno-occlusive disorder of unknown etiology occurs with a predeliction for young women.[20]

PRIMARY PULMONARY HYPERTENSION

A patient who develops pulmonary hypertension without evidence for heart, lung, or respiratory disease as a contributory cause is said to have "primary" pulmonary hypertension.[21] The term *primary pulmonary hypertension* simply reflects the temporary discontinuance of the search for an etiology. It is of interest, however, that an idiopathic form of the disease has been described with an autosomal dominant transmission.[22] In both familial and nonfamilial forms, it seems to have a predeliction for young women.[23,24]

In one kindred of primary pulmonary hypertension, a plasmin inhibitor has been found that should cause a decreased ability to lyse pulmonary emboli. It has been suggested that such a kindred would be at risk of developing an apparently idiopathic form of pulmonary hypertension from recurrent subclinical microemboli.[25] It has further been suggested that most patients with primary pulmonary hypertension have chronic unresolved microemboli.[26] Unfortunately, amelioration of this disease with chronic warfarin anticoagulation has not been described.

DIAGNOSIS OF PULMONARY HEART DISEASE

If the patient with evidence for pulmonary hypertension has no obvious predisposing cause, a diligent search should be conducted for occult heart or lung disease.

Very commonly it is the careful history and physical examination that direct the clinician to a diagnosis of underlying heart or lung disease. A history of chronic cough with sputum production, along with a description of the character of the sputum, may lead to the diagnosis of COPD or bronchiectasis. A history of sleep disturbance or narcolepsy may lead to a diagnosis of sleep apnea. The electrocardiogram, chest roentgenogram, echocardiogram, pulmonary function tests, and arterial blood gases, all may be critical in discovering an underlying cause. If the noninvasive work-up suggests pulmonary hypertension but fails to uncover an underlying cause, cardiac catheterization should be performed. The severity of the pulmonary hypertension usually should be documented by cardiac catheterization, and often it is advisable to test the reactivity of the pulmonary vascular resistance to drugs and oxygen.

HISTORY AND PHYSICAL EXAMINATION

Patients with secondary pulmonary hypertension generally present with clinical features reflecting the underlying heart or lung disease. To make a firm diagnosis of pulmonary heart disease it is necessary to exclude a cardiac shunt and left atrial hypertension as causative factors.

The symptoms of pulmonary hypertension reflect the inability to increase cardiac output during stress or exercise. Dyspnea on exertion, easy fatigability, chest pains, and syncope on exertion are common. Less common symptoms include cough, hemoptysis, and hoarseness caused by compression of the left recurrent laryngeal nerve by a dilated main pulmonary artery.

Except in acute pulmonary obstruction, any of the physical findings of pulmonary hypertension are apt to be found. The second heart sound may become narrowly split, with an increased intensity of the pulmonic component. A pulmonic ejection click and ejection murmur may develop. A high-pitched diastolic murmur of pulmonic regurgitation suggests severe pulmonary hypertension.

Physical findings specific for right ventricular involvement will develop as the pulmonary hypertension causes significant right ventricular dysfunction. As the right ventricle becomes hypertrophied and less compliant, the end-diastolic pressure rises and is reflected in a prominent presystolic jugular venous wave (a wave). A left parasternal or subxiphoid thrust may be noted and a fourth heart sound may be heard at the lower sternal edge. Unlike the more common fourth heart sound of left ventricular origin, this right-sided sound is expected to increase in intensity during inspiration. When the right ventricle fails and dilates, its filling pressure rises so that systemic venous hypertension develops. A right ventricular third heart sound and a tricuspid regurgitation murmur may be heard. Some of the findings of elevated venous pressure are common to both acute and chronic pulmonary heart disease. Distended neck veins are present. Complaints of right upper quadrant tenderness may be accompanied by a smooth, tender, liver edge and an increased span of liver dullness. Pedal edema and eventually ascites may develop.

In patients with severe emphysema and COPD, the physical findings of right ventricular disease are often obscured. The increased anteroposterior thoracic diameter is likely to make palpation and auscultation of right-sided findings difficult or impossible. Frequently in patients with severe emphysema and COPD, the right ventricular lift is better felt over the epigastrium, and on inspiration the right ventricular lift can often be felt in the left infracostal region. In this condition, the heart sounds, including right-sided S_3 and S_4, may be best heard to the left of the epigastrium. In severe emphysema, the overinflated lungs will diminish the span of hepatic dullness, while the flattened diaphragms may make even a normal-sized liver palpable below the right costal margin.

CHEST ROENTGENOGRAM

The chest roentgenogram must be carefully examined for abnormalities of the thoracic skeleton, pleura, and lung parenchyma, as well as the heart and pulmonary vasculature. Enlargement of central pulmonary arteries with "pruning" and attenuation of peripheral vessels is characteristic of pulmonary hypertension (Fig. 94.1).

Left heart chamber enlargement or valve calcification may point to a nonpulmonary source of right ventricular dysfunction.

Evidence for right ventricular and right atrial dilatation may also help establish the diagnosis of right-sided dysfunction. However, the overinflated lungs of COPD often obscure considerable cardiomegaly.

ELECTROCARDIOGRAM

Electrocardiographic evidence of right ventricular or of right atrial involvement may be the first clue of underlying pulmonary heart disease. Unfortunately, considerable right-sided dysfunction may exist without notable electrocardiographic findings.

The acute right ventricular strain of severe pulmonary embolism may be disclosed by the "McGinn-White" pattern of an S wave in lead I with a Q wave and inverted T wave in lead III. Less commonly the Q's and inverted T's may also be seen in lead II or aV_F, simulating a remote

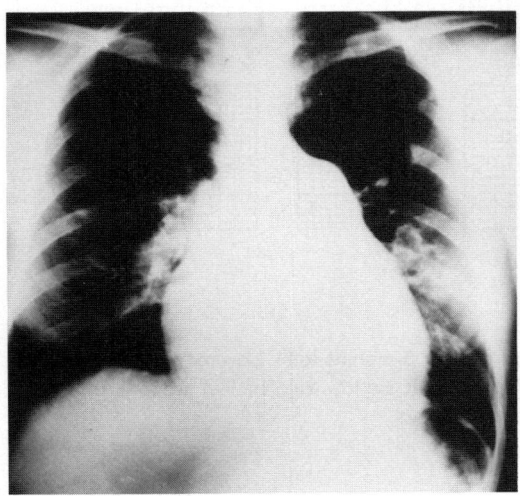
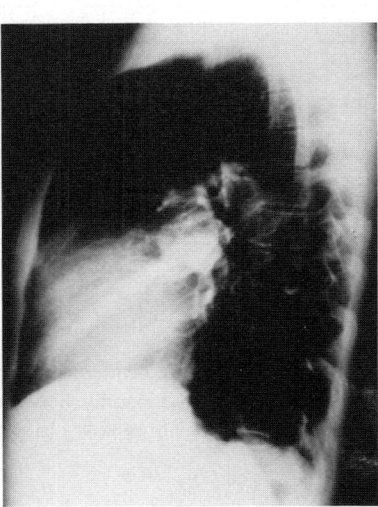

FIGURE 94.1 Chest roentgenograms (left, posteroanterior; right, lateral) of a patient with primary pulmonary hypertension. Note the enlarged central pulmonary arteries with attenuation of peripheral vessels. The lateral film demonstrates a markedly dilated right ventricle with filling of the retrosternal space.

inferior myocardial infarction. This pattern is not specific for acute right ventricular strain and is sometimes seen in more chronic forms of right ventricular dysfunction (Fig. 94.2).

In chronic right ventricular pressure overload, evidence for increased anterior and rightward QRS forces may develop with right axis deviation ($\geq 110°$) and R/S ratio ≥ 1 in lead V_1. Incomplete or complete right bundle branch patterns may also occur as manifestations of right ventricular hypertrophy or dilatation.

ECHOCARDIOGRAPHY

Echocardiographic findings in pulmonary hypertension include hypertrophy of the right ventricle (which may be misinterpreted as "asymmetric septal hypertrophy" as the right ventricular aspect of the intraventricular septum hypertrophies out of proportion to the posterior wall of the left ventricle). Dilatation of the right ventricle and atrium is usually observed; volume overload of the right ventricle may be identified by paradoxical septal motion. The diastolic (E to F) slope of the anterior mitral leaflet is usually diminished due to slow left atrial filling. Pulmonic valve motion may show characteristic abnormalities as well.[27] While the pulmonic valve changes are reasonably specific, they are insensitive.[28] Echocardiography would likely be more helpful in the assessment of pulmonary heart disease if the overinflated lungs of emphysema did not so often cause inadequate or suboptimal resolution. In such patients the most useful clinical information derived from echocardiographic analysis may be the exclusion of significant left-sided causes of pulmonary hypertension, such as severe left ventricular failure, occult mitral valve disease, or left atrial myxoma. Less commonly, evidence for a previously unsuspected intracardiac shunt will be uncovered by echocardiogram.

Doppler analysis has also proven useful in assessing the severity of concurrent mitral stenosis or regurgitation and in documenting the frequently associated pulmonic or tricuspid regurgitation. The Doppler technique may also allow approximate estimation of the pulmonary artery pressure by a variety of methods. The time to peak velocity of flow within the right ventricular outflow tract has been correlated with the mean pulmonary artery pressure[29] and the time to peak velocity in the main pulmonary artery has been correlated with the systolic pulmonary artery pressure.[30] The right ventricular and pulmonary artery systolic pressures may also be estimated by measuring the systolic gradient across an insufficient tricuspid valve.[31]

Additional information documenting the severity of right ventricular failure can be derived from radionuclide scans. Such scans are particularly useful for patients in whom adequate echocardiographic studies cannot be obtained; left ventricular volumes and function are often found to be normal and right ventricular volumes usually increased with evidence for poor right ventricular function.

CARDIAC CATHETERIZATION

Right-sided cardiac catheterization allows the measurement of cardiac output along with the pulmonary capillary wedge pressure, pulmonary arterial pressure, right ventricular pressure, and right atrial pressure. If the pressures seem lower than expected from the clinical presentation and noninvasive work-up, measurements should be repeated with exercise. If it is possible that such a patient is volume depleted, the pressures and cardiac output should be repeated after volume replacement. Frequently one can surmise that there is volume depletion from a very low right atrial pressure (0–2 mm Hg). If such low pressures are found with a low cardiac output, a volume challenge with 250 ml to 500 ml of saline is administered to raise the right atrial pressure to at least 5 mm Hg before assuming that the right-sided pressures are truly representative of the status of the pulmonary circulation.

Passive pulmonary hypertension secondary to pulmonary venous hypertension should reveal an elevated pulmonary capillary wedge pressure of ≥ 20 mm Hg with a pulmonary artery diastolic pressure of ≤ 5 mm Hg higher than the diastolic pulmonary wedge pressure. A diastolic gradient between the pulmonary capillary wedge pressure and the pulmonary artery pressure of more than 5 mm Hg denotes an elevation in pulmonary precapillary resistance consistent with pulmo-

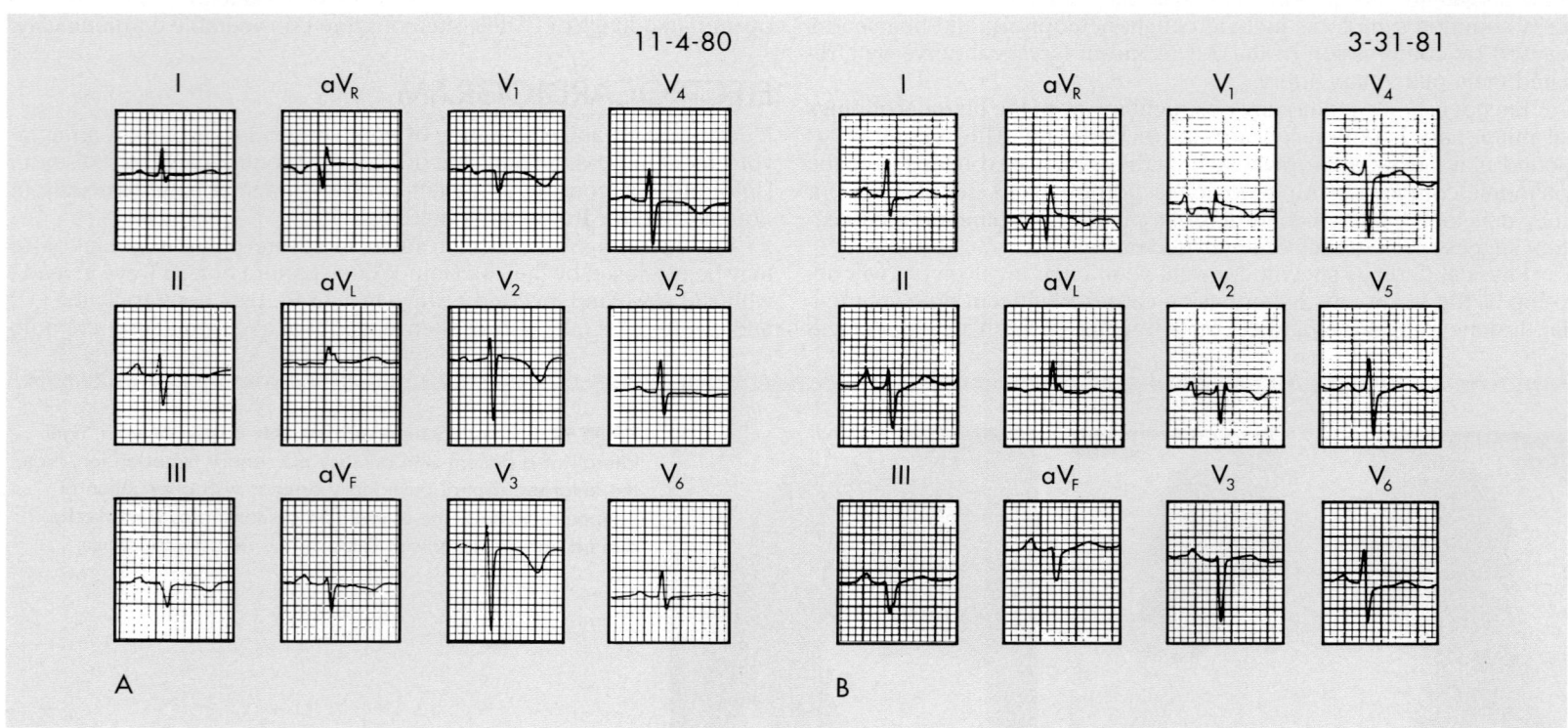

FIGURE 94.2 **A.** Electrocardiogram of patient with primary pulmonary hypertension and echocardiographic evidence of right ventricular hypertrophy and dilatation. Note S waves to V_6 and inverted T waves to V_5. This tracing also demonstrates a QS with an inverted T wave in lead III (S_1, Q_3, T_3). **B.** A repeat electrocardiogram performed 5 months later (several days before the patient's death) shows an rS in lead III, an R/S ratio of 1 in lead V_1, and right atrial abnormality (p-pulmonale).

nary disease or some other noncardiac cause of pulmonary hypertension.

Cardiac catheterization is often necessary to search for a possible congenital left-to-right shunt. This may be accomplished by performing appropriate indicator dilution curves, by searching for a "step-up" in right-sided oxygen content, or by passing the catheter through septal defects. It should be remembered, however, that in approximately 20% of individuals, any cause of pulmonary hypertension may result in a right-to-left shunt through a patent foramen ovale.

Pulmonary arteriograms are useful in excluding the possibility that unsuspected thromboembolism may be the cause of pulmonary hypertension. Unfortunately, in patients with severe pulmonary hypertension, pulmonary arteriography is not performed without significant risk. It is our practice to perform subselective pulmonary arteriograms. These localized and smaller injections appear to be better tolerated. If a patient has no evidence of emboli on several subselective views, the likelihood of massive or recurrent thromboembolism as a cause of pulmonary hypertension is essentially excluded. The role of magnification pulmonary wedge arteriograms is promising but has not been adequately assessed.[32]

If cardiac catheterization has failed to demonstrate pulmonary venous hypertension, left-to-right shunt, or pulmonary emboli, it may be assumed that the patient has primary pulmonary hypertension (Fig. 94.3). Cardiac catheterization may be of additional value in such patients for noting the response of their pulmonary vascular resistance and systemic vascular resistance to vasodilators. This may be done in the catheterization laboratory or in the intensive care unit with indwelling catheters.

MANAGEMENT OF PULMONARY HEART DISEASE
DECREASING PULMONARY HYPERTENSION

The most effective therapies for pulmonary heart disease are those that diminish pulmonary hypertension through the reduction of pulmonary vascular resistance and impedance to right ventricular outflow. It must be kept in mind that the reduction of pulmonary artery pressure brought about solely by lowering the cardiac output is unlikely to be of benefit.

Therapeutic measures that lower pulmonary hypertension may be considered in two categories: specific and general.

Whenever possible, *specific* therapy should be used to address the underlying cause of pulmonary hypertension, such as returning the patient to lower altitude, treating vasculitides with steroids or immunosuppressive therapy, surgical removal of a severely bronchiectatic lobe, surgical removal of unlysed central pulmonary emboli, and so on.

General therapeutic measures are applicable to most patients with pulmonary hypertension. These measures include oxygen, bronchodilators, avoidance of irritant inhalants, and the use of antibiotics for associated bronchitis. The arterial Po_2 should be kept at 60 mm Hg or above in order to lessen the degree of pulmonary hypertension and improve tissue oxygenation. Chronic domiciliary oxygen therapy should be used for patients with COPD who have hypoxemia at rest (with arterial $Po_2 < 60$ mm Hg) or who have polycythemia or pulmonary heart disease.[33] Continuous oxygen therapy seems to be more beneficial than nocturnal oxygen alone.[34] Apparently, those patients

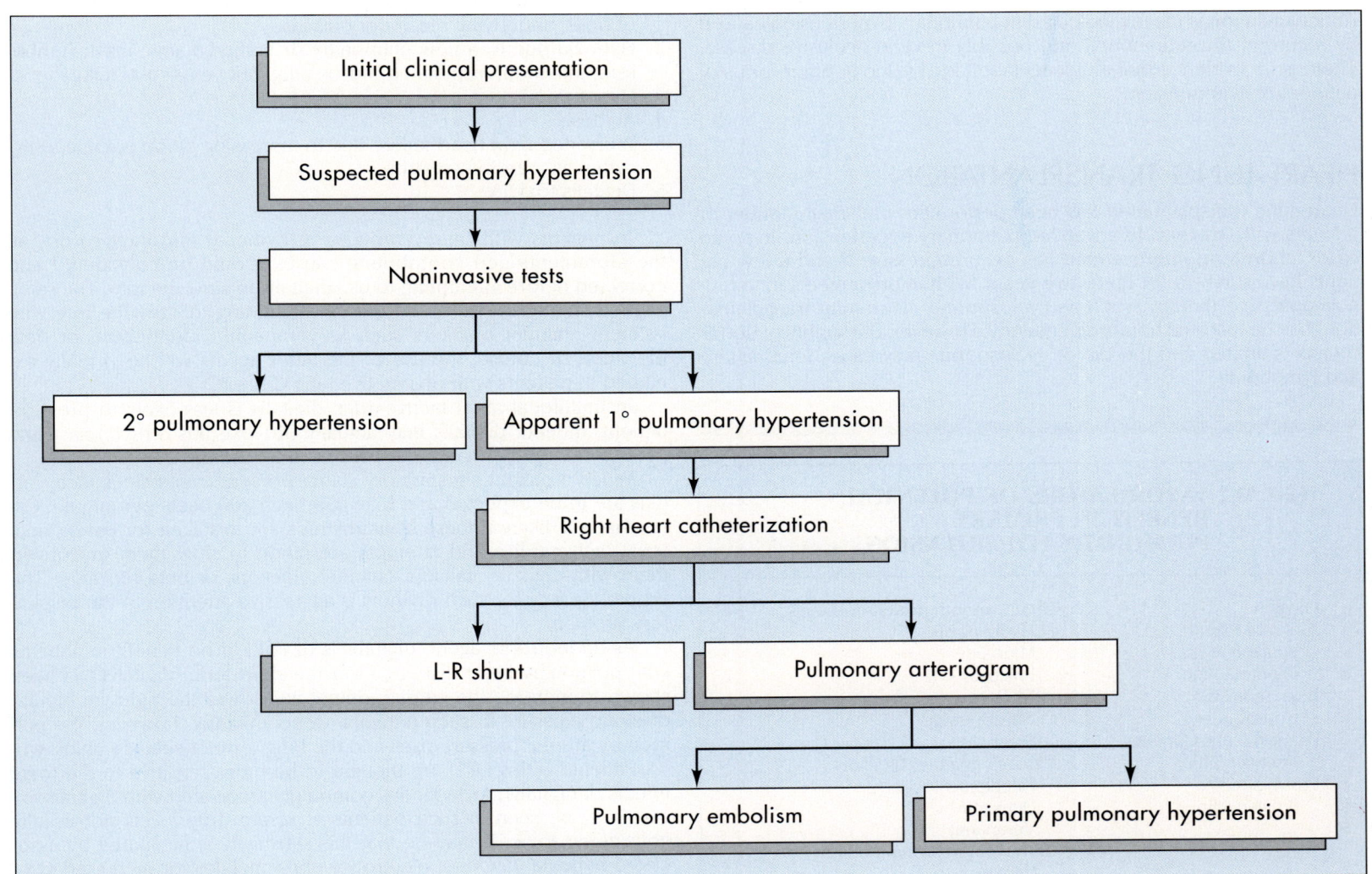

FIGURE 94.3 The interrelation of noninvasive testing and cardiac catheterization in the evaluation of patients with suspected pulmonary hypertension.

with COPD whose mean pulmonary artery pressures drop by more than 5 mm Hg in response to oxygen have a better prognosis than those whose pressures are less responsive.[35] Unfortunately, a similar benefit has not been demonstrated for patients with primary pulmonary hypertension.

Bronchopulmonary drainage, percussion, and ventilatory training have been advocated as adjunctive treatment in patients with COPD. These techniques are of no proven benefit.

In patients with polycythemia and hematocrits above 60%, phlebotomy has been demonstrated to diminish fatigue, headaches, and pulmonary artery pressure.[36] No evidence exists, however, that prognosis is improved.

Vasodilators have been tried in patients with pulmonary hypertension from a variety of causes. Except for the potential benefit of oxygen in COPD, there is little information on the long-term benefit of vasodilators in these patients. In some patients with primary pulmonary hypertension, the pulmonary vascular resistance has been reported to have been successfully lowered with a number of agents (Table 94.2). Unfortunately, in many patients, as the pulmonary arterial pressure drops, the cardiac output and systemic pressure also decrease. The pulmonary vascular resistance may alter but little. If coronary artery perfusion pressure drops, right ventricular ischemia and dysfunction may worsen.[37] It has been suggested that a greater relative drop in pulmonary vascular resistance as compared to systemic vascular resistance may be a useful index of potential therapeutic benefit.[38] Furthermore, it is not known whether immediate beneficial effect will predict long-term efficacy, or whether lack of such a short-term response means that long-term therapy is useless.

ANTICOAGULATION

Anticoagulation is clearly indicated in pulmonary hypertension caused by recurrent thromboemboli and possibly in veno-occlusive disease. There is no evidence that anticoagulation is of value in other forms of pulmonary hypertension.

HEART–LUNG TRANSPLANTATION

Heart–lung transplantation has been performed in a small number of patients with irreversible advanced pulmonary hypertension. In some cases, short-term improvement has been impressive,[39] and a few patients have survived for up to two years. With improvements in immunosuppressive therapy, such as cyclosporine, heart-lung transplantation may be resorted to more frequently. However, the supply of donor organs is limited and the use of cyclosporine may cause renal failure and lymphoma.

TABLE 94.2 VASODILATORS OF POTENTIAL BENEFIT IN PRIMARY PULMONARY HYPERTENSION

Oxygen	Direct smooth muscle relaxants
Alpha blockers	Hydralazine
Tolazoline	Minoxidil
Phentolamine	Prazosin
Beta agonists	Nitrates
Isoproterenol	Nitroprusside
Parasympathomimetics	Diazoxide
Acetylcholine	Calcium channel blockers
Prostaglandins	Nifedipine
Prostacyclin	Diltiazem
	Verapamil
	Converting enzyme inhibitor
	Captopril

DIURETICS

The use of diuretic therapy is particularly valuable when there is a component of passive pulmonary hypertension due to left ventricular failure. Otherwise, the reduction of central volume with diuretics may cause a lowering of cardiac output. Diuretics should be used with caution and only when systemic venous hypertension has risen enough to cause uncomfortable peripheral edema, effusions, or ascites. Diuretic therapy for edema formation should be reserved as a secondary adjunct to other means of improving respiratory function or lowering pulmonary arterial pressure. Mild peripheral edema may be accepted without resorting to diuresis.

Patients with COPD may develop inspissated bronchial secretions and worsened respiratory status with overly aggressive diuresis. In addition, excessive diuresis can be expected to lower the cardiac output and to decrease tissue perfusion and renal function. Ethacrinic acid may have the additional deleterious action of suppressing the stimulatory effect of carbon dioxide on the respiratory center.

If diuretics must be used in patients with severe lung disease, potassium chloride supplements are usually required to avoid bicarbonate excess, as well as hypokalemia.

DIGITALIS

Digitalis and other cardiac glycosides are most useful in controlling the ventricular rate during supraventricular tachycardias, especially atrial fibrillation and flutter. Whenever a patient with pulmonary heart disease develops a supraventricular tachycardia, the clinician must suspect one or more of the following causes:

1. Hypoxia and increased pulmonary hypertension due to worsening of basic underlying respiratory disease
2. Hypoxia due to a new pulmonary or hemodynamic insult (embolism, infection, inspissated mucus plug, left ventricular failure)
3. Hypokalemia
4. Acidosis
5. Worsened right heart failure due to increasing blood volume, polycythemia, cardiomyopathy
6. Digitalis toxicity

In patients with supraventricular arrhythmias and tachycardia, all the aforementioned contributing causes should be considered and corrected before attempting to use digitalis to slow the rate. The same caution should be exercised before attempting to slow the rate with calcium channel blockers such as verapamil or diltiazem, or beta blockers. Of course, the use of the latter agents will be virtually excluded in patients with obstructive lung disease.

In multifocal atrial tachycardia, digitalis is less likely to prove of benefit. Indeed, digitalis may actually provoke this arrhythmia; verapamil, on the other hand, has proven to be useful.

When a patient's respiratory status worsens, rapid sinus tachycardias are to be expected and may approach 200 beats per minute. Catastrophe is likely if these sinus rhythms are mistaken for paroxysmal atrial tachycardias and attempts are made to slow them or convert them with digitalis, calcium channel blockers, or beta blockers. The proper therapy for such rhythms is aggressive attention to the respiratory problem.

As an inotropic agent, digitalis is of little or no benefit in patients with pulmonary heart disease. Over the short term, digitalis has been shown to increase the cardiac output and lower the right ventricular diastolic pressure in such patients. Concomitantly, however, the pulmonary arterial pressure rises and the long-term effects are unknown.

Patients with COPD are thought to be more sensitive to the toxic effects of digitalis. Arrhythmias commonly associated with digitalis excess may be seen in such patients at serum drug levels not usually considered toxic. It may be that this sensitivity is facilitated by associated hypoxia, acidosis, electrolyte abnormalities, or increased sympathetic discharge. Indeed, it is likely that hypoxic stimulation of sympathetic drive is additive to the enhanced sympathetic tone induced by digitalis.

PULMONARY EMBOLISM

Pulmonary embolism is the most common cause of pulmonary heart disease. Among those patients with pulmonary embolism who have survived the first hour, the mortality rate for those who remain untreated is estimated to be 30%; this rate can be reduced to 8% with appropriate therapy.[4,40,41]

Pulmonary embolism differs from most causes of pulmonary heart disease in being abrupt in onset and less likely to be associated with severe pulmonary hypertension, even though the impedance to pulmonary blood flow may be greatly increased. When significant hypertension is found in acute pulmonary embolism, it seems to be more related to the associated hypoxia and humoral or neurohumoral factors.[42-44] For these reasons, the manifestations and diagnostic work-up of pulmonary embolism differ sufficiently from other causes of pulmonary heart disease to warrant separate discussion.

HISTORY AND PHYSICAL EXAMINATION

The most common symptoms of pulmonary embolism are dyspnea and chest pain; each is present in over 80% of documented cases. Cough and apprehension are each present in approximately 50% of cases. The most frequently encountered physical finding is tachypnea, with a respiratory rate at rest greater than 16 per minute. This nonspecific finding is very sensitive and is present in over 90% of cases.[45] The absence of tachypnea in a patient who has no reason for respiratory depression is strong evidence against the diagnosis of pulmonary embolism.

There are four ways in which pulmonary embolism may present; these clinical presentations are not mutually exclusive. They are (1) acute unexplained dyspnea, (2) pulmonary infarction or hemorrhage, (3) acute right ventricular failure, and (4) chronic pulmonary hypertension (Table 94.3).

If a patient presents only with acute unexplained dyspnea, the findings will be limited to shortness of breath and tachypnea. The electrocardiogram and chest roentgenogram are apt to be normal. Most of these patients will have a predisposition or risk factor for deep venous thrombosis and most will have arterial hypoxemia while breathing room air. These are the markers that often help in distinguishing such patients from those with hyperventilation syndrome and normal lungs.

Patients who present with pulmonary parenchymal injury will give some evidence of this damage. They may present many hours to several days after the initiating embolism, with pleuritic chest pain, cough, fever, and mild leukocytosis. Hemoptysis may occur. These patients often have a pleural or pleuropericardial friction rub, depending on which pleural surface is involved in the inflammatory process. These patients need not be dyspneic or hypoxic, and they may have no evidence of right ventricular failure if the embolism is not obstructing enough of the pulmonary vasculature. The chest roentgenogram will show a pulmonary infiltrate and usually a pleural effusion.[46] While careful fluoroscopy will demonstrate that the infiltrate has a pleural base, often the routine posteroanterior and lateral chest films will show a rounded infiltrate indistinguishable from a localized pneumonitis or atelectasis. Many such infiltrates are totally reversible and represent transient hemorrhagic injury without significant tissue necrosis.[47]

In the presence of previously adequate cardiac and pulmonary reserve, a pulmonary embolism must obstruct more than 60% of the total pulmonary vascular cross-sectional diameter in order for the patient to develop signs and symptoms of acute right ventricular failure. Pulmonary embolism that is severe enough to produce acute right ventricular failure usually causes severe dyspnea and air hunger. In such patients, hypoxia on room air is invariably present, and often intense. Chest pain of an anginal nature is frequent and may possibly be caused by ischemia of the acutely stressed right ventricle. Evidence for central venous hypertension will be manifested by distended neck veins and possibly a distended liver and peripheral edema if enough time has passed. Such massive pulmonary obstruction may present with cardiogenic shock, often with syncope or even cardiovascular collapse. Sudden cardiac death may occur, initially demonstrating electromechanical dissociation. A normal central venous pressure (less than 7 mm Hg) excludes massive pulmonary embolism as a cause of shock, unless the patient is also severely volume depleted.

Most rarely, patients will present with evidence for significant pulmonary hypertension and chronic dyspnea. This syndrome of chronic pulmonary heart disease may appear in patients who have had inadequate lysis of large thrombi despite therapy.[48] More likely it will develop among those with recurrent unrecognized or inadequately treated thromboembolism.

Undoubtedly, minor pulmonary embolism is often clinically silent or ignored. It may occur more often than previously suspected among those at high risk for venous thrombosis. Even severe pulmonary embolism is likely to go undetected in patients who have clouded sensorium or who are obtunded, or among those who have other diseases that may cause chest pain or dyspnea.[49]

PATHOPHYSIOLOGY

While pulmonary emboli may occur with a wide variety of materials (Table 94.4), the vast majority develop from venous thrombi. Most of these thrombi arise proximal to the knee, in the capacious deep veins of the thigh. They usually develop in patients whose legs have been relatively immobile for prolonged periods during which leg muscles have not been pumping to help move the columns of venous blood. Serial ^{125}I fibrinogen leg scans have detected thrombi in the valves of the soleal veins in from 45% to 70% of patients at prolonged bed rest or undergoing elective surgery with general anesthesia. In the majority of these patients, the process is limited to the calf veins; in as many as 20% the thrombi propagate above the popliteal veins into the deep veins of the thigh.[50,51]

As many as half of patients with proximal deep venous thrombosis remain asymptomatic and demonstrate no abnormality on physical examination.[52] Asymptomatic individuals may have either incomplete obstruction of the deep venous system or have a highly competent superficial venous system so that significant obstruction has not developed in the venous drainage of the lower extremity.

Many factors other than bed rest and immobility may predispose to deep venous thrombosis and subsequent thromboembolism (Table 94.5). Virchow first described venous thromboembolism; he also recognized the triad of risk factors that promote venous thrombosis.[53] The three factors that cause inappropriate clotting of venous blood are

TABLE 94.3 SYNDROMES OF PULMONARY EMBOLISM

Acute Unexplained Dyspnea	Acute Right Ventricular Failure
Dyspnea, tachypnea, most often hypoxemia	Dyspnea, tachypnea, hypoxemia Central venous hypertension Angina-like chest pain Possible syncope or cardiogenic shock
Pulmonary Infarction	
Pleurisy, cough, hemoptysis Mild fever and leukocytosis Pulmonary infiltrate and effusion Usually hypoxemia	**Chronic Pulmonary Heart Disease** Chronic dyspnea, hypoxemia, fatigue Severe pulmonary hypertension Chronic right-sided heart failure

venous endothelial injury, stasis of blood within the veins, and hypercoagulability of the blood.

Immobility, obesity, leg trauma, infection or surgery to the legs, long leg casts, systemic venous hypertension, proximal vein obstruction, and incompetent venous valves are among the factors that are likely to produce either venous endothelial injury or stasis of blood flow, or both.

The hemostatic system involves a complex dynamic interaction of vascular endothelium, platelets, the intrinsic and extrinsic coagulation cascades, and the fibrinolytic system. We know that each of these components is controlled by elements that either favor or inhibit clot formation or clot lysis. Hypercoagulability, therefore, may result from a predictably dizzying catalogue of abnormalities.[54] It is humbling to recognize that the myriad of facts now known about the hemostatic process is likely to be a small part of the whole. Among the recognized causes of hypercoagulability are polycythemia, thrombocytosis, sickle cell disease, estrogen therapy, and malignancies. Paradoxically, states associated with circulating "anticoagulants" are often associated with inappropriate coagulation. More recently, the clinical importance of deficiencies in antithrombin III has been emphasized.[55] Antithrombin III is a circulating glycoprotein that inhibits clotting factors and is necessary for control of the coagulation cascade. Patients with a genetic deficiency of, or an abnormal structure of, antithrombin III are at great risk of venous thromboembolism.

Antithrombin III deficiency may be due to an autosomal dominant trait or, less commonly, to a spontaneous mutation. Classically, type I disease is due to a deficiency in antithrombin III molecules. This form of deficiency is associated with a greater than 50% reduction in circulating immunologically assayed antithrombin III. Patients with type II abnormality are less common and exhibit a normal quantity of immunologically assayed antithrombin III, most of which fails to complex normally with serine proteases. Apparently, this form of the disease is due to synthesis and release of defective antithrombin III molecules. Type III abnormality involves yet another defect in which immunoassays and functional assays are both normal, but heparin fails to accelerate the rate of complexing between the antithrombin III and activated serine protease coagulant factors. Nephrotic syndrome, liver disease, estrogen therapy, disseminated intravascular coagulation, and even heparin therapy may cause acquired deficiencies of antithrombin III.

Deficiencies of other coagulation factors have also been implicated in venous thrombosis; these include hereditary abnormalities in plasminogen or fibrin and deficiencies in protein C, protein S, or venous endothelial plasminogen activator.

Patients with malignancies may have tumor emboli to the lung from direct extension from either the inferior or superior vena cava or from liver metastases growing into the hepatic veins. Patients with malignancy are also highly susceptible to venous thromboembolism due to a hypercoagulable state.[56]

DIAGNOSTIC PROCEDURES
IMPEDANCE PLETHYSMOGRAPHY

Impedance plethysmography is an easily performed, noninvasive procedure for the detection of thrombi in the large deep proximal veins of the thigh (Fig. 94.4). Since the majority of patients with thromboembolism have proximal deep venous thrombosis, this test is very useful in detecting silent thrombotic disease in patients with suspected pulmonary embolism. While over 90% of patients with pulmonary embolism have an identifiable risk factor for deep venous thrombosis, as many as 30% of patients with documented pulmonary embolism will have no

TABLE 94.4 POSSIBLE SOURCES OF PULMONARY EMBOLI

Thromboembolism from
    Deep veins of the thigh
    Prostatic or pelvic veins
    Vena cava, renal veins, hepatic veins
    Right atrium or ventricle
    Right-sided artificial valves
    Venous filters, ventriculoatrial shunts
Amniotic fluid and debris
Bone marrow and fat
Right atrial myxomata and other right-sided tumors
Malignancies invading the systemic venous circuit, especially hypernephroma
Right-sided valvular vegetations
Parasites
Talc and other debris used in illicit intravenous drugs
Catheter fragments
Right-sided artificial valve fragments
Air introduced with central venous catheterization or from traumatic venous laceration

TABLE 94.5 PREDISPOSITION TO VENOUS THROMBOSIS

Mechanisms of "Virchow's Triad"	Precipitating Causes
Endothelial injury	Trauma
	Inflammation
	Infection
	Hemodynamic stress
	Ischemia
Blood stasis	Immobility
	Obesity
	Heart failure
Hypercoagulable state	Pregnancy
	Oral contraceptives
	Cancer
	Polycythemia
	Nephrotic syndrome
	Thrombocytosis
	Sickle cell disease
	Deficiency of
	Antithrombin III
	Protein C or S
	Fibrin
	Plasminogen
	Plasminogen activator
	Lupus anticoagulant
	Paroxysmal nocturnal hemoglobinuria
	Thrombotic thrombocytopenic purpura (TTP)
	Heparin-induced thrombocytopenia
	Diabetes mellitus
	Hyperlipidemia
	Homocystinuria

evidence of proximal deep venous thrombosis by contrast venography.[57] Presumably, impedance plethysmography would also be normal in these individuals. Therefore, negative impedance plethysmograms should not dissuade the clinician from a diagnosis of venous thromboembolism when the clinical situation is otherwise suggestive.

LIQUID CRYSTAL COLOR THERMOGRAPHY

Liquid crystal color thermography has been used for the diagnosis of lower limb deep venous thrombosis.[58] In patients with deep venous thrombosis confirmed by contrast venography, the sensitivity was 97%. The predictive value of a negative thermogram was 96.5%. Although liquid crystal color thermography appears to be a promising technique in the diagnosis of deep venous thrombosis, further evaluation is required to assess its role in clinical practice.

ARTERIAL BLOOD GASES

The arterial blood gases in patients with acute pulmonary embolism who are breathing room air will usually demonstrate hypoxia and respiratory alkalosis.[59] However, 15% of patients with documented embolism will have an arterial Po_2 equal to or greater than 80 mm Hg.[60] The major use of arterial blood gases is to raise the clinician's suspicion of pulmonary embolism in a patient who is dyspneic or hyperventilating and has no other reason for hypoxia. Unexplained respiratory alkalosis in a patient with chronic obstructive pulmonary disease and prior hypercapnia should also raise the clinician's suspicion of pulmonary embolism.[61]

LABORATORY VALUES

Serum bilirubin, LDH, and SGOT determinations are of no value in the diagnosis of pulmonary embolism.[59] Plasma DNA is frequently elevated in pulmonary embolism, but a recent study did not find this test of any diagnostic usefulness.[62] Elevations in fibrinopeptide A and β-thrombulin are almost always present in patients with deep venous thrombosis and pulmonary embolism. Unfortunately, these elevations are nonspecific and unlikely to be clinically useful.

ELECTROCARDIOGRAM

The presence of right ventricular abnormality, as demonstrated by $S_1Q_3T_3$, right bundle branch block, right axis deviation, or right atrial abnormality, was found in only 26% of patients with pulmonary embolism in the Urokinase Pulmonary Embolism Trial.[63] Although these changes are, therefore, insensitive as well as nonspecific, they seem to be more commonly found in the electrocardiograms of patients with massive pulmonary embolism. Atrial fibrillation and other supraventricular arrhythmias may be seen, usually in those patients who have a prior predisposition to these arrhythmias.

CHEST ROENTGENOGRAM

The chest roentgenogram will demonstrate evidence for a pulmonary infiltrate in most patients with pulmonary injury. The majority of patients will demonstrate one or more abnormalities, including a pleural effusion, an infiltrate, atelectasis, or an elevated hemidiaphragm. Oligemic lung segments or abrupt arterial narrowing may also be seen in a minority of patients. Right ventricular dilatation or large central pulmonary arteries are less often noted.[46]

The most valuable role of the chest film is in the detection of other diseases that may mimic pulmonary embolism and in the proper interpretation of the lung perfusion scan.

LUNG SCANS

The lung perfusion scan is an extremely sensitive test for pulmonary embolism. A normal multiview perfusion scan (4 or more views) excludes the diagnosis of pulmonary embolism and further diagnostic procedures for thromboembolism are unnecessary.

Unfortunately, the abnormal lung scan is nonspecific and can only be interpreted with careful review of the chest roentgenogram and often with ventilation scans of the lungs.[64,65] Perfusion defects that are subsegmental or associated with roentgenographic abnormalities in the same area are highly nonspecific. If a defect is segmental or larger and ventilates normally, the likelihood of pulmonary embolism is much greater (Fig. 94.5). The probability is greatly increased if the chest film shows no corresponding defects and the clinical setting is consistent. In this latter circumstance, therapy for pulmonary embolism may be instituted without further corroboration of the diagnosis.

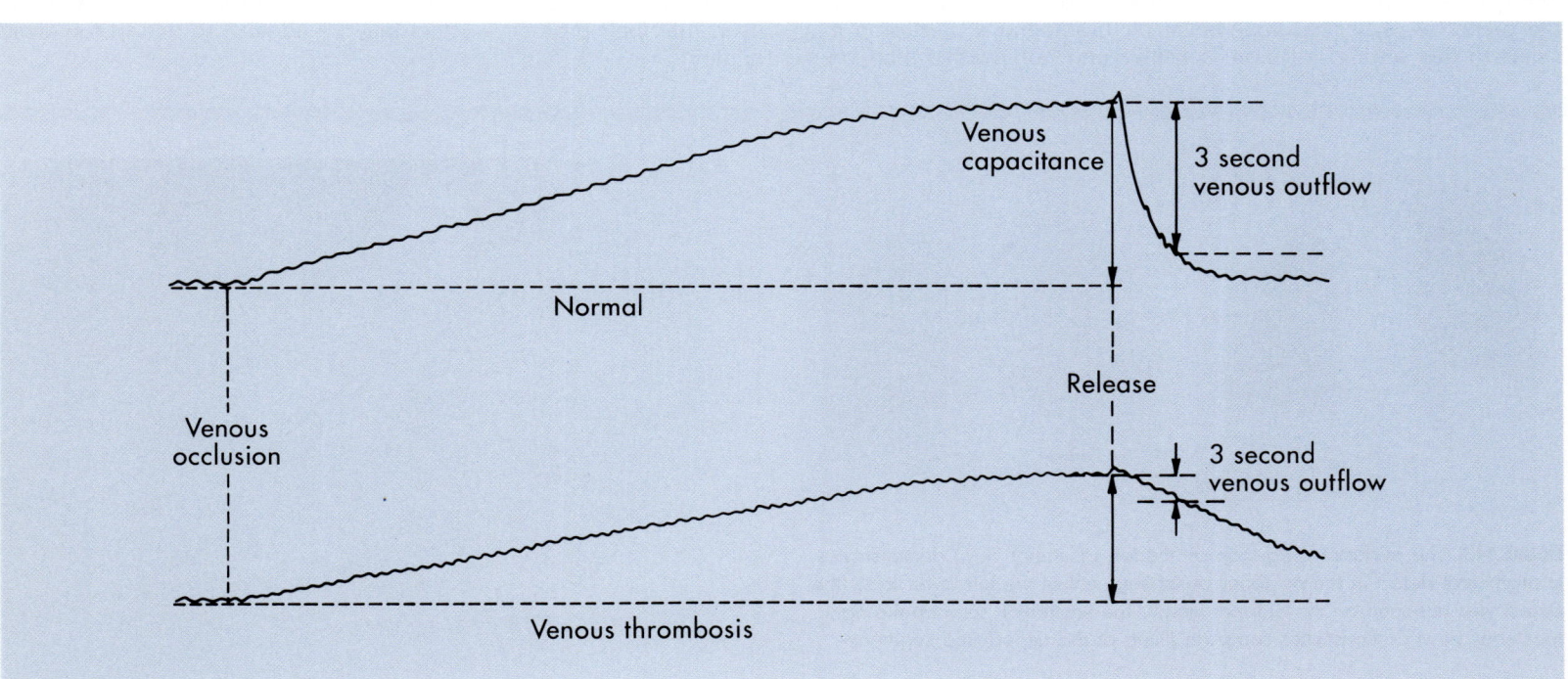

FIGURE 94.4 Typical impedance plethysmographic tracings. The 3-second venous outflow is reduced in the leg with recent deep venous thrombosis. (Wheeler HB, Anderson FA Jr: The diagnosis of venous thrombosis by occlusive impedance plethysmography. In Bernstein EF (ed): Noninvasive Diagnostic Techniques in Vascular Disease, 3rd ed, p 758. St Louis, CV Mosby, 1985. Reprinted by permission.)

PULMONARY ARTERIOGRAPHY

The most accurate procedure for establishing the diagnosis of pulmonary embolism is the pulmonary arteriogram. The visualization of small and nonoccluding emboli may be enhanced by obtaining selective arteriograms, by using cineangiographic techniques, or by selective and magnified views distal to balloon occlusion of smaller arteries. These specialized techniques are rarely necessary. Unfortunately, the invasive nature of the procedure, the potential complications of the radiographic dye load, and the cost preclude its routine use in all patients suspected of thromboembolism.

The arteriographic finding most specific for pulmonary embolism is the filling defect. Arterial "cut-offs" and "pruning" of vessels are highly consistent with the diagnosis, while oligemic lung segments, asymmetrical filling, and delay in lower zone filling or clearing are less reliable.[66]

A negative pulmonary arteriogram excludes the diagnosis of pulmonary embolism. Unfortunately, up to one third of these procedures yield equivocal results. The use of balloon occlusion arteriography can markedly reduce the number of equivocal studies (Fig. 94.6).[67] Digital subtraction angiography performed by injecting dye in the proximal (right atrial) port of an in-dwelling pulmonary artery catheter appears to give results comparable to conventional pulmonary arteriography.[68] Such studies may provide a reasonably accurate and often more convenient substitute to the conventional arteriogram; they are not likely, however, to decrease the cost or the morbidity of the procedure.

DIAGNOSTIC APPROACH

The diagnostic strategy for the work-up of possible pulmonary embolism depends on the urgency of the patient's clinical presentation and the strength of the clinician's suspicion.

In a patient with acute unexplained dyspnea and no predisposing risk for deep venous thrombosis, a normal chest roentgenogram and normal arterial P_{O_2} may be sufficient to allay the clinician's suspicion. Negative impedance plethysmograms of the lower extremities are often useful in further decreasing the likelihood of thromboembolism. Even though none of these noninvasive tests are specific or sensitive enough in themselves, their combined weight in this circumstance allows the clinician to proceed under the premise that pulmonary thromboembolism has been excluded.

If a patient with acute unexplained dyspnea has a predisposition to deep venous thrombosis, perfusion scans should be obtained even in the presence of normal impedance plethysmograms. Perfusion lung scans in this setting are more sensitive and noninvasive than venograms. They also carry lower morbidity and risk (one of the complications of venography is thrombosis!).

Patients with evidence for pulmonary parenchymal injury or right ventricular failure (without significant hypotension) should undergo lung perfusion scans, chest roentgenograms, and impedance plethysmograms or venograms. If these tests are congruent for venous thromboembolism, treatment may be instituted without obtaining pulmonary arteriograms. If the chest films are abnormal in the area of the perfusion abnormalities, or if the perfusion scans are equivocal (subsegmental defects), a ventilation scan is necessary.

In patients without hypotension, pulmonary arteriography is necessary only if the perfusion scans are equivocal. A pulmonary arteriogram may also be warranted if a scan consistent with pulmonary embolism is incongruent with the noninvasive tests, so that the clinician remains unconvinced.

In patients with right ventricular failure and shock, pulmonary arteriography should be resorted to early in the work-up, rather than delaying for perfusion scanning. Heparin therapy should be started when the diagnosis is first seriously entertained. Bleeding complications of pulmonary arteriography can be minimized by using antecubital venous cutdown for venous access. Alternatively, heparin anticoagulation can be reversed for a brief period with protamine.

PREVENTION OF VENOUS THROMBOSIS

The best management strategy for venous thromboembolism is the prevention and treatment of deep venous thrombosis. Patients at risk should be identified, and, when possible, risk factors for venous thrombosis should be reversed. If possible, leg exercises with repeated flexion and extension at the ankles and knees should be practiced by such patients. Mechanical devices have been developed that intermittently compress or that passively move the lower extremities during a period of enforced bed rest. Elastic stockings, when properly fitted and applied to provide a graded compression from ankle to thigh, decrease deep venous thrombosis in patients undergoing major surgery from 49% to 23% (as determined by fibrinogen ^{131}I).[69] These nonpharmacologic methods alone appear to provide inadequate prophylaxis for patients undergoing major surgery. There is reason to believe, however, that their protective effect may be additive to that of low-dose heparin.[70]

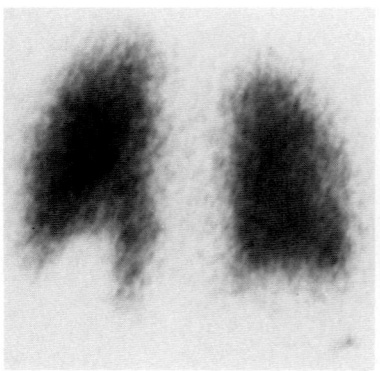
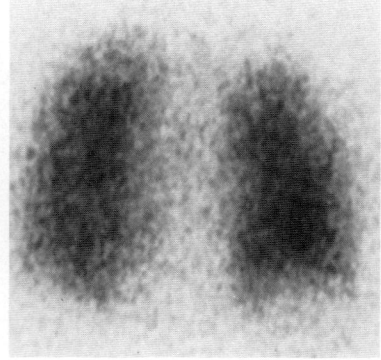

FIGURE 94.5 The perfusion lung scan on the left (posterior view) demonstrates a segmental defect in the posterior basal segment of the left lower lobe (the defect was not seen on the anterior views). The ventilation scan on the right (posterior view) demonstrates complete filling of this unperfused segment.

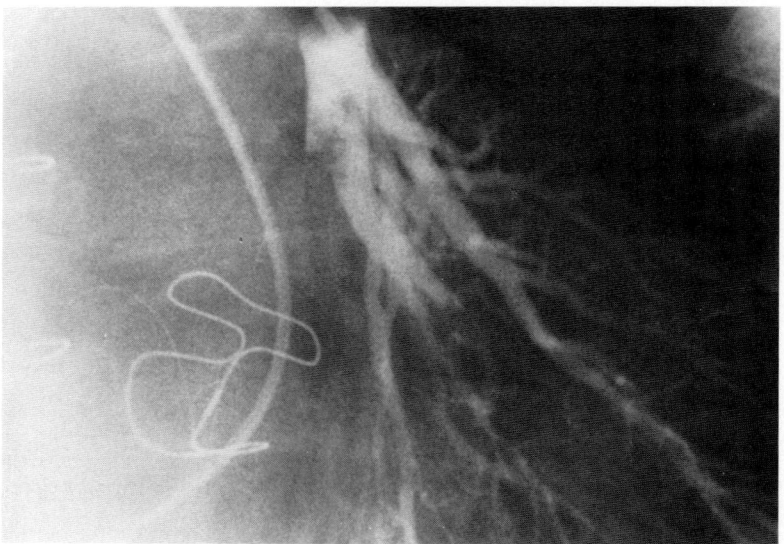

FIGURE 94.6 A balloon occlusion pulmonary arteriogram demonstrates intraluminal filling defects and cut-offs in the lower lobe vessels. These defects were poorly demonstrated on nonselective pulmonary arteriograms.

In many situations, low doses of heparin appear to prevent venous thrombosis effectively.[71] Even small doses of subcutaneous heparin (*i.e.*, 5,000 units q12h) appear to potentiate antithrombin III and thus neutralize the effect of activated factor X. A regimen of low-dose subcutaneous heparin has been demonstrated to decrease the incidence of positive venous scans in surgical patients, in patients with acute myocardial infarction,[72] and in other medical patients treated with bed rest.[73] Patients undergoing hip surgery or prostatectomy appear to be exceptions. In patients undergoing total hip replacement, higher doses of heparin to keep the activated partial thromboplastin time between 31.5 and 36 seconds appear to reduce the frequency of postoperative deep venous thrombosis.[74]

Other pharmacologic interventions that have been less successful in the prevention of deep venous thrombosis include dextran, dihyroergotamine mesylate (a potent venoconstrictor), and antiplatelet agents such as chloroquine sulfate (Plaquenil), aspirin, and sulfinpyrazone.

The most effective prophylaxis for deep venous thrombosis is oral warfarin therapy. Unfortunately, because of the risk of serious hemorrhage, particularly during the intraoperative period, full warfarin anticoagulation is usually reserved for the prevention of recurrent venous thrombosis after documented pulmonary embolism. Low-dose warfarin (keeping the prothrombin time 1.5 to 3.0 seconds above control) has been tried successfully in patients undergoing total hip replacement. Low-dose warfarin is given for one and a half to two weeks preoperatively, followed by full therapeutic doses as soon as possible after surgery.[75]

TREATMENT OF VENOUS THROMBOEMBOLISM
ANTICOAGULATION

The treatment for proximal deep venous thrombosis or for thromboembolism is intravenous heparin anticoagulation for 7 to 10 days, preferably by continuous intravenous infusion. Intravenous heparin is best monitored by maintaining the activated partial thromboplastin time at one and a half to two and a half times the control value. With this technique, major bleeding complications can be expected in 5% to 10% of patients, with an incidence of fatal hemorrhage of 0.6%. Patients most likely to have serious hemorrhagic complications on heparin therapy are women, patients over the age of 60 years, patients on other medications that may affect coagulation, and patients with other serious medical disorders.[76]

Treatment with oral warfarin is usually begun during the first week of heparin therapy and continued for 3 to 6 months or until the factors predisposing to venous thrombosis have resolved. In most studies, the incidence of recurrent thromboembolism is very low during warfarin therapy. Bleeding complications, however, can be expected to develop in from 21% to 38% of patients.[77,78] While low-dose heparin therapy carries no significant risk of bleeding, it has unfortunately been found ineffective in preventing recurrent thromboembolism. In patients with proximal deep venous thrombosis, the efficacy of subcutaneous heparin in preventing recurrence was improved by adjusting the 12-hour dose to prolong the activated partial thromboplastin time (at 6 hours after the dose) to one and a half times the control.[79] With this rather moderate dose, bleeding complications remained low. This method appears to be particularly useful in treating high-risk patients and patients in their first or third trimester of pregnancy (when the risk of teratogenicity and fetal or maternal injury from warfarin is at the highest).

Absolute contraindications to anticoagulation include hemorrhagic cerebrovascular accident within two weeks and recent neurosurgery or spinal or ocular surgery. Relative contraindications include other recent surgery, major trauma, recent gastrointestinal bleeding, severe hypertension, severe renal or hepatic failure, or other bleeding diatheses.

VENOUS INTERRUPTION

Interruption of the inferior vena cava may serve to protect patients with proximal deep venous thrombosis from recurrent thromboembolism. Patients who should be considered for venous interruption include those with serious contraindications to anticoagulation, those who have sustained a complication of anticoagulation, and those who have had recurrent thromboembolism despite apparently adequate anticoagulation.

The use of transvenously positioned filters has led to lower mortality rates (0.7%) and recurrence rates (3%) than those recorded for direct retroperitoneal or transabdominal vena caval interruptions.[80] The Kimray filter appears to offer advantages over the Mobin-Uddin umbrella in terms of higher patency rates at follow-up venography and lower rates of chronic venous stasis.

FIBRINOLYSIS

The routine use of fibrinolytic therapy for acute pulmonary embolism remains controversial. It is clear that the National Institutes of Health (NIH) trials of fibrinolytic therapy indicate a more rapid resolution of pulmonary emboli and an earlier return toward normal hemodynamics with the use of fibrinolytic agents than with heparin anticoagulation alone.[40,81] More importantly, however, fibrinolytic therapy did not decrease the mortality or apparent morbidity. In the two NIH trials, the follow-up lung perfusion scans showed no difference in the degree of embolic obstruction in the two groups by two weeks into therapy. One study reported that patients given fibrinolytic therapy had a higher measured diffusing capacity and estimated capillary blood volume at 1-year follow-up than those initially treated with anticoagulation alone. This may be interpreted as evidence for more complete resolution of microemboli and better capillary perfusion in patients treated initially with fibrinolytic therapy.[82] Nevertheless, there is no evidence that patient symptoms or prognosis is improved over those treated with conventional anticoagulation.

It has been suggested that fibrinolytic therapy may be useful in preventing complications of venous insufficiency in patients with proximal deep venous thrombosis.[83] While several studies have shown more complete resolution of venous thrombosis with fibrinolytic therapy,[84,85] long-term benefit has not yet been demonstrated. Thus, the role for fibrinolytic therapy remains doubtful in the management of routine venous thromboembolism.

The rate of significant bleeding complications in the NIH fibrinolysis trials was 45%. Lower rates have been reported in other studies. The high incidence of bleeding in the NIH trials has been attributed to the multiple arterial and venous punctures and invasive diagnostic procedures required in this group of patients. It is unfortunate that the critically ill, who are most likely to benefit from the head start in fibrinolysis offered by these agents, are also those most likely to require multiple punctures and invasive procedures.

Fibrinolytic therapy would appear to be most valuable in those patients with massive pulmonary embolism complicated by right ventricular failure and severe shock. Direct pulmonary embolectomy, if readily available, may be preferable in such critically ill patients as a more definitive procedure. If rapid surgical intervention cannot be performed or is contraindicated because of associated disease, fibrinolytic therapy should be strongly considered.

Absolute contraindications to fibrinolytic therapy include active internal bleeding, active intracranial processes, or cerebral vascular accident within two months. Relative contraindications include surgery, invasive biopsy, thoracentesis, paracentesis, or intra-arterial diagnostic procedure within ten days, as well as recent trauma, external sternal compression, infective endocarditis, and mitral valve disease with atrial fibrillation.

Tissue plasminogen activator is now being studied in acute myocardial infarction with intracoronary thrombosis.[86] This agent has a high affinity for fibrin and therefore converts plasminogen to plasmin within the fibrin clot rather than indiscriminately in the fluid phase. Whether this theoretical advantage will translate into lower bleeding complications and mortality remains to be seen; if it does, the resistance to the use of fibrinolysis in acute pulmonary embolism will decrease dramatically.

PULMONARY EMBOLECTOMY

Most patients who die from massive pulmonary embolism do so in the first few hours. For most of these unfortunate victims, there is insufficient time to confirm the diagnosis and place the patient on cardiopulmonary bypass. Therefore, the number of patients who will benefit from pulmonary embolectomy will remain small.

Candidates for emergency pulmonary embolectomy are those patients with cardiogenic shock resistant to volume expanders and requiring vasopressors; they should have an angiographic diagnosis of occluded central pulmonary arteries. If such patients have a serious contraindication to fibrinolysis, they must be considered even more strongly for surgical embolectomy.

Contraindications to pulmonary embolectomy include a pulmonary arterial systolic pressure of greater than 70 mm Hg (implying chronicity of the embolism), evidence of cardiac or pulmonary insufficiency before the thromboembolism, or absence of surgically accessible central emboli on angiographic study.[87]

Transvenous pulmonary embolectomy has been tried successfully using a specially designed catheter equipped with suction devices to entrap thromboemboli.[88,89] The catheter is manipulated through a femoral venotomy to the pulmonary artery. Emboli are aspirated into a cup at the catheter tip and withdrawn to the venotomy site. Multiple aspirations may be required. The role of this technique has not yet been established, but it is most attractive in that it can be employed immediately following angiography without instituting cardiopulmonary bypass.

Chronic pulmonary hypertension and pulmonary heart disease are uncommon after pulmonary thromboembolism.[48] Nevertheless, patients with massive unresolved or recurrent thromboembolism may suffer from severe dyspnea and hypoxia at rest. Elective pulmonary embolectomy should be considered in such patients if residual accessible thrombi can be angiographically demonstrated in central and lobar pulmonary artery branches. Considerable symptomatic improvement can be expected in such patients undergoing successful removal of obstructing emboli.[90]

REFERENCES

1. Chronic cor pulmonale: Report of an expert committee. Circulation 27:594, 1963
2. Lockhart A, Tzareva M, Nader F et al: Elevated pulmonary artery wedge pressure at rest and during exercise in chronic bronchitis: Fact or fancy. Clin Sci 37:503, 1969
3. Michelson N: Bilateral ventricular hypertrophy due to chronic pulmonary disease. Dis Chest 38:435, 1960
4. Dalen JE, Alpert JS: Natural history of pulmonary embolism. Prog Cardiovasc Dis 17:259, 1975
5. Chidsey CA, Kaiser GA, Sonnenblick EH et al: Cardiac norepinephrine stores in experimental heart failure in dogs. J Clin Invest 43:2386, 1964
6. McGregor M, Sniderman A: On pulmonary vascular resistance: The need for more precise definition. Am J Cardiol 55:217, 1985
7. Liebow AA, Hales MR, Lindskog GE: Enlargement of the bronchial arteries, and their anastomoses with the pulmonary arteries in bronchiectasis. Am J Pathol 25:211, 1949
8. Robin ED, Cross CE, Kroetz F et al: Pulmonary hypertension and unilateral pleural constriction with speculation on pulmonary vasoconstrictive substance. Arch Intern Med 118:391, 1966
9. Heath D, Edwards JE: The pathology of hypertensive pulmonary vascular disease. Circulation 18:533, 1958
10. Rabinovitch M, Haworth SG, Castaneda AR et al: Lung biopsy in congenital heart disease: A morphometric approach to pulmonary vascular disease. Circulation 58:1107, 1978
11. Robin ED: Some basic and clinical challenges in the pulmonary circulation. Chest 81:357, 1982
12. di Sant'Agnese PA, Talamo RC: Pathogenesis and pathophysiology of cystic fibrosis of the pancreas: Fibrocystic disease of the pancreas (Mucoviscidosis). N Engl J Med 277:1399, 1967
13. Faling LJ: Genetic influences in the development of emphysema in persons with normal serum proteins. Clin Chest Med 4(3):377, 1983
14. Cohen BH, Chase GA: Familial aggregation of chronic obstructive pulmonary disease: Epidemiological and genetic approaches. In Litwin SD (ed): Genetic Determinants of Pulmonary Disease. New York, Marcel Dekker, 1978
15. Kay JM, Smith P, Heath D: Aminorex and the pulmonary circulation. Thorax 26:262, 1971
16. Douglas JG, Munro JF, Kitchin AH et al: Pulmonary hypertension and fenfluramine. Br Med J 283:881, 1981
17. Garcia-Dorado D, Miller DD, Garcia EJ et al: An epidemic of pulmonary hypertension after toxic rapeseed oil ingestion in Spain. J Am Coll Cardiol 1(5):1216, 1983
18. Meyrick B, Reid L: Development of pulmonary arterial changes in rats fed Crotalaria Spectabilis. Am J Pathol 94:37, 1979
19. Heath D, Shaba J, Williams A et al: A pulmonary hypertension producing plant from Tanzania. Thorax 30:399, 1975
20. Wagenvoort CA, Wagenvoort N: The pathology of pulmonary veno-occlusive disease. Virchows Arch [A] 364:69, 1974
21. Fishman AP: Unexplained pulmonary hypertension. Circulation 65:651, 1982
22. Wagenvoort CA, Wagenvoort N: Primary pulmonary hypertension. Circulation 42:1163, 1970
23. Yu PN: Primary pulmonary hypertension: Report of six cases and review of the literature. Ann Intern Med 49:1138, 1958
24. Porter CM, Creech BJ, Billings FT Jr: Primary pulmonary hypertension occurring in twins. Arch Intern Med 120:224, 1967
25. Ingelsby TV, Singer JW, Gordon DS: Abnormal fibrinolysis in familial pulmonary hypertension. Am J Med 55:5, 1973
26. Fuster V, Steele PM, Edwards WD et al: Primary pulmonary hypertension: Natural history and the importance of thrombosis. Circulation 70:580, 1984
27. Nanda NC, Gramiak R, Robinson TI et al: Echocardiographic evaluation of pulmonary hypertension. Circulation 50:575, 1974
28. Algeo S, Morrison D, Ovitt T et al: Noninvasive detection of pulmonary hypertension. Clin Cardiol 7:148, 1984
29. Kitabatake A, Inoue M, Asao M et al: Noninvasive evaluation of pulmonary hypertension by a pulsed doppler technique. Circulation 68:302, 1983
30. Kosturakis D, Goldberg SJ, Allen HD et al: Doppler echocardiographic prediction of pulmonary arterial hypertension in congenital heart disease. Am J Cardiol 53:1110, 1984
31. Berger M, Haimowitz A, Van Tosh A et al: Quantitative assessment of pulmonary hypertension with tricuspid regurgitation using continuous wave doppler ultrasound. J Am Coll Cardiol 6:359, 1985
32. Stein PD: Wedge arteriography for the identification of pulmonary emboli in small vessels. Am Heart J 82:618, 1971
33. Stark RD, Finnegan P, Bishop JM: Long-term domiciliary oxygen in chronic bronchitis with pulmonary hypertension. Br Med J 3:467, 1973
34. Nocturnal Oxygen Therapy Trial Group: Continuous or nocturnal oxygen therapy in hypoxemic chronic obstructive lung disease: A clinical trial. Ann Intern Med 93:391, 1980
35. Ashutosh K, Mead G, Dunsky M: Early effects of oxygen administration and prognosis in chronic obstructive pulmonary disease and cor pulmonale. Am Rev Respir Dis 127:399, 1983
36. Weisse AB, Moschas CB, Frank MJ et al: Hemodynamic effects of staged hematocrit reduction in patients with stable cor pulmonale and severely elevated hematocrit levels. Am J Med 58:92, 1975
37. Hermiller JB, Bambach D, Thompson MJ et al: Vasodilators and prostaglandin inhibitors in primary pulmonary hypertension. Ann Intern Med 97:480, 1982
38. Rich S, Martinez J, Lamb W et al: Reassessment of the effects of vasodilator drugs in primary pulmonary hypertension: Guidelines to determining a vasodilator response. Am Heart J 105:119, 1983
39. Reitz BA, Wallwork JL, Hunt SA et al: Heart-lung transplantation: Successful therapy for patients with pulmonary vascular disease. N Engl J Med 306:557, 1982
40. The Urokinase Pulmonary Embolism Trial. Circulation (Suppl 2) 47:1, 1973
41. Alpert JS, Smith R, Carlson J et al: Mortality in patients treated for pulmonary embolism. JAMA 236:1477, 1976
42. Stein M, Levy SE: Reflex and humoral responses to pulmonary embolism. Prog Cardiovasc Dis 17:167, 1974
43. McIntyre KM, Sasahara AA: Hemodynamic and ventricular responses to pulmonary embolism. Prog Cardiovasc Dis 17:175, 1974
44. Alpert JS, Godtfredsen J, Ockene IS et al: Pulmonary hypertension secondary to minor pulmonary embolism. Chest 73:795, 1978
45. Bell WR, Simon TL, DeMets DL: The clinical features of submassive and massive pulmonary embolism. Am J Med 62:355, 1977
46. Moses DC, Silver TM, Bookstein JJ: The complementary roles of chest radiography, lung scanning, and selective pulmonary angiography in the diagnosis of pulmonary emboli. Circ Res 49:179, 1974
47. Dalen JE, Haffajee CI, Alpert JS et al: Pulmonary embolism, pulmonary hemorrhage, and pulmonary infarction. N Engl J Med 272:1278, 1965
48. Paraskos JA, Adelstein SJ, Smith RE et al: Late prognosis of acute pulmonary embolism. N Engl J Med 289:55, 1973

49. Freiman DG, Suyemoto J, Wessler S: Frequency of pulmonary thromboembolism in man. N Engl J Med 272:1278, 1965
50. Jeffrey PC, Immelman EJ, Banatar SR: Deep-vein thrombosis and pulmonary embolism: An assessment of the accuracy of clinical diagnosis. S Afr Med J 57:643, 1980
51. Sasahara AA, Sharma GVRK, Parisi AF: New developments in the detection and prevention of venous thromboembolism. Am J Cardiol 43:1214, 1979
52. Sevitt S, Gallagher N: Venous thrombosis and pulmonary embolism: A clinico-pathological study in injured and burned patients. Br J Surg 48:475, 1961
53. Virchow R: Cellular Pathology. London, Churchill, 1860
54. Schafer AI: The hypercoagulable states. Ann Intern Med 102:814, 1985
55. Hunter JH, Ferrech A, Ridley W et al: Familial antithrombin III deficiency. Q J Med 51:373, 1982
56. Gore JM, Appelbaum JS, Greene HL et al: Association between pulmonary embolism and occult malignancy. Ann Intern Med 96:556, 1982
57. Hull RD, Hirsh J, Carter CJ et al: Pulmonary angiography, ventilation lung scanning, and venography for clinically suspected pulmonary embolism with abnormal perfusion lung scan. Ann Intern Med 98:891, 1983
58. Sandler DA, Martin JF: Liquid crystal thermography as a screening test for deep vein thrombosis. Lancet 1:665, 1985
59. Szucs MM, Brooks HL, Grossman W et al: Diagnostic sensitivity of laboratory findings in acute pulmonary embolism. Ann Intern Med 74:161, 1971
60. Menzoian JO, Williams LF: Is pulmonary angiography essential for the diagnosis of acute pulmonary embolism? Am J Surg 137:543, 1979
61. Lippmann ML, Fein A: Pulmonary embolism in the patient with chronic obstructive pulmonary disease: A diagnostic dilemma. Chest 79:39, 1981
62. Lippmann ML, Morgan L, Fein A et al: Plasma and serum concentrations of DNA in pulmonary thromboembolism. Am Rev Respir Dis 125:416, 1982
63. Stein PD, Dalen JE, McIntyre KM et al: The electrocardiogram in acute pulmonary embolism. Prog Cardiovasc Dis 17:247, 1975
64. McNeil BJ: Ventilation-perfusion studies and the diagnosis of pulmonary embolism: Concise communication. J Nucl Med 21:319, 1980
65. Cheeley R, McCartney WH, Perry JR et al: The role of noninvasive tests versus pulmonary angiography in the diagnosis of pulmonary embolism. Am J Med 70:17, 1981
66. Dalen JE, Brooks HL, Johnson LW et al: Pulmonary angiography in acute pulmonary embolism: Indications, techniques, and results in 367 patients. Am Heart J 81:175, 1971
67. Benotti JR, Alpert JS, Dalen JE: Balloon occlusion pulmonary arteriography in the diagnosis of pulmonary embolism. Cathet Cardiovasc Diagn 10:519, 1984
68. Goodman PC, Zawadzki MB: Digital subtraction pulmonary angiography. Am J Radiol 139:305, 1982
69. Holford CP: Gradual compression for preventing deep venous thrombosis. Br Med J 2:969, 1976
70. Törngren S: Low dose heparin and compression stockings in the prevention of post-operative deep venous thrombosis. Br J Surg 67:482, 1980
71. Wessler S, Gitel SN: Low dose heparin: Is the risk worth the benefit? Am Heart J 98:94, 1979
72. Warlow C, Beattie AG, Terry G et al: A double blind trial of low dose of subcutaneous heparin in the prevention of deep vein thrombosis after myocardial infarction. Lancet 2:934, 1973
73. Halkin H, Goldberg J, Modan M et al: Reduction of mortality in general medical in-patients by low-dose heparin prophylaxis. Ann Intern Med 96:561, 1982
74. Leyvraz PF, Richard J, Bachmann F et al: Adjusted versus fixed-dose subcutaneous heparin in the prevention of deep-vein thrombosis after total hip replacement. N Engl J Med 309:954, 1983
75. Francis CW, Marder VJ, Evarts CM et al: Two-step warfarin therapy: Prevention of post-operative venous thrombosis without excessive bleeding. JAMA 249:374, 1983
76. Nelson PH, Moser KM, Stoner C et al: Risk of complications during intravenous heparin therapy. West J Med 136:189, 1982
77. Hull R, Delmore T, Genton E et al: Warfarin sodium versus low-dose heparin in the long-term treatment of venous thrombosis. N Engl J Med 301:855, 1979
78. Bynum LJ, Wilson JE: Low-dose heparin therapy in the long-term management of venous thromboembolism. Am J Med 67:553, 1979
79. Hull R, Delmore T, Carter C et al: Adjusted subcutaneous heparin versus warfarin sodium in the long-term treatment of venous thrombosis. N Engl J Med 306:189, 1982
80. Bomalaski JS, Martin GJ, Hughes RL et al: Inferior vena cava interruption in the management of pulmonary embolism. Chest 82:767, 1982
81. Urokinase-Streptokinase Embolism Trial: Phase 2 results: A cooperative study. JAMA 229:1600, 1974
82. Sharma GVRK, Burleson VA, Sasahara AA: Effect of thrombolytic therapy on pulmonary-capillary blood volume in patients with pulmonary embolism. N Engl J Med 303:842, 1980
83. Sasahara AA, Sharma GVRK, Tow DE et al: Clinical use of thrombolytic agents in venous thromboembolism. Arch Intern Med 142:684, 1982
84. Johansson L, Nylander G, Hedner U et al: Comparison of streptokinase with heparin: Late results in the treatment of deep venous thrombosis. Acta Med Scand 206:93, 1979
85. Watz R, Savidge GF: Rapid thrombolysis and preservation of valvular venous function in high deep vein thrombosis. Acta Med Scand 205:293, 1979
86. The TIMI Study Group: Special Report: The thrombolysis in myocardial infarction (TIMI) trial. N Engl J Med 312:932, 1985
87. Satter P: Pulmonary embolectomy: Indications and results. Eur Soc Cardiovasc Radiol 23:321, 1979
88. Heitala SO, Greenfield LJ: Percutaneous pulmonary embolectomy by the transvenous route. Eur Soc Cardiovasc Radiol 23:325, 1979
89. Greenfield LJ, Zocco JJ: Intraluminal management of acute massive pulmonary thromboembolism. J Thorac Cardiovasc Surg 77:402, 1979
90. Daily PO, Johnston GG, Simmons CJ et al: Surgical management of chronic pulmonary embolism. J Thorac Cardiovasc Surg 79:523, 1980

MYOCARDITIS

George Cherian ▪ M. Thomas Abraham

CHAPTER 95
VOLUME 2

Myocarditis is a focal or diffuse involvement of the heart muscle in an inflammatory process. It can result from a variety of common or rare infections, drugs, chemicals, or physical agents. The clinical picture generally depends on the location, extent, and rapidity of cardiac involvement. Focal involvement is usually subclinical unless an important area such as the conduction system is involved. Diffuse myocarditis also may be subclinical or may result in cardiac manifestations and heart failure of varying severity. Thus myocarditis, while often subclinical, can be the cause of electrocardiographic abnormalities, cardiomegaly, dysrhythmias, heart failure, or sudden death. There has been a resurgence of interest in myocarditis, which may be attributed to two observations. First, endomyocardial biopsy has shown an inflammatory infiltrate in a proportion of patients who present with unexplained severe heart failure, some of whom respond to immunosuppressive drug therapy.[1-4] This has necessitated a better understanding of the pathologic features of myocarditis. Second, it is being recognized that acute myocarditis can at times closely mimic myocardial infarction.[5,6]

VIRAL MYOCARDITIS
PATHOLOGY

The gross appearance of the heart and the inflammatory response are usually nonspecific and do not often allow an etiologic diagnosis. Thus the gross appearance may be similar in acute viral myocarditis and in toxic drug-induced myocarditis. It is not clear why there is predominant involvement of the heart muscle in some patients and of the pericardium in others.

A wide variety of viruses and viral diseases can result in myocarditis (Table 95.1). Coxsackievirus B is the most frequent cause of human myocarditis, while many of the other causes listed are rare. A few of the more important causes are discussed in greater detail later in this chapter.

MORPHOLOGIC FEATURES

The pathologic changes generally depend on the duration of the process. The lesions may involve not only the interstitium and cardiac muscle but also specialized tissue such as the conduction system. In adults, a fulminant course is rare, but when death occurs in a few days, the heart may appear to be entirely normal or may be flabby and slightly dilated with areas of subendocardial or intramyocardial hemorrhage. Areas of necrosis simulating myocardial infarction may be seen.[7] There is extensive cellular infiltration with marked destruction of myocardial cells. Acute inflammatory cells composed of polymorphonuclear leukocytes are uncommon in adults. At times the virus can be cultured from the myocardium.[8]

In the more common presentation, death following viral myocarditis occurs a few months or even 1 to 2 years after the initial infection. By this time there is marked dilatation of the cardiac chambers, varying degrees of left ventricular hypertrophy, and areas of endocardial thickening. The muscle is firm, and the cut surface shows strands of grayish fibrous tissue. Thickening of mitral valve leaflets and shortening of the chordae tendineae have been observed.[9] Thrombi in the atria and ventricles are less frequent than in dilated cardiomyopathy.[7] The inflammatory infiltrate is of the monocellular type, mainly with lymphocytes.[1,3,7,10]

TABLE 95.1 VIRUSES CAUSING MYOCARDITIS*

"Common" Agents	Uncommon Associations	Rare Associations
Coxsackievirus A	Infectious mononucleosis	Adenovirus
Coxsackievirus B†	Influenza	Arbovirus A (chikungunya)
Echovirus	Mumps	Arbovirus B (dengue)
	Mycoplasma pneumoniae‡	Cytomegalovirus
	Poliomyelitis	Herpes simplex
	Psittacosis (ornithosis)‡	Herpes zoster
	Rubella (German measles)	Rabies
	Viral hepatitis	Respiratory syncytial virus
		Rubeola (measles)
		Vaccinia
		Varicella (chickenpox)
		Variola (smallpox)
		Yellow fever

* Alphabetical listing. In most instances the myocarditis is subclinical. In some diseases histologic incidence is high in fatal cases. The rare causes are seldom of clinical significance.

† Accounts for about 50% of all cases.

‡ Classified here under viruses.

Viral myocarditis can cause transmural right and left ventricular necrosis without coronary narrowing.[6,11] Severe perimyocarditis in mice due to coxsackievirus infection can be limited to the right ventricle,[12] and left ventricular aneurysms have also been reported.[13]

Little is known about viral myocarditis in the fetus. Neonatal infections are widely disseminated, carry a high mortality, and seldom last more than 2 weeks; the changes at autopsy depend on the duration of the illness.[10]

PATHOGENESIS OF VIRAL MYOCARDITIS

Myofiber damage may be due to direct virus-mediated destruction and through immunologic cell-mediated mechanisms. B-cell responsiveness determines the capability to terminate viral replication, whereas T cells influence the severity of inflammation and myofiber injury.[10]

DIRECT DESTRUCTION. In the animal model, viruses can produce an early direct lysis of myocardial cells. Necrotic areas can develop before an inflammatory infiltrate is seen and in some areas without such a reaction. There are also areas of extensive necrosis without inflammation in immunosuppressed mice.[10]

CELL-MEDIATED DESTRUCTION. There is evidence in mice that myofiber damage can also result from a T cell–mediated reaction, and although several mechanisms are possible, cytotoxicity of T cells is the most likely.[10] Wong and co-workers[14] found virus-specific cytotoxic effector cells in the spleen of mice 7 days after infection with coxsackievirus B3. Coxsackievirus-infected myofibers were susceptible to destruction by the immune spleen cells. Other studies have shown that uninfected myocardial cells and fibroblasts can also be lysed *in vitro* by spleen cells. Thus, in mice, following a coxsackievirus B infection there is a cell-mediated immune response with the production of cytotoxic T cells. These have the capacity to damage both infected and uninfected myofibers. The nature of the antigen in the infected myofibers that is recognized by the effector T cells is not known. Studies indicate that the inoculation of mice with coxsackievirus B3 results in the appearance of new antigen(s) in cardiac tissue.[15]

HUMAN MYOCARDITIS. In one report, 10 patients with coxsackievirus B3/4, 4 with influenza, 4 with mumps, and 15 with cytomegalovirus (CMV) myocarditis were studied.[16] With the use of indirect immunofluorescent techniques, muscle-specific antisarcolemmal antibodies of the antimyolemmal type were found in 9 of the 10 patients with coxsackievirus B and in all with influenza and mumps myocarditis. By contrast, 13 of the 15 patients with CMV myocarditis lacked this antibody. Lymphocyte-mediated cytotoxicity against heterologous cardiac target cells was not observed.

Suppressor cell activity of patients with myocarditis has been shown to be significantly reduced, as is also true in some healthy controls.[17] There can be several explanations for this, as in some diseases such as systemic lupus erythematosus, in which serum factors can also lead to a reduced function of the suppressor compartment.[17]

It would appear that in coxsackievirus B myocarditis (and presumably with other viruses) there is an initial phase of direct virus-induced destruction of the myocardial fiber modified by the humoral immune system. This is followed by a T cell–mediated cytotoxic reaction probably in response to new antigen(s) in the myocardium. This cytotoxic reaction can affect both infected and noninfected myocardial cells.

DIAGNOSIS OF ACTIVE MYOCARDITIS BASED ON ENDOMYOCARDIAL BIOPSY

Multiple biopsies have shown concordance in histology obtained by biopsy and at autopsy, although sampling errors can occur.[3,18] The significance of inflammatory cells without evidence of necrosis is not clear. The morphologic criteria for the diagnosis of myocarditis depend on the following:

1. Evidence of recent damage to myocardial fibers manifested as myofibrillar degeneration, myocytolysis, or coagulative necrosis. Contraction band necrosis may occur but is frequently the result of handling of the biopsy specimen.
2. Inflammatory cells are present, especially in close relation to the damaged myocardial fibers. The value of quantification of the number of cells is debatable.[1,3,4,18] In areas of recent damage, neutrophils predominate to be later replaced by lymphocytes, macrophages, and plasma cells.
3. Evidence of repair is indicative of myocardial damage and is shown by the presence of granulation and young or mature scar tissue. This, too, is generally focal in distribution in keeping with the pattern of cell damage.
4. Other important changes include alteration in blood vessels, such as endothelial hyperplasia, minimal hemorrhages, or leakage of fibrin/fibrinogen.

Immunohistochemistry (to demonstrate B and T lymphocytes, T suppressive/cytotoxic cells, fibrin/fibrinogen, and immunoglobulin binding on muscle fibers) and ultrastructural studies (demonstration of viruses, structural myocardial fiber changes) have been used, but the mainstay of diagnosis at present is conventional light microscopy.

CLINICAL FEATURES

The spectrum of acute myocarditis is wide and varied (Table 95.2). At autopsy, evidence of myocarditis may be an incidental, noncontributory finding following an infective illness or may provide the only clue to an unexpected, sudden death. More commonly, electrocardiographic or chest film abnormalities may be detected during the routine evaluation in an infectious illness. In other patients there are cardiac symptoms and signs of varying severity.[19]

PRECEDING OR ACCOMPANYING VIRAL INFECTION

Although diseases such as mumps are obvious, others require a careful history, meticulous clinical examination, and related laboratory tests. With diseases such as coxsackievirus infection and related infections, there may be fever, sore throat, "common cold," cough, pleurodynia,

TABLE 95.2 SPECTRUM OF ACUTE MYOCARDITIS

Subclinical	Clinical
Abnormal electrocardiogram	Palpitation, tachycardia
Abnormal chest film	Arrhythmia, conduction defects
Unexpected sudden death	Chest pain: pleuropericardial, vague, ischemic
Noncontributory autopsy finding	Dyspnea, heart failure
	Fulminant heart failure
	Collapse: heart block, tamponade, shock
	Embolism: systemic, pulmonary
	Mitral ± tricuspid valvar regurgitation
	Chronic severe heart failure–chronic active myocarditis

abdominal pain, nausea, vomiting, diarrhea, or features of bronchitis or pneumonia. In one series, with myopericarditis due to coxsackievirus, 40% of patients had arthralgia and 60% had myalgia.[20] Fever, usually moderate, was present in 59% of patients, and 36% had a flulike illness. About 10% of patients had shotty lymphadenopathy (usually cervical and axillary), rash (most often morbilliform), orchitis, pneumonia, and pleural effusion. Phlebitis, hepatitis, nephritis, and encephalomyelitis each had an incidence of about 5%.[20] In another report, electrocardiographic changes of symptomless myocarditis were found in about one third of the young patients with influenza and echovirus infection who had severe myalgia at the onset of the illness.[10]

HEART RATE AND RHYTHM

Tachycardia disproportionate to the fever and palpitation may be the first indications of myocarditis. Various arrhythmias and conduction disturbances, some of little or no hemodynamic consequence and others causing a fatal outcome, may be present. These are outlined below under electrocardiographic changes. Ventricular premature beats are the most frequent abnormality and may be present in about one third of the patients during routine evaluation.[19] Rarely a dysrhythmic form of myocarditis is seen in which multiple, mixed, complex atrial and ventricular arrhythmias may be the only manifestation. This may require combination drug therapy.

CHEST PAIN

Chest pain is found in about two thirds of patients with viral myopericarditis and is present also in those without evidence of pericarditis. This pain may be pericardial, pleuropericardial, vague, or infrequently typical of myocardial ischemia and may even be associated with sweating, nausea, and vomiting (see discussion on differentiation from acute myocardial infarction). A pericardial rub is heard in about one third of patients.[21]

DYSPNEA AND HEART FAILURE

In the presence of lung involvement as in infection with *Mycoplasma pneumoniae,* the appearance or worsening of dyspnea may be due to myocarditis. The severity of heart failure varies. The cardiac impulse is displaced to the left, and careful inspection will reveal abnormal precordial pulsations at and medial to the apex. Such pulsations are often not palpable. Despite the tachycardia, the S_1 is muffled. A loud S_3 gallop is present. In a proportion of patients with more extensive cardiac enlargement, a soft apical systolic murmur may be heard. This is more often not pansystolic but the result of mitral regurgitation due to cardiac dilatation. In some, the murmur is typical of mitral regurgitation and may be difficult to distinguish from that of primary valvular regurgitation (see section on valvular regurgitation). In patients who have severe congestive heart failure, signs of tricuspid regurgitation may be present. The diastolic murmur of aortic regurgitation is not well documented, but this can conceivably occur, since viral antigens have been demonstrated in the aortic valve. In children, right-sided heart failure predominates with periorbital and peripheral edema, while in adults peripheral edema is rare. Complete recovery without residual changes demonstrated on the chest film or electrocardiogram is possible even in severe cases.[22]

FULMINANT HEART FAILURE

Coxsackievirus infection in the newborn is often rapidly fatal, and a similar course has been reported following echovirus infection.[9] The virus is often recovered from the myocardium. A rapidly progressive fulminant course is rare in adults but is well documented in myocarditis due to coxsackievirus[22] and other viruses such as influenza A.[8] Hemodynamic data are scarce. In one such instance the mean pulmonary capillary wedge pressure was 17 mm Hg to 20 mm Hg, mean right atrial pressure was 19 to 20 mm Hg, and the cardiac index was 1.17 to 1.47 liters/min/M2. There was no pericardial effusion.[8]

CIRCULATORY COLLAPSE

Occasionally circulatory collapse may result from complete atrioventricular block, ventricular tachycardia, or associated cardiac tamponade. Cardiogenic shock due to ventricular dilatation following aspiration of a large pericardial effusion has been reported in a patient with infective myocarditis.[23]

SUDDEN DEATH

Myocarditis is a cause of unexpected sudden death presumed to be due to a focal lesion causing a fatal ventricular arrhythmia. In one series, myocarditis accounted for 14% of unexpected sudden deaths. In another report, 17% of children through the age of 16 had died in this way and 53% were under 1 year of age.[9]

EMBOLISM

Systemic and pulmonary emboli have been reported in myocarditis and may be the presenting feature.

MITRAL AND TRICUSPID VALVULAR REGURGITATION

Patients with myocarditis in severe heart failure can present with mitral and tricuspid regurgitation.[21,22] The findings of mitral regurgitation can closely mimic those of primary valvular regurgitation.

ACUTE MYOCARDITIS MIMICKING MYOCARDIAL INFARCTION

Acute myocarditis can occasionally result in necrosis of significant regional segments of the myocardium with precordial pain, Q wave and ST-T wave changes on the electrocardiogram, rise in cardiac enzymes, and wall motion abnormalities with normal coronary arteries[5,24] and thus closely resemble acute myocardial infarction. We believe that acute myocarditis, particularly in young patients, is at times mistaken for acute myocardial infarction, and an awareness of this type of presentation is essential. One prospective study of 105 patients with acute myocardial infarction and controls matched for age and sex and living in the same geographic area showed no statistically valid association between virus infection and acute myocardial infarction.[25]

The presentation is usually in individuals who were previously healthy and has been well described in two reports.[5,24] The chest pain and electrocardiogram were typical of transmural acute myocardial infarction, and the cardiac enzyme levels were elevated. In the first patient a technetium-99m pyrophosphate scan done on the third hospital day showed intense uptake in the inferolateral wall of the left ventricle. In the second patient, two-dimensional echocardiography on the second day showed akinesis of the posterior, inferior, and anterolateral walls and apex. There was no pericardial effusion. Both patients had normal coronary arteries, and in one who had had an ergonovine injection there was no coronary spasm. Transmural right and left ventricular myocardial necrosis and scarring without significant coronary artery disease occurred in a 38-year-old man in whom coxsackievirus B1 antibodies were demonstrated.[6]

During acute myocarditis the electrocardiogram may show a pattern of transmural myocardial infarction with or without chest pain. Abnormal Q waves with poor R wave progression and elevation of the ST segment were found in 73% of patients with infective myocarditis who at admission were in congestive heart failure or shock.[26] The pain can be typical of acute myocardial infarction, including character, site, and radiation.[5] The peak levels of creatine kinase MB fraction (CKMB) may be higher and persist longer following acute myocarditis when compared with acute myocardial infarction.[27] This finding needs to be validated in a larger group of patients. The clinical pointers that are helpful in distinguishing acute myocarditis producing segmental necrosis from acute myocardial infarction due to coronary artery disease are outlined in Table 95.3.

NEONATAL MYOCARDITIS

In coxsackievirus infection in the newborn the onset may be sudden, with several newborns infected in the nursery, during the first 8 or 9 days of life. There may be preceding diarrhea. There is often lethargy, pallor, and at times mild cyanosis. The disease is often fatal; cyanosis with dyspnea and tachycardia are ominous signs. There may be circulatory collapse and systemic involvement of the central nervous system, liver, and kidneys.[20] There is usually cardiomegaly and liver enlargement. Fleeting systolic murmurs may be heard. The electrocardiogram shows ST-T changes and conduction abnormalities. Fever and circulatory collapse are prominent with echovirus infection.[9]

LABORATORY INVESTIGATIONS
DIAGNOSIS OF VIRAL DISEASE

When patients are first seen, throat swabs or washings and fecal or rectal swabs can be taken for tissue culture. Any infected tissue or pericardial fluid if aspirated should also be cultured. Paired sera should be drawn 2 weeks apart to detect a rise in antibody titer.

In general, virus can be isolated only if specimens are obtained during the first few days of the illness. Isolation from noncardiac tissue does not always mean that the virus was involved in the myocarditis. Tissue examination with light or electron microscopy may reveal characteristic changes in some diseases (*e.g.*, rabies). Viral antigens may be found in tissue, but nonspecific immunofluorescence can vitiate the results.

The clinical diagnosis usually depends on the detection of significant antibody titers. Ordinarily antibodies are not found until about 1 week after the onset of the illness. The early IgM antibody levels peak in 2 to 3 weeks and are later undetectable. IgG antibody peaks later and is the major component after the first month; it may be present for months or years.[28] The immunoglobulin class is thus of some help in determining the duration of the disease process.

The commonly used tests have included the detection and quantitation of complement-fixing, hemagglutination inhibiting, or neutralizing antibody in paired acute (less than 1 week) and convalescent (2 weeks or longer) sera. At least a fourfold rise indicates a recent infection. In general, the complement-fixing antibodies disappear in several weeks, while neutralizing antibodies persist for months to years.[28] The specificity of antibodies also varies greatly. For example the complement-fixing antibodies to coxsackievirus B lack specificity.[10] Newer radioimmunoassay and enzyme-linked immunosorbent assay (ELISA) procedures are useful in rapid identification, and polyvalent reagents can be used.

LABORATORY DATA

Slight to moderate leukocytosis with a neutrophil response is seen in about half the patients. The erythrocyte sedimentation rate is elevated in about 70% and rarely may exceed 80 mm/hr.[20] Changes in cardiac enzymes generally reflect the extent of cardiac damage. The pattern of enzyme elevation may be more prolonged, and this finding warrants further observations. There may be laboratory evidence of involvement of other organs such as the liver or kidneys or of the central nervous system.

CHEST FILM

Cardiac enlargement depends on the presence and severity of heart failure and of a pericardial effusion. In patients with moderate or severe myocarditis in heart failure there is generalized cardiomegaly with or without pulmonary venous congestion. Rarely, frank pulmonary edema may be found, and in a few patients there may be patchy pulmonary infiltration. There is only mild left atrial enlargement with congestive heart failure.

TABLE 95.3 DIFFERENTIATION OF ACUTE MYOCARDITIS MIMICKING ACUTE MYOCARDIAL INFARCTION

	Acute Myocarditis	Acute Myocardial Infarction
Age group	Also in children, adolescents, and young adults; common even under 30 years	Usually >40 years
Prior health	Usually normal	May have angina or predisposing diseases
Viral illness	Present	Absent
Chest pain	May be typical or absent; often atypical	Often typical
Multiorgan involvement	May be present	Absent
Pericardial effusion	Echo detected effusions in about one third Pericardial rub may persist for 7–10 days	Variable incidence Unusual for rub to persist
Electrocardiogram	Can be typical of acute myocardial infarction; changes tend to improve or disappear	Abnormalities tend to persist; normalization rare
Cardiac enzymes	CKMB values may be higher and persist longer	CKMB tends to rise early and disappear in 48 to 72 h
Cardiogenic shock	Uncommon	In 10% to 15%
Regional wall motion abnormalities	May be present, usually not persistent	Persist
Technetium scan	May be abnormal; abnormality may persist	Abnormal; not persistent
Convalescent exercise electrocardiogram	Normal	Often ischemic changes
Coronary angiography	Normal coronary arteries	Significant coronary artery disease
Late left ventricular angiography	Minimal wall motion abnormalities or normal	Significant wall motion abnormalities
Long-term prognosis	Good	Variable

ELECTROCARDIOGRAM

Electrocardiographic abnormalities are the mainstay in the diagnosis of myocarditis in asymptomatic patients. In the acute stage the electrocardiogram is always abnormal.[19,20] There is elevation of the ST segment with inversion or flattening of the T wave. The QT_c interval may be prolonged. The ST segment returns to the baseline in a few days, but the T wave changes may remain for weeks or months following severe myocarditis. Electrocardiographic changes usually resolve over a period of time. Transient abnormal Q waves or the pattern of myocardial infarction is occasionally seen.

Arrhythmias are present in about a third of patients, and most frequently these are ventricular premature beats, although ventricular tachycardia, ventricular fibrillation, atrial premature beats, atrial fibrillation, atrial flutter, and supraventricular tachycardia have all been reported. Bundle branch block and varying degrees of atrioventricular block may occur and, although usually transient, permanent complete atrioventricular block has been reported. In an elegant study on embryonic heart cell aggregates, Shrier and co-workers[29] have shown alterations in electrical parameters of heart cells following herpes simplex virus inoculation.

ECHOCARDIOGRAPHY

Echocardiography is valuable in the diagnosis and evaluation of myocarditis. Nieminen and associates have reported on serial echocardiographic observations in 68 consecutive patients with acute infectious myocarditis.[11] Those with mild myocarditis had only electrocardiographic abnormalities, those with moderate disease had abnormal precordial pulsations with a loud S_3 gallop, and those with severe myocarditis were in congestive heart failure. Wall motion abnormalities were present in all of the patients. With mild disease there was segmental hypokinesia, while with moderate myocarditis there was akinesia as well and the changes were more widespread. Patients in congestive heart failure had even more extensive akinetic or hypokinetic segments and at times dyskinesia. Patients with mild myocarditis showed no difference in the left ventricular diastolic diameter (LVIDd), left ventricular systolic diameter (LVIDs), or ejection fraction (EF), when compared with controls. There was an increase in the LVIDd and LVIDs measurements and a fall in the EF in both the moderate and severe group. The LVIDs was 55 ± 3 mm and the EF was $33 \pm 9\%$ in the severe group. In general, the site of the wall motion abnormalities correlated with the location of the T wave changes. Reversible transient "hypertrophy" has also been reported during acute myocarditis. This may be related to myocardial edema.

NUCLEAR IMAGING

TECHNETIUM-99m PYROPHOSPHATE SCAN. Technetium-99m pyrophosphate could be useful in the diagnosis of acute myocarditis since it is avidly taken up by the necrotic myocardium whether the necrosis is due to myocarditis or infarction,[5,12] and in pericarditis it is more likely to be positive at the time of ST segment elevation.[30] In experimental studies on mice, the maximum uptake is at about the seventh day, after which it generally fades.[11] In a patient with infective myocarditis admitted in cardiogenic shock, the scan was positive on the eighth hospital day and repeated studies showed persistence over the following 3½ years.[30]

GALLIUM-67 CITRATE SCAN. Myocardial gallium-67 uptake has been reported in some patients presenting with dilated cardiomyopathy[31] and in others with an inflammatory infiltrate on endomyocardial biopsy[32]; there was a response to immunosuppressive therapy in both groups. In the latter report the technetium-99m scan was negative.[32]

MYOSIN-SPECIFIC ANTIBODY. Radiolabeled antibody against cardiac myosin and antibody fragments (Fab[1,2]) specific for cardiac myosin have been used to image regions of necrosis following acute myocardial infarction.[33] Myosin-specific antibody has been found useful in differentiating between myocarditis and dilated cardiomyopathy.[34]

SEQUELAE AND FOLLOW-UP

The sequelae and follow-up depend on the severity of the initial myocarditis, persistence of cardiac failure, or presence of left ventricular dilatation or life-threatening ventricular arrhythmias.[35,36] Thus, of 20 patients who were admitted in cardiac failure or with cardiac enlargement, 10% died of heart failure; 63% with a left ventricular end-diastolic diameter greater than 5 mm on follow-up had life-threatening ventricular arrhythmias on ambulatory monitoring.[36] In another series, reduced work capacity was found in 40%.[21]

DEATH

Viral myocarditis is generally a mild benign disease ending in complete recovery. In newborns, however, mortality is high and may be about 50%.[10] Mortality may be as high as 33% in patients with congestive heart failure.[26] Death has been recorded due to viral myocarditis caused by adenovirus, coxsackieviruses A and B, hepatitis, infectious mononucleosis, influenza, mumps, poliomyelitis, rabies, smallpox, vaccinia, and varicella.[10] Undiagnosed myocarditis has been the cause in 14% to 17% of unexpected sudden deaths.[9]

CHRONIC HEART FAILURE

Persistent heart failure, which becomes progressively refractory to treatment, can follow acute myocarditis in about 20% of patients.[21,36] A proportion of patients with chronic heart failure show histologic evidence of an active inflammatory infiltrate, and some respond to immunosuppressive therapy.[1,4] Others progress to a clinical picture often indistinguishable from that of end-stage dilated cardiomyopathy. There are no well-documented reports of a subset of patients with proved acute myocarditis who "recovered" to a clinically normal state and later presented with dilated cardiomyopathy.

ARRHYTHMIAS

There are few studies on the follow-up of myocarditis using ambulatory monitoring. Eighteen such patients with severe myocarditis were followed for 49.1 ± 39.3 months, and five (28%) had ventricular tachycardia or coupled and multifocal ventricular premature beats.[36] Four of the five patients had an increased cardiothoracic ratio or left ventricular dilatation on echocardiography.

VENTRICULAR ANEURYSM

In acute myocarditis there are wall motion abnormalities[11] and at times transmural necrosis and scarring.[6] Ventricular aneurysms have been reported in experimental animals[13] and following rubella.[10] We have studied a 28-year-old patient who, following a flulike illness, presented with repeated episodes of ventricular tachycardia, left ventricular aneurysm, and normal coronary arteries.

CARDIOMEGALY

Cardiac enlargement may persist after acute myocarditis in 14% to 20% of patients with or without cardiac symptoms.[21]

PERSISTING ELECTROCARDIOGRAPHIC ABNORMALITIES

Persistence of electrocardiographic abnormalities is related to the severity of the myocarditis. T wave abnormalities were found during a 5-year follow-up in 21% to 27% of patients with past symptomatic myocarditis.[21] In a report from Japan, 13 patients who were all in congestive heart failure during the acute stage were followed for 5 years.[26] Of the nine patients with conduction abnormalities, atrioventricular block persisted in 40%; there was incomplete regression of right bundle branch block and fascicular block in four (44%), and return to normal in only three (33%). In 4 other patients who showed an infarct pattern with abnormal Q waves, poor R wave progression, and ST segment elevation, the electrocardiogram became normal in 2 months.

RECURRENT MYOPERICARDITIS
Myopericarditis due to coxsackievirus (and presumably others) can be complicated by recurrences over a period as long as 2 years and has been reported in 17% of patients in one series.[21]

CONSTRICTIVE PERICARDITIS
Constrictive pericarditis has been reported following coxsackievirus B infection and infectious mononucleosis and could occur with other viral diseases as well. Constriction may develop within months to years following the initial episode.

FOLLOW-UP CARE
Some patients with severe myocarditis and cardiac failure, particularly those with residual left ventricular dysfunction, may have serious arrhythmias and be at risk of sudden death. Such patients require ambulatory electrocardiographic monitoring and appropriate antiarrhythmic drugs.

DIFFERENTIAL DIAGNOSIS
The diagnosis of subclinical myocarditis requires an awareness of the association of myocarditis with certain infections and diseases. Most often in such cases the diagnosis is based on electrocardiographic changes. Differentiation of myocarditis from other conditions that present with cardiac failure, mitral regurgitation with or without tricuspid regurgitation, pericardial effusion, and ischemic chest pain is not always easy.

CARDIAC FAILURE IN INFANCY
In infants seen in cardiac failure, myocarditis must be distinguished from endocardial fibroelastosis, anomalous origin of left coronary artery, and glycogen storage disease. Endocardial fibroelastosis is characteristically associated with a marked increase in voltage, often with deep T wave inversion over the left chest leads in about 90% of patients. The apparent fall in the incidence of endocardial fibroelastosis and the epidemiologic, histologic, and viral studies suggest a possible role for viruses in the etiopathogenesis of this disorder. Anomalous origin of the left coronary artery is typically associated with an anterolateral infarct pattern on the electrocardiogram. In glycogen storage disease there is often generalized muscular weakness and macroglossia. The ventricular walls are thick on echocardiography, and the left ventricular cavity is small. The electrocardiogram usually shows left ventricular hypertrophy with strain pattern.

RHEUMATIC CARDITIS
Cardiomegaly, cardiac failure, or a pericardial rub does not occur in rheumatic carditis without a significant cardiac murmur, while in viral myocarditis all three singly or in combination are often present without any murmur. Arthralgia, and at times arthritis, may be present with viral fevers.[20] The murmur of aortic regurgitation and the soft mitral mid-diastolic Carey-Coombs murmur are not found in viral myocarditis. In viral myocarditis the murmur of mitral regurgitation when present is always associated with significant cardiomegaly, is less intense, and often decreases with vigorous diuretic therapy.

MITRAL REGURGITATION
Patients with myocarditis in whom the acute phase is missed can present in severe cardiac failure with signs of mitral regurgitation with or without tricuspid regurgitation. Such patients resemble others with primary valvular regurgitation as in chronic rheumatic heart disease. In rheumatic mitral regurgitation the degree of left atrial enlargement is greater and calcification of the valve may be present. Perhaps the most useful point is a significant decrease in the mitral murmur with a decrease in heart size following vigorous medical therapy in myocarditis.

PERICARDIAL EFFUSION
A pericardial effusion may mask the presence of associated myocarditis and its severity.[23] The increased movement of the heart within a moderate or large pericardial effusion may be mistaken on echocardiography for good contractions.[23] The elevated jugular venous pressure, tachycardia, hypotension, and cardiomegaly could be due in part to the myocarditis. Pulsus alternans is not found with pericardial effusion. The presence of an atrial gallop or a ventricular gallop favors myocarditis. Cardiac enzymes are often elevated in pericardial effusion as well.[27]

DILATED CARDIOMYOPATHY
The diagnosis of an antecedent and continuing myocarditis needs to be considered in patients presenting with dilated cardiomyopathy. A history of a viral or related illness, laboratory evidence for the same, and a brief illness would favor the diagnosis of myocarditis. The presence of an inflammatory infiltrate on cardiac biopsy suggests the diagnosis of chronic active myocarditis. End-stage dilated cardiomyopathy may be indistinguishable from the intractable failure of longstanding myocarditis.

MANAGEMENT
The management of acute myocarditis consists of general measures, management of complications, and specific therapy when possible. The treatment of cardiac failure, shock, and dysrhythmias has been discussed elsewhere, and only specific differences are mentioned here. Other measures, such as bed rest, which requires individualization, or pericardiocentesis, which may be dangerous, and the role of immunosuppressive therapy are discussed in greater detail. Clinical experience has shown that remarkable improvement is possible even in severe cases, and serial biopsy studies have revealed that myocytes presenting with myocytolytic changes can regain their normal architecture.[35] Hence no effort should be spared, and even heroic measures (e.g., intra-aortic balloon pumping) are justified in the critically ill patient. All patients receiving a diagnosis of myocarditis should be admitted to the hospital.

INTENSIVE CARE
There is a high incidence of sudden death in acute myocarditis.[9] Patients with hypotension, shock, severe cardiac failure, significant pericardial effusion at risk of tamponade, serious dysrhythmias, or atrioventricular conduction problems should be in an intensive cardiac care unit.

REST
Restriction of activities is indicated as long as there is active myocarditis or active concomitant disease. Reduction of a raised erythrocyte sedimentation rate could be helpful. In every case it is presumed that there is viral replication for up to 10 days, thus a 14-day period of bed rest from the onset of the viral illness would appear logical. Patients receiving a diagnosis of myocarditis based only on electrocardiographic changes during the course of an illness or those with no cardiac enlargement or failure should restrict their activities after discharge from the hospital as long as the electrocardiogram remains abnormal. Anything more than moderate physical exertion should be avoided. This may take up to 6 to 8 weeks. If the electrocardiogram normalizes or becomes stable, normal activities can be gradually resumed.

Patients with cardiomegaly or mild cardiac failure need further restrictions. Slow ambulation should start only after control of the failure. Marked restriction of activities should continue as long as there is improvement, and ideally patients in marked cardiac failure should have their activities severely restricted as long as they show signs of improvement. Some may return to normal, while others may show residual cardiomegaly or persistence of an abnormal electrocardiogram.

Once stabilized they should gradually return to activities that they can tolerate without disability. For some this may eventually mean a normal life, but for others it may entail varying degrees of restriction.

OXYGEN
Hypoxia is known to increase the incidence and severity of myocarditis in experimental studies and has been found to aggravate the myocarditis of influenza and poliomyelitis. Adequate oxygen therapy should be assured for patients in cardiac failure or those experiencing dyspnea or pulmonary complications such as infiltration, which may aggravate the hypoxia. Hyperbaric oxygen has been shown to enhance coxsackievirus B1 replication in mice.[9]

CARDIAC FAILURE
The general principles outlined elsewhere apply in acute myocarditis. Digitalis and diuretics are prescribed as required. An increased sensitivity to digitalis is often mentioned but seldom documented. In a patient likely to experience arrhythmias, adequate attention to the blood potassium level is essential. Blood digitalis assays are useful. We consider digitalis to be the first line of therapy. Patients in severe cardiac failure may require monitoring with a Swan-Ganz catheter. Preload- and afterload-reducing drugs, including sodium nitroprusside, may be essential. For some in shock, inotropic support with dobutamine or dopamine, occasionally volume loading, or intra-aortic balloon pumping may be indicated.

ARRHYTHMIAS
Ventricular arrhythmias are treated depending on their frequency and hemodynamic consequences. Atrial fibrillation and atrial flutter require treatment. There are no particular drugs that are favored over others, but the choice and dosage should take into account the presence of cardiac failure and the "pump" status of the patient. Temporary pacing should be done for complete atrioventricular block since this is an adverse prognostic sign in myocarditis. At times, a permanent pacemaker is required. Some patients have a tachycardia of 120 or more beats per minute without signs of cardiac failure. In such instances, if palpitation is a symptom, a small dose of a β-blocker such as propranolol, 10 mg three times a day, increased as required, can be tried cautiously.

PERICARDIAL EFFUSION/TAMPONADE
Patients with a pericardial effusion should be watched for signs of tamponade. The presence and severity of an underlying myocarditis may be masked by a tense effusion.[23] The heart is "flabby" in acute myocarditis, and, following the sudden removal of a large amount of fluid, the restricting influence of the pericardium is no longer present; the result can be rapid, progressive cardiac dilatation and fatal cardiogenic shock.[23] Thus with tamponade in acute myopericarditis, it would be prudent to aspirate only reasonable amounts of fluid slowly and to avoid removing all the fluid.

ANTICOAGULANTS
In acute myocarditis, anticoagulants are contraindicated when there is associated pericarditis and are indicated only when there has been systemic or pulmonary embolism. In acute myocarditis with severe heart failure, anticoagulants may be considered if a thrombus is demonstrated on two-dimensional echocardiography.

SPECIFIC THERAPY
Specific therapy where available should be used in cases of specific acute myocarditis such as psittacosis. Specific therapy for viral diseases is only evolving. Interferons are families of low molecular weight proteins produced in response to viral and other stimuli. They are released from infected cells and are thus available much earlier than antibody.

In vitro, they can inhibit the replication of virtually every type of virus. The role of interferon inducers and antiviral agents such as amantadine, vidarabine, idoxuridine, acyclovir, and methisazone will have to await further experience and clinical trials.

CORTICOSTEROIDS AND IMMUNOSUPPRESSIVE THERAPY
Viremia and replication of viruses in the myocardium lasts about 10 days in coxsackievirus and echovirus infections,[10] although at times they may persist longer. Corticosteroids and other immunosuppressive drugs should be avoided at least during the first 10 days. However, patients who are severely ill and unresponsive to conventional therapy should receive corticosteroids.[9] Severe, refractory cardiac failure in the acute stage and persistent heart failure and aggravation of cardiac failure are indications for immunosuppressive therapy as in chronic active myocarditis.

SPECIFIC VIRUS INFECTIONS
COXSACKIEVIRUS INFECTION
Coxsackievirus infection is recognized as the main cause of viral myocarditis. There are 24 types in group A and 6 in group B, but heart disease is mainly caused by coxsackievirus group B.[37] This group of enteroviruses has a worldwide distribution with both epidemic and sporadic infections. In temperate climates there is an increased incidence of infections in summer and early fall, but infections occur throughout the year in the tropics. Transmission of the infection is mainly through the fecal-oral route and is therefore increased by poor hygiene and a low socioeconomic status. Infection also spreads through the respiratory tract. With dissemination, the heart, central nervous system, pancreas, and testes can be involved. There may be generalized or focal myositis.

The bulk of coxsackievirus infections (50% to 80%) are asymptomatic, and many are undiagnosed febrile illnesses with or without respiratory symptoms, which often are mild. The manifestations may be those of a "common cold," pharyngitis, or gastroenteritis. Coxsackievirus infections are a common cause of benign meningitis. There may be a morbilliform or macular rash. Pleurodynia (Bornholm's disease) with a sudden sharp intercostal or abdominal pain, due mainly to muscle involvement, can be caused by coxsackievirus B or A or by echoviruses. The incubation period and the acute illness both last 2 to 6 days. The onset is usually acute with fever, and the pain is paroxysmal, with the initial episodes being more severe. Pleural rub is infrequent, and in about 25% of patients there may be localized tenderness and swelling.

In European coxsackievirus B5 epidemics, cardiac involvement varied from 5% to 12% and in sporadic cases coxsackievirus B infection was present in 30% to 39%.[38]

INFECTIOUS MONONUCLEOSIS
Electrocardiographic abnormalities have been noted in about 50% of patients with infectious mononucleosis, produced by the Epstein-Barr virus. The true incidence of myocarditis is not clear; autopsy reports vary widely. This is a disease found worldwide, affecting mostly adolescents and young adults; severe cardiac complications are rare even with myocarditis, and recovery is usually complete. Incomplete resolution is more common in older patients. Pericardial rub, heart failure, ST-T changes, presentation mimicking acute myocardial infarction, rare but fatal ventricular arrhythmia (even in young patients), varying degrees of atrioventricular block, persistent complete atrioventricular block, and constrictive pericarditis have all been reported.[21,39] Myocarditis is found in one third of the fatal cases, and atypical lymphocytes may be found in the myocardium along with other signs of myocarditis.

MYCOPLASMA PNEUMONIAE INFECTION

Cases of *M. pneumoniae* infection can present throughout the year, most of them involving children, adolescents, and young adults, and epidemics can occur every 2 to 4 years. Most members of a family may be involved. ST-T changes on the electrocardiogram without clinical cardiac involvement may be present in up to a third of the cases; they usually resolve in about 2 weeks, but at times may persist for a few months. Complete recovery is generally seen.[40] The electrocardiographic changes are more frequent in patients with myalgia. Pericarditis with effusion, significant myocarditis, and heart failure may be present. In the presence of dyspnea due to the pneumonia, it is not easy to diagnose heart failure due to myocarditis. A gallop rhythm indicates heart failure.

PSITTACOSIS (ORNITHOSIS)

Acute myopericarditis can occur in psittacosis, caused by *Chlamydia psittaci* and found predominantly in persons (including children) handling parrots, pigeons, and other fowl. The initial illness is most often asymptomatic or mild. Severe myalgia may be present. Pneumonitis and splenomegaly are common. Cardiac involvement is shown by precordial pain, cardiomegaly, and heart failure. In a series of nine patients, a pericardial rub was heard in two, cardiac enlargement was present in nine, and ST segment and T wave changes in eight and some had intraventricular conduction defects.[41] While in most cases there is complete recovery, in fatal cases the changes described under acute viral myocarditis are evident.

VIRAL HEPATITIS

Electrocardiographic abnormalities consisting of ST or T wave changes have been reported in 17.3% to 44% of patients. Bradycardia, junctional rhythm, ventricular premature complexes, atrial fibrillation, and prolongation of the QT_c interval have all been noted. The changes are usually transient but may rarely persist for some months. Asymptomatic myocarditis is rare, occurs during the first to the third week, and can result in heart failure and death.[21] A report on the autopsy findings in 30 patients who had both serum and viral hepatitis described electrocardiographic T wave changes, left axis deviation, and arrhythmias.[42] The electrocardiogram was normal in 5 of 13 patients with clinical cardiac involvement, including some with pulmonary edema. Petechial hemorrhage was the most common abnormality. It was frequently widespread, involving the subepicardial and subendocardial areas and the interventricular septum. All patients had a raised prothrombin time, and 24 (80%) had a serum bilirubin value exceeding 15 mg/dl. The inflammatory infiltrate consisted of "lymphocytes."[42]

UNSETTLED QUESTIONS AND RECENT OBSERVATIONS
VIRAL MYOCARDITIS AND DILATED CARDIOMYOPATHY

The clinical picture of severe heart failure in dilated cardiomyopathy may be indistinguishable from progressive heart failure following viral myocarditis, and since the initiating episode of myocarditis may be missed it is clear that some cases will masquerade as dilated cardiomyopathy. Studies of patients presenting with dilated cadiomyopathy demonstrated evidence of an inflammatory infiltrate in some, but the number of such patients is not known.[1] Mild viral myocarditis is a nonprogressive, self-limited condition and has not been shown to be responsible for progressive heart failure.[11] Considerable importance has been given to a report showing high titers of coxsackievirus B neutralizing antibody in patients with dilated cardiomyopathy.[43] In a disease without a clear onset, securing geographic controls matched for the seasonal variation of viral infections would be difficult. A study from Japan has shown raised complement-fixing and neutralizing antibody titers to many viruses when compared with controls, not only in dilated cardiomyopathy but also in hypertrophic cardiomyopathy as well.[28] Patients in cardiac failure are more susceptible to respiratory infections, and there is both experimental and clinical evidence that viral damage to the heart is more frequent with preexisting heart disease.[22] A causal role for viruses in dilated cardiomyopathy has yet to be proved.

FAMILIAL MYOCARDITIS

In one report, two families with dilated cardiomyopathy were studied.[32] The histologic diagnosis of myocarditis was documented in one patient. It was postulated that an infection in the presence of such an inherited defect could lead to severe, unchecked myocardial damage. Such families may be a distinct subset separate from other families with dilated cardiomyopathy due to specific structural or metabolic abnormalities.

VIRAL MYOCARDITIS AND "PERIPARTUM CARDIOMYOPATHY"

The frequency of myopericarditis following coxsackievirus infection increases during pregnancy.[10] The natural history of peripartum cardiomyopathy as described is similar to that of virus myocarditis.[44] There is a report of three patients in severe heart failure following infective myocarditis,[2] and we have treated two others with severe heart failure due to coxsackievirus B infection, all in the peripartum period. Interestingly, all five were treated with immunosuppressive therapy with a good response. We believe that a significant proportion of cases labeled "peripartum cardiomyopathy" may be due to viral myocarditis.

CAN VIRAL MYOCARDITIS RESULT IN CHRONIC VALVULAR HEART DISEASE?

The relationship of viral myocarditis and chronic valvular heart disease can be examined in experimental viral myocarditis, from evidence of endocarditis during acute viral myocarditis, from follow-up after viral myocarditis, and from evidence of past viral infections in patients with chronic valvular heart disease.[22,45]

Experimental studies have shown that viral infections can affect the endocardium and the valves.[22] Burch and associates have produced valvular endocarditis in 55% of mice and mural endocarditis in 50% following coxsackievirus B4 inoculation.[46] Significant valvulitis can be diagnosed from the presence of cardiac murmurs. Of 156 patients from various series with viral myocarditis, only 21% had a murmur during the acute stage (usually an apical short ejection murmur) and of our 26 patients, only two (7.6%) had significant murmurs.[22] There is thus a striking difference between the infrequent valve involvement in acute viral myocarditis and that in acute rheumatic carditis. With a variety of fatal viral infections, macroscopic, endocardial, or valvular involvement was present in only a minority of patients (12%).[22] In various reports, among 198 patients who were followed after viral myocarditis, only 10 (5%) have had persistent murmurs (short ejection systolic murmurs). At this writing there are no reports of any patients followed after acute viral myocarditis who required surgical correction for chronic valvular heart disease.[22]

CHRONIC ACTIVE MYOCARDITIS

The detection of unsuspected myocarditis by endomyocardial biopsy in patients presenting with dilated cardiomyopathy in severe heart failure has opened a new area of active investigation and hope.[1] The criteria for the biopsy diagnosis have been discussed in the section on pathology. The incidence of myocarditis in such patients has ranged from 9% to 63%.[47] The presence of an inflammatory infiltrate suggests an active, ongoing process. Immunosuppressive therapy has been tried in such patients because of the suspected role of immune mechanisms in the perpetuation of myocarditis.[1,2,4] Immunosuppressive therapy using prednisone with or without azathioprine results in a disappearance of the inflammatory infiltrate.[1-4] In some patients this is associated with a dramatic clinical and hemodynamic improvement with return to "normal" even after treatment is stopped.[1,4] In others, the initial improvement has been followed by clinical deterioration and reappearance of the changes noted on biopsy when immunosuppressive therapy is stopped, with, again, clinical and histologic improvement on reinstitution of immunosuppressive treatment. In a few, there is no clinical improvement despite disappearance of the inflammatory infiltrate and there is progression with increasing fibrosis.[1,3,4] Myocarditis has been classified as acute, rapidly progressive, or chronic,[3] or graded from 0 to 4 based on the biopsy findings.[4] In general, younger patients with a shorter duration of symptoms in weeks or months may do well, but as yet the clinical or histologic features of the subset of patients who can be confidently expected to improve on immunosuppressive therapy have not been defined.

MANAGEMENT

Chronic active myocarditis should be considered in patients with unexplained heart failure (usually of a rapid onset) or with an unexpected worsening of preexisting heart failure. Normally, therapy should start only after a biopsy diagnosis of active myocarditis, since repeat biopsies are necessary for following the response to therapy. The dosage and duration of treatment should be individualized. It is desirable to have controlled studies on the role of immunosuppressive therapy but such studies are unlikely to be available for some time. We recommend the following line of management. Prednisone alone has been used with success in isolated cases[1] including some of our own. The best results appear to be gained from a combination of prednisone 50 mg/M^2/day and azathioprine, 75 mg/M^2/day, maintained for 6 months with a careful follow-up of the hemoglobin and white blood cell count.[2] Some patients require much longer periods of treatment, and in others therapy may have to be resumed. A careful watch is kept on the clinical response. The biopsy is repeated at 1 month, 3 months, 6 months, and 1 year or whenever there is a clinical relapse. Tapering the dose and stopping or resuming therapy is decided based on the clinical status and the biopsy findings. Concomitant therapy for cardiac failure is gradually withdrawn depending on the patient's improvement.

Treatment with prednisone and azathioprine is generally given for at least 6 months. Treatment is continued or resumed if the clinical improvement has not stabilized, if there is a relapse with reappearance of an inflammatory infiltrate, or if there is persistence or reappearance of an inflammatory infiltrate on a routine follow-up biopsy. The therapy is stopped when the clinical status is stable and the biopsy is negative, but generally not earlier than 6 months; if there is no improvement in 3 months, despite the biopsy becoming negative; or should the patient's condition deteriorate during the period of immunosuppressive treatment.

NONVIRAL MYOCARDITIS

A variety of infections with other organisms can produce myocarditis (Table 95.4). Some of the bacterial, fungal, spirochetal, rickettsial, helminthic, and protozoal infections are important and are discussed in greater detail.

BACTERIAL MYOCARDITIS

Several bacterial infections can affect the myocardium (see Table 95.4). The most common are staphylococcal, pneumococcal, meningococcal, and streptococcal infections that result in myocardial microabscesses from which the organisms can be recovered. The course may be complicated by a suppurative pericarditis. Damage to the myocardium can also result from bacterial toxins (e.g., diphtheria) or hypersensitivity to bacterial products. Fatal infective endocarditis is consistently associated with myocarditis that is the result of coronary embolization, arteritis, or direct extension from the valves.

DIPHTHERIA

The disease is found worldwide in unimmunized populations. The exotoxin produces myocyte damage with granular and hyaline degeneration, and there may be extensive necrosis. There is a predilection for conduction tissue. In the later stages there is scarring of the myocardium. Myocarditis is present in about 70% of fatal cases and 20% of patients. Cardiac involvement occurs toward the end of the first week. There may be severe cardiac failure. The electrocardiogram shows ST segment and T wave changes. Conduction abnormalities were found in 72% of patients with myocarditis.[48] Bundle branch block carries about a 50% mortality, and complete heart block, 80% to 100%. Patients with only a first-degree atrioventricular block and T wave changes do well. The clinical features of acute myocardial infarction have been reported in a 13-year-old patient.[49] The electrocardiographic abnormalities may be slow to regress and may persist. Complete heart block may persist

TABLE 95.4 CAUSES OF NONVIRAL MYOCARDITIS

Bacterial	Mycotic	Protozoal
Actinomycosis*	Aspergillosis	Amebiasis
Brucellosis	Blastomycosis	Balantidiasis*
Clostridium infection*	Candidiasis	Chagas' disease
Diphtheria	Coccidioidomycosis	Leishmaniasis*
Gonococcus	Cryptococcosis	Malaria*
Infective endocarditis	Histoplasmosis	Naeglerial infection*
Melioidosis*	Sporotrichosis	Sarcosporidiosis*
Meningococcal infection		*Toxoplasmosis*
Pneumococcal infection	**Rickettsial**	
Salmonellosis	Q fever*	**Helminthic**
Staphylococcal infection	Rocky Mountain spotted fever	Ascariasis*
Streptococcal infection	Typhus—scrub	Cysticercosis*
Tuberculosis	Typhus—epidemic	Echinococcosis
Tularemia*		Filariasis
		Heterophyiasis*
Spirochetal		Paragonimiasis
Leptospirosis		Schistosomiasis*
Relapsing fever		Strongyloidiasis*
Syphilis		Trichinosis
		Visceral larva migrans

* Rare association. Protozoal and helminthic infections have certain geographic distributions.

or appear for the first time years later. Scarring of the myocardium can result in chronic heart failure. In general, survivors make a complete recovery. Antitoxin should be given as soon as the diagnosis of diphtheria is made. Among the antimicrobial agents, penicillin G is the drug of choice. Corticosteroids have been tried in conduction abnormalities. Pacing may be required.

STREPTOCOCCAL INFECTION
Apart from acute rheumatic fever, streptococcal infection can directly involve the heart as in scarlet fever with focal or diffuse infiltration of the myocardium. The myocarditis usually develops during the first week and resolves; but arrhythmias, conduction disturbances, and sudden death have been recorded.

MENINGOCOCCAL INFECTION
Myocardial involvement is common during fatal infections. There may also be circulatory collapse during fulminating meningococcemia as in the Waterhouse-Friderichsen syndrome. Meningococcal myocarditis can also result in arrhythmias, conduction disturbances, cardiac failure, and sudden death.

SALMONELLOSIS
Cardiac involvement in typhoid rarely attracts clinical attention, but cardiac enlargement in addition to electrocardiographic changes has been reported. The changes are usually ST segment and T wave changes that rarely last more than 1 week. Serious conduction abnormalities and arrhythmias are rare. Congestive heart failure from a rapidly progressing myocarditis can occur in seriously ill children and is associated with a high mortality. With *Salmonella* infection, endocarditis, mural thrombi, infected emboli, myocardial abscesses, and a purulent pericarditis can occur.

TUBERCULOSIS
Tuberculosis is one of the most common chronic bacterial diseases in some parts of the world and yet myocardial involvement is rare, with incidence at autopsy (excluding pericarditis) between 0.02% and 0.09%.[50,51] Tuberculoma and myocardial abscess formation can occur anywhere. A tendency for involvement of the superficial coronary arteries, sinoatrial node, and atrial conduction tracts has been noted.[51] Conduction abnormalities and arrhythmias are the most common mode of presentation.[50] The right side of the heart, especially the right atrium, is most commonly involved in miliary tuberculosis and infiltrative lesions. We have reported the case of an 18-year-old who presented in congestive cardiac failure, had signs of a right atrial mass that proved to be tuberculous on endomyocardial biopsy, and who recovered following resection and tuberculosis chemotherapy.[50]

FUNGAL MYOCARDITIS
Many fungal infections can involve the myocardium (see Table 95.4). These are rare except for opportunistic infections in patients who are immunosuppressed or seriously debilitated. Primary infection of the myocardium is uncommon; the disease spreads by way of small emboli from prosthetic or homograft valves. Thrombosis of the vessels, necrosis, and abscesses may be found. *Candida* and *Aspergillus* infections are the most frequent causes of fungal myocarditis.

ASPERGILLOSIS
Aspergillus species are found worldwide. The spores are ubiquitous and are constantly being inhaled. Aspergillosis is found predominantly in patients with chronic respiratory infection and in immunosuppressed individuals. The disease primarily affects the respiratory tract and lungs. Hematogenous spread occurs to the heart and other organs. There is vascular invasion of fungal mycelia, resulting in necrosis. Suppuration predominates and granulomas are rare.[52] The electrocardiogram may be normal or show T wave changes. Amphotericin B is the drug of choice.

CANDIDIASIS
There are several *Candida* species of which the most common is *C. albicans*. The source of infection in humans is usually from breaches of normal mucocutaneous barriers. Candidiasis is the most common opportunistic mycosis in the world, affecting patients on prolonged antibiotic therapy and immunosuppressed individuals, especially those on corticosteroids. Although *Candida* endocarditis is the most frequent cardiac manifestation, myocardial microabscesses, often multiple, can be found even in the absence of endocarditis.[53] Amphotericin B is used in treatment.

CRYPTOCOCCOSIS
Cryptococci are found worldwide. Serotype A, found in avian dung, is common in the United States, while serotypes B and C are seen particularly in southern California. The disease is largely airborne, particularly affecting those with disseminated malignancy. Hematogenous spread occurs from the lungs and particularly to the meninges. Granulomas and areas of fibrosis may occur in the heart with cardiomegaly and arrhythmias, particularly ventricular arrhythmias.[54]

SPIROCHETAL MYOCARDITIS
LEPTOSPIROSIS
Leptospiral myocarditis is found in 60% of fatal cases of leptospirosis. Epicardial hemorrhage may be found with subendocardial muscle necrosis and involvement of the papillary muscles. The infection, although uncommon, is found all over the United States and is more common in teenagers and young adults. Leptospirosis is generally acquired from contact with the urine of domestic animals and some wild animals, such as foxes. Swimming in contaminated water is a common source of infection. The onset is usually abrupt with fever, severe myalgia, and a characteristic conjunctival suffusion. The liver and kidneys are most frequently involved. Cardiac involvement is usually of little consequence, but at times atrial and ventricular arrhythmias, conduction problems, and rarely acute ventricular failure can occur.[55]

RELAPSING FEVER
Louse-borne relapsing fever is caused by the genus *Borrelia*. It is found in epidemic form following wars and in refugee camps, and an endemic form is seen in Ethiopia and parts of Sudan. Man is the only reservoir of infection. The onset is abrupt, and the brunt is borne by the liver, spleen, and myocardium; bleeding, which is often severe, occurs in about half the number affected.[56] Petechial hemorrhages are found in the heart. There is involvement of the small arterioles, with areas of necrosis. Prolongation of the QT_c interval is common (40%) as are atrioventricular conduction defects and arrhythmias. Death may be sudden.

SYPHILIS
Syphilitic myocarditis is rare. Congenital syphilis can result in a diffuse interstitial myocarditis. Adult syphilis results in gumma formation. The gummas have a predilection for the upper part of the ventricular septum and may cause atrioventricular conduction abnormalities.

RICKETTSIAL MYOCARDITIS
Rickettsial infections result in a vasculitis affecting mostly the small vessels with a mononuclear inflammatory infiltrate. Occlusive thrombi and hemorrhagic necrosis can occur. The vasculitis and multisystemic involvement are more severe with Rocky Mountain spotted fever. Cardiac involvement is usually mild, but fatalities from myocarditis have been reported.[57]

Q FEVER
Q fever is caused by *R. burnetii*. Endocarditis is common. Dyspnea may also be due to pneumonitis. The electrocardiogram may show ST segment and T wave changes, and ventricular tachycardia has been reported.[58] Petechial hemorrhages and foci of fibrosis may be found in the myocardium.

ROCKY MOUNTAIN SPOTTED FEVER
Rocky Mountain spotted fever is caused by *R. rickettsii*. Clinical myocarditis is not a prominent feature in patients with this disorder.[57]

SCRUB TYPHUS
Scrub typhus results from infection with *R. tsutsugamushi*. Myocarditis is common in these patients and the prognosis is good, although fatalities have been recorded in some epidemics. The vascular damage is less prominent, and necrosis is unusual.

HELMINTHIC MYOCARDITIS
A number of helminthic infestations can result in myocarditis (see Table 95.4). Many are rare causes of cardiac involvement, but some, such as trichinosis, hydatid disease, and visceral larva migrans can result in serious cardiac complications.[59]

CYSTICERCOSIS
Human infection with *Taenia solium* is found worldwide but is more common in Latin America and the Indian subcontinent. Heart involvement is rare (2% to 3%) and is more common in the left ventricle and interventricular septum. The larvae die in the myocardium; following tissue reaction, a cyst is formed. These cysts often calcify and rupture is uncommon.[59] Depending on their location, the cysts can give rise to symptoms and signs.

HYDATID DISEASE
Hydatid disease is found the world over but mostly in sheep-rearing countries and the tropics. The dog is the host, and the sheep is the usual intermediate host. Human infection is through dog feces. The oncospheres pass through the portal vein and lodge in various organs, particularly the liver, lung, and heart. Hydatid cysts are more common in the left ventricle and interventricular septum and infrequent in the atria.[59] Hydatid cysts in the heart may be silent and picked up on a routine chest film. They can produce symptoms and signs at their location or by rupture. Rupture may result in a serious or fatal anaphylactic reaction. These cardiac cysts tend to rupture early (38% in one series) probably due to cardiac movement. Rupture from the right ventricle is frequent. Rupture can result in shock, embolization, or pericardial tamponade followed by constrictive pericarditis.[60] Depending on their location, the cysts are treated by careful excision.

HETEROPHYIASIS
Flukes of the family Heterophyidae can cause a myocarditis. The eggs are trapped in the myocardium and cause capillary congestion, rupture, and hemorrhage.[59] The heart is enlarged, and there may be cardiac failure. At one time, this infestation accounted for 14% of cardiac deaths in the Philippines.

SCHISTOSOMIASIS
Schistosomiasis is endemic in certain parts of the Nile basin and the Orient. The ova embolize, and although direct myocardial involvement is rare, there is extensive pulmonary arteritis, thrombosis, and severe pulmonary hypertension. An inflammatory myocarditis has also been reported. The ova or the adult worm may be found in strategic cardiac locations and in one instance caused myocardial infarction.

TRICHINOSIS
Infection with *Trichinella spiralis* is common in Europe, the United States, Canada, and the Soviet Union but infrequent in the tropics. Although death is uncommon, myocarditis accounts for the majority of fatalities. The larval cysts are ingested in inadequately cooked pork products. After development, larval forms disseminate mostly to the skeletal and heart muscle and the central nervous system. In the majority of patients there are no symptoms, but there can be an acute trichinellotic syndrome with fever, muscle pain, periorbital edema, pneumonitis, and pleural involvement associated with eosinophilia and a rise in muscle enzymes.[61]

Unlike the situation in skeletal muscle, the larvae do not encyst in the myocardium. There is infiltration with lymphocytes and eosinophils with scattered hemorrhages and necrosis. Cardiac involvement is signaled by retrosternal pain and dyspnea, usually after the third week. There may be marked cardiomegaly, severe heart failure, and sudden death. The electrocardiographic changes are nonspecific. Mural endocarditis with thrombus formation can occur.[61] There is usually no residual cardiac damage. The diagnosis of trichinosis is based on skeletal muscle (calf) biopsy and skin tests. There may be a dramatic response to corticosteroids, which act by decreasing the host inflammatory respose. Prednisone is used in a dose of 60 mg/day. Thiabendazole is used to treat the helminthic infection.

TOXOCARIASIS (DOG AND CAT ROUNDWORM)
The dog and cat roundworm is found all over the world, and humans (usually children) may be accidental hosts by ingesting contaminated substances. The larvae migrate (visceral larva migrans) and while the liver is most commonly involved there can be myocarditis with granuloma development or an extensive inflammatory infiltrate resulting in cardiac failure and death. Corticosteroids have been used in treatment.

PROTOZOAL MYOCARDITIS
A variety of protozoal infections can include myocarditis as an important component of the systemic infection.[59] Some, such as Chagas' disease, are rampant in certain parts of the world, and others, such as toxoplasmosis, can result in significant cardiac disease. Other protozoal diseases rarely result in myocardial involvement (see Table 95.4).

ACUTE CHAGASIC MYOCARDITIS
American trypanosomiasis is an endemic infection of rural populations caused by *Trypanosoma cruzi*. It is transmitted by a blood-sucking insect of the subfamily Triatoma. The disease is mainly found in Central and South America. It is a major public health problem in Argentina, Brazil, and Chile where it is the most frequent form of heart disease. Although the parasite and insect are found in southwestern United States, human trypanosomiasis is notably lacking in these areas.

The infection is usually acquired during the early years of life, although it can occur at any time. Mucous membranes or the skin is infected by the excreta of the triatomes. The disease can also be transmitted by blood transfusion, congenital infection, from breast milk, or by contaminated food.[62] There is an acute phase of the disease separated from a chronic phase.

The acute phase is marked by a febrile illness; it mainly affects young children and is often unrecognized. Since the cheek is frequently the site of inoculation, there may be unilateral palpebral edema, hyperemia of the conjunctivae, and regional lymphadenopathy (Romaña's sign). The mortality is about 10%, due to heart failure or acute meningoencephalitis. At autopsy there is a severe, diffuse myocarditis, with parasites in the myocardial fibers and an infiltrate of lymphocytes, plasma cells, eosinophils, and macrophages.[62] In severe cases with failure of both left and right sides of the heart, the clinical manifestations are similar to those of other forms of acute myocarditis. Nonspecific electrocardiographic changes occur in a relatively large number of patients, with T wave changes and prolongation of PR and QT_c intervals. Premature beats, nodal rhythm, and conduction disturbances are rare. Intraventricular block is a poor prognostic sign. The acute stage subsides in 2 to 4 weeks. *T. cruzi* are found in the blood, and complement fixation tests may be negative in the early stages. The nitrofurazone derivatives have been superceded by the nitroimidazole compounds. These drugs are given orally and in the acute phase of Chagas' disease cause a rapid remission of fever as well as the symptoms and signs of parasitemia.

TOXOPLASMOSIS

Myocardial damage from this protozoon results from its presence in the myocardial fiber. *Toxoplasma gondii* has a worldwide distribution. The oocyst is passed in cat feces, and human infection is acquired from inadequately cooked meat or milk or from contact with pets. The localized form of toxoplasmosis can result in myocarditis. The infection is most commonly acquired *in utero;* it results in multisystemic involvement, and the heart is affected in about 50% of fatal cases. The adult form is uncommon, and it is more severe in immune deficiency states. The myocarditis may result in cardiac failure, pericarditis, and arrhythmias.[63] Even in mild cases the electrocardiogram may be abnormal. A combination of pyrimethamine and triple sulfonamides is effective in therapy.

AMEBIASIS

Entamoeba histolytica can spread from its habitat in the colon to cause liver abscesses. Rupture of an abscess in the left lobe occurs in 0.2% to 0.8% of cases; a suppurative pericarditis with trophozoites in the vegetations has been described.[59] Heart block has been reported. Emetine, metronidazole, and chloroquine are used in treatment.

MALARIA

Rarely, during the course of malaria, ST segment and T wave changes may be present. In fatal cases, and particularly those involving *Plasmodium falciparum* (malignant tertian), the myocardial capillaries may be stuffed with parasitized red blood cells and focal ischemic changes may be present.

MYOCARDITIS DUE TO BITES AND STINGS

Snakebites and stings from scorpions, wasps, and spiders can have profound cardiovascular effects.

SNAKEBITE. Snakebite can cause circulatory collapse, although the clinical picture is dominated by the neurotoxic, hematologic, and vascular complications of snake venom. Myocardial damage, ST segment depression, T wave changes, and intraventricular conduction defects have been reported as well as coronary artery thrombosis.

SCORPION STING. Myocarditis is one of the well-recognized complications of scorpion stings, and electrocardiographic abnormalities have been reported in 86% of patients.[64] These include prolongation of QT_c, ST segment, and T wave changes; atrial and ventricular tachycardia; ventricular and atrial premature beats; first-degree atrioventricular block; right bundle branch block; acute myocardial infarction or injury pattern; and transient left anterior fascicular block.[64] The changes have been attributed to direct effect of the venom, catecholamine release, disseminated intravascular coagulation, and electrolyte imbalances. Patients may present with hypertension or hypotension and pulmonary edema. Deaths are reported, especially in children.[65]

WASP AND SPIDER STING. These can result in hypotension, circulatory collapse, pulmonary edema, and arrhythmias. Clinical presentation like that of acute myocardial infarction has been reported following wasp sting.[66]

TOXIC MYOCARDITIS

Unlike hypersensitivity myocarditis, toxic drug-induced myocarditis is the result of a dose-related, cumulative damage to the myocardium. Higher doses over a short period of time give rise to acute changes that may be related to alterations in cellular metabolism, changes in cellular transport, or myocardial ischemia. The actual mechanism in most instances is not clear and is varied. Thus, emetine hydrochloride inhibits oxidative phosphorylation and cyclophosphamide produces multifocal ischemic necrosis from damage to the capillary endothelium, resulting in thrombosis.

Toxic myocarditis is characterized by multiple foci of change in various stages. There are areas of acute, extensive necrosis with a predominance of neutrophil infiltration and foci of healing, with fibroblasts and minimal monocellular reaction and an absence of eosinophils. Capillary microthrombi may be present. The endocardium and valves are generally spared, and the heart is not hypertrophied.[67]

The clinical presentation is with electrocardiographic abnormalities, arrhythmias, and hypotension. A variety of drugs including doxorubicin (Adriamycin), antimony, arsenicals, catecholamines, cyclophosphamide, daunorubicin, chloroquine, emetine, fluorouracil, lithium carbonate, paracetamol, and phenothiazines can result in toxic myocarditis. Digitalis and thyroid extract can produce an experimental myocarditis, but there is no evidence for a toxic myocarditis due to digitalis in humans.[67]

DOXORUBICIN

Doxorubicin (Adriamycin) inhibits nucleic acid synthesis. During the first few days there may be changes in the electrocardiogram with ST segment and T wave abnormalities and ventricular premature beats or supraventricular tachycardia. These are not dose related. Later, between 1 and 6 months of stopping therapy there is a rapid, severe biventricular failure that is relatively refractory to treatment. It is unusual to develop this complication with a total dose below 550 mg/M^2 but previous radiation and use of other cytotoxic drugs may induce cardiac changes at a lower dose. All chambers are dilated, and mural thrombi are frequent in both ventricles. The mitochondria are swollen, the cristae are disrupted, and there is marked reduction in myofibrillar bundles. Endomyocardial biopsy has shown a dose-related increase in the extent of myocyte damage beginning with a dose of about 240 mg/M^2.[68] However, the histologic changes may be too sensitive an index to use for tailoring the dose. Observation of heart size and for evidence of heart failure are good indicators, although some centers are using echocardiography or radionuclide ejection fractions to observe the results of this therapy.

CATECHOLAMINES

Catecholamines can cause an acute myocarditis. A direct toxic effect, tissue hypoxia, and platelet aggregation have all been suggested as possible mechanisms. Focal myocardial necrosis, severe myocytolysis, contraction band necrosis, epicardial hemorrhages, and an inflammatory infiltrate may be found. Arrhythmias are frequent.

CHLOROQUINE

There may be an idiosyncrasy to chloroquine, as with quinidine. The electrocardiographic changes are similar to those of emetine toxicity. Bradycardia, conduction abnormalities, and arrhythmias may be present.[69]

CYCLOPHOSPHAMIDE

High doses in excess of 45 mg/kg within 24 hours can result in a hemorrhagic myopericarditis. There are endocardial and epicardial

EMETINE

Cardiac toxicity is more frequent in ambulant patients, and during therapy bed rest should be advised. Emetine is contraindicated in patients with preexisting heart disease. Dehydroemetine is less toxic to the myocardium. There is mitochondrial swelling and cellular death.[71] The heart size is usually normal and cardiac enzymes may be elevated. The clinical manifestations of myocardial toxicity are hypotension, tachycardia, arrhythmias, and sudden death. The electrocardiogram usually shows T wave changes, the QT_c may be prolonged, and there may be ST segment changes. These changes generally regress in 1 to 2 months.

LITHIUM

Lithium carbonate is widely used in the treatment of manic-depressive disorders. Lithium prolongs repolarization, and T wave changes are frequent. Symptomatic sinus node dysfunction, supraventricular and ventricular arrhythmias, atrioventricular conduction abnormalities, and sudden death have been reported.[72]

Therapeutic levels of lithium can induce ventricular arrhythmias, and the dose should be carefully adjusted in patients with heart disease.

PHENOTHIAZINES

Therapy with phenothiazines (e.g., chlorpromazine, thioridazine) results in an alteration of cardiac catecholamines and an increase in the levels of circulating norepinephrine. Nonhomogeneous repolarization facilitates reentrant arrhythmias, so supraventricular tachycardia, ventricular tachycardia, and syncope can occur. The electrocardiogram may show prolongation of the PR and QT_c intervals and prominent U waves.[73] Quinidine and procainamide are avoided in therapy since they further decrease the conduction velocity, and lidocaine is preferred.

☐ HYPERSENSITIVITY MYOCARDITIS

Hypersensitivity myocarditis is not considered often enough in the differential diagnosis of a person presenting with nonspecific cardiac findings. The condition is both potentially reversible and, if unrecognized, lethal. The frequent eosinophilia, present with parasitic diseases common in some parts of the world, blunts the usefulness of this important finding in some geographic areas.

Hypersensitivity myocarditis is a form of delayed hypersensitivity mediated through chemically reactive metabolites. Most drug metabolites are univalent haptens, and this probably explains the infrequent occurrence of allergic drug reactions, since multivalent haptens are required to initiate antihapten antibodies. The drug would have been used without incident earlier by the individual, and the hypersensitivity drug reaction is not related to drug dosage nor is it a pharmacologic or toxic effect. Several drugs have been reported to produce hypersensitivity myocarditis (Table 95.5). Sometimes two or more drugs may be involved (e.g., methyldopa and hydrochlorothiazide). Most of the reports refer to sulfonamides, methyldopa, and penicillin.

MORPHOLOGIC FEATURES

The subject has been well reviewed by Fenoglio and associates.[74] At autopsy the heart is pale and flabby. Changes are found in both ventricles, especially in the subendocardial regions and the atria. The infiltrate shows a predominance of eosinophils along with lymphocytes and plasma cells and is mostly interstitial, although the perivascular areas, small arteries, arterioles, and veins are involved in a similar vasculitis. Focal myocytolysis is present, but the intact nuclei and cell membranes indicate a reversible process. Lesions are more or less of the same age. Extensive cellular necrosis, healing granulation tissue, and necrotizing vasculitis are conspicuous by their absence. Changes of myocardial infarction were not seen in the few patients who exhibited electrocardiographic change suggestive of infarction.[74]

CLINICAL FEATURES

Symptoms and signs of hypersensitivity are found in about 90% of patients. Fever with eosinophilia is the most frequent finding along with a rash and malaise. Cardiac findings are frequent but nonspecific. Tachycardia disproportionate to the fever, ventricular tachycardia, left bundle branch block, ST segment changes, and electrocardiographic changes of myocardial infarction have all been reported. Some of the changes may disappear and reappear. A mild rise in cardiac enzymes may be present with or without electrocardiographic changes of myocardial infarction. The patient may not appear to be critically ill, but death was sudden and unexpected in 83% of Fenoglio's cases.[74] Recent onset of nonspecific cardiac findings with symptoms and signs of drug allergy in a patient receiving a drug associated with hypersensitivity myocarditis should alert the physician to the possibility of this disorder.

TREATMENT

The offending drug should be withdrawn and supportive treatment for complications such as arrhythmias should be instituted. The patient should be managed in an intensive care area. Prednisone is administered in a dose of 40 mg to 60 mg/day, reduced in a few days, and continued for 10 to 14 days. Oral antihistamines have also been advocated.

GIANT CELL MYOCARDITIS

Giant cell myocarditis is associated with giant cells at the margins of serpiginous areas of myocardial necrosis. A histiocytic and eosinophilic infiltrate is found in the necrotic area. Both ventricles are affected along with the atria. No pericarditis or endocarditis is found.[75] The etiology is not certain, but an association with thymic tumors, thyroiditis, and sarcoid has been noted. The onset is usually sudden, with fever. The clinical course is rapid, much like that of fulminant viral myocarditis with extensive electrocardiographic changes, cardiac failure, and arrhythmias.

TABLE 95.5 DRUGS ASSOCIATED WITH HYPERSENSITIVITY MYOCARDITIS

Acetazolamide	Oxyphenbutazone
p-Aminosalicyclic acid	Penicillin*
Amitriptyline	Phenindione
Carbamazepine	Phenylbutazone
Chloramphenicol	Phenytoin
Chlorthalidone	Spironolactone
Chlortetracycline	Streptomycin
Hydrochlorothiazide	Sulfonamides*
Indomethacin	Sulfonylureas
Methyldopa*	Tetracycline

* More frequent association.

REFERENCES

1. Mason JW, Billingham ME, Ricci DR: Treatment of acute inflammatory myocarditis assisted by endomyocardial biopsy. Am J Cardiol 45:1037, 1980
2. Melvin KR, Richardson PJ, Olsen ECJ et al: Peripartum cardiomyopathy due to myocarditis. N Engl J Med 307:731, 1982
3. Fenoglio JJ Jr, Ursell PC, Kellogg CF et al: Diagnosis and classification of myocarditis by endomyocardial biopsy. N Engl J Med 308:12, 1983
4. Zee-Cheng CS, Tsai CC, Palmer DC et al: High incidence of myocarditis by endomyocardial biopsy in patients with idiopathic congestive cardiomyopathy. J Am Coll Cardiol 3:63, 1984
5. Desa'neto A, Bullington JD, Desser KB et al: Coxsackie B5 heart disease: Demonstration of infero-lateral wall myocardial necrosis. Am J Med 68:295, 1980
6. Saffitz JE, Schwartz DJ, Southworth W et al: Coxsackie viral myocarditis causing transmural right and left ventricular infarction without coronary narrowing. Am J Cardiol 52:644, 1983
7. Davies MJ: Myocarditis. In Pomerance A, Davies MJ (eds): The Pathology of the Heart, pp 193–210. London, Blackwell Scientific Publications, 1975
8. Engblom E, Ekfors TO, Meurman OH et al: Fatal influenza: A myocarditis with isolation of virus from the myocardium. Acta Med Scand 213:75, 1983
9. Noren GR, Kaplan EL, Staley NA: Nonrheumatic inflammatory diseases. In Adams FH, Emmanouilides GC, Moss AJ (eds): Heart Disease in Infants, Children and Adolescents, pp 576–594. Baltimore, Williams & Wilkins, 1983
10. Woodruff JF: Viral myocarditis. Am J Pathol 101:425, 1980
11. Nieminen MS, Heikkila J, Karjalainen J: Echocardiography in acute infectious myocarditis: Relation to clinical and electrocardiographic findings. Am J Cardiol 53:1331, 1984
12. Matsumori A, Kawai C, Sawada S et al: Experimental Coxsackie B3 perimyocarditis in the right ventricle in BALB/C mice: A one-year follow-up study. Jpn Circ J 44:842, 1980
13. El-Khatib MR, Chason JL, Lerner M: Ventricular aneurysms complicating Coxsackie virus Group B, Types 1 and 4 murine myocarditis. Circulation 59:412, 1979
14. Wong CY, Woodruff JJ, Woodruff JF: Generation of cytotoxic T lymphocytes during Coxsackie virus B-3 infection: II. Characterization of effector cells and demonstration of cytotoxicity against viral infected myofibers. J Immunol 118:1165, 1977
15. Paque RE, Gauntt CJ, Nealon TJ et al: Assessment of cell-mediated hypersensitivity against Coxsackie B3 viral-induced myocarditis utilizing hypertonic salt extracts of cardiac tissue. J Immunol 120:1672, 1978
16. Maisch B, Trostel-Soeder R, Stechemesser E et al: Diagnostic relevance of humoral and cell-mediated immune reactions in patients with acute viral myocarditis. Clin Exp Immunol 48:533, 1982
17. Eckstein R, Mempel W, Bolte HD: Reduced suppressor cell activity in congestive cardiomyopathy and in myocarditis. Circulation 65:1224, 1982
18. Dec CW Jr, Palacios IF, Fallon JT et al: Active myocarditis in the spectrum of acute dilated cardiomyopathies. N Engl J Med 312:885, 1985
19. Sainani GS, Dekate MP, Rao CP: Heart disease caused by Coxsackie virus B infection. Br Heart J 37:819, 1975
20. Hirschman SZ, Hammer GS: Coxsackie virus myopericarditis: A microbiological and clinical review. Am J Cardiol 34:224, 1974
21. Abelmann WH: Clinical aspects of viral cardiomyopathy. In Fowler NO (ed): Myocardial Diseases, pp 253–279. New York, Grune & Stratton, 1973
22. Cherian G, Krishnaswami S, Sukumar IP et al: Variations in the practice of cardiology: Some problems encountered in India. In Yu PN, Goodwin JF (eds): Progress in Cardiology, vol 9, pp 147–184. Philadelphia, Lea & Febiger, 1980
23. Timmis AD, Daly K, Monaghan M et al: Pericardiocentesis in myocarditis: The protective role of the pericardium in severe heart failure. Br Med J 287:1348, 1983
24. Chandraratna PAN, Nimalasuriya A, Reid CL et al: Left ventricular asynergy in acute myocarditis: Simulation of acute myocardial infarction. JAMA 250:1428, 1983
25. Griffiths PD, Hannington G, Booth JC: Coxsackie B virus infections and myocardial infarction: Results from a prospective epidemiologically controlled study. Lancet 1:1387, 1980
26. Take M, Sekiguchi M, Hiroe M et al: Long-term follow-up of electrocardiographic findings in patients with acute myocarditis proven by endomyocardial biopsy. Jpn Circ J 46:1227, 1982
27. Heikkila J, Karjalainen J: Acute pericarditis: Myocardial enzyme release is an evidence for myocarditis. J Am Coll Cardiol 5:490, 1985
28. Kitaura Y: Virological study of idiopathic cardiomyopathy. Jpn Circ J 45:279, 1981
29. Shrier A, Nahmias AJ, DeHaan RL: Herpes virus infection alters electrical parameters of heart cell aggregates. Am J Physiol 234:C169, 1978
30. Mitsutake A, Nakamura M, Inou T et al: Intense, persistent myocardial avid technetium-99m pyrophosphate scintigraphy in acute myocarditis. Am Heart J 101:683, 1981
31. O'Connell JB, Robinson JA, Henkin RE et al: Immunosuppressive therapy in patients with congestive cardiomyopathy and myocardial uptake of gallium-67. Circulation 64:780, 1981
32. O'Connell JB, Fowles RE, Robinson JA et al: Clinical and pathologic findings of myocarditis in the families with dilated cardiomyopathy. Am Heart J 107:127, 1983
33. Khaw BA, Beller GA, Haber E: Experimental myocardial infarct imaging following intravenous administration of iodine-131 labeled antibody (Fab^1)2 fragment specific for cardiac myosin. Circulation 57:743, 1978
34. Haber E: Personal communication, 1985
35. Sekiguchi M, Jiroe M, Take M: On the potentiality of myocardial cell regeneration: Ultrastructural observation employing serial endomyocardial biopsy in 9 cases of acute myocarditis. J Cell Mol Cardiol II (Suppl 3):21, 1979
36. Hayakawa M, Inoh T, Yokota Y et al: A long-term follow-up study of acute viral and idiopathic myocarditis. Jpn Circ J 47:1304, 1983
37. Kawai C, Matsumori A, Kitaura Y et al: Viruses and the heart: Viral myocarditis and cardiomyopathy. In Yu PN, Goodwin JF (eds): Progress in Cardiology, vol 7, pp 141–162. Philadelphia, Lea & Febiger 1978
38. Grist NR, Bell EJ: Editorial: Coxsackie viruses and the heart. Am Heart J 77:295, 1969
39. Frishman W, Kraus ME, Zabkar MAJJ et al: Infectious mononucleosis and fatal myocarditis. Chest 72:535, 1977
40. Ponka A: Carditis associated with *Mycoplasma pneumoniae* infection. Acta Med Scand 206:77, 1979
41. Sutton GC, Morrissey RA, Tobin JR Jr et al: Pericardial and myocardial disease associated with serologic evidence of infection by agents of the psittacosis-lymphogranuloma venereum group (Chlamydiaceae). Circulation 36:830, 1967
42. Bell H: Cardiac manifestations of viral hepatitis. JAMA 218:387, 1971
43. Cambridge G, MacArthur CGC, Waterson AP et al: Antibodies to Coxsackie B viruses in congestive cardiomyopathy. Br Heart J 41:692, 1979
44. Demakis JG, Rahimtoola SH, Sutton GC et al: Natural course of peripartum cardiomyopathy. Circulation 44:1053, 1971
45. Chandy KG, John TJ, Cherian G: Coxsackie viruses and chronic valvular heart disease. Am Heart J 100:578, 1980
46. Burch GE, DePasquale NP, Sun SC et al: Endocarditis in mice infected with Coxsackie virus B4. Science 151:447, 1966
47. Mason JW: Endomyocardial biopsy: The balance of success and failure. Circulation 71:185, 1985
48. Ledbetter MK, Cannon AB II, Costa AF: The electrocardiogram in diphtheritic myocarditis. Am Heart J 68:599, 1964
49. Class RN, Rivera-Callegos BT, Sanz-Malaga C: Diptheritic myocarditis simulating myocardial infarction. Am J Cardiol 16:580, 1965
50. Krishnaswami H, Cherian G: Right atrial tuberculoma: Report of a case with complete recovery. Thorax 39:550, 1984
51. Kinare SC: Interesting facets of cardiovascular tuberculosis. Indian J Surg 37:144, 1975
52. Williams AH: Aspergillus myocarditis. Am J Clin Pathol 61:247, 1974
53. Franklin WG, Simon AB, Sodeman TM: *Candida* myocarditis without valvulitis. Am J Cardiol 38:924, 1976
54. Jones I, Nassau E, Smith P: Cryptococcosis of the heart. Br Heart J 27:462, 1965
55. Edwards GA, Damm BM: Human leptospirosis. Medicine 39:117, 1960
56. Judge DM, Samuel I, Perine PL et al: Louse borne relapsing fever in man. Arch Pathol 97:136, 1974
57. Walker DH, Paletta CE, Cain BC: Pathogenesis of myocarditis in Rocky Mountain spotted fever. Arch Pathol Lab Med 104:171, 1980
58. Sheridan P, MacCraig JN, Hart RJC: Myocarditis complicating Q fever. Br Med J 2:155, 1974
59. Datta BN: Parasitic diseases of the heart. In Silver MD (ed): Cardiovascular Pathology, vol 2, pp 1153–1167. New York, Churchill Livingstone, 1983
60. Palant A, Deutsch V, Kishon Y et al: Pulmonary hydatid embolization: Report on 2 operated cases and review of published reports. Br Heart J 38:1086, 1976
61. Andy JJ, O'Connell JP, Daddario RC et al: Trichinosis causing extensive ventricular mural endocarditis with superimposed thrombosis. Am J Med 63:824, 1977
62. Amorim DD: Chagas' disease. In Yu PN, Goodwin JF (eds): Progress in Cardiology, vol 8, pp 235–279. Philadelphia, Lea & Febiger, 1979
63. Leak D, Meghji M: Toxoplasmic infection in cardiac diseases. Am J Cardiol 43:841, 1979
64. Kunhali K, Cherian G, Krishnaswami S et al: Left anterior fascicular block following scorpion sting. Indian J Chest Dis 21:86, 1979
65. Gueron M, Yaron R: Cardiovascular manifestations of severe scorpion sting. Chest 57:156, 1970
66. Levine HD: Acute myocardial infarction following wasp sting. Am Heart J 91:365, 1976
67. Fenoglio JJ Jr: The effects of drugs on the cardiovascular system. In Silver MD (ed): Cardiovascular Pathology, vol 2, pp 1085–1107. New York, Churchill Livingstone, 1983
68. Bristow MR, Mason JW, Billingham ME et al: Doxorubicin cardiomyopathy. Evaluation by phonocardiography, endomyocardial biopsy and cardiac catheterization. Ann Intern Med 88:168, 1978
69. Michael TAD, Aiwazzadeh S: The effects of acute chloroquine poisoning with special reference to the heart. Am Heart J 79:831, 1970
70. Appelbaum FR, Strauchen JA, Graw RC Jr et al: Acute lethal carditis caused by high dose combination chemotherapy. Lancet 1:58, 1976
71. Murphy ML, Bulloch RT, Pearce MB: The correlation of metabolic and ultrastructural changes in emetine myocardial toxicity. Am Heart J 87:105, 1974

72. Tilkian AG, Schroeder JS, Kao J et al: Effect of lithium on cardiovascular performance: Report on extended ambulatory and exercise testing before and during lithium therapy. Am J Cardiol 38:701, 1976
73. Fowler NO, McCall D, Chou TC et al: Electrocardiographic changes and cardiac arrhythmias in patients receiving psychotropic drugs. Am J Cardiol 37:223, 1976
74. Fenoglio JJ Jr, McAllister HA Jr, Mullick FG: Drug-related myocarditis: I. Hypersensitivity myocarditis. Hum Pathol 12:900, 1981
75. Davies MJ, Pomerance A, Teare RD: Idiopathic giant cell myocarditis: A distinctive clinicopathological entity. Br Heart J 37:192, 1975

RHEUMATIC FEVER

M. Thomas Abraham • George Cherian

CHANGING INCIDENCE

Over the past several decades there has been a sharp decline in the incidence of acute rheumatic fever (RF) and the severity of its manifestations in Western Europe, North America, and Japan. Over a period of 100 years, the reported incidence of acute RF in Denmark fell from 200 to 11/100,000.[1] In Malmo, Sweden, there was a reduction of 90% in incidence over a 25-year period from 1935 to 1960, 50% of which occurred before 1949, prior to the widespread use of antibiotics and corticosteroids.[2] Data from the United States show similar trends. The annual incidence of RF in Connecticut hospitals fell from 12.3/100,000 from 1934 to 1938 to 2.9/100,000 from 1968 to 1972.[3] Studies in Nashville, Tennessee, have shown an annual incidence of 6.4/100,000 in 1969.[4] Although it is true that the incidence of RF started to decline before the introduction of antibiotics, the major factor responsible for the dramatic fall in incidence over the past three decades is likely to be the widespread treatment of streptococcal infection.

Acute RF and rheumatic heart disease continue to be major public health problems in the heavily populated developing countries of Southeast Asia, China, Central and South America, the Middle East, and Africa, but precise incidence data are not available from many of these countries. A survey of RF in Sri Lanka revealed an annual incidence of 142/100,000 for the 5- to 19-year age group and 47/100,000 for the general population.[5] Rheumatic heart disease accounts for 25% to 50% of all cardiac admissions to hospitals in many of the developing countries.[5]

FACTORS INFLUENCING SUSCEPTIBILITY TO RHEUMATIC FEVER

STREPTOCOCCAL INFECTION

The streptococcal etiology of acute RF is universally accepted, and the epidemiology of acute RF parallels the epidemiology of streptococcal pharyngitis. Studies in military populations have shown that acute RF occurs in 3% of individuals with exudative streptococcal pharyngitis during epidemics.[6] The attack rate appears to be lower in civilian populations following sporadic streptococcal throat infections. Rheumatic fever does not follow streptococcal pyoderma, even when caused by organisms belonging to group A *Streptococcus,* and pharyngeal infections by streptococcal strains that usually cause pyoderma are not followed by acute RF. Changes in the virulence and pattern of prevalence of the various streptococci may be important in the falling incidence of acute RF.

AGE AND SEX

First attacks of acute RF occur most commonly in children between the ages of 6 and 15 years, with a peak at about 8 years. The disease is seldom seen in children under 3 years of age. Recurrences can occur at any age, with the rate falling steadily beyond adolescence.

Sex does not influence susceptibility to acute RF. However, it does seem to affect the manifestations of the disease, and chorea is more frequent in the female, especially after puberty.

SOCIOECONOMIC FACTORS AND THE AVAILABILITY OF MEDICAL CARE

The falling incidence of RF in the more affluent countries has closely paralleled improvements in the standard of living. Substandard, overcrowded housing with close person-to-person contact facilitates the spread of streptococcal infections. Materially disadvantaged groups of people even in affluent societies have a relatively high incidence of the disease. In New Zealand, acute RF is a major problem among the Maoris, who live in large family units, while among people of European descent the disease is exceedingly well controlled.[7]

Greater availability of medical care has been an important factor in reducing the incidence of acute RF. The incidence fell by 60% in districts of Baltimore in which there were comprehensive health care programs, while it remained unchanged or increased in the remainder of the city.

GENETIC FACTORS AND ETHNICITY

Familial clustering of RF is not infrequent, especially in areas where the disease is common. No definite pattern of inheritance has been identified in genetic studies, and often it is difficult to separate genetic from environmental factors. There is no racial predilection for RF.

GEOGRAPHY AND CLIMATE

Seasonal variations in the incidence of RF are less marked in the tropics. In the temperate zones, RF has a peak incidence in late winter and early spring. Prospective studies from India[8] and Kuwait[9] have shown that the frequency and severity of the various clinical manifestations differed little from those in studies reported from the United States.

PATHOLOGY
CARDIAC AND VASCULAR LESIONS

On gross inspection, the heart is often dilated with inflammation of the pericardium, myocardium, and endocardium. The pericardium is covered with a fibrinous exudate; small to moderate amounts of serosanguineous fluid may be present in the pericardial sac. The myocardium and valvular endocardium are edematous. Rows of typical small vegetations or verrucae (1 mm to 2 mm) are seen on the atrial surfaces of the atrioventricular valves and ventricular aspects of the semilunar valves, along the lines of valve closure. The endocardium of the left atrium above the base of the posterior mitral leaflet may be thickened, rough, and opaque (MacCallum's patch).

ASCHOFF NODULE

The pathognomonic tissue response in acute RF is represented by Aschoff nodules, which are found mainly in the mural endocardium but which also occur in the interstitium of myocardium adjacent to vascular channels and in the epicardium. During the earliest phase of development of the Aschoff nodule, collagen fibers in the affected areas become swollen, fragmented, and hypereosinophilic, with the ground substance between them showing basophilic swelling. The mass of altered collagen is referred to as "fibrinoid," which, in addition, contains fibrin, γ globulin, and certain other components of connective tissue. The mature Aschoff nodule, measuring less than 1 mm to 1 cm in length, consists of Aschoff cells, Anitschkow cells, plasma cells, lymphocytes, polymorphonuclear leukocytes, fibrinoid material, and focally swollen, fragmented, hypereosinophilic collagen. The arrangement and proportions of the various components vary with the stage of development of the nodule. Aschoff cells are large ovoid cells with indistinct borders containing abundant basophilic cytoplasm and from one to five nuclei. Anitschkow cells are small elongated cells with scanty eosinophilic cytoplasm and single nuclei. The nuclear chromatin of Anitschkow cells and some of the Aschoff cells is arranged into a dense central bar with serrated edges with fine strands extending to the nuclear periphery. These appearances have led to such descriptive terms as *owl-eye nuclei* and *caterpillar nuclei*, depending on the plane of histologic section.[10] Observations from ultrastructural studies are in keeping with the traditional view that Aschoff cells and Anitschkow cells are derived from multipotential mesenchymal cells.[10] A few damaged or normal cardiac muscle cells are present in some Aschoff nodules, particularly in their periphery. The nodules heal gradually leaving a fibrous scar.

The reported incidence of Aschoff nodules in left atrial appendages of patients undergoing mitral commissurotomy varies from 19% to 74%.[11] The Aschoff nodules may persist for many years after an attack of acute RF, and their presence is not necessarily indicative of recent or active carditis. They are found more frequently in younger patients and are more common in adults with mitral stenosis than in those with pure mitral regurgitation.[11]

PERICARDITIS

In fatal cases of acute RF, microscopic evidence of pericarditis is always present. Aschoff nodules may be found in the epicardium. Demonstration of IgG, IgM, C3, and fibrinogen on the pericardial surface by direct immunofluorescence has been reported.[12]

MYOCARDITIS

Myocardial involvement in acute RF is characterized by features of an interstitial myocarditis, in addition to the specific lesion, the Aschoff nodule. Myocardial fiber damage and occasionally frank necrosis of myocardial fibers may be present, particularly near the Aschoff nodules and around small blood vessels. Visible changes in the conduction system are rare.

ENDOCARDITIS

The left atrial endocardium generally shows extensive inflammatory changes. It is perhaps the most intensively involved part of the heart. The valvular endocardium shows edema and inflammatory cellular infiltration. The verrucae are composed of fibrinoid and thrombotic material including large numbers of degranulated platelets. Ultrastructural studies have demonstrated areas of endothelial denudation on valve surfaces that would expose collagen and other thrombogenic material in the subendothelial space directly to blood, thus encouraging further thrombosis. The endothelial changes may be important in the genesis of rheumatic valvular deformities.[10] As healing occurs, there is vascularization and fibrosis of the cusps.

VASCULITIS

The coronary arteries, aorta, pulmonary artery, and the smaller muscular arteries and arterioles all show evidence of inflammation, with the characteristic cellular infiltration and fibrinoid changes. Thrombosis of large coronary arteries is rare.

EXTRACARDIAC LESIONS

JOINTS

The affected joints show swelling of the articular and periarticular structures, serous effusion, and gross and histologic features of synovial inflammation; later, fibrinoid lesions with histiocytic granulomas may appear. The cartilage does not show erosion. The lesions heal without scarring or deformity of the joint.

SUBCUTANEOUS NODULES

Histologically, the nodules show a central area of fibrinoid necrosis surrounded by histiocytes, fibroblasts, and small round cells. There may be perivascular collections of lymphocytes and polymorphonuclear leukocytes. The lesions heal without residua.

CENTRAL NERVOUS SYSTEM

Pathologic changes reported in patients dying with rheumatic chorea include arteritis of small blood vessels, perivascular round cell infiltration, petechial hemorrhages, and cellular degeneration scattered throughout the cortex, cerebellum, and basal ganglia. No site is consistently involved, and Aschoff nodules are not found.

LUNGS

In cases of severe carditis, the lungs may be severely congested and covered with hemorrhagic spots. Microscopically, there is evidence of alveolitis with deposition of fibrin and hemosiderin within alveoli. It is now generally held that these nonspecific changes are merely manifestations of severe cardiac failure and pulmonary congestion.

ETIOLOGY AND PATHOGENESIS

A number of clinical, epidemiologic, and immunologic studies have firmly established the relationship between pharyngeal infection by group A streptococci and acute RF. Nevertheless, the evidence for the streptococcal etiology of RF is necessarily indirect, since the organism cannot be recovered from the lesions of acute RF and a satisfactory experimental model of the disease has not been produced. The major lines of evidence implicating group A *Streptococcus* in the etiology of acute RF have been extensively reviewed.[13]

Acute RF occurs in a susceptible individual only when there has been a preceding infection of the throat by group A streptococci for a sufficiently long period with a significant antibody response. The precise pathogenetic mechanisms whereby streptococcal pharyngeal infection leads to acute RF are not clearly understood despite decades of active research. The proposed mechanisms for pathogenesis of acute RF suggest that the disease may result from a persistent infection with streptococci or its variant forms, a direct toxic reaction to streptococcal products, or immunologically mediated tissue injury.

The pathologic features of lesions in acute RF are not in keeping with an infective origin. Isolation of β-hemolytic streptococci from heart valves of patients dying of acute RF has not been confirmed in later studies in which exogenous contamination was carefully avoided. It has been shown that L forms of certain serotypes of group A streptococci can destroy human cardiac cells in tissue culture.[14] The presence of streptococcal protoplasts in cardiac tissue of patients with RF has not been demonstrated.

Various streptococcal extracellular products have been shown to cause myocardial damage in experimental animals. Granulomatous lesions have been produced in rabbits by intravenous injections of group A streptococcal mucopeptide or peptidoglycan.[15] The fact that mucopeptide is not confined to streptococci raises doubts about its role in the pathogenesis of RF. A major argument against the role of streptococcal products in the pathogenesis stems from the observation that carditis is not seen at the time of streptococcal infection and becomes evident after a latent period of about 3 weeks.

IMMUNE MECHANISMS

There are several observations that lend support to the current view that imunologic mechanisms are involved in the pathogenesis of acute RF:

1. Acute RF is manifest after a latent period of about 3 weeks following an acute streptococcal infection. This latent period parallels the time period required for the development of an immune response.
2. In epidemics of streptococcal pharyngitis, the mean antibody response to several streptococcal antigens is higher in patients who develop acute RF than in those who do not.
3. Cardiac tissue from cases of fatal rheumatic myocarditis has shown myocardial and endocardial deposits of immunoglobulin and complement.[16]
4. Adequate penicillin therapy of streptococcal infection prevents the development of acute RF. This might imply that without a prolonged antigenic stimulus, acute RF does not occur.

HUMORAL IMMUNITY AND CROSS-REACTIVE ANTIGENS

Beginning in the early 1960s several workers have demonstrated evidence of immunologic cross-reactivity between antigenic components of group A streptococci and human tissues. Antigenic cross-reactivity has been demonstrated between streptococcal cell wall components and human cardiac myofibrils,[17] streptococcal cell membrane and human sarcolemmal membranes,[18] cell wall polysaccharide of group A streptococci and glycoproteins of cardiac valves,[19] streptococcal hyaluronate and human synovial tissue,[20] and streptococcal membrane and the neuronal cytoplasm of caudate and subthalamic nuclei.[21]

The observation that antigenic components of streptococci could elicit an antibody that bound to human tissues led to the search for and identification of such antibodies in patients with acute RF. Several workers have described heart-reactive antibodies in patients with acute RF that could be absorbed out by streptococcal cell wall extracts.[22] In contrast, heart-reactive antibodies found in the sera of patients with Dressler's syndrome, chagasic cardiomyopathy, postpericardiotomy syndrome, and cardiac transplant rejection cannot be removed by streptococcal components. Furthermore, serial determinations of heart-reactive antibodies have shown a positive correlation with the course of acute RF.[23]

The observed antigenic similarities between streptococcal and host tissue components could result in the production of antistreptococcal antibodies that lead to autoimmune damage to the host tissues and might explain the anatomical localization of lesions of acute RF. However, there is no direct proof that such antibody-mediated tissue injury is of primary importance in the pathogenesis of acute RF. The finding of similar cross-reactivity with a variety of tissues, including the heart, in bacteria other than streptococci, the large margin of error in the subjective fluorescent antibody technique used to demonstrate cross-reactivity, and the possibility that some of these reactions may be the result of nonspecific binding of immunoglobulins to Fc receptors present on the surface of the streptococcal cell wall and the tissue being examined cast doubt on the significance of antigenic cross-reactivity in the pathogenesis of acute RF.[14,24]

CELL-MEDIATED IMMUNITY

Attention has been directed to cellular immune mechanisms in acute RF. The Aschoff nodule, the pathognomonic histologic feature of RF, is a granulomatous lesion that is more likely to result from a cellular immune response. Studies of cellular reactivity to streptococcal membrane antigens using the leukocyte migration test have shown significant inhibition of cells from patients with RF compared with those from normal subjects.[25] The increased cellular reactivity persists for up to 5 years after the initial attack. A heightened lymphocyte blastogenic response to streptococcal antigens has been reported in patients with RF.[14] T cells obtained from guinea pigs immunized with streptococcal cell wall antigens have been shown to be cytotoxic to cultured guinea pig heart cells.[26] Hutto and Ayoub have shown that peripheral blood lymphocytes from patients with acute RF are cytotoxic to human cardiac cells grown in tissue culture.[27]

There appears to be an abnormal humoral and cellular response to streptococcal antigens in patients with acute RF. Humoral immune mechanisms might prepare the host's tissue for an autosensitization process and act in conjunction with sensitized cells to produce damage to the host's tissue.

SUSCEPTIBILITY TO ACUTE RF

A state of heightened antibody or B-cell responsiveness has been suggested as a cause for susceptibility to acute RF. Higher antibody response to influenza vaccine and isologous red blood cells has been observed in rheumatic patients compared with nonrheumatic subjects.[14] Patients with RF have also been shown to have a higher mean antibody response to several streptococcal antigens. Studies by Dudding and Ayoub have shown a sustained elevation of antibody to group A polysaccharide in a subset of patients with RF with valvular disease.[28] The question of altered immunoregulation in RF has been addressed by several workers. It appears that the immunologic hyperresponsiveness in some patients with RF could be due to diminished T suppressor cell function, either secondary to decreased T suppressor cell numbers or alternatively, to decreased suppressor receptor number or activation.[14]

CLINICAL FEATURES

The signs and symptoms of acute RF vary considerably, none of them being pathognomonic of the disease process. The clinical picture often overlaps with many other conditions, especially in the early stages. In 1944, T. Duckett Jones grouped the manifestations of acute RF into "major" and "minor" ones, based on their usefulness in diagnosis (see *Diagnosis*).

MAJOR CLINICAL MANIFESTATIONS
ARTHRITIS

Polyarthritis is the most common presenting manifestation of acute RF, especially in older children and adults, occurring in about 75% of patients. There has been little change in the incidence of this manifestation over the years. The latent period between the antecedent streptococcal infection and raised antibody titers is almost always found in patients with evidence of arthritis.

Typically the large joints are involved, in particular the knees, ankles, elbows, and wrists; however, almost any joint may be affected including the hips, spine, temporomandibular joints, and rarely the smaller joints of hands and feet. The classic picture is one of migratory polyarthritis, the joints being affected in quick succession and each affected joint showing signs of inflammation such as redness, swelling, and local heat for 24 hours to about a week; inflammatory features may last for 2 weeks to 3 weeks in one third of the patients. The affected joint may be exquisitely tender, and the pain is often disproportionate to the objective signs. Arthritis is generally milder and lasts for a shorter period in children. Apart from soft tissue swelling, no radiologic abnormalities are present and the arthritis subsides with no residual deformities, a possible exception being the very rare Jaccoud's arthritis, characterized by erosions of the metacarpal heads and deformities of the metacarpophalangeal joints resulting from periarticular fibrosis. The relationship of Jaccoud's arthritis to acute RF, seronegative rheumatoid arthritis, and chronic capsular fibrosis is not clear.

It appears that carditis occurs less frequently and is usually less severe in patients with severe polyarthritis than in those with milder joint manifestations. In a series reported by Feinstein and Spagnuolo, carditis was present in only 26% of patients with red, hot, swollen joints, in contrast to 96% of those with arthralgia alone.[29]

CARDITIS

Carditis is the most important manifestation of acute RF since it may result in permanent, disabling sequelae. The reported incidence of carditis in first attacks of acute RF varies from 40% to 51% in the United States and Canada and from 64% to 80% in the developing countries, although the difference is less apparent in later prospective studies.[30] As mentioned earlier, there appears to be an inverse relationship between the severity of arthritis and the frequency of carditis. It has also been pointed out that carditis occurs more frequently in younger patients.[29] The older the patient with a first attack of acute RF, the less likely he is to have carditis.

Features of carditis appear early in the course of acute RF, with significant murmurs being heard in 85% of patients by the second or third week of the illness. The severity of carditis varies considerably, ranging from subclinical inflammation to the fulminant form resulting in death during the acute phase. It is the general impression of most observers that there has been a notable decline in the incidence and severity of carditis over the past few decades.[31]

The unequivocal presence of one or more of the following features is essential for the diagnosis of carditis in a patient with suspected acute RF: (1) significant murmurs not previously present, (2) cardiomegaly, (3) cardiac failure, and (4) pericarditis.

CARDIAC MURMURS. Auscultatory signs of mitral and aortic regurgitation are frequently present, with the former being approximately three times more common. Involvement of the tricuspid valve is seldom recognized clinically during the acute phase. When the mitral valve is affected, as is the case in over 90% of patients with carditis, a high-pitched, blowing, pansystolic (or nearly pansystolic) murmur of moderate intensity is heard over the apex, often with radiation to the axilla. In some patients the murmur disappears altogether during recovery; in others it persists or increases. A third heart sound is often present, occasionally followed by an evanescent, low-pitched, mid-diastolic murmur of short duration (Carey-Coombs murmur) at the apex, attributed to swelling and stiffening of mitral valve leaflets, increased flow across the valve, and alteration in left ventricular compliance. The early diastolic decrescendo murmur of aortic regurgitation is present in fewer than a third of the patients and only intermittently in some.

CARDIAC ENLARGEMENT. Significant cardiomegaly occurs in just over 50% of patients with carditis and is a reliable indicator of the severity of cardiac involvement. The apical impulse may be diffuse and displaced downward. Cardiac enlargement on the chest film generally reflects dilatation of the left ventricle and left atrium and may, in some cases, be partly due to associated pericardial effusion. Serial radiologic and echocardiographic examination is useful in assessing prognosis and for follow-up.

CARDIAC FAILURE. Cardiac failure is relatively rare, occurring in less than 10% of patients with first attacks of acute rheumatic carditis.[32] Older children, adolescents, and adults with cardiac failure manifest the classic features. In contrast, the diagnosis of cardiac decompensation can be more difficult in the preschool child presenting with tachypnea, nausea and vomiting, a tender enlarged liver, and facial edema. Despite radiologic evidence of severe pulmonary venous congestion, paroxysmal dyspnea is often absent and the chest may be surprisingly clear on auscultation. Persistent tachycardia during sleep and a ventricular gallop rhythm are commonly present.

Persistent heart failure lasting for more than 12 weeks, ascribed in the past to chronic rheumatic carditis, is seldom seen nowadays, and when present may be due to severe mitral or aortic regurgitation or both (rather than due to myocarditis), requiring early surgical correction. Two-dimensional and Doppler echocardiography and radionuclide methods could be useful in separating patients with poor ventricular function (due to myocarditis) from those with severe valvar regurgitation. However, no recent data are available on the use of these noninvasive techniques during the acute phase of RF.

PERICARDITIS. Pericarditis, with a reported incidence of 5% to 10%,[30] generally occurs in association with severe carditis. It is clinically manifest by chest pain, a pericardial friction rub, or radiologic evidence of pericardial effusion. Chest pain is infrequent in young children with pericarditis. The chest film may show rapid fluctuations in heart size. Echocardiography is useful in confirming the presence of pericardial effusion and following its course. Pericardial effusion is seldom large and cardiac tamponade is extremely rare. The electrocardiogram may or may not show the typical ST segment and T wave abnormalities.

SUBCUTANEOUS NODULES

Subcutaneous nodules with a reported incidence of up to 30% in the past are seen less frequently, occurring in less than 10% of cases. Typically, these subcutaneous swellings measuring 0.5 cm to 2.0 cm are discrete, nontender, firm, and mobile and are located over the extensor surfaces of elbows, knees, ankles, and knuckles, the bony prominences such as the spinous processes of vertebrae, and the occipital region. They can be easily missed unless searched for carefully. They are usually multiple and may occur in crops.

Subcutaneous nodules appear relatively late in the course of the disease, often more than 3 weeks after the appearance of the other manifestations of RF and are thus not very helpful in the early diagnosis. The nodules seldom occur as an isolated manifestation and are most often seen in patients with severe or protracted carditis. In most cases they disappear in 1 or 2 weeks.

ERYTHEMA MARGINATUM

Erythema marginatum, the least frequent of the major manifestations, is a striking, evanescent rash seen in approximately 5% of patients with acute RF, usually in association with carditis.

The lesions, which occur mainly on the trunk, buttocks, and the proximal parts of the limbs, begin as mildly erythematous macules. The erythema extends peripherally; while the skin over the center of the macule returns to normal color. Thus the lesions appear as enlarging rings, or when they fuse they take on a serpiginous pattern. They are not itchy, are painless and nonindurated, and blanch on pressure. They can be elicited or accentuated by a hot bath and are difficult to see in dark-skinned races. Erythema marginatum usually occurs early in the course of acute RF but may recur intermittently for several months. Similar lesions have been reported in drug reactions, sepsis, and glomerulonephritis.

CHOREA

Over the past 30 years, the incidence of chorea in acute RF has fallen from around 50% to under 5% in most Western countries. Chorea has a predilection for females and is rare after puberty. There is generally a latent period of several months (most commonly 1 month to 3 months) between the preceding streptococcal infection and the appearance of chorea. Thus, when chorea appears, the other clinical manifestations of acute RF may have subsided and laboratory evidence of a recent streptococcal infection may no longer be demonstrable.

The onset of this neurologic disorder is usually insidious. Not uncommonly, emotional lability, irritability, and clumsiness are the earliest manifestations. These are followed by the appearance of choreiform movements, which typically are rapid, jerky, irregular, nonrepetitive, and purposeless. The involuntary movements, which may affect any muscle group but particularly those of the upper limbs and face, are worsened by excitement and fatigue and disappear during sleep.

Rapid changes in facial expression and grimacing are common. Speech, when affected, is halting and staccato. Characteristically there is generalized muscular hypotonia with varying degrees of weakness of affected muscles. Incoordination may be demonstrated if the patient is asked to carry out a specific action. Raising the arms overhead causes marked pronation of both hands (pronation sign). When the hands are held out in front there is flexion of wrists, hyperextension of metacarpophalangeal joints, and abduction of thumbs ("spooning"). When asked to squeeze the examiner's finger, the patient is unable to maintain a sustained grip (milkmaid's grip). When the patient is asked to protrude the tongue, it is shot out and withdrawn with high speed (jack-in-the-box tongue).

On an average, chorea lasts for 2 months to 4 months, although rarely it may persist for over 2 years. Development of rheumatic heart disease has been observed in nearly one fourth of the patients with pure chorea who are followed for 20 years.

MINOR CLINICAL MANIFESTATIONS

Fever, with no characteristic pattern, is almost always present for a week or so at the onset of acute RF, with the temperature rarely rising above 104°F (40°C). Low-grade fever may persist for 1 or 2 weeks. Not infrequently, anorexia, nausea, and vomiting are the presenting symptoms in the young child with carditis and heart failure. Abdominal pain attributed to mesenteric vasculitis or adenitis and epistaxis occur in less than 5% of patients. The so-called rheumatic pneumonia usually occurs in patients with severe carditis and heart failure and is rarely seen now. The radiologic features such as shifting areas of pulmonary infiltrates, patchy consolidation, and segmental atelectasis could well be related to the severe heart failure or an associated viral pneumonia. Mild normocytic normochromic anemia is common and improves once the inflammation subsides. Nonspecific ST-T changes and prolongation of the PR interval are common in acute RF as well as in other poststreptococcal states and carry no prognostic significance. A diagnosis of carditis should not be made on the basis of atrioventricular conduction abnormalities or other nonspecific electrocardiographic changes.

LABORATORY DATA
TESTS FOR ANTECEDENT STREPTOCOCCAL INFECTION

Laboratory data supporting a recent streptococcal infection or a history of recent scarlet fever are important in substantiating the diagnosis of acute RF as emphasized in the most recent revision of the Jones criteria.

THROAT CULTURE

All patients with suspected acute RF should have at least one properly obtained throat culture. Throat cultures are often negative by the time the clinical manifestations of acute RF appear. On the other hand, a positive culture for group A streptococcus may represent a carrier state (especially in children) rather than an active infection and thus may be of limited value.

TESTS FOR STREPTOCOCCAL ANTIBODIES

Demonstration of significant streptococcal antibody titers is more definitive evidence of an antecedent streptococcal infection. Among the various streptococcal antibody tests available, the well-standardized antistreptolysin-O (ASO) test is the most commonly used. The antibody titer usually begins to rise within 1 week to 2 weeks and reaches a peak in 3 weeks to 5 weeks after the infection, with the titers declining rapidly thereafter. Single titers of 333 Todd units/ml or more in children and 250 Todd units/ml or more in adolescents and adults indicate a recent streptococcal infection, as does a rise (or fall) of 2 dilutions or more on serial tests. Significant ASO titers are found in about 80% of patients early in the course of acute RF. Penicillin and corticosteroid therapy, differences in host response, and variation in streptolysin-O production among the various strains of streptococci are all important in determining the actual ASO response. In patients presenting with late manifestations such as chorea, ASO titers are often normal.

Additional streptococcal antibody tests, preferably anti-DNase B and antihyaluronidase, should be carried out in patients with suspected acute RF who have low or borderline ASO titers. It has been shown that serologic evidence of a recent streptococcal infection can be obtained in 95% of patients if three different antibody tests are employed.[33] Anti-DNase tends to remain raised longer than the other antibodies, and hence the test is particularly useful in patients seen some time after the onset of symptoms and in those presenting with chorea alone.

Other specific tests such as antistreptokinase and anti-NADase although useful are employed less commonly. The newer streptozyme test—a simple, rapid, inexpensive slide agglutination test that simultaneously determines antibodies to a variety of streptococcal extracellular antigens—appears to be highly sensitive, comparing favorably with the results of testing for two or three individual antibodies. Further data with regard to the specificity of the test and standardization are needed before the test can be accepted for general use.

TESTS FOR EVIDENCE OF ACTIVE INFLAMMATION (ACUTE PHASE REACTANTS)
ERYTHROCYTE SEDIMENTATION RATE

The erythrocyte sedimentation rate (ESR) is almost always accelerated in the presence of rheumatic activity unless suppressed by corticosteroids, salicylates, or other anti-inflammatory agents. It may be normal in patients with pure chorea or isolated erythema marginatum and in the presence of severe cardiac failure. On the other hand, anemia accompanying acute RF may result in a more rapid sedimentation rate. In general, the magnitude of increase in ESR parallels the intensity of the inflammatory reaction. A normal sedimentation rate in an untreated patient with suspected acute RF is uncommon.

C-REACTIVE PROTEIN

C-reactive protein (CRP, so named because of its reactivity with the C-polysaccharide of pneumococcus) is a unique β-globulin that appears in the blood during the course of any inflammatory condition. It can be measured semiquantitatively using a commercially available antiserum. According to some authors it reflects rheumatic activity more closely than the ESR since it is unaffected by factors such as anemia and changes in serum proteins and is particularly useful in monitoring patients for "rebounds" during withdrawal of suppressive drugs.[34] Like the ESR, it may be negative in isolated chorea and erythema marginatum and in patients on anti-inflammatory drugs. The main disadvantage of the test is its extreme sensitivity since the result may be positive even with mild inflammation of non rheumatic origin and heart failure regardless of its cause. The test is less widely used today than in the past.

OTHER TESTS

Other acute phase reactants include leukocyte count, Weltmann reaction, serum mucoprotein, serum hexosamine, and serum protein electrophoresis, none of which has gained wide usage.

DIAGNOSIS

The guidelines for RF originally proposed by Jones over 40 years ago have been widely accepted and have proved to be extremely useful, especially in avoiding overdiagnosis. According to the most recent revision of the Jones criteria, the presence of two major or one major and two minor manifestations indicates a high probability of RF, if supported by evidence of a preceding streptococcal infection (increased streptococcal antibody titers, positive culture for group A streptococci, recent scarlet fever) (Table 96.1). In the absence of such supportive evidence, the diagnosis of RF is doubtful, except in situations in which the disease is discovered after a long latent interval following the antecedent streptococcal infection (e.g., Sydenham's chorea, low-grade carditis).

It should be noted that all the major criteria are based essentially on clinical signs, and the importance of a careful physical examination cannot be overemphasized. The Jones criteria are at best a guide, not a rule, to the diagnosis of RF, which at times can be exceedingly difficult in view of the wide variations in the manifestations of the disease and the fact that many other conditions, some of them not so uncommon, may closely mimic RF. Uncritical application of the Jones criteria can lead to an erroneous diagnosis. It is conceivable that with strict adherence to the criteria the diagnosis would be missed in a few instances. Arthralgia coupled with abnormal laboratory test results may be the only manifestation present in a few patients with RF. On the other hand, with the decreasing frequency of subcutaneous nodules, erythema marginatum, and chorea, overdiagnosis is most likely to result from misinterpretation of the signs and symptoms of arthritis and carditis. It should be remembered that streptococcal infections are common and that they may precede an unrelated illness purely by chance.

None of the manifestations of acute RF is specific for the disorder, and a number of conditions presenting with fever, joint manifestations, and apparent cardiac involvement may cause diagnostic confusion.

Several disorders can closely simulate arthritis of acute RF. This is particularly true of acute reactive arthritis following infection elsewhere in the body as in the case of *Yersinia enterocolitica* and rubella infections. Collagen disorders such as rheumatoid arthritis and systemic lupus erythematosus with their multisystem involvement, Lyme arthritis, polyarthritis or arthralgia associated with viral hepatitis and sickle cell anemia, and gonococcal arthritis in the adolescent can pose problems in differential diagnosis.

Viral myopericarditis may mimic rheumatic myocarditis, as can atrial myxoma and infective endocarditis when associated with arthralgia, changing murmurs, and a high ESR. Innocent murmurs of childhood and murmurs due to congenital heart disease may be confused with those of acute rheumatic carditis.

TREATMENT

Treatment of acute RF is mainly supportive and should be tailored according to the severity of the various manifestations and the course of the illness. The various measures taken are aimed at eradication of streptococci from the throat, suppression of the inflammatory process, control of cardiac failure and chorea when present, and prevention of further recurrences of streptococcal throat infections.

ERADICATION OF RESIDUAL STREPTOCOCCI

All patients with acute RF, including those presenting with isolated chorea, should be given a therapeutic course of penicillin or a suitable alternative to eradicate residual group A streptococci in the throat, even when cultures are negative. The most commonly employed antibiotic regimens are outlined below:

1. A single intramuscular injection of benzathine penicillin G, 1.2 million units (600,000 units in children weighing less than 60 pounds)
2. Intramuscular injections of procaine penicillin, 600,000 units/day for ten days
3. Buffered penicillin G, 250,000 units orally, four times per day for ten days
4. Penicillin V, 250 mg, four times per day for ten days
5. Erythromycin, 250 mg, four times per day (40 mg/kg/day in children, not to exceed 1 g/day) for ten days, in patients who are allergic to penicillin.

BED REST

Although the value of prolonged bed rest in preventing the occurrence of carditis, or altering the severity and duration of the inflammatory process, has not been unequivocally proved, most physicians would consider it prudent to confine all patients with acute RF to bed for the first 3 weeks, when fever and arthritis are commonly present, and when carditis, if not already present, makes its appearance. By the end of 3 weeks, most patients presenting with arthritis are afebrile and free of joint symptoms. They may then gradually be allowed to ambulate and to resume normal activities after a further period of 3 weeks.

Patients with carditis but no definite cardiomegaly or evidence of cardiac failure are advised to rest in bed for an additional 1 or 2 weeks, while those showing cardiomegaly without cardiac failure should rest in bed for a full 6 weeks. Patients with carditis who develop cardiac failure are kept on strict bed rest until the failure is controlled. Restricted physical activities should continue until a month after anti-inflammatory treatment is stopped (*i.e.*, usually a total of 8 weeks to 12 weeks and occasionally longer).

A persistent, borderline, or mild elevation of the ESR seen in some patients, even after the clinical features of inflammation have completely subsided, should not be considered an indication for continued restriction of physical activity.

SUPPRESSION OF THE INFLAMMATORY PROCESS

There is little convincing evidence that either salicylates or corticosteroids, the anti-inflammatory agents most commonly employed in the treatment of acute RF, shorten the course of the illness, prevent the

TABLE 96.1 JONES CRITERIA (REVISED)

Major Manifestations	Minor Manifestations
Carditis	Fever
Polyarthritis	Arthralgia
Chorea	Previous rheumatic fever or rheumatic heart disease
Erythema marginatum	
Subcutaneous nodules	Acute-phase reactants: high erythrocyte sedimentation rate or positive C-reactive protein
	Prolonged PR interval

plus

Supporting evidence of a preceding streptococcal infection

(See text for details. Modified from ad hoc committee to revise the Jones Criteria (modified) of the council on rheumatic fever and congenital heart disease of the American Heart Association: Jones Criteria (revised) for guidance in the diagnosis of rheumatic fever. Circulation 32:664, 1965, by permission of the American Heart Association, Inc)

occurrence of carditis, or reduce the severity of residual cardiac damage. Nevertheless, their usefulness in controlling the inflammatory symptoms is unquestionable. Fever, arthritis, and pericarditis may respond dramatically, often with 24 to 48 hours; ESR begins to fall within a few days. Although there is no general agreement with regard to the choice and dosage of the anti-inflammatory agents, and the duration of treatment, most physicians tend to treat patients with carditis who have cardiomegaly or cardiac failure with corticosteroids. We find the following guidelines useful when planning treatment with anti-inflammatory agents for the various subsets of patients with acute RF.

1. Patients with arthralgia or mild arthritis and no evidence of carditis should initially be given simple analgesics (such as codeine) alone, especially when the diagnosis is in doubt, so as not to suppress the later appearance of definite arthritis or fever.
2. Patients with definite arthritis with or without associated mild carditis (no cardiomegaly or cardiac failure) should be treated with aspirin.
3. Patients with carditis and mild cardiomegaly but no cardiac failure (with or without arthritis) are usually treated with aspirin. It may become necessary to replace aspirin with corticosteroids in some of these patients, if the response to aspirin appears to be poor as evidenced by persistent tachycardia or fever or when toxic or near-toxic doses of aspirin are required to control the features of inflammation.
4. Patients with carditis and significant cardiomegaly with or without cardiac failure (with or without arthritis) should be treated with corticosteroids.
5. Patients with carditis and a long blowing apical systolic murmur with an intensity of grade 3 or more are usually treated with corticosteroids.
6. Patients with pericarditis are usually treated with corticosteroids, since the majority have cardiomegaly and cardiac failure.
7. Patients who develop carditis while on aspirin should be switched to corticosteroids.
8. Recurrent attacks of acute RF in patients with established rheumatic heart disease should be treated with corticosteroids. A diagnosis of carditis in these patients is often difficult.
9. Recurrent attacks of acute RF in patients with no evidence of carditis or established rheumatic heart disease can be treated with aspirin.
10. Anti-inflammatory agents are not indicated in patients with isolated chorea.

SALICYLATES

Salicylates, through their inhibitory effect on prostaglandin synthesis, suppress the inflammatory response. Aspirin is given in doses sufficient to control symptoms and to achieve a blood salicylate level of 20 mg to 35 mg/dl. Many physicians increase the dose of the drug until clinical manifestations of mild toxicity (hyperpnea, tinnitus, vertigo) appear. Blood levels of 20 mg to 25 mg/dl can usually be achieved with a dose of 90 mg to 120 mg/kg/day in children, and 6 to 8 g/day in adults given in six divided doses. The dose may be reduced to two thirds of the original once the clinical features of inflammation subside and halved when the acute phase reactants return to normal. The total duration of treatment with aspirin is usually 6 to 8 weeks, sometimes longer.

Prolonged high-dose therapy with blood salicylate levels over 25 mg/dl may result in mild, reversible hepatic injury, as reflected by elevated levels of serum transaminases. Side-effects such as nausea and vomiting can cause difficulties in maintaining an adequate dosage. The value of employing toxic or near-toxic doses of salicylates has been questioned by some authors,[35,36] who recommend a more modest dosage. A dose of 75 mg/kg/day in children and 900 mg every 3 to 4 hours in adults will usually achieve a serum salicylate level of 20 mg/dl, which is below the toxic range and usually effective.

Administration of the drug 30 minutes after meals and the use of an enteric-coated preparation are beneficial in reducing gastric irritation and bleeding. Administration of antacids renders the drug less effective.

CORTICOSTEROIDS

The United Kingdom and the United States joint trial of ACTH, aspirin, and cortisone in acute RF, using relatively low doses of corticosteroids, failed to show any advantage of corticosteroids with regard to residual cardiac damage at 1, 5, and 10 years after the initial attack, although each agent controlled the acute manifestations promptly and effectively.[37] Similar results were obtained at 1 year in two multicenter studies conducted on a smaller scale, in which prednisone in larger doses was used.[38,39] Other studies have been reported with results suggesting that corticosteroids in large doses given early in the course of the illness may still have some advantage over salicylates in reducing cardiac damage in patients with mild carditis. Most physicians currently limit the use of corticosteroids to patients with cardiomegaly or cardiac failure. In patients with severe acute rheumatic myocarditis or pancarditis, corticosteroids may be lifesaving.

ACTH is now seldom employed in the treatment of acute RF. Prednisone is generally preferred to other corticosteroids since it causes relatively fewer problems with electrolyte balance and is given initially in daily doses of 2.5 mg to 3.0 mg/kg in children and 60 mg to 120 mg in adults. We increase the dose if after a week the clinical or laboratory parameters do not show a significant improvement or if there is a worsening of the clinical or laboratory parameters following any subsequent reduction in dosage. The high-dose schedule of corticosteroid therapy is usually maintained for the first 1 to 3 weeks. Once the clinical and laboratory features of inflammation improve, the drug is tapered over a period of 2 weeks. While steroids are being withdrawn, aspirin, in standard doses as described previously, is added to the treatment in order to reduce the likelihood of a post-therapeutic rebound of rheumatic activity.

Side-effects with prolonged high-dose corticosteroid therapy include cushingoid changes, hypokalemia, salt and water retention, mild hypertension, toxic psychosis, and gastric ulceration. Striae, which may leave permanent scars, occur in nearly two thirds of patients and are particularly common in adolescent females.

The place of alternate-day high-dose corticosteroid therapy with its theoretical advantages and that of the newer nonsteroidal anti-inflammatory agents (*e.g.*, propionic acid derivatives) in the treatment of acute RF is not yet clear.

POST-THERAPEUTIC REBOUNDS

There may be a reactivation of the inflammatory process with reappearance of fever, arthralgia and arthritis, or abnormal laboratory test results, while the anti-inflammatory agents are being withdrawn or shortly thereafter. Occasionally these rebounds are more severe, especially in patients with severe carditis. Mild rebounds generally abate within a few days and require no more than simple analgesics or aspirin in small doses. In more severe cases, aspirin in full doses should be reinstituted and continued for a further 3 weeks to 4 weeks.

CONTROL OF CARDIAC FAILURE

Cardiac failure associated with acute rheumatic carditis can be controlled in most patients with conventional measures such as rest, salt restriction, digitalis, and diuretics. In some patients with resistant cardiac failure, vasodilator therapy may be indicated. In a small number of patients with severe mitral or aortic regurgitation (the valves often having been damaged during multiple recurrences previously) and severe intractable cardiac failure, valve replacement surgery carried out during the acute phase may be lifesaving.

MANAGEMENT OF CHOREA

Corticosteroids and salicylates do not affect the course of chorea and are not indicated unless there is clear evidence of concomitant carditis. Adequate rest in a quiet environment without physical or emotional stress and competent nursing care are essential. Chlorpromazine, 25 mg, phenobarbitone, 15 mg to 30 mg, or diazepam, 2 mg to 5 mg, given every 8 hours appear to be useful. Once improvement is apparent, patients are encouraged to resume normal physical activities.

RESIDUAL RHEUMATIC HEART DISEASE

Over the last few decades there has been a significant decrease in the morbidity and mortality from acute RF (especially in the affluent countries), owing to an unexplained decrease in the severity of the initial attack and even more importantly, to a reduction in the number of recurrences. In the preprophylaxis era, about 25% of patients were dead within 10 years of the initial attack of acute RF, and of the remainder, two thirds had heart disease.[40,41] In contrast, the death rate for patients on prophylaxis 7 to 10 years after onset is 1%, and two thirds have no residual heart disease.[37,42]

The incidence and severity of residual heart disease on follow-up appears to be clearly related to the severity of carditis during the acute attack. The long-term prognosis is excellent for patients who have no organic murmurs during the acute attack, provided recurrences of RF are prevented. In the United Kingdom–United States Cooperative Study, 94% of such patients were found to have normal hearts at 10-year follow-up.[37] With increasing severity of initial carditis, the prognosis becomes poorer, so that among patients who had cardiac failure or pericarditis during the acute attack, only 32% were without heart disease at 10 years.

In a 10-year follow-up study of 115 patients with RF on regular antibiotic prophylaxis, Tompkins and co-workers found disappearance of murmurs in 70% of patients with mitral regurgitation and in 27% of patients with aortic regurgitation.[43] In contrast, only 30% of patients with an initial murmur of mitral regurgitation were reported to have lost the murmur within 20 years in the pre-prophylaxis-era study of Bland and Jones.[41] The same authors found that 44% of their patients who were initially free of detectable heart disease developed significant murmurs over a 20-year follow-up period. In the United Kingdom–United States Cooperative Study, mitral stenosis, uncommon at 5 years, was definitely present in 18 of the 347 cases examined at 10 years.[37] On the other hand, Tompkins and co-workers found that none of their 115 patients on regular antibiotic prophylaxis developed mitral or aortic stenosis,[43] which would suggest that rheumatic mitral and aortic stenosis result from recurrent RF, perhaps subclinical in many cases, and hence are preventable.

PREVENTION
SECONDARY PROPHYLAXIS

The usefulness of long-term antibiotic prophylaxis in preventing recurrent attacks of RF is now firmly established. The death rate for patients on prophylaxis, 7 to 10 years after the onset of RF, has been reported to be 1%,[39] which is in marked contrast to a figure of about 25% in the preantibiotic era.[40,41] With monthly injections of benzathine penicillin G, a rate of less than one recurrence per 250,000 patient years has been observed in careful studies.

Once the diagnosis of acute RF has been established, and the patient has been given a therapeutic course of antibiotics to eradicate residual group A streptococci from the throat (as described in the section on treatment), long-term prophylaxis against recurrent streptococcal infections should be instituted. One of the following schedules may be employed for secondary prophylaxis:

1. Intramuscular injections of benzathine penicillin G, 1.2 million units every 4 weeks
2. Sulfadiazine, 0.5 g once a day for children under 60 pounds and 1 g once a day for all others
3. Buffered penicillin G, 200,000 to 250,000 units twice a day 30 minutes before or 1 hour after meals
4. Erythromycin, 250 mg, twice a day in patients allergic to penicillin and sulfonamides.

Benzathine penicillin is by far the most effective and reliable agent for long-term prophylaxis and is preferred in patients at high risk of developing recurrences and in those likely to be noncompliant on daily oral medication. It has been suggested that a 3-week schedule may be more effective in areas with a very high prevalence of streptococcal infections.[44] There have been studies indicating that penicillin levels fall more rapidly in adults.[45] Allergic reactions to benzathine penicillin are rare and are not more severe than those following other parenteral penicillins.

Although oral sulfadiazine and buffered penicillin are about equally effective in long-term prophylaxis, the latter is more commonly used at present. Prophylaxis with oral penicillin may cause emergence of resistant α-streptococci in the mouth, a potential hazard in patients with rheumatic valvular involvement. Patients on sulfadiazine should be monitored for development of side-effects. Sulfadiazine given during the last trimester of pregnancy can cause hyperbilirubinemia in the newborn. Poor compliance is a major problem in patients on long-term oral prophylaxis and is more common in females, adolescents, patients from large families, and those who were not hospitalized during the acute attack of RF and are not accompanied to the clinic by parents.[46] Serial determination of streptococcal antibody titer and spot checks of urine for the presence of penicillin are useful in assessing the efficacy of secondary prophylaxis. The many barriers to secondary prevention of acute RF encountered in the developing countries have been reviewed.[47]

There is little agreement with regard to the optimum duration of antistreptococcal prophylaxis. Ideally, in patients with rheumatic heart disease, penicillin should be continued indefinitely for maximal protection. Most often prophylaxis is discontinued when the patient reaches 30 years of age and 5 years have elapsed since the acute attack. A longer period of prophylaxis is indicated in patients who exhibit one of the following features and are thus at high risk of developing a recurrence: (1) recent episode of acute RF; (2) multiple recurrences in the past; (3) carditis during a previous attack; (4) presence of rheumatic heart disease; and (5) high risk of exposure to streptococcal infection at work (teachers, nurses, physicians, those in military service) or at home (mothers of young children, patients from crowded homes).

PRIMARY PROPHYLAXIS

Studies in military populations with a high frequency of streptococcal infections have shown that penicillin therapy can reduce the rate of occurrence of acute RF from 3.0% to 0.3%. Major factors that hamper successful prevention of first attacks of RF include the size of the population at risk, lack of public awareness that sore throats may lead to heart disease, inadequate primary health care facilities, and the imperfect methods for diagnosing streptococcal pharyngitis.[3]

A firm clinical diagnosis of streptococcal pharyngitis may not be easy when the classic features of fever, a fiery red throat with patches of exudate, and tender, enlarged cervical lymph nodes are not present. Furthermore, even some apparently mild streptococcal infections may be followed by RF. Therefore, throat cultures to exclude streptococcal infections are widely used in patients with an acute pharyngitis. Conjunctivitis, simple coryza, and hoarse throat are usually not associated with streptococcal infections; in patients presenting with these symptoms, cultures are not essential. In developing countries, cost factors seriously influence the decision whether to carry out cultures. It might be pointed out that in children immunized against diptheria, β-hemolytic *Streptococcus* is the chief, if not the only, bacterial cause of acute pharyngitis.

Penicillin remains the drug of choice in primary prophylaxis. Patients allergic to penicillin may be treated with a 10-day course of erythromycin. The sulfonamides, which suppress but do not eradicate group A streptococci from the throat, chloramphenicol, and the tetracyclines should not be used in the treatment of acute streptococcal pharyngitis. Drugs such as ampicillin, dicloxacillin, lincomycin, clindamycin, and cephalosporins, although effective, are not recommended and should be reserved for treatment of infections with bacteria other than β-hemolytic streptococci. The various antibiotic schedules effective in the treatment of streptococcal pharyngitis have been discussed elsewhere in this chapter.

STREPTOCOCCAL VACCINES

A satisfactory safe vaccine effective against at least the majority of the prevalent serotypes of group A streptococci has not yet been developed. Ideally, the vaccine should be highly antigenic yet free of cross-reactivity with cardiac tissues. Streptococcal M-proteins, the only antigens that stimulate protective antibodies, have been studied extensively and significant progress has been made in purification of M-proteins.

REFERENCES

1. DiSciascio G, Taranta A: Rheumatic fever in children. Am Heart J 99:635, 1980
2. Sievers J, Hall P: Incidence of acute rheumatic fever. Br Heart J 33:833, 1971
3. Markowitz M: The changing picture of rheumatic fever. Arthritis Rheum 20:369, 1977
4. Quinn RW, Federspiel C: The incidence of rheumatic fever in metropolitan Nashville. Am J Epidemiol 99:273, 1974
5. Community control of rheumatic fever in developing countries: I. A major public health problem. WHO Chron 34:336, 1980
6. Rammelkamp CH Jr, Denny FW Jr, Wannamaker LW: Studies on the epidemiology of rheumatic fever in the Armed Forces. In Thomas L (ed): Rheumatic Fever. Minneapolis, University of Minnesota Press, 1952
7. Stollerman GH: World Health Organization Western Pacific Seminar discusses prevention and control of cardiovascular diseases. Bull Int Soc Cardiol 10:8, 1969
8. Sanyal SK, Thapar MK, Ahmed SH et al: The initial attack of acute rheumatic fever during childhood in North India. Circulation 49:7, 1974
9. Majeed HA, Khan N, Dabbagh M et al: Acute rheumatic fever during childhood in Kuwait: The mild nature of the initial attack. Ann Trop Paediatr 1:13, 1981
10. Ferrans VJ, Roberts WC: Pathology of rheumatic heart disease. In Borman JB, Gotsman MS (eds): Rheumatic Valvular Disease in Children, pp 28–58. New York, Springer-Verlag, 1980
11. Virmani R, Roberts WC: Aschoff bodies in operatively excised atrial appendage and in papillary muscle: Frequency and clinical significance. Circulation 55:559, 1977
12. Persellin ST, Ramirez G, Motamed F: Immunopathology of rheumatic pericarditis. Arthritis Rheum 25:1054, 1977
13. McCarty M: The role of immunological mechanisms in the pathogenesis of rheumatic fever. In Read SE, Zabriskie JB (eds): Streptococcal Disease and the Immune Response, pp 13–21. New York, Academic Press, 1980
14. Barrett DJ: Pathogenesis of acute rheumatic fever. In Majeed HA, Yousof AM (eds): Research on Cardiac and Renal Sequelae of streptococcal Infections, pp 32–48. Munich-Deisenhofen, Dustri-Verlag, 1984
15. Rotta J, Bednar B: Biological properties of cell wall mucopeptide of hemolytic streptococci. J Exp Med 130:31, 1969
16. Kaplan MH, Bolande R, Rakita L et al: Presence of bound immunoglobulin and complement in the myocardium in acute rheumatic fever: Association with cardiac failure. N Engl J Med 271:637, 1964
17. Kaplan MH, Meyeserian M: An immunological cross reaction between Group A streptococcal cells and human heart tissue. Lancet 1:706, 1962
18. Zabriskie JB, Freimer EH: An immunological relationship between the group A *Streptococcus* and mammalian muscle. J Exp Med 124:661, 1966
19. Goldstein I, Halpern B, Robert L: Immunological relationship between streptococcal A polysaccharide and the structural glycoproteins of heart valve. Nature 213:44, 1967
20. Sandson J, Hammerman D, Janis R et al: Immunologic and chemical similarities between the *Streptococcus* and human connective tissue. Trans Assoc Am Physicians 81:249, 1968
21. Husby G, van de Rijn, Zabriskie JB et al: Antibodies reacting with cytoplasm of subthalamic and caudate nuclei neurons in chorea and acute rheumatic fever. J Exp Med 144:1094, 1976
22. Kaplan MH, Svec KH: Immunological relation of streptococcal and tissue antigens: III. Presence in human sera of streptococcal antibody cross-reactive with heart tissue: Association with streptococcal infection, rheumatic fever and glomerulonephritis. J Exp Med 119:651, 1964
23. Zabriskie JB, Hsuk C, Seegal BC: Heart reactive antibody associated with rheumatic fever: Characterization and diagnostic significance. Clin Exp Immunol 2:147, 1970
24. Ayoub EM: Immunological response to streptococcal infection. In Majeed HA, Yousof AM (eds): Research on Cardiac and Renal Sequelae of Streptococcal Infections, pp 15–25. Munich-Deisenhofen, Dustri-Verlag, 1984
25. Read SE, Fischetti VA, Utermohlen V et al: Cellular reactivity studies to streptococcal antigens: Migration inhibition studies in patients with streptococcal infections and rheumatic fever. J Clin Invest 54:439, 1974
26. Yang LC: Streptococcal-induced cell-mediated immune destruction of cardiac myofibers *in vitro*. J Exp Med 146:353, 1977
27. Hutto J, Ayoub EM: Cytotoxicity of lymphocytes from patients with rheumatic carditis to cardiac cells *in vitro*. In Read SE, Zabriskie JB (eds): Streptococcal Diseases and the Immune Response, p 733. New York, Academic Press, 1980
28. Dudding BA, Ayoub EM: Persistence of group A streptococcal antibodies in patients with rheumatic valvular disease. J Exp Med 128:1081, 1968
29. Feinstein AR, Spagnuolo M: The clinical patterns of acute rheumatic fever: A reappraisal. Medicine 41:279, 1962
30. Stollerman GH: Clinical manifestations of acute rheumatic fever. In Stollerman GH: Rheumatic Fever and Streptococcal Infection, pp 147–179. New York, Grune & Stratton, 1975
31. Cherian G, Koshi G, Chacko KA et al: Acute rheumatic fever and rheumatic carditis in India. In Hayase S, Murao S (eds): Proceedings of VIII World Congress of Cardiology, Tokyo, 1978, pp 514–516. Amsterdam, Excerpta Medica, 1978
32. Markowitz M, Gordis L: Clinical manifestations of acute rheumatic fever. In Markowitz M, Gordis L: Rheumatic Fever, 2nd ed. Philadelphia, WB Saunders, 1972
33. Bisno AL, Ofek I: Serologic diagnosis of streptococcal infection: Comparison of a rapid haemagglutination technique with conventional antibody tests. Am J Dis Child 127:676, 1974
34. Stollerman GH, Glick SJ, Patel D et al: Determination of C-reactive protein in serum as a guide to the treatment and management of rheumatic fever. Am J Med 15:645, 1953
35. Oakley CM: Acute rheumatic carditis. In Borman JB, Gotsman MS (eds): Rheumatic Valvular Disease in Children, pp 15–27. New York, Springer-Verlag, 1980
36. Hamdan JA, Manasra K, Ahmad M: Salicylate-induced hepatitis in rheumatic fever. Am J Dis Child 139:453, 1985
37. UK and US Joint Report: The natural history of rheumatic fever and rheumatic heart disease: Cooperative clinical trial of ACTH, cortisone and aspirin. Circulation 32:457, 1965
38. Combined Rheumatic Fever Study Group: A comparison of the effect of prednisone and acetylsalicylic acid on the incidence of residual rheumatic heart disease. N Engl J Med 262:895, 1960
39. Combined Rheumatic Fever Study Group: A comparison of short-term intensive prednisone and acetylsalicylic acid therapy in the treatment of acute rheumatic fever. N Engl J Med 272:63, 1965
40. Ash R: The first 10 years of rheumatic infection in childhood. Am Heart J 36:89, 1948
41. Bland EF, Jones TG: Rheumatic fever and rheumatic heart disease: A 20-year report on 1000 patients followed since childhood. Circulation 4:836, 1951
42. Wood HF, Feinstein AR, Taranta A: Rheumatic fever in children and adolescents, III. Comparative effectiveness of three prophylaxis regimens in preventing streptococcal infections and rheumatic recurrences. Ann Intern Med (Suppl 3) 60:31, 1964
43. Tompkins DG, Boxerbaum B, Liebman J: Long-term prognosis of rheumatic fever patients receiving regular intramuscular benzathine penicillin. Circulation 45:543, 1972
44. Padmavati S: Rheumatic fever and rheumatic heart disease in developing countries. Bull WHO 56:543, 1978
45. Raghuram TC, Brahmaji R: Serum penicillin levels in rheumatic heart disease. Ind Heart J 31:333, 1979
46. Gordis L, Markowitz M, Lilienfeld A: Why patients don't follow medical advice: A study of children on long-term antistreptococcal prophylaxis. J Paediatr 75:957, 1969
47. Markowitz M: Prevention of acute rheumatic fever and rheumatic heart disease. In Julian DG, Humphries JON (eds): Preventive Cardiology, pp 47–61. Scarborough, Ont, Butterworth, 1983

Restrictive and Obliterative Cardiomyopathy

Walter H. Abelmann

DEFINITION AND CLASSIFICATION

According to the definition and classification of the cardiomyopathies agreed on by the World Health Organization and the International Society and Federation for Cardiology in 1980, restrictive cardiomyopathy is one of three forms of cardiomyopathy, the other two being dilated and hypertrophic cardiomyopathy.[1] To quote from this report: "Endomyocardial scarring usually affects either one or both ventricles and restricts filling. Involvement of the atrioventricular valves is common but the outflow tracts are spared. Cavity obliteration is characteristic of advanced cases."

By definition, this entity includes endomyocardial fibrosis and Löffler's cardiomyopathy (endocarditis parietalis fibroplastica), for the latter of which the term *eosinophilic endomyocardial disease* was proposed. Again, by definition, restrictive physiology associated with heart muscle disease of known cause or associated with systemic disorders was excluded, such conditions falling into the category "specific heart muscle disease." Inasmuch as one of the classic forms of restrictive physiology, amyloid heart disease, falls into this latter category and impairment of filling or diastolic function is not infrequently encountered in several other specific heart muscle diseases, the present review will also include consideration of such conditions; they are also of considerable importance to the clinician in the assessment and differential diagnosis of individual patients.[2]

Increasing attention has focused on abnormalities of diastolic function in dilated[3] and hypertrophic[4] cardiomyopathies, and also in other forms of heart disease, such as hypertensive,[5] aortic valvular,[6] and ischemic heart disease.[7] This review, however, does not consider alterations of diastolic function in situations in which the primary defect is hypertrophy or impaired systolic function. In other words, whereas restrictive physiology may be associated with many forms of heart disease and much of what is said about altered diastolic function and myocardial compliance may also apply to other forms of cardiomyopathy, the focus here is on restrictive cardiomyopathy.

CLINICAL OVERVIEW

Restrictive cardiomyopathy, as well as specific heart muscle disease with predominantly restrictive physiology, is relatively rare. The other forms of cardiomyopathy—dilated and hypertrophic, as well as specific heart muscle disease with systolic dysfunction and/or arrhythmias or conduction disturbances—are encountered much more frequently. The clinician should suspect restrictive cardiomyopathy when encountering a patient with manifestations of congestive heart failure in the presence of a small or only slightly enlarged heart, a presentation raising the question of constrictive pericarditis, which remains the principal differential diagnosis. The restrictive physiology is attributable to impaired diastolic function, associated with decreased distensibility of either or both ventricles during diastole, secondary to increased stiffness of the heart (*i.e.*, decreased compliance). This change may be secondary to changes in the endocardium, the myocardium, or both.

The purest forms of restrictive cardiomyopathy (Table 97.1) are idiopathic myocardial fibrosis, endomyocardial fibrosis associated with eosinophilia or Löffler's disease, and endomyocardial fibrosis unassociated with eosinophilia, primarily seen in the tropics. The most frequent cause of relatively pure restrictive pathophysiology in the West, however, remains amyloid heart disease. Among other diseases of the myocardium that may present as restrictive cardiomyopathy are hemochromatosis, sarcoid heart disease, neoplasms, Fabry's disease, and, predominantly in the young, fibroelastosis.

After a consideration of the characteristics and determinants of normal and abnormal diastolic function, both physiologic and pathologic, the clinical presentation, natural history, diagnosis, and when available, treatment of these disorders is discussed.

NORMAL AND ABNORMAL DIASTOLIC FUNCTION

During diastole or the filling period, it is the function of the ventricles to receive blood from the atria and to expand from the relatively small end-systolic volume to an end-diastolic volume appropriate to permit expulsion of an adequate stroke volume during the following systole. Diastole is classically considered to be passive, albeit to some extent aided by atrial systole. Diastolic filling is dependent on prompt relaxation of the myocardium, now considered an active process, as well as on appropriate distensibility or compliance of the inactive myocardium and its supporting structures. The normal pressure–volume relationships during diastole are illustrated in Figure 97.1, *A*. It is seen that over a considerable filling volume, the diastolic pressure rises but little. Let, however, ventricular distensibility or compliance be decreased (Fig. 97.1, *B*), and a greater diastolic filling pressure will be needed to accommodate a given volume. It is also evident from this figure that, whereas a normal ventricle may accommodate a large stroke volume at only moderately elevated end-diastolic pressure, the steeper pressure–volume relationship of a stiff ventricle does not permit a large

TABLE 97.1 MYOCARDIAL DISEASES THAT MAY MANIFEST PREDOMINANTLY RESTRICTIVE PATHOPHYSIOLOGY

Löffler's eosinophilic endomyocardial disease
Tropical endomyocardial fibrosis
Idiopathic myocardial fibrosis
Amyloidosis
Hemochromatosis
Sarcoidosis
Scleroderma
Pseudoxanthoma elasticum
Fabry's disease
Gaucher's disease
Endocardial fibroelastosis
Carnitine deficiency
Neoplastic heart disease
Carcinoid heart disease
Radiation heart disease

stroke volume at normal diastolic pressures. As Figure 97.1 also clearly indicates, for a given end-diastolic volume, the end-diastolic pressure of a stiff ventricle is always greater than for the normal ventricle. Putting it another way, in the stiffer or less compliant heart, the ventricle can fill with normal end-diastolic volume only by means of developing a higher end-diastolic pressure. Thus, even when systolic function is preserved, the end-diastolic pressure is elevated, resulting in elevated filling pressures (*i.e.*, elevated pulmonary capillary and venous pressures in the case of the left ventricle and elevated central venous pressure in the case of the right ventricle).

In principle, only the left ventricle, only the right ventricle, or both ventricles may manifest decreased compliance (*i.e.*, impaired diastolic function). As a rule, however, since the cause is usually a diffuse morbid process, both ventricles are affected.

Basically, there are two mechanisms by which the diastolic function of the ventricles can be altered. First, the constitutive properties of the ventricles may be altered so as to decrease ventricular compliance. Second, the physicochemical processes determining ventricular relaxation may be altered so as to prolong or delay relaxation.

Alterations of the constitutive properties of the ventricles may be limited to the pericardium, leading to constrictive pericarditis, a condition that here concerns us only in regard to differential diagnosis. It may be limited to the endocardium, as in endocardial fibroelastosis, which, on occasion, may indeed alter compliance. Altered ventricular compliance in the absence of impaired systolic function, however, is most frequently associated with diffuse interstitial or replacement fibrosis,[8,9] or then with infiltration by or deposition of foreign materials such as amyloid,[10] hemosiderin (hemochromatosis),[11] or ceramide trihexoside.[12] Ventricular compliance is also decreased in concentric hypertrophy,[13] in healing myocardial infarction,[14] and perhaps in myocardial edema.[15]

The clinical and hemodynamic syndrome of restrictive cardiomyopathy, however, has also been observed in the absence of histopathologic evidence of endocardial or myocardial abnormalities (*i.e.*, without significant fibrosis, infiltration, or deposition).[16] This is the case in idiopathic restrictive cardiomyopathy[9] and in concentric hypertrophy.[13] This has led to the hypothesis that abnormalities of the cytoskeleton or interstitium may be involved. Indeed, alterations of the collagen matrix have been described in cardiac hypertrophy.[17]

Decreases of ventricular compliance associated with impaired ventricular relaxation due to presumed changes in physicochemical processes have been observed in ischemia, either transient or prolonged,[18] in calcium overload,[4] in volume overloading,[19] in vagal stimulation,[20] and in hyperosmolality.[21]

Of great clinical importance is the recognition that decreased ventricular compliance may result in circulatory congestion, a state closely paralleling that seen in constrictive pericarditis, closely resembling congestive heart failure, even though myocardial contractility and hence the systolic function of the heart may be preserved.

INCIDENCE AND PREVALENCE

Among the three forms of cardiomyopathy, restrictive cardiomyopathy is the least frequent form in developed countries, comprising generally less than 5% of all cardiomyopathies. Endomyocardial fibrosis, however, has a significantly higher prevalence in tropical regions, comprising 14% in Uganda and 10% in Nigeria of patients dying of heart failure; in the Ivory Coast this disease accounted for 20% of deaths due to heart failure in individuals under age 40.[22]

PATHOLOGIC MANIFESTATIONS

As a rule, both ventricles are affected, although the process may predominate in either the right or the left ventricle. Notwithstanding manifestations of congestion in both pulmonary and systemic circulations, the heart tends to be normal in size or only slightly dilated. There may be mild to moderate thickening of the free wall of either or both ventricles. The pericardium is normal, as are the endocardium and cardiac valves, with the exception of endomyocardial fibrosis, in which both endocardium and atrioventricular valves are affected. In restrictive cardiomyopathy in general, but especially in endomyocardial fibrosis, the ventricular cavities may be reduced in size, partly by retraction of the apex toward the base, partly by mural thrombi, which may also be found in the atria.

The histopathology may reveal nonspecific interstitial and perivascular fibrosis (Fig. 97.2). A mild to moderate degree of fiber hyper-

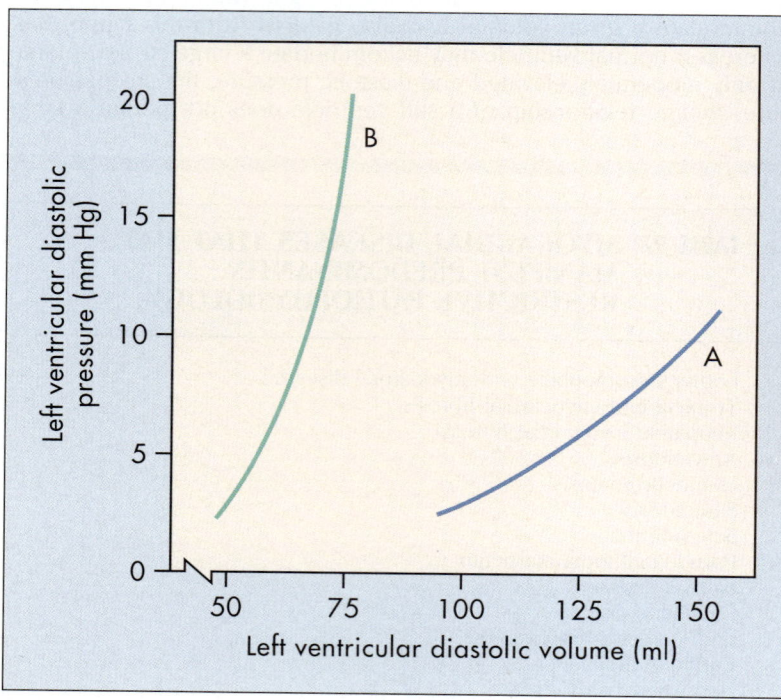

FIGURE 97.1 The relationship of diastolic pressure to diastolic volume: (A) in a normal (compliant) and (B) in a restricted (stiff) left ventricle.

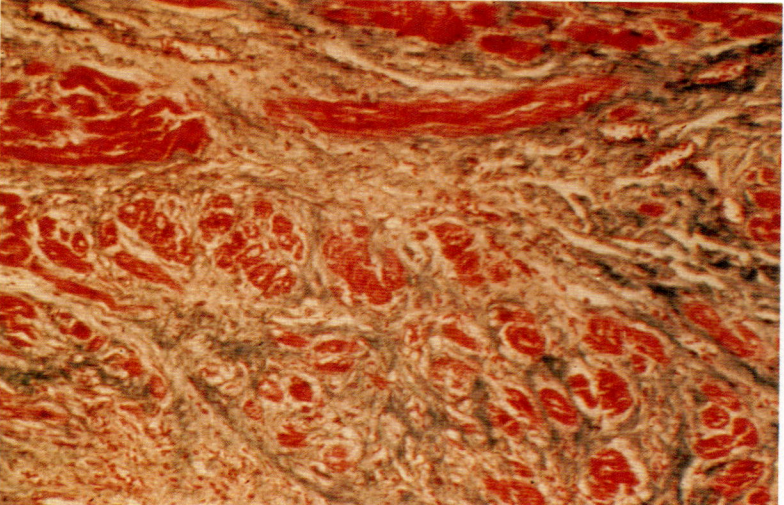

FIGURE 97.2 Microscopic section from the left ventricle in a case of idiopathic diffuse myocardial fibrosis. The few residual myofibers are surrounded by fibrous tissue. (Masson trichrome, × 500).

trophy may be seen. Specific lesions or deposits may be found in restrictive cardiomyopathy associated with specific heart muscle disease. The pathologic changes or deposits may be unevenly distributed. Thus, if endomyocardial biopsy is to be representative and identify a specific process, if present, it must include multiple samples from different sites.

HEMODYNAMICS

Restrictive cardiomyopathy has characteristic, albeit nonspecific, hemodynamic features that are a result of the reduced ventricular compliance and abnormalities of diastolic function. The most frequent abnormality of ventricular pressure tracings is the so-called dip-plateau or square root sign (Fig. 97.3): the right and/or left ventricular pressure tracings manifest a deep early diastolic decline, followed by a rapid rise to a plateau in early to mid diastole.[10] The atrial pressure tracings display a prominent y descent, followed by a rapid rise and plateau, which, together with the usually rapid x descent, form the characteristic M- or W-shaped waveform. Less frequently, the early diastolic dip is absent; early diastolic pressure is elevated and rises gradually to higher abnormal levels during diastole.[23] The more common, first pattern is identical to that seen in constrictive pericarditis[24]; the second pattern resembles that of cardiac tamponade.[24]

In constrictive pericarditis, secondary to limitation of diastolic filling, the right ventricular systolic pressure tends to be less than 40 mm Hg, so that the right ventricular diastolic pressure is usually one third or more of the systolic pressure. Also, classically, when both ventricles are involved, the right and left ventricular filling pressures tend to equalize.[23] Furthermore, this equalization persists or is even accentuated during interventions such as exercise, which may be a valuable diagnostic test.

Unlike constrictive pericarditis, which tends to equalize ventricular filling pressures, restrictive cardiomyopathy tends to preserve or even accentuate (e.g., during exercise or after contrast ventriculography) the difference between right and left ventricular filling pressures (see Fig. 97.3). In pure restrictive cardiomyopathy, systolic function is preserved, that is, ejection fraction and cardiac output are within normal limits or only slightly decreased.

CLINICAL MANIFESTATIONS

If idiopathic restrictive cardiomyopathy is defined as cardiomyopathy of unknown cause with abnormal diastolic function but preserved systolic function, and endomyocardial fibrosis is excluded, the literature contains only few well documented cases.[8,9] They were adults ranging from 23 to 77 years of age, who presented primarily with congestive heart failure or because of chest pain, often of several years' duration. Physical examination most frequently revealed an elevated jugular venous pressure and evidence of pulmonary and systemic congestion. Gallop sounds and murmurs of mitral and tricuspid regurgitation were heard in some patients. Several had atrial arrhythmias, atrial fibrillation was frequent, and the brady-tachycardia syndrome as well as complete heart block were also observed. By roentgenography, enlargement of the cardiac silhouette was not unusual, but by echocardiography left ventricular enlargement was unusual, whereas atrial and right ventricular enlargement were more common.

LABORATORY STUDIES

There are no specific laboratory tests except those for systemic disorders associated with restrictive cardiomyopathy. Electrocardiograms may manifest low voltage when infiltration or deposition is extensive; even local processes may be associated with conduction disturbances, ranging from first-degree atrioventricular (AV) block to complete heart block. There may also be atrial or ventricular arrhythmias or both. Regional fibrosis or deposition may result in loss of precordial R waves or other changes simulating myocardial infarction. Echocardiography,[25] gated blood pool scans, and contrast ventriculography are valuable in determining that systolic function is maintained, that ventricular chambers are at most mildly dilated, and that atria are dilated. Computerized tomography (CT) scans or magnetic resonance imaging may be more sensitive in detecting thickened or abnormal pericardium.

As already mentioned, right- and left-sided heart catheterization permits the detection of dominance of restriction or abnormal diastolic function. As a matter of fact, it is often the early diastolic dip and end-diastolic plateau, along with elevated but divergent left and right ventricular filling pressures in the presence of normal systolic function, that first lead to the diagnosis of restrictive cardiomyopathy (see Fig. 97.3).

Endomyocardial biopsy may be a most valuable procedure in the evaluation of a patient suspected of having restrictive cardiomyopathy.[26] In good hands, this procedure carries a very low risk, although biopsy of the left ventricle is more likely to result in significant arrhythmias. As a rule, the morbid process affects both ventricles, so that a biopsy of the right ventricular septum is sufficient. In order to achieve representative sampling of myocardium, however, at least four to five biopsies should be performed. Biopsies are most valuable in the detection of specific heart muscle disease, such as amyloidosis (Fig. 97.4), hemochromatosis, sarcoid, Fabry's disease, and endomyocardial fibrosis. Often, biopsy will demonstrate only nonspecific fibrosis. Special stains for specific heart muscle disease should always be per-

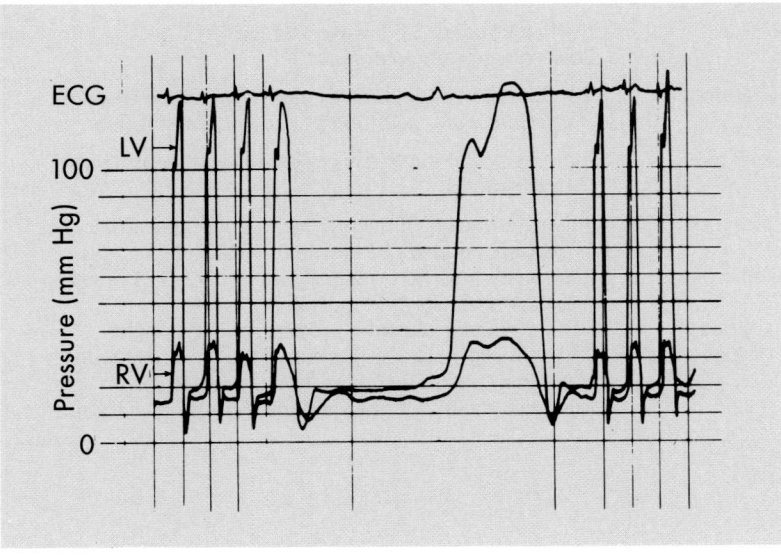

FIGURE 97.3 Simultaneous recordings of left ventricular (LV) and right ventricular (RV) pressures from a patient with idiopathic restrictive cardiomyopathy. Note the early diastolic dip and plateau and the near-equilibration of the elevated diastolic pressures of both ventricles. The diastolic pressure of the left ventricle exceeds that of the right. (Benotti JR, Grossman W, Cohn PF: Clinical profile of restrictive cardiomyopathy. Circulation 61:1206, 1980)

formed (*i.e.*, Congo red, iron stains). If the biopsy reveals only normal myocardium, constrictive pericarditis should be strongly suspected, although sampling errors must always be kept in mind.

DIFFERENTIAL DIAGNOSIS

The most important differential diagnosis is with constrictive pericarditis (Table 97.2).[27-29] In the majority of cases, a good physical examination, supplemented by a chest roentgenogram and echocardiograms, will make this differentiation possible. In some cases, cardiac catheterization may be necessary. Many of the clinical and hemodynamic differences between restrictive cardiomyopathy and constrictive pericarditis have already been mentioned.

Coronary angiography and ventriculography[30] may be useful in the differential diagnosis, as may CT scanning.[31] Endomyocardial biopsy is an important recent addition to our diagnostic approach. When multiple samples of myocardium are unremarkable, a diagnosis of constrictive pericarditis is favored. The demonstration of a specific infiltrative process essentially rules out constrictive pericarditis.

One must keep in mind that constrictive pericarditis and myocardial fibrosis may coexist,[32] especially in radiation heart disease.[33] A small subset of patients, notwithstanding all diagnostic procedures, may still have to come to exploratory thoracotomy.

TREATMENT

There is no specific medical therapy for restrictive cardiomyopathy. In the absence of contraindications, anticoagulation as well as antiplatelet drugs are recommended to prevent the formation and propagation of intracardiac thrombi. Agents that reduce the heart rate, such as β-adrenergic blockers, are contraindicated, inasmuch as tachycardia may be needed to compensate for a reduced stroke volume. Caution must also be exercised with regard to diuretics and vasodilators, because elevated filling pressures may be needed to maintain a normal cardiac output.

Since abnormal left ventricular diastolic function in patients with hypertrophic cardiomyopathy has been shown to be improved by ni-

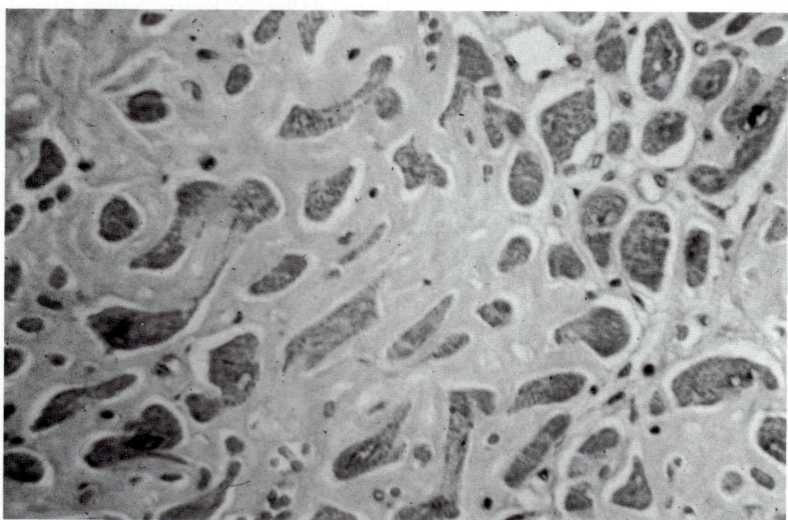

FIGURE 97.4 Microscopic section from the left ventricle in a case of diffuse amyloidosis. Note that each myofiber is encased by amyloid. (H&E, × 800)

TABLE 97.2 DIFFERENTIAL DIAGNOSIS OF RESTRICTIVE CARDIOMYOPATHY FROM CONSTRICTIVE PERICARDITIS

	Constrictive Pericarditis	Restrictive Cardiomyopathy
Physical Examination	Medium- to high-pitched diastolic sound about 0.12 second after S_2 ("pericardial knock") Murmurs rare	Low-pitched diastolic sound about 0.12 second after S_2 (third heart sound or protodiastolic sound) Murmurs of AV valve regurgitation
Electrocardiogram	Low voltage	LVH, secondary ST-T wave changes Low voltage (amyloidosis)
Roentgenogram	Normal cardiac silhouette, pericardial calcification, little or no pulmonary vascular redistribution	Configuration of left ventricular prominence or mild cardiomegaly, pulmonary vascular redistribution
Echocardiogram	Pericardial thickening, small to moderate pericardial effusion, reduced cavitary dimensions	Increased wall thickness consistent with ventricular hypertrophy
Cardiac Catheterization	Square root sign almost always; ventricular and atrial pressures equal and elevated in diastole. Pulmonary systolic pressure exceeds right ventricular end-diastolic pressure by ≤30%–50%. Diastolic pressures increase further but remain nearly equal with volume loading, leg elevation, or exercise Kussmaul's sign (80%) Pulsus paradoxus (<20%)	Square root sign frequently; ventricular and atrial pressures equal and elevated in diastole. Pulmonary systolic pressure commonly ≥2–3 times right ventricular end-diastolic pressure Left ventricular diastolic pressure exceeds right ventricular diastolic pressure by ≥5 mm Hg with volume loading, leg elevation, or exercise. Kussmaul's sign and pulsus paradoxus usually absent.

(After Benotti JR, Grossman W: Restrictive cardiomyopathy. Annu Rev Med 35:113, 1984)

fedipine, in doses that did not depress systolic function,[4] a trial of calcium channel blockers may be warranted in patients with restrictive cardiomyopathy, at least of the idiopathic type.

SPECIFIC FORMS OF RESTRICTIVE CARDIOMYOPATHY

ENDOMYOCARDIAL FIBROSIS WITH OR WITHOUT EOSINOPHILIA

In 1936, Löffler described a form of endocardial disease associated with eosinophilia, which he called endocarditis parietalis fibroplastica and which became known as Löffler's endomyocardial disease. Originally seen in Switzerland, this disease has been reported from many countries in the temperate zone.[34-37]

In 1946, Bedford and Konstam drew attention to a form of heart disease of unknown etiology occurring in Africa that subsequently became known as endomyocardial fibrosis and was found to be widespread in tropical regions throughout the world. Although it was long thought that these were two different forms of heart disease, the tropical form generally without eosinophilia and the temperate zone form associated with eosinophilia, more recently it has become clear that pathologically and clinically these two entities are essentially identical. Thus, a unitarian concept of endomyocardial fibrosis has evolved.[38] As a bridge, associated eosinophilia has been reported occasionally from tropical countries and noneosinophilic endomyocardial fibrosis (EMF) has been seen in the West.[38]

LÖFFLER'S ENDOMYOCARDIAL DISEASE

Endomyocardial disease has been reported in association with significant eosinophilia of almost any etiology, including idiopathic (hypereosinophilia syndrome), parasitic disease, periarteritis nodosa, asthma, neoplasms, Hodgkin's disease, and eosinophilic leukemia.[38-40] Eosinophilia always precedes the heart disease, and a pathogenetic role has been attributed to it. Furthermore, cardiac manifestations have been associated with a characteristic morphologic abnormality of eosinophils, namely degranulation, which appears to occur after their release from the bone marrow. Heart disease is related quantitatively to the number of degranulated eosinophils and to the duration of their presence. Thus, Spry and associates[41] concluded that the presence of more than 10^9 degranulated eosinophils per liter of blood for several weeks constitutes a risk factor for endomyocardial disease. Although the mechanism by which eosinophils become degranulated, and the mechanisms by which these altered eosinophils produce changes in endocardium and myocardium remain unknown, some potentially relevant information is accumulating. The degranulated eosinophils manifest an increased capacity to bind IgG, increased oxygen metabolism, and increased eosinophil peroxidase, the last of which has cytotoxic properties. Indeed, direct toxic effects of eosinophils on rat myocytes *in vitro* have been reported.[42]

Eosinophilic endomyocardial disease shows a predilection for males and is rare in childhood. Three clinical presentations have been distinguished.[38] Patients may present with acute thromboembolic events in the systemic circulation, fever, and pulmonary, gastrointestinal, or renal manifestations. Or, patients may present with progressive congestive heart failure. Finally, there are patients with persistent eosinophilia, who eventually develop evidence of cardiac involvement. As a rule, both ventricles are involved.

Characteristically, the cardiac disease has a long asymptomatic phase, during which signs of heart disease may also be absent, and both electrocardiogram and chest roentgenogram may be normal. Right and/or left ventricular third heart sounds are common, and, as the disease advances, murmurs of mitral and/or tricuspid insufficiency are not infrequent. At this stage, cardiomegaly may become evident on the chest roentgenogram. Eventually, the full-blown picture of decompensated restrictive cardiomyopathy may develop, with markedly distended neck veins, rapid Y descent, and anasarca. Systemic microemboli may give rise to retinal lesions[43] and also to peripheral splinter hemorrhages.[44]

Cardiac arrhythmias and conduction disturbances may occur but tend to be late manifestations. Nonspecific electrocardiographic abnormalities may be seen early.

Pathologic findings closely resemble those of endomyocardial fibrosis (Fig. 97.5), as do hemodynamic and echocardiographic studies. Two-dimensional echocardiograms[45] demonstrate normal to small ventricles, enlarged atria, obliteration of one or both ventricular apices by echogenic material, and preservation of ventricular systolic function. The AV valves and papillary muscles may be involved.

There is no specific medical therapy. Endocardiectomy and replacement of AV valves are appropriate surgical approaches. Laser photoablation of pathologic endocardium has been proposed.[46]

TROPICAL ENDOMYOCARDIAL FIBROSIS

Endomyocardial fibrosis was first reported as a heart failure of unknown cause in West African troops and in natives of Uganda. It has also become known as Davies' disease.[47] It is endemic in Uganda and western Nigeria, and it has also been described from the Sudan, the Congo, Kenya, Tanzania, and Ceylon, South India, Thailand, Malaya, Brazil, Venezuela, and Colombia.

The etiology of endomyocardial fibrosis remains unknown, although the unitary hypothesis of pathogenesis of endomyocardial fibrosis postulates a major etiologic role of degranulated eosinophils.[38] The general absence of eosinophilia in cases of tropical endomyocardial fibrosis has been attributed to the advanced stage in which the affected patients seek medical attention. Malnutrition has been considered as playing a contributory etiologic role, as has viral infection. A postulated etiologic role for serotonin, which occurs in high concentration in the plantain (banana) diet of East and West African natives, has not been borne out.

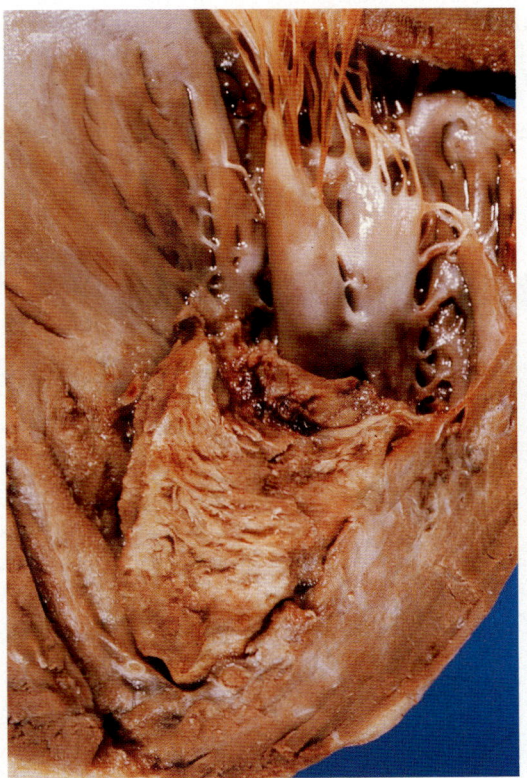

FIGURE 97.5 The left ventricle from a case of Löffler's eosinophilic endomyocardial disease. Note the endomyocardial fibrosis and apical thrombus.

The earliest stage of this disease has been described as a pancarditis, usually occurring in childhood, which may persist for weeks and/or recur subsequently, especially in the rainy season.

Tropical endomyocardial disease is generally detected only in the late stages, when it tends to present as restrictive cardiomyopathy, with dyspnea, fatigue, or ascites and edema predominating. It affects children and young adults, without predilection for sex. Endomyocardial fibrosis is frequently seen in association with malnutrition or parasitic infections, especially malaria and filariasis. Although both ventricles are affected in three fourths of the cases, endomyocardial fibrosis may be predominantly right ventricular (20% of cases) or left ventricular (5%).[44] Periorbital edema and parotid swelling may occur. Mitral murmurs are rare, as are mural thrombi and emboli (see Fig. 97.5). Arrhythmias, most often of supraventricular origin, and pericardial effusions may be seen.

Pathologically, endomyocardial lesions are found in one or both ventricles and in the AV valves and their supporting structures. In the left ventricle, the scar tissue is limited to the inflow tract but may extend to or be limited to the apex. The posterior mitral cusp and its attachments may be fused and present as a sheet of white fibrous tissue extending from the atrium to the apex. The fibrotic process may extend into the myocardium, to one third to one half of its thickness. Right ventricular involvement is more variable, is often patchy, and may extend into the outflow tract. The anterior mitral leaflet, as well as the tricuspid valve leaflets, tends to be preserved. The right ventricle, and more rarely the left ventricle, may become partly obliterated by fibrous tissue; adherent mural thrombi may further reduce ventricular cavities. One then may speak of obliterative cardiomyopathy. Emboli, however, are rare. One or both atria may become quite dilated.

When endomyocardial fibrosis involves predominantly the right ventricle, the clinical presentation is that of right ventricular failure with tricuspid insufficiency, elevated venous pressure, hepatomegaly, ascites, and edema, which may include the face. Pulmonary congestion is absent, and left ventricular filling pressures and pulmonary arterial pressures may be normal. Angiocardiography may reveal obliteration of the right ventricular apex and reduction of the size of the right ventricle, with marked enlargement of the right atrium.[48] Although the heart may not be enlarged overall, a pericardial effusion may be present. The differential diagnosis from constrictive pericarditis and rheumatic heart disease may be difficult.

Pure left ventricular involvement, which is rare, presents as mitral insufficiency. Inasmuch as the posterior leaflet is primarily affected, the regurgitation occurs predominantly early in systole and results in an early systolic murmur, a loud S_3, and even an opening snap.[49] There may be significant pulmonary hypertension.

When both ventricles are involved, which is the rule, the presentation is that of restrictive cardiomyopathy. When the heart is small, the differential diagnosis from constrictive pericarditis may be difficult. When the heart is moderately enlarged, other forms of cardiomyopathy may have to be considered.

Hemodynamic studies may reveal the classic picture of restrictive cardiomyopathy.[48,50,51] The left ventricular angiocardiograms are characterized by a small left ventricle and frequent apical obliteration. Right ventricular involvement is often characterized by a high degree of obliteration not only of the apex but also of the body of the chamber. The right atrium as a rule is markedly enlarged.[48]

M-mode echocardiography[52] (Fig. 97.6) reveals exaggerated thickening and motion of the anterior right ventricular wall, paradoxical septal motion, and some increase in right ventricular end-diastolic dimension. In contrast, the left ventricular end-diastolic dimension may be decreased. A pericardial effusion may be present. Two-dimensional echocardiography may demonstrate obliteration of the apex of either ventricle and atrial enlargement.[51] Atrial arrhythmias are frequent.[53]

Endomyocardial biopsy is valuable for confirmation of the diagnosis, but in a typical case it is not considered essential.[51]

There is no specific medical therapy for endomyocardial fibrosis. Surgical treatment, comprising endocardiectomy and replacement or repair of the affected AV valve, has become well established, with good clinical results.[54,55] Postoperative complete heart block may require a permanent pacemaker.[56]

AMYLOID HEART DISEASE

Amyloidosis is considered a disorder of the immune system characterized by antigenic stimulation of the reticuloendothelial system, resulting in the deposition of amorphous extracellular material in many tissues. Cardiac amyloidosis frequently manifests as congestive heart failure, especially in elderly patients. Cardiac arrhythmias and conduction disturbances are frequent. When deposition of amyloid is diffuse,

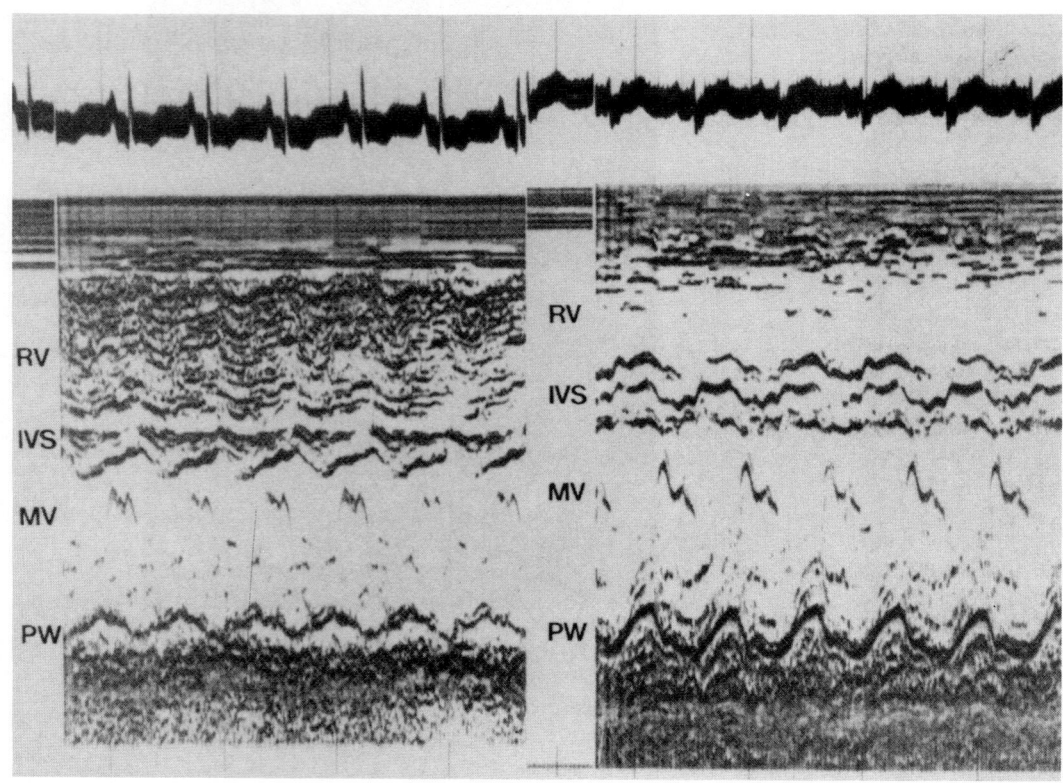

FIGURE 97.6 Preoperative and postoperative M-mode echocardiograms of the right and left ventricles from a patient with endomyocardial fibrosis. Preoperatively, the right ventricle is filled with dense echoes. (*RV*, right ventricle; *IVS*, interventricular septum; *MV*, mitral valve; *PW*, posterior wall). (Laing HC et al: Endomyocardial fibrosis in a European woman and its successful surgical treatment. J Thorac Cardiovasc Surg 74:803, 1977)

it leads to the syndrome of the "stiff heart,"[10] which must be distinguished from other forms of restrictive cardiomyopathy and from constrictive pericarditis.[23]

CLASSIFICATION OF AMYLOIDOSIS

Amyloidosis has been classified according to clinicopathologic criteria or patterns of distribution of amyloid.[57] The clinicopathologic classification distinguishes primary amyloidosis with deposits predominantly in the heart, lungs, gastrointestinal tract, skeletal muscle, and skin from secondary amyloidosis, with deposits mainly in liver, spleen, kidneys, and adrenals. Amyloidosis associated with multiple myeloma has a distribution similar to that of primary amyloidosis. The classification according to patterns of distribution[57] distinguishes pattern I (with involvement of tongue, gastrointestinal tract, heart, skeletal and smooth muscle, skin and nerves) from pattern II (with involvement of liver, spleen, kidneys, and adrenals) and also provides for a mixed pattern I and II and a localized form with deposits limited to a single tissue or organ.

The biochemical and immunologic identification of several different types of amyloid fibril proteins has rendered possible a rational classification of amyloidosis.[58] An immunoglobulin light-chain protein, AL, is found in primary amyloidosis and in plasma cell dyscrasias. Senile amyloid, AS, is primarily localized in the heart (ASc) or brain (ASb). Protein AA is associated with secondary amyloidosis. Protein AF, related to prealbumin, is present in familial amyloid polyneuropathy, which includes the Portuguese form (type I), which is associated with cardiac involvement.

PATHOGENESIS

Amyloid deposits in tissue consist primarily of aggregates of rigid, linear, nonbranching protein fibrils. The amyloid protein is thought to originate from plasma cells, which give rise to circulating amyloid precursors, the concentration of which is increased in acute and especially in chronic inflammatory diseases and also increases with age. The immune system is thought to play a role as well.[58]

PATHOLOGY

SENILE CARDIAC AMYLOIDOSIS. Amyloid deposits in the heart are not infrequent in subjects over the age of 50 and may be seen in over half of hearts over the age of 60.[59] Although in the majority of cases these deposits are limited to the atria, in about one third of cases the ventricles and one or more valves are involved. Although cardiac deposits of amyloid in the elderly population are not generally associated with evidence of heart disease, atrial fibrillation and congestive heart failure have been shown to have a higher incidence in patients with senile cardiac amyloidosis than in a control population.

AMYLOID HEART DISEASE. Although cardiac involvement is the rule in primary amyloidosis, it is not infrequent in amyloidosis secondary to myeloma and other chronic disease. Mild to moderate increase in size and weight of the heart is the rule. Amyloid deposits may be seen in endocardium (including valves), myocardium, or pericardium, as well as in intramural coronary arteries and veins. In advanced stages, the cardiac chamber walls are thickened and stiff and the cut surface appears pale and waxy. When deposits are patchy, they appear as grayish streaks or nodules. Histopathologically, the deposits may surround bundles of muscle fibers, may surround individual myofibers, or may replace myofibers (Fig. 97.4). The conduction system may be involved.[60]

CLINICAL MANIFESTATIONS

Amyloid heart disease most commonly is encountered in one of four presentations, or a combination thereof.

PRESENTATION AS RESTRICTIVE CARDIOMYOPATHY. The patient develops gradually progressive congestive heart failure, with a normal to only slightly enlarged heart, with chronically distended neck veins, and, occasionally, a positive Kussmaul's sign, as well as low voltage on the electrocardiogram. The differential diagnosis is with other causes of restrictive cardiomyopathy and with constrictive pericarditis, and many such patients have undergone unnecessary exploratory thoracotomy.

PRESENTATION AS VALVULAR HEART DISEASE. When endocardial deposits of amyloid involve cardiac valves—most commonly the AV valves—and interfere with their function, rheumatic or other valvular disease or even dilated cardiomyopathy with mitral and tricuspid regurgitation may be mimicked.

PRESENTATION AS ISCHEMIC HEART DISEASE. Atypical chest pain, sometimes resembling angina pectoris, abnormal Q waves, poor progression of precordial R waves, or patterns of inferior myocardial infarction may lead to the diagnosis of ischemic heart disease. This may be associated with deposits limited to the myocardium or with actual involvement of coronary arteries.[61]

PRESENTATION AS ISOLATED CARDIAC ARRHYTHMIA OR CONDUCTION DISTURBANCES. Atrial and/or ventricular arrhythmias are frequent, with ventricular premature beats occurring in over half the cases. Some degree of heart block is seen in 10% to 30% of cases, with right or left bundle branch block being noted less frequently. It has been difficult to relate such manifestations to the distribution of amyloid in the heart.[60] Cardiac arrhythmias associated with amyloid disease tend to be refractory to therapy and are especially common in association with digitalis.[62] Sudden death is not uncommon. A rare complication is intracardiac thrombosis and embolization to either the systemic or pulmonary circulation.[63]

Although cardiac manifestations may precede manifestations of the systemic disease, the latter may give rise to the first signs and symptoms or may dominate. Such manifestations may give valuable hints as to the etiology of the heart disease. Noteworthy is orthostatic hypotension, which occurs in 10% to 15% of patients and is attributable to involvement of the adrenals and the autonomic nervous system.[64]

DIAGNOSIS

As is evident from the previous discussion, the cardiac manifestations of amyloidosis are not specific. The newer, noninvasive tests have added to our ability to define and quantitate the anatomical and functional manifestations but also have not yielded any specific diagnostic features.[65] Echoes from myocardium infiltrated with amyloid may be dense and produce a "speckled" pattern, which is presumptive evidence of cardiac amyloidosis (Fig. 97.7).[66] However, this appearance is not specific and may also be seen in endomyocardial fibrosis and other infiltrative disorders.

Thus, a definite diagnosis can be made only by means of a cardiac biopsy. The endomyocardial approach is considered the safest and most effective.[23,67] Because of the often uneven distribution of amyloid deposits, multiple biopsies increase the likelihood of detection. When amyloidosis is primary, its detection is especially important in patients presenting with the stiff heart syndrome, in order to prevent thoracotomy for presumed constrictive pericarditis. When amyloid heart disease is secondary to systemic amyloidosis, biopsy of other tissues, especially liver, kidney, rectal mucosa, or tongue, may permit a presumptive cardiac diagnosis. When senile amyloidosis coexists with ischemic heart disease, the diagnosis becomes especially difficult, if not impossible.

Although the usual hematoxylin-eosin stain of biopsy material may suggest the presence of amyloid, special stains are indicated when amyloid is suspected. Congo red stain with polarized light microscopy, demonstrating birefringence, and thioflavin stain with fluorescence microscopy are commonly used, but the sensitivity and specificity of these methods remain under dispute.[68] Electron microscopy is a valuable adjunct, revealing a typical appearance of amyloid fibrils interposed between connective tissue fibrils and the plasma membrane.

TREATMENT

There is no specific therapy for cardiac amyloidosis.

HEMOSIDEROSIS AND HEMOCHROMATOSIS

Hemosiderosis is defined as increased iron deposits in multiple organs without cirrhosis, whereas the coexistence of such deposits with hepatic cirrhosis is known as hemochromatosis.[69] Deposits of iron in the heart are always associated with extracardiac deposits, but the latter are not necessarily associated with significant cardiac involvement. When cardiac iron deposits are extensive, supraventricular arrhythmias and/or clinical congestive heart failure may result. The presentation is usually that of dilated cardiomyopathy with systolic dysfunction, but diastolic dysfunction may coexist and, occasionally, the presentation is that of restrictive cardiomyopathy.[11,70] Inasmuch as myocardial iron deposits can be reduced therapeutically, hemochromatosis heart disease is a form of cardiomyopathy for which there is specific therapy[71]; hence its recognition becomes clinically important.

PATHOGENESIS

Abnormal iron deposits in organs and tissues may result from excessive oral or parenteral administration of iron. Thus, hemochromatosis heart disease is almost the rule in patients who have received more than 100 blood transfusions for causes other than acute blood loss.[69] Congenital and acquired anemias, associated with defects of erythrocytes or erythrocyte production, may result in abnormal storage of iron, secondary to increased gastrointestinal absorption and decreased utilization of iron or hemolysis. Chronic diseases of the liver may result in increased iron deposits in tissues. Primary hemochromatosis is a recessive genetic disorder, linked with chromosome 6 and associated with HLA antigens[72] and with increased gastrointestinal absorption of iron.

There has been considerable controversy about the question of whether deposition of iron in myocardium *per se* is a cause of cardiac dysfunction. Thus, a study of 211 autopsy cases of iron storage disease revealed an equal incidence of heart failure in cases of hemochromatosis and advanced and early hemosiderosis.[73] Furthermore, chronic administration of iron to experimental animals failed to produce clinical heart disease.[74] However, subsequent clinical and postmortem studies suggest that there is a quantitative relationship between the amount of iron deposited in myocardium and myocardial dysfunction.[69,75]

PATHOLOGY

Iron has a predilection for active, contracting myofibers. Iron deposits are more extensive in the ventricles than in the atria; less iron is deposited in the conducting system. Deposits are most frequent in the subepicardium and then the subendocardium; they are sparse in the mid zone. In the myocyte, iron is initially deposited around the nucleus but later fills most of the cell, leading ultimately to degeneration and fibrosis. Myocardial deposits may be visible on gross inspection of the cut cardiac surface.

CLINICAL MANIFESTATIONS

After a long asymptomatic course, the usual cardiac manifestations are those of a dilated cardiomyopathy, characterized by exertional dyspnea, orthopnea, and peripheral edema. The manifestations of right-sided heart failure often dominate over those of left-sided heart failure. Congestive heart failure secondary to hemochromatosis tends to be refractory to conventional therapy. A few cases of restrictive cardiomyopathy secondary to iron deposits have been reported[11,70] with presentations that suggested constrictive pericarditis.

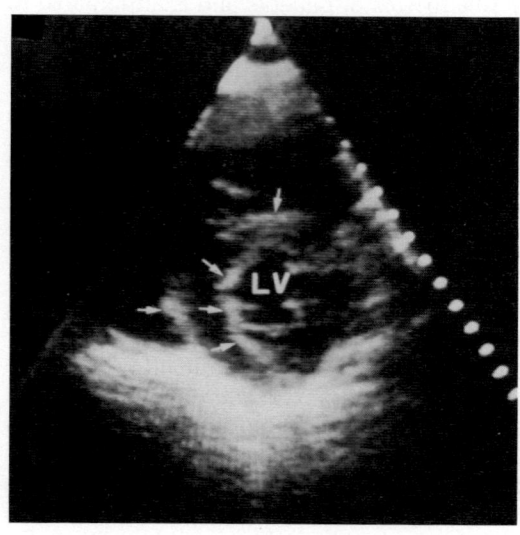
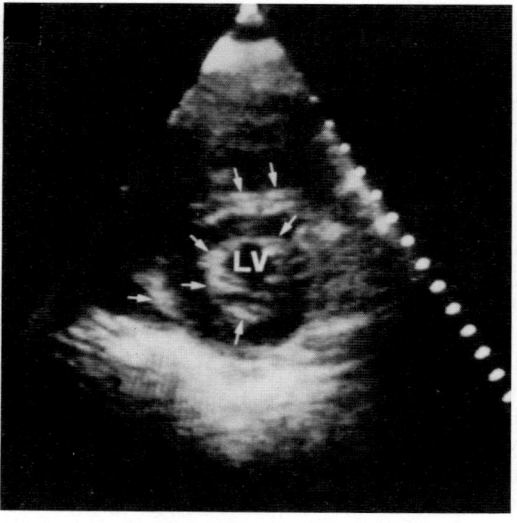

FIGURE 97.7 Two-dimensional short axis views of the left ventricle (*LV*) just below the tips of the mitral leaflets in diastole (*left panel*) and systole (*right panel*) in a patient with systemic amyloidosis. The ventricular walls are thickened, showing areas of intense echoes (*white arrows*) resulting in a "granular sparkling" appearance characteristic but not diagnostic of amyloid infiltration. The decreased voltage on the electrocardiogram in association with increased wall thickness also is compatible with an infiltrative process. (Come P (ed): Diagnostic Cardiology. Philadelphia, JB Lippincott, 1985)

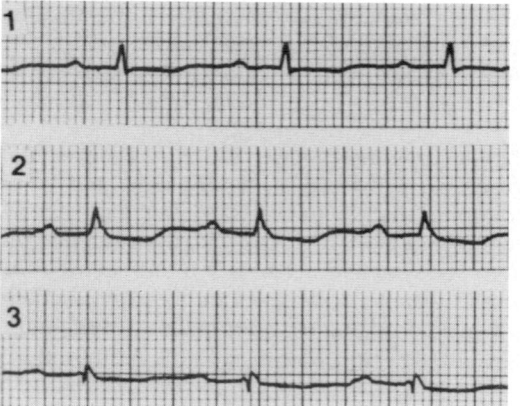
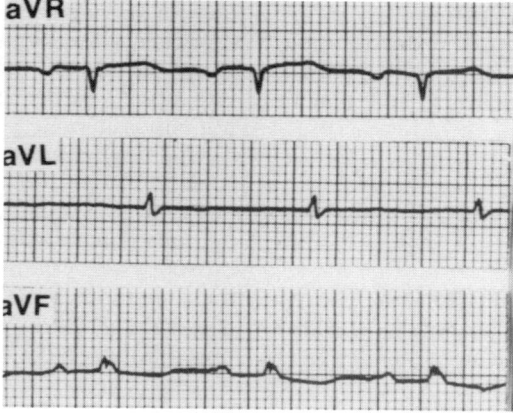

DIAGNOSIS

A presumptive diagnosis of hemochromatosis may be made when bronze discoloration of the skin, diabetes mellitus, and cirrhosis of the liver coexist, when there is a family history of hemochromatosis, or when a patient has received more than 100 blood transfusions. The suspicion is confirmed when plasma iron levels are elevated in the presence of a normal or low total iron binding capacity and when the serum ferritin level is elevated. Biopsy of skin or liver may yield confirmation. Absolute proof of cardiac involvement may require endomyocardial biopsy.

TREATMENT

Repeated phlebotomies have been demonstrated to be of both hemodynamic and clinical benefit[71,76] and thus are the therapy of choice (Fig. 97.8). In patients with hemochromatosis secondary to anemia treated with multiple transfusions, however, this approach is not feasible. Chelation with agents such as deferoxamine has been suggested.[77] In a patient with hemosiderosis who is on chronic dialysis, combined treatment with hemofiltration and deferoxamine was effective.[78]

FABRY'S DISEASE

Fabry's disease, or angiokeratoma corporis diffusum universale, is an inherited disorder of glycolipid metabolism. It is an X-linked deficiency of α-galactosidase A, a lysosomal enzyme required for glycosphingolipid metabolism. Absence of this enzyme results in intracellular accumulation of the neutral glycolipid trihexosyl ceramide, especially in the kidneys, myocardium, and skin. Glycolipid also accumulates in myocardium, conduction system, valves (especially the mitral valve[12,79]), and vascular endothelium. Small arteries may become occluded. The cardiovascular disease is seen predominantly in males. Congestive heart failure, myocardial ischemia, and hypertension are among the clinical manifestations. Electrocardiographic changes are nonspecific and include arrhythmias and conduction defects. Increased thickness of the left ventricular wall may be seen echocardiographically.

As a rule, the myocardial deposits result in congestive cardiomyopathy, but instances of obstructive and restrictive cardiomyopathy have been reported.[80] A definite diagnosis can be made by endomyocardial biopsy. No specific therapy is known.

GAUCHER'S DISEASE

This inherited deficiency of β-glucosidase is characterized by impaired metabolism of glycosyl ceramide, resulting in accumulation of cerebrosides in brain, liver, spleen, lymph nodes, bone marrow, and myocardium. Myocardial deposits may reduce ventricular compliance, but clinical heart disease is rare.[81]

ENDOCARDIAL FIBROELASTOSIS

Primary endocardial fibroelastosis, a hyperplasia of elastic tissue of the endocardium, is a disease of infancy and early childhood. It usually resembles a dilated cardiomyopathy but merits brief mention here because of the occasional occurrence of a "contracted" form, in which the left ventricle is normal in size or hypoplastic.[82] Endocardial fibroelastosis usually involves the left ventricle, the left atrium, or both, and rarely the right ventricle. The endocardial surface is covered with a homogeneous, white, glistening layer. In some cases, the mitral and, more rarely, the aortic valve is involved. Endocardial elastic fibers are not only increased in number but are intrinsically abnormal.[83] The etiology remains unknown, although many causes have been proposed. There is increasing evidence for an infectious etiology,[84] but the disease may have many causes.

Hemodynamically, there is a tendency to decreased systolic function, although cardiac output and stroke volume are usually within normal limits. Occasionally, elevated filling pressures may be associated with normal systolic function[85] and right ventricular and right atrial pressure tracings of the restrictive type have been described.[86] The usual presentation, during the first year of life, is heart failure, with cardiomegaly and pulmonary congestion, electrocardiographic evidence of left ventricular hypertrophy, and, less frequently, arrhythmias or conduction disturbances. Rarely, there may be evidence of myocardial infarction. The contracted form is more likely to occur in newborns with evidence of right ventricular hypertrophy,[82] elevated left atrial pressure, and pulmonary hypertension.

In the differential diagnosis, Pompe's disease, myocarditis, anomalous coronary artery, endomyocardial fibrosis, and dilated cardiomyopathy must be considered. The prognosis is generally poor.

CARNITINE DEFICIENCY

In 1973, Engel and Angelini[87] first reported a syndrome of progressive skeletal myopathy with lipid vacuoles on muscle biopsy, associated with deficiency of carnitine, a cofactor essential for the transport of long-chain fatty acids into mitochondria for oxidation. Depletion of carnitine interferes with mitochondrial oxidation of fatty acids and results in accumulation of lipids in the cytoplasm.[88] Although the usual presentation is that of dilated cardiomyopathy with congestive heart

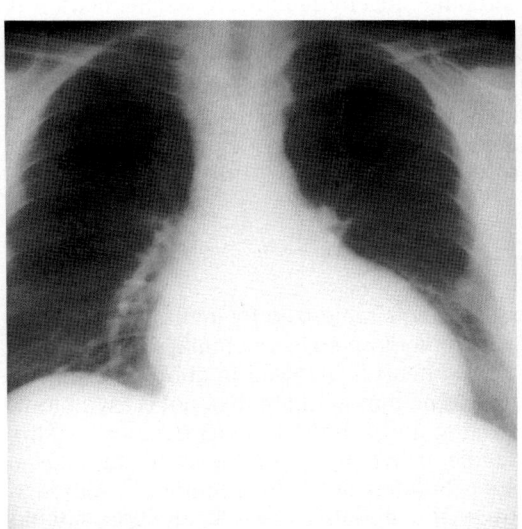 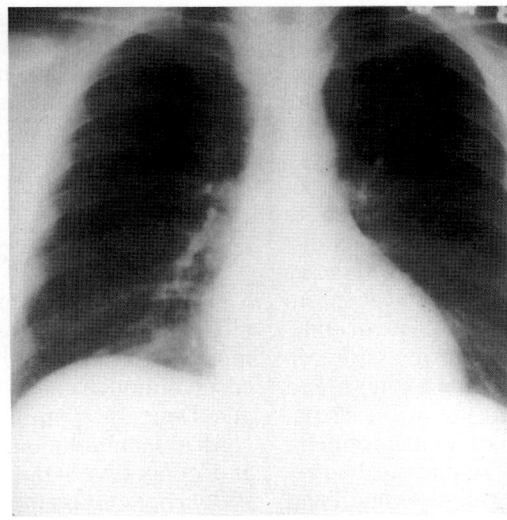

FIGURE 97.8 Roentgenograms of the chest, posteroanterior view, from a 36-year-old man with hemochromatosis, before (*left*) and 16 months after (*right*) start of therapy with monthly phlebotomies. Note the reduction in cardiac size after therapy.

failure, a family has been reported recently in which four of five children developed cardiomyopathy.[89] Three of these patients died suddenly; two were found to have concentric hypertrophy and one had dilated hypertrophy at autopsy. Endocardial fibroelastosis was evident in all three. In one of these, as well as in one of the surviving siblings, severe plasma and tissue deficiency of carnitine was demonstrated. The surviving affected sibling was treated with L-carnitine, 3 g/day orally, and manifested improved myocardial function and reduced heart size.

An alertness to this potentially treatable form of endocardial fibroelastosis appears warranted in cases of familial cardiomyopathy and/or endomyocardial biopsy revealing endocardial fibroelastosis.

PSEUDOXANTHOMA ELASTICUM

Pseudoxanthoma elasticum, also known as Grönblad-Strandberg syndrome, is a rare inherited disorder of connective tissue characterized by thickened, yellowish, sagging skin. In the rare cases of cardiac involvement, fibrous thickening of the atrial and/or ventricular endocardium has been described, sometimes involving the AV valves. Occasionally, there may be intimal fibrosis of coronary arteries. One case of restrictive cardiomyopathy in a 39-year-old woman, proved by cardiac catheterization and later autopsy, has been reported[90]; the pathologic anatomy as well as manifestations closely resembled those of endomyocardial fibrosis. No specific therapy is known.

SCLERODERMA HEART DISEASE

Progressive systemic sclerosis (PSS), or scleroderma, is a chronic disease of connective tissue, characterized by progressive edema and thickening and tightening of the skin involving the trunk; it is often associated with Raynaud's phenomenon. Other target organs include lungs, gut, kidney, heart, and pericardium. It must be emphasized that in patients with localized scleroderma (i.e., sclerodactyly or acrosclerosis) visceral involvement is a late phenomenon.

The etiology of scleroderma is unknown, and the pathogenesis is uncertain. A comprehensive theory of pathogenesis has been proposed by Campbell and Le Roy[91] on the basis of a study of 261 cases. It was proposed that scleroderma is a disease of small arteries, 150 μm to 500 μm in diameter. Initially, there is an inflammatory mononuclear reaction around these vessels, leading to proliferation of endothelial cells, medial myofibroblasts, and interstitial fibroblasts, with production of excessive amounts of collagen and mucopolysaccharides. As a result, the interstitium, as well as the vascular intima, becomes stiff and indurated. Eventually, blood flow is reduced, leading to degenerative changes in distal tissues. The organic vascular lesions in turn stimulate spasm, which results in further decrease in perfusion and further tissue damage.

Soma Weiss and associates, in 1943, first drew attention to myocardial fibrosis in scleroderma. Subsequently, the recognition of widespread vascular lesions in scleroderma led to the view that all myocardial lesions are secondary to vascular lesions.[92] A more recent analysis of 52 patients with progressive systemic sclerosis by Bulkley and associates[93] failed to demonstrate any association of myocardial necrosis and fibrosis with lesions in either the extramural or intramyocardial coronary arteries. The demonstration of contraction band necrosis suggested that the lesions might be due to intermittent vascular spasm (i.e., an "intramyocardial Raynaud's phenomenon."") Most recently, Follansbee and associates[94] studied 26 patients with progressive systemic sclerosis by means of thallium scans at maximal exercise and after redistribution. Abnormal thallium scans were found in 20 patients, although only 6 had clinical evidence of cardiac involvement. Eighteen patients had fixed perfusion defects, and 10 patients had reversible defects; of the latter, 7 underwent cardiac catheterization and all had normal coronary angiograms. Evidently, then, ischemia is an important pathogenetic factor in the myocardial lesions of progressive systemic sclerosis and spasm may play a major contributory role.

Scleroderma heart disease manifests primarily as pericarditis or congestive heart failure. Although usually a late manifestation, cardiac involvement may be the first clinical evidence of scleroderma. Cardiac manifestations often are secondary to renal involvement and systemic hypertension or to pulmonary involvement and pulmonary hypertension. Echocardiographic studies have reported data compatible with restrictive heart disease.[95]

The direct effects of drugs used in the therapy for scleroderma on the heart have not been studied.

NEOPLASTIC DISEASE

Primary tumors of the heart, as well as extracardiac tumors extending or metastasizing to the heart, may infiltrate the myocardium, result in restrictive physiology, and thus present as restrictive cardiomyopathy. Although, as a rule, this is a late phenomenon and hence the diagnosis of neoplastic disease is likely to have been made earlier, occasionally restrictive cardiomyopathy may be the first presentation.[96]

Often, pericardium and endocardium are involved as well, contributing to the restriction. Displacement of the heart by an extrinsic tumor may also result in restrictive physiology, masquerading as cardiac tamponade.[97]

Congestive heart failure is not uncommon in patients with neoplastic involvement of the heart.[98,99] Only rarely, however, has the pathophysiology been evaluated, so that a reliable estimate of the frequency of restrictive cardiomyopathy is not possible. Furthermore, inasmuch as the pericardium is often involved as well, and a pericardial effusion may be present, the clinical picture may be a composite result of both restrictive and constrictive physiology.

It must be emphasized, however, that tumors involving the heart only uncommonly present as restrictive cardiomyopathy and most frequently are silent or result in arrhythmias, conduction disturbances, intracavitary obstruction, or pericardial disease.

When tumors encroach on either the right or left ventricular cavity, they may take up much of this cavity and lead to obliterative cardiomyopathy. This occurs in some cases of rhabdomyoma, the most common primary cardiac tumor in infancy and childhood; it is only rarely encountered in adults. Multiple masses may obliterate much of either the right or the left ventricular cavity. Surgical treatment may be attempted.

Fibroma of the heart, although most frequent in childhood, also occurs in adults. This is generally a solitary tumor, usually in a ventricle, and it may arise from the septum. Obliteration may lead to congestive heart failure. Sudden death may occur, secondary to encroachment on or actual invasion of the conduction system.

Among metastatic tumors of the heart, melanoma, carcinoma of the thyroid or lung, and sarcoma most frequently involve the heart.[99] A cardiac arrhythmia, especially of supraventricular origin, is the most frequent clinical manifestation of cardiac metastases, heart failure being second. Leukemia and malignant lymphoma may involve the myocardium as well as the pericardium, usually by direct extension.[100] Inasmuch as systemic manifestations of neoplastic disease usually predominate, involvement of the heart is easily overlooked and discovered only at autopsy.

SARCOID HEART DISEASE

Sarcoidosis is a systemic disease characterized by infiltration of multiple organs with noncaseating granulomatous inflammation, leading to replacement fibrosis.[101,102] The heart is involved in about one fifth of cases, although cardiac involvement more often than not is asymptomatic. Depending on the location and extent of the cardiac lesions, the cardiac manifestations include arrhythmias, conduction disturbances, and congestive heart failure. Sudden death is common.[103] Although systolic function is more often impaired than diastolic function, sarcoid heart disease may cause restrictive cardiomyopathy. Rarely, ventricular aneurysms, secondary to transmural involvement, may occur.[104] The most frequent form of sarcoid heart disease, however, is cor pulmonale secondary to pulmonary involvement. The diagnosis of myocardial involvement may be made by endocardial biopsy and corticosteroid therapy may be beneficial.[105] Because of the frequency of sudden death in patients with arrhythmias and conduction disturbances, prophylactic insertion of an artificial pacemaker has been recommended.

CARCINOID HEART DISEASE

In about half the patients with malignant carcinoid tumors and hepatic metastasis, there is involvement of the heart. Carcinoid heart disease comprises fibrous endocardial plaques, predominantly of the right side of the heart, involving both the pulmonic and tricuspid valves and resulting in pulmonic stenosis and tricuspid regurgitation; less frequently, the left side is involved. These lesions do not represent metastases but have been attributed to serotonin and other substances secreted by the tumor. The clinical picture and features of diagnostic studies are dominated by right-sided heart failure secondary to pulmonic stenosis and tricuspid insufficiency. Restrictive cardiomyopathy has been reported in a patient following replacement of the pulmonic and tricuspid valves, leading to death 22 months after operation.[106]

RADIATION-INDUCED HEART DISEASE

Radiation-induced heart disease most frequently involves the pericardium alone, either acutely or chronically; it may lead to constrictive pericarditis.[33] In its most severe form, however, it may involve the myocardium. Myocardial fibrosis may be severe and result in restriction, which may become clinically evident only after pericardiectomy. Endocardial involvement is rare and usually not severe. Mitral and aortic insufficiency have been seen rarely.

REFERENCES

1. Report of the WHO/ISFC task force on the definition and classification of cardiomyopathies. Br Heart J 44:672, 1980
2. Abelmann WH: Classification and natural history of primary myocardial disease. Prog Cardiovasc Dis 27:73, 1984
3. Grossman W, McLaurin LP, Rolett EL: Alterations in left ventricular relaxation and diastolic compliance in congestive cardiomyopathy. Cardiovasc Res 13:514, 1979
4. Lorell BH, Paulus WJ, Grossman W et al: Modification of abnormal left ventricular diastolic properties by nifedipine in patients with hypertrophic cardiomyopathy. Circulation 65:499, 1982
5. Hirota Y: A clinical study of left ventricular relaxation. Circulation 62:736, 1980
6. Grossman W, McLaurin LP, Stefadouros M: Left ventricular stiffness associated with chronic pressure and volume overloads in man. Circ Res 35:793, 1974
7. Mann T, Goldberg S, Mudge GH Jr et al: Factors contributing to altered left ventricular diastolic properties during angina pectoris. Circulation 59:14, 1979
8. Benotti JR, Grossman W, Cohn PF: Clinical profile of restrictive cardiomyopathy. Circulation 61:1206, 1980
9. Siegel RJ, Shah PK, Fishbein MC: Idiopathic restrictive cardiomyopathy. Circulation 70:165, 1984
10. Chew C, Ziady GM, Raphael MJ et al: The functional defect in amyloid heart disease: The "stiff heart" syndrome. Am J Cardiol 36:438, 1975
11. Cutler DJ, Isner JM, Bracey AW et al: Hemochromatosis heart disease: An unemphasized cause of potentially reversible restrictive cardiomyopathy. Am J Med 69:923, 1980
12. Ferrans VJ, Hibbs RG, Burda CO: The heart in Fabry's disease: A histochemical and electron microscopy study. Am J Cardiol 24:95, 1969
13. Grossman W, McLaurin LP, Moos SP et al: Wall thickness and diastolic properties of the left ventricle. Circulation 49:129, 1974
14. Hood WB Jr, Bianco JA, Kumar R et al: Experimental myocardial infarction: IV. Reduction of left ventricular compliance in the healing phase. J Clin Invest 49:1316, 1970
15. Pogatsa G, Dubecz E, Gabor G: The role of myocardial edema in the left ventricular diastolic stiffness. Basic Res Cardiol 71:263, 1976
16. McManus BM, Bren GB, Robertson EA et al: Hemodynamic cardiac constriction without anatomic myocardial restriction or pericardial constriction. Am Heart J 102:134, 1981
17. Caulfield JB: Morphologic alterations of the collagen matrix with cardiac hypertrophy. Perspect Cardiovasc Res 7:167, 1983
18. Gaasch WH, Bing OHL, Franklin A et al: The influence of acute alterations in coronary blood flow on left ventricular diastolic compliance and wall thickness. Eur J Cardiol 7(suppl):147, 1978
19. McCullagh WH, Covell JW, Ross J Jr: Left ventricular dilatation and diastolic compliance changes during chronic volume overloading. Circulation 45:943, 1972
20. Bianco JA, Freedberg LE, Powell WJ Jr et al: Influence of vagal stimulation on ventricular compliance. Am J Physiol 218:264, 1970
21. Templeton GH, Mitchell JH, Wildenthal K: Influence of hyperosmolality on left ventricular stiffness. Am J Physiol 222:1406, 1972
22. World Health Organization: Cardiomyopathies: Report of a WHO expert committee. WHO Tech Rep Ser 697:7, 1984
23. Meaney E, Shabetai R, Bhargava V et al: Cardiac amyloidosis, constrictive pericarditis, and restrictive cardiomyopathy. Am J Cardiol 38:547, 1976
24. Hancock EW: Subacute effusive-constrictive pericarditis. Circulation 43:183, 1971
25. Mehta AV, Ferrer PL, Pickoff AS et al: M-mode echocardiographic findings in children with idiopathic restrictive cardiomyopathy. Pediatr Cardiol 5:273, 1984
26. Ferriere M, Donnadio D, Gros B et al: Biopsie endoventriculaire droite: Indications et résultats: Cent seize observations. Presse Méd 14:773, 1985
27. Shabetai R: The Pericardium, p 432. New York, Grune & Stratton, 1981
28. Anderson PAW: Diagnostic problem: Constrictive pericarditis or restrictive cardiomyopathy? Cathet Cardiovasc Diagn 9:1, 1983
29. Benotti JR, Grossman W: Restrictive cardiomyopathy. Ann Rev Med 35:113, 1984
30. Chang LWM, Grollman JH Jr: Angiocardiographic differentiation of constrictive pericarditis and restrictive cardiomyopathy due to amyloidosis. AJR 130:451, 1978
31. Isner JM, Carter BL, Bankoff MS et al: Differentiation of constrictive pericarditis from restrictive cardiomyopathy by computed tomographic imaging. Am Heart J 105:1019, 1983
32. Levine HD: Myocardial fibrosis in constrictive pericarditis: Electrocardiographic and pathologic observations. Circulation 48:1268, 1973
33. Stewart JR, Fajardo LF: Radiation induced heart disease: An update. Progr Cardiovasc Dis 27:173, 1984
34. Chusid MJ, Dale DC, West BC et al: The hypereosinophilic syndrome: Analysis of 14 cases with review of the literature. Medicine 54:1, 1975
35. Davies J, Spry CJF, Vijayaraghavan G et al: A comparison of the clinical and cardiological features of endomyocardial disease in temperate and tropical regions. Postgrad Med J 59:179, 1983
36. Chew CYC, Ziady GM, Raphael MJ et al: Primary restrictive cardiomyopathy: Non-tropical endomyocardial fibrosis and hypereosinophilic heart disease. Br Heart J 39:399, 1977
37. Parillo JE, Borer JS, Henry WC et al: The cardiovascular manifestations of the hypereosinophilic syndrome: Prospective study of 26 patients, with review of the literature. Am J Med 67:572, 1979
38. Olsen EGJ, Spry CJF: Relation between eosinophilia and endomyocardial disease. Progr Cardiovasc Dis 27:241, 1985
39. Jaski BE, Goetzl EJ, Said JW et al: Endomyocardial disease and eosinophilia. Circulation 57:824, 1978
40. Fauci AS, Harley JB, Roberts WC et al: The idiopathic hypereosinophilic syndrome: Clinical, pathophysiologic and therapeutic considerations. Ann Intern Med 97:78, 1982
41. Spry CJF, Davies J, Tai P-C et al: Clinical features of fifteen patients with hypereosinophilic syndrome. Q J Med 52:1, 1983
42. Spry CJF, Tai P-C, Davies J: The cardiotoxicity of eosinophils. Postgrad Med J 59:147, 1983
43. Chaine G, Davies J, Kohner EM et al: Ophthalmological abnormalities in the hypereosinophilic syndrome. Ophthalmology 89:1348, 1982
44. Davies J, Spry CJF, Sapsford R et al: Cardiovascular features of eleven patients with eosinophilic endomyocardial disease. Q J Med 52:23, 1983
45. Acquatella H, Schiller NB, Puigbo JJ et al: Value of two-dimensional echocardiography in endomyocardial disease with and without eosinophilia: A clinical and pathologic study. Circulation 67:1219, 1983
46. Isner JM, Michlewitz H, Clarke RH et al: Laser photoablation of pathological endocardium: In vitro findings suggesting a new approach to the surgical treatment of refractory arrhythmias and restrictive cardiomyopathy. Ann Thorac Surg 39:201, 1985
47. Connor DH, Somers K, Hutt MSR et al: Endomyocardial fibrosis in Uganda (Davies' disease): II. Am Heart J 75:107, 1968
48. Hess OM, Turina M, Senning A et al: Pre- and postoperative findings in patients with endomyocardial fibrosis. Br Heart J 40:406, 1978
49. Fowler JM, Somers K: Left ventricular endomyocardial fibrosis and mitral incompetence. Lancet 1:227, 1968
50. Bertrand E, Renambot J, Chauvet J et al: Sur 14 cas de fibrose endocardique constrictive (ou fibrose endo-myocardique). Arch Mal Coeur 68:625, 1975
51. Fawzy ME, Ziady G, Halim M et al: Endomyocardial fibrosis: Report of eight cases. J Am Coll Cardiol 5:983, 1985
52. George BO, Gaba FE, Talabi AI: M-mode echocardiographic features of endomyocardial fibrosis. Br Heart J 48:222, 1982
53. Somers K, Gunstone RF, Patel AK et al: Atrial arrhythmias in endomyocardial fibrosis. Cardiology 57:369, 1972

54. Metras D, Coulibaly AO, Ouattara K et al: Endomyocardial fibrosis: Early and late results of surgery in 20 patients. J Thorac Cardiovasc Surg 83:52, 1982
55. Moraes CR, Buffolo E, Lima R et al: Surgical treatment of endomyocardial fibrosis. J Thorac Cardiovasc Surg 85:738, 1983
56. Dubost CH, Progent C, Gerbaux A et al: Surgical treatment of constrictive fibrous endocarditis. J Thorac Cardiovasc Surg 82:585, 1981
57. Isobe T, Osserman EF: Patterns of amyloid and their association with plasma-cell dyscrasia, monoclonal immunoglobulins and Bence Jones protein. N Engl J Med 290:473, 1974
58. Glenner GG: Amyloid deposits and amyloidosis: The β-fibrilloses. N Engl J Med 302:1283, 1980
59. Pomerance A: Cardiac pathology in the elderly. Cardiovasc Clin 12:9, 1981
60. Ridolfi RL, Bulkley BH, Hutchins GM: The conduction system in cardiac amyloidosis: Clinical and pathologic features of 23 patients. Am J Med 62:677, 1977
61. Roberts WC, Waller BF: Cardiac amyloidosis causing cardiac dysfunction: Analysis of 54 necropsy patients. Am J Cardiol 52:137, 1983
62. Rubinow A, Skinner M, Cohen AS: Digoxin sensitivity in amyloid cardiomyopathy. Circulation 63:1285, 1981
63. Barth RF, Willerson JT, Buja LM et al: Amyloid coronary artery disease, primary systemic amyloidosis and paraproteinemia. Arch Intern Med 126:627, 1970
64. Kyle RA, Bayrd ED: Amyloidosis: Review of 236 cases. Medicine 54:271, 1975
65. Borer JS, Henry WL, Epstein SE: Echocardiographic observations in patients with systemic infiltrative disease involving the heart. Am J Cardiol 39:184, 1977
66. Siqueira-Filho AG, Cunha CLP, Tajik AJ et al: M-mode and two-dimensional echocardiographic features in cardiac amyloidosis. Circulation 63:188, 1981
67. Schroeder JS, Billingham ME, Rider AK: Cardiac amyloidosis: Diagnosis by transvenous endomyocardial biopsy. Am J Med 59:269, 1975
68. Lie JT: Amyloidosis and amyloid heart disease. Primary Cardiol 8:75, 1982
69. Buja LM, Roberts WC: Iron in the heart: Etiology and clinical significance. Am J Med 51:209, 1971
70. Nody AC, Bruno MS, DePasquale NP et al: Fulminating idiopathic hemochromatosis presenting as constrictive pericarditis. Ann Intern Med 83:373, 1975
71. Short EM, Winkle RA, Billingham ME: Myocardial involvement in idiopathic hemochromatosis: Morphologic and clinical improvement following venesection. Am J Med 70:1275, 1981
72. Edwards CQ, Dadone MM, Skolnick MH et al: Hereditary hemochromatosis. Clin Hematol 11:411, 1982
73. MacDonald RA, Mallory GK: Hemochromatosis and hemosiderosis: Study of 211 autopsied cases. Arch Intern Med 105:686, 1960
74. MacDonald RA: Hemochromatosis: A perlustration. Am J Clin Nutr 23:592, 1970
75. Arnett EW, Nienhuis AW, Henry WL et al: Massive myocardial hemosiderosis: A structure-function conference at the National Heart and Lung Institute. Am Heart J 90:777, 1975
76. Dabestani A, Child JS, Henze E et al: Primary hemochromatosis: Anatomic and physiologic characteristics of the cardiac ventricles and their response to phlebotomy. Am J Cardiol 54:153, 1984
77. Ley TJ, Griffith D, Niehuis AW: Transfusion hemosiderosis and chelation therapy. Clin Hematol 11:437, 1982
78. McCarthy JT, Libertin CR, Mitchell JC et al: Hemosiderosis in a dialysis patient: Treatment with hemofiltration and deferoxamine chelation therapy. Mayo Clin Proc 57:439, 1982
79. Desnick RJ, Blieden LC, Sharp HL et al: Cardiac valvular anomalies in Fabry disease: Clinical, morphologic and biochemical studies. Circulation 54:818, 1976
80. Colucci WS, Lorell BH, Schoen FJ et al: Hypertrophic obstructive cardiomyopathy due to Fabry's disease. N Engl J Med 307:926, 1982
81. Smith RRL, Hutchins GM, Sack GH et al: Unusual cardiac, renal and pulmonary involvement in Gaucher's disease: Interstitial glucocerebroside accumulation, pulmonary hypertension, and fatal bone marrow embolization. Am J Med 65:352, 1978
82. Tingelstad JB, Shiel RO'M, McCue CM: The electrocardiogram in the contracted type of primary endocardial fibroelastosis. Am J Cardiol 27:304, 1971
83. Martinez-Hernandez A, Starcher BC: Elastic fibers in endocardial fibroelastosis. Arch Pathol 94:431, 1972
84. Factor SM: Endocardial fibroelastosis: Myocardial and vascular alterations associated with viral-like muscle particles. Am Heart J 96:791, 1978
85. McLoughlin TG, Schiebler GL, Krovetz LJ: Hemodynamic findings in children with endocardial fibroelastosis: Analysis of 22 cases. Am Heart J 75:162, 1968
86. Yu PN, Cohen J, Schreiner BF Jr et al: Hemodynamic alterations in primary myocardial disease. Progr Cardiovasc Dis 7:125, 1964
87. Engel AG, Angelini C: Carnitine deficiency of human skeletal muscle with associated lipid storage myopathy: A new syndrome. Science 173:899, 1973
88. DiMauro S, Trevisan C, Hays A: Disorders of lipid metabolism in muscle. Muscle Nerve 3:369, 1980
89. Tripp ME, Katcher ML, Peters HA et al: Systemic carnitine deficiency presenting as familial endocardial fibroelastosis: A treatable cardiomyopathy. N Engl J Med 305:385, 1981
90. Navarro-Lopez F, Llorian A, Ferrer-Roca O et al: Restrictive cardiomyopathy in pseudoxanthoma elasticum. Chest 78:113, 1980
91. Campbell PM, Le Roy EC: Pathogenesis of systemic sclerosis: A vascular hypothesis. Semin Arthritis Rheum 4:351, 1975
92. Sackner MA, Heinz ER, Steinberg AJ: The heart of scleroderma. Am J Cardiol 17:542, 1966
93. Bulkley BH, Ridolfi RL, Salyer WR et al: Myocardial lesions of progressive systemic sclerosis: A cause of cardiac dysfunction. Circulation 53:483, 1976
94. Follansbee WP, Curtiss EI, Medsger TA Jr et al: Physiologic abnormalities of cardiac function in progressive systemic sclerosis with diffuse scleroderma. N Engl J Med 310:142, 1984
95. Eggebrecht RF, Kleiger RE: Echocardiographic patterns in scleroderma. Chest 71:47, 1977
96. Kaplan A, Cohen J: Restrictive cardiomyopathy as the presenting feature of reticulum cell sarcoma. Am Heart J 77:307, 1969
97. Wynne J, Markis JE, Grossman W: Extrinsic compression of the heart by tumor masquerading as cardiac tamponade. Cathet Cardiovasc Diagn 4:81, 1978
98. Mahaim I: Les Tumeurs et les Polypes du Coeur: Etude Anatomico-clinique, p 568. Lausanne, F. Roth & Cie, 1945
99. McAllister HA Jr, Fenoglio JJ Jr: Tumors of the cardiovascular system. Atlas of Tumor Pathology, second series, fascicle 15, p 111. Washington DC, Armed Forces Institute of Pathology, 1978
100. McDonnell PJ, Mann RB, Bulkley BH: Involvement of the heart by malignant lymphoma: A clinicopathologic study. Cancer 49:944, 1982
101. Roberts WC, McAllister HA, Ferrans VJ: Sarcoidosis of the heart: A clinicopathologic study of 35 necropsy patients (Group I) and review of 78 previous described necropsy patients (Group II). Am J Med 63:86, 1977
102. Silverman KJ, Hutchins GM, Bulkley BH: Cardiac sarcoid: A clinicopathologic study of 84 unselected patients with systemic sarcoidosis. Circulation 58:1204, 1978
103. Bulkley BH, Rouleau JR, Whitaker JK et al: The use of ^{201}thallium for myocardial perfusion imaging in sarcoid heart disease. Chest 72:27, 1977
104. Ahmed SS, Rozenfort R, Taclob LT et al: Development of ventricular aneurysm in cardiac sarcoidosis. Angiology 28:323, 1977
105. Lorell B, Alderman EL, Mason JW: Cardiac sarcoidosis: Diagnosis with endomyocardial biopsy and treatment with corticosteroids. Am J Cardiol 42:143, 1978
106. McGuire MR, Pugh DM, Dunn MI: Carcinoid heart disease: Restrictive cardiomyopathy as a late complication. J Kans Med Soc 79:661, 1978

GENERAL REFERENCES

Goodwin JF: Obliterative and restrictive cardiomyopathies, In Hurst JW (ed): The Heart, Arteries and Veins, 5th ed, pp 1580–1590. New York, McGraw Hill, 1978

Johnson RA, Palacios I: Nondilated cardiomyopathies. Adv Intern Med 30:243, 1984

Shabetai R: Cardiomyopathy: How far have we come in 25 years, how far yet to go? J Am Coll Cardiol 1:252, 1983

Wheeler R, Abelmann WH: Cardiomyopathy associated with systemic diseases. Cardiovasc Clin 4:283, 1972

Ziady GM, Oakley CM, Raphael MJ et al: Proceedings: Primary restrictive cardiomyopathy. Br Heart J 37:556, 1975

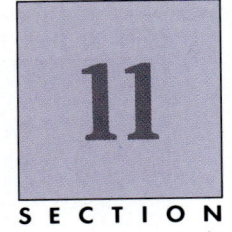

SECTION 11

Section Editor
Elliot Rapaport, MD

Congenital Heart Disease in the Adult

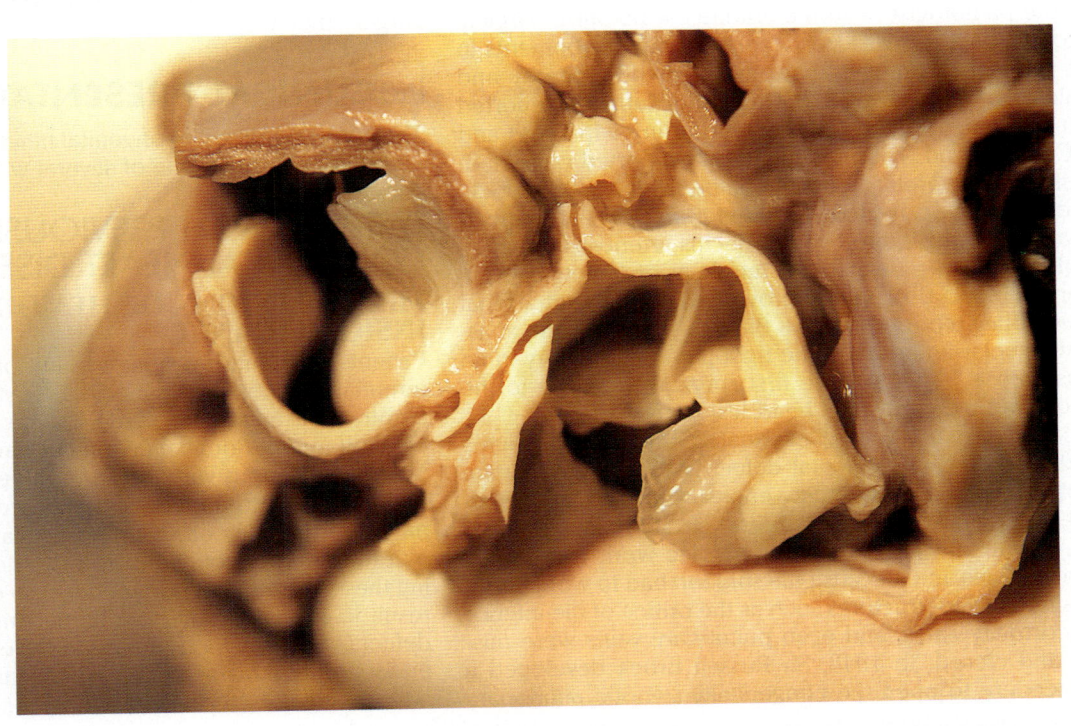

THE ADULT WITH SURGICALLY CORRECTED CONGENITAL HEART DISEASE: THE UNNATURAL HISTORY

Melvin D. Cheitlin

HISTORY

In no field in medicine have more dramatic advances been made in the last 50 years than in the recognition and surgical correction of patients with congenital heart disease. Until mid 20th century, congenital heart disease was rarely recognized during life and therefore was a matter of interest only to the pathologist or to the erudite cardiologist. Surgical treatment for congenital heart disease depended on developments in anesthesia and surgical techniques that permitted thoracotomy and finally cardiopulmonary bypass. In 1939, Gross and Hubbard[1] reported the first ligation of a patent ductus arteriosus, and in 1945 Gross and Hufnagel[2] and Crafoord and Nylin[3] independently reported correction of coarctation of the aorta. Helen Taussig together with Alfred Blalock, in a brilliant and innovative advance, developed the concept of creating an additional defect in acquired patent ductus arteriosus to establish a left-to-right shunt in patients with tetralogy of Fallot, thus increasing pulmonary blood flow and improving the peripheral arterial saturation. In 1945, they reported the first Blalock-Taussig shunt, anastomosing the left subclavian artery to the right pulmonary artery in an end-to-side anastomosis.[4] This was the first surgical approach to the most common of cyanotic congenital heart lesions.

These surgical procedures were all extracardiac. Other procedures were developed to correct atrial septal defect (ASD) in the beating heart. Under hypothermia, the systemic venous return could be suddenly occluded, the right atrium opened, and an atrial septal defect rapidly sutured. The time available for intracardiac work was strictly limited to several minutes, and because the surgeon had to work under this time constraint, diverse structures such as the orifice of the inferior vena cava, the coronary sinus, and even pulmonary veins were mistaken for ASDs and closed. In 1948, Sir Russell Brock developed a closed heart procedure to open the congenitally stenotic pulmonary valve.[5]

Repair of intracardiac defects of all varieties was not possible until 1953 when John Gibbon of Philadelphia introduced the first successful pump oxygenator for extracorporeal cardiopulmonary support.[6] Since then, innovative operative techniques have been developed that have made correction or palliation of almost all types of congenital heart disease feasible. At the present time, the most common reason for a patient's being inoperable is that there are no pulmonary arteries of sufficient size to accept the shunt or that there is irreversible pulmonary vascular disease with severe pulmonary hypertension. Now that heart–lung transplantation has been developed, even these problems are not beyond hope of operative intervention.

Until recently, the area of congenital heart disease has been of interest to pediatric cardiologists and to a few adult cardiologists. Congenital heart disease is relatively infrequent and occurs in approximately 8 in 1000 live births.[7] In the past, only a few lesions were seen with any frequency by the internist or the adult cardiologist and therefore deemed of importance: ASD, patent ductus arteriosus, interventricular septal defect, Ebstein's disease, and occasionally pulmonary atresia. With operative intervention, many patients with congenital heart disease are now entering adulthood and should pass to the care of the adult cardiologist and the internist. Also, many patients with complicated congenital heart lesions are living to reproductive age, and because their offspring have a greater chance of having congenital heart disease, the prevalence of congenital heart disease may increase in the future. It is therefore important that cardiologists and internists be aware of how these people will present to them and what problems peculiar to either their native disease or the disease as modified by surgery they will be expected to recognize and treat.

CLINICAL PRESENTATION

The adult patient with congenital heart disease will present to internists and cardiologists in one of several ways.[8]

PATIENTS WITH PREVIOUSLY UNRECOGNIZED CONGENITAL HEART DISEASE

MINOR LESIONS OF HEMODYNAMIC INSIGNIFICANCE

Patients with minor lesions present problems of recognition and differential diagnosis. A right-sided aortic arch can be mistaken for a paratracheal mass. The bicuspid aortic valve can present with a systolic ejection murmur or an ejection click and mild aortic insufficiency. The pulmonary venous varix can present as a "solitary pulmonary nodule" and even lead to unnecessary thoracotomy. The patient with a coronary artery-to-pulmonary artery fistula can present with a continuous murmur and be thought to have a patent ductus arteriosus. Recognizing these lesions is important because over time the natural course can result in serious problems. The patient with a small ventricular septal defect (VSD) or a bicuspid aortic valve requires prophylaxis to prevent endocarditis, a major danger. The bicuspid aortic valve can also calcify after the age of 40 years, resulting in severe calcific aortic stenosis.

MAJOR LESIONS OF HEMODYNAMIC SIGNIFICANCE

Patients with major lesions present problems in diagnosis and management. Seeing adults and even elderly patients with ASD, Ebstein's disease, or even coronary artery anomalies is not uncommon. Identifying such patients allows for appropriate recommendations for management.

PATIENTS WITH RECOGNIZED, UNOPERATED LESIONS

SURGERY NOT INDICATED

No surgery is indicated in some patients with congenital lesions. This includes most patients with Ebstein's disease and elderly patients with small patent ductus arteriosus or ASD or even with large ones if asymptomatic.

SURGERY NOT POSSIBLE

By far the most difficult group of patients to manage are those in whom surgery is not possible. The most common problem is that of the patient with atrial defect, ventricular defect, or patent ductus arteriosus and severe pulmonary hypertension due to pulmonary vascular disease. Management of complications of polycythemia due to arterial desaturation, paradoxic systemic emboli, right heart failure, chest pain, syncope, and arrhythmias challenges the most sensitive and expert physician.

PATIENTS WITH PREVIOUS OPERATIVE INTERVENTIONS

Patients who have had operative interventions are becoming the most common group the internist or the adult cardiologist will see and about whom we have the least information. Operative interventions may be of three types: palliative surgery, total physiologic correction, and surgical cure. Theoretically, problems would be expected only in the group with palliative surgery. If the last two categories were correctly labeled (total physiologic correction, surgical "cure"), patients in these categories might be considered normal with the prognosis of a normal person of the same age. As we learn more about these patients, it is apparent that the "unnatural history" of these repaired lesions is still not completely known. Also apparent is that many of these patients have problems either unchanged by the surgery or actually related to the surgical repair. The last category, those with surgical cure, is the smallest and probably can be applied with confidence only to many of those with repair of patent ductus arteriosus and to some with repair of ASD. All others should be considered as still having some potential problem and followed indefinitely. The rest of the chapter addresses this last category, that of the patient who has had operative intervention.

OUTCOMES OF OPERATIVE CORRECTION

Patients who have operative correction of a congenital heart lesion can have *complete correction without sequelae*, a result that is unusual; or *correction of the lesion with uncorrected residual problems due to the congenital heart lesion*. Examples of postsurgical residual problems are the residual pulmonary vascular disease after closure of patent ductus arteriosus or VSD and the arterial abnormality left by repair of a previous Blalock-Taussig, Potts, or Waterston-Cooley shunt.

RESIDUAL ABNORMALITY AFTER REPAIR

Examples of residual abnormalities left after repair are residual right ventricular outflow tract obstruction after correction of tetralogy of Fallot, residual shunt after repair of VSD or ASD, residual aortic valve obstruction or regurgitation after commissurotomy for aortic stenosis, residual hypertension after coarctation repair, and pulmonary valve regurgitation after repair of pulmonary valvular stenosis.

ABNORMALITIES PRODUCED BY SURGERY

At times, serious problems are produced by the operation. Patients with onlay patch repair of the right ventricular outflow tract in tetralogy of Fallot can develop aneurysms of the patch. The unrecognized anomalous origin of the left anterior descending coronary artery from the right coronary artery, which crosses the outflow tract of the right ventricle, can be injured during repair of tetralogy of Fallot, resulting in a large anterior wall myocardial infarction.

ABNORMALITIES THAT DEVELOP ON LATE FOLLOW-UP AS A RESULT OF SURGERY

Conduits with and without prosthetic valves have been observed to calcify, and there has been degeneration and calcification of the heterograft valves. Onlay patches and the right ventricular outflow tract can also calcify. Atrial and ventricular arrhythmias related to surgical incision of atrium and ventricle as well as atrioventricular and bundle branch block have been seen.

ABNORMALITIES OF VENTRICULAR FUNCTION

Abnormalities of ventricular function may be secondary to the underlying congenital heart disease, due to some problem occurring during surgery, or due to the nature of the repair that appears only on later follow-up. Patients with ASDs with apparently normal left ventricle preoperatively may appear postoperatively with left ventricular dysfunction and congestive heart failure. Presumably these patients have had an intraoperative event, possibly ischemia related to inadequate myocardial protection or air or thromboembolism that resulted in left ventricular damage. Patients with repair that leaves the anatomical right ventricle as the systemic ventricle, as occurs in transposition of the great vessels with the Mustard or Senning procedure, may have a ventricle that may not be capable of sustaining systemic pressures over many years and therefore may eventually result in congestive heart failure.

LONG-TERM EXPERIENCE AFTER OPERATIVE INTERVENTION

According to Hoffman and Christianson, ASD, VSD, patent ductus arteriosus, pulmonary stenosis, and coarctation of the aorta make up about 60% of all hemodynamically important congenital heart lesions.[9] If one adds aortic stenosis and tetralogy of Fallot, coronary cameral or coronary arteriovenous (AV) fistulas, pulmonary AV fistulas, pulmonary atresia, and Ebstein's disease, the vast majority of lesions the adult cardiologist would see are covered. In 1982, McNamara and Latson[10] estimated that one half to two thirds of these patients will have undergone operative repair, with a 5% mortality, so that about 8,500 new patients will reach adulthood per year in the United States.

There are, of course, many other important lesions that have been repaired and that may be of importance to the adult cardiologist and internist in the future. Many of the patients with right-to-left shunts who were repaired in infancy are not included in the previous list: transposition of the great vessels, tricuspid atresia, total anomalous pulmonary venous drainage, and the left heart hypoplastic syndromes. Without surgery most of these patients die early in life, usually within the first two years, and almost none survives to adulthood. For all except perhaps the left heart hypoplastic syndromes, there are now successful operative repairs or palliations possible. Since these are more uncommon lesions and for the most part the repairs have been successful only in the last 10 to 20 years, we have not yet had sufficient time for these patients to present in any number to the adult cardiologist. For this reason, the following discussion reviews mostly the results seen after operative intervention in the common lesions.

PATENT DUCTUS ARTERIOSUS

Experience with ligation of patent ductus arteriosus since it was first repaired in 1938 has been the longest, and in many ways the results have been the most successful. In the absence of previous left ventricular dilatation or pulmonary hypertension, successful ligation of the patent ductus arteriosus can result in what is closest to a "cure" with a normal life expectancy without complications. Adult patients with repaired patent ductus arteriosus have had resolution of symptoms if these were present preoperatively.[11] If the left-to-right shunt was significant and the main pulmonary artery and ascending and transverse aortas are distended, these usually remain enlarged. The heart size, on the other hand, usually decreases promptly unless pulmonary hypertension persists because of an elevated vascular resistance. The electrocardiogram (ECG) also returns toward normal rapidly. A residual short systolic ejection murmur at the base can be present. In the past, recanalization of the ligated ductus has occurred, but with the present technique of triple ligation this should be rare.[12] Residual pulmonary vascular disease probably will not regress[13] and, as in VSD, can progress despite successful ligation of the ductus (Fig. 98.1). If the ductus is successfully ligated, prophylaxis for infective endocarditis is no longer required 6 months after surgery.

INTERATRIAL SEPTAL DEFECT

With the exception of mitral valve prolapse and bicuspid aortic valve, in my experience interatrial septal defect is the most common congenital heart lesion seen in the adult. In the infant and child, VSD and patent ductus are more common, but because of the high incidence of spontaneous closure of these lesions during infancy, they are less frequently seen in the adult than is ASD. Before cardiopulmonary bypass was available, operative closure was accomplished under hypothermia and by an atrial "well" technique in the beating heart. With these techniques, surgery was rushed and frequently resulted in a failure to close the defect successfully or in other complications associated with suture of orifices other than the defect. At present, all defects are closed under direct vision, with the patient on cardiopulmonary bypass, and the perioperative mortality in these patients is under 1%, even in older patients as long as no other procedures such as coronary bypass surgery for coronary disease are necessary.[14] With ostium primum defects and sinus venosus defects, the operation requires insertion of a patch. In sinus venosus defect, there are frequently associated lesions, such as mitral and tricuspid valve abnormalities with valvular regurgitation and anomalously draining pulmonary veins, which result in slightly more difficult surgery and more frequent residual defects.

Most young patients recognize few symptoms. In patients over 40 to 50 years of age, two thirds to three quarters are symptomatic preoperatively, with fatigability, shortness of breath, signs of elevated pulmonary artery pressure, atrial arrhythmias, or congestive heart failure.[15] Postoperatively, the vast majority of the patients improve symptomatically.[14,16] This is also true of younger patients who may not have recognized symptoms on limited activity before surgery. The heart size decreases after surgery, mostly due to a decrease in right ventricular volume with some decrease in the size of the pulmonary vessels. There is frequently a residual faint systolic ejection murmur because the main pulmonary artery may still remain abnormally dilated. The tricuspid diastolic flow rumble along the left sternal border should disappear. Most often the second sound remains split but postoperatively moves normally with respiration. In the ostium primum defect, there is frequently residual mitral regurgitation from an abnormal clefting of the mitral valve. The ECG frequently returns toward normal. Clark and associates[17] noted that the R' in lead V_1 decreases within the first 6 months postoperatively in 84% of patients. The marked left axis deviation in the ostium primum defect does not change.

Residual abnormalities can be found on late evaluation after surgical repair. About 5% to 23% of patients with ASDs have clinically recognized atrial arrhythmias.[17-19] When measured, sinoatrial dysfunction can be found in one half to three quarters of the patients with ASDs preoperatively. Atrial flutter or fibrillation is a rhythm that may occur long after successful repair of the ASD. Even without preoperative evidence of atrial arrhythmias, patients with repaired ASDs can develop these arrhythmias late after closure. This is probably related to damage done to the atrial conduction tracts and the sinoatrial node due to the atriotomy and the placement of the vena caval sumps for cardiopulmonary bypass. Brandenburg and co-workers[18] showed that in those patients who had preoperative episodes of atrial tachyarrhythmias, such as paroxysmal atrial tachycardia, supraventricular tachycardia, atrial flutter, and atrial fibrillation, the majority continued to have these arrhythmias on follow-up after closure of the ASD. Junctional rhythms and sick sinus syndrome are more common after repair of sinus venosus defects. Because of the possibility of damage to the atrioventricular node and bundle of His, occasional atrioventricular block is seen after repair of ostium primum defect.

The incidence of residual atrial defects with left-to-right shunting has been estimated at about 5% to 10%[20] but has been reported as high as 35%.[21,22] These are usually small incidental shunts with pulmonary-to-systemic blood flow ratios rarely greater than 1.5 to 1. In those patients with preoperative pulmonary hypertension, the pulmonary artery pressure drops on repair of the ASD in proportion to the decrease in pulmonary blood flow. In those with an increase in pulmonary vascular resistance, there usually is no change in calculated pulmonary vascular resistance postoperatively. On occasion, even after successful closure, pulmonary vascular resistance may increase late postoperatively.[20] Pulmonary vascular disease is very unusual in children, usually occurring between the ages of 20 and 40 years. Past the age of 40 years, if pulmonary vascular resistance is still low it is much less likely to progress.

Graham and colleagues[23] have shown that right ventricular volume decreases postoperatively if the ASD is closed in infancy, but with closure occurring in older children and adults, the right ventricular diastolic volume may remain significantly larger than is normal. Al-

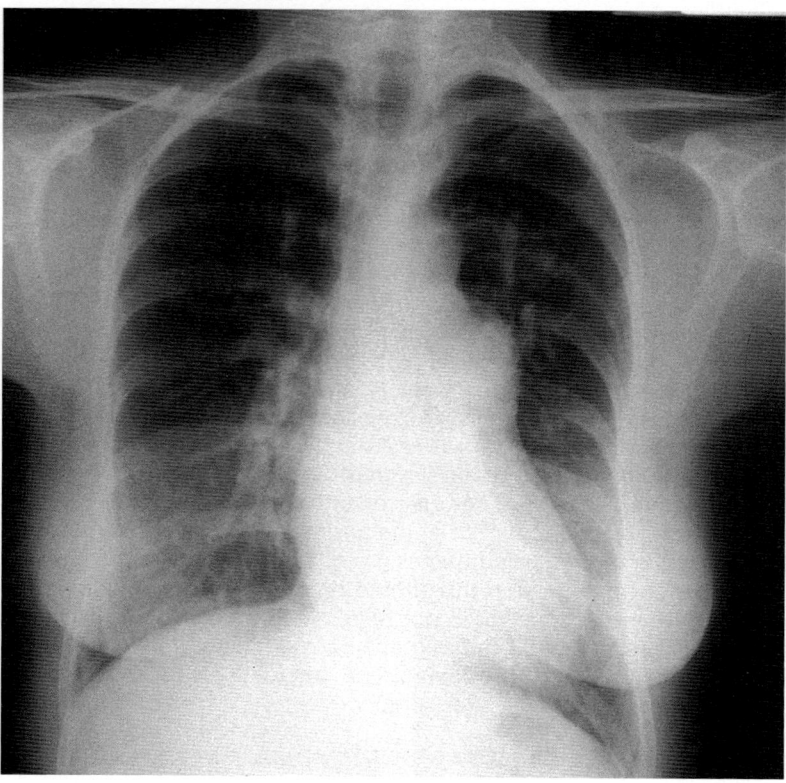

FIGURE 98.1 Chest roentgenogram, posteroanterior projection of a 30-year-old woman with elevated pulmonary vascular resistance due to a patent ductus arteriosus ligated in childhood. Pulmonary hypertension secondary to progressive pulmonary vascular disease has continued. Note the enlarged main pulmonary artery and primary pulmonary branches with clear peripheral lung fields.

though the right ventricle characteristically decreases in volume, the right atrium and major pulmonary arteries do so to a lesser extent. Liberthson and associates[24] showed that the majority of symptomatic patients had right ventricular dysfunction by radioisotope techniques measuring systolic and diastolic right ventricular volumes. No patient developed right ventricular dysfunction postoperatively, but only half of the patients with preoperative right ventricular dysfunction had improved right ventricular dysfunction postoperatively. The patients with persistent symptoms continued to have abnormal right ventricular function.

Epstein and associates[25] showed that patients with repaired ASD were not able to increase cardiac output maximally with exercise to the same extent achievable by normal patients the same age; this occurred in 7 of the 12 patients who had ASD repair after age 11. The ultimate significance of these findings to the patient is unclear, since the majority of symptomatic patients improve with surgery and life expectancy returns toward normal.[16]

Since there is no jet lesion in ostium secundum defects, there is no increase in susceptibility to infective endocarditis. Antibiotic prophylaxis is therefore not deemed necessary even after repair, and this is probably true even if a patch is used.[26] Mitral valve prolapse is reportedly common in patients with secundum ASDs; this may be related to the distortion of the left ventricle by the enlarged right ventricle, thus disturbing the posteromedial papillary muscle support and resulting in prolapse during systole. The right ventricle returns toward normal on closing the defect, and the mitral valve prolapse therefore may be decreased. If mitral valve prolapse or the murmur of mitral regurgitation due to clefting of the mitral leaflet in ostium primum defect continues to be present postoperatively, prophylaxis to prevent infective endocarditis is still clearly indicated.

INTERVENTRICULAR SEPTAL DEFECT

Patients with interventricular septal defect have been surgically corrected since the earliest days of cardiopulmonary bypass surgery. Originally, all defects were closed with a patch through a right ventriculotomy, but later, to avoid right ventricular free wall damage, a transatrial approach was developed. After it was shown that a large number of interventricular septal defects in infants, even large ventricular septal defects, closed spontaneously, the number of operative repairs has decreased.

Symptomatic patients who had operative repair of interventricular septal defect are almost universally improved symptomatically. McNamara and Latson[10] report that 90% of the postoperative patients in their study were in Class I or II 4 to 13 years after repair of the VSD. Whether this means the patients will do well long term is questionable since 60% of McNamara and Latson's patients with a postoperative peak systolic pressure of greater than 60 mm Hg were in this group. Frequently there is a residual systolic murmur, usually an ejection murmur, but at times this may be pansystolic, which in 14% to 25% of reported series[27] is associated with a usually small residual left-to-right shunt from incomplete closure of the defect. Less than 10% of these are functionally significant, but even a small defect can form the basis for continued danger from infective endocarditis.

Postoperatively the heart size usually decreases as a result of diminished volume overload of the left ventricle. The pulmonary arterial vessels may continue to be prominent, especially in those patients with an elevated pulmonary vascular resistance. If the pulmonary vascular resistance is increased preoperatively, it usually does not decrease after surgery. The pulmonary artery systolic pressure will drop proportionately to the decrease in pulmonary blood flow achieved by closing the shunt. Unfortunately, patients with elevated pulmonary vascular resistance can develop progressive pulmonary hypertension as pulmonary vascular resistance continues to increase even after successful repair. Progressive pulmonary hypertension tends to be unusual if the patient was repaired at 2 years of age or younger but is unpredictable in patients repaired after this age.[28,29]

Friedli and co-workers[28] reported that of patients with pulmonary vascular resistance greater than one third of systemic vascular resistance operated on after 2 years of age, only 1 patient showed reduction of pulmonary vascular resistance to normal and 16 patients showed no change 1 to 7 years postoperatively. The 7 late deaths in the series were presumably due to Eisenmenger's syndrome.

The electrocardiogram shows right bundle branch block 90% of the time in those repaired through a ventriculotomy and somewhat less commonly in those who are repaired transatrially.[30] Although the main right bundle branch and even the bifurcation of the bundle of His have been the site of injury in the early operative days of VSD repair, this occurs rarely now. Right bundle branch block is usually due to injury to the peripheral right bundle branches and therefore probably has little prognostic significance as far as the development of advanced heart block on follow-up is concerned. If pulmonary hypertension persists, right ventricular hypertrophy usually persists although it may be difficult to detect in the presence of right bundle branch block. Echo Doppler study is a better way of detecting residual pulmonary hypertension, especially if there is Doppler-detected tricuspid regurgitation where the gradient from right ventricle to right atrium can be added to the systemic venous pressure and an estimate of right ventricular systolic pressure obtained. In the absence of pulmonary stenosis, this is equal to the pulmonary artery systolic pressure. The persistence of right ventricular hypertrophy on echocardiography is further evidence of residual pulmonary hypertension.

Sudden death has been reported in these patients. In the Joint Study of the Natural History of Congenital Heart Disease,[31] there were 17 late deaths, most of them sudden deaths, among the 385 patients surviving VSD repair. The mechanism for these sudden deaths is uncertain. McNamara and Latson[10] believe that most occur in patients with residual pulmonary hypertension, but it is possible that the right ventricular scar permits a substrate for ventricular tachycardia. Bharati and Lev[32] have suggested that sudden death due to late injury to the conduction system may occur either directly or as a result of blockage to lymphatic drainage of the heart and subsequent endocardial fibroelastosis.

Left ventricular function has been examined by radioisotope ventriculography in patients with ventricular septal defects before and after repair. Jarmakani and associates[33] reported 23 patients studied 1 to 5 years after repair. The mean age at surgery was 5.4 years. They reported an increase in left ventricular diastolic volume, an increase in left ventricular mass, and a decrease in ejection fraction compared to the normal. Subsequently, the same group reported that this did not occur in patients operated on in infancy.[34] Otterstad and co-workers[35] reported exercise tests and hemodynamic studies in 17 patients before and 11 to 21 years after repair. Resting values were normal, but with exercise there was subnormal increase in left and right ventricular cardiac output as well as an abnormal increase in right and left ventricular end-diastolic pressure. There was no correlation with symptoms, the age at repair, or the size of the shunt. Of most interest was that Otterstad and associates also studied 35 patients with smaller interventricular septal defects with shunts deemed not large enough to require repair and found on follow-up the same pattern of left and right ventricular dysfunction with subnormal left ventricular fractional shortening and velocity of contractile fiber shortening (VCF) on echocardiography, suggesting the possibility that a longstanding VSD even with a small shunt may lead to disturbed systolic function and reduced compliance of both ventricles. This is consistent with the finding of Jablonsky and associates,[36] who studied 17 patients with VSD and pulmonary-to-systemic blood flow ratios less than 2:1 by gated radioisotope ventriculography at rest and exercise, and showed that patients with VSD could not increase ejection fraction with exercise as could the normal person. They also studied 12 patients after VSD repair 9 to 22 years previously and showed that these patients also did not increase left ventricular ejection fraction with exercise.

In the United States, about 3% of patients with VSDs will develop aortic regurgitation, either with supracristal VSD and prolapse of the aortic valve, especially the right coronary cusp, or from a separate abnormality of the aortic valve such as a bicuspid aortic valve. The aortic regurgitation can be progressive if it is independent of the VSD even if the VSD is closed. With supracristal VSD and the aortic regurgitation caused by prolapse due to lack of support of the right coronary cusp, there is evidence that the aortic regurgitation may not progress if the ventricular septal defect is repaired.[37]

Finally, the matter of prophylaxis to prevent infective endocarditis must be addressed. Currently, prophylaxis is not considered to be necessary if there is no evidence for residual left-to-right shunt by 3 to 6 months postoperatively.

PULMONARY VALVE STENOSIS

In 1948, Sir Russell Brock[5] operated on a patient with pulmonary stenosis. Once cardiopulmonary bypass was available, all surgery in pulmonary valvular stenosis was done on bypass through a pulmonary artery incision. In our experience, there is almost always some pulmonary regurgitation present postoperatively. Since the pulmonary artery pressure is low, the diastolic gradient causing the pulmonary regurgitation is small, and the murmur characteristically is short, low frequency, and decrescendo, and starts appreciably after the aortic component of the second heart sound. Generally there is still a short systolic ejection murmur present, and an ejection click may still be present since the poststenotic dilatation does not disappear postoperatively. Frequently the right ventricle enlarges after surgery, probably related to the pulmonary regurgitation. Right ventricular hypertrophy on the ECG regresses, but usually there is at least a late right and anterior electrical force resulting in an rSr' in lead V_1.

Most patients do very well with relief of pulmonary valve stenosis on follow-up. In my experience, there are no late atrial or ventricular arrhythmias seen in patients with good relief of the obstruction. There are two residual defects that may affect long-term follow-up: residual pulmonary valve stenosis and the development of right ventricular volume overload due to the pulmonary regurgitation. In the Joint Study of Congenital Heart Disease, only 10 of 294 patients who had surgery for valvular pulmonary stenosis had a transpulmonic valve peak systolic pressure gradient of 50 mm Hg or more.[38] In these patients it is possible that late ventricular arrhythmias may be a problem.

The other residual is that of pulmonic valvular regurgitation. I have seen two patients with uncomplicated repair of valvular pulmonary stenosis who have developed severe tricuspid regurgitation on follow-up, resulting in severe increases in right atrial pressure and systemic venous congestion. Later, there was a decrease in right ventricular forward output requiring tricuspid valve anuloplasty and, in one patient, tricuspid valve replacement. If there is a patent foramen ovale, a right-to-left shunt and cyanosis can occur. It is possible that patients with longstanding pulmonary valve stenosis can have, preoperatively, right ventricular subendocardial myocardial fibrosis. Whether this has long-term significance after repair is at present unknown.

At present, most patients with pulmonary valve stenosis have been managed by balloon valvuloplasty with success equivalent to that of surgery; how this will change the picture given above is not known.[39] Finally, since all these patients have residual pulmonary regurgitation, prophylaxis to prevent infective endocarditis is indicated.

AORTIC STENOSIS

Valvular aortic stenosis can result from a unicuspid valve, a bicuspid valve usually with myxomatous change, a unicuspid valve or a bicuspid valve with "fused" commissure, or an acommissural valve. These valves have been opened by commissurotomy under direct vision with successful elimination of the gradient postoperatively. Occasionally there will be aortic regurgitation postoperatively. The left ventricular hypertrophy on ECG will regress and the majority of symptomatic patients will become asymptomatic.

The prognosis of these patients, however, is guarded. Hsieh and associates[40] reported 59 patients who had aortic valvotomy before 1968. All were older than 1 year of age at the time of operation, and the mean follow-up time was 17.7 years. Of these, 46 patients are still living, 26 (57%) are 30 to 40 years old, and 6 (13%) are older. By actuarial analysis, survival was 94% at 5 years and 27% at 22 years. Of 13 patients who died, 7 died suddenly. Reoperation was carried out on 21 patients (36%), 3 of whom died. Actuarial analysis showed a chance of reoperation of 2% at 5 years and 44% at 22 years. Bacterial endocarditis occurred on four occasions in 3 patients, with an incidence of 3.8 episodes per thousand patient-years. Actuarial analysis of death, reoperation, or complication indicated the probability of being free of such an episode as 93% at 5 years but only 39% at 22 years. These findings point out that valvuloplasty for valvular aortic stenosis is a temporizing procedure with continuing problems for the patient.

Whitmer and co-workers[41] exercised children with valvular and discrete subvalvular aortic stenosis before and 3 to 30 months after surgery, and showed that the ST segment depression with exercise that occurred before surgery was much improved or absent postoperatively. They considered this evidence of relief of obstruction. In patients with discrete membranous subvalvular aortic stenosis, there is also good evidence that obstruction can be relieved by surgery. Ashraf and associates[42] reported on follow-up of 32 patients with discrete subaortic membranous stenosis that there were 4 recurrences, and 17 other patients had excision myotomy, also with 3 recurrences. The actuarial survival rate was 88% for 10 years. Reoperation was performed in 10 patients, 7 for recurrence and 3 for aortic valve replacement for preexisting aortic regurgitation that had progressed since the first procedure.

Recently, balloon valvuloplasty has been applied in the treatment of patients with valvular aortic stenosis. This technique may be especially important in neonates in congestive heart failure with severe aortic stenosis.[43] The long-term prognosis of patients treated with balloon valvuloplasty is not known.

Patients with valvular aortic stenosis have been shown to have residual subendocardial left ventricular fibrosis.[44] How this will affect the future course of these patients is unknown, but it is clear that valvulotomy for aortic stenosis is a temporizing procedure, with most of these patients having further problems, probably resulting in aortic valve replacement in the future. Unfortunately, these patients tend to have small aortic valve rings, so that only a small prosthetic valve may be inserted. This can result, even with a well-functioning valve, in moderate prosthetic valvular stenosis, a condition that has been termed *prosthetic valve mismatch*. Patients with surgically released aortic valvular or subvalvular stenosis still have abnormal valves that require antibiotic prophylaxis to prevent infective endocarditis.

COARCTATION OF THE AORTA

Coarctation of the aorta was first repaired by Crafoord and Nylin in 1945[3] by resection and end-to-end anastomosis. At present there are several other surgical techniques, such as graft interposition, aortoplasty, and, in infants, subclavian artery flap aortoplasty.

Coarctation of the aorta in infants is frequently associated with other defects such as patent ductus arteriosus, VSD, and valvular and subvalvular aortic stenosis. These infants frequently present in heart failure and have a high mortality at surgery. There is also an incidence of mitral valve abnormality, but this is rarely hemodynamically significant. The patient with isolated coarctation of the aorta is usually asymptomatic when the diagnosis is made, usually by physical examination.

There have been many reports of large series of patients with long-term follow-up after surgery indicating good relief of obstruction with a normalization of blood pressure.[45,46] A good result may be defined as a gradient of 10 mm Hg or less between the systolic blood pressure of the arm and that of the leg. However, in all of these studies, residual problems have been frequent, and late mortality, mainly related to cardiovascular disease, is not insignificant.

One problem in estimating the recurrence rate of coarctation postoperatively is in separating recurrence from an initially inadequate operation. In most studies, 10% to 20% of patients with good postoperative relief of obstruction continue to have resting hypertension postoperatively. The reappearance of the gradient is most common when a patient is under the age of 1 year when operated on,[47] and recurrence of coarctation occurs in 3% to 17.5% of patients, depending on the type of surgical repair possible.[46] The frequency with which systemic hypertension returns late after surgery increases with increasing age of patient at surgery.[46,48]

Treadmill exercise testing has been recommended to uncover inadequate coarctation repair, since it has been noted that even with normal systolic blood pressure at rest, on exercise patients who had coarctation repair have an abnormally higher systolic pressure than normal persons.[49] This appears to be due to the increased cardiac output ejected into a moderately restricted proximal aorta that is stiffer than normal. Unless the resting arm-to-leg systolic gradient is abnormal, elevation of systolic pressure with exercise does not identify the patients with an inadequate surgical repair.[50]

There are other residual abnormalities that cause problems in patients with coarctation repair. Of patients with coarctation of the aorta, 50% to 85% have a bicuspid aortic valve that can either be the cause of the aortic regurgitation or, later in life, the basis for the development of calcific aortic stenosis. It can also be the site of infective endocarditis. Aneurysms can occur around the site of the coarctation, in the cranial circulation, or even at other sites in the aorta distant from the coarctation. These aneurysms can rupture, causing cerebral hemorrhage and death, and this can occur some time after successful coarctation repair.[51] Late dissection of the aorta can occur, usually proximal to the coarctation site. Schneeweiss and co-workers[52] have reported intramural coronary small vessel disease. Abnormal thallium-201 myocardial perfusion has been seen in patients with coarctation of the aorta, suggesting, again, small vessel abnormality.[53]

Clarkson and associates[46] reported the late outcome (10 to 28 years postoperatively) of 160 patients ages 1 to 54 years with surgical repair of the aorta. They found that the 20-year survival of patients operated on between the ages of 1 and 19 was slightly less than the normal population (95% vs. 97%). In the group operated on between the ages of 20 and 39 years, the probability of survival was slightly less, but in those 40 years of age and older the discrepancy between the patients' 15-year survival (52%) and the general population (81%) was marked. There were 19 late deaths (12%), 79% of which were due to cardiovascular disease. Thirteen patients had a poor result, 11 because of recoarctation and 2 because of a complication at the site of repair. In most patients the blood pressure became normal for the first 5 to 10 years after surgery, but when followed longer, the proportion with hypertension increased. The likelihood of being alive without complications and with a normal blood pressure was 69% at 10 years, 65% at 15 years, and 20% at 25 years postoperatively.

Because of the belief that a Dacron onlay patch repair of the coarctation site would leave the posterior wall intact to grow and allow creation of a normal aortic lumen as the child grew, in many centers this became the operation of choice, rather than resection of the coarctation with end-to-end anastomosis. Unfortunately, in follow-up, there has been an alarming incidence of both true and false aneurysms at the site of patch repair. In a report by Clarkson and co-workers,[54] an aneurysm was found in 5 of 38 patients in whom a Dacron onlay patch graft was used either as primary repair or to renew an earlier repair, an actuarial incidence of 38%, at 14 years. There have been reports of late rupture of these aneurysms, so they should be repaired.[55]

Because of these residual lesions and problems, all patients with coarctation should be followed even after successful repair and evaluated for recoarctation, the development of systemic hypertension, which should be immediately treated, and covered with prophylactic antibiotics to prevent infective endocarditis.

TETRALOGY OF FALLOT

Palliative shunting by anastomosing the right subclavian artery to the right pulmonary artery (the Blalock-Taussig shunt) was the first operation applicable to tetralogy of Fallot. Subsequently, other types of palliative operations, such as the Potts shunt (left pulmonary artery to descending aorta) and Waterston-Cooley shunt (right pulmonary artery to ascending aorta), have been introduced. Palliative partial correction was afforded by the Brock procedure, which consisted of a right ventricular infundibulectomy, which increased pulmonary blood flow. The palliative procedures increase the arterial oxygen saturation and do improve exercise tolerance.[56]

On follow-up of patients with palliative shunts, the major problem is that patients outgrow the shunt, become progressively cyanotic and arterially desaturated, and have to have a second shunt or total correction. The most serious long-term problem has been the development of pulmonary vascular disease, most frequently with the Potts and the Waterston-Cooley procedures and least frequently with the Blalock-Taussig shunt (Fig. 98.2). Over many years all of these palliative shunts are plagued by the development of pulmonary vascular disease, infective endarteritis, cerebrovascular accidents, and death at attempted total repair. Bertranou and colleagues[57] studied all published autopsy

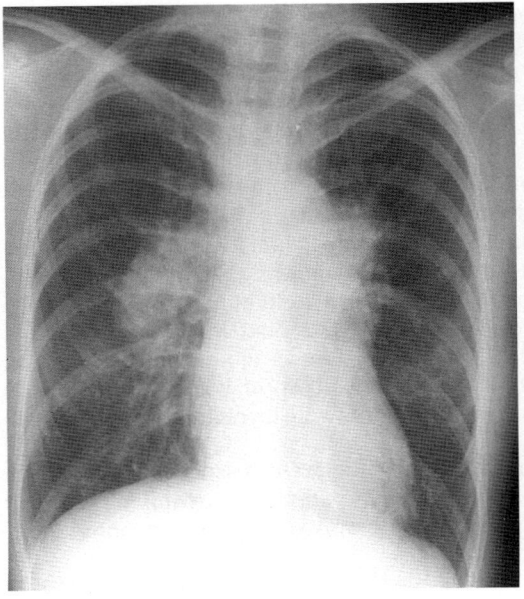
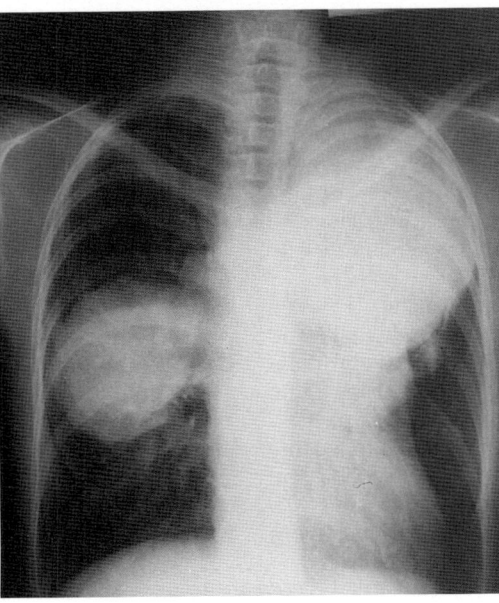

FIGURE 98.2 Thirty-year-old woman with tetralogy of Fallot who had bilateral Blalock-Taussig shunts in 1948. Posteroanterior projection of chest roentgenogram on the left in 1965 and on the right in 1971. There are aneurysms of both right and left pulmonary arteries with severe pulmonary hypertension and pulmonary vascular disease. In 1972 the patient died of rupture of the left pulmonary aneurysm.

cases of patients with tetralogy of Fallot dying without surgery and reported the survival to be 35% at 1 year and 10% at 25 years. In 350 patients with tetralogy of Fallot and palliative surgery, Presbitero and co-workers[56] reported a 10-year survival of 87% and a 25-year survival of 50%.

At present, total correction, that is, relief of the right ventricular outflow tract obstruction consisting of infundibulectomy or pulmonic valvulotomy, at times with an onlay patch across the right ventricular outflow tract, together with patch closure of the VSD, is the procedure of choice. In Presbitero and colleagues' study,[56] 106 patients had had total correction, and their actuarial survival curves compared to the palliated group were significantly better. At 20-year follow-up postoperatively, these patients had an almost normal life expectancy for the age group.

A variety of late problems have been noted with complete correction. Those patients who have had a right ventriculotomy have a high incidence of right bundle branch block. Even with transatrial repair of the VSD, the incidence of right bundle branch block is high, probably due to the infundibular muscle resection, which causes peripheral right bundle branch block.[58] Injury to the conduction system occurs, as shown by electrophysiologic studies. Neches and associates[59] reported a high incidence of electrophysiologic abnormalities, with 20% having prolonged HV intervals and 23% of the patients developing second-degree atrioventricular block on atrial pacing with rates below 160 beats/min. Two thirds of the patients had some form of conduction abnormality. The development of late high-degree atrioventricular block has been rare, but the future significance of the high incidence of conduction system damage is unknown.

Residual VSD with left-to-right shunting occurs in a minority of patients. Joransen and colleagues[60] reported follow-up catheterization of 132 patients with repaired tetralogy of Fallot and found 12 (9%) with a significant residual VSD. In addition, incomplete resection of right ventricular infundibulum was common. Resting right ventricular systolic pressure was less than 80 mm Hg in 100 patients and was from 80 mm Hg to 150 mm Hg in the other 32 patients. Exercise at catheterization was done in 34 patients and was abnormal in 17 (50%). Therefore, the incidence of residual defects was high.

Although most patients with tetralogy of Fallot who have been completely repaired are asymptomatic or only minimally symptomatic; exercise studies in patients have shown limited ability to increase cardiac output compared to normal[25,61,62] and have a decreased exercise capacity compared to normal.

Ventricular function has been studied by radionuclide study. Early studies reported abnormalities of left ventricular function.[63,64] More recently, studies of adolescents and adults with repaired tetralogy of Fallot have shown a normal left ventricular function and normal ejection fraction, as well as normal increase in ejection fraction with exercise in the majority of patients.[64-66] When there has been a longstanding palliative shunt with left ventricular dilatation or residual large left VSD with a large left-to-right shunt, then left ventricular function can be decreased.[64] On the other hand, right ventricular function, probably as a result of right ventriculotomy, possibly with an onlay patch or with possible residual right ventricular outflow tract obstruction, frequently has been abnormally low. Often an abnormally low right ventricular ejection fraction is found, with a further decrease on exercise.[66,67] There is some evidence that the right ventricular ejection fraction at rest and with exercise is more likely to be normal in those patients with repair done before the age of 2 years.[68]

James and associates[69] showed an inverse relationship between maximal working capacity and the age at surgery in both male and female patients. Furthermore, although some patients had ventricular arrhythmias at rest on ambulatory ECG monitoring, on exercise testing in some patients ventricular arrhythmias became more frequent. Garson and co-workers[70] studied 104 patients with treadmill testing, using the Bruce protocol, 7 years after repair. Of these patients, 14% had premature ventricular contractions (PVCs) on the resting ECG and 30% developed PVCs on exercise. Patients with exercise arrhythmias were older, were tested longer after their surgery, and had a higher right ventricular systolic pressure and right ventricular end-diastolic pressure than those without arrhythmias.

Burns and colleagues[71] reported 44 adult patients with tetralogy of Fallot studied a mean of 14 years after repair and found that 50% had multiform repetitive PVCs or increased PVCs during the exercise or on recovery from the exercise on ambulatory ECG monitoring or treadmill testing. They found that these patients had a higher right ventricular systolic pressure, lower cardiac index, and more often a residual left-to-right shunt or abnormally low left ventricular ejection fraction.

Garson and associates[72] reported 233 patients with repair of the tetralogy of Fallot at a median age of 9.7 years, with 26 surgical deaths (11.1%), 12 late cardiac deaths (5.9%), and 3 noncardiac deaths (1.3%) in a mean follow-up of 5.2 years. Of the 12 cardiac deaths, 8 occurred suddenly, and all had a documented right ventricular systolic pressure above 60 mm Hg and PVCs. Their conclusion was that late death after repaired tetralogy of Fallot was due to ventricular tachyarrhythmias, and the patients at greatest risk were those with PVCs and an incomplete right ventricular infundibular resection leaving them with a right ventricular systolic pressure above 60 mm Hg.

Garson and colleagues[73] have reported retrospective evidence that antiarrhythmic drugs that successfully suppress ventricular arrhythmias can decrease the incidence of sudden death in these patients. Finally, Hu and co-workers[74] have reported surgical correction of tetralogy of Fallot in 30 patients 40 to 60 years of age with low operative mortality (3%) and with 110-month follow-up and gratifying long-term results.

Most patients with resection of the right ventricular infundibulum and enlargement of the pulmonic ring with an onlay patch will have postoperative pulmonic valvular regurgitation. In the relatively short-term follow-up available, this volume load of the right ventricle is handled well. Whether this will remain benign when we have long-term follow-up remains to be seen. Occasionally aneurysms have formed at the site of the outflow tract onlay patch (Figs. 98.3, 98.4). Certainly, all patients with repaired tetralogy of Fallot should continue to receive antibiotics to prevent infective endocarditis.

TRANSPOSITION OF THE GREAT VESSELS

The other lesions characterized by right-to-left shunting in the presurgical era have had a poor prognosis, with little chance of survival beyond infancy or certainly childhood. With transposition of the great vessels, surgical procedures resulting in physiologic correction of the defect were introduced in 1959 by Senning[75] and in 1964 by Mustard.[76] An arterial anatomical "switch" operation was introduced by Jatene in 1976.[77] The patients were usually 1 year of age and almost always under 5 years of age at the time of repair. At present, we are seeing more patients with these complex congenital heart lesions entering adulthood as a result of these surgical procedures. Furthermore, the surgical techniques have undergone change more recently, which may influence the late result, so it is even more difficult to know what the post-repair course will be. Furthermore, these lesions of necessity have one or more other defects, some of which, like the patent ductus arteriosus or VSD, are compensating for the major lesion and allowing mixing of systemic and pulmonary venous return and therefore survival of the child. These other lesions may vary from patient to patient and can affect survival and possibly the postsurgical natural history. In many series, double-outlet right ventricle is included, especially when the VSD is committed to the pulmonary artery. Patients with left ventricular outflow tract obstruction are also included. These patients are not a homogeneous group, which may account for the variability of both perioperative and late results. There is almost no information concerning series of patients reaching adulthood, so our information is mainly derived from series of patients still in childhood or adolescence.

Most infants with transposition of the great vessels have had a procedure at an early age to increase interatrial venous mixing. Earliest was the Blalock-Hanlon atrial septectomy done in the beating heart.

Later, Rashkind introduced a catheter–balloon procedure whereby the membrane of the foramen ovale is ruptured, thus allowing for interatrial mixing of pulmonary and systemic venous return.

The Mustard operation corrects the effects of transposition of the great vessels by constructing an intra-atrial baffle, usually using pericardium, which directs the pulmonary venous return through the tricuspid valve and to the aorta and the systemic venous return through the mitral valve and to the lungs, thus physiologically "correcting" the lesion. The Senning procedure accomplishes the same end by ingeniously refolding the atrium and atrial septum in an origami-type correction.

Patients have done exceedingly well considering the extremely poor prognosis before surgical correction. The patients are usually acyanotic and report normal activity with little limitation. The major problems found are occasional obstruction of the superior vena cava or pulmonary venous return by the baffle. This can be detected by two-dimensional Doppler echocardiography[78] and is usually recognized within several years of surgery. Leakage of the baffle is not unusual, especially when detected with contrast by two-dimensional echocardiography. There are frequently residual defects, including obstruction of left ventricular outflow tract due to incomplete resection, continued left-to-right shunting through the incompletely closed VSD, or, more ominously, the murmur of tricuspid regurgitation, possibly meaning dilatation and failure of the systemic right ventricle.[79]

Flinn and associates[80] reported on the pooled ECG and clinical data on 372 patients with transposition of the great vessels who had survived the Mustard procedure for at least 3 months. The mean age at surgery was 2 years and the mean follow-up period was 4.5 years. Simple transposition of the great vessels was present in 70% of patients and complex forms in 28%. The major problem was that the resting heart rates were slower than normal for age-matched normal children, and although 76% of the patients had sinus rhythm during the first year after the operation, this declined to only 57% by the end of the eighth postoperative year. There were increasing numbers of patients with junctional rhythm. During the 16 years of follow-up, 39 patients received pacemakers, at a mean interval of 1.8 years after surgery, and 25 patients (7%) died, 9 of them suddenly. The cumulative survival rate was 91% at 11 years and 71% at 15 years, and no strong risk factors for sudden death were recognized.

Physiologic and electrophysiologic studies have been reported in patients who had the Senning procedure, and the short-term results have been excellent. George and co-workers[81] reported 35 patients with simple and 10 patients with complex transposition of the great vessels who were repaired with the Senning procedure. There were infrequent patients with right ventricular dysfunction, arrhythmias, or baffle obstruction, and 4 deaths, 3 in the complex group. These good results were similar to those reported previously by Byrum and associates.[82]

Late arrhythmias have been a persistent problem after the Mustard procedure. Hayes and Gersony[83] reported 95 patients after Mustard correction followed by ECG and 24 followed by ambulatory ECG. At the time of discharge, 20% had atrial arrhythmias. By the sixth year, 75% had atrial arrhythmias. The most common arrhythmia was junctional rhythm. Supraventricular tachycardia in the context of a tachyarrhythmia–bradyarrhythmia syndrome was seen in 8 of 10 patients. Complete heart block was not seen. Pacemakers were needed in 6 patients, and the incidence of death in this series was 3%.

A major problem after the Mustard and Senning procedures is that the right ventricle remains the systemic ventricle. In simple transposition of the great vessels, the majority of patients 1 year after Mustard procedure have a decreased right ventricular ejection fraction averaging 43% to 47%.[84] The normal value is 65%. If the VSD is closed at the time of the Mustard procedure, the right ventricular ejection fraction is lower.[79] Benson and colleagues[85] showed an abnormal right ventricular ejection fraction response with no change or a decrease in ejection fraction during exercise in 9 of 15 asymptomatic patients studied 3.5 to 15 years after Mustard procedure. In a later study, Hurwitz and co-workers,[86] using radionuclide ventriculography in 14 infants 3 years after Mustard procedure, showed a normal right ventricular ejection fraction of 0.57% ± 0.8%. Mathews and associates[87] reported exercise studies in 21 patients with transposition of the great vessels a mean of 9 years after the Mustard procedure. The patients were all clinically well, without complaints of exercise intolerance. Exercise tolerance was diminished in half the patients and arrhythmias were provoked in over 70% during or after the exercise. The most serious arrhythmias produced were multifocal PVCs.

The Jatene or "arterial switch" operation was designed for patients with transposition of the great vessels and VSD where the venous switch operation had a high mortality. For a simple transposition of the great vessels, the Jatene procedure has an operative mortality higher

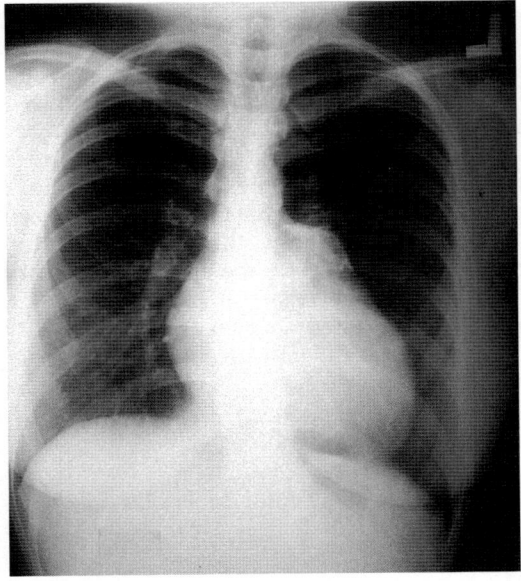

FIGURE 98.3 Chest roentgenogram, posteroanterior projection of an asymptomatic 27-year-old woman with tetralogy of Fallot, repaired at the age of 7. There is an aneurysm of the right ventricular outflow tract onlay patch. Note the calcification in the aneurysm.

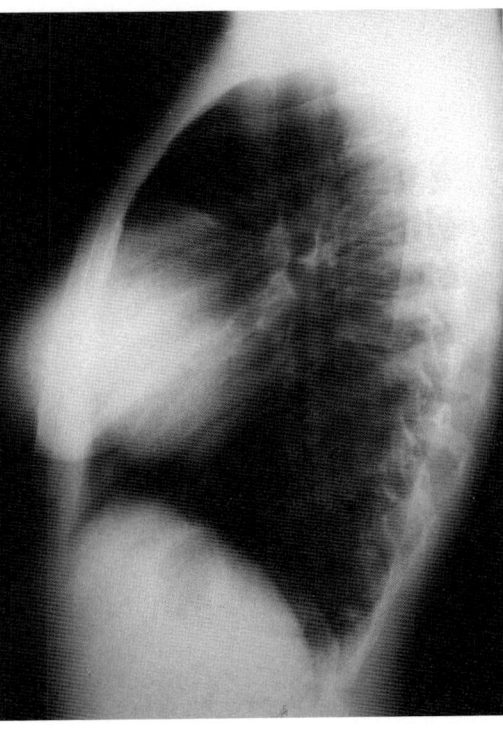

FIGURE 98.4 Chest roentgenogram, left lateral projection. Same patient as in Figure 98.3.

than with the Mustard or Senning procedure, 10% to 17% at best.[88] The great advantage of the Jatene procedure is that the atria are not disturbed and the left ventricle becomes the systemic ventricle, thus eliminating the problem of late failure of the systemic right ventricle seen in the venous switch operations. To avoid the problem of failure of the anatomical left ventricle when it suddenly becomes the systemic ventricle, a two-stage procedure was developed. The first stage bands the pulmonary artery to increase the left ventricular wall tension and stimulate left ventricular hypertrophy, and at a later time the arterial switch operation is accomplished. Lange and associates[89] have reported on all 16 of the children having this two-stage correction for simple transposition of the great vessels, with late cardiac catheterization data in 12. The follow-up was 6 months to 7 years. None have had coronary or myocardial insufficiency after an adaptation phase of 6 months after the anatomical correction. No arrhythmias attributable to the anatomical correction were seen. The only residual was mild right ventricular hypertension due to residual stenosis from the band site. The other residual is the dilatation of the pulmonary root, which, after the arterial switching operation, becomes the aortic root. Bical and co-workers[90] reported on 50 patients with transposition of the great vessels and VSD who also had an arterial switch operation and closure of the VSD. Of these 50 patients, 39 had preliminary pulmonary artery banding. The perioperative mortality was 32%. All 31 survivors did well and were in sinus rhythm during a follow-up period of 31 ± 14 months. Left ventricular function was normal. Stenosis of the right ventricular outflow tract occurred in 7 patients, 5 of whom required reoperation.

Borow and associates[91] evaluated left ventricular contractile function after the arterial switch operation and found the left ventricular function by end-systolic pressure dimension and wall stress shortening relationships to be normal. Martin and colleagues[92] reported on 92 survivors of the arterial switch correction of transposition of the great vessels during a 3-year follow-up period. There have been no cases of arrhythmic death or symptomatic arrhythmias requiring treatment. Postoperative ECG's show 60% to be free of arrhythmias. Supraventricular premature beats increased from 4.9% preoperatively to 23% postoperatively. One patient had acquired complete heart block. It appears that serious arrhythmias are fewer in the arterial switch operation than in the venous switch operation.

The short-term outlook for patients with postoperative correction of transposition of the great vessels has been very good. Patients with the arterial switch operation repair have normal systemic left ventricles and fewer arrhythmias. Whether this will continue to be true as larger series are followed into adulthood remains to be determined.

TRICUSPID ATRESIA

In tricuspid atresia there is a failure of the tricuspid valve to develop so that there is no connection from right atrium to right ventricle. All the systemic venous return entering the right atrium goes through the patent foramen ovale or an ASD into the left atrium, where it mixes with pulmonary venous return and is distributed by the left ventricle to both lungs and systemically. Among the several variations of tricuspid atresia are those where the blood goes through a VSD to the residual outflow tract of the right ventricle into the pulmonary artery, and another group with an absence of VSD. These patients have only a potential right ventricle without a lumen, and blood flow to the pulmonary artery is through a patent ductus or through bronchial collateral vessels. Finally, there are two groups of tricuspid atresia, according to arterioventricular concordance or discordance.

Physiologically, tricuspid atresia is characterized by a nonfunctioning or abnormally functioning right ventricle, a common mixing of systemic and pulmonary venous return at the left atrial level, and a single pumping chamber at the left ventricle. Many patients have had a systemic arterial-to-pulmonary artery shunt created to increase pulmonary blood flow and systemic arterial saturation. These shunts include the Blalock-Taussig, Waterston-Cooley, and the Glenn procedure, the latter consisting of anastomosing the superior vena cava directly to the right pulmonary artery.

Since the entire systemic and pulmonary blood flow is handled by the left ventricle, left ventricular failure is a frequent occurrence and has limited the success of shunting procedures. The Glenn procedure was designed to decrease the volume of blood pumped by the left ventricle, but it had limited success due to increasing pulmonary vascular resistance in the right lung and the development of pulmonary arteriovenous shunting.[93]

In 1971, Fontan and Baudet introduced a procedure designed to direct all systemic venous return either directly into the pulmonary artery or, in a modification in those with an adequate right ventricle with VSD, from right atrium to right ventricle.[94] The absolute prerequisite for this to be successful is a normal low pulmonary vascular resistance. This was accomplished with a valved Dacron shunt, and originally a valve was placed in the inferior vena cava.

Long-term follow-up in large numbers of patients with tricuspid atresia is not yet available, but recently Girod and associates[95] have published the largest follow-up on 32 patients with tricuspid atresia who have survived the Fontan procedure for at least 1 year. The mean follow-up period was 8.9 years (range, 7–16 years). At the time of surgery, the patients' ages ranged from 4 years to 36 years, and 20 had had previous systemic-to-pulmonary artery shunts. There were 5 late deaths, mostly associated with progressive obstruction of the conduit with or without an attempted reoperation. In spite of the problems of the 27 survivors, 26 are New York Heart Association Class I or II, and only one is Class III.

The problems that must be evaluated in these patients in the future are

1. Pulmonary artery obstruction remaining from the previous systemic-to-pulmonary artery shunt.
2. Progressive obstruction of the conduit. Originally this was a Dacron graft with a heterograft valve. Due to the development of the fibrin peel termed *neointima*, obstruction over the years has been frequent (6 of the 32 above-reported patients). To avoid this, aortic homografts have been used, as well as direct wide anastomoses between the right atrium and the pulmonary artery.
3. Atrial arrhythmias, including supraventricular tachycardia, atrial fibrillation and atrial flutter, have been seen. In some patients these are handled well hemodynamically; in others, the loss of atrial contraction has resulted in marked hemodynamic deterioration and death.
4. Residual left-to-right shunts, either through residual atrial defects or left ventricular to pulmonary artery residual flow. Alteration of technique will reduce these problems.
5. Cyanosis can be due to the above problem or result from the development of pulmonary arteriovenous fistulas and intrapulmonary shunting in about 25% of patients with the Glenn procedure and is also now seen with the passage of time in the Fontan procedure.[93] The exact reasons for these pulmonary arterial fistulas are unknown but may be related to the nonpulsatile flow, the known redistribution of blood flow to the lung bases versus the apices, or to other unknown factors.
6. Systemic venous congestion due to some increase in pulmonary vascular resistance or minimal obstruction of conduit. The long-term effect on hepatic function is unknown.
7. Mitral valve prolapse and mitral regurgitation.
8. Left ventricular dysfunction of unknown etiology.[96]

The ultimate problems when such patients enter adulthood are yet to be determined.

EBSTEIN'S ANOMALY

Ebstein's anomaly, characterized by the displacement of the attachment of the posterior or septal leaflet of the tricuspid valve into the right ventricle, results in a portion of the anatomical right ventricle lying above the tricuspid valve and becoming "atrialized." Frequently there are additional anomalies such as ASDs and atrioventricular bypass tracts, which are almost always right-sided. Occasionally, additional lesions are present, such as right ventricular outflow tract obstruction or patent ductus arteriosus. In those patients with ASD, a right-to-left shunt and cyanosis are common.

The disease is characterized by a high frequency of atrial arrhythmias, predominantly paroxysmal supraventricular tachycardia, but also atrial fibrillation and atrial flutter, and a lesser number of patients with paroxysmal ventricular tachycardia or ventricular fibrillation, probably arising from the abnormal right ventricle. Sudden death related to these arrhythmias is not unusual.

The natural course of patients with Ebstein's anomaly is variable, and prognosis does not depend on the degree of malformation of the right heart.[97] Kumar and associates[98] reported that, in the absence of associated defects other than ASD, 70% of infants with Ebstein's anomaly survived the first two years, and half survived to the age of 13. Patients surviving childhood can have a long, uncomplicated course, dying in old age, or can gradually decompensate, developing severe tricuspid regurgitation and congestive heart failure or progressive arrhythmias. Sudden death has been reported in up to 20% of patients, usually older children and adults.

Surgical correction is not usually necessary in the majority of patients with Ebstein's anomaly. Surgery is considered only when the patient has uncontrollable tachyarrhythmias or severe or progressive cyanosis or becomes functional New York Heart Association Class III or IV. The surgery usually is either tricuspid valvuloplasty or creation of a monocusp valve using the large anterior leaflet, usually with closure of the patent foramen ovale or ASD and plication or occasional excision of the atrialized portion of the right ventricle. If repair of the valve is not possible, tricuspid valve replacement has been performed.

In a report by Oh and colleagues,[99] valvuloplastic repair was possible in 42 (84%) of 50 patients. Only 8 patients required valve replacement with a bioprosthesis. If a bypass tract is identified, ablation is attempted, usually with identification of the site by intraoperative electrophysiologic mapping.

In a report of an international study by Watson[100] in 1974, the mortality rate for tricuspid valve replacement was 56% in patients under 15 years of age and 33% in patients over age 15. In later series, the perioperative mortality has been lower. Silver and associates[101] surveyed 13 reports in the literature in which 160 patients with Ebstein's anomaly survived surgery. The perioperative mortality in these patients was 11%. In a report by Oh of 50 patients with Ebstein's anomaly, there were 4 perioperative deaths (7%) and 3 late deaths.[99]

Late results of surgery in Ebstein's anomaly reveal improvement of functional classification in most. In Oh's series,[99] 88% were New York Heart Association functional Class II to IV preoperatively, and on follow-up of 1 month to 144 months (mean, 33 months) there were 3 deaths, all sudden. Of the remaining 41 patients, 11 (27%) continued to have symptomatic arrhythmias, and 30 had no symptoms. In the literature review by Silver and co-workers,[101] 87% were New York Heart Association functional Class III or IV preoperatively. Of the 78 patients where follow-up duration was reported, 43 (55%) had been followed up to 5 years, 18 (23%) 10 years, and 17 (22%) up to 15 or more years. Postoperative functional classification was reported in 94 patients, and 93 were in New York Heart Association functional Class I or II.

Patients at risk of late sudden death after surgery are not predictable from the functional classification or the types of arrhythmias that they had before surgery. In Oh's study,[99] of the 5 patients who died suddenly, 4 had had ventricular tachycardia or ventricular fibrillation perioperatively, suggesting ventricular arrhythmic instability. It is possible that electrophysiologic studies postoperatively will identify these patients.

CONCLUSION

Many obvious questions still remain regarding the course of patients who have congenital heart disease who have been operated on. The ability of the anatomical right ventricle to sustain a normal cardiac output against systemic vascular resistance so that the patient lives a normal life span is still uncertain. The effect of regression of right ventricular or left ventricular hypertrophy and the effect of residual fibrosis in these ventricles on the long-term contractility of the ventricle are still undetermined. The effect of atriotomy and ventriculotomy scar on the development of late arrhythmias, including conduction defects, is also still unknown.

The long-term durability of conduits and bioprosthetic valves is questionable (Figs. 98.5, 98.6). In 148 patients with right heart conduits inserted between 1971 and 1983, Jonas and co-workers[102] in 1985 reported 34 valve conduits requiring replacement, all for obstruction. The actuarial freedom from conduit replacement was 81% at 5 years, 61% at 7 years, and 0 at 10 years for valve conduits. Those with nonvalve conduits were 100% operation-free at 4 years.

It is clear that the natural course of the patient with congenital heart disease who has had surgical intervention is still being elucidated.

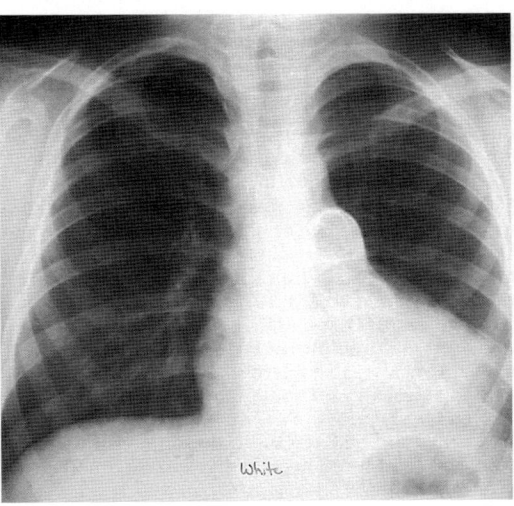

FIGURE 98.5 Chest roentgenogram, posteroanterior projection, in a 15-year-old boy with pulmonary atresia and an aortic homograft conduit from the right ventricle to the pulmonary artery. Note the calcification of the entire graft.

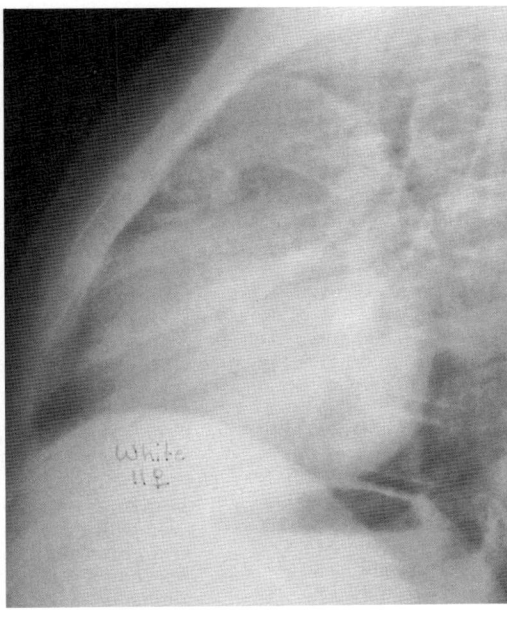

FIGURE 98.6 Chest roentgenogram, left lateral projection. Same patient as in Figure 98.5.

REFERENCES

1. Gross RE, Hubbard JP: Surgical ligation of a patent ductus arteriosus: Report of first successful case. JAMA 112:729, 1939
2. Gross RE, Hufnagel CA: Coarctation of the aorta: Experimental studies regarding its surgical correction. N Engl J Med 233:287, 1945
3. Crafoord C, Nylin G: Congenital coarctation of the aorta and its surgical treatment. J Thorac Surg 14:347, 1945
4. Blalock A, Taussig HB: The surgical treatment of malformations of the heart in which there is pulmonary stenosis or pulmonary atresia. JAMA 128:189, 1945
5. Brock RC: Pulmonary valvulotomy for the relief of congenital pulmonary stenosis: Report of three cases. Br Med J I(4562):1121, 1948
6. Gibbon JH Jr: Application of a mechanical heart and lung apparatus to cardiac surgery. Minn Med 37:171, 1974
7. Neill CA: Etiology of congenital heart disease. Cardiovasc Clin 4(3):137, 1972
8. Cheitlin MD: Congenital heart disease in the adult. Modern Concepts of Cardiovascular Disease 55:20, 1986
9. Hoffman JIE, Christianson R: Congenital heart disease in a cohort of 19,502 births with long-term follow-up. Am J Cardiol 42:641, 1978
10. McNamara DG, Latson LA: Long-term follow-up of patients with malformations for which definitive surgical repair has been available for 25 years or more. Am J Cardiol 50:560, 1982
11. Fisher RG, Moodie DS, Sterba R et al: Patent ductus stenosis in adults—Long-term follow-up: Nonsurgical versus surgical treatment. J Am Coll Cardiol 8:280, 1986
12. Jones JC: Twenty-five years' experience with the surgery of patent ductus arteriosus. J Thorac Cardiovasc Surg 50:149, 1965
13. Neutze JM: Follow up of high resistance patients after shunt surgery. NZ Med J (Cardiac Suppl) 64:37, 1965
14. Nasrallah AT, Hall RJ, Garcia E et al: Surgical repair of atrial septal defect in patients over 60 years of age. Circulation 53:329, 1976
15. Craig RJ, Selzer A: Natural history and prognosis of atrial septal defect. Circulation 37:805, 1968
16. St John Sutton MG, Tajik AJ, McGoon DC: Atrial septal defect in patients ages 60 years or older: Operative results and long-term postoperative follow-up. Circulation 64:402, 1981
17. Clark DS, Hirsch HD, Tamer DM et al: Electrocardiographic changes following surgical treatment of congenital cardiac malformations. Prog Cardiovasc Dis 17:451, 1975
18. Brandenburg RO Jr, Holmes DR Jr, Brandenburg RO, McGoon DC: Clinical follow-up study of paroxysmal supraventricular tachyarrhythmias after operative repair of a secundum type atrial septal defect in adults. Am J Cardiol 51:273, 1983
19. Bink-Boelkens MTE, Velvis H, Homan van der Heide JJ et al: Dysrhythmias after atrial surgery in children. Am Heart J 106:125, 1983
20. Gersony WM, Krongrad E: Evaluation and management of patients after surgical repair of congenital heart diseases. Prog Cardiovasc Dis 18:39, 1975
21. Young D: Later results of closure of secundum atrial septal defect in children. Am J Cardiol 31:14, 1973
22. Arnfred E: The significance of the radiological examination in evaluating the results of surgical treatment of atrial septal defects. J Cardiovasc Surg 8:230, 1967
23. Graham TP Jr, Cordell GD, Bender HW Jr: Ventricular function following surgery. In Kidd BSL, Rowe RD (eds): The Child With Congenital Heart Disease After Surgery, pp 277–293. Mount Kisco, NY, Futura, 1976
24. Liberthson RR, Boucher CA, Strauss HW et al: Right ventricular function in adult atrial septal defect: Preoperative and postoperative assessment and implications. Am J Cardiol 47:56, 1981
25. Epstein SE, Beiser GD, Goldstein RE et al: Hemodynamic abnormalities in response to mild and intensive upright exercise following operative correction of an atrial septal defect or tetralogy of Fallot. Circulation 47:1065, 1973
26. Morriss JH, McNamara DG: Residuae, sequelae, and complications of surgery for congenital heart disease. Prog Cardiovasc Dis 18:1, 1975
27. Keith JD: Ventricular septal defect. In Keith JD, Rowe RD, Vlad P (eds): Heart Disease in Infancy and Childhood, 3rd ed, pp 320–379. New York, Macmillan, 1978
28. Friedli B, Kidd BSL, Mustard WT, Keith JD: Ventricular septal defect with increased pulmonary vascular resistance: Late results of surgical closure. Am J Cardiol 33:403, 1974
29. DuShane JW, Krongrad E, Ritter DG et al: The fate of raised pulmonary vascular resistance after surgery in ventricular septal defect. In Kidd BSL, Rowe RD (eds): The Child With Congenital Heart Disease After Surgery, pp 299–312. Mount Kisco, NY, Futura, 1976
30. Subramanian S: Ventricular septal defect: Problem of repair in infancy. In Kidd BSL, Rowe RD (eds): The Child With Congenital Heart Disease After Surgery, pp 11–24. Mount Kisco, NY, Futura, 1976
31. Weidman WH, Blount SG, DuShane JW et al: Clinical course in ventricular septal defect. Circulation (Suppl I)56:I-56, 1977
32. Bharati S, Lev M: Sequelae of atriotomy and ventriculotomy on the endocardium, conduction system and coronary arteries. Am J Cardiol 50:580, 1982
33. Jarmakani JM, Graham TP Jr, Canent RV Jr et al: The effect of corrective surgery on left heart volume and mass in children with ventricular septal defect. Am J Cardiol 27:254, 1971
34. Cordell D, Graham TP Jr, Atwood GF et al: Left heart volume characteristics following ventricular septal defect closure in infancy. Circulation 54:294, 1976
35. Otterstad JE, Simonsen S, Erikssen J: Hemodynamic findings at rest and during mild supine exercise in adults with isolated, uncomplicated ventricular septal defects. Circulation 71:650, 1985
36. Jablonsky G, Hilton JD, Liu PP et al: Rest and exercise ventricular function in adults with congenital ventricular septal defects. Am J Cardiol 51:293, 1983
37. Glasser SP, Cheitlin MD, McCarty RJ et al: Thirty-two cases of interventricular septal defect and aortic insufficiency: Clinical, hemodynamic and surgical features. Am J Med 53:473, 1972
38. Nugent EW, Freedom RM, Nora JJ et al: Clinical course in pulmonary stenosis. Circulation (Suppl I)56:I-38, 1977
39. Pepine CJ, Gessner IH, Feldman RL: Percutaneous balloon valvuloplasty for pulmonic valve stenosis in the adult. Am J Cardiol 50:1442, 1982
40. Hsieh K-S, Keane JF, Nodas AS et al: Long-term follow-up of valvotomy before 1968 for congenital aortic stenosis. Am J Cardiol 58:338, 1986
41. Whitmer JT, James FW, Kaplan S et al: Exercise testing in children before and after surgical treatment of aortic stenosis. Circulation 63:254, 1981
42. Ashraf H, Cotroneo J, Dhar N et al: Long-term results after excision of fixed subaortic stenosis. J Thorac Cardiovasc Surg 90:864, 1985
43. Brown JW, Robison RJ, Waller BF: Transventricular balloon catheter aortic valvotomy in neonates. Ann Thorac Surg 39:376, 1985
44. Cheitlin MD, Robinowitz M, McAllister H et al: The distribution of fibrosis in the left ventricle in congenital aortic stenosis and coarctation of the aorta. Circulation 62:823, 1980
45. Maron BJ, Humphries JO, Rowe RD et al: Prognosis of surgically corrected coarctation of the aorta. A 20 year postoperative appraisal. Circulation 47:119, 1973
46. Clarkson PM, Nicholson MR, Barratt-Boyes BG et al: Results after repair of coarctation of the aorta beyond infancy: A 10 to 28 year follow-up with particular reference to late systemic hypertension. Am J Cardiol 51:1481, 1983
47. Nanton MA, Olley PM: Residual hypertension after coarctatectomy in children. Am J Cardiol 37:769, 1976
48. Menasche PH, Blondeau P, D'Allaines C et al: Resultats lointains de la correction chirugicale de la coarctation de l'aorte. Etude de 90 malades opérés depuis 1 á 15 ans. Arch Mal Coeur 71:181, 1978
49. Freed MD, Rocchini A, Rosenthal A et al: Exercise-induced hypertension after surgical repair of coarctation of the aorta. Am J Cardiol 43:253, 1979
50. Markel H, Rocchini AP, Beekman RH et al: Exercise-induced hypertension after repair of coarctation of the aorta: Arm versus leg exercise. J Am Coll Cardiol 8:165, 1986
51. Shearer WT, Rutman JY, Weinberg WA et al: Coarctation of the aorta and cerebrovascular accident: A proposal for early corrective surgery. J Pediatr 77:1004, 1970
52. Schneeweiss A, Sherf L, Lehrer E et al: Segmental study of the terminal coronary vessels in coarctation of the aorta: A natural model for study of the effect of coronary hypertension on human coronary circulation. Am J Cardiol 49:1996, 1982
53. Kimball BP, Shurvell BL, Mildenberger RR et al: Abnormal thallium kinetics in postoperative coarctation of the aorta: Evidence for diffuse hypertension-induced vascular pathology. J Am Coll Cardiol 7:538, 1986
54. Clarkson PM, Brandt PWT, Barratt-Boyes BG et al: Prosthetic repair of coarctation of the aorta with particular reference to Dacron onlay patch grafts and late aneurysm formation. Am J Cardiol 56:342, 1985
55. Ala-Kulju K, Järvinen A, Maamies T et al: Late aneurysms after patch aortoplasty for coarctation of the aorta in adults. Thorac Cardiovasc Surg 31:301, 1983
56. Presbitero P, D'Antonio P, Brusca A et al: Prognosis of Fallot's tetralogy after palliative operations: 10–25 years follow-up. Pediatr Cardiol 4:175, 1983
57. Bertranou EG, Blackstone EH, Hazelrig JB et al: Life expectancy without surgery in tetralogy of Fallot. Am J Cardiol 42:458, 1978
58. Horowitz LN, Simson MB, Spear JF et al: The mechanism of apparent right bundle branch block after transatrial repair of tetralogy of Fallot. Circulation 59:1241, 1979
59. Neches WH, Park SC, Mathews RA et al: Tetralogy of Fallot: Postoperative electrophysiologic studies. Circulation 56:713, 1977
60. Joransen JA, Lucas RV Jr, Moller JH: Postoperative haemodynamics in tetralogy of Fallot. A study of 132 children. Br Heart J 41:33, 1979
61. Wessel HU, Cunningham WJ, Paul MH et al: Exercise performance in tetralogy of Fallot after intracardiac repair. J Thorac Cardiovasc Surg 80:582, 1980
62. Reybrouck T, Weymans M, Stijns H et al: Exercise testing after correction of tetralogy of Fallot: The fallacy of a reduced heart rate response. Am Heart J 112:998, 1986
63. Jarmakani JM, Graham TP Jr, Canent RV et al: Left heart function in children with tetralogy of Fallot before and after palliative or corrective surgery. Circulation 46:478, 1972
64. Rocchini AP, Keane JF, Freed MD et al: Left ventricular function following attempted surgical repair of tetralogy of Fallot. Circulation 57:798, 1978
65. Rosing DR, Borer JS, Kent KM et al: Long-term hemodynamic and electrocardiographic assessment following operative repair of tetralogy of Fallot.

66. Reduto LA, Berger HJ, Johnstone DE et al: Radionuclide assessment of right and left ventricular exercise reserve after total correction of tetralogy of Fallot. Am J Cardiol 45:1013, 1980
67. Graham TP Jr, Cordell D, Atwood GF et al: Right ventricular volume characteristics before and after palliative and reparative operation in tetralogy of Fallot. Circulation 54:417, 1976
68. Borow KM, Green LH, Castaneda AR et al: Left ventricular function after repair of tetralogy of Fallot and its relationship to age at surgery. Circulation 61:1150, 1980
69. James FW, Kaplan S, Schwartz DC et al: Response to exercise in patients after total surgical correction of tetralogy of Fallot. Circulation 54:671, 1976
70. Garson A Jr, Gillette PC, Gutgesell HP et al: Stress-induced ventricular arrhythmia after repair of tetralogy of Fallot. Am J Cardiol 46:1006, 1980
71. Burns RJ, Liu PP, Druck MN et al: Analysis of adults with and without complex ventricular arrhythmias after repair of tetralogy of Fallot. J Am Coll Cardiol 4:226, 1984
72. Garson A Jr, Nihill MR, McNamara DG et al: Status of the adult and adolescent after repair of tetralogy of Fallot. Circulation 59:1232, 1979
73. Garson A Jr, Randall DC, Gillette PC et al: Prevention of sudden death after repair of tetralogy of Fallot: Treatment of ventricular arrhythmias. J Am Coll Cardiol 6:221, 1985
74. Hu DCK, Seward JB, Puga FJ et al: Total correction of tetralogy of Fallot at age 40 years and older: Long-term follow-up. J Am Coll Cardiol 5:40, 1985
75. Senning Å: Surgical correction of transposition of the great vessels. Surgery 45:966, 1959
76. Mustard WT, Keith JD, Trusler GA et al: The surgical management of transposition of the great vessels. J Thorac Cardiovasc Surg 48:953, 1964
77. Jatene AD, Fontes VF, Paulista PP et al: Anatomic correction of transposition of the great vessels. J Thorac Cardiovasc Surg 72:364, 1976
78. Smallhorn JF, Gow R, Freedom RM et al: Pulsed Doppler echocardiographic assessment of the pulmonary venous pathway after the Mustard or Senning procedure for transposition of the great arteries. Circulation 73:765, 1986
79. Hagler DJ, Ritter DG, Mair DD et al: Right and left ventricular function after the Mustard procedure in transposition of the great arteries. Am J Cardiol 44:276, 1979
80. Flinn CJ, Wolff GS, Dick M II et al: Cardiac rhythm after the Mustard operation for complete transposition of the great arteries. N Engl J Med 310:1635, 1984
81. George BL, Laks H, Klitzner TS et al: Results of the Senning procedure in infants with simple and complex transposition of the great arteries. Am J Cardiol 59:426, 1987
82. Byrum CJ, Bove EL, Sondheimer HM et al: Hemodynamic and electrophysiologic results of the Senning procedure for transposition of the great arteries. Am J Cardiol 58:138, 1986
83. Hayes CJ, Gersony WM: Arrhythmias after the Mustard operation for transposition of the great arteries: A long-term study. J Am Coll Cardiol 7:133, 1986
84. Graham TP Jr, Atwood GF, Boucek RJ Jr et al: Abnormalities of right ventricular function following Mustard's operation for transposition of the great arteries. Circulation 52:678, 1975
85. Benson IN, Bonet J, McLaughlin P et al: Assessment of right ventricular function during supine bicycle exercise after Mustard's operation. Circulation 65:1052, 1982
86. Hurwitz RA, Caldwell RL, Girod DA et al: Ventricular function in transposition of the great arteries: Evaluation by radionuclide angiocardiography. Am Heart J 110:600, 1985
87. Mathews RA, Fricker FJ, Beerman LB et al: Exercise studies after the Mustard operation in transposition of the great arteries. Am J Cardiol 51:1526, 1983
88. Castaneda AR, Norwood WI, Jonas RA et al: Transposition of the great arteries and intact ventricular septum: Anatomical repair in the neonate. Ann Thorac Surg 38:438, 1984
89. Lange PE, Sievers HH, Onnasch DGW et al: Up to 7 years of follow-up after two-stage anatomic correction of simple transposition of the great arteries. Circulation (Suppl I)74:I-47, 1986
90. Bical O, Hazan E, Lecompte Y et al: Anatomic correction of transposition of the great arteries associated with ventricular septal defect: Midterm results in 50 patients. Circulation 70:891, 1984
91. Borow KM, Arensman FW, Webb C et al: Assessment of left ventricular contractile state after anatomic correction of transposition of the great arteries. Circulation 69:106, 1984
92. Martin RP, Radley-Smith R, Yacoub MH: Arrhythmias before and after anatomic correction of transposition of the great arteries. J Am Coll Cardiol 10:200, 1987
93. Cloutier A, Ash JM, Smallhorn JF et al: Abnormal distribution of pulmonary blood flow after the Glenn shunt or Fontan procedure: Risk of development of arteriovenous fistulae. Circulation 72:471, 1985
94. Fontan F, Baudet E: Surgical repair of tricuspid atresia. Thorax 26:240, 1971
95. Girod DA, Fontan F, Deville C et al: Long-term results after the Fontan operation for tricuspid atresia. Circulation 75:605, 1987
96. Graham TP Jr, Franklin RCG, Wyse RKH et al: Left ventricular wall stress and contractile function in childhood: Normal value and comparison of Fontan repair versus palliation only in patients with tricuspid atresia. Circulation (Suppl I)74:I-61, 1986
97. Nihoyannopoulos P, McKenna WJ, Smith G et al: Echocardiographic assessment of the right ventricle in Ebstein's anomaly: Relation to clinical outcome. J Am Coll Cardiol 8:627, 1986
98. Kumar AE, Fyler DC, Miettinen OS et al: Ebstein's anomaly: Clinical profile and natural history. Am J Cardiol 28:84, 1971
99. Oh JK, Holmes DR Jr, Hayes DL et al: Cardiac arrhythmias in patients with surgical repair of Ebstein's anomaly. J Am Coll Cardiol 6:1351, 1985
100. Watson H: Natural history of Ebstein's anomaly of tricuspid valve in childhood and adolescence. An international co-operative study of 505 cases. Br Heart J 36:417, 1974
101. Silver MA, Cohen SR, McIntosh CL et al: Late (5 to 132 months) clinical and hemodynamic results after either tricuspid valve replacement or anuloplasty for Ebstein's anomaly of the tricuspid valve. Am J Cardiol 54:627, 1984
102. Jonas RA, Freed MD, Mayer JE Jr et al: Long-term follow-up of patients with synthetic right heart conduits. Circulation (Suppl II)72:II-77, 1985

CORONARY ARTERIAL ANOMALIES

Melvin D. Cheitlin

Coronary arterial origin and distribution have a wide range of variability considered to be within normal limits. For instance, the posteroinferior aspect of the left ventricle is supplied primarily by the right coronary artery (right dominant distribution) in about 75% to 80% of human hearts, by the left circumflex system (left dominant distribution) in about 10% to 15%, and by branches of both the right coronary artery and left circumflex system (balanced distribution) in about 5% to 10%.[1] The origin of the right conal artery is usually from the proximal right coronary artery but in 20% to 50% of hearts can arise from a separate ostium. There are also variations in the number and distribution of obtuse marginal vessels and septal perforating vessels. These variations are so common as to be considered normal. When the origin or distribution of the coronary arteries markedly differs from this normal range, it is considered to be a coronary artery anomaly.

The exact incidence of coronary anomalies in the population is unknown. Many coronary anomalies produce no hemodynamically significant problems and have been called "minor" anomalies. These are frequently overlooked in a routine autopsy done on a patient who has died of unrelated causes. They also frequently cause no physical signs or changes in routine laboratory studies such as chest roentgenogram, electrocardiogram, or echocardiogram. The information on frequency of coronary artery anomalies comes from autopsy series such as that reported in 1956 by Alexander and Griffith, who found 54 cases of coronary anomalies in 18,950 autopsies (0.3%).[2] There are also clinical series reported that are obviously weighted toward anomalies with pathophysiologic significance and coronary arteriographic series that are weighted toward anomalies resulting in clinical symptoms such as angina pectoris or physical findings such as murmurs.

In a series of all stillborns and children up to 15 years of age autopsied in a given area of Czechoslovakia with a population of 1,220,000, there were 3969 stillborn children, with 81 (2.1%) having a congenital heart defect, and 470,188 live-born children, with 1008 (0.21%) having a congenital heart defect. There were congenital heart defects found in 6.2% of all autopsied children, and of 1090 with congenital heart defects, 0.6% had a coronary artery anomaly.[3]

In the coronary arteriographic literature, the incidence of coronary anomalies varies from 0.6% to 1.55% of all patients catheterized. The largest series, reported by Hobbs and associates,[4] comes from the Cleveland Clinic and consisted of 38,703 coronary arteriographies between 1972 and 1978, with 601 patients (1.55%) having coronary anomalies; of these, 523 (87%) were anomalies of origin and distribution, and 78 (13%) were coronary arterial fistulas. Baltaxe and Wixson[5] reported 1000 consecutive coronary angiograms in patients with angina pectoris and found nine congenital coronary anomalies (0.9%). In a paper reporting coronary arteriography in 120 consecutive patients 35 years of age or younger who had suffered a myocardial infarction, five (4%) had major coronary anomalies.[6]

The rarity of coronary artery anomalies does not negate their importance. Cardiologists must be aware of the possibility of coronary anomalies in the differential diagnosis of angina pectoris, myocardial infarction, cardiac syncope, or sudden death in a young person. Coronary anomalies are important in the differential diagnosis of the continuous murmur. During coronary arteriography, the possibility of coronary anomaly arises when a myocardial territory is not supplied by any visualized coronary vessel. When there is complete absence of the left anterior descending or left circumflex coronary arteries, although complete obstruction is a possibility, the question should always be raised of the possibility of a coronary artery arising anomalously from the aorta, and a separate origin of the vessel should be sought. Cusp injection or power aortic root injection can be used to detect the origin of the anomalous coronary artery.

To the cardiovascular surgeon, the presence of a coronary anomaly is important even if the coronary anomaly is not the reason for the cardiac surgery. The classic illustration of this is the origin of the left anterior descending coronary from the right coronary artery with passage across the anterior wall of the right ventricular outflow tract. With a right ventriculotomy, severing of the left anterior descending coronary artery may occur and most often leads to death of the patient or, at the very least, a large anterior wall myocardial infarction. Of obvious importance is the high takeoff of the coronary artery from the ascending aorta above the level of the aortic ring. Low cross-clamping of the aorta or a low aortotomy for aortic valve replacement can be disastrous in these cases. Also, failure to perfuse the separate orifice of the left anterior descending coronary artery can cause disastrous myocardial damage during bypass surgery. The anomalous origin of the left circumflex artery from the right sinus of Valsalva with passage posterior to the aorta, if not recognized, can result in accidental ligation of the circumflex coronary artery with myocardial infarction during valve replacement.

Ogden classified coronary anomalies according to his understanding of their clinicopathologic significance into the following[7]:

1. Minor coronary variations, including most of the abnormalities of origin from the aorta
2. Major distribution coronary anomalies, including coronary arterial fistulas and origin of the coronary anomaly from the pulmonary artery
3. Secondary coronary anomalies, including variations seen in tetralogy of Fallot, transposition, corrected transposition, truncus arter-

TABLE 99.1 CLASSIFICATION OF CORONARY ARTERIAL ANOMALIES

Class	Anomalies
I	Anomalies of origin or distribution
II	Abnormal communications between coronary arteries and cardiac chambers (coronary arteriovenous or coronary-cameral fistulas) or coronary great vessel fistulas
III	Coronary artery hypoplasia or atresia
IV	Coronary artery aneurysms
V	Coronary arterial variations secondary to a primary intracardiac defect

(Adapted from Hobbs RJ, Millit HD, Raghavan PV et al: Congenital coronary anomalies: Clinical and therapeutic implications. Cardiovasc Clin 12:43, 1982)

iosus, and pulmonary atresia as well as dysplasia of the coronary artery seen in supravalvular aortic stenosis and coronary arterial fistulas.

A classification of coronary anomalies is presented in Table 99.1.

ANOMALIES OF ORIGIN OR DISTRIBUTION OF THE CORONARY ARTERY (FIGS. 99.1, 99.2)

The coronary ostial buds form about the seventh month of gestation, shortly after conotruncal partitioning. Most aberrant vessels can be explained by various patterns of abnormal persistence and eradication of these angioblastic aortic buds.[8] Because the arterial distribution on the epicardial surface of the ventricle is dependent on the position of the ventricular chambers, many coronary anomalies with ectopic origins have normal coronary distributions on the surface of the ventricle.

The pathophysiologic significance of anomalously originating vessels depends on whether coronary blood flow can increase in response to myocardial oxygen demand. If it can, the anomaly is "minor" and without clinical significance. If for any reason it cannot (e.g., owing to obstruction because of its origin or course or to low perfusion pressure due to origin from the pulmonary arterial bed or obstruction due to hypoplasia), then myocardial ischemia and angina pectoris or myocardial infarction, arrhythmias, and sudden death can result. In Ogden's classification these abnormalities of origin and distribution from the aorta were all considered to be without significance to blood flow and benign and, therefore, minor anomalies.

ECTOPIC ORIGIN FROM AORTIC SINUS

ECTOPIC ORIGIN OF LEFT MAIN CORONARY ARTERY FROM RIGHT SINUS OF VALSALVA OR RIGHT CORONARY ARTERY (SINGLE CORONARY ARTERY WITH RIGHT CORONARY ARTERY DISTRIBUTION)

In Hobbs's series, ecotopic origin of the left main coronary artery from the right sinus of Valsalva or the right coronary artery constituted 0.02% of the 38,703 coronary arteriographic studies on patients and 1.5% of the coronary anomalies; it is a rare lesion. In this lesion there are four patterns of coronary distribution (see Fig. 99.1, A):

1. The left main coronary artery passes obliquely posteriorly behind the right ventricular outflow tract to the position where the normally arising left main artery divides into the left anterior descending artery and the left circumflex artery.
2. The left main coronary artery passes anteriorly over the right ventricular outflow tract to the interventricular groove, where it divides into the left anterior descending and left circumflex coronary arter-

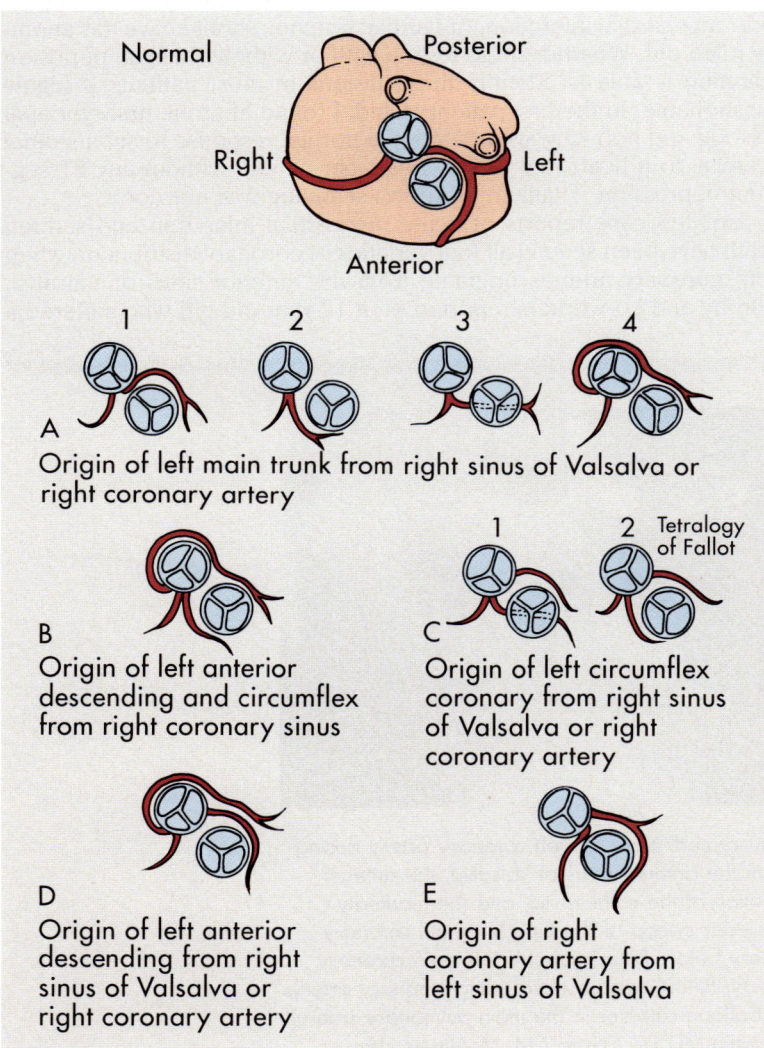

FIGURE 99.1 The coronary arterial anomalies of ectopic origin from the aortic sinus. See text for discussion.

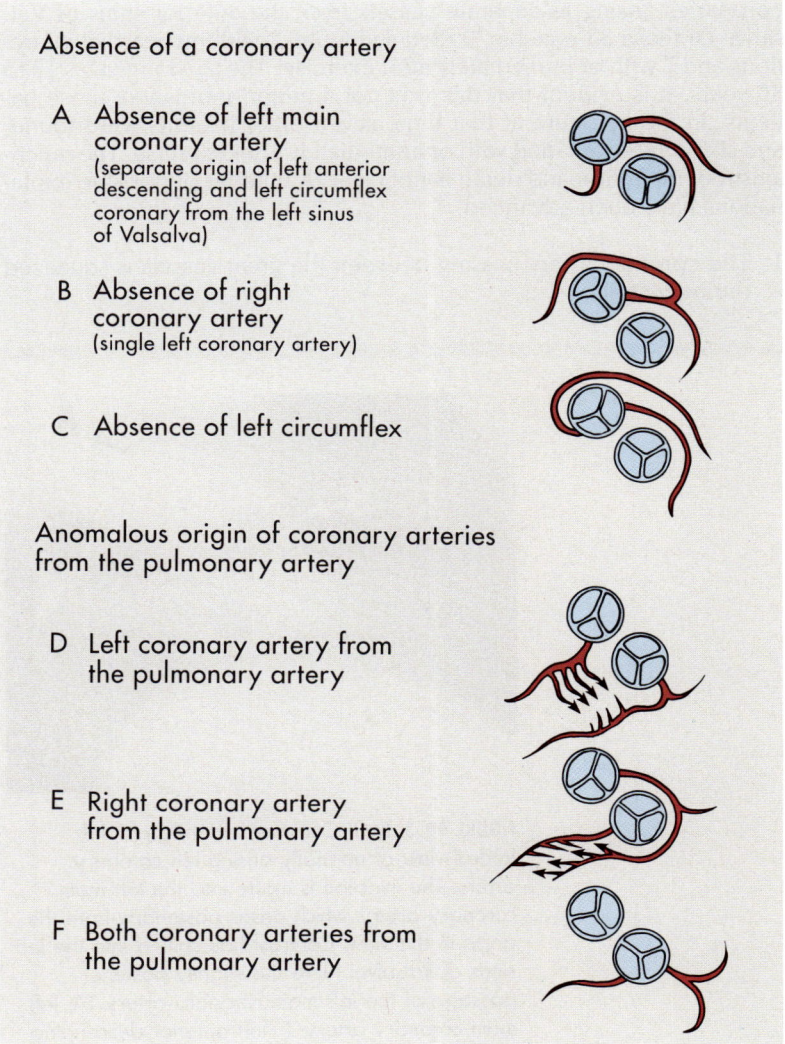

FIGURE 99.2 The coronary arterial anomalies of absence of a coronary artery and of anomalous origin of coronary arteries from the pulmonary artery. See text for discussion.

ies. The left circumflex passes posteriorly to the atrioventricular (AV) groove.
3. The left main coronary artery passes intramurally through the subendocardial region of the crista supraventricularis and then surfaces in the proximal interventricular sulcus, dividing into the left anterior descending coronary and the circumflex coronary arteries.
4. The left main coronary artery arises to the right of the right coronary artery and passes posteriorly around the aorta to the left, where it divides into the left anterior descending and left circumflex coronary arteries.

Ishikawa and Brandt recently reported the angiographic definition of the four anomalous courses taken by the left main coronary artery arising from the anterior sinus of Valsalva, usually in the right anterior oblique and left anterior oblique views.[9] A caudal anterior loop indicates a septal course with the left main coronary artery passing intramyocardially and running along the crista supraventricularis; a cranial posterior loop is seen when the left main coronary artery passes to the left and posteriorly behind the right ventricular outflow tract; a cranial anterior loop is seen when the left main coronary artery passes anteriorly over the right ventricular outflow tract; and a caudal posterior loop is seen when the left main coronary artery passes to the right behind the aorta.

In an autopsy study from the Armed Forces Institute of Pathology in 1974, 33 instances of the left main coronary artery arising from the anterior sinus of Valsalva were found (Fig. 99.3).[10] There were 14 instances of both arteries arising as a single vessel (single coronary artery of the right coronary distribution) and 19 instances of the right and left coronaries arising as separate vessels from the anterior sinus of Valsalva. Of these 33 patients, 9 died suddenly: 2 with myocardial infarctions and 7 with or immediately after exercise. The age range was 13 to 36 years. It is evident that this was not a minor anomaly in these patients. In the literature at that time, seven other patients were found, and six of the seven died with or immediately after exercise. The mechanism of infarction and death is not clear. A number of possible explanations have been advanced:

1. The coronary artery passing between the great vessels is squeezed during systole.
2. The coronary artery is kinked during systole.
3. The oblique takeoff of the vessel causes a slitlike orifice capable of collapsing in a valvelike fashion with activity and an increase in size of the aorta and pulmonary artery (Fig. 99.4).
4. Coronary spasm occurs.
5. The left anterior descending and circumflex arteries appear to be smaller than normal in these patients, and perhaps these smaller arteries are incapable of increasing myocardial blood flow in response to increases in demand.

Of these explanations, it is unlikely that the low-pressure pulmonary artery can compress the left coronary vessel distended by systemic pressure, but kinking is possible. Also, some of these coronary arteries pass intramurally posteriorly so that the origin and initial portion of the coronary vessel is in the wall of the aorta, presumably subjected to compression with exercise. At postmortem examination, the orifice of the ectopically arising coronary artery is slitlike, with the common wall of the coronary artery and aorta acting as a flap that can close with stretching of the artery on expansion of the aorta (Fig. 99.5). This seems to be the most likely explanation for sudden calamitous ischemia. Bloomfield and associates have reported systolic compression by angiography in the right coronary artery arising from the left sinus of Valsalva as it passes behind the right ventricular outflow tract.[11] The possibility of coronary spasm has not been ruled out in these patients.

Whatever the mechanism, cardiac syncope, sudden death, angina pectoris, and massive myocardial infarction have all been seen in this anomaly. For this reason, any child or young person with angina pectoris, myocardial infarction, or cardiac syncope should have this anomaly ruled out. Whether stress testing with or without thallium perfusion scanning is able to identify these lesions in most patients is highly questionable. In the first patient tested, I found after the first syncopal episode and non–Q wave infarction a normal response to submaximal exercise to a heart rate of 150 beats per minute without any ST segment depression. Thallium perfusion scanning was not done.

Isolated case reports of acute myocardial infarction and sudden death have been seen in all four varieties of coronary distribution when both coronary arteries originate from the anterior sinus of Valsalva. Murphy and co-workers reported on a 12-year-old girl who suffered a

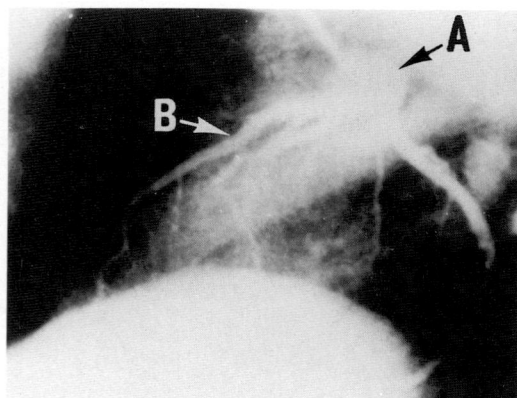 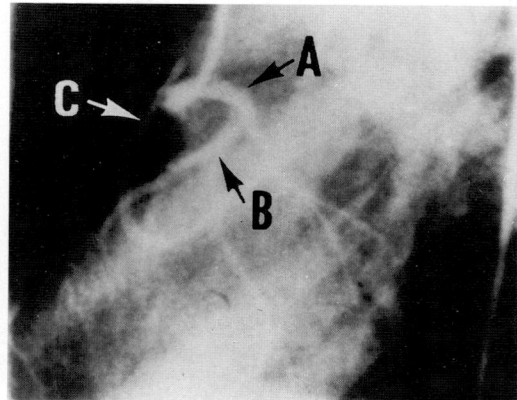

FIGURE 99.3 (Left) Coronary arteriogram, left lateral view of normally arising left coronary artery. The injection is made into the left main coronary artery, which arises posteriorly from the aorta in this view. Contrast has spilled into the left sinus of Valsalva. Note the slightly posterior passage of the left main coronary artery. (A, left main coronary artery; B, left anterior descending coronary artery) (Right) Coronary arteriogram, left lateral view of injection into the left main coronary artery. The patient is a 15-year-old boy who suffered a sudden cardiac arrest and was resuscitated. Note the left coronary artery arising from the anterior sinus of Valsalva, the anterior position of the catheter tip, and the markedly posterior sweep of the long left main coronary artery before bifurcation. (A, left main coronary artery; B, left anterior descending coronary artery; C, balloon catheter in the main pulmonary artery) (Cheitlin MD, De Castro CM, McAllister HA: Sudden death as a complication of anomalous left coronary origin from the anterior sinus of Valsalva. Circulation 50:780, 1974. Used by permission of the American Heart Association, Inc)

myocardial infarction and on coronary arteriography had an anomalous left coronary artery that passed posterior to the aorta with systolic compression of the vessel as it passed in this anomalous course.[12] I have recently seen a patient with exertional angina pectoris and syncope who had a thallium defect at the apex, a markedly abnormal stress test with deep ST segment depression, and the left main coronary artery passing anterior to the right ventricular outflow tract (Figs. 99.6, 99.7). Following bypass surgery, there is no longer a thallium defect. It is, therefore, possible that all of the abnormal distributions can be associated with sudden catastrophic myocardial ischemia.

Echocardiography with special attention paid to the origin of coronary vessels from the aorta may be most helpful as a noninvasive test in detecting this lesion, whereas stress testing may be negative. The use of thallium testing in these patients has not been well investigated. Liberthson recently reported a 54-year-old woman with angina pectoris at rest with a diagnosis of ectopic origin of the left coronary artery from the proximal right coronary artery suggested by two-dimensional echocardiography who had an abnormal pacing stress test and anterolateral perfusion thallium defect with redistribution at rest.[13] Bypass surgery resulted in a reversal of the ischemic studies and the relief of signs and symptoms. Whenever the diagnosis is suspected, coronary angiography is the only certain way to rule out this potentially fatal anomaly.

With discovery of this anomaly, when there is no other explanation for the clinical evidence of ischemia, it is recommended that surgery be performed. There have been reports of a few patients who have undergone such operations. Davia and associates reported a patient who had the valvelike common wall between the coronary artery and the heart removed, leaving the patient with a funnel-like opening into the left and right coronary artery. An 8-year follow-up reported the patient to be asymptomatic.[14] Coronary vein bypass grafting has also been performed in these patients.[15] Because most of the patients with this anomaly and myocardial ischemia or sudden death have been in the second and the third decades of life, the presence of the anomaly alone is sufficient evidence to explain symptoms. In older patients in whom this anomaly is found together with coronary artery disease, the patient's symptoms may be due to the coronary artery disease rather than to the anomaly, and his care should proceed on this basis.

ECTOPIC ORIGIN OF LEFT ANTERIOR DESCENDING ARTERY FROM RIGHT SINUS OF VALSALVA

Although ectopic origin of the left anterior descending artery from the right sinus of Valsalva (see Fig. 99.1, C) occurs as an isolated finding, it is distinctly rare. In Hobbs's series this was found in 0.03% of patients and 2.2% of coronary anomalies.[4] Dalal and colleagues, in 8000 arte-

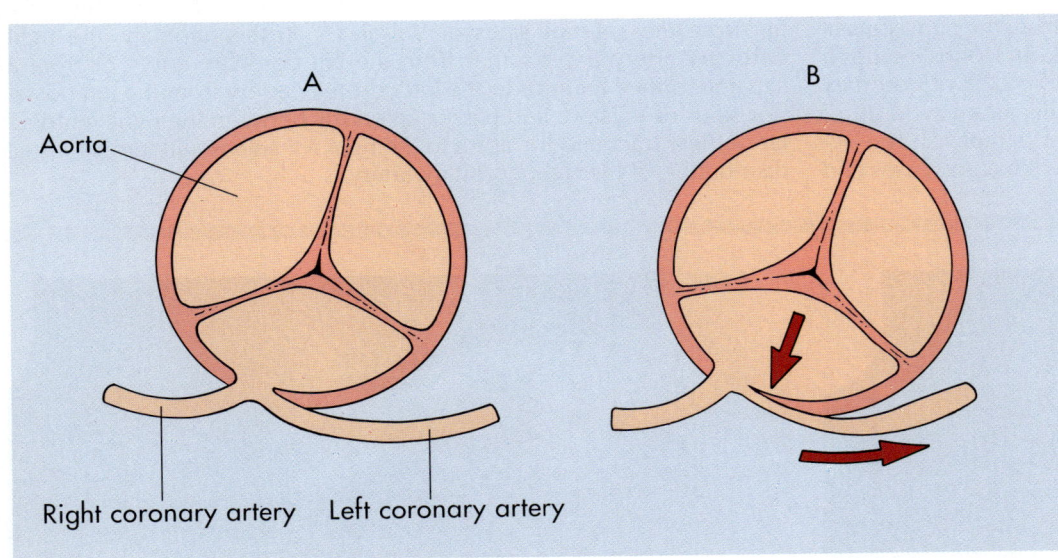

FIGURE 99.4 A. Diagram of cross section of aortic root at the level of the coronary ostia in a patient with the left coronary artery arising from the anterior sinus of Valsalva. B. Proposed mechanism of the ostial closure with expansion of the aorta and pull on the left coronary artery. Note the postulated flaplike closure of the ostium by the coronary arterial wall. Arrow is sinus and suggests outward force causing flaplike closure of ostium; arrow along left coronary artery suggests pulling force possibly causing collapse of orifice. (Modified from Cheitlin MD, De Castro CM, McAllister HA: Sudden death as a complication of anomalous left coronary origin from the anterior sinus of Valsalva. Circulation 50:780, 1974. Used by permission of the American Heart Association, Inc)

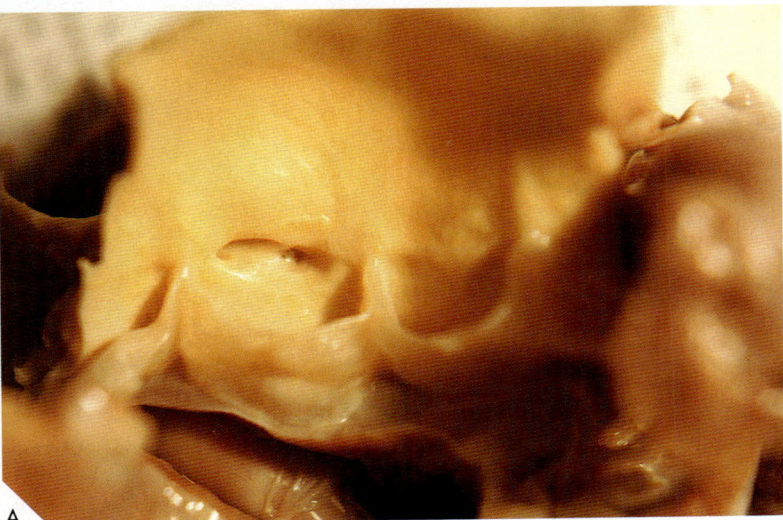

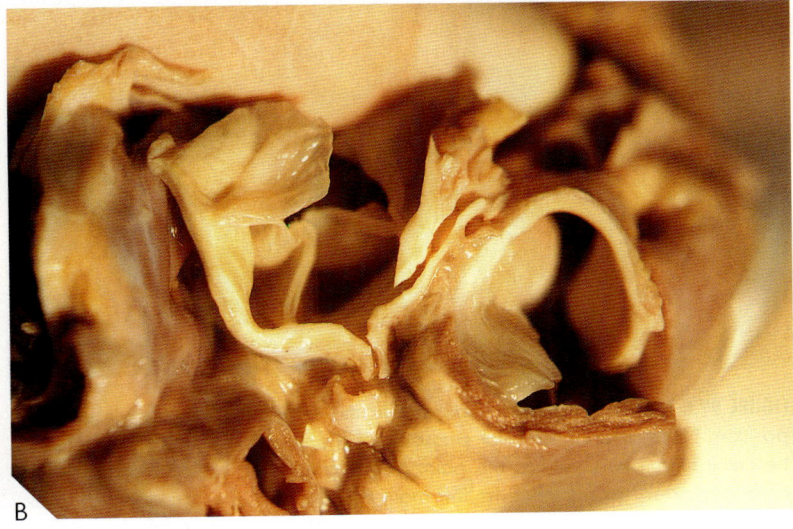

FIGURE 99.5 A. Aortic root showing anterior sinus of Valsalva with both right and left coronary ostia. The right coronary appears as a black dot to the right of the obliquely arising left coronary artery. B. Same specimen as in part A. Aortic and pulmonary arteries cut transversely at the level of the coronary ostia. Note the anterior take-off of the right coronary artery perpendicular to the aortic wall and the obliquely posterior take-off of the left coronary artery as it passes posterior to the right ventricular outflow tract.

riograms, reported a single instance of this anomaly in a 52-year-old man with coronary atherosclerosis in his circumflex and right coronary arteries.[16] Engle and colleagues, in 4250 coronary arteriographic patients, found three cases of left anterior descending artery originating from the right coronary artery as the only anomaly.[17] Ogden, in his review of 224 cases of coronary artery anomalies, documented ten cases, six arising from the right coronary artery and four from the right sinus of Valsalva.[7] No case of this anomaly has been reported to cause symptoms.

This anomaly occurs in as many as 6% of patients with tetralogy of Fallot.[18] In a review of the literature, McManus and colleagues reported a total of 3204 patients with tetralogy of Fallot at surgery, at angiography, and at postmortem examination with 106 (3%) having coronary anomalies.[19] The most frequent coronary anomaly was left anterior descending artery arising from the right coronary artery (81 of 106 coronary anomalies). There were also 19 single right and left coronary arteries. The major danger in this anomaly is the inadvertent sectioning of the left anterior descending coronary artery during the right ventriculotomy.[20] Because of the increased incidence of coronary anomalies among these patients, special attention must be given to identifying this problem preoperatively by coronary angiography.

ECTOPIC ORIGIN OF LEFT CIRCUMFLEX CORONARY ARTERY FROM RIGHT SINUS OF VALSALVA OR RIGHT CORONARY ARTERY

Probably the most common congenital coronary artery anomaly is ectopic origin of the left circumflex coronary artery from the right sinus of Valsalva or right coronary artery (see Fig. 99.1, D). In Hobbs's series it occurred in 0.45% of all patients and constituted 29.2% of coronary artery anomalies.[4] Page and co-workers found this anomaly in 20 of 2996 patients (0.67%) undergoing coronary arteriography.[21] The ectopic vessel arises from the right sinus of Valsalva in half the cases and from the right coronary artery in the other half. The circumflex artery always passes posteriorly around the aorta in arriving at its usual position in the anterior atrioventricular sulcus to distribute to the usual circumflex territory (Fig. 99.8). Page and associates decribed a helpful finding in raising suspicion of this anomaly in the right anterior oblique ventriculogram: that of the opacification of the circumflex artery in profile behind the aortic root as it passes posteriorly (Fig. 99.9).[21] This is confirmed when, with injection of contrast agent into the left main coronary artery, only the distribution of the left anterior descending coronary is seen. In Page's patients all had coronary obstructive disease to explain their angina pectoris or myocardial infarction. Sudden death[22] and myocardial infarction[23] in the distribution of the anomalous left circumflex coronary artery, which was widely patent, has been reported so that myocardial ischemia can be related to this coronary anomaly as well. With mitral valve replacement, inadvertent occlusion of this anomalous artery by suture has occurred, resulting in a posteroinferior myocardial infarction.[24]

ECTOPIC ORIGIN OF RIGHT CORONARY ARTERY FROM LEFT SINUS OF VALSALVA

In Hobbs's series, ectopic origin of the right coronary artery from the left sinus of Valsalva (see Fig. 99.1, E) occurred in 0.13% of patients and accounted for 8.3% of all coronary anomalies.[4] In our series with associates from the Armed Forces Institute of Pathology, we found 18 patients with this anomaly without coronary obstructive disease at the same time that we found 33 patients with the left coronary artery arising from the anterior sinus of Valsalva.[10] In this anomaly, the right coronary artery arises either from the left coronary artery or from a separate orifice anterior to the left coronary artery from the left posterior sinus of Valsalva and passes anteriorly between the right ventricular outflow tract and the aorta to the right AV sulcus and into the usual distribution of the right coronary artery.

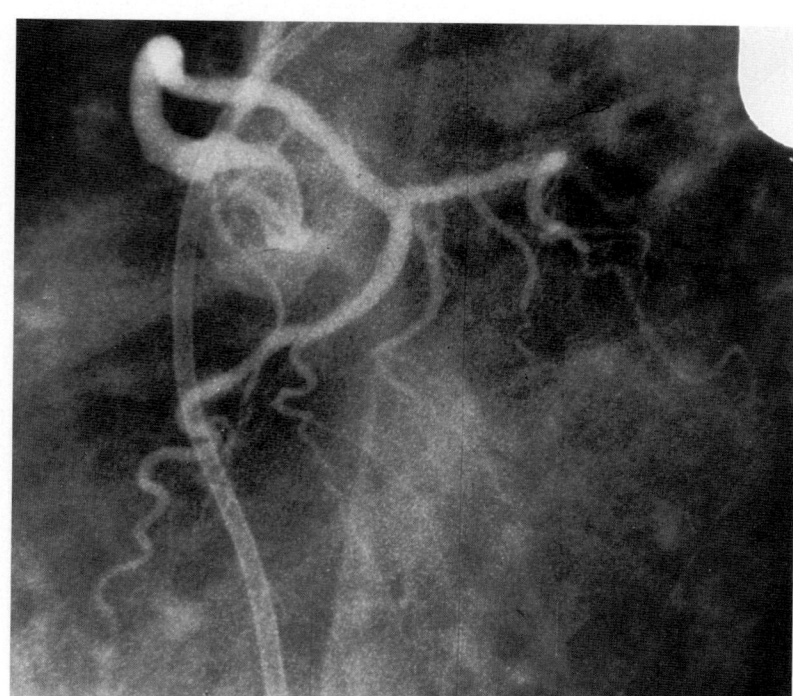

FIGURE 99.6 Coronary arteriogram, cine-frame, high left anterior oblique position. Note anterior superior passage of the very long left coronary artery before it turns posteriorly to the point of bifurcation. Note that a septal coronary artery arises from the left main coronary artery. The artery passes from the anterior sinus of Valsalva anteriorly over the right ventricular outflow tract before bifurcating. The patient had angina pectoris, and an anterior apical perfusion defect was found by thallium perfusion scintigraphy. The second catheter is through the right ventricular outflow tract into the main pulmonary artery.

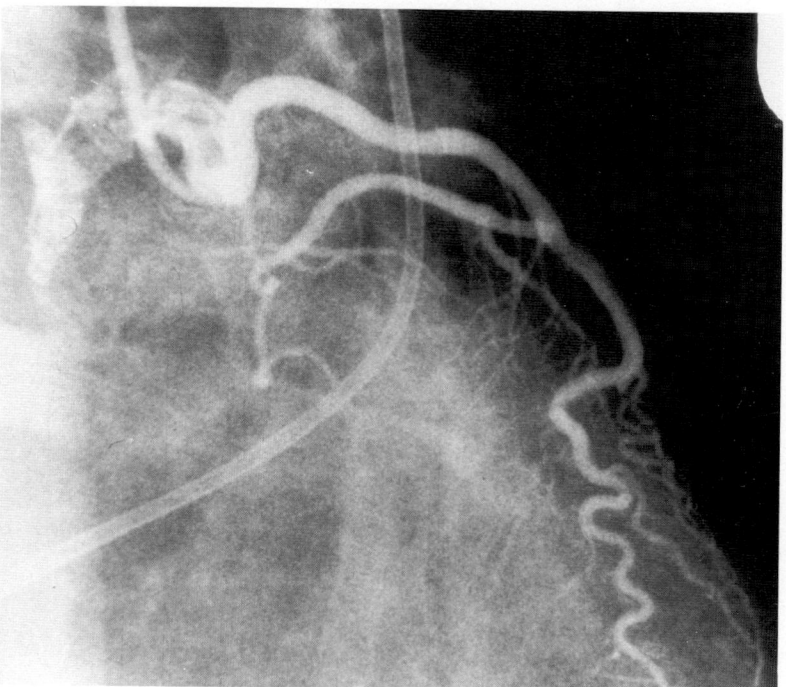

FIGURE 99.7 The same patient as in Fig. 99.6. Coronary arteriogram, cine-frame, in the right anterior oblique view. Note anterior superior passage of the left main coronary artery. Also, note the septal artery arising from the long left main coronary artery. The second catheter is in the main pulmonary artery.

In our cases, there were no instances of unexplained sudden death. We saw a patient with acute inferior wall myocardial infarction with this anomaly and no obstructive disease. Since this report there have been a number of case reports of angina pectoris, myocardial ischemia, and atrioventricular conduction defects,[25,26] as well as sudden death in a 9-month-old infant reported by Liberthson and colleagues.[27]

Of ten autopsy patients with this anomaly, Roberts and colleagues reported three patients with clinical problems: one with recurrent ventricular tachycardia, one with typical angina pectoris, and one with sudden death.[28] The mechanism they described was similar to that described in the anomalously arising left coronary artery from the anterior sinus of Valsalva, that is, the slitlike orifice with the obliquely anteriorly passing right coronary artery resulting in sudden occlusion with exercise and expansion of the aorta or right ventricular outflow tract. Bypass surgery has been done in some of these patients with relief of angina pectoris.[29]

ECTOPIC ORIGIN OF CORONARY ARTERIES FROM THE AORTA

There is some variation of the position of the coronary ostia within respective sinuses of Valsalva. Banchi showed that in normal hearts the left coronary artery arose at the level of the free margin of the aortic cusps in 48%, above the cusps in 34%, and below the cusps in 18%.[30] The right coronary artery arose 71% at the cusps, 19% above, and 10% below. Occasionally the ostia arise higher than the level of the cusps, up to 2 cm above the cusps. In Hobbs's series a high right coronary artery takeoff was found in 0.18% of patients and 11.3% of coronary anomalies, whereas the high takeoff of the left coronary artery was found in 0.02% of patients and 1.3% of coronary anomalies.[4] This high takeoff creates problems in engaging the ostium at coronary arteriography. If the ostium is very high, a low aortotomy could accidentally sever the coronary artery. There have been occasional reports of an

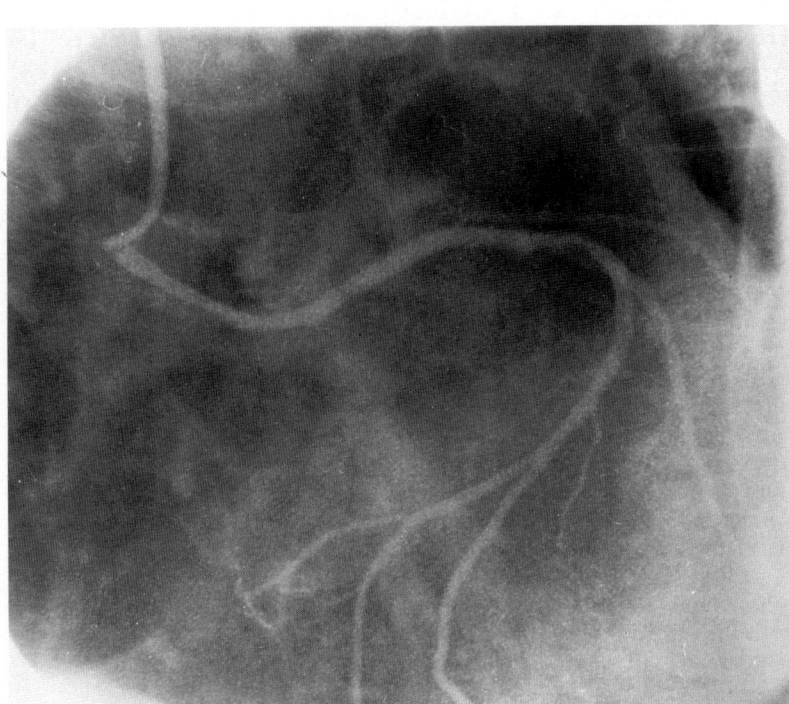

FIGURE 99.8 Coronary arteriogram, cine-frame, left anterior oblique view. Note the catheter in the left circumflex coronary artery arising from the right sinus of Valsalva and passing to the right and posteriorly before arriving in the left atrioventricular sulcus and giving off the obtuse marginal branches. There was a separate left anterior descending coronary artery coming off the left coronary sinus of Valsalva in the usual position; it is not shown.

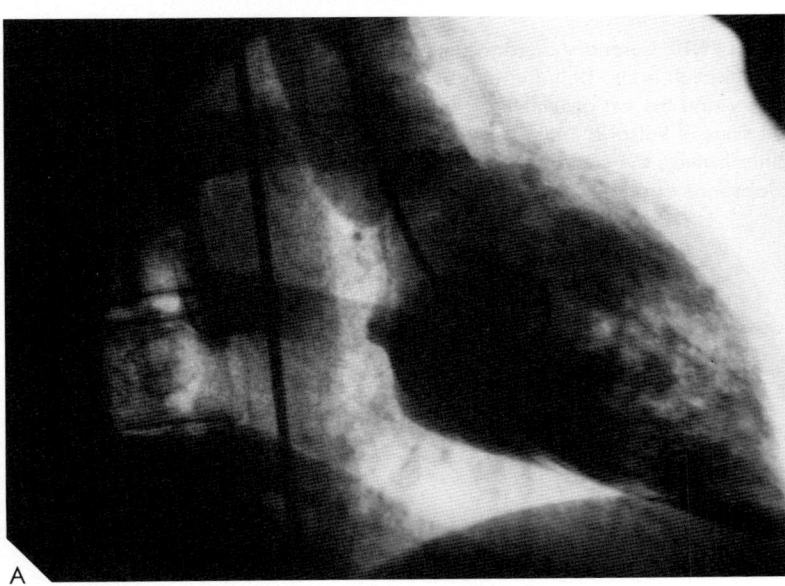
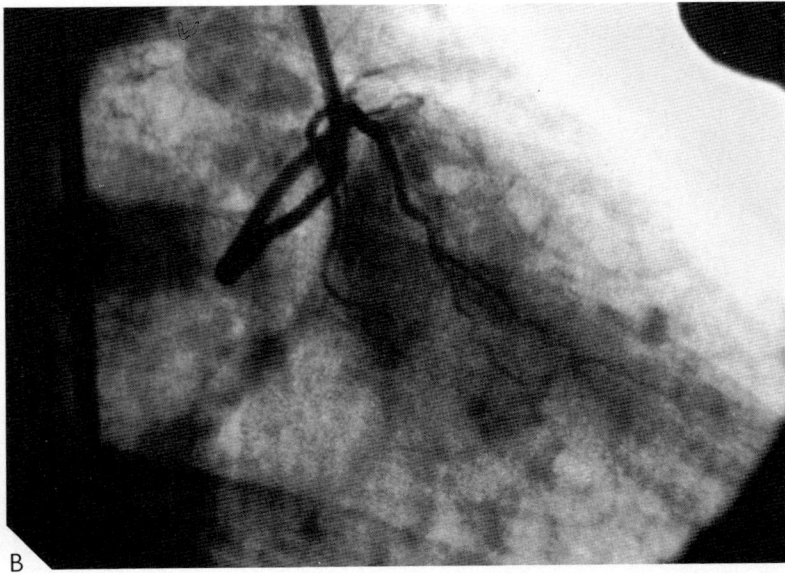

FIGURE 99.9 A. Left ventricular angiocardiogram in the right anterior oblique projection. Patient has left circumflex coronary artery arising anomalously from the anterior sinus of Valsalva and passing rightwardly and posteriorly around the aorta. Note the opacified left circumflex artery on end just to the left of the aortic root. **B.** Coronary arteriogram in right anterior oblique projection (same patient). Injection into the left circumflex coronary artery arising from the anterior sinus of Valsalva.

anomalous coronary artery that arises from the innominate artery.[31] Blake and associates reported such a patient and concluded that his was really a heart with aortic atresia and a partially transposed aorta so that the "single coronary artery" arising from the innominate artery was really the hypoplastic ascending aorta giving rise to the coronary arteries.[32] On occasion, a right coronary artery can arise well above the left sinus of Valsalva, a problem for the coronary arteriographer.[33]

ABSENT CORONARY ARTERIES

The left main coronary artery is absent in 0.47% of patients and accounted for 30.3% of the coronary anomalies in Hobbs's series.[4] Schlesinger found a separate ostium for a left anterior descending artery and for a left circumflex artery from the aorta in 2 of 1000 consecutive autopsies.[34] In this anomaly, the left anterior descending and left circumflex coronary arteries arise as separate ostia from the left posterior sinus of Valsalva (see Fig. 99.2, A). Differentiation of this anomaly from that of a very short left main coronary artery is difficult (Fig. 99.10). On coronary arteriography, both anomalies can result in opacification of only the left anterior descending artery or only the left circumflex artery and lead to the mistaken conclusion that one of the coronaries is completely occluded. This anomaly is seen with a dominant left coronary artery (44%), with aortic valve disease, and with bicuspid aortic valve (17%).[4] During surgery, if this is not recognized, failure to perfuse one of the orifices could result in myocardial infarction.[35]

With absent right coronary artery from the anterior sinus of Valsalva, the right coronary artery arises as a branch of the left coronary artery and passes either anteriorly or posteriorly to the aorta to supply the territory of the right coronary artery (Fig. 99.2, B). In other cases, there is a single right coronary artery that gives rise to the left coronary artery.[36] These cases have been referred to as cases of a left main coronary that arises from the right coronary artery or from the anterior sinus of Valsalva. There have been reports of myocardial infarction and sudden death with single coronary arteries.[37,38] Lipton and co-workers have, on the basis of the angiographic appearance, proposed a classification based on the site of origin and the anatomical distribution of the branches.[39] They pointed out that the cross-sectional area of the single coronary artery is only 50% of the combined cross-sectional area of the normal two-coronary artery system. Rarely, congenital atresia of the left coronary ostium occurs, usually resulting in severe myocardial ischemia and infarction in the distribution of the left coronary artery in infancy.[40,41]

Absence of the left circumflex coronary artery (see Fig. 99.2, C) is a very rare anomaly (0.008% of patients in Hobbs's series[4]) and is compensated for by the right coronary artery, which crosses the crux of the posterior heart and ascends in the left atrioventricular sulcus to supply the territory of the left circumflex artery. Regarding other case reports claiming total absence of the left circumflex coronary artery,[40,42] there is the possibility that the anomalously arising left circumflex artery was not found.[43] However, Bestetti and colleagues have reported a 12-year-old girl who died with dilated cardiomyopathy, presumably unrelated, who had anatomically proven absence of the left circumflex coronary artery without a compensating continuation of the right coronary artery in the left AV sulcus.[44]

ABNORMAL CORONARY ORIGINS FROM THE PULMONARY ARTERY

ANOMALOUS LEFT CORONARY ARTERY ORIGINATING FROM THE PULMONARY ARTERY

A left coronary artery originating from the pulmonary artery (ALCAPA; see Fig. 99.2, D) is one of the most frequently recognized coronary artery anomalies, resulting in severe myocardial ischemia and early death. In Wesselhoeft and associates' review of the literature,[45] 90% of the patients were symptomatic and died within the first year of life, which explains why in Hobbs's series,[4] a coronary arteriographic series in adults, this anomaly occurred in only 0.003% of patients and represented only 0.17% of coronary artery anomalies.

ALCAPA is certainly the most important clinical coronary artery anomaly in infancy. Only 10% of patients live to adulthood. The first case of ALCAPA was described by Abbott in 1908 in a 60-year-old woman who died in an accident.[46] In 1933 Bland, White, and Garland described the clinical diagnostic features of this disorder.[47]

At birth the left coronary artery arises from the pulmonary artery and is perfused under the high pulmonary artery pressure owing to the high pulmonary vascular resistance present in the fetus and the infant. After birth the pulmonary vascular resistance falls, and the left coronary artery is perfused under the low pressure of the pulmonary artery, resulting in myocardial ischemia of the anterolateral wall and usually massive myocardial infarction. There is frequently dilatation of the left ventricle, the murmur of mitral insufficiency, and death either suddenly with an arrhythmia or as a result of severe congestive heart failure (Fig.

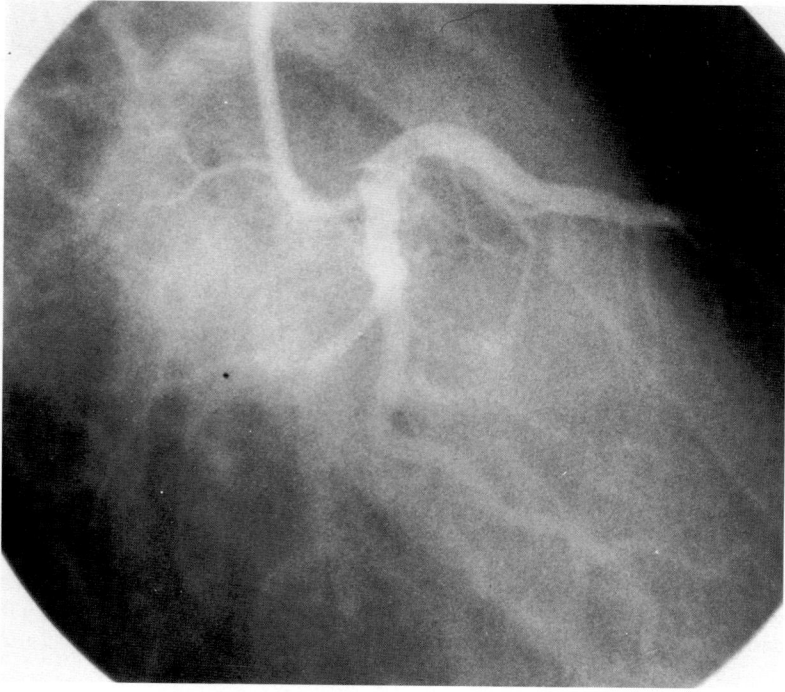

FIGURE 99.10 Coronary arteriogram, cine-frame, right anterior oblique view. The injection is into both the orifices of the left anterior descending coronary artery and the left circumflex artery, which are side-by-side, arising from the left sinus of Valsalva. Note the absence of a left main coronary artery. In other frames, the contrast spills directly into the left coronary sinus, and there is absence of any evidence of a left main coronary artery.

99.11). If the perfusion pressure of the left coronary artery remains elevated until extensive collaterals form between the normally arising right coronary artery and the left coronary artery, depending on the flow and the relative resistances of pulmonary and coronary vascular beds, there will be maintenance of myocardial flow and survival into childhood and adulthood.[48] Wilson and associates, in a survey of the literature, reported 44 patients living beyond the first decade, 41% of whom had the diagnosis made postmortem.[49] Many lacked symptoms during life, and those who died did so suddenly at a mean age of 35 years. In those diagnosed during life, the mean age of diagnosis was 29 years.

At catheterization there is often a marked increase in flow in the right coronary artery with resultant dilatation of the right coronary artery. Because pulmonary vascular resistance is usually lower than coronary vascular resistance, there is flow away from the myocardial bed into the pulmonary artery, a left-to-right shunt. This was first suggested in 1885 by Brooks[50] and later in 1958 by Edwards.[51] This low-resistance runoff to the pulmonary artery was first demonstrated by Sabiston and associates and can result in a continuous murmur with diastolic accentuation along the left sternal border.[52] Stress testing and thallium perfusion studies have demonstrated myocardial ischemia.[53] In medically treated patients there is a high incidence of myocardial infarction, poor left ventricular function, arrhythmia, and even sudden death. This can occur even in adults who have been asymptomatic throughout childhood. With two-dimensional echocardiography, it has been possible to raise suspicion of this anomaly and even to visualize the origin of the left coronary artery from the pulmonary artery.[54,55] The most common finding on echocardiography is the dilatation of the right coronary artery because of increased coronary flow.[55] A lung scan that reveals the myocardium is excellent evidence for anomalous origin of the left coronary artery from the pulmonary artery.[56]

Because of the poor prognosis with medical management in these patients, surgical correction on discovery of the lesion has been recommended.[57] In patients under 1 year of age, surgery has been attended by poor results. In a report by Driscoll and colleagues, only two of eight patients operated on under 1 year of age survived.[58] Laborde and associates attempted transplantation or grafting of the left coronary artery to the aorta in 20 consecutive patients. Under 1 year of age, four of five died; after 1 year of age, the mortality was only 15%.[59] As a result of this experience, Driscoll and associates as well as Laborde and associates[59] have recommended delay of surgery if at all possible until the patient is 12 to 18 months old. After this age, on identification of the lesion surgical correction should be undertaken.

Surgical approaches have varied from simple ligation of the left coronary artery to stop the "coronary steal"[48,60] to reconstitution of a "two-coronary system." This has been accomplished by grafting of the aorta to the left coronary artery using the subclavian artery,[61] by creating a transpulmonary artery tunnel from the aorta to the left coronary artery,[62] by ligating the left coronary artery and performing a saphenous vein bypass graft to the left anterior ascending coronary artery, and finally by transplanting the left coronary artery to the aorta.[63,64] In the older patient, these techniques are successful with decreased symptomatology and reversal of evidence of myocardial ischemia as manifested by absence of angina pectoris and reversal of the abnormal exercise ST segment depression and abnormal thallium perfusion scan.[59,65] Postoperatively the collaterals eventually disappear, and the right coronary artery may regress to normal size.

Much rarer than anomalous origin of the left coronary from the pulmonary artery is the anomalous origin of the anterior descending or left circumflex artery from the pulmonary artery.[66,67] There have been occasional case reports of this very rare condition, usually found in children or young adults with increasing angina pectoris. These lesions have also been approached with bypass surgery with success.[68]

RIGHT CORONARY ARTERY ORIGINATING FROM THE PULMONARY ARTERY

Origin of the right coronary artery from the pulmonary artery (see Fig. 99.2, *E*) is much more unusual than origin of the left coronary artery from the pulmonary artery. In 1982 there had been over 200 cases described in the literature in which the left coronary artery arose from the pulmonary artery and only 23 in which the right coronary artery arose from the pulmonary artery.[69] This lesion was originally described by Brooks in 1886,[50] before the origin of the left coronary artery from the pulmonary artery had been described, and it was thought to be benign. In most patients the anomaly was discovered incidentally or by the presence of a continuous murmur. On review of the cases reported, there have been instances of angina pectoris, life-threatening arrhythmias, and even sudden death in 4 of the 23 cases.[70] Successful repair with reimplantation in the aorta or ligation with saphenous vein bypass grafting has been reported.[71]

ANOMALOUS ORIGIN OF BOTH CORONARY ARTERIES FROM THE PULMONARY ARTERY

The least common of the coronary artery anomalies arising from the pulmonary artery is that of both arteries arising from the pulmonary artery (see Fig. 99.2, *F*). Because of the low pulmonary artery perfusion pressure, this condition is compatible with only a short life.[72,73] Occasionally patients with large ventricular septal defects or truncus

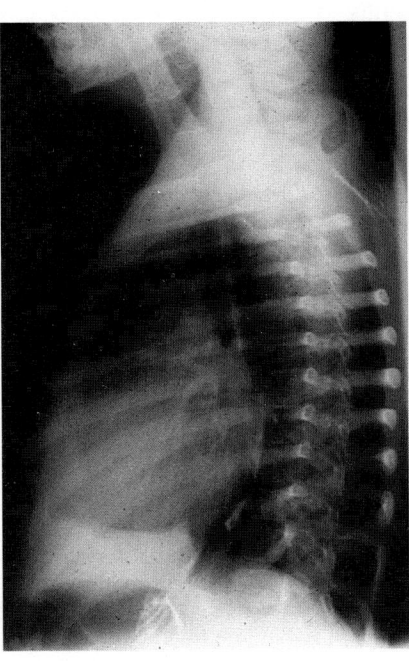
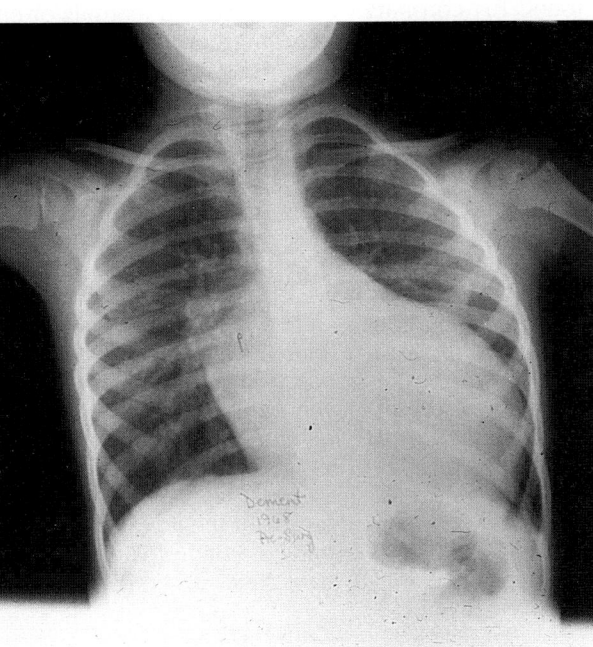

FIGURE 99.11 Chest roentgenogram, left lateral view in the left panel and anterior-posterior projection in the right panel. The patient was a five-year-old boy with left coronary artery arising anomalously from the pulmonary artery. Patient had congestive heart failure and severe mitral insufficiency. Note the markedly enlarged and aneurysmal left ventricle and the large left atrium. There is also pulmonary venous redistribution.

arteriosus with pulmonary hypertension and both coronary arteries arising from the pulmonary artery have lived into childhood and even adulthood. Although there have been attempts to correct this defect, to date none has been successful.[73,74]

CORONARY ARTERY FISTULAS

Coronary artery fistulas, after the anomalously arising left coronary artery from the pulmonary artery, are the most common congenital coronary anomalies resulting in pathophysiologic problems. Coronary fistulas were first described in 1865 by Krause.[75] The incidence of coronary fistula is estimated to be 1 in 50,000 children with congenital heart disease.[76] In Hobbs and associates' report of 55,856 coronary arteriographic patients, 101 patients (or 0.2%) were found to have coronary fistulas.[77] Fistulas can occur between any of the coronary arteries and any cardiac chamber (coronary-cameral fistulas) (Fig. 99.12). Coronary artery fistulas can drain into the main pulmonary artery, coronary veins including coronary sinus (coronary AV fistulas), and other rarer sites such as the superior vena cava, bronchial arteries, and right pulmonary artery.

The etiology of congenital coronary-cameral fistulas, according to Grant, is the persistence of embryonic arterioluminal sinusoids connecting primitive epicardial coronary vessels with the cardiac chambers.[78] Normally these embryonic arteriocameral connections decrease in size until finally they are represented as thebesian veins and the sinusoids. Coronary artery-to-pulmonary artery fistulas are probably the result of accessory coronary arteries that arise from angioblastic anlage in the pulmonary artery in the presence of normally arising coronary arteries from the aorta with intercoronary anastomoses.[79]

In large series of patients it appears that both sexes are equally affected. The site of origin of the fistulas, the number of fistulas, and the site into which the fistulas empty have been reported by pooling reports in the literature of all reported cases. Levin and associates reported on the largest number of coronary artery fistulas (363 cases) in 1978.[80] Of those cases, 181 (50%) arose from the right coronary artery, 151 (42%) from the left coronary artery, and 19 (5%) from both vessels. In 12 cases (3%) the vessel of origin was not specified. The site of drainage occurred into the right ventricle in 150 cases (41%), the right atrium in 94 cases (26%), the pulmonary artery in 63 cases (17%), the coronary sinus in 23 cases (7%), the left atrium in 18 cases (5%), the left ventricle in 11 cases (3%), and the superior vena cava in four cases (1%). It is apparent that the fistulas arose from each of the coronaries with about the same frequency and emptied into the systemic venous side of the circulation in over 90% of cases.

Of interest is the report of Hobbs and colleagues from the Cleveland Clinic who, in the course of a 10-year period, found 101 coronary artery fistulas in 55,856 patients undergoing coronary arteriography.[77] In this study, the site of drainage was into the pulmonary artery in 65.6% of cases, the left ventricle in 17.2%, the left atrium in 6.6%, the right atrium in 7.4%, and the right ventricle in only 3.3%. Only 58.2% drained into the right side of the heart and 41.8% into the left. One hundred ten fistulas were classified as small, three as medium, and nine as large. This series found the incidental coronary fistulas by coronary arteriography. As compared with coronary fistulas in general, in this series there was a high incidence of pulmonary artery drainage and left ventricular drainage.

With drainage into the systemic venous side of the circulation, there is a constant left-to-right shunt from the systemic-pressure coronary artery into the low-pressure, right-sided chambers with the formation of a continuous murmur. The continuous murmur is also present when the fistulas empty into the left atrium. The majority of reported patients have continuous murmurs, but this might be misleading because those with continuous murmurs are more likely to have their fistulas discovered. In one report of 56 patients, 70% had continuous murmurs.[81] The vast majority of the patients with very small fistulas did not have continuous murmurs. In Hobbs's series, for instance, only 3% had a continuous murmur.[77] When the fistulas drain into the left ventricle, there may only be a diastolic murmur and the hemodynamics of a large aortic-to-left-ventricular shunt, which simulates the hemodynamics of aortic insufficiency.[82,83]

The pathophysiology of the coronary-cameral fistula depends on the size of the shunt. If it is large, and frequently it is in children with coronary-cameral fistulas and coronary AV fistulas, there is aneurysmal dilatation of the proximal feeding coronary artery as well as any venous structure into which it drains (coronary vein or coronary sinus).[84] The coronary arterial end of the fistula tends to be larger than the drainage end. Diagnosis can be suggested by physical examination. If a continuous murmur is heard at the base of the chest, the drainage area is likely to be into the pulmonary artery, and the differential diagnosis is that of patent ductus arteriosus and aorticopulmonary window. In fact, the first coronary artery fistula diagnosed in a live patient was by Björk and Crafoord, who mistakenly operated on the patient for patent ductus arteriosus and found by exploration a coronary artery-to-pulmonary artery fistula.[85]

A subtle auscultatory clue to differentiating coronary-to-pulmonary-artery fistula from patent ductus arteriosus is the peaking of the continuous murmur in mid-diastole with the coronary-to-pulmonary-artery fistula rather than at the second sound as occurs in patent ductus arteriosus. Yuqing and Ruping have reported coronary-cameral fistulas draining into the right and left ventricles with large left-to-right shunts and aneurysmal dilatation and tortuosity of the coronary arteries so massive that protrusions of the right cardiac border and ovoid opacities superimposed on the cardiac silhouette in the lateral chest film could be seen.[86] The best noninvasive way of identifying the larger coronary artery fistulas may be by two-dimensional echocardiography and Doppler studies.[87] Both the enlarged proximal coronary artery and the turbulence and jet of the blood entering the low-pressure chamber can be visualized by echocardiographic Doppler techniques.[88] In some instances even the dilated coronary artery can be visualized as well as the enlarged coronary sinus into which the fistula empties.[89] The most common presentation is that of an asymptomatic patient with a continuous murmur or a coronary artery fistula found accidentally during coronary arteriography.[84] Complications from coronary arterial fistulas have been reported:

Myocardial ischemia with angina, presumably related to the coronary steal pathophysiology[84,90]
Myocardial infarction[91]
Coronary aneurysmal dilatation[92]
Dyspnea and left heart failure secondary to the left-to-right shunt[84,93]
Elevation of pulmonary vascular resistance and pulmonary hypertension[94]
Infective endocarditis or endarteritis[95,96]
Rupture of the coronary artery fistula and hemopericardium[97]

Angina pectoris has been reported in 18.4% of the cases in the literature as collected by Wilde and Watt.[84] There have been patients with coronary arterial fistulas with ischemia, as manifested by angina pectoris, exercise ST segment depression, and thallium perfusion abnormalities, who have had these abnormalities reversed with ligation of the fistulas.[98] Many of the patients with angina have had coronary arterial disease in addition to the fistulas (Fig. 99.13).[91] There is a question as to whether the coronary arterial lesions were secondary to intimal injury due to the abnormal flow patterns caused by the coronary fistula.[91] Myocardial infarction in patients without arterial obstruction is very rare.

Congestive heart failure is limited to patients with large left-to-right shunts, mainly infants and young children or the elderly, in whom there are possibly other reasons for the heart failure. In Wilde and Watt's review of the literature, 75% of the patients presented signs and symptoms of congestive heart failure. How often progression of the left-to-right shunt is seen is unknown. Most studies with repeat catheterizations have shown no increase in the size of the shunt.[99] There are a few reported instances of spontaneous closure of the coronary arterial fistula.[100] In most series, the young patients tended not to have symptoms and the older patients had symptoms but these were not definitely from the coronary arterial fistulas.

Pulmonary hypertension is also unusual and is seen only with large left-to-right shunts.[101] Infective endocarditis is unusual, occurring in 3% to 4% of cases,[84] and the complication of rupture of the coronary fistula is very rare.

With small fistulas, the complications listed above have been unusual. Recommendations as to the indication for surgical repair of these fistulas vary in the literature from surgical closure on identifying the fistula to repair in only those with large shunts or with symptoms definitely related to the fistulas.[77,81,84,93] Surgical repair consists of ligation of the low-pressure side of the fistulous connection if there is a single orifice. Frequently this requires bypass surgery, opening the cardiac chamber and oversewing the fistula's orifice. If there are multiple connections, ligation nearer the origin at the coronary artery is recommended, but if the proximal coronary artery will be compromised, then ligation with bypass of the coronary artery is recommended.[84] Although ligation of the low-pressure side of congenital fistulas is usually not successful with other congenital AV fistulas because recurrence is high, the recurrence rate with this approach for coronary arterial fistulas has been extremely low.[102] Surgical mortality in those not having additional cardiac lesions has been very low.

There is little doubt that patients with large left-to-right shunts should have them repaired. There is also little argument that patients with angina pectoris or demonstrable ischemia in areas related to the fistula should have the fistula repaired. The major question arises with the small coronary arterial fistula in the asymptomatic patient. This includes most of the patients with coronary-artery-to-pulmonary-artery fistulas. It is my present opinion that these patients should be followed medically. This opinion has been reinforced by the report in Hobbs and colleagues, whose 101 patients had mostly small asymptomatic fistulas.[77] Ninety-eight fistulas (97%) were discovered as incidental findings at the time of catheterization and had not been clinically suspected. Ninety of these patients were treated medically, and eleven underwent surgery. Follow-up ranged from 1 to 11 years. Thirty of the patients subsequently died of associated cardiac disease, but no deaths were attributed to the coronary artery fistulas. During follow-up none of the medically treated patients developed symptoms or complications as a result of the coronary fistula. Eight of the patients had subsequent catheterizations and had no change in the size of the left-to-right shunt. The only recommendation for the medically treated patient with coronary arterial fistula is that of antibiotics at the time of dental procedures or bacteremia from other causes to decrease the chance of infective endarteritis.

CORONARY ARTERY HYPOPLASIA OR ATRESIA

The dominant left coronary system supplying the entire left ventricle and septum together with a diminutive right coronary artery with branches to the right atrium and right ventricular free wall and no branches to the left ventricle is a common normal variant. Hypoplasia of the left coronary artery is much rarer, especially in adults. This simulates a single right coronary artery, except that a diminutive left coronary arterial system is present.[40] Usually the patients are infants. Patients in the seventh or eighth decade have been described with this lesion, usually at postmortem examination after sudden death.[41]

CORONARY ARTERY ANEURYSM

Nonfistulous coronary artery aneurysms result from atherosclerosis, mycotic aneurysm in endocarditis, inflammatory processes such as mucocutaneous lymph node syndrome and periarteritis nodosa, traumatic aneurysm, and congenital coronary aneurysm. In a study by Daoud and associates, of 89 postmortem cases of coronary arterial aneurysms reported up to 1963, only 16 were thought to be congenital.[103] Since the advent of coronary arteriography, there are many more cases being described during life.[104] Occasionally these aneurysms can be enormous, distorting the cardiac silhouette on chest roentgenogram (Fig. 99.14).[105] Congenital aneurysms can be asymptomatic and have been discovered during coronary arteriography to investigate a distorted cardiac silhouette or have resulted in myocardial ischemia

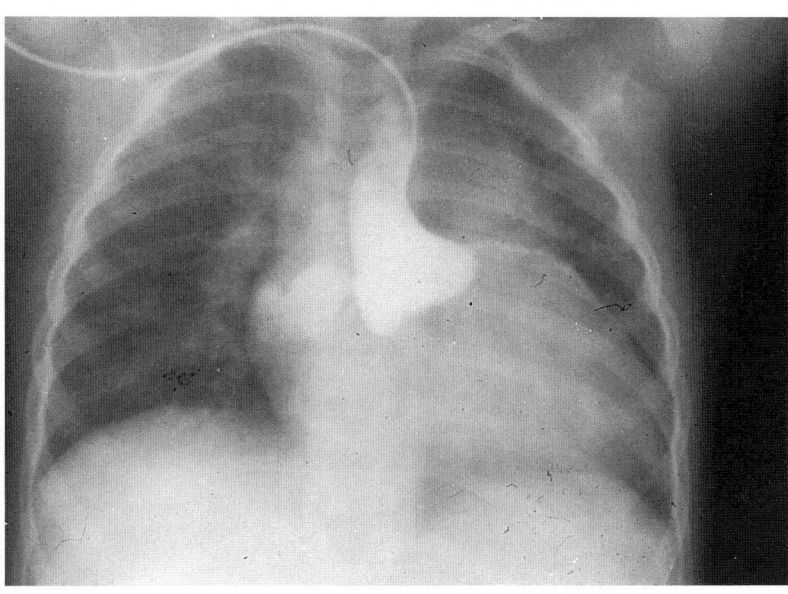

FIGURE 99.12 Aortogram, posteroanterior projection. The patient was a two-year-old boy with a continuous heart murmur along the left sternal border. Contrast is seen in the root of the aorta with the right coronary artery fistula and contrast entering the right atrium. Note the distal right coronary artery is normal in size and course.

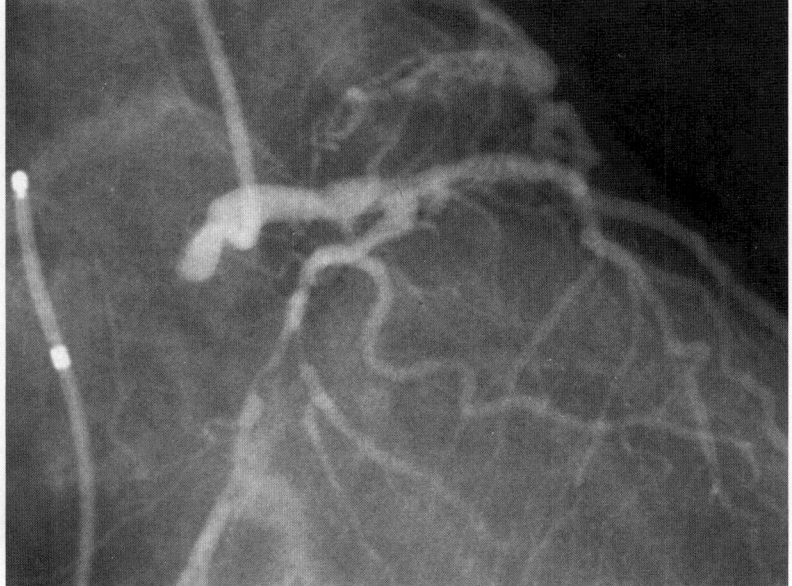

FIGURE 99.13 Coronary arteriogram, cine-frame, right anterior oblique position. The catheter is in the left coronary artery. Note the fistulous vessels arising from the left anterior descending coronary artery and emptying into the main pulmonary artery. Note the high-grade obstructive disease in the branches of the circumflex coronary artery. The patient was a 65-year-old woman with extensive coronary artery disease, angina pectoris, and no murmurs.

and myocardial infarction due to thrombus with or without distal embolism (Fig. 99.15).[106] Coronary artery aneurysms should be considered in the evaluation of children and young patients with chest pain. Systolic and diastolic murmurs have been described. The chest x-ray film can reveal masses due to their large size or, on occasion, ringlike calcifications due to calcification of the aneurysmal wall.[107,108] When the aneurysm is discovered, saphenous vein bypass grafting with ligation and exclusion of the aneurysm may be the best approach in symptomatic cases.[109] There have been reports of progression of the coronary aneurysm formation even after bypass grafting.[110]

CORONARY ARTERIAL VARIATIONS SECONDARY TO A PRIMARY INTRACARDIAC DEFECT

The pattern of coronary arterial origin and distribution varies from the usual pattern in patients with various cardiac congenital anomalies. The anomalous origin of the left anterior descending coronary artery from the right coronary artery in tetralogy of Fallot has been mentioned. The coronary arterial origin and distribution varies from the normal in patients with corrected transposition of the great arteries, truncus arteriosus, dextrocardia, and situs inversus viscerum. Rarely, the coronary ostia can be occluded or markedly obstructed in patients with congenital aortic valve abnormalities. Two such cases were reported by Gibson and colleagues in young patients with aortic valve disease resulting in both aortic stenosis and aortic insufficiency with membrane-like obstruction of the left coronary cusp.[111] In some cases these obstructive membranes were thought to represent a forme fruste of supraventricular membranous aortic stenosis. Surgical removal of these obstructions has been performed successfully.[112]

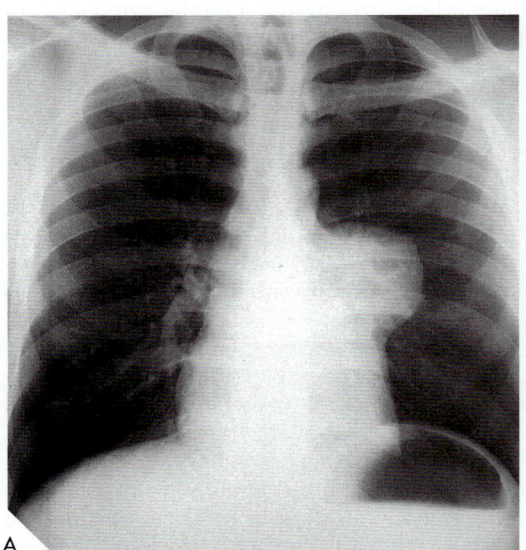
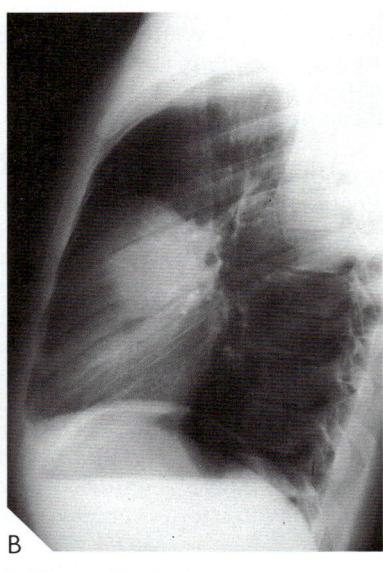
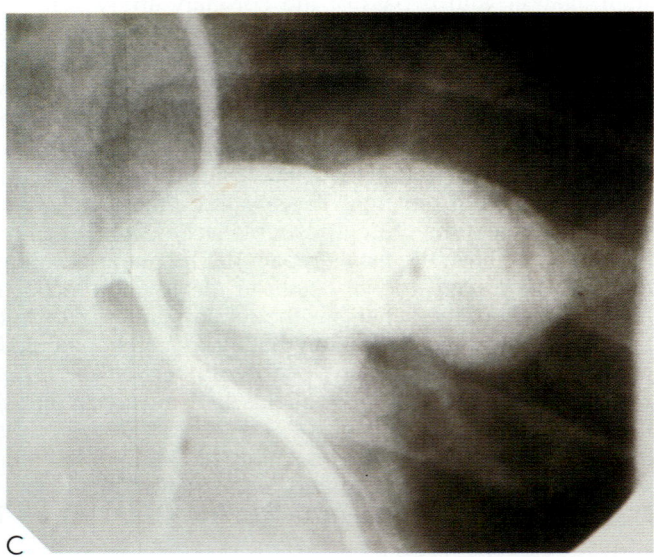
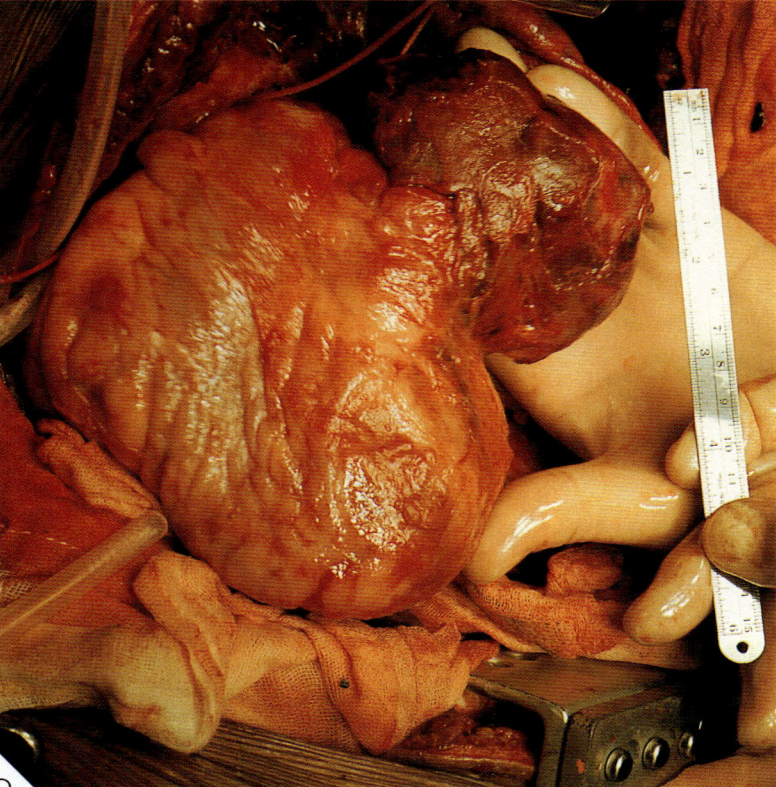

FIGURE 99.14 **A.** Posteroanterior anterior chest roentgenogram of a 21-year-old asymptomatic man with a congenital coronary artery aneurysm arising from the origin of the left anterior descending coronary artery. **B.** Left lateral chest roentgenogram. Note mass in middle mediastinum. **C.** Coronary arteriogram. Injection into left coronary artery in shallow left anterior oblique projection. Note large opacified aneurysm arising from origin of left anterior descending coronary artery with circumflex coronary continuing normally. **D.** Coronary aneurysm at the time of surgery. Large coronary aneurysm is in the surgeon's hand.

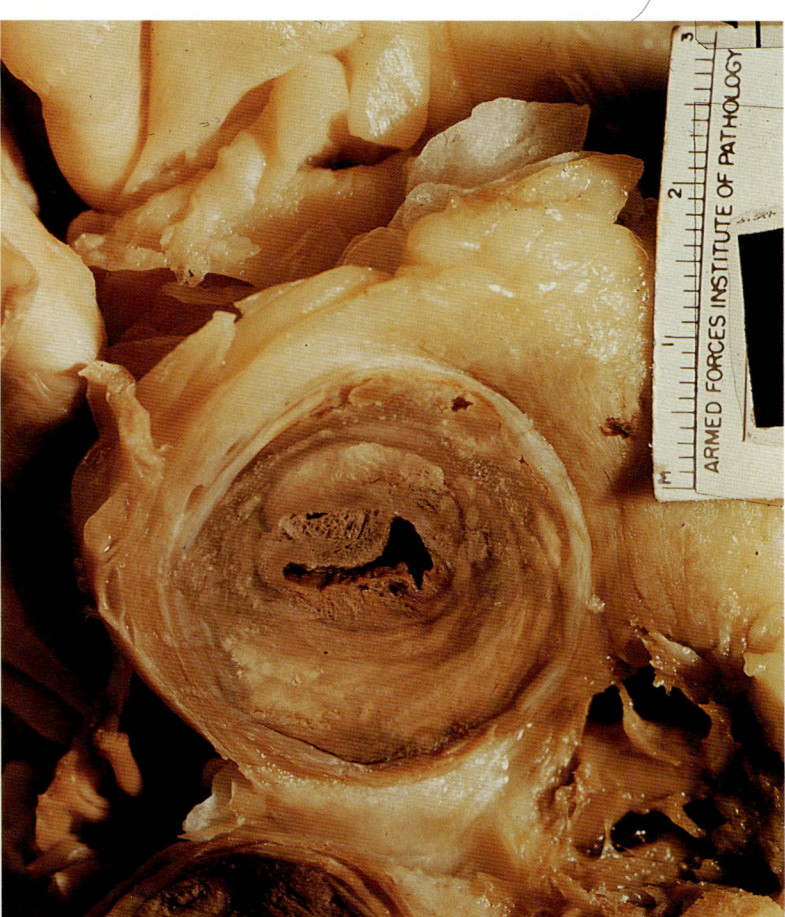

FIGURE 99.15 Cross-section of a congenital coronary aneurysm in a 2-year-old child. Note the laminated thrombus almost filling the lumen. (From Virmani R, Forman MB (eds): Nonatherosclerotic Ischemic Heart Disease. New York, Raven Press, 1989, by permission).

REFERENCES

1. Baroldi G, Scomazzoni G: Coronary circulation in the normal and the pathologic heart, p 26. AFIP Monograph, Washington, DC, U.S. Government Printing Office, 1967
2. Alexander R, Griffith O: Anomalies of the coronary arteries and their clinical significance. Circulation 14:800, 1956
3. Samanek M, Goetzova J, Benesova D: Distribution of congenital heart malformities in an autopsied child population. Int J Cardiol 8:235, 1985
4. Hobbs RJ, Millit HD, Raghavan PV et al: Congenital coronary anomalies: Clinical and therapeutic implications. Cardiovasc Clin 12:43, 1982
5. Baltaxe HA, Wixson D: The incidence of congenital anomalies of the coronary arteries in the adult population. Radiology 122:47, 1977
6. Glover MV, Kuber MT, Warren SE et al: Myocardial infarction before age 36: Risk factor and arteriographic analysis. Am J Cardiol 49:1600, 1982
7. Ogden JA: Congenital anomalies of the coronary arteries. Am J Cardiol 25:474, 1970
8. Lurie PR, Takahashi M: Abnormalities and diseases of the coronary vessels. In Moss AJ, Adams FH, Emmanoulides GC (eds): Heart Disease in Infants, Children, and Adolescents, p 501. Baltimore, Williams & Wilkins, 1983
9. Ishikawa T, Brandt PWT: Anomalous origin of the left main coronary artery from the right anterior aortic sinus: Angiographic definition of anomalous course. Am J Cardiol 55:770, 1985
10. Cheitlin MD, DeCastro CM, McAllister HA: Sudden death as a complication of anomalous left coronary origin from the anterior sinus of Valsalva. Circulation 50:780, 1974
11. Bloomfield P, Erhlich C, Folland ED et al: Anomalous right coronary artery: A surgically correctable cause of angina pectoris. Am J Cardiol 51:1235, 1983
12. Murphy DA, Roy DL, Sohal M et al: Anomalous origin of left main coronary artery from anterior sinus of Valsalva with myocardial infarction. J Thorac Cardiovas Surg 75:282, 1978
13. Liberthson RR, Zaman L, Weyman A et al: Aberrant origin of the left coronary artery from the proximal right coronary artery: Diagnostic features and pre- and post-operative course. Clin Cardiol 5:377, 1982
14. Davia JE, Green DC, Cheitlin MD et al: Anomalous left coronary artery origin from the right coronary sinus. Am Heart J 108:165, 1984
15. Donaldson RM, Raphael MJ, Yacoub MH et al: Hemodynamically significant anomalies of the coronary arteries. Thorac Cardovasc Surg 30:7, 1982
16. Dalal JJ, West RO, Parker JO: Isolated anomaly of the left anterior descending coronary artery. Cathet Cardiovasc Diagn 10:189, 1984
17. Engle HJ, Torres C, Page HL Jr: Major variations in anatomical origin of the coronary arteries: Angiographic observation in 4,250 patients without congenital heart diseases. Cathet Cardiovasc Diagn 1:157, 1975
18. Meng CLL, Eckner FAO, Lev M: Coronary artery distribution in tetralogy of Fallot. Arch Surg 90:363, 1965
19. McManus BM, Waller BF, Jones M et al: The case for preoperative coronary angiography in patients with tetralogy of Fallot and other complex congenital heart diseases. Am Heart J 103:451, 1982
20. Dabizzi RP, Caprioli O, Aiazzi L et al: Distribution and anomalies of coronary arteries in tetralogy of Fallot. Circulation 61:95, 1980
21. Page HL Jr, Engel HJ, Campbell WB et al: Anomalous origin of the left circumflex coronary artery. Circulation 50:768, 1974
22. Patterson FK: Sudden death in a young adult with anomalous origin of the posterior circumflex artery. South Med J 75:748, 1982
23. Edelstein J, Juhasz RS: Myocardial infarction in the distribution of a patent anomalous left circumflex coronary artery. Cathet Cardiovasc Diagn 10:171, 1984
24. Morin D, Fischer AP, Sohl BE et al: Iatrogenic myocardial infarction. A possible complication of mitral valve surgery related to anatomical variation of the circumflex coronary artery. Thorac Cardiovasc Surg 30:176, 1982
25. Isner JM, Shen EM, Martin ET et al: Sudden unexpected death as a result of anomalous origin of the right coronary artery from the left sinus of Valsalva. Am J Med 76:55, 1984
26. Benge W, Martins JB, Funk DC: Morbidity associated with anomalous origin of the right coronary artery from the left sinus of Valsalva. Am Heart J 99:46, 1980
27. Liberthson RR, Gang DL, Custer J: Sudden death in an infant with aberrant origin of the right coronary artery from the left sinus of Valsalva of the aorta: Case report and review of the literature. Pediatr Cardiol 4:45, 1983
28. Roberts WC, Siegel RJ, Zipes DP: Origin of the right coronary artery from the left sinus of Valsalva and its functional consequences: Analysis of 10 necropsy patients. Am J Cardiol 49:863, 1982
29. Brandt B III, Martins JB, Marcus ML: Anomalous origin of the right coronary artery from the left sinus of Valsalva. N Engl J Med 309:596, 1983
30. Banchi A: Morfologia della arteriae coronariae cordis. Arch Ital Anat Embriol 3:87, 1904
31. Davis JS, Lie JT: Anomalous origin of a single coronary artery from the innominate artery. Angiology 28:775, 1977
32. Blake HA, Manion WC, Mattingly TW et al: Coronary artery anomalies. Circulation 30:927, 1964
33. Yans J, Kumar SP, Kwatra M: Anomalous origin of the right coronary artery above the left sinus of Valsalva. Cathet Cardiovasc Diagn 4:407, 1978
34. Schlesinger MJ, Zoll PM, Wessler S: The conus artery: A third coronary

artery. Am Heart J 38:823, 1949
35. Ogden JA: Anomalous aortic origin: Circumflex, anterior descending or main left coronary arteries. Arch Pathol 88:323, 1969
36. Hillestad L, Eie H: Single coronary artery. Acta Med Scand 189:409, 1971
37. Allen GL, Snider TH: Myocardial infarction with a single coronary artery. Arch Intern Med 117:261, 1966
38. Warren SE, Alpert JS, Vieweg WVR et al: Normal single coronary artery and myocardial infarction. Chest 72:540, 1977
39. Lipton MJ, Barry WH, Obrez I et al: Isolated single coronary artery: Diagnosis, angiographic classification, and clinical significance. Radiology 130:39, 1979
40. Byrum CJ, Blackman MS, Schneider B et al: Congenital atresia of the left coronary ostium and hypoplasia of the left main coronary artery. Am Heart J 99:354, 1980
41. Van der Hauwaert L, Dumoulin M, Moerman P: Congenital atresia of the left coronary ostium. Br Heart J 48:298, 1982
42. Barresi V, Susmano A, Colandrea MA et al: Congenital absence of the circumflex coronary artery. Am Heart J 86:811, 1973
43. Donaldson RM, Raphael MJ: Missing coronary artery: Review of technical problems in coronary arteriography resulting from anatomical variants. Br Heart J 47:62, 1982
44. Bestetti RB, Costa RB, Oliveira JSM et al: Congenital absence of the circumflex coronary artery associated with dilated cardiomyopathy. Int J Cardiol 8:331, 1985
45. Wesselhoeft H, Fawcett JS, Johnson AL: Anomalous origin of the left coronary artery from the pulmonary trunk. Its clinical spectrum, pathology, and pathophysiology. Based on a review of 140 cases with seven further cases. Circulation 38:403, 1968
46. Abbott ME: Congenital cardiac disease. In Osler W (ed): Modern Medicine, vol IV, p 323. Philadelphia, Lea and Febiger, 1908
47. Bland EF, White PD, Garland J: Congenital anomalies of coronary arteries: Report of an unusual case associated with cardiac hypertrophy. Am Heart J 8:787, 1933
48. Nadas A, Gamboa R, Hugenholtz P: Anomalous left coronary artery originating from the pulmonary artery. Circulation 29:167, 1964
49. Wilson CL, Dlabal PW, Holeyfield RW et al: Anomalous origin of left coronary artery from pulmonary artery. Case report and review of literature concerning teen-agers and adults. J Thorac Cardiovasc Surg 73:887, 1977
50. Brooks HSJ: Two cases of an abnormal coronary artery arising from the pulmonary artery. J Anat Physiol 20:26, 1886
51. Edward JE: Anomalous coronary arteries with special reference to arteriovenous-like communications. Circulation 17:1001, 1958
52. Sabiston DC, Neill C, Taussig H: The direction of blood flow in anomalous left coronary artery arising from the pulmonary artery. Circulation 22:591, 1960
53. Finley JP, Howman-Giles R, Gilday DL et al: Thallium-201 myocardial imaging in anomalous left coronary artery arising from the pulmonary artery. Am J Cardiol 42:675, 1978
54. Fisher EA, Sepehri B, Lendrum B et al: Two-dimensional echocardiographic visualization of the left coronary artery in anomalous origin of the left coronary artery from the pulmonary artery. Circulation 63:698, 1981
55. Caldwell RL, Hurwitz RA, Girod DA et al: Two-dimensional echocardiographic differentiation of anomalous left coronary artery from congestive cardiomyopathy. Am Heart J 106:710, 1983
56. Sfakianakis ON, Damoulaki-Sfakianaki E, McLead RE et al: Anomalous origin of the left coronary artery diagnosed by a lung scan. N Engl J Med 296:675, 1977
57. LaPorta AJ, Suy-Verburg RM, Stalpaert G et al: The spectrum of clinical manifestations of anomalous origin of the left coronary artery and surgical management. J Pediatr Surg 14:225, 1979
58. Driscoll DJ, Nihill MR, Mullins CT et al: Management of symptomatic infants with anomalous origin of the left coronary artery from the pulmonary artery. Am J Cardiol 47:642, 1981
59. Laborde F, Marchand M, Leca F et al: Surgical treatment of anomalous origin of the left coronary artery in infancy and childhood: Early and late results in 20 consecutive cases. J Thorac Cardiovasc Surg 82:423, 1981
60. Sabiston DC, Floyd WL, McIntosh HD: Anomalous origin of the left coronary artery from the pulmonary artery in adults. Arch Surg 97:963, 1968
61. Stephenson LW, Edmunds LH Jr, Freidman S et al: Subclavian left coronary artery anastomosis (Meyer operation) for anomalous origin of the left coronary artery from the pulmonary artery. Circulation 64(suppl II):130, 1981
62. Takeuchi S, Imamura H, Katsumoto K et al: New surgical method for repair of anomalous left coronary artery from pulmonary artery. J Thorac Cardiovasc Surg 78:7, 1979
63. Moodie DS, Fyfe D, Gill CC et al: Anomalous origin of the left coronary artery from the pulmonary artery (Bland-White-Garland syndrome) in adult patients: Long-term follow-up after surgery. Am Heart J 106:381, 1983
64. Grace RR, Angelini P, Cooley DA: Aortic implantation of anomalous left coronary artery arising from the pulmonary artery. Am J Cardiol 39:608, 1977
65. Arciniegas E, Furooki AZ, Hakimi M et al: Management of anomalous left coronary artery from the pulmonary artery. Circulation 62(suppl I):182, 1980
66. Tamer DF, Mallom SM, Garcia OL et al: Anomalous origin of the left anterior descending coronary artery from the pulmonary artery. Am Heart J 108:341, 1984
67. Ott DA, Cooley DA, Pinsky WW et al: Anomalous origin of circumflex coronary artery from right pulmonary artery. J Thorac Cardiovasc Surg 76:190, 1978
68. Evans JJ, Phillips JF: Origin of the left anterior descending coronary artery from the pulmonary artery. J Am Coll Cardiol 3:219, 1984
69. Coe JY, Radley-Smith R, Yacoub M: Clinical and hemodynamic significance of anomalous origin of the right coronary artery from the pulmonary artery. Thorac Cardiovasc Surg 30:84, 1982
70. Lerberg DB, Ogden JA, Zuberbuhler JR et al: Anomalous origin of the right coronary artery from the pulmonary artery. Am Thorac Surg 27:87, 1979
71. Mintz GS, Iskandrian AS, Bemis CE et al: Myocardial ischemia in anomalous origin of the right coronary artery from the pulmonary trunk. Am J Cardiol 51:610, 1983
72. Keeton BR, Keenan DJM, Monro JL: Anomalous origin of both coronary arteries from the pulmonary trunk. Br Heart J 49:397, 1983
73. Goldblatt E, Adams APS, Ross IK et al: Single-trunk anomalous origin of both coronary arteries from the pulmonary artery. Thorac Cardiovasc Surg 87:59, 1984
74. Bharati S, Szarnicki RJ, Popper R et al: Origin of both coronary arteries from the pulmonary trunk associated with hypoplasia of the aortic tract complex: A new entity. J Am Coll Cardiol 3:437, 1984
75. Krause W: Über den Ursprung einer akzessorischen A. coronaria aus der a pulmonalis. Z Rationall Med 24:225, 1865
76. Wenger NK: Rare causes of coronary heart disease. In Hurst JW (ed): The Heart, p 1348. New York, McGraw-Hill, 1978
77. Hobbs RE, Millit HD, Raghavan PV et al: Coronary artery fistulae: A 10-year review. Cleve Clin Q 49:191, 1982
78. Grant RT: Development of cardiac coronary vessels in the rabbit. Heart 13:261, 1926
79. Gobel FL, Anderson CF, Baltaxe HA et al: Shunts between the coronary and pulmonary arteries with normal origin of the coronary arteries. Am J Cardiol 25:655, 1970
80. Levin DC, Fellows KE, Abrams HL: Hemodynamically significant primary anomalies of the coronary arteries. Circulation 58:25, 1978
81. Urrutia-S CO, Falaschi G, Ott DA et al: Surgical management of 56 patients with congenital coronary artery fistulae. Ann Thorac Surg 35:300, 1983
82. Vogelbach K-H, Edmiston WA, Stenson RE: Coronary artery-left ventricular communications: A report of two cases and review of the literature. Cathet Cardiovasc Diag 5:159, 1979
83. Arani DT, Greene DG, Klocke FJ: Coronary artery fistulas emptying into the left heart chambers. Am Heart J 96:438, 1978
84. Wilde P, Watt I: Congenital coronary artery fistulae: Six new cases with a collective review. Clin Radiol 31:301, 1980
85. Björk G, Crafoord C: Arteriovenous aneurysm of the pulmonary artery simulating patent ductus arteriosus Botalli. Thorax 2:65, 1947
86. Yuqing L, Ruping D: Radiologic diagnosis of coronary artery fistula—with emphasis on the evaluation of plain film manifestation. Chin Med J [Engl] 92:589, 1979
87. Yoshikawa J, Katao H, Yanagihara K et al: Noninvasive visualization of the dilated main coronary arteries in coronary artery fistulas by cross-sectional echocardiography. Circulation 65:600, 1982
88. Miyatake K, Okamota M, Kinoshita N et al: Doppler echocardiographic features of coronary arteriovenous fistulae in complementary roles of cross sectional echocardiography and the Doppler technique. Br Heart J 51:508, 1984
89. Rodgers DM, Wolf NM, Barrett MJ et al: Two-dimensional echocardiographic features of coronary arteriovenous fistulae. Am Heart J 104:872, 1982
90. Housman LB, Morse J, Litchford B et al: Left ventricular fistula as a cause of intractable angina pectoris. Successful surgical repair. JAMA 240:372, 1978
91. Yamabe H, Fujitani K, Mizutani T et al: Two cases of myocardial infarction with coronary arteriovenous fistulae. Jpn Heart J 24:303, 1983
92. Meyer MH, Stephenson HE, Ketas TE et al: Coronary artery resection for giant aneurysmal enlargement and arteriovenous fistulae. Am Heart J 74:603, 1967
93. Liberthson RR, Sagar K, Berkoben JP et al: Congenital coronary arteriovenous fistula: Report of 13 patients, review of the literature, and delineation of management. Circulation 59:849, 1979
94. Davidson PH, McCrackan BH, McIlveen JJS: Congenital coronary arteriovenous aneurysm. Br Heart J 17:569, 1955
95. Taber RE, Gale MH, Lam CR: Coronary artery-right heart fistulas. J Thorac Cardiovasc Surg 53:84, 1967
96. Rittenhouse EA, Doty DB, Ehrenhaft JL: Congenital coronary artery-cardiac chamber fistula. Ann Thorac Surg 20:468, 1975
97. Habermann JH, Howard ML, Johnson ES: Rupture of the coronary sinus with hemipericardium. A rare complication of coronary arteriovenous fistula. Circulation 28:1143, 1963
98. Raffer SF, Oetgen WJ, Weeks KD Jr et al: Thallium-201 scintigraphy after surgical repair of hemodynamically significant primary coronary artery anomalies. Chest 81:687, 1982
99. Francis CK, Sacheti CK, Cohen RB: Fistulous communication between the left coronary artery and main pulmonary artery: A thirteen-year follow-up.

Cathet Cardiovasc Diag 5:357, 1979
100. Griffiths SP, Ellis K, Hordof AJ et al: Spontaneous complete closure of a congenital coronary artery fistula. J Am Coll Cardiol 2:1169, 1983
101. Trejo Gutierrez JF, Cecena LE, Abad AZ et al: Fistula arteriovenosa coronaria, estudio de 14 casos. Arch Inst Cardiol Mex 55:153, 1985
102. Lowe JE, Oldham HN Jr, Sabiston DC Jr: Surgical management of congenital coronary artery fistulas. Ann Surg 194:373, 1981
103. Daoud AS, Pankin D, Tulgan H et al: Aneurysms of the coronary artery—report of ten cases and review of the literature. Am J Cardiol 11:228, 1963
104. Sebra-Gomes R, Somerville J, Ross DN et al: Congenital coronary artery aneurysms. Br Heart J 36:329, 1974
105. Lim CH, Tan NC, Tan L et al: Giant congenital aneurysm of the right coronary artery. Am J Cardiol 39:751, 1977
106. Ebert PA, Peter RH, Gunnells JC et al: Resecting and grafting of coronary artery aneurysm. Circulation 43:593, 1971
107. Andersen M, Wennevold A: Aneurysms of the hepatic artery and of the left coronary artery with myocardial infarction: Report of a fatal case in a 14-year-old boy. Scand J Thorac Cardiovas Surg 5:172, 1971
108. Wilson CS, Weaver WF, Zeman ED et al: Bilateral nonfistulous congenital coronary arterial aneurysms. Am J Cardiol 35:319, 1975
109. Ghahrani A, Iyengar R, Cunha D et al: Myocardial infarction due to congenital coronary arterial aneurysm (with successful saphenous vein bypass graft). Am J Cardiol 29:863, 1972
110. Mattern AL, Baker WP, McHale JJ et al: Congenital coronary aneurysms with angina pectoris and myocardial infarction treated with saphenous vein bypass graft. Am J Cardiol 30:906, 1972
111. Gibson R, Nihill MR, Mullins CE et al: Congenital coronary artery obstruction associated with aortic valve anomalies in children: Report of two cases. Circulation 64:857, 1981
112. Josa M, Danielson GK, Weidman WH et al: Congenital ostial membrane of left main coronary artery. J Thorac Cardiovas Surg 81:338, 1981

CYANOTIC CONGENITAL HEART DISEASE

Mary Allen Engle

CHAPTER 100

VOLUME 2

Physical disability and premature death are the lot of the cyanotic person unless the condition can be relieved by surgery and complications prevented or ameliorated by medical measures. If death from hypoxia or cardiac failure does not occur early in infancy, the surviving child or adult can expect the following. Breathlessness and easy fatigue result from exertion-limit activities. Growth rate is usually impaired. Cyanosis and clubbing are cosmetic handicaps, as is scoliosis, which by adolescence is common and is sometimes rapidly progressive. In addition to the risk of infective endocarditis, there is a special hazard of cerebral complication in the form of brain abscess or cerebrovascular thrombosis or embolism. Poor dental structure with defective enamel and dental caries contributes to the risk of brain abscess. Polycythemia is associated with headache and with problems of bleeding or clotting. Some men with breakdown of excess red blood cells have hyperuricemia and suffer gout. If the hypoxic, polycythemic woman is able to become pregnant, she has a greater than average risk that the pregnancy will result in abortion or in a baby with intrauterine growth retardation who may also have congenital heart disease. Cardiac failure or renal impairment is a late consequence of the unrelieved cardiac burden and hypoxia. Sudden death is not an uncommon event in cyanotic patients with Ebstein's anomaly or with pulmonary vascular obstructive disease, or in patients with unstable rhythm or conduction occurring naturally or postoperatively. However, the outlook for these patients has improved during the last several decades.

The year 1985 marked the 40th anniversary of a new way of life for most "blue" babies. In 1945 Drs. Blalock and Taussig reported on an operation that changed Eileen Saxon's color from blue to pink and stopped her suffering from the attacks of paroxysmal dyspnea and deep cyanosis that had characterized her few months of life. This miracle transpired as a result of teamwork that combined the diagnostic acumen of Dr. Helen Taussig and the surgical skill of Dr. Alfred Blalock.[1] These two doctors from Johns Hopkins Hospital had the courage to apply Dr. Taussig's ideas about increasing deficient pulmonary blood flow and Dr. Blalock's experimentally tested technique of vascular anastomoses. Their collaboration led to the development of two interdependent new specialities: pediatric cardiology and cardiovascular surgery. Improvements in diagnostic techniques and in medical and surgical capabilities leapfrogged over the next decades. Teams expanded to include pediatric and medical cardiologists, cardiovascular surgeons, anesthesiologists, radiologists, physiologists, pathologists, pharmacologists, nurse specialists, respiratory therapists, technicians, social workers, and experts in rehabilitation. Centers of excellence concentrated human skills and physical facilities to make optimal care available on a 24-hour-a-day basis. The patients with cyanotic congenital heart disease who have benefited range from the high-risk newborn with critically severe malformation to the older patient who survived into adult life either because of the relatively mild nature of his malformation or as the result of previous palliative surgical intervention.

The state of the art in rendering care to the cyanotic patient has developed to a high level. Palliative procedures to increase[1-4] or to decrease[5] pulmonary blood flow, as the case required, or to improve venous mixing[6,7] or to reroute venous return[8,9] were followed by reparative surgery designed to correct or to relieve the malformation.[10-20] Only a few anomalies are still beyond such help. For the last 15 years, skills in diagnosis and in operative and perioperative management[21,22] allow open heart surgery to be carried out safely even in the neonate.[23,24]

Accomplishments overall have been assessed by evaluation of early and long-term results of management.[25] Dr. Taussig set the example for this by directing attention not only to the expected good results of operation but also to recognition and treatment or prevention of undesirable sequelae or complications.[26,27] Although the great majority of patients enjoy considerable benefit from surgery, only rarely is "total correction" of the malformation a reality.

DIAGNOSTIC CATEGORIES

Cyanotic congenital heart disease can be divided into categories based on the degree of pulmonary blood flow, excessive or deficient, and on the pressure in the pulmonary circuit. In all anomalies in which there is cyanosis, some abnormal communication exists that permits right-to-left shunting at one or more of these levels: atrial, ventricular, or vascular (venous return or arterial outlet). However, it is the status of pulmonary blood flow that to a great extent determines the ability of that person to survive, to function, and to undergo cardiac surgery. The chest film provides valuable information about pulmonary vasculature.

EXCESSIVE PULMONARY BLOOD FLOW

Excessive pulmonary blood flow in the cyanotic person implies that there is both right-to-left and left-to-right shunting. This occurs when the great arteries or the pulmonary veins are transposed or malposed; when there is common mixing because of a single atrium, ventricle, or aorticopulmonary trunk; or when there is hypoplastic left heart syndrome (HLHS).

When a large intracardiac or extracardiac communication exists and the capacity of the pulmonary bed and the left side of the heart is unrestricted and the pulmonary vascular resistance is unusually low, the pulmonary flow may be torrential, increased fourfold or fivefold. The lungs are literally flooded. Such a state is not a steady one. Either death occurs or some adjustments take place that limit the excessive pulmonary flow to a near normal amount or even restrict it so that it is less than normal. These adjustments occur through the development of pulmonary stenosis, pulmonary arterial obstruction, or spontaneous decrease in size or closure of the defect. One or the other of these limiting factors may be present at birth or may develop during the childhood years. Once established, that adaptation may continue stable or may progress. Thus, a condition with no visible cyanosis at birth may convert to a cyanotic one, or a mildly cyanotic condition can become more deeply so through the mechanism of these adaptations. In the overall consideration of cyanotic heart disease in general and of any one patient in particular, this spectrum of changes in the pulmonary flow, pressure, and resistance should be borne in mind.

The ease of bidirectional mixing and the resistance to pulmonary flow (precapillary and postcapillary) determine the volume of pulmonary blood flow, and this in turn affects the degree of cyanosis. When there is no obstruction to flow or to mixing, then the lower the pulmonary resistance, the greater the pulmonary flow in relation to the systemic flow, and the higher the oxyhemoglobin saturation of the admixed blood which reaches the aorta. Such a patient is apt to present in cardiac failure early in infancy and to be only minimally cyanotic. He has hyperkinetic pulmonary hypertension. An infant with complete transposition of the great arteries (CTGA) and a large ventricular septal defect (VSD) typically presents in this way (Fig. 100.1). In contrast, the most deeply cyanotic patients with increased pulmonary blood flow have obstruction to mixing or to pulmonary venous return, or both. Examples are the newborn infant with transposed great arteries and an otherwise normal heart (Fig. 100.2) or the infant with obstructed anomalously draining pulmonary veins and a small, patent foramen ovale (PFO).

In anomalies with increased pulmonary flow, pulmonary arterial pressure is elevated. The presence of either pulmonary stenosis or of pulmonary vascular obstruction of slight to moderate degree lessens somewhat the excessive pulmonary flow. Increasing amounts of pulmonary stenosis or of vascular obstruction convert this anomaly into a situation with deficient pulmonary flow, the second category to be discussed below.

DEFICIENT PULMONARY BLOOD FLOW

Deficient pulmonary blood flow in the cyanotic patient signifies impairment of flow to or through the lungs.

WITHOUT PULMONARY HYPERTENSION

When flow *into* the lungs is interfered with, the precapillary pulmonary arterial pressure is normal or less than normal. Usually obstruction to pulmonary flow is in the form of pulmonary stenosis or atresia. However, sometimes the obstruction is more proximal in the heart in the form of tricuspid stenosis, atresia, or insufficiency. Rarely the pulmonary circuit is bypassed by anomalous drainage of caval blood into the left atrium[28] or by a pulmonary arteriovenous fistula.[29]

The most common malformation in this group, at all ages, is the tetralogy of Fallot (Fig. 100.3). Severe pulmonary stenosis or atresia

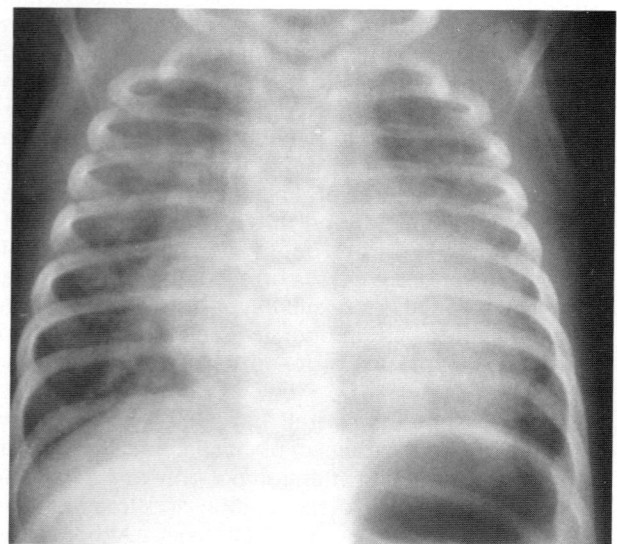

FIGURE 100.1 CTGA with large VSD. Cardiomegaly and increased pulmonary arterial markings in a minimally cyanotic 3-month old boy in cardiac failure. His auscultatory findings of holosystolic murmur at the lower left sternal border indicated that he had a VSD. The absence of a convex main pulmonary artery in the presence of increased pulmonary blood flow suggested that the pulmonary artery was misplaced and perhaps, therefore, transposed. Echocardiography and cardiac catheterization confirmed the diagnoses of large VSD and CTGA.

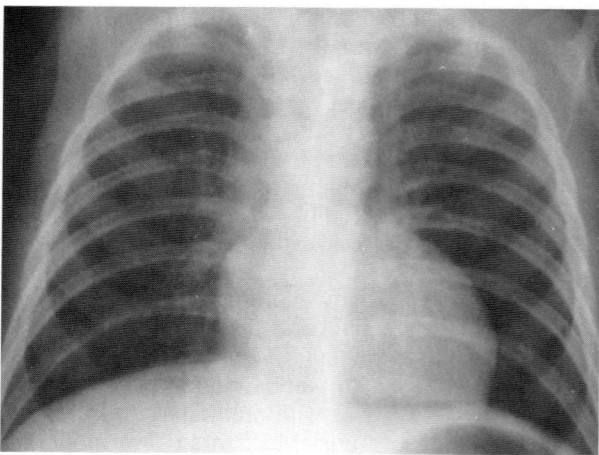

FIGURE 100.2 CTGA without other anomalies. This chest film is from a newborn infant with deep cyanosis and tachypnea but no heart murmur. Note the slight cardiomegaly, narrow base of the heart, and dense hilar markings. The concavity in the region of the main pulmonary artery is due to displacement of the pulmonary artery, which is transposed. Early recognition of this condition in the first hours of life permits treatment before hypoxia, acidosis, and cardiac failure occur.

coexists with a large, high, saddle-shaped VSD. Right ventricular (RV) hypertrophy follows as a consequence of these two abnormalities. Overriding of the aorta results from its unprotected position above the VSD. Some conditions with shunting at the ventricular level mimic a tetralogy. In these, severe pulmonary stenosis or atresia is present together with a single ventricle, atrioventricular septal defect, VSD with a double-outlet right ventricle (DORV), or with transposed great arteries. Other conditions with cyanosis and decreased pulmonary flow are less likely to be confused with tetralogy. These include severe pulmonic stenosis or atresia with intact ventricular septum (Fig. 100.4) and PFO or atrial septal defect (ASD); rudimentary RV with tricuspid and pulmonic stenosis or atresia (Fig. 100.5); and Ebstein's anomaly of tricuspid valve with PFO or ASD.

WITH PULMONARY HYPERTENSION AT THE SYSTEMIC LEVEL

In deficient pulmonary blood flow with pulmonary hypertension there is obstruction to flow *through* the lungs, and the pulmonary hypertension is due to pulmonary vascular obstruction. This obstruction is usually in the precapillary bed, in the arterioles and pulmonary arteries. Distal to the capillaries, obstruction in the form of stenosis of pulmonary veins or within the left atrium can occur. Pathologically, changes of graded severity are present in the intima, media, and adventitia of small pulmonary arteries and, as the obstructive–obliterative process worsens, in the larger pulmonary vessels as well.[30,31] The term "Eisenmenger syndrome" encompasses those malformations with intracardiac or extracardiac communication between the two circulations and

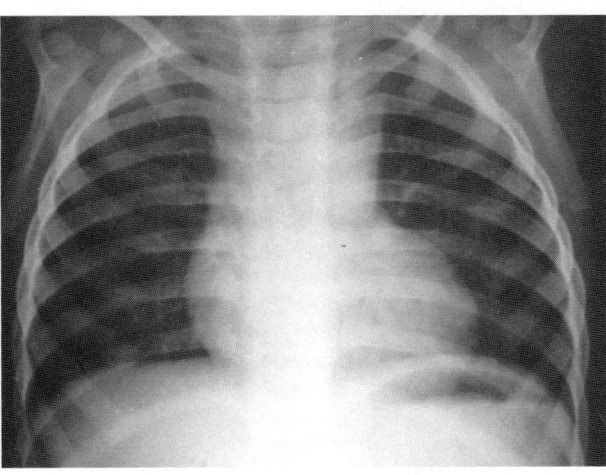

FIGURE 100.3 Tetralogy of Fallot. Roentgenogram shows average-sized, boot-shaped heart with concave main pulmonary artery segment and scant pulmonary arterial markings. The base of the heart is not narrow, a feature in a cyanotic newborn that distinguishes tetralogy from CTGA.

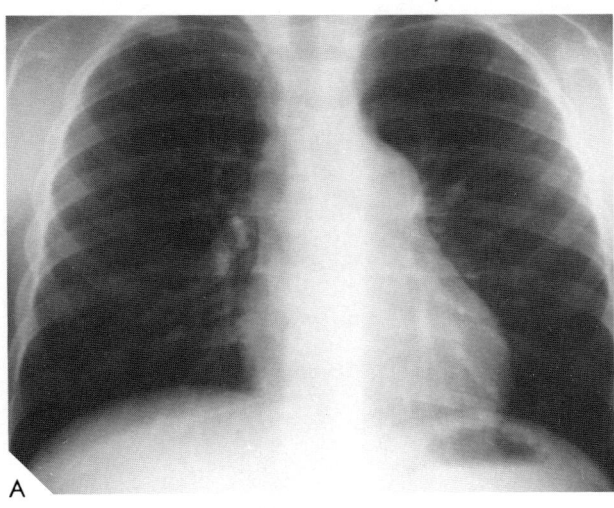
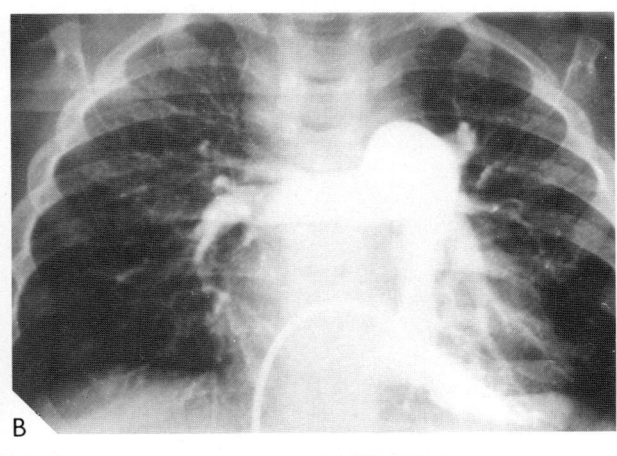
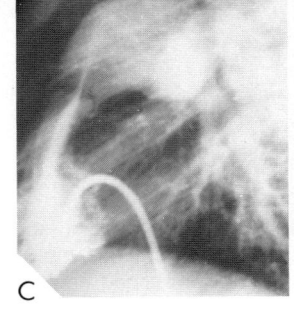
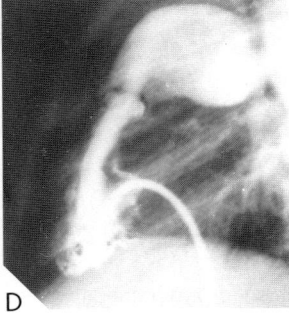

FIGURE 100.4 Valvular pulmonic stenosis with PFO. **A.** Roentgenogram shows average-sized heart with prominent, convex main pulmonary artery. Pulmonary arteries are visible in the hilar regions but are sparse in the middle and outer thirds of the lung fields. **B.** Selective right ventricular angiocardiogram opacifies the right ventricle with hypertrophied walls and the main pulmonary artery and branches. The poststenotic dilatation of the main pulmonary artery accounts for the convex prominence of the left heart border on roentgenogram (**A**). **C** and **D** are lateral films that show (**C**) the narrow jet through the central small orifice of the radiolucent, thickened, stenotic pulmonary valve. In **D** the column of blood traversing the narrow opening has widened. Poststenotic dilatation is evident on lateral views, as well as frontal. There is very little evidence in early systole (**C**) or late systole (**D**) of accompanying infundibular hypertrophy.

resistance to pulmonary blood flow that is equal to, or in excess of, systemic vascular resistance. Within the heart, the shunt site originally described by Eisenmenger was a VSD, but right-to-left shunting in the presence of high pulmonary vascular resistance can also occur with absence of the ventricular septum or through connections at the atrial level through a PFO or ASD (Fig. 100.6). At the aorticopulmonary level, the shunt sites include truncus arteriosus, aorticopulmonary window, and patent ductus arteriosus. In all of these situations except the last, cyanosis is of equal distribution over the body. However, when shunt reversal occurs through a patent ductus arteriosus distal to the left subclavian artery, venous blood preferentially enters the descending aorta and there is differential cyanosis of the toes and lower part of the body in comparison with the face and fingers.

METHODS OF DIAGNOSIS

Accurate diagnosis is based on a synthesis of details from informative, noninvasive techniques and from cardiac catheterization with contrast visualization. The cyanotic patient may need this full diagnostic evaluation in anticipation of surgery, and often it is used as well in the analysis of postoperative results. Usually cardiac catheterization is repeated no more than once after operation, whereas the noninvasive diagnostic

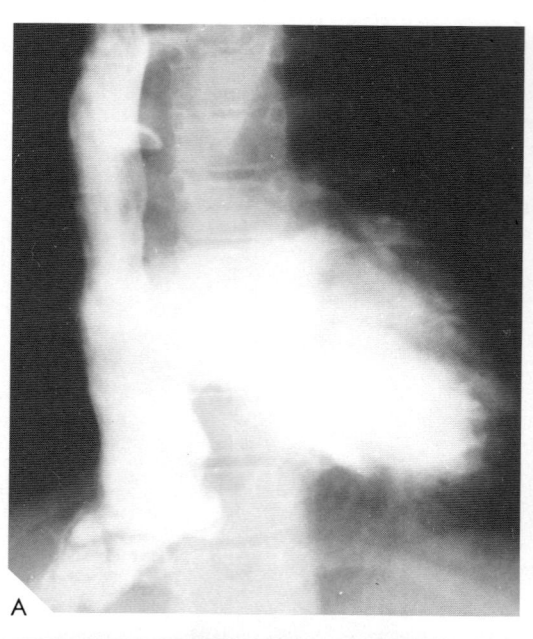
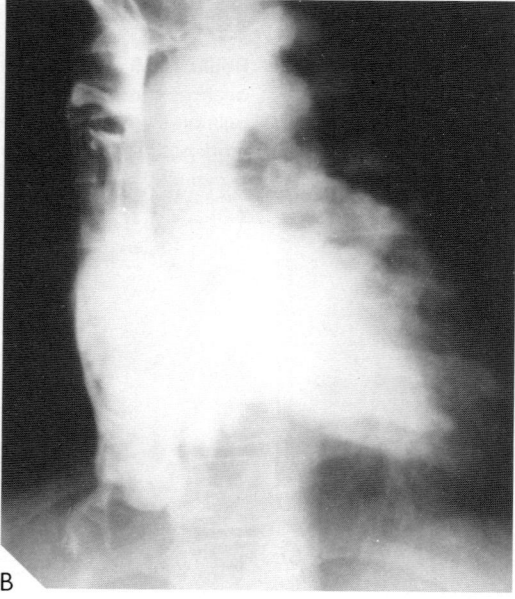

FIGURE 100.5 Tricuspid atresia with rudimentary right ventricle and left Blalock–Taussig anastomosis. Digital subtraction angiocardiogram from right cephalic vein shows the physiology and anatomy of tricuspid atresia early in sequence (**A**) and later (**B**). In **A**, contrast medium in superior vena cava refluxes into the dilated inferior vena cava, and the combined caval blood enters the right atrium and crosses immediately through an atrial septal defect to the left atrium and left ventricle. In **B** the ascending aorta fills next and arches to the left. The left subclavian artery (*arrow*) has been turned down and anastomosed to the left pulmonary artery, which opacifies faintly. Rudimentary right ventricle is not seen clearly in these films.

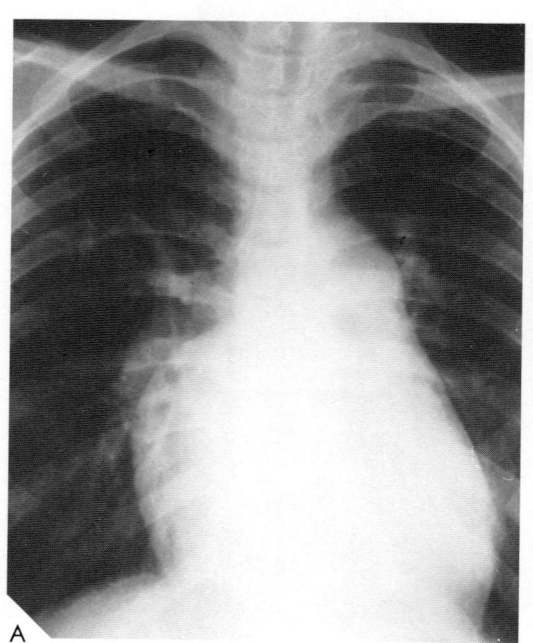
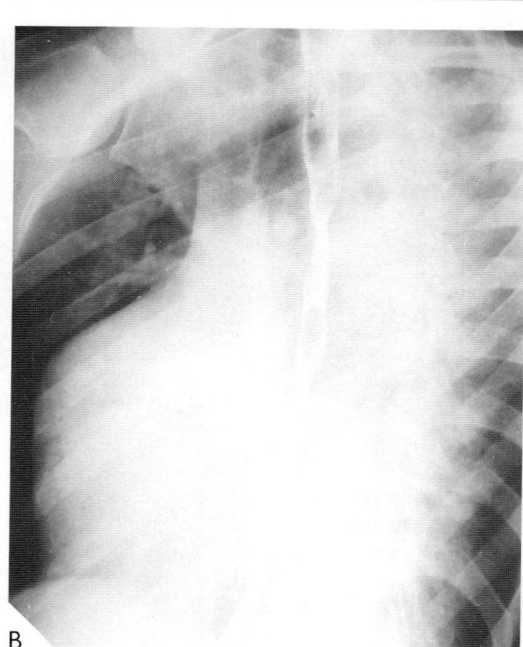
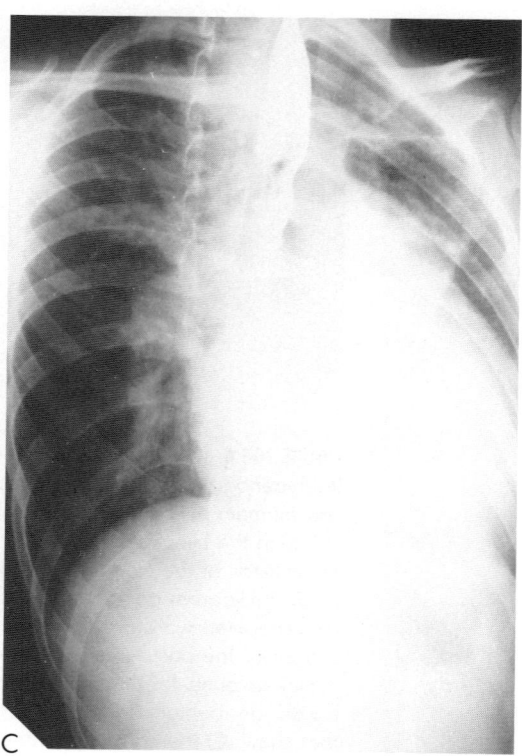

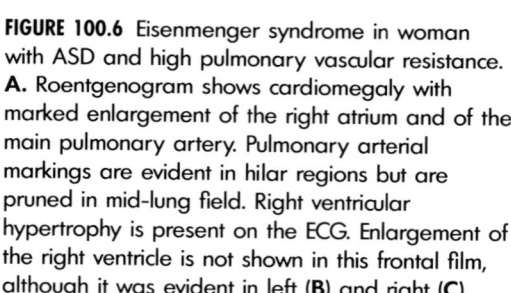

FIGURE 100.6 Eisenmenger syndrome in woman with ASD and high pulmonary vascular resistance. **A.** Roentgenogram shows cardiomegaly with marked enlargement of the right atrium and of the main pulmonary artery. Pulmonary arterial markings are evident in hilar regions but are pruned in mid-lung field. Right ventricular hypertrophy is present on the ECG. Enlargement of the right ventricle is not shown in this frontal film, although it was evident in left (**B**) and right (**C**) anterior-oblique views. Barium swallow shows left aortic arch and no evidence of left atrial enlargement. **B.** Left anterior-oblique view shows marked anterior enlargement of the heart due to increased size of the right atrium and ventricle. Normal esophagram. **C.** Right anterior-oblique view shows enlargement of the anterior (right) ventricle. Normal esophagram shows no evidence of left atrial enlargement.

studies are useful in life-long follow-up. Such long-term follow-up is advisable, not only for the benefit of that individual patient but also as a means of continually improving methods of care.

NONINVASIVE STUDIES

The least invasive study is the history, including family history of congenital heart disease. The mother's health during pregnancy is usually described as "fine." Cyanosis at birth that does not clear in a few hours raises the suspicion of cyanotic congenital heart disease and calls for transfer to a pediatric cardiac center for diagnosis and treatment. If the blue baby who is a few months old has trouble with feedings because he gets tired and short of breath and he breathes rapidly even at rest, one suspects that cardiac failure is developing. If his breathing is easy at rest but he has episodes on slight provocation of deep cyanosis, labored respirations, and great anxiety, he is probably having a "tet spell," an attack of paroxysmal dyspnea in a baby with tetralogy of Fallot or similar physiology. During such a spell, infundibular spasm seems to occur, and when one listens with a stethoscope, the murmur of pulmonic stenosis has disappeared. The mother usually finds that putting the baby on her shoulder in a knee-chest position comforts him. The toddler and young child spontaneously assume a knee-chest position when they squat to rest. Cardiac failure does not occur in patients with simple tetralogy of Fallot or single ventricle with severe pulmonic stenosis; therefore, a history of treatment for cardiac failure directs one's attention to a different category of cyanotic congenital heart disease.

To the time-honored noninvasive techniques of history, physical examination, electrocardiogram (ECG), and cardiac series of chest roentgenograms has been added the especially valuable tool of echocardiography. Recording of the M-mode and two-dimensional (2-D) sound beam as it is reflected from cardiac chambers, valve, arterial roots, and the ventricular septum has provided a new dimension and refinement to judging cardiac structure and function. Addition of continuous and pulsed-wave Doppler methodology helps to estimate flows and pressures. Just as the correlation of phonocardiography with findings at cardiac catheterization and angiocardiography strengthened the accuracy of the physician's interpretation of heart sounds and murmurs, so does the correlation of echocardiography and angiocardiography enhance the accuracy of auscultatory, ECG, and roentgenographic interpretation. Specific questions, such as that of aortic–mitral valve continuity, presence or absence of the ventricular septum, or septal–aortic continuity, can often be answered using ultrasound. Other frequently used diagnostic techniques in the evaluation of the cyanotic patient are continuous ECG monitoring for disturbance of rhythm and conduction, and standardized tests of exercise function to assess physical performance. In older children and adults, radionuclide cineangiocardiography is useful for left and right ventricular function and aortic regurgitation.[32] In some circumstances, right-to-left or left-to-right shunt can also be detected. Magnetic resonance imaging[33] is one of the newest diagnostic techniques to show cardiac anatomy and flow through shunts and conduits.

INVASIVE TECHNIQUES

Invasive techniques of cardiac catheterization with contrast visualization utilizing biplane cineangiocardiograms or cut film in simultaneous biplane standard and angled projections affords detailed analysis of shunt site and size, as well as the other abnormalities that are associated with, or a consequence of, that particular cyanotic patient's anomaly (Figs. 100.4, 100.7, 100.8). Ventricular performance is evaluated at the same study. Recording of His bundle electrograms and electrical pacing permit analysis of disturbed cardiac rhythm and conduction, which may be abnormal as part of the anomaly (*e.g.*, in "corrected" transposition with ventricular inversion) or as a result of surgery.

Digital subtraction angiocardiography[34] is a minimally invasive diagnostic study that reduces both radiation to the patient and the dose of contrast medium used. A mask of the unopacified heart is made and subtracted electronically from the image recorded after contrast medium has been injected into a peripheral vein or a vessel nearer the heart or a cardiac chamber or artery. Images of diagnostic quality are obtained.

In the operating room, electrophysiologic mapping of the conduction system and echocardiography are sometimes called on as diagnostic tools. Lung biopsy may be needed for evaluation of the pulmonary vascular bed in patients with pulmonary hypertension.

STEPS IN DIAGNOSIS
PRELIMINARY CLASSIFICATION

A systematic approach to diagnosis and differential diagnosis of the cyanotic patient begins with the history plus findings on physical examination and addition of clues from selected studies until certain possibilities are eliminated and a most likely diagnosis is reached and defined so that appropriate management can follow.

The next step is to identify cardiac and visceral situs by physical examination, roentgenogram, ECG, and echocardiogram. In the normal situation (situs solitus), the cardiac apex and stomach are on the left, and the liver, inferior vena cava, and right atrium are on the right. The reverse situation is situs inversus with dextrocardia. Cyanotic anomalies in these two situations tend to be more straightforward and therefore easier to analyze than when there is discordance of cardiac position and abdominal viscera: levocardia with situs inversus, mesocardia with situs solitus or inversus, dextrocardia with situs solitus, or malposition with visceral heterotaxy (scrambled relation of viscera). In those situations, anomalies of systemic and pulmonary venous return, defective or absent cardiac septa, and transposed arteries are common. Associated conditions of splenic agenesis (bilateral right-sidedness) or of polysplenia (bilateral left-sidedness) should be suspected.

If the heart is in the right side of the chest (dextrocardia), one must determine whether that position is due to cardiac displacement, to rotation (dextroversion), or to inversion of cardiac chambers (mirror-image dextrocardia). The form of the P wave in lead 1 of the ECG is a help here: if there is normal sinus mechanism, upright P indicates that the right atrium is on the right side; the heart is dextrorotated. Inverted P indicates inversion of the atria with the anatomical right atrium on the left. If there is a changing P-wave pattern or if the P wave is biphasic or of other unusual contour, then the pacemaker is ectopic and further analysis of atrial situs cannot be made from the ECG.

When visceroatrial situs has been determined, the ECG assumes additional diagnostic value in evaluation of cardiac chambers affected by the anomaly. Most cyanotic malformations are associated with hypertrophy of the RV. When the RV is concentrically hypertrophied (RVH) without dilatation and RV systolic pressure is at a systemic level (as in tetralogy of Fallot), the ECG shows right-axis deviation and R-S reversal in V leads. When RV pressure is greater than systemic, R wave voltage increases to more than 10 mm in V, ST segments become depressed, and T waves are deeply inverted in right precordial leads (RV "strain").[35] For the pressure to be greater in the right than in the left ventricle, the ventricular septum must be intact or a VSD is restrictive. Pure severe pulmonic stenosis with intact ventricular septum and PFO is the leading diagnostic possibility when RV strain is found. The next most likely diagnosis is primary pulmonary hypertension with PFO. Conduction delay over the RV or incomplete or complete right bundle branch block (IRBBB or CRBBB) suggests in the unoperated patient that the volume of the RV is increased, as in Ebstein's anomaly of the tricuspid valve or in total anomalous pulmonary venous return (TAPVR).

In the newborn, absence of the expected RV forces implies that the RV is rudimentary. Left ventricular hypertrophy (LVH) indicates that the LV has a pressure or volume load that is greater than normal. Inversion of T waves in V_5 and V_6 in the undigitalized patient is referred to as LV "strain," a more serious degree of LV overburden. Wide-notched P waves signify left atrial abnormality, whereas high, peaked waves indicate right atrial hypertrophy.

Acceleration or prolongation of atrioventricular conduction has specific significance. For instance, Wolff–Parkinson–White syndrome occurs not uncommonly in Ebstein's anomaly. High-grade or complete heart block is rare in the cyanotic patient unless he has "corrected" transposition of the great arteries. The mean electrical axis is usually to the right with pure RVH. Left-axis deviation is associated with lack of development of the RV or with a single ventricle. A superior axis (around −90°) suggests an atrioventricular septal defect.

With the questions of visceroatrial situs and of cardiac conduction and hypertrophy settled, it is time to classify the patient according to pulmonary blood flow and pressure. The intensity and timing of the pulmonic closure component of the second heart sound offer the best way to judge presence or absence of pulmonary hypertension, while the best guide to status of pulmonary blood flow is a well-penetrated chest roentgenogram (see Figs. 100.1 through 100.4, 100.6).

In the frontal film, attention is paid to the contour of the main pulmonary artery, as well as to the main branches in the hilar area and to the degree of vascularity in the middle and outer thirds of the lung fields. Concavity in the region of the main pulmonary artery means that the artery is hypoplastic (as in severe tetralogy, see Fig. 100.3), absent (as in pulmonary atresia), or misplaced (as in transposition, see Figs. 100.1 and 100.2, or in truncus arteriosus). Prominent convexity of the main pulmonary artery may be due either to poststenotic dilatation distal to valvular pulmonic stenosis (see Fig. 100.4) or to the opposite situation in which there is increased flow or pressure in the main pulmonary artery (see Fig. 100.6).

Perusal of the hilar regions and the rest of the lung fields helps to decide which of these situations prevails. Enlarged pulmonary arterial markings in the hilar areas and mid-lung fields that extend to the outer third are seen with increased pulmonary arterial flow (see Fig. 100.1), while with pulmonary vascular obstruction, the right and left pulmonary arteries appear cut off in mid-lung field, and the periphery is clear (see Fig. 100.6). Stippled, punctate markings radiating from the hilar regions suggest that pulmonary venous return is obstructed, whereas a hazy perihilar appearance of fluffy areas suggests pulmonary edema. In the cyanotic infant in heart failure, such edema may be localized to the right upper lobe. Kerley B lines above the diaphragm signifying lymphatic and pulmonary venous congestion are present less often in the infant or child with pulmonary venous hypertension than they are in the adolescent and adult.

Small pulmonary artery branches in the hilar regions and unusually radiolucent lung fields are evidence of impairment to blood flow *into* the lungs and hence indicate pulmonary stenosis or atresia (see Fig. 100.3). When hilar pulmonary arterial markings are scant or absent but a lacy appearance of small vessels is seen in the lung fields, one thinks

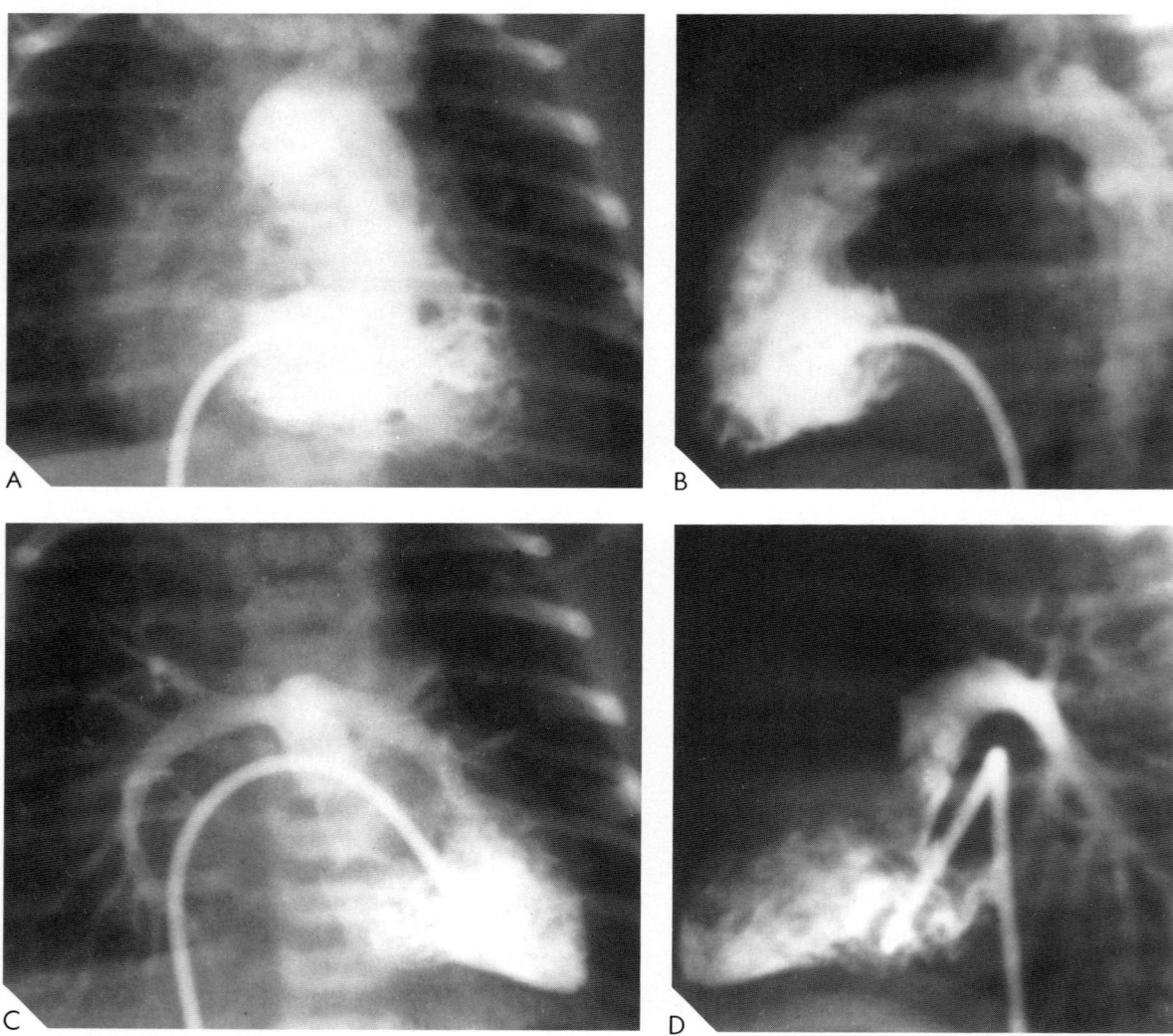

FIGURE 100.7 Complete d-transposition of the great arteries. Selective angiocardiograms in frontal and simultaneous lateral views on left and right with injection into right ventricle (**above, A** and **B**) and left ventricle (**below, C** and **D**). From the right ventricle the transposed anterior aorta fills. From the left ventricle the posteriorly transposed pulmonary artery fills. Some contrast medium refluxes into the left atrium. Through a small VSD, a faint shunt of opacified blood enters the right ventricle and the transposed aorta.

of pulmonary atresia and collateral circulation to the lungs from the systemic circulation. Barium swallow often confirms the presence of these vessels as they leave the anterior part of the descending aorta and indent the esophagus forward as they enter the lung fields to merge with pulmonary arteries.

On the cardiac series of chest roentgenograms, one also obtains information concerning overall heart size, specific cardiac chamber enlargement, and aortic size. With barium swallow in each view, one can tell whether the aorta arches to the right, as it does in about 25% of patients with tetralogy or truncus (see Fig. 100.8), or normally to the left, where it descends, and whether there are retroesophageal vessels. Displacement of the barium-filled esophagus by an enlarged left atrium does not often occur in the cyanotic patient. If present, this finding suggests abnormality of the left atrioventricular valve or excessive pulmonary blood flow and venous return, just as in the noncyanotic person.

Correlating this information, we can place the cyanotic patient into one of the two main diagnostic categories: high pulmonary flow or low flow. In the latter situation, we need to distinguish low pressure and resistance from high resistance. Then we proceed further to refine the diagnosis.

DIFFERENTIAL AND DEFINITIVE DIAGNOSIS

Table 100.1 summarizes some of the noninvasive techniques and the information that assists the physician in making the differential diagnosis of the cyanotic anomalies.

EXCESSIVE PULMONARY BLOOD FLOW

CHARACTERISTICS. Physical examination of the cyanotic infant with increased pulmonary blood flow reveals a tachypneic infant who may be in respiratory distress and cardiac failure. The volume-overloaded heart is enlarged and overly active. Children who survive this period usually show grooving of the rib cage at the level of the diaphragm as a sequel of chronic respiratory effort. A precordial bulge is due to underlying ventricular enlargement. It is rare to find a cyanotic adult who still has a large left-to-right shunt. Most have converted to the Eisenmenger syndrome by late adolescence or early adulthood. Anomalous unobstructed pulmonary venous return is the most likely diagnosis if a cyanotic adult has increased pulmonary blood flow.

Since some pulmonary hypertension is present with excessive pulmonary flow, the pulmonic component of the second sound is accentuated and often occurs early so that S_2 is narrowly split. When the great arteries are transposed or there is a truncus arteriosus, the loud second sound at the second left interspace is the aortic or truncus closure sound. In these anomalies, the systolic cardiac murmur is most often due to an associated VSD or to excess flow across the pulmonary outflow tract. An early diastolic murmur at the base is heard when a semilunar valve is incompetent, for instance in truncus valve regurgitation or pulmonary hypertension with pulmonic valve insufficiency.

The ECG usually reflects both pressure and volume overload of the RV and shows right-axis deviation with RV hypertrophy and intraventricular conduction delay.

Roentgenograms show pulmonary arterial congestion and cardiomegaly. Particular attention is paid to the base of the heart, which is deformed by the abnormal arterial or venous trunks. In the newborn, for instance, a narrow basal shadow in frontal view (see Fig. 100.2) that widens to double that size in the right anterior oblique view is almost pathognomonic of complete d-transposition of the great arteries. A big vascular collar at the base of the heart on both sides is caused by anomalous drainage of the pulmonary veins to a left vertical vein and so around to the dilated right superior vena cava and right atrium ("figure of eight," "snowman," or "cottage loaf" sign). If the dilatation involves only the superior vena cava on the right, one suspects that vessel as the point of entry of the pulmonary veins. Abnormally wide aortic shadow in all views suggests a truncus.

Echocardiographic analysis together with cardiac catheterization and selective injection of contrast medium serves to define the often complex anatomy and hemodynamics of these cyanotic patients with bidirectional shunting.

SPECIFIC MALFORMATIONS. In the newborn, the most common anomaly in this category is complete d-transposition of the great arteries, wherein the systemic and pulmonic circuits are independent because the great arteries arise from the wrong ventricles (see Fig. 100.7). Survival depends on some shunt mechanism for mixing of ox-

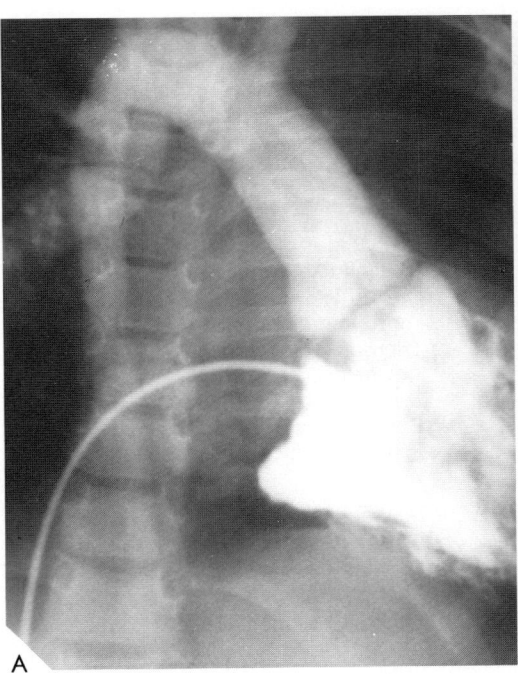
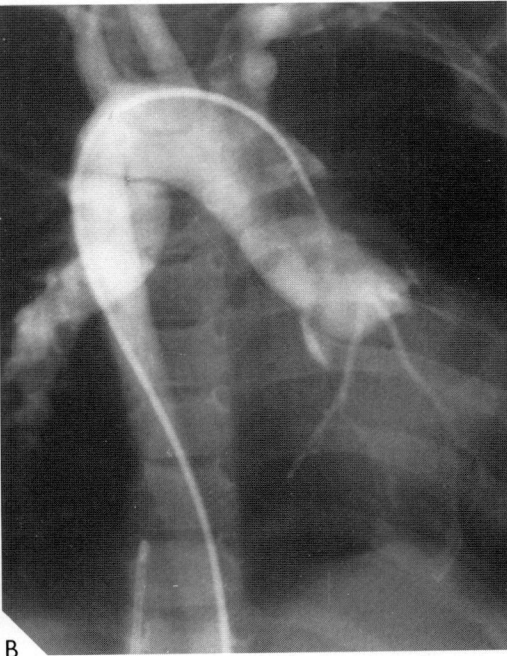
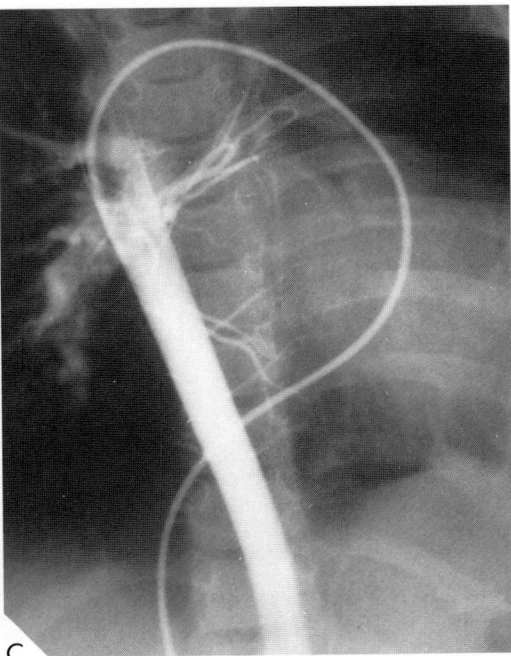

FIGURE 100.8 Truncus arteriosus and single ventricle. **A.** Ventricular injection shows the right aortic arch and the descending aorta with an anomalous vessel coursing from the region of the transverse arch into the right lung field. **B.** Selective injection into the base of the aorta (truncus) identifies more clearly the anomalous vessel, which takes the course of a right pulmonary artery. **C.** Opacification of the right descending aorta shows opacification of the vessel entering the lower portion of the right lung.

ygenated and desaturated blood. Blood that is directed to the lungs tends to be "trapped" in the left heart–pulmonary circuit so that pulmonary flow comes to exceed systemic flow, and both pulmonary arterial and venous pressures are elevated. Usually the newborn's heart is otherwise normal, with only a PFO and patent ductus; thus, little mixing of the circuits occurs. The infant is deeply cyanotic, tachypneic, soon acidotic, and unlikely to survive beyond the first few hours or days. However, if there is a VSD large enough to equalize the systolic pressure in the right and left ventricles and to permit unobstructed mixing of venous and arterial blood, the effect of the disproportionately large volume that circulates through the lungs and is oxygenated is to minimize or even obscure the cyanosis. Such a baby often leaves the newborn nursery unrecognized, only to return in a few weeks in cardiac failure (see Fig. 100.1).

Other transposition complexes that fall into this cyanotic group of anomalies with increased pulmonary flow and streaming of some unoxygenated blood into the aorta include "corrected" or l-transposition (when the aorta is anterior and to the left of the pulmonary artery and the ventricles and their atrioventricular valves are inverted) with overriding aorta and the types of double-outlet right ventricle (DORV) and double outlet left ventricle (DOLV). The Taussig–Bing[36,37] anomaly is a form of DORV with the VSD in relation to the pulmonary artery, which then receives oxygenated blood streaming from the LV and has a higher oxygen concentration than the aorta. With DORV, the VSD may be infracristal, intracristal, or supracristal, may be muscular, or may be multiple, while the great arteries may have their normal anteroposterior relation, be side to side, or in a position of d- or l-transposition. The functional result of these various arrangements may be similar, with cyanosis and increased pulmonary flow, but the defined anatomy makes a considerable difference in expectation of favorable result of surgery.

No one of these unusual transpositional complexes nor the conditions to be discussed below (truncus arteriosus, single ventricle) is common. But they are of uncommon interest because of the challenge they pose for understanding the anatomy and function and for planning surgical repair. In each of them, the pulmonary artery and the aorta, if unobstructed, have the same pressure. Unless some degree of pulmonic stenosis exists, pulmonary vascular resistance is likely to be

TABLE 100.1 NONINVASIVE TECHNIQUES IN DIFFERENTIAL DIAGNOSIS OF COMMON CYANOTIC CONGENITAL ANOMALIES

Anomaly	S_2P	ECG	Roentgenogram C/T	MPA	PULM VASC	Other	Echo Confirmation
Excessive Pulmonary Flow							
CTGA	↑	RAD, RVH	↑	Concave	↑	Narrow base, frontal wide base, RAO	Aortic root anterior to PA; two simultaneous roots, long axis
TAPVR	↑	RAD, RAE, RVCD	↑	Convex	↑	Vascular collar if drains to SVC or left vertical vein	Lack of pulmonary veins entering LA
Common atrium	↑	RVH, RAD or	↑	Convex	↑		Absence of atrial septum
Ventricle	↑	Variable	↑	Variable	↑		Absence of ventricular septum
Truncus	↑	CVH, RVH, or LVH	↑	Variable	↑		One trunk above VSD or single ventricle
Deficient Pulmonary Flow							
Without Pulmonary Hypertension							
Tetralogy	↓	RAD, RVH	N	Concave	↓	Boot-shaped heart	High VSD. Overriding aorta, larger than PA. Narrow RV outflow tract.
Tet-like*	↓	RAD, RVH	N	Concave	↓		Depends on individual anomaly
PS with intact ventricular septum and PFO, ASD	↓	RVS	N or ↑	Convex	↓		Hypertrophy RV wall and septum. P valve sometimes thick, immobile. Contrast echo RA → LA.
Tricuspid atresia or stenosis	↓	LAD, LVD	N	Concave	↓		Absence of tricuspid valve echo. Small RV; average MPA. Contrast echo RA → LA. VSD by echo dropout or Doppler.
Ebstein's anomaly	↓	RAD, low voltage, RVCD	N or ↑	Concave	↓	RAE	Tricuspid valve distal in RV. Dilated proximal RV. Contrast echo RA → LA.
Pulmonary AV fistula	N or ↓	RAD, RVH	N or ↑	Convex	↓		Contrast echo PA → LA. Image of fistula or dilated veins by LA.
With Pulmonary Hypertension at Systemic Level							
Eisenmenger syndrome (PVO & ASD, VSD, or A-P connection)	↓	RAD, RVH	N or ↓	Convex	↓	In outer lung fields	Systolic time intervals. Hypertension pulmonary trunk. Hypertension RV. Contrast echo R → L through communication.

S_2P, second heart sound, pulmonic component; ECG, electrocardiogram; C/T, cardiothoracic ratio; MPA, main pulmonary artery; PULM VASC, pulmonary vascularity; CTGA, complete transposition of great arteries; RAD, right-axis deviation; RVH, right ventricular hypertrophy; RAO, right anterior-oblique view; PA, pulmonary artery; TAPVR, total anomalous pulmonary venous return; RAE, right atrial enlargement; RVCD, right ventricular conduction delay; SVC, superior vena cava; LA, left atrium; CVH, combined ventricular hypertrophy; LVH, left ventricular hypertrophy; VSD, ventricular septal defect; PFO, patent foramen ovale; RA, right atrium; ASD, atrial septal defect; RVS, right ventricular strain; RV, right ventricle (ventricular); LAD, left-axis deviation; LVD, left ventricular dominance; PVO, pulmonary vascular obstruction; A-P, aortico-pulmonary connection; ↑, increased; ↓, decreased; N, normal.

70% or more of systemic resistance by early childhood. This is an unfavorable situation for undertaking surgery, since elevated pulmonary vascular resistance is unlikely to decline and is apt to continue to rise even after surgical repair.

Classification of *truncus arteriosus* into four types, based on point of origin of the pulmonary arteries, assumed practical significance when it became possible in some carefully selected patients to remove the pulmonary arteries from the truncus and anastomose them to the distal end of a valved conduit.[16] The proximal end of the conduit, sewn into the outflow tract of the RV, creates a new pulmonary outflow tract. The VSD is closed with a patch so that LV blood exits through the truncus valve into the aorta, which has been oversewn where the pulmonary arteries had arisen. The types of truncus are identified by selective injections of contrast medium into the truncus just above the valve or selectively into the vessels as they leave the ascending or descending arches of the truncus (see Fig. 100.8).[38]

Type I truncus, in which the common pulmonary trunk exits from the lateral aspect of the trunk near the truncus valve, is more common than the other types and lends itself more easily to repair. In type II, there is separate take off of right and left pulmonary arteries from the posterior aspect of the ascending trunk; they are not in continuity. Type III is more complicated, since the pulmonary arteries arise from the lateral aspects of the ascending aorta or from brachiocephalic arteries or a ductus-like structure from the transverse arch (see Fig. 100.8). Type IV truncus resembles the condition of pseudotruncus arteriosus, a variant of tetralogy of Fallot. In both, the lung vessels derive from systemic arteries leaving the descending aorta, but in type IV truncus, no remnant of pulmonary arteries is found.

Some patients have unusual vascular arrangements that do not fit neatly into this classification but are atypical or hybrids. Pulmonary vascular supply to the two lungs may be different; the vessels to one lung may not connect with the other; there may be only a single pulmonary artery. Edwards and McGoon considered these many variations and reclassified the condition in which there is "absence of anatomic origin from the heart of the pulmonary arterial supply."[39] That reclassification has clinical significance for repair. Of 262 such patients, 64% had confluence of right and left pulmonary arteries, 3% had nonconfluence, 24% had no pulmonary arteries, and 9% had unilateral absence of a pulmonary artery.[40]

At the time of study it is important when considering surgery to determine not only pulmonary resistance and flow, the points of origin of the pulmonary arteries and their continuity or discontinuity with one another, but also to identify where the truncus arises in relation to the RV or LV, the presence of a ventricular septum and size of the defect, and the question of truncus valve insufficiency or stenosis, and the origins of the coronary arteries.

Definition of the type of *single ventricle* has assumed practical significance with the early success of the Fontan procedure[17] or of placing a synthetic septum in selected patients.[18] The most common type of single ventricle is that with two atria and inversion of the atrioventricular valves, which communicate with one ventricle that is an inverted LV with an outlet chamber that resembles a RV infundibulum or conus. The great arteries are usually in l-transposition relationship but may be d-transposed, side by side, or in the normal relationship. Obstruction to flow may occur at an atrioventricular valve, within the ventricle at the bulboventricular foramen leading to the outlet chamber, in the valves, or in the great arteries themselves. There may be a common truncus (see Fig. 100.8). Each of these possibilities must be carefully evaluated in diagnosis of the patient with a single ventricle.

Common atrium is even more unusual. It is sometimes found in patients with Ellis–van Creveld syndrome. The patient's clinical findings may mimic those of an ASD, except for mild cyanosis and superior axis and an ectopic atrial pacemaker on the ECG. The echocardiogram is diagnostic because of the absence of septal echoes. Structure and function of the atrioventricular valves and presence of pulmonary hypertension are evaluated at this study. Determination of systemic venous return (by catheterization from the left arm as well as from the leg) and of pulmonary venous drainage (by selective injection into the pulmonary artery) is needed in planning repair.

TAPVR is another uncommon condition that is amenable to surgery.[15] Its rarity is indicated by Rowe's report that it occurred once in 6825 live births surveyed in Auckland, New Zealand.[41] The anomaly constituted 1% of the autopsied specimens from newborns with congenital heart disease at Johns Hopkins.[41] Mitchell did not list the malformation in the report of a cooperative, prospective study of the outcome of 56,109 births in 12 centers in the United States with an incidence of congenital heart disease of 0.814%.[42] Fyler reported a 2% incidence of this anomaly in the critically ill infants in the first month of life in the New England Regional Infant Cardiac Program, in which the emphasis was on detection and treatment of the sick newborn with heart disease.[43] Lack of obstruction to the anomalously draining pulmonary veins favors survival beyond the age of one year. Then the condition is much more benign and resembles a simple ASD in its manifestations and suitability for surgery.

Darling and co-workers divided the anomalies of drainage of all the pulmonary veins according to their point of juncture with the right atrium or a tributary thereof.[44] In decreasing order of frequency, there are four groups: supracardiac, cardiac, infracardiac, and mixed. Echocardiography can identify the lack of entry of pulmonary veins into the left atrium and can sometimes locate the anomalous channel and point of entry. At cardiac catheterization, the condition is recognized by the identity of oxyhemoglobin saturation in the right and left sides of the heart. The type of drainage is determined by selectively injecting contrast medium into the main pulmonary artery and observing the confluence of pulmonary veins and their course above or below the diaphragm to the point of abnormal entry. Any narrowing in the path of drainage or obstruction to flow from the right atrium into the left atrium through the ASD and thus into the systemic circulation is analyzed by this visualization and by measurement of pressures and oxyhemoglobin saturation in the pulmonary artery, cavae, and chambers of the right side of the heart. When the right side of the heart is markedly dilated, the volume of the left atrium and ventricle appears small by comparison, but it is usually adequate to support the full systemic flow after repair. Selective LV injection and echocardiographic appearance help to evaluate ventricular size.

The HLHS functionally mimics the condition of TAPVR and is at least eight times as common in the cyanotic newborn who appears gray, tachypneic, and often shocky. Echocardiography has become useful in identifying the components of the underdeveloped mitral and aortic valves, LV, and ascending aorta. The distinguishing features of HLHS on ultrasound are the absence of echoes or the small amplitude of echoes from the mitral valve and the absence or the unusually small size of the LV, aortic valve, and aortic root. The left atrium is usually large, and the atrial septum often bows into the right atrium.

Very few infants survive beyond the first days or weeks of life. Norwood has pioneered a sequence of operations that afford palliation for some babies.[20]

DEFICIENT PULMONARY BLOOD FLOW WITHOUT PULMONARY HYPERTENSION

It was for many of this group of cyanotic patients with reduced pulmonary flow and low pressure that shunt procedures to increase pulmonary blood flow proved to be so helpful and opened the field of surgery on blue babies.

CHARACTERISTICS. The patient's history frequently reveals easy respirations when quiet but quick dyspnea on exertion and squatting to rest.

Physical examination of the patient with right-to-left shunting and severe valvular or subvalvular pulmonary stenosis reveals generalized cyanosis and small size for age. The stethoscope detects diminution and delay of the pulmonic component of the second heart sound (S_2P). It may even be inaudible so that only the sound of aortic closure is heard at the apex and base of the heart. The systolic murmur in these cyanotic patients is due to pulmonic stenosis, not to the septal defect. It is a crescendo–decrescendo, ejection-type systolic murmur, maximal in the second left interspace (the pulmonary area), and it radiates along the course of pulmonary blood flow such that it is audible over the lung fields posteriorly. An early systolic ejection sound signifies valvular pulmonic stenosis, although this helpful sign may be absent when the stenosis is severe. With pulmonary atresia, no cardiac murmur is heard, but over the lung fields anteriorly or posteriorly, on one or both sides, one may hear a continuous murmur of collateral circulation due to systemic arteries anastomosing with intrapulmonary arteries (pseudotruncus arteriosus). Cardiac diastolic murmurs are unusual in cyanotic persons. An early decrescendo diastolic murmur is heard when there is pulmonary regurgitation. A scratchy diastolic murmur at the lower left sternal border is audible in some patients with Ebstein's anomaly of the tricuspid valve.

Electrovectorcardiography depicts the hypertrophy of the RV and shows "strain" if the RV systolic pressure is greater than the systemic pressure. If the RV is rudimentary or underdeveloped, there is absence of the expected RV forces. CRBBB with low voltage is typical in Ebstein's anomaly.

Radiologic confirmation of decreased pulmonary blood flow is the hypovascularity of the lung fields, which appear unusually radiolucent. If there is infundibular stenosis with hypoplasia of the main pulmonary artery, the heart appears boot-shaped with a concave outflow tract (see Fig. 100.3). On the other hand, if the stenosis is purely valvular, there is poststenotic dilatation of the main pulmonary artery and often of the left main branch (see Fig. 100.4). The cardiothoracic ratio is average unless the ventricular septum is intact and the RV pressure is much higher than the systemic pressure.

Echocardiography in the patient with tetralogy shows that RV and LV chambers are of equal size, that there is a ventricular septum with a high VSD, and in patients in whom there is overriding of the aorta, that there is discontinuity between septum and the aortic root. Sweep of the transducer from mitral valve to aorta shows these structures to be in continuity, thus minimizing a possible DORV. In general, the larger the aortic root, the smaller the pulmonary anulus in a tetralogy; thus, determination of size of the aortic root helps in this assessment of severity of the anomaly. The narrowed infundibulum is usually evident.

In the differential diagnosis of tetralogy from other tetralogy-like malformations, it is noteworthy that with pulmonic stenosis and intact septum, there is septal–aortic continuity. Tricuspid atresia with rudimentary RV is characterized by absence of tricuspid echoes and presence of a small RV chamber, while in Ebstein's anomaly there are recorded abnormal displacement and movement, as well as delay of closure, of the tricuspid valve.

These preliminary determinations help to plan the cardiac catheterization with contrast visualization. When the pressure in the RV is measured to be at a systemic level, the patient is positioned and injections are made selectively to distinguish tetralogy of Fallot from those conditions that mimic it.

SPECIFIC MALFORMATIONS. *Tetralogy of Fallot* consists of a high VSD, large enough to equalize systolic pressure in the two ventricles at a systemic level, in conjunction with pulmonic stenosis of such severity that the pressure in the pulmonary artery is normal or less than normal. When the diagnosis of tetralogy is established, analysis is made of the many features that are important in planning surgery. At catheterization (Fig. 100.9), one evaluates (1) the presence and the severity of subvalvular, valvular, and supravalvular pulmonic stenosis; (2) proximity of the infundibular stenosis to the pulmonary valve; (3) size of the pulmonary anulus and (4) of the main pulmonary artery and the two branches and whether there is normal continuity; (5) the presence of branch stenosis; (6) the location of the VSD, which is almost always infracristal but may be intracristal and is rarely multiple; (7) the degree of overriding of the aorta; and (8) the origin and course of the coronary arteries. Important too is the determination of any systemic blood supply to the lungs. Sometimes one pulmonary artery arises from the aorta rather than from the RV like its mate. If a shunt procedure has been performed previously, that too is analyzed for patency and for pressure in the pulmonary artery beyond the anastomosis, as well as for any distortion or complications such as kinking[45] or aneurysmal dilatation. Often one finds pulmonary hypertension following a large Potts anastomosis (descending aorta to left pulmonary artery).[2] In an unusual variant of tetralogy, there is absence of the pulmonary valve and aneurysmal dilatation of the main pulmonary artery and branches. The obstruction is at the anulus. A diastolic murmur is prominent. Moderate pulmonary hypertension is often found.

If there is *tricuspid atresia* (see Fig. 100.5), one determines the adequacy of right atrial outlet to the left atrium and the outflow from the LV; whether there is any obstruction to aortic flow at the cardiac level or beyond; whether there is a large VSD or a small and restrictive VSD for communication of the LV with the rudimentary RV; the size and tripartite nature (inflow, midportion, infundibulum) of the RV chamber; size of the pulmonary anulus and vessels; and any systemic blood supply to the pulmonary artery, either native or surgically created (see Fig. 100.5). Echocardiography guides and supplements the cardiac catheterization with angiocardiography.

With severe *pulmonic stenosis* and intact septum (see Fig. 100.4) or with a small VSD, the systolic pressure in the RV exceeds that in the left and may soar to over 200 mm Hg. The wall, septum, and crista supraventricularis are greatly hypertrophied. The RV usually is of adequate size but in the newborn may be rudimentary. Rarely it is greatly dilated. There may be secondary tricuspid regurgitation. In the newborn, the pulmonary valve may be dysplastic or atretic.

In *Ebstein's anomaly of the tricuspid valve*, the degree of downward displacement of the tricuspid valve and the portion of the RV that is atrialized are analyzed by echocardiography and cardiac catheterization, since these features determine severity. Intracardiac recording of the ECG aids in distinguishing the point of change of atrialized RV and atrium.

The condition of *anomalous systemic venous return to the left atrium* may occur alone or as part of a more complex anomaly. As an isolated event it is associated with cyanosis but no heart murmur, ECG abnormality, or cardiomegaly. A straight, vertical shadow at the base of the heart on the left suggests a left superior vena cava or vertical vein. Usually that structure drains into the coronary sinus, but it may enter the left atrium. If one suspects anomalous systemic venous drainage, it can be identified by selective injection from the arms and from below the diaphragm.

Pulmonary arteriovenous fistula may present at birth as critically severe congenital heart disease[29] or it may be so mild in its physiologic consequences as to escape recognition. In the severe form a large fistulous connection steals blood away from the main or a major pulmonary artery into a large pulmonary vein or an extension of the left atrium itself. The volume-loaded heart fails. One needs a high index of suspicion even to consider this rare diagnosis and to recognize it on echocardiography[29] and at cardiac catheterization. Injection of contrast material into the pulmonary artery depicts the shunt of blood into the pulmonary veins and left atrium. Interruption of the fistula can be lifesaving.

DEFICIENT PULMONARY FLOW WITH PULMONARY HYPERTENSION AT THE SYSTEMIC LEVEL

The correlation on physical examination of the right-to-left shunting and elevated pulmonary pressure and vascular resistance is accentuation of the pulmonic component of the S_2 (S_2P). S_2P occurs earlier than normal so that S_2 is narrowly split or single. Sometimes there is a murmur of pulmonic insufficiency: a high-pitched, decrescendo diastolic murmur occurring in early and mid-diastole along the left sternal border and heard better with the patient supine than upright. There may be no systolic murmur at all or a short early systolic murmur at the upper or lower sternal border. Occasionally an early systolic ejection sound is heard. There is an RV tap.

The heart is not much enlarged until it decompensates. The RV hypertrophy is reflected on the ECG. Radiographically there is enlargement of the pulmonary arterial tree up to the point of precapillary obstruction. This gives the effect of abrupt "pruning" of the pulmonary vascularity in the middle and outer thirds of the lung fields, while the hilar region appears full and the main pulmonary artery is unusually convex. Echocardiography shows hypertrophy and dilation of the RV and septum, as well as the relation of the ventricular septum, aortic root, and mitral valve. Usually the abnormal connection between the two circulations is large and can be imaged echocardiographically, whether at the atrial, ventricular, or aorticopulmonary level. Doppler studies identify the level of shunt.

When the cyanotic patient is shown by noninvasive methods to have the Eisenmenger reaction, we do not recommend cardiac catheterization and angiocardiography. He is not a candidate for cardiac surgery. While surgery has little if anything to offer, under medical management he may be remarkably free from symptoms and may lead a quietly active life as an adult.[46]

MANAGEMENT

Today's population of patients born with a form of cyanotic heart disease consists of a mix of unoperated patients ranging from severe to mild, as well as a variety of postoperative children and adults with a wide spectrum of functional and anatomical results. Management is individualized and is based on accurate diagnosis and regular reassessment of that patient and of the changing trends in therapy.

In his lifetime of care, the cyanotic patient's primary physician, cardiologist, and cardiovascular surgeon provide a cooperating continuum with different responsibilities at different times. In consultation with the patient's physician, the cardiologist provides definitive diagnosis, prevention, and treatment of complications, cardiologic care during surgery, as well as systematic long-term follow-up. Reminders of the importance of antibiotics in therapeutic doses at the time of oral or genitourinary surgery help prevent infective endocarditis.[47] Counseling for schooling, job selection, recreation, marriage, and family begins early and continues lifelong. I consider that our goals are to encourage that person to perform near the peak of his capacity and to be a well-adjusted, effective member of society. To be competitive in the job market, the person born with a cardiac defect meets a certain reluctance of the employer toward hiring the "handicapped." Therefore, we should not only help the adolescent and adult to be as nearly normal as modern medicine and surgery permit, but we should also encourage him to be the best prepared for his job that he can be.

Any hope for lasting benefit from management of the cyanotic patient involves cardiac surgery. Consummate skill and continuing commitment to improvement of results are required of the cardiovascular surgeon, who must understand and strive to repair the great variety of abnormalities of structure and function that constitute cyanotic con-

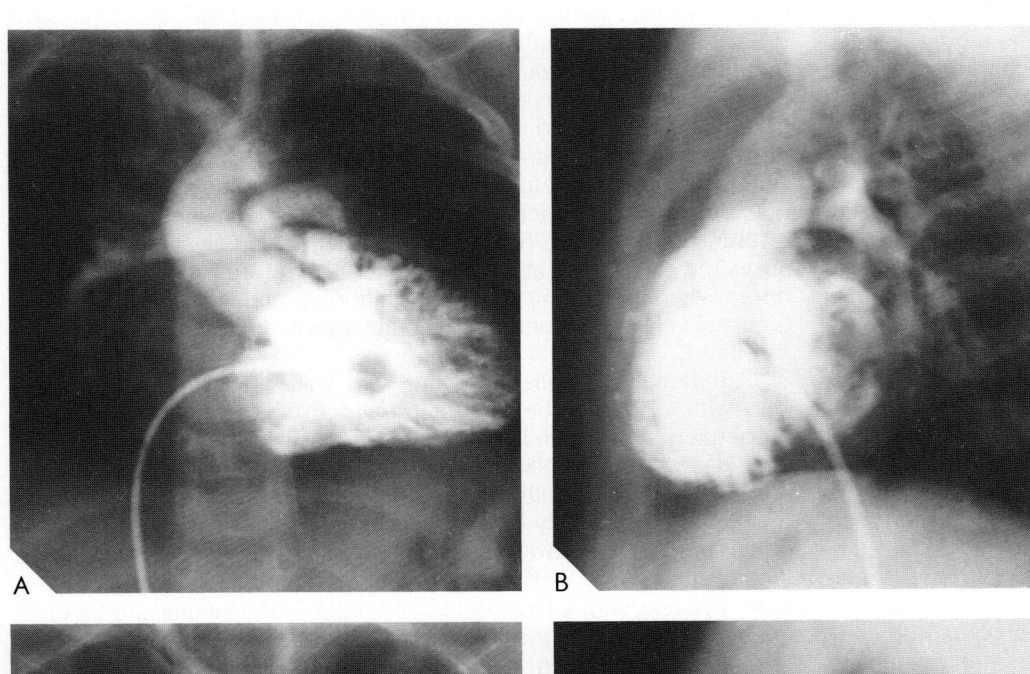
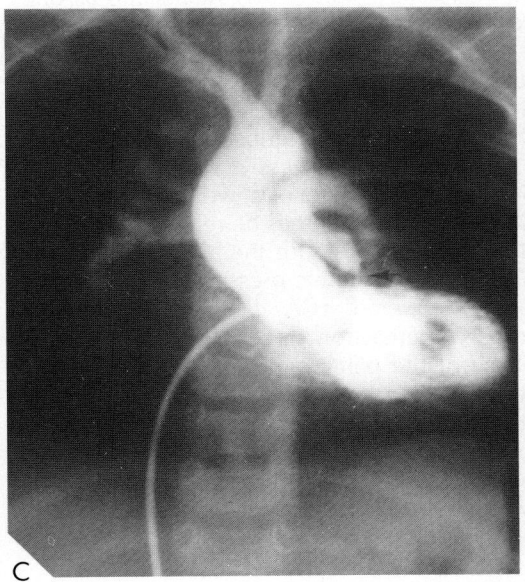
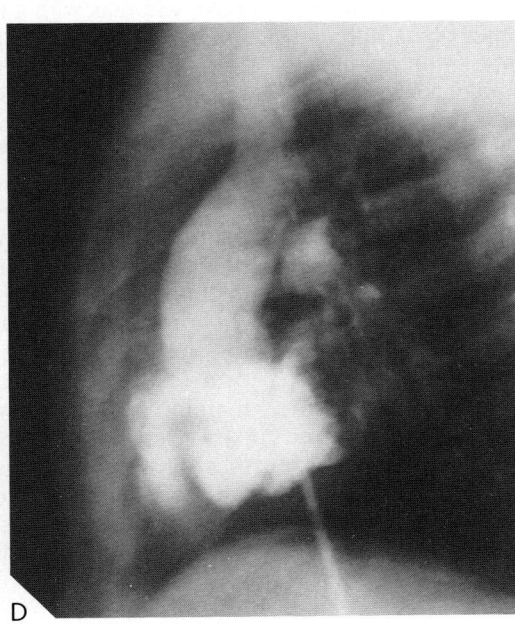

FIGURE 100.9 Tetralogy of Fallot. Selective RV angiocardiogram in simultaneous frontal (**A**) and lateral (**B**) projections shows equal opacification of the large, overriding aorta that arches to the left and of the infundibular narrowing (*arrow*), infundibular chamber, small pulmonary anulus, and hypoplastic main pulmonary artery and more nearly normal-sized, confluent right and left pulmonary arteries. In lateral view, **B**, the high VSD is opacified as systemic venous blood shunts right to left into the left ventricle posteriorly.

Selective LV injection (**C** and **D**) shows dense opacification of the large aorta and of the small pulmonary artery. Extreme infundibular pulmonic stenosis (*arrow*) is seen even better than on RV injection (**A** and **B**). In lateral projection, **D**, the VSD is opacified by blood shunting into the right ventricle.

genital heart disease. Consideration and planning for cardiac surgery and the perioperative management of the patient are a shared medical and surgical cardiologic responsibility, wherein skills and experience are joined to ensure a favorable outcome. Meticulous attention to detail is just as important in the intensive care unit after surgery as it is in the operating room. The younger and smaller the subject, the less room there is for small error or for deviation from the guidelines for care previously agreed upon and regularly in use by the team.

Our present attitude about the indications for the time of surgery for patients with the most common of the cyanotic malformations follows. For the unusual anomalies, similar principles apply. Each patient is judged individually, but in general, if the anatomy is suitable for open repair at low risk, we believe that definitive repair is preferable to early palliation followed by later open heart surgery. Short-term results thus far support this concept.

EXCESSIVE PULMONARY BLOOD FLOW
PALLIATION

Palliation for this group consists of two types of procedures. One is the creation of an ASD either medically by the Rashkind technique of balloon atrial septostomy[7] in the newborn or surgically, later on, by the Blalock–Hanlon procedure of atrial septectomy.[6] The purposes are to improve interatrial mixing and relieve obstruction to pulmonary venous return in patients with complete transposition of the great arteries or pulmonary veins. For the newborn infant under the age of 2 weeks who has CTGA, the Rashkind procedure is lifesaving. Benefit usually lasts for several months. When the baby begins to become more cyanotic, tachypneic, and polycythemic, he should be operated upon before he is severely ill with cardiac failure, pulmonary edema, or cerebrovascular accident. He then should undergo surgical rerouting of venous return to the heart by the Mustard procedure[9] or the Senning operation[8] or the arterial switch operation introduced by Jatene.[19] The choice of the type of operation will become easier when long-term results accumulate. Long-term experience with the Mustard operation[48] with our patients at The New York Hospital–Cornell University Medical College has shown that infants can undergo open repair at the same low risk and with the same good expectation of improvement as the older child. Most of our patients are operated on around the age of 4 to 6 months. Follow-up into adolescence and young adulthood has continued to show favorable outcome.

For sick infants with TAPVR, we believe that early open repair is preferable to preliminary palliation by balloon septostomy or atrial septectomy.

The other palliative operation for cyanotic infants with increased pulmonary flow is that of pulmonary arterial banding.[5] This is utilized in babies with excessive pulmonary flow and uncontrollable cardiac failure in an effort to gain a better balance of systemic and pulmonary flow. It is also employed, albeit infrequently, in some babies with early evidence of elevated pulmonary vascular resistance in an attempt to protect the pulmonary bed. Subjects who are candidates for pulmonary artery banding include those with any of the transposition complexes in association with a large VSD, those with a single ventricle without pulmonary stenosis, and those with common truncus arteriosus.

In these patients with cyanotic heart disease, it is difficult to place the pulmonary artery band if there is an anomalous or posterior location of the pulmonary artery; it is also more difficult than in the simple VSD to know how tight the band should be. Too loose a band means an ineffective operation with the high risk that accompanies any surgery on a sick patient that does not help. Too tight a band causes deepening of cyanosis and increase in polycythemia. Pericardial adhesions make later surgery difficult. Additional problems encountered when later repair is attempted concern not only the tightness but also the width of the band and its location on the artery. Often it is necessary to repair and to enlarge the constricted artery. The position of the band too close to the pulmonary valve causes damage to the leaflets as they open. Migration of the band to the bifurcation obstructs flow to one or both pulmonary artery branches, which then do not enlarge with growth of the patient.

Against these problems of banding the pulmonary artery must be weighed the risks and rewards of early open heart surgery in the cyanotic patient with the anomalies mentioned above. If the risks seem equal or less with the direct approach, we favor repair over surgical palliation and subsequent open operation. There is a distinct benefit to growth and development that comes with early disappearance of a right-to-left shunt.

OPEN REPAIR

Open repair for patients with CTGA is of two types, the venous switch (Mustard[9] or Senning[8] procedure) and the arterial switch of Jatene.[19] Our experience has been chiefly with the first of these.[48]

The Mustard procedure physiologically corrects the condition of transposition of the great arteries by rerouting the systemic and pulmonary venous returns within the atrium. The atrial septum is excised and a pericardial patch is emplaced so that the blood in the cavae and coronary sinus drains into the new physiologic "right" atrium, mitral valve, LV, and so to the pulmonary artery. Pulmonary venous blood enters the new physiologic "left" atrium (previous anatomical right atrium) and crosses the tricuspid valve to be pumped by the RV into the aorta. The Senning procedure uses the patient's own atrial wall to reroute systemic and pulmonary venous return.

Early problems following these procedures consist of damage to the conduction system with arrhythmias, and later the "sick sinus syndrome," superior vena caval obstruction, pulmonary venous obstruction, inadequacy of size of the new right or left atrium, shriveling of the patch, leaks about the patch, and tricuspid insufficiency. Each problem has been analyzed and is now to a large extent preventable. However, development of superior vena caval obstruction several months after surgery has continued to occur in some of our infants after the Mustard operation. Supraventricular arrhythmias have been reduced to a low level in both of these repairs at the atrial level. Questions still to be answered concern what will happen to the new atria and to the venous return when the patient grows to adulthood, and whether the RV and tricuspid valve can function efficiently for decades at a systemic pressure level.

Additional anomalies together with CTGA pose other problems. VSD with CTGA can be small and restrictive and of little physiologic consequence, or it can be large and of considerable significance. The large defect permits mixing so that the baby is not deeply cyanotic, but it is also associated with the early onset of severe pulmonary vascular obstruction. In a study of lung specimens of 200 patients with TGA, only 9 of 107 (8.4%) with intact septum or a small VSD demonstrated greater than grade 2 (Heath and Edwards[30]) pulmonary vascular disease, whereas with a large defect, 37 of 93 (40%) infants and 26 of 35 (75%) children over the age of one year had greater than grade 2 changes. A large patent ductus arteriosus was similarly harmful in this regard: all five infants under one year who had grade 3 or grade 4 changes had a large patent ductus arteriosus. The conclusions drawn were that the large VSD or patent ductus arteriosus should be closed before the age of 6 months to prevent progressive damage.[49]

In TGA, a small amount of pulmonic stenosis, which is usually subpulmonic and often dynamic,[50] can sometimes be relieved at the time of venous switch operation. It is favorable for the arterial switch procedure to prepare the LV to bear a systemic pressure.[19]

For the more anatomical repair of TGA, Jatene[19] carried out a transfer of aorta with coronary arteries from its point of origin in the RV over to the transected base of the pulmonary artery. Arterial blood thereby reached the systemic circulation. The distal end of the pulmonary artery was sewn onto the proximal portion of the transected aorta, thus allowing venous blood to flow into the pulmonary circulation. For the procedure to succeed, the LV must be hypertrophied, as it is in the neonate or in patients with pulmonic stenosis, either native or surgically induced by banding the pulmonary artery.

The arterial switch procedure is being carried out in a few centers such as those in Sao Paulo,[19] London,[51] and Boston[52] with decreasing mortality and increasing success.

Rare in CTGA are other complicating anomalies such as coarctation of the aorta, rudimentary RV, and tricuspid atresia. Coarctation should be repaired early, and the other two conditions call for palliation if atrial mixing is inadequate. If the pulmonary flow is really excessive, pulmonary banding may help as palliation.

The other malformation in the transposition complexes, or conotruncal positional anomalies, with DORV or DOLV with and without ventricular inversion, has been treated with some success as ingenious techniques have been utilized to interrupt the shunt at the ventricular level and to direct the blood flow in a physiologic direction.[53] Repair depends on the location of the VSD in relation to the great arteries (subaortic, subpulmonic, uncommitted) and on the degree of rotation of the great arteries in relation to one another and the ventricular septum. The surgeon may use the Rastelli procedure of an external valved conduit or an internal interventricular rerouting by a hammock-like synthetic prosthesis. For example, the cyanotic child with Taussig–Bing anomaly (DORV and subpulmonic VSD) may undergo open heart surgery with a hammock-like patch to interrupt the ventricular shunt and to connect the overriding pulmonary artery to the LV, leaving the aorta arising from the RV. Functionally the condition would thus be a complete transposition. But a Mustard or Senning procedure carried out at the same operation reroutes the venous return so as to correct the flow of blood physiologically.

Truncus arteriosus can be repaired by the Rastelli procedure[16] even in early infancy[54] when the baby's cardiac failure has been treated and the anatomy defined. When a synthetic valved conduit is used, later operation in childhood to place a larger external valved conduit is a necessary sequel to early surgical success. Not only does that conduit fail to grow, but it can also become obstructed by compression or development of an internal peel.[55,56] Surgical planning requires preoperative delineation of the relation of the truncus to the RV or LV, the take-off of the pulmonary arteries, and the question of truncus insufficiency or stenosis. Type I truncus in which the pulmonary arteries emerge from the left basal aspect of the trunk in a nearly normal position is fortunately the most common type, since it presents fewer difficulties in placing a graft with a valve to create an outflow from the RV to the pulmonary artery than do types II and III, in which the pulmonary arteries arise separately and more remotely. Type IV truncus without any pulmonary arteries but with systemic arterial supply from the descending aorta may defy attempts at repair, but often the collateral circulation is adequate for growth, minimal cyanosis, and quiet activities. Severe truncus insufficiency can be relieved by replacing the truncus valve. High pulmonary vascular resistance, greater than 70% of systemic, renders the patient with truncus inoperable.

There is discussion about operation on selected patients with single ventricle without pulmonary vascular obstruction.[57] Some can be helped by a Fontan operation[17] and some by septation of the ventricle. The latter surgical candidates have two atrioventricular valves with separate attachment of papillary muscles so that a prosthetic septum can be constructed to allow blood to flow in the physiologic direction to the great arteries. The cardiac conduction system is anomalous and tends to run, not posteroinferiorly distal to the tricuspid valve, but anterosuperiorly and in relation to the bulboventricular foramen. Intraoperative mapping of conduction pathways may add to the safety of this operation by avoidance of heart block. Since no growth of the prosthetic septum can be anticipated, it seems advisable for such surgery to be deferred until after the age of 5 years. Until then, banding of the pulmonary artery might be considered as a temporary measure to cut down excessive flow.

Common atrium can be successfully repaired with a large patch after precise definition of the points of entry of each pulmonary vein and cava and identification of the coronary sinus. Often there are bilateral superior cavae; the anomalous left cava then may drain into the coronary sinus as it usually does, or may drain into the left side of the common atrium while anomalous pulmonary veins drain into the right side of the common atrium. Therefore, it is essential that drainage of systemic and of pulmonary veins be accurately identified in the operating room before the large patch is sewn in to create two atria appropriately related to the atrioventricular valves. The mitral valve is usually malformed but rarely functionally incompetent or stenotic.

Patients with TAPVR present as symptomatic infants in two ways. One presentation is that of a sick, slightly cyanotic, distressed baby in cardiac failure with a volume-overloaded right heart, flooded lungs, some pulmonary hypertension, and slight or no obstruction to pulmonary venous drainage. The other is as a deeply cyanotic, dyspneic baby with a small heart and obstructed pulmonary venous outlet. Both presentations are true cardiac emergencies that call for prompt recognition and immediate diagnostic studies followed by open heart surgery to reunite the pulmonary veins with the left atrium and to close the ASD. There is then about a 75% chance of survival and of lasting improvement.[15,58] When the suture line in the left atrium is extended maximally to include the left atrial appendage, the risk of the anastomosis' becoming obstructive as the child grows into childhood is minimized. Consistently successful surgery in these infants is too recent for long-term follow-up of the effects of growth.

About 10% of patients with TAPVR do not get into such difficulty early in life, probably because there is no obstruction to the anomalously draining veins and because the pulmonary vascular bed is compliant enough to accept a large volume without pulmonary hypertension. For this group of patients, open repair can be scheduled electively. We prefer to do this after the age of 5 or 6 years to ensure as large an anastomosis as possible.

Infants with the HLHS have little chance for salvage unless there is some additional malformation that permits a sufficiently large ascending aorta to supply adequate coronary and cerebral arterial circulation. Then creation of an ASD can relieve some of the obstruction to pulmonary venous outflow, and banding the pulmonary artery can bring pulmonary flow into better balance with systemic flow. For those newborn infants with the usual HLHS with mitral and aortic atresia, diminutive LV, and stringlike ascending aorta, Norwood[20] devised two-stage palliation. The procedure is being carried out in only a few centers, with limited success. The first palliation accomplishes unobstructed mixing of pulmonary venous return with systemic venous return at the atrial level by excising the septum primum. The main pulmonary artery is transected and oversewn with a Goretex patch. The patent ductus is ligated and transected at the aortic orifice. The aorta distal and proximal is incised and the distal aorta enlarged with a Goretex patch. Thus, the aorta is enlarged. The proximal main pulmonary artery is anastomosed to the ascending aorta and the Goretex patch. To provide pulmonary blood flow, a 4-mm Goretex tube graft is interposed between the innominate artery and the right pulmonary artery. Physiologically the infant has a common atrium, single RV, and a truncus arteriosus with limited pulmonary blood flow. If the baby survives and grows, a second palliation is needed to maintain adequacy of flow into the systemic and pulmonary circulations.

DEFICIENT PULMONARY BLOOD FLOW WITHOUT PULMONARY HYPERTENSION

PALLIATION

Palliation by a shunt to increase pulmonary flow is indicated for the symptomatic infant with tetralogy who has hypercyanotic spells or is polycythemic but who has unfavorable anatomy for open repair owing to marked hypoplasia of the RV outflow tract and pulmonary anulus and arteries. Palliation is also indicated for infants with severe pulmonic stenosis together with (1) rudimentary RV or (2) with single ventricle or (3) with CTGA and VSD. For some of these infants who are helped by a shunt to increase pulmonary flow, there is hope for reparative operation a few years later. If that is not possible, it is comforting to know that benefit from a first palliative operation can last for many years and that there are other shunt procedures available if the early one is outgrown.

Favored by most as choice of shunt for large babies and children is the Blalock–Taussig end-to-side anastomosis of subclavian to pulmonary artery.[1] This has provided the most satisfactory long-term results with only a small risk of pulmonary hypertension and with relative ease of take-down at later open heart surgery. However, in the first month of life, there is still difficulty with patency of the anastomosis when a small subclavian artery is turned down to a hypoplastic pulmonary artery. The Blalock–Taussig operation is sometimes modified by use of a Goretex tube interposed between the innominate or subclavian artery and the main or branch pulmonary artery, thus abolishing the need to interrupt the subclavian artery.

The Glenn anastomosis[3] of the superior vena cava to the right pulmonary artery offers an alternative way to augment pulmonary flow. This shunt tends to "shrivel" as time passes owing to the development of an arteriovenous fistula in the right lower lobe, development of venous collaterals between the superior and inferior vena cava, expansion of the bronchial arterial flow to the lungs, or recanalization of the connection between the superior vena cava and right atrium.[59,60] We reserve it for specially selected anomalies, such as tricuspid atresia when a Fontan procedure is a possibility in the future. Because of the problem of kinking and even of interruption of continuity of the right pulmonary artery when the ascending aorta is anastomosed to it (Waterston shunt[45,61]), we do not recommend this procedure unless there is no alternative.

If a different shunt procedure is needed and the baby has a left descending aorta, a Potts anastomosis of measured diameter (no more than 5 mm) can be made between the descending aorta and the adjacent left pulmonary artery. If this shunt is not too large initially and does not grow too large, it provides relatively equal blood flow to both lungs without pulmonary hypertension, cardiac failure, or interruption of continuity of pulmonary arteries. Take-down of this anastomosis at later repair is more difficult than tying off a Blalock–Taussig shunt but is less difficult than take-down of a Waterston shunt when the right pulmonary artery must be patched to enlarge it or restore continuity.[61]

Thus far we have considered surgical palliation for these symptomatic babies. Medical palliation sometimes buys time until the infant grows a bit and becomes a better candidate for open repair. If he is anemic, iron therapy may be instituted and then discontinued when the hemoglobin reaches 15 g to 17 g and the hematocrit is 48 to 50. To persist in iron supplementation beyond this mildly polycythemic level is to run the risk of excessive polycythemia and its consequences.

Another medical measure that may temporarily relieve the hypercyanotic spells that are attributed to infundibular spasm is use of the β-blocker, propranolol. The liquid preparation is given orally four times daily, beginning at a dose of 1 mg/kg/day and doubling or tripling that amount if necessary.

OPEN REPAIR

Open repair is our preference over palliation for the patient with tetralogy of Fallot (see Fig. 100.9) who has favorable anatomy and in whom the pulmonary anulus and pulmonary artery are at least one third the size of the aorta. This operation can be carried out in the infant with severe symptoms, but for the minimally symptomatic baby or toddler, operation can usually be deferred until the age of 2 or 3 years. Some patients are older than that when first referred to a cardiac center. Some have already had one or more shunt procedures. These patients may range in age from preschoolers to adults. All are candidates for open repair[62,63] unless the anatomy of the pulmonary tree is unsuitable or there is some other noncardiac contraindication to surgery.

Open repair through a right ventriculotomy consists first of relief of the obstruction by resection of infundibular fibromuscular stenosis and incision along the lines of fusion of pulmonary valve cusps, and second, of closure of the VSD with a patch, taking care to avoid the conduction system. The hypoplastic outflow tract of the RV usually needs to be enlarged by a roofing patch, which sometimes extends through the pulmonary anulus and out onto the main pulmonary artery to enlarge these areas if they appear to restrict pulmonary flow. Pressure measurements in the operating room help to judge this point. It is desired that the RV systolic pressure be reduced to less than 70% of the systemic pressure and that the pressure in the main pulmonary artery be normal. In exceptional cases, pulmonary hypertension after repair is due to previously unrecognized peripheral pulmonary stenosis or hypertensive vascular changes related to a previous large systemic-to-pulmonary artery shunt. Preoperative cardiac catheterization may not detect these abnormalities when the patient has low pulmonary flow. Relief of the proximal pulmonary stenosis and establishment of full pulmonary flow may unmask them.

Clinical results of open repair of tetralogy of Fallot usually are excellent from the patient's point of view, but the preexisting anatomy determines how "corrective" the operation is. The child whose anatomy has the least derangement from the normal (discrete infundibular pulmonary stenosis, normal-sized pulmonary anulus and pulmonary arteries, and minimal overriding of the aorta) may indeed be totally corrected and have no murmur, with normal pressures, ECG, and heart size thereafter. His repair results in complete closure of the VSD by the patch, without heart block, and in complete resection of the infundibular stenosis without damage to the valve and with no systolic pressure gradient between the RV and pulmonary artery. This is the uncommon tetralogy.

Much more often there are multiple areas of stenosis with hypoplasia from the outflow tract through the pulmonary arterial branches. The pulmonary valve may be incompetent after its incision. It is incompetent when the outflow tract of the RV must be enlarged by a patch that extends through the valve ring and out onto the main pulmonary artery. Even then, the systolic pressure gradient measured in the operating room between the RV and pulmonary artery branches often is not abolished. The pulmonary insufficiency that is a necessary consequence of this enlargement is usually well tolerated if there is no large residual left-to-right shunt through an incompletely closed VSD and no obstruction distally to pulmonary blood flow. Sometimes the abnormally functioning pulmonary valve needs to be replaced when right ventricular function is severely compromised.[64]

Postoperative complete heart block that was a problem in the early days of open heart surgery for tetralogy has largely been prevented by proper placement of stitches to avoid the conduction bundle in the danger zone in the posteroinferior rim of the defect. Another potential problem is the postoperative pattern in the ECG of left anterior hemiblock (left-axis deviation and RBBB). Occurrence of ventricular premature beats or tachycardia spontaneously or on exercise carries a risk of sudden death.[63]

We favor early repair in children with tetralogy. They have the benefit early of being acyanotic and of having no impairment to growth that can be attributed to cyanosis or to a surgically created left-to-right shunt. Early repair also forestalls problems that are acquired and that make the anatomy worse as the patient grows older, problems such as progressive subvalvular pulmonic stenosis or even atresia. Initial reparative surgery avoids the problems mentioned above that may occur in long-term follow-up of systemic-to-pulmonary artery shunts.

Patients with *pseudotruncus arteriosus*, that form of tetralogy with pulmonary atresia and systemic blood supply to the pulmonary artery branches, usually get along moderately well through infancy and childhood. Their open repair by the Rastelli procedure[16] is best deferred until later childhood or adolescence, because part of the repair concerns the introduction of a homograft vessel and valve or of a Dacron conduit with porcine valve to establish a route of blood flow to the pulmonary arteries. Since there will be no growth of the graft and since late conduit obstruction is a frequent problem, it is preferable to wait, if the patient's condition permits, until a graft can be inserted that is large enough that it will not later restrict pulmonary flow. Repair then involves ligation of large vessels of collateral circulation near the aorta and closure of the VSD. Long-term results are similar to those of other forms of truncus arteriosus, with problems of acquired obstruction of the conduit.[55,56]

Patients with *tetralogy-like lesions* are candidates for open heart surgery if the team is fully cognizant of the anatomy and thoroughly experienced with techniques of repair of these unusual situations.

Patients with *pulmonic stenosis, intact ventricular septum,* and *defective atrial septum* should undergo open repair when the diagnosis is made, since the stenosis must be severe in order for the right-to-left shunt at the atrial level to be established. Commonly the stenosis is purely valvular (see Fig. 100.4) and is relieved through a pulmonary arteriotomy by incising out to the pulmonary anulus along the lines of fusion. Unless the right ventricular systolic pressure measured in the operating room after the valvotomy is still elevated to near systemic levels, it is not necessary to do an infundibular resection, since that secondary form of obstruction in the outflow tract of the ventricle subsides spontaneously as hypertrophy regresses after an effective valvotomy.[65] Long-term results have shown lasting relief of obstruction without recurrence. A murmur of pulmonary insufficiency is audible in about one quarter of the patients postoperatively, but the insufficiency appears of little physiologic consequence.

The technique of balloon angioplasty at cardiac catheterization recently introduced by Kan has provided a prompt drop in the pressure gradient during the half hour or so of measurements in the catheterization laboratory.[66] When carried out by experienced catheterizing teams, the procedure has low risk, as does open heart surgical repair, and should provide the same relief of symptoms and regression of RV hypertrophy. The benefits are the absence of a scar on the chest and the short hospital stay without the discomfort of recovery from surgery.

Pure pulmonary atresia with intact ventricular septum is a difficult lesion to treat. It poses a different problem depending on whether the right ventricle is of adequate size or not. Sometimes it is considerably enlarged; at other times it is markedly underdeveloped. If the judgment is that the ventricle is too small to receive and discharge a full complement of systemic venous return, we believe that an attempt to create an opening into the pulmonary artery has little chance of success and that a shunt procedure should be undertaken as the initial procedure.

Many children with *tricuspid atresia* and patent pulmonary arteries benefit from the Fontan operation,[67] which in effect utilizes the hypertrophied right atrium to be the right side of the heart, both as receptacle and pump, to send blood to the lungs where the resistance is low. The ASD is closed and the right atrium is connected to the RV if it is adequate in size or to the main pulmonary artery through a valved conduit. Sometimes the atrial appendage is sewn directly to the pulmonary artery without a conduit. If a large VSD is present, it is closed. Signs of systemic venous congestion, with hepatomegaly, ascites, and edema, have been a frequent postoperative problem, but usually they resolve with time and with the use of diuretics.

Certain patients with *Ebstein's anomaly of the tricuspid valve* who are markedly symptomatic and have great cardiomegaly experience symptomatic improvement and a decrease in heart size by insertion of an artificial tricuspid valve near the tricuspid anulus.[13,68] Care must be exercised to avoid damage to the conduction tissue near the coronary sinus and central fibrous body. The trade-off for this relief is the presence of an artificial valve with its own problems of anticoagulation, possible pulmonary embolism, and infection. We believe the indications for surgery should be strong before this procedure is undertaken, since many persons with Ebstein's anomaly live a long and full life, on ordinary activity, without symptoms or arrhythmia, despite the presence of considerable cardiomegaly.

Partial or total anomalous systemic venous drainage is one of the rarest of all the conditions discussed herein. It can be treated successfully by interrupting the abnormal connection into the left atrium and redirecting the flow to the right side of the heart.

Pulmonary arteriovenous fistula, when large, is amenable to repair by interruption of the abnormal connection.

DEFICIENT PULMONARY BLOOD FLOW WITH PULMONARY HYPERTENSION AT THE SYSTEMIC LEVEL

There is no surgery for patients with the Eisenmenger syndrome except for heart-lung transplantation. Medical measures to relieve symptoms and to prolong life include erythropheresis for excessive polycythemia and treatment of cardiac failure when that occurs. Some children, adolescents, and young adults remain remarkably free of symptoms for many years.[56]

THE CYANOTIC NEONATE

It is important to acknowledge that not all blue babies have cyanotic congenital heart disease. Differential diagnosis in the newborn includes peripheral and pulmonary reasons for the blue appearance.[69]

Peripheral cyanosis comes from excess extraction of oxygen by the tissues, such that capillary blood approaches the lower oxygen content of systemic veins rather than arteries. Extremities are cool and capillary refill sluggish. It often occurs in a setting of low cardiac output or shock. In contrast, the baby with central cyanosis is warm and has good capillary refill and cyanosis of the lips, as well as of the fingers and toes. Arterial blood gases and pH help in this distinction.

To separate pulmonary from cardiac causes of cyanosis, arterial blood gases are also a help. Pulmonary hypoperfusion or ventilation–perfusion imbalance is the basis for cyanosis of pulmonary origin. A problem that involves both the lungs and the heart is persistent pulmonary hypertension, sometimes called persistent fetal circulation.[70] For reasons not yet understood, newborns with this condition maintain high pulmonary vascular resistance and have resultant shunting of systemic venous blood right to left through the fetal passages of PFO and patent ductus arteriosus. Just as the cause is unknown, so is the specific and optimal treatment. These are tachypneic, distressed infants who benefit from care in a neonatal intensive care unit. This is true as well for the persistently cyanotic newborn suspected to have congenital heart disease.[71]

REFERENCES

1. Blalock A, Taussig HB: The surgical treatment of malformations of the heart in which there is pulmonary stenosis or pulmonary atresia. JAMA 128:189, 1945
2. Potts WJ, Smith S, Bigson S: Anastomosis of the aorta to a pulmonary artery. JAMA 132:627, 1946
3. Glenn WWL, Patino JF: Circulatory bypass of the right heart: I. Preliminary observation on direct delivery of vena caval blood into pulmonary arterial circulation: Azygos vein–pulmonary artery shunt. Yale J Biol Med 27:147, 1954
4. Waterston DJ: Treatment of Fallot's tetralogy in children under 1 year of age. Rozhl Chir 41:181, 1962
5. Muller WH JR, Damman JF Jr: Treatment of certain malformations of the heart by the creation of pulmonary stenosis to reduce pulmonary hypertension and excessive pulmonary blood flow. Surg Gynecol Obstet 95:213, 1952
6. Blalock A, Hanlon CR: The surgical treatment of complete transposition of the aorta and the pulmonary artery. Surg Gynecol Obstet 90:1, 1950
7. Rashkind WJ, Miller WW: Creation of an atrial septal defect without thoracotomy. JAMA 196:991, 1966
8. Senning A: Surgical correction of transposition of the great vessels. Surgery 45:966, 1959
9. Mustard WT: Successful two-stage correction of transposition of the great vessels. Surgery 55:469, 1964
10. Brock RC: Pulmonary valvulotomy for the relief of congenital pulmonary stenosis: Report of three cases. Br Med J 1:1121, 1948
11. Sellors TH: Surgery of pulmonary stenosis: A case in which the pulmonary valve was successfully divided. Lancet 1:988, 1948
12. Lillehei CW, Cohen M, Warden HE et al: Direct vision intracardiac surgical correction of the tetralogy of Fallot, pentalogy of Fallot, and pulmonary atresia defects. Report of first 10 cases. Ann Surg 142:418, 1955
13. Lillehei CW, Gannon PG: Ebstein's malformation of the tricuspid valve. Method of surgical correction utilizing a ball-valve prosthesis and delayed closure of atrial septal defect. Circulation 31:1, 1965
14. Ross DN, Somerville J: Correction of pulmonary atresia with homograft aortic valve. Lancet 2:1446, 1966
15. Dillard DH, Mohri H, Hessel EA II et al: Correction of total anomalous pulmonary venous drainage in infancy utilizing deep hypothermia with total circu-

latory arrest. Circulation 35 & 36 (Suppl I):105, 1967
16. Rastelli GC, Titus JL, McGoon DC: Homograft of ascending aorta and aortic valve as a right ventricular outflow: An experimental approach to the repair of truncus arteriosus. Arch Surg 95:698, 1967
17. Fontan F, Baudet E: Surgical repair of tricuspid atresia. Thorax 26:240, 1971
18. Sakakibara S, Tominaga S, Imai Y et al: Successful total correction of common ventricle. Chest 61:192, 1972
19. Jatene AD, Fontes VF, Paulista PP et al: Anatomic correction of transposition of the great vessels. J Thorac Cardiovasc Surg 72:366, 1976
20. Norwood WI, Kirklin JK, Sanders SP: Hypoplastic left heart syndrome: Experience with palliative surgery. Am J Cardiol 45:87, 1980
21. Coceani F, Olley PM: The response of the ductus arteriosus to prostaglandins. Can J Physiol Pharmacol 51:220, 1973
22. Olley PM, Coceani F, Bodach E: E-type prostaglandins: A new emergency treatment for cyanotic congenital heart malformations. Circulation 55:728, 1976
23. Barratt-Boyes BG, Simpson MM, Neutze JM: Intracardiac surgery in neonates and infants using deep hypothermia. Circulation 43, No. 1:25, 1971
24. Castaneda AR, Lamberti J, Sade RM et al: Open-heart surgery during the first three months of life. J Thorac Cardiovasc Surg 68:719, 1974
25. Engle MA, Perloff JK (eds): Congenital Heart Disease After Surgery, p 419. New York, Yorke Medical Books, 1983
26. Taussig HB, Crawford H, Pelargonio S et al: Ten to thirteen year follow-up on patients after a Blalock-Taussig operation. Circulation 25:630, 1962
27. Taussig HB, Crocetti A, Eshaghpour E et al: Long-time observations on the Blalock-Taussig operation: I. Results of first operation. Johns Hopkins Med J 129:243, 1971
28. Maillis MS, Cheng TO, Neyer JF et al: Cyanosis in patients with atrial septal defect due to systemic venous drainage into the left atrium. Am J Cardiol 33:674, 1974
29. Fried R, Amberson JB, O'Loughlin JE et al: Congenital pulmonary arteriovenous fistula producing pulmonary arteriovenous steal syndrome. Pediatr Cardiol 2:313, 1982
30. Heath D, Edwards JE: The pathology of hypertensive pulmonary vascular disease: A description of six grades of structural changes in the pulmonary arteries with special reference to congenital cardiac septal defects. Circulation 18:533, 1958
31. Rabinovitch M, Reid LN: Quantitative structural analysis of the pulmonary vascular bed in congenital heart defects. Cardiovasc Clin 11:149, 1981
32. Treves S, Royal H, Babchyck B: Pediatric nuclear cardiology. Cardiovasc Clin 11:247, 1981
33. Pohost GM, Ratner AV: Nuclear magnetic resonance: Potential applications in clinical cardiology. JAMA 251:1304, 1984
34. Levin AR, Goldberg HL, Borer JS et al: Digital angiography in the pediatric patient with congenital heart disease: Comparison with standard methods. Circulation 68:374, 1983
35. Engle MA, Ito T, Lukas DS et al: Electrocardiographic evaluation of pulmonic stenosis. J Pediatr 57:171, 1960
36. Taussig HB, Bing RJ: Complete transposition of the aorta and a levoposition of the pulmonary artery. Am Heart J 37:551, 1949
37. Van Praagh R: What is the Taussig-Bing malformation? Circulation 38:445, 1968
38. Levin DC, Baltaxe HA, Goldberg HP et al: The importance of selective angiography of systemic arterial supply to the lungs in planning surgical correction of pseudotruncus arteriosus. AJR 121:606, 1974
39. Edwards JE, McGoon DC: Absence of anatomic origin from heart of pulmonary arterial supply. Circulation 47:393, 1973
40. Berry BE, McGoon DC, Ritter DG et al: Absence of anatomic origin from heart of pulmonary arterial supply: Clinical application of classification. J Thorac Cardiovasc Surg 68:119, 1974
41. Rowe RD, Mehrizi A: Total anomalous pulmonary venous drainage. In The Neonate with Congenital Heart Disease, pp 80, 219-230. Philadelphia, WB Saunders Co, 1968
42. Mitchell SC, Korones SB, Berendes HW: Congenital heart disease in 56, 109 births: Incidence and natural history. Circulation 43:323, 1971
43. Fyler DC, Parisi L, Berman MA: The regionalization of infant cardiac care in New England. Cardiovasc Clin 4:339, 1972
44. Darling RD, Rothney WB, Craig JM: Total pulmonary venous drainage into the right side of the heart. Lab Invest 6:44, 1957
45. Tay DJ, Engle MA, Ehlers KH et al: Early results and late developments of the Waterston anastomosis. Circulation 50:220, 1974
46. Young D, Mark H: Fate of the patient with the Eisenmenger syndrome. Am J Cardiol 28:658, 1971
47. Prevention of bacterial endocarditis: A statement for health professionals prepared by the Committee on Rheumatic Fever and Infective Endocarditis of the Council of Cardiovascular Disease in the Young. Circulation 70:1123A, 1984
48. O'Loughlin JE, Engle MA, Gay WA Jr et al: Modified Mustard operation for simple and complex transposition of the great arteries: 5 to 11 year follow-up. In Engle MA, Perloff JK (eds): Congenital Heart Disease After Surgery, pp 210-226. New York, Yorke Medical Books, 1983
49. Newfeld EA, Paul MH, Muster AJ et al: Pulmonary vascular disease in complete transposition of the great arteries: A study of 200 patients. Am J Cardiol 34:75, 1974
50. Robinson PF, Wyse RKH, Macartney FJ: Left ventricular outflow tract obstruction in complete transposition of the great arteries with intact ventricular septum: A cross sectional echocardiography study. Br Heart J 54:201, 1985
51. Yacoub MH, Arensman FW, Keck E et al: Fate of dynamic left ventricular outflow tract obstruction after anatomic correction of transposition of the great arteries. Circulation 68(Suppl II):56, 1983
52. Castaneda AR, Norwood WJ, Jonaska-Colon SD et al: Transposition of the great arteries and intact ventricular septum: Anatomical repair in the neonate. Ann Thorac Surg 38:438, 1984
53. Mazzucco A, Faggian G, Stellin G et al: Surgical management of double-outlet right ventricle. J Thorac Cardiovasc Surg 90:29, 1985
54. Sharma AK, Brown WJ, Mee RBB: Truncus arteriosus: A surgical approach. J Thorac Cardiovasc Surg 90:45, 1985
55. McGoon D: Long-term effects of prosthetic materials. In Engle MA, Perloff JK (eds): Congenital Heart Disease After Surgery, pp 177-201. New York, Yorke Medical Books, 1983
56. Jonas RA, Freed MD, Mayer JE Jr et al: Long-term follow-up of patients with synthetic right heart conduits. Circulation 72(Suppl II):77, 1983
57. Edie RN, Ellis K, Gersony WM et al: Surgical repair of single ventricle. J Thorac Cardiovasc Surg 66:350, 1973
58. Hawkins JA, Clark EB, Doty DB: Total anomalous pulmonary venous connection. Ann Thorac Surg 36:548, 1983
59. Mathur M, Glenn WWL: Long-term evaluation of cava-pulmonary artery anastomosis. Surgery 74:899, 1973
60. Glenn WWL: Superior vena cava-pulmonary anastomosis. Ann Thorac Surg 37:9, 1984
61. Gay WA Jr, Ebert PA: Aorta-to-right pulmonary artery anastomosis causing obstruction of the right pulmonary artery. Ann Thorac Surg 16:402, 1973
62. Fuster V, McGoon DC, Kennedy MA et al: Long-term evaluation (12 to 22 years) of open heart surgery for tetralogy of Fallot. Am J Cardiol 46:635, 1980
63. Garson A Jr, Nihill MR, McNamara DG et al: Status of the adult and adolescent after repair of tetralogy of Fallot. Circulation 59:1232, 1979
64. Bove EL, Kavey R-EU, Byrum CJ et al: Improved right ventricular function following pulmonary valve replacement for residual pulmonary insufficiency or stenosis. J Thorac Cardiovasc Surg 90:50, 1985
65. Engle MA, Holswade GR, Goldberg HP et al: Regression after open valvotomy of infundibular stenosis accompanying severe valvular pulmonic stenosis. Circulation 17:862, 1958
66. Kan J, White RI Jr, Mitchell SE et al: Percutaneous balloon valvuloplasty: A new method for treating congenital pulmonary valve stenosis. N Engl J Med 9:540, 1983
67. Mair DD, Rice MJ, Hagler DJ et al: Outcome of the Fontan procedure in patients with tricuspid atresia. Circulation 72(Suppl II):88, 1985
68. Mair DD, Seward JB, Driscoll DJ et al: Surgical repair of Ebstein's anomaly: Selection of patients and early and late operative results. Circulation 72(Suppl II):70, 1985
69. Engle MA, O'Loughlin JE: The infant with cyanotic congenital heart disease. In Fortuin NJ (ed): Current Therapy in Cardiovascular Disease 1984-1985, pp 158-164. Philadelphia, BC Decker, 1984
70. Linday LA, Ehlers KH, O'Loughlin JE et al: Noninvasive diagnosis of persistent fetal circulation versus congenital cardiovascular defects. Am J Cardiol 52:847, 1983
71. Engle MA: Cyanotic congenital heart disease. Am J Cardiol 37:283, 1976

INTERATRIAL SEPTAL DEFECT IN THE ADULT

Melvin D. Cheitlin • Elliot Rapaport

INCIDENCE AND CLASSIFICATION

Interatrial septal defect (IASD) is not the most common congenital heart defect found in the adult. If mitral valve prolapse is excluded as a strictly defined "congenital defect," the bicuspid aortic valve occurring in 1% to 2% of the population has this honor. The IASD, however, is certainly the most frequently seen, previously undetected, hemodynamically significant, congenital cardiac lesion in the adult.

In infancy and childhood the IASD comprises 7% to 25% of diagnosed congenital cardiac lesions, far less than the most common lesion—the interventricular septal defect.[1-3] In the adult patient IASDs are seen more frequently than interventricular septal defects for several reasons. Many interventricular septal defects spontaneously close in infancy and childhood, whereas at least after the first year of age, IASDs rarely close.[4] Also, because of the usually benign asymptomatic course of even patients with large left-to-right shunts, and the subtle physical findings, many children and young adults are not identified as having IASDs.

Pathologically, there are three types of congenital IASDs: (1) ostium secundum, (2) ostium primum, and (3) sinus venosus (Fig. 101.1). The blown-open foramen ovale may be considered a fourth IASD.

The ostium secundum defect arises as a result of the failure of the septum secundum to develop sufficiently to cover the ostium secundum opening in the septum primum. It is characterized by an opening in the atrial septum in the area of the foramen ovale of varying size, at times with multiple openings but always with an inferior rim of septum above the floor of the atrium. Although abnormalities of the mitral valve such as mitral valve prolapse have been described with IASD,[5] usually the atrioventricular valves are normal.

The ostium primum defect is a result of failure of the embryonic endocardial cushion to contribute to closure of the inferior portion of the atrial septum. Pathologically, it is characterized by an opening of varying size at the inferior portion of the atrial septum, with no rim of atrial tissue above the floor of the atrium at the level of the mitral and tricuspid valves. Characteristically, the course of the His bundle is displaced and elongated because of this defect. Frequently, other associated defects result from failure of the endocardial cushions to contribute normally to the development of the heart, such as clefting of the anterior leaflet of the mitral valve, abnormal chordal attachments to the ventricular septum, and clefting of the septal leaflet of the tricuspid valve, resulting in mitral and/or tricuspid valve insufficiency. If there is failure to contribute to closure of the membranous ventricular septum, an accompanying ventricular septal defect can result. The full expression of failure of the endocardial cushions to function properly is the total atrioventricular canal.

The sinus venosus defect probably results from a failure of the sinus venosus and proximal portions of the superior and inferior vena cava to be properly incorporated into the fetal right atrium.[6] It is characterized by a defect of variable size, usually at the superior-posterior portion of the atrial septum. Frequently there is accompanying partial anomalous pulmonary venous drainage, especially from the right upper lung into the base of the superior vena cava or the right atrium. More unusually, the defect can be low in the atrial septum near the entrance of the inferior vena cava.

The blown-open foramen ovale is not strictly a congenital IASD but more of an acquired lesion, resulting in shunting of blood at the atrial level. An anatomically patent foramen ovale exists in from 12% to 25% of all adult hearts and is the result of failure of the secundum septum to fuse to the primum septum over the foramen ovale.[6] Patients with right-sided heart failure may elevate right atrial pressure above that in the left atrium and create a right-to-left shunt through a patent foramen ovale. In addition, however, with increases in left atrial pressure, the membrane of the foramen ovale can be stretched and become incompetent, resulting in an opening between the left and right atria. Although this is uncommon, such an increase in left atrial pressure can result from mitral valve disease, especially mitral stenosis. Under these circumstances, mitral stenosis with a left-to-right shunt at the atrial level occurs and is known as Lutembacher's syndrome.

Lutembacher described the coexistence of mitral stenosis with atrial septal defect. Some of these cases may have represented patients with mitral stenosis and blown-open formen ovale as described above. Other cases represented patients with a classic pure secundum atrial septal defect in whom the soft apical diastolic rumble from increased tricuspid valve flow was misinterpreted as indicating the coexistence of mitral stenosis. Still other cases were observed during the period in which rheumatic fever and rheumatic valvulitis was far more common than it is today; these patients had associated rheumatic mitral valve deformity and atrial septal defect in which an apical diastolic rumble was present but in which hemodynamically significant mitral stenosis was absent. There remain a few patients with true atrial septal defect and rheumatic mitral stenosis. In these patients the presence of a gradually developing hemodynamically significant mitral stenosis resulted in an elevation of left atrial pressure and, because of the presence of a large communication between the atria and right ventricular dysfunction, comparable elevations in right atrial and central venous pressure as well. These patients have enormous left-to-right shunts with marked pulmonary blood flow associated with the peripheral symptoms of congestive heart failure, which reflects high right ventricular filling pressure with good right ventricular systolic pump function.[7] The studies of Nadas and Alimurung,[8] however, clearly have shown that Lutembacher's syndrome is an unusual disorder.

PATHOPHYSIOLOGY

All types of IASD are characterized by a left-to-right shunt as long as pulmonary vascular resistance is not severely elevated. Left and right atrial pressures are essentially equalized whenever a large defect exists in the atrial septum. The amount of blood that enters the right ventricle contrasted to the left ventricle during diastolic filling will be a function of the relative compliances of the two ventricles. The more distensible right ventricle fills to a greater extent at the same common filling pressure than the thicker left ventricle. The difference in the two outputs is the difference between the pulmonary and systemic blood flow and, therefore, the left-to-right shunt. Although the relative ventricular compliance is the determining factor, it should be noted that in the usual case of atrial defect because of streamlining of returning pulmonary venous blood flow, a greater proportion of blood having coursed through the right lung enters the right atrium compared with the pulmonary blood flow that has traversed the left lung.

The magnitude of the left-to-right shunt depends on the size of the defect and the relative compliance of the right and left ventricles in diastole. Arterial saturation remains normal in the low pressure IASD[9]; however, small amounts of right-to-left shunting can be seen across the IASD with two-dimensional echocardiographic bubble-contrast studies.

Because of the IASD and the left-to-right shunt, there is an increased end-diastolic right ventricular volume, with blood entering the right ventricle from both systemic venous return to the right atrium and pulmonary venous return to the left atrium across the IASD. During inspiration more of the right ventricular diastolic filling comes from the systemic venous return, and during expiration more is derived from the pulmonary venous return across the IASD. There is, therefore, a constant increased right ventricular diastolic volume, resulting in constant increased right ventricular stroke volume compared with left ventricular stroke volume. An increase in size of the right atrium and right ventricle and an increase in pulmonary blood flow result, enlarging pulmonary arteries and veins.

With increased flow, the calculated pulmonary vascular resistance is usually normal or low with opening of more of the potential vascular beds in the lung. Because of this, the pulmonary artery pressure remains normal in the large majority of patients with IASD. In a small number of patients with IASD and large left-to-right shunts, pulmonary vascular disease develops, resulting in increased pulmonary vascular

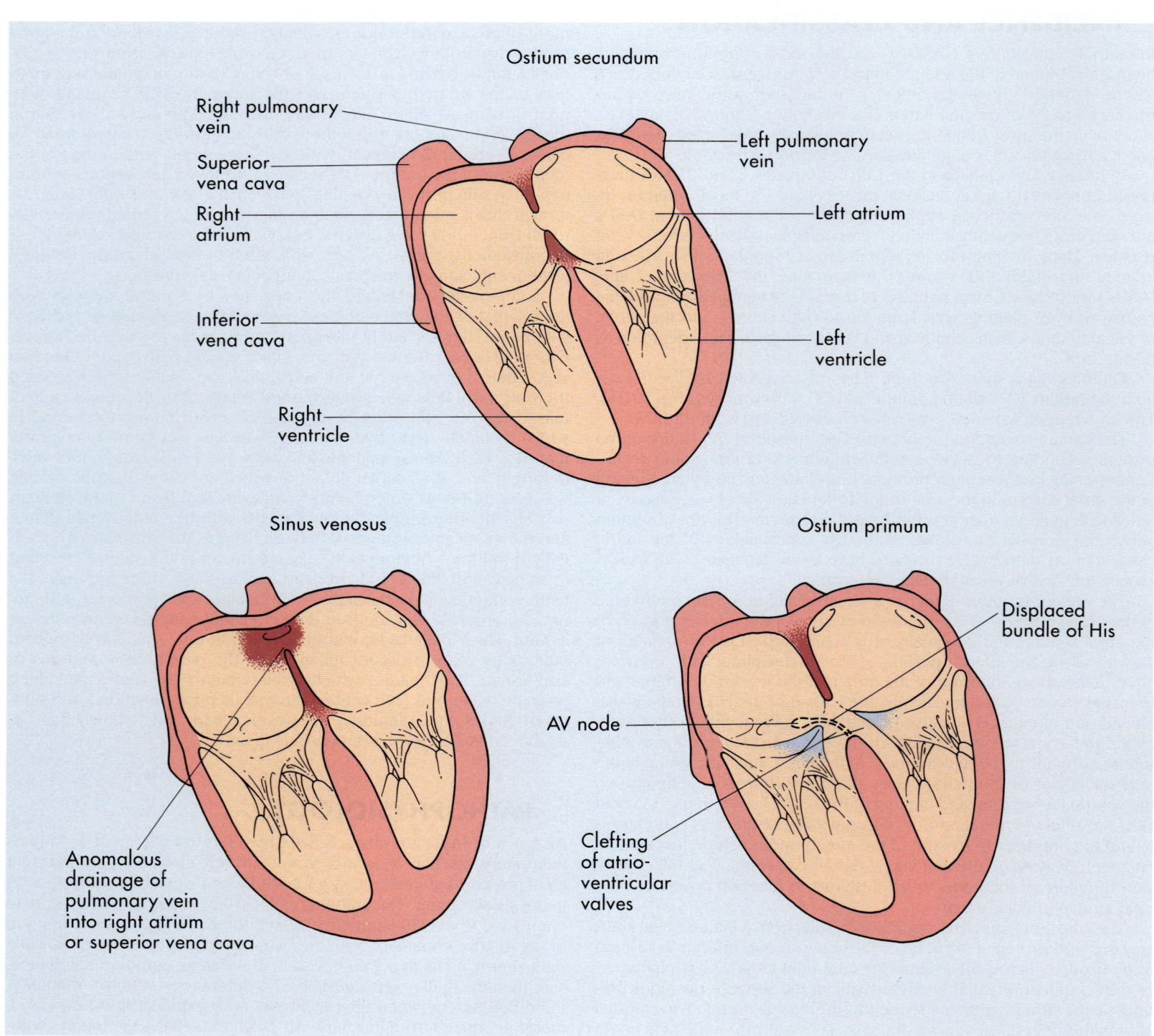

FIGURE 101.1 Diagrams of the three types of interatrial septal defects. See text for discussion.

resistance and pulmonary hypertension. Patients with pulmonary vascular disease and resultant severe pulmonary hypertension in association with an atrial septal defect demonstrate decreasing magnitude of left-to-right shunt as pulmonary vascular disease develops. This is probably related to decreasing diastolic compliance of the right ventricle associated with developing right ventricular hypertrophy. Eventually the shunt becomes predominantly right-to-left with systemic arterial desaturation and cyanosis. It is of interest that these patients for the most part have normal atrial pressures despite the presence of an elevated end systolic right ventricular volume. Similarly, patients with severe pulmonic valve stenosis associated with atrial septal defect, which can result in large right-to-left atrial shunts, also tend to have normal right atrial pressure. These data suggest that failure of the right ventricle in atrial septal defect is manifested by a progressive decrease in right ventricular stroke output, resulting in a decreasing left-to-right and eventual right-to-left atrial shunt. However, atrial filling pressure generally stays within the normal range.

In contrast, patients with large atrial septal defects may in later years develop elevation in left ventricular end-diastolic pressure which in turn will be mirrored by a comparable rise in left atrial and, therefore, right atrial and central venous pressure. These patients maintain a large left-to-right shunt with a low pulmonary vascular resistance but have associated high atrial pressures and large pulmonary blood flows. In a sense, these cases are representative of left ventricular diastolic pump dysfunction. It has been postulated that these cases may arise because of a reversed "Bernheim effect," in which the interventricular septum has been pushed into the left ventricular cavity by the markedly enlarged right ventricle with subsequent decrease in diastolic compliance of the left ventricle. On occasion, patients developing atrial fibrillation will manifest high atrial pressures and systemic congestion, reflecting the inability of the left ventricle to fill adequately under these circumstances. The situation is perhaps summarized by pointing out the interesting paradox that right ventricular failure in atrial septal defect is reflected primarily by increasing systolic right ventricular pump dysfunction with a decreasing right ventricular stroke output and resultant right-to-left shunt, while left ventricular failure is manifested primarily by alterations in left ventricular filling characteristics, high common atrial pressures, high central venous pressures, and systemic congestion, but with a large left-to-right shunt and essentially normal or low pulmonary vascular resistance.[10]

The pathologic changes that lead to pulmonary vascular disease in patients with large left-to-right shunts, presumably due to the increased pulmonary blood flow persistent over a number of years, have been described by Heath and Edwards[11] and amplified and extended by Reid and colleagues.[12,13] The changes consist of extension of the smooth muscle in the media abnormally into the intra-acinar pulmonary arteries, failure of the media of the preacinar arteries to regress normally, a decreased number of the pre- and intra-acinar vessels than in the normal lung, and finally morphologic changes of obliterative vascular disease with intimal thickening, hyalinization, and fibrosis and angiomatoid and plexiform lesions ultimately leading to arterial necrosis.

CLINICAL PICTURE AND DIAGNOSIS
HISTORY AND PHYSICAL EXAMINATION

The young patient with even a large IASD with large left-to-right shunt is frequently asymptomatic, since this right ventricular volume load is well tolerated. On careful questioning, the patient may not be able to engage in strenuous sports requiring sustained, high-level exercise. Because the patient has had the problem since birth, activities requiring this level of sustained exercise are frequently avoided, and the patient does not recognize any limitations or symptoms. As patients reach the fourth decade, exercise capacity decreases, and an increasing proportion of them become symptomatic with decreased exercise tolerance, easy fatigability, dyspnea on exertion, atrial tachyarrhythmias such as paroxysmal atrial fibrillation, and ultimately congestive heart failure.[14,15] By the sixth decade practically all patients have symptoms. In patients with pulmonary vascular disease, which rarely occurs before age 20 and will have occurred by age 40 to 50 or not at all,[14] symptoms occur earlier and are those of decreasing exercise capacity, fatigability, shortness of breath, and those symptoms associated with pulmonary hypertension and arterial desaturation such as polycythemia, an anginal type of chest pain, arrhythmias, syncope on exertion, hemoptysis, and cyanosis.

On physical examination there may be evidence of increased precordial and parasternal right ventricular activity by palpation. The increased right ventricular stroke volume results in a systolic ejection murmur at the second interspace at the left sternal border, which is usually grade III on a scale of VI or less but in about 5% of cases can be grade IV accompanied by a thrill. This murmur is a right ventricular systolic ejection murmur and is similar to that heard as an innocent murmur.

When the systolic ejection murmur in the second and third left interspace is associated with a thrill in a patient with atrial defect, there is usually a measurable systolic pressure gradient across the pulmonary valve. This mild pulmonary valve stenosis is totally functional in the sense that it is created by the enormous pulmonary blood flow. Once pulmonary blood flow is reduced, as by surgical closure of the atrial defect, the gradient disappears along with the thrill and loud ejection murmur.

The large, relatively constant right ventricular stroke volume into the dilated pulmonary arterial bed results in delayed pulmonary valve closure and, therefore, a relatively wide splitting of S_2. The splitting persists throughout respiration, even with changes in position such as sitting and standing, in which right ventricular venous return is usually decreased and normal splitting disappears. This is a characteristic finding of all left-to-right shunting at the atrial level and is the most important finding suggesting IASD, since it is present about 85% of the time. The pulmonary component of S_2 is of normal intensity except in pulmonary hypertension in which the intensity increases. With the large main pulmonary artery, splitting of S_1 with the second component having a high-frequency clicking sound is not unusual. Although this has been called the sound of increased tricuspid closure, it is more likely a pulmonary ejection click.

The presence of the physical findings of mitral valve prolapse, that is, a nonejection click or clicks with or without a late systolic murmur at the apex, has been described in patients who have a secundum IASD.[16] Liberthson and co-workers have described an increasing incidence of mitral valve prolapse with age in a retrospective study of 498 patients with secundum IASD. The incidence was 0.4% in 213 patients under age 21 years, 2% in 187 patients age 21 to 49 years, and 15% in 98 patients age greater than 50 years.[17] At times the findings of prolapsed mitral valve are the most prominent physical findings in these patients, and the IASD is discovered only when a chest film or echocardiogram is done, since the characteristic findings of IASD, that is, the widely split second sound and systolic ejection murmur at the base, may not be prominent.

With increased diastolic blood flow across the tricuspid valve in young patients there is frequently a middiastolic, low-frequency murmur along the left sternal border at the third and fourth interspace, but hearing this in an older adult is most unusual.

With the ostium primum defect and the clefting of the atrioventricular valves, either tricuspid or mitral insufficiency can be heard. Because the clefting is most prominent in the aortic leaflet of the mitral valve, the jet of mitral insufficiency frequently goes directly through the low-lying defect in the atrial septum into the right atrium. For this reason, the murmur of mitral insufficiency is frequently heard well at the apex but radiates well to the lower left sternal border and is often confused with the murmur of a ventricular septal defect.

The systemic venous pressure is normal until congestive heart failure occurs, when both pulmonary venous and systemic venous pressures rise together. Since a large IASD makes the two atria common chambers, there can be subtle abnormalities of the systemic venous waves but the mean pressures in the two atria are the same. Since there is increased right atrial filling even during systole in an IASD with a large left-to-right shunt, the cervical venous V wave can be abnormally prominent and even be higher than the A wave—a distinct abnormality.

With pulmonary vascular disease, right ventricular hypertrophy occurs with a forceful sustained right ventricular lift, and the pulmonary component of S_2 becomes prominent. The murmur of pulmonary valvular insufficiency and tricuspid insufficiency can occur with severe pulmonary hypertension. In this case because of the huge pulmonary arteries, the pulmonary S_2 can remain widely split even with severe pulmonary hypertension. Clubbing and cyanosis finally occur with the development of right-to-left shunt and arterial desaturation.

LABORATORY FINDINGS
CHEST FILM

With a small IASD and a small left-to-right shunt no abnormalities may be seen. With a large left-to-right shunt the right side of the heart, mainly the right ventricle but also the right atrium, may be dilated. The main pulmonary arteries and pulmonary vascular markings are increased in size and are more prominent than normal peripherally in the lung fields (Figs. 101.2, 101.3). Occasionally with sinus venosus defects, anomalous pulmonary venous drainage into the superior vena cava can be seen. Even with moderate size left-to-right shunts the chest film is within normal limits in about 15% of cases.

With pulmonary vascular disease and pulmonary hypertension, the heart can become somewhat smaller in volume as the left-to-right shunt decreases and right ventricular hypertrophy occurs. The main pulmonary artery and pulmonary arterial markings become extremely large centrally and may even develop calcification due to the presence of pulmonary arterial atherosclerosis. These large central arteries are in sharp contrast to the diminished pulmonary vascular markings and the clear lateral third of the lung fields, a condition described as "pruning" of the pulmonary vascular tree (Figs. 101.4, 101.5).

ELECTROCARDIOGRAM

With the diastolic enlargement of the right ventricle there is increased prominence of the normal rightward and anterior terminal forces due to depolarization of the outflow tract of the right ventricle and crista supraventricularis. This is common to all types of IASDs with left-to-right shunts and results in an rSR' in V_1, a QR in aV_R, and an S wave in leads V_1 and V_6. Contrary to the normal variant with an rSR' in V_1, the R' in IASD is usually larger than the R wave. This is frequently termed *incomplete right bundle branch block*, but vectorially these terminal forces are not slowed and most probably represent just a delayed depolarization of the dilated right ventricle. Occasionally there will be true right bundle branch block with delayed terminal right anterior forces.

With the ostium primum defect because of the abnormally long His bundle, the branches of the posterior fascicle have a shorter distance to ventricular muscle than those of the left anterior fascicle. This results in a sequence of ventricular activation seen in left anterior hemiblock in which the posteroinferior left ventricle is depolarized before the anterolateral left ventricular wall, resulting in terminal forces that are leftward and superior. This results in severe left axis deviation in the frontal plane and simulates "left anterior hemiblock." Severe left axis deviation occurs in the vast majority of ostium primum defects and should be the primary reason for suspecting an ostium primum defect in a patient with IASD.

The electrocardiographic findings of the sinus venosus defect are similar to those of the secundum defect. In a study of 40 patients with sinus venosus defects, Davia and co-workers found that 40% had abnormal P wave vectors with abnormal left axis deviation of the P wave,

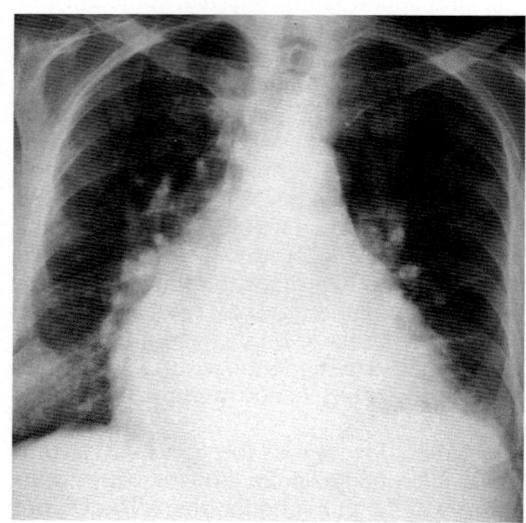

FIGURE 101.2 Chest roentgenogram, posteroanterior projection in a 70-year-old man with a history of heart failure for 10 years. Thought to have cardiomegaly, he was found to have a large secundum atrial septal defect with a pulmonary blood flow three times systemic blood flow. Notice generalized cardiomegaly and increased pulmonary vascularity.

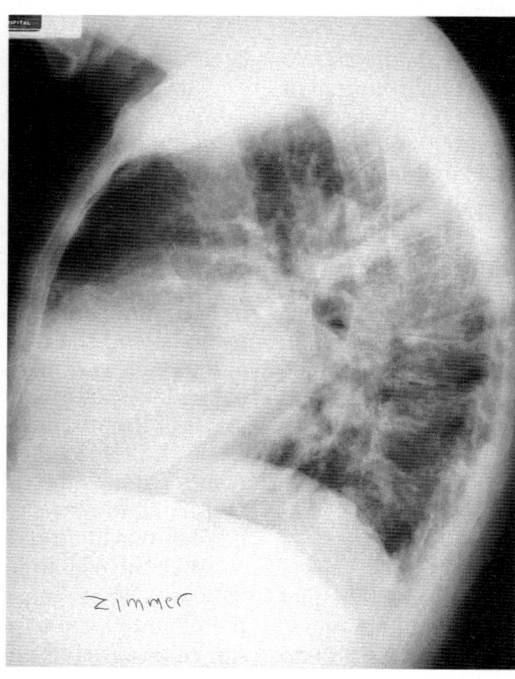

FIGURE 101.3 Chest roentgenogram, left lateral projection. Same patient as Fig. 101.2. Notice retrosternal filling by enlarged right ventricle and very large right pulmonary artery as it passes behind the ascending aorta.

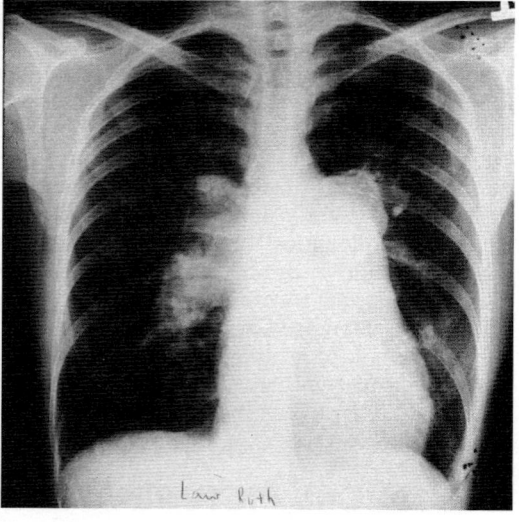

FIGURE 101.4 Chest roentgenogram, posteroanterior projection. The patient is a 40-year-old cyanotic woman with a large secundum interatrial septal defect with no residual left-to-right shunt and a large right-to-left shunt at the atrial level. Note the massive enlargement of the main pulmonary artery as well as the primary proximal pulmonary artery branches. This is in contrast to the absence of pulmonary vascular markings in the lateral one-third of the lung fields ("pruning of pulmonary vessels"). Note calcification in main pulmonary artery and right pulmonary artery, consistent with atherosclerosis and severe, chronic pulmonary hypertension.

indicating a low atrial pacemaker.[18] This finding should alert the clinician to a possible sinus venosus defect with accompanying partial anomalous pulmonary venous drainage.

ECHOCARDIOGRAPHY

M-mode and two-dimensional echocardiography have characteristic abnormalities making the diagnosis of IASD possible with a high degree of accuracy. The right ventricle is dilated as is the right atrium in IASD. The left ventricle is small compared with the right ventricle, and the interventricular septum is flattened in diastole, resulting in the "paradoxical" septal motion in systole seen in the M-mode echo. With two-dimensional echocardiography the right ventricular outflow tract and main pulmonary artery and bifurcation of the pulmonary artery are enlarged. In the apical four-chamber view, especially in the subcostal view, it is possible to image the IASD and determine its position in the atrial septum (Figs. 101.6, 101.7). Although pulmonary veins can be imaged as they come into the left atrium, it is usually not possible to image anomalously draining pulmonary veins. Such can be inferred if they drain into the coronary sinus by the presence of the huge coronary sinus.

With the injection of aerated saline or contrast medium, microbubbles appear on the echocardiogram and can be seen to cross the IASD after injection. These bubbles can be seen to cross to the left atrium, even in patients with large left-to-right shunts and normal pulmonary vascular resistance, and help identify the level of the left-to-right shunt. Among the available echocardiographic approaches to the diagnosis of atrial septal defect, two-dimensional contrast echocardiography appears to be the most sensitive. With Doppler ultrasound, abnormal turbulence can be detected at the septum and the relative magnitude of the shunt estimated by comparing right ventricular stroke volume with left ventricular stroke volume.

RADIOISOTOPE SHUNT STUDY

With bolus injections into the internal jugular vein, red blood cells tagged with technetium-99m can be imaged as they pass through the right and left sides of the heart. Normally both sides of the heart are seen in sequence because by the time the left side is imaged, the right side is cleared of radioactivity. In atrial septal defects, the radioactive tracer passes across the defect back into the right atrium, short-circuiting the systemic circulation and resulting in rapid and prolonged

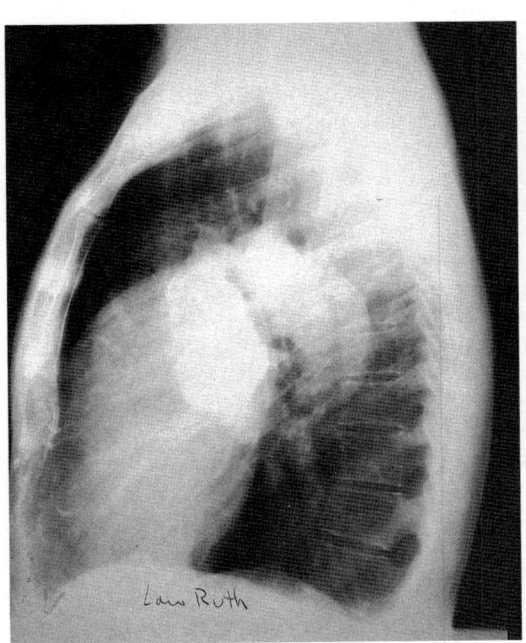

FIGURE 101.5 Chest roentgenogram, left lateral projection. Same patient as in Fig. 101.4. Note severe enlargement of the right ventricle retrosternally as well as the massive enlargement of the pulmonary arteries.

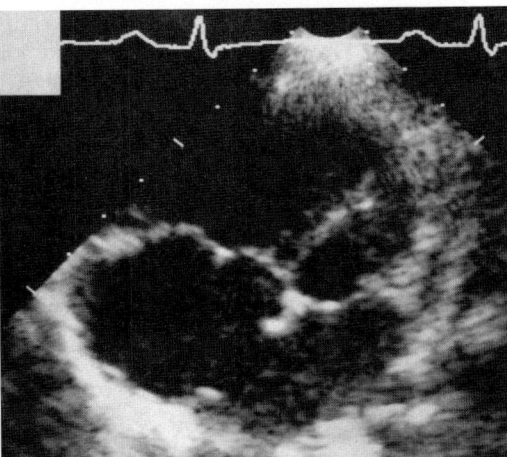

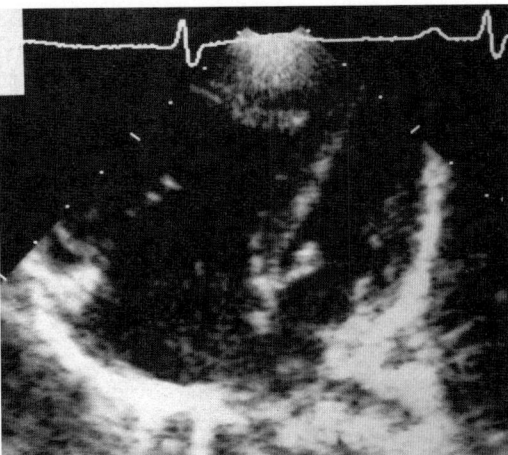

FIGURE 101.6 Two-dimensional echocardiogram of a patient with a secundum interatrial septal defect. Note the echogenic inferior run of the atrial septum in both right and left panels. Both are four-chamber views with slightly different angles showing echo dropout in the middle of the interatrial septum.

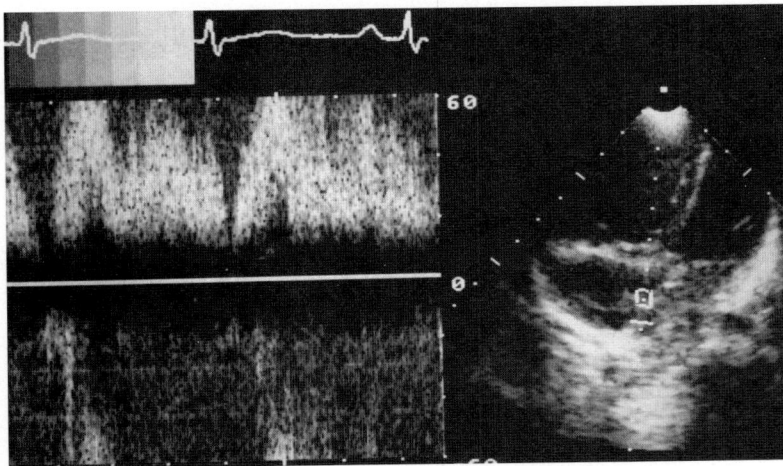

FIGURE 101.7 Two-dimensional Doppler echocardiogram: pulsed mode with Doppler cursor at the atrial septal defect. Left panels show disturbed velocities throughout cardiac cycle with peaks in systole and diastole, consistent with atrial septal defect with left-to-right shunt.

recirculation to the lungs, whose washout is slowed proportionally to the magnitude of the shunt. On the first-pass radionuclide angiogram, the usual three distinct phases of right side of the heart, lungs, and left side of the heart merge, owing to the rapid recirculation through the right heart, and the distinct left-sided heart image is obscured by the presence of radioactive tracer in the right side of the heart and lungs.[19]

With the first-pass technique, it is possible to image the time activity or "concentration" curve as the radioactivity passes through the lungs. The component of the washout curve due to recirculation can be extracted from the curve using gamma variate analysis, and when compared with the area of the systemic flow component, the size of the left-to-right shunt can be determined. Using this technique, Alderson and associates showed a good correlation between the radionuclide and oxymetric measurement of the shunt.[20]

COMPUTED TOMOGRAPHY AND MAGNETIC RESONANCE IMAGING

Both computed tomography and magnetic resonance imaging can visualize the IASD in both size and position. Magnetic resonance imaging is particularly valuable because of the lack of radiation and because the ability to image pulmonary veins and detect anomalous veins, especially the site of their drainage, is better than with catheterization and angiography.[21]

CATHETERIZATION AND ANGIOGRAPHY

Until the development of two-dimensional echocardiography and the more advanced imaging techniques, the definitive way to diagnose IASD was at catheterization. Here the demonstration of a left-to-right shunt by oxygen step-up or the early appearance of inhaled hydrogen establishes the presence of a left-to-right shunt at the atrial level. It is important to obtain blood samples for oxygen saturation both low and high in the superior vena cava, to detect anomalous pulmonary venous drainage into and above the superior vena cava. It should be remembered that an oxygen step-up in the right atrium is not pathognomonic of IASD (see Table 101.1).

Frequently it is possible to pass the catheter through the IASD into the left atrium and out into a pulmonary vein. It is also possible to enter the anomalously draining pulmonary vein and establish the level of the vena cava or right atrium into which it drains.

Right-sided heart pressures are usually normal, and with a large IASD there is usually no difference in the mean pressure between left and right atria. With large left-to-right shunts and high right ventricular stroke volumes, systolic pressure gradients of 5 mm Hg to 15 mm Hg can occur across the right ventricular outflow tract and pulmonary valve as measured by fluid-filled catheters. On occasion we have seen gradients up to 40 mm Hg without pulmonary valve disease.

With the development of pulmonary vascular disease, pulmonary hypertension and finally congestive heart failure, along with elevation of left and right ventricular end-diastolic and right atrial pressures, occur.

TABLE 101.1 DIFFERENTIAL DIAGNOSIS OF OXYGEN STEP-UP IN THE RIGHT ATRIUM

1. Anomalous pulmonary venous drainage to the right atrium or coronary sinus with and without atrial septal defect
2. Coronary arteriovenous fistula
3. Coronary right atrial fistula
4. Sinus of Valsalva aneurysm with rupture into the right atrium
5. Interventricular septal defect with tricuspid insufficiency
6. Left ventricular-to-right atrium tunnel
7. Dissection of aorta with rupture into the right atrium
8. Mitral atresia with a left-to-right shunt at the atrial level

Angiocardiography is valuable in detecting the exact position of the IASD in the septum but is rarely necessary. In the past, IASD has been imaged by injections into the pulmonary artery with follow-through in the left anterior oblique position. At present it is preferable to make the injection into the left atrium or right upper pulmonary vein and to image in the left anterior oblique position with a 15° cephalad angulation. This images the atrial septum on end. If a sinus venosus defect is present, angiography with injection into the pulmonary artery in the anteroposteral position will help to detect anomalous pulmonary venous drainage.

DIAGNOSIS OF ATRIAL SEPTAL DEFECT

The diagnosis of atrial septal defect is frequently made following history and physical examination together with the routine chest film and electrocardiogram. The typical patient with ostium secundum defect is likely to be relatively asymptomatic or may express some easy tiredness and fatigability and at times a history of some shortness of breath on exertion. On physical examination, a parasternal lift, with a widely split and fixed S_2 together with a relatively soft grade II/VI pulmonic systolic ejection murmur, is the usual finding. Additionally, some patients may demonstrate a soft tricuspid diastolic flow murmur along the lower sternal border. The chest film demonstrates increased pulmonary vascularity, reflecting the increase in pulmonary blood flow and volume. The main pulmonary artery segment is prominent, and there is usually enlargement of the right ventricle and right atrium. Left atrial size, however, is usually normal. The electrocardiogram classically shows an incomplete right bundle branch block, and in the usual secundum ostium defect this is often associated with a right axis deviation in the frontal plane leads. The above findings have in the past generally been supplemented by performance of cardiac catheterization to permit a definitive diagnosis. However, in a number of centers, when a clinical picture has been classic, patients have been scheduled for surgical correction without prior cardiac catheterization or selective angiography. With the advent of M-mode, two-dimensional, and contrast echocardiography, the diagnosis is readily confirmed, and at times, therefore, patients again will be scheduled for surgical closure without cardiac catheterization. The advantage of the catheterization technique is that it not only permits demonstration of the defect through angiographic studies or through passage of the catheter through the defect but also permits one to evaluate the magnitude of the left-to-right shunt and to evaluate the status of the pulmonary circulation. The left-to-right shunt in the usual secundum patient is simply the difference between the pulmonary and the systemic blood flows, and this can provide meaningful information relative to the desirability of surgical closure. In this connection, it usually is unnecessary to perform some of the tests described earlier, such as a radioisotope shunt study, computed tomography, or magnetic resonance imaging. These more sophisticated tests should be reserved for use in patients in whom the clinical presentation is atypical.

DIFFERENTIAL DIAGNOSIS

The differential diagnosis of oxygen step-up in the right atrium is shown in Table 101.1. The usual clinical problems that need differentiation from IASD are the following:

1. Innocent murmur. Systolic ejection murmurs without organic disease are common in children and in young adults. The systolic murmur is similar to that of the IASD; however, the S_2 is normally split or can be made to come together on sitting, standing, or Valsalva maneuver. There are no clicks or diastolic murmurs, and the chest film and echocardiogram are normal.
2. Mild valvular pulmonic stenosis. The presence of an ejection click and a large main pulmonary artery but normal peripheral pulmonary vascular markings help to differentiate this problem.
3. Patients with high cardiac output such as is seen in thyrotoxicosis,

severe anemia, and pregnancy can all have systolic ejection murmurs that can be confused with atrial septal defects.
4. Pectus excavatum and narrow anteroposterior diameter chest ("pancake" heart). A basilar systolic ejection murmur is common as is an apparently enlarged cardiac silhouette on the chest film.
5. Anomalous pulmonary venous drainage with intact atrial septum. A systolic ejection murmur is common in this situation. These patients are more likely to have a normally split S_2. At times one can see the anomalous vein on the chest film. This is especially true in the scimitar syndrome with total anomalous right pulmonary venous drainage into the inferior vena cava.
6. Other diseases frequently misdiagnosed in the adult patient with an IASD include
   a. Mitral stenosis because of the similarity in clinical and laboratory findings:
      1) Right ventricular hypertrophy
      2) Opening snap mistaken for widely split S_2
      3) Tricuspid diastolic murmur mistaken for murmur of mitral stenosis
      4) Enlarged pulmonary vessels seen in both
      5) rSR' in V_1 seen in both
   b. Cardiomyopathy and coronary artery disease, especially in elderly patients.

COURSE AND NATURAL HISTORY

The majority of IASDs in infants are not discovered since in the infant the compliances of right and left ventricles are similar and, therefore, there is little left-to-right shunting. As the child grows and the right ventricular compliance becomes greater than the left, the left-to-right shunt increases, and by the time the child is 3 to 5 years of age, there is a large left-to-right shunt, and all the signs given above have developed.

Usually the patient does not recognize symptoms during childhood and early adulthood, even with a huge left-to-right shunt. It is not unusual for the patient to feel better and recognize a greater exercise tolerance after surgical repair, compared with the preoperative condition. There is also excellent evidence that the ability to achieve normal maximal exercise capacity and maximal increase in cardiac output is impaired with a significant atrial septal defect. In the fourth decade, symptoms of decreasing exercise tolerance, fatigability, and dyspnea on exertion begin. In 15% to 20% of patients atrial arrhythmias occur, including atrial fibrillation, atrial tachycardia and flutter, and sick sinus syndrome. Beyond the age of 50 to 60 years, there is increasing symptomatology and the development of congestive heart failure and the vast majority of patients are symptomatic.[22] The possible reasons for this increasing symptomatology are the development of right ventricular dysfunction and decrease in left ventricular compliance due to hypertension, left ventricular hypertrophy, and myocardial ischemia, resulting in an increased left-to-right shunt.

The reasons for the development of pulmonary vascular disease in some but not other patients with ostium secundum atrial septal defects is unknown. It is almost never seen in patients under the age of 20 who live at sea level, whereas it is seen significantly before the age of 20 among patients who live at high altitudes. If it is going to occur, it will almost always occur before age 40. It appears that pulmonary vascular disease also seems to develop more commonly in women than in men.

There is massive enlargement of the proximal pulmonary arteries, clear peripheral lung fields, right ventricular hypertrophy, decrease in left-to-right shunting, and finally reversal of the shunt with right-to-left shunting and hypoxemia and its consequence, polycythemia (see Figs. 101.4, 101.5).[23] Chest pain possibly due to right ventricular myocardial ischemia, hemoptysis, arrhythmias, and sudden death are all seen. The time of death in these patients is usually in the fourth to sixth decades.

Of all patients with defects causing left-to-right shunts and finally pulmonary vascular disease and reversal of the shunt, these patients have the largest pulmonary arteries because the high flow and low pressure earlier in life have kept the histology of the pulmonary artery normal. With the large ventricular septal defect and patent ductus arteriosus and pulmonary vascular disease, the pulmonary artery is accustomed to high pressures and has "arterialized" with a change in media and histology toward that of the aorta. Therefore the dilatation of the pulmonary artery with severe pulmonary vascular resistance increase is less dramatic. With the high pulmonary artery pressure there is the development of atherosclerosis and calcification in the pulmonary arteries; and with polycythemia, thrombosis can occur in the pulmonary arteries, further restricting the lumen.

The development of pulmonary vascular disease markedly affects life expectancy in patients with atrial septal defect. In the data reported by Dalen and colleagues on the outcome of 48 patients with atrial septal defects diagnosed by cardiac catheterization between 1945 and 1956, 21 of 23 patients with normal vascular resistance were still alive in 1966, whereas only 5 of 20 with pulmonary vascular disease were alive.[24]

The mortality rate in patients with IASD has been calculated in the past, and the best summary of these data is in Campbell's paper published in 1970.[14] With most patients now being operated on, it is impossible to get a better estimate of the survival curve and the natural history of patients with an IASD. Campbell found the annual mortality rates to be low in the first 2 decades, at 0.6% to 0.7%. The annual mortality rose in successive decades from 2.7% in the third decade to 7.5% in the sixth. The mean age at death was 37.5 ± 4.5 years; three fourths of the patients were dead by age 50, and 90% by age 60.

INDICATIONS FOR SURGERY

A significant proportion of infants will demonstrate spontaneous closure of a secundum atrial septal defect. This will usually occur before the age of 4, and, therefore, surgical closure before this age is rarely indicated.[25] Once a child has reached school age, however, it is unlikely that spontaneous closure will occur. Therefore, such children should have routine closure of their atrial defect when it is discovered even though the children may be asymptomatic, provided the defect is of hemodynamic significance. In a sense, this is performed for prophylactic purposes, namely, to prevent the subsequent development in early adulthood of pulmonary vascular disease and the resultant decrease in longevity that will occur when this complication ensues. Additionally, closure prevents the late development of "left ventricular failure" and should be accompanied in most patients by a normal expected longevity. Since surgery can be carried out with less than 1% operative risk, this would seem to be a wise course in essentially all patients with a secundum atrial septal defect in whom the pulmonary blood flow is more than one and a half times the systemic blood flow and pulmonary vascular resistance is essentially in the normal range or reduced.

Because of increasing symptomatology with a large left-to-right shunt in later life, IASD should be closed even in older patients if there are no complicating problems. The mortality in operative closure in this group of older patients is acceptably low if one eliminates patients having concomitant procedures such as coronary arterial saphenous vein bypass grafting or valve replacement. In both the Nasrallah[22] and the St. John Sutton series[26] there was a marked improvement in symptoms postoperatively in patients over 60 to 65 years of age. Also, compared with an age-adjusted general population, there was a similar long-term survival after the IASD was corrected.

An exception to the above recommendation is the asymptomatic older patient with a sinus venosus defect, anomalously draining pulmonary veins, and a small left-to-right shunt. Operation in these patients requires patching the defect to include the anomalous vein on the left side of the patch and frequently also requires enlarging the superior vena cava with an onlay patch. Since this surgery can result in compromise of the superior vena cava or occasionally in tearing loose of the patch with misdirection of the venous return into the left atrium and cyanosis, if the shunt is small—less than 1.8:1—undertaking closure is probably not advisable.

When the pulmonary vascular resistance approaches systemic vascular resistance, that is, when there is Eisenmenger's syndrome with an IASD, there is generally little hope that there will be reduction in pulmonary vascular resistance if the shunt is closed. Since the atrial septal defect can be repaired without injury to the right ventricle, some have advocated the closure of the atrial defect with pulmonary vascular disease when the pulmonary artery pressure is not tremendously high and the principal problem to the patient is related to arterial hypoxemia and consequent polycythemia. Under these circumstances the defect can be closed, resulting in an increase toward normal of the arterial P_{O_2} and saturation. The price paid is that now, with exercise, all the systemic venous return must go through the lung, and with exercise the pulmonary artery pressure will rise higher than before surgery and thus put an increased afterload burden on the right ventricle, possibly resulting in right ventricular failure.

With the ostium primum defect, repair of the cleft in the aortic leaflet is undertaken with care not to create greater mitral insufficiency than before surgery. If this occurs the patient will be much worse off, with severe mitral insufficiency into the left atrium and pulmonary venous chamber without runoff to the right atrium. Therefore, the left atrial pressure will increase, and the patient will be more symptomatic than before surgery. Care must also be taken in these cases not to injure the atrioventricular node or His bundle; with present awareness of the problem this is a rare complication of surgery.

POSTSURGICAL REPAIR HISTORY

Almost all younger patients with atrial septal defects are asymptomatic before closure, even though after closure many feel better than they did before. A large proportion of symptomatic patients over the age of 65 years are symptomatically improved after closure of the atrial septal defect.[22,25,26] Problems have been seen, however, after repair of the defect at any age.

Recurrence of atrial arrhythmias occurs mainly in those patients who have had preoperative atrial arrhythmias. In a study by Brandenburg and co-workers[27] of 188 patients aged 44 years and older with isolated IASD, 27 (14%) had documented paroxysmal atrial tachyarrhythmias preoperatively, and 16 had paroxysmal atrial fibrillation. In a 1½ to 25-year postoperative follow-up (mean 12 years) of 16 patients with preoperative paroxysmal atrial fibrillation, 14 (88%) continued to have increasingly frequent paroxysmal atrial fibrillation.

Occasionally these arrhythmias will occur for the first time after repair has been accomplished; thus, atrial arrhythmias may be present in 15% to 23% of patients with "repaired" IASD. Of all patients older than age 60 the frequency of atrial arrhythmias may be as high as 50%.[28] It is therefore not warranted to tell the patient that the defect is being closed to prevent atrial arrhythmias.

Despite marked symptomatic improvement and increased exercise capacity postoperatively, there is good evidence that right ventricular function is not normal with exercise. Thus, the patient with repaired IASD may not be able to achieve maximum cardiac output and maximum exercise equivalent to a normal person of the same sex and age.[29] The right ventricular wall motion and ejection fraction have been measured by radioisotope techniques, and these studies have indicated a reduced ejection fraction and right ventricular wall motion.[30] Liberthson and associates[31] studied 20 adults with IASD. In all 20 the right ventricle was dilated preoperatively. In 9 asymptomatic patients, aged 18 to 45 years (mean 25 years), the right ventricular wall motion was normal preoperatively and in all patients remained normal. In 11 patients, aged 36 to 63 years (mean 52 years), there was moderate-to-severe right ventricular hypokinesia preoperatively. All had functional class II–III symptoms, and 6 had atrial fibrillation. The pulmonary to systemic blood flow ratio and systolic pulmonary arterial pressure were similar in the two groups. Symptoms and right ventricular size improved postoperatively in all 11 patients, but only 1 had normal postoperative right ventricular function and became asymptomatic. It thus appears that right ventricular dysfunction may be present in some patients before surgery, and in those patients the right ventricular function may not become normal after surgery.

A residual left-to-right shunt can occur and if this is sought can be found in 7% to 30% of cases; however, it almost never is as large as preoperatively.[2,32]

Interatrial conduction defects can be demonstrated with electrophysiologic studies,[33] and patch detachment with right-to-left shunt can occur. With residual mitral insufficiency a jet impingement on the septal patch and even severe hemolysis can occur. If there is no residual jet lesion from mitral insufficiency, then prophylaxis for infective endocarditis is not necessary in these patients.

REFERENCES

1. Hoffman JIE: Natural history of congenital heart disease. Circulation 37:97, 1968
2. McNamara DG, Latson LA: Long-term follow-up of patients with malformation for which definitive surgical repair has been available for 25 years or more. Am J Cardiol 50:560, 1982
3. Kitada M, Nakajima S, Uheda K et al: The natural history of congenital heart disease in young adults. Jpn Circ J 46:1246, 1982
4. Mody MR: Serial hemodynamic observation in secundum atrial septal defect with special reference to spontaneous closure. Am J Cardiol 32:978, 1973
5. Roberts WC: Cardiac valvular residua and sequelae after operation for congenital heart disease. Am Heart J 106:1181, 1983
6. Schrire V, Vogelpoel L: Atrial septal defect. Am Heart J 68:263, 1964
7. Rapaport E, Rabinowitz M, Haynes FW et al: Clinical and hemodynamic observations in Lutembacher's syndrome. Acta Cardiol 9:594, 1954
8. Nadas AS, Alimurung MM: Apical diastolic murmurs in congenital heart disease. Am Heart J 43:691, 1952
9. Levin AR, Spach MS, Boineau JF et al: Atrial pressure–flow dynamics in atrial septal defects (secundum type). Circulation 37:476, 1968
10. Tikoff G, Schmidt AM, Kuida H et al: Heart failure in atrial septal defect. Am J Med 39:533, 1965
11. Heath D, Edwards JE: The pathology of hypertensive pulmonary vascular disease. Circulation 18:533, 1958
12. Hislop A, Haworth SG, Shinebourne EA et al: Quantitative structural analysis of pulmonary vessels in isolated ventricular septal defect in infancy. Br Heart J 37:1014, 1975
13. Rabinovitch M, Haworth SG, Castenada AR et al: Lung biopsy in a morphometric approach to pulmonary vascular disease. Circulation 58:1107, 1978
14. Campbell M: Natural history of atrial septal defect. Br Heart J 32:820, 1970
15. Craig RJ, Selzer A: Natural history and prognosis of atrial septal defects. Circulation 37:805, 1968
16. Betriu A, Wigle ED, Felderhof DH et al: Prolapse of the posterior leaflet of the mitral valve associated with secundum atrial septal defect. Am J Cardiol 35:363, 1975
17. Liberthson RR, Boucher CA, Fallon JT et al: Severe mitral regurgitation: A common occurrence in the aging patient with secundum atrial septal defect. Clin Cardiol 4:229, 1981
18. Davia JE, Cheitlin MD, Bedynek JD: Sinus venosus atrial septal defect: Analysis of fifty cases. Am Heart J 85:177, 1973
19. Dollery CT, West JB, Wikken DEL et al: Regional pulmonary blood flow in patients with circulatory shunts. Br Heart J 23:225, 1961
20. Alderson PO, Jost RG, Strauss AW et al: Radionuclide angiocardiography: Improved diagnosis and quantification of left-to-right shunts using area ratio technique in children. Circulation 51:1136, 1975
21. Higgins CB, Byrd BF, Farmer DW et al: Magnetic resonance imaging in patients with congenital heart disease. Circulation 70:851, 1984
22. Nasrallah AT, Hall RJ, Garcia E et al: Surgical repair of atrial septal defect in patients over 60 years of age: Long-term results. Circulation 53:329, 1976
23. Young D, Mark H: Fate of the patient with the Eisenmenger syndrome. Am J Cardiol 28:658, 1971
24. Dalen JE, Haynes FW, Dexter L: Life expectancy with atrial septal defect: Influence of complicating pulmonary vascular disease. JAMA 200:112, 1967
25. Cockerham JT, Martin TC, Gutierrez FR et al: Spontaneous closure of secundum atrial septal defect in infants and young children. Am J Cardiol 52:1267, 1983
26. St. John Sutton MG, Abdul AJ, McGoon DC: Atrial septal defect in patients ages 60 years or older: Operative results and long-term postoperative follow-up. Circulation 64:402, 1981
27. Brandenburg RO Jr, Holmes DR Jr, Brandenburg RO et al: Clinical follow-up of paroxysmal supraventricular tachyarrhythmias after operative repair of a secundum type atrial septal defect in adults. Am J Cardiol 51:273, 1983
28. Bink-Boelkens MT, Velvis H, Homan vander Heide JJ et al: Dysrhythmias after atrial surgery in children. Am Heart J 106:125, 1983

29. Epstein SE, Beiser GD, Goldstein RE et al: Hemodynamic abnormalities in response to intense upright exercise following operative correction for atrial septal defect and tetralogy of Fallot. Circulation 47:1065, 1973
30. Graham TP Jr: Ventricular performance in adults after operation for congenital heart disease. Am J Cardiol 50:612, 1982
31. Liberthson RR, Boucher CA, Strauss HW et al: Right ventricular function in adult atrial septal defect. Am J Cardiol 47:56, 1981
32. Santoso T, Meltzer RS, Castellanos S et al: Contrast echocardiographic shunts may persist after atrial septal defect repair. Eur Heart J 4:129, 1983
33. Karpawich PP, Antillon JR, Cappola PR et al: Pre- and postoperative electrophysiologic assessment of children with secundum atrial septal defect. Am J Cardiol 55:519, 1985

Ductus Arteriosus and Ventricular Septal Defect in the Adult

CHAPTER 102
VOLUME 2

Warren G. Guntheroth

Ductus arteriosus and ventricular septal defect are two congenital cardiovascular anomalies with abnormal connections between the systemic and pulmonary circulation at levels reflecting arterial pressure, in contrast to atrial septal defects and pulmonary venous anomalies that connect at venous pressure levels. The ductus arteriosus is universally present prior to birth, but normally should close in the first day of life and become the ligamentum arteriosus. The modifying term *patent* is unnecessary when referring to the persistence of the ductus after birth.[1] For both a ductus arteriosus and a ventricular septal defect (VSD) the size of the connection between the systemic and pulmonary circulation varies widely from individual to individual, and therefore the pressure that is transmitted between the two circuits. The natural history of ductus arteriosus and VSD is similar because of the potential for high-pressure transmission from the systemic to the pulmonary circulation, which could lead to the development of pulmonary vascular obstruction, or Eisenmenger's syndrome. Consequently, most adults are in one of three categories, presenting with (1) a mild condition produced by a small connection with low pressure and with little symptomatology, (2) status postoperative repair of the ductus arteriosus or VSD, and (3) Eisenmenger's syndrome. The intermediate forms are rarely seen in adulthood, making the possibility or necessity of surgical correction uncommon in the adult age-group.

The cause of the ductus arteriosus or VSD in over 90% of cases is unknown. Although both connections are present in fetal life, the VSD is closed in the process of organogenesis, usually by the third month of gestation. The ductus arteriosus however should normally remain patent until the first day after birth; its persistence may reflect prematurity, or in most cases, a congenital anomaly not unlike that of the VSD. Generally, there is no genetic pattern to either defect, but a rare familial constellation can be demonstrated. Mostly the appearance of these defects is sporadic, and although the chance of having a second sibling with congenital heart disease is increased five to ten times over that of the general population, the higher rate appears to reflect a maternal milieu, rather than mendelian inheritance. Factors in the maternal history of importance include rubella in the first trimester for the ductus and maternal alcohol abuse during pregnancy for the VSD. If the mother has congenital heart disease, the chance of the infant also having congenital heart disease is substantially higher, directly related to the severity of the residual heart disease in the mother.

The ductus arteriosus constitutes approximately 10% of all congenital heart disease and has a significantly higher incidence in females (70% of the total). VSD is the most common of all forms of congenital heart disease, excluding the bicuspid aortic valve, and represents approximately 20% of all children with congenital heart disease. The figure is perhaps as high as 30% in the newborn and as low as 10% in an adult population with congenital heart disease.[2] The ratio of males to females in the population with VSD is approximately 1.

PATHOLOGIC ANATOMY

During fetal life the ductus bypasses the pulmonary circulation by connecting the main pulmonary artery to the descending aorta, with a relatively smooth arch. In the older child or adult with a smaller ductus, the aortic arch is smooth, and the ductus, similar to a ligamentum arteriosus, does not substantially alter the normal contours of either the pulmonary artery or the aorta. The length and width of the ductus varies considerably; additional variations include aneurysms, and in the older patient there may be calcification of the duct wall. This calcification can make the surgical interruption of the ductus more difficult.

VSDs vary not only in size but also in location. The majority (65%) occur in the membranous septum[3] (Fig. 102.1). The membranous septal defects are subaortic and somewhat posterior, toward the tricuspid valve. About 30% of the VSDs are in the muscular septum, and these are approximately equally divided between those in the posterior muscular septum, toward the tricuspid valve, and those in the more apical septum. Approximately 5% of the patients with VSD will have it localized in the subpulmonary position in the right ventricular infundibulum, also described as supracristal, in contrast to the membranous defects, which are subcristal. The importance of the supracristal defect lies in its involvement in herniation of the right coronary cusp of the aortic valve, inducing aortic insufficiency. Approximately 3% may have multiple defects. It is possible, although rare, to have a communication between the left ventricle and the right atrium in the relatively small area of membranous septum that normally divides these two chambers.

Clearly, almost half of VSDs will close spontaneously.[3] It has been suggested that the closure represents a delayed partition that should have been complete *in utero*,[4] but considering that this should occur in the first trimester of gestation, it is difficult to think of partitioning in the same sense as closure of the ductus arteriosus after birth. The membranous defects close in some individuals through involvement of the tricuspid valve. The process is assumed to involve endothelial roughening by the jet of the left-to-right shunt, both on the rim of the defect and on the tricuspid valve leaflet that is adjacent, leading to adhesion between the two surfaces and eventual fibrosis. Some have asserted that this is practically the only method of spontaneous closure of the VSD.[5] The tricuspid valve normally is sufficiently redundant that no disabling effects are observed on the valve function. There is a second category of membrane formation that may accrete in the same fashion as the membrane in subaortic stenosis.[3] The pathogenesis is thought to be accumulation of platelets on the roughened endothelium of the margin of the defect, and accumulation of a daily, microscopic increment over a period of months leads to membrane formation. If this is examined anatomically during its formation, it will frequently appear to be aneurysmal; this aneurysmal membrane is thought to be the source of an early systolic click that predicts the spontaneous closure of a VSD. Muscular septal defects can also close spontaneously through accretion of platelets and fibrin, followed by fibrosis. We found that the size of the defect did not affect the rate of spontaneous closure.[3]

In the adult with a large VSD without pulmonary stenosis there will always be evidence of pulmonary hypertension, and usually Eisenmenger's syndrome, with all of the associated pathology of pulmonary vascular obstruction, including medial hypertrophy of the arteries and intimal hyperplasia; terminally there may be intravascular clotting and pulmonary infarction. It should be noted that the original description of the anatomy of the Eisenmenger complex included an overriding aorta, but the name Eisenmenger's syndrome applies to the circumstances of pulmonary hypertension of an obstructive nature regardless of the precise anatomy of the aortic root and may also be applied to a ductus arteriosus with pulmonary hypertension. It also should be understood that most of the membranous defects are subaortic, and the decision as to where the septum should be in relationship to the aortic root in those individuals with a very large subaortic defect is somewhat

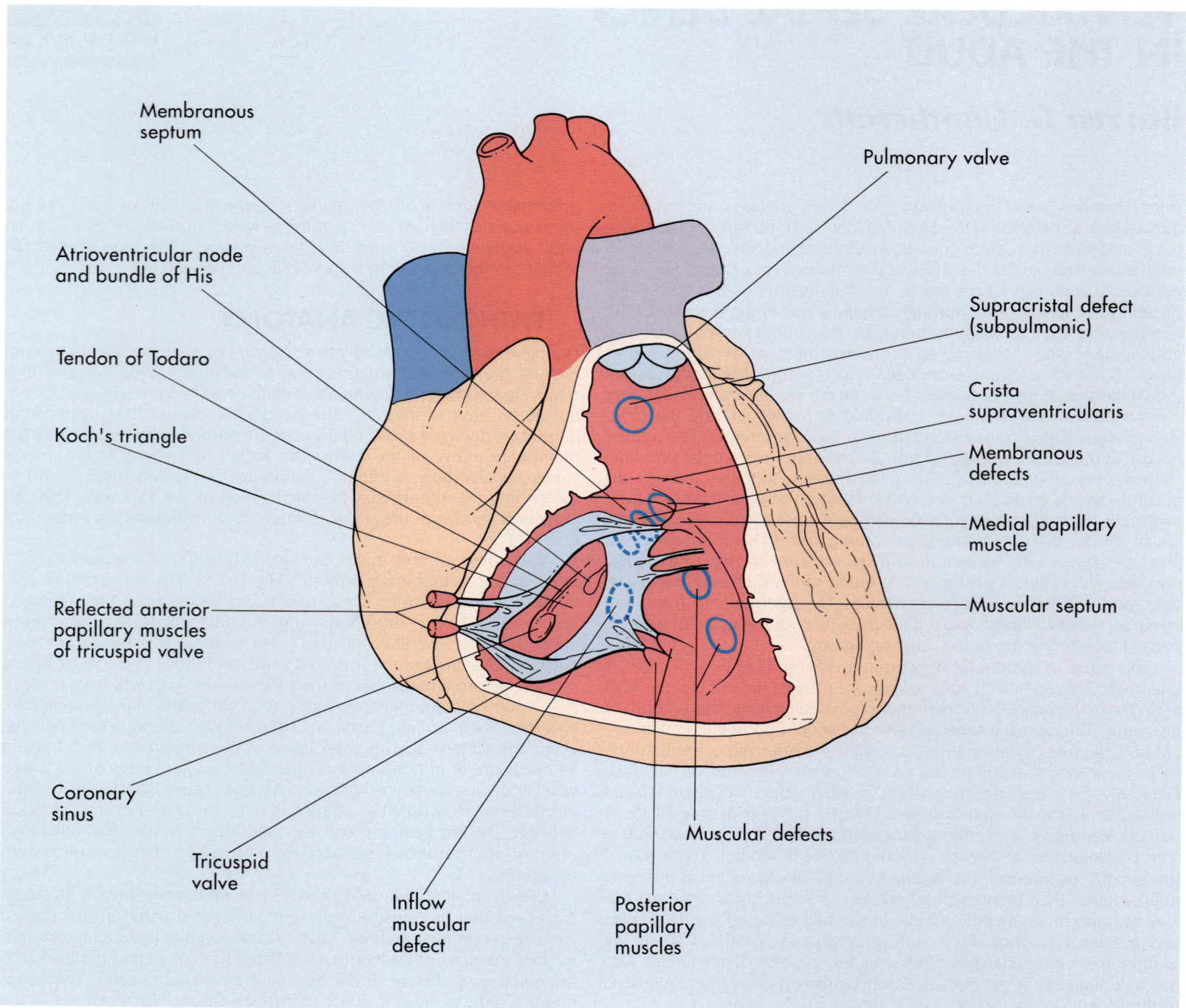

FIGURE 102.1 Drawing of the ventricular septum and location of the common defects. The tricuspid valve has been removed to allow visualization of a membranous inflow septal defect. Muscular septal defects can occur in many locations, but the supracristal or subpulmonic defects create special problems (see text). (Modified from Dillard DH, Miller DW Jr: Atlas of Cardiac Surgery. New York, Macmillan, 1983)

subjective and is best judged by lateral angiocardiography,[6] or by echocardiography.

The VSD can accompany many other congenital cardiac anomalies, including pulmonary stenosis, in which case tetrad of Fallot may be diagnosed. Kjellberg and colleagues[7] hypothesized that the presence of the VSD interfered with the normal location of the crista supraventricularis, the septal or the parietal band, or both; right ventricular hypertrophy would necessarily involve the crista, causing increasing infundibular stenosis in some patients with a VSD.

Aortic insufficiency, judged at autopsy, may represent a herniation of the right coronary cusp in the subpulmonary (supracristal) VSD but more commonly is associated with a membranous VSD and does not usually involve herniation. In the subpulmonary VSD, the cusp herniation may partially occlude the defect.

A VSD in association with congenitally corrected transposition of the great arteries (also known as levo-TGA or ventricular inversion) constitutes a serious anatomical problem for the surgeon because of the change in position of the conducting system, not to mention the coronary distribution and the fact that the mitral and tricuspid valves are also switched. Additionally, the effects of the abnormality on the endocardial cushion apparently expose the atrioventricular (AV) node to distortion and cumulative injury, resulting in AV block even without surgery.

The presence of either a VSD or ductus arteriosus will increase the chances of other congenital defects. For example, several centers (including ours) have found genitourinary tract abnormalities in approximately 10% of patients with a VSD.

PATHOLOGIC PHYSIOLOGY

The small ductus arteriosus will have relatively little hemodynamic impact on the young adult. The run-off from the aorta into the pulmonary artery will be small, by definition, so that the pulse pressure will not be altered significantly, nor will the pulmonary blood flow be increased by much. Similarly, since the increase in pulmonary venous return to the left atrium will be small, the left atrial pressure is not significantly increased and there is no increase in transudation in the pulmonary microcirculation. Consequently, these individuals will not have histories of frequent pneumonia in childhood, which the large ductus will create. The pressure gradient between the aorta and the pulmonary artery will be continuous, during both systole and diastole, and will produce the characteristic crescendo systolic phase and a decrescendo diastolic phase, unless the shunt is so very small that the total acoustical energy will be inadequate for the murmur to be audible at the chest wall. Some have pointed out that the diastolic flow through the ductus is coincident with the normal period of coronary blood flow and may therefore steal from the latter. This has been postulated as a cause for congestive failure in the older patient, even though the ductus is small. However, the appearance of congestive failure in that age-group may occur with or without a ductus, and the argument for mandatory surgical closure of the small duct is not supported by objective data.

The small ventricular septal defect also involves a large pressure gradient between the left and right ventricles and will produce a high velocity jet that can be heard at the chest wall as a high-pitched pansystolic murmur. Generally, it is held that these small VSDs produce the loudest murmurs, but if they are small enough they may produce sufficiently little acoustical energy as to be quite soft in intensity. With Doppler studies, we have documented small defects with inaudible murmurs and have observed the progression from a fairly loud pansystolic murmur to a soft murmur during spontaneous closure of the defect. The pansystolic nature of the murmur of a VSD can be predicted from the pressure gradients between the two ventricles, which will develop with isovolumic systole before the aortic and the pulmonary valves open (Fig. 102.2). Consequently, the murmur of a VSD will have an early onset and may be labeled a regurgitant systolic murmur, as opposed to the ejection murmurs of aortic or pulmonary stenosis. Only tricuspid regurgitation and mitral regurgitation will produce similar timing and quality of murmurs, but mitral regurgitation will appear at the apex, and tricuspid regurgitation, although sharing the location of the left sternal border with a VSD, will usually have a lower pitch, because the velocity is much lower in the patient who has no elevation of right ventricular pressure.

A large ductus arteriosus will usually be accompanied by severe pulmonary hypertension in the adult, and the continuous, machinery-like murmur of the smaller ductus will have disappeared. The flow will be confined largely to systole in those patients with high pulmonary artery pressures, but in whom a left-to-right shunt persists. The systolic murmur will be crescendo. The diastolic component is inaudible, and the flow can be demonstrated to be attenuated during diastole by Doppler technique.[8] In advanced stages of Eisenmenger's syndrome, the shunt can be entirely right-to-left, and there will be differential cyanosis, with greater cyanosis and clubbing of the toes than of the right hand. Confirmation can be provided by analysis of arterial blood gases from the femoral artery compared with the right brachial artery.

The large VSD in the adult with Eisenmenger's syndrome will have little, if any, left-to-right shunt and consequently will rarely demonstrate much in the way of a systolic murmur. The left ventricular inflow murmur of "relative mitral stenosis" that is seen with large left-to-right shunts is not present. Needless to say, the patient with Eisenmenger's syndrome will have a loud, single S_2 but neither a ductus arteriosus or a VSD will cause loud murmurs, and clinically it will be difficult to distinguish these conditions from idiopathic pulmonary hypertension, ex-

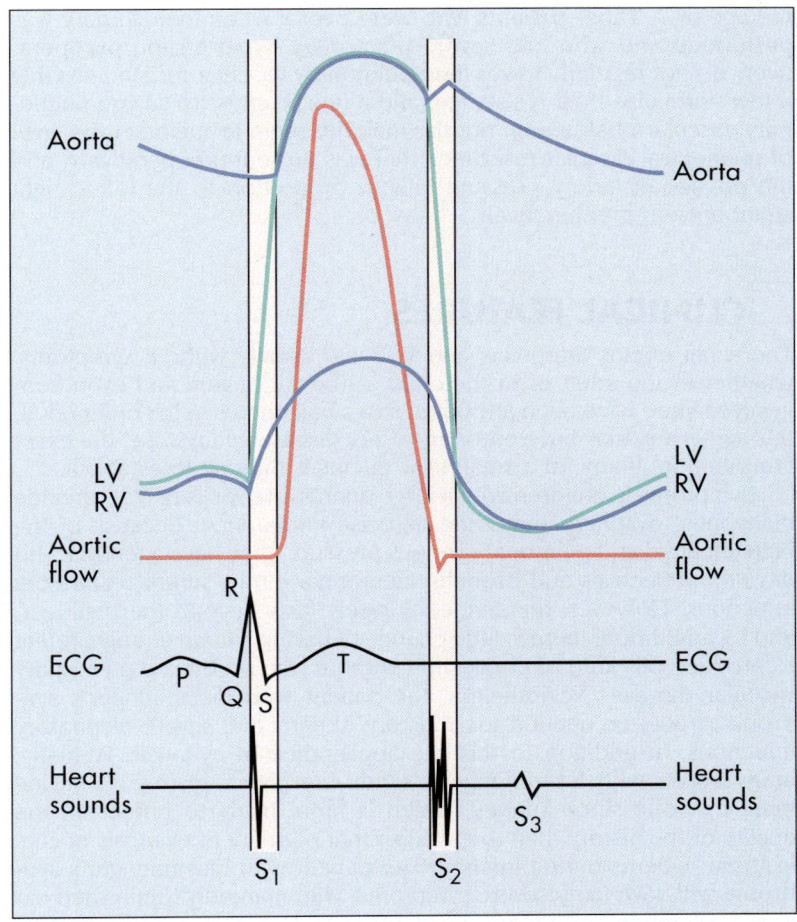

FIGURE 102.2 Diagram of the pressures in the right and left ventricle during a cardiac cycle. Pressure rises during isovolumic systole (*shaded interval*), prior to opening of the aortic and pulmonic valves and prior to onset of aortic flow. If a small VSD is present, the pressure in the left ventricle will quickly exceed that in the right and the flow across the defect will begin prior to ejection. The result is an early-onset, usually pansystolic murmur.

cept for a history of an earlier murmur from those patients whose pulmonary hypertension originated from a ductus arteriosus and VSD.

One effect of the presence since birth of a large ductus arteriosus or VSD has been asserted to be small body size. The assumption was made that the inefficiency of the circulation produced by the defects would interfere with normal height and weight development. However, the course during childhood is one that involves congestive failure only for the first year; if the subject survives, height is not particularly affected and the weight is affected predominantly in the first year. When small stature is encountered, it is more likely to be a coincidence, or to be secondary to a process that is more general, such as that found in the fetal alcohol syndrome and chromosomal problems such as Down's syndrome.

The postoperative patient whose VSD has been closed will commonly demonstrate right bundle branch block. Most often this is produced by the ventriculotomy and represents a parietal block that has no known disadvantage, except for obscuring true right ventricular hypertrophy on the electrocardiogram (ECG). In a smaller percentage, the right bundle branch block may follow injury of the moderator band or of the more central right bundle. These latter injuries have been reported to be associated with an increased risk of late, complete AV block, but the evidence has not been consistent. The assumption that these patients would behave in a manner similar to the adult infarction patient who suffered conduction disturbances of two of the three bundles and was a candidate for elective pacing in anticipation of complete AV block has not been confirmed.

Some patients after surgical repair of a VSD appear to have no pulmonary hypertension at rest, but moderate levels of hypertension have been recorded with exercise.[9] This seems to be particularly true for those subjects who had surgical repair later in life, particularly after the age of 7. Those patients who were over 2 when their surgery was performed and who had severe pulmonary hypertension preoperatively do not regularly lower their pulmonary vascular resistance. Only a few normalize their resistance, and a few progress to severe pulmonary vascular obstruction, but the majority seem to maintain the level of pulmonary vascular resistance that was present preoperatively, and the pulmonary artery pressure falls in proportion to the left-to-right shunt present preoperatively.

CLINICAL FEATURES

The small ductus arteriosus and VSD are usually without symptoms, whether in the adult or in the child. Although angina and even congestive failure have been attributed to a small ductus in the older adult, this age-group may have coronary artery disease in any case; the exact contribution, if any, of a small-flow ductus is difficult to establish.

Symptoms in children with a large ductus arteriosus or VSD include tachypnea, dyspnea, and some exercise intolerance. Because of the high left atrial and pulmonary venous pressure, they have a tendency to develop atelectasis and bronchopneumonia during minor respiratory infections. However, this tendency rarely lasts beyond the first year, and by adulthood, there is little chance of having a large enough defect to produce this kind of congestion without also producing pulmonary vascular disease. Nevertheless, the patient with Eisenmenger's syndrome should be queried for a history of early and severe respiratory infections, in addition to the late appearance of cyanosis. Actually, many adults with Eisenmenger's syndrome give a history as having been cyanotic since infancy, which is more likely to reflect on the quality of the history than to establish that permanent cyanosis occurs in these patients during infancy. The patient with Eisenmenger's syndrome will have fairly severe symptoms, with markedly diminished exercise tolerance, air hunger, headaches, and an increasing frequency of hemoptysis. Wood found that a third of his patients with Eisenmenger's syndrome had hemoptysis by the time they were 24 years of age, and by age 40, 100% had hemoptysis.[10] In his entire series, 29% of patients with Eisenmenger's syndrome had hemoptysis as the cause of death. Angina with exertion has been relatively frequent in some patients, and arrhythmias have been a significant problem in a few.

The small ductus arteriosus produces a murmur at the second left interspace with onset in early systole with gradual crescendo up to the S_2, followed, without interruption, by a decrescendo diastolic murmur. This murmur was first described by Gibson in 1900[11] and is frequently described as a machinery-like, continuous murmur. In the small ductus, the second sound is normal and inspiratory splitting will usually be obscured by the murmur. There will be no inflow murmur at the apex of the "relative mitral stenosis" type seen in childhood with large ductus flow, and their pulses and pulse pressure will be relatively normal.

The large ductus in the adult will present physical findings that are little different from those of any other patient with Eisenmenger's syndrome, and on auscultation they will be indistinguishable from those who have idiopathic pulmonary hypertension. The second sound will be loud and usually palpable, and splitting will rarely be appreciable. There may be an ejection click, reflecting the large main pulmonary artery reaching its elastic limit during systole. Since there is no runoff during diastole owing to the high pulmonary resistance, the peripheral pulses are not exaggerated. If a diastolic murmur is audible, it is likely to represent pulmonary insufficiency, rather than the diastolic flow through the ductus, which is the first physical sign to disappear with increasing pulmonary vascular resistance. Tricuspid regurgitation may occur with evidence of congestive failure, and since the rightsided heart pressures will be systemic, the murmur will be of early onset and high pitched, resembling a VSD. There may be differential cyanosis and clubbing, which can be appreciated more readily if the subject is quite warm, allowing peripheral vasodilatation to exaggerate the right-to-left shunt, which will increase the differential cyanosis between the feet and right hand.

The physical findings with a small VSD will be similar to those found in childhood—an early onset, blowing systolic murmur at the lower left sternal border that is more or less pansystolic. Some of the smaller, muscular defects however will be maximal halfway toward the apex and may be mistaken for mitral regurgitation. However, if the precordium is mapped out carefully with a stethoscope, it will be appreciated that the maximal intensity is not truly apical but between the apex and lower left sternal border. Also, these murmurs from muscular defects are not usually pansystolic but will end somewhat before the aortic closure. The S_2 will be normal in splitting and in intensity, and there will be no left ventricular inflow murmur with the small shunt. An early systolic click may be audible, suggesting that the defect is in the process of spontaneous closure through aneurysmal membrane formation. The click coincides with the maximal excursion of the membrane during early systole. The small VSD murmur will have a high-pitched, blowing quality, distinguishable from the murmur of tricuspid regurgitation, which will be more medium pitched and somewhat decrescendo in timing with normal right ventricular pressures. The large VSD with pulmonary hypertension in the adult will be indistinguishable from any other form of pulmonary hypertension. The few patients who develop infundibular pulmonary stenosis will have an ejection murmur rather than a pansystolic murmur and the S_2 will be single, and the pulmonary component will be inaudible or of low intensity. The increasing incidence of aortic insufficiency with age may create some difficulty in separating the patient with aortic insufficiency from those with pulmonary insufficiency secondary to pulmonary hypertension. The presence of a wide pulse pressure is an obvious clue for those with more advanced aortic insufficiency. The presence of a modest-sized VSD with aortic insufficiency may produce the combination of a systolic and diastolic murmur that superficially suggests a ductus arteriosus, but the VSD with aortic insufficiency will have a "to-and-fro" murmur. The VSD component produces an early-onset, plateau-shaped systolic murmur, compared with the crescendo systolic ductal murmur. The diastolic murmur of aortic insufficiency is characteristically high-pitched, compared with the diastolic phase of the ductal murmur.

The large VSD with Eisenmenger's syndrome may have murmurs of pulmonic insufficiency and tricuspid regurgitation. Late in the course, systemic hypertension is not unusual in Eisenmenger's syndrome and may or may not be associated with polycythemia.

ELECTROCARDIOGRAPHY

The ECG for either a small ductus arteriosus or VSD may be normal. For those defects that are between small and moderate size, a mild increase in left ventricular voltages may be seen, reflecting the fact that only the left ventricle has an increased volume for either of these anomalies. In the child with a moderate left-to-right shunt through either ductus arteriosus or VSD, a pattern that was once known as "left ventricular diastolic overload" may be found, consisting of relatively large Q and R waves over the left precordium, accompanied by prominent T waves. The large ductus arteriosus or VSD in adults however will usually reveal only right ventricular hypertrophy with Eisenmenger's syndrome, and the pattern of combined ventricular hypertrophy (Fig. 102.3) that is characteristic of large left-to-right shunts in childhood will rarely be found in the adult. In younger patients, the large shunt with high pressure will have both left ventricular hypertrophy due to the diastolic load of increased volume and right ventricular hypertrophy due to the increased systolic load faced by the right ventricle, ejecting against a substantially elevated pulmonary artery diastolic pressure. The adult patient with Eisenmenger's syndrome will simply have marked right ventricular hypertrophy, sometimes with "strain" with a wide QRS-T angle, and a T vector that is sometimes leftward and posterior in contrast to the anterior and rightward QRS vector. Right atrial hypertrophy may be suggested by p-pulmonale.

In the postoperative adult after ductus arteriosus division, the ECG will usually be normal, but in the postoperative VSD patient there will be right bundle branch block in the majority of instances. This does not indicate that the right bundle branch block followed interruption of the main right bundle but more likely the block followed the right ventriculotomy, causing a parietal block of no particular significance.

RADIOLOGY

Chest roentgenograms in the patient with a small ductus arteriosus or VSD will be similar, with a heart size that is normal or only slightly increased; if there is enlargement, it will usually be due to slight increase in size of the left atrium and left ventricle. In those instances of somewhat larger flow, but small enough to maintain normal pressures in the pulmonary circulation, the pulmonary blood flow may be modestly exaggerated, as deduced from the pulmonary vascular markings. Pulmonary venous congestion will not be present in this adult group, nor will it be present with Eisenmenger's syndrome. In the stable forms of Eisenmenger's syndrome the heart will usually be small, since there is no increase in volume work, but the main pulmonary artery will be very prominent, and frequently, but not invariably, the central hilar vessels will be enlarged, producing a "pruned tree" appearance. Later, with the development of pulmonary insufficiency and tricuspid regurgitation, the heart may be quite large. If there is aortic insufficiency associated with the VSDs, then left ventricular enlargement will be observed. Occasionally, a right aortic arch may be seen in the patient with a VSD, but rarely with a ductus patient with Eisenmenger's syndrome. In general, the appearance for the large ductus with Eisenmenger's syndrome will be indistinguishable from that of the VSD, except that the aortic knob on the left, in its usual site, will be prominent in the ductus (Fig. 102.4). Calcification may be seen in the ductus arteriosus, providing an additional clue to the diagnosis. In the VSD postoperative adult, the heart size will usually be normal, particularly if the surgical correction was done fairly early in childhood; but for those in whom it was done in late adolescence, it is common to find persistence of some chamber enlargement (particularly the left atrium and left ventricle).

ECHOCARDIOGRAPHY

The small ductus in the adult will be difficult to image with the echo, but Doppler interrogation will find the ductal turbulence quite easily

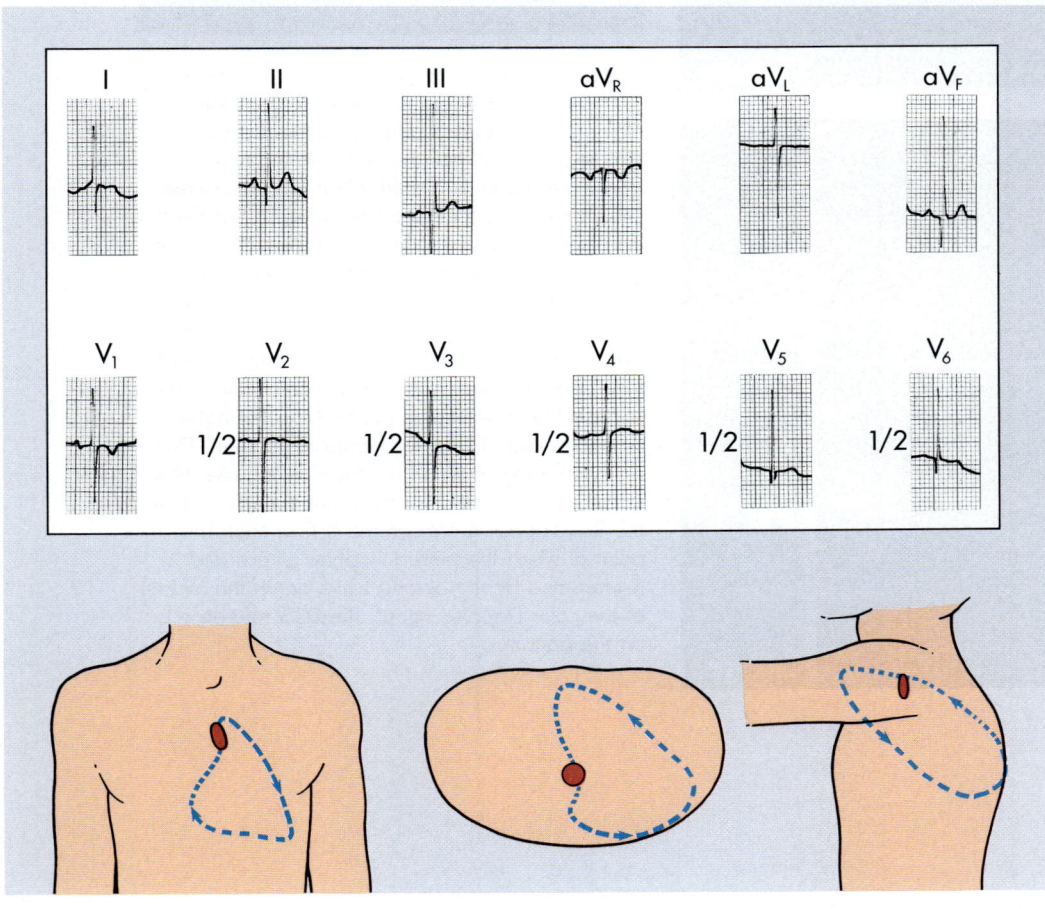

FIGURE 102.3 ECG and vectorcardiogram (Frank system) in a child with a moderately large VSD. The "fat loops" in the vectorcardiogram are characteristic of combined ventricular hypertrophy with left ventricular dominance. (Modified from Guntheroth WG: Pediatric Electrocardiography. Philadelphia, WB Saunders, 1965)

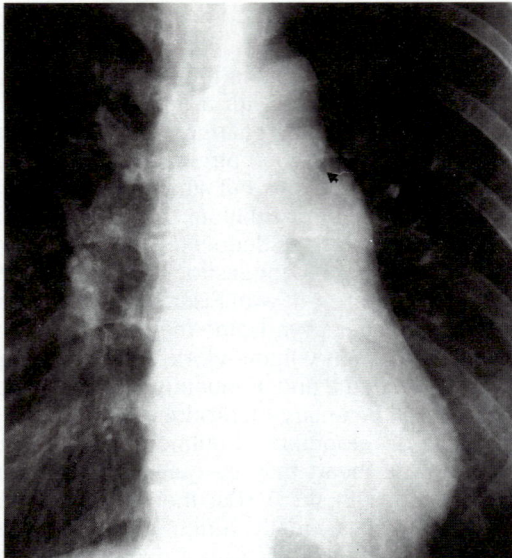

FIGURE 102.4 A chest roentgenogram in a young woman with a ductus arteriosus and pulmonary hypertension. There was still a small left-to-right shunt at the time of this film. Note the prominence of the aortic knob, consistent with the earlier large recirculation that was carried by the aorta, in addition to the pulmonary vessels.

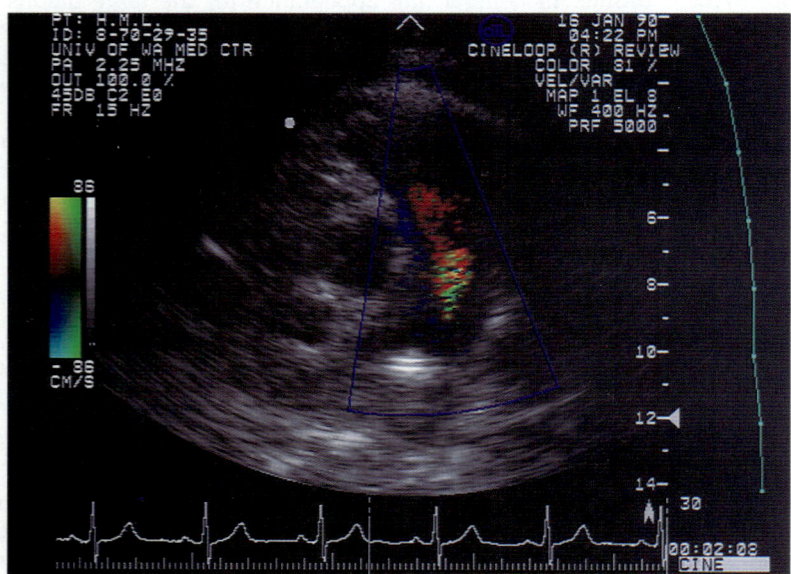

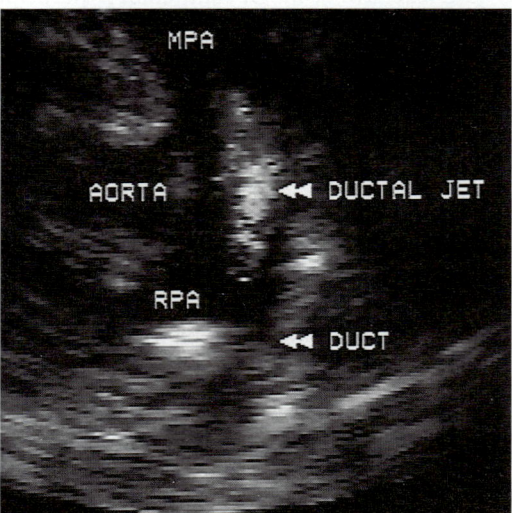

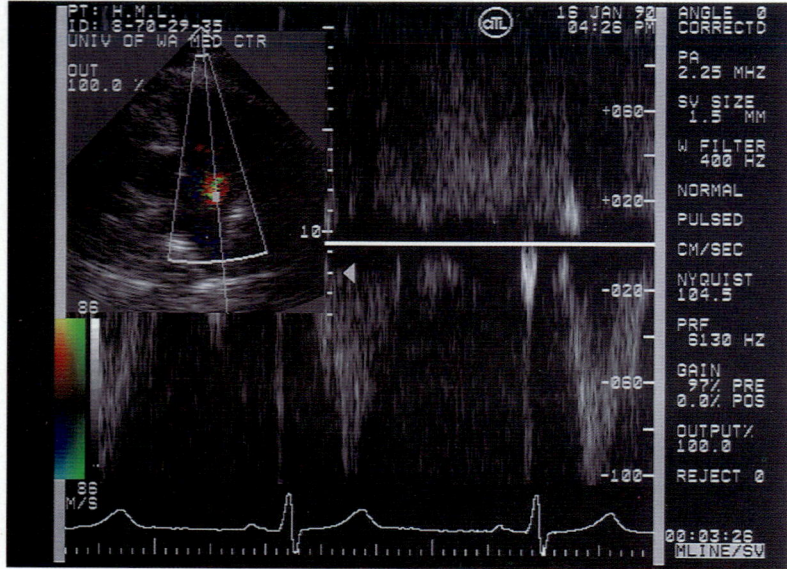

FIGURE 102.5 A. Freeze-frame of a color-coded Doppler echocardiogram from a 24-year-old woman with a ductus arteriosus. The red color indicates that the flow is coming toward the transducer, which is placed in the left parasternal short axis plane for the aortic valve; i.e., at the left parasternal margin at the third left interspace. The green and yellow dots indicate turbulent flow. Note that the diastolic flow extends back almost to the pulmonary valve. **B.** Black and white print of part A with labels. (*MPA*, main pulmonary artery; *RPA*, right pulmonary artery) **C.** Composite screen relating the conventional pulsed Doppler (right) and color-coded Doppler (upper left corner). The right ventricular ejection produces a negative flow in the main pulmonary artery, but during diastole the flow is positive (above the 0-flow line). The point at which the pulsed Doppler is recorded is represented by the oblong white dot in the middle of the color Doppler signal. The ECG reference is on the bottom.

when directed to the site of the left pulmonary artery from the parasternal short axis approach. The typical Doppler signal seen in the main pulmonary artery with systolic and diastolic turbulence is shown in Figure 102.5, the systolic flow is directed peripherally, but the diastolic flow is directed back toward the pulmonary valve. This flow disturbance in the main pulmonary artery may be absent in the very small shunt. However, when the ductus orifice is approached, continuous turbulent flow toward the transducer can be recorded. Similarly, on the aortic arch side of the ductus arteriosus, approached from the suprasternal notch, ductal flow can be recorded directly at its aortic orifice. The Doppler findings thus are significantly different from those of an aortic-pulmonary window. In the larger ductus, the duct itself can be imaged, and depending on the size of the left-to-right shunt and pulmonary hypertension, the left atrium and left ventricle may be enlarged. In the presence of pulmonary hypertension, however, the left-sided chambers will not be enlarged and the pulmonary artery may be, as well as the right atrium and right ventricle in later stages of the Eisenmenger's syndrome. If there is no pulmonary hypertension, the flow in the pulmonary artery will show both systolic and diastolic turbulence, but with increasing pulmonary vascular resistance, there will be attenuation of the diastolic flow.[8] Various echocardiographic clues to the presence of pulmonary hypertension are available such as flattened *a* waves, midsystolic closure of the pulmonic valve, increased ratio of preejection period to ejection time for the right ventricle, increased acceleration of flow in the pulmonary artery by Doppler studies,[12] and increased interval between the pulmonic closure and tricuspid opening, derived from either the echocardiogram[13] or the Doppler studies.[14] If tricuspid regurgitation is present, the peak velocity of the regurgitant jet can be used to predict the right ventricular–right atrial pressure gradient, and thereby the right ventricular systolic pressure.[12]

Small VSDs, those less than 2 mm in diameter, cannot be imaged by present technique. However, the jet is easily found by pulsed or color-coded Doppler, exploring with the 2D echocardiogram, bearing in mind that the defect may be in the muscular septum as well as in the membranous septum and inflow as well as outflow tracts of the right ventricle. The jet produces turbulent flow in the right ventricle and will be directed toward the transducer on the anterior chest wall, producing a positive flow pattern in the usual graphic presentation (Fig. 102.6). The 2D echocardiogram may demonstrate a partial occlusion of the septal defect by part of the tricuspid valve apparatus. In our opinion, the echo-Doppler study is now sufficiently specific and sensitive that there is little reason for cardiac catheterization in the small VSD or ductus arteriosus. In the presence of pulmonary hypertension, the VSD is likely to be large and easily appreciated by echocardiography, whereas there may be little flow through it by Doppler. The presence or absence of right ventricular outflow tract obstruction is of considerable importance since an adult with that plus a VSD is still a candidate for surgical repair, because this constitutes tetrad of Fallot. Systolic turbulence in the main pulmonary artery with a high velocity jet from the right ventricle rules out Eisenmenger's syndrome and establishes pulmonic stenosis. The Doppler examination also will provide evidence of insufficiency of the tricuspid, pulmonary, and aortic valves, all of which may be involved with a VSD, the first two in Eisenmenger's syndrome, and the last in any-aged subject with a VSD. The Doppler is particularly useful in the small muscular VSD with a pansystolic blowing murmur close to the apex that might be confused with mitral regurgitation. In mitral regurgitation, the regurgitant jet is directed posteriorly, in contrast to the anterior direction of the VSD jet.[15]

The echocardiogram and Doppler studies may also detect two other coincidental lesions that could potentially be corrected in patients that otherwise might be deemed inoperable Eisenmenger's syndrome, mitral stenosis, and cor triatriatum. Both of these conditions produce pulmonary hypertension secondary to pulmonary venous hypertension. We have encountered the former condition complicating a VSD in a young woman; both the mitral stenosis and the VSD were corrected at surgery.

CATHETERIZATION AND ANGIOCARDIOGRAPHY

The clinical appearance of a small ductus arteriosus or VSD is sufficiently unambiguous that cardiac catheterization and angiocardiography are not indicated, particularly if echocardiographic evidence is supportive. The findings by Doppler echocardiography are sufficiently specific that there is even less reason for considering an invasive study. If catheterization is deemed warranted in an individual, a step-up in oxygen saturation at the pulmonary artery level or ventricular level, in the ductus arteriosus and VSD, respectively, is examined for. Pulmonary vascular resistance should be calculated, and assuming a normal

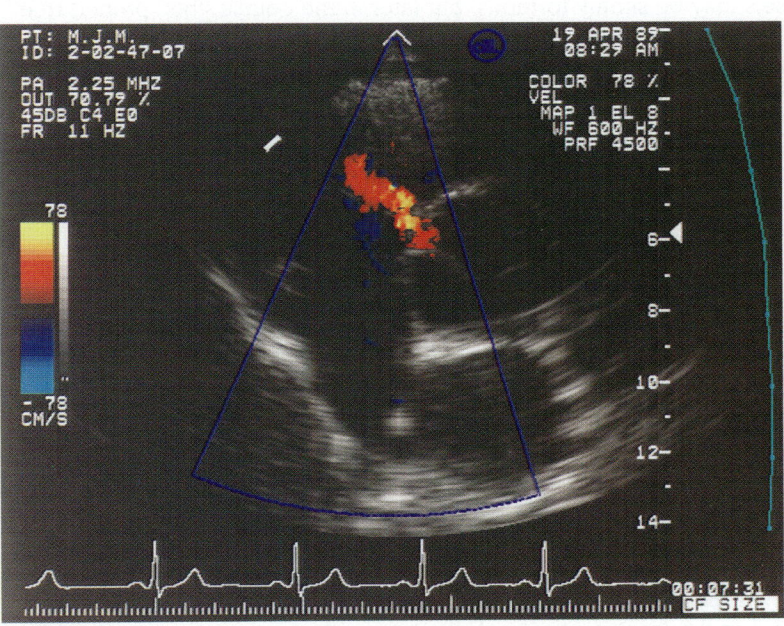
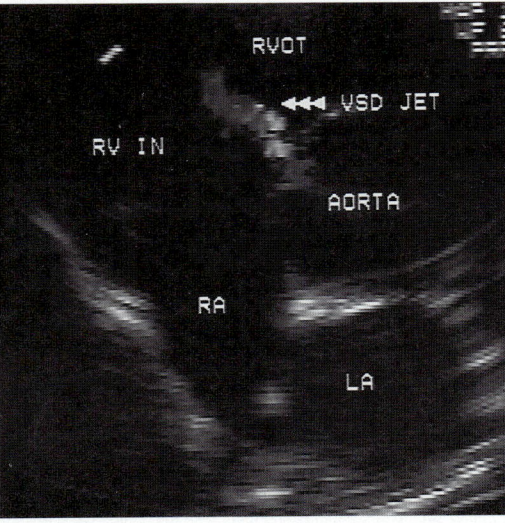

FIGURE 102.6 A. Freeze-frame of a color-coded Doppler echocardiogram from a 26-year-old man with a small membranous defect in the interventricular septum, immediately below the aortic annulus. The echocardiogram is from the left parasternal short axis view of the aortic valve. The flow is into the right ventricle and produces a red color, indicating that the flow is toward the transducer on the precordium. **B.** Black and white print of part A. (LA, left atrium; RA, right atrium; RVOT, right ventricular outflow tract; RVIN, right ventricular inflow)

systemic resistance, the ratio between the pulmonary and systemic vascular systems is a sound basis for determining normal versus increased resistance; the ratio is probably more reliable than the actual calculation of resistance in units or dynes seconds cm^{-5}. In the smaller ductus arteriosus and VSD, it would be surprising for the catheter to pass through the shunt, but if it does, the course of the catheter is relatively specific for either a ductus arteriosus or VSD. Angiocardiography will rarely be necessary and not particularly revealing unless the injection is made on the systemic side. This requires the addition of an arterial approach, and the small but real risk of femoral arterial impairment. For a ductus, the injection should be at the top of the aortic arch, and the filming should be in sufficient obliquity to maximize the aortic arch, without overlap of the ascending and descending aorta. For the small VSD, the filming should be done in a plane that is aligned to the plane of the ventricular septum. The plane of the ventricular septum usually runs at a 30° to 45° angle with the true anteroposterior orientation, and more than one injection may be required for optimal visualization.[16] For either the ductus or VSD, a hydrogen electrode recording from below and at the site of the suspected shunt will be diagnostic (Fig. 102.7).[17] That is not to say that this is required for a secure diagnosis, but the method is somewhat more sensitive than oximetry for small left-to-right shunts.

For large shunts, or more likely large anatomical connections but with Eisenmenger's syndrome in the adult, the indication for invasive study is the possibility of operability. This is not an endorsement of repeated cardiac catheterizations in the patient with Eisenmenger's syndrome, since there is little to encourage the belief that pulmonary vascular obstruction is reversible after the first 4 or 5 years of life. There may be rare exceptions, such as the patient with a ductus arteriosus whom we reported[18] whose early right-to-left shunt from pulmonary hypertension was related to chronic lung disease of the premature infant and in whom the resistance fell markedly after the first couple of years of life, allowing a resumption of left-to-right shunting and surgical closure. For an adult who has the physical findings of Eisenmenger's syndrome, the risks of catheterization are substantial and should not be entered into for a repeat confirmation of inoperability unless there is a significant possibility of an additional lesion that might produce pulmonary venous hypertension, such as a cor triatriatum or mitral stenosis. The search for a drop in resistance with the administration of 100% FIo$_2$, or the administration of a vasodilator such as tolazoline, is not an adequate indication for catheterization if the patient is clearly cyanotic at rest. Such a patient can be confirmed as having a significant right-to-left shunt by the simple laboratory test of a hematocrit or hemoglobin determination. If the hematocrit is five points above the normal of 45% for male and 40% for female, there is almost certainly a significant right-to-left shunt and there is little logic for heart catheterization, particularly recatheterization in an individual who has had a complete study with pulmonary wedge pressure measurements on an earlier study. An elevated pulmonary wedge pressure should be interpreted with some caution since the pulmonary arterial tree in advanced Eisenmenger's syndrome has a rather abrupt narrowing of diameter between the major arteries and arterioles and may make a true wedge pressure determination somewhat difficult. An apparent elevation in wedge pressure should be confirmed by wedging in more than one lobe. In some patients, the foramen ovale may be patent, permitting direct measurement of the left atrial and pulmonary vein pressures, which can rule out mitral stenosis or cor triatriatum. Again, echocardiography should be able to rule out these causes of increased "wedge" pressure.

For the adult with a large ductus arteriosus, confirmation of a right-to-left shunt does not require catheterization but can be demonstrated by comparison of a femoral artery blood gas study with that of the right brachial artery. However, even that is not required if the patient has cyanosis in the lower extremity, particularly if confirmed by an elevated hematocrit.

Occasionally, borderline cases of high resistance but significant left-to-right shunt, with a ratio of pulmonary to systemic flow of 1.5:1 to 2:1 by oximetry require additional information. The use of 100% FIo$_2$ to search for an increase in left-to-right shunting and a decrease in pulmonary vascular resistance is useful, although its application to patients who are clearly cyanotic at rest is of dubious validity. Similarly, tolazoline is widely used as an indicator of a component of the pulmonary vascular resistance that is reactive, rather than fixed pulmonary vascular obstruction. Of considerable importance is the avoidance of catheterization data from acute situations involving pulmonary disease, such as pneumonia or atelectasis, which assuredly will increase the resistance to blood flow in the lungs.

If angiocardiography is added to the catheterization in patients with an Eisenmenger's syndrome, it should be done with caution, since sudden death is not rare in that situation. Use of the newer contrast agents that involve un-ionized iodine compounds is indicated to reduce the risks, and digital subtraction angiography should be considered to permit the use of lesser amounts of the agent. The angiocardiographic appearance of the pulmonary vascular tree should be examined. In early stages of pulmonary vascular obstruction, the vessels may be simply tortuous, but later in the course, the "pruned tree"

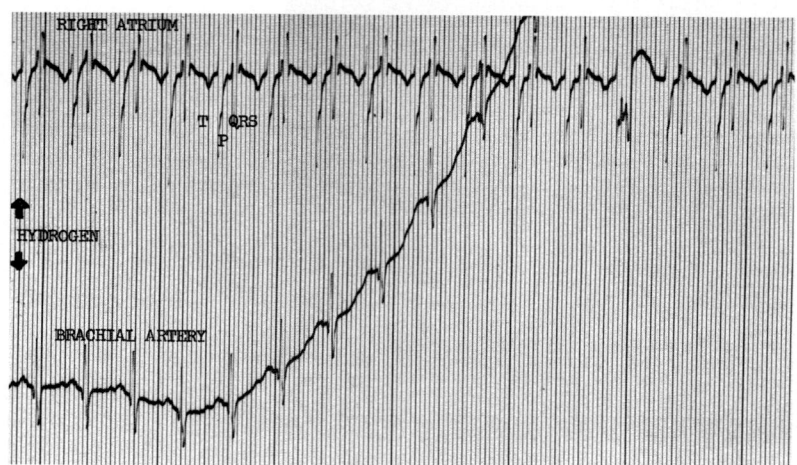
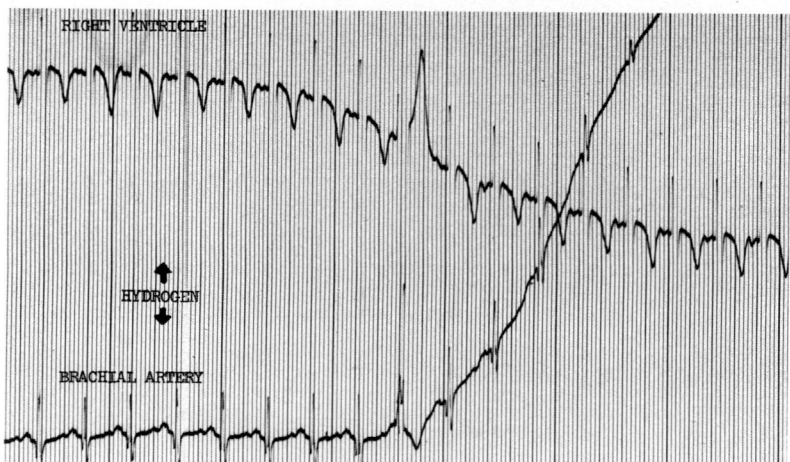

FIGURE 102.7 Hydrogen electrode records from an exploring catheter in the right atrium **(left)** and right ventricle **(right)**, compared with an electrode in the brachial artery. Inhalation of hydrogen is indicated by arrows. The typical intracavitary ECG complexes identify the location of the exploring electrode: large atrial complexes are above, and ventricular complexes are below. There is no change in potential in the right atrium, upstream of the VSD, but when the exploring electrode is in the right ventricle, the potential changes well before the change in the brachial artery, confirming the presence of a VSD. (Arcasoy MM, Guntheroth WG, Mullins GL: Simplified intravascular hydrogen electrode method. Am J Dis Child 104:349, 1962. Copyright © 1962, American Medical Association)

of abrupt transition from large to small caliber pulmonary arteries may appear.

If hypotension develops during the catheterization or angiography, an α-agonist such as phenylephrine may be helpful, or atropine can be used if bradycardia is present.

In the instance of an adult who has acquired infundibular stenosis resulting in tetrad of Fallot,[6] careful angiographic demonstration of the anatomy of the right ventricular outflow tract, as well as the site of the VSD, should be obtained. In addition, evaluation of the course of the coronary arteries is important and may require selective injection, but simple aortic root injection may be satisfactory to rule out a major coronary branch running across the right ventricular outflow tract where a surgeon might contemplate ventriculotomy.

COURSE AND COMPLICATIONS

The adult with a ductus arteriosus or VSD will usually have established the course of the disease by the time the cardiologist sees him as an adult. This course reflects the initial severity of the condition, namely the size of the early connection between the systemic and pulmonary circulations. The small connections will demonstrate a relatively benign course, uncomplicated by pulmonary vascular disease or congestive heart failure. For these patients the most significant complication is that of infective endocarditis. Fortunately, the site of endocarditis in patients with a small ductus arteriosus or VSD is usually in the right side of the heart, and embolization to the systemic circulation is then unusual. The ductus may become directly infected, which in some instances can lead to closure of the ductus by vegetations, although there are less benign outcomes of such a process. The cumulative risk of endocarditis has been advanced as grounds for surgical approach to the ductus with some logic, since Campbell estimated that the risk of infectious endocarditis was probably 1% per year.[19] However, the logic for surgery for small VSDs is less certain, although the risk of endocarditis is 0.6% per year.[20] Whether, in the postoperative patient, the right ventriculotomy and some distortion of the endothelium of the two outflow tracts may constitute hazards of equal importance, in general and with reference to endocarditis, remains to be seen. I have not found it a compelling argument to close small VSDs surgically as a routine. In particular this approach seems unwarranted given the cumulative rate of spontaneous closure of small VSDs, a process that is by no means confined to infancy. It has been evident for many years that adult cardiologists saw far fewer VSDs than their colleagues in pediatric cardiology, and the difference could not be accounted for by early demise or surgery. I have personally observed four young adults who had spontaneous closure of their small VSDs in their late teens. An unsightly median sternotomy scar can have more impact on the life of a young adult than might be imagined by individuals with little contact with this sensitive age group. Otterstand and colleagues found that adults with small VSDs had disturbed systolic function and limited working capacity, but they found similar—and worse—function in postoperative VSD patients.[21]

Surgical intervention is an important consideration for those patients with aortic insufficiency and a modest-sized VSD. There is an assumption in the literature that the course of the aortic insufficiency can be interrupted by early closure of the septal defect, but documentation is missing. Herniation of the right coronary cusp through the subpulmonary defect is certainly understandable, but the majority of individuals with aortic insufficiency, which involves as many as 6% of all VSDs,[22] show no clear relationship to either a subpulmonary defect or particularly large defects, and early closure of a small VSD may not alter the course of the aortic insufficiency. In fact, I have seen rare instances of young adults whose VSD was closed surgically but in whom aortic insufficiency was initiated by a mishap of a suture of the defect involving one of the coronary cusps. Another uncommon but serious postoperative problem in the young adult may be the requirement of a pacemaker for injury to the conduction system, resulting in complete AV block.

The development of infundibular pulmonary stenosis in the patient with a VSD may protect from pulmonary vasculature obstruction and create a tetrad of Fallot in the young adult. These patients are surgical candidates, and when they become cyanotic it is time to consider repair before polycythemia becomes a major factor.[6]

Pulmonary vascular obstruction is a complication of most larger ductus arteriosus and VSDs that survive to adulthood. The development is accelerated by living at high altitude. Pregnancy is quite hazardous to the female with Eisenmenger's syndrome, particularly at the time of delivery and shortly thereafter. The product of the pregnancy is at substantially increased risk of having congenital defects, including cardiac disease, and there is a fairly high rate of spontaneous abortion and of low birth weight infants if they survive until term.

Survival with Eisenmenger's syndrome until the 20s is not at all rare, but after age 30 there are relatively few recorded cases of survival. There are only a handful of patients in the world's literature who have survived beyond 40 years of age, although at least one has been reported to have survived until 63 years of age.[23] Hemoptysis takes a substantial toll, increasingly so after 25 years of age. Hypotension after some fairly minor procedures has been reported, including cardiac catheterization. Whether having a VSD or an atrial septal defect in the presence of Eisenmenger's syndrome is an advantage or not has been argued. The assumption is, if there is no communication between the two circuits and some event produces an acute increase in pulmonary vascular resistance, there will be inadequate venous return to the left side of the heart, and therefore inadequate cardiac output and shock and death may follow. In the presence of a communication between the two sides, such as a VSD or ductus, the right side of the heart can assist in providing perfusion pressure for the systemic circulation, although at the expense of a falling oxygen saturation.

The development of polycythemia is usually associated with symptoms of hypoxia, such as headache, which has led many centers to advocate venesection to lower the hematocrit. It is assumed that the reduced hematocrit will optimize delivery of oxygen to the periphery, but this argument fails to take into account picking up adequate oxygen during passage through the lung. If venesection is done, it must be done with replacement of the blood by either plasma or equivalent fluids, which will remain intravascular, as opposed to saline or lactated Ringer's solution. If no replacement is given for the blood, a hypercoagulable state develops acutely and the patient is at increased risk for cerebrovascular accidents. Having begun venesection, it will be necessary to continue this indefinitely, and the expense and unpleasantness are not trivial over a prolonged period. I have not elected to perform venesection in patients who had polycythemia except when it was accompanied by congestive heart failure. In that instance there can be little question that a reduction in viscosity below the level of 60% will reduce the work of the heart. Avoiding sodium in the replacement fluid is crucial in that situation.

In patients with polycythemia and cyanosis, a right-to-left shunt is present and consequently the danger of a cerebral abscess should be kept in mind. The development of neurologic signs, and even nonspecific changes in personality or somnolence, when accompanied by fever, should arouse suspicion and lead to consultation with a neurosurgeon or neurologist. These abscesses do not invariably require surgical drainage however, and in at least one instance in my experience, treatment was instituted early enough that the small abscess never liquefied; with intensive chemotherapy, the patient made a complete recovery without surgery. Still, most instances of cerebral abscess will require surgical drainage, in addition to intensive chemotherapy.

Management of the adult with a small ductus or VSD includes recommendations for physical exertion. There are no grounds for restricting the patients with small defects, and physical conditioning is as helpful to those individuals as it is for any one. Patients with Eisenmenger's syndrome, on the other hand, are at risk of sudden death with overexertion, and the patient should be counseled to exercise only up to the point of breathlessness and to avoid situations that do not permit the individual to set his own pace.

Prophylaxis against infective endocarditis is as important and probably more so for the adult than for the child with these congenital heart problems. Although for many decades, cardiologists seemed to be aware of oral sepsis as the most significant factor for endocarditis, following the unfortunate, anecdotal assertion by Kelson and White[24] that a high percentage of patients with endocarditis had had an extraction, the emphasis switched to a preoccupation with extractions and other dental procedures. In a survey of the literature, a total of 1,323 cases were found and an incidence of prior dental procedures of only 3.6%.[25] Earlier, Lewis and Grant[26] described the invasion of commensal organisms from the mouth, particularly *Streptococcus viridans*, as "almost physiological." Since the frequency of bacteremia after chewing is approximately the same as after an extraction, and considering the frequency of chewing versus an extraction, it can be argued that endocarditis, even following an extraction for an infected tooth, is approximately 900 times more likely to have resulted from the bacteremia from chewing rather than from the extraction. It seems much more productive for the physician to emphasize excellent dental care and hygiene for the individual with heart disease than to be excessively preoccupied with chemoprophylaxis, particularly the use of parenteral antibiotics.[25] For one thing, it is difficult for the vast majority of the world's population with heart disease to obtain parenteral antibiotics, and the net result inhibits dental care for these patients, who need it more than the average person. The British committee on prevention of endocarditis has recommended the administration of 3 g of amoxicillin as a single oral dose 30 to 60 minutes prior to an extraction or other major dental procedure, to be supervised by the dentist.[27] The absorption of amoxicillin is excellent; it is very little bound by protein, and the dosage recommended provides for at least 8 hours of bactericidal serum levels. This recommendation seems to be a significant improvement in terms of practicality, compared with the parenteral regimen of the American Heart Association.

Surgical intervention for patients with Eisenmenger's syndrome who have a ductus arteriosus or VSD should not be undertaken because of the high risk and the absence of any substantial benefit. Even if the patient survived closure of the defect, the change in pulmonary artery pressure would reflect only that of the left-to-right shunt existing prior to surgery; a patient with Eisenmenger's syndrome would not have a significant left-to-right shunt but would have a right-to-left shunt of varying size. Cardiac transplantation alone would have a similar lack of rationale, and the only reasonable procedure is a heart and lung transplantation. This is currently available in only a few centers.

Finally, the acquired VSD deserves surgical consideration, whether due to trauma or infarction. Clearly, it makes no sense to close a defect following an infarction if there is global or major dysfunction of the left ventricle, but if the defect is large and the evidence exists for reasonable performance of the left ventricle, then prompt closure may be lifesaving.

REFERENCES

1. Marquis RM, Godman MJ: Nomenclature of the ductus arteriosus. Br Heart J 49:288, 1983
2. Hoffman JIE: Natural history of congenital heart disease: Problems in its assessment with special reference to ventricular septal defects. Circulation 37:97, 1968
3. Moe DG, Guntheroth WG: Spontaneous closure of uncomplicated ventricular septal defect. Am J Cardiol 60:674, 1987
4. Mitchell SC, Berendes HW, Clark WM: The normal closure of the ventricular septum. Am Heart J 73:334, 1967
5. Anderson RH, Lenox CC, Zuberbuhler JR: Mechanisms of closure of perimembranous ventricular septal defect. Am J Cardiol 52:341, 1983
6. Guntheroth WG, Kawabori I, Baum D: Tetralogy of Fallot. In Adams FH, Emmanouilides GC (eds): Heart Disease in Infants, Children, and Adolescents, 3rd ed, p 217. Baltimore, Williams & Wilkins, 1983
7. Kjellberg SR, Mannheimer E, Rudhe V et al: Diagnosis of Congenital Heart Disease, 2nd ed. Chicago, Year Book Medical Publishers, 1959
8. Stevenson JG, Kawabori I, Guntheroth WG: Non-invasive detection of pulmonary hypertension in patent ductus arteriosus by pulsed Doppler echocardiography. Circulation 60:355, 1979
9. Maron BJ, Redwood DR, Hirshfield JW et al: Postoperative assessment of patients with ventricular septal defect and pulmonary hypertension: Response to intense upright exercise. Circulation 48:864, 1973
10. Wood P: The Eisenmenger syndrome. Br Med J 2:701, 1958
11. Gibson GA: Persistence of the arterial duct and its diagnosis. Edinburgh Med J 8:1, 1900
12. Hatle L, Angelsen B: Doppler Ultrasound in Cardiology, 2nd ed, pp 170, 257–258. Philadelphia, Lea & Febiger, 1985
13. Stevenson JG, Kawabori I, Guntheroth WG: Noninvasive estimation of peak pulmonary artery pressure by M-mode echocardiography. J Am Coll Cardiol 4:1021, 1984
14. Hatle L, Angelsen BAJ, Tromsdal A: Noninvasive estimation of pulmonary artery systolic pressure with Doppler ultrasound. Br Heart J 45:157, 1981
15. Stevenson JG, Kawabori I, Guntheroth WG: Differentiation of ventricular septal defects from mitral regurgitation by pulsed Doppler echocardiography. Circulation 56:14, 1977
16. Bargeron LM Jr, Elliott LP, Soto B et al: Axial cineangiography in congenital heart disease. Circulation 56:1075, 1084, 1977
17. Arcasoy MM, Guntheroth WG, Mullins GL: Simplified intravascular hydrogen electrode method. Am J Dis Child 104:349, 1962
18. Kawabori I, Morgan BC, Guntheroth WG: Reversal of "inoperable" pulmonary hypertension. Am Heart J 89:775, 1975
19. Campbell M: Natural history of persistent ductus arteriosus. Br Heart J 30:40, 1968
20. Otterstad JE, Nitter-Hauge S, Myrhe E: Isolated ventricular septal defect in adults. Br Heart J 50:343, 1983
21. Otterstad JE, Simonsen S, Erikssen J: Hemodynamic findings at rest and during mild supine exercise in adults with isolated, uncomplicated ventricular septal defects. Circulation 71:650, 1985
22. Corone P, Doyon E, Gaudeau S et al: Natural history of ventricular septal defect: A study involving 790 cases. Circulation 55:908, 1977
23. Warnes CA, Boger JE, Roberts WC: Eisenmenger ventricular septal defect with prolonged survival. Am J Cardiol 54:460, 1984
24. Kelson SR, White PD: Notes on 250 cases of subacute bacterial endocarditis studied and treated between 1927 and 1939. Ann Intern Med 26:40, 1945
25. Guntheroth WG: How important are dental procedures as a cause of infective endocarditis? Am J Cardiol 54:797, 1984
26. Lewis T, Grant RT: Observations relating to subacute infective endocarditis. Heart 10:21, 1923
27. Simmons NA: The antibiotic prophylaxis of infective carditis. Lancet 2:1323, 1982

CONGENITAL VALVULAR AND OTHER ISOLATED OBSTRUCTIVE LESIONS IN THE ADULT

Mary J. H. Morriss • Dan G. McNamara

Until recent years, patients with congenital malformations of the heart accounted for a very small percentage of adult patients evaluated for heart disease. Because infants and young children with lethal anomalies such as transposition, truncus, tetralogy of Fallot, and total anomalous pulmonary venous return are being saved by early medical and surgical treatment, these salvaged patients are entering adult life by the thousands each year. Among some 22,000 infants born each year with congenital heart disease, we estimate that about 60% of them (13,500) have an anomaly that would likely lead to their death if left untreated. Fully 80% of these infants (10,750) now recover as a result of modern medical and surgical treatment, and, allowing for late deaths in childhood, 90% of them (9675) will likely enter adult life. Cardiac centers for pediatric patients have been active in infant diagnosis and surgical treatment for about 20 years; thus, these patients are just now beginning to enter the realm of the internist and cardiologist responsible for the adult patient. Some of these patients are cured; others, although much improved, require continued follow-up. In a small percentage, the surgical result is poor, and the patients require additional treatment to be able to lead independent and productive lives.

In this chapter we consider the obstructive congenital lesions occurring at valves and elsewhere in the heart and vessels, and include obstructive lesions that persist despite surgery as well as those lesions that result from the operation. These lesions can be categorized as follows:

1. Obstruction to systemic venous return
2. Obstruction to emptying of the right side of the heart
3. Obstruction to pulmonary venous return
4. Obstruction to emptying of the left side of the heart

OBSTRUCTION TO SYSTEMIC VENOUS RETURN

Congenital systemic venous obstruction is not a known isolated defect producing symptoms, in spite of numerous embryologic variations that affect venous return. Acquired systemic venous obstruction may result from surgical repair of transposition of the great arteries by the Mustard or Senning technique. The superior vena cava and, less often, the inferior vena cava may become stenosed as a result of redirecting the orifices of the vena cavae to the systemic venous side of the baffle. Obstruction to vena caval return, although unusual, may be recognized in the early postoperative period, is usually isolated, and gradually subsides. If only the superior vena cava is obstructed, the connecting azygous system shunts venous return to the unobstructed inferior vena caval route.

It is not yet known whether late-onset superior vena cava obstruction will be an important problem in the adult who has had a Mustard repair in childhood, although recorded residual mean gradients as high as 11 mm to 16 mm Hg between superior vena cava and systemic venous atrium seem to be well tolerated.[1] Superior vena caval obstruction clinically presents with facial swelling, distended cervical veins, and prominence of the venous pattern on the upper torso as well as chylous pleural effusions attributed to high venous pressure transmitted to the lymphatic ducts as they drain into subclavian or internal jugular veins. Surgical repair can be accomplished with a high success rate. Late-onset superior vena caval obstruction has been described after presumed contraction of the pericardial baffle following endocarditis.[2] Partial superior vena caval obstruction allowing jugular venous stasis and thrombosis has accounted for one documented case of fatal pulmonary embolus.[3] The problem of venous stasis and SVC thrombosis is aggravated if a transvenous pacing wire is inserted to treat dysrhythmias in the postoperative Mustard patient.

OBSTRUCTION TO RIGHT VENTRICULAR INFLOW

Isolated congenital tricuspid stenosis is seldom encountered; most cases involve adults who have had confirmation of the congenital etiology by visualization of the valve at surgery. Degenerative changes on the congenitally stenotic tricuspid valve render this anomaly very rare in the child.

Obstruction at the tricuspid valve level produces the rare form of pure right-sided heart failure with jugular venous distention, prominent venous *a* waves (during sinus rhythm), hepatomegaly, and peripheral edema, without orthopnea, cough, or rales in the lung. Auscultatory findings may be confused with those of mitral stenosis, but careful attention to several differences may help in making the correct bedside diagnosis. With congenital isolated tricuspid valve stenosis, an opening snap is not present, nor is a diastolic thrill, although a prominent late diastolic rumble, scratchy and of high frequency with characteristic increase in intensity during inspiration, is heard at the lower left sternal border. The electrocardiogram in sinus rhythm shows right atrial enlargement but no right ventricular hypertrophy. Radiographic prominence of the border of the right side of the heart secondary to increased right atrial size is expected. Elevation of right atrial pressure at catheterization, especially the *a* wave, is usual, and the diastolic gradient across the tricuspid valve may be only slight because the large systemic venous reservoir allows a dissipation of right atrial pressure in tricuspid stenosis, much more so than does the limited left atrial reservoir allow a diffusion of left atrial pressure. Tricuspid valvotomy has been performed in this condition and provides the few direct observations of valve anatomy.[4]

Other forms of right ventricular inlet obstruction may also be apparent in adult life, with some forms acquired from surgical management of congenital heart disease. Satisfactory repair of complete atrioventricular (AV) canal in childhood may leave a patient with obstruction at the level of the tricuspid valve, particularly in the patient who has required tricuspid valve replacement. If tricuspid valve replacement in childhood has been necessary or if tricuspid annuloplasty has been required to improve right AV valve insufficiency after repair of other congenital defects such as tetralogy of Fallot, survival to adulthood with late manifestation of AV valve stenosis may occur. The attendant high risks of thromboembolism and endocarditis of prosthetic tricuspid valves are well known.

Obstruction at the tricuspid valve seen in association with Ebstein's anomaly is usually coupled with significant valve insufficiency, although rarely the obstruction may seem to be the dominant feature. It must be remembered that isolated tricuspid valve stenosis can be mimicked by the more common conditions of constrictive pericarditis and right atrial myxoma.

RIGHT VENTRICULAR OBSTRUCTIVE MUSCLE BUNDLE

Intracavitary obstruction to egress of blood from the right ventricle can occur at several levels (Fig. 103.1). The anomalous muscle bundle effecting a "double chambered right ventricle" and producing outflow obstruction in the sinus portion of the right ventricle occurs in 20% of patients as an isolated defect. In the other 80% it is associated with ventricular septal defect distal to the stenosis. The site of obstruction is well beneath the area of the infundibulum and anatomically quite unlike the obstruction of pure infundibular stenosis involving the crista supraventricularis or that associated with tetralogy of Fallot.

The anomalous muscle band traverses the cavity of the right ventricle, extending from the anterior wall of the ventricle to the crista or that portion of the ventricular septum just below the crista, dividing the cavity into a proximal high pressure chamber and a distal low pressure chamber. Progression in the degree of obstruction at this level has been demonstrated by serial catheterization in childhood and is estimated to be part of the natural history in up to 50% of cases.[5,6]

Clinical findings in patients with isolated right ventricular muscle bundle are indistinct from infundibular subvalve obstruction. Some clinicians confuse the auscultatory findings with those of a small ventricular septal defect. A harsh systolic murmur is heard at the lower left sternal border, with increasing length and intensity of the murmur and development of a systolic thrill paralleling increasing degrees of obstruction. Unlike pulmonic valve stenosis, an ejection click is absent.

Electrocardiographic findings can be normal in spite of significant outflow obstruction, with the lack of recognizable right ventricular hypertrophy attributed to the relatively small size of the proximal high pressure chamber. A pattern of right ventricular hypertrophy with prominent R waves over the right-sided chest lead V_{4R} without deep S waves over the left side of the chest has been described also in this anomaly.[7]

Cardiac catheterization should confirm the level of obstruction, and in all patients undergoing catheterization right ventricular pressure measurements should be made at the inflow area, apex of the ventricle, and outflow areas to avoid missing this diagnosis by recording right ventricular pressure only distal to the obstruction in the low-pressure chamber. Biplane angiography can successfully outline the obstruction, recognizing that the stenosis may be seen in only one projection and missed in the other owing to variations in the location of these muscle bundles. On the anteroposterior view the muscle bundle may produce a filling defect in systole that appears to separate the right ventricle into two chambers approximately equal in size, whereas in the lateral view the filling defect caused by the hypertrophied band appears to originate in the area of the crista but to follow an oblique course caudally and ventrally.

Recognition of double-chamber right ventricle may be possible with two-dimensional echocardiography when a thickened protrusion in the body of the ventricle is seen and further confirmation of the obstructive nature of the echocardiographic finding with Doppler studies is possible. Surgical correction is available for this defect, using the same indications used for relief of comparable degrees of infundibular obstruction.

INFUNDIBULAR PULMONARY STENOSIS

The outflow portion of the right ventricle between the crista supraventricularis and the pulmonary valve is referred to as the infundibulum. Infundibular pulmonic stenosis, occurring when there is stenosis of any part of this chamber, can be discrete or diffuse (see Fig. 103.1). Infundibular obstruction is most commonly seen as part of tetralogy of Fallot; however, primary infundibular stenosis can occur in isolation. Discrete infundibular obstruction is produced by a thick fibrous band situated at the junction of the right ventricular cavity and the outflow tract, with a well-defined infundibular chamber resulting. Less com-

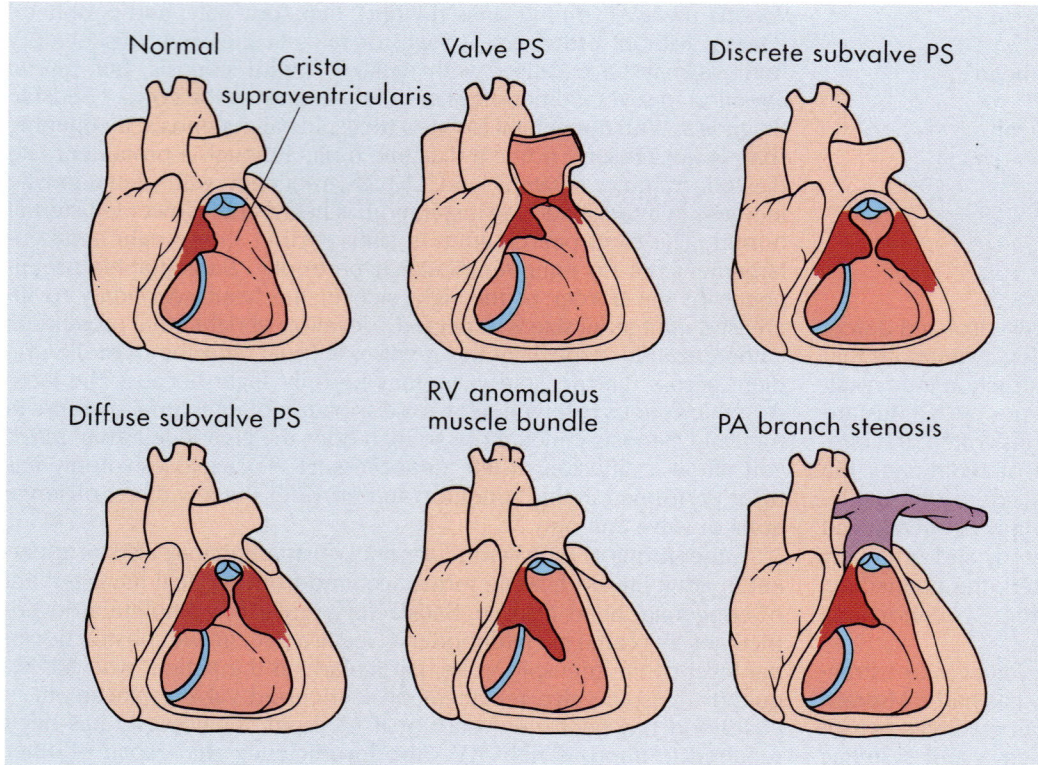

FIGURE 103.1 Anatomical sites at which obstruction to right ventricular outflow may occur. (PS, pulmonary stenosis; RV, right ventricular; PA, pulmonary artery)

monly, a more diffuse obstruction occurs secondary to marked muscular hypertrophy in the outflow portion of the ventricle and produces a narrowed area variable in length immediately beneath the pulmonary valve or lower in the infundibulum.

The physiologic effect of discrete infundibular obstruction mirrors that of valve pulmonic stenosis and relates to the degree of severity of outflow obstruction. A more dynamic obstruction can result when diffuse muscular infundibular narrowing is present and the outflow gradient can be measurably increased with provocative measures such as exercise or isoproterenol infusion. Subvalve pulmonary obstruction is possibly more likely to progress in severity than is isolated pulmonary valve obstruction.

Symptomatology is usually minimal unless significant obstruction is present and causes fatigue, exertional dyspnea, chest pain, or syncope. Congestive heart failure is rare, and onset carries a poor prognosis.

Physical findings may not be specific for this defect but when properly interpreted can suggest the degree of obstruction. Characteristically, when a systolic ejection murmur is heard lower on the chest than that usually attributed to pulmonary valve stenosis, subvalve obstruction should be considered. Locating the maximal intensity of the murmur at the third or fourth left interspace may suggest discrete low infundibular obstruction and the murmur might be difficult to distinguish from that produced by a ventricular septal defect. The murmur may have its maximal intensity at the third left interspace, a position often shared by the harsh murmur generated by isolated pulmonary valve stenosis, and correlate with the site of obstruction, being greatest just below the level of the pulmonary valve. The murmur becomes harsher and longer and more encompassing of the second aortic sound with increasing degrees of obstruction and thus is contrasted with the diminishing outflow murmur that is described when progressive infundibular obstruction occurs in tetralogy of Fallot. Outflow tract obstruction prolongs the right ventricular ejection time and is reflected in a widely split second heart sound with a diminished pulmonary component. A palpable thrill is present with all but the mildest degrees of obstruction. The ejection sound frequently occurring with valve stenosis is never encountered with isolated subvalve obstruction.

When the radiographic examination is not normal, the diagnosis of infundibular pulmonic stenosis may be suggested by viewing a bulge produced by an infundibular chamber along the left mid segment of the heart border in the anteroposterior or right anterior oblique view, which, because of its position, is not confused with poststenotic dilatation of the pulmonary artery segment. The electrocardiogram often dependably shows right ventricular hypertrophy, which correlates with the degree of stenosis.

Echocardiographic recognition of infundibular pulmonary stenosis previously centered around the M-mode feature of fluttering of the pulmonary valve leaflets due to their position upstream from the turbulence, which was not a feature of pulmonary valve stenosis. Two-dimensional echocardiography now allows visualization of the correct site of obstruction and the nature of the obstruction, that is, discrete or diffuse.

Pressure gradients obtained at cardiac catheterization can be diagnostic if an infundibular chamber pressure curve can be demonstrated. On pullback from the pulmonary artery there is no systolic pressure gradient measured across the pulmonary valve, but upon entering the infundibular chamber, the diastolic pressure drops and is the same as the diastolic pressure in the body of the right ventricle while the systolic pressure is elevated proximal to the infundibular obstruction. The short length of the infundibular chamber and the fact that the catheter holes may span the site of obstruction account for the failure to record these three different pressure areas in cases of isolated infundibular pulmonic stenosis. Right ventricular angiography will allow visualization of the location and severity of the infundibular stenosis and exclude an anomalous muscle bundle as the cause of the subvalve obstruction.

Treatment of infundibular pulmonic stenosis remains surgical, again with indications similar to those used in considering surgical candidacy when isolated pulmonary valve stenosis is found. It remains to be proven whether catheter techniques of balloon dilatation of isolated subvalve pulmonic stenosis will be safe and effective.

PULMONARY VALVE STENOSIS

Pulmonary valve stenosis, along with aortic stenosis and coarctation of the aorta, is one of the more common obstruction-producing forms of congenital heart disease that allows for patient survival well into adulthood.[8] A small number of infants with severe valvular pulmonic stenosis cannot be expected to reach adult years without operation. On the other hand, as suggested by the natural history study of this defect, mild pulmonary valve stenosis may have little hemodynamic effect and may not progress in severity.[9] Lack of progression is less well defined in children and adolescents who have at least moderate pulmonary valve obstruction. Persons who had pulmonary valvotomy for severe pulmonary valve stenosis in childhood will continue to need surveillance in adult years, since there is the possibility that operative relief will again be required for residual or progressive right ventricular outflow obstruction. A population of particular interest will be those patients who have undergone transvenous balloon catheter pulmonary valvuloplasty. The long-term results of this method must be defined, especially since surgical valvotomy has been one of the safest and most successful heart operations. Progressive right ventricular outflow obstruction in adulthood might be seen in patients who during infancy or childhood had conduit reconstruction of the right ventricular outflow tract as part of the repair of the congenital heart defect (*e.g.*, truncus arteriosus, pulmonary atresia). The peculiar phenomenon of formation of a luminal peel within the conduit may produce outflow obstruction over time, and conduits placed in childhood may become obstructive during pubertal growth or after attainment of adult size.

Pulmonary valve stenosis is the most common form of isolated right ventricular outflow obstruction and is virtually always congenital (see Fig. 103.1). A rare exception is the acquired obstruction due to carcinoid syndrome. Another infrequent acquired pulmonic valve stenosis is attributed to endemic rheumatic fever when rheumatic involvement of other valves is invariably present. The congenitally stenotic pulmonary valve typically has fused commissures of varying thickness and rigidity, with the most severe deformity consisting of an igloo configuration with central orifice and conical shape. There is a tendency of the valve orifice to enlarge somewhat as body size increases; however, this is offset by progressive thickening and fibrosis of the valve, which effectively reduce the orifice size. Calcification of the valve is usually seen only in adults who have had long-standing valvular obstruction. A more atypical valve dysplasia is described in isolation and in Noonan's syndrome, when Turner phenotype, normal chromosomes, and pulmonary valve stenosis are associated; in this anomaly the leaflets are often myxomatous, rigid, and limited in their lateral movement and less suitable anatomically for surgical valvotomy.

In most cases, the physical examination in a patient with pulmonary valve stenosis points to the valve as the site of obstruction. A systolic ejection sound, louder in expiration, is the most distinctive feature of the auscultation and is thought to be generated by the sudden excursion of the thickened pulmonary valve. The presence of this ejection click, although not invariably found, implies the valvular site of obstruction. It does not necessarily signify that important obstruction is present, and in the presence of more severe obstruction the click moves closer to the first heart sound, making discrimination from the first heart sound impossible. The severity of obstruction is frequently suggested by physical examination. A systolic thrill palpable in the pulmonic area, usually at the second left intercostal space, is present in all but the mildest obstruction and signifies an outflow gradient of approximately 25 mm Hg or more. A harsh systolic ejection murmur is heard in the same area with the intensity and length of the murmur increasing as obstruction becomes more severe. Prolongation of the right ventricular ejection time delays the second component of the second heart sound (P_2) and widens the splitting of the second heart sound in this anomaly. A long systolic murmur that peaks late in systole and extends up to or beyond the aortic component of the second heart sound (A_2) is a reliable indicator of severe pulmonary valve stenosis and is of greater usefulness than the width of splitting of the second heart sound. Poor compliance of a hypertrophied right ventricle may be inferred when prominent *a* waves are seen on inspection of the jugular venous pulse, when a prominent fourth heart filling sound is heard, and with palpation of a parasternal right ventricular lift, which is usually sustained.

Symptoms, if present, correlate with at least moderate severity of obstruction. Mild exertional dyspnea and fatigue due to inability to increase pulmonary flow may be the only complaints even with severe pulmonary stenosis. Angina, syncope, and cyanosis, possible with right-to-left atrial shunting through a patent foramen ovale, are seen only with severe pulmonary stenosis. Overt congestive heart failure, rare in childhood, is described in adulthood when tricuspid valve incompetence occurs. The lung hypoplasia seen in some adult patients with this condition is not implicated as the reason for symptoms.[10]

Radiographic findings are rarely specific for diagnosis of this anomaly and do not predict well the severity of valve involvement. Heart size and pulmonary vascular markings are generally normal in childhood, although increased heart size is common after 30 years of age. A large main pulmonary artery segment or left pulmonary artery attributed to poststenotic dilatation may be visible at the upper left border of the heart but correlates better with age than with severity. Valve calcification is seen only in adults who have had longstanding obstruction. The electrocardiogram is generally consistent in allowing quantitation of the severity of stenosis. Important pulmonary stenosis is reflected in electrocardiographic changes of right-axis deviation, right atrial enlargement, and right ventricular hypertrophy; when right precordial leads are interpreted to show a QR pattern with inverted T waves and ST segment depression, severe pulmonary stenosis is present. Echocardiographic confirmation of the valvular site of obstruction can be obtained, and Doppler-signal quantification of the expected gradient is possible.

Cardiac catheterization and angiography confirm the severity and site of obstruction, and therapeutic intervention has become available recently. Wood's classification[11] is useful in discussing severity and is based on the measured peak right ventricular pressure alone at catheterization, leading to designation as mild (right ventricular pressure less than 50 mm Hg), moderate (right ventricular pressure 50 mm–100 mm Hg), and severe (right ventricular pressure greater than 100 mm Hg). A mean systolic gradient across the valve of at least 10 mm Hg can be used to define a case of isolated pulmonary valve stenosis. Measurements of peak gradients across the stenotic valve must be interpreted with consideration of the conditions during which these measurements are made. Validation of the interpretation of these measurements depends on normal cardiac output, since the pressure gradient will be markedly affected (as a square function) by changes in cardiac output. Angiography may help in distinguishing a thickened pulmonic valve that domes in systole from a more dysplastic valve exhibiting thickened, more immobile leaflets with accompanying annular stenosis and narrowed sinuses. Infundibular narrowing acquired secondary to the valve obstruction should also be identified, since it may require additional surgical resection.

Therapeutic pulmonary valvuloplasty by means of catheter balloon dilatation has been described recently in children and in adult patients.[12,13] Adolescent and adult patients may require a dilatation technique using two balloons placed side by side because of the larger annulus size (Fig. 103.2). The risk of catheter occlusion of a stenotic valve during cardiac catheterization is still respected, but selected patients, even those with severe valve obstruction, may be found to benefit when pulmonary valve stenosis is relieved by this technique. Short-term follow-up suggesting sustained relief of obstruction is encouraging. There are concerns that when a severely dysplastic valve is identified, balloon dilatation will not be effective.

Symptomatic adults with pulmonary valve stenosis have been considered to be candidates for surgical valvotomy, in which an incision is made in the pulmonary artery and the valvotomy is performed from above the valve. Additional infundibular obstruction can be resected through the valve, and valvectomy of a severely dysplastic valve with patch enlargement of annular stenosis is employed if indicated. If preoperative right ventricular pressure is suprasystemic, an outflow patch is more likely to be required in order to successfully relieve the obstruction. Valvotomy or valvectomy renders the valve insufficient, but the resulting pulmonary insufficiency is usually well tolerated.

Earlier intervention in patients with pulmonary valve stenosis may be indicated if percutaneous valvuloplasty procedures are determined to be safe and efficacious, with preservation of right ventricular function assured. Bacterial endocarditis, although rare in this malformation, has been described, and prophylaxis against this condition is recommended.

PULMONARY ARTERY BRANCH STENOSIS

Stenosis in the pulmonary artery is usually congenital and may occur at any site distal to the valve, from the main pulmonary artery to the peripheral branches (see Fig. 103.1). There may be a single stenosis or multiple sites of stenosis in the pulmonary arterial tree. As with other forms of right ventricular outflow obstruction, the principal hemodynamic burden is that of right ventricular pressure overload, with the clinical severity related to the degree of obstruction. The feasibility of surgery and the surgical approach are dictated by the nature of the obstruction. Multiple peripheral pulmonary stenoses or coarctations of the pulmonary arteries are characteristically seen in patients with congenital rubella syndrome or as part of Williams' syndrome (see Fig. 103.8) in conjunction with mental retardation, with characteristic facies, and supravalve aortic stenosis[14]; up to two thirds of cases are associated with other forms of congenital heart disease. In general, when there are discrete areas of stenosis the distal vessel beyond the obstruction exhibits poststenotic dilatation and may become thin walled and aneurysmal, with the potential for erosion and rupture into small bronchi, resulting in hemoptysis. In other cases, the narrowed area may be elongated, with a more diffuse hypoplasia of the pulmonary arteries and no areas of poststenotic dilatation.

Differentiation of this site of obstruction from other sites of right ventricular outflow obstruction is not simple, based on auscultation alone. However, the absence of a systolic ejection click and wide transmission of the systolic murmur to the axillae and back or the presence of a continuous murmur may suggest peripheral pulmonic stenosis.

The electrocardiogram reflects the degree of right ventricular hypertrophy fairly reliably. The peculiar additional feature of left-axis deviation may be seen when this lesion is part of the rubella syndrome. The chest film is remarkable in its lack of main pulmonary artery dilatation. Cardiac catheterization confirms the distal site of obstruction with careful withdrawal tracings from the wedge positions to the main pulmonary artery and knowledge that the main pulmonary artery pressure proximal to the obstruction is similar to that in the right ventricle, with high systolic pressure and low diastolic pressure.[15] Angiocardiography is the single most useful method for confirming the diagnosis, allowing visualization of the severity and location of obstruction.

Proximal obstructions are able to be approached surgically with pulmonary angioplasty, but in general this form of pulmonary stenosis is less amenable to surgical correction, particularly if numerous areas of coarctation occur. The newer approach to relief of obstruction via catheter balloon angioplasty is still investigative.

PULMONARY VEIN OBSTRUCTION

Obstruction of the lumen of one or more pulmonary veins near their connection to the left atrium, while rare, occurs nevertheless in adults either as an isolated anomaly or in association with other cardiac malformations, causing important signs of pulmonary venous obstruction ranging from a chronic cough and exertional shortness of breath to frank pulmonary edema (Fig. 103.3). Obstruction of pulmonary veins can also result from extrinsic compression on one or more veins from adjacent primary malignancy, metastatic disease, or sclerosing mediastinitis.

Surgical repair of stenosis of individual pulmonary veins has been rather disappointing, unlike surgical repair of stenosis of the common pulmonary vein. We have had experience with one adult patient, a 30-year-old woman, in whom balloon dilatation of the stenotic areas was performed by Dr. Charles E. Mullins, but despite initial obliteration of the pressure gradient, the procedure proved to be only partially and temporarily successful.

Acquired pulmonary vein obstruction in the adult patient requires explanation, particularly in the setting of postoperative atrial baffle repair (Mustard or Senning operation) of anomalies such as transposition of the great arteries (Fig. 103.4). Patients who have had intra-atrial baffle repair for transposition of the great arteries may exhibit postoperative pulmonary venous obstruction, thought to be more common if Dacron material rather than pericardium is used for baffle construction. When acute, this problem complicates the early postoperative course and requires prompt revision. Pulmonary venous obstruction occurring several weeks or months after this operation has also been reported to develop even after postoperative heart catheterization demonstrated no pulmonary venous obstruction.[16] The possible mechanisms include formation of a neointima, baffle contraction, kinking of

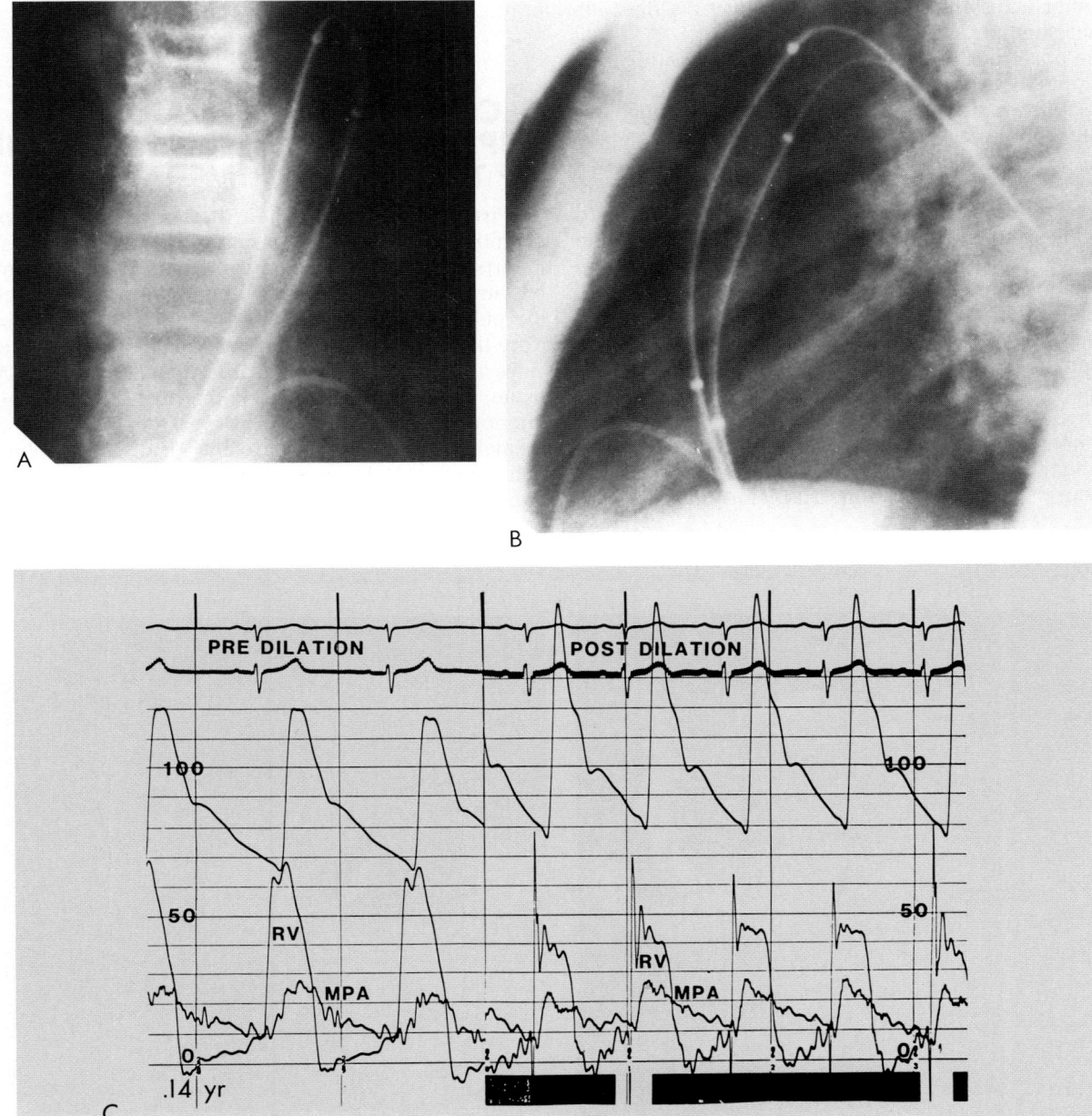

FIGURE 103.2 A and **B.** Pulmonary valve dilation technique in the older patient may require the use of two balloon dilatation catheters placed side by side. The balloons are inflated with dilute contrast material and are visible here on anteroposterior and lateral cine frames while dilatation is performed. **C.** Pressure tracing before dilation with gradient of 52 mm Hg. Right ventricular (RV) pressure 70/0,8; pulmonary artery (MPA) pressure 18/9. Pressure tracing post dilation with gradient of 20 mm Hg. Right ventricular pressure 45/0,5; pulmonary artery pressure 25/10. Note that there has been a significant change in simultaneously measured femoral artery pressure.

the baffle, development of adhesions between the atrial wall and the baffle, and simply growth of the patient. These events in a previously asymptomatic postoperative patient may cause symptoms of pulmonary venous obstruction later in life.

A similar problem can occur in a patient who has undergone operation for correction of total anomalous pulmonary venous return, especially if correction was performed in infancy or early childhood. Presumably, the anastomotic site between the common pulmonary venous chamber and left atrium fails to grow. In the adult who has had surgical repair of one of these defects, pulmonary symptoms such as exercise-induced coughing or wheezing may mimic pneumonia, asthma, or reactive airway disease and should raise the question of pulmonary venous obstruction. Chest radiographs exhibiting prominent unilateral or bilateral venous markings should suggest pulmonary venous obstruction, but films are often misread as pulmonary parenchymal disease. On physical examination, this diagnosis may be further suspected when either a distant continuous murmur or a diastolic murmur is heard, but often no murmur is audible.

Diagnosis of late-onset postoperative pulmonary venous obstruction might be confirmed by two-dimensional echocardiogram with abnormally high velocity flow pattern detected by Doppler, although this is accomplished much more easily in the thin-chested child than in the adult subject. Diagnosis may require cardiac catheterization and angiography in order to be certain of the precise site of the obstruction. The surgical result in transposition of the great arteries with Mustard repair should be highly successful if no pulmonary venous obstruction exists, providing the patient has sinus rhythm, no pulmonary hypertension or pulmonary stenosis preoperatively, and good ventricular function on ultrasound study afterwards. Thus, in the patient with the above criteria, important exercise intolerance either by history or by exercise stress test should alert the physician to the suspicion of pulmonary vein stenosis.

The same can be said for the patient with postoperative total anomalous pulmonary venous return. Since those patients can be cured by surgery, any impairment, including symptoms of exercise-induced dyspnea, cough, or wheezing, should raise the suspicion of pulmonary venous obstruction.

The clinical and noninvasive suspicion and identification of pulmonary venous obstruction can be very difficult. The difficulty is great in the young pediatric patient as well as in the adult. Although the young child is easier to examine by ultrasound as well as by auscultation, the adult can more readily describe the symptoms of exercise-induced breathing difficulty and fatigue that might provoke more prompt action. Likewise, mere "right heart" catheterization is inadequate for the diagnosis. It may be necessary to probe each of the pulmonary veins by retrograde catheter—aorta, right ventricle, "right atrium" (new pulmonary venous atrium), and pulmonary veins. Also, measurement of parameters of cardiac function under resting conditions alone may fail to identify the problem.

Surgical revision of the Mustard procedure consists of enlargement of the pulmonary venous atrium by sewing in a gusset in the atrial wall. Removal or replacement of the intra-atrial baffle is rarely necessary. Revision of the pulmonary venous anastomosis can be accomplished in reoperation for anomalous venous return.

COR TRIATRIATUM AND SUPRAVALVULAR STENOSING RING OF THE LEFT ATRIUM

Cor triatriatum occurs when there is partitioning of the left upper chamber of the heart and results during embryogenesis from failure of incorporation of the common pulmonary venous chamber into the true left atrium.[17] In this anomaly, the upper (proximal) chamber receives the pulmonary veins and is separated by a fibromuscular diaphragm from the lower (distal) chamber, which communicates with the mitral valve and from which the left atrial appendage arises. A patent foramen ovale, when present, connects the right atrium to the true left atrium inferior to the membrane. However, an atrial septal defect may communicate with either the proximal or distal chamber. Obstruction to pulmonary venous drainage results from small restrictive openings in the diaphragm. The degree of obstruction depends upon the effective orifice size and determines the age at clinical presentation. Severe

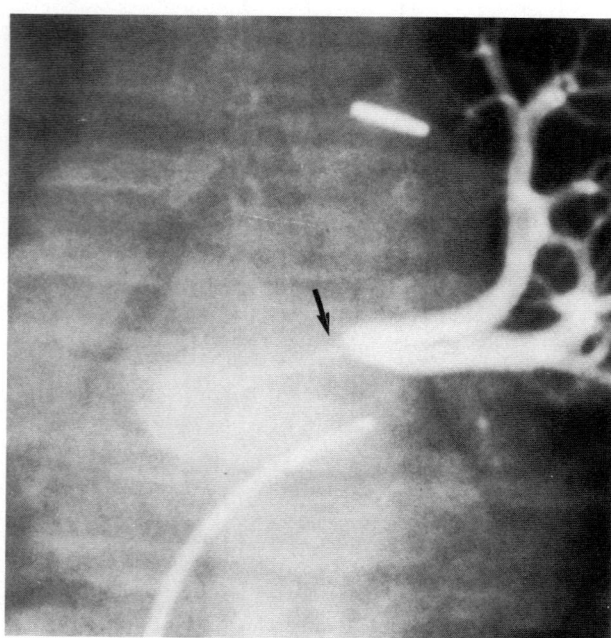

FIGURE 103.3 Severe obstruction to the left upper pulmonary vein demonstrated with a jet of contrast entering the left atrium (arrows) at the narrowed junction of the pulmonary vein to the left atrium. The transseptal catheter used for injection has been pulled back into the left atrium.

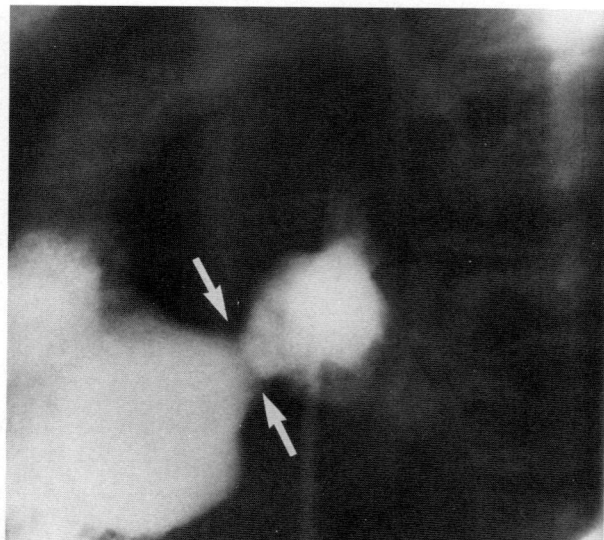

FIGURE 103.4 Pulmonary venous obstruction occurring after the Mustard operation. The newly created channel between the pulmonary veins and the pulmonary venous atrium is significantly narrowed (arrows), giving a "dumb-bell" appearance to the pulmonary venous atrium.

pulmonary venous obstruction causes symptoms in early infancy, but initial appearance of signs and symptoms in the presence of milder obstruction may be delayed until adulthood.

The clinical and hemodynamic presentation in isolated cor triatriatum resembles that of mitral stenosis, except that the murmur of cor triatriatum is less distinctive and often absent. Because of the rarity of the congenital lesion, the diagnosis is often overlooked. Patients complain of exertional dyspnea and shortness of breath, cough, wheezing, and frequent pulmonary infections. Less commonly, patients present with pulmonary edema, syncope with effort, or manifestations of low cardiac output.

The chest radiograph is interpreted to show cardiomegaly and pulmonary venous congestion, but radiographs are commonly misinterpreted as pulmonary parenchymal disease. Electrocardiographic evidence for right ventricular hypertrophy and right atrial enlargement is seen.

Auscultation consistently yields an increased pulmonic component to the second heart sound and a nonspecific systolic murmur; the presence of a mid or late diastolic murmur unassociated with the opening snap heard in acquired mitral stenosis may be of further diagnostic value. There are reports of patients with cor triatriatum who have no audible murmur.

This malformation can be detected from the apical or subcostal plane on two-dimensional echocardiogram,[18] which is considered by some to be a tool superior to selective pulmonary artery angiography in this condition. At catheterization the pulmonary venous obstruction is reflected in the elevated pulmonary artery and pulmonary artery wedge pressures. Technically good angiography can outline the diaphragm dividing the accessory chamber from the true left atrium. When the filling defect of the membrane cannot be seen, the obstruction may be suspected only when there is a prolonged transit time of the contrast through the lungs, with opacification first of the pulmonary venous chamber and later filling of the true left atrial chamber to which the left atrial appendage connects. Although the pulmonary hypertension seen in this condition is usually reversible and secondary to pulmonary venous obstruction, true pulmonary vascular disease may be present and a large bolus pulmonary artery angiogram to visualize the membrane may prove to be dangerous. The safety of the echocardiogram, as well as its high sensitivity and specificity for identifying cor triatriatum, renders ultrasound the better means to diagnose this anomaly. Cardiac catheterization (excluding pulmonary artery selective angiography) is needed largely to exclude other anomalies. One common associated anomaly is drainage of the left upper pulmonary vein into the left innominate vein. Another is patent ductus arteriosus. Echocardiographic demonstration of these anomalies may be readily achieved in the child but is technically difficult in the adult.

Surgical excision of the membrane is best performed using total cardiopulmonary bypass by entering the pulmonary venous chamber and removing the obstructing septum from above to allow free passage of pulmonary venous blood through the left atrium. If this is accomplished, relief of pulmonary hypertension will result, and follow-up catheterization has documented this benefit in individual patients.

Another malformation obstructing pulmonary venous return is supravalve mitral ring.[19] This malformation may be isolated but usually accompanies other congenital heart anomalies, such as ventricular septal defect, or is seen as part of the constellation of multiple sites of left-sided heart obstruction (Shone's syndrome). In this condition, a shelf-like ring produces obstruction just above the mitral annulus. In contrast to cor triatriatum, no separation into two distinct chambers is produced and the obstruction is found distal to the left atrial appendage.

Cardiac myxoma, usually left atrial in origin, must be considered in the differential diagnosis of the adult patient with clinical obstruction to pulmonary venous return or left ventricular filling. Myxoma is covered elsewhere in this volume and is acquired rather than congenital, but the manifestations may mimic pulmonary disease.

MITRAL VALVE STENOSIS

Mitral valve stenosis in the adult population is, of course, the result of acquired rather than congenital disease. Reported series of congenital mitral stenosis uniformly describe the early age of recognition of this anomaly, its rarity as an isolated defect, and its poor prognosis, with high mortality in infancy and childhood.[20,21] The anatomy of the congenitally malformed mitral valve is usually diffusely abnormal, with either small anulus, thickened valve leaflets, shortened chordae tendineae, or decreased interpapillary muscle distance or papillary muscle fusion (parachute mitral valve), all contributing to obstruction to left ventricular inflow. The natural history of severe congenital mitral stenosis is such that survival to adulthood without successful valvotomy or valve replacement in childhood is unlikely, but mild forms are becoming recognized with the aid of ultrasound. The expanded role of echocardiography in diagnosis of congenital heart disease may yield information about milder forms of mitral stenosis that may not be of the severity previously thought typical of congenital mitral stenosis and that may not produce symptoms until after puberty. For example, the frequently abnormal mitral valve structures known to be associated with aortic coarctation[22] may become functionally obstructive and produce signs of mitral stenosis in adulthood.

Mitral stenosis may be important in the adult in the setting of congenital heart disease when it is acquired after surgical repair of congenital defects. When repair of the AV canal has been performed in childhood, insufficient tissue may be available to allow reconstruction of a well-functioning left AV valve, and this valve may become an important site of obstruction in later years. If mitral insufficiency has been previously improved with surgical annuloplasty or valve replacement, mitral stenosis in the adult can be a long-term sequela to surgery.

Clinical symptoms are shared by all forms of mitral stenosis and relate to the severity of obstruction rather than to its location or cause, congenital or acquired. Left atrial, pulmonary venous, and pulmonary capillary pressure are elevated and produce symptoms of increased work and effort of breathing, with later pulmonary edema interfering with gas exchange in the lungs manifest as increased $PaCO_2$ and decreased PaO_2. Hemoptysis due to rupture of thin-walled bronchial veins, chest pain, and thromboembolism, particularly when atrial fibrillation is present, are other symptoms seen in the adult with mitral stenosis. Sudden hoarseness may result when the recurrent laryngeal nerve is compressed by a large left atrium or stapled by the large left atrium and dilated pulmonary artery. By the time right-sided heart failure secondary to mitral valve stenosis develops, the condition is very far advanced.

On physical examination, shared features of low cardiac output, tachypnea, and auscultatory evidence of a loud pulmonary closure sound, pulmonary insufficiency murmur, and separate rumbling, low-frequency, diastolic murmur of mitral valve stenosis may be common to all forms of mitral stenosis. The less pliable, relatively immobile leaflets of the congenitally abnormal valve rarely produce an opening sound. Likewise, the presence of a diastolic murmur is less predictable in the congenital form than in acquired mitral stenosis.

Moderate to severe mitral stenosis is reflected on the electrocardiogram by left atrial enlargement when the patient is in sinus rhythm. Right-axis deviation and right ventricular hypertrophy are present when significant pulmonary hypertension is produced by the left-sided heart obstruction, and they are roughly predictive of severity. Radiographic evidence of left atrial enlargement with elevation of the left mainstem-bronchus, a "double density" atrial shadow, and straightening of the border of the left side of the heart due to enlargement of the left atrial appendage are apparent in anteroposterior films, whereas displacement of the barium-filled esophagus in the lateral view is commonly seen. Pulmonary edema producing prominent venous markings and visible Kerley B lines correlates with left atrial pressure in excess of 20 mm to 25 mm Hg.

Mitral valve morphology may be better defined by echocardiogram than by angiography, although assessment of severity of obstruction is best defined by the catheterization measurement of mitral valve area, as well as pulmonary wedge or left atrial to left ventricular *a* wave gradient. Angiographic detail of mitral valve anatomy is difficult to obtain, although exclusion of cor triatriatum and the rarely recognized supravalvular stenosing ring may further suggest the valvular site of obstruction. The enlarged left atrium, slow clearance of contrast from the left atrium, annulus size, and thickened valve leaflets may be apparent, and angiographic features identifying the parachute mitral valve deformity are described.[23]

For significant mitral stenosis, operation is necessary. Valvotomy or reconstruction of the valve, even with residual gradient or resultant mitral incompetence, may be a surgical result preferable to valve replacement, particularly in the young patient, with valve replacement postponed until later years if at all possible.[24]

SUBVALVULAR AORTIC STENOSIS

Subvalvular aortic obstruction in the left ventricular outflow tract accounts for about 10% of patients with obstruction to left ventricular ejection. Discrete obstruction due to a membranous diaphragm beneath the aortic valve is thought to be more common than a diffuse fibromuscular tunnel obstruction, with intermediate forms between these two types more difficult to classify. Other less common lesions produce isolated subaortic stenosis, including anomalous muscle bundles of the left ventricular outflow tract,[25] abnormalities of mitral valve insertion or formation with accessory tissue,[26-28] and rare left ventricular obstructive tumors.

Left ventricular obstruction may result from the disproportionate thickening of the septal wall, which is one feature of the more diffuse cardiomyopathy seen in familial primary hypertrophic cardiomyopathy or as a transient form in infants born to diabetic mothers.[29] Subaortic stenosis as a part of more complex congenital heart lesions, for example, narrowing of the outflow tract by abnormal attachments of the mitral valve in complete AV canal, will not be covered here.

Discrete subvalvular aortic stenosis resulting from a thin membranous structure closely adherent to or just a few millimeters below the aortic valve is usually distinguished from obstruction longer in length and more removed from the aortic valve, referred to as a fibromuscular collar,[30] and further contrasted to the even more elongated tunnel obstruction in which the outflow tract hypoplasia is frequently associated with a small aortic annulus. The major distinctions among these forms of obstruction relate to the length and anatomical features of the narrowing, since surgical outcome will be greatly influenced by these features.

The discrete membranous diaphragm is usually thin, averaging 1 mm to 2 mm in thickness, and is usually situated above the muscular portion of the outflow tract, most commonly just below the aortic valve, and may be attached to one of the cusps of the aortic valve. The membrane extends to the superior part of the anterior mitral valve leaflet, but attachments to the mitral valve are absent or minimal. Left ventricular hypertrophy is seen, but with less narrowing of the left ventricular outflow tract in spite of significant obstruction at the level of the membrane. Most importantly, surgical removal of this more accessible form of subvalvular obstruction can be successfully performed with permanent relief.

Classification of the other less discrete forms of subvalvular obstruction is more difficult, since the pathology may be similar and simply variable in degree. When the obstruction is not a thin and discrete membrane, it may take the form of a thicker, more fibrous ring at a lower site 1 cm or more below the aortic valve and may be accompanied by further narrowing of the outflow tract extending an additional 1 cm to 2 cm below the ring. The membrane is attached to the anterior leaflet of the mitral valve, there is a more diffuse fibromuscular narrowing of the outflow tract, and with most severe forms, hypoplasia of the aortic annulus; underdevelopment of the ascending aorta or mitral valve may further contribute to the severity of anatomical narrowing.

The ineffectiveness of surgical techniques for relief of the more diffuse forms of subvalvular aortic stenosis is recognized. Operation is by way of aortotomy with exposure of the outflow tract from above after retraction of the aortic valve leaflets. The surgical risk is increased owing to known but not completely avoidable complications. Operative damage to the mitral valve, surgical complete heart block, and creation of a ventricular septal defect have all been described after the extensive subvalvular resection required to afford relief of obstruction.

When subvalvular aortic stenosis is associated with other defects, recognition may be difficult and diagnosis may not be made until after correction of the associated anomalies. In the adult population, patients with subvalvular aortic stenosis as their major diagnosis may be seen in several clinical settings, such as after repair of coarctation or other forms of left-sided heart obstruction, with a history of prior operation for subvalvular aortic stenosis resulting in recurrent or poorly relieved obstruction, or with the history of a murmur previously thought to represent an insignificant ventricular septal defect but with the onset of syncope, electrocardiographic evidence of left ventricular hypertrophy, or the appearance of a new murmur of aortic insufficiency.

Clinical differentiation of subvalvular aortic stenosis from valvular aortic stenosis may be difficult. A harsh systolic ejection murmur, often accompanied by a thrill, is common to both, with radiation of the murmur along the upper right sternal border and into the carotids and suprasternal notch. The murmur of discrete subvalvular obstruction is not infrequently loudest at the mid left sternal border and when radiation is minimal may be confused with the murmur of an isolated ventricular septal defect. A systolic ejection sound (aortic click) is rarely heard with isolated subvalvular aortic stenosis, and its presence on auscultation should raise the question of associated aortic valve abnormality. A murmur of aortic insufficiency is thought to be heard more commonly in patients with subvalvular rather than valvular aortic stenosis and is attributed to leaflet damage resulting from the high velocity jetting of blood through the narrow subvalvular area, causing wear and tear of the valve.[31] A mid-diastolic murmur interpreted to be secondary to interference with left ventricular filling when there is encroachment of the stenosis on the mitral valve has reportedly disappeared after successful operation in selected patients.

The chest radiograph is seldom helpful in implicating the subvalvular area as the site of obstruction. Because subvalvular obstruction, when recognized, is often severe, there may be cardiomegaly, particularly when aortic insufficiency is present, and accentuated pulmonary venous markings. Dilatation of the aortic root is not uncommon but correlates more with additional aortic insufficiency; valve calcification, if present, is specific for valve involvement. The electrocardiographic evidence of left ventricular hypertrophy and left ventricular strain suggests severe obstruction; however, the unreliability of these parameters and the absence of these findings even with documentation of severe aortic stenosis are described for subvalvular as well as valvular stenosis. Regression of left ventricular hypertrophy after successful resection of a discrete subvalvular aortic membrane is described.[32]

Echocardiography may be particularly useful in distinguishing among types of aortic stenosis. The distinctive pattern of early aortic valve semiclosure on M-mode echocardiogram has been recognized as a feature of subvalvular aortic stenosis.[33] The potential for identifying the thin subvalvular membrane by two-dimensional echocardiogram is becoming well recognized when the imaging plane is able to be directed perpendicular to the membrane, but diagnosis may be more difficult when the membrane is extremely thin, adherent to the aortic valve, or when associated defects of the heart are present. Visualization of the more markedly hypoplastic subvalvular area resulting from tunnel stenosis is more easily accomplished.

Cardiac catheterization and angiography are used in further assessment of the location and severity of aortic stenosis. Pressure recordings performed with angiographic catheter withdrawal across the outflow tract may not clearly define the subvalvular area as the site of obstruction unless there is a sufficiently long subvalvular area and a subvalvular chamber can be identified. A single gradient at the level of a discrete subvalvular membrane may mimic an aortic valve gradient. Selective left ventricular angiography best defines the nature of subvalvular aortic stenosis. A thin, linear filling defect just below the aortic valve can be identified with quality studies (Fig. 103.5) and differentiated from the long, tubular narrowing producing relatively fixed obstruction during all phases of the cardiac cycle typical of the diffuse subvalvular obstruction. Further recognition of a narrow aortic anulus, hypoplasia of the ascending aorta, and left ventricular midcavity obliteration may be seen with diffuse forms of subvalvular outflow obstruction. Rare impingement of anomalous mitral valve tissue causing subvalvular obstruction, as well as filling defects secondary to tumor masses, may identify these other causes of subvalvular obstruction.

Features of subvalvular aortic stenosis that are often emphasized are the progressive nature of the obstruction and the damage to the aortic valve over time. In view of these considerations, operation for removal of a discrete subvalvular aortic membrane may be undertaken earlier, with less stringent criteria based on outflow gradient alone when compared with aortic valve stenosis, and the natural history of progressive aortic insufficiency may be improved by early surgical repair of subvalvular aortic stenosis.

Operation for more diffuse subvalvular obstruction is not performed electively but is necessitated by the more severe outflow obstruction produced, even though surgery is not only more hazardous but less successful. Significant residual gradients are found after surgery in many cases, and recurrent stenosis, in spite of earlier favorable operative relief, is not uncommon. In only rare instances is surgical relief of subvalvular diffuse obstruction more than palliative. Reoperation with more drastic attempts at outflow tract reconstruction has been described, such as placement of a conduit from the left ventricular apex to the descending aorta[34] and the Rastan aortoventriculoplasty for enlarging the outflow tract, which necessitates prosthetic valve replacement.[35] There seems to be a particularly high incidence of bacterial endocarditis in patients with subvalvular aortic stenosis, with vegetations occurring on the aortic valve upstream from the subvalvular obstruction. Endocarditis prophylaxis is therefore critical in these patients.

AORTIC STENOSIS

The most common site at which obstruction to left ventricular outflow occurs is at the level of the aortic valve. Congenital aortic valve stenosis accounts for approximately 5% of patients with congenital heart disease. The strong male preponderance, estimated to be 4:1, is well known but unexplained. Calcific aortic stenosis in the adult, once considered to be mostly rheumatic or atherosclerotic in origin, is now widely accepted to have developed on a congenitally deformed valve in the great majority of cases, if not all. The most common anomaly of the valve leading to fibrosis and eventual calcification is bicuspid aortic valve (Fig. 103.6). The frequency of occurrence of the congenitally bicuspid aortic valve may be underestimated.[36] Its presence is rarely detected in childhood, and even in the adult it often remains unrecognized until fibrosis and calcification take place, producing stenosis. Thus, for many generations calcific aortic stenosis was assumed to be acquired because of the late onset and lack of signs or symptoms in the child. The majority of bicuspid aortic valves become stenotic by the fifth or sixth decade.

Anatomical variations in valve structure that produce obstruction to left ventricular outflow are several. Severe obstruction in infants under one year of age is most often due to unicuspid or dome-shaped valve. These malformations may form a continuum with the hypoplastic left heart syndrome, and mortality in infancy is high even when operative relief of valve obstruction is attempted. In other forms of aortic stenosis, the valve is thickened, and varying degrees of commissural fusion and development are recognized. The most common malformation identified is the bicuspid aortic valve with fusion of the commissures and an eccentric orifice between the left coronary and noncoronary cusps.[37] Rarely, the valve may have three fused cusps with a single central orifice.[38]

The principal hemodynamic effects of aortic valve stenosis result from incomplete opening of the valve with systolic overload imposed on the left ventricle, resulting in increased left ventricular pressure, production of an outflow gradient, increased left ventricular wall tension with resultant hypertrophy of the ventricle, and a relative mismatch of coronary flow to left ventricular myocardial demand, which can be worsened in the adult who has additional anatomical narrowing of coronary vessels.[39]

Definition of the severity of aortic stenosis is not based on the

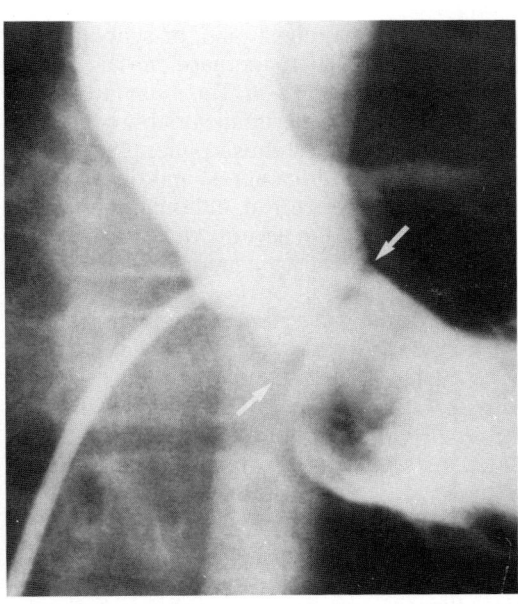

FIGURE 103.5 Discrete subvalvular aortic membrane producing left ventricular outflow obstruction is seen as a filling density (arrows) after left ventricular angiography.

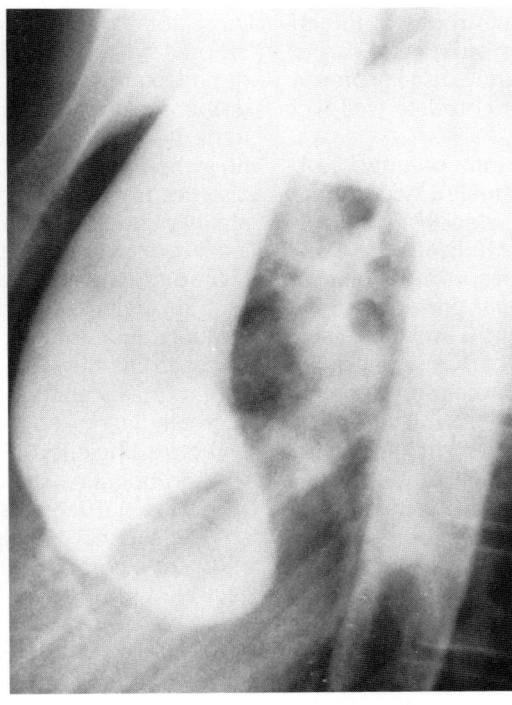

FIGURE 103.6 Bicuspid aortic valve seen "en face" after aortic root angiography shows doming of the aortic valve with the negative washout produced from nonopacified blood ejected from the left ventricle.

single measurement of left ventricular outflow gradient measured at catheterization. The Gorlin and Gorlin formula for calculating valve orifice size relates the valve gradient to the measured output across the valve.[40] A modest pressure gradient becomes highly important in the presence of a low cardiac output and less significant if the output is elevated at the time the left ventricular–to–aortic gradient is measured. Based on these considerations, when the aortic valve area is reduced from the normal 2.6 cm^2 to 3.5 cm^2 area (not indexed)[41] to less than 0.5 cm^2/m^2 (indexed area), the obstruction is critical.[42] The manual of operations from the collaborative natural history study of congenital defects used as a working definition of severe aortic stenosis the presence of at least one of the following two criteria: left ventricular strain pattern present on the electrocardiogram together with a peak systolic gradient of more than 40 mm Hg, or peak systolic gradient in excess of 80 mm Hg.[43]

The physical examination of the patient with aortic valve stenosis virtually always allows accurate anatomical diagnosis but often is not as predictive of the severity in the child as it usually is in the adult. A left ventricular lift is felt on palpation, and a systolic thrill is present in all but the mildest degrees of outflow obstruction correlating with gradients of 25 mm Hg or greater. The thrill is felt in the primary aortic area at the upper right sternal border and also in the suprasternal notch and carotid arteries. A systolic ejection click focuses on the mobile aortic valve as the site of left ventricular outflow obstruction and is heard at the apex or at the upper right sternal border in most cases of congenital aortic valve stenosis and does not vary with the respiratory cycle, which helps to distinguish it from a pulmonary valve ejection sound. The absence or disappearance of an aortic ejection click correlates with fibrosis and calcification. The harsh loud ejection murmur at the base radiates like the thrill to the neck, and in most cases becomes harsher, longer, and peaks later as the obstruction progresses until the onset of reduced left ventricular force of contraction. An early diastolic murmur of aortic insufficiency is seldom heard in patients with aortic valve stenosis but is found in a high percentage of patients with a subvalvular membrane stenosis. The presence of a fourth heart sound also is found when more left ventricular failure ensues.[44] The value of recognition of the slow upstroke of the carotid pulse is more useful in clinical diagnosis in the adult population than it is in childhood. With important degrees of valve obstruction, the aortic valve is held open longer to allow left ventricular ejection, and there is a delay in valve closure, resulting in narrow splitting or even paradoxical splitting of the second heart sound.

On chest film the heart size is usually normal or only minimally enlarged, since the concentric left ventricular hypertrophy in the absence of dilatation does not produce radiographic evidence of cardiomegaly. Poststenotic dilatation of the ascending aorta is usually present but may be either striking or absent and does not correlate well with the severity of obstruction.

The electrocardiogram correlates roughly with the severity of obstruction, although it is well recognized that a normal or near normal electrocardiogram does not exclude severe aortic stenosis. High-voltage QRS complexes in the lateral precordial leads indicating left ventricular hypertrophy are present in varying degrees in most patients with important aortic valve stenosis. The additional presence of left ventricular strain, that is, ST segment depression and T wave inversion in the lateral precordial leads, reliably indicates severe stenosis. In adolescents and young adults a normal electrocardiogram does not exclude a high left ventricular–to–aortic pressure gradient. A particularly good predictor of severity exists when ischemic changes not found on resting electrocardiogram are found during exercise testing in young persons, since these are said to indicate a valvular gradient 50 mm Hg or greater.[45]

The echocardiographic features of aortic stenosis on M mode were recognized to consist of multiple diastolic valve echoes generated by the thickened leaflets, an eccentric point of closure of the valve, and concentric hypertrophy of the left ventricle. With two-dimensional studies, the movement of the abnormal valve is seen as it domes in systole, and leaflet separation can be measured. Additional features of dilation of the aortic root, annulus size, recognition of the presence of a bicuspid aortic valve, the degree of hypertrophy of the ventricle, and exclusion of other sites of left ventricular obstruction are all useful. A clinically useful formula to predict left ventricular (LV) pressure[46] is based on the ratio of the thickness of the left ventricular posterior wall in systole to the left ventricular cavity size in systole and is expressed as

$$\text{LV pressure (mm Hg)} = 225 \times \frac{\text{LV systolic wall thickness (mm)}}{\text{LV end-systolic diameter (mm)}}$$

The coexistence of aortic insufficiency increases the end-systolic diameter and may result in underestimation of left ventricular pressure. By pulsed Doppler ultrasound one can more reliably estimate the outflow gradient from the velocity of the jet of blood through the narrowed orifice and, in addition, can detect aortic insufficiency.

Cardiac catheterization is usually undertaken to assess the severity of aortic stenosis, since the clinical diagnosis of the structural anomaly is known. Catheterization in preparation for surgery is carried out when aortic stenosis is estimated to be severe, when ischemic changes are found on the electrocardiogram, when a history of syncope or presyncope is elicited, when a positive exercise test is obtained, or when chest pain occurs with exercise. At the time of catheterization, a reliable measurement of cardiac output must be obtained and used with the measurement of peak gradient to determine the severity of obstruction by valve area calculations. When the stenotic orifice precludes easy passage of the retrograde catheter, the transseptal approach to the left ventricle allows measurement of left ventricular pressure with simultaneous pressure measurements recorded from above the aortic valve. Angiography allows visualization of the thickened valve leaflets, excursion of the valve, degree of left ventricular wall thickening, and the poststenotic dilatation of the aortic root. The jetting of contrast through the eccentric orifice is seen after left ventricular angiogram.

It is recognized by cardiologists that aortic stenosis is not a stable disease, and one should expect progression in the degree of left ventricular obstruction due to increase in cardiac output occurring with growth, as well as further deformity of the valve promoted by abnormal mechanical wear and tear.[47] All young patients recognized to have congenital malformation of the aortic valve will require lifelong follow-up. Absence of clinical symptoms in the presence of a diagnosis of aortic valve disease is not unusual. When symptoms do occur, there is most notably fatigue, exertional dyspnea, chest pain, or syncope. Exertional syncope is attributed to the inability to increase cardiac output during exercise owing to fixed severe obstruction. The main fear in this lesion is sudden death, since its incidence has been variably predicted to be 1% to 19%.[48,49] Sudden death in aortic stenosis patients who have no symptoms and a normal electrocardiogram at rest and during exercise has not been documented to have occurred, although the unreliability of noninvasive testing in assessing the severity of aortic stenosis leads to recommendations for cardiac catheterization and close follow-up of patients because of this concern.

Management of patients with aortic valve stenosis includes the recommendation for strict observance of endocarditis prophylaxis. When endocarditis complicates the course of these patients, clinically significant mortality and morbidity occur and the need for operative therapy is greatly increased owing to valve dysfunction, generally resulting in aortic insufficiency. Pediatric cardiologists recommend that patients with aortic valve stenosis avoid strenuous exercise, and competitive sports are not recommended.[50]

The surgical treatment of aortic stenosis must be individualized to allow for a correctly timed procedure that will treat symptoms but also best allow preservation and function of the native valve in order to avoid or defer prosthetic valve replacement. All surgery on the aortic valve is best considered to be palliative. Young patients under 20 years of age are free of valve calcification, and valvotomy can be performed for the relief of stenosis. Successful valvotomy depends further on the number of valve cusps, degree of valve thickening, and annulus size. The use of cardiopulmonary bypass with direct inspection of valve anatomy at surgery provides for the best decision about how surgical technique can relieve obstruction without creating significant valve regurgitation.[51] Acceptance of residual aortic stenosis or aortic insufficiency after surgery is preferable to valve replacement in young patients. The average age at which valvotomy has been required in patients with congenital aortic valve stenosis is approximately 11 to 14 years, with predictions that if commissurotomy for aortic stenosis is required in the first 2 decades of life, aortic valve replacement will be required subsequently but generally can follow valvotomy by at least 9 years.[52] Valve replacement is necessary when it is impossible to reconstruct the existing valve and an accompanying procedure to enlarge the aortic annulus to enable insertion of a larger, less obstructive valve may be necessary. The less thrombogenic tissue valves were enthusiastically promoted in past years; however, the rapid rate of deterioration in function of these valves, along with accelerated calcification in younger patients, renders them poorly suitable for implantation in all but elderly patients. The St. Jude bileaflet valve is popular for valve replacement at present, but long-term anticoagulation must be conducted. Endocarditis prophylaxis is as important postoperatively as it is preoperatively. Since multiple surgical procedures are likely to be required in patients born with congenital deformity of the aortic valve, careful assessment for surgery must be conducted with a view to relief of symptoms, choice of procedure, and preservation of ventricular function. The newer techniques of balloon dilatation of stenotic heart valves at the time of catheterization have been applied in a limited way to relieve aortic valve obstruction and may be developed further if this intervention proves to be safe, but they offer lasting advantage only when the aortic valve is not calcified, and they may be more beneficial in childhood (Fig. 103.7).

SUPRAVALVULAR AORTIC STENOSIS

Supravalvular aortic stenosis is produced by an abrupt narrowing in the ascending aorta immediately distal to the aortic valve. The anomaly is

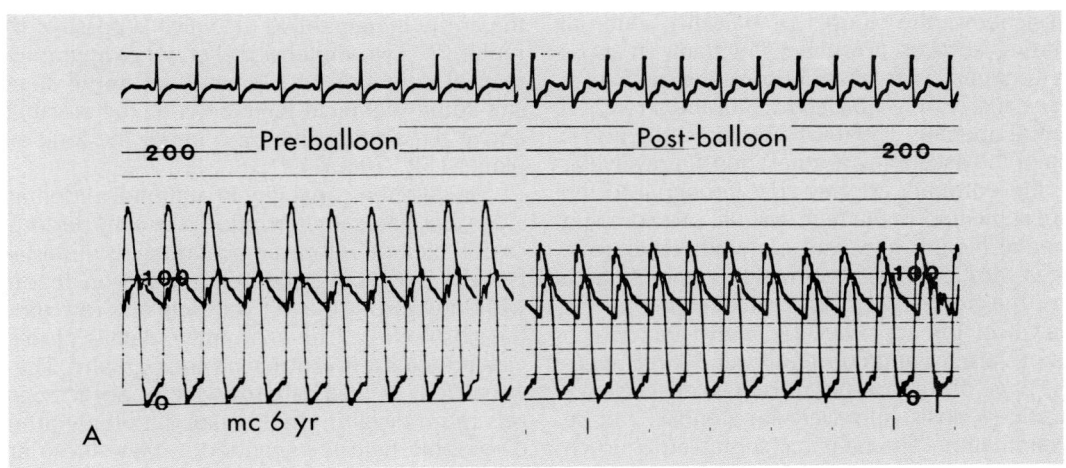

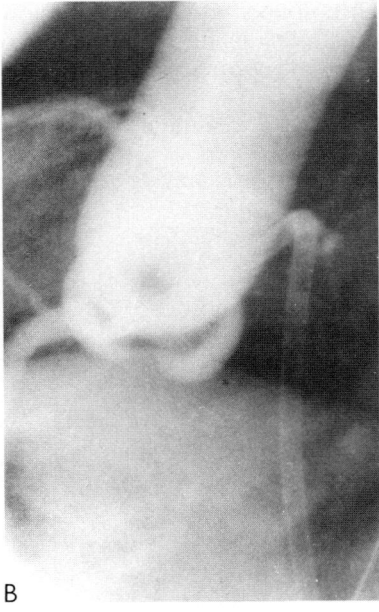

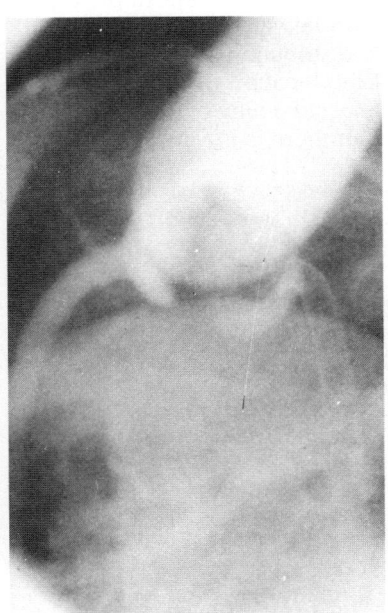

FIGURE 103.7 A. Pressure tracings obtained before and after balloon dilation of a congenitally stenotic aortic valve. The predilation gradient was recorded to be 60 mm Hg (left ventricular pressure 160/0,18; aortic pressure 100/78). After balloon dilation, the gradient was reduced to 20 mm Hg (left ventricular pressure 120/0,18; aortic pressure 100/65). **B.** Angiographic appearance of stenotic valve before dilation is viewed on the left, with the negative jet of blood passing through the narrowed orifice. After dilation, on the right, a wider stream of nonopacified blood is seen, with apparent enlargement of the orifice.

frequently associated with other congenitally constricted arteries, including multiple pulmonic arterial branch stenoses and stenoses of branches of the aorta. Two major syndromes involving supravalvular aortic stenosis are known and consist of a nonfamilial form with abnormal ("elfin") facies and mental retardation (Williams' syndrome)[53] and a familial form thought to be autosomal dominant in inheritance but with the gene variably expressed among family members.[54,55] Sporadic forms are also described, and a small number of cases have been associated with congenital rubella syndrome or found in patients with a body habitus resembling Marfan's disease. Up to 40% of patients with supravalvular aortic stenosis have the constellation of findings described by Williams, including mental retardation, peculiar facies, narrowing of peripheral systemic and pulmonary arteries, strabismus, inguinal hernia, and abnormal dentition; these patients are easily recognized by their distinctive appearance (Fig. 103.8). An intrauterine metabolic defect involving a sensitivity of developing tissues to vitamin D has been implicated in the causation of this syndrome. In the familial form a generalized arterial disease affecting large arteries is linked with the supravalvular aortic stenosis, and family members may have related conditions of varying severity.

Three types of supravalvular stenosis are described,[56] the most common of which is the hourglass narrowing produced by extreme thickness of the media just above the sinuses of Valsalva; external deformation of the ascending aorta is not always evident on gross inspection. Occurring less frequently is an obstruction at the same level as the hourglass deformity caused by a fibrous membrane stretched across the aorta with a central opening. The third type of obstruction is a more uniform hypoplasia of the ascending aorta. When supravalvular aortic stenosis is present, the coronary arteries arise proximal to the obstruction, where they are subjected to the high systolic pressure and become tortuous, with medial hypertrophy and early atherosclerotic changes. In some instances, aortic valve abnormalities coexist as a result of direct adhesion of the free edges of the valve leaflets to the wall of the aorta at the level of the supravalvular narrowing, which serves to block the sinuses of Valsalva and coronary ostia. Aortic aneurysm formation distal to the zone of stenosis has also been described.[57]

Like other forms of aortic stenosis, supravalvular stenosis can be suspected from clinical examination. The palpable suprasternal notch and carotid artery thrill accompanying supravalvular stenosis are much more prominent than that found with aortic valve stenosis. A harsh, loud systolic murmur follows the same distribution as the thrill and is transmitted into the neck. Because of the location of the obstruction above the valve, there is more preferential streaming of the high-velocity jet toward the innominate vessel than there is in valvular stenosis. This results in an inequality of pulse volume and blood pressure between the arms, with higher systolic pressure and wider pulse pressure in the right arm than in the left. This phenomenon has been termed the Coanda effect. It produces an average systolic blood pressure 18 mm Hg higher in the right arm than in the left.[58] The aortic valve closure sound is louder than normal in some patients and inexplicably diminished in others. An aortic ejection click is not heard in these patients, a fact that helps to distinguish this anomaly from valvular aortic stenosis in the child but may be of less help in the adult patient when the ejection sound of valve stenosis disappears with the onset of leaflet calcification. The coexistence of right ventricular outflow obstruction may account for an additional murmur of pulmonary stenosis, or even a continuous murmur when pulmonary branch stenosis is present. Bruits over the abdomen can suggest other large-vessel narrowing, such as renal artery stenosis.

By chest radiograph cardiac silhouette is frequently normal, but compared with aortic valve stenosis the ascending aorta is not so dilated. The electrocardiogram shows left ventricular hypertrophy. Biventricular hypertrophy may be manifest if pulmonary stenosis is part of the syndrome, depending on the relative severity of the two. Echocardiography can identify this form of left ventricular outflow obstruction, as well as help to exclude other forms. Imaging of narrowing of the aortic lumen above the valve is possible by M-mode echocardiography.[59,60] Two-dimensional echocardiography has improved the accuracy of detection of supravalvular aortic stenosis, although there are still some technical limitations to the feasibility of imaging the aorta above the aortic valve from either the long axis or subcostal imaging planes (Fig. 103.9).[61,62]

Despite the capability in anatomical definition that ultrasound provides, cardiac catheterization is usually performed to assess the degree of obstruction before surgical repair is undertaken. A pressure gradient is measured above the aortic valve on recordings as the catheter is withdrawn from the left ventricle and into the ascending aorta, across the obstruction. The anatomical details of the constriction are further viewed after left ventricular angiography. The length of obstruction is visualized, as well as narrowing of aortic segments or branching vessels more distal in origin, including renal artery stenosis when the radiographic field is expanded to view these areas. Coronary anatomy can be defined with the appearance of tortuous large vessels; a small left coronary vessel that fills slowly may raise the suspicion of additional obstruction to the orifice of this vessel due to an underdeveloped left coronary cusp blocking the entrance into the left sinus of Valsalva.

Surgical treatment of supravalvular aortic stenosis is less satisfac-

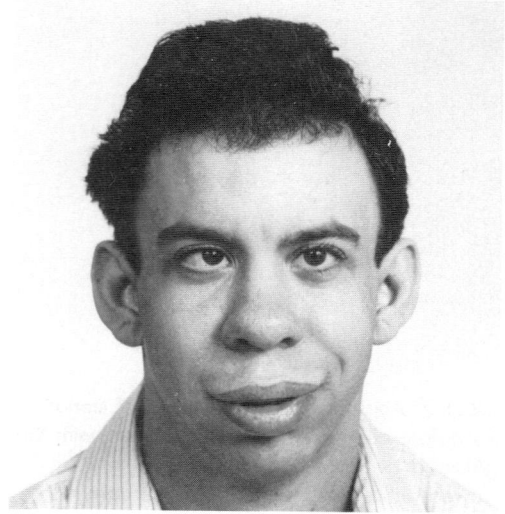

FIGURE 103.8 Adult male (25 years) with Williams' syndrome has typical facies and strabismus.

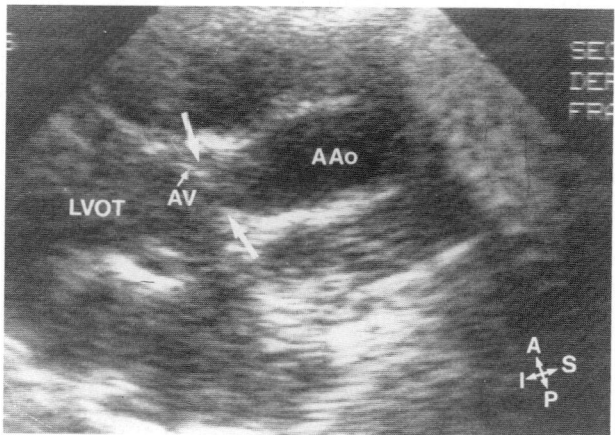

FIGURE 103.9 Long-axial two-dimensional echocardiogram recorded in a patient with discrete supravalvular aortic stenosis and infolding just above the aortic valve (arrow). (AV, aortic valve; LVOT, left ventricular outflow tract; AAo, ascending aorta.)

tory than that of aortic valve or membranous subvalvular stenosis, but there are some very good surgical results.[63] However, when the aorta is diffusely hypoplastic, surgical relief of obstruction is unsatisfactory. In this case, patching the area of proximal obstruction serves only to displace the pressure gradient more distally; in these instances, prosthetic replacement of a long segment of aorta may be necessary. When the more common form of discrete supravalvular narrowing is recognized, a good surgical outcome can be effected by partial resection of the constrictive ridge and by widening the aorta with a diamond-shaped or oval patch graft during operation with cardiopulmonary bypass. Less frequently, resection of the narrowed segment and primary anastomosis has been performed. All approaches are complicated when there is obstruction to coronary ostia or additional abnormalities of the aortic valve with valve edges adherent to the supravalvular area. In these latter instances the uncertain outcome calls for stricter criteria for surgical repair, with the recognition that prosthetic valve replacement or coronary bypass techniques may be necessary.

COARCTATION OF THE AORTA

Coarctation of the aorta refers to the congenital anomaly producing obstruction to aortic flow from a membrane-like occlusion within the lumen of the thoracic aorta. Surgical treatment has been available for 40 years, but indications for and timing of surgery have changed during this period of time and the surgical techniques from which to choose have increased. This lesion has a male/female sex preponderance of 2:1. It also occurs in at least 20% of patients with Turner's syndrome and XO karyotype. Bicuspid aortic valve is the most common associated cardiac lesion in 85% of patients. The frequency of extracardiac lesions, such as aneurysm of the circle of Willis, while less well defined, is probably low and may be a problem acquired with age. Patients with coarctation are usually identified in childhood, but the diagnosis is sometimes first made in early adult years. In any patient with hypertension in the upper extremities, the anomaly should be excluded by feeling for femoral pulses. The poor natural history, with average age of death at 35 years, has been improved considerably by expert surgical repair, preferably performed in childhood.

Anatomical features of isolated coarctation consist of a shelflike thickening on the posterolateral wall of the aorta opposite the ductus arteriosus or ligamentum. The obstruction is most commonly in a "juxtaductal" location distal to the origin of the left subclavian artery.[64] Rarely, the left subclavian may arise distal to the coarctation. The frequency of associated cardiac defects is high in infants with congestive heart failure and most often includes large ductus arteriosus or large ventricular septal defect.[65] These defects seldom allow survival of the surgically untreated patient into adult life. The most common associated anomaly, bicuspid aortic valve, has no functional importance in the infant. The frequent mitral valve lesions may be benign phenomena detected only by echocardiogram or left ventricular angiogram, but some produce severe mitral valve stenosis and dominate the clinical picture.

Latency of symptoms attributed to coarctation is the general rule. Most patients come to attention when referred for evaluation of a heart murmur or hypertension. Headaches secondary to coarctation are rare, and if severe and unrelenting suggest the possibility of cerebral arterial aneurysm. Normal blood flow to lower extremities is provided by collateral circulation; thus signs of claudication and cool lower extremities are rare. More commonly, leg complaints relate to compression of nerve roots by enlarged anterior spinal arteries with resultant complaints of paresthesias and numbness.

Coarctation of the aorta is typically a very obvious clinical diagnosis if the blood pressure is measured in both arms and at least one leg.[66] The severity of upper extremity hypertension depends on the degree of obstruction and the amount of collateral circulation. Large, numerous collaterals may prevent severe elevation of arm blood pressure even if the coarctation is very severe. A mildly stenotic area of coarctation does not stimulate the development of large collaterals and does not cause severe hypertension. The combination of congestive heart failure and coarctation, especially in the infant, is usually associated with very severe systemic hypertension that subsides as the failure diminishes with time or anticongestive medical therapy. Proximity of the origin of the left subclavian artery to the site of coarctation may render left arm pulses and blood pressure lower than right arm pressures and intermediate between right arm and leg pressures. When one or both subclavian arteries arise distal to the coarctation, physical examination should also reflect this fact and can make careful examination even more specific in recognizing these additional anatomical details. Frequently, bounding carotid pulses are visible and a thrill is palpable in the suprasternal notch and in the carotids. Collateral vessels may be palpable over the back and give rise to systolic or continuous murmurs. The murmur generated by the coarctation itself can vary from a short, nonspecific systolic murmur heard with maximum intensity at the mid left sternal border or in the left infraclavicular area or over the back or axilla to a continuous murmur caused by a persistent systolic and diastolic gradient across the narrow lumen. Additional systolic, diastolic, or continuous murmurs from collaterals, associated aortic valve abnormalities, and mitral valve malformations can be found. A systolic ejection click can be produced by excursion of a bicuspid aortic valve but can also be heard when the ascending aorta is dilated and the aortic valve is normally tricuspid. Indirect evidence of hypertension can be inferred when resistance to ventricular filling results in an audible apical fourth heart sound and when the first component of the second heart sound has an increased intensity. Clinical signs of congestive heart failure are rare with isolated coarctation beyond the newborn period and before 40 years of age.

The electrocardiogram can be normal, but the expected left ventricular hypertrophy or even left ventricular strain pattern can occur.

Chest radiograph rarely is interpreted to show cardiomegaly, but inspection for rib notching due to erosion of the inferior rib margins may be a clue to overdeveloped collateral vessels. The classic "3" sign along the left upper border of the mediastinal shadow is produced by prestenotic and poststenotic dilatation of the aorta above and below the coarcted area. The "reversed 3" sign refers to identation of the barium-filled esophagus reflecting the same prestenotic and poststenotic dilatation on its medial side.

Two-dimensional echocardiographic imaging of the aorta from the suprasternal notch is reliable in demonstrating coarctation in many patients. The coarctation may be in an "atypical" plane, and a scan of ascending aorta, transverse aorta, and descending aorta must be conducted, with careful identification of aortic branching, until a convincing area of decreased diameter is found in the usual location.[67] Vigorous pulsation of the aorta proximal to the obstruction and reduced aortic pulsation below are further confirmatory evidence that coarctation is present. Alterations in Doppler flow pattern give additional useful information. The frequently associated bicuspid aortic valve is also demonstrable by echocardiography.

The necessity of adjunctive cardiac catheterization has been debated, since isolated coarctation can be a diagnosis obvious on physical examination, and the "usual" location can be suggested when typical radiographic findings are viewed. In the past, proponents of catheterization justified the need to define the anatomy of the coarctation with the opinion that surgical repair would be facilitated if a discrete coarctation were found and that if a long-segment hypoplasia were identified and graft replacement were necessary, this knowledge might influence the timing of surgery. Rarely a patient was subjected to thoracotomy without catheterization only to encounter an abdominal coarctation. With the further availability of two-dimensional echocardiography and visualization of the anatomy of coarctation, catheterization was felt to be unnecessary in many centers and was reserved for patients in whom coarctation was complicated by associated defects. The therapeutic role of catheterization in management has gained recent popularity with the technique of balloon dilatation in the setting of native coarctation as well as postoperative restenosis (Fig. 103.10).[68] It is not yet known whether the injury to the vessel after angioplasty will allow a later incidence of recurrence or even aneurysm formation. The long-term follow-up of patients will establish candidacy for this technique as well as the safety and long-term results and will need to be compared with the established benefits of surgical repair.

Coarctation of the aorta was one of the defects of the heart first corrected by operation, with earliest surgical reports in the mid-1940s. The optimal timing of surgery is still often debated. Elective surgery in infancy is thought to be associated with a high risk of restenosis most apparent on long-term follow-up with significant residual coarctation occurring in up to 42%.[69] To avoid the high risk of reoperation, elective surgical repair later in life was felt to be preferable but has resulted in chronic postoperative hypertension as a direct correlate of age of repair. Considering these factors and the data on normal growth of the aorta, the ideal time for elective surgical repair of aortic coarctation is probably age 5 years.[70,71] The question has been raised about the candidacy for surgery of patients over age 40 who have established hypertension and a higher operative risk; however, even in this age-group surgical intervention has significant benefit and age alone should not disqualify any individual patient. The chief risks of coarctation with severe hypertention—hypertensive encepholopathy, cerebral hemorrhage, and left ventricular failure—may all be improved by surgical repair. The risk of bacterial endocarditis is probably not altered by surgical intervention.

Techniques available for surgery (Fig. 103.11) with discrete obstruction have included resection with end-to-end anastomosis and patch angioplasty. Interposition of a Dacron tube graft may be necessary when a long coarcted segment is excised. The technique of subclavian flap repair in infants and children may be neither adaptable nor necessary for repair in adults.[72]

Postoperative management after coarctation repair involves recognition of two problems unique to this defect: paradoxical hypertension and the syndrome of mesenteric arteritis. Both problems have an increased incidence in older patients who had had longstanding hypertension. When satisfactory relief of coarctation is achieved, paradoxical increase in blood pressure, often to levels exceeding preoperative levels, may be documented immediately after surgery. This hypertension has been attributed to a hyperactivity of the sympathetic nervous system during the first 24 hours followed by activation of the plasma renin–angiotension system within the next 2 to 3 days after surgery. Treatment of hypertension in the immediate postoperative period should be vigorous to effect diastolic blood pressures below 100 mm Hg, since postoperative hypertension may also contribute to the development of mesenteric arteritis.[73] The clinical picture of mesenteric arteritis involves recognition of abdominal pain, ileus, and vomiting, with progression in rare cases to intestinal necrosis. The reported incidence after coarctation surgery may be as high as 28% and is felt to have a direct relationship to the presence of and degree of postoperative hypertension. The mechanism of this syndrome has been thought to be reactive vasospasm of intestinal arterial vessels caused by reestablishment of pulsatile flow and exacerbated by hypertension after coarctation repair.[74] Severe necrotizing panarteritis will require bowel resec-

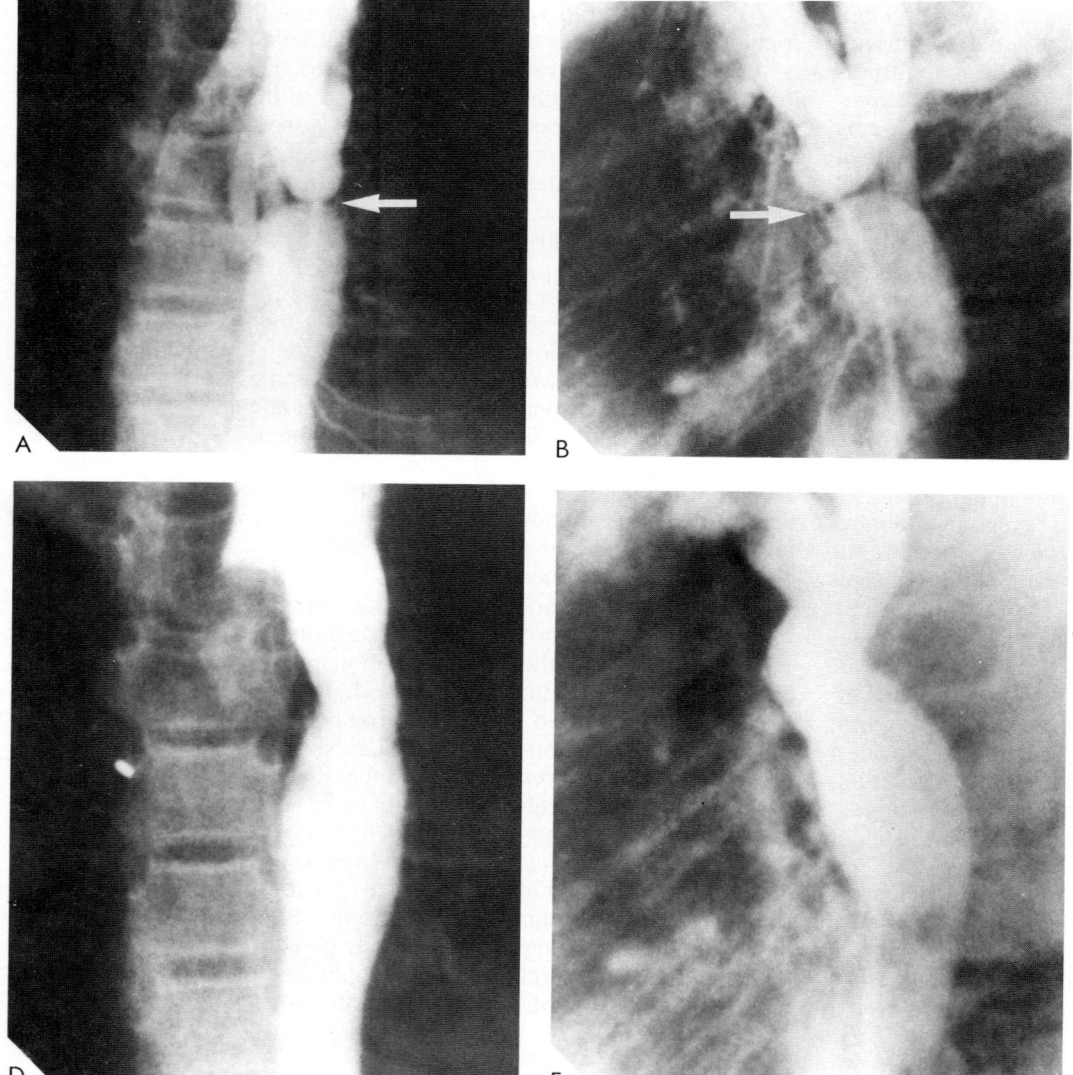

FIGURE 103.10 Dilation of native coarctation of the aorta in a teenage patient. Predilation angiograms are recorded in anteroposterior (AP) and lateral views with a "marker" catheter to allow measurements to direct the choice of balloon size. Tight "waisting" is seen (arrows) in AP (**A**) and lateral (**B**) views before dilation. **C.** The balloon is viewed, with waisting (arrow) at the site of tight coarctation visible during inflation in the AP view. Postdilation angiogram in the same patient confirms significant widening of the aorta in AP (**D**) and lateral (**E**) views after dilation of the coarcted segment.

tion and is a life-threatening complication. Routine postoperative management is best conducted with intravenous fluids for 48 to 72 hours postoperatively, nasogastric drainage, and very slow introduction of oral fluid intake and feeding when bowel sounds are active and blood pressure is medically controlled with parenteral drugs. Surgical relief of coarctation is effective in reestablishing normal aortic flow and equalizing blood pressure above and below the obstructive segment in all age groups and should be performed electively any time significant coarctation is recognized beyond early childhood. Lifelong observation for hypertension and rarer complications with endocarditis or aortic disruption is required.

CONCLUSION

The internists and cardiologists who look after adults are beginning to see a large number of patients with unoperated congenital heart anomalies and even more with postoperative congenital heart disease.

Lesions that are obstructive to systemic or pulmonary venous return or to right or left ventricular ejection are virtually all amenable to surgical repair, although some are very mild and call for no surgical treatment or special precaution other than the need for endocarditis prophylaxis and occasional check-ups.

Postoperative congenital heart disease is a new form of heart disease that often is not recognized by physicians who have not been active in a pediatric cardiology diagnostic and surgical center. The signs and symptoms that these patients have are unlike those in the unoperated patient, and most of these patients, while improved, need continued cardiac observation and care for their lifetime, including surveillance for arrhythmia.

Clinically, many of the congenital obstructive lesions (typically pulmonary or aortic stenosis) in the adult are very obvious on physical examination because of the loud murmur. However, other obstructive lesions may be difficult to recognize, especially the ones that were quiescent and thus overlooked in childhood and then became severe in adult life. In anomalies such as cor triatriatum, flow across the stenotic orifice may be so reduced that the murmur is faint. A very faint or absent murmur in the patient with cough and dyspnea on effort with rales in the lungs is likely to point more toward lung disease than heart disease. In order to separate the two, the electrocardiogram is helpful. In the anomalies that cause severe obstruction to pulmonary venous return, the electrocardiogram typically shows severe right ventricular hypertrophy by electrocardiogram, while in lung disease the electrocardiogram is normal or shows only mild right ventricular hypertrophy.

A number of benign obstructive anomalies may be encountered in the adult who is asymptomatic and requires no special treatment or precaution; however, it is just as important to recognize benign congenital heart disease as it is to diagnose the serious conditions. Physicians must allow the patient with a benign defect to have a normal life, free from the anxiety that can be produced by too much medical attention or too frequent check-ups.

The adult patient with congenital heart disease, benign or otherwise, who has been attending cardiac clinics for many years may have been questioned so often about symptoms that the history taking has convinced the patient that symptoms are to be expected. If the patient has not been treated normally by parents, teachers, neighbors, and

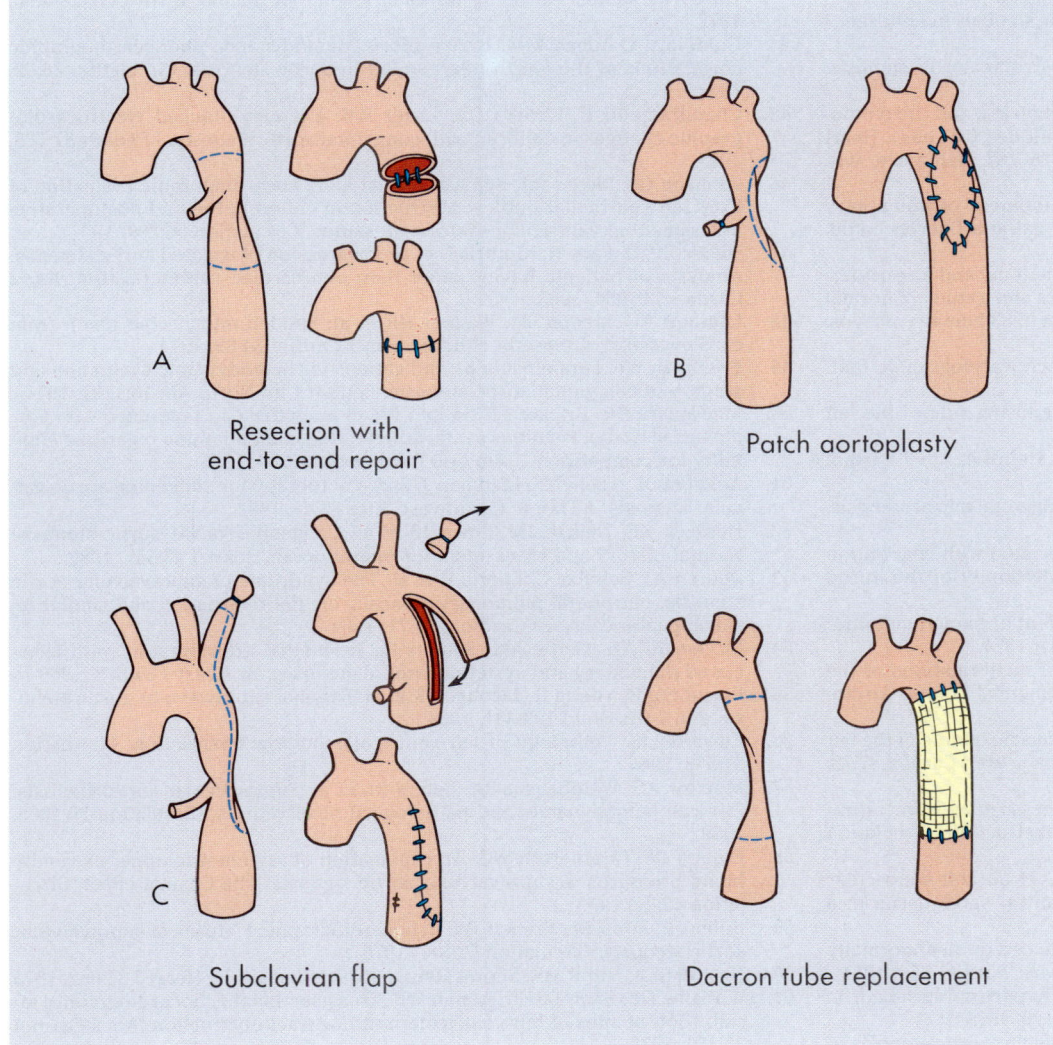

FIGURE 103.11 Diagram of the several available methods of surgical repair of coarctation of the aorta.

physicians, it may require some reassurance and explanation to the patient to encourage a healthy, independent, and responsible adult life.

Management of adult patients with isolated congenital and valvular lesions requires cooperation between pediatric and adult cardiologists to interpret the previous history of the patient, the natural history of the defect, and the expectations for favorable hemodynamic balance in adult life.

REFERENCES

1. El-Said GM, Mullins CE, Nihill MR et al: Hemodynamic and angiographic changes after Mustard operation for transposition of the great arteries. Eur J Cardiol 3:3, 1975
2. Mazzei EA, Mulder DG: Superior vena cava syndrome following complete correction (Mustard repair) of transposition of the great vessels. Ann Thorac Surg 11:243, 1971
3. Shah-Mirany J, Mirhoseini M, Head LR: Fatal pulmonary embolism from jugular veins following benign superior vena cava syndrome. Ann Thorac Surg 11:238, 1971
4. Keefe JF, Wolk M, Levine HJ: Isolated tricuspid valvular stenosis. Am J Cardiol 25:252, 1970
5. Hartmann AF Jr, Tsifutis A, Arvidsson H et al: The two-chambered right ventricle. Circulation 26:279, 1962
6. Hartmann AF, Goldring D, Carlsson E: Development of right ventricular obstruction by aberrant muscle bands. Circulation 30:679, 1964
7. Rowland TW, Rosenthal A, Casteneda AR: Double-chamber right ventricle: Experience with 17 cases. Am Heart J 89:455, 1985
8. Johnson LW, Grossman W, Dalen JE et al: Pulmonic stenosis in the adult. N Engl J Med 287:1159, 1972
9. Levine OR, Blumenthal S: Pulmonic stenosis. Circulation 31,32 (Suppl 3):III-33, 1965
10. deTroyer A, Yernault JC, Englert M: Lung hypoplasia in congenital pulmonary valve stenosis. Circulation 56:647, 1977
11. Wood P: Diseases of the Heart and Circulation, p 501. London, Eyre & Spottiswoode, 1968
12. Pepine CJ, Gessner IH, Feldman RL: Percutaneous balloon valvuloplasty for pulmonic valve stenosis in the adult. Am J Cardiol 50:1442, 1982
13. Rocchini AP, Kueselis DA, Crowley D et al: Percutaneous balloon valvuloplasty for treatment of congenital pulmonary valvular stenosis in children. J Am Coll Cardiol 3:1005, 1984
14. Williams JCP, Barratt–Boyes BG, Lowe JB: Supravalvular aortic stenosis. Circulation 24:1311, 1961
15. Emmanoulides GC: Obstructive lesions of the right ventricle and the pulmonary arterial tree. In Moss AJ, Adams FH, Emmanouilides GC (eds): Heart Disease in Infants, Children and Adolescents, pp 226–257. Baltimore, Williams & Wilkins, 1977
16. Driscoll DJ, Nihill MR, Vargo TA et al: Late development of pulmonary venous obstruction following Mustard's operation using a Dacron baffle. Circulation 55:484, 1977
17. VanPraagh R, Corsini I: Cor triatriatum: Pathologic anatomy and a consideration of morphogenesis based on 13 postmortem cases and a study of normal development of the pulmonary vein and atrial septum in 83 human embryos. Am Heart J 78:379, 1969
18. Moodie DS, Hagler DJ, Ritter DG: Cor triatriatum: Echocardiographic findings. Mayo Clin Proc 51:289, 1976
19. Manubens R, Krovetz LJ, Adam P: Supravalvular stenosing ring of the left atrium. Am Heart J 60:286, 1960
20. Van der Horst RL, Hastreiter AR: Congenital mitral stenosis. Am J Cardiol 20:773, 1967
21. Collins–Nakai R, Rosenthal A, Casteneda AR et al: Congenital mitral stenosis. Circulation 56:1039, 1977
22. Rosenquist GC: Congenital mitral valve disease associated with coarctation of the aorta: A spectrum that includes parachute deformity of the mitral valve. Circulation 49:985, 1974
23. Macartney FJ, Scott O et al: Diagnosis and management of parachute mitral valve and supravalvular mitral ring. Br Heart J 36:641, 1974
24. Carpentier A, Branchini B, Cour JC et al: Congenital malformations of the mitral valve in children: Pathology and surgical treatment. J Thorac Cardiovasc Surg 72:854, 1976
25. Moularet AJ, Oppenheimer-Dekker A: Anterolateral muscle bundle of the left ventricle, bulboventricular flange and subaortic stenosis. Am J Cardiol 37:78, 1976
26. Cooperberg P, Hazell S, Ashmore PG: Parachute accessory anterior mitral valve leaflet causing left ventricular outflow tract obstruction. Circulation 53:908, 1976
27. Mathewson JW, Reimenschneider TA, McGough EC et al: Left ventricular outflow tract obstruction produced by redundant mitral valve tissue in a neonate. Circulation 53:196, 1976
28. Bjork V, Hultquist G, Lodin H: Subaortic stenosis produced by an abnormally placed anterior mitral valve leaflet. J Thorac Cardiovasc Surg 41:659, 1961
29. Gutgesell HP, Mullins CE, Gillette PC et al: Transient hypertrophic subaortic stenosis in infants of diabetic mothers. J Pediatr 89:120, 1976
30. Newfeld EA, Muster AJ, Paul MH et al: Discrete subvalvular aortic stenosis in childhood. Am J Cardiol 38:53, 1976
31. Morrow AG, Fort L, Roberts WC et al: Discrete subaortic stenosis complicated by aortic valvular regurgitation. Circulation 31:163, 1965
32. Kelly DT, Wulfsberg E, Rowe RD: Discrete subaortic stenosis. Circulation 46:309, 1972
33. Davis RM, Feigenbaum M, Chang S et al: Echocardiographic manifestations of discrete subaortic stenosis. Am J Cardiol 33:277, 1974
34. Norman JC, Nihill MR, Cooley DA: Valved apico-aortic composite conduits for left ventricular outflow obstructions. Am J Cardiol 45:1265, 1980
35. Rastan H, Koncz J: Aortoventriculoplasty: A new technique for the treatment of left ventricular outflow tract obstruction. J Thorac Cardiovasc Surg 71:920, 1976
36. Roberts WC: The congenitally bicuspid aortic valve: A study of 85 autopsy cases. Am J Cardiol 26:72, 1970
37. Hallman GL, Cooley DA: Aortic stenosis. In Hallman GL, Cooley DA (eds): Surgical Treatment of Congenital Heart Disease, p 60. Philadelphia, Lea & Febiger, 1975
38. Ellis FH, Kirklin JW: Congenital valvular aortic stenosis: Anatomic findings and surgical technique. J Thorac Cardiovasc Surg 43:199, 1962
39. Buckberg G. Eber L, Herman M et al: Ischemia in aortic stenosis: Hemodynamic prediction. Am J Cardiol 35:778, 1975
40. Gorlin R, Gorlin SG: Hydraulic formula for calculation of area of stenotic mitral valve, other cardiac valves and central circulatory shunts. Am Heart J 41:1, 1951
41. McMillan IRR: Aortic stenosis: A postmortem cinephotographic study of valve action. Br Heart J 17:56, 1955
42. Friedman WF, Benson LN: Aortic stenosis. In Moss AJ, Adams FH, Emmanouilides GC (eds): Heart Disease in Infants, Children and Adolescents, p 172. Baltimore, Williams & Wilkins, 1983
43. Vijayan A, Vlad P, Lambert EC et al: Serial data in cases of valvar and subvalvar aortic stenosis at the Children's Hospital of Buffalo. Birth Defects 8:60, 1972
44. Goldblatt A, Augen MM, Braunwald E: Hemodynamic-phonocardiographic correlations of the fourth heart sound in aortic stenosis. Circulation 26:92, 1962
45. Chandramouli B, Ehruko DA, Lauer RM: Exercise induced electrocardiographic changes in children with congenital aortic stenosis. J Pediatr 87:725, 1975
46. Johnson GL, Meyer RA, Schwartz DC et al: Echocardiographic evaluation of fixed left ventricular outflow obstruction in children: Pre and postoperative assessment of ventricular systolic pressures. Circulation 56:299, 1977
47. Nestico P, DePace N, Kimbris D et al: Progression of isolated aortic stenosis: Analysis of patients having more than one cardiac catheterization. Am J Cardiol 52:1054, 1983
48. Lambert EC, Menon VA, Wagner HR et al: Sudden unexpected death from cardiovascular disease in children. Am J Cardiol 34:89, 1974
49. Friedman WF, Pappelbaum SJ: Indications for hemodynamic evaluation and surgery in congenital aortic stenosis. Pediatr Clin North Am 18:1207, 1971
50. McNamara DG, Bricker JT, Galioto FM et al: Bethesda Conference #16: Cardiovascular abnormalities in the athlete: Recommendations regarding eligibility for competition. J Am Coll Cardiol 6(6):1204, 1985
51. Ankeney JL, Tzeng TS, Liebman J: Surgical therapy for congenital aortic valvular stenosis. J Thorac Cardiovasc Surg 85:41, 1983
52. Hossack KF, Neutze JM, Lowe JB et al: Congenital valvar aortic stenosis: Natural history and assessment for operation. Br Heart J 43:561, 1980
53. Beuren AJ, Schulze C, Eberle P et al: The syndrome of supravalvular aortic stenosis, peripheral pulmonary stenosis, mental retardation and similar facial appearance. Am J Cardiol 13:471, 1964
54. McDonald AH, Gerlis AM, Somerville J: Familial arteriography with associated pulmonary and systemic arterial stenoses. Br Heart J 31:375, 1969
55. Eisenberg R, Young D, Jacobson R et al: Familial supravalvular aortic stenosis. Am J Dis Child 108:341, 1964
56. Edwards JE: Pathology of left ventricular outflow obstruction. Circulation 31:586, 1965
57. Morrow AG, Waldhausen JA, Peters RL et al: Supravalvular aortic stenosis: Clinical, hemodynamic and pathological observations. Circulation 20:1003, 1959
58. French JW, Guntheroth WG: An explanation of asymmetric upper extremity blood pressures in supravalvular aortic stenosis: The Coanda effect. Circulation 42:31, 1970
59. Bolen JL, Popp RL, French JW: Echocardiographic features of supravalvular aortic stenosis. Circulation 52:817, 1975
60. Nasrallah A, Nihill MR: Supravalvular aortic stenosis. Br Heart J 37:662, 1975
61. Williams DE, Sahn DJ, Friedman WF: Cross-sectional echocardiographic localization of sites of left ventricular outflow tract obstruction. Am J Cardiol 37:250, 1976
62. Sahn DJ, Anderson F: Supravalvular aortic stenosis. In Sahn DJ, Anderson F

63. Rastelli GC, McGoon DC, Ongley PA et al: Surgical treatment of supravalvular aortic stenosis. J Thoracic Cardiovasc Surg 51:873, 1966
64. Edwards JE: Malformations of the thoracic aorta. In Gould SE (ed): Pathology of the Heart and Blood Vessels, p 422. Springfield, IL, Charles C Thomas, 1968
65. Becker AE, Becker MJ, Edward JE: Anomalies associated with coarctation of aorta: Particular reference to infancy. Circulation 41:1067, 1970
66. McNamara DG, Rosenberg HS: Coarctation of the aorta. In Watson H (ed): Textbook of Paediatric Cardiology, pp 175–223. London, Lloyd-Luke Medical Books, 1968
67. Weyman AE, Caldwell RL, Hurwitz RA et al: Cross-sectional echocardiographic detection of aortic obstruction: II. Coarctation of the aorta. Circulation 57:498, 1978
68. Lock JE, Bass JL, Amplatz K et al: Balloon dilation angioplasty of aortic coarctations in infants and children. Circulation 68:109, 1983
69. Hesslein PS, McNamara DG, Morriss MJH et al: Comparison of resection versus patch aortoplasty for repair of coarctation in infants and children. Circulation 64:164, 1981
70. Moss AJ, Adams FH, O'Loughlin BJ et al: The growth of the normal aorta and of the anastomotic site in infants following surgical resection of coarctation of the aorta. Circulation 19:338, 1959
71. Liberthson RR, Pennington DG, Jacobs ML et al: Coarctation of the aorta: Review of 234 patients and clarification of management problems. Am J Cardiol 43:835, 1979
72. Waldhausen JA, Nahrwold DL: Repair of coarctation of the aorta with a subclavian flap. J Thorac Cardiovasc Surg 51:532, 1966
73. Rocchini AP, Rosenthal A, Barger C et al: Pathogenesis of paradoxical hypertension after coarctation resection. Circulation 54:382, 1976
74. Ho ECK, Moss AJ: The syndrome of "mesenteric arteritis" following surgical repair of aortic coarctation. Pediatrics 49:40, 1972

PULMONARY VASCULAR DISEASE IN ADULTS WITH CONGENITAL HEART DISEASE

CHAPTER 104
VOLUME 2

Joseph S. Alpert • James E. Dalen

Pulmonary vascular disease is one of the most serious complications of congenital heart disease. The presence of this complication may eliminate the possibility of corrective surgery and lead to shortened life expectancy. As pulmonary vascular disease develops in patients with congenital cardiac lesions and a left-to-right shunt, pulmonary arterial pressure gradually increases *pari passu* with increasing pulmonary vascular resistance. As pulmonary vascular resistance and pressure rise, the magnitude of the left-to-right shunt decreases, eventually becoming insignificant in volume. At this point in the natural history of pulmonary vascular disease, there is often a small right-to-left shunt of approximately the same magnitude as the small left-to-right shunt (so-called balanced shunting). Further progression of pulmonary vascular disease leads to an increase in the magnitude of the right-to-left shunt with resultant systemic arterial hypoxemia and clinical cyanosis, the so-called Eisenmenger *reaction*. The term Eisenmenger's *syndrome* is often used instead of Eisenmenger's reaction. Strictly speaking, the syndrome refers to the original combination of lesions described by Eisenmenger: ventricular septal defect (VSD), overriding aorta, severe pulmonary vascular disease, and a right-to-left shunt.[1] In this chapter, Eisenmenger's syndrome refers to this combination of abnormalities, whereas Eisenmenger's reaction implies severe pulmonary vascular disease with resultant right-to-left shunting of blood in a patient with a congenital cardiac defect.

Normally, the resistance to blood flow across the pulmonary vascular bed is low, one twelfth of the resistance across the systemic vascular bed. The mean pulmonary arterial pressure in normal persons is only 12 ± 2 mm Hg.[2] The resistance across the pulmonary vascular bed is calculated by measuring the pulmonary blood flow and the mean pulmonary artery (PA) and mean left atrial (LA) or confirmed mean pulmonary capillary (PC) wedge pressure. Two different units have been used: dynes-sec-cm^{-5} (dsc) and resistance units/m^2. The pulmonary vascular resistance is measured in dynes-sec-cm^{-5} by multiplying the pressure gradient across the pulmonary vascular bed (PA mean pressure minus mean LA or PC wedge pressure) by a constant 80 and dividing by the total pulmonary blood flow in liters per minute. The normal pulmonary vascular resistance by this calculation is less than 120 dsc. A simpler formula consists of dividing the pressure gradient (PA mean pressure minus mean LA or PC wedge pressure) by the pulmonary blood flow expressed as liters/m^2. The normal pulmonary vascular resistance is less than 3 units/m^2. The low resistance of the pulmonary vascular bed is the result of the thin media of the precapillary pulmonary arterioles compared with the thicker media of systemic arterioles.

As pulmonary vascular disease develops, the pulmonary arterioles undergo a variety of changes that lead to thicker walls and hence higher vascular resistance (see below). Measured pulmonary vascular resistance increases progressively with worsening pulmonary vascular disease. Ultimately, pulmonary vascular resistance equals or even exceeds systemic vascular resistance. Patients with Eisenmenger's reaction have pulmonary vascular resistance that equals or exceeds systemic vascular resistance.

PATHOLOGY AND PATHOPHYSIOLOGY OF PULMONARY VASCULAR DISEASE

Pulmonary vascular disease involves three alterations in the normal microscopic architecture of the pulmonary vascular bed: increased muscularity of small pulmonary arteries; intimal hyperplasia, scarring and, at times, vessel thrombosis; and reduced number of intra-acinar arteries.[3-8] Increased muscularity of small pulmonary arteries is undoubtedly a response of vascular smooth muscle to increased wall tension secondary to increased intraluminal pressure, that is, pulmonary hypertension. Moreover, pulmonary arterial smooth muscle is found more distally in the vascular bed of pulmonary hypertensive persons than in normotensive subjects. The increase in pulmonary arterial muscle mass is due to hyperplasia rather than hypertrophy, with the new smooth muscle cells formed locally from mesenchymal cells.

Intimal hyperplasia, fibrosis, and vessel thrombosis are prominent histologic features of advanced pulmonary vascular disease. As intimal thickening progresses, intimal cells are replaced by hyalinized, collagenous tissue leading to what is termed "onion-skin" lesions. Thrombosis of small pulmonary arteries may be followed by recanalization. Intimal hyperplasia and fibrosis appear to be the result of intimal injury secondary to increased hydrostatic shear forces generated within the vessel lumen by pulmonary hypertension.

Patients with severe pulmonary vascular disease demonstrate decreased numbers of intra-acinar pulmonary arteries accompanied by increased pulmonary arterial smooth muscle volume and extent.[6,7] It is unknown whether arteries already in existence disappear or whether new arteries fail to form. Some authorities favor the first mechanism as the most likely explanation for the decreased number of intra-acinar arteries.

In 1958, Heath and Edwards[9] introduced the first comprehensive histologic classification of pulmonary vascular disease, which has subsequently been modified.[4] Six grades of worsening pathologic change have been identified, as shown in Table 104.1. Grade I consists of vascular smooth muscular hypertrophy in small pulmonary arteries. In grade II, smooth muscle hypertrophy and mild to severe intimal hyperplasia occur. Grade III changes consist of replacement of intimal cells by hyalinized, collagenous tissue leading to "onion-skinning" of the small pulmonary arteries. In grade IV patients, so-called plexiform lesions are observed. These consist of locally dilated segments of small pulmonary arteries with thin, damaged walls and large numbers of intraluminal cellular septae, giving the arterial lumen the appearance of being filled with capillary-like channels. Grade V changes consist of grade IV changes combined with extensive fibrosis of the media and intima of small pulmonary arteries. Thin-walled vessels often rupture, producing small foci of hemosiderosis. Grade VI changes involve an acute arteritis with fibrinoid necrosis (Table 104.1). The higher histologic grades of pulmonary vascular disease severity correlate with increasingly severe hemodynamic and angiographic evidence[10] of pulmonary vascular disease and pulmonary hypertension (Table 104.2). Virmani and Roberts[4] have classified the anatomical changes of pulmonary vascular disease into three grades. Grade I changes consist of medial thickening, grade 2 changes are defined as medial thickening and intimal thickening, and grade 3 changes consist of medial and intimal thickening plus plexiform lesions.

Increased flow, increased pressure, embolism, thrombosis, hyp-

TABLE 104.1 MODIFIED HEATH-EDWARDS HISTOLOGIC CLASSIFICATION OF PULMONARY VASCULAR DISEASE

Grade	Change	Grade	Change
I	Vascular smooth muscle hypertrophy in small pulmonary arteries	IV	Plexiform lesions—dilated segments of artery with intraluminal capillary-like channels
II	Vascular smooth muscle hypertrophy and intimal hyperplasia in small pulmonary arteries	V	Grade IV changes plus extensive fibrosis of the media and intima of small pulmonary arteries
III	Intimal hyperplastic cells replaced by collagen producing an "onion-skin" appearance of small pulmonary arteries	VI	Acute arteritis with fibrinoid necrosis

TABLE 104.2 A COMPARISON OF ANGIOGRAPHIC, HEMODYNAMIC, AND HISTOLOGIC FEATURES OF PULMONARY VASCULAR DISEASE

Angiographic Features	Group A: Normal Hemodynamics	Group B: ↑ Flow Normal Pressure	Group C: ↑ Flow ↑ Pressure	Group D: ↑ PVR	Group E: Pulmonary Venous Hypertension
Resistance to hand injection	Low	Low	Low to moderate	Increased	Variable
Reflux of contrast	Rare	Rare	Frequent (27%)	Usual (63%)	Occasional (10%)
Proximal muscular arteries (1–2 mm)	Straight	Dilated	Dilated ± tortuous	Dilated, tortuous	Dilated or constricted
Tapering of muscle arteries	Even, gradual	Even, rapid	Uneven, rapid	Uneven, rapid; beading	Even, rapid (lower lobes)
Supernumerary vessels (monopedial branching)	Numerous from elastic and muscular arteries	Numerous, dilated	Reduced, especially from elastic arteries	Reduced to sparse or absent	Reduced, constricted
Capillary blush	Full, granular blush around each artery	Full, granular	Full reticular-granular (18%)	Sparse, patchy (94%)	Sparse-full, coarse, reticular (18%)
Small veins (1–2 mm)	Narrow, orderly arborization	Dilated	Dilated	Normal	Dilated
V/A diameter ratio; mean ± SD	V/A = 1.04 ± 0.28	V/A = 0.99 ± 0.23	V/A = 0.87 ± 0.18	V/A = 0.93 ± 0.22	V/A = 1/43 ± 0.33 ($P < 0.001$)
Heath-Edwards histology grade	Normal to I	Normal to II	Normal to early III	Early III, late III, IV, and V	II to early III

↑ increased; PVR, pulmonary vascular resistance; V, vein; A, artery. (Modified from Nihill MR, McNamara DG: Magnification pulmonary wedge angiography in the evaluation of children with congenital heart disease and pulmonary hypertension. Circulation 58:1094, 1978. By permission of the American Heart Assoc, Inc)

oxia, acidosis, and a number of vasoactive substances are all capable of producing pulmonary hypertension by a variety of mechanisms. Common to all etiologies of pulmonary hypertension is the concept that pulmonary hypertension begets more pulmonary hypertension. Initially, pulmonary hypertension leads to endothelial cell injury secondary to increased intraluminal hydrostatic shear forces applied to the endothelium. Endothelial proliferation results. At the same time, increased wall tension within the pulmonary arteries leads to vascular smooth muscle hyperplasia. Both of these processes progressively restrict the lumen of small pulmonary arteries, leading to increased vascular resistance and further elevation of pulmonary arterial pressure. A vicious cycle is engendered, with sustained pulmonary hypertension leading to continuing endothelial injury and vascular smooth muscle hyperplasia, which in turn lead to worsening pulmonary hypertension. Hypoxia, acidosis, embolism, *in situ* thrombosis, and release of various vasoactive substances, such as platelet-associated thromboxane A_2,[5] may in part or in concert aggravate pulmonary hypertension by increasing pulmonary vascular resistance. Eventually, arteries that lack smooth muscle layers dilate, thrombose, or rupture, with resultant cellular repair and proliferation leading to dilatation or plexiform lesions.

Early in the course of pulmonary vascular disease, pulmonary vasoconstriction plays an important role in the genesis of pulmonary hypertension. Late in the natural history of pulmonary vascular disease, fixed, nonreactive, anatomical obstruction predominates. Increased flow, increased pressure, or both occur commonly in the pulmonary circulation of patients with congenital heart disease and left-to-right shunts. The cycle just described is initiated, leading to gradually progressive pulmonary vascular disease. The various pulmonary hypertensive factors cited above can be additive. Thus, a patient with a large patent ductus arteriosus (PDA) (increased pulmonary arterial pressure *and* flow) will develop pulmonary vascular disease at an earlier age and of greater severity than a patient with a large atrial septal defect (ASD) (increased pulmonary flow only). Similarly, patients with congenital heart disease and left-to-right shunts who live at higher elevations will have moderate arterial hypoxemia, and they develop pulmonary vascular disease at an earlier age than patients with similar defects living at sea level.[11] The rate of development of pulmonary vascular disease differs markedly from person to person despite similar congenital defects and similar magnitude of left-to-right shunts. It has been suggested that pulmonary arterial smooth muscle vascular reactivity differs from person to person, accounting for this spectrum of severity of pulmonary vascular disease. Similar differences in vascular smooth muscle reactivity have been observed in the systemic circulation of patients with essential hypertension.

PRIMARY PULMONARY HYPERTENSION

Some persons develop severe pulmonary hypertension in the absence of a left-to-right shunt, that is, despite the absence of congenital heart disease. Such patients are believed to have pulmonary vasculature that is particularly reactive, leading to the vicious spiral of pulmonary vasoconstriction and hypertension under circumstances that do not affect the pulmonary circulation of the vast majority of the population. Patients with this form of idiopathic pulmonary hypertension are said to have "primary" pulmonary hypertension (PPH), that is, pulmonary hypertension in the absence of cardiovascular or pulmonary disease. PPH is an uncommon process; it may be suspected clinically, but the diagnosis should be made only when all other forms of pulmonary hypertension are excluded.

ETIOLOGY

Although several mechanisms have been advanced to explain the etiology of PPH, none has been proven. PPH may represent a broad spectrum of disease states with a common clinical and pathologic end point. The possible importance of a thromboembolic etiology for PPH has been difficult to determine. It has been argued that PPH may result from recurrent episodes of asymptomatic pulmonary embolism.[12] However, a number of pathologic studies have demonstrated clear-cut differences between patients with PPH and patients with chronic pulmonary embolism. Moreover, thromboemboli found in patients with PPH are usually of recent origin in contrast to emboli noted in patients with chronic pulmonary embolism, in whom the emboli are in various stages of organization.

In Europe a number of persons taking the diet pill preparation aminorex fumorate developed pulmonary hypertension.[13] The clinical course was similar to that of PPH, except that regression of the disease process was reported with cessation of the drug.

Other etiologic possibilities have been suggested. Raynaud's phenomenon has been observed in approximately 30% of patients with PPH and has raised the possibility that PPH may be a form of collagen vascular or autoimmune disease.[14] Cases of PPH coexisting with postnecrotic hepatic cirrhosis have been observed, suggesting that a vasculitis might be responsible.[15] Female hormones may play a role, since the disease occurs 4.5 times more frequently in women than in men. The histologic changes observed in the pulmonary vasculature of patients with PPH resemble those already described in patients with Eisenmenger's syndrome.

CLINICAL FEATURES

Symptoms usually develop between the ages of 15 and 40. However, the disorder has been reported in infants and young children. Unfortunately, most patients come to medical attention late in the course of their illness when severe pulmonary hypertension has resulted in right ventricular failure.[16]

Dyspnea is by far the most common symptom in patients with PPH. Other frequently noted symptoms include easy fatigability, syncope, precordial chest pain, and weakness. Angina-like chest pain may occur. The mechanism of this chest pain is unknown, although it may be due to ischemia of the right ventricular subendocardium and/or distention of the pulmonary artery. Other symptoms that may be observed include palpitations, cough, hemoptysis, anxiety, depression, and psychosis.

The clinical signs observed are the result of pulmonary hypertension, right ventricular pressure overload, and resultant hypoxia. Cyanosis is sometimes noted, although it is usually mild and peripheral. Clubbing is a rare finding. The systemic blood pressure is low with a small pulse pressure. The jugular veins are distended, and there are prominent *a* waves reflecting forceful right atrial contraction. If tricuspid regurgitation is present there may also be prominent *v* waves.[16]

A forceful right ventricular heave is usually appreciated, and a pulmonary artery pulsation is often felt in the second left intercostal space. On auscultation, S_1 is usually normal, followed by a high-pitched, clicking, pulmonary ejection sound, followed closely by a soft systolic flow murmur. A characteristic auscultatory finding is accentuated intensity of the pulmonic component of S_2, which is often narrowly split. There is usually a prominent right ventricular S_4. Murmurs of pulmonic regurgitation or tricuspid regurgitation may be present. S_3 may be heard when right ventricular failure develops. Other physical findings of right-sided failure, including hepatomegaly, peripheral edema, or ascites, may be present.[16]

LABORATORY EVALUATION

The electrocardiogram reveals right ventricular hypertrophy and may demonstrate right atrial enlargement. Normal sinus rhythm is usually present.

Arterial blood gas analysis frequently reveals hypoxia; if hypoxia is persistent, secondary polycythemia may develop. When right-sided heart failure is present, abnormalities of liver function may be detected.

The chest film in PPH reveals prominent dilatation of the main and central pulmonary arteries with marked pruning of the peripheral pulmonary vasculature. There may also be radiographic evidence of right ventricular and right atrial enlargement. The aorta is usually small. Survival in PPH correlates inversely with the size of the main pulmonary artery.

Echocardiography documents an enlarged right ventricle, small left ventricle, and thickened interventricular septum. If the pulmonic valve is visualized, it usually shows attenuation of the a wave dip and midsystolic notching. The E-F slope of the mitral valve may be reduced, reflecting diminished left ventricular compliance secondary to the reverse Bernheim phenomenon. Lung scanning is usually nonspecific or normal and may be hazardous late in the course of the disease.

The definitive diagnosis of PPH is made by cardiac catheterization and pulmonary angiography. Catheterization of the right side of the heart reveals elevated pulmonary and right ventricular pressures; in some patients, pulmonary pressures may be as high as 200/110 mm Hg. The pulmonary vascular resistance is extremely high, usually reaching 750 dsc to 1000 dsc. Cardiac output is usually depressed. When left-sided heart pressures are measured, they are normal or low, although measuring an accurate pulmonary capillary wedge pressure may be difficult. Pulmonary angiography demonstrates large central pulmonary arteries with marked peripheral tapering. Emboli are not seen.

DIAGNOSIS

The diagnosis of PPH is a diagnosis of exclusion. It is imperative that diagnostic efforts be vigorously pursued in patients with severe pulmonary hypertension to ensure that no patient with secondary pulmonary hypertension is erroneously classified as having PPH.

TREATMENT

No effective treatment for PPH is available. It is logical to expect that pulmonary vasodilating agents might decrease right ventricular afterload and thus augment right ventricular emptying in patients with PPH, thus improving symptoms resulting from low cardiac output and right ventricular failure. Indeed, there have been numerous reports indicating the beneficial effects of various vasodilators in selected cases of PPH. Although some anecdotal reports are encouraging, others are less so, and the success of these agents has been controversial.[17-25] One retrospective series supports the use of life-long anticoagulation therapy with warfarin in patients with PPH.[12,26]

Recent observations support the concept of prolonged therapy with high-dose calcium channel blockade (up to 720 mg/day diltiazem or 240 mg/day nifedipine) for patients with PPH. Patients who responded demonstrated sustained reduction in pulmonary arterial pressure together with regression of right ventricular hypertrophy.[27] Prolonged intravenous infusions (1–25 months) of prostacyclin can also reduce pulmonary vascular resistance and improve tissue oxygen delivery in patients with PPH.[28] Exercise tolerance improves in patients responding to prolonged prostacyclin infusion, but the natural history does not seem to be affected. Some observations suggest that patients with PPH and Raynaud's phenomenon are particular likely to respond to vasodilator therapy.[29] Another interesting but as yet unproven form of therapy in patients with PPH consists of concomitant administration of thromboxane synthetase inhibitors and calcium channel blockade.[30] This form of oral therapy seeks to reduce levels of vasoconstricting thromboxane and increase levels of prostacyclin while relaxing pulmonary vascular smooth muscle with calcium channel blockade. The long-term effects of such therapy are as yet unknown.

Not all patients with PPH respond to calcium channel blockade. Indeed, some persons develop a decrease in cardiac output with concomitant right ventricular dysfunction during such therapy.[31] Since some patients with PPH appear to have recurrent thromboembolic events as the cause of pulmonary hypertension, anticoagulation would seem to be the best therapy for these patients. Other patients apparently develop pulmonary hypertension as a result of pulmonary vasoconstriction and are best suited for vasodilator therapy. Lung scanning may help to differentiate vasoconstrictive from thromboembolic disease and thus guide therapy.[32]

NATURAL HISTORY OF PULMONARY VASCULAR DISEASE

Although it was once believed that patients with Eisenmenger's reaction had a grave prognosis, more recent series have demonstrated that despite functional limitations, most of these patients lead active lives with little risk of death or other complication before the third decade of life.[33] Survival beyond 50 years of age is very uncommon. Once balanced shunting or net right-to-left shunting develops, operative mortality for closure of the congenital defect is high and postoperative functional results are poor. Pulmonary vascular disease usually fails to regress postoperatively, and right ventricular failure supervenes, leading to further deterioration in exercise tolerance.

Patients with Eisenmenger's reaction complain of dyspnea and fatigue. Some also report chest discomfort of uncertain etiology. Death in Eisenmenger's patients is usually the result of their heart disease or its complications.

Complications of Eisenmenger's reaction include right ventricular failure with or without syncope, arrhythmias, pulmonary infarction with or without hemorrhage, paradoxical embolism, brain abscess, bacterial endocarditis, spontaneous abortions, and gout. Many of these complications are life threatening and require urgent therapy. Terminal events include fatal arrhythmias, heart failure, pulmonary infarction and hemorrhage, brain abscess, and infectious endocarditis.

CLINICAL FEATURES

Patients with severe pulmonary vascular disease usually complain of effort intolerance with dyspnea on exertion and undue fatigue. Syncope also occurs commonly, but chest pain is less frequent. The physical examination is strikingly abnormal in these patients; central cyanosis, digital clubbing, a prominent right ventricular lift and pulmonary arterial impulse, and a loud P_2 are almost always present. Jugular venous filling is normal with a prominent a wave in patients without right ventricular failure. Patients with right ventricular failure may demonstrate jugular venous distention with cv waves secondary to tricuspid regurgitation. A normal or slightly reduced arterial pulse contour is observed in most patients with Eisenmenger's reaction. A right ventricular S_3 is commonly present.

The electrocardiogram invariably demonstrates one of the patterns of right ventricular hypertrophy. Depending on the underlying congenital cardiac defect, associated left ventricular hypertrophy may also be observed. The chest roentgenogram confirms the presence of an enlarged right ventricle and central pulmonary arteries. The peripheral lung fields are often oligemic in patients with advanced pulmonary vascular disease. Abnormalities of cardiac chamber size are common and depend on the underlying form of congenital heart disease. Echocardiographic examination confirms the presence of right ventricular and pulmonary arterial enlargement. Tricuspid or pulmonic valvular regurgitation is often present. The pulmonic valve tracing demonstrates the loss of the right atrial kick.

Common hemodynamic features of the Eisenmenger reaction regardless of etiology include arterial hypoxemia, markedly elevated pulmonary arterial pressure and pulmonary vascular resistance, and normal or modestly elevated left ventricular filling pressures. Right atrial hypertension may result from right ventricular failure. Erythrocytosis is commonly present. Balanced shunting or net right-to-left shunting of blood is observed.

A number of noninvasive cardiac techniques can be employed to estimate the severity of pulmonary vascular disease in patients with congenital cardiac defects. Echocardiography with Doppler studies and magnetic resonance images both give reasonable estimates of the severity of pulmonary hypertension.[34-36]

Therapeutic management of patients with Eisenmenger's reaction is limited largely to medical therapy. Correction of the congenital cardiac defect carries a prohibitive risk without much chance for improvement in symptoms postoperatively. However, patients with moderately severe pulmonary vascular disease (pulmonary vascular resistance of 600 dsc to 800 dsc or more) and a net left-to-right shunt may benefit from closure of their congenital cardiac defect. Complete resolution of pulmonary vascular disease following successful surgery is unlikely, and such patients invariably demonstrate residual cardiac disability. Combined heart and lung transplantation has been performed in a small number of these patients with occasional survival beyond 3 years. There are multiple problems associated with heart and lung transplants, and this therapeutic modality should still be considered experimental.

Medical therapy for patients with Eisenmenger's reaction and right ventricular failure consists of digitalis, diuretics, and supplemental inspiratory oxygen as well as decreased activity. On occasion, cautious administration of vasodilators (*e.g.*, nifedipine, diltiazem) or angiotensin converting enzyme inhibitors is of benefit in these patients. Some clinical observations suggest that continuous supplemental inspiratory oxygen therapy improves survival in children with Eisenmenger's reaction.[37] Oxygen administration leads to systemic vasoconstriction and modest reductions in cardiac output in these patients, which may limit the benefit of this therapy in some patients.[38] Regular phlebotomy is performed in order to maintain the hematocrit under 60%. Patients who require frequent phlebotomy may require supplemental iron to prevent iron deficiency. Some authorities advocate prophylactic anticoagulation with warfarin to prevent pulmonary arterial thrombosis in patients with Eisenmenger's reaction; however, no convincing data are available to suggest improvement in long-term prognosis with anticoagulation therapy. Antibiotic prophylaxis against infectious endocarditis should be administered scrupulously.

CONGENITAL CARDIAC LESION ASSOCIATED WITH PULMONARY VASCULAR DISEASE

Any cardiac defect that permits left-to-right shunting may lead to the development of pulmonary vascular disease. In infants, the most common congenital defects associated with pulmonary vascular disease are complete transposition of the great arteries with VSD, PDA, large VSD, truncus arteriosus, and complete atrioventricular (AV) canal defect.

In adults, normally all cases of severe pulmonary vascular disease secondary to congenital heart disease are in patients with VSD, ASD, PDA, and incomplete AV canal defect (ostium primum defects). The distribution of congenital cardiac defects in 91 cases of Eisenmenger's reaction reported by Brammell and co-workers[39] is shown in Table 104.3.

PULMONARY VASCULAR DISEASE IN PATIENTS WITH VENTRICULAR SEPTAL DEFECT

Eisenmenger's original patient had a VSD, an overriding aorta, severe pulmonary vascular disease, and a right-to-left shunt.[1] This is the true definition of Eisenmenger's syndrome or complex. In current usage, the associated overriding aorta is not required and any patient with a VSD and severe pulmonary vascular disease leading to a net right-to-left shunt is said to have Eisenmenger's syndrome.

VSD is the most common congenital cardiac defect to be associated with pulmonary vascular disease. Pulmonary vascular disease develops at an earlier age in patients with VSD than in persons with ASD. The explanation for this observation rests with the synergistic effect of increased flow *and* pressure in producing pulmonary vascular disease. Patients with ASD have increased flow alone in the pulmonary vascular bed.

In general, the larger the VSD the more likely the patient is to develop pulmonary vascular disease at an early age.[40] However, anecdotal case reports attest to exceptions to this rule, that is, patients with small VSDs who develop Eisenmenger's reaction. VSDs commonly decrease in size as patients grow older. In fact, a substantial percentage of VSDs close spontaneously during childhood or early adult life.[41] Thus, Eisenmenger's reaction in association with VSD is rarely seen in persons born with a small or moderate size VSD. These latter persons usually demonstrate decreasing pulmonary pressures and flow that occur *pari passu* with decreasing VSD size. If pulmonary vascular resistance is normal in childhood, pulmonary vascular disease rarely occurs during adult life. In one follow-up study,[41] pulmonary vascular disease developed in only 1% of unoperated patients who had normal pulmonary vascular resistance when they were first seen.

CLINICAL FEATURES
HISTORY

Patients with Eisenmenger's syndrome (VSD, pulmonary vascular disease, and right-to-left shunting) usually have a history of a conspicuous murmur heard in early infancy. Inadequate medical attention or rapid progression of pulmonary vascular disease results in failure to correct the VSD surgically before severe pulmonary vascular disease develops. Eisenmenger's reaction, when it occurs in VSD patients, usually develops during childhood, although occasional patients have been reported with this complication occurring during infancy.

Patients with Eisenmenger's syndrome complain of dyspnea, fatigue, and occasionally hemoptysis and/or exertional chest discomfort in the absence of significant coronary arterial obstruction. The onset of right ventricular failure with peripheral edema, anorexia, and ascites marks the beginning of a rapid phase of deterioration that leads to death. Cerebral abscess or thrombosis may occur secondary to erythrocytosis, and syncope is relatively rare. Infective endocarditis is a constant risk.

PHYSICAL EXAMINATION

Symmetric cyanosis and clubbing are the hallmarks of Eisenmenger's syndrome. Cyanosis tends to increase with exertion as patients grow older. The carotid pulse is normal or modestly decreased in volume. Jugular venous pressure may be normal with only a slight increase in *a* wave amplitude in patients with right ventricular compensation. As right ventricular dilatation and failure develop, the amplitude of the *a* wave increases and a marked *cv* wave may appear as a result of the

TABLE 104.3 CAUSES OF EISENMENGER'S REACTION: COLORADO GENERAL HOSPITAL 1950–1965

Defect	No. of Cases	Age at Diagnosis (Mean Range)
Ventricular septal defect	51	9.2 yr (2 mo–35 yr)
Patent ductus arteriosus	17	11.6 yr (2 mo–37 yr)
Secundum atrial septal defect	9	20.8 yr (6 yr–36 yr)
Endocardial cushion defect	5	5.2 yr (19 mo–10 yr)
Combined lesions	9	5.6 yr
Total	91	

(Brammel HL, Vogel JHK, Pryor R et al: The Eisenmenger syndrome: A clinical and physiologic reappraisal. Am J Cardiol 28:679, 1971)

development of tricuspid valve regurgitation. Jugular venous pressure is increased in persons with right ventricular decompensation.

Initially, the hemodynamic overload of VSD is borne by the left ventricle, leading to hypertrophy and dilatation of that chamber. As pulmonary vascular disease and pulmonary hypertension develop, concomitant right ventricular hypertrophy is observed. Therefore, palpation of the precordium of a patient with Eisenmenger's syndrome reveals evidence of increased left *and* right ventricular size. A pulsation over the dilated pulmonary artery is often felt as well.

As pulmonary vascular disease develops and right ventricular systolic pressure increases, the gradient that leads to systolic flow across the VSD lessens. Consequently, the characteristic holosystolic murmur of the VSD decreases in length. As pulmonary vascular disease worsens, the murmur becomes shorter and crescendo–decrescendo in shape and eventually disappears. The blowing early diastolic murmur of pulmonic regurgitation (Graham Steell) or the systolic murmur of tricuspid regurgitation may be heard. Forward flow into the dilated pulmonary artery of patients with Eisenmenger's syndrome may be accompanied by an early systolic click. The second heart sound is usually single (P_2) and loud in patients with Eisenmenger's syndrome.

ELECTROCARDIOGRAPHY
The electrocardiogram of patients with Eisenmenger's syndrome usually demonstrates both left and right ventricular hypertrophy. The pattern of right ventricular hypertrophy may be subtle (S_1, S_2, S_3 and terminal R in AVR) or obvious (large RS in lead V_1). Right-axis deviation is the rule.

CHEST ROENTGENOGRAPHY
Chest roentgenography in patients with Eisenmenger's syndrome demonstrates left and usually right ventricular enlargement. The left and right atria are also often enlarged. The aortic knob is normal or small, and the main pulmonary artery and its main branches are dilated. The peripheral lung fields are hyperlucent as a result of marked tapering of the distal pulmonary arteries. If severe pulmonary vascular disease has been present since infancy or early childhood, left atrial and left ventricular enlargement may be absent, and the only abnormalities seen on the chest film are large central pulmonary arteries and hyperlucency of the peripheral lung fields.

ECHOCARDIOGRAPHY
Echocardiographic examination usually demonstrates four-chamber enlargement in patients with Eisenmenger's syndrome. Left and right ventricular wall thicknesses are increased. The VSD itself is usually visible. Contrast echocardiography with microbubble contrast agents (*e.g.*, boluses of agitated sterile saline solution) demonstrate right-to-left shunting. Doppler studies can demonstrate severe pulmonary hypertension, right-to-left shunting of blood, and pulmonic or tricuspid regurgitation in patients with Eisenmenger's syndrome.

CARDIAC CATHETERIZATION
Conventional cardiac catheterization and angiography are associated with higher risks of complications and thus should be avoided unless absolutely indicated. Cardiac catheterization and angiography, however, confirm abnormalities previously demonstrated by clinical and noninvasive examination. The presence of balanced or net right-to-left shunting of blood, the size of the VSD itself, and the severity of pulmonary vascular disease can be directly or indirectly demonstrated at catheterization. In patients with VSD and marked pulmonary hypertension, it is often useful to determine the response of pulmonary arterial pressure to inspiration of 100% oxygen. If pulmonary artery pressure falls markedly and if a substantial net left-to-right shunt across the VSD can be documented, surgical closure of the defect may be undertaken, albeit at higher than normal risk. A fall in pulmonary arterial pressure secondary to breathing 100% oxygen implies the presence of a substantial element of pulmonary vasoconstriction, which *may* decrease following successful closure of the VSD.

THERAPY
Management of patients with severe pulmonary vascular disease and right-to-left shunting of blood has been outlined above. It consists of supportive therapy (oxygen, diuretics, anticoagulants, prophylactic antibiotics, phlebotomy) and, occasionally, judicious administration of vasodilators such as captopril or hydralazine or calcium-entry blocking agents. Surgical closure of the VSD is rarely if ever undertaken unless a substantial portion of the increased pulmonary vascular resistance is the result of vasoconstriction.

PULMONARY VASCULAR DISEASE IN PATIENTS WITH PATENT DUCTUS ARTERIOSUS

In the series of 91 cases of Eisenmenger's reaction reported from the Colorado General Hospital (1950–1965), PDA was the second most common lesion, accounting for 17 cases.[34] Given the ease of recognition of PDA and the general acceptance that the diagnosis of PDA is an indication for surgery, the number of PDAs presenting in adult life has decreased.

As in the case of VSD, pulmonary vascular disease occurs at an early age and is related to the size of the defect.[42] When the ductus is short and wide, it offers little resistance to flow from the aorta. In this circumstance, the pulmonary circulation is subjected to systemic pressure from the onset. The result may be a very large left-to-right shunt, leading to left ventricular failure. However, if the fetal pattern of pulmonary vasculature persists in patients with a large ductus, the pulmonary blood flow may not increase, and pulmonary vascular disease is present in the early postnatal period.

Controversy persists as to the pathogenesis of pulmonary vascular disease in PDA patients when it is detected in adult life. The pulmonary vascular disease may be an acquired complication of increased pulmonary blood flow as in patients with secundum ASD, or it may have been present from the early postnatal period. Favoring the latter possibility is the fact that adult PDA patients with pulmonary vascular disease often present without signs of left atrial, left ventricular, and ascending aortic enlargement by electrocardiography, echocardiography, or plain film. This, coupled with the lack of a history of congestive heart failure (CHF) in infancy, is strong evidence that these patients have not been subjected to increased pulmonary blood flow but rather have had pulmonary vascular disease from earliest life.

It seems likely that both mechanisms may occur. However, regardless of mechanism, the presence of severe pulmonary hypertension after 2 years of age nearly always reflects severe, irreversible pulmonary vascular disease.[43]

The incidence of pulmonary vascular disease in patients with PDA has been estimated to be about 10%.[44] Pulmonary vascular disease has been reported to be more frequent in PDA patients residing at high altitude,[45] indicating the impact of mild hypoxia as in patients with ASD.[11]

CLINICAL FEATURES
HISTORY
The adult presenting with PDA complicated by pulmonary vascular disease may have a history of CHF in infancy if a large left-to-right shunt was present through the ductus. In such cases, a murmur is likely to have been noted. In patients in whom pulmonary vascular disease has been present since an early age, a murmur may not have been noted, and patients may have been nearly asymptomatic during childhood. There may be a history of maternal rubella.

Most PDA patients with pulmonary vascular disease are symptomatic, with dyspnea and decreased exercise tolerance. The other symptoms of pulmonary vascular disease, chest pain, hemoptysis, palpitations, and syncope, may also be present. A symptom peculiar to PDA with pulmonary vascular disease, leg fatigue without significant dyspnea, may be present in patients with a right-to-left shunt.[46] With marked enlargement of the pulmonary artery, hoarseness due to compression of the left recurrent laryngeal nerve may be present.

PHYSICAL EXAMINATION
The most prominent cardiac findings are those of a closely split, loud, and often palpable S_2 and a parasternal heave. PDA patients with pulmonary vascular disease lose the diastolic component of the classic continuous murmur of PDA when the level of pulmonary arterial diastolic pressure reaches aortic diastolic pressure. Therefore, these patients have a systolic murmur only if they still have a left-to-right shunt; when there is only right-to-left shunting, there is no murmur.[47] The neck veins display a prominent A wave and are distended if right ventricular failure is present.

A distinct finding in PDA patients with right-to-left shunting from the pulmonary artery to the descending aorta is differential cyanosis. The feet demonstrate cyanosis and clubbing while the hands remain normal. Given the close proximity of the PDA to the left subclavian artery, the left hand, and especially the left thumb, may be cyanotic and clubbed while the right hand is normal.[46]

ELECTROCARDIOGRAPHY
The electrocardiogram demonstrates right atrial and right ventricular hypertrophy. If there has been a large left-to-right shunt in the past, there may be evidence of combined ventricular hypertrophy.

CHEST ROENTGENOGRAPHY
PDA patients with pulmonary vascular disease rarely show marked cardiac enlargement. The main chamber enlargement is the right ventricle, with prominent central pulmonary arteries with distal tapering. The PDA may be calcified and seen on chest film, especially in those over 30 years of age.

If there is radiographic evidence of enlargement of the left ventricle, left atrium, and ascending aorta, it is likely that there was a significant left-to-right shunt in the past.

ECHOCARDIOGRAPHY
The left atrium, left ventricle, and ascending aorta are normal unless there has been a large left-to-right shunt. The right ventricle is enlarged, and the pulmonary valve echo lacks an atrial kick. The PDA may be visualized by two-dimensional echocardiography. Pulsed Doppler echocardiography is very useful in detecting pulmonary hypertension in patients with PDA. In uncomplicated PDA, flow through the ductus is easily detected throughout systole and diastole. In the presence of pulmonary hypertension, flow through the ductus is significantly shortened during diastole.[48]

CARDIAC CATHETERIZATION
The diagnosis of PDA is often apparent from the course of the right-sided heart catheter as it passes from the pulmonary artery through the ductus into the descending aorta. A left-to-right shunt may be detected by a step-up in oxygen content in the pulmonary artery[49] or by indicator dilution techniques. In advanced pulmonary vascular disease, there may be no evidence of a left-to-right shunt but rather arterial desaturation (particularly in the descending aorta) due to right-to-left shunting. The diagnosis of PDA may be further documented by angiography, which may also confirm the presence of pulmonary hypertension by demonstrating absence or limitation of shunting from the aorta to the pulmonary artery during diastole.

Pulmonary artery pressure and calculated pulmonary vascular resistance reflect the severity of pulmonary vascular disease. Pulmonary artery pressure is often at systemic levels.

NATURAL COURSE AND THERAPY
The presence of pulmonary vascular disease limits life expectancy and, when severe, contraindicates surgical correction. Supportive medical therapy as with VSD, secundum ASD, and primum ASD complicated by pulmonary vascular disease is indicated.

SECUNDUM ATRIAL SEPTAL DEFECT WITH PULMONARY VASCULAR DISEASE

Of the congenital cardiac defects that may lead to pulmonary vascular disease, secundum ASD is the lesion most likely to be first detected in adult life. In a series of 412 patients with ASD seen at the Peter Bent Brigham Hospital and Children's Hospital (PBBH-CHMC) from 1948 to 1977, 45% of defects were first detected after age 20 and 25% of patients were older than 30.[50] The other lesions associated with pulmonary vascular disease (VSD, PDA, and ostium primum defect) are far more likely to have signs and symptoms leading to diagnosis in infancy or childhood.

The reason that secundum ASD is less likely to be diagnosed in childhood is that patients with ASD may be asymptomatic or their mild dyspnea on exertion and decreased exercise tolerance may be overlooked. The systolic murmur may be assumed to be a functional murmur in a patient who is asymptomatic or has modest symptoms.

Unlike the other congenital defects, pulmonary vascular disease rarely occurs before age 20 in patients with uncomplicated secundum ASD. In the 331 patients with ASD in the PBBH-CHMC series who underwent catheterization, there was a clear relationship between age and pulmonary vascular resistance. Of 147 patients catheterized before age 20, 94% had normal pulmonary vascular resistance (<2 units/m^2). Of those catheterized after age 20, only 55% had normal pulmonary vascular resistance.[50] This fact, coupled with serial cardiac catheterizations in which patients with ASD progressed from normal to near normal pulmonary vascular resistance to severe pulmonary vascular disease, makes it clear that pulmonary vascular disease is an acquired complication of ASD.[51]

Furthermore, it is difficult, if not impossible, to predict which patients with ASD will develop pulmonary vascular disease in adult life. Some patients with ASD survive to the eighth decade without developing pulmonary vascular disease, while others present with incapacitating pulmonary vascular disease in the third or fourth decade.

Patients with small ASDs (<1 cm^2) do not have a significant left-to-right shunt[52] and therefore are not at risk of developing pulmonary vascular disease.[53] In patients with an ASD of sufficient size to permit a left-to-right shunt, the size of the defect and the magnitude of the left-to-right shunt are not related to the probability of developing pulmonary vascular disease.

One clue to the pathophysiology of pulmonary vascular disease in patients with ASD is the observation that pulmonary vascular disease occurs at an earlier age in ASD patients who reside at modest elevation (>4000 feet). Of 49 patients with ASD who resided at sea level, only 6% developed pulmonary hypertension (mean pulmonary artery pressure > 35 mm Hg) before age 20. However, 21% of 53 patients living at elevations greater than 4000 feet had pulmonary hypertension before age 20.[11]

It seems likely that the mild hypoxemia associated with living at altitudes greater than 4000 feet leads to pulmonary vasoconstriction with a subsequent increase in pulmonary artery pressure. Sustained vasoconstriction may lead to medial hyperplasia in the small pulmonary arteries and thus initiate the changes in the media and adventitia that are associated with progressive pulmonary vascular disease.

The factors that initiate pulmonary vascular disease in patients with ASD living at sea level are uncertain. Unlike patients with large VSDs or a large PDA, the pulmonary circulation is not exposed to increased pressure prior to the development of pulmonary vascular disease. In patients with ASD, the development of pulmonary vascular disease must be a response to the exposure of the pulmonary vascular bed to the prolonged high-flow state associated with left-to-right shunting. It has been suggested that pulmonary vascular disease in patients with ASD begins with changes in the intima, in contrast to pulmonary vascular disease in VSD, which begins with medial hyperplasia. As pulmonary vascular disease progresses in patients with ASD, the changes in the intima and media become comparable to those of patients with VSD or PDA complicated by pulmonary vascular disease.

The later onset of pulmonary vascular disease in patients with ASD as compared with that in patients with VSD and PDA is almost certainly due to the fact that patients with ASD are not exposed to high pressure in the pulmonary circulation prior to the development of pulmonary vascular disease. The reason that some patients with large pulmonary blood flow secondary to ASD develop pulmonary vascular disease and others do not is unknown. It is possible that the process begins with pulmonary vasoconstriction in susceptible patients with reactive pulmonary vascular smooth muscle. The occurrence of pulmonary vascular disease in only some patients with ASD is similar to the situation that occurs in patients with tight mitral stenosis. Some of these latter patients develop reactive pulmonary vascular disease while the majority have only passive pulmonary hypertension without pulmonary vascular disease.[54]

CLINICAL FEATURES

HISTORY

Nearly all patients with ASD complicated by pulmonary vascular disease present with symptoms, the most common of which are dyspnea and decreased exercise tolerance. Unlike ASD with normal pulmonary artery pressure, dyspnea in patients with pulmonary vascular disease is frequently progressive and severe and is usually the reason that the patient seeks medical attention. Patients may have been asymptomatic or only mildly symptomatic in childhood. They may give a history of having a heart murmur; however, in most cases the diagnosis of ASD has not been suspected until the patient presents with significant symptoms.

Patients with pulmonary vascular disease are nearly twice as likely to have palpitations due to atrial arrhythmias and chest pain than patients without pulmonary vascular disease.[50] Chest pain in patients with pulmonary vascular disease is similar to angina pectoris except that it lasts longer and is often noted when the patient is fatigued, rather than during exertion. Hemoptysis and syncope are late findings in patients with advanced pulmonary vascular disease. Patients with severe pulmonary vascular disease with the Eisenmenger reaction may report intermittent cyanosis.

PHYSICAL EXAMINATION

The characteristic flow murmur associated with ASD is present in more than 90% of patients but may be softer and shorter than in patients without pulmonary vascular disease. Fixed splitting is present in the majority but is more narrowly split than in uncomplicated ASD. The P_2 is prominent and may be palpable. A flow murmur across the tricuspid valve is rarely present. A prominent parasternal heave is present in almost all cases.

An S_4 gallop and a prominent a wave in the jugular pulse are commonly noted. In the presence of severe pulmonary vascular disease with the Eisenmenger reaction, a murmur of pulmonic insufficiency may be present, and cyanosis and clubbing may be evident.

ELECTROCARDIOGRAPHY

The electrocardiogram may demonstrate atrial fibrillation or flutter if pulmonary vascular disease is present. In the PBBH-CHMC series, atrial fibrillation or flutter was present in only 7% of those patients whose pulmonary resistance was less than 2 units/m^2 but in 22% of those with increased pulmonary vascular resistance.[50]

In addition to the usual electrocardiographic findings seen in ASD, incomplete right bundle branch block and/or right-axis deviation, the R or R' in lead V_1 may be especially prominent in the presence of pulmonary hypertension. In the PBBH-CHMC series, of 86 patients in whom the R wave in V_1 was less than or equal to 5 mV, only one patient had severe elevation of pulmonary vascular resistance, whereas 6 of 10 patients with an R wave of greater than 20 mV had severe pulmonary vascular disease (pulmonary vascular resistance $\geq$ 7 units/m^2).[50]

CHEST ROENTGENOGRAPHY

The roentgenographic findings in patients with ASD complicated by pulmonary vascular disease are similar to those described for patients with VSD complicated by pulmonary vascular disease, except the left ventricle and left atrium are small or normal in patients with ASD. The predominant findings are a large right ventricle and enlarged central pulmonary arteries with tapering of the distal pulmonary arteries. The lung fields may be hyperlucent secondary to pruning of the distal pulmonary arteries. The aortic knob is small or normal.

ECHOCARDIOGRAPHY

Secundum ASD is suggested on M-mode echocardiography by the presence of a dilated right ventricle with paradoxical (*i.e.*, anterior) or flattened systolic motion of the interventricular septum (right ventricular volume overload). In patients with pulmonary hypertension, the anterior motion of the interventricular septum is very abrupt in early systole. The presence of right-to-left shunting can be detected by injecting saline into the venous circulation. The echo-producing bubbles will be detected in the left atrium. The secundum defect is often directly visualized by two-dimensional echocardiography and can be distinguished from an ostium primum defect.

CARDIAC CATHETERIZATION

The diagnosis of ASD is confirmed at cardiac catheterization by detecting a step-up in oxygen content of at least two volumes percent between the right atrium and the cavae,[55] by passing a catheter through the defect from the right atrium to the left atrium, or by indicator dilution techniques.[49]

The presence of pulmonary vascular disease is recognized by measuring pulmonary artery pressure and pulmonary blood flow and calculating pulmonary vascular resistance. Pulmonary hypertension is a common complication of secundum ASD. In one series of 239 patients with confirmed ASD, pulmonary arterial mean pressure exceeded 35 mm Hg in 21%, was borderline elevated (26 mm–35 mm Hg) in 12%, and normal ($\leq$25 mm Hg) in 67%.[11] Thus, the incidence of pulmonary hypertension was 21% to 33% depending on definition. In the PBBH-CHMC series of 311 patients with ASD, 31% had a pulmonary arterial mean pressure in excess of 20 mm Hg.[50] In the majority of cases of pulmonary hypertension in patients with ASD, a significant left-to-right shunt is still present. Therefore, the pulmonary blood flow is increased, and the calculated pulmonary vascular resistance is only modestly elevated (3–6 units/m^2). Pulmonary hypertension in this circumstance is hyperkinetic and is not a manifestation of fixed, irreversible pulmonary vascular disease. Pulmonary wedge angiography in these patients reveals dilatation of the elastic and transitional arteries together with dilatation and tortuosity of all vessels.[10]

Significant pulmonary vascular disease is present when pulmonary hypertension is associated with a pulmonary blood flow that is near normal or only slightly increased. In this circumstance, the pulmonary vascular resistance is markedly elevated to more than 6 units to 8 units/m^2. In the PBBH-CHMC series, 10% of the patients had severe pulmonary vascular disease (pulmonary vascular resistance > 7 units/m^2).[50] With the most severe form of pulmonary vascular disease, the Eisenmenger reaction is evident from the lack of a net left-to-right shunt, with arterial desaturation due to a right-to-left shunt. The Eisenmenger reaction was noted in 6% to 13% of patients with ASD in a collected series reported by Cherian and co-workers.[56]

NATURAL COURSE AND THERAPY

It is clear that the presence of pulmonary vascular disease decreases the life expectancy of patients with ASD. In a series of 48 patients with secundum ASD who were followed for 10 to 20 years, 23 patients had no evidence of pulmonary vascular disease at initial cardiac catheterization. Twenty-one of these patients were alive and well at follow-up. However, only 5 of 20 patients with PVD (pulmonary arterial mean pressure > 25 mm Hg and pulmonary vascular resistance > 120 dsc) were alive at follow-up 10 to 20 years later. Of the 15 deaths in the patients with pulmonary vascular disease, 6 occurred during surgical correction, and 9 patients died of their heart disease without surgery.[51]

Surgical correction of ASD not complicated by pulmonary vascular disease carries a very low risk. In the PBBH-CHMC series, there was only one death among 187 patients operated on between 1961 and 1977.[50] The operative mortality for repair of secundum ASD in patients over 60 years of age is also low.[57,58] The hemodynamic results and prognosis of such patients are excellent.[44]

However, if surgery is performed in ASD patients with pulmonary vascular disease, the surgical risk is increased,[51] and the outcome is uncertain. In ASD patients with Eisenmenger's reaction, surgical repair is contraindicated because of the high operative risk and the fact that there is no hemodynamic benefit to be gained from closure of the defect. The primary benefit of surgical repair of ASD is to decrease pulmonary blood flow by preventing left-to-right shunting. In patients with Eisenmenger's reaction there is no significant left-to-right shunt; therefore, there is no benefit to surgical closure.

In ASD patients with pulmonary vascular disease with a persistent left-to-right shunt, the decision for surgical correction is difficult. If the pulmonary hypertension is hyperkinetic, that is, if the pulmonary vascular resistance is only modestly elevated (<6 units/m^2), surgery is usually advisable. However, when pulmonary vascular disease is more advanced with pulmonary vascular resistance > 6 units/m^2, the risk of surgery is increased and there is a definite possibility that pulmonary vascular disease will progress despite successful surgical correction. Steele and co-workers[59] reported the results of surgery in 26 ASD patients who had a total pulmonary resistance greater than or equal to 7 units/m^2. They reported excellent results for surgical correction of patients with total pulmonary resistance less than 14 units/m^2, whereas of five patients with total pulmonary resistance greater than 14 units/m^2, four died, and one had progression of symptoms at follow-up.

We conclude that surgical correction of ASD is complicated and results are often poor when pulmonary vascular resistance exceeds 600 dsc (6 units/m^2). The decision for surgical correction in patients with severe pulmonary vascular disease, that is, when pulmonary vascular resistance is greater than 600 dsc, must be individualized on the basis of the magnitude of pulmonary blood flow, age, and associated disease.

Although the prognosis for ASD patients with severe pulmonary vascular disease is compromised, they may survive for a decade or more with medical therapy.[51] In addition to conventional therapy with digitalis and diuretics, chronic anticoagulation should be considered. Anticoagulation therapy sufficient to keep the prothrombin time 1.2 to 1.4 times control[60] should be instituted to prevent pulmonary embolism in patients who are immobile as a result of advanced disease or who have a history of venous thromboembolism. Patients with right-to-left shunting are at risk of paradoxical embolism[61] and should be treated with anticoagulants. The incidence of atrial fibrillation or flutter increases with age and with pulmonary vascular disease. Therefore, patients with ASD complicated by atrial fibrillation, even those who have had successful surgical closure, require chronic anticoagulation to prevent systemic embolism.[62] Some investigators believe that chronic anticoagulation is indicated to prevent progression of pulmonary vascular disease and in-situ pulmonary artery thrombosis. The efficacy of anticoagulation in this regard has not been established.

Agents that preferentially cause vasodilatation of the pulmonary circulation would be of potential benefit to the ASD patient with pulmonary vascular disease if the pulmonary vascular disease is not fixed. At the present time, there are insufficient data to recommend vasodilator therapy in patients with pulmonary vascular disease.[63] If vasodilators are used in patients with pulmonary vascular disease, they must be used with caution. An abrupt decrease in systemic vascular resistance can lead to an equally abrupt decrease in pulmonary blood flow with resultant increased arterial desaturation.[64]

PULMONARY VASCULAR DISEASE IN PATIENTS WITH PARTIAL ATRIOVENTRICULAR CANAL DEFECTS

Patients with complete AV canal defects, with atrial and ventricular defects together with abnormalities of the mitral and tricuspid valves, are highly symptomatic in early life and frequently develop severe pulmonary vascular disease in the first year of life. Such patients rarely survive to adult life without surgical correction of the defect.[65]

When the AV canal defect is incomplete and the ventricular septum is intact, survival to adult life is far more likely. Incomplete AV canal defects, also known as ostium primum defects, consist of a low-lying ASD, a complete or incomplete cleft of the mitral valve, and in some cases a cleft or other abnormality of the tricuspid valve.

Primum ASDs are much less frequent than secundum ASDs and are far more likely to become symptomatic at an early age. In the Mayo Clinic series of patients undergoing surgery for congenital heart disease, secundum defects were four times as common as primum defects.[66] Of 397 patients with secundum ASDs, 65% were repaired in adult life. Only 15% of 101 patients with primum defects were operated on in adult life.[66]

Ostium primum defects become symptomatic at an earlier age because the left-to-right shunt tends to be larger than with secundum defects and because of the associated mitral regurgitation with its impact on pulmonary venous pressure. The incidence of significant pulmonary vascular disease is much higher in primum defects than with secundum defects. In a series of 91 patients with Eisenmenger's reaction (pulmonary vascular resistance > 800 dsc) from the Colorado General Hospital, 9 patients had secundum ASD while 5 had ostium primum defects.[39] Given the much higher incidence of secundum defects, patients with ostium primum defects were overrepresented in the population of patients with the Eisenmenger reaction.

Furthermore, pulmonary vascular disease may occur at a much younger age in patients with primum defects. All five of the patients with Eisenmenger reaction in the Colorado General Hospital series were younger than age 14.[39]

The reasons for the higher incidence of pulmonary vascular disease and its appearance at a younger age in patients with primum defect are uncertain; however, it is very likely that the associated mitral regurgitation is an important factor. Significant mitral regurgitation leads to pulmonary venous hypertension, which causes passive pulmonary arterial hypertension and in some cases can lead to reactive pulmonary hypertension secondary to pulmonary vasoconstriction.[54]

Once the process of pulmonary vascular disease begins with medial hyperplasia, it may progress to intimal thickening and plexiform lesions, as in patients with other forms of congenital heart disease.[4]

CLINICAL FEATURES
HISTORY

Unlike patients with secundum ASD, patients with pulmonary vascular disease secondary to ostium primum defects will nearly always have been symptomatic during childhood. Many will have a history of CHF during infancy, as is the case with adults with pulmonary vascular disease secondary to VSD or PDA. Patients with pulmonary vascular disease due to ostium primum defects are highly symptomatic, with dyspnea and decreased exercise tolerance and palpitations. In addition, they may demonstrate symptoms associated with advanced pulmonary vascular disease (*e.g.*, syncope, chest pain, and hemoptysis).

PHYSICAL EXAMINATION

Approximately 30% of patients with ostium primum ASD have the stigmata of Down's syndrome. It is estimated that 30% to 40% of all patients with Down's syndrome have congenital heart disease and that in half of these cases the lesion is an ostium primum defect.[67] The prevalence of Down's syndrome may be even higher in adults with ostium primum defects because the defect may not be corrected in childhood in some patients with mental retardation associated with Down's syndrome.

On cardiac examination, the findings are similar to secundum ASD with pulmonary vascular disease: a systolic murmur at the pulmonic area with fixed but narrow splitting of S_2. The P_2 is loud and may be palpable. A prominent parasternal heave is present. The additional finding in primum defects is a systolic murmur, often with a thrill due to mitral regurgitation. A murmur of tricuspid insufficiency may be present owing to a cleft in the tricuspid valve or to functional tricuspid insufficiency secondary to right ventricular failure. A murmur of pulmonary insufficiency may be present with severe pulmonary hypertension.

The neck veins demonstrate prominent *a* waves as well as *v* waves if tricuspid regurgitation is present, and the central venous pressure is elevated in the presence of right ventricular failure. If the Eisenmenger reaction is present, right-to-left shunting will lead to central cyanosis and clubbing.

ELECTROCARDIOGRAPHY

The characteristic findings in ostium primum defect are incomplete right bundle branch block with left-axis deviation (left anterior hemiblock). In patients with normal sinus rhythm, the majority have first degree AV block.[68] Atrial fibrillation or flutter may be present in older patients. The R wave in lead V_1 is prominent with pulmonary hypertension.

CHEST ROENTGENOGRAPHY

Unlike secundum ASD, in which chamber enlargement is confined to the right ventricle, patients with ostium primum defects have four-chamber enlargement and therefore significant cardiomegaly. The aortic knob is small or normal. The proximal pulmonary arteries are enlarged with distal tapering as with other causes of pulmonary vascular disease.

ECHOCARDIOGRAPHY

M-mode echocardiography reveals a dilated right ventricle and evidence of right ventricular volume overload as in secundum ASD. The mitral valve is noted to be abnormally close to the interventricular septum, and the tricuspid valve may appear to lie within both ventricles. The primum defect and the cleft mitral valve are well visualized by two-dimensional echocardiography. Pulmonary hypertension is recognized by abrupt anterior movement of the intraventricular septum in early systole and loss of the atrial kick in the pulmonic valve echo. Right-to-left shunting can be detected by injection of saline into the venous circulation.

CARDIAC CATHETERIZATION

A step-up in oxygen content at the atrial level is to be expected as in the case of secundum ASD.[49] Large v waves may be present in the left atrial pressure tracing. The diagnosis of the ostium primum defect is confirmed by left ventricular cineangiography, which demonstrates mitral regurgitation and the characteristic "goose neck" appearance of the elongated narrow left ventricular outflow tract.[68,69]

As in the case of secundum ASD, the presence of pulmonary vascular disease is determined by measuring pulmonary arterial pressure and blood flow and calculating pulmonary vascular resistance. In some patients, pulmonary vascular resistance may remain normal even in adult life.[49]

With progressive pulmonary vascular disease, pulmonary arterial pressure increases, pulmonary blood flow decreases, and pulmonary vascular resistance increases. With the Eisenmenger reaction, the net shunt is right to left with resultant systemic desaturation.

NATURAL COURSE AND THERAPY

The only definitive therapy for ostium primum defects is surgical correction. In the absence of pulmonary vascular disease, the operative mortality is low and the results are excellent. Hynes and co-workers[68] reported the results of surgical correction in 47 adults with ostium primum defects. The operative mortality rate was 6.4%, and only 2 patients required mitral valve replacement. All surviving patients had class I or II disease at follow-up.

As in secundum defects, the risks of surgery increase and the benefits decrease in the presence of pulmonary vascular disease. Surgery is contraindicated in the presence of severe, fixed pulmonary vascular disease.

The fate of the patient with pulmonary vascular disease secondary to ostium primum defect is similar to that of the patient with pulmonary vascular disease secondary to secundum ASD. However, in addition to the complications of pulmonary vascular disease, the patient with an ostium primum defect is also compromised by left ventricular failure secondary to mitral regurgitation when it is present. Medical therapy is primarily supportive, as outlined for secundum ASD.

REFERENCES

1. Eisenmenger V: Die angeborenen Defecte der Kammerscheidwand der Herzens. Z Klin Med 32:1, 1897
2. Dexter L: Pulmonary vascular disease in acquired and congenital heart disease. Arch Intern Med 139:922, 1979
3. Edwards JE: Functional pathology of the pulmonary vascular tree in congenital cardiac disease. Circulation 15:164, 1957
4. Virmani R, Roberts WC: Pulmonary arteries in congenital heart disease: A structure-function analysis. In Roberts WC (ed): Congenital Heart Disease in Adults, pp 455–500. Philadelphia, FA Davis, 1979
5. Hoffman JIE, Rudolph AM, Heymann MA: Pulmonary vascular disease with congenital heart lesions: Pathologic features and causes. Circulation 64:873, 1981
6. Rabinovitch M, Haworth SG, Castenada AR et al: Lung biopsy in congenital heart disease: A morphometric approach to pulmonary vascular disease. Circulation 58:1107, 1978
7. Rabinovitz M, Castenada AR, Reid L: Lung biopsy with frozen section as a diagnostic aid in patients with congenital heart defects. Am J Cardiol 47:77, 1981
8. Hutchins GM, Ostrow PT: The pathogenesis of the two forms of hypertensive pulmonary vascular disease. Am Heart J 92:797, 1976
9. Heath D, Edwards JE: The pathology of hypertensive pulmonary vascular disease: A description of six grades of structural changes in the pulmonary arteries with special reference to congenital cardiac defects. Circulation 18:533, 1958
10. Nihill MR, McNamara DG: Magnification pulmonary wedge angiography in the evaluation of children with congenital heart disease and pulmonary hypertension. Circulation 58:1094, 1978
11. Dalen JE, Bruce RA, Cobb LA: Interaction of chronic hypoxia of moderate altitude on pulmonary hypertension complicating defect of the atrial septum. N Engl J Med 266:272, 1962
12. Fuster V, Edwards W: Idiopathic pulmonary hypertension: The importance of a thromboembolic etiology. Am J Cardiol 49:986, 1982
13. Gurtner HP: Pulmonary hypertension, "plexogenic pulmonary arteriopathy" and the appetite depressant drug aminorex: Post or propter? Bull Eur Physiol Mol Resp 15:897, 1979
14. Wolcott G, Burchell HB, Brown AL: Primary pulmonary hypertension. Am J Med 49:70, 1970
15. Segel N, Kay JM, Bayley TJ et al: Pulmonary hypertension with hepatic cirrhosis. Br Heart J 30:575, 1968
16. Alpert JS, Braunwald E: Primary pulmonary hypertension. In Braunwald E (ed): Heart Disease. Philadelphia, WB Saunders 1980
17. Shettigar UR et al: Primary pulmonary hypertension: Favorable effect of isoproterenol. N Engl J Med 295:1414, 1976
18. Ruskin JM, Hutter AM: Primary pulmonary hypertension treated with oral phentolamine. Ann Intern Med 90:772, 1979
19. Rubin LJ, Peter RH: Oral hydralazine therapy for primary pulmonary hyper-

tension. N Engl J Med 302:69, 1980
20. Klinke WD, Gilbert JACC: Diazoxide in primary pulmonary hypertension. N Engl J Med 302:91, 1980
21. Leier CV et al: Captopril in primary pulmonary hypertension. Circulation 67:155, 1983
22. Camenni F et al: Primary pulmonary hypertension: Effects of nifedipine. Br Heart J 44:352, 1980
23. Landmark K et al: Verapamil and pulmonary hypertension. Acta Med Scand 204:299, 1978
24. Kambara H et al: Primary pulmonary hypertension: Beneficial therapy with diltiazem. Am Heart J 101:230, 1981
25. Watkins DW et al: Prostacyclin and prostaglandin E for severe idiopathic pulmonary artery hypertension. Lancet 1:1083, 1980
26. Cohen M, Edwards WD, Fuster V: Regression in thromboembolic type of primary pulmonary hypertension during 2½ years of antithrombotic therapy. J Am Coll Cardiol 7:172, 1986
27. Rich S, Brundage BH: High-dose calcium channel-blocking therapy for primary pulmonary hypertension: Evidence for long-term reduction in pulmonary arterial pressure and regression of right ventricular hypertrophy. Circulation 76:135, 1987
28. Jones DK, Higenbottam TW, Wallwork J: Treatment of primary pulmonary hypertension with intravenous epoprostenol (prostacyclin). Br Heart J 57:270, 1987
29. Fisher J, Mack RJ, Likier HM et al: Nifedipine in pulmonary arterial hypertension: Importance of Raynaud's phenomenon. Chest 92:400, 1987
30. Rich S, Hart K, Kieras K et al: Thromboxane synthetase inhibition in primary pulmonary hypertension. Chest 91:357, 1987
31. Packer M, Medina N, Yushak M: Adverse hemodynamic and clinical effects of calcium channel blockade in pulmonary hypertension secondary to obliterative pulmonary vascular disease. J Am Coll Cardiol 4:890, 1984
32. Rich S, Pietra GG, Kieras K et al: Primary pulmonary hypertension: Radiographic and scintigraphic patterns of histologic subtypes. Ann Intern Med 105:499, 1986
33. Young D, Mark H: Fate of the patient with Eisenmenger syndrome. Am J Cardiol 28:658, 1971
34. Come PC: Echocardiographic recognition of pulmonary arterial disease and determination of its cause. Am J Med 84:384, 1988
35. Bouchard A, Higgins CB, Byrd BF et al: Magnetic resonance imaging in pulmonary arterial hypertension. Am J Cardiol 56:938, 1985
36. von Schulthess GK, Fisher MR, Higgins CB: Pathologic blood flow in pulmonary vascular disease as shown by gated magnetic resonance imaging. Ann Intern Med 103:317, 1985
37. Bowyer JJ, Busst CM, Denison DM et al: Effect of long-term oxygen treatment at home in children with pulmonary vascular disease. Br Heart J 55:385, 1986
38. Packer M, Lee WH, Medina N et al: Systemic vasoconstrictor effects of oxygen administration in obliterative pulmonary vascular disorders. Am J Cardiol 57:853, 1986
39. Brammell HL, Vogel JHK, Pryor R et al: The Eisenmenger syndrome: A clinical and physiologic reappraisal. Am J Cardiol 28:679, 1971
40. Engle MA, Kline SA: Ventricular septal defect in the adult. In Roberts WC (ed): Congenital Heart Disease in Adults, pp 279–310. Philadelphia, FA Davis, 1979
41. Corone P, Doyon F, Gaudeau S et al: Natural history of ventricular septal defect: A study involving 790 cases. Circulation 55:908, 1977
42. Kelly DT: Patent ductus arteriosus in adults. In Roberts WC (ed): Congenital Heart Disease in Adults, pp 316–321. Philadelphia, FA Davis, 1979
43. Rabinovitch M, Keane JF, Norwood WI et al: Vascular structure in lung tissue obtained at biopsy correlated with pulmonary hemodynamic findings after repair of congenital heart defects. Circulation 69:655, 1984
44. McNamara DG, Latson LA: Long-term follow-up of patients with malformations for which definitive surgical repair has been available for 25 years or more. Am J Cardiol 50:560, 1982
45. Espino-Vela J, Cardonas N, Cruz R: Patent ductus arteriosus. Circulation 38(suppl 5):45, 1968
46. Perloff JK: Patent ductus arteriosus. In Perloff JK: The Clinical Recognition of Congenital Heart Disease, pp 524–560. Philadelphia, WB Saunders, 1978
47. Harvey WP: Auscultatory features of congenital heart disease. In Roberts WC (ed): Congenital Heart Disease in Adults, pp 53–90. Philadelphia, FA Davis, 1979
48. Stevenson JG, Kawabori I, Guntheroth WG: Noninvasive detection of pulmonary hypertension in patent ductus arteriosus by pulsed Doppler echocardiography. Circulation 60:355, 1979
49. Dalen JE, Grossman W: Shunt detection and measurement. In Grossman W: Cardiac Catheterization and Angiography, pp 131–143. Philadelphia, Lea & Febiger, 1980
50. Hamilton WT, Haffajee CI, Dalen JE et al: Atrial septal defect secundum: Clinical profile with physiologic correlates in children and adults. In Roberts WC (ed): Congenital Heart Disease in Adults, pp 267–277. Philadelphia, FA Davis, 1979
51. Dalen JE, Haynes FW, Dexter L: Life expectancy with atrial septal defect. JAMA 200:112, 1967
52. Dexter L: Atrial septal defect. Br Heart J 18:209, 1956
53. Andersen M, Lyngborg K, Moller I et al: The natural history of small atrial septal defects: Long-term follow-up with serial heart catheterizations. Am Heart J 92:302, 1976
54. Dalen JE, Dexter L, Ockene IS et al: Precapillary pulmonary hypertension: Its relationship to pulmonary venous hypertension. Trans Am Clin Climatol Assoc 86:207, 1974
55. Dexter L et al: Studies of congenital heart disease: II. The pressure and oxygen content of blood in the right auricle, right ventricle, and pulmonary artery in control patients, with observations on the oxygen saturation and source of pulmonary "capillary" blood. J Clin Invest 26:554, 1947
56. Cherian G, Uthaman CB, Durairaj M et al: Pulmonary hypertension in isolated secundum atrial septal defect: High frequency in young patients. Am Heart J 105:952, 1983
57. St. John Sutton M, Tajik AJ, McGoon DC: Atrial septal defect in patients 60 years or older: Operative results and long-term postoperative follow-up. Circulation 64:402, 1981
58. Nasrallah AT, Hall RJ, Garcia E et al: Surgical repair of atrial septal defect in patients over 60 years of age: Long-term results. Circulation 53:329, 1976
59. Steele PM, Fuster V, Ritter DG et al: Secundum atrial septal defect with pulmonary vascular obstructive disease: Long-term follow-up and prediction of outcome after surgical correction (abstr). J Am Coll Cardiol 1:663, 1983
60. Hall RD, Raskob GE, Hirsh J et al: A cost-effectiveness analysis of alternative approaches for long-term treatment of proximal venous thrombosis. JAMA 252:235, 1984
61. Meister SG, Grossman W, Dexter L et al: Paradoxical embolism: Diagnosis during life. Am J Med 53:292, 1972
62. Forfang K, Simonsen S, Andersen A et al: Atrial septal defect of secundum type in the middle aged: Clinical results of surgery and correlations between symptoms and hemodynamics. Am Heart J 94:44, 1977
63. Friedman WF, Heiferman MF: Clinical problems of postoperative pulmonary vascular disease. Am J Cardiol 50:631, 1982
64. Krongrad E, Helmholz F, Ritter DG: Effect of breathing oxygen in patients with severe pulmonary vascular disease. Circulation 47:94, 1973
65. Newfeld EA, Sher M, Paul MH et al: Pulmonary vascular disease in complete atrioventricular canal. Am J Cardiol 39:721, 1977
66. Danielson GK, McGoon DC: Surgical considerations in treating adults with congenital heart disease. In Roberts WC (ed): Congenital Heart Disease in Adults, pp 543–562. Philadelphia, FA Davis, 1979
67. Crone RK, Gang DL: Down's syndrome and patent ductus arteriosus: Case records of the Massachusetts General Hospital. N Engl J Med 312:497, 1985
68. Hynes JK, Tajik AJ, Seward JB et al: Partial atrioventricular canal defect in adults. Circulation 66:284, 1982
69. Criley JM, French WJ: Cardiac catheterization in adults with congenital heart disease. In Roberts WC (ed): Congenital Heart Disease in Adults, pp 173–212. Philadelphia, FA Davis, 1979

ECHOCARDIOGRAPHY IN CONGENITAL HEART DISEASE

Kyung J. Chung • David J. Sahn

During the past decade, advances in ultrasound instrumentation and their application to image cardiac structures made major contributions to pediatric cardiology. Cross-sectional, M-mode, and Doppler echocardiography can be utilized to define cardiac anatomy, function, and blood-flow patterns noninvasively. The major diagnostic challenge of echocardiography is to define complex cardiac anomalies in newborn infants and to assess the cardiac output and the pressure gradient across stenotic valves and to estimate the pulmonary vascular resistance in children undergoing major cardiac surgery. Once the patient is substantially beyond infancy, most congenital cardiac anomalies have already been diagnosed and corrected. However, certain cardiac diseases become apparent in older children, and other conditions that may not warrant early surgery, such as aortic valve stenosis, need serial follow-up, since they may change with time and growth.

A major area for echocardiography in older children and adults with congenital heart disease is that of postoperative anatomical and functional assessment to evaluate and follow residua of corrective or palliative surgery. Lastly, changes in immigration have brought to many United States centers increasing numbers of adults with complicated congenital heart disease from Latin America and Asia. In this chapter we review echocardiographic and Doppler methods and their use in adults with congenital heart disorders both before and after surgery.

SHUNT LESIONS

Simple shunt lesions can be detected with echocardiography; some may present in the adult.

ATRIAL SEPTAL DEFECT

M-mode echocardiographic features of atrial septal defect have been described extensively.[1,2] These are indirect parameters and depend upon the hemodynamic status of the right ventricle. Right ventricular chamber dilatation and abnormal ventricular septal motion are the key findings. These echocardiographic findings are very sensitive to right ventricular volume overload but are not specific for atrial septal defect. Similar findings can be seen in patients with tricuspid regurgitation, pulmonary regurgitation, or right ventricular dysfunction. However, hemodynamically significant atrial septal defects almost always show M-mode patterns of right ventricular volume overload.

Two-dimensional echocardiography has the advantage that it visualizes the atrial septum directly.[3-6] The optimum view to examine the atrial septum is the subcostal four-chamber view, which can still often be used in adults. From these views, one can eliminate the potential errors created by echocardiographic dropout in precordial or apical views. From apical views, the ultrasound beam is parallel to the orientation of the atrial septum, especially the posterior portion of the atrial septum, and therefore is often associated with artifactual septal dropout of this region. In the subcostal view, sound energy is perpendicular to the septum. Lastly, right parasternal views have also been helpful for imaging the atrial septum.

There are three major types of atrial septal defect. Secundum type atrial septal defect, the most common type, is due to defect of the septum primum and is located in the central portion or fossa ovalis area (Fig. 105.1). Primum, or partial endocardial cushion type, atrial septal defect is due to the defect in the atrioventricular canal portion of the atrial septum, and the lower margin of the defect extends to the inlet ventricular septum and atrioventricular valves. Primum atrial septal defect is almost always associated with the atrioventricular valve deformities, especially cleft mitral valve. Sinus venosus–type defects are usually located in the high portion of the atrial septum at the junction of the superior vena cava and the right atrium and are often associated with anomalous return of the right upper lobe pulmonary vein into the right atrium (Fig. 105.2, A).

By examining the entire atrial septum, one can easily diagnose atrial septal defect if the size of the defect is within the range of echocardiographic resolution (>3 mm). From the subcostal view, all types of atrial septal defects can be searched for if one finds the superior vena cava, inferior vena cava, and carefully scans for the atrial septal area. As described above, apical and precordial views have their drawbacks because of their beam angle. Secundum atrial septal defect can be falsely diagnosed as a result of a lack of ultrasound reflection from this thin fossa ovalis area. However, primum-type atrial septal defect can be seen easily from these views, since it is located low in the atrial septum and there is alignment of the atrioventricular valves.

Injection of saline or indocyanine green into a peripheral vein creates echo-dense contrast and has been helpful in detecting a right-to-left shunt in patients with atrial septal defect, since a small amount of right-to-left shunting is present, especially with a Valsalva maneuver, in the majority of patients with atrial septal defect even if they have a net left-to-right shunt.[7-10] Also, a left-to-right shunt at the atrial level may be detected by negative contrast effect (an echo-free area) in the right atrium induced by the nonopacified bloodstream across the atrial septal defect.[11]

With the two-dimensional echocardiographic imaging and Doppler, flow through an atrial septal defect can be localized by placing the pulsed Doppler sample volume in the right atrium.[12,13] In patients with atrial septal defects, characteristic audio and spectral signals are obtained. Flow from the left to right through an atrial septal defect is toward the transducer, and the flow pattern is a low-velocity (60–80 cm/sec) turbulent flow starting in early systole with increasing velocity at end-systole and continuing through to diastole. The second peak of velocity occurs during diastole with atrial contraction (Fig. 105.2, B). In patients in whom two-dimensional image quality is inadequate to visualize the atrial septum, Doppler echocardiography guided by two-dimensional imaging can confirm the presence of left-to-right shunting at this level. The flow velocity through an atrial defect must be differentiated from the superior vena caval flow, which may have a similar direction and pattern. The velocity of the vena caval flow may be distinguished from atrial septal defect by the different locations of the sample volume compared with atrial septal defect. Also, velocity increases during inspiration with the vena caval flow, whereas it may vary less with inspiration in atrial septal defect. Increased flows are also recorded across the tricuspid and pulmonary valves in atrial septal defect patients.

Recent interest has been focused on quantitative measurement of cardiac output by Doppler echocardiography.[14-17] This method has potential advantages, since it can measure pulmonary and systemic blood flow, calculating the magnitude of left-to-right shunt (Qp/Qs). Valdes–Cruz and Sahn[14] and their co-workers have worked extensively in applying Doppler echocardiography to cardiac flow measurement in animal models of atrial septal defect and in clinical settings. Systemic flows were measured from the ascending aorta, while pulmonary blood flow was determined from sample volumes positioned in the main pulmonary artery. A Doppler examination of Qp/Qs in animal models was correlated well to measurements with the electromagnetic flow meter. In clinical settings, however, errors can be made as a result of suboptimal imaging quality for vessel diameter and marked spectral dispersion in pulmonary velocity curves with turbulence resulting from increased pulmonary blood flow. With substantial improvement of imaging capability with higher-frequency transducers, multiple sampling areas, and continuing efforts to avoid potential sources of error, a noninvasive modality to quantitate pulmonary and systemic flow in patients with atrial septal defect is still possible using Doppler echocardiography. New color flow-imaging techniques (see below) can also directly image the interatrial shunt (Fig. 105.3).

VENTRICULAR SEPTAL DEFECTS

Ventricular septal defect is the most common form of congenital heart disease, accounting for 25% of congenital heart disease in children. Ventricular septal defect may occur as an isolated lesion or as a part of complex cardiac anomaly. The clinical manifestations of simple ventricular septal defect depend on the size of the defect and the pulmonary vascular resistance. Children with a small ventricular septal defect are asymptomatic and the lesion is often found incidentally during routine physical examination. There is no evidence of electrocardio-

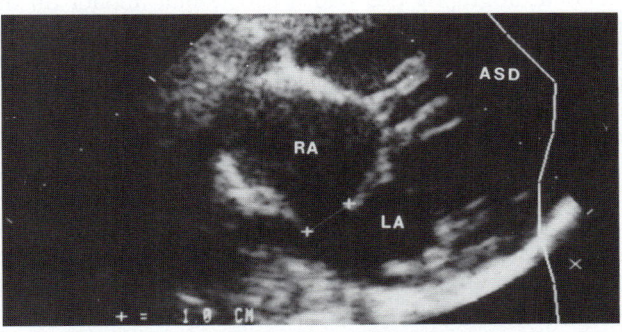

FIGURE 105.1 Subcostal view two-dimensional image of a secundum atrial septal defect 1 cm in diameter. (*RA*, right atrium; *LA*, left atrium.)

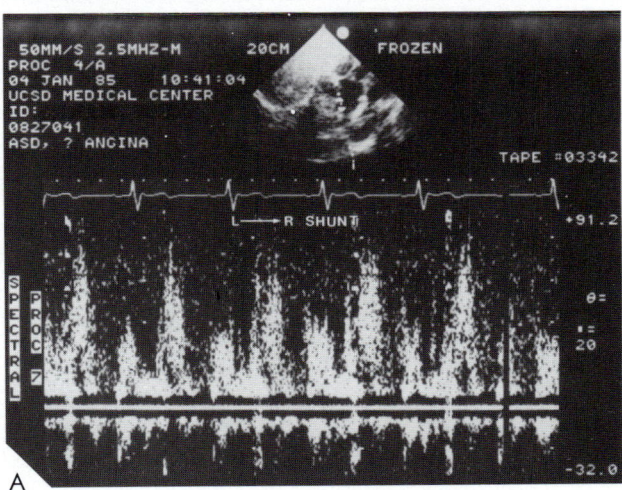

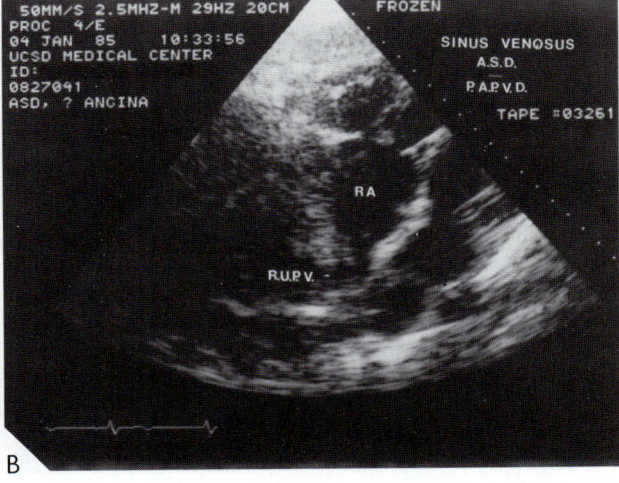

FIGURE 105.2 A. Superiorly tilted subcostal view in an adult images the right upper pulmonary vein (*RUPV*) draining directly into the right atrium. The patient had an associated sinus venosus atrial septal defect not imaged on this particular stop frame. **B.** Doppler interrogation of the area of the high atrial septal defect and the anomalous right upper pulmonary vein shows turbulent and elevated-velocity flow coming toward the transducer in late systole and early diastole, characteristic of a left-to-right shunting atrial defect.

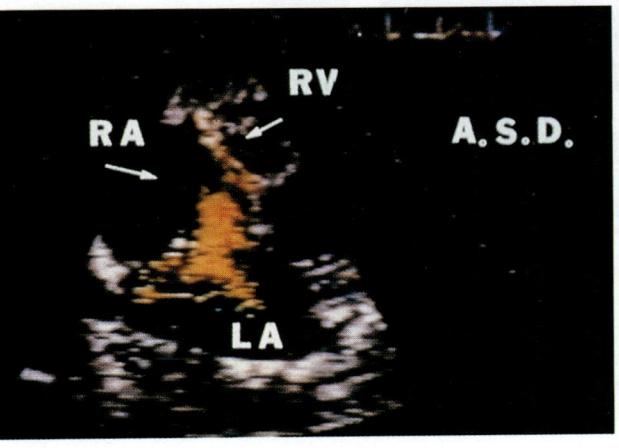

FIGURE 105.3 Stop-frame image from a two-dimensional flow mapping study. Velocities toward the transducer are color encoded in increasing brightnesses of red to orange. This late systolic frame shows the direct imaging of left-to-right shunt flow across a secundum atrial septal defect. (*RV*, right ventricle; *RA*, right atrium; *LA*, left atrium.)

graphic or chest film abnormalities in these children; in contrast, when the defect is large, the symptoms and signs are present during infancy, requiring invasive diagnostic studies and often surgical intervention. Small ventricular septal defects require no surgical intervention; however, bacterial endocarditis prophylaxis is mandatory because endocardial changes may predispose to cardiac infection. Therefore, it is important to identify ventricular septal defect for proper management.

There are several types of ventricular septal defect: perimembranous; muscular (single or multiple); atrioventricular canal type; subpulmonary; and malalignment. Ventricular septal defects of the atrioventricular canal and the malalignment types are almost always large and can be detected by two-dimensional echocardiography without difficulty. Atrioventricular canal type defect is best seen in an apical four-chamber view. Malalignment type (as in tetralogy of Fallot) and perimembranous defects are best seen in both parasternal and subcostal long-axis views. Two-dimensional echocardiography is not as reliable in detecting ventricular septal defects of subpulmonary or muscular types, with the exception of large ones (Fig. 105.4). In small children, ventricular septal defects of these types (diameter greater than 2–3 mm) can usually be detected using four-chamber long-axis or short-axis or subcostal views.[18] In older patients especially, the reliability of two-dimensional echocardiography for imaging small membranous or muscular ventricular septal defects is very limited.[19–21]

Very recent developments in ultrasound instrumentation have provided a combination of two-dimensional imaging with noninvasive real-time analysis of blood-flow patterns using Doppler methods.[22,23] The newest techniques, overlaying Doppler flow information onto the two-dimensional image using a color flow map, provides us with more accurate anatomical and physiologic information to describe cardiac anomalies.[24–26] Disturbance of the circulation by high-velocity turbulent flow through a ventricular septal defect can be detected and localized by Doppler. Figure 105.5 presents one such example in a patient who is suspected clinically of having a ventricular septal defect, but the defect was not visualized on the two-dimensional echocardiogram because of its size and location (muscular ventricular septal defect). Using Doppler methods with the color flow mapping, it was easy to localize the area of defect (see Fig. 105.5).

Obviously, in substantial ventricular septal defects, left ventricular and atrial size are increased.[27,28] Methods have also been described for calculating Qp/Qs in ventricular septal defects by using aortic flows by Doppler for Qs and mitral flows by Doppler for Qp.[14]

AORTIC STENOSIS

Echocardiography has had a substantial impact on diagnosing and measuring the severity of aortic stenosis. Although M-mode echocardiography has been used to assess the severity of aortic stenosis, it can provide only qualitative assessment.[29–32] Even the qualitative diagnosis of aortic stenosis can be difficult in patients with aortic stenosis associated with other cardiac anomalies, such as mitral stenosis or coarctation of the aorta. M-mode echocardiographic findings are thickening of the valve leaflets, shown as multiple echoes during diastole. M-mode echocardiography has also been used to estimate the left ventricular (LV) to aortic (AO) gradient indirectly by a method combining the thickness of the left ventricular wall (LVTs) and the diameter of the left

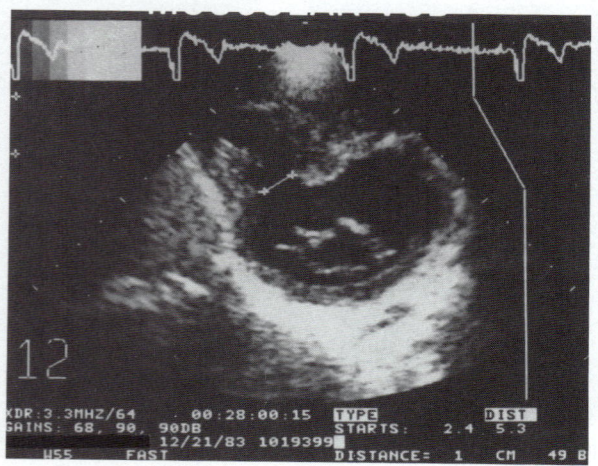

FIGURE 105.4 Short-axis two-dimensional image at the level of the mitral valve shows imaging and measurement of a muscular ventricular defect that enters the right ventricle just to the right of the moderator band. This is a large muscular ventricular septal defect.

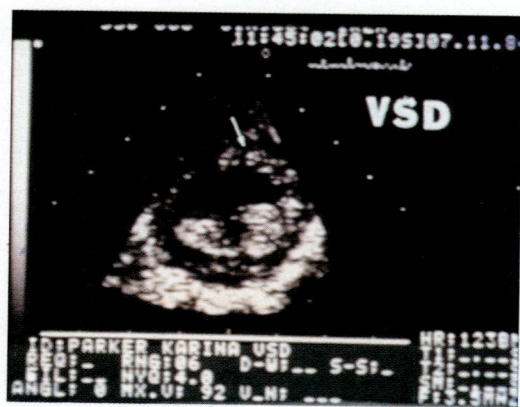 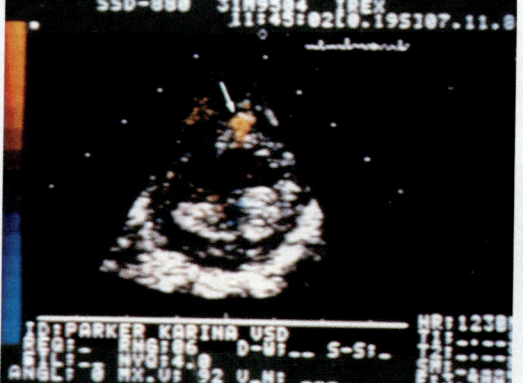 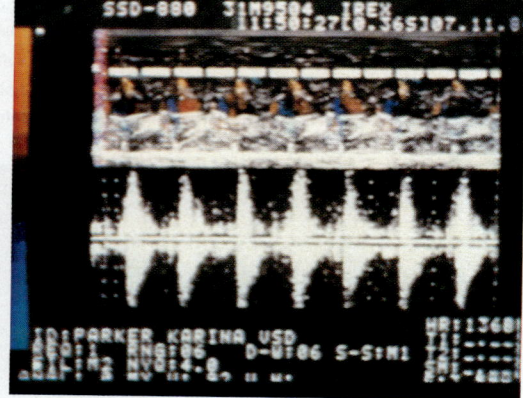

FIGURE 105.5 In the short-axis view (left), a muscular ventricular septal defect is barely resolved and delineated by the arrow. The flow map two-dimensional echocardiogram (center) shows the left-to-right shunt flow coming through the defect into the right ventricle. It was only after the shunt flow was imaged that the underlying ventricular septal defect was noted on the two-dimensional echocardiogram. When a single sample volume is placed within the imaged shunt flow, the characteristic MQ-mode with flow traversing the septum from left to right is obtained, and the characteristic spectrum of high-velocity systolic flow is shown (right).

ventricular chamber (LVDs) at end-systole. A formula has been derived using these two parameters and a constant factor $(225)^{29,31}$.

LV peak systolic pressure (SP) − systolic blood pressure (BP)

$$= \frac{LVTs}{LVDs} \times 225 - \text{systolic BP} = LV - AO \text{ gradient}$$

The reliability of this technique is variable. Most investigators agree that this formula is inaccurate if the left ventricle is dilated or a patient has systemic hypertension, for instance due to coarctation of the aorta. In any case, echocardiographic left ventricular hypertrophy is an important indicator of the hemodynamic status in the left ventricle. Serial measurement of the left ventricular wall thickness may predict the progression of aortic stenosis in the patient.

In contrast to the complex nature of right ventricular outflow tract morphology, the left ventricular outflow tract is larger and has simpler anatomy, and two-dimensional echocardiography is able to provide significant anatomical detail in left ventricular outflow tract obstruction. Initial two-dimensional echocardiographic studies of valvular aortic stenosis by Weyman and co-workers[33] indicated that the degree of aortic stenosis could be estimated by measuring maximum leaflet separation during systole as the diameter between the inner surface of the leaflets imaged by two-dimensional echocardiography in long-axis view (Fig. 105.6). More recently, DeMaria and associates[34] suggested that intercusp distance during systole by two-dimensional echocardiography correlated poorly with the aortic valve area or peak transvalvular gradient measured during cardiac catheterization. Errors in estimating the severity of valve disease in his experience were due to inadequate imaging of the aortic orifice by two-dimensional echocardiography or to situations in which the patient had a calcified aortic valve or low cardiac output state.

The usefulness of two-dimensional echocardiography in quantitative evaluation of aortic stenosis is still uncertain. However, the applications of Doppler echocardiography, especially continuous Doppler, are promising for assessing the severity of aortic stenosis quantitatively. With obstruction to blood flow through the stenotic valve, there is an increased maximal velocity of the flow distal to the obstruction.[35-39] As initially suggested by Hatle,[35] measuring the maximal velocity with Doppler echocardiography, peak transvalvular aortic gradient can be estimated using a modified Bernoulli equation: peak gradient $= 4 \times V^2$ (V = maximal velocity). A normal aortic flow pattern in the ascending aorta shows a rapid upstroke and a downward slope during systole with a narrow spectral width due to laminar flow during systole. Disturbed flow due to aortic stenosis can be detected in the ascending aorta, but there is also a high-velocity laminar flow jet present in the aorta. In order to accurately estimate the pressure gradient, it is necessary to have the ultrasound beam as parallel as possible to the direction of the jet ($<20°$), and one must record the maximum Doppler flow signal by listening to the audio signal and by monitoring the peak flow velocity on the spectral display (see Fig. 105.6). Hatle and co-workers,[35] using continuous-wave Doppler, reported that there was a close relationship between the peak systolic pressure gradient obtained by Doppler techniques and the pressure obtained during cardiac catheterization. Stamm[36] and Oliveira-Lima[37] and their co-workers have also confirmed Hatle's observations. The Doppler measured gradient accurately separated those patients with significant aortic ste-

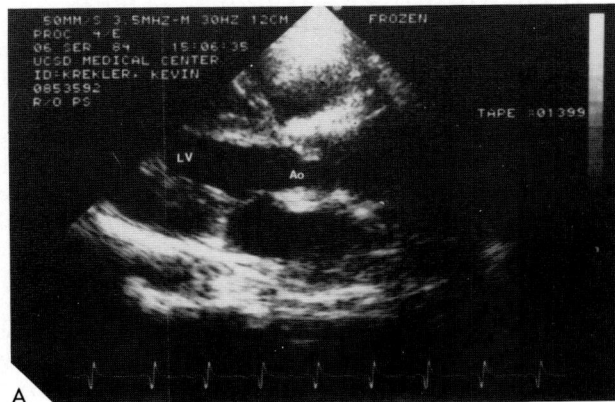
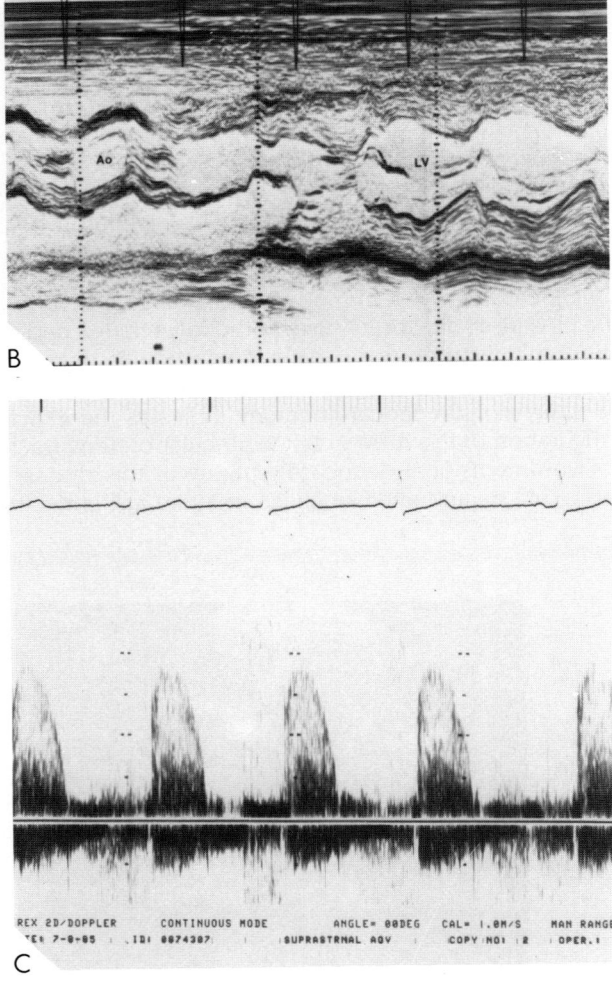

FIGURE 105.6 A domed aortic valve is visualized in a long-axis view (**A**) that also shows the degree of left ventricular (LV) hypertrophy. The characteristic M-mode sweep from the redundant thickened aortic valve into the left ventricle is shown in **B**. Suprasternal notch interrogation using continuous Doppler velocimetry shows peak systolic velocities almost 4 m/sec in **C**, corresponding with moderate to severe valvular aortic stenosis.

nosis (gradient > 50 mm Hg) from those with less severe aortic stenosis. Despite its good correlation with the cardiac catheterization gradient, the Doppler method still has problems related to its accuracy for predicting transvalvular pressure gradient. Doppler echocardiography may overestimate standard catheter laboratory pressure gradients, since it uses the maximal velocity value, which represents maximal instantaneous pressure differences between the left ventricle and the ascending aorta during systole, whereas in most of the cardiac catheterization laboratories, the gradient reported is between the peak left ventricle and peak aorta pressure (peak-to-peak). The difference between the two methods is greater in patients with mild to moderate aortic stenosis. Doppler estimation may be 20 mm to 30 mm Hg higher than peak-to-peak catheterization gradient. Underestimation of the aortic valve gradient has also been a dilemma. This often results from failure to obtain maximal velocity. If the Doppler beam becomes more perpendicular to the jet, there is marked decrease of the Doppler-derived velocity than true velocity. Use of color flow mapping may further improve the accuracy of Doppler evaluation of aortic stenosis by visually indicating the direction of the jet across the valve. Visualization of the jet may allow more accurate use of angle corrections for determination of peak velocity.

The gradient across the aortic valve is also dependent upon the stroke volume. Thus, in patients with low cardiac output, the gradient may be smaller despite significant aortic stenosis.

A cardiac output measurement by Doppler methods, thermodilution, or Fick's methods, combined with a pressure gradient measured by Doppler methods, will, therefore, provide the most accurate noninvasive assessment of the degree of aortic stenosis.

SUBAORTIC STENOSIS

Subaortic obstruction is uncommon in neonates or young children. It is, however, recognized in older children and young adults, often as a progressive disease. Echocardiography has been effective in differentiating the characteristics of subaortic stenosis and is, in fact, superior to angiography for this diagnosis.

Discrete subaortic stenosis accounts for 8% to 10% of all causes of congenital aortic stenosis.[40,41] This lesion consists of a thin, membranous diaphragm or a fibrous ridge encircling the left ventricular outflow tract immediately beneath the aortic valve; secondary muscular hypertrophy may coexist with this disease. Associated cardiac defects are often present and may obscure the signs of subaortic stenosis.[41-43]

Discrete subaortic stenosis has been studied by both M-mode and two-dimensional echocardiography. M-mode echocardiographic findings are premature closure of the aortic valve, aortic valve flutter, and a linear echocardiographic structure in the left ventricular outflow tract.[44,45] Although these findings suggest subaortic stenosis, they are nonspecific. Two-dimensional echocardiography indicates the exact location and configuration of this form of left ventricular outflow tract obstruction.[42,46] Two-dimensional echocardiography in this disease entity often shows a thin, membrane-like linear structure just beneath the aortic valve (Fig. 105.7). This membrane is usually attached anteriorly to the ventricular septum and posteriorly to the anterior leaflet of the mitral valve. The aortic valve structure may be slightly thickened or normal.

Discrete subaortic stenosis is often associated with other congenital cardiac defects such as ventricular septal defect, patent ductus arteriosus, coarctation of the aorta, idiopathic hypertrophic subaortic stenosis, endocardial cushion defect, or other mitral valve abnormalities.[41,43] Therefore, typical clinical and catheterization findings of discrete subaortic stenosis may often be masked by, or become apparent after correction of, other associated lesions. Because two-dimensional echocardiography can demonstrate the subaortic membrane precisely, this is probably the procedure of choice in patients who are suspected of having left ventricular outflow tract obstructive lesions. Doppler can be used to assess the severity or to detect and follow the course of associated or resultant aortic valve insufficiency.

POSTOPERATIVE ECHOCARDIOGRAPHIC EVALUATION

Postoperative cardiac evaluation is rather complicated because the natural anatomy of disease has been changed by extensive surgical reconstruction. Therefore, a reliable serially applicable noninvasive method, such as echocardiography, seems to be an ideal test to assess the anatomical and functional residua after surgery. Postoperative evaluation with echocardiographic methods in patients with simple lesions and the examinations after the surgical repair of tetralogy of Fallot, transposition of the great arteries (Mustard or Senning operation) or a Fontan procedure for tricuspid atresia or single ventricle are endeavors requiring the use of echocardiography and Doppler techniques.

INTRA-ATRIAL BAFFLE PROCEDURE

The intra-atrial baffle operation (atrial switch procedure) by the Senning or Mustard technique is a widely accepted procedure for d-transposition of great arteries. In order to evaluate the results of such operations, long-term hemodynamic and anatomical follow-up is necessary in these patients. Newer techniques of arterial switching are being applied in infants, but most Mustard patients are now close to adulthood. Common postoperative complications of the intracardiac baffle procedure by either Senning or Mustard operation are pulmonary venous or systemic vena caval obstruction, right ventricular dysfunction, cardiac arrhythmia, and tricuspid valve regurgitation.[47-51] By far, venous obstructions are the most common postoperative problems, and the clinical symptoms and signs of baffle obstruction may be slow and progressive. Serial cardiac catheterization is used routinely on these patients. Therefore, a noninvasive technique for evaluating venous pathways ought to be desirable not only as a means of diagnosing obstructions but also as a safe method for obtaining longitudinal data. Several reports are available describing techniques for assessment of systemic vena caval and pulmonary venous obstruction after surgical repair of the transposition of the great arteries. Chin and co-workers[52]

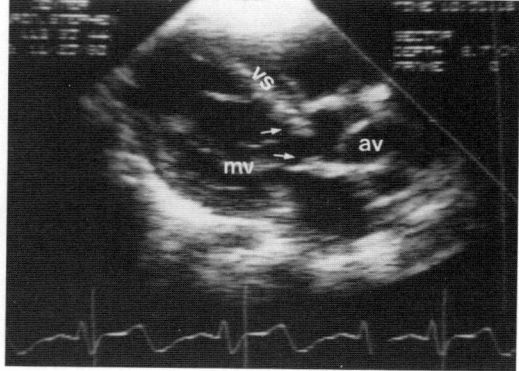

FIGURE 105.7 Long-axis view shows the septal (vs) and mitral valve (mv) components of a subaortic membrane. This fibromuscular cuff of obstructive tissue was located inferior to the aortic valve (av).

recently reported the two-dimensional echocardiographic appearance of caval and pulmonary venous pathways after the baffle procedure and established the normal values for the caval and pulmonary venous pathway dimensions (Figs. 105.8, 105.9). Also, systemic venous obstruction has been evaluated by two-dimensional contrast and pulsed Doppler echocardiography.[53] So far, none of these methods provides quantitative assessment of the degree of the obstructions; rather these methods provide qualitative information on the caval obstruction.

Because of the nature of these surgeries, a main concern is physiologic adaptation of the anatomical right ventricle and tricuspid valve to the systemic pressure, in addition to the patency of the systemic and pulmonary venous channels. Although two-dimensional echocardiography can directly visualize both ventricles, postoperative assessment is limited mainly to the left ventricle because of the more complicated anatomical configuration of the right ventricle. The complex of the inflow, body, and outflow parts of the systemic right ventricle and its position right beneath the sternum prevent accurate measurement of the dimensions by echocardiography, thus compromising functional

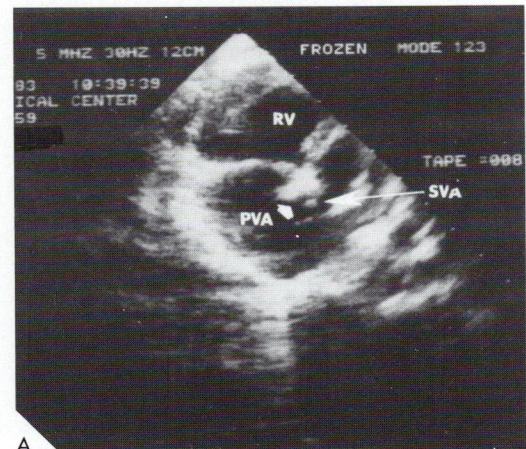
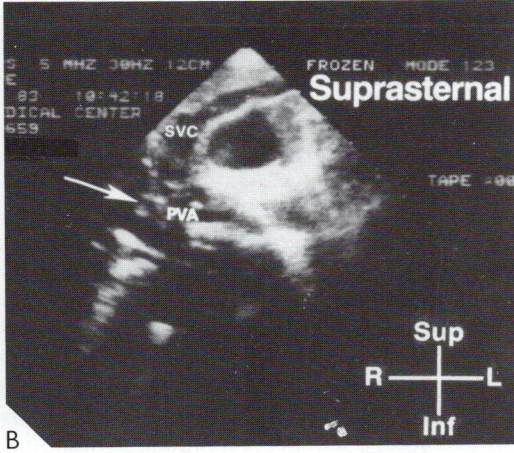

FIGURE 105.8 Apex view (**A**) shows a break in the baffle between the systemic venous atrium (*SVA*) and the pulmonary venous atrium (*PVA*), which wraps around it from the pulmonary veins into the right ventricle (*RV*) after a Mustard repair for transposition. Suprasternal imaging (**B**) shows the superior vena cava (*SVC*) descending, and a similar interruption associated with the baffle into the pulmonary venous atrium is visualized. This represents the area of the baffle leak.

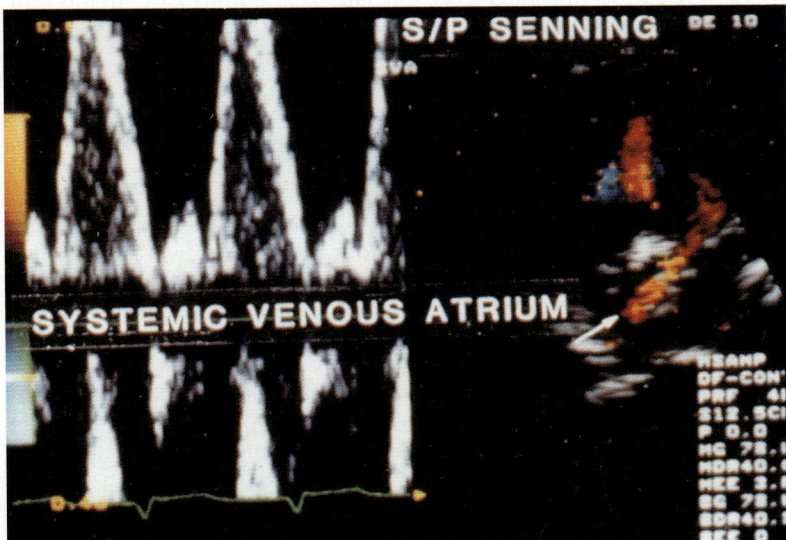
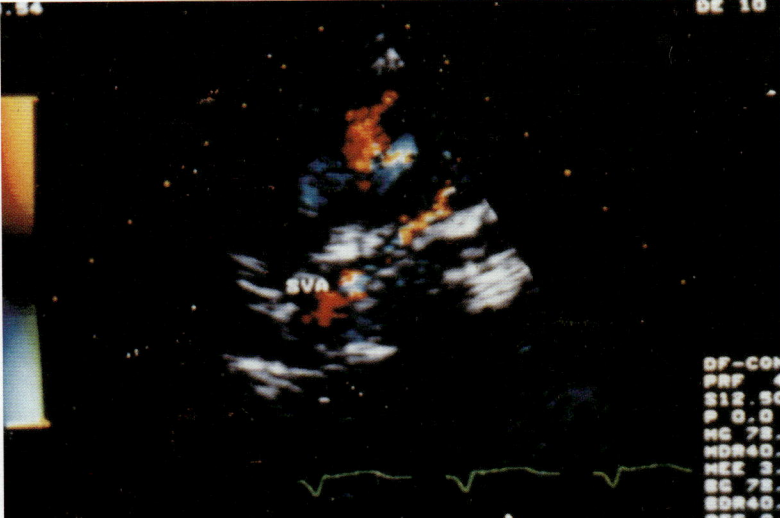
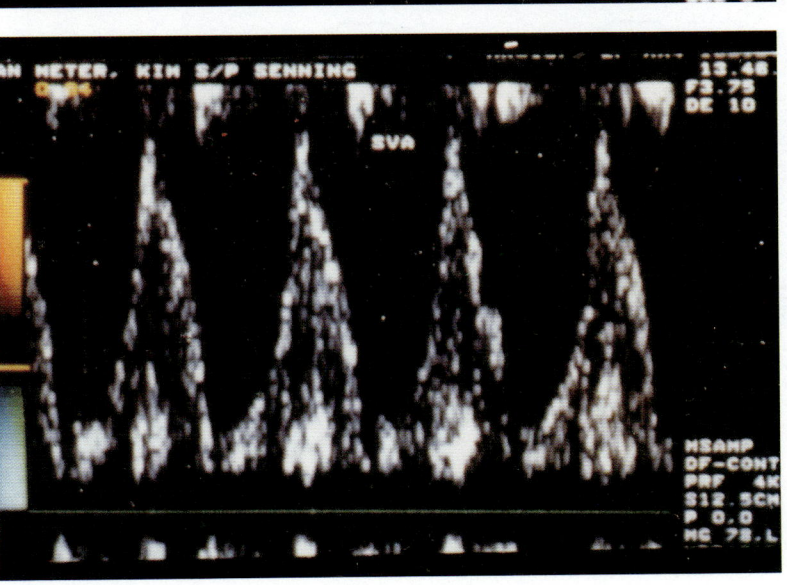

FIGURE 105.9 Color flow imaging has been helpful in determining flow in the pathways after atrial switching for transposition, defining the flow velocity distribution in both the pulmonary venous and systemic venous inflows. The example above shows narrowing of the systemic venous inflow with an increase in late diastolic velocity documenting mild systemic inflow obstruction of superior caval inflow in a patient after Senning repair.

assessment of this systemic ventricle. Left ventricular function and configuration in postoperative transposition may depend upon left ventricular pressure influenced by pulmonary arterial pressure or left ventricular outflow tract obstruction. With physiologic inversion of ventricular function in d-transposition of the great arteries, the ventricular septal function is committed to the systemic right ventricle, a change from its normal commitment to the left ventricle in normally related great arteries. Two-dimensional echocardiograms display posterior systolic bowing of the ventricular septum.[47,54] Before surgical intervention, reversal of ventricular septal bowing may be caused by left ventricular hypertension (pressure) due to a large ventricular septal defect, a patent ductus arteriosus, or left ventricular outflow tract obstruction. Reversal of posterior systolic bowing after an atrial switch operation is the indicator of a venous left ventricular hypertension due to pulmonary arterial hypertension (pulmonary venous obstruction or obstructive pulmonary vascular disease) or left ventricular outflow tract obstruction. Structural abnormalities of the ventricular outflow tract can usually be assessed by imaging this area.[55]

Tricuspid valve regurgitation and right ventricular dysfunction occur in patients with a d-transposition of great arteries after surgical repair. The systemic load and surgical insult to the right ventricle and tricuspid valve seem to be the cause and may progress as the child grows. Doppler echocardiography has the major role in determining the status of tricuspid valve regurgitation. With the aid of color Doppler echocardiography, it is feasible to assess the degree of a regurgitant volume by two-dimensional Doppler echocardiographic methods. Significant morbidity and mortality from tricuspid regurgitation and right ventricular failure have been reported. A recent report suggests that in a group of postoperative patients with d-transposition of the great arteries, the right ventricle responded to afterload stress with a smaller increase in minute work index than did the left ventricle in postoperative tetralogy of Fallot, ventricular septal defect, or control groups. The abnormal response of the transposition patient may indicate a predisposition to substantially late ventricular dysfunction.[48]

FONTAN PROCEDURE

Systemic venous atrial to pulmonary artery connections by Fontan procedure and their modifications have been used for correction of various congenital heart diseases, mainly for tricuspid atresia or a single ventricle. This continuity between the atrium and pulmonary artery has been accomplished either by direct anastomosis over the right atrial appendage and pulmonary artery or by valved or nonvalved conduits between the right atrium and pulmonary artery or the right ventricular outflow portion. Although the overall results of this operation have been encouraging and most patients have improved clinical symptoms and signs, the long-term results have not been adequately assessed.[56] There is increasing concern about the long-term outcome of the procedure, with particular regard to ventricular function after exercise and the continued patency of the systemic venous connection to the pulmonary artery. Significant abnormalities in cardiac hemodynamics at rest, which become more significant with exercise, have been shown at cardiac catheterization and radionuclide ventriculography in asymptomatic patients who had undergone a successful Fontan operation.[56,57] Recently, Hagler and co-workers[58] reported methods for functional assessment of the Fontan operation by echocardiography and Doppler. Postoperative assessment by M-mode and two-dimensional echocardiography demonstrated normal or mildly reduced left ventricular function in most patients. In the majority of patients, a typical flow pattern was observed in the pulmonary artery by pulsed Doppler echocardiography, with a predominant diastolic flow and accentuation by atrial systole somewhat similar to the venous flow pattern observed in the superior vena cava. "Abnormal" flow patterns (disorganized systolic flow, absence of atrial waves, and little or no increase with inspiration) were observed in patients with reduced ventricular function or residual shunts. Atrioventricular valve insufficiency (usually mitral insufficiency in tricuspid atresia patients) by Doppler methods were present in some. Despite these echocardiographic abnormalities, most patients had satisfactory clinical courses.

Noninvasive assessment of venous to pulmonary artery continuity is rather limited because of the various surgical modifications of this technique. Combined use of two-dimensional echocardiography and Doppler methods most likely provides the best noninvasive method for detection of obstructions and for detection of residual right-to-left shunt at the atrial level.

POSTOPERATIVE TETRALOGY OF FALLOT

A number of patients have now grown to be adults, status postoperative for repair of tetralogy of Fallot. A variety of electromechanical residua exist in these patients. It is common during two-dimensional imaging to visualize the enlarged aorta and the subaortic patch material as bright and somewhat echogenic. The assessment of residual ventricular defects is usually best accomplished in such patients by interrogating the area around the patch for Doppler velocities.

Right ventricular enlargement, continued paradoxical septal motion, and echocardiographic right ventricular hypertrophy are likewise common in such patients. The right ventricular outflow tract has

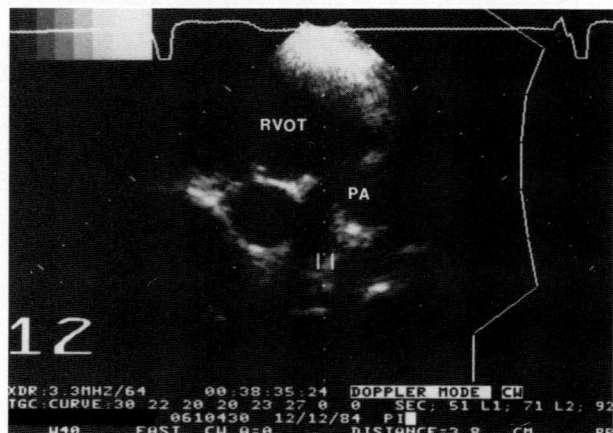
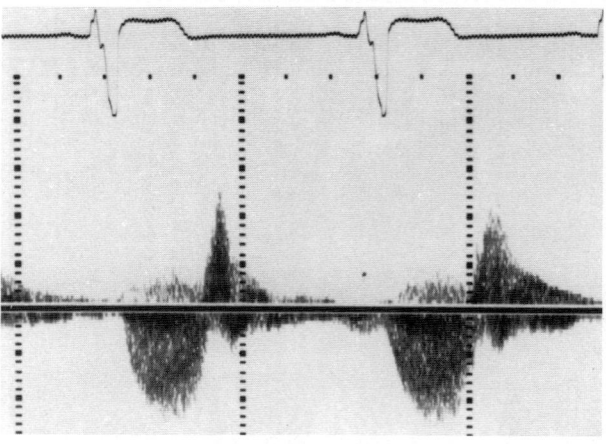

FIGURE 105.10 Short-axis view shows aneurysmal dilatation of the right ventricular outflow tract (RVOT) into a narrow pulmonary artery (PA) bifurcation. Continuous Doppler interrogation over this reconstructed right ventricular outflow tract after tetralogy repair shows high-velocity systolic and diastolic flow characteristic of mild residual pulmonary stenosis and pulmonary insufficiency.

usually been reconstructed by an outflow patch, or sometimes even a conduit, and can be interrogated for evaluation of residual pulmonic stenosis and insufficiency (Fig. 105.10). Wide open pulmonary insufficiency or aneurysmal dilatation of the right ventricular outflow tract is not uncommon in such patients even though they may be asymptomatic.

Finally, in assessing the adequacy of the tetralogy results, it is important to judge right ventricular pressure. There are two major ways to accomplish this by Doppler echocardiographic techniques in such patients. The first is using the Bernoulli gradient methods for looking at residual pulmonic stenosis (Fig. 105.11). The second involves a modification of the work by Hatle, recently reported by Yock and Popp[59] from Stanford. These authors have reported on the evaluation of velocities in tricuspid insufficiency as estimators of right ventricular pressure and have added on central venous pressure to right ventricle/right atrium gradient calculated by a Bernoulli method as an estimate of right-sided heart pressures. Obviously, a patient with tetralogy of Fallot might have elevated right-sided heart pressures because of vascular disease induced by previous shunting or because of residual right ventricular outflow tract obstruction. Nonetheless, as an overall index of the intensity of right ventricular hypertension, the tricuspid insufficiency method appears reliable in our hands, and most patients with status tetralogy of Fallot repair do have tricuspid insufficiency.

IMPORTANCE OF ESOPHAGEAL ECHO IN PERIOPERATIVE AND POSTOPERATIVE MANAGEMENT

In recent years intense interest has developed in the utility of esophageal echo. Despite its semi-invasive nature, it has an outstanding capability for defining cardiac anatomy, both intraoperatively and postoperatively. This attribute is especially important for the evaluation of adults, where imaging, especially in the postoperative period, may be inadequate for defining pulmonary venous inflow, systemic venous inflow, or extracardiac conduits. In addition, the finer points of complex anatomy in patients being considered for Fontan correction may not be well enough imaged by external echocardiography to allow comprehensive noninvasive diagnosis.[60-62] This situation may also call for esophageal echo.

For evaluation of congenital heart disease, this test plays an important part in the assessment of atrial anatomy, mitral and tricuspid valve function (Fig. 105.12), and the integrity of septal patches. Esophageal echo is particularly useful with postoperative outpatient adults needing visualization of areas difficult to see from the chest wall (Fig. 105.13). We believe that, despite its slightly invasive nature, transesophageal scanning will find an expanding role in the evaluation of adults with congenital heart disease.

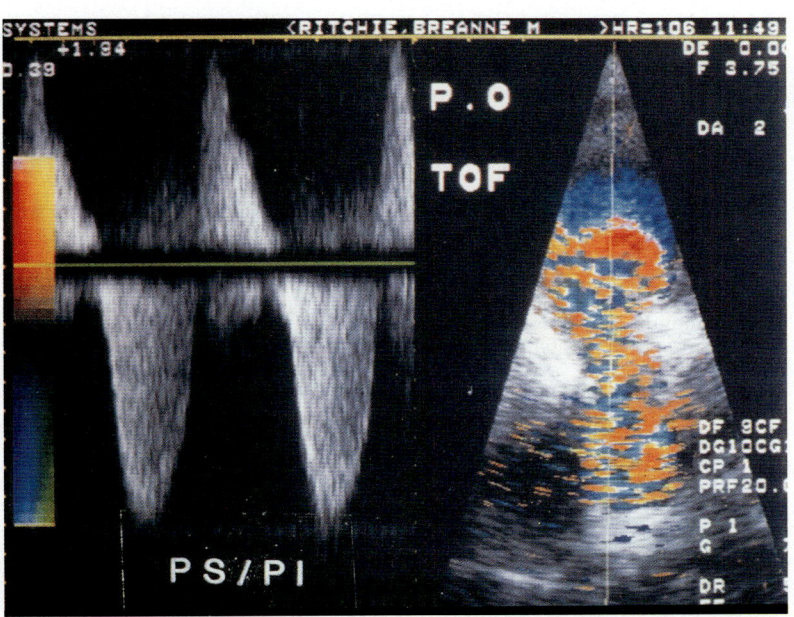

FIGURE 105.11 Color flow mapping has also been useful in defining the position and nature of flow in extracardiac conduits. This figure delineates flow acceleration and turbulence in an extracardiac conduit with moderate residual pulmonary outflow obstruction and pulmonary insufficiency; this is characteristic of an adequate result after tetralogy repair.

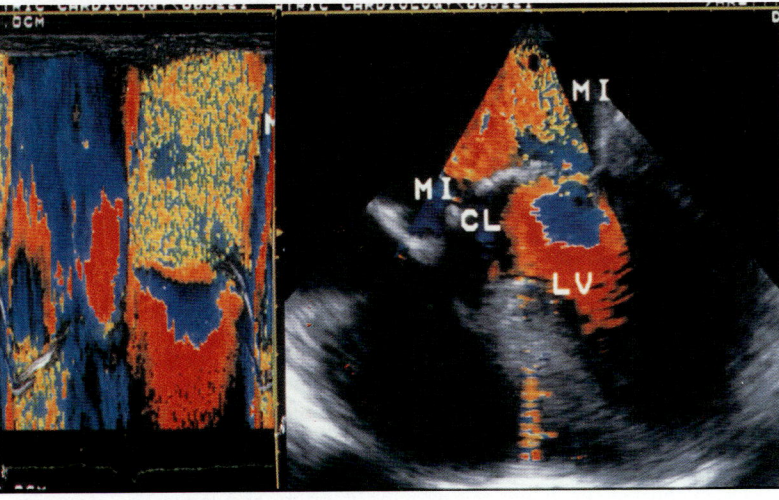

FIGURE 105.12 This transesophageal view documents mitral insufficiency in a patient after repair of atrioventricular septal defect. A pattern of holosystolic mitral insufficiency is seen against the lateral wall but does not appear to originate through the area of the cleft in the valve. Most surgeons prefer not to obliterate the cleft because it is a true commissure in a trileaflet atrioventricular valve.

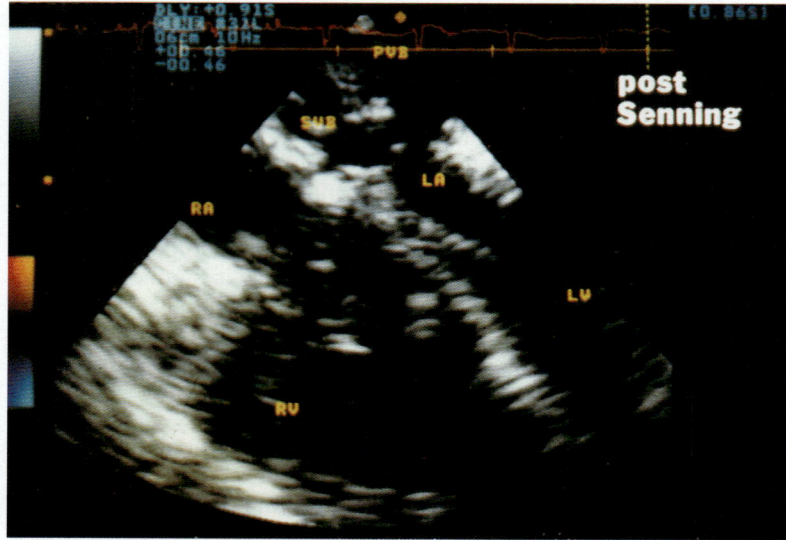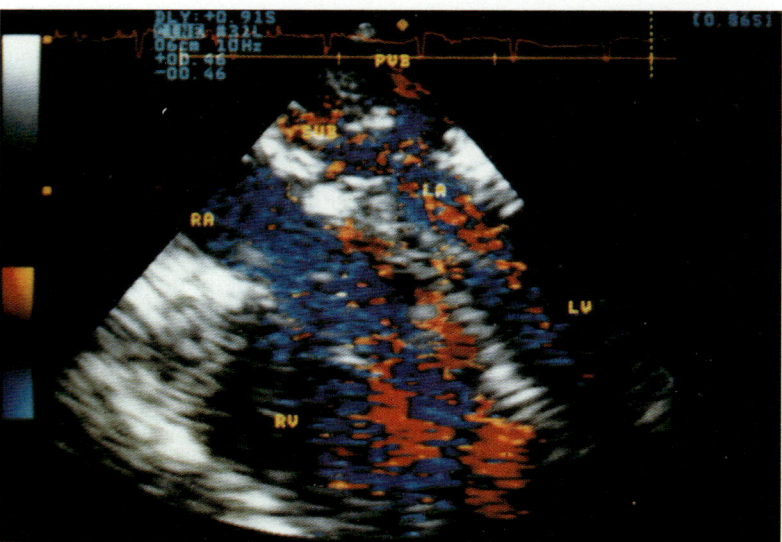

FIGURE 105.13 This transesophageal image shows narrowing of the inlet of the superior vena cava into the systemic venous atria, with aliasing and turbulence visualized on the color flow map. The pulmonary venous atrium as viewed from the esophagus appears wide open with a smooth, laminar, nonobstructed flow.

REFERENCES

1. Diamond MA, Dillon JC, Haine CL et al: Echocardiographic features of atrial septal defect. Circulation 43:129, 1971
2. Tajik AJ, Gau GT, Ritter DG et al: Echocardiographic pattern of right ventricular diastolic volume overload in children. Circulation 46:36, 1972
3. Dillon JC, Weyman AE, Feigenbaum H et al: Cross-sectional echocardiographic examination of the interatrial septum. Circulation 55:115, 1977
4. Bierman FZ, Williams RG: Subxiphoid two-dimensional imaging of the interatrial septum in infants and neonates with congenital heart disease. Circulation 60:80, 1979
5. Matsumoto M: Ultrasonic features of interatrial septum: Its motion analysis and detection of its defect. Jpn Circ J 37:1382, 1973
6. Sanders SP: Echocardiography and related techniques in the diagnosis of congenital heart defects. Echocardiography 1:185, 1984
7. Serruys PW, VanDenBrand M, Hugenholtz PF et al: Intracardiac right-to-left shunts demonstrated by two-dimensional echocardiography. Br Heart J 42:429, 1979
8. Valdes–Cruz LM, Pieroni DR, Roland JMA et al: Echocardiographic detection of intracardiac right-to-left shunts following peripheral vein injections. Circulation 54:558, 1976
9. Seward JB, Tajik AJ, Hagler DJ et al: Peripheral venous contrast echocardiography. Am J Cardiol 39:202, 1977
10. Fraber TD, Harris PJ, Hehar VS et al: Detection and exclusion of interatrial shunts by two-dimensional echocardiography and peripheral venous injection. Circulation 59:379, 1979
11. Weyman AE, Wann LS, Caldwell RL et al: Negative contrast echocardiography: A new method for detecting left-to-right shunts. Circulation 59:498, 1979
12. Minagoe S, Tei C, Kisanuki A et al: Noninvasive pulsed Doppler echocardiographic detection of the direction of shunt flow in patients with ASD: Usefulness of the right parasternal approach. Circulation 71:745, 1985
13. Goldberg SJ, Areias JC, Spitaels SEC et al: Use of time interval histographic output from echo-Doppler to detect left-to-right shunts. Circulation 58:147, 1978
14. Valdes–Cruz LM, Sahn DJ: Two-dimensional echo Doppler for noninvasive quantitation of cardiac flow: A status report. Modern Concepts Cardiovasc Dis 51:123, 1982
15. Meijboom EJ, Valdes–Cruz LM, Horowitz S et al: A two-dimensional Doppler echocardiographic method for calculation of pulmonary and systemic blood flow in a canine model with a variable-sized left-to-right extracardiac shunt. Circulation 68:437, 1983
16. Valdes–Cruz LM, Horowitz S, Mesel E et al: A pulsed Doppler echocardiographic method for calculating pulmonary and systemic blood flow in atrial level shunts: Validation studies in animals and initial human experience. Circulation 69:80, 1984
17. Kitabatake A, Inoue M, Asa M et al: Noninvasive evaluation of the ratio of pulmonary to systemic flow in atrial septal defect by duplex Doppler echocardiography. Circulation 69:73, 1984
18. Bierman FZ, Fellows K, Williams RG: Prospective identification of ventricular septal defects in infancy using subxiphoid two-dimensional echocardiography. Circulation 62:807, 1980
19. Snider AR, Silverman NH, Schiller NB et al: Echocardiographic evaluation of ventricular septal aneurysms. Circulation 59:920, 1979
20. Cheatham JP, Latson LA, Gutgesell HP: Ventricular septal defect in infancy: Detection with two-dimensional echocardiography. Am J Cardiol 47:85, 1981
21. Sanders SP: Echocardiography and related techniques in the diagnosis of congenital heart defects. Echocardiography 1:333, 1984
22. Stevenson JG, Kawaboi I, Dooley T et al: Diagnosis of ventricular septal defect by pulsed Doppler echocardiography. Circulation 58:322, 1978
23. Magherim A, Azzolina G, Wiechmann V: Pulsed Doppler echocardiography for diagnosis of ventricular septal defects. Br Heart J 43:143, 1980
24. Miyatake K, Okamoto M, Kinoshita N et al: Clinical applications of a new type of real-time two-dimensional Doppler flow imaging system. Am J Cardiol 54:857, 1984
25. Sahn DJ: Real-time two-dimensional Doppler echocardiography flow mapping. Circulation 71:849, 1985
26. Hishimura RA, Miller FA, Callahan MJ et al: Doppler echocardiography: Theory, instrumentation, technique, and application. Mayo Clin Proc 60:321, 1985
27. Lewis AB, Takahashi M: Echocardiographic assessment of left-to-right shunt volume in children with ventricular septal defect. Circulation 54:78, 1976
28. Lester LA, Vitullo D, Sodt P et al: An evaluation of the left atrial/aortic root ratio in children with ventricular septal defect. Circulation 60:364, 1979
29. Gewifz MH, Werner JC, Kleinman CS et al: Role of echocardiography in aortic stenosis: Pre- and post-operative studies. Am J Cardiol 43:69, 1979
30. Blackwood RA, Bloom KR, Williams CM: Aortic stenosis in children: Experience with echocardiographic predictions of severity. Circulation 57:263, 1978
31. Schwartz A, Vignola PA, Walker HJ et al: Echocardiographic evaluation of fixed left ventricular outlet obstruction in children. Circulation 56:299, 1977
32. Bass JL, Einzig S, Hong CY et al: Echocardiographic screening to assess the severity of congenital aortic valve stenosis in children. Am J Cardiol 44:82, 1979
33. Weyman AE, Feigenbaum H, Nurwitz RA et al: Cross-sectional echocardiographic assessment of the severity of aortic stenosis in children. Circulation 55:773, 1977
34. DeMaria AN, Joye JA, Bommer W et al: Value and limitations of cross-sectional echocardiography of the aortic valve in the diagnosis and quantification of valvular aortic stenosis. Circulation 62:304, 1980
35. Hatle L, Angelson BA, Tromsdal A: A noninvasive assessment of aortic stenosis by Doppler ultrasound. Br Heart J 43:284, 1980
36. Stamm RB, Martin P: Quantification of pressure gradients across stenotic valves by Doppler ultrasound. J Am Coll Cardiol 2:707, 1983
37. Oliveira–Lima C, Sahn DJ, Valdes–Cruz LM et al: Prediction of the severity of left ventricular outflow tract obstruction by quantitative two-dimensional echocardiographic Doppler studies. Circulation 68:348, 1983
38. Berger M, Berdoff RL, Gallerstein PE et al: Evaluation of aortic stenosis by continuous wave Doppler ultrasound. J Am Coll Cardiol 3:150, 1984
39. Hatle L, Angelsen B: Doppler Ultrasound in Cardiology: Physical Principles and Clinical Applications, 2nd ed, p 124. Philadelphia, Lea & Febiger, 1985
40. Katz NM, Buckley MJ, Liberthson RR: Discrete membranous subaortic stenosis: Report of 31 patients, review of the literature, and delineation of management. Circulation 56:1034, 1977
41. Newfeld EA, Muster AJ, Paul MH et al: Discrete subvalvular aortic stenosis in childhood: Study of 51 patients. Am J Cardiol 38:53, 1976
42. Chung KJ, Fulton DR, Kreidberg et al: Combined discrete subaortic stenosis

with ventricular septal defects in infants and children. Am J Cardiol 53:1429, 1984
43. Chung KJ, Manning JA, Gramiak R: Echocardiography in coexisting hypertrophic subaortic stenosis and fixed left ventricular outflow tract obstruction. Circulation 49:673, 1974
44. Popp RL, Silverman JF, French JW et al: Echocardiographic findings in discrete subvalvular aortic stenosis. Circulation 49:226, 1974
45. Krueger SK, French JW, Farber AD et al: Echocardiography in discrete subaortic stenosis. Circulation 59:506, 1979
46. Weyman AE, Feigenbaum H, Hurwitz RA et al: Cross-sectional echocardiography in evaluating patients with discrete subaortic stenosis. Am J Cardiol 37:358, 1976
47. Bierman FZ: Two-dimensional echocardiography in the older child. J Am Coll Cardiol 5:375, 1985
48. Borow K, Keane JF, Castaneda AR et al: Systemic ventricular function in patients with tetralogy of Fallot, ventricular septal defect and transposition of the great arteries repaired during infancy. Circulation 64:878, 1981
49. Parrish MD, Graham TP, Bender HW et al: Radionuclide angiographic evaluation of right and left ventricular function during exercise after repair of transposition of the great arteries: Comparison with normal subjects and patients with congenitally corrected transposition. Circulation 67:178, 1983
50. Marx GR, Hongen TJ, Norwood WI et al: Transposition of the great arteries with intact ventricular system: Results of Mustard and Senning operations in 123 consecutive patients. J Am Coll Cardiol 1:476, 1983
51. Chung KJ, Hesselink JR, Chernoff HL et al: Digital subtraction angiography in patients with transposition of the great arteries after surgical repair. J Am Coll Cardiol 5:113, 1985
52. Chin AJ, Sanders SP, Williams RG et al: Two-dimensional echocardiographic assessment of canal and pulmonary venous pathways after the Senning operation. Am J Cardiol 52:118, 1983
53. Silverman NH, Snider AR, Colo S et al: Superior vena caval obstruction after Mustard's operation: Detection by two-dimensional contrast echocardiography. Circulation 64:392, 1981
54. VanDoesburg NH, Bierman FZ, Williams RG: Left ventricular geometry in infants with d-transposition of the great arteries and intact interventricular system. Circulation 68:733, 1983
55. Marino B, Simone GD, Pasquini et al: Complete transposition of the great arteries: Visualization of left and right outflow tract obstruction by oblique subcostal two-dimensional echocardiography. Am J Cardiol 55:1140, 1985
56. Sanders SP, Wright GB, Keane JF et al: Clinical and hemodynamic results of the Fontan operation for tricuspid atresia. Am J Cardiol 49:1733, 1982
57. Torso SD, Kelly MJ, Kalff V et al: Radionuclide assessment of ventricular contraction at rest and during exercise following the Fontan procedure for either tricuspid atresia or single ventricle. Am J Cardiol 55:1127, 1985
58. Hagler DJ, Seward JB, Tajik AM et al: Functional assessment of the Fontan operation: Combined M-mode, two-dimensional and Doppler echocardiographic studies. J Am Coll Cardiol 4:756, 1984
59. Yock P, Popp R: Noninvasive estimation of right ventricular systolic pressure. Circulation 70:657, 1984
60. Takamoto S, Kyo S, Adachi H et al: Intraoperative color flow mapping by real time two-dimensional echocardiography for evaluation of valvular and congenital heart disease repairs. J Cardiovasc Surg 90:802, 1985
61. Seward JB, Khandheria BK, Oh JK et al: Transesophageal echocardiography: Technique, anatomic correlations, implementation and clinical applications. Mayo Clin Proc 63:649, 1988
62. Ritter SB, Hillel Z, Narang J, Lewis D, Thys D: Transesophageal real time Doppler flow imaging in congenital heart disease: Experience with new pediatric transducer probe. Dynamic Cardiovasc Imaging 2:92, 1989

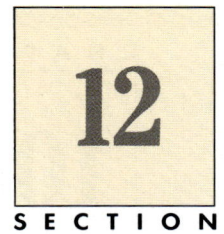

SECTION 12

Section Editor
Melvin D. Cheitlin, MD

Other Disorders of the Cardiovascular System

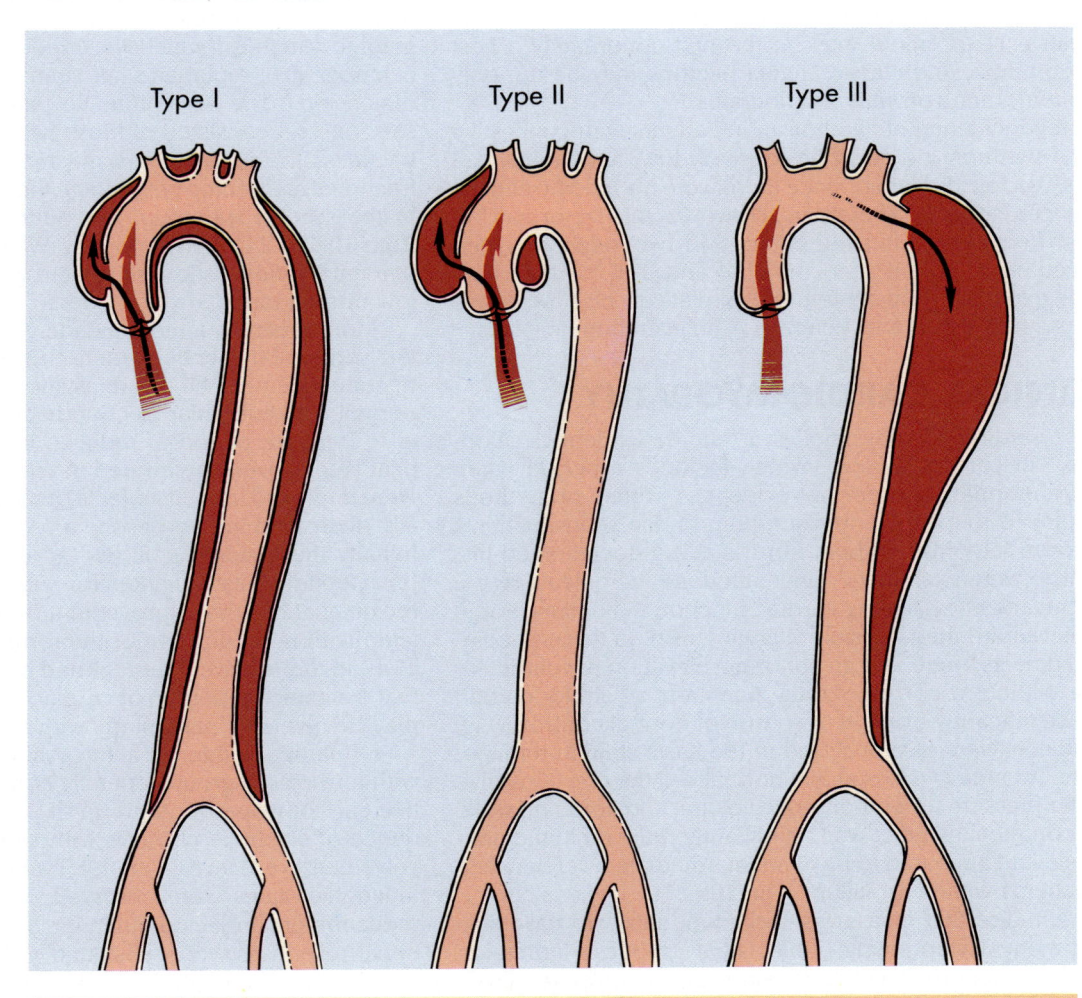

Alcohol and the Heart

Timothy J. Regan

Disease of heart muscle related to alcoholism has gained renewed recognition in the past several decades. Reports from several urban centers in England and the United States have described patients with low-output heart failure who did not appear to have nutritional, cardiovascular, or coronary risk factors as a background. These patients were characterized by a long-term history of ethanol abuse.[1,2]

As with other causes of primary myocardial disease, a diffuse abnormality of the myocardium is present, unrelated to coronary atherosclerosis, arterial hypertension, or valvular or congenital heart disease. Although symptoms of congestive heart failure may be the most common presentation in myocardial disease of multiple etiologies, congestive heart failure may occur in less than half of the patients when seen initially.[3] In a study of 55 patients with congestive failure, 11 had coexisting cardiac arrhythmias. In a significant proportion, arrhythmias without congestive heart failure may be the first abnormality. Chest pain is not uncommon, and classic angina pectoris may be the only symptom despite normal coronary arteriograms.

For a time the incidence of alcoholism in patients with congestive cardiomyopathy was considered to be relatively low, and virtually all cases were classified as idiopathic, since there were no specific clinical markers or myocardial tissue alterations. However, this factor has become the most frequent identifiable etiology in two series reported from referral centers in recent years, at 21%[4] and 32%.[5] A high incidence would be expected from centers with a relatively high incidence of alcoholism, such as urban and Veterans Administration hospitals.

SUBCLINICAL CARDIOMYOPATHY

The concept of cardiomyopathy implies a time-dependent development of disease in cardiac muscle, which includes a period when symptoms and abnormal signs are not evident. A variety of methods have been employed to examine this question. In one series, patients with biopsy-proven fatty liver without fibrosis and a documented history of alcoholism were examined.[6] Since afterload increments represent a feasible means of evaluating cardiac function in humans, aortic pressure was elevated during infusion of angiotensin. In these noncardiac alcoholic subjects, there was an abnormal elevation of ventricular filling pressure without a corresponding increment of stroke output, which differed significantly from the response of normal controls (Fig. 106.1). The subjects were also analyzed in the basal state in terms of contractile state. An index was used that normalized the first derivative of left ventricular pressure for end-diastolic volume and aortic diastolic pressure. This contractility index was significantly reduced in the noncardiac alcoholic and appeared to be at an intermediate level between normals and patients with heart failure (Fig. 106.2).

Noninvasive studies that measure systolic time intervals have also confirmed that many asymptomatic subjects have modest depression of left ventricular function. These techniques in particular require a stable state for valid quantification. Thus, measurements need to be made after dissipation of the neurohumoral alterations associated with the postethanol state, which may mask a depressed functional state of the myocardium. These may not be evident clinically and may require a week or more for restoration of the basal state. Since clinical evidence of cardiac decompensation is relatively rare in the premenopausal female, a study of male and female cirrhotics averaging 39 years of age was performed.[7] These subjects were age-matched and had equivalent degrees of cirrhosis by biopsy. Significant abnormalities of the time intervals were present in the males (Fig. 106.3), while female alcoholics exhibited no significant abnormality.

In addition, high-fidelity electrocardiograms showed abnormalities that were not readily observed on conventional electrocardiograms. The PRc, QRS, and QTc were prolonged in the alcoholic group as a whole, and the septal Q wave was frequently absent. There was also increased notching and slurring on the QRS complex consistent with a primary myocardial disease process. These conduction changes appeared unlikely to be due to increased ventricular mass, since heart size was within normal limits.

In an M-mode echocardiographic study of 22 asymptomatic chronic alcoholics, cardiac dimensions were adjusted for age and body surface area. Sixty-eight percent of these asymptomatic subjects demonstrated significant increases in at least one of the echocardiographic variables, which included left ventricular mass and diastolic chamber size, septal and left ventricular wall thickness, and left atrial dimension.[8] The asymptomatic patients were subclassified into two sets; one set consisted of those with an increased left ventricular wall thickness to radius ratio, a mean increase 16% above normal, and a fractional shortening percentage that was in the upper range of normal. In the second subgroup, left ventricular diastolic dimension ranged from 10% to 24% above normal. Wall thickness to radius ratio and the percent fractional shortening were within normal limits, although in the low normal range.

More recently, a radionuclide gated heart scan was used to assess left ventricular ejection fraction in subjects admitted to an alcohol treatment center.[9] Of the 18 asymptomatic subjects, 13 showed a subnormal left ventricular ejection fraction in the basal state. Following a 4- to 9-month period of reduced intake of alcohol or abstinence, repeat studies were performed in ten of the subjects. Ejection fractions were improved in four subjects, remained unchanged in four, and actually decreased in two despite a reduction in reported alcohol intake. Initially these subjects all had an elevated serum level of γ-glutamyl transpeptidase as a marker for substantial recent ethanol intake. On reexamination, the improvement in ejection fraction generally correlated with normalization of the serum concentrations of this enzyme. Thus, in this relatively short period of abstinence these findings suggest that a significant degree of cardiac dysfunction in the subclinical state may be reversed, particularly with longer term abstinence.

Of particular interest is the evaluation of cardiac status in patients with cirrhosis, a group generally considered to be resistant to congestive cardiomyopathy. A group of 37 subjects who had histologic evidence of alcoholic cirrhosis without symptoms or signs of cardiac involvement were investigated.[10] Two distinct patterns of left ventricular functional status were observed. More than half the subjects had a reduction of cardiac output in the basal state, and left ventricular functional responses were substantially depressed during volume loading or increase of afterload. There was no significant stroke work increment in response to these interventions, in contrast to the increase seen in control subjects.

The other subgroup was characterized by an elevation of cardiac output in the basal state in association with a diminished peripheral arterial resistance. This high-output state has been found to be independent of significant anemia, arterial hypoxia, or thiamine deficiency. A neurohumoral mechanism may be operative, since in the presence of portal systemic shunts of blood flow, high blood glucagon levels have been reported in the peripheral circulation, which may alter the hemodynamics in a manner similar to that of the high-output group. Despite these considerations, the responses to afterload increments suggested that the cardiac output elevation was secondary to the diminished peripheral resistance and not related to a primary hypercontractile state. In these patients, stroke work failed to increase during afterload increments.

A lowered systemic vascular resistance in cirrhotic subjects has been considered to be a potential basis for the relative rarity of congestive cardiomyopathy in this group of subjects. However, since the majority of alcoholics with cirrhosis have a normal peripheral vascular resistance, this rationale appears to be unlikely. Nutritional factors have a potential bearing on this question. As liver disease progresses, important nutritional deficiencies may occur that may influence the appearance of some of the components of cardiomyopathy, including synthesis and degradation of collagen in the interstitium and the development of cardiac hypertrophy. Moreover, genetic factors that may control development of disease in a given organ undoubtedly vary from one patient to another.

Since subclinical dysfunction is present in many patients with cirrhosis, the possibility that unusual circulatory stresses may result in

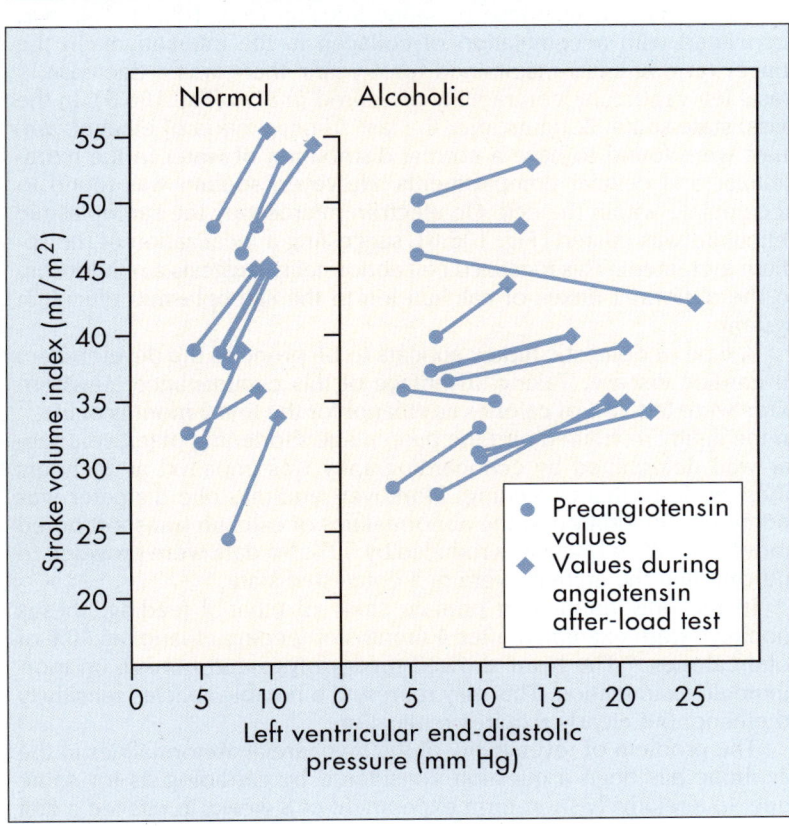

FIGURE 106.1 Left ventricular response to angiotensin in normals and alcoholics without clinical evidence of cardiac disease. The latter exhibited a nearly threefold rise of ventricular end-diastolic pressure but only a minimal stroke output increment. Mean values are depicted in heavy lines. (Modified from Regan TJ, Levinson GE, Oldewurtel HA et al: Ventricular function in noncardiacs with alcoholic fatty liver. Role of ethanol in the production of cardiomyopathy. J Clin Invest 48:397, 1969)

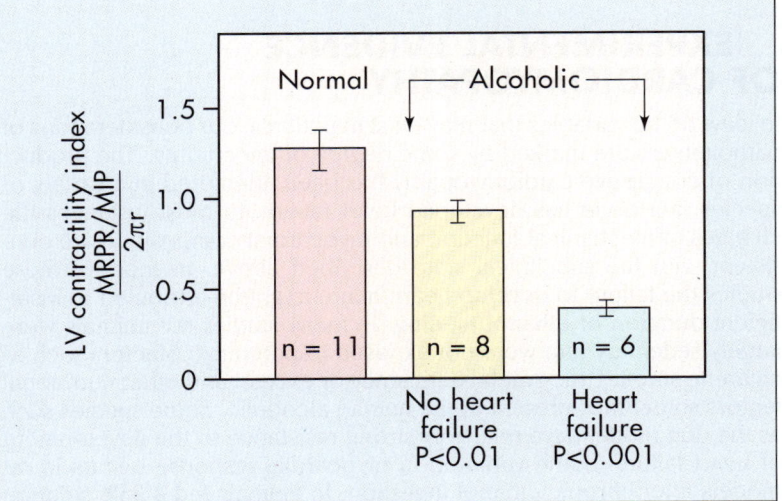

FIGURE 106.2 The contractility index at rest in the noncardiac alcoholic was significantly reduced below that of the normal but is higher than in alcoholic subjects who developed clinical evidence of heart disease. (MRPR, maximum rate of pressure rise; MIP, maximum isovolumic pressure; r, radius.) (Modified from Regan TJ, Levinson GE, Oldewurtel HA et al: Ventricular function in noncardiacs with alcoholic fatty liver. Role of ethanol in the production of cardiomyopathy. J Clin Invest 48:397, 1969)

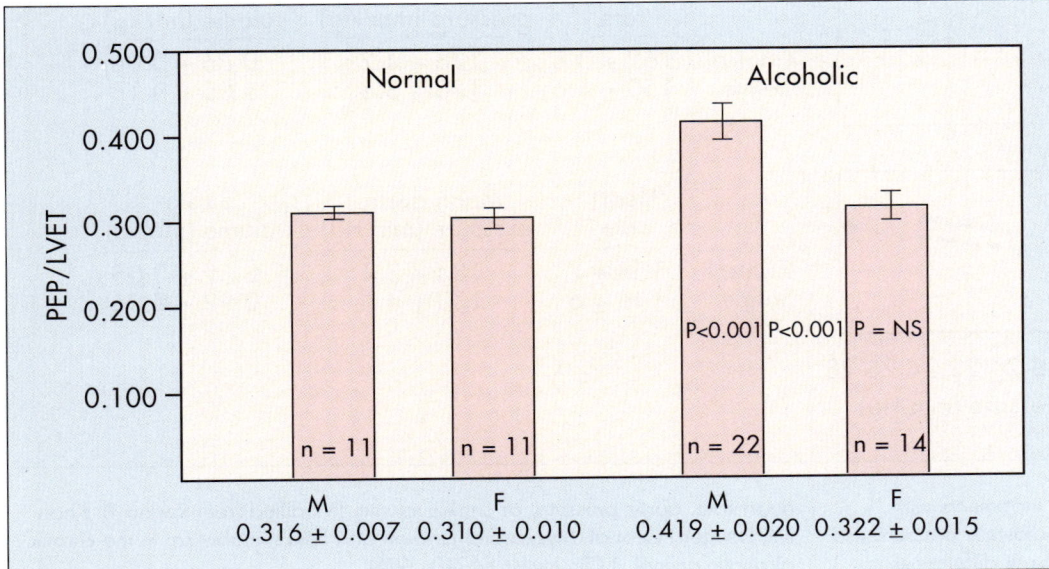

FIGURE 106.3 Sex and preclinical cardiac malfunction: systolic time intervals in males and females with biopsy-proven cirrhosis. Only males had abnormal intervals, approximating those reported for noncirrhotic alcoholics without clinical evidence of heart disease. (PEP, pre-ejection period; LVET, left ventricular ejection time)

cardiac decompensation must be kept in mind. Thus, during surgical interventions in which large vascular shunts are actually introduced in patients with cirrhosis, pulmonary congestion may be an important complication. The likelihood of excessive leakage of albumin from capillary beds in cirrhosis suggests a factor that may promote pulmonary congestion during acute volume expansion, particularly if renal excretory responses are subnormal.[11]

A pathologic counterpart to these observations has been reported in a series of 43 noncardiac cirrhotics, free of other etiologies for heart disease.[12] Widespread focal myocardial fibrosis of the heart that did not correlate closely with heart weight was noted in 22 of 43 alcoholic patients at autopsy.

EXPERIMENTAL EVIDENCE OF CARDIOMYOPATHY

In view of the variables that may exist in patients, our considerations of pathogenesis are marked by some degree of uncertainty. The production of congestive cardiomyopathy has been attempted in a variety of species, but none has developed heart failure. In most instances the changes in mechanical function and myocardial composition are consistent with the subclinical state described above. In most of these studies the failure to develop heart failure might be attributed to insufficient duration of ethanol feeding. In many studies the animals were largely sedentary and were not exposed to potential cofactors such as cigarette smoke, trace metal deficiency or excess, and other nutritional factors sometimes present in the human alcoholic. Some species such as the dog model have relatively strong resistance to the development of heart failure. Some variation in myocardial response occurs in rat models after chronic ethanol ingestion. In animals fed a 25% solution of ethanol over a 7-month period, a decrease in ventricular contractile force was reported as early as 4 months after the onset of feeding, a change unaffected by vitamin supplementation.[13] More recently, animals fed an isocaloric liquid diet in which ethanol accounted for 39% of calories showed no abnormality in basal function of the isolated heart after 10 months. However, the response of left ventricular systolic pressure and its first derivative during a challenge with sympathomimetic agents showed a definite decline compared with controls.[14] The most notable metabolic aberration was impaired binding and uptake of calcium by the isolated sarcoplasmic reticulum, which may have explained the subnormal contractile response to the catecholamine.

In two studies using the canine model, mechanical abnormalities have been demonstrated using two different techniques. In the mongrel dog fed a 25% solution for 29 months, in vivo functional abnormalities were not observed.[15] However, the force-velocity relationship (V_{max}) was significantly impaired in the glycerinated heart muscle preparation. The authors confirmed the calcium-transport abnormalities noted in the previous study. Although high-energy phosphate content of tissue homogenates was normal, a decrease of isocitric dehydrogenase activity was observed with significant depression of myocardial respiratory rate in response to several substrates. In the second series of mongrel dogs, ethanol was fed as 36% of total calories for a period of up to 4 years.[16] After 12 months there was a decrease in left ventricular compliance in response to saline infusion (Fig. 106.4). This was associated with accumulation of collagen in the interstitium. In the longer term animals maintained for 4 years, there was a decrease in basal left ventricular contractility measured in vivo (Fig. 106.5). In the basal state some 32 hours after the last administration of ethanol, animals were found to have a normal distribution of water in the extracellular and cellular compartments. However, sodium was found to accumulate within the cell. On electron microscopy the sarcoplasmic reticulum was dilated (Fig. 106.6), suggesting a localization of the sodium increment. This localized cell abnormality suggests a relationship to the abnormal fluxes of calcium ion in the sarcoplasmic reticulum system.

A type of domestic turkey appears to be prone to the development of cardiac disease. Taking advantage of this circumstance, newborn birds were fed 25% of calories as ethanol for the first 2 months of life.[17] In the lightly restrained bird the percentage shortening of left ventricular wall determined by echocardiography was impaired at 24 hours after the last ethanol feeding. Moreover, end-diastolic diameter was increased. In addition to the abnormalities of calcium transport noted above, Na^+-K^+-ATPase was reduced by 50%. No data were provided to indicate that the animals were in a congested state.

In the only nonhuman primate study of ethanol feeding, rhesus monkeys were examined after 4 months of feeding ethanol as 40% of total calories.[18] The heart showed myocytolysis and fibrosis on morphologic examination. This may represent a notable species sensitivity to ethanol but clearly requires replication.

The problem of reversibility of the myocardial abnormalities in the alcoholic has been a question considered by cardiologists for some time. In a relatively short-term experiment of 8 weeks in rats fed a diet comprising 25% ethanol daily,[19] abnormalities of mitochondrial respiration were exhibited, similar to those described in the canine model.[15]

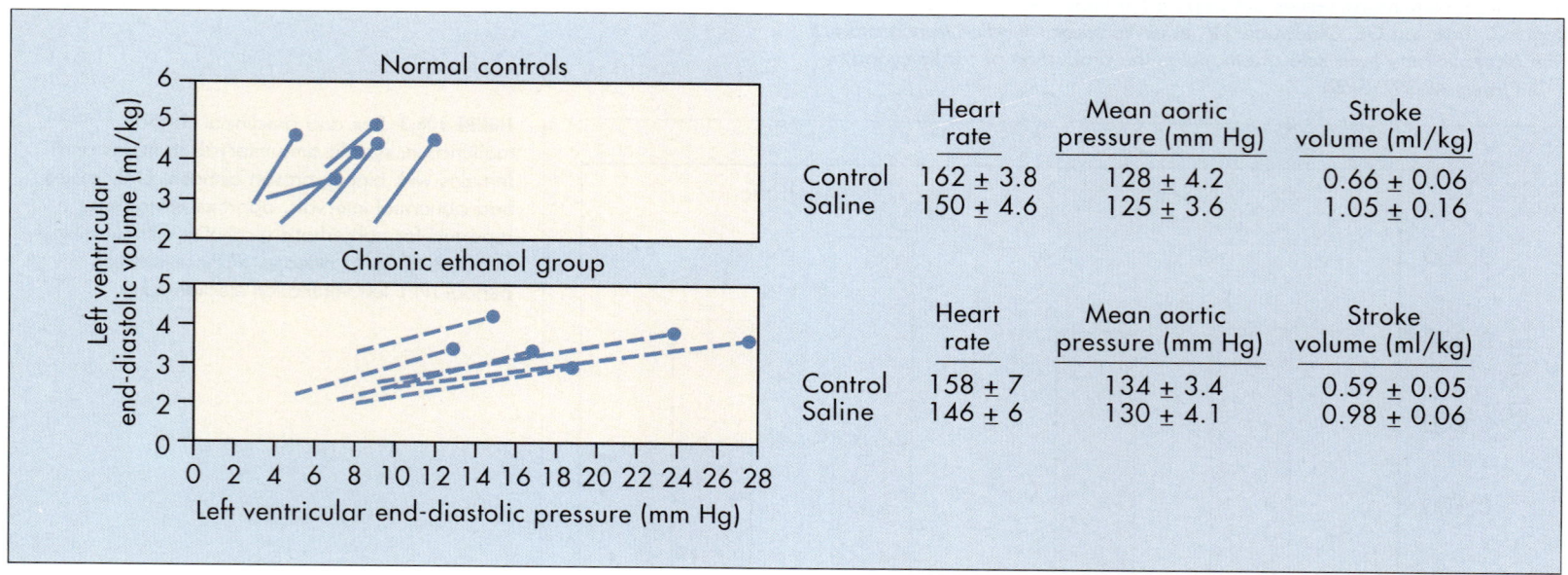

FIGURE 106.4 The response of the left ventricle to volume increments with normal saline was marked by a significantly higher end-diastolic pressure rise in animals on the chronic ethanol regimen, without significant differences in heart rate, aortic pressure, or stroke volume. (Modified from Regan TJ, Khan MI, Ettinger PO et al: Myocardial function and lipid metabolism in the chronic alcoholic animal. J Clin Invest 54:740, 1974)

After a period of 8 weeks of abstinence, respiration in the mitochondria was returned to near normal levels, and abnormalities of maximal developed tension as well as rate of tension development were largely reversed. A similar restoration to normal has been observed after a 10-month period in which ethanol accounted for 39% of calories.[14] Biochemical and mechanical abnormalities were found to be normalized 6 months after removal of alcohol from the diet.

HEART FAILURE

When the subclinical abnormalities of the heart in the alcoholic progress to a symptomatic state, the type of presentation may vary as with other primary myocardial diseases. Symptoms are most commonly related to heart failure in the initial abnormality, although this occurs in a minority of patients.[3] Complaints of weakness and easy fatigability may be part of the early symptomatology, although these complaints may be related at least in part to skeletal muscle changes due to alcoholism. A history of exertional or nocturnal dyspnea reflects the progression to pulmonary congestion. Since the addicted person may frequently delay seeking medical assistance for weeks to months, evidence of right-sided heart failure is not uncommon, with distended jugular veins, enlarged, tender liver, as well as edema of the dependent portions of the body.

Varied degrees of cardiomegaly may be present. In some, the cardiac enlargement may be relatively minor, while more substantial cardiomegaly occurs in patients who have mitral regurgitation secondary to papillary muscle insufficiency as part of the cardiomyopathic process. An early diastolic gallop is usually heard but is not invariable at this stage of the disease. An atrial gallop may be heard as an isolated finding or associated with an S_3 sound. The murmur of mitral regurgitation is usually well differentiated from that related to rheumatic valvular disease. The murmur is characteristically confined to a portion of systole, is only rarely pansystolic, and as a rule changes as cardiac compensation is restored.

The progression from a subclinical stage into cardiac decompensation is illustrated in Figure 106.7. This patient received the amount of Scotch to which he was accustomed on a daily basis and was ambulatory and in a well-nourished state during this period. Although he never developed evidence of pulmonary congestion, after 8 weeks he showed some of the peripheral manifestations of early cardiac decompensation, with increase in circulation time and venous pressure as manifestations of an enhanced central volume. A modest degree of sinus tachycardia was associated with reversal of the normal diurnal pattern of urine excretion. After 16 weeks a diastolic gallop was first heard at the apex. This persisted for several weeks until ethanol consumption was interrupted. The abnormalities exhibited in Figure 106.7 spontaneously reverted to normal over the subsequent few weeks without the need for cardiac medication.

The electrocardiogram at this time may be relatively normal or show nonspecific changes. A majority of patients have a diminished or absent septal Q wave at this stage.[7] Poor progression of the R wave across the precordium is fairly common, particularly as the disease advances, presumably as a result of progression of ventricular pathology and conduction delay. Evidence of left ventricular and atrial enlargement is common, but left anterior hemiblock occurs in a minority

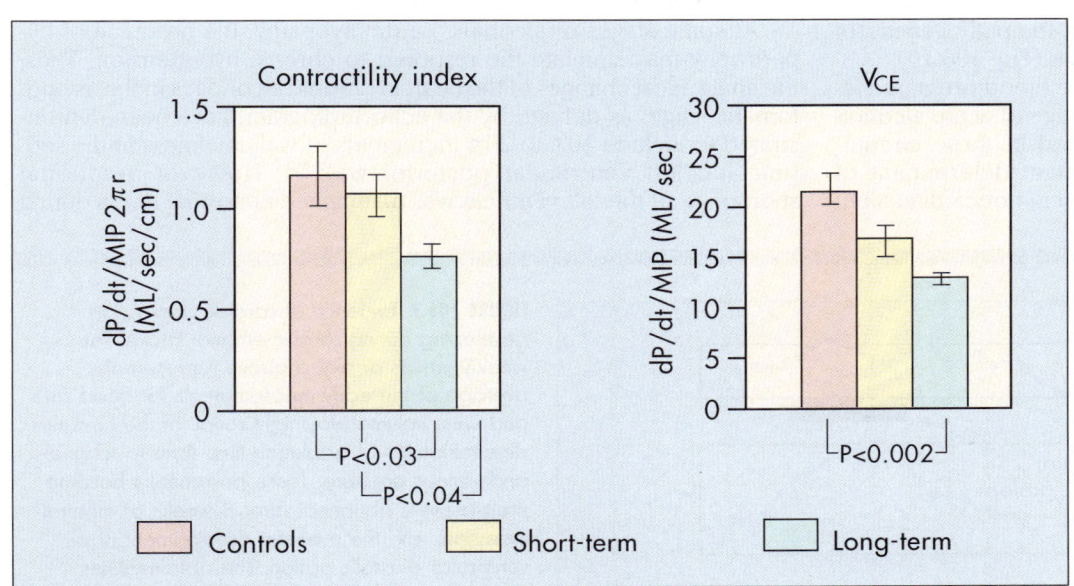

FIGURE 106.5 The index of myocardial contractility (**left panel**) was significantly lower than the control value only in the long-term alcoholic group. Similarly, the velocity of the contractile element (V_{CE}) (**right panel**) was also reduced in the long-term group. (MIP, maximal isovolumic pressure; ML/sec, muscle lengths/sec; P, probability) (Modified from Regan TJ, Thomas G, Harder B et al: Progression of myocardial abnormalities in experimental alcoholism. Am J Cardiol 46:233, 1980)

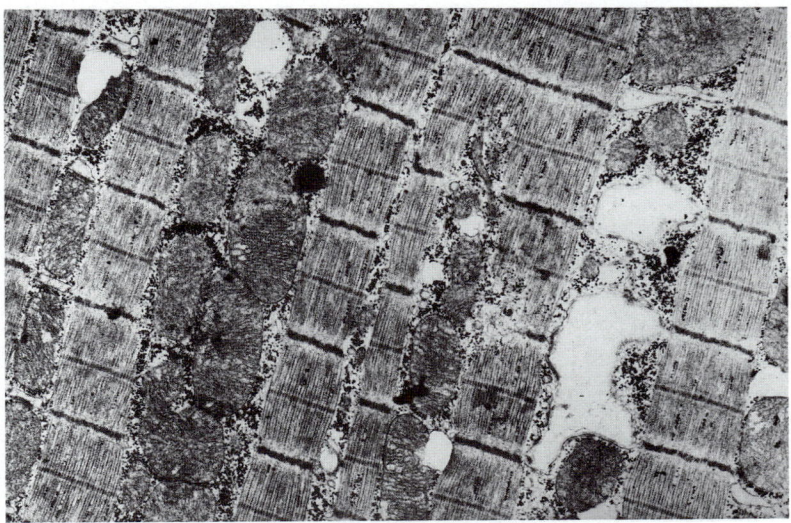

FIGURE 106.6 This electron micrograph from the left ventricular myocardium of a long-term alcoholic animal illustrates the dilated sarcoplasmic reticulum system. There is an occasional lipid body, but the mitochondria appear to be within the limits of normal. Glycogen particles are diffusely distributed. (Regan TJ, Thomas G, Harder B et al: Progression of myocardial abnormalities in experimental alcoholism. Am J Cardiol 46:233, 1980)

of the patients, while left or right bundle branch block appears in approximately 10%.

Hemodynamics in the patient who presents with chest pain or palpitations as the initial symptomatology may be expected to differ from those of the patient with exertional dyspnea.[20] The former have been reported to have an increase of left ventricular end-diastolic pressure at rest despite a slight but significant reduction of end-diastolic volume when studied in a stable state (Fig. 106.8). The ejection fraction may be normal, but measurements of contractility index and relaxation have revealed substantial reductions in this group of patients with normal heart size (Fig. 106.9). In a subset of patients without symptoms related to heart failure, there was an increase of left ventricular end-diastolic volume despite a similar level of end-diastolic pressure, while the contractility indices were not notably different. In patients who presented with exertional dyspnea and varying degrees of cardiomegaly, there were the expected higher levels of end-diastolic pressure and volume and a further modest reduction of ejection fraction and the contractility indices. Those heart failure subjects who presented with mitral regurgitation were compared with nonalcoholics who had similar degrees of mitral regurgitation. In the latter, cardiac function was virtually normal, whereas there was severe depression of left ventricular function in the alcoholic, presumably due to the effect of ethanol on left ventricular performance.

ROLE OF ARTERIAL HYPERTENSION

Fowler originally observed that in nearly one quarter of patients with primary myocardial disease, casual readings of arterial blood pressure were elevated at some time during the period of observation.[2] The elevation of blood pressure was transient and disappeared when treatment of heart failure was effective. However, the role of transient blood pressure elevations must be considered in the pathogenesis of the cardiac syndromes associated with alcoholism (Fig. 106.10).

In noncardiac alcoholics, a majority may have blood pressure elevation in the late intoxication-early withdrawal stage of acute alcoholism.[21] While heart failure has not been reported in these circumstances, acute hypertension may be an important determinant of cardiac decompensation. A study was undertaken in noncardiac alcoholics to assess the effects of inebriation and the postintoxication period on the level of arterial pressure in relation to cardiac function as compared with recovery levels. The hypertension was not related to a high-output state, since peripheral arterial resistance was substantially elevated.[22] High plasma levels of aldosterone and renin, as well as urinary catecholamines, correlated with this vasoconstrictor response. A decline of these hormones as blood pressure spontaneously normalized is compatible with this interpretation. However, changes in the intrinsic nerve activity of the arterial wall smooth muscle may be an important determinant of this response. As noted by Altura and colleagues, the response of the smooth muscle to adrenergic stimulation may vary with different stages of alcohol intake,[23] and an increased sensitivity to the neurotransmitter norepinephrine may have contributed to the observed rise of peripheral vascular resistance.

While reduced levels of circulating magnesium ion can elicit arterial vasoconstriction,[24] the levels of magnesium were in the low normal range in the transient hypertensive group but did not differ from those in the normotensive alcoholic.[22] This does not exclude a change in smooth muscle magnesium levels and an effect on cell calcium activity.

Despite the observation that these chronic ethanolic subjects can have an acute hypertensive response to acute intoxication, the left ventricular dimensions by echocardiography were normal in the acute hypertensives as well as in the normotensive alcoholic group.

It is unknown whether fixed hypertension can develop in persons who have frequent vasoconstrictive responses to ethanol withdrawal. Studies of cardiac function in alcoholic patients, when carried out days to weeks after the last ethanol consumption, have shown normal arterial pressure in the preclinical state,[6] mild failure,[25] or severe heart failure after compensation.[26] Moreover, in none of these studies were such consequences of hypertension as retinopathy reported.

At some stages of alcoholic cardiomyopathy, the presence of hypertrophy may simulate the response to chronic hypertension. Thus, the anatomical changes of the heart in chronic alcoholics in the asymptomatic stage, as defined by the echocardiogram, have been demonstrated to include 10% to 20% increments of wall thickness in the septum and left ventricular posterior wall.[8,27] However, fractional shortening of the left ventricle was maintained at normal levels during

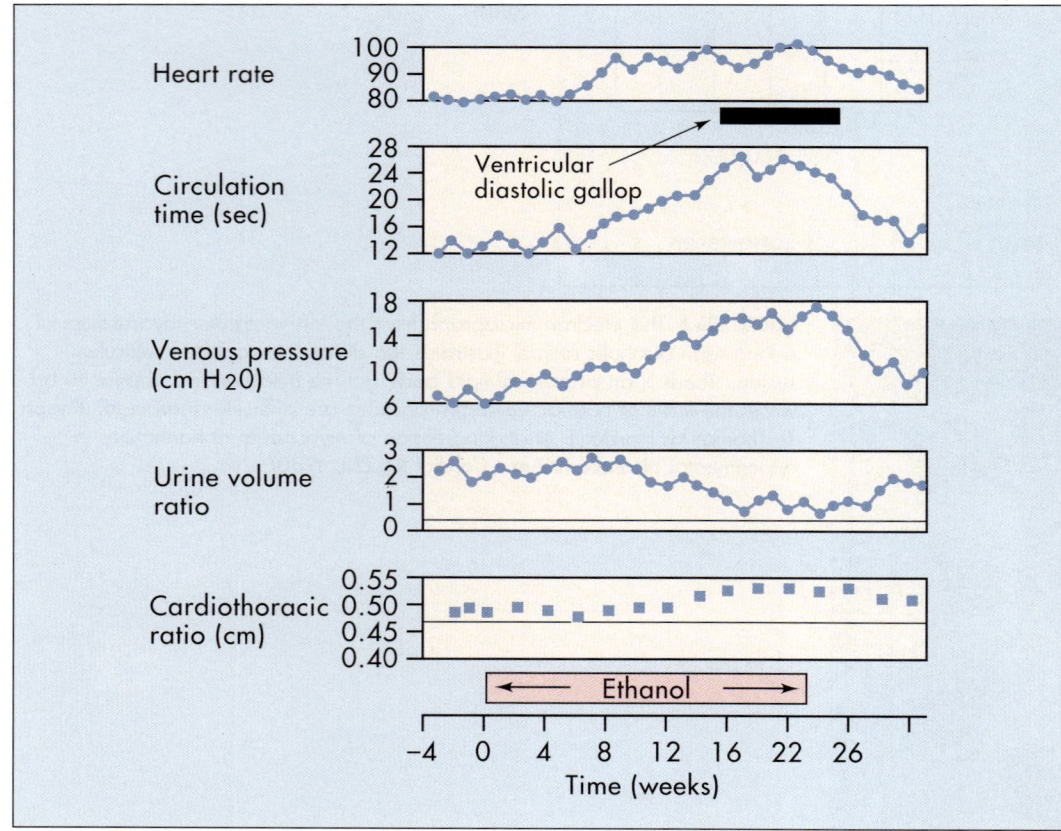

FIGURE 106.7 Evidence of cardiac depression developing during chronic ethanol intake. The weekly values depicted above represent the average of the daily measurements for heart rate and urine volume (day/night ratio), of the biweekly determinations of circulation time (arm-to-tongue), and venous pressure. These parameters became progressively abnormal after 8 weeks of ethanol ingestion, with the eventual development of a ventricular diastolic gallop. The abnormalities disappeared after interruption of alcohol intake. (Modified from Regan TJ, Levinson GE, Oldewurtel HA et al: Ventricular function in noncardiacs with alcoholic fatty liver. Role of ethanol in the production of cardiomyopathy. J Clin Invest 48:397, 1969)

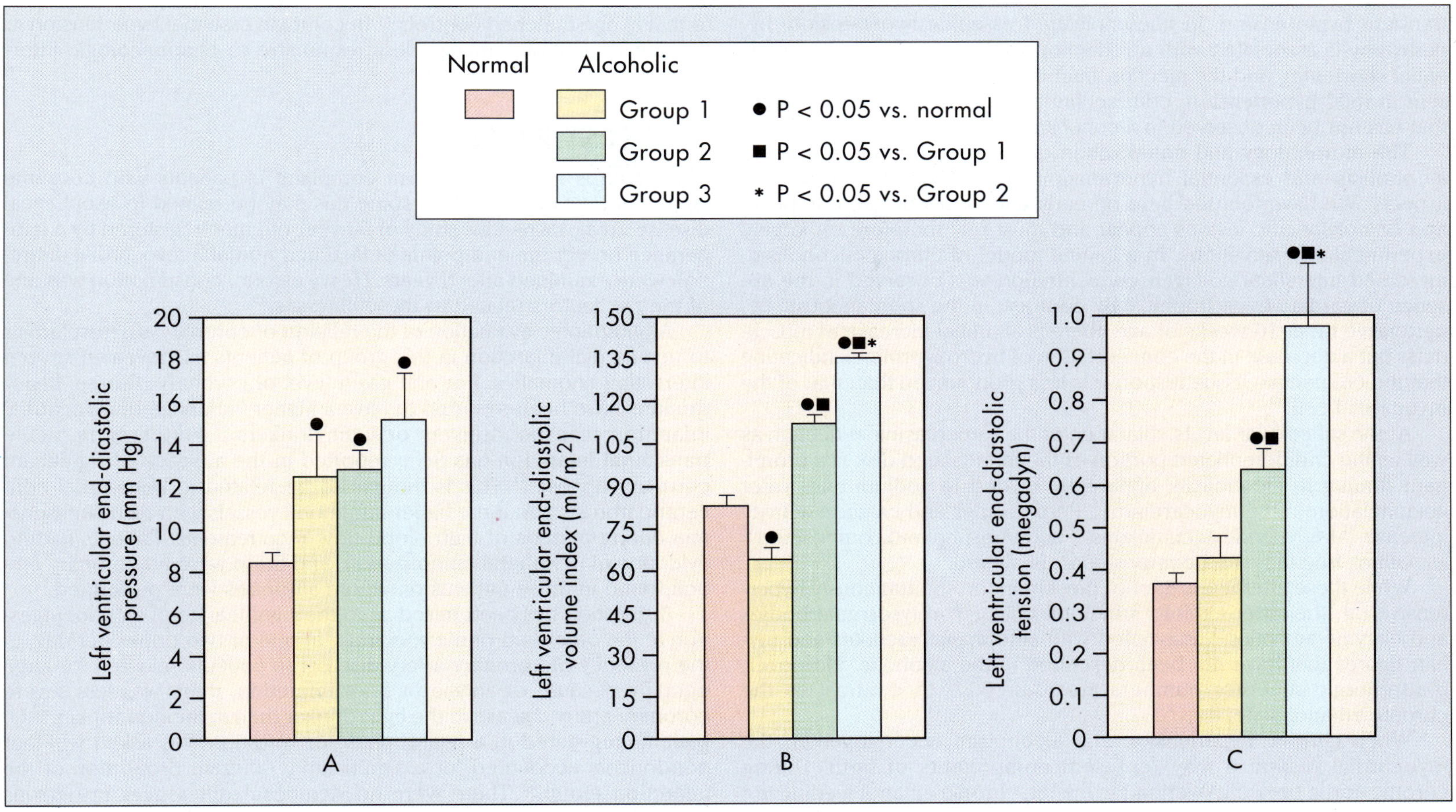

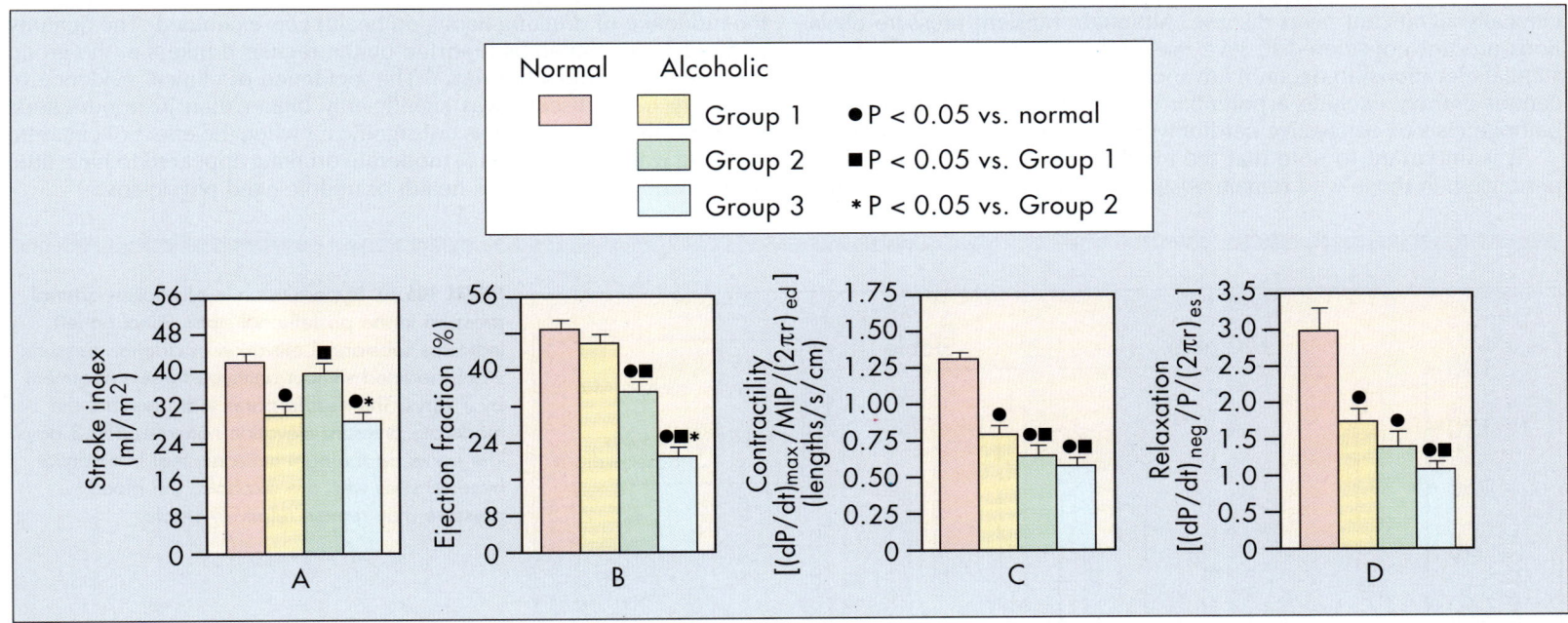

FIGURE 106.8 Left ventricular end-diastolic (**A**) pressure, (**B**) volume index, and (**C**) tension in normals and alcoholic patients (group 1, presence of chest pain or palpitations with normal heart size; group 2, same as group 1; group 3, exertional dyspnea with varied degree of cardiomegaly. Whereas the end-diastolic pressure is elevated in all three patient groups to essentially similar levels, the volume and tension indicate a progressive increase over the levels noted in normals. Compared with the patients in groups 2 and 3, the end-diastolic tension in group 1 patients remains at the normal level. (Modified from Ahmed SS, Levinson GE, Fiore JJ et al: Spectrum of heart muscle abnormalities related to alcoholism. Clin Cardiol 3:335, 1980)

FIGURE 106.9 Left ventricular systolic parameters (**A**) stroke index, (**B**) ejection fraction, (**C**) contractility, and (**D**) relaxation in alcoholic (group 1, presence of chest pain or palpitations with normal heart size; group 2, same as group 1; group 3, exertional dyspnea with varied degree of cardiomegaly) and normal subjects. A progressive decline is noted in the "indices" of left ventricular contraction. The ejection fraction is unchanged from the normal in group 1 only. An increase in the end-diastolic volume in group 2 normalizes the stroke output, but the ejection fraction declines. Further increase in end-diastolic volume in group 3 fails to increase the stroke index, and the ejection fraction is further reduced. (Modified from Ahmed SS, Levinson GE, Fiore JJ et al: Spectrum of heart muscle abnormalities related to alcoholism. Clin Cardiol 3:335, 1980)

transient hypertension. In uncomplicated essential hypertension, hypertrophy is associated with a reduction in the velocity of circumferential shortening and the ejection fraction.[28] When hypertrophy is absent in mild hypertension, contractility may be increased,[29] an effect that has not been observed in alcoholism.[6,8,27]

The morphology and composition of the myocardium in chronic alcoholism and essential hypertension appear to differ in several aspects. We have focused here on early alterations before complication or nonspecific lesions appear and must rely therefore on largely experimental observations. In a canine model of chronic alcoholism, increased interstitial collagen concentration was observed in the absence of cardiac hypertrophy.[14] By contrast, in the spontaneously hypertensive rat at 16 weeks of age, there is an initial increase of muscle mass but a decrease in the concentration of hydroxyproline, indicating that the connective tissue response is less pronounced than that of the myocardial cell.[30]

At the subcellular levels, dilatation of the sarcoplasmic reticulum as well as the undifferentiated portion of the intercalated disk is a prominent finding in alcoholism, apparently related to sodium and water accumulation in the myocardium.[16] Peroxisomes and catalase activity increase,[31] triglyceride accumulates,[32] and phospholipid composition[32] as well as free fatty acid composition[33] is altered.

While these alterations are not present in the spontaneously hypertensive rat, the latter exhibits structural changes in lysosomal bodies and enzyme activities[34] associated with autophagic vacuoles and myelin figures that have not been described in the alcoholic. Moreover, β-adrenergic receptor numbers are reduced,[35] in contrast to the chronic ethanol state.[36]

When chronic hypertension and alcoholism occur together, the myocardial response may represent components of both. During chronic aortic pressure overload in the rat, chronic ethanol feeding did not interfere with the normal hypertrophic response.[37]

The clinical observation[2,10] that cardiomyopathy is unusual in patients with chronic cirrhosis may clarify the relevance of hypertension to the development of the cardiomyopathic state. The largest transient elevations of systemic arterial pressure have been reported in persons with compensated cirrhosis.[21] It would thus appear that this intermittent peripheral arterial response may commonly be unassociated with clinically significant heart disease. Although transient pressure elevations are not considered to give rise to myocardial disease,[28] if substantial elevations do occur in advanced subclinical heart disease, one cannot entirely exclude a potential role for this phenomenon in the pathogenesis of congestive cardiomyopathy in chronic alcoholism.

It is important to note that the incidence of chronic essential hypertension in those who remain abstinent for a year is, at 10%, similar to that in age-matched controls.[21] In contrast, essential hypertension in the active alcoholic appears less responsive to pharmacologic intervention.[38]

CHEST PAIN

Chest pain is not an infrequent complaint in patients who consume large amounts of alcohol. In some this may be related to esophageal disease. In a prospective study of 50-year-old men registered by a temperance board, the end-points of fatal and nonfatal myocardial infarction were examined after 9 years. Heavy alcohol consumption was one of the risk factors related to these illnesses.[39]

Angiographic evaluation of the relation of coronary atherosclerosis to myocardial infarction in this group of patients has revealed several interesting anomalies. For any given level of coronary disease, heavy drinkers have been reported to have a higher incidence of myocardial infarction than nondrinkers or light drinkers.[40] Furthermore, acute transmural infarction has been reported in the absence of significant coronary disease.[41] This is thought to be related to periarterial concentric fibrosis about the larger intramural vessels with resultant ischemia during periods of high blood-flow requirements. Patients had no evidence of peripheral embolization, and there were no coronary emboli found in those patients on whom autopsies were performed.

A question has been raised as to the significance of alcohol ingestion at the other end of the spectrum, at one or two drinks per day, in the presence of coronary artery disease. In patients selected for angiography because of angina or prior infarction, there was less severe coronary artery disease in the light drinker than in the nondrinker.[42] Of patients registered in a health plan, the question was asked whether nondrinkers accounted for a significantly different proportion of the infarction group.[43] There were no significant differences in persons under the age of 64. Above this age, patients who did not use alcohol had a significantly higher incidence of myocardial infarction, a phenomenon particularly evident in women. There was, however, no difference in the incidence of out-of-hospital sudden death in the same population.

In contrast to these findings is a prospective study of physicians who were first seen as medical students and followed to midlife when the influence of drinking habits on health was examined. The quantity of alcohol consumed as reported by the regular drinkers in the group averaged two drinks per day.[44] The incidence of clinical evidence of coronary heart disease was significantly higher than in nondrinkers; however, the difference was not significant when the effect of cigarette smoking was removed. Thus, moderate drinking appeared to have little or no evident effect on the health of middle-aged physicians.

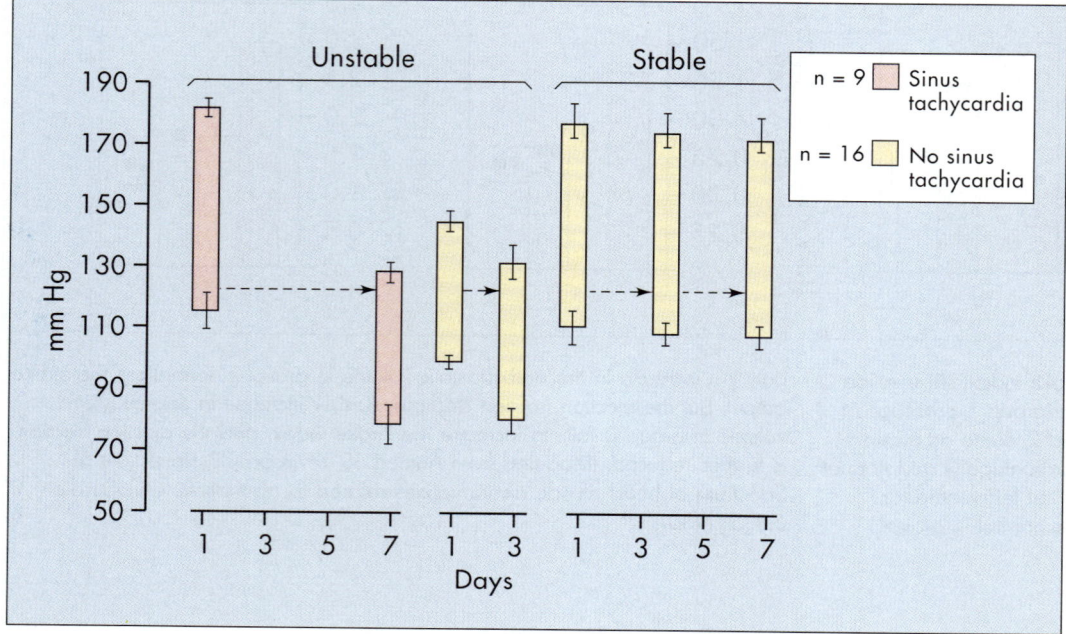

FIGURE 106.10 Hypertension in alcoholics: arterial pressure in the postethanol state. Panel on left indicates substantial elevation of arterial pressure, which declined without antihypertensive treatment by 7 days. The middle panel indicates that the moderate pressure elevation normalized in 3 days. The panel on the right indicates that in essential hypertensives who are alcoholic, the blood pressure may remain relatively stable.

The mechanism postulated for the preventive effect of ethanol on atherosclerosis is related to its known properties of increasing high-density lipoprotein (HDL) levels. However, recently the subspecies of these lipoproteins were assayed in persons drinking modest amounts of alcohol and compared with periods when these same persons were abstinent.[45] HDL_3 levels were elevated by ethanol. However, HDL_2, the moiety that regulates efflux of cholesterol from the coronary arteries, was not affected.

COURSE OF CONGESTIVE CARDIOMYOPATHY

Individual case reports have indicated the potential for recovery from mechanical cardiac dysfunction when the patient ceases alcohol consumption. In some, the improved mechanical function could readily be attributed to restoration of normal sinus rhythm. The inherent difficulties of clinical evaluation have precluded a randomized study, but the outlook is generally considered to be poor in those who continue to ingest substantial amounts of ethanol. In a European study, 42 of 108 patients with a diagnosis of congestive cardiomyopathy were considered to be alcoholic and continued to be actively so.[46] Two thirds of these subjects were dead within 3 years, while of the nonalcoholics, one third had died.

The effects of abstinence presumably depend upon the stage of the cardiac disease at which the patients behavior is altered. Although there are no definitive answers, three studies strongly suggest a beneficial effect of interrupting alcohol intake. In a small series, all ten patients who stopped drinking survived a decade of follow-up.[47] In a study of 31 alcoholics in the United States, follow-up over several years indicated that none of the 12 who stopped alcohol consumption succumbed, while there were 19 deaths in those who persisted in their addiction.[48] This clinical investigation was particularly suggestive because the subjects in both groups had similar degrees of cardiomegaly and congestive heart failure on entrance into the study.

In a larger series of 64 alcoholic subjects, one third were apparently persuaded to abstain.[49] During the subsequent 4 years, the mortality rate in the latter was 9% in contrast to those who remained actively alcoholic and succumbed at an incidence of 57%. It should be pointed out that many in the surviving group did not improve their clinical cardiac status. As in hepatic cirrhosis, the response to abstinence may not be fully reversible after many years of toxic injury. In the main these studies support the view that ethanol is a major etiologic element in this disease.

DYSRHYTHMIAS

Arrhythmias are another manifestation of heart disease related to alcoholism. The presence of arrhythmias in subjects without overt cardiomyopathy or enlarged heart but with a background of alcoholism has been described during acute intoxication. The cardiac event developing in these circumstances is probably often misdiagnosed as idiopathic, since little or no clinical evidence of heart disease remains after resolution of the rhythm problem, and the extent of alcohol use may be unrecognized.

In a report of patients admitted to an emergency room, 32 separate symptomatic dysrhythmic episodes requiring hospitalization occurred in 24 patients who drank heavily and habitually with superimposition of heavy ingestion before the arrhythmia.[50] Atrial fibrillation was the most common arrhythmia (Fig. 106.11). Sinus rhythm was restored spontaneously in some but usually required cardioversion or pharmacologic intervention. Recurrence of the syndrome during subsequent episodes of intoxication was associated with the same arrhythmia as during the original episode. Plasma electrolytes were usually normal. The frequent weekend or holiday presentations suggested the term "holiday heart syndrome," representing an acute cardiac rhythm disturbance with heavy ethanol consumption in a person without other clinical evidence of heart disease and disappearing without evident residua on abstinence.

One to two weeks after restoration of normal sinus rhythm, these patients were found to have abnormal systolic time intervals consistent with subclinical mechanical dysfunction. On high-speed electrocardiogram, moderate conduction delays were found and were considered to be the background for the induction of acute arrhythmias.[50] An anatomical substrate is suggested by dilatation of the intercalated disk, the low-resistance pathways between cardiac cells, observed in a chronic animal model (Fig. 106.12).

The phenomenon of the holiday heart has been reproduced in the electrophysiology laboratory. In 11 subjects who abused alcohol but had no clinical evidence of heart disease, atrial fibrillation was inducible without acute ethanol administration in four and in another four only during its use.[51] The arrhythmogenic potential of this substance has been emphasized in an analysis of 40 patients with new-onset atrial fibrillation. Among patients under 65 years of age, alcohol was considered to be causative or contributory in approximately two thirds.[52]

Although an accurate estimate of the incidence of arrhythmias in the population addicted to alcohol is not available, Holter monitor evaluation of successive patients during the intoxication and early withdrawal stages is of interest.[53] Subjects in whom the admission electrocardiogram revealed arrhythmias or evidence of cardiac ischemia were excluded. Of the 60 patients monitored during the initial 12 or 14 hours, 12 patients were identified who had high composite arrhythmia scores due mainly to the presence of ventricular premature contractions. Biochemical assays of the serum revealed high plasma catecholamine concentrations. The observation that propranolol was effective in controlling the arrhythmias suggested a probable role for the sympathetic nervous system. It should be noted that dysrhythmias seem to appear without evident electrolyte disorder, but such disorders may be an important factor in some patients.

Sporadic reports of sudden death from medical examiners suggest that a small fraction of the addicted are at risk for cardiac arrest. In an examination of the causes of sudden unexpected death in a 15- to 49-year-old Finnish population, 5.2% of deaths were attributed to alcoholism.[54] Fatty liver was the principal pathologic finding in a series from Baltimore, Maryland, but there was no detailed histologic investigation of the heart.[55] A similar phenomenon has been subsequently observed in a predominantly rural population.[56] This medical examiner's series consisted of 411 sudden deaths over a 4-year period in subjects with fatty liver and population characteristics that mirrored those of the general alcohol-abusing population. A majority had modest blood ethanol levels.

More suggestive is a series of autopsies on 50 persons, 30 of whom had died suddenly.[57] Historical data indicated that all had been chronic alcoholics for years, and 17 of 30 had alcoholemia at the time of death. Compared with controls who were considered to have died from lethal alcohol intoxication, the sudden death group had greater degrees of myocardial hypertrophy and foci of fibrosis and necrosis, as well as mononuclear cell infiltration.

An additional variable that is relevant to arrhythmogenesis is the sleep apnea and oxygen desaturation that have been described in asymptomatic persons at blood ethanol levels above 80 mg/dl.[58] This phenomenon requires investigation in terms of its cardiac effects in chronic alcoholics.

DIAGNOSIS

Since the cardiovascular system may be affected by chronic alcohol abuse in a variety of ways, a careful historical inquiry is essential in patients with unexplained abnormalities related to transient hypertension, arrhythmias, chest pain, or any degree of cardiac decompensation.

Clinical reports of cardiomyopathy have emphasized the difficulty in obtaining a history of alcoholism. There is a male predominance, and suggestive diagnostic aspects include social disruption, accident proneness, and a family history of chronic alcohol abuse. The major positive diagnostic feature is the history of ethanol ingestion in intoxicating amounts for many years, frequently marked by periods of spree drinking. Often this information can be obtained only through persistent questioning over many visits with the patient or by communication with relatives.

Difficulties with quantification of alcohol intake in personal interviews are well illustrated by the experience with assessment of known alcoholics interviewed during their weekly visits to a liver clinic.[59] A majority of patients with alcohol in the urine convincingly denied intake approximately 50% of the time. Twenty-five percent denied drinking every time they were questioned.

Six alcoholic drinks per day for many years has been suggested[60] to increase cardiovascular mortality in an epidemiologic survey; alcoholic patients with congestive cardiomyopathy usually give histories of heavier consumption. In considering the incidence of heart disease in alcoholics, the widely held assumption that extracardiac disease such as cirrhosis is not usually associated with clinically evident heart disease, as well as the converse relationship, should be recognized. Whether this represents differential organ sensitivity or a protective effect of impaired hepatic function on development of cardiac disease is unknown.

In terms of variables in addition to ethanol abuse that may affect the development of cardiomyopathy, several factors have been considered to be potentially important. In contrast to liver disease, clinically evident malnutrition is usually not present in the cardiac patient. In females, the disease is rare before menopause. It should also be noted that a genetic predisposition has been evaluated in the terms of the HLA antigens.[61] Examination of two loci (A and B) revealed no significant differences compared with controls. Cigarette smoking is very common in the person addicted to alcohol. Since myopathic responses to chronic cigarette smoking have been seen experimentally,[62] this factor may be of more importance in pathogenesis than generally recognized.

A variety of biochemical changes may occur in the alcoholic that can be reflected in abnormalities of blood composition.[63] Mean corpuscular volume of red cells may be increased as well as liver enzyme concentrations. Albumin and urea may be reduced while HDL may be enhanced. In terms of cardiac enzymes, creatine phosphokinase and lactic dehydrogenase concentrations have been examined; no diagnostic changes in these isoenzymes have been detected despite the presence of subclinical cardiac abnormalities or frank heart failure.[64] Moreover, circulating heart antibodies as detected by immunofluorescent methods were not present in patients with alcoholic cardiomyopathy,[65] in contrast to the recognized immunologic entities, such as Dressler's syndrome. In examination of biopsy specimens from patients or autopsy tissue preparations, no distinctive features have been revealed in patients with alcoholic heart disease as compared with results in those with other causes of congestive cardiomyopathy.[66] Early in the prefailure stage there would appear to be dilatation of the

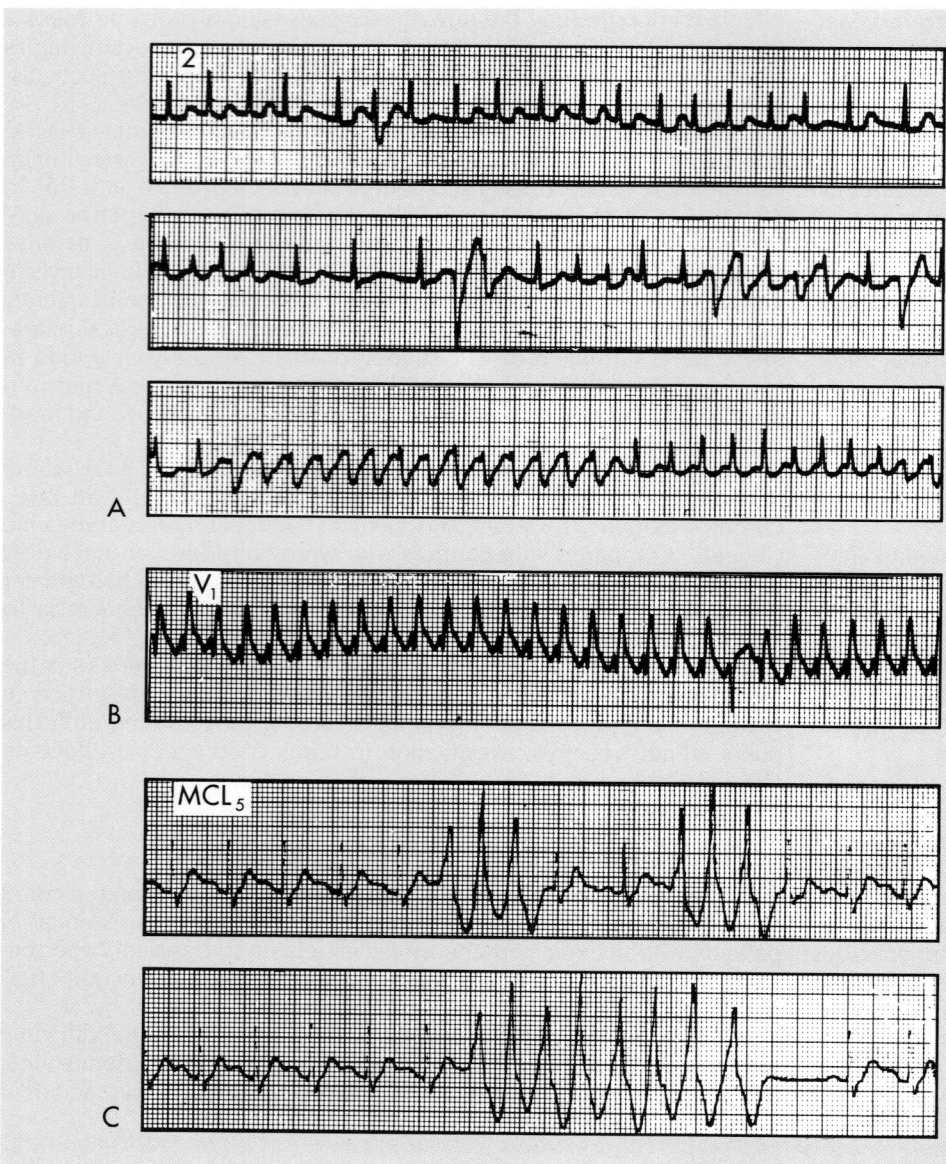

FIGURE 106.11 Electrocardiograms of illustrative cases. **A.** Atrial fibrillation is seen in top strip with one aberrant (Ashman) beat (the sixth). Within 10 minutes (next two strips), the rate accelerated with runs of wide complexes (?aberration or ventricular tachycardia) at rate of 240/min. **B.** Atrial flutter with 1:1 conduction (verified later by carotid massage) at rate of 250/min with right bundle branch block aberration. A single normally conducted beat is seen (C). Runs of ventricular tachycardia 1 minute following the end of a treadmill stress test (both strips). (Regan TJ, Ettinger PO: Varied cardiac abnormalities in alcoholics. Alcoholism: Clin Exp Res 3:40, 1979. Reproduced with permission)

sarcoplasmic reticulum and the undifferentiated portion of the intercalated disk,[67] but these events apparently are obscured at later stages when considerable myocytolysis may be seen. Increased amounts of fibrous tissue, which are usual findings, may appear as an increase in the interstitial collagen component or replacement of myocardial fibers.[66] Small vessels are usually normal, but in fibrous areas the vessels may occasionally show more thickening. These vascular abnormalities may be secondary in nature.

Skeletal muscle is a readily available tissue for biopsy in identification of the alcoholic, and its examination has perhaps been underutilized. In subjects without acute muscle symptomatology, those drinking more than 100 g alcohol per day for longer than 3 years developed atrophy of striated muscle fibers. This affects predominantly type 2B fibers, which are dependent on anaerobic glycolytic metabolism. There was no evident damage to mitochondria, and the patients had no complicating endocrine diseases that might similarly affect muscle fibers.[68]

MANAGEMENT

Therapy depends on the state of cardiac disease when the patient is first seen. During the first episode of low-output heart failure, if the patient has not been symptomatic for a long time and has only modest cardiomegaly without severe pulmonary edema, he may be managed initially by diuretics to correct the volume overload; bed rest is also advised. There is presumably a role for preload- and afterload-reducing agents as the disease progresses, but controlled studies on long-term efficacy have not been reported. Paradoxically, oral ethanol has been used therapeutically in acute heart failure at a dose of 0.9 g/kg body weight.[69] Systemic and pulmonary wedge pressures were significantly reduced without a change in stroke volume or cardiac output. Efficacy presumably depended upon the substantial reduction of systemic vascular resistance. The failure of stroke volume to increase acutely in response to ethanol as it does in response to other agents that reduce afterload could well be related to the negative inotropic action of ethanol. Moreover, this response contrasts with the increase of ejection fraction in cardiac patients seen after a 700- to 900-calorie breakfast.[70]

It should be noted that in the absence of a substantially increased peripheral resistance in heart failure, the negative inotropic action of ethanol may dominate. Thus, a progressive rise of left ventricular end-diastolic pressure and volume has been observed without a significant change of peripheral resistance (Fig. 106.13).

Digitalis can be most useful in the control of atrial fibrillation or sinus tachycardia and contributes to the management of congestive heart failure in advanced stages of the disease. Although long-term bed rest has been suggested as perhaps aiding in management,[71] the most important feature of institutionalization is the enforced abstinence from alcohol.

In terms of long-term management, abstinence from alcohol is mandatory. As with other addicted persons association with groups focused on this purpose is strongly encouraged. Some patients may require supervised treatment with disulfiram (Antabuse) to discourage intake of alcohol. However, the use of Antabuse for alcoholism in cardiac patients may be associated with complications in view of the fact that dopamine β-hydroxylase, which is involved in the synthesis of norepinephrine in the heart, is inhibited by this agent.[72] In the event of an Antabuse–alcohol reaction, an inhibitor of alcohol dehydrogenase, 4-methylpyrazole, has shown promise.[73] The rapid accumulation of acetaldehyde is reversed, and thus symptoms such as flushing and tachycardia are attenuated.

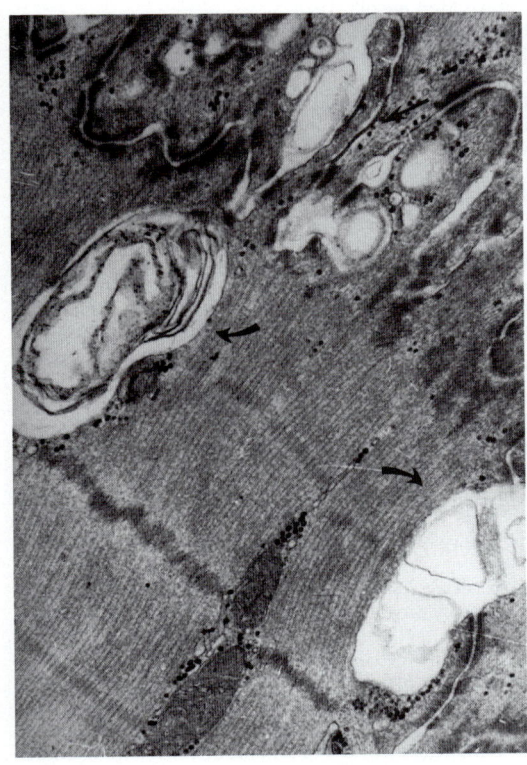

FIGURE 106.12 Intercalated disk of alcoholic dog. Cystic areas of dilatation of undifferentiated regions are apparent (curved arrows). A nexus (straight arrow) appears normal. (Ettinger PO, Wu CF, DeLaCruz C Jr et al: Arrhythmias and the "holiday heart": Alcohol-associated cardiac rhythm disorders. Am Heart J 91:66, 1976. Reproduced with permission)

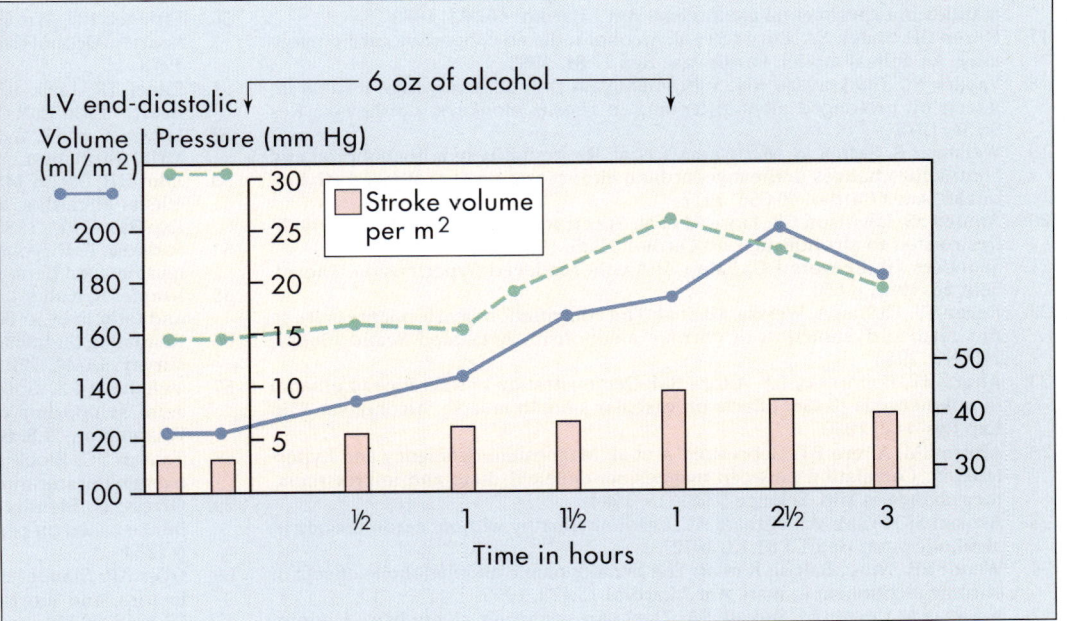

FIGURE 106.13 These observations made during ingestion of 6 oz of Scotch by an alcoholic patient with cardiac decompensation reveal a depressant effect on the left ventricle at a dose that has no effect in the noncardiac alcoholic. (Modified from Regan JJ, Haider B: Ethanol abuse and heart disease. Circulation 44:957, 1971)

REFERENCES

1. Evans W: The electrocardiogram of alcoholic cardiomyopathy. Br Heart J 21:445, 1959
2. Fowler NO, Gueron M, Rowlands DT Jr: Primary myocardial disease. Circulation 23:498, 1961
3. Shirey EK, Proudfit WL, Hawk WA: Primary myocardial disease: Correlation with clinical findings, angiographic and biopsy diagnosis. Am Heart J 99:198, 1980
4. Fuster V, Gersh BJ, Giuliani ER et al: The natural history of idiopathic dilated cardiomyopathy. Am J Cardiol 47:525, 1981
5. Schwarz F, Mall G, Zebe H et al: Determinants of survival in patients with congestive cardiomyopathy: Quantitative morphologic findings and left ventricular hemodynamics. Circulation 70:923, 1984
6. Regan TJ, Levinson GE, Oldewurtel HA et al: Ventricular function in noncardiacs with alcoholic fatty liver: Role of ethanol in the production of cardiomyopathy. J Clin Invest 48:397, 1969
7. Wu CF, Sudhakar M, Jaferi G et al: Preclinical cardiomyopathy in chronic alcoholics: A sex difference. Am Heart J 91:281, 1976
8. Mathews EC Jr, Gardin JM, Henry WL et al: Echocardiographic abnormalities in chronic alcoholics with and without overt congestive heart failure. Am J Cardiol 47:570, 1981
9. Read R, Bell J, Batey R: Cardiac function assessed by gated heart pool studies in an alcohol clinic population: A preliminary study. Alcoholism: Clin Exp Res 8:467, 1984
10. Ahmed SS, Howard M, ten Hove W et al: Cardiac function in alcoholics with cirrhosis: Absence of overt cardiomyopathy—Myth or fact? J Am Coll Cardiol 3:696, 1984
11. Epstein M, Schneider N, Befeler B: Relationship of systemic and intrarenal hemodynamics in cirrhosis. J Lab Clin Med 89:1175, 1957
12. Steinberg JD, Hayden MT: Prevalence of clinically occult cardiomyopathy in chronic alcoholism. Am Heart J 101:461, 1981
13. Maines JF, Aldinger EE: Myocardial depression accompanying chronic consumption of alcohol. Am Heart J 73:55, 1967
14. Segel LD, Rendig SV, Mason DT: Alcohol-induced cardiac hemodynamic and Ca^{2+} flux dysfunctions are reversible. J Mol Cell Cardiol 13:443, 1981
15. Sarma JSM, Shigeaki I, Fischer R et al: Biochemical and contractile properties of heart muscle after prolonged alcohol administration. J Mol Cell Cardiol 8:972, 1976
16. Thomas G, Haider B, Oldewurtel HA et al: Progression of myocardial abnormalities in experimental alcoholism. Am J Cardiol 46:233, 1980
17. Noren GR, Staley NA, Einzig S et al: Alcohol-induced congestive cardiomyopathy: An animal model. Cardiovasc Res 17:81, 1983
18. Vasdev SC, Chakravarti RN, Subrahmanyam D et al: Myocardial lesions induced by prolonged alcohol feeding in rhesus monkeys. Cardiovasc Res 9:134, 1975
19. Weishaar R, Sarma JS, Maruyama Y et al: Reversibility of mitochondrial and contractile changes in the myocardium after cessation of prolonged ethanol intake. Am J Cardiol 40:556, 1977
20. Ahmed SS, Levinson GE, Fiore JJ et al: Spectrum of heart muscle abnormalities related to alcoholism. Clin Cardiol 3:335, 1980
21. Saunders JB, Beevers DG, Paton A: Alcohol-induced hypertension. Lancet, Sept 26, 1981, p 654
22. Regan TJ, Pathan A, Weisse AB et al: The contribution of arterial pressure to the cardiac dysfunction of chronic alcoholism. Acta Med Scand [Suppl] 703:273, 1986
23. Altura BT, Pohorecky LA, Altura BM: Demonstration of tolerance to ethanol in non-nervous tissue: Effects on vascular smooth muscle. Alcoholism: Clin Exp Res 4:62, 1980
24. Altura BM, Altura BT, Gebrewold A et al: Magnesium deficiency and hypertension: Correlation between magnesium-deficient diets and microcirculatory change in situ. Science 223:1315, 1984
25. Asokan SK, Frank MJ, Witham AC: Cardiomyopathy without cardiomegaly in alcoholics. Am Heart J 84:13, 1972
26. Wendt VE, Wu C, Balcon R et al: The hemodynamic and metabolic effects of chronic alcoholism in man. Am J Cardiol 15:175, 1965
27. Askanas A, Udoshi M, Sadjadi SA: The heart in chronic alcoholism: A noninvasive study. Am Heart J 99:9, 1980
28. Dunn FG, Chandraratna PAN, DeCarvalho JGR et al: Pathophysiological assessment of hypertensive heart disease with echocardiography. Am J Cardiol 39:789, 1977
29. Dreslinski GR, Messerli FH, Dunn FG et al: Patterns of left ventricular adaptation in borderline and mild essential hypertension: Echocardiographic findings. Chest 80:592, 1981
30. Tomanek RJ, Hovanec JM: The effects of long-term pressure-overload and aging on the myocardium. J Mol Cell Cardiol 13:471, 1981
31. Kino M: Chronic effects of ethanol under partial inhibition of catalase activity in the rat heart: Light and electron microscopic observations. J Mol Cell Cardiol 13:5, 1981
32. Regan TJ, Khan MI, Ettinger PO et al: Myocardial function and lipid metabolism in the chronic alcoholic animal. J Clin Invest 54:740, 1974
33. Lange LG, Sobel BE: Myocardial metabolites of ethanol. Circ Res 52:479, 1983
34. Tomanek RJ, Trout JJ, Lauva IK: Cytochemistry of myocardial structures related to degenerative processes in spontaneously hypertensive and normotensive rats. J Mol Cell Cardiol 16:227, 1984
35. Yamada S, Ishima T, Tomita T et al: Alterations in cardiac alpha and beta adrenoreceptors during the development of spontaneous hypertension. J Pharmacol Exp Ther 228:454, 1984
36. Segel ID, Mason DT: Beta-adrenergic receptors in chronic alcoholic rats. Cardiovasc Res 16:34, 1982
37. Whitman V, Schuler HG, Musselman J: Effects of chronic ethanol consumption on the myocardial hypertrophic response to a pressure overload in the rat. J Mol Cell Cardiol 12:519, 1980
38. Saunders JB, Bannan LT, Beevers DG et al: Alcohol and hypertension. Lancet, Feb 13, 1982, p 401
39. Wilhelmsen L, Wedel H, Tibbin G: Multivariate analysis of risk factors for coronary heart disease. Circulation 48:950, 1973
40. Deutscher S, Rockette HE, Krishnaswami V: Evaluation of habitual excessive alcohol consumption on myocardial infarction risk in coronary disease patients. Am Heart J 108:988, 1984
41. Regan TJ, Wu CF, Weisse AB et al: Acute myocardial infarction in toxic cardiomyopathy without coronary obstruction. Circulation 51:453, 1975
42. Barboriak JJ, Anderson AJ, Hoffman RG: Interrelationship between coronary artery occlusion, high-density lipoprotein cholesterol, and alcohol intake. J Lab Clin Med 94:348, 1979
43. Klatsky AL, Friedman GD, Siegelaub AB: Alcohol use and cardiovascular disease: The Kaiser–Permanente experience. Circulation 64 (Suppl III):32, 1981
44. Thomas CB, Santora PB, Schaffer JW: Health of physicians in midlife in relation to use of alcohol: A prospective study of a cohort of former medical students. Johns Hopkins Med J 146:1, 1980
45. Haskell WL, Camargo C Jr, Williams PT et al: The effect of cessation and resumption of moderate alcohol intake on serum high-density-lipoprotein subfractions: A controlled study. N Engl J Med 310:805, 1984
46. Bory M, Mancini C, Djiane P et al: Les myocardiomyopathies ethyliques. Nouv Presse Med 6:295, 1977
47. Koide T, Kato A, Takabatake Y et al: Variable prognosis in congestive cardiomyopathy: Role of left ventricular function, alcoholism, and pulmonary thrombosis. Jap Heart J 21:451, 1980
48. Shugoll GI, Bowen PJ, Moore P et al: Follow-up observations and prognosis in primary myocardial disease. Arch Intern Med 129:67, 1972
49. Demakis JG, Proskey A, Rahimtoola SH et al: The natural course of alcoholic cardiomyopathy. Ann Intern Med 80:293, 1974
50. Ettinger PO, Wu CF, DeLa Cruz C Jr et al: Arrhythmias and the "holiday heart": Alcohol-associated cardiac rhythm disorders. Am Heart J 95:555, 1978
51. Engel TR, Luck JC: Effect of whiskey on atrial vulnerability and "holiday heart." J Am Coll Cardiol 1:816, 1983
52. Lowenstein SR, Gabow PA, Cramer J et al: The role of alcohol in new-onset atrial fibrillation. Arch Intern Med 143:1882, 1983
53. Zilm DH, Jacob MS, MacLeod SM et al: Propranolol and chlordiazepoxide effects of cardiac arrhythmias during alcohol withdrawal. Alcoholism: Clin Exp Res 4:400, 1980
54. Sarkioja T, Hirvonen J: Causes of sudden unexpected deaths in young and middle-aged persons. Forensic Sci Int 24:247, 1984
55. Kramer K, Kuller L, Fisher R: The increasing mortality attributed to cirrhosis and fatty liver in Baltimore (1957–1966). Ann Intern Med 69:273, 1968
56. Randall B: Sudden death and hepatic fatty metamorphosis: A North Carolina survey. JAMA 243:1723, 1980
57. Velisheva LS, Goldina BG, Boguslavsky VI: Proceedings: USA-USSR First Joint Symposium on Sudden Death, DHEW Publication No. (NIH) 78-1470. Washington, U.S. Government Printing Office, 1978
58. Taasan VC, Block AJ, Boysen PG et al: Alcohol increases sleep apnea and oxygen desaturation in asymptomatic men. Am J Med 71:240, 1981
59. Orrego H, Blendis LM, Blake JE et al: Reliability of assessment of alcohol intake based on personal interviews in a liver clinic. Lancet, Dec 22/29, 1979, p 1354
60. Dyer AR, Stamler J, Paul O et al: Alcohol consumption, cardiovascular risk factors, and mortality in two Chicago epidemiologic studies. Circulation 56:1067, 1977
61. Kachru RB, Proskey AJ, Telischi M: Histocompatibility antigens and alcoholic cardiomyopathy. Tissue Antigens 15:398, 1980
62. Ahmed SS, Torres R, Regan TJ: Interaction of chronic cigarette and ethanol use on myocardium. Clin Cardiol 8:129, 1985
63. Morgan MY: Markers for detecting alcoholism and monitoring for continued abuse. Pharmacol Biochem Behav 13:1, 1980
64. Fink R, Marjot DH, Rosalki SB: Detection of alcoholic cardiomyopathy by serum enzyme and isoenzyme determination. Ann Clin Biochem 16:165, 1979
65. Trueman T, Thompson RA, Cummins P et al: Heart antibodies in cardiomyopathies. Br Heart J 46:296, 1981
66. Olsen EGJ: The pathology of cardiomyopathies: A critical analysis. Am Heart J 98:385, 1979
67. Ferrans VJ, Buja M, Roberts WC: Cardiac morphologic changes produced by ethanol. In Rothschild MA, Oratz M, Schreiber SS (eds): Alcohol and Abnormal Protein Biosynthesis: Biochemical and Clinical, pp 139–185. New York, Pergamon Press, 1975

68. Martin FC, Slavin G, Levi AJ et al: Investigation of the organelle pathology of skeletal muscle in chronic alcoholism. J Clin Pathol 37:448, 1984
69. Greenberg BH, Schultz R, Grunkemeier GL et al: Acute effects of alcohol in patients with congestive heart failure. Ann Intern Med 97:171, 1982
70. Brown JM, White CJ, Sobol SM et al: Increased left ventricular ejection fraction after a meal: Potential source of error in performance of radionuclide angiography. Am J Cardiol 51:1709, 1983
71. McDonald CD, Burch GE, Walsh JJ: Alcoholic cardiomyopathy managed with prolonged bed rest. Ann Intern Med 74:681, 1971
72. Sauter AM, Boss D, von Wartburg JP: Reevaluation of the disulfiram-alcohol reaction in man. Q J Stud Alcohol 38:1680, 1977
73. Lindros KO, Stowell A, Pikkarainen P et al: The disulfiram (Antabuse)-alcohol reaction in male alcoholics: Its efficient management by 4-methylpyrazole. Alcoholism: Clin Exp Res 5:528, 1981

Cardiovascular Injury as the Internist Sees It

Melvin D. Cheitlin

THE IMPORTANCE OF CARDIOVASCULAR TRAUMA

Cardiovascular trauma has been recognized for millenia and until this century was believed to be almost invariably fatal. As late as 1888, Dr. Billroth wrote that "the surgeon who touched the heart lost the respect of his colleagues."[1] Dr. D. H. Williams of Chicago and later Washington, D.C., first successfully sutured the pericardium of a 24-year-old man stabbed in the heart in 1893, but he did not report it until 1897.[2] The first report of successful suturing of a stab wound of the right ventricle was by Rehn in 1896.[3] It was not until the development of techniques for blood replacement, endotracheal intubation, ventilatory support, and the discovery of antibiotics that significant advances were made in the treatment of cardiovascular trauma.

As is frequently the case, advances in the treatment of vascular and cardiac injury were made during wartime: World War II, where for the first time significant salvage of patients who suffered abdominal and thoracic wounds was possible; the Korean War, where techniques for repair of vascular injuries were developed; and the Vietnam War, where the principle of rapid evacuation by helicopter from the site of injury to the place where definitive surgical treatment was accomplished. Results of these advances can be seen in the mortality figures.[4] Whereas survival after an abdominal thoracic wound was a rarity in the Civil War, the mortality from thoracic abdominal wounds steadily decreased in World War I with blood transfusion and in World War II with modern thoracic operative techniques, blood transfusion, and antibiotics. In the Korean War, amputation ceased to be the treatment for peripheral arterial injuries and vascular repair was routinely accomplished. Finally, in Vietnam, rapid evacuation to definitive treatment facilities resulted in a mortality of less than 1% in any casualty found alive on the field.

Most of the approaches to the management of casualties and surgical techniques developed during wartime have been applied to the treatment of civilian cardiovascular injury. Major metropolitan areas have literally become battlefields where penetrating injuries from knives and bullets are a nightly occurrence and are seen and treated in almost every emergency room. The other great source of mayhem on the human body is the escalating use and abuse of motor vehicles resulting in accidents, especially those involving drivers under the influence of alcohol. In many urban communities, the techniques of rapid evacuation, either by emergency squads capable of sophisticated resuscitation in the field or by helicopters, has been adapted from the battlefield.

Since cardiovascular trauma is mostly the province of the surgeon in the acutely injured patient, or even the pathologist, this chapter will concentrate on the problems of cardiovascular trauma presented to the internist and cardiologist and will deal very little with the acute problems that are managed mostly by surgeons. The problems, therefore, are for the most part those of recognition and diagnosis of the type and severity of injury and the assessment of the proper treatment, including the indications for and timing of operative repair.

PHYSICAL CAUSES OF TRAUMA

Cardiovascular trauma can be physically produced by a variety of forces:

1. Penetrating injuries
   Low-velocity injuries (*e.g.*, knife, shrapnel, and flying objects)
   High-velocity injuries (*e.g.*, gunshot wounds)
2. Nonpenetrating injuries
   Deceleration and acceleration injuries (*e.g.*, fall from a height, motor vehicle accidents)
   Chest compression or crush injury (*e.g.*, steering wheel injury or crush injury by heavy object falling on the body)
   Blast and concussion
   Lower body compression (*e.g.*, cave-in of a sand pit)
   Electrical injury
   Environmental injuries (*e.g.*, cold and heat)

Injury of tissue is caused by the delivery of energy to the tissues by physical force contacting the body. With missile injury the damage depends on (1) the mass of the missile, (2) the shape and tumbling characteristics of the missile, and (3) the velocity of the missile.

In general, low-velocity missiles cause little damage away from the actual track of the object, and the damage is related to the structures directly injured by the missile. The characteristic low-velocity injury is the knife wound, but slowly moving missiles, such as shrapnel or low-velocity pellets or bullets, are in the same category. Rapidly losing velocity, their energy spent, they may come to rest and become the source of intracardiac foreign objects. Moving slowly, they can be reflected off bones and even tissue planes, abruptly changing the course of their path through the body. For this reason, it is not always possible to determine the pathway of the object after it has penetrated the body and, therefore, to tell when the heart has been injured by simply noting the point of penetration. Low-velocity objects, such as needles, bullets, or shrapnel, can also come to rest in veins or arteries and travel from these points either centripetally or centrifugally, embolizing to points in the body distant from their point of entry.

High-velocity missiles release energy on contact with the body according to the equation

$$KE = \frac{M(V_1^2 - V_2^2)}{2G}$$

where KE = kinetic energy, M = missile mass, V_1 = entrance velocity of the missile, V_2 = exit velocity of the missile, and G = gravity constant. Penetration of tissue by a moving object results in a cylinder of energy around the pathway, released to the tissues in the form of heat and gaseous expansion. This results in tissue necrosis in a cylinder at a variable distance from the missile track.[5] In addition to this energy release, the size of the missile track is determined by characteristics of the missile itself and how it is tumbling when it enters the body. The "dumdum" bullet, which is designed to expand on contact, creates a very large missile track and area of injury.

It is relatively easy to understand direct injury due to thoracic compression or the heart's striking the spine or sternum. Deceleration injury to the cardiovascular system occurs as a result of sudden deceleration of the body at the time of impact, for instance, in a motor vehicle accident. The organs, including the heart and great vessels, still moving at the original velocity of the vehicle, strike the rib cage or spine, resulting in myocardial contusion and laceration. The vascular structures (veins, aorta, and great vessels) are variably restrained by the intercostal vessels and the great vessels of the arch, and differential movement at points of attachment can result in laceration.[6] The inferior vena cava as it penetrates the hiatus of the diaphragm and enters the right atrium represents such a point of possible differential movement and is the site of laceration. The exact mechanism of laceration of the aorta in motor vehicle accidents with steering-wheel injuries is still controversial. Originally it was thought that the heart continued to move and that the arch held by the great vessels was relatively stationary. For this reason, the most frequent sites of laceration would be at the root of the aorta where it is attached to the heart and at the distal arch near the ligamentus arteriosus, where differential movement would be the greatest. These are indeed the two most frequent sites of laceration. Animal experiments with dogs and primates subjected to sudden sternal compression similar to that seen in motor vehicle accidents with steering wheel injuries have shown, with high-speed arteriography, a marked displacement of the heart out of the middle mediastinum into the right or left chest, or markedly inferiorly or superiorly, thus placing great stress on the same sites.[7]

Finally, compressive injuries to the abdomen and lower extremities, such as those seen when a person is suddenly buried by a dirt slide, cause a marked compression of veins and arteries, causing a sudden increase in venous return to the heart. At the same moment, there is a marked increase in systemic vascular resistance, causing a marked impedance to left ventricular ejection. Together, these forces can cause ventricular, atrial, or even valvular rupture.

Another important feature of an injury is the exact time in the cardiac cycle where the injury is imposed. In animal experiments, it has been shown that myocardial contusion and laceration are much more likely to occur when the injury is delivered in diastole rather than in systole.[8] In diastole, the ventricular mass of the heart is greatest and the wall's firmness and elasticity are least. In systole, ventricular mass is smallest and the heart muscle is resilient and firm and capable of moving away from the force, thus limiting the distortion of the wall for any given force.

PATHOLOGIC CLASSIFICATION OF CARDIAC TRAUMA

Cardiovascular trauma can be divided into (1) penetrating injuries and (2) nonpenetrating injuries. Any cardiovascular structure can be injured, and although pericardial tamponade is more frequent in penetrating than in nonpenetrating injury, any structure—pericardium, atrium, ventricle, atrial and ventricular septa, papillary muscles, valves, coronary vessels, aorta, great arteries, and veins—can be contused or lacerated by either penetrating or nonpenetrating injuries. In 1958, Parmley, Manion, and Mattingly published their experience with nonpenetrating cardiovascular trauma from the Armed Forces Institute of Pathology, a referral point collecting specimens from all over the world contributed by Armed Forces hospitals, Veterans' Administration hospitals, and, more recently, from many other civilian sources and community and university hospitals.[9,10]

In any pathology collection, the types of trauma seen are weighted toward the most serious injuries, since death is the ticket by which the patients entered the study. For this reason, the most common lesion by far is laceration of cardiac chambers and myocardial contusion; only a small number of the other injuries to valves, ventricular septa, coronary arteries, and great vessels are seen. In a clinical practice, most patients with injury severe enough to cause chamber laceration will have multiple injuries and die. To be seen in a clinical series, the patient has to survive long enough to reach the emergency room. For this reason, clinical series from trauma centers will have a much larger percentage of suspected myocardial contusion and other less common injuries, such as valvular, coronary, and great vessel injuries.

THE ACUTELY INJURED PATIENT WITH THORACOABDOMINAL INJURY

The patient is frequently brought to the emergency room by ambulance. Typically with trauma sufficient to cause cardiac injury the patient has multiple system injuries. In the acutely injured patient, rapid assessment must be performed, evaluating the adequacy of airway and respiration, systemic blood pressure, and cardiac output. Presence of cyanosis, the type and depth of respiration, and the possible presence of tension pneumothorax should be rapidly assessed. Establishment of an adequate airway and respiration and gaseous exchange may require an airway, a tracheostomy, or intubation and assisted ventilation.[11]

If the patient has neither pulse nor blood pressure, cardiac resuscitation should be started, including the rapid establishment of large-bore intravenous access with at least two 16-gauge intravenous needles or catheters inserted. Crystalloids can be started but should be rapidly replaced by blood or colloids such as dextran until blood is obtained. This is especially important if blood loss is evident, but even without an obvious site of blood loss, 2 liters of fluid should be infused rapidly in the presence of shock.

Rapid assessment of venous pressure, either by inspection of the neck veins or measurement of central venous pressure by catheter, should be done. If central venous pressure is elevated and if a wound capable of resulting in cardiac tamponade is possible, a presumptive diagnosis should be made and acted upon.

Life-threatening arrhythmias should be immediately treated. If asystole is present, isoproterenol may be started while a temporary pacemaker is placed. If there is ventricular tachycardia or ventricular fibrillation, cardioversion or defibrillation with 200 to 400 wattseconds should be performed immediately.

Once respiratory and circulatory support is adequately established, a rapid history can be obtained. Details of the injury from the patient or witnesses should be ascertained, including descriptions of the time and place of the accident; the type of gun, knife, or other weapon responsible for the injury; the position of the patient in the motor vehicle (whether the patient was a driver or where in the vehicle the patient was sitting); and the type of accident (whether it was a head-on or rear-end collision). A past history of cardiovascular disease, such as angina or an old myocardial infarct, may be important. A history of drugs, alcohol, or medications that the patient may have been taking might explain arrhythmias or electrocardiographic changes. Similarly, a history of previously known heart murmurs might explain the presence of a heart murmur and thus avoid unnecessary diagnostic studies.

A rapid physical examination assessing the presence and site of contusions and entrance and exit wounds of missiles should be done.

Examination of the head and neck for cranial and cervical injury is especially important. Palpation for depressed cranial fractures should be performed, as well as examination for evidence of blood or spinal fluid in the nose or ear canal. The height of the central venous pressure; the presence of a point of maximal impulse (PMI) and abnormal ventricular lifts; pericardial friction rubs; the quality of the heart sounds; the presence of gallops, murmurs, and rales; and the presence of pulsus alternans or pulsus paradoxus should all be noted. Abdominal and extremity injury and the presence and adequacy of arterial pulses should be recorded. The color of the face (cyanosis, pallor) and extremities (rubor or pallor) can be clues to respiratory problems or to a recognition of peripheral arterial or venous injury. A rapid neurologic examination for the state of consciousness, cranial nerve abnormalities, pupillary and extraocular eye movements, movements and strength of all extremities, and the presence and quality of the tendon reflexes should be made.

Laboratory examination studies should include a hemoglobin, hematocrit, serum electrolytes, urinalysis, and arterial blood gases; a chest x-ray study looking for fractured ribs, sternum, clavicle, or spine, pneumomediastinum or pneumothorax, pleural effusion, pulmonary edema or contusion, the position and size of the cardiac silhouette, and width of the superior mediastinum, and sharpness of the aortic knob, evidence of abdominal contents above the diaphragm; and an abdominal flat plate looking for air under the diaphragm or air or fluid in the peritoneal cavity. If head injury is present, a computed tomography scan (if available) of the head should be obtained.

CARDIOVASCULAR INJURIES

Cardiac injury occurs in about 3% of all patients with thoracoabdominal wounds.[12] Mortality of penetrating wounds depends on the mechanism of injury, whether high or low velocity, as well as the accompanying injuries, and varies from 65% to 80%, with gunshot wounds being the most lethal.[13] Once the patient reaches the hospital alive, mortality varies from 5% to 30%.[14] With recent reports of penetrating cardiac wounds the mortality is still in the area of 30%.[15]

PENETRATING CARDIAC INJURY AND PERICARDIAL TAMPONADE

Pericardial tamponade is mostly seen with penetrating thoracic or upper abdominal injuries although occasionally it can be seen after nonpenetrating injury with laceration of a cardiac chamber or coronary artery or vein. Tamponade depends on a relatively intact pericardium and, therefore, is less often seen with marked disruption of the pericardium. In these cases the patient presents with hemothorax and exsanguination. Paradoxically, the presence of cardiac tamponade, most often due to laceration of the right ventricle or right atrium, results in a slowing down of the bleeding into the pericardium from those low-pressure chambers and maintenance of the circulation long enough for the patient to get to the hospital. Laceration of the left ventricle is more likely to result in severe tamponade and death. The presence of an elevated central venous pressure by examination or measurement in a person with a thoracoabdominal injury should be interpreted as possible cardiac tamponade. The differential diagnosis includes right heart failure as a result of right ventricular injury, with or without tricuspid insufficiency, and previous heart disease with right ventricular failure.

If the patient has a penetrating injury that could have caused tamponade and the patient is pulseless, in shock, or pulseless without blood pressure, a thoracotomy should be performed in the emergency room in order to have any hope of success.[14-17] Under these circumstances transportation to the operating room, with its attendant delay, dooms the patient. If the patient is hemodynamically stable but the central venous pressure is elevated with penetrating injury that could have caused tamponade, pericardiocentesis with a large-bore needle has been advocated. If the injury is a low-velocity injury with a small-bladed weapon, where slow bleeding and gradual tamponade have occurred, occasionally this will be successful definitive therapy. With rapid bleeding, intrapericardial blood clotting occurs, and the pericardiocentesis may be negative or inadequate, and tamponade frequently recurs even if it is initially successful. In a series of 459 cases of penetrating wounds of the heart, unsuccessful pericardiocentesis occurred 25% of the time.[13] For this reason, these patients are taken immediately to the operating room for thoracotomy for exploration of the pericardium and heart and suture of the laceration and ligation or repair of the bleeding arteries or veins.[16]

In pericardial tamponade the filling of the right ventricle is maintained only by increased venous pressure, which is initially generated by increased venous tone as a result of increased sympathetic nervous system activity and later by expansion of the blood volume. In this situation, if the patient is anesthetized and sympathetic tone withdrawn, cardiovascular collapse can occur.[14] For this reason, the patient's chest should be shaved, prepped, and draped, and the surgical team set for immediate thoracotomy before anesthesia is given.

Unlike cardiac tamponade occurring in the course of acute and chronic pericardial disease where the elevated central venous pressure is always present as the first sign of developing tamponade, in the acutely injured patient where the intravascular volume may be low due to hemorrhage, pericardial tamponade may manifest itself only by a marked drop in stroke volume and blood pressure; the neck veins may not be visible. For this reason, in a thoracoabdominal injury where pericardial tamponade is possible, rapid blood replacement should be given, and if the blood pressure doesn't return toward normal after estimated blood loss is replaced, thoracotomy should be done since tamponade is frequently the cause. In most instances where blood replacement is adequate, the neck veins become distended and the blood pressure may still remain low where tamponade is present.[18,19]

With penetrating cardiac injury on presentation to the emergency room, three categories of patients have been defined predicting the management and mortality[20]:

1. The lifeless, pulseless patient without blood pressure. These patients should have emergency thoracotomy. They have a reported mortality of about 50%,[16] which is also our experience at San Francisco General Hospital.
2. The hypotensive patient with progressive hemorrhage and acute tamponade. This is the most frequent group requiring immediate pericardiocentesis or thoracotomy, or both, with a resultant mortality of about 25%.[16]
3. The normotensive patient with a cardiac wound that has spontaneously sealed, without tamponade or with only a gradually progressive tamponade. This is the least common presentation. With proper recognition and treatment, the patients have a very low mortality.

A note of caution is necessary in the acutely injured patient who has received massive amounts of fluids and blood during the resuscitation: if there has been over-replacement of fluid or if there is preexisting cardiac disease, right ventricular infarction, or myocardial contusion, the patient may develop an elevated central venous pressure on the basis of overtransfusion or myocardial failure. Where there is overtransfusion in a patient with a normal heart, there are frequently rales, a third heart sound, and a murmur of tricuspid or mitral insufficiency. On measurement, the cardiac output is higher than normal, and the stroke volume is excellent with bounding pulses with a normal or high systolic blood pressure. When myocardial failure is present, the pulse may be thready and small with other signs of failure, such as rales and pulmonary congestion on chest x-ray, pulsus alternans, and an S_3 gallop. In these situations an echocardiogram can be extraordinarily helpful for differential diagnosis, demonstrating fluid in the pericardium, signs of tamponade, such as collapse of right atrium or right ventricle, and good left ventricular contraction in the case of tamponade and poor ventricular contraction with or without fluid in the pericardium in the case of myocardial injury.

OTHER PERICARDIAL INJURY

Laceration of the pericardium with rupture of a portion or of the entire heart into the left pleural cavity has been seen. Often trauma severe enough to cause herniation of the heart is associated with massive cardiac laceration and is usually fatal. It is not unusual to find laceration of the pericardium incidentally at the time of surgery or angioplasty. Occasionally, just laceration of the pericardium with herniation of the heart is seen. From 1937 to 1982, 142 cases were found in the literature, with 99 survivors.[21] Pericardial laceration with cardiac herniation can be suspected by physical examination with displacement of the point of maximal impulse to the left and displacement of the cardiac silhouette into the left chest. On chest x-ray film, if laceration with herniation is diagnosed, thoracotomy with replacement of the heart and repair of the pericardium should be done. If there is no displacement of the heart, usually the diagnosis is not made, but in the absence of bleeding or other evidence of compromise, no treatment is needed. If a portion of the heart such as the left atrial appendage is herniated, repair is imperative since the heart can herniate and become incarcerated.[22]

Pericarditis is not uncommon with acute injury and is manifested by chest pain, frequently pleuritic, and a pericardial friction rub with or without tamponade. On echocardiography, fluid may be, but is not necessarily, present. In the absence of pericardial tamponade or severe pain no treatment is necessary. If pain is present, analgesics and anti-inflammatory agents, such as aspirin or indomethacin, are frequently effective.

The late development of pericarditis or so-called post-traumatic pericarditis is not uncommon and is probably related to autoimmune injury due to trauma to the heart and pericardium with development of antibodies and then antibody–antigen complement fixation with pericardial injury.[23] This can occur from five days to six months post-injury, can result in pericardial effusion and even tamponade, and can be recurrent.

Most often blood in the pericardium is quickly resorbed without residual damage. On occasion, pericardial injury probably associated with bleeding and extensive tissue necrosis can later result in a thickened, constrictive pericarditis presenting months or years later.[24] If constrictive pericarditis with or without calcification is present and hemodynamically significant, pericardiectomy should be performed.

CARDIAC LACERATION

Cardiac laceration is usually the result of penetrating injury although it can occur with nonpenetrating trauma (Figs. 107.1 to 107.4). The chambers most vulnerable to laceration, because of their positions, are the right ventricle and intracardiac portion of the great vessels in 40% to 60% of cases, left ventricle, and then right atrium. The left atrium is the least often lacerated.[15,16,19,25]

Earlier reports indicated that stab wounds to the heart were the most frequent causes of lacerations seen clinically. In later series, gunshot wounds are becoming more frequent.[25] With laceration of the thin-walled, low-pressure, right atrium and right ventricle with subsequent tamponade, there is often a slowing and cessation of bleeding, allowing for longer survival and, therefore, greater opportunity for definitive therapy. With relief of the pericardial tamponade by needle aspiration, however, there is danger of bleeding restarting, and frequently tamponade recurs. With a simple small perforation, it is true that a laceration may stop bleeding and be treatable by pericardiocentesis. However, most often it is necessary to suture the laceration through open thoracotomy.

Suture of a laceration of the ventricle leaves a scar, which, if small enough, will not interfere with ventricular function. If the injury is large enough, or if a coronary artery is damaged, a true aneurysm can result at the site of laceration repair. If the laceration continues to bleed but the clot is contained by adherent pericardium, a false aneurysm can result (Figs. 107.1 to 107.4). When these are found, repair is essential since late rupture can occur.

MYOCARDIAL CONTUSION

Myocardial contusion is most frequently seen in civilian life as a result of motor vehicle accidents, and it is certainly the most frequent cardiovascular trauma seen at the present time. The term *myocardial contusion* implies myocardial necrosis with or without hemorrhage into the myocardium. For many years it has been recognized that fatal arrhythmias can occur with sudden chest injury as a result of a blow or sudden compression. Postmortem examinations in these cases may reveal no

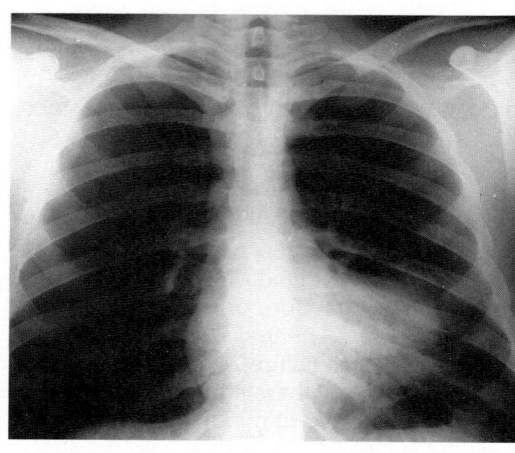

FIGURE 107.1 Chest roentgenogram, posteroanterior view, one month after injury. The patient was a 20-year-old man, stabbed in the left chest. A 2-cm laceration of the left ventricle was repaired by primary suture in an emergency thoracotomy. Notice the bulge along the left cardiac border. (Fowler NO: Cardiac Diagnosis and Treatment, 3rd ed. Hagerstown, MD, Harper & Row, 1980)

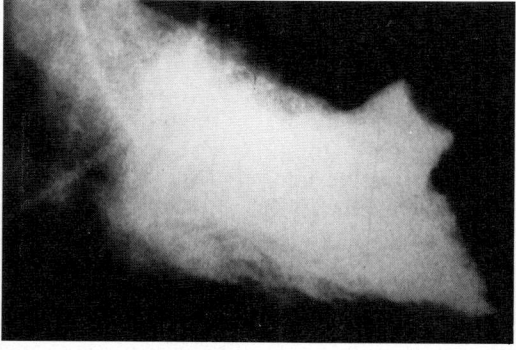

FIGURE 107.2 Frame from a cineangiogram, injection in left ventricle, right anterior oblique view (same patient as in Fig. 107.1). Ventricle is in diastole. Note the protruding lumen of the false aneurysm. This was present both in systole and diastole. The outer wall of the false aneurysm is not seen. (Fowler NO: Cardiac Diagnosis and Treatment, 3rd ed. Hagerstown, MD, Harper & Row, 1980)

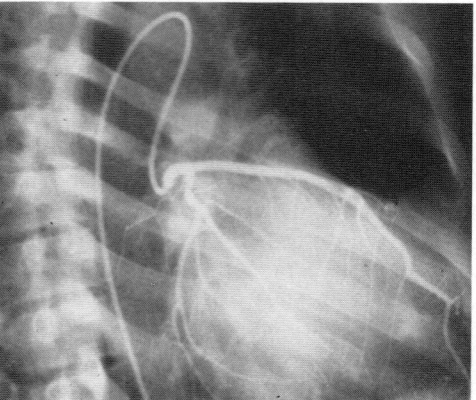

FIGURE 107.3 Coronary arteriogram, right anterior oblique view (same patient as in Fig. 107.1). Injection into the left coronary artery. Note abrupt cutoff of diagonal branch (*arrow*) due to ligation of bleeding artery at surgery. Note absence of vessels over false aneurysm. (Fowler NO: Cardiac Diagnosis and Treatment, 3rd ed. Hagerstown, MD, Harper & Row, 1980)

injury to the myocardium. With contusion, hemorrhage into the myocardial tissue might be expected, but in these cases there may be no sign at all of myocardial injury. Such cases have been referred to as *commotio cordis* and are probably the result of low energy imparted to the ventricle at a vulnerable time in the cardiac cycle, causing ventricular tachycardia and ventricular fibrillation.[26,27]

INCIDENCE

The true incidence of myocardial contusion is unknown. In patients dying after major thoracoabdominal trauma, the autopsy incidence of myocardial contusion is about 15%.[28] In other series the incidence reported has been 9% to 76%.[29,30] Myocardial contusion is undoubtedly more common than we suspect, but since there is no "gold standard" for the diagnosis in the patient who survives, we do not truly know the incidence.

CLINICAL PICTURE

Myocardial contusion occurs as the result of a direct blow to the myocardium due to compressive injury or to the heart's striking the chest cage in a deceleration or acceleration injury. In either case, intramyocardial hemorrhage and necrosis occur. The consequence of this necrosis with release of potassium, myocardial enzymes, and other intracellular contents into the interstitial space results in problems similar to those seen with myocardial necrosis due to myocardial infarction caused by coronary artery disease. These complications are arrhythmias, myocardial rupture, myocardial dysfunction with congestive heart failure, and ventricular aneurysm.

The patient likely to have myocardial contusion usually has had severe compressive or crushing injury or been in a deceleration or acceleration accident.[31,32] The "steering wheel injury" is the most common cause of myocardial contusion in the United States. There is frequently multisystem trauma and not infrequently multiple fractured ribs.[33] It has been said that patients with fracture of the sternum or of the first or second ribs are most likely to have cardiac trauma.[34] Other crush injuries, such as being struck by a ball, crushed against a wall, or crushed under a log or under a fallen car or other object, have also been reported. Although it is common that there be obvious chest wall injury such as bruises or lacerations, it is also not uncommon for cardiac contusion to be present with little sign of external injury to the chest or precordial area. This is especially true in deceleration injuries where at speeds as low as 20 mph myocardial contusion can occur with no signs of external chest wall injury.[30]

DIAGNOSIS

The diagnosis can most easily be made when there are signs of myocardial necrosis and cardiac dysfunction that are new for the patient following an appropriate degree of trauma. The patient may have no physical findings indicating cardiac damage. There may be a pericardial friction rub. If myocardial damage is severe, signs of heart failure may be present, including pulmonary rales and S_3 gallop, small pulse pressure consistent with a decreased stroke volume, pulsus alternans, elevation in central venous pressure with right ventricular injury, or the murmur of tricuspid or mitral insufficiency with cardiac dilatation. Chest pain is common but is usually confused with chest wall pain due to the injury. Others have described discomfort consistent with angina, but it is always difficult to differentiate pain due to myocardial contusion from angina in a patient with underlying coronary artery disease who now has increased myocardial oxygen demand because of tachycardia, hypertension, and increased sympathetic tone and catecholamines post-trauma. The chest x-ray film can be helpful in demonstrating injury to the chest wall cage, multiple rib fractures, or fracture of the sternum, all of which are frequently seen with myocardial contusion. If there is marked left ventricular dysfunction, Kerley-B lines, pulmonary vascular redistribution, and even pulmonary edema can be seen. If myocardial laceration has occurred or in instances of old myocardial contusion, occasionally the distortion of the cardiac silhouette consistent with ventricular aneurysm can be seen (see Fig. 107.1). Distortion of the cardiac silhouette can be due to adhesions after thoracic injury so definitive studies such as echocardiography, radioisotope angiography, computed tomography, or cardiac angiography are necessary before making the diagnosis of aneurysm (Fig. 107.5).

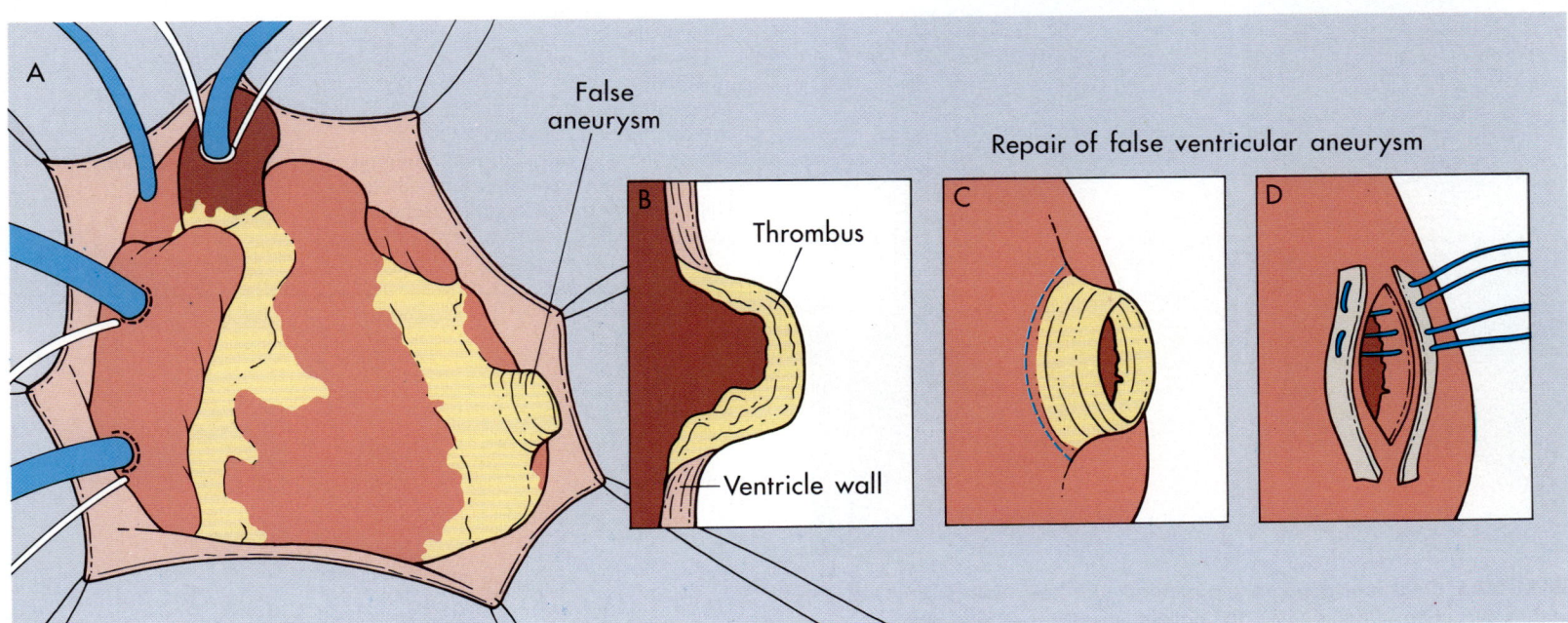

FIGURE 107.4 Drawing of findings at surgical repair of false aneurysm of the left ventricle (same patient as Fig. 107.1). Sutures from the original repair of the left ventricular laceration had torn loose. Organized thrombus and collagen formed the wall of the aneurysm (W). (LV, left ventricular wall; C, organized thrombus.) Repair accomplished by mattress sutures with Teflon bolstering strips. (Modified from Fowler NO: Cardiac Diagnosis and Treatment, 3rd ed. Hagerstown, Harper & Row, 1980)

LABORATORY DATA
ELECTROCARDIOGRAPHIC CHANGES
The electrocardiogram may demonstrate signs of an acute myocardial injury with ST segment elevation, T wave inversion, and even Q wave formation, all consistent with an acute myocardial infarction.[28,29] In these cases there is again difficulty in separating contusion from an acute myocardial infarction with underlying coronary artery disease. Also, rarely, the coronary artery can be contused and an intra-arterial clot formed, creating an acute myocardial infarction. More commonly, the electrocardiogram shows only nonspecific ST wave changes or only T wave changes.[30]

ARRHYTHMIAS
Arrhythmias are also common, and although premature ventricular contractions are the most common arrhythmia, every conceivable arrhythmia has been described: all of the atrial and ventricular tachyarrhythmias, including idioventricular rhythms, atrial and ventricular tachycardia, and atrial and ventricular fibrillation, as well as conduction defects, such as right and left bundle branch block, and all degrees of atrioventricular block and all types of fascicular block, as well as simply prolonged QT interval.[29,30]

The presence of arrhythmias after severe abdominal or thoracic trauma occurs in approximately three fourths of patients when monitored and has been reported as evidence of the frequency of myocardial contusion.[35] Unfortunately, there are many possible causes of arrhythmia and electrocardiographic changes after trauma (Table 107.1) other than myocardial contusion. The presence of serious ventricular arrhythmias after trauma is important enough, especially if associated with other signs of myocardial dysfunction, to justify monitoring the patient in an intensive care unit for 24 to 48 hours. Arrhythmias such as ventricular tachycardia or ventricular fibrillation, as well as less important arrhythmias such as atrial flutter and atrial fibrillation, are managed in the same way they would be when occurring after a myocardial infarction. With hemodynamic instability, electrical cardioversion is mandatory. Without hemodynamic instability, medical management with appropriate antiarrhythmic drugs should be carried out. Lesser arrhythmias such as premature atrial contractions, short bursts of paroxysmal atrial tachycardia, or premature ventricular contractions need be treated only if the arrhythmia is causing symptoms or if the arrhythmia is associated with ventricular dysfunction. If the patient is asymptomatic, then treatment has not been shown to be necessary.

CARDIAC ENZYMES
Serum glutamic oxaloacetic transaminase (SGOT), lactate dehydrogenase (LDH), creatine kinase (CK), and CK isoenzymes are all frequently elevated after acute trauma. The most specific enzyme for myocardial necrosis is that of MB isomer of creatine kinase (CK-MB). In a series of 78 patients with blunt thoracic trauma, 24% had serum MB-CK $\geq$ 6% of total CK activity; 36% had $\leq$6% MB-CK; and 40% had no CK-MB activity. Electrocardiographic changes occurred in 89% of the patients with an elevated CK-MB and in 32% of patients without elevated CK-MB. Eleven patients died, and five had macroscopic cardiac injury. All five of these patients had had serum MB-CK activity.[36]

The presence of MB isoenzyme is not pathognomonic of myocardial injury, however, since it is also found in other tissues, especially small bowel, urinary bladder, and liver, and in small amounts in skeletal muscle and other tissues.[37] If skeletal muscle injury is extensive, the MB isoenzyme of CK can be elevated also. For practical purposes, if the MB isoenzyme of CK is elevated in the presence of other evidence of myocardial contusion, this must be considered as good evidence for the presence of myocardial contusion.[36,38]

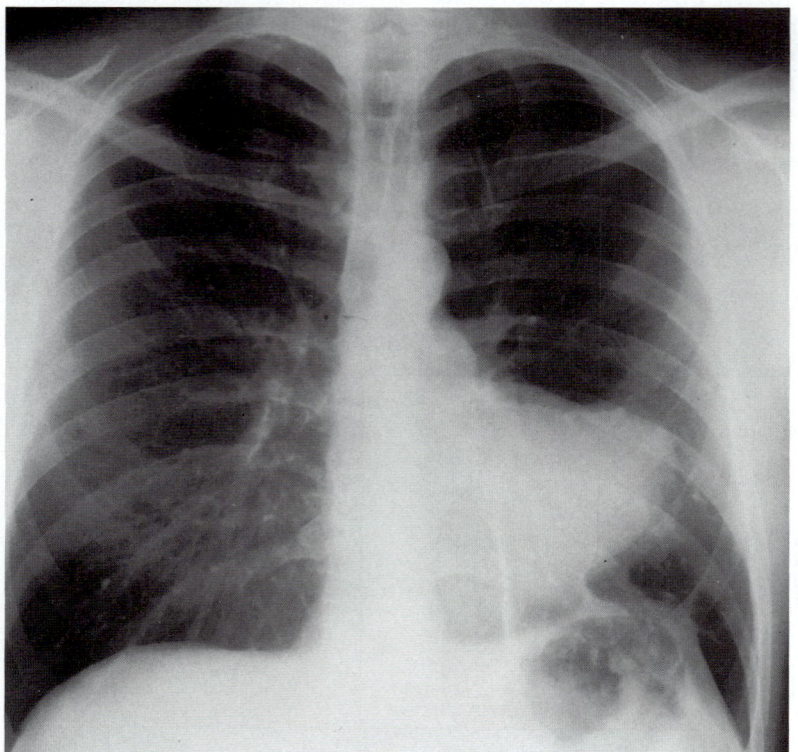

FIGURE 107.5 Chest roentgenogram, posteroanterior view. Note similarity of cardiac silhouette to Figure 107.1. The patient was a 33-year-old man, stabbed in the left chest. This film was taken 2 weeks after injury. On catheterization there were no coronary artery injuries, and ventriculography showed normal right and left ventricular chambers in systole and diastole. The cardiac silhouette distortion is due to adhesions and old hematoma after thoracotomy.

TABLE 107.1 CAUSES OF ARRHYTHMIA AFTER TRAUMA

Contusion
Electrolyte shifts (potassium, magnesium)
Blood gas alterations
    Hypoxia
    Hypercarbia
    Acidosis
Drugs and alcohol
Preexisting heart disease
Catecholamine and autonomic nervous system stimulation, both sympathetic and parasympathetic
Hypotension and myocardial ischemia
Central nervous system injury

ECHOCARDIOGRAPHY

M-mode echocardiography is not very helpful in detecting a myocardial contusion. Two-dimensional echocardiography, which can visualize a large percentage of the left ventricle and right ventricle, is much more likely to be helpful. In animal experiments, myocardial contusion results in hypokinesis or akinesis of that segment of the injured wall.[39] There is a lack of systolic thickening and even diastolic expansion in the area of contusion. There tends also to be a change in myocardial echodensity, possibly due to hemorrhage or edema, and even a thickening of the wall with diastole, possibly due to edema.[39,40] An approximate ejection fraction can be calculated by the two-dimensional echo and can be helpful in estimating ventricular function.

How good the two-dimensional echo will be in ruling out myocardial contusion is not known. The presence of a wall motion abnormality is not pathognomonic of myocardial contusion. It could be due, for instance, to underlying cardiac disease. In the study by King and his associates,[41] of 1771 consecutive trauma victims hospitalized, 147 had clinical evidence of blunt chest trauma. Three had unequivocal evidence of myocardial trauma, and all three had elevated CK-MB isoenzyme. Of 144 patients, 121 had an elevated CK, and 15 had identifiable CK-MB fraction elevation. Two-dimensional echocardiograms were done on these 15 patients, and seven had abnormalities (47%), six with wall motion abnormalities and one with a pericardial effusion.

If a ventricular aneurysm is present, this can usually be detected by two-dimensional echo.

RADIOISOTOPE ANGIOGRAPHY

Blood pool studies with technetium-99 pyrophosphate red cell labeling can be done noninvasively.[42] With this technique, the ejection fraction can be obtained as well as wall motion abnormalities localized including ventricular aneurysms.[43,44] This technique is less likely to be helpful in the emergency room and more likely to be helpful on the wards. Sutherland and co-workers[45] reported 77 patients with multisystem trauma, including severe blunt chest injury, prospectively evaluated by radionuclide angiography. No patient had a clinical history of heart disease. Of these patients, 42 (53%) had focal abnormalities of wall motion, 27 involving right ventricle, 7 left ventricle, and 7 biventricular, and only one involving the septum. Ejection fractions were lower in those with than in those without wall motion abnormalities. Repeat scintigraphic examination at a later date showed improvement or resolution of abnormalities in 84% of the patients.

TECHNETIUM-TAGGED PYROPHOSPHATE SCANNING

^{99m}Technetium-tagged pyrophosphate or "hot spot" scanning is useful in detecting areas of myocardial necrosis. The pyrophosphate forms an apatite with calcium in necrotic tissue, thereby tagging it with radioisotope. This area of increased radioactivity is detected by scintillation cameras and can be localized to specific areas of the heart.[44,46] In experimental animals, this has been a useful way of localizing and quantifying myocardial contusion[47] while in humans it has been less helpful, apparently because of the frequency of chest wall injury and necrosis, all of which also can concentrate pyrophosphate. In experimental myocardial contusion, pyrophosphate sequestration in contused myocardium occurs within two hours.[47] Since right ventricular injury is most common and since the right ventricle is applied closely to the sternum, it is possible that this injury would be frequently missed and interpreted as chest wall, not myocardial, injury.

MAGNETIC IMAGING AND COMPUTED TOMOGRAPHY SCANNING

Whether magnetic imaging and computed tomography (CT) scanning will be helpful in detecting myocardial contusion is unknown. With the ability to detect myocardial edema and hemorrhage with nuclear magnetic resonance (NMR) and a change in density of myocardium with CT scanning, it is likely to be a useful technique for the identification of myocardial contusion where it is available.

To really test the value of all these tests in identifying myocardial contusion, a prospective study where these tests were done and then the heart pathologically examined would be necessary. Because of the relative infrequency of these traumatic problems and the low incidence of death after survival for a time in the hospital, there are few studies with significant numbers of autopsies. The best of these studies is that of Potkin and associates[35] who did electrocardiograms, 24-hour electrocardiograms, CK-MB enzymes, and pyrophosphate scanning on over 100 consecutive patients with significant abdominal or thoracic trauma. They found that 70% had ECG changes, 73% had a dysrhythmia on 24-hour ECG monitoring, 27% had Lown grade 3 or more arrhythmias, 72% had CK-MB > 6 units, 27% had CK-MB $\geq$ 2% of total CK-MB, and 2% had positive pyrophosphate scans. Only 15 patients died but none of cardiovascular trauma. At autopsy, five had myocardial contusion and ten did not. There were no differences in ECG or rhythm abnormalities, CK-MB, or pyrophosphate scanning between those with and those without myocardial contusion at autopsy.

MANAGEMENT

Myocardial contusion should be suspected where the traumatic incident is severe enough to be possibly associated with contusion. It is important to be particularly suspicious of all patients with multiple rib fractures and sternal fractures. One must look for signs of myocardial injury by changes in cardiac function or the presence of a pericardial friction rub. Electrocardiograms, a long rhythm strip, and CK-MB isoenzymes every 6 hours for three times should be obtained. If there is clinical suspicion of cardiac contusion or abnormal ECG or CK-MB elevation, a two-dimensional echo should be obtained. The patient should be monitored for 24 to 48 hours in an intensive care unit.

If there is the possibility of severe cardiac dysfunction with failure, for instance, pulmonary rales, interstitial pulmonary congestion or edema on chest x-ray film, poor myocardial contraction by echo, or decreased ejection fraction by echo or radioisotope angiogram, then the patient should be managed with hemodynamic monitoring using a Swan-Ganz catheter placed in the pulmonary artery. Hemodynamic monitoring makes it possible to differentiate pulmonary contusion, where the pulmonary artery wedge pressure is low, from myocardial contusion and congestive heart failure where the pulmonary artery wedge pressure would be high. If the right atrial and right ventricular filling pressure is high and the pulmonary artery wedge pressure is normal, the diagnosis of right ventricular contusion can be made.

Treatment should be considered for symptomatic arrhythmias or those causing hemodynamic instability. The effects of poor left ventricular function, such as pulmonary edema or low cardiac output, should be treated. The treatment of myocardial dysfunction and pulmonary congestion is similar to the treatment of poor left ventricular function with acute myocardial infarction and may require diuretics and preload and afterload reduction, as well as inotropic agents, such as dopamine and dobutamine. The use of these drugs is dictated by the measured hemodynamic parameters of left ventricular function and the effects of the drugs evaluated immediately by remeasuring these hemodynamics.

PROGNOSIS AND LATE COMPLICATIONS

Contusion or laceration can result in an area of myocardial fibrosis with akinesia or hypokinesia or even ventricular aneurysm (see Figs. 107.1 to 107.4) similar to that seen after an acute myocardial infarction. Most of these patients do very well if they survive the first few days. Extensive cardiac damage sufficient to cause chronic congestive heart failure can occur, but this is distinctly unusual. Most patients with myocardial injury that extreme do not survive the initial hospitalization. Those who do survive frequently compensate for the myocardial damage very well. In general, the prognosis is better for a given degree of myocardial injury after contusion than the same amount of myocardial damage after an acute myocardial infarction. Trauma patients are for the most part young with normal hearts before the trauma and do not have extensive coronary artery disease that could be the source of problems in the future. At San Francisco General Hospital we have found that once the patient has survived the first few days after myocardial contusion, there have been very few late, functionally important sequelae. Whether arrhythmias can be established permanently as a result of myocardial contusion is not known. However, there is no reason why localized myocardial damage, for whatever reason, could not change the sequence of depolarization and repolarization in such a way as to allow for the development of reentrant or automatic rhythms.

INTRACARDIAC INJURIES

Although the individual lesions will be discussed as separate entities, it is not infrequent that several intracardiac injuries coexist, for instance, injury to the aortic valve and an aortic-to-right-ventricular fistula or a ventricular septal defect, mitral insufficiency, and so forth. The combination of lesions lends its own findings and pathophysiologic problems to the patient's clinical picture. It is also not unusual for one lesion with striking physical findings, such as a ventricular septal defect and a loud systolic murmur, to overshadow a second important injury, such as mitral insufficiency. For this reason, with any intracardiac injury, a complete study with right and left heart catheterization is necessary before surgery. How this may change with the information obtained with two-dimensional echocardiography, Doppler techniques, and rapid CT scanning is unknown, but at the present time, complete catheterization and angiography should be done before surgery is undertaken.

SEPTAL DEFECTS

Both atrial septum and ventricular septum can be ruptured with either penetrating or nonpenetrating injuries.[48-50] Probably because of its protected position behind the sternum, the atrial septum is much less often involved than the ventricular septum. Another factor making atrial septal defect difficult to detect is the relative benignity of the physical findings in atrial septal defect. With a left-to-right shunt at the atrial level, there is a right ventricular volume overload causing right ventricular hyperactivity, but the murmur that develops is mainly a systolic ejection murmur over the right ventricular outflow tract related to the increased right ventricular stroke volume. The other important physical finding is the widely split S_2, again related to the large right ventricular stroke volume, but how soon this develops after acute production of an atrial septal defect in the adult is not known. It is possible that the widely split S_2 results from the large capacity pulmonary arteries and delay in "hang out" time to close and tense the pulmonary valve, resulting in the delayed P_2. This enlargement of capacitance of pulmonary arteries takes time to develop; it is not present when the atrial septal defect is acutely formed.

Rupture of the ventricular septum can occur at any place in the septum with penetrating injuries.[48,49] With nonpenetrating injuries, resulting mainly from crush or deceleration accidents, the ventricular septum is either immediately lacerated or ruptures later as a consequence of myocardial contusion with necrosis of the ventricular septum.[50] In this circumstance the development of the rupture can occur three days to a week or even two after the injury.

With interventricular septal rupture, there is the development of a left-to-right shunt, the magnitude of which is determined by the size of the defect and the relative resistance of the two circuits, the pulmonary vascular and the systemic vascular beds. Since the patient is usually normal before injury, the pulmonary vascular resistance is normal, that is, very low compared to the systemic vascular resistance. For this reason, the left-to-right shunt tends to be large even with relatively small defects. The left-to-right shunt increases pulmonary blood flow and, therefore, volume-loads the left ventricle. If the defect is large enough, the pressures in the right ventricle and left ventricle must equilibrate, and the volume of the shunt and pulmonary blood flow are determined by the relative resistances of the circuits. If the defect is very large, the lungs are flooded, the left ventricle fails, and the patient has pulmonary edema and usually dies.

If the shunt is smaller and the pulmonary blood flow is on the order of two to three times systemic blood flow, the left ventricle can usually handle this marked increase in flow and sustain forward stroke volume as well as the large left-to-right shunt, with or without signs of congestive heart failure.

The diagnostic clue to this problem is the development of a new systolic murmur at some time after the injury. Location of the murmur depends on the site of the defect and the direction of the jet. The murmur is often at the left sternal border but may be closer to or at the apex, depending on where the defect is in the septum. The murmur is most often regurgitant, pansystolic, and loud, usually accompanied by a systolic thrill. The loudness of the pulmonic second sound depends on the pulmonary artery pressure, which is determined by the size of the defect, the volume of the left-to-right shunt, and the pulmonary vascular resistance. If the pulmonary artery pressure is high, then the pulmonic second sound will be increased, and in addition to left ventricular overactivity, there will be a right ventricular lift along the left sternal border and precordium.

The chest x-ray film frequently shows pulmonary congestion or pulmonary edema and may show increase in all pulmonary vascular markings because of the left-to-right shunt. The electrocardiogram is of little diagnostic help, but the two-dimensional echocardiogram can make the diagnosis with increase in left ventricular volume, possibly increase in left atrial size, increase in the size of the right ventricular outflow tract, and enlargement of the major pulmonary arteries. With a bubble-contrast study, a jet of unopacified blood can be seen to enter the right ventricular blood pool opacified by the cloud of injected microbubbles; thus, the location and size of the defect can be approximated rather well.

Treatment of this problem depends on the size of the shunt and on whether the cardiac function is being compromised. If the shunt is small, there may be no congestive heart failure. Conventional management with digitalis and diuretics will frequently be all that is necessary in the patient with mild congestive heart failure. If the patient is in severe congestive heart failure, preload and afterload reduction with nitroprusside can be extremely useful, decreasing left atrial pressure and even the size of the left-to-right shunt by decreasing the systemic vascular resistance. Others have recommended intra-aortic balloon pumping with reduction of left ventricular systolic impedance and decrease in the left-to-right shunt. If this is necessary as a temporizing procedure, then the patient needs surgery.

Since these defects are known to decrease spontaneously in size or even to close, if the patient is hemodynamically stable, a period of medical management is indicated.[51] If the patient fails to respond to medical management as outlined above, surgical closure of the ventricular septal defect is recommended. If the left-to-right shunt continues to be large or the patient is functionally impaired by the large shunt over a period of 3 to 6 months, elective closure of the defect is indicated.

VALVULAR INJURIES

Any valve can be damaged by either penetrating or nonpenetrating injury with the development of varying degrees of valvular insufficiency. In penetrating injuries the pulmonary valve is more frequently injured than in nonpenetrating injuries where it is rarely involved. In nonpenetrating injury the aortic, tricuspid, and mitral valves can all be torn. In my experience, in mitral insufficiency the papillary muscles are torn more often than the valve leaflet is ruptured. In aortic valve injury, the leaflet itself is torn, either at or behind the leading edge of the cusp, most frequently near the commissure.

The hemodynamic consequences of valvular injury are those of acute valvular insufficiency. With acute valvular insufficiency, the regurgitant volume increases the diastolic size of the ventricle. With increase in the ventricular volume without time for ventricular hypertrophy, wall stress is increased, and congestive heart failure occurs. The sudden increase in the ventricular volume within the noncompliant pericardium results in further elevation in ventricular diastolic filling pressure and atrial pressure. The actual increase in ventricular and atrial volume acutely is small enough so that the cardiac size on chest roentgenogram may not increase markedly and actually may still be within normal limits. Venous hypertension and congestion, however, are frequent in the face of the apparently "normal" cardiac size, resulting in the clinical picture of acute valvular insufficiency.

TRICUSPID INSUFFICIENCY

With tricuspid insufficiency the compliance of the right atrium and systemic veins makes for varying degrees of elevation of the cervical venous wave. With wide open tricuspid insufficiency, the v wave can be dramatic.[52] With lesser degrees, the v wave may just be more prominent than the a wave, which is distinctly abnormal, but the overall venous pressure may not be elevated. Since the right atrial–systemic venous bed is very compliant, there can be significant tricuspid insufficiency with or without significant elevation in the venous pressure.[52]

The murmur of tricuspid insufficiency is variable, from the typical pansystolic murmur along the left sternal border, which may or may not increase with inspiration, to a systolic ejection murmur along the left sternal border, to no murmur at all. On palpation the volume-loaded right ventricle may cause parasternal precordial lift. Echocardiography can help make the diagnosis by demonstrating enlargement of the right ventricle and right atrium with paradoxical motion of the ventricular septum, especially on the M-mode echocardiogram.[53,54] Doppler echocardiography can be very helpful in finding the presence of tricuspid insufficiency when the diagnosis is obscure.

Repair of the tricuspid valve is necessary only if the patient has signs, after treatment, of the consequences of severe elevation of the systemic venous pressure such as hepatomegaly with liver function abnormalities, ascites, or intractable peripheral edema. Also, if there is any left heart disease or increase in pulmonary vascular resistance, the forward flow through the lungs may be impaired and the left ventricular output will be limited. If these persist after conventional medical management, the tricuspid valve can be repaired or, if necessary, replaced.

MITRAL VALVE INSUFFICIENCY

In nonpenetrating injury, mitral valve insufficiency is often a consequence of left ventricular wall or papillary muscle damage.[55] It is suspected by the development of a pansystolic murmur at some time after the trauma. If papillary muscle rupture has occurred, the murmur can appear immediately. If there is necrosis of the left ventricular wall or papillary muscle, or both, without rupture, the murmur can appear later. The diagnosis is suspected by the development of a systolic murmur. The signs are those of mitral insufficiency with a hyperactive, volume-loaded left ventricle. The consequences are those of left ventricular failure with an increased left atrial and pulmonary capillary pressure with or without the ability to increase effective forward cardiac output.[56] Echocardiography can help quantify the degree of mitral insufficiency by showing enlargement of the left ventricle and left atrium and now by Doppler techniques, demonstrating the extent of the penetration into the left atrium of the regurgitant jet. If the insufficiency is minimal, no treatment other than antibiotic prophylaxis to prevent infective endocarditis is indicated. If the mitral insufficiency is severe, medical management including digitalis, diuretics, and nitroprusside for preload and afterload reduction is indicated. If the patient has severe mitral insufficiency and does not respond rapidly to the measures listed above, then surgery, usually with mitral valve replacement, is indicated.[56,57]

AORTIC VALVE INSUFFICIENCY

Aortic insufficiency results from a tear of one or more of the aortic cusps.[58] The degree of aortic insufficiency is variable but is usually severe. The findings are typical of acute aortic insufficiency, that is, the diastolic murmur of aortic insufficiency along the left sternal border and the peripheral signs of aortic insufficiency. These signs are minimal if the leak is small. If the degree of aortic insufficiency is severe and acute, some of the peripheral signs of severe aortic insufficiency will be masked by the decrease in forward stroke volume and by the high left ventricular filling pressure; for instance, the systolic blood pressure may not be high and the diastolic pressure may not be very low because it cannot drop lower than the elevated left ventricular end-diastolic pressure.[59] Since the left ventricle is filling from both the left atrium and aorta, the left ventricular filling pressure rapidly increases during diastole, frequently exceeding the left atrial pressure in mid-diastole and closing the mitral valve prematurely. This early closure of the mitral valve can be detected on two-dimensional echocardiography. The consequence of this is the muffling of the first heart sound with severe elevations in left ventricular filling pressure, left atrial and pulmonary capillary pressure elevation, and the physical and roentgenographic signs of pulmonary congestion and edema. The pulmonary artery pressure is also increased, and there may be a loud pulmonic second sound and even right heart failure. With tachycardia, the loud pulmonic second sound and the short, lower-pitched diastolic murmur may be mistaken for a first heart sound and a systolic ejection murmur. For this reason, listening to the murmur and simultaneously feeling the pulse or watching the electrocardiogram is important when a patient is found to have a murmur post-traumatically to make sure of the proper timing of the murmur.

With severe acute aortic insufficiency, the collapsing quality of the carotid pulse and the to-and-fro murmur on compression of the femoral artery (Duroziez's sign) still should be present even without other signs that are dependent on the wide pulse pressure. Echocardiography and Doppler cardiography can be helpful in identifying the presence of aortic sufficiency and quantifying it, as can radioisotope nuclear angiography in estimating the magnitude of the regurgitant volume.

Treatment depends on the magnitude of the aortic insufficiency. If it is minimal, no treatment may be necessary. If left ventricular failure has occurred, conventional treatment with diuretics and digitalis is sufficient at times. If the patient is in acute pulmonary edema, preload and afterload reduction with nitroprusside is frequently helpful. In this problem, aortic balloon counterpulsation is contraindicated. If the patient responds to medical management and the degree of aortic insufficiency is not severe, the patient should be managed as for aortic insufficiency from other causes. If the aortic insufficiency is massive and has produced the clinical picture of acute aortic insufficiency, valve replacement should be done as soon as possible.[58]

PULMONIC VALVULAR INSUFFICIENCY

The pulmonary valve is very rarely injured in nonpenetrating trauma but can be lacerated in penetrating wounds. Laceration of the pulmonic valve results in pulmonic valvular insufficiency characterized by the typical murmur and signs of right ventricular volume overload. In the presence of normal pulmonary arterial pressure, the murmur of pulmonic valvular insufficiency starts after the aortic component of the second heart sound and is perceptibly separated from it. Because the diastolic pressure gradient between the pulmonary artery and the right ventricle is small, the murmur tends to be low-pitched, rumbling, and short. If the pulmonary artery pressure is high, the murmur is indistinguishable from that of aortic insufficiency. If the regurgitant volume is large, there may be the signs of right ventricular volume overload, a lifting precordium, and right-sided S_3 and S_4 gallops. If the right ventricle dilates, tricuspid insufficiency can result. Usually even severe pulmonic valvular insufficiency is well tolerated and by itself rarely needs surgical repair.

INTRACARDIAC FISTULAS

Fistulous communications between high-pressure and low-pressure chambers can and most often do result from penetrating injury[60] but have also been reported after nonpenetrating injury.[61] The usual fistulas are between the aorta and the right ventricle, the right atrium, or occasionally the pulmonary artery.[62]

In general, fistulas from the aorta to the pulmonary artery are heard along the upper left sternal border, and fistulas from the aorta to the right ventricle are heard along the mid and lower left sternal border. Fistulas from the aorta to the right atrium are heard along the lower left sternal border, or even loudest at the right sternal border. Fistulas between the aorta and low-pressure pulmonary artery, right atrium, and right ventricle result in a left-to-right shunt and a continuous murmur. Fistulas with the left atrium, which are extremely rare, do not result in a left-to-right shunt but increased left ventricular volume overload. If the shunt is large, there are signs of increased aortic runoff simulating those of aortic insufficiency, increased pulmonary blood flow, right-sided and left-sided ventricular hyperactivity, and finally signs of left-sided with or without right-sided congestive heart failure. If the shunt is large and causes hemodynamic decompensation, immediate repair is required.[62]

CORONARY ARTERY INJURIES

The coronary arteries can be injured, usually by penetrating injuries but also occasionally by nonpenetrating trauma.[63,64] The coronary arteries can be lacerated or occluded by thrombus or dissection.[65,66] As previously stated, injury can form a false or true aneurysm and form fistulas either with the coronary veins or with any cardiac chamber. The coronary arteries can be occluded by emboli originating from intracardiac thrombus formed after myocardial contusion.

With laceration of a coronary artery, there is usually bleeding into the pericardium and pericardial tamponade (see Fig. 107.3). The electrocardiogram may demonstrate an acute myocardial infarction, may show ST or T wave changes only, or even be normal.[63,65] The lacerated coronary artery is usually discovered at the time of emergency thoracotomy to relieve the tamponade and at that time is usually ligated. If the territory supplied by the coronary is large enough and there has been no electrocardiographic evidence of acute myocardial infarction, and if facilities are available for coronary bypass surgery, attempts have been made to repair the artery or to perform saphenous vein bypass grafting to prevent myocardial infarction. The usual requirement for emergency surgery at odd hours without the bypass team available as well as the acute development of an acute myocardial infarction usually results in the ligation of the bleeding vessel. Since the patient is frequently young without other coronary disease, if he survives the resulting myocardial infarction and if the resulting infarction does not severely reduce left ventricular function the patient may do well.

The development of a coronary arteriovenous or coronary-cameral fistula after injury, usually penetrating injury, results in the development of a continuous murmur, frequently with diastolic accentuation.[67] Most frequently the coronary cameral fistulas have been between the right coronary artery and the right atrium or right ventricle.[68] Occasionally the left anterior descending coronary artery can develop a fistulous communication with the left ventricle and, rarely, with the left atrium. The size of the shunt frequently is not great in the beginning but can remain stable over a time, increase, or decrease. As the shunt increases, the flow into the proximal coronary artery must increase proportionately. If this occurs, with maintenance of the coronary pressure normal distal to the fistula, there will be no myocardial ischemia as a result of this coronary "steal." If the shunt into the low-resistance chamber is large enough and the flow into the proximal coronary artery cannot proportionately increase, the pressure distal to the shunt will drop, with the possible development of myocardial ischemia, especially with activity.[69] Under these circumstances, the patient will develop angina pectoris or may develop myocardial infarction. In these circumstances, the fistula should be closed surgically. If the patient is asymptomatic, a thallium perfusion study or radioisotope nuclear wall motion study with exercise can demonstrate the development of ischemia on exercise. If this occurs, closure of the fistula is indicated. If the patient is asymptomatic and there is stability of a small left-to-right shunt and no false aneurysm is associated with the fistula, the major danger is that of infective endarteritis, and antibiotics should be given for prophylaxis. It is probable that abnormal flow over time will generate a larger proximal coronary artery and possible that atherosclerosis may be accelerated at or just beyond the level of the shunt. This has been used as an indication for surgical correction but in fact is still largely theoretic. Many patients do very well over a period of many years with coronary arteriovenous or cameral fistulas. Bravo and associates reported a patient with a traumatic coronary arteriovenous fistula followed for 20 years without change in the size of the shunt or angiographic anatomy.[70]

CORONARY ARTERY INJURY AND THROMBOSIS

Coronary artery injury and thrombosis are not unusual in gunshot wounds with pathways that come near but do not directly lacerate the artery. On the other hand, very rarely a nonpenetrating injury, usually a crush injury, can result in direct trauma to the coronary artery with subsequent thrombosis and myocardial infarction.[65,71] To be sure that this is due to coronary thrombus and not to direct myocardial contusion and necrosis, coronary artery occlusion must be demonstrated by angiography[64] or at postmortem examination. Although it is possible that some of the occlusions seen by coronary arteriography were in reality spasms of the injured artery, thrombosis in the coronary artery has been described in young people with crush injuries at postmortem examination. When it does occur, the patient usually has the consequences of acute coronary occlusion, that is, a transmural myocardial infarction, because the injury commonly occurs in previously normal patients who have not had the development of collateral vessels. Under these circumstances, treatment should be that of a patient who has had a transmural myocardial infarction. Removal of the clot or bypass grafting is usually not effective since the acute infarction is already completed. The rarity of this phenomenon is seen in the fact that in the 1958 report of the Armed Forces Institute of Pathology (AFIP) of 546 cases of nonpenetrating cardiovascular trauma, weighted toward severe injuries, there were no cases of coronary thrombosis.[9] In fact, when an acute myocardial infarction is seen after an accident, it is far more common for it to be the result of underlying coronary artery disease with myocardial infarction precipitated by the excitement of the accident or, possibly, by the higher coagulative state present postinjury than due to either myocardial contusion or coronary injury.

INJURY TO THE GREAT VESSELS

Any vessel, artery or vein, can be injured either by penetrating or nonpenetrating injury.[72] Injuries to the arteries and veins can be either laceration, thrombosis, aneurysm formation, or arteriovenous fistulous formation.

The most important injury to the aorta is that of laceration.[6,73] Penetrating injury with aortic laceration frequently results in rapid exsanguination. In deceleration injuries, differential movement of the aorta during the acute deceleration or with marked displacement of the heart out of the middle mediastinum places great stress on the ascending aorta at its root and the descending aorta just beyond the take-off of the left subclavian artery at the level of the ligamentus arteriosus. Laceration and even complete disruption of the aortic intima and media can occur. If the adventitia also ruptures, rapid exsanguination occurs, and the patient is dead within minutes.[6] If the rupture occurs in the ascending aorta, since it is intrapericardial there are no structures resisting rupture, and with 200 ml to 300 ml of blood rapidly filling the pericardial space, tamponade occurs and the patient dies. For this reason, it is most unusual to see a survivor with rupture of the ascending aorta, and I have seen just two cases in 35 years.

When the descending aorta ruptures and the adventitia does not, bleeding into the adventitia is contained by the pleura and other mediastinal tissues, and a false aneurysm can develop without rupturing (Figs. 107.6 and 107.7).[74] The ends of the aortic rupture can retract, and the continuity of the blood flow is maintained by the walls of the false aneurysm only.

In the AFIP experience, 15% of the patients with aortic rupture with nonpenetrating injury lived long enough to reach the hospital.[6] We have seen many instances of patients with aortic transection and false aneurysm who have survived years after their accidents and been discovered accidentally on chest x-ray film taken for an unrelated reason. At times there is calcification in the false aneurysm visible on the x-ray film.

The diagnosis should be suspected in any patient with major thoracoabdominal injury or in a deceleration accident, especially if there was steering wheel compression of the chest. The usual patient has multiple rib fractures and sternal fractures. In such cases, chest x-ray study as close to the posterior–anterior position as possible should be obtained. Bleeding into the mediastinum usually causes widening of the superior mediastinal shadow. Frequently there is loss or distortion of the paraspinal stripe of the descending aorta, and bleeding over the cap of the lung and arch makes the superior aortic arch margin indistinct (see Fig. 107.6). If rupture has occurred into the left pleural cavity, pleural effusion may be present. Shift of the trachea to the right can also be caused by the mediastinal hematoma.[75]

On physical examination, there are frequently no signs attributable to the rupture. Occasionally there may be dissection of the blood in the adventitia with compression of the aorta. At times this involves one or more of the great branches of the aorta. In these instances there may be a systolic murmur heard well in the back, similar to that of coarctation of the aorta, and the femoral pulses may be decreased.

If aortic rupture is suspected, an immediate aortogram should be obtained (see Fig. 107.7).[75] If the patient is hemodynamically stable, the aorta is ruptured, and there are no contraindications such as myocardial failure or neurologic injury, immediate repair should be done.[73,74] If the patient is in a facility where this cannot be done and is stable, blood pressure should be lowered and cardiac contractility decreased with a combination of nitroprusside and beta blockade and the patient immediately transported to a facility where the surgery can be done.[76]

In the instances where aortic rupture occurred weeks, months, or years before, a decision must be made as to whether the repair should be done. The studies addressing this problem show that late aortic rupture is not unusual and late symptoms or late increase in aortic aneurysmal size can occur which later leads to surgical correction.[77] For this reason, when an aortic rupture with false aneurysm is discovered, no matter when it occurred, the rupture should be repaired.[78]

Aortic venous fistulas with either the inferior vena cava or the innominate vein or superior vena cava have been seen with penetrating injuries, the most common of which have occurred during surgery for herniated nucleus pulposus with accidental perforation of the abdominal aorta and subsequent rupture of the false aneurysm into the inferior vena cava.[79] In this instance, the patient frequently has a huge shunt, left ventricular volume overload, and congestive heart failure. This catastrophe is suspected when a continuous murmur is heard over the abdomen and back. Smaller arteries can be involved in perforating injuries, causing various sized shunts. All of these are characterized by loud, continuous bruits and, when discovered, should be repaired.

False aneurysms of branches of the aorta and extremity arteries are also usually the result of penetrating injury. Because of their proclivity

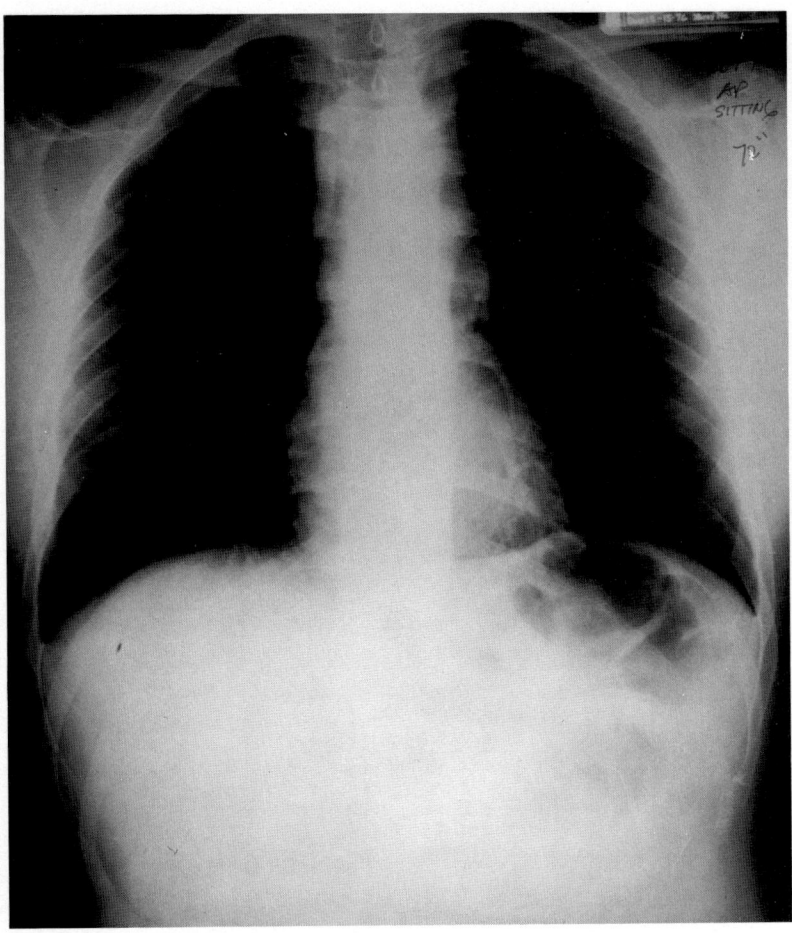

FIGURE 107.6 Chest roentgenogram, anteroposterior sitting portable view at 72 inches. Patient is a 24-year-old man involved as the driver in a head-on automobile collision. The patient struck his chest on the steering wheel. Note the normal cardiac silhouette, the widened upper mediastinal shadow, and the distorted descending aortic stripe consistent with aortic rupture.

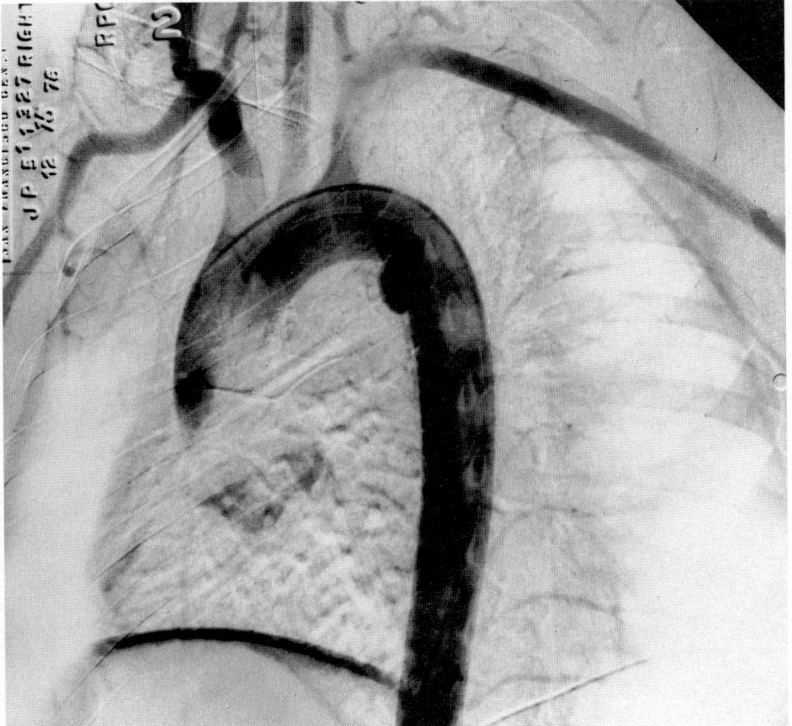

FIGURE 107.7 Retrograde aortogram, subtraction film, left anterior oblique view. Same patient as Figure 107.6. Note catheter in the ascending aorta. Contrast has almost washed out of the root of the aorta. The great vessels are normally arising. At the isthmus of the aorta, medially there is a bulge of contrast into the false aneurysm. At surgery there was partial laceration of the descending aorta, which was repaired with a short graft.

to enlarge and finally rupture, they should be repaired when discovered.

Thrombosis of arteries either as a result of penetrating or nonpenetrating injury usually causes acute ischemia of the organs supplied by the artery.[80] If this involves the limbs, a sudden, cold, pulseless extremity results; when this occurs, immediate surgery to remove the clot or bypass the obstruction and revascularize the organ is indicated. If the thrombosed vessel has not produced acute ischemia or symptoms, usually it will not be discovered, and, if there are no immediate clinical consequences, need not be repaired at that time.

RETAINED FOREIGN BODIES

Low-velocity missiles, on penetrating the body, frequently lose momentum and come to rest within the body. Foreign bodies can penetrate the heart and lodge within the cardiac muscle or within any of the cardiac chambers. Foreign bodies can also lodge in veins or arteries and migrate (Figs. 107.8 and 107.9).[81] With systemic venous entry, the foreign body can migrate into the right heart and frequently lodges in a branch of the pulmonary artery.[82] With penetration of the pulmonary venous circuit, the foreign body can migrate into the left heart and then embolize into the arterial tree, lodging in any branch.[83] Such cases of migrating foreign bodies in the cardiovascular system are well documented.

Foreign bodies retained within the heart can cause several problems. The entrance of the foreign body can directly damage any of the intracardiac structures. Low-velocity penetrating injuries can carry bacterially contaminated foreign material into the body, which can result in septic abscesses within the body, including in the heart. At times the foreign bodies within the pericardium can also result in recurrent pericarditis that resolves only on removal of the foreign body. If the foreign body is lodged within the myocardium, it frequently becomes encapsulated with fibrous tissue and remains inert for years. On occasion the foreign body can erode nearby structures, for instance the coronary artery, causing occlusion or aneurysm formation. Finally, the presence of the foreign body intraluminally frequently results in fibrin deposit with subsequent embolization.

The presence of a retained foreign body that is not infected raises the question of whether it is necessary to remove it. Bland and Beebe reported 40 patients with intracardiac foreign bodies followed from World War II for a period of 20 years.[84] On follow-up examination, there were a number who had had complications involving embolization and erosion of bronchus with subsequent pneumonectomy. Of the 40 patients, 30 had neurasthenic problems related to the knowledge of the presence of an intracardiac foreign body. Their conclusion was that if the foreign body was 1 cm or larger, the psychological burden of retaining such a foreign body in the heart made its removal worthwhile.

IATROGENIC CARDIOVASCULAR INJURIES

By far the fastest growing literature in the area of cardiovascular trauma is that due to the increasing development and use of invasive techniques, both diagnostic and therapeutic. With needles blindly placed within the body and catheters introduced through these needles, there have been increasing numbers of reports of arterial and venous laceration, thrombosis, arteriovenous fistulas, and "lost" catheters (Figs. 107.10 and 107.11).[85-88] Techniques have been developed to remove

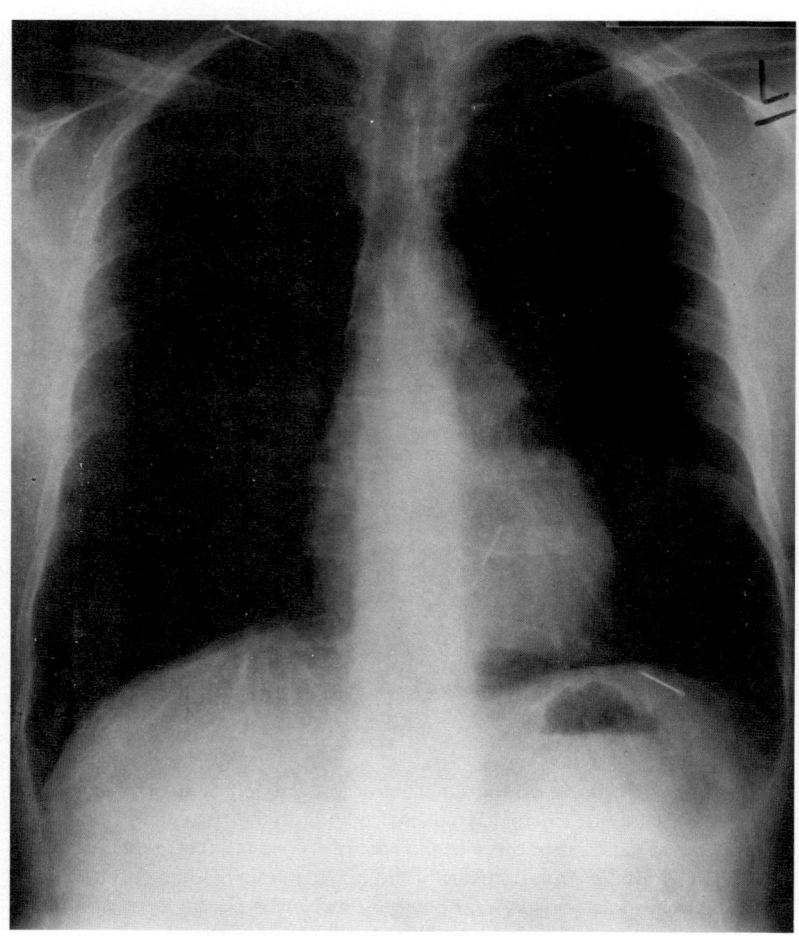

FIGURE 107.8 Chest roentgenogram, posteroanterior view. The patient was a 42-year-old psychotic man who inserted sewing needles into his peripheral veins. These migrated into the right heart and out into the lung. Notice two needles within the cardiac silhouette and one needle apparently just below, actually in the lung behind the dome of the left hemidiaphragm.

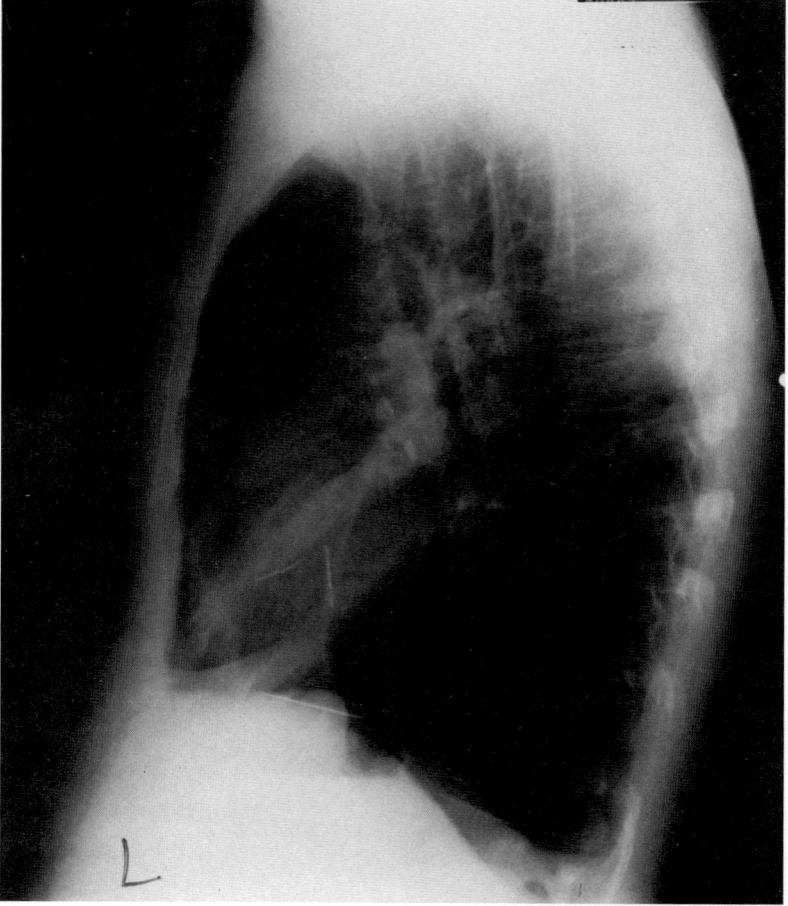

FIGURE 107.9 Chest roentgenogram, left lateral view (same patient as Fig. 107.8). Notice two sewing needles within the cardiac silhouette and one at the base of the left lung.

these lost segments of cut-off polyethylene tubing and other types of catheters with special snare catheters.[89] With needle biopsy techniques, false aneurysms and arteriovenous fistulas of the renal artery have been reported.[90] With the transseptal technique of left heart catheterization, the accident of passing the needle into the root of the aorta can result in an aortic-to-right atrial fistula or into the pericardium resulting in pericardial tamponade.[91]

Needle punctures of the chest wall, done to enter the left ventricle and measure the left ventricular pressure and to perform pericardiocentesis, have resulted in lacerations of the left and right ventricles with resultant pericardial tamponade. Electrophysiologic studies with placement of multiple stiff catheters in the right atrium across the tricuspid valve into the right ventricle and into the coronary sinus have resulted in occasional perforation of the right atrium, right ventricle, and coronary sinus. Finally, percutaneous placement of catheters into subclavian veins or internal jugular veins has resulted in multiple complications, some noncardiovascular, such as pneumothorax or chylothorax, and some involving the cardiovascular system, such as tearing of the subclavian artery or carotid artery, with hemorrhage and even exsanguination. With increasing invasive techniques, such as balloon angioplasty and valvuloplasty, closure of atrial defects, patent ducti with catheter techniques, and embolization of arteriovenous fistulas with plastic balls or wire coils, we can expect to see a variety of interesting and novel cardiovascular traumatic complications in the future.

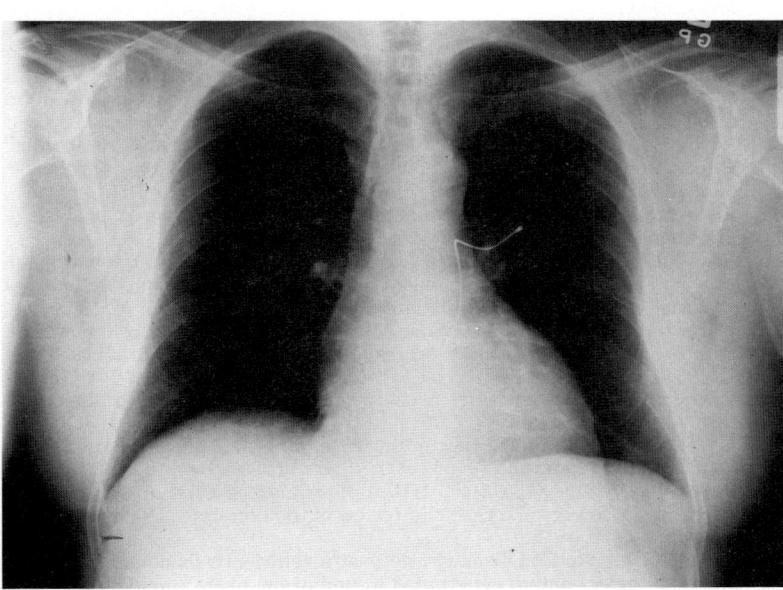

FIGURE 107.10 Chest roentgenogram, posteroanterior view. Patient was a 54-year-old man who had a temporary pacing catheter placed through the femoral vein for complete heart block. The catheter was inadvertently cut and eventually migrated with its distal end in the left pulmonary artery. The catheter was later removed with a snare catheter nonoperatively.

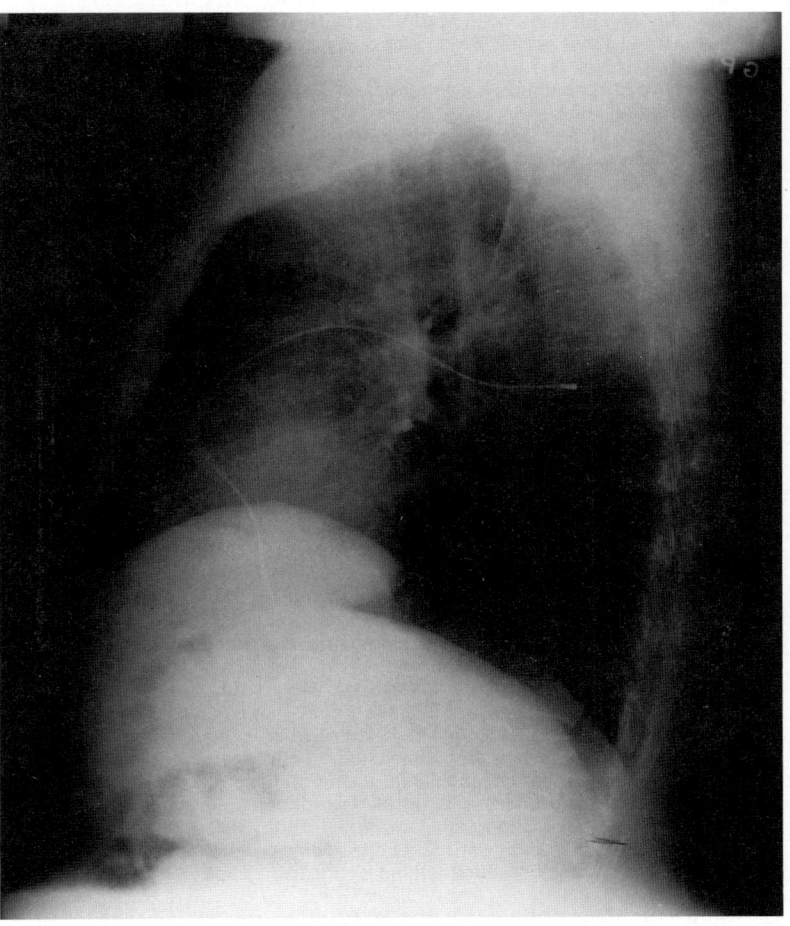

FIGURE 107.11 Chest roentgenogram, left lateral view. Notice catheter from inferior vena cava through the right heart, out into the left distal pulmonary artery.

REFERENCES

1. Elsberg CA: Ueber Herzwunden und Herznaht. Bruns-Beitrag zur Khnische Chirurgie 25:433, 1899
2. Williams DH: Stab wound of the heart and pericardium—Suture of the pericardium, recovery, patient alive three years afterward. Med Rec 51:437, 1897
3. Rehn E: Fall von penetrirender stech verletzung des rechten Henzen-Herznaht. Zentralbl Chir 23:1048, 1896
4. Brewer LA III: Wounds of the chest in war and peace, 1943–1968. Ann Thorac Surg 7:387, 1969
5. Amato JJ, Rich NM: Temporary cavity effects in blood vessel injury by high velocity missiles. J Cardiovasc Surg (Torino) 13:147, 1972
6. Parmley LF, Mattingly TW, Manion WC, Jahnke EJ Jr: Nonpenetrating traumatic injury of the aorta. Circulation 17:1086, 1958
7. Cooper GJ, Maynard RL, Pearce BP et al: Cardiovascular distortion in experimental nonpenetrating chest impacts. J Trauma 24:188, 1984
8. Lau IV: Effect of timing and velocity of impact on ventricular myocardial rupture. J Biomech Eng 105:1, 1983
9. Parmley LF, Manion WC, Mattingly TW: Nonpenetrating traumatic injury of the heart. Circulation 18:371, 1958
10. Parmley LF, Mattingly TW, Manion WC: Penetrating wounds of heart and aorta. Circulation 17:953, 1958
11. Trunkey DD, Cheitlin MD: Chest trauma. In Mills J, Ho MT, Trunkey DD (eds): Current Emergency Diagnosis and Treatment, p 241. Los Altos, CA, Lange, 1983
12. Reul GJ Jr, Mattox KL, Beall AC Jr, Jordan GL Jr: Recent advances in the operative management of massive chest trauma. Ann Thorac Surg 16:52, 1973
13. Sugg WL, Rea WJ, Ecker RR et al: Penetrating wounds of the heart. An analysis of 459 cases. J Thorac Cardiovasc Surg 56:531, 1968
14. Borja AR, Lansing AM, Randsdell HT Jr: Immediate operative treatment for stab wounds of the heart. Experience with fifty-four consecutive cases. J Thorac Cardiovasc Surg 59:662, 1970
15. Taveres S, Hankins JR, Moulton AL et al: Management of penetrating cardiac injuries: The role of emergency room thoracotomy. Ann Thorac Surg 38:181, 1984

16. Robbs JV, Baker LW: Cardiovascular trauma. Curr Probl Surg 21:1, 1984
17. Rohman M, Ivatury RR, Steichen FM et al: Emergency room thoracotomy for penetrating cardiac injuries. J Trauma 23:570, 1983
18. Trinkle JK, Toon RS, Frantz JL et al: Affairs of the wounded heart: Penetrating cardiac wounds. J Trauma 19:467, 1979
19. Demetriades D, Van der Veen BW: Penetrating injuries of the heart: Experience over two years in South Africa. J Trauma 23:1034, 1983
20. Steichen FM, Dargan EL, Efron G et al: A gradual approach to the management of penetrating wounds of the heart. Arch Surg 103:574, 1971
21. Clark DE, Wiles CS III, Lim MK et al: Traumatic rupture of the pericardium. Surgery 93:495, 1983
22. Mattila S, Silvola H, Ketonen P: Traumatic rupture of the pericardium with laceration of the heart. Case report and review of the literature. J Thorac Cardiovasc Surg 70:495, 1975
23. Engle MA, McCabe JC, Ebert PA, Zabriskie J: The post-pericardiotomy syndrome and antiheart antibodies. Circulation 49:401, 1974
24. Sbokos CG, Karayannocos PE, Kontaxis A et al: Traumatic hemopericardium and chronic constrictive pericarditis. Ann Thorac Surg 23:225, 1977
25. Feliciano DV, Bitondo PA-C, Mattox KL et al: Civilian trauma in the 1980's. A 1-year experience with 456 vascular and cardiac injuries. Ann Surg 199:717, 1984
26. Frazer M, Mirchandani H: Commotio cordis, revisited. Am J Forensic Med Pathol 5:249, 1984
27. Viano DC, Artiman CG: Myocardial conduction system dysfunction from thoracic infarct. J Trauma 18:452, 1978
28. DeMuth WE Jr, Baue AE, Odom JA Jr: Contusion of the heart. J Trauma 7:443, 1967
29. Kissane RW: Traumatic heart disease: Nonpenetrating injuries. Circulation 6:421, 1952
30. Doty DB, Anderson AE, Rose EF et al: Cardiac Trauma: Clinical and experimental correlation of myocardial contusion. Am Surg 180:452, 1974
31. Lasky II, Nahum AM, Siegel AW: Cardiac injuries incurred by drivers in automobile accidents. J Forensic Sci 14:13, 1969
32. Poole GV, Myers RT: Morbidity and mortality rates in major blunt trauma to the upper chest. Ann Surg 193:70, 1981
33. Hipona FA, Paredes S: The radiologic evaluation of patients with chest trauma. Med Clin North Am 59:65, 1975
34. Hamilton JRL, Dearden C, Rutherford WH: Myocardial contusion associated with fracture of the sternum: Important features of the seat belt syndrome. Injury 16:155, 1984
35. Potkin RT, Werner JA, Trobaugh GB et al: Cardiac contusion. Evaluation of noninvasive tests of cardiac damage in suspected cardiac contusion. Circulation 66:627, 1982
36. Kettunen P: Cardiac damage after blunt chest trauma, diagnosis using CK-MB; enzymes and electrocardiogram. Int J Cardiol 6:355, 1984
37. Tsung SH: Creatine kinase isoenzyme patterns in human tissue obtained at surgery. Clin Chem 22:172, 1976
38. Kumar SA, Puri VK, Mittal VK, Cortez J: Myocardial contusion following nonfatal blunt chest trauma. J Trauma 23:327, 1983
39. Pandian NG, Skorton DJ, Doty DB, Kerber RE: Immediate diagnosis of acute myocardial contusion by two-dimensional echocardiography: Studies in a canine model of blunt chest trauma. J Am Coll Cardiol 2:488, 1983
40. Miller A, Seward JB, Gersh BJ et al: Two-dimensional echocardiographic findings in cardiac trauma. Am J Cardiol 50:1022, 1982
41. King RM, Mucha P Jr, Seward JB et al: Cardiac contusion: A new diagnostic approach utilizing two-dimensional echocardiography. J Trauma 23:610, 1983
42. Hurley DP, Mena I, Miranda R, Nelson RJ: Myocardial dysfunction following blunt chest trauma. Arch Surg 118:1384, 1983
43. Fenner JE, Knopp R, Lee B et al: The use of gated radionuclide angiography in the diagnosis of cardiac contusion. Ann Emerg Med 13:688, 1984
44. Simon TR, Parkey RW, Lewis SE: Role of cardiovascular nuclear medicine in evaluating trauma and the postoperative patient. Semin Nucl Med 13:123, 1983
45. Sutherland GR, Driedger AA, Halliday RL et al: Frequency of myocardial injury after blunt chest trauma as evaluated by radionuclide angiography. Am J Cardiol 52:1099, 1983
46. Brantigan CO, Burdick D, Hopeman AR, Eisman B: Evaluation of technetium scanning for myocardial contusion. J Trauma 18:460, 1978
47. Downey F, Chagrasulis R, Fore D, Parmley LF: Accumulation of technetium-99m stannous pyrophosphate in contused myocardium. J Nucl Med 18:1171, 1977
48. Sinha SN, Bhattacharya SK, Mymin D et al: Ventricular septal defects due to penetrating injuries of the heart. Can Med Assoc J 107:1182, 1972
49. Asfaw I, Thomas NW, Arbulu A: Interventricular septal defects from penetrating injuries of the heart. A report of 12 cases and review of the literature. J Thorac Cardiovasc Surg 69:450, 1975
50. Inoue K, Suma J, Taguchi K, Otoda M: Nonpenetrating ventricular septal defect and ventricular septal aneurysm—A case study and review of the literature. Jpn J Thorac Surg 28:112, 1975
51. Midell AI, Replogle R, Bermudez G: Spontaneous closure of a traumatic ventricular septal defect following a penetrating injury. Ann Thorac Surg 20:339, 1975
52. Mary DA, Day JB, Pakrashi BC, Ionescu MI: Isolated tricuspid incompetence after penetrating trauma. Am J Cardiol 31:752, 1973
53. Kessler KM, Foianini JF, Davia JE, Cheitlin MD: Tricuspid insufficiency due to nonpenetrating trauma. Am J Cardiol 37:442, 1976
54. Shukhzadeh A, Langbehn RF, Ghabrisi P et al: Chronic traumatic tricuspid insufficiency. Clin Cardiol 7:299, 1984
55. Cuadros CL, Hutchinson JE III, Mogtader AH: Laceration of a mitral papillary muscle and the aortic root as a result of blunt trauma to the chest. Case report and review of the literature. J Thorac Cardiovasc Surg 88:134, 1984
56. Mazzucco A, Rizzoli G, Faggian G et al: Acute mitral regurgitation after blunt chest trauma. Arch Intern Med 143:2326, 1983
57. Harada M, Osawa M, Kosukegawa K et al: Isolated mitral valve injury from nonpenetrating cardiac trauma. J Cardiovasc Surg 18:459, 1977
58. McIlduff JB, Foster ED: Disruption of a normal aortic valve as a result of blunt chest trauma. J Trauma 18:373, 1978
59. Najafi H, Dye WS, Javil H et al: Rupture of an otherwise normal aortic valve. Report of two cases and review of the literature. J Thorac Cardiovasc Surg 56:57, 1968
60. Thandroyen FT, Matisonn RE: Penetrating thoracic trauma producing cardiac shunts. J Thorac Cardiovasc Surg 81:569, 1981
61. DeSa'Neto A, Padnick MB, Desser KB, Steinhoff NC: Right sinus of Valsalva—Right atrial fistula secondary to nonpenetrating chest trauma. Circulation 60:205, 1979
62. Rayner AVS, Fulton RL, Hess PJ, Daicoff GR: Post-traumatic intracardiac shunts. Report of two cases and review of the literature. J Thorac Cardiovasc Surg 73:728, 1977
63. Rea WJ, Sugg WL, Wilson LC et al: Coronary artery laceration: An analysis of 22 patients. Ann Thorac Surg 7:518, 1969
64. Gaspard P, Clermont A, Villard J, Amiel M: Non-iatrogenic trauma of the coronary arteries and myocardium: Contribution of angiography—Report of six cases and literature review. Cardiovasc Intervent Radiol 6:20, 1983
65. Wainwright RJ, Edwards AC, Maisey MN, Sowton E: Early occlusion and late stricture of normal coronary artery following blunt chest trauma. Chest 78:796, 1980
66. Fischer H: Accidental injuries of the coronary vessels. Review of the literature. Attuel Traumatol 9:49, 1979
67. Liberthson RR, Barron K, Hawthorne JW et al: Traumatic coronary arterial fistula. A case report and review of the literature. Am Heart J 86:817, 1973
68. Reyes LH, Mattox KL, Gaasch WH et al: Traumatic coronary artery–right heart fistula. Report of a case and review of the literature. J Thorac Cardiovasc Surg 70:52, 1975
69. Jones RC, Jahnke EJ: Coronary artery–atrioventricular fistula and ventricular septal defect due to penetrating wound of the heart. Circulation 32:995, 1965
70. Bravo AJ, Glancy DL, Epstein SE, Morrow AG: Traumatic coronary arteriovenous fistula. A 20 year follow-up with serial hemodynamic and angiographic studies. Am J Cardiol 27:673, 1971
71. Oliva PB, Hilgenberg A, McElroy D: Obstruction of the proximal right coronary artery with acute inferior infarction due to blunt chest trauma. Ann Intern Med 91:205, 1979
72. Symbas PN, Kourias E, Tyras DH, Hatcher CR Jr: Penetrating wounds of great vessels. Ann Surg 179:757, 1974
73. Turney SZ, Altar S, Ayella R et al: Traumatic rupture of the aorta. A five-year experience. J Thorac Cardiovasc Surg 72:727, 1976
74. Bochly K, Perry JF Jr, Strate RG, Fisher RP: Salvageability of patients with post-traumatic ruptures of the descending thoracic aorta in primary trauma center. J Trauma 17:754, 1977
75. Marsh DG, Sturm JT: Traumatic aortic rupture: Roentgenographic indications for angiography. Ann Thorac Surg 21:337, 1976
76. Aronstam EM, Gomez AC, O'Connell TJ, Geiger JP: Recent surgical and pharmacologic experience with acute dissecting and traumatic aneurysm. J Thorac Cardiovasc Surg 59:231, 1970
77. Fleming AW, Green DC: Traumatic aneurysms of the thoracic aorta. Ann Thorac Surg 18:91, 1974
78. Midgley F, Behrendt DM: Surgical repair of chronic post-cardiac aneurysms of the aortic arch. J Thorac Cardiovasc Surg 67:229, 1974
79. Spittell JA Jr, Palumbo PJ, Love JG et al: Arteriovenous fistula complicating lumbar-disk surgery. N Engl J Med 268:1162, 1963
80. Thompson JE: Acute peripheral arterial occlusion. N Engl J Med 290:950, 1974
81. Symbas PN, Harlaftis N: Bullet emboli in the pulmonary and systemic arteries. Ann Surg 185:318, 1977
82. Schechter DC, Gilbert L: Injury of the heart and great vessels due to pins and needles. Thorax 24:246, 1969
83. Moncades R, Maluga T, Unger E et al: Migrating trauma—Cardiovascular foreign bodies. Circulation 57:186, 1978
84. Bland EF, Beebe GW: Missiles in the heart: A twenty year follow-up report of World War II cases. N Engl J Med 274:1039, 1966
85. Borja AR, Masri Z, Shruck L, Pejo S: Unusual and lethal complications of infraclavicular subclavian vein catheterization. Int Surg 57:42, 1972
86. Rich NM, Hobson RW, Fedde CW: Vascular trauma secondary to diagnostic and therapeutic procedures. Am J Surg 128:715, 1974

87. Senno A, Schweitzer P, Merrill C et al: Arteriovenous fistulas of the internal mammery artery: Review of the literature. J Cardiovasc Surg 16:296, 1975
88. Doering RB, Stemmer EA, Cornelly JE: Complication of indwelling venous catheterization. With particular reference to catheter embolus. Am J Surg 114:259, 1967
89. Curry JL: Recovery of detached intravascular catheter or guide wire fragments. Am J Roentgen Radium Ther Nucl Med 105:894, 1969
90. Leiter E, Gribetz D, Cohen S: Arteriovenous fistula after percutaneous needle biopsy—Surgical repair with preservation of renal function. N Engl J Med 287:971, 1972
91. Enghoff E, Cullhead I: Experiences with transseptal left heart catheterization: A review of 454 studies. Am Heart J 81:398, 1971

Diseases of the Aorta and Peripheral Arteries

John A. Spittell, Jr • Peter C. Spittell

Acquired diseases of the aorta and peripheral vessels are the result of a broad spectrum of etiologic factors, including aging, atherosclerosis, hypertension, infection, inflammatory disorders, degenerative diseases, and trauma.

Arteries normally undergo structural changes with age, including an increase in thickness of the intimal area, a loss of elasticity, an increase in calcium content, and an increase in diameter.[1] Alone, these changes are usually of no consequence, except when widening of the aged aorta at the root leads to aortic insufficiency or is complicated by rupture of the aorta. The aging process is best considered a "physiologic arteriosclerosis," representing more of an adaptive response of the vessel wall to hemodynamic stress[2] than a manifestation of atherosclerosis.

Atherosclerosis is a very prevalent and complex disease and is the result of multiple etiologic factors. It is characterized by the focal accumulation of lipid, carbohydrate, blood products, fibrous tissue, and calcium deposits first in the intima of arteries[1] and resulting in the complications of arterial occlusion, aneurysm formation, and atheroembolism.

Hypertension is a well-known risk factor in the development of atherosclerosis. It also accelerates the process of atherosclerosis and the structural changes of aging, as well as other degenerative arterial diseases. Hypertension is the most common etiologic factor in aortic dissection and may play a role in the formation and rupture of some arterial aneurysms.[3,4]

Infection of the aorta and peripheral vessels, most commonly bacterial or fungal, can result in the formation of a mycotic aneurysm or infection of an existing aneurysm. Syphilitic aortitis and aneurysm, although less common, must be kept in mind when ascending aortic aneurysm and aortic valve regurgitation are seen.

Inflammatory disorders involving the aorta and peripheral vessels are typically seen in the arteritides, which characteristically have a wide variety of overlapping systemic and vascular manifestations.

Degenerative diseases, other than atherosclerosis, include Mönckeberg's sclerosis, cystic medial necrosis, and cystic degeneration of the popliteal artery.

Trauma, either blunt or penetrating, to the aorta and peripheral vessels can result in transection, occlusion, or aneurysm. Blunt trauma to the aorta occurs with sudden deceleration or crush injuries. Acute or chronic blunt trauma of the hand may cause arterial occlusion.[5] Penetrating trauma from puncture or laceration of the artery may result in massive hemorrhage, dissection, occlusion, or subsequent false aneurysm formation.

DISEASES OF THE AORTA

Atherosclerosis is the most common cause of occlusive peripheral arterial disease, being more frequent in the abdominal aorta and arteries of the lower extremities than in the upper extremities. Risk factors commonly implicated in the development of atherosclerosis of peripheral vessels are the same as for coronary artery disease and include hypertension, cigarette smoking, diabetes mellitus, hyperlipidemia, and genetic factors.

"Fatty streaks," are said to be the first macroscopic lesion of atherosclerosis. The earliest microscopic change is said to be "intimal proliferation of smooth muscle cells," presumably derived from the media of the artery.[6] Both "fatty streaks" and smooth muscle cell proliferation are more common at aortic branch points, which have been shown to be sites of increased endothelial damage.[1]

Current experimental evidence indicates that both lipid transport and platelet interaction with the arterial wall play important roles in the pathogenesis of atherosclerosis. The basic mechanisms of atherogenesis are an active area of research; the apolipoproteins, particularly apolipoprotein A-1 appear to be related to the ability of high-density lipoprotein cholesterol to remove cholesterol from the cell.[7]

The major critical events in the pathogenesis of atherosclerosis include the following:

1. Hemodynamic stress, endothelial injury, and platelet interaction with the arterial wall
2. Smooth muscle cell proliferation
3. Lipid and lipoprotein entry and accumulation
4. Altered mechanisms of lipid removal
5. Fibrosis and development of thrombi
6. Ulceration, calcification, and/or aneurysm formation.

ANEURYSMAL DISEASE
ETIOLOGY
Atherosclerosis is the most common cause of aneurysmal disease of the aorta, thus aneurysms are more common in males (5:1) and are rare in patients under 50 years of age. Other causes of aneurysmal disease include inherited disorders of connective tissue (the Marfan syndrome and Ehlers-Danlos syndrome), syphilis and other infections, arteritis, and trauma.

Regardless of etiology, the development of an aneurysm is related to weakening of the media of the artery. The atherosclerotic process causes weakening of the aortic wall, degeneration of the media, and localized dilatation. Hypertension often coexists and contributes to weakening of the aortic wall and expansion of the aneurysm.[4] Once started, the process of dilatation tends to be progressive because the lateral pressure increases with widening of the lumen (Bernoulli theorem) and slowing of flow. This contributes to the formation of laminated mural thrombus, which may embolize into the distal arterial circulation.[5]

THORACIC AORTA

Approximately 25% of all atherosclerotic aneurysms involve the thoracic aorta, most commonly, the aortic arch and descending thoracic aorta. Cystic medial necrosis, frequently associated with the Marfan syndrome, can result in aneurysmal disease involving the ascending aorta. Luetic aneurysms involving the ascending aorta are less common today, largely due to effective antibiotic therapy of early syphilis. Traumatic aneurysms, secondary to rapid deceleration or blunt injuries of the chest, usually occur just distal to the origin of the left subclavian artery as a sequel to incomplete rupture of the aorta at the isthmus. Moderate to severe hypertension has been implicated as a major etiologic factor in some aneurysms of the ascending aorta.[3,4]

Most patients with aneurysms of the thoracic aorta are asymptomatic. Signs or symptoms of thoracic aortic aneurysm, when present, are related to the size and location of the aneurysm and are usually caused by impingement on adjacent structures such as the innominate veins, superior vena cava, recurrent laryngeal nerve, trachea, and/or esophagus. Therefore, the patient may present with the manifestations of superior vena cava syndrome, hoarseness, respiratory obstruction, or dysphagia. Additional symptoms include cerebral ischemia secondary to partial obstruction of aortic arch vessels, anterior chest pain, shortness of breath, and posterior thoracic pain. Aortic valvular insufficiency can result from progressive dilatation of the aortic root.

Often, aneurysms of the thoracic aorta are first noted on a chest roentgenogram. They must be considered in the differential diagnosis of any mediastinal mass. Aortic angiography is the definitive diagnostic procedure and should be done prior to surgical repair. Recent reports suggest that two-dimensional echocardiography is useful in visualizing the thoracic aorta,[8,9] but computed tomography with intravenous contrast enhancement will likely become the standard imaging procedure.[10]

Prognosis of thoracic aortic aneurysms is largely related to size, with those greater than 6 cm in diameter being more prone to rupture. In the study by Joyce and colleagues, the survival of persons with untreated thoracic aortic aneurysm was 68% in 3 years, 50% in 5 years, and 30% in 10 years; symptomatic aneurysms were more prone to rupture than those that were asymptomatic. Additional factors that worsened the prognosis included diastolic hypertension, and associated coronary and cerebrovascular disease.[11] In a more recent study, Bickerstaff and associates found that rupture of a thoracic aortic aneurysm was associated with long-standing hypertension in every instance.[12]

Because of the poor prognosis for untreated thoracic aortic aneurysm, surgical resection is the treatment of choice, unless the patient is not an acceptable surgical risk for other reasons. Current indications for surgical treatment of thoracic aortic aneurysm include a symptomatic aneurysm, an enlarging aneurysm, an aneurysm greater than 6 cm in diameter, coexistent hypertension, and traumatic aneurysm.

Because of the frequency of aortic dissection and rupture in the patient with the Marfan syndrome, Gott and coworkers[13] recommend prophylactic repair, even in asymptomatic cases, when the aortic root diameter reaches 6 cm.

Aortic injuries associated with severe blunt chest trauma and sudden deceleration are common. In one autopsy series of fatal automobile accidents, rupture of the thoracic aorta, usually at the isthmus, was found in one sixth of all victims.[14] Aortic rupture is the most common traumatic condition of the thoracic aorta encountered clinically[2] and results from the sudden torsion that occurs with sudden deceleration such as occurs in motor vehicular accidents or falls from heights and from the blunt chest trauma that may occur in vehicular accidents or blast injuries.

The aortic rupture in sudden deceleration varies from incomplete laceration to complete transection. With horizontal deceleration injuries, 80% of aortic ruptures occur at the aortic isthmus just distal to the origin of the left subclavian artery, near the attachment of the ligamentum arteriosum. The shearing force is maximum at this point because the proximal thoracic aorta is fixed by the brachiocephalic vessels and the distal thoracic aorta is fixed by intercostal arteries and pleural reflections, making the isthmus the most mobile portion of the aorta. Traumatic rupture of the ascending aorta is more common with vertical deceleration injuries. Other sites where traumatic aortic rupture occasionally occurs include the supravalvular portion of the ascending aorta, the origin of the innominate artery, the aortic arch, and the abdominal aorta.

Traumatic rupture of the aorta should be suspected in all motor vehicular accidents, in falls from a height, and with blunt chest trauma. Approximately two thirds of persons with aortic rupture have evidence of other thoracic trauma including chest, pulmonary, or cardiac contusions, rib or vertebral fractures, and hemorrhagic pleural effusions.[15] Clues to traumatic aortic rupture are a history of sudden deceleration and/or chest trauma, rib or sternal fractures, evidence of fluid in the left chest, and hypertension in the arms[16] and decreased or absent pulses in the legs.

A chest roentgenogram is abnormal in over 90% of patients with traumatic rupture of the thoracic aorta, the most common finding being mediastinal widening (Fig. 108.1). Other radiologic findings supportive of the diagnosis include a shift of the trachea to the right, blurring of the normally sharp aortic outline, an apical cap obscuring the medial margin of the upper lobe of the left lung, depression of the left mainstem bronchus, and a left pleural effusion.

Although 80% of patients with traumatic aortic rupture die instantly, Parmley and colleagues[17] estimated that as many as 20% of patients may survive long enough to permit diagnosis and treatment.

The key to diagnosis is a high degree of suspicion. If aortic rupture is a possibility, prompt aortography is indicated.

Definitive therapy for traumatic rupture of the thoracic aorta is prompt surgical resection of the lacerated area and replacement with a graft. Prompt recognition and operation for ruptured thoracic aorta has resulted in a survival of 75% to 80% of patients with this injury who reach the hospital alive.[18,19]

In the case of those patients who survive their injuries and present later with a traumatic thoracic aortic aneurysm, surgical therapy is preferred because of the unpredictable course of the lesion and the relatively low risk of surgical resection.[2]

Surgical repair of thoracic aortic aneurysm is dependent on its size and location. Extracorporeal circulation with hypothermia and myocardial protection is required in repair of ascending aortic and aortic arch aneurysms. The repair of descending thoracic aortic aneurysms involves cross-clamping of the aorta just distal to the left subclavian artery with the attendant risk (4% to 18%) of spinal cord ischemia with resultant paraplegia. Resection of these aneurysms should thus be done expeditiously, using current techniques for temporarily bypassing the thoracic aorta. Operative mortality is generally less than 10%.[20]

Following successful surgical repair and in those patients with contraindications to surgical therapy, medical management of associated hypertension is very essential.[3]

ABDOMINAL AORTA

The abdominal aorta is the most common site for the development of aneurysms with approximately three fourths of all atherosclerotic aneurysms being located here.[21] Males are affected more frequently than females in a ratio of 9:1. The majority of patients are 60 to 70 years old, but 20% of patients are over 70. Eighty percent to 90% of aortic aneurysms are in the abdominal aorta, most of which occur distal to the origin of the renal arteries. Two percent to 5% of abdominal aortic aneurysms are suprarenal and most commonly are the result of distal extension of a thoracic aneurysm (thoracoabdominal aneurysm).[21] Mycotic aneurysms and dissecting aneurysm are occasionally seen in the abdominal aorta, but atherosclerosis is by far the most common etiologic factor.

Some aneurysms begin in an area of dense atheroma where atherosclerosis has destroyed elastic elements of the media with resultant weakening of the aortic wall producing a fusiform or less often a saccular aneurysm. As the aorta widens, tension in the wall of the aorta increases at constant arterial pressure (law of Laplace). As noted previously, systemic hypertension enhances aneurysm formation.[4]

Several recent studies suggest that a tendency toward aneurysm formation in the abdominal aorta may be inherited. Johansen and Koepsell noted that first-degree relatives of a person with an abdominal aortic aneurysm have an estimated 11.6-fold increased risk of developing an aortic aneurysm when compared to control subjects.[22] Tilson and Seashore have concluded from their studies of families with abdominal aortic aneurysms that there are both sex-linked and autosomal patterns operative in the inheritance of the tendency to develop an aortic aneurysm.[23]

More than one half of the patients with an abdominal aortic aneurysm are asymptomatic.[5] Occasionally, awareness of abdominal pulsation, a sensation of abdominal fullness, and back or flank pain are presenting complaints. Careful physical examination will reveal an expansile pulsatile mass in the abdomen. Tenderness of the aneurysm on palpation suggests recent enlargement or impending rupture of the aneurysm. Rupture of the aneurysm causes severe pain in the abdomen and back with radiation into the flanks, genitals, or legs with associated hypotension.

The diagnosis of abdominal aortic aneurysm may be confirmed on roentgenograms of the lumbar spine in about 85% of cases, but abdominal ultrasound is the best method to detect and determine the size of an abdominal aortic aneurysm (Fig. 108.2).[24] The normal aortic diameter is 2 cm at the celiac axis and 1.8 cm below the renal axis, with clinically significant abdominal aneurysms measuring 4 cm or more in diameter.

Excretory urography is a useful part of the evaluation of the patient with an abdominal aortic aneurysm, if there is no medical urgency. It will identify preoperatively any important renal anomaly (such as horseshoe kidney) that may complicate surgery and any ureteral encroachment by the aneurysm. In the hypertensive patient, clues to significant associated renovascular disease may be noted.

Aortography is not necessary in the majority of patients with an abdominal aortic aneurysm. It is useful, however, to delineate any associated significant peripheral, renal, or mesenteric occlusive disease if there are symptoms or physical findings to suggest their presence and/or need for repair at the time of surgical repair of the aortic aneurysm.

The prognosis for untreated abdominal aortic aneurysm is closely related to size and natural history of the aneurysm. In a review of 24,000 autopsies, Dearling and co-workers[25] found that aneurysms 10 cm or greater had 60% incidence of rupture, aneurysms 7 cm to 10 cm had 45% incidence of rupture, and aneurysms 4 cm to 7 cm had 25% incidence of rupture. In a more recent study of 296 patients with an

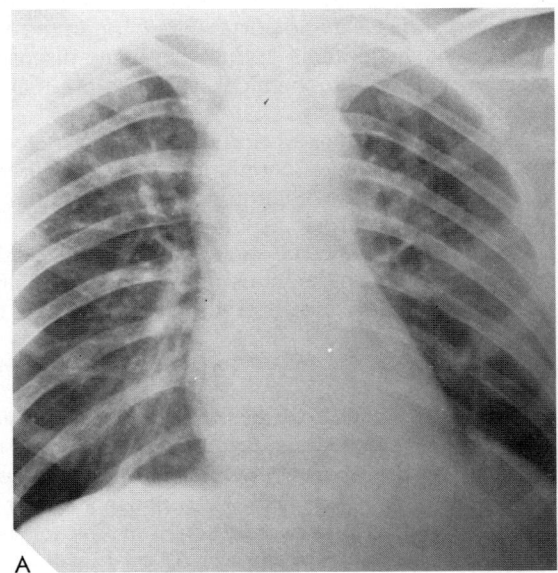
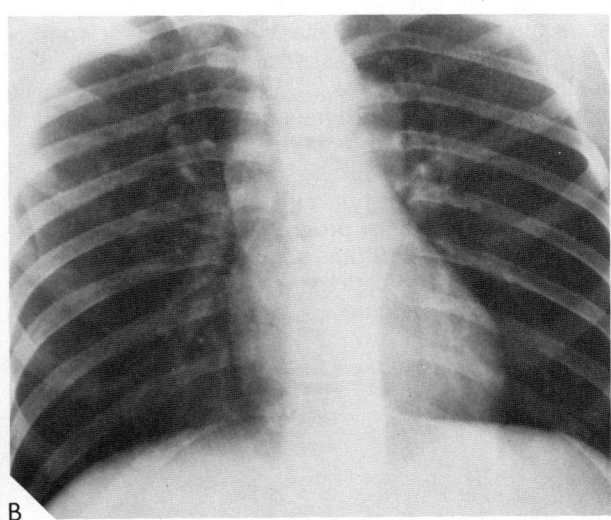
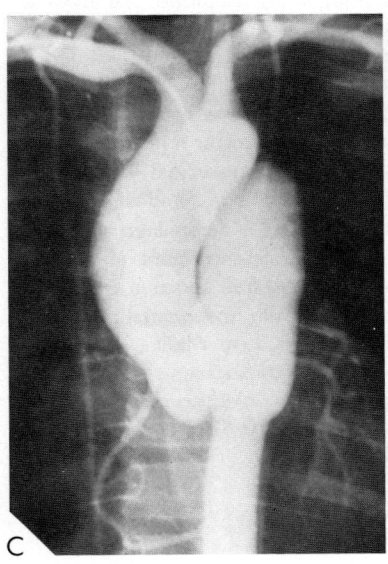
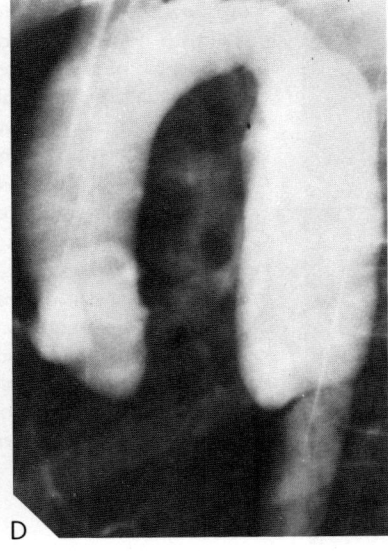

FIGURE 108.1 A. Chest film of 12-year-old girl involved in automobile accident. Severe chest injury; note questionably widened superior mediastinum. **B.** Twelve days later, after surgery for pelvic fractures, mediastinum is widened and arch is prominent. **C** and **D.** Anteroposterior and lateral views of thoracic aortogram show false aneurysm at site of laceration. At operation, there was circumferential intimal laceration with only adventitial tissue containing aneurysm, which was successfully repaired. (Fulton RE, Stanson AW, Forbes GS et al: Vascular imaging. In Juergens JL, Spittell JA Jr, Fairbairn JF II (eds): Peripheral Vascular Diseases, 5th ed. Philadelphia, WB Saunders, 1980, by permission of Mayo Foundation)

abdominal aortic aneurysm, Bicherstaff and colleagues reported an overall incidence of rupture of 20.3%; rupture occurred in only two aneurysms smaller than 5 cm in diameter.[26]

Rupture into the free peritoneal space is usually fatal, but most abdominal aneurysms rupture retroperitoneally, initially with temporary containment of the hemorrhage with an average of 24 hours between rupture and death, thus allowing time for diagnosis and surgical intervention. Additional clinical presentations associated with rupture include gastrointestinal bleeding secondary to erosion into the gastrointestinal tract, most commonly into the duodenum, and acute right-sided heart failure caused by rupture of the aneurysm into the adjacent inferior vena cava, creating an aortocaval fistula.

Atheroembolism is an occasional complication of abdominal aortic aneurysm and presents a distinctive clinical picture of livedo reticularis, blue toes, hypertension, and renal insufficiency; all of the clinical features are caused by arteriolar embolization by atheromatous debris from the laminated thrombus within the aneurysm. Prompt recognition of the symptom-complex is important because resection of the aneurysm is the only effective treatment.

Elective surgical resection is indicated in most patients with aneurysm diameter 4.5 cm or greater, in the absence of other significant medical problems.[27] Surgical mortality in good risk patients is approximately 3%. The operative technique consists of replacement of the aneurysm with a prosthetic graft to restore arterial continuity. Remaining aneurysmal wall and retroperitoneum are closed over the graft, which helps to prevent the complication of erosion into the gastrointestinal tract.

Age and preexisting cardiac, pulmonary, cerebrovascular, and/or renal diseases add to the risk of operation. Currently, operative mortality is most often secondary to coronary artery disease with associated myocardial ischemia and poor left ventricular function.[28] Hence particular attention to cardiac status, with assessment of exercise tolerance, is helpful in evaluating the operative risk of the patient with an aortic aneurysm. Coronary arteriography is not needed in every patient but is carried out as in any patient with symptomatic coronary artery disease.

In the patient who is a poor surgical risk, aneurysms in the range of 5 cm in diameter can be observed, but regular evaluationultrasound measurement should be done and any progressive enlargement or the development of tenderness or symptoms should evoke reconsideration of surgical resection. Even in patients with poor left ventricular function, large or symptomatic aneurysms can be resected by supporting the patient in the early postoperative period with intra-aortic balloon counterpulsation.[29]

Late complications of aneurysmectomy occur in about 8.5% and include occlusion of the prosthetic graft (4%), stenosis (0.6%), false aneurysm formation (3%), enteric fistula formation (1%), and infection (3%).[30] The need for effective control of systemic hypertensinfarction, stroke, and recurrent aneurysm formation in hypertensive persons.[31]

AORTIC DISSECTION

Aortic dissection with a frequency of 2000 new cases in the United States each year is the most common catastrophic illness involving the aorta, being more frequent than ruptured abdominal aortic aneurysm.[32]

The exact cause of aortic dissection is not known, but multiple factors may be involved. Recent opinions cast doubt on the causal relationship between cystic medial necrosis and aortic dissection. Indeed the histopathologic changes seen in patients with cystic medial necrosis do not differ significantly from the changes seen in age-matched controls,[33] and recent investigations suggest that these changes result from a process of injury and repair consequent to hemodynamic forces.[34] Systemic hypertension is almost invariably an antecedent (in 94%) and may play a role in initiating the intramural hematoma, as well as having a direct weakening effect on the aortic media.[35] The causative role of hypertension is supported by the finding that coarctation of the aorta predisposes to aortic dissection.[36] Other major risk factors are the Marfan syndrome, and for type I and type II dissection, congenitally bicuspid or unicommissural aortic valves.[37]

In the Marfan syndrome, the histopathologic changes in the aorta have not been found to differ from those seen in controls.[33,34] Thus, the aneurysmal disease and aortic dissection in the Marfan syndrome and perhaps other heritable connective tissue diseases affecting the aorta may be due to a biochemical derangement that is not manifested by histologic alterations.[2]

Additional causes of aortic dissection include trauma associated with sudden deceleration injuries, as well as direct trauma to the arterial wall associated with intra-aortic balloon pumping[38] or arterial cannulation during cardiac operation.[39]

There is an increased incidence of aortic dissection in pregnancy; 50% of all aortic dissections in females under 40 years of age occur during pregnancy, most commonly in the third trimester.[21] This sug-

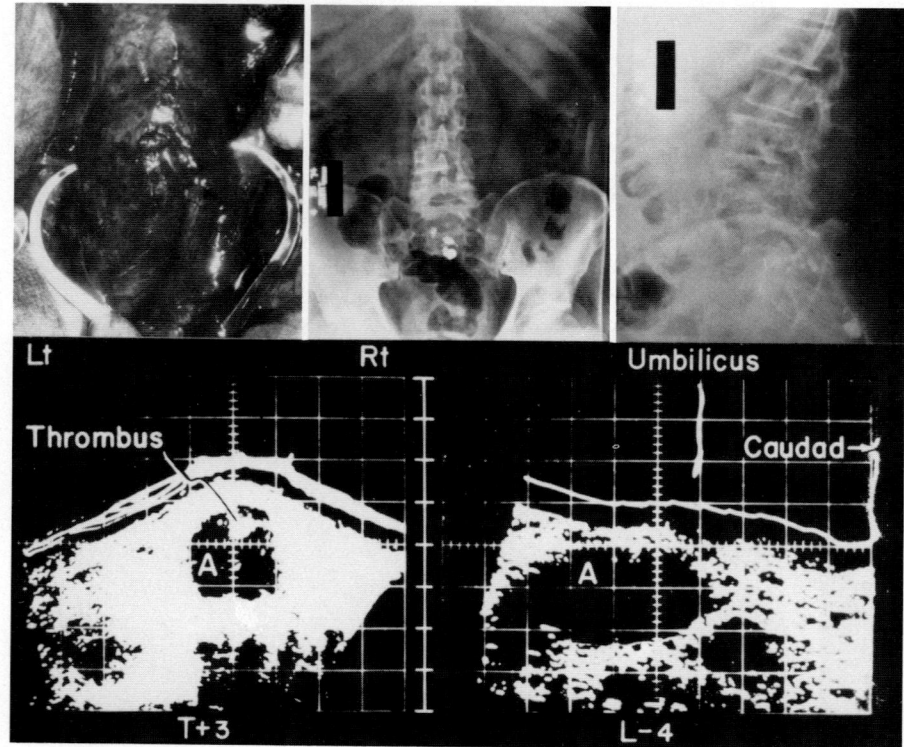

FIGURE 108.2 Correlation of abdominal aortic aneurysm size by surgical, roentgenographic, and ultrasound measurements. Caliper measurement of external transverse aneurysm diameter at time of surgery (upper left). Anteroposterior lumbar spine film (upper middle). Aneurysm is seen as midline soft tissue density. Transverse aneurysm diameter was 6.9 cm. Lateral lumbar spine film (upper right). Aneurysm could not be adequately visualized. The lower left scan shows a bi-stable ultrasound transverse scan 3 cm above umbilicus (T + 3). Internal aneurysm (A) diameter is easily seen. Outer margin of aneurysm wall is not well differentiated from adjacent structures. Internal aneurysm diameter measured 6.0 cm; anteroposterior diameter was 7.1 cm. The lower right scan shows a longitudinal bi-stable ultrasound scan of aneurysm 4 cm to left of umbilicus (L-4). Outer wall of aneurysm can be identified. Anteroposterior internal aneurysm diameter determined in this view is 7.4 cm. Umbilicus is marked as reference point. As one moves caudad to umbilicus, smaller echo-free space is separated from main aneurysm. This is consistent with aneurysmal dilatation of left common iliac artery. Grid scale is 3 cm. Midline vertical and longitudinal scales are divided into 0.6 cm segments. (Maloney JD, Pairolero PC, Smith BF et al: Ultrasound evaluation of abdominal aortic aneurysms. Circulation 56(suppl II):80, 1977, by permission of American Heart Association, Inc.)

gests that there may be an endocrine factor in some cases of aortic dissection, although many of the women had hypertension.

Aortic dissection traditionally results from a transversal intimal tear, which allows the pulsatile force of the aortic lumen to be transmitted, producing longitudinal tearing of the aortic media. The intimal tear is found in the ascending portion of the aortic arch in 90% of patients, usually within 2.0 cm of the aortic valve. Less frequent locations of the intimal tear include the descending aorta and the transverse aortic arch. Rare cases of aortic dissection do not have an associated intimal tear, either proximally or distally, raising the question of whether the intimal tear is the primary event or is secondary to the development of an intramural hematoma in the media. Even more rarely the intimal tear originates in an ulcerated atheromatous plaque, although this is seen almost exclusively with dissection in the descending aorta.[40]

Once initiated, the dissection may extend proximally and or distally. When the dissection encounters branches of the aorta, it may occlude them, extend into their walls, or pass around their origins. Reentry of the dissection through a second more distal intimal tear is most common in the iliac arteries. Rupture of the external layer of the dissection into a body cavity or space is the most common cause of death in aortic dissection; congestive heart failure usually due to aortic regurgitation is the second most common cause of death.

The classification of aortic dissection is based on the fact that over 95% of all dissections arise in one of two locations: (1) the ascending aorta within several centimeters of the aortic valve and (2) the descending thoracic aorta, usually just beyond the origin of the left subclavian artery at the site of the ligamentum arteriosum.

DeBakey and associates[41] proposed the following original classification for aortic dissection (Fig. 108.3):

Type I: The dissection arises in the ascending aorta and extends distally.
Type II: The dissection is limited to the ascending aorta.
Type III: The dissection arises at or just distal to the origin of the left subclavian artery and extends distally or rarely retrogradely into the arch of ascending aorta.

A fourth type has been proposed to include iatrogenic retrograde dissection during intra-arterial catheterization or cannulation.

For clinical purposes, since types I and II have a similar prognosis, there are really only two types; those with the tear in the ascending aorta and those with the tear in the descending aorta, also called "proximal" and "distal," respectively.[42] The peak incidence of aortic dissection is in the 5th to 7th decades, and it is more common in males than in females (2 to 3:1); although the incidence is equal between males and females in persons under 40 years of age due to the occurrence of aortic dissection occurring in females during pregnancy.

Aortic dissection should always be considered in any patient who presents with chest pain, but classic presentation is a sudden onset of excruciating pain, usually beginning in the anterior chest radiating to the back and moving distally as the dissection progresses. The pain is described as often "ripping," "tearing," or "stabbing." It is very suggestive that a patient experiencing such pain who appears to be in shock but has moderate or even severe hypertension has aortic dissection. Cardiac murmurs are usually heard at the base of the heart and may be systolic, diastolic, or both. A diastolic murmur of aortic regurgitation indicates involvement of the ascending aorta and is heard in over 50% of patients with type I dissections. Other cardiovascular findings include tachycardia, friction rubs, bruits, changes in arterial pulses, and, occasionally, distention of neck veins. Peripheral pulse deficits may be transitory owing to decompression of the hematoma into the true lumen.

Neurologic deficits, more common with proximal dissections, are seen in 40% or more of patients and include cerebrovascular accident, disturbances of consciousness, ischemic paraparesis, and ischemic peripheral neuropathy.[43]

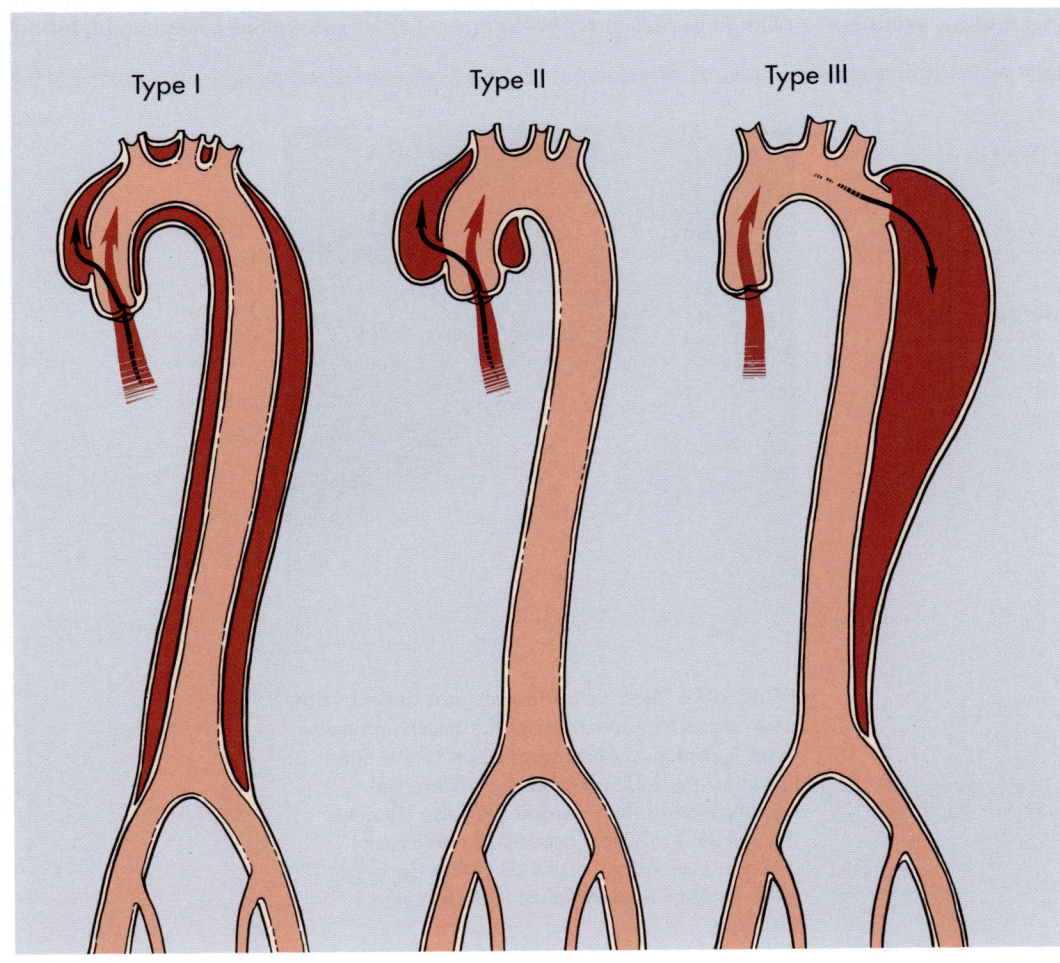

FIGURE 108.3 Classification of aortic dissection. Type I: primary tear in ascending aorta and dissection involving aortic arch and distal aorta for a variable distance. Type II: dissection involving only ascending aorta. Type III: primary tear in subclavian artery, extending distally for a variable distance. (Modified from DeBakey ME, Henly WS, Cooley DA et al: Surgical management of dissecting aneurysms of the aorta. J Thorac Cardiovasc Surg 49:130, 1965)

Signs that may be seen rarely in aortic dissection include pulsation of one of the sternoclavicular joints,[44] Horner's syndrome secondary to compression of the superior cervical ganglion, vocal cord paralysis, and pleural effusion (more common on the left). If the dissection has extended into the abdominal aorta, it is usually tender and its pulsation widened.[2]

Laboratory studies are not very helpful in acute aortic dissection. There may be a mild to moderate leukocytosis. Serum lactate dehydrogenase and bilirubin levels are sometimes increased because of blood sequestered within the false lumen, but serum glutamic oxaloacetic transaminase and creatine phosphokinase values are usually normal. Disseminated intravascular coagulation has been reported rarely.

The most common electrocardiographic (ECG) pattern is left ventricular hypertrophy from systemic hypertension. Acute ischemic changes can be seen if the dissection has involved the coronary ostia, and the ECG changes of acute pericarditis can be seen if there has been leakage of blood into the pericardium.[2] Arrhythmias of any type may be seen but are not common.

The diagnosis of aortic dissection can be elusive unless suspected from the history. The availability of effective therapy makes it important not only that the diagnosis be made promptly but also that the location of the primary intimal tear be determined. Although angiography is the definitive test for determining the site of the intimal tear, certain findings on physical examination suggest involvement of the ascending aorta (type I):

1. Initial pain in the anterior chest
2. Aortic diastolic murmur
3. Pericardial friction rub
4. Decreased or absent blood pressure or pulses in right arm
5. Decreased right carotid artery pulsation
6. Evidence of myocardial ischemia or infarction on ECG
7. The Marfan syndrome.

Chest roentgenography may aid in the diagnosis of dissecting aneurysm (Table 108.1).[45] An abnormally widened supracardiac aortic contour and mediastinal widening may be seen. This finding is particularly useful if an earlier chest roentgenogram is available for comparison. If the aortic knob is calcified, a wide separation of the intimal calcification from the adventitial border ("calcium sign") is virtually pathognomonic, particularly when seen in the lateral projection. Chest roentgenograms may be normal in 20% of cases so a normal chest roentgenogram does not exclude aortic dissection. Fluoroscopy may show that the pulsations in an abnormally widened aorta are diminished or absent over an area of dissection.

Two-dimensional echocardiography may show a widened aortic root, delineate the dissecting hematoma, and even demonstrate the intimal flap.[46]

Computed tomography with intravenous contrast enhancement may be of benefit as an initial diagnostic procedure when aortic dissection is suspected. It is quite reliable in demonstrating the dissection; however, it will not demonstrate sites of reentry in the lower thoracic or abdominal aorta, aortic regurgitation, or involvement of branches of the aorta.

Aortography is the definitive diagnostic procedure and is essential to localize the site of origin of the dissection and to delineate the extent of the dissection as well as the circulation to vital organs. Diagnostic aortographic features include opacification of the false lumen, deformity of the true lumen by the false lumen, widening of the aorta, narrowing or occlusion of branches of the aorta, and presence of an intimal flap (Fig. 108.4).[5]

Initially, the patient suspected of having aortic dissection should be placed in an intensive care unit for close observation, appropriate monitoring, and pharmacologic therapy. Initial objectives are to control pain and hypertension with pharmacologic therapy. Both two-dimensional echocardiography and computed tomography are useful noninvasive tests to confirm the diagnosis if they are available without delay. However, to obtain a definitive diagnosis and to plan definitive management, thoracic aortography should be carried out urgently and then continued pharmacologic management, surgical treatment, or both can be instituted.

Medical management (Table 108.2) of aortic dissection, originally proposed by Wheat and associates,[47] is aimed at lowering the rate of change of pressure development (dP/dt) as well as lowering the blood

TABLE 108.1 ROENTGENOGRAPHIC FINDINGS IN 74 CASES OF THORACIC AORTIC DISSECTION

Finding	No. Patients	%
Abnormalities in region of aortic knob	49	66
Change from previous films	9*	47*
Irregular aortic contour	28	38
Discrepancy in diameters of ascending and descending aorta	25	34
Pleural effusion		
Left	15	
Bilateral	4	
Right	1	
Indistinct aortic margin	13	18
Mediastinal widening	8	11
Displacement of calcified intima	5	7
Negative chest or nonspecific findings	13	18

* Previous films were available in 19 cases.

(Earnest F, Muhm JR, Sheedy PF: Roentgenographic findings in thoracic aortic dissection. Mayo Clin Proc 54:43, 1979, by permission of Mayo Foundation)

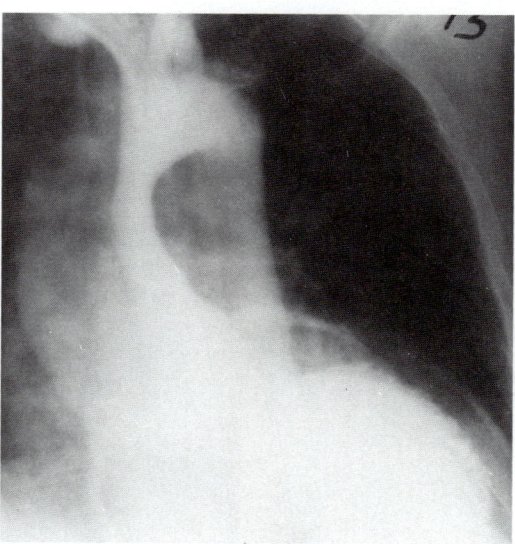

FIGURE 108.4 Thoracic aortogram in a patient with acute dissecting aneurysm of the ascending aorta (type I) demonstrating compression of the true lumen by the false channel and differential opacification of the true and the false channels. (Spittell JA Jr: Clinical aspects of aneurysmal disease. Curr Probl Cardiol 5:1, 1980. Copyright © 1980 by Year Book Medical Publishers, Inc., Chicago)

pressure. β-blockade is essential if sodium nitroprusside is used to control hypertension since the latter can cause an increase in left ventricular ejection velocity, which is an undesirable affect in aortic dissection.[48]

It is generally accepted that in type I and II dissections results with surgical therapy are better than those with medical therapy.[49,50] The best therapy of type III dissection is less clear. Some recommend 2 to 3 weeks of pharmacologic therapy followed by surgical repair if the dissection becomes stable and the patient's general condition does not contraindicate surgery. Others recommend long-term medical therapy with regular periodic evaluation for evidence of any progression of dissection or development of saccular aneurysm, both of which are indications for surgery. In summary, surgical results are superior to medical therapy in proximal dissection while decisions for medical or surgical therapy are individualized in most cases of uncomplicated distal dissection.

The objectives of surgical therapy include excision of the intimal tear, obliteration of the entrance into the false lumen, repair of aortic regurgitation (if present), and restoration of patency to any major arteries occluded by the dissection.[51]

Postoperatively, long-term medical therapy of hypertension is essential since hypertension and left ventricular ejection velocity play an important role in the recurrence of aortic dissection. Regular evaluation including a chest roentgenogram is desirable several times a year initially and later once or twice a year.

AORTITIS

Inflammatory changes can occur in the wall of the aorta in response to any type of injury; therefore, aortitis refers to a group of disorders with diverse etiologies.

GIANT CELL ARTERITIS

The etiology of giant cell arteritis (granulomatous arteritis, cranial arteritis, temporal arteritis) is unknown, but some believe it to be a generalized form of vascular inflammation akin to the collagen vascular diseases.[52] The disease characteristically involves medium-sized arteries, but the aorta and its major branches are involved in approximately 15% of cases.[53]

Pathologically, the arteritis involves isolated segments of the aorta and its major branches. The morphologic alterations noted in affected arteries suggest some form of immunologic reaction, possibly against the elastic lamina of the arterial wall. With widespread but segmental vascular involvement the disease is distributed in "skip areas" and is "patchy," thus limiting the value of arterial biopsy in areas not clinically involved.

The involved aorta may undergo generalized dilatation with resultant formation of saccular aneurysm or dissection hematoma.

Clinically, giant cell arteritis is a subacute or chronic inflammatory process with local and systemic manifestations. It occurs most commonly in persons older than 55 years and affects females more frequently than males (1.5 to 3:1).[52]

Headache is the most common symptom and is characteristically severe and throbbing. The symptom-complex of polymyalgia rheumatica with general malaise may precede, accompany, or be present without the headache. Jaw pain with chewing, anorexia, weight loss, and fever are other frequent symptoms. When the disease involves the aorta or its major branches, ischemic symptoms of the upper or lower extremities may be prominent or even the major complaint of the patient.

On physical examination, the temporal arteritis are involved in 50% to 75% and examination of the involved arteries may show tenderness, swelling, and erythema of the overlying skin along with thickening, nodularity, and reduced or absent pulsation of the involved artery.

Laboratory findings suggestive of giant cell arteries include a rapid erythrocyte sedimentation rate (ESR) (often >100 mm/hr) and a moderate normochromic normocytic anemia.

The major complication of giant cell arteritis is blindness secondary to ischemic optic neuritis, ischemic retrobulbar neuritis, or occlusion of the central retinal artery.[52] Extensive involvement of the thoracic aorta can result in occlusion of one or more branches of the aortic arch, dilatation or saccular aneurysm of the aorta, or even aortic dissection.

The diagnosis of giant cell arteritis should be suspected in any elderly patient with an otherwise unexplained ESR, anemia, headache, and/or weight loss. The diagnosis is typically made by biopsy of a superficial temporal artery; however, in cases with larger vessel and aortic involvement, angiography may show segmental involvement, an absence of irregular ulcerating plaques, and an anatomical distribution more typical of arteritis (usually involving the brachial, axillary, and subclavian arteries). An important point in differential diagnosis is that polyarteritis nodosa and Takayasu's disease tend to affect younger individuals. Also, renal artery involvement is rarely seen in giant cell arteritis, in contrast to Takayasu's disease. Management of the patient with giant cell arteritis is prompt administration of corticosteroids in adequate doses (beginning with 45 mg to 60 mg of prednisone daily) to suppress the arteritis. Arterial changes are reversible with adequate therapy, but with failure to suppress the rapid ESR there may be progressive involvement of the aorta and resultant dissection or rupture. Fortunately, giant cell arteritis usually runs a self-limited course up to many months so that eventually most patients can be gradually weaned from corticosteroid therapy after the disease is suppressed.

TAKAYASU'S DISEASE

In contrast to giant cell arteritis, Takayasu's disease ("pulseless disease") is most common in persons from 20 to 50 years old with 90% of patients being under 30 years old[50] and in up to 75% of patients onset of the arteritis is in the teenage years. It affects females more commonly than males (8.5:1).

Takayasu's arteritis is characterized by marked intimal proliferation and fibrosis along with fibrous scarring of the media. It is the intimal proliferation that accounts for the obliterative changes in the aorta and involved arteries. The arteritis most commonly involves the aortic arch and its major branches, extending in most patients to the descending aorta and its branches, the process being most marked at the points of origin of arteries from the aorta (Fig. 108.5). The pulmonary artery is involved in up to 50% of cases.[54]

The onset of Takayasu's arteritis in more than one half of patients is characterized by fever, anorexia, malaise, weight loss, night sweats, and fatigue, but the true nature of the disease often goes unrecognized

---

TABLE 108.2 PHARMACOLOGIC TREATMENT PROGRAM FOR ACUTE DISSECTING ANEURYSM

Hypertensive Patients

Trimethaphan or sodium nitroprusside intravenously until oral drugs control blood pressure
Propranolol, 20 mg four times daily

Normotensive Patients

Propranolol, 1 mg intramuscularly every 4 to 6 hours or 20 mg orally every 6 hours until the signs and symptoms of the occlusive arterial phase develop. The initial "systemic phase" subsides and is followed by a latent period when there may be signs and symptoms related to inflammatory changes within affected vessels. The occlusive arterial phase is characterized principally by ocular disturbances and marked diminution or disappearance of the pulses in the upper extremities; clinical manifestations vary and reflect arterial insufficiency to the involved end organs. Cerebrovascular insufficiency, arterial insufficiency of the upper or lower extremities, and/or mesenteric arterial insufficiency may be seen, depending on the location of the arteritis and aortitis. A "reversed coarctation" may be seen with weak pulses and low blood pressure in the upper extremities and elevated blood pressure in the lower extremities. Hypertension is the result of acquired aortic coarctation and/or involvement of the renal arteries by the arteritis.

Laboratory evaluation of Takayasu's disease is usually remarkable for a rapid ESR, mild anemia of chronic disease (during the systemic phase), and elevated levels of IgG.

The clinical diagnosis of Takayasu's disease is made by aortography, with the characteristic findings being an irregular intimal surface, segmental narrowing of a variable length of descending or abdominal aorta, and/or narrowing of the origin of major branches of the aorta.[2] Rarely, Takayasu's arteritis can affect the aortic root and cause both aortic valvular insufficiency and coronary ostial involvement. Additional findings that may be seen include post-stenotic dilatations, saccular aneurysms, and, of course, complete arterial occlusion. The most common cause of death in Takayasu's disease is heart failure.

In the early "systemic phase" of the disease, therapy with corticosteroids, at times combined with anticoagulant therapy, is effective in controlling systemic and ischemic symptoms and may result in return of pulses. In the later occlusive phase, surgical bypass of the obstruction may be necessary to relieve significant cerebral or limb ischemia or the hypertension caused by renal artery stenosis.[52,55] Best results of arterial surgery in Takayasu's disease are achieved when it is performed after the activity of the disease is suppressed.

SYPHILITIC AORTITIS AND ARTERITIS

Syphilitic aortitis is relatively rare today, owing to the aggressive and effective antibiotic treatment of syphilis in its early stages. Luetic aortitis is the direct result of spirochetal infection of the aortic media during the initial infection with subsequent inflammation and scarring of the media, adventitia, and vasa vasorum. The aortic wall becomes progressively weakened by the inflammatory process and fibrosis. The result is a characteristic wrinkling of the intima as a late manifestation 10 to 30 years after the initial infection. An obliterative type of luetic arteritis (small vessel lesions) can occur in any stage of acquired or congenital syphilis.

Syphilitic aortitis most commonly involves the ascending aorta and, in order of decreasing frequency, the aortic arch, and the descending thoracic aorta.[2] The infection may extend into the aortic root, producing the aortic valvular regurgitation so often seen with syphilitic aneurysms of the ascending aorta.

Syphilitic aneurysms are most commonly saccular and are usually located in the ascending aorta, where they, like other thoracic aortic aneurysms, may cause symptoms by compression of other mediastinal structures or by bony erosion. Although rare, syphilitic abdominal aortic aneurysms occur, most commonly at the T-12 to L-2 level in patients under 50 years of age. This is in contrast to atherosclerotic abdominal aortic aneurysms, which are seen in older persons and are typically located below the origin of the renal arteries.

Luetic aortitis, unless complicated, is usually asymptomatic.[2] The diagnosis of syphilitic aortitis is suggested by a history of and positive serologic tests for syphilis, as well as the presence of other manifestations of tertiary lues (seen in 10% to 30% of patients with cardiovascular syphilis). The chest roentgenogram may show an ascending aortic aneurysm and extensive calcification of the ascending aorta. The calcification most suggestive of syphilitic aortitis is linear calcification of the ascending aorta; the calcification seen with other types of aortitis does not usually involve the ascending aorta.

The prognosis for patients with syphilitic aortitis is about the same as that for the general population,[56] whereas the prognosis for those with syphilitic aortic aneurysm is poor, especially when the lesion is large enough to cause symptoms.[57]

Preventive therapy with antibiotics is the most important aspect in the treatment of syphilitic aortitis. Once aneurysm or aortic regurgitation occur, therapy is the same as for such a lesion when it is due to other causes, along with appropriate antiluetic antibiotic therapy.

OTHER AORTIC INFECTIONS

Bacterial or fungal infection of the aortic wall is most common in the ascending aorta[58]; in fact, the aorta is the artery most often involved with mycotic aneurysm.[59]

Mycotic aneurysm is the original term used by Osler to describe localized dilatation of the aortic or any arterial wall caused by sepsis. It is thought that the hematogenous spread of bacteria in septicemia or infective endocarditis causes "seeding" of the aortic wall, producing an endaortitis. Fusiform, saccular, or false aneurysms result. Alternatively, infection may complicate a preexisting atherosclerotic aneurysm, but the incidence of this is rare (about 1.2 cases/year).[58] *Staphy-*

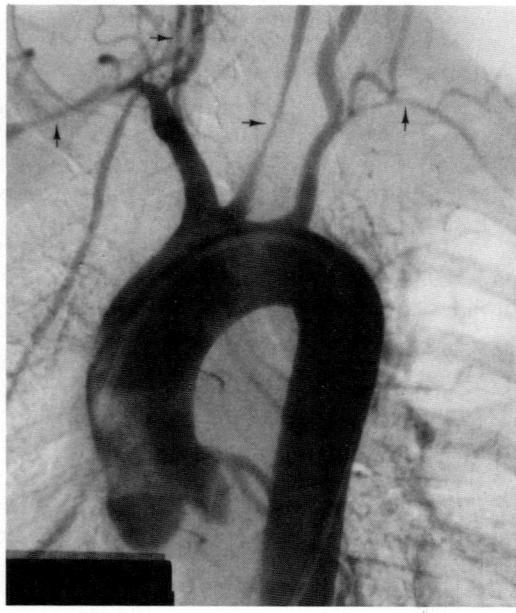

FIGURE 108.5 Arch aortogram in 28-year-old woman with idiopathic medial aortopathy and arteriopathy (Takayasu's disease). Note severe narrowing of both common carotid arteries (*horizontal arrows*) and both subclavian arteries (*vertical arrows*). Left axillary artery is occluded in mid course. (Sheps SG, McDuffie FC: Vasculitis. In Juergens JL, Spittell JA, Fairbairn JF (eds): Peripheral Vascular Diseases, 5th ed. Philadelphia, WB Saunders, 1980, by permission of Mayo Foundation)

lococcus is the most common infecting organism[60]; *Salmonella* species, *Streptococcus*, *Pseudomonas*, and anaerobes are involved less frequently. Rarely, fungal infection with *Candida* or *Aspergillus* may occur. The natural history of mycotic aneurysm is one of progressive expansion, thinning of the aneurysm wall, and eventual rupture.

The clinical manifestations of an infected aneurysm are those of a bloodstream infection; mycotic aneurysms usually do not produce signs unless they encroach on a surrounding structure or it ruptures. Therefore, the finding of a tender, pulsatile abdominal or extremity mass in a patient with a febrile illness should raise the suspicion of mycotic or infected aneurysm.

Diagnosis is generally made with aortography although ultrasound, gallium scanning, and computerized tomography with intravenous contrast enhancement may serve as useful screening procedures.

Treatment of mycotic aneurysm includes appropriate antibiotic chemotherapy and wide surgical excision.

THE ARTERITIS OF RHEUMATIC DISEASE

The cardiovascular system is involved as one of the major secondary targets of rheumatoid arthritis. Small and medium-sized arteries are most commonly involved by the vasculitis. Although unproven, it is thought the vasculitis is of immune complex origin.[61] In acute rheumatic fever, both arteries and veins are sometimes the site of the acute vasculitis. Aortic involvement in rheumatoid arthritis and rheumatic fever is a panaortitis, involving the intima, media, and adventitia.[62] The involved arteries may develop an acute necrotizing vasculitis that may be complicated by thrombosis resulting in myocardial infarction, cerebrovascular occlusive disease, mesenteric infarction, and Raynaud's phenomenon.[63] Interestingly, these vascular changes are most often encountered in patients receiving steroid therapy,[61] but the significance of this association is unknown.

Other uncommon forms of aortitis include that seen with ankylosing spondylitis and relapsing polychondritis.

PERIPHERAL ARTERIAL DISEASE

Peripheral arterial disease, whether occlusive, aneurysmal, or vasospastic, is generally not difficult to diagnose. The extremities are easy to examine, and symptoms of peripheral arterial disease, if present, are fairly distinctive.

Examination of the peripheral arterial system should include an evaluation of the pulsations and character of the upper extremity arteries (subclavian, brachial, radial, and ulnar), the abdominal aorta, and the lower extremity arteries (femoral, popliteal, dorsal pedis, and posterior tibial).

If occlusive arterial disease is suspected in either the upper or the lower extremity, auscultation over the major arteries for bruits may elicit helpful confirmation.[64] Furthermore, the degree of any ischemia can be roughly estimated by the observation of any pallor that develops with elevation (Table 108.3) and the time required for return of color and filling of veins with dependency after elevation (Table 108.4).

When there are symptoms or signs of peripheral arterial disease in an upper extremity the adequacy of the circulation in the hand can be easily assessed by the Allen test (Fig. 108.6).[65] In addition, the existence of compression of the subclavian artery in the thoracic outlet should be evaluated by the thoracic outlet maneuvers (Figs. 108.7 through 108.9).

Additional objectivity in the diagnosis of peripheral arterial disease has been added by the development of noninvasive methods applicable to occlusive arterial disease, aneurysmal disease, and vasospasm.

For occlusive arterial disease in the lower extremity, systolic brachial and ankle blood pressures, taken in the supine position, can be readily made with a hand-held Doppler flow detector and a standard arm blood pressure cuff. Normally the supine systolic pressure at the ankle equals or exceeds that at the brachial level, while in the case of occlusive arterial disease the systolic pressure at the ankle is reduced. By determining the systolic brachial and ankle pressures before and after standard exercise (we use walking on a treadmill at 2 miles per hour at a 10% grade for 5 minutes if the patient's symptoms permit), not only is the detection of occlusive arterial disease more sensitive[66] but also one can develop some standards of quantification (Table 108.5) and get a more accurate estimate of functional disability imposed by the occlusive disease than the medical history provides. During the standard exercise, ECG monitoring for any ischemic change is desirable because of the frequency of significant coronary artery disease in patients with intermittent claudication. In the case of occlusive arterial disease in the upper extremity, systolic pressures in the arms can be similarly determined. Occlusive arterial disease in the digits can be determined by measuring the systolic pressure (using a Doppler flow detector distal to an occluding cuff) or by plethysmographic methods.[67] By performing the thoracic outlet maneuvers as described and by measuring brachial artery pressures with a hand-held Doppler detector, objective confirmation of the presence or absence of thoracic outlet compression can be obtained.

Although arteriography is the only diagnostic procedure that demonstrates the location of occlusive arterial disease and its extent and the character of the arterial circulation proximally and distally, it is usually only necessary when restoration of pulsatile flow is being considered or the etiology of the occlusive arterial disease is uncertain.

As in the case of abdominal aortic and iliac artery aneurysms, ultrasound is the diagnostic method of choice for femoral and popliteal artery aneurysms.[68]

TABLE 108.3 GRADING OF ELEVATION PALLOR*

Grade of Pallor	Duration of Elevation
0	No pallor in 60 seconds
1	Definite pallor in 60 seconds
2	Definite pallor in less than 60 seconds
3	Definite pallor in less than 30 seconds
4	Pallor on the level

* Elevation of extremity at angle of 60 degrees above the level.

(Spittell JA Jr: Recognition and management of chronic atherosclerotic occlusive peripheral arterial disease. Mod Concepts Cardiovasc Dis 50:19, 1981, by permission of American Heart Association, Inc.)

TABLE 108.4 COLOR RETURN (CR) AND VENOUS FILLING TIME (VFT)

Finding	Time for CR (sec)	VFT (sec)
Normal	10	15
Moderate ischemia	15–20	20–30
Severe ischemia	40+	40+

(Spittell JA: Recognition and management of chronic atherosclerotic occlusive peripheral arterial disease. Mod Concepts Cardiovasc Dis 50:19, 1981, by permission of American Heart Association, Inc.)

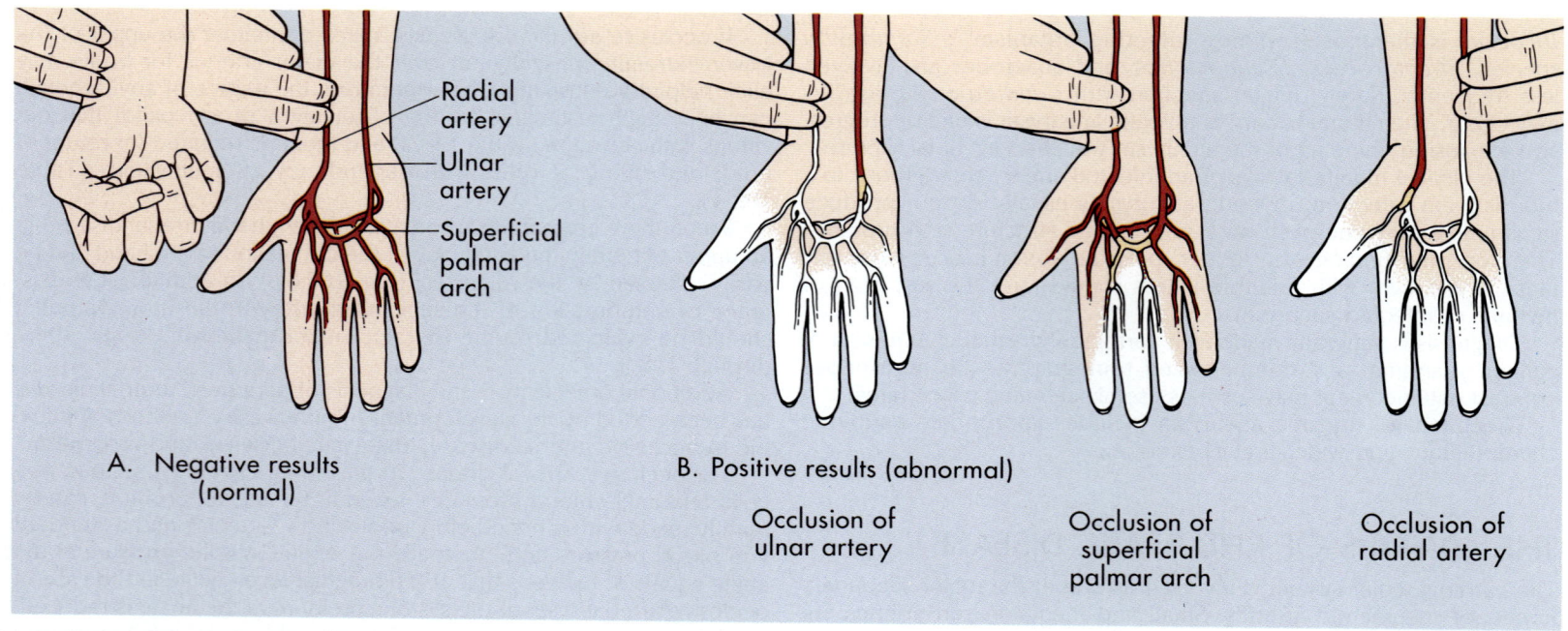

FIGURE 108.6 Allen test. **A.** Normal (negative) result, indicating patency of ulnar artery and superficial palmar arch. **B.** Abnormal (positive) result due to occlusion of ulnar artery (**left**), radial artery (**right**), and superficial palmar arch (**center**). (Modified from Spittell JA Jr: Occlusive peripheral arterial disease: Guidelines for office management. Postgrad Med 71:137, 1982)

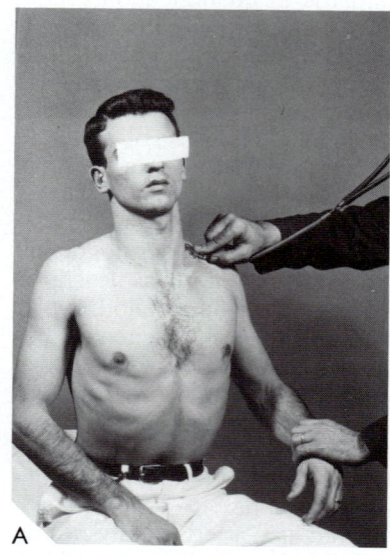
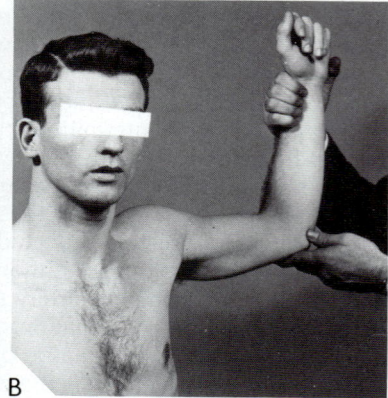

FIGURE 108.7 A. Costoclavicular maneuver, active. Auscultation over subclavian artery, above or below midportion of clavicle, may reveal systolic bruit as artery is compressed. Radial pulse and bruit over subclavian artery disappear when complete compression of subclavian artery occurs. **B.** Costoclavicular maneuver, passive. (Fairbairn JF II, Campbell JK, Payne WS: Neurovascular compression syndrome of the thoracic outlet. In Juergens JL, Spittell JA, Fairbairn JF II (eds): Peripheral Vascular Diseases, 5th ed, pp 629–653. Philadelphia, WB Saunders, 1980, by permission of Mayo Foundation)

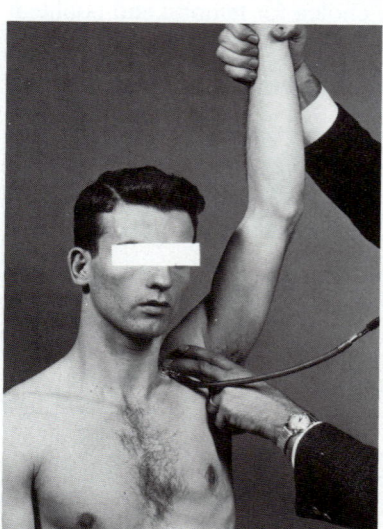

FIGURE 108.8 Hyperabduction maneuver. Axillary artery may be completely or incompletely compressed by maneuver. In the latter case, bruit may be heard above or below clavicle or, on occasion, deep in axilla. (Fairbairn JF II, Campbell JK, Payne WS: Neurovascular compression syndrome of the thoracic outlet. In Juergens JL, Spittell JA, Fairbairn JF II (eds): Peripheral Vascular Diseases, 5th ed, pp 629–653. Philadelphia, WB Saunders, 1980, by permission of Mayo Foundation)

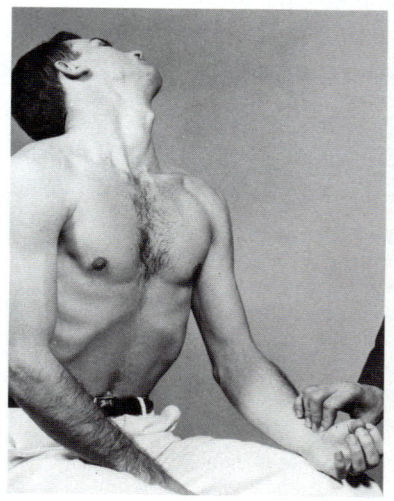

FIGURE 108.9 Scalene or Adson maneuver. This test is used in both cervical rib or anomalous first thoracic rib syndrome and scalenus anticus syndrome. Auscultation over subclavian artery being tested may reveal bruit when artery is partially compressed. (Fairbairn JF II, Campbell JK, Payne WS: Neurovascular compression syndrome of the thoracic outlet. In Juergens JL, Spittell JA Jr, Fairbairn JF II (eds): Peripheral Vascular Diseases, 5th ed, pp 629–653. Philadelphia, WB Saunders, 1980, by permission of Mayo Foundation)

Noninvasive testing is also available for documentation of a vasospastic disorder and for serial evaluation of the effect of therapy. The vasospastic response to cold can be demonstrated by measuring the skin temperature of the digits before and after their immersion in ice water for 30 seconds.[69] In the normal person the digital skin temperatures return to the preimmersion level in 3 to 10 minutes while in the vasospastic disorders the time required to reach preimmersion temperatures exceeds 10 minutes.

OCCLUSIVE PERIPHERAL ARTERIAL DISEASE

Both acute and chronic occlusive peripheral arterial disease can result in loss of digits or limbs. In acute arterial occlusion the outcome depends on prompt recognition, restoration of adequate circulation, and prevention of injury to the ischemic limb, as well as on the type of arterial occlusion (embolic or thrombotic), its location, and associated cardiac or systemic disease. Recognition of chronic occlusive arterial disease, even when asymptomatic, is important since much of the limb loss that occurs results from trauma that is preventable by patient education.[70]

The etiology of occlusive peripheral arterial disease is diverse (Table 108.6). Acute peripheral arterial occlusion can be the initial manifestation of cardiac or systemic disease and at times may be the principal manifestation of acute aortic dissection. Although arteriosclerosis is by far the most common cause of occlusive peripheral arterial disease, the less common types of occlusive arterial disease often present important therapeutic opportunities; they are more easily recognized if thought of, and features that should bring them to mind are listed in Table 108.7.

The clinical presentation of a person with an acute peripheral arterial occlusion may include any or all of the 5 Ps—pain, pallor, paresthesia, pulselessness, paralysis—in varying degrees. At times, abrupt shortening of the claudication distance in the patient with symptomatic occlusive arterial disease will be the only symptomatic evidence of an acute arterial occlusion.

The hallmark of symptomatic occlusive arterial disease is intermittent claudication, and it is as typical in its occurrence with walking and relief with standing still as angina pectoris is with exertion or stress. With care, the many musculoskeletal and neurologic conditions that may be confused with intermittent claudication (Fig. 108.10) can be differentiated by history alone. If not, and findings on physical examination do not settle the issue, noninvasive testing can be of great assistance. When ischemia becomes more severe the patient with chronic occlusive peripheral arterial disease may develop ischemic pain at rest; this is usually in the toes and/or foot, is worse at night, and is relieved temporarily by dependency. In the ischemic limb, trauma can lead to ischemic ulceration, which is typically a painful ulceration with a discrete edge covered with eschar or having a pale base; ischemic ulceration most often occurs on the toes, the heel, or the foot (Fig. 108.11).

Although most occlusive peripheral arterial disease is atherosclerotic and therefore seen in persons over 40 years of age often with associated hyperlipidemia, diabetes, and other manifestations of atherosclerosis (coronary artery disease and cerebrovascular disease), several of the uncommon types of occlusive disease deserve special mention because of their unique clinical features.

Thromboangiitis obliterans (Buerger's disease) is a distinct clinical entity. It involves small and medium-sized arteries and veins of both the upper and lower extremities of young persons, mostly males, who smoke. The criteria for making a diagnosis of thromboangiitis obliterans are shown in Table 108.8. Of interest, some recent work suggests that it may be an autoimmune disorder.[71]

Popliteal artery entrapment typically occurs in young persons and may present the unique feature of calf claudication with walking but not with running[72]; this is probably due to the differences in degree, location, and/or duration of calf muscle tension in running and walking.

In the upper extremity, chronic occupational occlusive arterial disease in the hand deserves mention because of the large number of occupations (Table 108.9) in which recurrent blunt trauma to the palm of the hand can result in occlusive disease in portions of the palmar arch or in the arch itself. Usually the dominant hand is the one involved. The presenting symptoms may be Raynaud's phenomenon, persistent coldness, pain and/or cyanosis, and ischemic ulceration of the involved fingers.

The symptoms of the patient with thoracic outlet compression vary from none to intermittent "claudication" of the arm and forearm, Raynaud's phenomenon, and/or severe ischemia of the hand or fingers, depending on the location and extent of the arterial occlusion, which is usually embolic from thrombus at the site of subclavian artery compression. If a cervical or abnormal first rib is the cause of the thoracic outlet compression, it often can be palpated in the supraclavicular fossa.

One other uncommon but important type of occlusive arterial disease that can present as either acute or chronic arterial insufficiency is ergotism. This is usually the result of misuse of ergot-containing suppositories in the person with migraine, so the history of either should alert the clinician to this possibility. The manifestations may be seen in the upper or lower extremities and tend to be symmetrical. The arteriographic picture of ergotism is distinctive (Fig. 108.12).

TABLE 108.5 NONINVASIVE LABORATORY ASSESSMENT OF ARTERIAL INSUFFICIENCY OF THE LEGS

Degree of Arterial Insufficiency	Standard Exercise		Systolic Blood Pressure Index*	
	Claudication	Duration (min)	Before Exercise	After Exercise
Minimal	0	5	Normal to mild	Abnormal
Mild	+	5	>0.8	>0.5
Moderate	+	<5	<0.8	<0.5
Severe†	+	<3	<0.5	<0.15

* Systolic pressure index is obtained by dividing the systolic ankle blood pressure by the systolic brachial blood pressure, both measured in the supine position (normal, 0.95 or greater).

† Often the systolic ankle blood pressure is less than 50 mmHg.

(Spittell JA Jr: Recognition and management of chronic atherosclerotic occlusive peripheral arterial disease. Mod Concepts Cardiovasc Med 50:19, 1981, by permission of American Heart Association, Inc.)

TABLE 108.6. CLASSIFICATION OF OCCLUSIVE ARTERIAL DISEASE

I. Acute Arterial Occlusion
  A. Thrombotic arterial occlusion secondary to:
    1. Atherosclerosis
      a. Arteriosclerosis obliterans
      b. Atherosclerotic aneurysm
    2. Thromboangiitis obliterans (Buerger's disease)
    3. Arteritis due to:
      a. Connective tissue diseases
      b. Giant cell (temporal or cranial) arteritis
      c. Takayasu's arteritis
    4. Myeloproliferative disease
      a. Polycythemia vera
      b. Thrombocytosis
    5. Hypercoagulable states
      a. Complicating neoplastic disease
      b. Complicating ulcerative bowel disease
      c. Idiopathic ("simple") arterial thrombosis
    6. Trauma
      a. Arterial puncture and arteriotomy
      b. Secondary to fractures and bone dislocations
      c. Arterial entrapment
        1) Lower extremity: adductor tendon compression of superficial femoral artery; popliteal artery entrapment
        2) Upper extremity: thoracic outlet compression; "crutch" thrombosis
      d. Frostbite
  B. Embolic arterial occlusion (arising from thrombi of):
    1. Cardiac origin
      a. Valvular heart disease, including valvular prostheses
      b. Acute myocardial infarction
      c. Myocardial aneurysm
      d. Atrial fibrillation
      e. Cardiomyopathy
      f. Infective endocarditis
      g. Left-sided myxoma
    2. Proximal atherosclerotic plaques or arterial narrowing
    3. Proximal arterial aneurysms
      a. Atherosclerotic
      b. Post-stenotic dilatation
      c. Fibromuscular dysplasia
  C. Miscellaneous causes
    1. Arterial spasm, secondary to:
      a. Ergotism
      b. Trauma of blunt or penetrating type
      c. Intra-arterial injections
    2. Aortic dissection
      a. Luminal compression (by extension of the dissection into branch(es) of the aorta)
      b. Occlusion at site of reentry of dissection
    3. Foreign bodies
      a. Bullet embolism
      b. Guide wires and catheters

II. Chronic Arterial Occlusive Disease
  A. Arteriosclerosis obliterans
  B. Thromboangiitis obliterans (Buerger's disease)
  C. Arteritis
    1. Connective tissue disorders
    2. Giant cell (temporal or cranial) arteritis
    3. Takayasu's disease
  D. Trauma
    1. Blunt trauma: chronic occupational arterial occlusion in the hand
    2. Arterial entrapment: superficial femoral artery; popliteal artery
  E. Congenital arterial narrowing

(Spittell JA Jr: Office and bedside diagnosis of occlusive arterial disease. Curr Probl Cardiol 8:1, 1983. Copyright © 1983 by Year Book Medical Publishers, Inc., Chicago)

TABLE 108.7 CLINICAL FEATURES SUGGESTING UNCOMMON TYPES OF OCCLUSIVE ARTERIAL DISEASE

1. A person younger than age 40
2. Acute ischemia in the absence of prior evidence of occlusive arterial disease
3. Occlusive arterial disease confined to the upper extremity
4. Digital occlusive arterial disease, particularly if accompanied by systemic symptoms

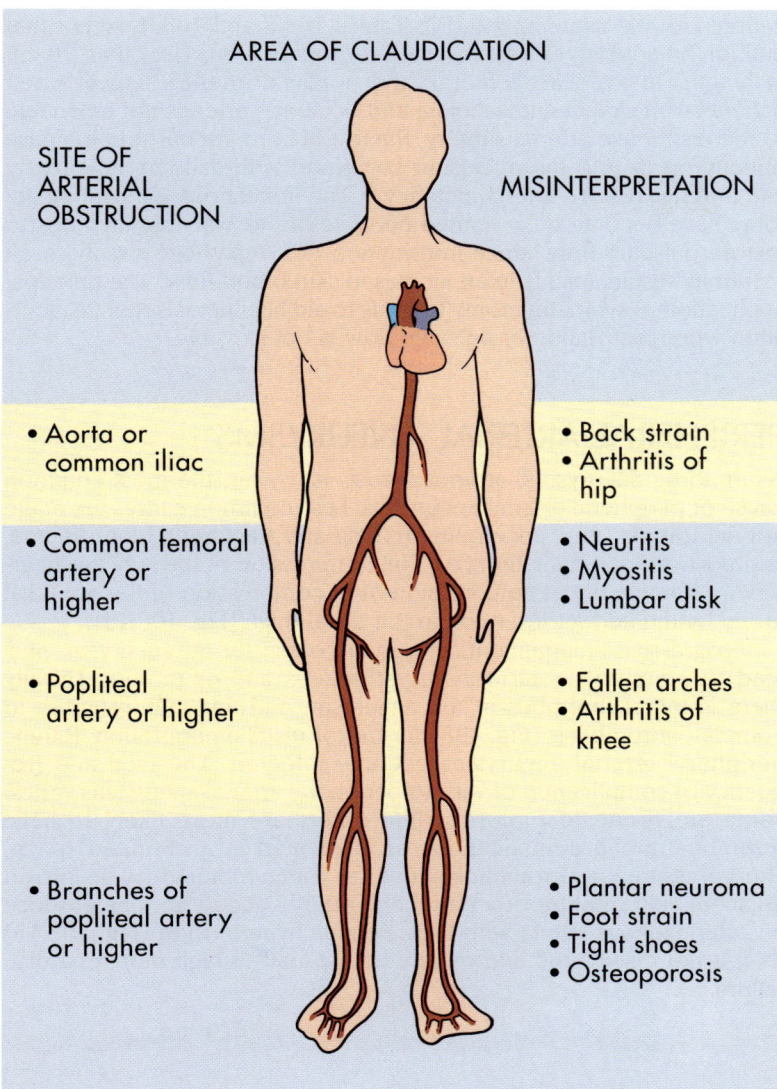

FIGURE 108.10 Common misinterpretation of claudication. Neurologic and musculoskeletal disorders are often incorrectly diagnosed as cause of patient's pain. Careful evaluation of mode of onset and relief will usually clarify distress as intermittent claudication. (Modified from Gifford RW Jr, Hurst JW: A note on the location of intermittent claudication. GP 16:89, 1957)

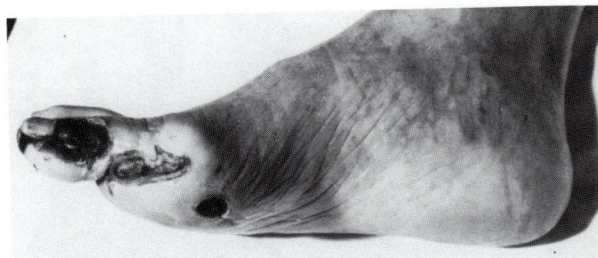

FIGURE 108.11 Ischemic ulceration of the first toe and adjacent part of the foot in a person with arteriosclerosis obliterans.

TABLE 108.8 THROMBOANGIITIS OBLITERANS (BUERGER'S DISEASE): CRITERIA FOR DIAGNOSIS

Age: <30 years

Sex: Males most often

Habits: Smoker

History:
Superficial phlebitis
Raynaud's phenomenon
Claudication, arch or calf

Physical Examination:
Small arteries involved
Upper extremity involved

Laboratory Findings:
Blood sugar and lipids normal

Roentgenogram:
No arterial calcification

(Spittell JA Jr: Some uncommon types of occlusive peripheral arterial disease. Curr Probl Cardiol 8:1, 1983. Copyright © 1983 by Year Book Medical Publishers, Inc., Chicago)

TABLE 108.9 OCCUPATIONS IN WHICH CHRONIC (TRAUMATIC) OCCLUSIVE ARTERIAL DISEASE OF THE HAND HAS BEEN SEEN

Farmer: tools and tractor steering wheel
Laborer: air hammer
Carpenter: hand tools
Mechanics: wrenches; "hammerhand"
Truck drivers: levers, valves, and steering wheel
Butcher: hand tools
Creamery worker: "hammerhand" on milk can lids
Forestry worker: chain saw
Packing house worker: "hammerhand"
Pharmacist: loosening bottle caps
Obstetrician: outlet forceps

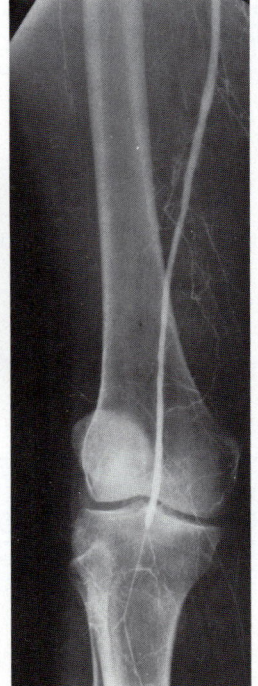

FIGURE 108.12 Arteriogram showing intense spasm of the distal popliteal artery of 55-year-old woman with calf claudication of acute onset due to ergotism from the misuse of ergot-containing suppositories for her migraine headaches. (Spittell JA Jr: Some uncommon types of occlusive peripheral arterial disease. Curr Probl Cardiol 8:1, 1983. Copyright © 1983 by Year Book Medical Publishers, Inc., Chicago)

Regardless of the etiology of occlusive peripheral arterial disease, conservative measures are a basic part of proper management. The importance of avoidance of vasoconstrictive influences such as cold and certain pharmacologic agents (β-blocking drugs, ergot preparations) as well as the complete cessation of smoking should be understood by the patient. Although smoking has an adverse effect on all types of occlusive arterial disease, the patient with thromboangiitis obliterans can be virtually assured that the activity and progression of the disease will stop with cessation of smoking (and resume if the use of tobacco is resumed). For the patient with intermittent claudication a walking program—to the point of symptoms—several times a day may over a period of weeks result in a significant increase in the walking distance. Presently available vasodilators are not effective in the management of intermittent claudication,[73] but preliminary reports[74] indicate that pentoxifylline (a methyl xanthine with multiple effects)[75] may improve the walking distance of some patients with intermittent claudication. The dosage of pentoxifylline is 400 mg, three times daily, taken orally with meals.

In acute arterial occlusion not amenable to embolectomy or thrombectomy, thrombolytic therapy may be useful in selected cases but the usual side-effects and complications of the thrombolytic therapy are limiting factors. Antithrombotic therapy has not been shown to have value in occlusive arterial disease except for the prevention of recurring embolic or thrombotic arterial occlusion.

In the nondiabetic patient with atherosclerotic occlusive arterial peripheral arterial disease whose only symptom is intermittent claudication, restoration of pulsatile flow is elective, with its indication being disabling claudication (Table 108.10). On the other hand, when the ischemia is severe enough to cause pain at rest, when there is ischemic ulceration, or when the patient is a diabetic with symptomatic occlusive arterial disease, restoration of pulsatile flow is indicated because of the increased risk of limb loss in these circumstances (Table 108.11). The availability of percutaneous balloon angioplasty provides a means of restoring pulsatile arterial blood flow with reduced morbidity, mortality, and cost when compared with arterial surgery[76]; the indications are the same as listed in Tables 108.8 and 108.9 except that balloon angioplasty is best reserved for focal lesions (less than 10 cm in length) in the iliac, femoral, and popliteal arteries.[77] In selected patients with significant ischemia and occluded arteries not amenable to reconstructive arterial surgery, the use of intra-arterial streptokinase directly on or into the occlusion combined with balloon angioplasty can at times restore arterial patency.[78] The indications for sympathectomy have become quite limited because of the available methods to restore pulsatile flow, since interruption of sympathetic supply to an extremity results mainly in an increased skin blood flow. The principal application of sympathectomy today is to aid healing of ischemic ulceration when restoration of pulsatile flow is not possible.

PERIPHERAL ARTERIAL ANEURYSMS

As in aortic aneurysms, arteriosclerosis is, by far, the most common cause of peripheral arterial aneurysms. Less common causes are acute arterial trauma (*e.g.*, penetrating trauma and fractures), blunt trauma, and post-stenotic dilatation (*e.g.*, in compression of the subclavian artery in thoracic outlet compression or in compression of the popliteal artery by the adductor tendon in the distal thigh [Fig. 108.13]).

Progressive enlargement, the usual course for an aneurysm, may lead to pressure on surrounding structures and/or rupture. Usually there is mural thrombus in the aneurysm, and this may progress to complete thrombosis (Fig. 108.14) and/or distal embolization. Rarely, peripheral arterial aneurysms become infected. The type and frequency of complication of various peripheral arterial aneurysms varies; some are prone to rupture, while others are more likely to have thromboembolic complications or, if located in a confined space, exert pressure on surrounding structures. Since rupture may be into an adjacent vein, rupture of a peripheral arterial aneurysm may produce an arteriovenous fistula with local venous hypertension (Fig. 108.15) and, if not discovered and repaired, may lead to high output cardiac failure.

TABLE 108.10 CHRONIC ATHEROSCLEROTIC OCCLUSIVE ARTERIAL DISEASE AND INTERMITTENT CLAUDICATION

Restoration of pulsatile flow to limb elective because
1. It does not affect longevity or ameliorate coronary or cerebrovascular disease.
2. The incidence of severe ischemia is relatively low.
3. Runoff should be adequate.
4. Complications of the procedure, although infrequent, do occur.
5. Reocclusion may occur.

(Spittell JA Jr: Peripheral vascular disease: Advances in diagnosis and management. Cardiology Series (Baylor College of Medicine) 7(2):1, 1984)

TABLE 108.11 CHRONIC ATHEROSCLEROTIC OCCLUSIVE ARTERIAL DISEASE AND REST PAIN OR ISCHEMIC ULCERATION

Restoration of pulsatile flow indicated because
1. The incidence of limb loss is relatively high without treatment.
2. It may permit a lower level of amputation.
3. The risks of the procedure are less than is the risk of amputation.

(Spittell JA Jr: Peripheral vascular disease: Advances in diagnosis and management. Cardiology Series (Baylor College of Medicine) 7(2):1, 1984)

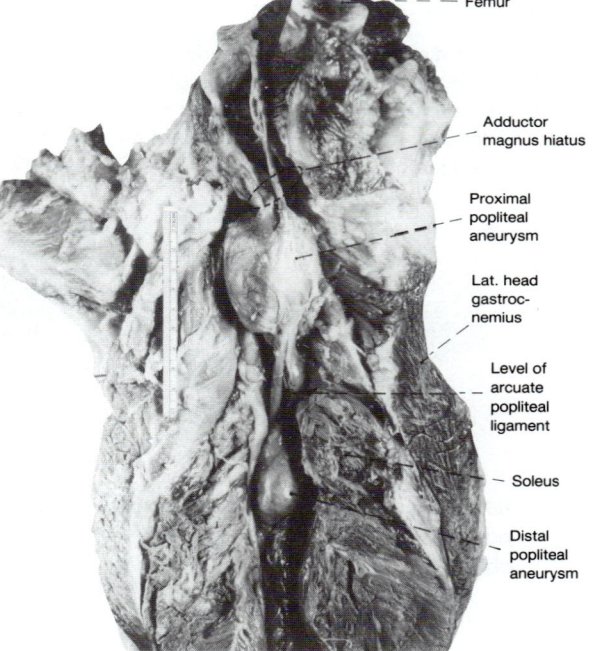

FIGURE 108.13 Photograph of popliteal fossa in dissected amputated limb of patient having proximal and distal popliteal aneurysms. (Gedge SW, Spittell JA Jr, Ivins JC: Aneurysms of the distal popliteal artery and its relationship to the arcuate popliteal ligament. Circulation 24:270, 1961, by permission of American Heart Association, Inc.)

In the extremities the most common aneurysms encountered are those of the femoral and popliteal arteries. They are vastly more common in men and, being atherosclerotic in type, are bilateral in more than one half of cases. In more than 40% of patients with a popliteal aneurysm there are aneurysms of other arteries, usually the abdominal aorta, iliac, or femoral arteries.[79] They are easily detected by careful palpation of the groin, adductor canal, and popliteal space; confirmation of the diagnosis or differentiation from other masses is most expediently achieved with ultrasound.[68] Surgical therapy gives best results before complications of the aneurysm have occurred.[79]

Aneurysms of the upper extremity are uncommon and usually are the result of blunt trauma (e.g., of the palm of the hand) or penetrating trauma or in the subclavian artery result from (post-stenotic dilatation) compression of the artery between the uppermost rib and clavicle.[80]

Splenic artery aneurysm deserves mention because it is the only aneurysm seen more commonly in women. The most common clinical manifestation is a curvilinear shadow of calcification on roentgenograms that include the left upper abdominal quadrant (see Fig. 108.15, A). Another distinctive feature is the unexplained tendency of splenic artery aneurysms to rupture in the third trimester of pregnancy.[81] In patients who are otherwise well, particularly if of childbearing age, elective resection of splenic artery aneurysms seems appropriate.

Renal artery aneurysms, although uncommon and usually asymptomatic, come to the clinician's attention most often on arteriograms carried out in hypertensive patients. The principal complication is thromboembolic, resulting in renal ischemia although rupture does occur rarely, and like aneurysm of the splenic artery, most often occurs during pregnancy. Surgical resection is advised when the renal artery aneurysm is symptomatic, causing documented renovascular hypertension, or is present in a woman of childbearing age.[82]

VASOSPASTIC DISORDERS

The vasospastic disorders (Table 108.12) are poorly understood and frequently overlooked.[83] Both Raynaud's phenomenon and livedo reticularis occur as primary disorders or secondary manifestations of other, often serious diseases. Acrocyanosis, which at times may be confused with the cyanotic phase of Raynaud's phenomenon, is a benign almost constant coldness and bluish discoloration of the hands and fingers and occasionally the feet and toes. Reflex sympathetic dystrophy, basically a neurologic disorder, is included because of the frequency of vasospastic manifestations as a part of the clinical picture. Chronic pernio occurs in persons with either a hyperreactive vascular system or local sensitivity to cold; repeated vasospasm, resulting from reaction to cold, is responsible for the clinical features.

The differentiation of vasospastic disorders from occlusive arterial disease is usually not difficult (Table 108.13). The vasospastic disorders involve small arteries and arterioles and hence their hallmarks are changes in skin color and temperature rather than intermittent claudication and gangrene.

Raynaud's phenomenon, the most common vasospastic disorder, may be defined as brief and intermittent color changes (triphasic usually—pallor, cyanosis, rubor) of the digits due to constriction of small arteries and arterioles, precipitated by exposure to cold or stress. Primary Raynaud's phenomenon is a relatively benign disorder while Raynaud's phenomenon that is secondary in type may be a clinical clue to an important underlying or causative factor (Table 108.14). The differentiation of Raynaud's disease from secondary Raynaud's phenomenon (Table 108.15) is thus of more than academic importance. Initial evaluation of the patient with Raynaud's phenomenon should include those things listed in Table 108.16. If no secondary cause is

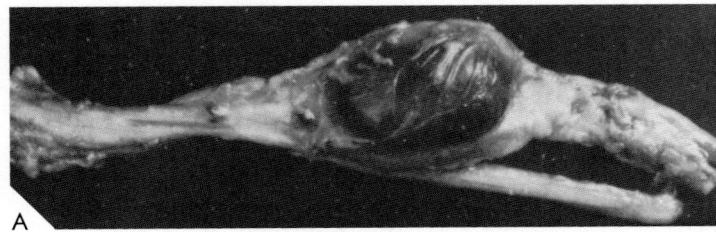
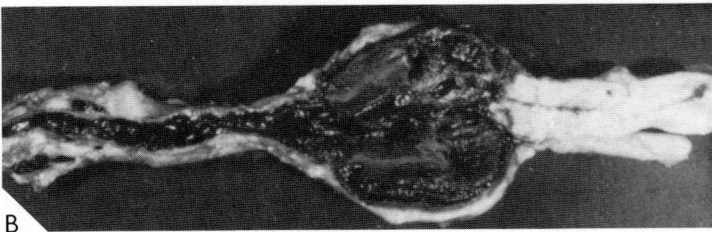

FIGURE 108.14 **A.** Arteriosclerotic aneurysm of popliteal artery. **B.** Specimen opened; complete filling of aneurysm and portion of artery distal to aneurysm by thrombus may be noted. (Spittell JA Jr, Wallace RB: Aneurysms. In Juergens JL, Spittell JA Jr, Fairbairn JF II (eds): Peripheral Vascular Diseases, 5th ed, pp 415–439. Philadelphia, WB Saunders, 1980, by permission of Mayo Foundation)

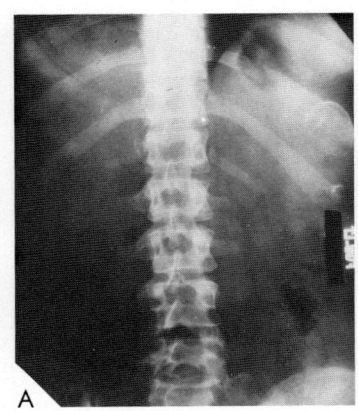
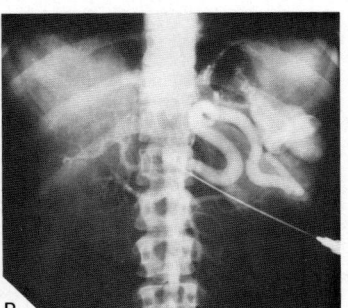
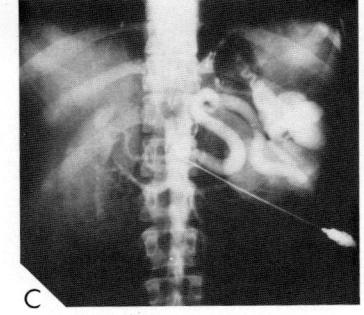
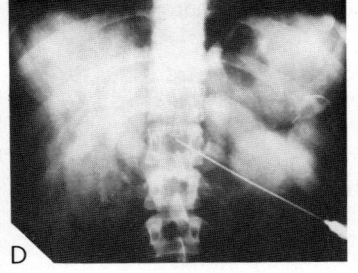

FIGURE 108.15 **A.** Roentgenogram of the abdomen showing crescentic areas of calcification in the left upper quadrant. **B.** Aortogram showing enlarged tortuous splenic artery and opacification within the calcified areas. **C.** Aortogram following second injection of dye. There is opacification of the venous aneurysm adjacent and medial to the calcium-containing aneurysms. **D.** Roentgenogram taken 10 seconds after the one represented in **C**, showing enlarged splenic and portal veins. (Cassel WG, Spittell JA Jr, Ellis FH Jr et al: Arteriovenous fistula of the splenic vessels producing ascites. Circulation 16:1077, 1957, by permission of the American Heart Association, Inc.)

TABLE 108.12 VASOSPASTIC DISORDERS

Raynaud's phenomenon
  Primary (Raynaud's disease)
  Secondary
Livedo reticularis
  Primary
  Secondary
Acrocyanosis
Reflex sympathetic dystrophy
Chronic pernio

TABLE 108.13 DIFFERENTIAL DIAGNOSIS OF VASOSPASTIC AND OCCLUSIVE ARTERIAL DISEASE

Finding	Vasospastic Disorders	Occlusive Arterial Disease
Arteries involved	Small	All
Color changes	+	±
Claudication	−	+
Absent pulses	−	+
Ischemic ulceration	±	±
Major gangrene	−	±

(Spittell JA Jr: The vasospastic disorders. Curr Probl Cardiol 8:1, 1984. Copyright © 1984 by Year Book Medical Publishers, Inc., Chicago)

TABLE 108.14 CONDITIONS THAT MAY CAUSE SECONDARY RAYNAUD'S PHENOMENON

After Trauma
Related to occupation
  Pneumatic hammer disease
  Occupational occlusive arterial disease of the hand
  Occupational acro-osteolysis
  Vasospasm of typists and pianists
Following injury or operation

Neurologic Conditions
Thoracic outlet syndrome
Carpal tunnel syndrome
Other neurologic diseases

Occlusive Arterial Disease
Arteriosclerosis obliterans
Thromboangiitis obliterans
Postembolic or post-thrombotic arterial occlusion

Miscellaneous Conditions
Scleroderma
Lupus erythematosus
Rheumatoid arthritis
Dermatomyositis
Fabry's disease
Paroxysmal hemoglobinuria
Cold agglutinins or cryoglobulinemia
Primary pulmonary hypertension
Myxedema
Associated with certain neoplasms
Associated with hepatitis B antigenemia
Pheochromocytoma
Ergotism
After combination chemotherapy for testicular cancer

(Modified from Spittell JA Jr: Vasospastic disorders: Recognition and management. Cardiovasc Clin 10:279, 1980)

TABLE 108.15 DIFFERENTIAL DIAGNOSIS OF PRIMARY AND SECONDARY RAYNAUD'S PHENOMENON

Features	Suggestive of	
	Raynaud's Disease	Secondary Raynaud's Phenomenon
Sex	F	M
Age at onset	<40 yr	>40 yr
Bilateral involvement	+	±
Ischemic changes	−	+
Systemic symptoms	−	+
Asymmetric involvement	−	+

(Spittell JA Jr: Vasospastic disorders: Recognition and management. Cardiovasc Clin 10:279, 1980)

TABLE 108.16 RECENT RAYNAUD'S PHENOMENON EVALUATION

History:
Drugs

Examination:
Thoracic Outlet Compression
Allen's test

Laboratory Studies:
Complete blood cell count
Sedimentation rate
Protein electrophoresis
Antinuclear antibody
Cold agglutinins
Cryoglobulin
Urinalysis
Other "indicated" by history of physical findings

TABLE 108.17 MANAGEMENT OF RAYNAUD'S PHENOMENON

Protection from cold
No tobacco
Avoid drugs that may cause vasoconstriction
  β-Blockers
  Ergot preparations
Vasodilator
  Prazosin
  Nifedipine
Biofeedback
Sympathectomy

found, observation of the patient for at least 2 years is necessary before a diagnosis of primary Raynaud's phenomenon (Raynaud's disease) can be made with reasonable certainty. The management of Raynaud's phenomenon is shown in Table 108.17. Biofeedback is especially useful in young persons or for those whose occupation does not permit pharmacologic therapy. Sympathectomy is infrequently needed today and is generally reserved for the young person with Raynaud's disease who is seriously inconvenienced by vasospasm that cannot otherwise be controlled.

Livedo reticularis (Fig. 108.16), like Raynaud's phenomenon, can be primary or it can be secondary to a number of underlying conditions (Table 108.18). The purplish mottling due to spasm of the dermal arterioles is most often seen in the lower extremities and is more prominent in a cold environment. Recurrent ulceration about the ankles may occur in primary livedo. Evaluation of the patient with new livedo reticularis must take into consideration the various causes of secondary livedo listed in Table 108.18. Management consists of treating any underlying disorder and the measures listed for Raynaud's phenomenon, except that biofeedback and sympathectomy have not been used.

The least common and most innocuous of the vasospastic disorders is acrocyanosis. It is always primary, but the cause is not known. After a right-to-left shunt and methemoglobinemia have been excluded, the patient can be reassured and usually no other therapy is necessary.

Reflex sympathetic dystrophy is probably a neurologic disorder, usually following trauma. Although pain is the predominant symptom, edema, warmth, hyperhidrosis, coldness, and color changes are also common features. The vasospastic features respond nicely to therapy with prazosin, facilitating restoration of the patient to normal activity.

As mentioned, the pernio syndrome results from local cold injury. It is classified as shown in Table 108.19. Pernio is initiated by abnormal reaction of the blood vessels to changes in environmental temperature. In chronic pernio (Fig. 108.17), repeated exposure to cold in a susceptible person, usually a woman, results in erythematous, cyanotic, hemorrhagic, and/or ulcerative lesions of the toes during the colder months. The lesions stop during warm weather. Early experience with prazosin has shown it to be remarkably effective in chronic pernio.

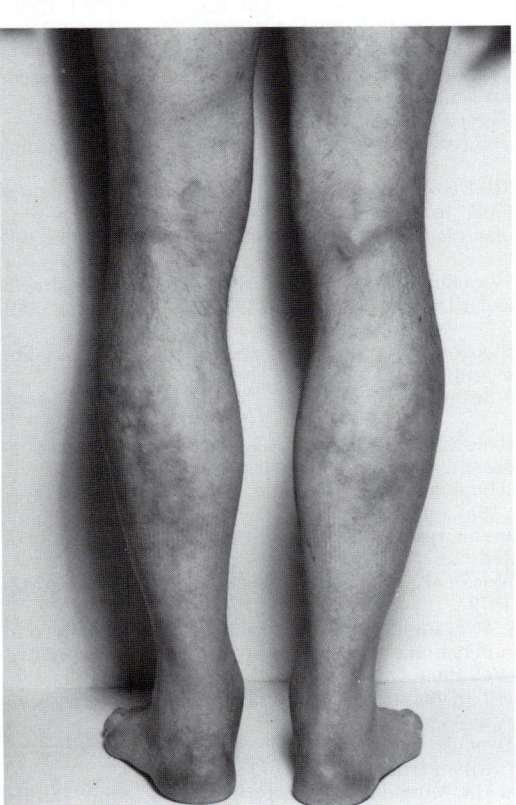

FIGURE 108.16 Livedo reticularis of lower extremities.

TABLE 108.18 CLASSIFICATION OF LIVEDO RETICULARIS

I. Primary (Idiopathic) Livedo Reticularis
II. Secondary Livedo Reticularis
   A. Connective tissue diseases
   B. Vasculitis
   C. Myeloproliferative disorders
   D. Dysproteinemias
   E. Atheroembolism (cholesterol embolization)
   F. After cold injury
   G. Use of amantadine hydrochloride (Symmetrel)
   H. Reflex sympathetic dystrophy

(Spittell JA Jr: Vasospastic disorders. Cardiovasc Clin 13:75, 1983)

TABLE 108.19 CLASSIFICATION OF PERNIO SYNDROME

I. Acute Pernio (local cold injury)
II. Chronic Pernio (chronic chilblains; erythrocyanosis)
III. Trench Foot and Immersion Foot (combination of acute and chronic pernio)

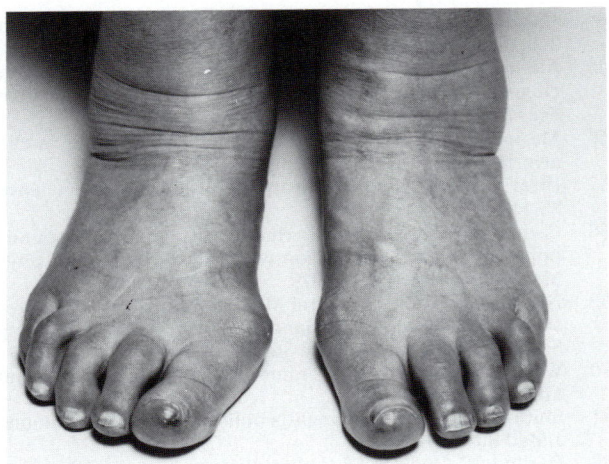

FIGURE 108.17 Chronic pernio: blue toes and blisters in a 70-year-old woman with a history of repeated cold injury. (Spittell JA Jr: The vasospastic disorders. Curr Probl Cardiol 8:1, 1984. Copyright © 1984 by Year Book Medical Publishers, Inc., Chicago)

REFERENCES

1. Fuster V, Kottke BA, Juergens JL: Atherosclerosis. In Juergens JL, Spittell JA Jr, Fairbairn JF (eds): Peripheral Vascular Diseases, 5th ed, pp 219–235. Philadelphia, WB Saunders, 1980
2. Spittell JA Jr, McGoon DC: Acquired diseases of the thoracic aorta. In Brandenburg RO, Fuster V, Giuliani ER et al (eds): Cardiology: Fundamentals and Practice, pp 1718–1731. Chicago, Year Book Medical Publishers, 1987
3. Roberts WC: The hypertensive diseases: Evidence that systemic hypertension is a greater risk factor to the development of other cardiovascular diseases than previously suspected. Am J Med 59:523, 1975
4. Spittell JA Jr: Hypertension and arterial aneurysm. J Am Coll Cardiol 1:523, 1983
5. Spittell JA Jr: Clinical aspects of aneurysmal disease. Curr Probl Cardiol 5:1, 1980
6. National Heart and Lung Institute Task Force on Arteriosclerosis: Arteriosclerosis (DHEW publication No. [NIH] 72-219), vol 2. Washington, DC, US Government Printing Office, 1971
7. Maciejko JJ, Holmes DR, Kottke BA et al: Apolipoprotein A-1 as a marker of angiographically assessed coronary artery disease. N Engl J Med 309:385, 1983
8. DeMaria AN, Bommer W, Neuman A et al: Identification and localization of aneurysms of the ascending aorta by cross-sectional echocardiography. Circulation 59:755, 1979
9. Mintz GS, Kotler MN, Sejal BL et al: Two-dimensional echocardiographic recognition of the descending thoracic aorta. Am J Cardiol 44:232, 1979
10. Sanders JH Jr, Lalave S, Neiman HL et al: Thoracic aortic imaging without angiography. Arch Surg 114:1326, 1979
11. Joyce JW, Fairbairn JF, Kincaid OW et al: Aneurysms of the thoracic aorta: A clinical study with special reference to prognosis. Circulation 29:176, 1964
12. Bicherstaff LK, Pairolero PC, Hollier LH et al: Thoracic aortic aneurysms: A population-based study. Surgery 92:1103, 1982
13. Gott VL, Pyeritz RE, Magovern GJ et al: Surgical treatment of aneurysms of the ascending aorta in the Marfan syndrome. N Eng J Med 314:1070, 1986
14. Greendyke RM: Traumatic rupture of aorta: Special reference to automobile accidents. JAMA 195:527, 1966
15. Fleming AW, Green DC: Traumatic aneurysms of the aorta: Report of 43 patients. Ann Thorac Surg 18:91, 1974
16. Fox S, Pierce WS, Waldhausen JA: Acute hypertension: Its significance in traumatic aortic rupture. J Thorac Cardiovasc Surg 77:622, 1979
17. Parmley LF, Mattingly TW, Manion WC: Penetrating wounds of the heart and aorta. Circulation 17:956, 1958
18. Kirsh MM, Bechrendt DM, Orringer MB et al: The treatment of acute traumatic rupture of the aorta: A 10-year experience. Ann Surg 184:308, 1976
19. Ayella RJ, Hankins JR, Turney SZ et al: Ruptured thoracic aorta due to blunt trauma. J Trauma 17:199, 1974
20. DeBakey ME, McCollum CH III: Diseases of the aorta. In Chung EK (ed): Quick Reference to Cardiovascular Diseases, 2nd ed, pp 325–337. Philadelphia, JB Lippincott, 1983
21. Slater EE, DeSanctis RW: Diseases of the aorta. In Braunwald E (ed): Heart Disease, A Textbook of Cardiovascular Medicine, pp 1597–1632. Philadelphia, WB Saunders, 1980
22. Johansen K, Koepsell T: Familial tendency for abdominal aortic aneurysms. JAMA 256:1934, 1986
23. Tilson MD, Seashore M: Fifty families with abdominal aortic aneurysms in two or more first-order relatives. Am J Surg 147:551, 1984
24. Maloney JD, Pairolero PC, Smith BF et al: Ultrasound evaluation of abdominal aortic aneurysms. Circulation 56(suppl II):80, 1977
25. Dearling RC, Messina CR, Brewster DC et al: Autopsy study of unoperated abdominal aortic aneurysms: The case for early resection. Circulation 56(suppl II):161, 1977
26. Bicherstaff LK, Hollier LH, Van Peenen HJ et al: Abdominal aortic aneurysms: The changing natural history. J Vasc Surg 1:6, 1984
27. Joyce JW: Aneurysmal disease. In Spittell JA Jr (ed): Clinical Vascular Disease, pp 89–101. Philadelphia, FA Davis, 1983
28. Brown OW, Hollier LH, Pairolero PC et al: Abdominal aortic aneurysm and coronary artery disease: A reassessment. Arch Surg 116:1484, 1981
29. Hollier LH, Spittell JA, Puga F: Intra-aortic balloon counterpulsation as an adjunct to aneurysmectomy in high-risk patients. Mayo Clin Proc 56:565, 1981
30. Thompson WM, Johnsrude RS, Jackson DC et al: Late complications of abdominal aortic reconstructive surgery: Roentgen evaluation. Ann Surg 185:326, 1977
31. Hollier LH, Kazmier FJ, Plate G et al: Influence of concomitant hypertension on late morbidity and mortality after aortic aneurysm repair (abstr). J Am Coll Cardiol 5:488, 1985
32. Wolfe WJ, Moran JF: The evolution of medical and surgical management of aortic dissection. Circulation 56:503, 1977
33. Hasleton PS, Leonard JC: Dissecting aortic aneurysm: A clinicopathological study: II. Histopathology of the aorta. Q J Med 48:63, 1979
34. Schlatman TJM, Becker AE: Pathogenesis of dissecting aneurysm of the aorta: Comparative histopathologic study of the significance of medial changes. Am J Cardiol 39:21, 1977
35. Roberts WC: Aortic dissection: Anatomy, consequences and causes. Am Heart J 101:195, 1981
36. Fukuda T, Tadavarthy SM, Edwards JE: Dissecting aneurysm of the aorta complicating aortic valvular stenosis. Circulation 53:169, 1976
37. Larson EW, Edwards WE: Risk factors for aortic dissection: A necropsy study of 161 cases. Am J Cardiol 53:849, 1984
38. Lefemine AA, Kosowksy B, Madoff I et al: Results and complications of intra-aortic balloon pumping in surgical and medical patients. Am J Cardiol 40:416, 1977
39. Nicholson WJ, Crawley IS, Logue RB et al: Aortic root dissection complicating coronary bypass surgery. Am J Cardiol 41:103, 1978
40. Hirst AE et al: Dissecting aneurysms of the aorta: A review of 505 cases. Medicine 37:217, 1958
41. DeBakey ME, Henly WS, Cooley DA et al: Surgical management of dissecting aneurysms of the aorta. J Thorac Cardiovasc Surg 49:130, 1965
42. Slater EE, DeSanctis RW: The clinical recognition of dissecting aortic aneurysm. Am J Med 60:625, 1976
43. Moersch FP, Sayre GP: Neurologic manifestations associated with dissecting aneurysm of the aorta. JAMA 144:1141, 1950
44. Logue RB, Sikes C: New sign in dissecting aneurysm of the aorta: Pulsation of sternoclavicular joint. JAMA 148:1209, 1952
45. Earnest F IV, Muhm JR, Sheedy PF: Roentgenographic findings in thoracic aortic dissection. Mayo Clin Proc 54:43, 1979
46. Victor MF, Mintz GS, Kotler MN et al: Two dimensional echocardiographic diagnosis of aortic dissection. Am J Cardiol 48:1155, 1981
47. Wheat MW Jr, Palmer RF, Bartley TD et al: Treatment of dissecting aneurysms of the aorta without surgery. J Thorac Cardiovasc Surg 50:364, 1965
48. Palmer RF, Lasseter KC: Letter to the editor: Nitroprusside and aortic dissecting aneurysm. N Engl J Med 294:1403, 1976
49. Appelbaum A, Karp RB, Kirklin JW: Ascending vs. descending aortic dissections. Ann Surg 183:296, 1976
50. Miller DC, Stinson DB, Oyer PE et al: Operative treatment of aortic dissections: Experience with 125 patients over a 16-year period. J Thorac Cardiovasc Surg 78:305, 1979
51. Spittell JA Jr, Wallace RB: Dissecting aneurysm of the aorta (dissecting hematoma, aortic dissection). In Juergens JL, Spittell JA Jr, Fairbairn JF II (eds): Peripheral Vascular Diseases, 5th ed, pp 403–413. Philadelphia, WB Saunders, 1980
52. Sheps GG, McDuffie FC: Vasculitis. In Juergens JL, Spittell JA Jr, Fairbairn JF II (eds): Peripheral Vascular Diseases. 5th ed, pp 493–553. Philadelphia, WB Saunders, 1980
53. Klein RG, Hunder GG, Stanson AW et al: Large artery involvement in giant cell (temporal) arteritis. Ann Intern Med 83:806, 1975
54. Lupi E et al: Pulmonary artery involvement in Takayasu's arteritis. Chest 67:1, 1975
55. Ishikawa K: Survival and morbidity after diagnosis of occlusive thromboaortopathy (Takayasu's disease). Am J Cardiol 47:1026, 1981
56. Rich C Jr, Webster BL: The natural history of uncomplicated syphilitic aortitis. Am Heart J 43:321, 1951
57. Kampmeier RH: Saccular aneurysms of the thoracic aorta: A clinical study of 633 cases. Ann Intern Med 12:624, 1938
58. Edwards JE: Manifestations of acquired and congenital diseases of the aorta. Curr Probl Cardiol 3:7, 1979
59. Mundth ED, Darleny RC, Alvarado RH et al: Surgical management of mycotic aneurysms and the complications of infection in vascular reconstructive surgery. Am J Surg 117:460, 1969
60. Anderson CB, Butcher HR Jr, Ballinger WF: Mycotic aneurysms. Arch Surg 109:712, 1974
61. Conn DL, McDuffie FC, Dyck PJ: Immunopathologic study of sural nerves in rheumatoid arthritis. Arthritis Rheum 15:135, 1972
62. Heggtveit HA, Henbnigar GR, Morrione TG: Panaortitis. Am J Pathol 42:151, 1963
63. Robbins SL, Cotran RS: Diseases of the blood vessels. In Robbins SL, Cotran RS (eds): The Pathologic Basis of Disease, pp 593–642. Philadelphia, WB Saunders, 1979
64. Carter SA: Arterial auscultation in peripheral vascular disease. JAMA 246:1682, 1981
65. Allen EV: Thromboangiitis obliterans: Methods of diagnosis of chronic occlusive arterial disease distal to the wrist with illustrative cases. Am J Med Sci 178:237, 1932
66. Marinelli MR, Beach KW et al: Noninvasive testing vs clinical evaluation of arterial disease. JAMA 241:2031, 1979
67. Hirai M: Cold sensitivity of the hand in arterial occlusive disease. Surgery 85:140, 1979
68. Carpenter JR, Hattery RR, Hunder GG et al: Ultrasound evaluation of the popliteal space: Comparison with arthrography and physical examination. Mayo Clin Proc 51:498, 1979
69. Nielson SL, Nobin BA, Hirai M et al: Raynaud's phenomenon in arterial obstructive disease of the hand demonstrated by locally provoked cooling. Scand J Thorac Cardiovasc Surg 12:105, 1978
70. Weis AJ, Fairbairn JF II: Trauma, ischemic limbs and amputation. Postgrad Med 43:111, 1968
71. Spittell JA Jr: Thromboangiitis obliterans—an autoimmune disorder? N Engl J Med 308:1157, 1983
72. Darling RC, Buckley CJ, Abbott WM et al: Intermittent claudication in young athletes: Popliteal artery entrapment syndrome. J Trauma 14:543, 1974

73. Coffman JD: Drug therapy: Vasodilator drugs in peripheral vascular disease. N Engl J Med 300:713, 1979
74. Porter JM, Cutler BS, Lee VY et al: Pentoxifylline efficacy in the treatment of intermittent claudication: Multicenter controlled double blind trial with objective assessment of chronic occlusive arterial disease patients. Am Heart J 104:66, 1982
75. Spittell JA Jr: Pentoxifylline and intermittent claudication. Ann Intern Med 102:126, 1985
76. Doubilet P, Abrams HL: The cost of underutilization: Percutaneous transluminal angioplasty for peripheral vascular disease. N Engl J Med 310:95, 1984
77. Position paper: Percutaneous transluminal angioplasty. Ann Intern Med 99:864, 1983
78. Hess H, Ingrisch H et al: Local low-dose thrombolytic therapy of peripheral arterial occlusions. N Engl J Med 307:1627, 1983
79. Wychulis AR, Spittell JA Jr, Wallace RB: Popliteal aneurysms. Surgery 68:942, 1970
80. Pairolero PC, Walls JT, Payne S et al: Subclavian-axillary artery aneurysms. Surgery 90:757, 1981
81. Stanley JC, Frye WJ: Pathogenesis and clinical significance of splenic artery aneurysms. Surgery 76:898, 1974
82. Hubert HP, Pairolero PC, Kazmier FJ: Solitary renal artery aneurysm. Surgery 88:557, 1980
83. Spittell JA Jr: The vasospastic disorders. Curr Probl Cardiol 8:1, 1984

CARDIAC NEOPLASMS

Emilio R. Giuliani • Jeffrey M. Piehler

Cardiac tumors have been the focus of study by physicians for centuries. It was not until the modern era of cardiac surgery, however, that the study of these neoplasms was raised from the academic to the therapeutic level. Pathologic descriptions of cardiac tumors were recorded as early as the 16th century.[1] The first antemortem diagnosis of a primary cardiac tumor was recorded in 1935.[2] Crafoord, in 1954, reported the first successful removal of an atrial myxoma using extracorporeal circulation.[3] Advances in intracardiac operative techniques have permitted resection of the majority of primary cardiac tumors with an acceptable low mortality. Since the majority of these tumors are benign and resection frequently leads to a complete cure and restoration of normal life expectancy, it is incumbent on the physician to identify these tumors and identify them prior to any major or serious complication.

Fortunately, along with advances in operative technique have been advances in diagnostic techniques, particularly in noninvasive procedures such as cardiac ultrasound, computed tomography, and magnetic resonance imaging that make the diagnosis of cardiac tumors not only relatively simple and safe but also highly accurate.

Primary cardiac neoplasms, that is, tumors that originate in the heart itself, can be either benign or malignant (Table 109.1). The incidence of such tumors has been reported as 0.001% to 0.5% in unselected autopsy series.[4] It is estimated that approximately 80% of all primary neoplasms are benign and, therefore, potentially curable.[5]

The heart can also be affected by secondary neoplasms. These are largely malignant tumors that have either metastasized to the myocardium via hematogenous or lymphogenous routes or have extended directly into the myocardium from the surrounding intrathoracic structures. These tumors, secondary cardiac neoplasms, are many times more common than primary cardiac tumors.

BENIGN PRIMARY CARDIAC TUMORS
CARDIAC MYXOMAS

Cardiac myxoma is by far the most common primary cardiac tumor and accounts for approximately 50% of all such lesions. These tumors have been encountered in all age-groups; the majority, however, are diagnosed between the third and sixth decades of life. They seem to occur more frequently in women and are rare in children. Familial myxomas have been reported; however, considering the rarity of this tumor, it is difficult to document familial patterns.

For many years there has been a divergence of opinion regarding the exact nature of atrial tumors. Two views are held. One possibility is that these tumors are really thrombi swollen by the imbibition of plasma and are in various stages of organization. The other possibility is that these tumors are true neoplasms. Most recent evidence supports the latter view on the basis of these characteristic findings: the gross appearance of the tumor, the microscopic appearance of the tumor, the systemic effects caused by the presence of the tumor, recurrence, and invasiveness.

Approximately 75% of cardiac myxomas originate in the left atrium, 20% occur within the right atrium, and the remaining tumors appear equally distributed within the two ventricles. The tumors arise from the endocardial surface of the cardiac chamber, and the majority arise from the intra-atrial septum. When the tumor originates within the ventricular chambers, it almost always begins in the free wall. The vast majority of myxomas are single, but they may be multiple, occurring in one or more chambers. Approximately 10% of the reported cases of atrial myxoma are bilateral. Recurrence of tumor is rare. A few reported cases of invasion of the tumor and the occasional reported recurrence suggest that these tumors may, indeed, have some low-grade malignant features.

The clinical features of atrial myxoma are the result of obstruction of blood flow by the tumor, tumor mobility, embolization, and nonspecific systemic effects from the presence of the tumor.[6] Many tumors are asymptomatic and are identified, incidentally, at autopsy. The duration of symptoms depends on the rate of growth of the tumor. The specific cardiac chamber in which a myxoma is located also has a profound effect on the presenting clinical picture.

The constitutional manifestations, which occur in over 90% of patients, are due to the presence of the tumor and are independent of the location of the tumor.[7,8] The most frequently seen systemic symptoms are weight loss, fatigue, fever, and arthralgias. Less commonly encountered are rashes, clubbing of the fingers, and Raynaud's phenomenon.[9]

The abnormalities found on laboratory investigation include anemia, which is frequently hemolytic, elevated sedimentation rate, leukocytosis, thrombocytopenia, polycythemia, and hypergammaglobulinemia.[7-10] The elevated immunoglobulins are usually of the IgG fraction.[11] Although actual circulating immune complexes have not been identified, the association of elevated immunoglobulins and hypocomplementemia strongly suggests the presence of a tumor-specific antigen–antibody complex that activates complement pathways.[12] Such complexes and the systemic reaction to them probably explain the symptoms that suggest collagen vascular disease (most usually vasculitis) with which patients with myxoma are known to present.[13]

The exact etiology of these constitutional symptoms and laboratory abnormalities is unclear. In general, however, all of these reverse on removal of the tumor.[13,14] In some cases, the constitutional manifestations of myxoma dominate the clinical picture.

As stated, constitutional symptoms associated with myxoma are independent of tumor location within the heart. On the other hand, the sequela of emboli, obstruction, or tumor mobility is dependent on the location of the tumor within the heart.

LEFT ATRIAL MYXOMAS

In addition to the systemic symptoms noted above, symptoms of mitral valve obstruction are often present and may be acute or chronic. Symptoms include positional dyspnea, orthopnea, and paroxysmal nocturnal dyspnea. These symptoms are the result of increased left atrial pressure that is reflected as an increase in pulmonary venous pressure and pulmonary congestion. Syncope may be the result of complete transitory obstruction of the mitral valve. If the obstruction is of long duration, then secondary pulmonary hypertension may develop with right ventricular hypertrophy and, ultimately, right ventricular failure.

Rarely, the tumor may obstruct the pulmonary veins draining into the left atrium. In this case the clinical symptoms are similar to those of obstruction at the mitral valve level.

Systemic embolization of tumor fragments has been reported in 30% to 60% of patients with left atrial myxomas (Table 109.2).[7,9,15,16] The symptoms that result cannot be distinguished from acute arterial insufficiency of other etiologies. The embolic material can be either thrombus or actual tumor fragments. The diagnosis of a myxoma can be made by histologic examination of the removed embolized material.[17-20] The embolus is usually relatively small; however, instances of embolization of the entire tumor mass have been reported.[20] Tumor emboli have been noted at virtually all systemic locations,[16] although they most frequently are detected in the brain, kidney, lower extremities, or aortoiliac region.[18] Multiple sites of embolization are frequent.[21] Coronary embolization is infrequent.[22]

Cerebrovascular embolization occurs most often (see Table 109.2).[23] It is not unusual for the first clinical manifestation of a myxoma to be a cerebrovascular event. When the emboli are small, they present as transient ischemic attacks,[23,24] and when larger, they take the form of cerebral infarction with completed stroke.

The fate of the tumor fragment, which embolizes to the cerebral vessel within the central nervous system, remains controversial.[25,26] Two late complications have been observed. In rare instances, the tumor fragment may continue to grow and, therefore, present as an expanding intracranial mass.[23,27,28] A more unusual delayed complication is the development of vascular aneurysms at the site of the embolus.[25,26,29] These aneurysms have been shown to enlarge progressively and occasionally rupture.[30,31] Aneurysmal changes in the cerebral vasculature in patients with atrial myxoma have been detected angiographically.[32] The exact mechanism of aneurysm formation is not known. Although it is obvious that an occasional patient may develop a

TABLE 109.1 PRIMARY CARDIAC NEOPLASMS

I. Benign
  A. Myxoma
  B. Fibroma
  C. Rhabdomyoma
  D. Rare tumors
II. Malignant
  A. Sarcoma(s)
    1. Muscle
    2. Vascular
    3. Connective tissue
  B. Rare tumors

TABLE 109.2 CLINICAL PROFILE OF 30 PATIENTS WITH LEFT ATRIAL MYXOMAS

Symptom	No. Patients	Percent
Emboli	11	37
Cerebral	6	
Peripheral	4	13
Multiple	1	
Syncope	4	13
Arthralgia and/or myalgias	4	13
Weakness and anorexia	15	50
Weight loss	10	33
4 to 55 pounds	1	
Cough	8	27
Hemoptysis	3	10
Fever	6	20

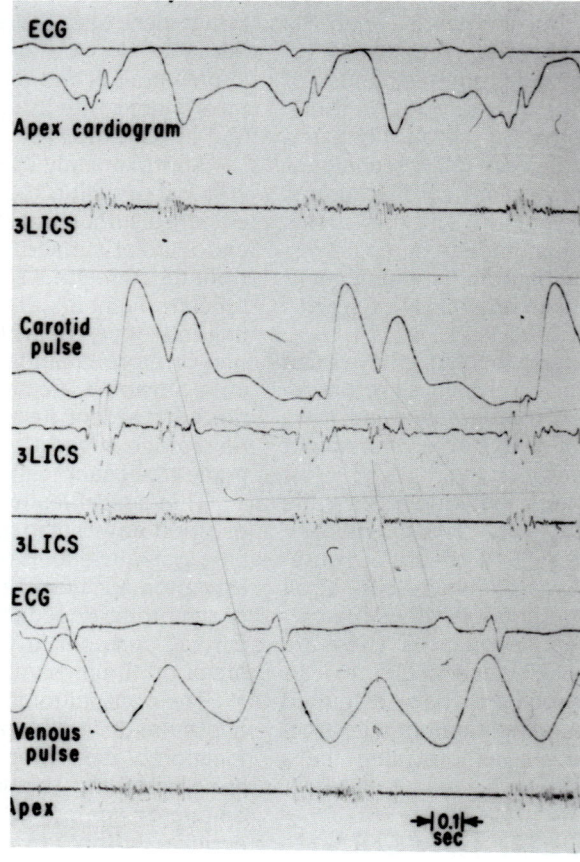

FIGURE 109.1 Cardiac recordings of a 39-year-old woman with left atrial myxoma. Note typical vibrations on the phonocardiogram during isovolumic contraction (S_1 to onset of ejection) and during isovolumic relaxation (P_2 to early diastolic sound—tumor plop). Characteristic notching is noted on the upstroke of the apex cardiogram. (Zitnik RS, Giuliani ER, Burchell HB: Left atrial myxoma: Phonocardiographic clues to diagnosis. Am J Cardiol 23:588, 1969)

delayed neurologic complication of embolization of a tumor fragment years after resecting a primary tumor, clinical experience has demonstrated that these complications are indeed rare, and that cerebral angiography is not necessary in every case with atrial myxomas.[25]

CLINICAL EXAMINATION. The physical findings in patients with left atrial myxoma vary with the pathophysiology produced by the tumor.[6] When the tumor obstructs the inflow to the left ventricle, the findings are similar to those of mitral stenosis. The first heart sound is usually loud and widely split. Frequently, an early diastolic sound termed the *tumor plop* is noted (Fig. 109.1). This transient sound presumably results from the sudden impact of the tumor against the endocardial wall with tensing of the tumor stalk.[33,34] This "tumor plop" follows the second heart sound at an interval intermediate between that of an opening snap and a third heart sound. The sound is of lower frequency than the usual opening snap; however, in many instances, such a differentiation can be quite difficult. The murmur is a diastolic low frequency rumble comparable to that heard in rheumatic valvular mitral stenosis. In contrast to rheumatic mitral stenosis, the obstruction can be intermittent; therefore, the auscultatory findings are intermittent—a clue to the presence of a left atrial myxoma. With longstanding obstruction to left ventricular inflow, pulmonary vascular changes occur and ultimately pulmonary hypertension develops. When this occurs, the pulmonary component of the second heart sound is accentuated.[35] Ultimately, the right side of the heart fails and all the findings of right ventricular failure become evident. In cases in which the tumor interferes with mitral valve closure or the valve is damaged by the tumor, the typical apical pansystolic murmur of mitral insufficiency can be noted. On occasion, the quality of the murmur will vary with body position presumably due to movement of the tumor.

NONINVASIVE TESTING. The electrocardiographic findings in patients with left atrial myxoma are nonspecific and reflect changes in chamber size and hypertrophy of the chamber walls.[7,35] The majority of patients are in normal sinus rhythm, although atrial fibrillation or flutter is sometimes encountered. Occasionally left ventricular hypertrophy predominates in patients with mitral regurgitation. In patients with pulmonary hypertension, right ventricular hypertrophy is present.

Plain chest roentgenograms can be normal or can reveal findings compatible with chronic mitral valvular dysfunction; that is, mild to moderate left atrial enlargement, pulmonary vascular congestion, and left ventricular enlargement. A giant left atrium is an unusual roentgenographic feature in patients with myxoma and is a helpful differentiating clue between myxoma and chronic mitral valvular disease.[35] Presumably, the pathophysiologic changes induced by the tumor occur at a more rapid rate than that from chronic mitral valvular dysfunction, and thus there is insufficient time for atrial dilation to develop. Occasionally, calcification of a myxoma (Fig. 109.2) can be visualized on the plain chest roentgenogram, although this feature is usually better appreciated by fluoroscopic examination where the movement of the tumor can be seen.[36] The finding of calcification within the left atrium is, of course, not pathognomonic of the left atrial myxoma. A wide variety of cardiac tumors are known to become calcified. In addition, many other pericardiac structures (*e.g.*, cardiac valves, intraluminal thrombi, atrial walls, and coronary arteries) are known to calcify, and these must be distinguished from a primary tumor with calcification.

Echocardiography presently is the preferred laboratory technique for diagnosis of left atrial myxomas.[7,37] Other invasive diagnostic modalities such as angiocardiography are rarely required for diagnosis or for preoperative surgical guidance.[38] When cardiac catheterization is required in the presence of a known left atrial myxoma, knowledge of the location of the tumor and its point of attachment, as determined from echocardiographic studies, can be helpful in preventing dislodgement of tumor fragments by catheters. In general, two-dimensional echocardiography is more accurate in making the diagnosis of left atrial myxoma than its M-mode counterpart.

By the M-mode technique, atrial myxomas are usually visualized only if the tumor prolapses into the mitral valve during diastole.[37,39] This event is visualized as dense echoes posterior to the anterior leaflet of the mitral valve shortly after valvular opening (Fig. 109.3). The tumor presence may also create slowing of anterior leaflet closure. During systole, the tumor is usually confined totally to the left atrium above the valve and, therefore, is not readily seen. False negative M-mode examinations can be obtained in cases of sessile or nonprolapsing tumors that do not project into the mitral funnel.[39,40] A second cause of a false-negative M-mode examination is the failure of the tumor to produce the characteristic echoes presumably because of the acoustic density of the mass.[41] False-positive examinations result from the presence of other conditions that produce multiple echoes behind the anterior mitral valve leaflet during diastole, such as bacterial vegetations (Fig. 109.4), redundant myxomatous valve leaflets, flail posterior leaflet, and mitral ring calcification. In general, these conditions can be distinguished from myxoma based on the absence of mass echoes in the left atrium or by additional studies leading to the correct diagnoses.

Two-dimensional echocardiography (Fig. 109.5) is superior to M-mode echocardiography in diagnosis and, therefore, for preoperative evaluation of patients with intracardiac tumors. In contrast to the M-mode technique, two-dimensional studies offer an accurate assess-

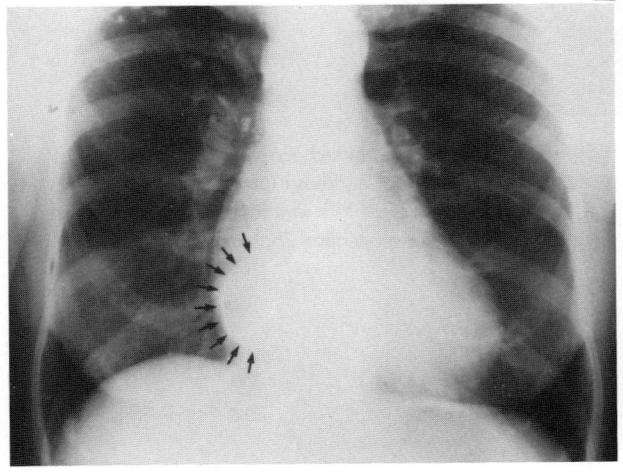

FIGURE 109.2 Chest roentgenogram of a calcified right atrial myxoma (arrows) that was successfully removed.

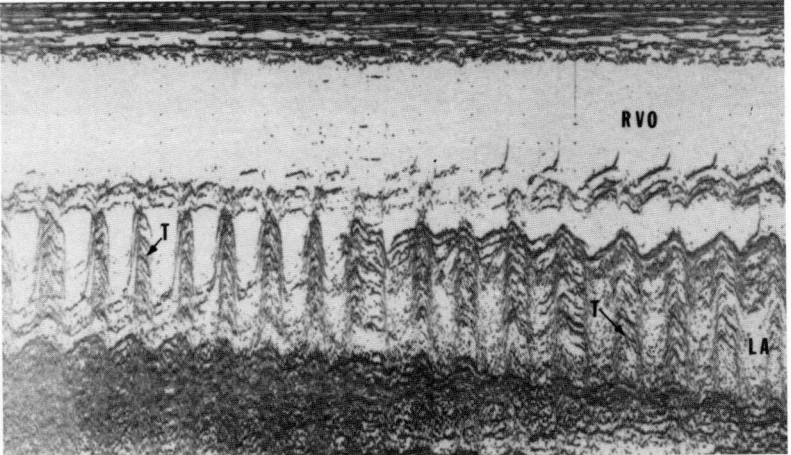

FIGURE 109.3 Apex to base scan of 64-year-old man who presented with chronic congestive failure. T with arrow points to abnormal echo due to atrial tumor prolapsing through mitral funnel on the left and in the left atrium on the right. (*RVO*, ventricular outflow tract; *LA*, left atrium) (Giuliani ER: Role of echocardiographic studies in the ambulatory patients. In Brandenburg RO (ed): Office Cardiology, pp 103–123, 1980. Philadelphia, FA Davis)

ment of tumor size, point of attachment to the cardiac wall, degree of tumor mobility, and effect of the tumor on cardiac function. The two-dimensional method is more sensitive in the detection of small tumors,[42] is able to visualize tumors that do not encroach on the mitral funnel, and provides visualization of all four cardiac chambers to assess the possibility of multiple tumors. Nevertheless, unfavorable acoustic density of some tumors can result in false-negative two-dimensional studies as well.[41] In addition, the improved visualization of the entire left atrium by the two-dimensional technique allows the differentiation of tumor from the more prevalent intra-atrial thrombus, which can produce a similar mass effect. A thrombus frequently produces a layered echo appearance, allowing one to distinguish the two conditions.[43] The visualization of an intra-atrial mass with characteristic tumor echoes is sufficient diagnosis for surgical intervention. Cardiac catheterization with associated contrast studies should be considered in patients in whom the diagnosis is not clear from echocardiographic examination or in those patients who are considered to have associated cardiac disease.

Left atrial myxomas have been successfully diagnosed using gaited radionuclide cardiac imaging.[44] The tumor creates a filling defect with different locations or size during systole and diastole corresponding to tumor movement. In general, radionuclide imaging is less sensitive than echocardiographic procedures; however, there have been instances in which tumors were detected by radionuclide techniques and missed echocardiographically, perhaps due to acoustic qualities of the mass. It has been suggested that these two studies complement each other and that together they form a highly specific combination of diagnostic modalities with value both in preoperative diagnosis as well as in postoperative follow-up and family screening.[45]

Myxomas have also been detected by computed tomographic scanning.[46] Although experience with this modality in the diagnosis of myxomas has not been extensive, with technological advancement leading to increasing resolution an important role may well be recognized.

Magnetic resonance imaging is the latest imaging technique available. This modality was not readily applicable to cardiac disorders because of motion artifacts. With successful gating mechanisms, this may prove to be the most sensitive and specific modality for identifying cardiac tumors.

INVASIVE TESTING. Intracardiac pressure tracings are frequently abnormal in patients with myxoma but are rarely of diagnostic value. Right-sided cardiac catheterization usually reveals elevations in pulmonary arterial and pulmonary capillary wedge pressures compatible with obstruction to the left-sided blood flow. Left atrial or pulmonary capillary wedge pressure tracings can demonstrate a rapid y descent resulting from the sudden decrease in left atrial volume concomitant with prolapse of the tumor through the mitral valve. A nonprolapsing tumor, on the other hand, can result in obstruction to blood flow throughout the cardiac cycle and, therefore, result in a slow y descent. Frequently, a large v wave is noted in the left atrial pressure tracing reflecting either associated mitral insufficiency from the tumor's interference with val-

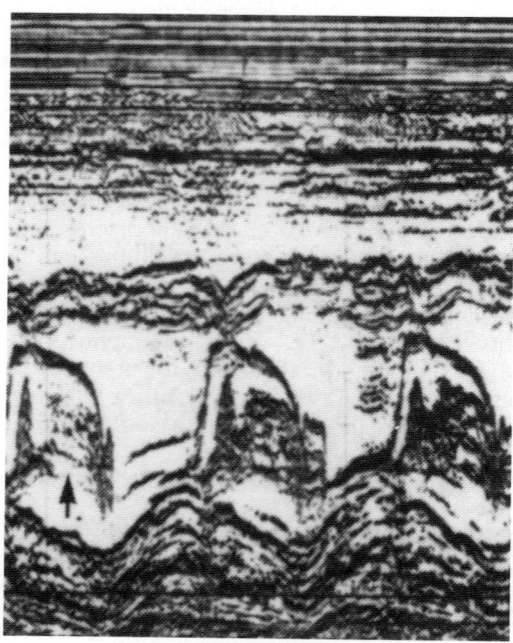
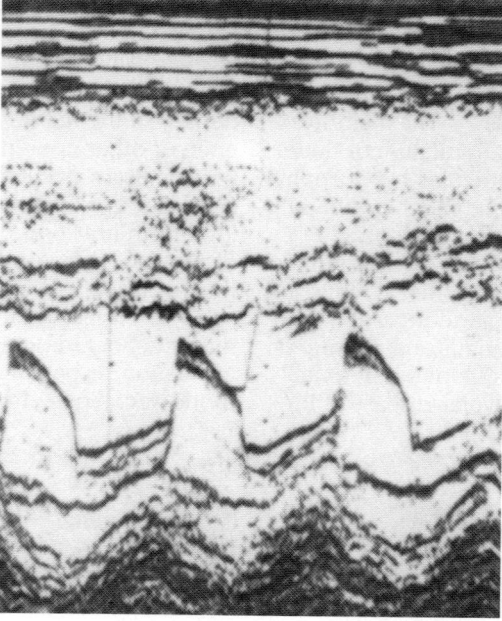

FIGURE 109.4 These two mitral valve echograms were obtained 24 hours apart in a 30-year-old man with *Hemophilus parainfluenzae* endocarditis. Left tracing shows a large mass of shaggy echoes (vegetation) compatible with left atrial myxoma. The second echo (*right panel*) was obtained after the patient complained of pain in the left leg and the left femoral pulse was absent. There is complete disappearance of the abnormal echoes, and at surgery a large mass of vegetation was recovered from the left femoral artery. (Roy P, Tajik AJ, Giuliani ER et al: Spectrum of electrocardiographic findings and bacterial endocarditis. Circulation 53(suppl III):474, 1978, by permission of the American Heart Association, Inc)

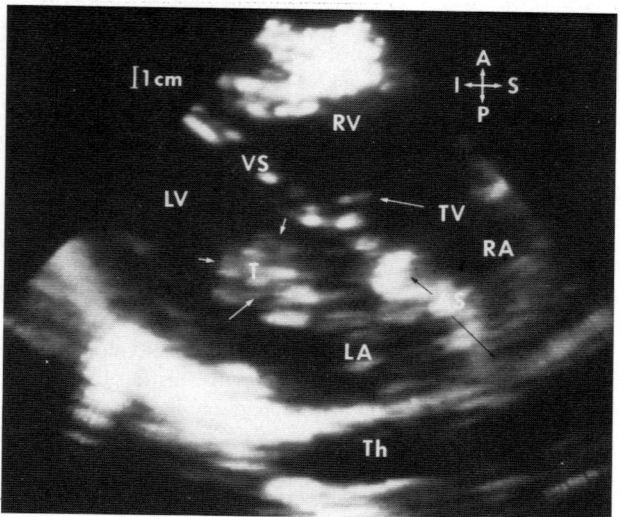

FIGURE 109.5 Four-chamber echocardiographic section of patient with a left atrial myxoma (arrows). (RV, right ventricle; VS, ventricular septum; LV, left ventricle; TV, tricuspid valve; RA, right atrium; LA, left atrium; Th, thoracic aorta)

vular closure or the compromise of the left atrial capacity by the tumor mass. A prolapsing tumor can also be associated with a notch in the ascending limb of the left ventricular pressure tracing resulting from a sudden drop in ventricular volume associated with movement of tumor into the left atrium during ventricular systole.

Before the advent of highly accurate noninvasive methods, cardiac angiography was the primary diagnostic modality for left atrial myxomas as well as other cardiac tumors.[47] Although it is not currently used as the first diagnostic study, the angiographic appearance of cardiac tumors should be appreciated since occasionally the diagnosis is not fully appreciated prior to invasive cardiac catheterization.

Tumors create a filling defect in the dye opacification, and frequently tumor movement can be easily appreciated. The exact point of origin of the tumor often cannot be appreciated angiographically. False-positive studies are frequently the result of intracardiac thrombus; however, valvular vegetations, septal aneurysms, and unusual streaming of nonopacified blood can also result in the appearance of a mass effect.[48]

Occasionally, there is sufficient mitral valvular insufficiency to result in opacification of the left atrium via a left ventricular injection. More frequently, pulmonary arterial injections with filming during the levo phase will be more profitable in identifying left atrial tumors. Because of the threat of tumor embolization, transseptal heart studies should be avoided.

DIFFERENTIAL DIAGNOSIS. The most frequent presentation is the patient whose symptoms are related to mechanical interference of mitral valve function and, therefore, mitral stenosis is the most important lesion to consider in the differential diagnosis (Table 109.3). Features in the patient's history and physical examination help to distinguish between mitral stenosis and left atrial myxoma. With the introduction of cardiac ultrasound, the clinical suspicion of left atrial myxoma can now be readily confirmed.

When systemic symptoms predominate and are associated with multiple systemic emboli, the most frequent initial diagnosis is infective endocarditis. When these symptoms are associated with an elevated sedimentation rate in a patient with a heart murmur, then the diagnosis of infective endocarditis must be considered and excluded. In a patient who has not received antibiotics, two separate sets of negative blood cultures satisfactorily excludes the diagnosis of infective endocarditis, and the echocardiographic features of a left atrial myxoma clarify the cause of the patient's problem. It must be remembered that on rare occasions infection may complicate an atrial myxoma. The mere documentation of a tumor does not exclude infective endocarditis, particularly in the patient with systemic symptoms.

Vasculitis is frequently suspected in patients with fever, elevated sedimentation rate, rashes, joint pains, and multiple systemic small arterial aneurysms. Again, a high index of suspicion in the presence of cardiac findings should alert the physician and allow him to make the correct diagnosis and verify this by echocardiographic examination.

RIGHT ATRIAL MYXOMAS

Constitutional symptoms are frequently associated with right atrial myxoma and, at times, may dominate the clinical picture. Nondiagnostic laboratory abnormalities are seen with right atrial myxomas similar to those described in patients with left atrial myxomas.

Right atrial myxomas, as they enlarge, impinge on the tricuspid valve and interfere with its normal function. Generally, the result is obstruction to atrial outflow, resulting in an elevated atrial pressure that may manifest itself with elevation of central venous pressure (elevated jugular venous pressure). When the tumor has been present for an extended period, hepatomegaly, peripheral edema, and ascites develop.[49] Obstruction can also lead to low cardiac output expressed as fatigue, exertional dyspnea, and occasionally cyanosis. When the obstruction is transient and complete, it can produce syncope.

The resultant elevated right atrial pressure may lead to opening of the foramen ovale with subsequent right to left shunting.[50] This, at times, can be significant and be associated with polycythemia. Paradoxical emboli have been reported.[51]

Tumor fragments frequently embolize and lodge in the pulmonary circuit. The fact that the symptoms of pulmonary embolism are less frequent than symptoms of systemic emboli from the left tumor probably reflects a greater tolerance of the lungs to such insults. Recurrent pulmonary emboli, however, can lead to pulmonary hypertension and, ultimately, to right-sided heart failure. Heart failure is usually of relatively short duration and nonresponsive to usual treatment.

TABLE 109.3 DIFFERENTIATING FEATURES BETWEEN LEFT ATRIAL MYXOMA AND MITRAL VALVE DISEASE

	Myxoma	Mitral Valve Disease
History	Short duration	Chronic
	Associated constitutional symptoms	None
	History of syncope	Unusual
	History of rheumatic fever unusual	Common
Symptoms	Occasionally episodic	Progressive
	Onset sudden	Gradual
Physical Examination	Tumor "plop"	Opening snap
	Murmurs vary with position	Murmurs constant
	Associated valve disease rare	Often
ECG	Sinus rhythm	Atrial fibrillation
Chest Roentgenogram	Tumor calcification	Valve calcification
	Small left atrium	Left atrium enlarged
Echocardiogram		
M-mode	Echoes within "mitral funnel"	Abnormal leaflet and motion of both leaflets
	Leaflets normal except for E-F slope of anterior leaflet	
2D	Mobile mass within left atrium usually attached to fossa ovalis	Abnormal leaflets with limited motion
		Large left atrium

CLINICAL EXAMINATION. The clinical findings are dependent on the severity and the type of tricuspid dysfunction produced. When the tumor is primarily obstructive, the findings are those of tricuspid stenosis. These findings include a slow y descent in the elevated jugular venous pressure pulse,[50] presystolic murmur in patients with sinus rhythm, and an early mid-diastolic murmur in patients with atrial fibrillation. The characteristics of the murmurs are that they are best heard along the left lower sternal border and occasionally along the right lower sternal border and that they increase in intensity during the inspiratory phase of respiration. Quite rarely, an early diastolic sound corresponding to the "tumor plop" of the left atrial myxoma has been documented. When the tumor prevents normal closure of the tricuspid valve, then the classic murmur of tricuspid insufficiency is present. Occasionally, calcified right atrial tumors have been known to destroy the tricuspid valve, producing severe tricuspid regurgitation.

NONINVASIVE TESTING. The electrocardiographic findings are frequently normal.[51] The abnormalities, when present, are nonspecific and include changes of right atrial hypertrophy, right axis deviation, low voltage, right bundle branch block, and atrial fibrillation.[51]

The chest roentgenogram is frequently normal but may show signs of right ventricular and/or right atrial dilatation. Occasionally, calcification of a right atrial myxoma is seen.[52]

Echocardiography remains the diagnostic procedure of choice. With the use of M-mode techniques (Fig. 109.6), the myxoma is seen as a mass of echoes posterior to the anterior leaflet of the tricuspid valve, often appearing after a brief delay from onset of ventricular diastole.[53,54] These findings can be produced by any tumor mass, such as vegetations of infective endocarditis, atrial thrombi, and instrumental gain artifacts. An experienced echocardiographer, however, can distinguish between these possibilities.

Two-dimensional echocardiographic examination has many advantages.[55] It permits complete examination of the heart and of the full extent and motion of the tumor that is not readily apparent by M-mode. Right atrial thrombus (Fig. 109.7) must be considered, but usually characteristic findings make diagnosis easy.

INVASIVE TESTING. Various cardiac catheterization pressure wave tracing abnormalities are present depending on the pathophysiology produced. If the tumor traverses rapidly through the tricuspid valve, then a rapid y descent is seen. A notch in the upstroke of the right ventricular pressure curve, similar to that described in left atrial myxoma,[56] reflects tumor displacement from the right ventricle into the right atrium. If a right atrial tumor is suspected or known, then contrast angiography should be done with injection into the vena cava. Catheter manipulation within the right atrium should be avoided to avoid embolization of tumor fragments.

DIFFERENTIAL DIAGNOSIS. The diagnosis most frequently entertained in patients with right atrial myxoma includes rheumatic tricuspid stenosis, infective endocarditis, constrictive pericarditis, vasculitis, and carcinoid heart disease.

Rheumatic tricuspid valve disease is almost always associated with mitral and/or aortic valve disease. It is extremely rare for it to occur as an isolated lesion. Thus the differential diagnosis between rheumatic tricuspid valve disease and right atrial myxoma should be quite easy. In a patient with findings of tricuspid valve obstruction in the absence of associated mitral valve disease and/or aortic valve disease the possibility of right atrial myxoma should immediately be evident. Patients with right atrial myxoma usually are in normal sinus rhythm. Patients with rheumatic tricuspid stenosis usually have atrial fibrillation because of the associated mitral valve disease. The conditions of chronic constrictive pericarditis, chronic cor pulmonale, Ebstein's anomaly, carcinoid heart disease, and other unusual causes of right-sided heart disease can be readily identified by adequate two-dimensional echocardiographic studies.

VENTRICULAR MYXOMAS

Ventricular myxomas constitute less than 10% of all myxomas.[57] The diagnosis of both right and left ventricular myxomas is made by echocardiography.[58]

Left ventricular myxomas represent approximately 5% of all myxomas and lead to symptoms of syncope, chest pain, and findings similar to valvular aortic stenosis because they frequently obstruct the left ventricular outflow tract.[59,60]

Right ventricular myxomas may interfere with either pulmonary valve or tricuspid valve function and usually present as either exertional dyspnea or syncope.[61,62]

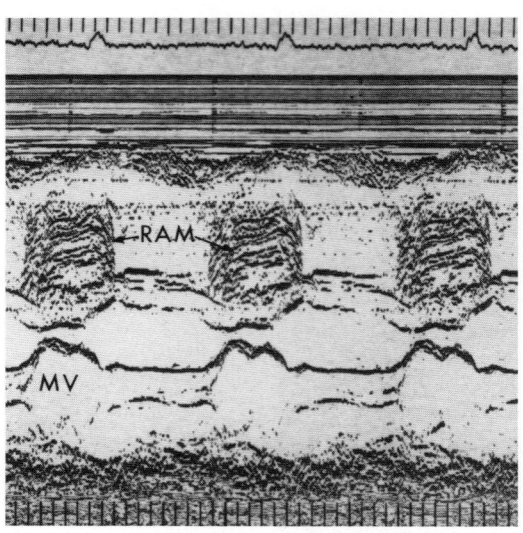

FIGURE 109.6 M-mode echogram obtained through the ventricular chambers demonstrating a mass of echoes filling the tricuspid valve (arrows). This patient at surgery had a large right atrial myxoma (RAM). Electrocardiogram is at top of tracing for reference. (Giuliani ER, Nasser FN: Two-dimensional echocardiography in acquired heart disease. Current Probl Cardiol 5:28, 1981. Copyright © 1981 by Year Book Medical Publishers, Inc, Chicago)

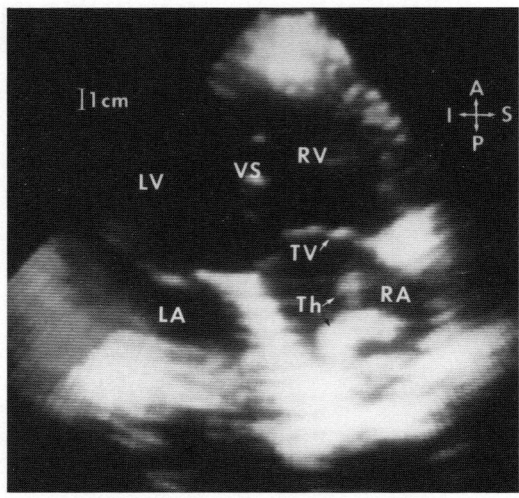

FIGURE 109.7 Echocardiogram of patient with large right atrial mass. This represented thrombus material (Th). (RV, right ventricle; TV, tricuspid valve; RA, right atrium; LA, left atrium; LV, left ventricle; VS, ventricular septum)

SURGICAL TREATMENT

Myxomas are potentially lethal benign neoplasms that may be associated with local and systemic complications. Virtually all myxomas can be resected surgically, and surgery offers the only acceptable form of treatment. In a patient with no prior history of cardiac disease in whom a typical myxoma is diagnosed by two-dimensional echocardiographic techniques, surgery is undertaken promptly without additional invasive studies. This avoids the risk of tumor embolization related to catheter manipulation and minimizes the delay between diagnosis and operation.[63] Asymptomatic coronary artery disease represents the only pathology that would be inapparent to the operating surgeon under these conditions. Symbas and associates[64] have emphasized a significant mortality between the time of diagnosis and operative intervention due to massive embolization or total obstruction to intracardiac blood flow. Such observations emphasize the importance of promptly operating on any patient in whom the diagnosis of intracardiac myxoma has been made.

Operations for myxomas are all performed via a median sternotomy using standard cardiopulmonary bypass techniques. The general principles of surgical management of these lesions include avoiding undue manipulation of the heart, which could lead to tumor embolization during the procedure; attempting to excise the endocardial origin of the tumor in an effort to prevent recurrence; careful removal of any loose tumor fragments from the cardiac chambers after the tumor has been removed; and careful inspection of the cardiac valves that have been in contact with the tumor to determine if traumatic damage has occurred. The use of cardioplegic arrest provides a quiet operating field that enhances the probability of removing the friable tumors intact.

The approach to the tumors should be individualized, taking into account the tumor location and size. A small left atrial tumor arising from the area of the fossa ovalis can be approached through the right atrium with en bloc excision of the tumor and its point of attachment to the atrial septum. The resulting atrial septal defect can be closed with either a pericardial or a prosthetic patch. Larger left atrial myxomas arising from the septum are often best evaluated through separate incisions into each atrium, whereby the point of attachment can be clearly delineated from the left side and the septal resection carried out from the right side. Left atrial tumors arising from other than the atrial septum can be approached through the left atrium. For these tumors, it would seem prudent to remove the endocardium at the point of insertion of the tumor stalk and to consider coagulating this area as well in an effort to minimize the chance of tumor recurrence.

Right ventricular tumors can be approached either through a right ventriculotomy or through the right atrium with exposure through the tricuspid valve, depending on the exact location of the tumor. In general, a full-thickness excision of the ventricular wall at the point of tumor origin would not appear to be warranted; however, an excision of a portion of the endocardium in this region should be attempted. Left ventricular myxomas can be most safely approached through either the mitral or the aortic valve, depending on tumor location. Associated valvular pathology may require valvular replacement or annuloplasty at the time of tumor removal.

The results of surgical resection of cardiac myxomas are excellent.[65] Operative mortality is below 5%. Immediate hemodynamic improvement is noted, the risk of embolism is eliminated, and the constitutional symptoms usually completely resolve. The issue of tumor recurrence was initially emphasized by Read and associates.[66] Subsequent long-term follow-up of patients with resected myxomas reveals a recurrence rate of less than 5%. Resection of point of origin of the tumor would appear to be an important factor in minimizing the chance of recurrence. Nevertheless, all patients with resected myxomas should have periodic echocardiographic follow-up in order to assess possible recurrence as well as the development of a new tumor.

LESS COMMON BENIGN CARDIAC TUMORS

A rhabdomyoma is another benign cardiac tumor that represents either a localized form of cardiac glycogenosis or a malformation (hamartoma). The tumor may be single or multiple and involve any portion of the heart. It is the most common cardiac tumor encountered in infants and in children. It is rarely seen in adults.[67,68] The tumors vary in size and produce symptoms by either obstructing intracardiac blood flow or interfering with normal cardiac conduction. Rarely, a diffuse form may lead to heart failure. Approximately 30% of cases are associated with tuberous sclerosis. The diagnosis can be made by echocardiography or angiography. The mortality of rhabdomyoma in infancy is high. Because the tumors are often multiple, approximately 90%, no operative management was initially recommended. However, since the tumors have little propensity for further growth, surgical resection, even if subtotal, often produces gratifying symptomatic improvement. Successful resection of these tumors has been performed in children as young as 12 days of age.[68] For those children with tuberous sclerosis, this becomes the most important factor in determining ultimate prognosis.[69]

Fibromas are benign tumors that can be found at any age and may involve any portion of the heart but seem to have a predilection for cardiac valves.[70] In contrast to rhabdomyomas, these tumors are virtually always solitary. The tumor is most often located in the left ventricular free wall (Fig. 109.8) or interventricular septum. When they involve the valves in children, they are distributed equally among all valves, but in adults, the aortic valve is primarily involved.

The symptoms produced by these tumors are dependent on the valve involved and on the extent of involvement. The most common presentation is heart failure owing to significant valvular dysfunction or to impairment in ventricular function. Significant arrhythmias are found in approximately one third of the cases; sudden death is common. Two-dimensional echocardiographic and angiographic examinations are essential for the diagnosis.

Using current techniques of cardiopulmonary bypass, the resection of even large intramural cardiac fibromas is feasible. Usually, a dissect-

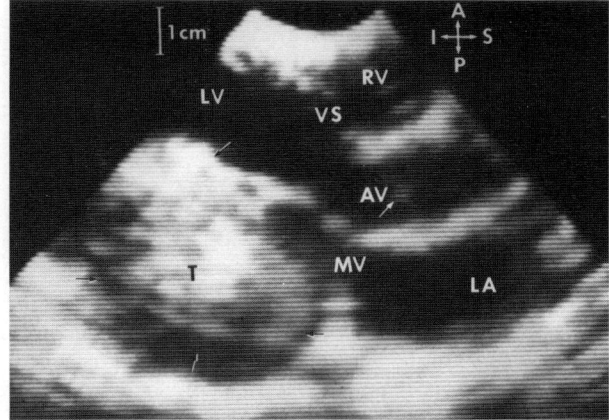

FIGURE 109.8 Echocardiographic long axis view of left ventricle showing a large left ventricular tumor (fibroma) in a young patient. Tumor (T) is identified, and the extent of tumor involvement (small arrows) is shown. (LV, left ventricle; VS, ventricular septum; RV, right ventricle; AV, aortic valve; MV, mitral valve; LA, left atrium)

ing plane between the tumor and adjacent myocardium can be established. In many cases, the tumor can be enucleated and myocardial integrity re-established without the need for prosthetic material.

Resection of septal tumors is considerably more challenging than the resection of tumors involving the left ventricular free wall. Although complete resection of the fibroma is the therapeutic goal of the cardiac surgeon, excellent palliation has been obtained by removal of only that portion of the tumor that interferes with valvular or left ventricular function. It has been pointed out, however, that the potential for sudden death in these patients probably remains. The long-term outcome for patients who have had myocardial fibromas completely resected appears to be excellent.

Mesotheliomas are tumors that are observed almost always in adults and predominately in women. These tumors are very rare. Clinically, they present with symptoms of syncope due to partial or complete atrial ventricular block. The tumors are found almost always in the atrial ventricular node area, although microscopic foci are seen in other areas of the heart.

Papillary fibroelastomas are rare, benign tumors that originate either in cardiac valves or adjacent endocardium.[71] The aortic valve is most frequently involved in adults in whom these tumors are encountered. When they occur on the atrioventricular valves, they originate from the atrial surface generally. These tumors are usually incidental findings at postmortem examination. They can occasionally interfere with valve function and produce mild aortic regurgitation or mild mitral regurgitation. Surgical resection of a symptomatic papillary fibroelastoma would appear indicated.

MALIGNANT CARDIAC TUMORS

Sarcomas of the heart represent virtually all the primary malignant tumors affecting adults; malignant tumors in infants and children are exceedingly uncommon.[68,71] Sarcomas of the heart may arise from any tissue including the muscle, vascular, connective, or adipose tissue. They are most common in early adult life and appear to have a predilection for men in the middle third of life. These tumors infiltrate the heart extensively and often extend locally into the pericardium and surrounding structures. Over three fourths of the tumors have distant metastasis at the time of discovery.[72]

The sarcomas generally manifest themselves through cardiac symptoms. Congestive heart failure can be the result of tumor infiltration of the myocardium, infiltration of the cardiac valves interfering with normal function, or growth into the cavity interfering with progress of blood flow. Extracardiac extension may result in pericardial effusion and acute cardiac tamponade. Symptoms resulting from metastasis may be the first manifestation of a primary malignant cardiac tumor. Angiosarcomas involve primarily the right atrium and most often adult males (Fig. 109.9).[73–75] Rhabdomyosarcomas and fibrosarcomas, on the other hand, appear to affect the two sexes equally and to have no predilection for a particular cardiac chamber or structure.

The diagnosis is based on clinical and echocardiographic findings. All treatment has been palliative. No patient has been cured with these primary malignant neoplasms. Primary surgical resection of the tumors has been reported; however, the role of surgery in the management of these patients remains to be established.[76,77]

The incidence of cardiac metastases discovered at autopsy in patients dying of malignancies varies from 1% to 20%.[78,79] Clinically, the incidence of metastatic cancer to the heart is increasing, presumably because of improved survival rates associated with palliative treatment of the primary tumors.

Although malignant melanoma has, by far, the greatest propensity to metastasize to the heart,[80] in terms of absolute numbers in clinical encounters the most common primary foci are bronchogenic carcinoma (Fig. 109.10), carcinoma of the breast, lymphoma, and leukemia. These four groups of cancer account for the majority of cardiac metastasis that are seen today.

Tumor spread to the heart occurs by three mechanisms: (1) direct extension from adjacent intrathoracic structures, (2) hematogenous spread, and (3) lymphatic spread. Direct extension to the heart occurs most frequently in patients with bronchogenic carcinoma and other mediastinal tumors. Direct extension, however, can also occur via the great vessels such as hypernephroma extending up the inferior vena cava to the right side of the heart. Hematogenous metastases can occur, theoretically, from any malignancy. Since the myocardium has the greatest blood supply, this area is the most frequently involved with blood-borne metastases. Hematogenous spread appears to occur equally to the right and left ventricle. Extensive mediastinal lymph node metastases can lead to lymphatic stasis. Tumor then propagates in a retrograde fashion into the heart, which has an abundant lymphatic network. Cardiac metastases occur most commonly in a patient with widespread metastatic disease. Rarely, is it the sole organ for metastases and is cardiac involvement the first manifestation of the malignancy.

The majority of myocardial metastases are asymptomatic. The metastatic lesions are usually small and do not interfere with ventricular systolic function. The tumors, however, may increase in size and interfere with myocardial function to the point of congestive heart failure. The metastases may also interfere with normal conduction. Electrocar-

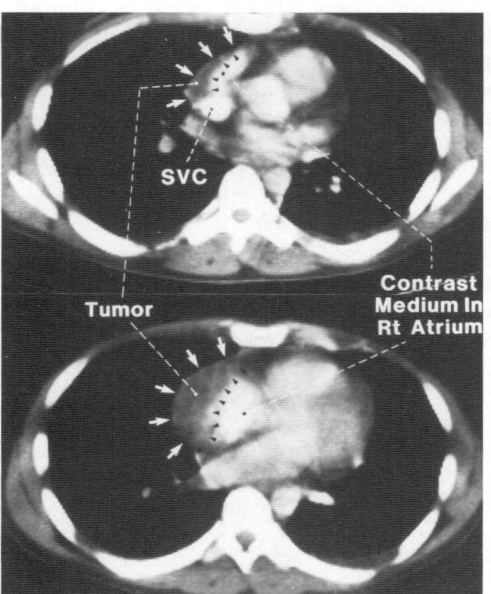

FIGURE 109.9 CT scan of a young man with angiosarcoma of the right atrium. This mass was not seen at the time of two-dimensional echocardiography. Patient died within 3 months of diagnosis and following surgery and chemotherapy.

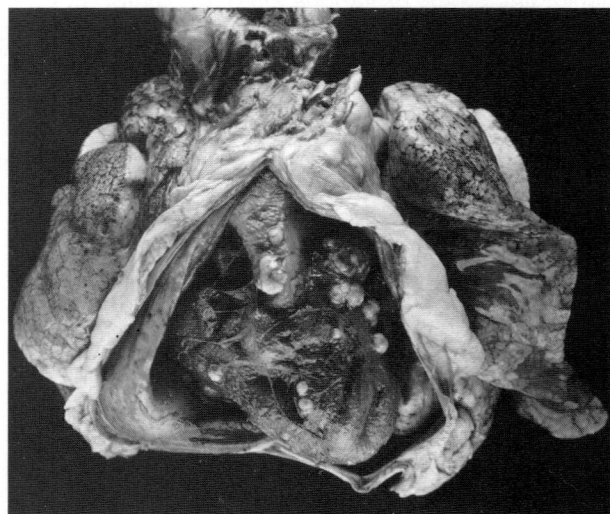

FIGURE 109.10 Pathologic specimen of a 63-year-old man with carcinoma of the left main bronchus showing extension to the pericardium. There was 2000 ml of blood within the pericardial sac. Note metastasis on epicardial surface and also to the mediastinum, ribs, and pancreas.

diographic changes and arrhythmias are common, the most common being atrial fibrillation. Pericardial involvement with the development of pericardial effusion is a common clinical presentation (Fig. 109.11), and occasionally the diagnosis can be made by withdrawing pericardial fluid and subjecting it to cytologic examination. Pericardial constriction has been noted due to extensive growth of the tumor or to pericardial tamponade. More commonly, however, it is a complication of roentgen therapy. Occasionally, a distant tumor can metastasize and embolize to a coronary artery, producing a clinical picture of acute myocardial infarction.

The presence of cardiac metastases should be suspected on a basis of the patient's tumor cell type and cardiac examination. The diagnosis can usually be confirmed by two-dimensional examination.

Treatment of a patient with metastatic cardiac disease is purely palliative.

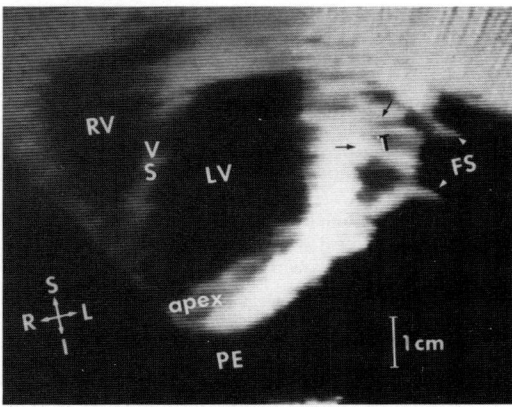

FIGURE 109.11 Modified four-chamber tomographic view of patient with large pericardial effusion. Patient had a mastectomy several years previously for adenocarcinoma. Note large tumor mass within the pericardial space and attached to the epicardium (T and arrows and also the fibrinous strands [FS] extending from the tumor). In this case, the diagnosis of a metastatic tumor to the pericardium was possible. (RV, right ventricle; VS, ventricular septum; LV, left ventricle; PE, pericardial effusion) (Giuliani ER, Nasser FN. Two-dimensional echocardiography in acquired heart disease. Curr Probl Cardiol 5:28, 1981. Copyright © 1981 by Year Book Medical Publishers, Inc, Chicago)

REFERENCES

1. Columbos MR: Pathology of cardiac tumors. Am J Cardiol 21:315, 1968
2. Barnes AR, Beaver DE, Snell AM: Primary sarcoma of the heart. Am Heart J 9:40, 1939
3. Crafoord C: Discussion. In CR Tarm (ed): International Symposium on Cardiovascular Surgery: Studies in Physiology, Diagnosis, and Techniques, p 202. Philadelphia, WB Saunders, 1955
4. McCallister HA, Fenoglio JJ: Tumors of the cardiovascular system. In Atlas of Tumor Pathology, fascicle 15, 2nd series. Washington, DC, Armed Forces Institute of Pathology, 1978
5. Richardson JV, Brandt B, Doty DB et al: Surgical treatment of atrial myxomas: Early and late results of 11 operations and review of the literature. Ann Thorac Surg 28:354, 1979
6. Zitnik RS, Giuliani ER: Clinical recognition of atrial myxomas. Am Heart J 80:680, 1979
7. Sutton MGS, Mercier LA, Giuliani ER et al: Atrial myxomas: A review of clinical experience in 40 patients. Mayo Clinic Proc 55:371, 1980
8. Goodwin JF: Diagnosis of left atrial myxoma. Lancet 1:464, 1963
9. Peters MN, Hall RJ, Cooley DA et al: The clinical syndrome of atrial myxomas. JAMA 230:695, 1974
10. Selzer A, Sakai FJ, Popper RW: Protean clinical manifestations of primary tumors of the heart. Am J Med 52:9, 1972
11. Glasser SP, Bedynek JL, Hall RJ et al: Left atrial myxoma: Report of a case involving hemodynamic, surgical, histologic, and histochemical characteristics. Am J Med 50:113, 1971
12. Byrd WE, Matthews OP, Hunt RE: Left atrial myxoma presenting as a systemic vasculitis. Arthritis Rheum 23:240, 1980
13. Huston KA, Combs JJ, Lie JT et al: Left atrial myxoma simulating peripheral vasculitis. Mayo Clin Proc 53:752, 1978
14. Kaminsky ME, Ehlers KH, Engle MA et al: Atrial myxoma mimicking a collagen disorder. Chest 75:93, 1979
15. O'Neil MB, Grehl TM, Hurley EH: Cardiac myxomas: A clinical diagnostic challenge. Am J Surg 138:68, 1979
16. Silverman J, Olwin JS, Graettinger JE: Cardiac myxomas with systemic embolization: Review of the literature and report of a case. Circulation 26:99, 1962
17. Koikkalainen K, Kostianen S, Luosto R: Left atrial myxoma revealed by femoral embolectomy. Scand J Thorac Cardiovasc Surg 11:33, 1979
18. Bradham RR, Gregorie HB, Howell JS et al: Aortic obstruction from embolizing cardiac myxoma. J Scand Med Assoc 75:7, 1979
19. Schweiger MJ, Hafer JG, Brown R et al: Spontaneous cure of infected left atrial myxoma following embolism. Am Heart J 99:630, 1980
20. Yeoh NT, Clegg JF: Massive embolism from cardiac myxoma. Angiology 32:819, 1981
21. Rajpal RS, Leibsohn JA, Liekweg WG et al: Infected left atrial myxoma with bacteremia simulating infective endocarditis. Arch Intern Med 139:1176, 1979
22. Frenay JJ, Bonte J, Franken P et al: Left atrial myxoma with left retinal emboli, right hemiparesis and myocardial infarction: Neurologic and echocardiographic diagnosis: Surgical treatment. Acta Neurol Belg 81:215, 1981
23. Sankok BA, VonEstorff I, Giuliani ER: CNS embolization due to atrial myxoma: Clinical features and diagnosis. Arch Neurol 37:485, 1980
24. Yarnell PR, Spann JF, Dougherty J et al: Episodic central nervous system ischemia of undetermined cause: Relation to occult left atrial myxoma. Stroke 2:35, 1971
25. Sankok BA, VonEstorff I, Giuliani ER: Subsequent neurological events in patients with atrial myxoma. Ann Neurol 8:305, 1980
26. Roeltgen DP, Weimer GR, Patterson LF: Delayed neurologic complications of left atrial myxoma. Neurology 31:8, 1981
27. Frank RA, Shalen PR, Harvey DG et al: Atrial myxoma with intellectual decline and cerebral growths on CT scan. Ann Neurol 5:396, 1979
28. Raukin LI, Desousa AL: Metastatic atrial myxoma presenting as intracranial mass. Chest 74:451, 1978
29. Burton C, Johnston J: Multiple cerebral aneurysms and cardiac myxoma. N Engl J Med 282:35, 1970
30. Desousa AL, Muller J, Campbell R et al: Atrial myxoma: A review of the neurological complications, metastases, and recurrences. J Neurol Neurosurg Psychiatry 41:1119, 1978
31. Price DL, Harris JL, New PFH et al: Cardiac myxoma: A clinicopathologic and angiographic study. Arch Neurol 23:558, 1970
32. Stoane L, Allen JH, Collins HA: Radiologic observations in cerebral embolization from left heart myxomas. Radiology 87:262, 1966
33. Bass NM, Sharratt GJP: Left atrial myxoma diagnosed by echocardiography with observation on tumor movement. Br Heart J 35:1332, 1973
34. Martinez-Lopez JI: Sounds of the heart in diastole. Am J Cardiol 34:594, 1974
35. Harvey WP: Clinical aspects of cardiac tumors. Am J Cardiol 21:328, 1968
36. Davis G, Kincaid O, Hallermann F: Roentgen aspects of cardiac tumors. Semin Roentgenol 4:384, 1969
37. Schattenberg T: Echocardiographic diagnosis of left atrial myxoma. Mayo Clin Proc 43:620, 1968
38. Dunningan A, Oldham HN, Serwer GA et al: Left atrial myxoma: Is cardiac catheterization essential? Am J Dis Child 135:420, 1981
39. Giuliani ER, Lemur F, Schattenberg T: Unusual echocardiographic findings in a patient with left atrial myxoma. Mayo Clin Proc 53:469, 1978
40. Chadda KD, Pochaczevsky R, Gupta PD et al: Nonprolapsing atrial myxoma: Clinical, echocardiographic, and angiographic correlations. Angiology 29:179, 1978
41. Come PC, Riley MF, Markis JE et al: Limitations of echocardiographic techniques in evaluation of left atrial masses. Am J Cardiol 48:947, 1981
42. Lappe D, Bulkley BH, Weiss JL: Two-dimensional echocardiographic diagnosis of left atrial myxoma. Chest 74:55, 1978
43. Echt DS, Green SE, Popp RL: Advancing the diagnosis of left atrial myxoma. Chest 82:522, 1982
44. Pitcher D, Wainwright R, Brennand-Roper D et al: Cardiac tumors: Noninvasive detection and assessment by gated cardiac blood poor radionuclide imaging. Br Heart J 44:143, 1980
45. Pohost GM, Pastore JO, McKusick KA et al: Detection of left atrial myxoma by gated radionuclide cardiac imaging. Circulation 55:88, 1977
46. Sutton D, Al-Kutoubi MA, Lipkin DP: Left atrial myxoma diagnosed by computerized tomography. Br J Radiol 55:80, 1982

47. Steinberg I, Miscall L, Redo F et al: Angiocardiography in diagnosis of cardiac tumors. Am J Roentgenol 91:364, 1964
48. Abrams HC, Adams DF, Grant HA: The radiology of tumors of the heart. Radiol Clin North Am 9:299, 1971
49. Talley RC, Baldwin BJ, Symbas PN et al: Right atrial myxoma: Unusual presentation with cyanosis and clubbing. Am J Med 48:256, 1970
50. Meyers SM, Shapiro JE, Barresi V et al: Right atrial myxoma with right-to-left shunting and mitral valve prolapse. Am J Med 62:308, 1977
51. Goldschlager A, Popper R, Goldschlager N et al: Right atrial myxoma with right-to-left shunt and polycythemia presenting as congenital heart disease. Am J Cardiol 30:82, 1972
52. Steiner RE: Radiologic aspects of cardiac tumors. Am J Cardiol 21:344, 1968
53. Yuste P, Asin E, Cerdan FJ et al: Echocardiogram in right atrial myxoma. Chest 69:94, 1976
54. Pernod J, Piwnica A, Duret JC: Right atrial myxoma: An echocardiographic study. Br Heart J 40:201, 1978
55. Roudaul R, Pouget B, Videan P et al: Right atrial myxoma in an asymptomatic child: Echocardiographic diagnosis. Eur Heart J 1:453, 1980
56. Sung RJ, Ghahramani AR, Mallon SM et al: Hemodynamic features of prolapsing and non-prolapsing left atrial myxoma. Circulation 51:342, 1975
57. McCallister HA: Primary tumors and cysts of the heart and pericardium. Curr Probl Cardiol 4(2):1, 1979
58. Ports TA, Schiller NB, Strunk BL: Echocardiography of right ventricular tumors. Circulation 56:439, 1977
59. dePaiva EC, Macreira-Coelho E, Amram SS et al: Intracavitary left ventricular myxoma. Am J Cardiol 20:260, 1967
60. Meller J, Teichholz LE, Pichard AD et al: Left ventricular myxoma: Echocardiographic diagnosis and review of the literature. Am J Med 63:816, 1977
61. Zager J, Smith JO, Goldstein S et al: Tricuspid and pulmonary valve obstruction relieved by removal of a myxoma of right ventricle. Am J Cardiol 32:101, 1973
62. Synder NS, Smith DC, Lau FY et al: Diagnostic feature of right ventricular myxoma. Am Heart J 91:240, 1976
63. Pindyck F, Peirce EC, Baron MG et al: Embolization of left atrial myxoma after transseptal cardiac catheterization. Am J Cardiol 30:569, 1972
64. Symbas PN, Hatcher CR, Gravanis MB: Myxoma of the heart: Clinical and experimental observations. Ann Surg 183:470, 1976
65. Miller JI, Mankin HT, Broadbent JC et al: Primary cardiac tumors: Surgical considerations and results of operation. Circulation 45(suppl)I:134, 1972
66. Read RL, White HJ, Murphy ML et al: The malignant potentiality of left atrial myxoma. J Thorac Cardiovasc Surg 68:857, 1974
67. Fenoglio JJ, McCallister HA, Ferrans VJ: Cardiac rhabdomyoma: A clinicopathologic and electron microscopic study. Am J Cardiol 38:241, 1976
68. Arciniegas E, Hakimi M, Farooki ZQ et al: Primary cardiac tumors in children. J Thorac Cardiovasc Surg 79:591, 1980
69. House S, Forbes N, Stewart S: Rhabdomyoma of the heart: A diagnostic and therapeutic challenge. Ann Thorac Surg 29:373, 1980
70. Williams DB, Danielson GK, McGoon DC et al: Cardiac fibroma: Long-term survival after excision. J Thorac Cardiovasc Surg 84:230, 1982
71. Shub C, Tajik AJ, Seward JB et al: Cardiac papillary fibroelastomas: Two-dimensional echocardiographic recognition. Mayo Clin Proc 56:629, 1981
72. Silverman NA: Primary cardiac tumors. Ann Surg 191:127, 1980
73. Strohl KP: Angiosarcoma of the heart. Arch Intern Med 136:929, 1976
74. Glancy DL, Morales JB, Roberts WC: Angiosarcoma of the heart. Am J Cardiol 21:413, 1968
75. Rossi NP, Koischos JM, Aschenbrener CA et al: Primary angiosarcoma of the heart. Cancer 37:891, 1976
76. Schwartz JE, Schwartz GP, Judson PL et al: Cardiovasc Dis Bull Texas Heart Inst 6:413, 1979
77. Baldelli P, DeAngeli D, Dolara A et al: Primary fibrosarcoma of the heart. Chest 62:234, 1972
78. Haufling SM: Metastatic cancer to the heart: Review of the literature and report of 127 cases. Circulation 22:474, 1960
79. Malaret GE, Aliaga P: Metastatic disease to the heart. Cancer 22:457, 1968
80. Smith LH: Secondary tumors of the heart. Rev Surg 33:223, 1976

SECTION 13

Section Editor
Melvin D. Cheitlin, MD

Secondary Disorders of the Heart

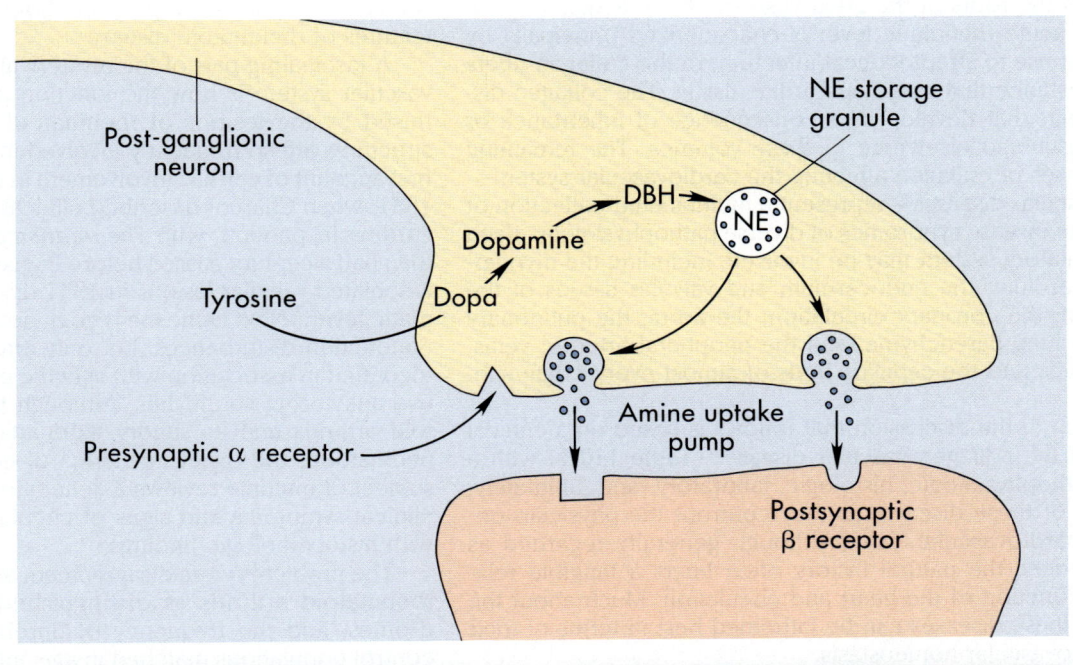

COLLAGEN DISEASES AND THE HEART

Jonathan L. Halperin

CHAPTER 110
VOLUME 2

As an essential structural element of all tissues of the circulatory system, collagen fibers may participate in a host of pathologic processes. Diseases of cardiovascular collagen may be primary and inherited or secondary and acquired. The genetically transmitted disorders of connective tissue are rare lesions of collagen chemistry closely related to other disorders of elastic tissue and mucopolysaccharides. In these cases, the skeletal framework of the heart is unable to bear the dynamic stress of cyclic heart action and degeneration occurs in valvular architecture and the roots of the great vessels. Of the acquired rheumatic diseases, acute rheumatic fever is characterized principally by damage, in response to streptococcal infection, to the collagen fibers and ground substance that make up cardiac tissue. The collagen diseases of the heart that develop as a consequence of inheritance or infection are discussed elsewhere in these volumes. The remaining secondary diseases of collagen affecting the cardiovascular system—the collagen vascular diseases—represent a multifaceted collection of connective tissue disease syndromes of diverse pathophysiology. Each part of the circulatory system may be involved, including the myocardium; the pericardium; the endocardium and valvular tissues of the cardiac skeleton; the coronary circulation; the aorta; the pulmonary vasculature and lung parenchyma; and the peripheral arteries, veins, arterioles, venules, and the capillary beds of almost every organ subsystem.

The approach in the discussion that follows is based on a clinical classification of the collagen vascular diseases (Table 110.1) with a view toward pathophysiologic, histologic, laboratory, and, ultimately, clinical aspects of these diseases as they confront the physician oriented toward cardiovascular care. Although generally regarded as rheumatic disorders, the natural history often bears a tangible relationship to the function of the heart and circulation. Much about the mechanisms of these diseases can be fathomed best in terms of their impact on cardiovascular homeostasis.

RHEUMATOID ARTHROPATHY
RHEUMATOID ARTHRITIS

A discussion of the cardiovascular manifestations of connective tissue disease appropriately begins with the syndrome of rheumatoid arthritis. In many respects, rheumatoid arthritis may be viewed as the prototype collagen vascular disease, although several of the other "rheumatoid diseases" have scant articular manifestations and most involve a host of connective tissues other than simply the collagen fiber produced by fibroblasts. The spectrum of cardiovascular involvement in rheumatoid arthritis is protean, and it may come to involve virtually all tissues of the cardiovascular system, including the pericardium, myocardium, coronary arteries, conducting system, endocardium, and valves, in addition to the aorta and peripheral vessels. Because the lungs are commonly involved in rheumatoid arthritis, clinical manifestations may take the form of pulmonary heart disease as well.

Part of this diversity derives from the complex relationship between our notion of the pathophysiology of this disease and observed histopathologic features. The blood of most patients with rheumatoid arthritis contains a heterogeneous group of antibodies specific for IgG, designated rheumatoid factors, apparently generated as a result of chronic antigenic stimulation. Whereas such "seropositivity" may develop transiently in patients with acute rheumatic fever, infective endocarditis or other types of sustained infection, rheumatoid factors generally disappear as the inciting cause is overcome and progressive arthritis does not develop. How rheumatoid factors form is not known, but these antibodies are not typically present in the sera of patients with degenerative osteoarthritis and even the continued detection of rheumatoid factor in the serum does not generally lead to the development of rheumatoid arthritis. Nevertheless, immunologic factors play an essential role in the development of both the synovial and cardiovascular features of rheumatoid disease.

A fascinating part of the mystery about involvement of the cardiovascular system is how the function of the heart is seldom compromised by the lesions of rheumatoid arthritis when its component structures are so frequently involved in the inflammatory process. The first account of cardiac involvement in rheumatoid arthritis appeared in 1881, when Charcot described clinical and necropsy evidence of pericarditis in patients with *rheumatisme articulaire chronique*.[1] More than half a century passed before Baggenstoss and Rosenberg reported associated valvular lesions in 1941 distinct from the sequelae of rheumatic fever.[2] Next came the recognition of electrocardiographic (ECG) conduction disturbances, but only after this type of defect had been identified in association with specific pathologic changes of seronegative ankylosing spondylitis. Although the systemic nature of rheumatoid arthritis and its sundry extra-articular manifestations were well understood, the exact incidence of cardiovascular changes was the subject of multiple reviews a generation ago, and it became clear that clinical symptoms and signs of circulatory disorders poorly correlate with histopathologic findings.[3,4]

The problems were disagreement about the criteria for diagnosis of rheumatoid arthritis as distinguished from other rheumatoid syndromes, and the frequency of unrelated cardiovascular disease in control populations matched in age and sex. As corticosteroid therapy became widespread, the importance of separating the cardiovascular effects of this class of medications was emphasized. One study of 254 patients with rheumatoid arthritis and an equal number of control patients with other diseases showed evidence of congestive heart failure in nearly 10% of rheumatoid arthritis patients as compared with only 1% of controls.[4] Angina pectoris was four times more common, left ventricular enlargement nearly twice as common, and enlargement of the right ventricle or either atrium about five times more common in the patients with rheumatoid arthritis. Cardiac murmurs were noted ten times as often, although murmurs were identified in fewer than 10% of the rheumatoid patients.

Overall, rheumatoid heart lesions were thought to occur in approximately one third of patients with rheumatoid arthritis, taking the form of pericarditis, myocarditis, endocarditis with valvulitis, and coronary arteritis, but clinical features were regarded as nondiagnostic. A retrospective study of 62 autopsied patients with peripheral rheumatoid arthritis compared the findings to those in twice as many patients from the general necropsy population matched for age and sex, and found an 82% incidence of heart disease in the rheumatoid population, as against 66% in the control group.[3] Clinical evidence of heart disease was recorded in two thirds of the rheumatoid population, nearly twice the prevailing rate in most clinical series. Indeed, over half of the rheumatoid patients displayed cardiac lesions at autopsy that could not be correlated with other illness or therapy, as compared with a small fraction of the control group, and the postmortem incidence of such lesions was considerably greater than the incidence of clinical manifestations attributable to them. Nevertheless, in 27% of the patients with rheumatoid arthritis with clinical cardiac disease, the only cardiac lesions evident at autopsy were those related to rheumatoid disease. Most strikingly, in 8 of the 62 cases (13%) the cause of death was apparently rheumatoid heart disease.

The diversity of histologic and clinical features of cardiovascular involvement in rheumatoid arthritis is also related to the manner in which humoral and cellular immunity interact in the pathophysiology of this disease. The most characteristic pathologic lesion of rheumatoid arthritis is the nodular granuloma (Fig. 110.1), which occurs in cardiovascular tissue in rough proportion to the severity of the rheumatoid disease and is usually associated with diffusely distributed rheumatoid nodules in the subcutaneous tissues and elsewhere. Such nodules rarely compromise cardiac function and, indeed, were present in only 2 of the 62 autopsied cases just mentioned. Interstitial inflammatory changes of connective tissue seem more common, consisting of round cell infiltration, edema, and fibrosis, which have a particular predilection for the pericardium, where the disease may be even more extensive than in synovial tissues. The progression of interstitial disease to secondary amyloid deposition is relatively uncommon except in advanced cases, where abnormalities of cardiac diastolic function may be sufficiently severe to result in restrictive cardiomyopathic physiology that is difficult to distinguish from chronic pericardial constriction.

Coronary arteritis may be diffuse, but small vessels are mainly affected by intimal proliferation; neither commonly produces clinically significant myocardial ischemia. Particularly challenging today is the interaction between the atherogenic and thrombogenic impact of corticosteroid exposure in patients with coronary syndromes and rheumatoid arthritis.

CLINICAL FEATURES

PERICARDITIS. It should not be surprising that as a serosal surface the pericardium more commonly becomes involved in the inflammatory process of rheumatoid arthritis than the myocardium, endocardium, or vascular structures of the heart. In most patients with rheumatoid arthritis, however, pericarditis has little clinical impact and generally goes undetected during the patient's lifetime. The diagnosis of rheumatoid pericarditis is made in barely 2% of adults with rheumatoid arthritis; yet the rate rises to 6% in patients with juvenile rheumatoid arthritis (Still's disease) and 10% of patients with arthritis crippled enough to require hospitalization.[5,6] It has been said of pericardial disease in general that the frequency of diagnosis is proportional to the clinician's index of suspicion and diligence of examination. Auscultation of pericardial friction rub or echocardiographic features of pericardial effusion have been reported in approximately 30% of patients with rheumatoid arthritis in several studies.[7,8] In cases with subcutaneous rheumatoid nodules, echocardiographic signs of pericardial involvement are found in 50%, which matches the incidence in some necropsy series.[3,4,9]

TABLE 110.1 COLLAGEN DISEASES INVOLVING THE CARDIOVASCULAR SYSTEM

I. Rheumatoid Arthropathy
   A. Rheumatoid arthritis
      1. Adult form
      2. Juvenile rheumatoid arthritis (Still's disease)
   B. Seronegative spondyloarthropathy
      1. Ankylosing spondylitis
      2. Reiter's disease
      3. Behçet's disease
      4. Psoriatic arthritis
      5. Intestinal arthritides
II. Vasculitis Syndromes
   A. Systemic lupus erythematosus
   B. Diffuse vasculitides
      1. Periarteritis nodosa
      2. Mucocutaneous lymph node syndrome (Kawasaki disease)
      3. Allergic angiitis and granulomatosis (Churg-Strauss syndrome)
      4. Hypersensitivity vasculitis
      5. Wegener's granulomatosis
      6. Giant cell arteritis
      7. Takayasu's aortopathy
   C. Diverse disorders associated with vasculopathy
      1. Vasculitides of acute rheumatic fever
      2. Cryoglobulinemia
      3. Thromboangiitis obliterans (Buerger's disease)
      4. Hereditary angioedema
III. Sclerosing Syndromes
   A. Scleroderma
      1. Progressive systemic sclerosis
      2. CREST variant
   B. Polymyositis-dermatomyositis complex
      1. Polymyositis
      2. Dermatomyositis
      3. Overlap syndromes
   C. Mixed connective tissue disease

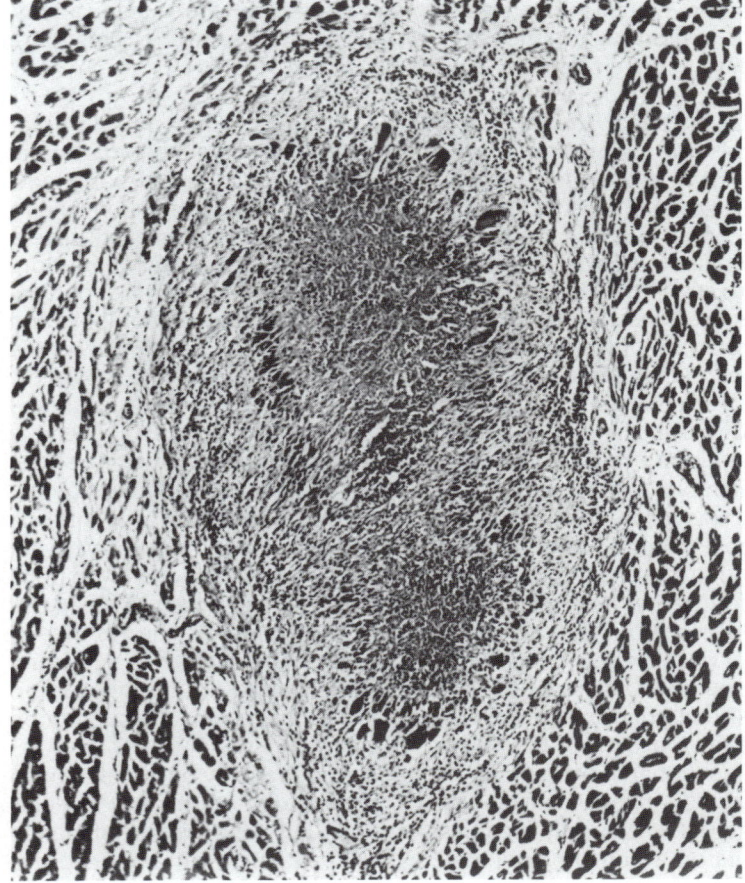

FIGURE 110.1 Rheumatoid granuloma in a section of myocardium. A central zone of fibrinoid necrosis is surrounded by histiocytes and fibroblasts as well as interspersed multinucleated giant cells. The outer zone of fibrosis contains chronic inflammatory cells (H&E, X35) (McAllister HA: Collagen vascular diseases and the cardiovascular system. In Silver MD (ed): Cardiovascular Pathology. New York, Churchill Livingstone, 1983)

Pathophysiologically, acute fibrinous rheumatoid pericarditis reveals the inflammatory interplay of leukocytes and immune complexes. The pericardial fluid contains low levels of glucose, hemolytic complement (CH50), and C3 and elevated levels of lactic dehydrogenase, γ-globulin, and cholesterol; rheumatoid factor may also be detected. Histologically, there is evidence of plasma cell infiltration and deposition of immunoglobulins with cytoplasmic inclusion of immune complexes, but rheumatoid granulomas are unusual. More commonly, the inflammatory changes are nonspecific, including adhesions and pericardial scarring.

It is important to distinguish rheumatoid pericarditis from viral, tuberculous, and drug-induced varieties. The anti-inflammatory drug phenylbutazone has been associated with a pericarditis syndrome,[10] and sustained corticosteroid therapy may dramatically alter the clinical features of tuberculosis.[11] Pericardial involvement may even be the first manifestation of rheumatoid disease. More often, symptoms of chest and shoulder pain in patients with rheumatoid arthritis are mistaken for articular discomfort or masked by analgesic or anti-inflammatory medication.

Compressive complications of rheumatoid pericarditis, acute cardiac tamponade, and chronic constrictive pericarditis are uncommon, but the latter appears more often. Both can be fatal if not treated vigorously. Neither tamponade nor constriction seem to respond regularly to intensive corticosteroid or cytotoxic medication and invasive approaches are usually required. Cases of cardiac compression may take the form of effusive-constrictive pericarditis in which fluid becomes loculated by pericardial adhesions, making needle aspiration or catheter drainage incompletely effective. In such cases, pericardiectomy may be called for. Despite the antithrombotic effects of many salicylates and certain other nonsteroidal anti-inflammatory medications, acute hemorrhagic pericarditis producing tamponade by hemopericardium is quite rare.

MYOCARDIAL INVOLVEMENT. Disease of cardiac muscle associated with rheumatoid arthritis takes three forms: granuloma formation, myocarditis, and amyloid deposition. These varied pathologic processes and the superimposed effects of drugs and infection lead to myocardial changes evident at autopsy in 19% of patients with severe rheumatoid arthritis.[3] Cardiac enlargement has been described more frequently in patients with rheumatoid arthritis than in control populations evaluated by electrocardiography, chest roentgenography, and necropsy. In practice, however, rheumatoid arthritis usually spares the myocardium even when the fibrous tissues of the heart are involved.

Most echocardiography literature has focused on pericardial and endocardial changes. Some studies, however, have reported lower diastolic closure rates of the anterior mitral valve leaflet in patients with rheumatoid arthritis and suggested that abnormal ventricular compliance was responsible.[9] Congestive symptoms were present in only one of those patients, however, and hemodynamic measurements were not provided to corroborate the ultrasound findings. Subsequently, careful M-mode echocardiographic measurements in 35 consecutive patients with rheumatoid arthritis were published to emphasize the absence of mitral valve leaflet abnormalities except as a rare event.[12] In the future, the sound beam might bounce the other way again, but to date no consistent abnormalities of left ventricular dimensions or wall motion have been described in patients with this disease.

Functional indices of left ventricular contractility have never been measured systematically in cases of rheumatoid arthritis, but it seems unlikely that clinically significant systolic left ventricular dysfunction occurs on a primary myopathic basis. In patients with advanced disease, congestive symptoms and signs may develop with or without ECG or roentgenographic features of cardiomegaly or echocardiographic correlates of impaired diastolic myocardial relaxation. Complicating factors abound in such devastating cases, although an early retrospective study found no higher incidence of hypertension in patients with rheumatoid arthritis than in a control population.[3] Coronary atherosclerosis may be more frequent, but whether myocardial infarction develops any more often seems more a matter of belief than epidemiologic certainty.

Before 1980, histopathologic diagnosis required postmortem examination, since catheter-directed endomyocardial biopsy was not practically available. In most cases studied at autopsy, myocardial involvement had been unrecognized during life. The lesions are characterized by nonspecific inflammatory changes involving interstitial infiltration by lymphocytes, plasma cells, histiocytes, and fibroblasts. Eosinophilic infiltration and localized intramyocardial vasculitis are the exception rather than the rule, and patients displaying these changes may have had superimposed hypersensitivity responses to drugs or viral infection. When Lebowitz identified rheumatoid myocarditis in 19% of cases at autopsy, most patients had had associated active arthritis, endocarditis, pericarditis, or peripheral vascular changes suggesting a particularly severe form of the disease.[3]

Myocardial granulomas may be encountered in patients with advanced subcutaneous nodular rheumatoid arthritis, and amyloid infiltration sometimes develops in patients with longstanding disease. Both are rare complications, and with the latter there is almost always involvement of other organs such as the spleen, liver, and kidneys as well. Isolated cardiac amyloidosis has been described, and the availability of endomyocardial biopsy of the interventricular septum may allow more accurate estimation of the incidence of amyloidosis in the living rheumatoid population.

In patients presenting with clinical manifestations of cardiomyopathy in the presence of rheumatoid arthritis, evaluation is directed mainly to excluding reversible contributory factors such as abnormal fluid accumulation, hypertension, pulmonary involvement, ischemia, and rhythm disturbances. Management then entails application of conventional modalities for treating heart failure, including sodium restriction, diuretic agents, digitalis glycosides, and judicious administration of vasodilator drugs. Congestive rather than hypoperfusive manifestations tend to predominate in those occasional patients with clinically apparent involvement of cardiac muscle by rheumatoid disease, and some have suggested that drugs reducing preload through venodilation (such as the organic nitrate class) may be better tolerated and of generally greater clinical value than afterload-reducing substances. The angiotensin-converting enzyme inhibitors are often effective hemodynamically, but adverse reactions to captopril (particularly leukopenia, azotemia, and proteinuria) may be more frequent in patients with active connective tissue disease than in other forms of congestive heart failure.[13]

ENDOCARDIAL AND VALVULAR INVOLVEMENT. Like rheumatoid myocarditis, the histologic pattern of endocardial involvement in rheumatoid arthritis is generally nonspecific. There is infiltration of lymphocytes, histiocytes, plasma cells, and occasionally eosinophils accompanying collagen deposition, fibrosis, and calcific sclerosis. Valvular involvement is more prominently characterized by formation of granulomas that morphologically resemble the rheumatoid nodules encountered in subcutaneous tissue and, less commonly, in the respiratory, intestinal, musculoskeletal, reticuloendothelial, and hematopoietic systems. Valvular granulomas have been described in approximately 3% of patients with rheumatoid arthritis at autopsy, but in most of these cases the size and location of the lesion do not produce clinical features of valve dysfunction.[3,14] The order of frequency of involvement of the cardiac valves—mitral the highest, then aortic, tricuspid, and pulmonic—parallels that in rheumatic fever, and it is virtually impossible to distinguish valvular disease related to rheumatoid arthritis from rheumatic heart disease following streptococcal infection, without histologic examination of the involved tissue. In rheumatoid arthritis, nodular granulomas usually occur in the annular skeleton and basal attachments of the leaflets.[15] When the matrix of the leaflets becomes involved, a thin margin of normal tissue usually remains at the surface in contact with the circulation, unlike the situation in rheumatic valvular disease in which the entire thickness of the leaflet is affected without preservation of a capsule of normal valvular tissue. Several patients with involvement of all four cardiac valves have been described; in these cases, valves in the left side of the heart were more extensively involved than those in the right side.[16,17] Hemodynamically, left-sided involvement also tends to cause more impairment of valvular function than rheumatoid lesions in the right side of the heart.

As in other forms of rheumatoid heart disease, clinical features occur less frequently than histologic abnormalities. Congestive symptoms are cardinal, but auscultatory clues may be misleading. Coexisting problems such as anemia or hypertension may distort cardiac murmurs, and auscultatory findings are commonly absent altogether in patients showing necropsy evidence of granulomatous involvement of valvular tissue. The hemodynamic consequences may reflect either valvular regurgitation or stenosis. Those studies noting reduced diastolic closing velocity of the mitral leaflets on echocardiographic examinations have raised the possibility that this controversial finding reflects subclinical valvular disease rather than an abnormality of myocardial function.[9] Indeed, although rarely severe, mitral stenosis due to rheumatoid arthritis is one of the few nonrheumatic causes of this valvular abnormality most cardiologists ever face. It is actually more routine to encounter patients with features of both rheumatic and rheumatoid cardiac valvular disease, and in some of these cases valvular surgery is required.[18] Although bleeding complications may develop more frequently in patients with rheumatoid arthritis subjected to cardiac valve replacement, these have not been defined in statistically meaningful terms.

DISEASE OF THE CONDUCTING SYSTEM. The first report of complete heart block due to rheumatoid granulomatous involvement of the conduction pathways appeared in 1959[19]; since that time about 24 cases have been described. Complete atrioventricular dissociation, therefore, must be called a rare complication of rheumatoid arthritis, and its incidence in patients hospitalized with the disease has been estimated at less than 0.1%.[20] Other than direct involvement of the conducting system with granulomas, pathologic processes producing cardiac conducting system disease include extension of the inflammatory process from the base of the aortic or mitral valve leaflets, amyloidosis, or acute hemorrhage into a rheumatoid nodule. It is important in interpreting the older literature to bear in mind the distinction between peripheral rheumatoid arthritis and seronegative ankylosing spondylitis, because clinically significant disease of the conducting system is far less common in the former than the latter.

In patients with rheumatoid arthritis, although progression to complete heart block seldom occurs, lesser degrees of conduction delay are encountered fairly frequently. The most common abnormality is first-degree atrioventricular block, which occurred eight times more frequently in one series of patients with rheumatoid arthritis than in a control population.[4] Left bundle branch block occurred four times more often in the rheumatoid population, but the opposite was true of right bundle branch block. Although right bundle branch block developed in 1% or 2% of the control group, it was not described in any of the 254 patients with rheumatoid arthritis. Management of patients with symptomatic bradycardia resulting from involvement of the conducting system generally entails the use of permanent cardiac pacemakers. There is every reason to believe that this mode of therapy is as effective for patients with rheumatoid arthritis and advanced conducting system disease as for other pacemaker candidates, but the possibility of progressive endocardial fibrosis generally demands selection of a pacing system permitting repeated evaluation of output and sensing characteristics and the capability of reprogramming these parameters to meet changing patient needs defined by repeated analyses over the course of months and years. Whether patients with rheumatoid heart disease requiring pacemakers also represent a subset with significant myocardial diastolic compliance abnormalities able to benefit from dual-chamber stimulation has not yet been clarified.

Other than conduction system disorders, patients with rheumatoid arthritis occasionally display abnormalities of impulse generation in the form of sinoatrial block, wandering atrial pacemaker, and atrial fibrillation. Preexcitation related to a paranodal accessory pathway of atrioventricular conduction has been described in rare patients with rheumatoid arthritis, although no causal relationship has been suggested and the association seems incidental. Ventricular extrasystoles occurred in twice as many patients with rheumatoid arthritis as in the control population in the study mentioned above,[4] but there has been no proof of a specific association between rheumatoid arthritis and malicious ventricular dysrhythmias or sudden cardiac fibrillatory death.

CORONARY ARTERY DISEASE. Still another area of rheumatoid heart disease filled with controversy is the problem of myocardial ischemia due to coronary artery disease. The major autopsy studies of a generation ago were unanimous in finding more frequent coronary artherosclerosis in patients with rheumatoid arthritis than in matched control populations.[3,4] Moreover, histologic evidence of coronary arteritis has been reported in approximately 20% of autopsied cases, presenting a second mechanism of arterial narrowing.[21] Peripheral vasospastic events such as Raynaud's phenomenon are considerably less common in patients with rheumatoid arthritis than in those with systemic sclerosis or systemic lupus erythematosus, and there is little reason to believe that vasotonic events are of importance in limiting coronary blood flow in patients with rheumatoid arthritis. Corticosteroid therapy is thought to accelerate the progression of the atherosclerotic process through a variety of mechanisms, and it was a long-held view that patients with rheumatoid arthritis, even at relatively young ages, were at risk of developing myocardial ischemia on the basis of coronary obstructive disease. In the 254 cases described by Cathcart and Spodick, angina pectoris occurred four times more often in patients with rheumatoid arthritis than in the reference population.[4] In a total of 19 separate studies published since 1941 and encompassing over 900 patients, the incidence of coronary atherosclerosis at autopsy approaches 40%.[22] In 16% of these autopsied cases, there was also evidence of myocardial infarction. In all, about 25% of myocardial infarctions in patients with rheumatoid arthritis proved fatal. These facts stand in contrast to more recent observations showing significantly lower morbidity and mortality from myocardial infarction in 62 patients with rheumatoid arthritis (matched for age, sex, and coronary risk factors with an equal number of autopsied control patients) reported in 1974.[22] It has been speculated that the antithrombotic effects of nonsteroidal anti-inflammatory and salicylate medications commonly given for rheumatoid arthritis may explain this more favorable outcome. Although coronary arteritis is found fairly frequently at autopsy (in about 1 of 5 patients)[21] and intimal inflammation may lead to severe narrowing or occlusion of the lumen, myocardial necrosis resulting from this form of vascular involvement seems relatively rare.

Myocardial revascularization surgery is performed quite commonly in patients with coexisting coronary atherosclerotic lesions and rheumatoid arthritis, and the clinical course of these patients is not appreciably different from the remainder of the coronary bypass population. The effectiveness of aspirin therapy in reducing the rate of postoperative vein graft occlusion in the general population subjected to this revascularization procedure[23] argues strongly that this form of therapy be continued in patients with rheumatoid arthritis undergoing coronary bypass surgery.

SERONEGATIVE SPONDYLOARTHROPATHY

This group of syndromes is reminiscent of rheumatoid arthritis except for the absence of rheumatoid factor in serum and a predilection of arthropathy for the sacroiliac and lumbosacral joints as well as the articulations of the spine. The disorders occur predominantly in men. The prototype syndome is ankylosing spondylitis; with the frequency of cardiac involvement less in Reiter's disease, Behçet's syndrome, psoriatic arthritis, and the intestinal arthritides. It has been theorized that a genetically determined abnormal host response to a variety of infectious processes, the portals of entry for which include the intestinal and genitourinary tracts, is the fundamental abnormality in these diseases.

A remarkable association has been found between the occurrence of seronegative spondyloarthropathy and histocompatibility antigen HLA-B27, which occurs in approximately 5% in the normal population but in over 90% of patients with ankylosing spondylitis or Reiter's disease, in over 80% of patients with spondyloarthropathy complicating intestinal inflammation, in 50% of patients with psoriatic arthritis, and in a similar proportion of patients with iritis.[24,25] In general, cardiac involvement in patients with seronegative spondyloarthropathy is most frequent in the presence of HLA-B27 positivity.

ANKYLOSING SPONDYLITIS

It has long been known that ankylosing spondylitis is frequently accompanied by abnormalities of the proximal aorta. These may consist of dilatation of the aortic valve annulus, fibrous thickening and focal inflammation of the aortic valve cusps that prolapse into the left ventricular cavity, dilatation of the sinuses of Valsalva, and degenerative changes of the elastic tissue of the aortic media. The lesions are similar to those encountered in luetic aortitis except for their proximity to the valve ring. The thickening and foreshortening of the aortic valve cusps and the displacement and dilatation of aortic valve ring may result in severe aortic regurgitation. Occasionally, the fibrotic changes may extend into the endocardium at the base of the anterior mitral valve leaflet and the upper portion of the interventricular septum, but mitral regurgitation is an unusual development. Although fibrosis of the proximal His-Purkinje apparatus of the conducting system has been known since this syndrome was distinguished from rheumatoid arthritis, it has been rather recently that the frequency of cardiac conduction disturbances has been recognized. The importance of ankylosing spondylitis as a cause of severe conduction disturbance is evident in the observation that the prevalence of ankylosing spondylitis in men with permanent cardiac pacemakers is 15 times greater than in the general population.[26] Histologically, the myocardial lesions themselves are fairly nonspecific, with features of fibrosis, perivascular lymphocytic infiltration, and accumulation of ground substance. Cardiac enlargement and hypertrophy are rather frequently encountered and the left ventricle may be dilated even in the absence of aortic insufficiency. The fibrotic process may also obliterate the pericardial cavity, but clinical evidence of pericarditis is unusual in ankylosing spondylitis.[27,28]

Spondylitis of the axial skeleton may be accompanied by fever and accelerated erythrocyte sedimentation rate, but the serologic abnormalities encountered in rheumatoid arthritis are absent. Active myocarditis may appear before aortic regurgitation or conduction disturbances become manifest. The clinical syndrome is generally characterized by chest pain, pericardial friction rub, sinus tachycardia, cardiomegaly, and ECG features of first-degree atrioventricular block. Cardiac functional abnormalities are seldom encountered before the onset of rhythm disturbances or aortic insufficiency, and it thus becomes difficult to assess the impact of the disease on myocardial performance without the confounding influence of these factors. It is worth emphasizing that cardiac manifestations of the disease may precede articular findings so that the development of aortic regurgitation or complete heart block in a middle-aged male demands consideration of ankylosing spondylitis in the differential diagnosis. Valvular regurgitation develops gradually, but in many patients atrioventricular block becomes advanced without manifestations of incompetence of the left ventricular outflow tract. It has been stated that aortic regurgitation relates to the duration of clinical spondylitis and the degree of peripheral joint involvement. In patients with spondylitis for more than 30 years, 10% had evidence of a valvular lesion; this figure rose to 18% when peripheral arthropathy was also evident.[29]

Cardiac auscultatory findings include tamborous accentuation of the aortic component of the second heart sound, and the soft decrescendo diastolic murmur is usually unaccompanied by systolic ejection murmur in this early stage. The sound of aortic valve closure may be diminished in intensity when regurgitation becomes more severe and harsh systolic ejection murmurs then become apparent. At this time, usually several years after the onset of the condition, the Austin Flint murmur may develop as more severe aortic insufficiency impinges on the excursion of the anterior mitral leaflet. Management of regurgitation involves administration of vasodilator medication in addition to digitalis and diuretic agents, and aortic valve replacement has been accomplished successfully in a limited number of cases.

Atrioventricular block occurs to some extent in as many as 20% of patients with ankylosing spondylitis, and about a fourth of these develop complete heart block.[29] The majority of these conduction disturbances occur as intermittent phenomena. Almost equally common are intraventricular conduction disturbances, but these are generally permanent once they develop. Cardiac pacemakers have been implanted routinely in the presence of high-grade atrioventricular block, often without the diagnosis of ankylosing spondylitis having been recognized initially.

REITER'S DISEASE

The acute illness produced by Reiter's disease usually consists of nonspecific urethritis, migratory polyarthritis, conjunctivitis, balanitis, and keratoderma blenorrhagica. Although initial episodes may subside spontaneously, recurrences occur in patients with HLA-B27 antigen positivity, resulting in painful deformation of the feet and axial skeleton. Atrioventricular block and aortic valvular incompetence are the most frequent cardiac manifestations. The histopathology of the disease is quite similar to that encountered in ankylosing spondylitis. It may not be surprising, therefore, that conducting system disease has been described in Reiter's disease as well.[30-34]

BEHCET'S DISEASE

Cardiac involvement has rarely been described in patients with Behçet's disease, which is another of the seronegative spondyloarthropathies. The clinical syndrome is characterized by aphthous ulceration of the buccal mucosa, thrombophlebitis, and genital ulcers as well as arthropathy involving the hands. Cardiac involvement has been reported in fewer than 20 cases, the most frequent manifestations of which were rhythm disturbance, pericarditis, and myocarditis. Histologically, the features consist of inflammatory cell infiltration and fibrosis of left ventricular myocardium, but the pathophysiology of the disorder is poorly understood. In one reported case of Behçet's disease, conducting system involvement was associated with rupture of an aneurysm of the sinus of Valsalva into the left ventricular cavity.[35-39]

VASCULITIS SYNDROMES
SYSTEMIC LUPUS ERYTHEMATOSUS

Although only 1 of the 14 preliminary criteria for the diagnosis and classification of systemic lupus erythematosus describes cardiac involvement, the frequency of cardiac lesions in this multisystemic disease is generally recognized by the present generation of physicians. Still, it is an intriguing statement about parochial subspecialization that the rheumatologist sees the incidence of "lupus carditis" as decreasing with the earlier discovery of mild cases of systemic lupus erythematosus, while the cardiologist finds evidence of heart involvement increasing as methodology becomes more sophisticated. In truth, improvements in diagnostic methods in both fields have brought the frequency of clinical recognition of cardiac involvement in lupus erythematosus into line with that found at autopsy.

The basic anatomical lesion of systemic lupus erythematosus is microvasculitis, and this is accompanied by the presence in serum of antibodies to various components of the cell nucleus—antinuclear antibodies. The pathogenesis of the disease seems to involve formation of immune complexes consisting of these antibodies combined with circulating antigen and complement that become deposited in microvascular endothelium, producing a variety of hyperimmune phenomena. Immunohistologic studies of cardiac tissue obtained at necropsy in patients with advanced systemic lupus erythematosus have disclosed evidence of IgG deposition in 90% of specimens.[40] These deposits were granular (suggesting immune complex aggregates) and occur predominantly in the walls of pericardial and myocardial vessels. Direct immunofluorescence studies of valvular tissue and associated vegetations reveal IgG and complement components in these stroma as well. Some discrepancy has been observed between the patterns of immunopathologic involvement and other features of interstitial inflammation, which has been taken as evidence that these are not simultaneous processes. Anti-heart antibodies have been identified in the sera of some patients with lupus erythematosus, but the detection of these antibodies has not been correlated with either the frequency or the severity of cardiac lesions identified clinically or histologically.[41] Presently, it is the belief that these antibodies represent a response to persistent release of myocardial antigens into the circulation rather than a cause of cardiac inflammation.

Attention was drawn to the heart in systemic lupus erythematosus in 1924 when Libman and Sacks first described the associated nonbacterial endocarditis characterized by verrucous valvular vegetations.[42] Clinical evidence of cardiac involvement is seldom florid, but some astute physicians have identified features of cardiac disease in over 50% of patients.[43] Although the frequency of Libman-Sacks endocarditis at autopsy ranges widely (from 3% to 74%), some evidence of lupus carditis may be found in the vast majority of cases examined. On average, the typical endocarditic lesions of systemic lupus erythematosus have been identified in approximately 50% of patients with fatal disease.[44]

Since the advent of corticosteroid therapy, the cardiovascular manifestations of systemic lupus erythematosus have changed dramatically. It would initially seem remarkable, therefore, that Libman-Sacks endocarditis, albeit morphologically altered, is still encountered in about half the cases of corticosteroid-treated systemic lupus erythematosus.[44] As in patients not subjected to this form of therapy, each of the four cardiac valves may become involved in the pathologic process.[43,45,46] With the advent of corticosteroids, valvular lesions are now virtually confined not only to the left side of the heart but in particular to the posterior portion of the mitral valve apparatus. Partial healing of the verrucous lesions occurs in over half the corticosteroid-treated patients, but subsequent calcification of the annular region is now encountered far more often (if, indeed, this ever occurred prior to corticosteroid intervention). Just as is true for lupus endocarditis, pericarditis appears to occur with nearly equal frequency in both corticosteroid-treated and untreated patients with systemic lupus erythematosus, while the nature and extent of pericardial involvement is substantially different in the two groups. With the advent of corticosteroid therapy, pericarditis became more fibrous than fibrinous and infective pericarditis has increased substantially in incidence. In contrast, the frequency of lupus myocarditis has declined noticeably since the advent of corticosteroid therapy and myocardial inflammatory changes, when present, are seldom as severe as those encountered in non-corticosteroid-treated patients. There is no appreciable difference in the frequency of conducting system abnormalities, and those cardiac rhythm disturbances that develop in patients with active lupus myocarditis or pericarditis seem to improve somewhat as corticosteroid therapy is instituted.[47]

Corticosteroids have their impact on the heart in systemic lupus erythematosus in other ways as well. The deposition of subepicardial fat is considerably greater in corticosteroid-treated patients, particularly when this form of therapy has been given long enough to produce clinical features of Cushing's syndrome. Systemic hypertension is now common in patients with corticosteroid-treated lupus erythematosus, and this seems to correlate with the presence of left ventricular hypertrophy. These abnormalities were infrequent when the disease followed its natural course. In patients with systemic lupus erythematosus, corticosteroids play a role alongside renal involvement in the development of hypertension. Congestive heart failure is also aggravated by corticosteroid therapy, particularly when renal function is compromised and in the presence of hypertension, anemia, endocarditis, or myocarditis. It is remarkable, indeed, that congestive heart failure was an unusual manifestation of systemic lupus erythematosus prior to the corticosteroid era.[44]

Most important in this interaction between treatment and the cardiovascular picture of systemic lupus erythematosus is the accelerated development of coronary atherosclerosis, which was virtually unheard of in patients before the development of corticosteroid drugs. A landmark report from the National Heart, Lung and Blood Institute found that in 42% of cases treated with long-term corticosteroid medication, the lumen of at least one of the three major coronary arteries was obstructed more than 50% by atherosclerotic plaque, despite an average patient age of only 35 years.[44] The development of symptomatic myocardial ischemia and myocardial infarction in young women with corticosteroid-treated systemic lupus erythematosus is now common, and this, perhaps more than any other aspect of the disease, has altered the spectrum of cardiac involvement. Extensive atherosclerosis was extremely rare prior to the corticosteroid era, even though lipid disturbances associated with the nephrotic syndrome occurred. Whether the corticosteroids themselves accelerate the progression of the atherosclerotic process or whether the risk-enhanced state engendered by their use, mediated by diabetes, thrombosis, hypertension, or altered lipid metabolism, is responsible remains enigmatic. The lesions themselves appear morphologically indistinguishable from more senescent forms of atherosclerosis, and management proceeds along similar lines. Whether aggressive efforts to ameliorate these risk factors when they are produced by corticosteroids in patients with systemic lupus erythematosus will have an impact on the coronary manifestations of the disease also remains unsettled.

CLINICAL FEATURES

PERICARDITIS. Evidence of pericarditis has been described in approximately 70% of autopsies of patients with systemic lupus erythematosus, and it appears that this is the most common cardiac lesion associated with the disease.[48,49] Clinical studies lend support to this contention, although the disorder is not always identified ante mortem. Chest pain, usually of pleuritic character, is described by almost 50% of patients, and it has been reported as the chief presenting complaint in over 15%.[43] Inflammation of the pericardium may be either focal or diffuse and fibrous or fibrinous; effusions may be serous or sanguinous, but the protein content is generally high and complement activity is low.[50,51] LE cells have occasionally been described in the pericardial fluid. Histologically, the pericardium shows various stages of connective tissue necrosis in the acute stage and fibrosis with adhesions in the chronic phase. These manifestations seem substantially affected by corticosteroid therapy.[44] Acute pericarditis may be associated with voluminous pericardial effusions, occasionally leading to cardiac tamponade. Constrictive pericarditis, however, occurs rarely, and a remitting, episodic course is the rule.[52] Drug-induced lupus erythematosus is frequently accompanied by pericarditis, particularly when the antiarrhythmic agent procainamide or the vasodilator hydralazine is responsible.[53,54]

Once clinically suspected on the basis of symptoms of pleuritic or positional chest or shoulder pain, dyspnea, and other manifestations of active disease in a patient with systemic lupus erythematosus, the diagnosis of pericarditis can be supported by physical findings of tachycardia and pericardial friction rub in most, but not all, cases. ECG abnormalities generally involve sinus tachycardia, atrial arrhythmias, depression of the PR segment, and varied anomalies of the TU repolarization complex. Echocardiography has proven the most sensitive diagnostic method, but signs of pericardial effusion or pericardial thickening appear in a large number of cases without symptomatic cardiac involvement.[55] When pericardial effusion is large enough, the development of cardiac tamponade may proceed gradually or develop as an abrupt event, at times as a consequence of intrapericardial hemorrhage. Because corticosteroid therapy of systemic lupus erythematosus has become standard practice, the incidence of superimposed infectious pericardial disease appears to have increased,[44] and tuberculous pericarditis in such patients may pose vexing problems of evaluation and management.

The treatment of pericarditis in patients with systemic lupus erythematosus has not been evaluated rigorously. Most clinicians believe that symptomatic acute pericarditis warrants aggressive treatment with anti-inflammatory medication; concern about associated antithrombotic effects of some available drugs and the danger of hemopericardium remains a worrisome but largely theoretic consideration. Corticosteroid therapy seems beneficial, and large doses are indicated in patients with hemodynamic compromise from pericardial effusion or when concomitant myocarditis exists. Caution has been advocated when pericardiocentesis is performed in patients with lupus pericarditis because of apparently greater hazards of hemorrhagic complications,[56] and it may be prudent in such cases to leave a drainage catheter in place for several hours following the procedure. Repeated pericardiocentesis may thereby be obviated. Surgical pericardiectomy is seldom required since very few cases of chronic constriction due to systemic lupus erythematosus have been reported.

MYOCARDITIS. In the pre-corticosteroid era, infiltration of myocardial tissue by lymphocytes and plasma cells was detected at autopsy in between 20% and 75% of patients with systemic lupus erythematosus.[48,57] With earlier identification of systemic lupus and the advent of corticosteroid medication, this figure has fallen to less than 10%.[44] Foci of myocardial necrosis are more common, but the basis for these may be either inflammatory or ischemic, perhaps related to accelerated atherosclerosis. Microvascular arteriopathy of myocardial vessels takes the form of segmental arteritis and periarteritis of vessels 0.1 mm to 1.0 mm in diameter and luminal occlusion may accompany these changes with fibrosis of subserved tissue. Cardiac enlargement may be encountered along with disproportionate tachycardia or gallop rhythm; these changes may occur in as many as 12% to 25% of all patients with lupus erythematosus at some point in the course, but the clinical diagnosis of lupus myocarditis occurs in substantially fewer than 10%.[58]

ECG manifestations include abnormalities of repolarization and disturbances of impulse generation and propagation. The inflammatory process may involve the conducting system of the heart, leading in milder cases to prolongation of the PR interval and in more advanced cases to complete heart block.[43,44] Echocardiographic studies have detected a reduction in left ventricular systolic function in some series,[59] but it is difficult to exclude ischemic factors related to coronary atherosclerotic disease. It must also be emphasized that the deleterious effects of hypertension, fluid retention, and uremia make clinical congestive heart failure more common than true lupus myocarditis.

Despite a number of adverse aspects, corticosteroid therapy in high doses is indicated in patients with myocarditis complicating systemic lupus erythematosus. Corticosteroid medication was accompanied by improvement in congestive heart failure in nearly 90% of cases in a report issued over 30 years ago.[60] Addition of digitalis, diuretics, and vasodilator medication may also be warranted, and temporary inotropic support with catecholamine compounds may be beneficial in acute management.

ENDOCARDITIS. The characteristic Libman-Sacks form of endocarditis was described even before the diagnostic criteria for systemic lupus erythematosus were defined, and the earliest observations of vegetative endocardial lesions in patients with this disease appeared in the literature at the turn of the century.[61] The verrucous valvular lesions themselves may vary widely in size from little more than 1 mm to clusters of over 5 mm in diameter (Fig. 110.2). The lesions contain granular basophilic material designated "hematoxylin bodies" within the cytoplasm and may be located anywhere on the endocardial surface of the heart, but there is a predilection for the angles between the cusps and annuli of the atrioventricular valves, the fornix of the posterior mitral leaflet, and the chordal attachments. Mitral valve involvement is much more frequent than aortic valve involvement and, with the advent of corticosteroid therapy, valves in the right side of the heart are less frequently involved than those in the left side of the heart.[44] Although the lesions themselves are found rather frequently, it is uncommon for valve function to be adversely affected. Systolic and diastolic murmurs over the mitral area may vary in loudness with the course and activity of the systemic disease, but anemia, tachycardia, fever, and pleuropericardial friction rubs are confounding factors in interpretation. Hemodynamically significant valvular regurgitation is uncommon, but occasional cases have required valve replacement surgery.[62,63]

In the corticosteroid era, histologic evidence of endocarditis occurs in approximately 50% of cases, usually when pericarditis is also present.[44] In the majority of cases the ventricular aspect of the posterior mitral leaflet is affected and the vegetation may extend onto adjacent mural endocardium, causing adherence of the papillochordal apparatus. Even so, clinically significant mitral incompetence is uncommon, and, when present, it is difficult to exclude hypertension and ischemia related to coronary atherosclerosis as contributing factors. Left atrial enlargement is identified echocardiographically more often in patients with systemic lupus erythematosus than in matched control patients,[55] and it is conceivable that newer methods of echo-

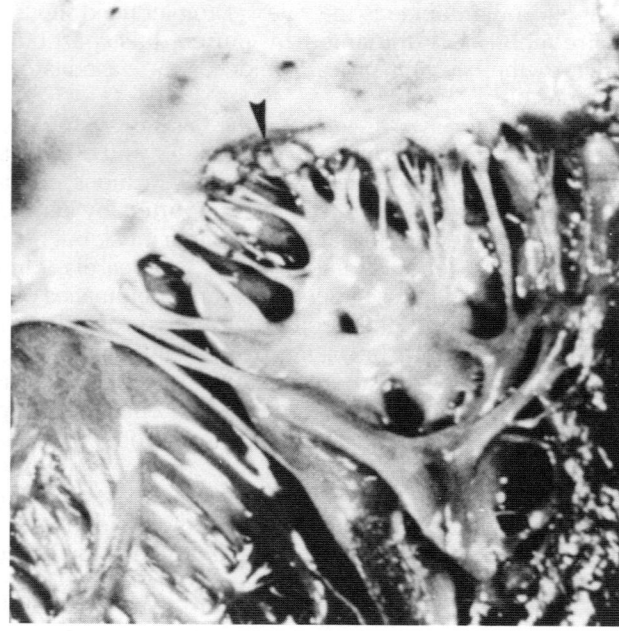

FIGURE 110.2 Verrucous endocarditis of Libman and Sacks involving the chordal attachments of an atrioventricular valve in a patient with systemic lupus erythematosus. The vegetations are usually 1 to 4 mm in diameter, may occur in clusters, and involve mural endocardium as well as valvular tissue. (McAllister HA: Collagen vascular diseases and the cardiovascular system. In Silver MD (ed): Cardiovascular Pathology. New York, Churchill Livingstone, 1983)

Doppler evaluation may detect milder degrees of mitral regurgitation in patients with verrucous lupus endocarditis.

ELECTROPHYSIOLOGIC DISTURBANCES. ECG abnormalities develop at some time during the clinical course of most patients with systemic lupus erythematosus if one includes nonspecific T wave changes, which is the most common disturbance.[43,45] Histologic findings in patients with conducting system disease in the presence of systemic lupus erythematosus more commonly reflect coronary atherosclerosis or vasculitis involving the sinoatrial or atrioventricular nodal arteries than active myocarditis, but progressive fibrosis of the conducting system is fairly common in chronic cases.[44] Atrial and ventricular tachyarrhythmias have been described, particularly in association with myopericarditis. Recently, conduction disturbances have attracted greater attention because of reports of several cases of complete heart block and a lupus-like syndrome in infants born to mothers with active systemic lupus erythematosus.[64,65] Indeed, at partum, fetal bradycardia in a patient with systemic lupus erythematosus should raise the possibility of this condition in addition to other causes of fetal distress.

CORONARY ARTERY DISEASE. Chest pain in patients with systemic lupus erythematosus more commonly results from pericarditis than myocardial ischemia. Although acute myocardial infarction was a rare complication in the pre-corticosteroid era it now represents a major cause of premature mortality in the lupus population for reasons addressed earlier in this section. It has been clearly demonstrated that, on the whole, young adult patients with systemic lupus erythematosus have more severe coronary atherosclerotic lesions than age- and sex-matched control patients, but not all victims of the disease show this predisposition to coronary atherosclerosis during corticosteroid treatment. This difference seems mainly related to serum cholesterol concentration and arterial blood pressure, but other factors, such as nephrotic syndrome, are clearly important as well. Lupus patients with more severe forms of coronary obstructive lesions are also those with greater histologic evidence of chronic pericardial and endocardial inflammation, suggesting that the inflammatory process may play a role in the progression of this form of coronary atherosclerosis.[66] In practice, accelerated coronary atherosclerosis must be distinguished from epicardial and intramyocardial forms of coronary arteritis. In over 50% of cases studied at autopsy, the lumens of some intramural coronary arteries appear narrowed by cellular intimal fibrous tissue and perivascular fibrosis is present in some cases.[44] In general, the vascular involvement is focal, not associated with inflammatory cells, and rarely accompanied by necrosis of subserved myocardium.

Clinical myocardial infarction occurs almost exclusively in patients with coronary atherosclerosis and still represents a rare complication of coronary arteritis. Corticosteroid therapy, therefore, is generally withheld in patients with systemic lupus erythematosus who develop acute myocardial infarction unless there is evidence of active disease elsewhere. Management proceeds along the conventional lines for coronary atherosclerotic disease, involving nitrate, β-adrenergic antagonist, and calcium antagonist medications in conjunction with progressive supervised exercise and risk-factor modification. When symptoms prove refractory, coronary angiography and myocardial revascularization may be performed successfully. Specific guidelines for the use of these invasive procedures in patients with coronary complications of systemic lupus erythematosus, however, have not yet been established. Several cases have been reported in which percutaneous transluminal coronary angioplasty has been performed, but the use of this modality in such patients has had limited application.

CORONARY ARTERITIS

Necrotizing vasculitis is a common feature of many immune complex diseases of connective tissue. The clinical manifestations of these diffuse vasculitides may be produced by infectious agents such as the hepatitis B virus or bacterial endocarditis, in which persistent antigenemia results in specific autoimmune phenomena and immune complex formation. In most vasculitides, however, the etiology is unknown and classification is based on clinical and histologic features, depending mainly on the size and location of involved vessels, the activity of inflammation, and the morphologic characteristics of the vascular lesions themselves (Fig. 110.3). It is impractical in this context to present a comprehensive classification of vasculitis, but those most frequently producing cardiac involvement include periarteritis nodosa, the mucocutaneous lymph node syndrome of Kawasaki, the allergic granulomatosis of Churg and Strauss, hypersensitivity vasculitis, Wegener's granulomatosis, temporal or giant cell arteritis, Takayasu's aortopathy, and the arteritis accompanying acute rheumatic fever. Overlapping syndromes may be produced in drug-induced vasculitis and mixed connective tissue disease. Coronary arteritis has also been rarely associated with such diverse disorders as cryoglobulinemia, thromboangiitis obliterans, and hereditary angioedema, which can be conceived collectively only as they seem to involve an interplay of the immune properties of circulating blood with the molecular ultrastructure of collagen.[67-69]

The host of clinical manifestations is so varied as to defy categorization, but attention will be devoted first to the periarteritis syndromes, followed by arteritis of medium-sized vessels and hyperimmune microarteriopathy. It should be emphasized, however, that the discussion focuses on coronary vasculitis, which should be suspected in a patient with known systemic vasculitis who develops palpitations, syncope, angina pectoris, or congestive heart failure. Indeed, coronary arteritis must be a leading consideration whenever a young person without risk factors for premature coronary atherosclerosis develops myocardial ischemia or infarction. Sometimes, these are the earliest manifestations of a lethal collagen disease.

PERIARTERITIS NODOSA

Periarteritis nodosa may present a highly variable clinical picture related to involvement of the muscular arteries and adjacent veins, occasionally arterioles and venules, but not capillary vessels. Necrotizing inflammation is segmental with a predilection for branch points, and small aneurysms may develop, complicated by thrombosis or rupture. Acute inflammatory changes predominantly consist of polymorphonuclear leukocytic infiltration, while mononuclear cells dominate the chronic lesions. Coronary involvement is fairly frequent, and myocardial infarction is an important cause of death in these cases. When patients with periarteritis nodosa survive ischemic insult, myocardial fibrosis and left ventricular dysfunction might ensue, aggravated by hypertension, which commonly occurs as a consequence of renal disease. Pericarditis is less important in periarteritis nodosa than in rheumatic arthritis or systemic lupus erythematosus, and endocardial lesions are quite uncommon.

The disease itself has sundry manifestations, occurring over a wide range of ages and characterized by multisystemic malfunction and a highly variable course ranging from fulminant illness to a remitting syndrome lasting months or years. Cardiac involvement most commonly takes the form of congestive heart failure and hypertension, to which renal disease is contributory. Coronary arteritis develops frequently, but angina pectoris is rare in proportion to the frequency of myocardial infarction. Because nervous tissue is rather frequently involved in periarteritis nodosa, it has been suggested that a disproportionate number of myocardial ischemic events in patients with polyarteritis nodosa are clinically silent. The coronary vessels are second only to renal vessel involvement in periarteritis nodosa, and aneurysm formation, thrombosis, and active arteritis may coexist. Coronary arteritis has been described in 60% of patients with periarteritis nodosa studied at necropsy and in nearly all cases the large epicardial vessels were affected.[70] Intramural coronary arteries and arterioles were inflamed in about 40% of the cases. Myocardial infarction may be evident in as many as two thirds of cases, most of which show histologic evidence of coronary arteritis, but the correspondence is not uniform.[71]

Cardiovascular mortality is also related to aneurysmal rupture and hemorrhage into the gastrointestinal tract or pericardium; cardiac arrhythmias and advanced pericardial disease occasionally produce fatality. Acute pericarditis is generally fibrinous, and uremia may be an important contributing factor. Hemopericardium sometimes represents a cause of acute cardiac tamponade in patients with periarteritis nodosa. Even without large pericardial effusion, however, the development of acute pericarditis in patients with this connective tissue disorder has been viewed as an ominous sign and usually occurs in the preterminal phases of the inflammatory disease. Left ventricular hypertrophy occurs mainly in association with systemic hypertension, but myocarditis has been described, seemingly of minimal clinical importance. Although conducting system involvement has been reported, clinically significant bradyarrhythmias are uncommon in periarteritis nodosa. Atrial tachyarrhythmias, however, are encountered fairly frequently.[68,72-74]

In general, the management of cardiac complications in patients with periarteritis nodosa is directed toward symptomatic relief and aggressive therapy of the underlying disease with corticosteroid or cytoxic medications. Because of the generally poor prognosis, however, there has been little experience with invasive therapeutic approaches involving catheterization or surgical techniques.

KAWASAKI DISEASE

The mucocutaneous lymph node syndrome first described in Japanese children resembles the juvenile form of periarteritis nodosa. Although still predominantly encountered in Japan, Kawasaki disease has become increasingly recognized in other parts of the world. This acute febrile illness with mucocutaneous lesions and cervical lymphadenopathy may occasionally involve severe arteritis of the large epicardial coronary arteries, as well as other organs, resulting in rapid clinical deterioration or death from myocardial infarction or cardiac arrhythmias. Males are affected somewhat more frequently than females and seem more prone in particular to coronary complications. Clinical and histopathologic changes typically relate to the duration of illness and may take the form of myocarditis or a spectrum of coronary arterial lesions ranging from aneurysmal dilatation to luminal obstruction. Myocarditis predominates in the early stages of the disease, with clinical, ECG, radiographic, or echocardiographic manifestations becoming apparent in approximately 50% of cases. Myocarditis is accompanied by pericarditis in less than 10% of cases, and endocarditis is even more unusual.[75] Panarteritis of the coronary arteries and inflammation of their vasa vasorum is thought responsible for aneurysm formation, which may also occur in limb arteries, occasionally leaving chronic aneurysmal dilatation after the acute illness recedes. Hepatitis B–associated antigens are found in the sera of a substantial number of patients and this antigen has been identified in the vascular lesions themselves along with immunoglobulin and complement.[76,77] In most cases, signs of myocardial inflammation resolve after about 3 weeks, just about the time coronary aneurysms develop. It should be emphasized, however, that the occurrence of coronary aneurysm does not correlate with the presence of signs of myocarditis and that myocarditis occurs with nearly equal frequency in patients developing aneurysms as in patients without aneurysm formation.

Shortly after Weyman and associates first reported noninvasive visualization of the left main coronary artery by two-dimensional echocardiography, Matsu and co-workers described echocardiographic features of coronary artery aneurysms in patients with Kawasaki disease.[78,79] Subsequently, many additional papers have appeared describing two-dimensional echocardiographic demonstration of coronary arterial aneurysms in patients with this disease.[80-82] The sensitivity of noninvasive diagnosis in the hands of experienced examiners may approach 100%, while specificities in one study were 64% and 46% for aneurysms in the left and right coronary arteries, respectively.[81]

Cineangiographic studies have revealed coronary aneurysm formation in approximately 20% of patients with Kawasaki disease.[82,83] Aneu-

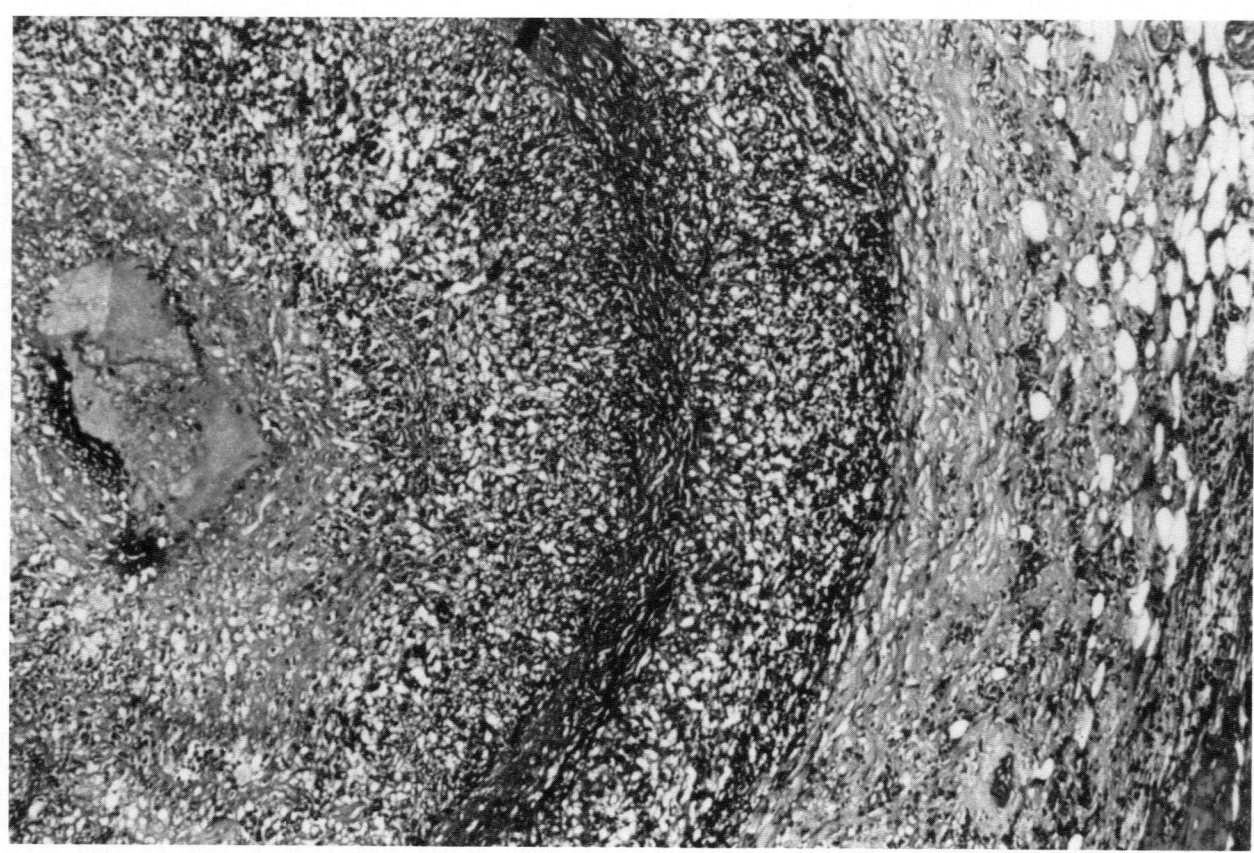

FIGURE 110.3 Section of a coronary artery from a patient with systemic vasculitis complicating rheumatoid arthritis. There is dense inflammatory cell infiltration, fragmentation of the internal elastic lamina, and intraluminal thrombosis. (Courtesy of Dr. Bruce I. Goldman)

rysms of the coronary arteries are most commonly sacculofusiform rather than purely saccular, tubular, or fusiform. The majority of these cases develop cardiovascular symptoms, including myocardial infarction in one third. Typical symptoms of myocardial infarction may not occur, and the major symptom appears to be congestive heart failure without clear history of acute infarction. A pattern of myocardial infarction on the ECG generally develops, if at all, within the first year and sudden death is most frequently encountered within 2 months of the onset of Kawasaki disease. In about a third of patients with coronary aneurysms, these lesions regress as the clinical manifestations of disease resolve, but 8% or 10% of affected vessels may develop stenotic obstructions.[83] Although the mechanism of progressive coronary obstruction remains unclear, intimal thickening and superimposed thrombus formation within the aneurysmal sac may be contributory.

Angiography characteristically displays multiple small aneurysms at the branch points of the coronary vessels. Half the patients with coronary involvement display mitral regurgitation, and left ventricular function is generally more severely impaired in these cases.[84] Severe involvement of multiple coronary vessels, extensive infarction pattern, low electrocardiographic QRS voltage, conduction disturbances, and severe congestive heart failure are markers of particularly poor prognosis. Myocardial ischemia and mitral valve annular dilatation seem pathogenetically related to the development of mitral regurgitation, and Kawasaki disease has now been clearly established as a form of acquired valvular disease in young children. As in the adult atherosclerotic population, the prognosis of left main coronary artery obstruction is generally poor and this abnormality is associated with reduced left ventricular ejection fraction, enlarged left ventricular end-diastolic volume, and clinical features of dilated cardiomyopathy. Left coronary involvement is more likely to be symptomatic, and this group is prone to the development of left ventricular functional abnormalities, myocardial infarction, and mitral regurgitation.

The management of patients with Kawasaki disease in the early stage is highly subjective, and studies comparing different treatment approaches must generally be faulted for a lack of randomized, controlled design. Corticosteroid therapy is not generally favored and should, perhaps, be avoided. On the other hand, aspirin is said to be helpful in preventing aneurysm development.[85] Antianginal medication in the form of organic nitrates is a mainstay for the control of active myocardial ischemia. Calcium channel antagonists are now used with increasing frequency, but caution has been advocated with the use of both these and β-adrenergic antagonist agents, particularly in the presence of congestive heart failure.

Coronary artery bypass graft surgery is sometimes employed in children with coronary pathology related to Kawasaki disease; yet the rate of saphenous vein graft occlusion is fairly high, approaching 30% in small series.[85,86] It has not been concluded, therefore, whether coronary surgery is effective as a mode of therapy for this disease, but congestive heart failure has been reported to improve dramatically after mitral valve replacement in occasional patients. Antithrombotic medication in the form of aspirin, dipyridamole, warfarin, or a combination of these agents has been advocated, but the usefulness of this form of therapy in modifying the long-term prognosis after surgery remains undetermined. Increasing experience is accumulating in Japan with the use of percutaneous transluminal coronary recanalization using urokinase in Kawasaki disease, but this has not yet been sufficiently extensive to justify conclusions regarding the effectiveness of the technique.

ALLERGIC ANGIITIS AND GRANULOMATOSIS
The necrotizing vasculitis described by Churg and Strauss in 1951[87] may involve vessels of the heart in a fashion quite similar to that of periarteritis nodosa except for a greater tendency to granuloma formation, eosinophilia, and pulmonary vasculitis. Lung involvement is usually predominant, however, often with atopy and severe bronchospastic episodes. Clinically, syndromes of necrotizing polyangiitis frequently overlap, incorporating features of hypersensitivity vasculitis, and Wegener's granulomatosis. Cardiomyopathy has been described in association with this condition, however, and diagnosis is often delayed because coexisting pulmonary pathology masks congestive dyspnea. Endomyocardial biopsy may produce nonspecific results, compatible with idiopathic dilated myopathy although occasional intramyocardial vessels display immunoglobulin deposits. The response to corticosteroid therapy is variable, and, indeed, this form of therapy has been anecdotally associated with the development of myocardial failure. In corticosteroid-treated patients with dilated cardiomyopathy, mural thromboembolic events may herald the end stage of disease.[88–92]

WEGENER'S GRANULOMATOSIS
Target organs of the necrotizing granulomatous vasculitis described by Wegener are the kidney and respiratory systems. Occasional cases of cardiovascular involvement have been reported, which serve to emphasize the potential for disseminated disease. The most common histologic cardiac abnormalities are pericarditis and coronary arteritis, which seem to occur with equal frequency. In one reported case, vasculitis of the left anterior descending coronary artery was associated with sudden death due to cardiac rhythm disturbance. Cardiac tachyarrhythmias, however, are usually of supraventricular origin and more benign. Complete heart block has also been described. In most cases, the clinical picture is dominated by the involvement of respiratory and renal tissue, particularly as these represent the sine qua non for diagnosis. Dramatic remission has been reported after treatment with cyclophosphamide, indicating the importance of accurate and early diagnosis of this condition.[91,93–97]

GIANT CELL ARTERITIS
Also designated cranial or temporal arteritis, this vasculopathy commonly affects older individuals, producing granulomatous lesions consisting of multinucleated giant cells with patchy, segmental involvement accompanied by thrombosis of the aorta and proximal arteries. Aneurysm formation and dissection can occur and involvement of the carotid, vertebral, axillosubclavian, and ophthalmic arteries is most frequent. Thrombotic occlusions of the coronary, iliac, and mesenteric vessels also produce morbidity and mortality. Often accompanying giant cell arteritis is the polymyalgia rheumatica syndrome in which cardiac involvement may take the form of myocarditis (usually clinically inapparent) or coronary arteritis. The essential clinical point is that myocardial infarction preceded by polymyalgia rheumatica, weight loss, headache, fever, or anemia in an elderly patient must raise the diagnostic possibility of giant cell arteritis. In such cases, the erythrocyte sedimentation rate is typically persistently elevated. The response to corticosteroid medication may be dramatic, but chronic maintenance therapy is often required on an alternate-day or other periodic dosage regimen.[98–102]

TAKAYASU'S ARTERITIS
Takayasu's aortopathy, also known as the aortic arch syndrome and pulseless disease, represents a granulomatous vasculitis of the aorta and proximal arteries that may occur in several forms, usually in females. Pulmonary artery involvement is evident histologically in about half the cases. Although cardiopulmonary symptoms are fairly uncommon, cardiac manifestations take the form of aortic regurgitation and, rarely, coronary arterial involvement. Diagnosis is usually suggested by ischemic symptoms involving the cerebral vasculature or the upper extremities, and laboratory comformation usually depends on aortography. Serologic studies produce variable results and are thus unreliable aids to diagnosis. The response to corticosteroid medication, however, seems most favorable when an accelerated erythrocyte sedimentation rate reflects active inflammatory disease. Both successful surgical revascularization of occluded arterial segments and balloon angioplasty have been described.[103–107]

SCLEROSING SYNDROMES
SCLERODERMA

Progressive fibrosis of the skin is the hallmark of the sclerosing syndromes, but it has been clear for nearly 50 years that these diseases can be more than skin deep. The pathophysiology involves a poorly understood interplay of fibroblast stimulation, microvascular architecture, and the chemistry of collagen itself, leading to sclerotic skin, abnormal enteric motility, and Raynaud's phenomenon. The spectrum of disease ranges from localized to generalized forms, and the prognosis depends on the extent of visceral involvement, particularly of the lungs, kidneys, and heart. At the extremes of this span are two very different conditions: (1) a limited cutaneous form in which visceral fibrosis is mild or occurs after decades of disease, and (2) an often lethal form of aggressive systemic sclerosis with early visceral involvement. Although specific serum markers have not been identified for patients with scleroderma, SCL-70 antinuclear antibodies and anticentromere antibodies have been found in the sera of patients with related syndromes.[108]

Whether the gradual vascular obliteration that seems at the root of scleroderma involves a defect of collagen, abnormal fibroblast regulation, or a primary immunologic process is not known, but distinctive microvascular lesions have been identified, generally involving vessels 150 μm to 500 μm diameter. A mononuclear cell inflammatory infiltrate develops in the perivascular space, and it is believed that tissue factors are generated that stimulate fibroblasts and disrupt vascular endothelial function, resulting in chemotaxis, vasospasm, and intravascular thrombosis. Intense proliferation of the intimal layer of small arteries may lead to renal failure, systemic and pulmonary hypertension, and digital infarction. The functional attenuation of the microvasculature in scleroderma is associated with abnormal capillary loops evident on nail bed microscopy. The pattern of sclerotic skin changes roughly parallels the distribution of arteriovenous anastomoses (glomus bodies) in the thermoregulatory skin. The histologic appearance of pulmonary arteriolar thickening resembles changes in primary pulmonary hypertension. In the kidneys, mainly the interlobular arteries and glomerular basement membrane are affected and malignant nephrosclerosis may precede the development of systemic hypertension in patients with scleroderma.

The most frequent cardiovascular manifestation is cutaneous vasospasm, which may take the form either of episodic attacks of Raynaud's phenomenon characterized by well-demarcated pallor, cyanosis, and rubor or of persistent acrocyanosis. The mechanism by which these forms of cutaneous ischemia develop has not been established and may be different from the pathophysiology of idiopathic Raynaud's disease in patients without connective tissue abnormalities. Most patients with symmetrical symptoms of temperature sensitivity in the hands and feet with or without color changes show neither serologic abnormalities nor sclerosing features. On the other hand, a disturbance of autonomic control of the microcirculation emphasizes the importance of vasoregulatory tissue as a target organ in systemic sclerosis. Raynaud's phenomenon occurs about five times more frequently in females than males and may affect as many as 10% of the normal female population. The idiopathic form of cutaneous vasospasm is statistically associated with migraine headaches and variant angina due to coronary vasospasm. In these cases, structural abnormalities of the digital arterioles are generally not evident except in severely advanced cases. On the other hand, patients with Raynaud's phenomenon secondary to the sclerosing syndromes frequently display digital arterial occlusion due to thrombotic or immunologic processes resulting in endothelial thickening. Ischemic attacks in these patients may be the result of normal vasoconstrictor responses imposed on an already compromised circulation, but abnormal vasomotor responsiveness is also an important factor. Skin blood vessels in patients with scleroderma demonstrate hypersensitivity to serotonin,[109] an effect that might be exaggerated at lower temperatures.[110] In patients with Raynaud's phenomenon secondary to collagen vascular disease, intraluminal thrombosis may prompt the release of serotonin from platelets, contributing to ischemic symptoms, and elevated plasma β-thromboglobulin levels indicate increased platelet activation *in vivo*. *In vitro*, enhanced platelet aggregation in response to adenosine diphosphate has been described in patients with severe symptoms. Damage to vascular endothelium might exaggerate the vasoconstriction mediated by serotonin released from platelets; some of the therapeutic efficacy of reserpine in these cases could result from its action in depleting serotonin in addition to its more widely recognized sympatholytic effects. Case reports of clinical improvement in patients with vascular and renal crises of scleroderma through the use of the angiotensin-converting enzyme inhibitor captopril may actually result from potentiation of the vasodilator effects of bradykinin, the metabolism of which is also inhibited by this drug. There is no direct evidence, however, that the bradykinin–killikrein system is abnormal in patients with Raynaud's phenomenon due to scleroderma.

Arteriographic studies of patients with scleroderma have demonstrated digital arterial occlusions in over 90% of cases.[111] Some patients with Raynaud's phenomenon associated with the sclerosing syndromes have elevated levels of plasma fibrinogen that may result in abnormally high blood viscosity, particularly at lower temperatures.[112] In addition to endothelial thickening, extravascular interstitial tissue pressure may be elevated in the digits of patients with scleroderma, and external compression may tend to precipitate vessel closure and vasospastic symptoms. Subcutaneous tissue pressure measured directly in patients with skin manifestations of scleroderma averaged 25 mm Hg in one study, vastly greater than the average of 4 mm Hg in normal subjects.[113] This increased extravascular compressive force could provoke vessel closure particularly when the intraluminal pressure is diminished distal to an obstruction.

The coronary circulation seems affected mainly in terms of autoregulation. Intramyocardial blood flow is abnormal both at rest and after exercise in the majority of patients with diffuse systemic sclerosis, and it is tempting to link this phenomenon pathophysiologically with the dramatic constriction of renal, pulmonary, and cutaneous beds that follows peripheral cold exposure in patients with this disease.[114,115] That the abnormality is not fundamentally linked with sympathetic nervous system activity was shown as early as 1929 by Lewis in studies demonstrating cold-provoked vasospasm of the digits after sympathetic blockade in patients with scleroderma.[116] It is conceivable that the local vascular abnormality is one of intimal scarring and obliteration of the microvasculature related to endothelial injury, mesenchymal proliferation, and fibrosis, but the inciting cause—be it infectious, immunologic, enzymatic, or ischemic—remains a complete mystery.

Anecdotal case descriptions of sclerosing syndromes with cardiac disease have appeared since the last quarter of the 19th century, but the heart was not recognized as a common target organ in scleroderma until the report of Weiss and associates in 1943.[117] Although clinical congestive heart failure, cardiomegaly, ECG abnormalities, and sudden death were recognized thereafter and pathologic studies revealed myocardial fibrosis distinct from that seen in advanced ischemic heart disease, the nature of primary cardiac disease in scleroderma has remained enigmatic. In general, cardiac manifestations may be produced by concomitant renal and pulmonary pathology, but the specific feature of myocardial fibrosis has been described in approximately 50% of postmortem examinations.[118,119] The cardiomyopathy that occurs in patients with scleroderma seems a consequence of both microvascular insufficiency and fibrosis, leading most often to clinical features of congestive heart failure and conducting system abnormalities.

Myocardial fibrosis has been identified in 12% to 81% of autopsies with systemic sclerosis.[120,121] This variability is partly related to the broad spectrum of clinical illness. The myocardial lesion itself has features of contraction band necrosis and replacement fibrosis, distributed throughout ventricular walls in over half the cases, while extramural coronary arteries are generally patent. Symptomatic cardiac involvement is considerably less frequent, however, and when present it generally indicates a poor prognosis for survival. Histologic changes are the rule in patients with ventricular arrhythmias and conduction disturbances, congestive heart failure, angina pectoris, and sudden death. It has been proposed that intermittent vasospastic phenomena are responsible for this unique form of myocardial sclerosis as a result of recurrent ischemia.

Pericardial disease may take both acute and chronic forms even in the absence of uremia, but endocardial involvement seldom has clinical significance. Usually clinically silent, pericardial involvement is rather frequently identified histologically, and evidence of pericardial disease in scleroderma has been reported in 33% to 72% of autopsy cases.[118,122,123] When azotemia is excluded as a contributing factor, slightly more than half the patients with scleroderma show histologic evidence of pericarditis, as compared with approximately 12% of matched controls.[118] Pericarditis becomes clinically apparent in 5% to 15% of the patients with clinical scleroderma, but echocardiographic evidence of pericardial effusion has been reported in over 40% of an unselected series of patients with advanced disease.[124] A similar incidence has been encountered in the less devastating CREST variant (an acronym for the syndrome of calcinosis, Raynaud's phenomenon, esophageal dysfunction, sclerodactyly, and telangiectasia). It should be emphasized that fewer than one third of patients with echocardiographic features of pericardial effusion display clinical evidence of pericarditis.[123]

CLINICAL FEATURES

PERICARDITIS. Pericarditis itself may be a recurrent problem in patients with systemic sclerosis, and an effusive picture is the rule. The fluid may be either transudative or exudative, and this seems to correlate with the activity of disease in other organ systems. Like the blood serum, the fluid generally does not display the characteristic abnormality of immune complex or complement activation. Development of clinical pericardial disease is seldom directly responsible for mortality, but chronic pericarditis and congestive heart failure seem to predict the early progression of renal failure and identify a subgroup with relatively poor prognosis, particularly when pericardial effusions are large. It has been speculated that the reduction in cardiac output and associated systemic hemodynamic abnormalities that accompany chronic cardiac compression by large pericardial effusion may aggravate abnormalities of renal perfusion in these cases.

To repeat Osler's often quoted description, patients with advanced scleroderma seem "encased in an ever-shrinking, slowly contracting skin."[125] It is notable, therefore, that constrictive pericarditis is distinctly uncommon. The rare acute compressive syndromes are generally amenable to pericardiectomy. In other respects, management of pericardial disease in scleroderma consists of the administration of anti-inflammatory medications, although many of the nonsteroidal agents, such as indomethacin, may have direct adverse affects on renal hemodynamics. Intravascular volume must be carefully monitored. Administration of corticosteroid medication has not been systematically evaluated, although therapy in fairly high doses has been recommended with close observation of renal function.

MYOCARDIAL DISEASE. Although pericardial and myocardial involvement in scleroderma occur with approximately equal frequency, the prognosis when these two processes become symptomatic is distinctly different. The 7-year survival rate of patients with progressive systemic sclerosis and clinical evidence of pericarditis is 30% to 35%, while for patients with congestive heart failure, survival through this interval is unusual.[126] Since the lumens of the epicardial coronary arteries are seldom obstructed except by associated atherosclerotic disease, the myocardial pathology in systemic sclerosis is a consequence of disturbed microcirculation and fibrosis. Other than congestive heart failure, the disorder may take the form of cardiac conduction disturbances, ECG abnormalities, exertional chest pain, and sudden death. Exertional dyspnea may be a consequence of elevated left ventricular filling pressure or pulmonary involvement, and right ventricular failure may occur as a feature of cor pulmonale. Myocardial dysfunction may also occur as a result of arterial hypertension, which seems to correspond with vasospastic crises. Nevertheless, the symptoms of myocardial involvement are generally those of congestive cardiomyopathy, the onset of which may be insidious or fulminant. It should be noted that cardiac disease may become clinically manifest prior to cutaneous manifestations in one fourth to one third of cases of progressive systemic sclerosis and that myocarditis has been a suspected contributory process in some cases.[117,127]

Echocardiographic studies have shown a variety of abnormalities in patients with scleroderma other than the pericardial findings mentioned above. Left ventricular hypertrophy may occur in the absence of hypertension in a fairly large number of patients, and pulmonary hypertension clearly occurs in the absence of left heart failure. A more fundamental abnormality of myocardial diastolic relaxation is suggested by the occurrence in approximately one third of patients of abnormal closing velocity of the mitral apparatus during this phase of the cardiac cycle in the absence of mitral stenosis. Mitral valve prolapse is occasionally encountered in patients with the sclerosing syndromes, but this association seems lower than that of mitral prolapse with innocent forms of cutaneous vasospasm.[124,128,130]

It should be stressed that myocardial fibrosis is not diagnostic of scleroderma, and this may be found in other forms of myocarditis, in muscular dystrophy, in rheumatic heart disease, in mucopolysaccharidosis, and following cardiac surgery, radiation exposure, or drug toxicity, including that associated with methysergide. A more distinctive pathologic entity, contraction banded necrosis, first described in 1968, has been found in approximately one third of patients with scleroderma and seems to correlate more closely with the clinical manifestations of cardiac disease.[119] The specific myofibrillar eosinophilic degeneration that this lesion represents has been thought to result from repeated coronary reperfusion following intermittent vasospastic ischemia. The histologic lesion can be produced by temporary coronary artery occlusion in dogs, and the same lesion has been identified within a month of cardiac surgery in patients without evident systemic sclerosis.[119,129] The lesion is occasionally encountered in the periphery of myocardial infarction following atherosclerotic coronary events as well as in other forms of acute disease producing destruction of cardiac tissues, such as myocarditis and direct electrical injury.[130] The eosinophilic bands seem to represent condensation of contractile elements in myocardial cytoplasm between areas of increased granularity. Abnormal mitochondria appear along with loss of nuclear material, but there is a relative paucity of inflammatory cells. Vascular endothelial integrity is destroyed, with leakage of blood products into the interstitial space. The fundamental question—whether the formation of contractile band necrosis is related to a structural abnormality of myocardial collagen—is still unanswered.

CORONARY PERFUSION DISTURBANCES. Myocardial perfusion imaging using thallium-201 scintigraphy has proven a sensitive index of abnormal coronary vasomotor regulation in patients with systemic sclerosis, in whom cold-provoked and exercise-induced perfusion defects have been identified.[131,132] In a study of 26 patients with diffuse scleroderma, 6 had clinical evidence of cardiac involvement, while 20 had abnormal thallium perfusion images, including 10 with reversible exercise-induced defects and 18 with fixed abnormalities (8 had both).[114] Seventy percent of the patients with exercise-related defects had normal coronary arteriography, but left and right ventricular ejection fractions at rest were lower in these patients than in those with normal thallium images during exercise (Fig. 110.4). The study did not include a matched control population, however, and it is difficult to dissociate factors confounding interpretation of these findings, such as pulmonary vascular disease.

Coronary vascular abnormalities, although infrequent in the extramural vessels, are occasionally encountered in the intramural arteries. Vascular narrowing, fibrosis, fibrinoid necrosis, and concentric intimal hypertrophy have been described more frequently in patients with systemic sclerosis than in a control population, and these lesions are reminiscent of those encountered in the kidneys and other organs.[131] The intramural arterioles may also be responsible for conducting system disease, including the complete heart block described by Lev and coworkers.[133] This postulate stands in contrast, however, to the paucity of small vessel pathology in some reported series.

The principles of management for patients with scleroderma and myocardial disease have not been specifically defined, and therapy must be individualized on the basis of predominant clinical features. For patients with congestive heart failure, therapy with digitalis, diuretics, and vasodilator agents is employed. It is essential that blood pressure be controlled, and the converting enzyme inhibitor captopril has been found effective in this setting. Correction of hypertension may be associated with prompt relief of vasospastic phenomena in the cutaneous vascular beds,[134] and it is intriguing to speculate that this might ameliorate myocardial vasospastic factors as well. β-Adrenergic antagonist drugs should generally be avoided because of their potential to exacerbate peripheral, if not coronary, vasospasm, unless severe hypertension is present in the systemic arterial bed, since this is often mediated by renin and may respond remarkably well to the institution of a member of this class of drugs. It is the absence of vasoconstrictor properties and effective amelioration of angiotensin-mediated hypertension and sodium retention related to mineralocorticoid activity that have brought converting enzyme inhibition such rapid acceptance in clinical practice. Early reports that colchicine might retard the progression of fibrosis have yet to clearly verify a role for this agent in patients with myocardial involvement.

COR PULMONALE. Renal failure and obliterative pulmonary vascular disease leading to hemodynamic collapse may occasionally be the clinical presentation of untended scleroderma, and at this stage the disease is usually refractory to treatment. That pulmonary vasotoxicity is a pertinent factor is suggested by the observation that amelioration of pulmonary hypertension is most likely to develop during treatment with the calcium channel antagonist nifedipine in patients who also suffer from Raynaud's phenomenon. Whether this vasodilator response is related directly to excitation–contraction coupling in vascular smooth muscle[135] or to an intermediating effect on platelet aggregation[136] remains speculative. Right ventricular enlargement is the most frequent feature of pulmonary heart disease.

When conduction disturbances develop, cardiac pacing may be appropriate, and it is fortunate that endocardial fibrosis is not a dominant feature of the disease. Nevertheless, endocardial pacing thresholds may be expected to deteriorate over time, and pacing systems capable of dealing with this should generally be selected. Ventricular arrhythmias may be particularly menacing in patients with myocardial sclerosis, particularly since antiarrhythmic medication is often poorly tolerated by patients with scleroderma. Guidelines for treatment of ventricular ectopic activity in this setting, therefore, are generally an extension of the approach employed in patients with atherosclerotic ischemic heart disease.

In essence, the relationship between histopathologic evidence of structural microvascular disease and functional disturbances of microvascular control (manifested as vasospasm) remains at the core of the uncertainty surrounding the involvement of the heart in scleroderma and related sclerosing syndromes. Do recurrent episodes of ischemia produce progressive myocardial fibrotic changes? Is structural abnormality of the intramural coronary vessels, like that encountered in the pulmonary and renal circuits, similarly preceded by a period of inflammation? Cytotoxic activity has been identified in the serum of some patients with systemic sclerosis, and there is speculation that endothelial damage caused by these substances produces increased vascular permeability. Exudation of plasma proteins into the interstitial space

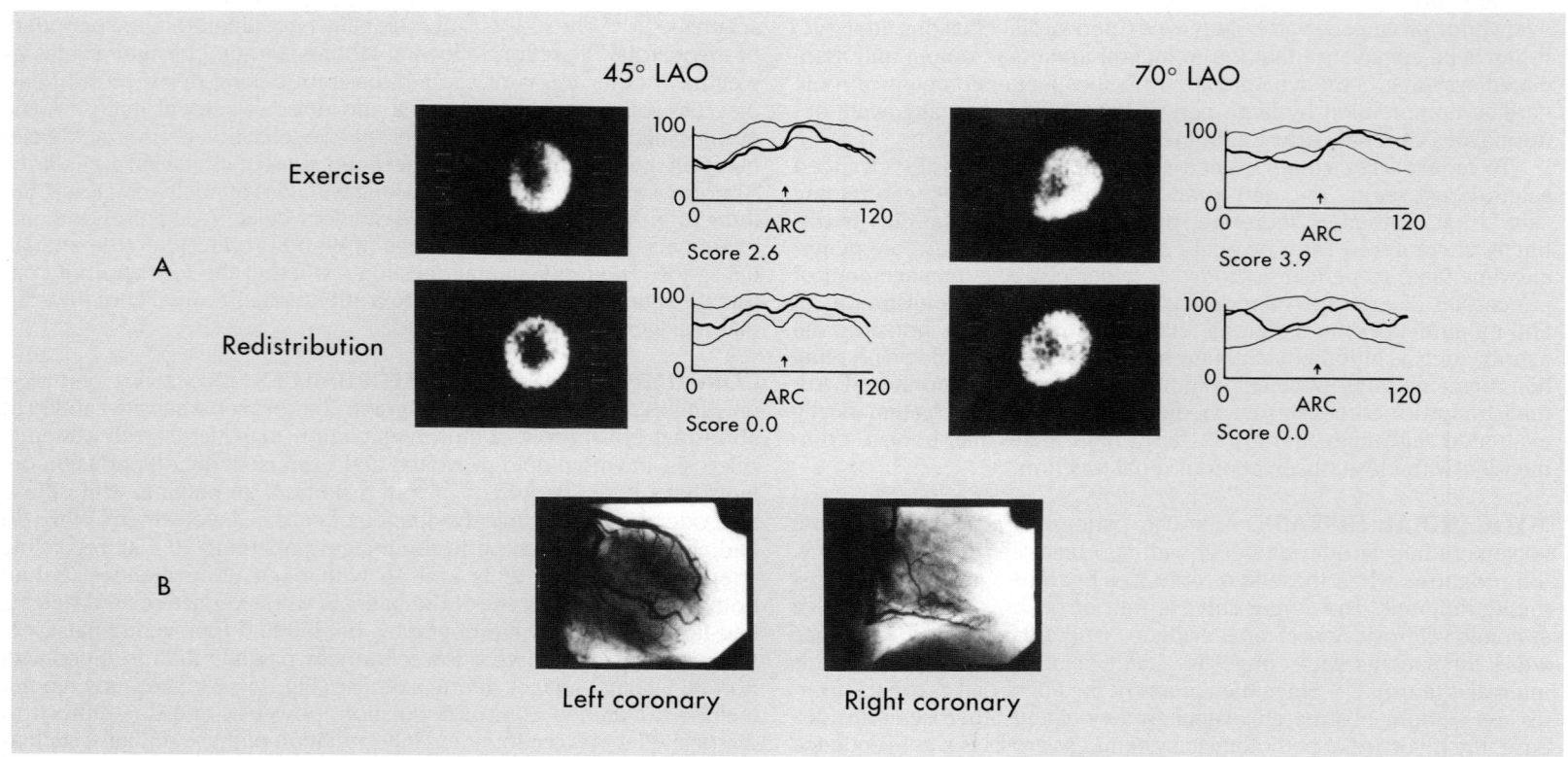

FIGURE 110.4 Thallium scans with circumferential-profile curves (**A**) and coronary angiograms (**B**) in a patient with an exercise-induced defect. Scans are shown in the 45° and 70° left anterior oblique (LAO) projections. The exercise (EXER) images show a perfusion abnormality of the septum and anteroseptal wall, confirmed by the circumferential-profile curves. The redistribution (REDIST) scans show nearly complete normalization of these defects. The angiograms (subsequently obtained) are normal. (Follansbee WP, Curtiss EI et al: Physiologic abnormalities of cardiac function in progressive systemic sclerosis with diffuse scleroderma. N Engl J Med 310:142–148, 1984. Reprinted by permission)

might result in stimulation of fibroblast collagen synthesis. Whether this is the mechanism of "scleroderma heart" has yet to be determined.

THE POLYMYOSITIS–DERMATOMYOSITIS COMPLEX

Polymyositis and related inflammatory disorders of skeletal muscle are recognized with increasing frequency. Rather than diseases of specific etiology, these autoimmune disorders are better regarded as syndromes that may occur in isolation or in association with other collagen vascular diseases, systemic infections, or malignancy. Clinical and laboratory features overlap with those of several of the rheumatic diseases so as to blur the distinction from periarteritis nodosa, systemic lupus erythematosus, or scleroderma to name a few. A particularly striking feature, however, is usually myopathy, and the frequency of histologic inflammation in patients with skeletal muscle weakness is astounding. The pathologic picture includes infiltration of mononuclear inflammatory cells and destruction of muscle fibers. This myolytic process is in unstable equilibrium with a regenerative one involving the synthesis of myofibrils from a proliferative sarcolemma. In addition to muscular changes, the endothelia of microcirculatory vessels, including capillaries, become involved in proliferative fibrosis. The resulting intimal thickening is similar to that in scleroderma and systemic lupus erythematosus and may be a factor in vasospastic or thrombotic vascular occlusion.[137]

Polymyositis was first described by Wagner in 1886,[138] and cardiac involvement was reported by Oppenheim in 1899.[139] Despite its obvious muscular persuasion, the heart was classically regarded as infrequently involved in polymyositis. There is an increasing body of evidence, however, that the heart is commonly affected by diseases in the polymyositis–dermatomyositis complex. Noninvasive cardiac diagnostic studies of 21 patients with polymyositis in Washington found ECG conduction abnormalities in 50%. Phonocardiographic ejection clicks and systolic murmurs were present in 33% and echocardiographic mitral valve prolapse in 50%.[140] Cardiac lesions have been identified most frequently in the conducting system of the myocardium, but pericarditis occurs as well. Valvular and coronary structures are generally spared, although certain overlap syndromes are characterized by endocarditis or arteritis. Degeneration of collagen and replacement by inflammatory fibrosis is particularly prominent in the area of the sinoatrial node but also occurs in the remainder of the specialized conducting tissue. Other parts of atrial and ventricular myocardium may become inflamed, fibrotic, or frankly necrotic with evolution of creatine phosphokinase into serum, producing the clinical findings of subacute myocarditis or cardiomyopathy. ECG and echocardiographic abnormalities are more frequent than reported symptomatic disturbances, but deaths related to cardiac arrhythmias or congestive heart failure are conspicuous both in the literature and in practice.[141] Prognosis generally depends on associated diseases, and death is most often related to metastatic malignancy, pneumonitis, or sepsis.

CLINICAL FEATURES

Females predominate in a ratio of 2:1 as victims of the polymyositis–dermatomyositis syndromes and average about 50 years of age. Cardiovascular symptoms have been reported in 10% to 15% of cases and include palpitations, chest pain, congestive dyspnea, and edema.[142] The clinical importance of myocarditis is emphasized in a report of 16 autopsies at the Johns Hopkins Hospital, where the incidence of myocarditis was 25%, and congestive heart failure had been clinically apparent in each of these four cases.[143] Vasculopathy is particularly prominent in childhood forms of the disease. At any age, however, immune complex deposition within the intramuscular vessels, loss of capillaries, and endothelial thickening may contribute to myocardial ischemia and necrosis. The myocardial isoenzyme of creatine phosphokinase (CPK-MB) activity is substantially elevated in the majority of patients with active polymyositis, and this seems roughly to coincide with the severity of myocardial dysfunction.[137] Atrioventricular and fascicular conduction blocks have been reported repeatedly in polymyositis, and there appears to be some correlation between the severity of skeletal muscular and myocardial involvement.[142,143] Pericarditis, although relatively rare, may take the form of an intermittent acute illness or subside incompletely leaving persistent symptoms and signs of serosal irritation. Although pulmonary fibrosis can occur and pneumonitis is common, these generally relate to the severity of muscular weakness and typical cor pulmonale is distinctly rare.

Both corticosteroid and immunosuppressive drugs have been touted as effective in the management of patients with syndromes in the polymyositis–dermatomyositis complex, but controlled trials are virtually nonexistent. Nonsteroidal anti-inflammatory medication is generally relegated to controlling symptoms of pericarditis, while prednisone is regarded as the drug of choice in active systemic polymyositis.[144]

MIXED CONNECTIVE TISSUE DISEASE

Given the tendency of disorders in the polymyositis–dermatomyositis complex to display clinical features overlapping with other connective tissue diseases, particularly systemic lupus erythematosus and progressive systemic sclerosis, mixed connective tissue disease was not recognized as a discrete clinical entity until 1972.[145] Indeed, mixed connective tissue disease is principally characterized by the overlapping clinical manifestations of systemic lupus erythematosus, progressive systemic sclerosis, and polymyositis, and patients frequently develop clinical features of each of these three connective tissue diseases. Unique to the mixed syndrome, however, is the association with high titers of circulating antibodies to nuclear ribonucleoprotein. In addition, fluorescent antinuclear antibody is almost always present in a speckled pattern. Beyond these distinctive serologic features, mixed connective tissue disease is also notable for the frequency and spectrum of cardiovascular involvement. This has been the subject of two reviews involving a total of 55 patients with clinical and laboratory features of the disease who underwent cardiovascular evaluation by noninvasive or invasive means.[146,147] Nearly 90% of the patients were female, ranging in age from 1 to 64 years, and averaging 33 years. Arthritis or arthralgias, myositis, abnormal esophageal motility, lymphadenopathy, and hypergammaglobulinemia were frequent clinical features. Cardiovascular manifestations included Raynaud's phenomenon, pulmonary hypertension, pericarditis, mitral valve prolapse, intimal hyperplasia of coronary arteries, and myocarditis. At the symptomatic level, dyspnea was described in 55% of cases, but in the majority this was attributed to restrictive pulmonary pathology. Thirty-nine percent of patients reported chest pain, related either to mitral valve prolapse, pericarditis, angina pectoris, or musculoskeletal factors. Nineteen percent complained of palpitations, and 9% experienced syncope or presyncope. Edema was described by 24% of the patients in one series but in none of those in another.

In the largest published series, two thirds of patients with mixed connective tissue disease had abnormalities on cardiovascular physical examination.[148] Nearly half had cardiac murmurs, usually of ejection character, and a fourth of the population had fourth heart sounds, as opposed to only 5% with ventricular diastolic (S_3) gallops. Twenty-one percent had abnormally loud pulmonary valve closure sounds compatible with pulmonary hypertension, 16% had the midsystolic click of mitral valve prolapse, 8% had pericardial friction rub, 10% had jugular venous distention, 13% had systemic hypertension, and there was objective evidence of edema in 8%.

The ECG was abnormal in two thirds of the cases. The most common findings were right ventricular hypertrophy, right atrial abnormalities, intraventricular conduction disturbances, and repolarization abnormalities, including those of acute myopericarditis. Left ventricular hypertrophy and left atrial abnormalities were infrequent findings, almost exclusively associated with systemic hypertension. Chest roentgenograms displayed abnormalities referrable to the cardiovascular system in slightly more than one fourth of patients with mixed connective tissue disease, usually in the form of cardiomegaly related to right ventricular enlargement or of pericardial effusion. Roentgenographic features of chronic pulmonary hypertension were rarely observed. Echocardiographic studies revealed pericardial abnormalities in about a third of cases, usually effusion. Right ventricular enlargement was slightly less frequent, and left ventricular dilatation was distinctly unusual. Hypertrophy generally correlated with hypertension. Mitral valve prolapse was present in about 25% of the cases (more than twice as often as in a matched control population), but the reason for this association is quite unclear. This frequent disorder may contribute to chest pain, extrasystoles, and cardiodynamic symptoms that may overlap with other aspects of the disease.

Radionuclide ventriculography usually does not demonstrate systolic wall motion abnormalities, and left ventricular ejection fraction is generally maintained within the normal range.[147] Hemodynamic measurements have been systematically made in relatively few patients. One series of 17 cases was notable for mean pulmonary artery pressure averaging 10 mm Hg to 15 mm Hg above normal as a consequence of modestly elevated pulmonary arteriolar resistance, but right-sided heart pressures in diastole remained in the normal range except in severe cases.[148] Pulmonary hypertension is related to intimal proliferation of small pulmonary arteries and arterioles and involves fibrinous microthrombi probably arising *in situ* rather than as a consequence of embolization from sources in the right side of the heart or peripheral veins. Parenchymal pulmonary fibrosis and lymphocytic infiltration are of lesser importance in raising the pulmonary vascular resistance. Pulmonary capillary wedge pressure is usually maintained in the normal range.

Intimal hyperplasia may also occur in coronary arteries, but this is not the rule. Several cases of mixed connective tissue disease involving children and young adults have been characterized by chest pain, fever, tachycardia, progressive congestive heart failure, and ventricular arrhythmias leading to death.[148,149] Clinically evident myocarditis remains less frequent than histologic abnormalities, but severe dilated cardiomyopathy has been reported in association with a variety of connective tissue disease syndromes. Conduction abnormalities include atrioventricular block and infranodal bundle branch blocks, particularly when there is apparent flair of systemic vasculitis in patients with mixed connective tissue disease, but conducting system abnormalities are not routinely encountered.

Although overlap syndromes must be expected to display clinical diversity in terms of cardiovascular involvement, manifestations of mixed connective disease in the heart seem mainly to involve neighboring pericarditis with or without pericardial effusion, mitral valve prolapse, intimal hyperplasia of coronary arteries, perivascular leukocytic myocardial infiltrates, and pulmonary hypertension. The frequency of an associated condition such as coronary atherosclerosis and systemic hypertension is such that cardiac changes may be due to a combination of variables. The natural history of mixed connective tissue disease, like the other collagen vascular syndromes thus seems inexorably linked with the function of the circulatory system.

REFERENCES

1. Charcot JL: Clinical Lectures on Senile and Chronic Diseases, vol 95, p 172. London, Sydenham Society, 1881
2. Baggenstoss AH, Rosenberg EF: Cardiac lesions associated with chronic infectious arthritis. Arch Intern Med 67:241, 1941
3. Lebowitz WB: The heart in rheumatoid arthritis (rheumatoid disease): A clinical and pathological study of 62 cases. Ann Intern Med 58:102, 1962
4. Cathcart ES, Spodick DH: Rheumatoid heart disease: A study of the incidence and nature of cardiac lesions in rheumatoid arthritis. N Engl J Med 266:959, 1962
5. Kahn AH, Spodick DH: Rheumatoid heart disease. Semin Arthritis Rheum 1:327, 1972
6. Leitman PS, Bywaters EGL: Pericarditis in juvenile rheumatoid arthritis. Pediatrics 32:855, 1963
7. Kirk J, Cosh J: The pericarditis of rheumatoid arthritis. Q J Med 38:397, 1969
8. Schorn D, Hough IP, Anderson IF: The heart in rheumatoid arthritis: An echocardiographic study. S Afr Med J 50:8, 1976
9. Bacon PA, Gibson DG: Cardiac involvement in rheumatoid arthritis: An echocardiographic study. Ann Rheum Dis 33:20, 1974
10. Spodick DH: Acute Pericarditis, p 97. New York, Grune & Stratton, 1959
11. Goyette EM: Treatment of tuberculous pericarditis. Prog Cardiovasc Dis 3:141, 1960
12. Davia JE, Cheitlin MD, DeCastro CM et al: Absence of echocardiographic abnormalities of the anterior mitral valve leaflet in rheumatoid arthritis. Ann Intern Med 83:500, 1975
13. Romankiewicz JA, Brogden RN, Heel RC et al: Captopril: An update and review of its pharmacologic properties and therapeutic efficacy in congestive heart failure. Drugs 25:6, 1983
14. Sokoloff L: Cardiac involvement in rheumatoid arthritis and allied disorders: Current concepts. Mod Concepts Cardiovasc Dis 33:847, 1964
15. Roberts WC, Kehoe JA, Carpenter DF et al: Cardiovascular lesions in rheumatoid arthritis. Arch Intern Med 122:141, 1968
16. Carpenter DF, Goden A, Roberts WC: Quadrivalvular rheumatoid heart disease associated with left bundle branch block. Am J Med 43:922, 1967
17. Waaler E: The visceral lesions of rheumatoid arthritis. Acta Rheum Scand 13:20, 1967
18. Bortolotti U, Valente M, Agozzino L et al: Rheumatoid mitral stenosis requiring valve replacement. Am Heart J 107:1049, 1984
19. Handforth CP, Woodbury JFF: Cardiovascular manifestations of rheumatoid arthritis. Can Med Assoc J 80:86, 1959
20. Lever MA, Cosh J: Complete heart block in rheumatoid arthritis. Ann Rheum Dis 42:389, 1983
21. Cruickshank B: Heart lesions in rheumatoid disease. J Pathol Bacteriol 76:223, 1958
22. Davis RF, Engleman EG: Incidence of myocardial infarction in patients with rheumatoid arthritis. Arthritis Rheum 17:527, 1974
23. Chesebro JH, Clements IP, Fuster V et al: A platelet-inhibitor drug trial in coronary-artery bypass operations: Benefit of perioperative dipyridamole and aspirin therapy on early postoperative vein-graft patency. N Engl J Med 307:73, 1982
24. Moll JMH: Ankylosing Spondylitis. Edinburgh, Churchill Livingstone, 1980
25. Dausset J, Svejgaard A: HLA and Disease. Copenhagen, Munksgaard/Williams & Wilkins, 1977
26. Bergfeldt L: HLA-B27-associated rheumatic diseases with severe cardiac bradyarrhythmias. Am J Med 75:210, 1983
27. Bergfeldt L, Edhag O, Vedin L et al: Ankylosing spondylitis: An important cause of severe disturbances of the cardiac conduction system. Prevalence among 223 pacemaker treated men. Am J Med 73:187, 1982
28. Bergfeldt L, Edhag O, Vallin H: Cardiac conduction disturbances, an underestimated manifestation in ankylosing spondylitis. Acta Med Scand 212:217, 1982
29. Graham DC, Symthe HA: The carditis and aortitis of ankylosing spondylitis. Bull Rheum Dis 9:171, 1958
30. Cosh JA, Barritt DW, Jayson MI: Cardiac lesions of Reiter's syndrome and ankylosing spondylitis. Br Heart J 35:553, 1973
31. Paulus HE, Pearson CM, Pitts W Jr: Aortic insufficiency in five patients with Reiter's syndrome: A detailed clinical and pathologic study. Am J Med 53:464, 1972
32. Rossen RM, Goodman DJ, Harrison DC: A-V conduction disturbances in Reiter's syndrome. Am J Med 58:280, 1975
33. Hassel D, Heinsimer J, Califf RM et al: Complete heart block in Reiter's syndrome. Am J Cardiol 15:967, 1984
34. Ruppert GB, Lindsay J, Barth WF: Cardiac conduction abnormalities in Reiter's syndrome. Am J Med 73:335, 1982
35. Nojiri C, Endo M, Koyanagi H: Conduction disturbance in Behçet's disease. Chest 86:636, 1984
36. Higashihara M, Mori M, Takeuchi A et al: Myocarditis in Behcet's disease. J Rheumatol 9:630, 1982
37. Comess KA, Zibelli LR, Gordon D et al: Acute, severe aortic regurgitation in Behçet's syndrome. Ann Intern Med 99:639, 1983
38. Schiff S, Moffatt R, Mandel WJ et al: Acute myocardial infarction and recurrent ventricular arrhythmias in Behçet's syndrome. Am Heart J 103:438, 1982
39. Scarlett JA, Kistner ML, Yang LC: Behçet's syndrome report of a case associated with pericardial effusion and cryoglobulinemia treated with indomethacin. Am J Med 66:146, 1979
40. Bidani AK, Roberts JL, Schwartz MM et al: Immunopathology of cardiac lesions in fatal systemic lupus erythematosus. Am J Med 69:849, 1980
41. Das SK, Cassidy JT: Antiheart antibodies in patients with systemic lupus erythematosus. Am J Med Sci 265:275, 1973
42. Libman E, Sacks B: A hitherto undescribed form of valvular and mural endocarditis. Arch Intern Med 33:701, 1924
43. Hejtmancik MR, Wright JC, Quint R et al: The cardiovascular manifestations of systemic lupus erythematosus. Am Heart J 68:119, 1964

44. Bulkley BH, Roberts WC: The heart in systemic lupus erythematosus and the changes induced in it by corticosteroid therapy. Am J Med 58:243, 1975
45. Shearn MA: The heart in systemic lupus erythematosus. Am Heart J 58:452, 1959
46. Brigden W, Bywaters EG, Lessof MH et al: The heart in systemic lupus erythematosus. Br Heart J 22:1, 1960
47. Soffer LJ, Elster SK, Hammerman DJ: Treatment of acute disseminated lupus erythematosus with corticotropin and cortisone. Arch Intern Med 53:503, 1954
48. Klemperer P, Pollack AD, Baehr G: Pathology of disseminated lupus erythematosus. Arch Pathol 32:569, 1941
49. Marks AD: The cardiovascular manifestations of systemic lupus erythematosus. Am J Med Sci 264:255, 1972
50. Cohen AS, Canoso JJ: Pericarditis in the rheumatologic diseases. In Spodick DH (ed): Pericardial Diseases, pp 237–255. Philadelphia, FA Davis, 1976
51. Kinney E, Wynn J, Hinton DM et al: Pericardial fluid complement: Normal values. Am J Clin Pathol 72:972, 1979
52. Yurchak PM, Levine SA, Gorlin R: Constrictive pericarditis complicating disseminated lupus erythematosus. Circulation 31:113, 1965
53. Browning CA, Bishop RL, Heilpern RJ et al: Accelerated constrictive pericarditis in procainamide-induced systemic lupus erythematosus. Am J Cardiol 53:376, 1984
54. Carey RM, Coleman M, Feder A: Pericardial tamponade: A major presenting manifestation of hydralazine-induced lupus syndrome. Am J Med 54:84, 1973
55. Chia BL, Evelyn PKM, Feng PH: Cardiovascular abnormalities in systemic lupus erythematosus. J Clin Ultrasound 9:237, 1981
56. Dubois EL: The clinical picture of systemic lupus erythematosus. In Dubois EL (ed): Lupus Erythematosus: A Review of the Current Status of Discoid and Systemic Lupus Erythematosus and Their Variants, pp 265–275, 402–404. Los Angeles, University of Southern California Press, 1974
57. Griffith GC, Vural IL: Acute and subacute disseminated lupus erythematosus: Correlation of clinical and post-mortem findings in eighteen cases. Circulation 3:492, 1951
58. Chang RW: Cardiac manifestations of SLE. Clin Rheum Dis 8:197, 1982
59. del Rio A, Vazquez JJ, Sobrino JA et al: Myocardial involvement in systemic lupus erythmatosus. Chest 74:414, 1978
60. Harvey A, Shulman LE, Tumulty PA et al: Systemic lupus erythematosus: Review of the literature and clinical analysis of 138 cases. Medicine 33:291, 1954
61. Osler W: On the visceral manifestations of the erythema group of skin disease. Am J Med Sci 127:1, 1904
62. Shulman HJ, Christian CL: Aortic insufficiency in systemic lupus erythematosus. Arthritis Rheum 12:138, 1969
63. Paget SA, Bulkley BH, Brauer LE et al: Mitral valve disease of systemic lupus erythematosus: A cause of severe congestive heart failure reversed by valve replacement. Am J Med 59:134, 1975
64. Esscher E, Scott JS: Congenital heart block and maternal systemic lupus erythematosus. Br Med J 1:1235, 1979
65. Hess EV, Spencer-Green G: Congenital heart block and connective tissue disease. Ann Intern Med 91:645, 1979
66. Haider YS, Roberts WC: Coronary arterial disease in systemic lupus erythematosus. Am J Med 70:775, 1981
67. Grey HM, Kohler PF: Cryoimmunoglobulins. Semin Hematol 10:87, 1973
68. Parrillo JE, Fauci AS: Necrotizing vasculitis, coronary angiitis and the cardiologist. Am Heart J 99:547, 1980
69. Harrington TM, Torretti D, Pytko VF et al: Hereditary angioedema and coronary arteritis. Am J Med 287:50, 1984
70. Holsinger DR, Osmundson PJ, Edwards JE: The heart in periarteritis nodosa. Circulation 25:610, 1962
71. Zeek PM: Periarteritis nodosa: A critical review. Am J Clin Pathol 22:777, 1952
72. Zeek PM: Medical progress: Periarteritis nodosa and other forms of necrotizing angiitis. N Engl J Med 248:764, 1953
73. Alarcon-Segovia D, Brown AL: Classification and etiologic aspects of necrotizing angiitides: Analytic approach to a confused subject with a critical review of the evidence for hypersensitivity in polyarteritis nodosa. Mayo Clin Proc 39:205, 1964
74. James TN, Birk RE: Pathology of the cardiac conduction system in polyarteritis nodosa. Arch Intern Med 117:561, 1966
75. Hiraishi S, Yashiro K, Oguchi K et al: Clinical course of cardiovascular involvement in the mucocutaneous lymph node syndrome. Am J Cardiol 47:323, 1981
76. Duffy J, Lidsky MD, Sharp JT et al: Polyarthritis, polyarteritis and hepatitis B. Medicine 55:19, 1976
77. Michalak T: Immune complexes of hepatitis B surface antigen in the pathogenesis of periarteritis nodosa: A study of seven necropsy cases. Am J Pathol 90:619, 1978
78. Weyman AE, Feigenbaum H, Dillon JC et al: Non-invasive visualization of the left main coronary artery by cross-sectional echocardiography. Circulation 54:169, 1976
79. Matsu H, Matsumoto S, Hamanaka Y: Echocardiographic features of coronary artery aneurysms in acute febrile mucocutaneous lymph node syndrome (MCLS) (in Japanese). Jpn Soc Ultrasound 31:139, 1977
80. Yoshikawa J, Yanagihara K, Oaki T et al: Cross-sectional echocardiographic diagnosis of coronary artery aneurysms in patients with the mucocutaneous lymph node syndrome. Circulation 59:133, 1979
81. Shimazu S, Kiyosawa S, Hamaoka K et al: Two-dimensional echocardiography of coronary arterial lesions with MCLS, in special reference to the comparison with coronary angiography (in Japanese). Acta Paediatr Jpn 83:1632, 1979
82. Kiyosawa N, Onouchi Z, Haba S et al: A study of the indication for coronary angiography in patients with MCLS. Pediatr Jpn 21:55, 1980
83. Onouchi Z, Shimazu S, Kiyosawa N et al: Aneurysms of the coronary arteries in Kawasaki disease. Circulation 66:6, 1982
84. Kitamura S, Kawashima Y, Kawachi K et al: Left ventricular function in patients with coronary arteritis due to acute febrile mucocutaneous lymph node syndrome or related diseases. Am J Cardiol 40:156, 1977
85. Nakanishi T, Takao A, Nakazawa M et al: Mucocutaneous lymph node syndrome: Clinical, hemodynamic and angiographic features of coronary obstructive disease. Am J Cardiol 55:662, 1985
86. Kitamura S, Kawachi K, Harima R et al: Surgery for coronary heart disease due to mucocutaneous lymph node syndrome (Kawasaki disease). Am J Cardiol 51:444, 1983
87. Churg J, Strauss L: Allergic granulomatosis, allergic angiitis and periarteritis nodosa. Am J Pathol 27:277, 1951
88. Sokolov RA, Rachmaninoff N, Kaine HD: Allergic granulomatosis. Am J Med 32:131, 1962
89. Varriale P, Minoque WF, Alfenito JC: Allergic granulomatosis: Case report and review of the literature. Arch Intern Med 113:235, 1964
90. Chumbley LC, Harrison EG, DeRemee RA: Allergic granulomatosis and angiitis (Churg-Strauss syndrome): Report and analysis of 30 cases. Mayo Clin Proc 52:477, 1977
91. Fauci AS, Wolff SM: Wegener's granulomatosis: Studies in 18 patients and a review of the literature. Medicine 52:535, 1973
92. Wishnick MM, Valensi Q, Doyle EF et al: Churg-Strauss syndrome. Am J Dis Child 136:339, 1982
93. Wegener F: Uber generlisierte, septische Gafasserkran Kungen. Verh Dtsch Gesamte Pathol 29:202, 1936
94. Gatenby PA, Lytton DG, Bulteau VG: Myocardial infarction in Wegener's granulomatosis. Aust NZ J Med 6:336, 1976
95. Fauci AS, Haynes BF, Katz P et al: Wegener's granulomatosis: Prospective clinical and therapeutic experience with 85 patients for 21 years. Ann Intern Med 98:76, 1983
96. Rosenberg DM, Weinberger SE, Fulmer JD et al: Functional correlates of lung involvement in Wegener's granulomatosis. Am J Med 69:387, 1980
97. Forstot JZ, Overlie PA, Neufeld GK et al: Cardiac complications of Wegener's granulomatosis: A case report of complete heart block and review of the literature. Semin Arthritis Rheum 10:148, 1980
98. Klein RG, Hunder GG, Stonson AW et al: Large artery involvement in giant cell (temporal) arteritis. Ann Intern Med 83:806, 1975
99. Austen WG, Blennerhassett MB: Giant cell aortitis causing an aneurysm of the ascending aorta and aortic regurgitation. N Engl J Med 272:80, 1965
100. Paulley JW: Coronary ischemia and occlusion in giant cell (temporal) arteritis. Acta Med Scand 208:257, 1980
101. Martin JF, Kittas C, Triger DR: Giant cell arteritis of coronary arteries causing myocardial infarction. Br Heart J 43:487, 1980
102. How J, Strachan RW: Aortic regurgitation as a manifestation of giant cell arteritis. Br Heart J 40:1052, 1978
103. Lande A, LaPorta A: Takayasu arteritis: An arteriographic-pathological correlation. Arch Pathol Lab Med 100:437, 1976
104. Cipriano PR, Silverman JF, Perlroth MG et al: Coronary arterial narrowing in Takayasu's aortitis. Am J Cardiol 39:744, 1977
105. Lupi-Herrera E, Sanchez-Torres G, Marcushamer J et al: Takayasu's arteritis: Clinical study of 107 cases. Am Heart J 93:94, 1977
106. Sunamori M, Hatano R, Yokokawa T et al: Aortitis syndrome due to Takayasu's disease: A guide for the surgical indication. J Cardiovasc Surg 17:443, 1976
107. Bloss RS, Duncan JM, Cooley DA et al: Takayasu's arteritis: Surgical considerations. Ann Thorac Surg 27:574, 1979
108. Tan EM, Rodnan GP, Garcia I et al: Diversity of antinuclear antibodies in progressive systemic sclerosis: Anticentromere antibody and its relationship to CREST syndrome. Arthritis Rheum 23:617, 1980
109. Winkleman RK, Goldyne ME, Linscheild RL: Hypersensitivity of scleroderma cutaneous vascular smooth muscle to 5-hydroxytryptamine. Br J Dermatol 95:51, 1976
110. Vanhoutte PM, Janssens WJ: Thermosensitivity of cutaneous vessels and Raynaud's disease. Am Heart J 100:263, 1980
111. Dabich L, Bookstein JJ, Zweifler A: Digital arteries in patients with scleroderma. Arch Intern Med 130:708, 1972
112. Pringle R, Walder DN, Weaver JPA: Blood viscosity and Raynaud's disease. Lancet 1:1086, 1965
113. Sodeman WA, Burch GE: Tissue pressure: An objective method of following skin changes in scleroderma. Am Heart J 17:21, 1939
114. Follansbee WP, Curtiss EI, Medsger TA et al: Physiologic abnormalities of cardiac function in progressive systemic sclerosis with diffuse scleroderma. N Engl J Med 310:142, 1984
115. LeRoy CE. Editorial: The heart in systemic sclerosis. N Engl J Med 310:188,

116. Lewis T: Experiments relating to the peripheral mechanism involved in spasmodic arrest of the circulation of the fingers, a variety of Raynaud's disease. Heart 15:7, 1929
117. Weiss S, Stead E, Warren J et al: Scleroderma heart disease. Arch Intern Med 71:749, 1943
118. Botstein GR, LeRoy CE: Primary heart disease in systemic sclerosis (scleroderma): Advances in clinical and pathologic features, pathogenesis, and new therapeutic approaches. Am Heart J 102:913, 1981
119. Reichenbach DD, Benditt EP: Myofibrillar degeneration: A response of the myocardial cell to injury. Arch Pathol 85:189, 1968
120. D'Angelo WA, Fries JF, Masi AT et al: Pathologic observations in systemic sclerosis (scleroderma): A study of fifty-eight autopsy cases in fifty-eight matched controls. Am J Med 46:428, 1969
121. Bulkley BH, Ridolfi RL, Salyer WR et al: Myocardial lesions of progressive systemic sclerosis: A cause of cardiac dysfunction. Circulation 53:483, 1976
122. Sackner MA, Heinz ER, Steinberg AJ: The heart in scleroderma. Am J Cardiol 17:542, 1966
123. McWhorter JE, LeRoy EC: Pericardial disease in scleroderma (systemic sclerosis). Am J Med 57:566, 1974
124. Smith JW, Clements PJ, Levisman J et al: Echocardiographic features of progressive systemic sclerosis (PSS): Correlation with hemodynamic and postmortem studies. Am J Med 66:28, 1979
125. Osler W: On diffuse scleroderma: With special reference to diagnosis, and to the use of the thyroid-gland extract. J Cutan Genitourinary Dis 16:49, 1898
126. Medsger IA, Masi AT: Survival with scleroderma: II. A life-table analysis of clinical and demographic factors in 358 male US veteran patients. J Chron Dis 26:647, 1973
127. Oram S, Strokes W: The heart in scleroderma. Br Heart J 23:243, 1961
128. Weiss S, Zyskind Z, Rosenthal T et al: Cardiac involvement in progressive systemic sclerosis (PSS): An echocardiographic study. Rheumatology 39:190, 1980
129. Herdson PB, Sommers HM, Jennings RB: A comparative study of the fine structure of normal and ischemic dog myocardium with special reference to early changes following temporary occlusion of a coronary artery. Am J Pathol 46:367, 1965
130. Jennings RB, Sommers HM, Herdson PB et al: Ischemic injury of myocardium. Ann NY Acad Sci 156:61, 1969
131. Campbell PM, LeRoy EC: Pathogenesis of systemic sclerosis: A vascular hypothesis. Semin Arthritis Rheum 4:351, 1975
132. Alexander EL, Firestein GS, Leitl G et al: Scleroderma heart disease: Evidence for cold-induced abnormalities of myocardial function and perfusion. Arthritis Rheum 24(suppl 4):S58, 1981
133. Lev M, Landowne M, Matchar JC et al: Systemic scleroderma with complete heart block. Am Heart J 72:13, 1976
134. Whitman HH, Case DB: New developments in the treatment of scleroderma. Drug Therapy 6:97, 1981
135. Creager MA, Pariser KM, Winston EL et al: Nifedipine-induced fingertip vasodilatation in patients with Raynaud's phenomenon. Am Heart J 108:370, 1984
136. Malamet R, Wise RA, Ettinger WH et al: Nifedipine in the treatment of Raynaud's phenomenon. Am J Med 78:602, 1985
137. Bradley WG: Inflammatory Disease of Muscle, p 1255. Baltimore, Williams & Wilkins, 1958
138. Wagner E: Fall von acuter polymyositis. Dtsch Arch Klin Med 40:241, 1886
139. Oppenheim H: Zur dermatomyositis. Berl Klin Wochenschr 36:805, 1899
140. Gottdiener JS, Sherber HS, Hawley RJ et al: Cardiac manifestations in polymyositis. Am J Cardiol 41:1141, 1978
141. Haupt HM, Hutchins GM: The heart and cardiac conduction system in polymyositis-dermatomyositis: A clinicopathologic study of 16 autopsied patients. Am J Cardiol 50:998, 1982
142. Sharratt GP, Danta G, Carson PHM: Cardiac abnormality in polymyositis. Ann Rheum Dis 36:575, 1977
143. Kehoe RF, Bauernfeind R, Tommaso C et al: Cardiac conduction defects in polymyositis. Ann Intern Med 94:41, 1981
144. Bohan A, Peter JB, Bowman RL et al: A computer assisted analysis of 153 patients with polymyositis and dermatomyositis. Medicine 56:255, 1977
145. Sharp GC, Irvin WS, Tan EM et al: Mixed connective tissue disease: An apparently distinct rheumatic disease syndrome associated with a specific antibody to an extractable nuclear antigen (ENA). Am J Med 52:148, 1972
146. Oetgen WJ, Mutter ML, Lawless OJ et al: Cardiac abnormalities in mixed connective tissue disease. Chest 83:185, 1983
147. Alpert MA, Goldberg SH, Singsen BH et al: Cardiovascular manifestations of mixed connective disease in adults. Circulation 68:1182, 1983
148. Whitlow PL, Gilliam JM, Chubick A et al: Myocarditis in mixed connective tissue disease: Association of myocarditis with antibody to nuclear ribonuclear protein. Arthritis Rheum 23:808, 1980
149. Howard JP: Mixed connective tissue disease in a child. J Ky Med Assoc 87:601, 1980

PREGNANCY IN THE CARDIAC PATIENT

John H. McAnulty • James Metcalfe
Kent Ueland

The cardiovascular changes that occur during pregnancy allow the uterus and developing fetus to receive an adequate blood supply and permit other organs of the body to adapt to the pregnancy. The mother and fetus are so dependent on these alterations that both are potentially at risk from maternal heart disease. This is particularly true for the fetus in that a restriction in maternal cardiac output preferentially results in a limitation of uterine blood flow. In this chapter we will summarize the important cardiovascular changes occurring with pregnancy, discuss the recognition and management of maternal heart disease, and review the importance of specific maternal cardiovascular lesions for pregnancy.

MATERNAL CARDIOVASCULAR CHANGES DURING NORMAL PREGNANCY
CARDIAC OUTPUT

The most remarkable change occurring with pregnancy is the 40% increase in resting cardiac output above the nonpregnant value.[1] Most of this increment is achieved early in pregnancy, with peak values at 15 to 20 weeks (Fig. 111.1). Because cardiac output is dependent on venous return, it is influenced by the position of the woman while the measurement is taken, particularly late in pregnancy; women who are at full term may actually have a fall in cardiac output below postpartum levels when they are supine and the pregnant uterus interferes with venous return to the heart.[2] The initial rise in cardiac output is due mainly to an increase in stroke volume, which then falls; the heart rate increases progressively throughout most of pregnancy. The cardiac output varies dramatically at the time of labor. With each uterine contraction, it can increase by 25%, probably as the result of augmentation of venous return as blood is squeezed from the uterus. These changes may be affected by the type of anesthesia used in labor. Immediately after delivery, cardiac output increases by 60% to 80%, again depending on the type of anesthesia used.[3] The magnitude of change is less in patients who are delivered by cesarean section. The cardiac output falls during the two-week postpartum period but continues to be greater than normal during that time.

The woman's hemodynamic response to exercise is altered during pregnancy. In general, cardiac output is higher at any given external work load. As is the case at rest, tachycardia becomes increasingly important in maintaining cardiac output as pregnancy advances.

The increase in cardiac output during pregnancy is associated with a gradual increase in maternal oxygen consumption to a level that is 20% above that of the nonpregnant state. Because the increase in cardiac output occurs earlier and is proportionately greater than the increase in oxygen consumption, the systemic arteriovenous oxygen difference falls by 20% to 40% early in pregnancy and widens to nonpregnant levels at term.

The mechanism by which these changes occur is not fully under-

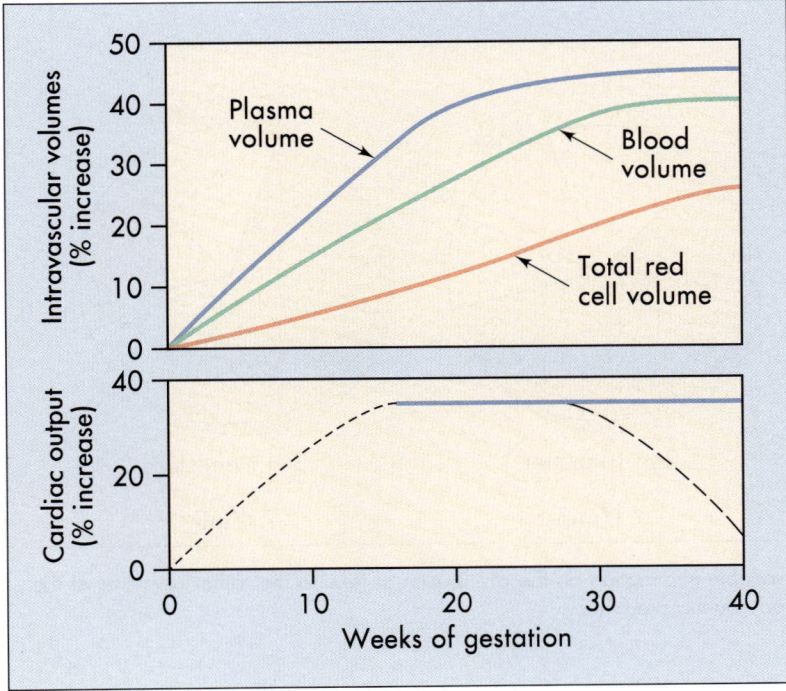

FIGURE 111.1 Schematic representations of the percent increases in cardiac output and intravascular volumes that occur during pregnancy. Plasma volume increases by approximately 50% and total red cell volume by approximately 25%, causing a resultant 40% increase in total blood volume. Cardiac output increases by 40% above nonpregnant levels, reaching its maximum by the twentieth week of pregnancy. The dashed line indicates the susceptibility of cardiac output to a decrement in venous return, most noticeable in the supine position and becoming more pronounced as pregnancy advances.

stood. They are associated with changes in volume, venous tone, vascular resistance, and myocardial performance.

BLOOD VOLUME

The blood volume increases progressively throughout pregnancy to a value that is 40% above the nonpregnant level by term. Early in pregnancy this is due to an increase in plasma volume and it is associated with an increase in red blood cell mass later in pregnancy (see Fig. 111.1). In an average pregnancy, there is a gradual accumulation of 500 mEq to 900 mEq of sodium and total body water increases by 6 to 8 liters, most of which is extracellular.[4]

VASCULAR CAPACITY AND PERIPHERAL VASCULAR RESISTANCE

The increased intravascular volume is associated with an increase in venous capacity due to relaxation of the great veins during pregnancy, apparently the result of the direct action of progesterone.[5,6] This allows peripheral blood pooling and prevents congestion of the pulmonary vascular system.

Systolic and diastolic blood pressures fall during pregnancy, particularly in the first two trimesters. This is due to a fall in systemic vascular resistance that exceeds the degree of increase in cardiac output. The distribution of blood flow also changes during pregnancy, probably the result of local alterations in the vascular resistance (Fig. 111.2). This permits increased blood flow to the pregnant uterus and the breasts; flow to the kidneys is also increased.

VENTRICULAR SIZE AND FUNCTION

Changes in left ventricular diastolic function have been demonstrated with systolic time intervals and echocardiography;[7-10] the most prominent is an increase in left ventricular end-diastolic volume. This is apparently due to structural alteration in the muscle rather than an increase in distending pressure: it can be reproduced in guinea pigs by administration of estrogen.[11] The constant variation in preload and afterload during pregnancy makes evaluation of the inotropic state of the heart difficult. In general, the indices of contractility, including ejection fraction and the velocity of circumferential fiber shortening, do not change during pregnancy.

MATERNAL HEART DISEASE
RECOGNITION

It can be particularly difficult to recognize cardiovascular disease during pregnancy. While dyspnea, fatigue, chest discomforts, orthopnea, palpitations, peripheral edema, and syncope are frequently associated with cardiac disease, each can be a normal symptom or sign in a healthy pregnant woman. The same is true for pedal edema, an S_3 gallop, a systolic ejection murmur, and rales. Awareness of these symptoms and signs that accompany the maternal physiologic changes in pregnancy is essential in order to avoid overdiagnosis. However, there are symptoms and signs that cannot be considered normal during pregnancy and dictate the need for further evaluation (Table 111.1). While a diastolic murmur is appropriately listed as an abnormality requiring further evaluation, it is important to exclude benign explanations. These include the continuous bruit due to increased blood flow to the breasts, the "mammary souffle," and venous hums, which can be affected with ipsilateral neck vein compression. Cardiomegaly by examination or chest x-ray film is an important finding but can be confused with displacement of the heart to the left by the elevated diaphragm in late pregnancy.

MANAGEMENT

Whenever possible, the definition and management of heart disease should begin prior to pregnancy. The physician who is responsible for the management of a woman with heart disease should take the initiative in discussing contraception, the implications of pregnancy, and the long-term plan for motherhood, as well as the place of cardiac surgery in her life plan. Genetic counseling is of particular importance when one parent has a congenital cardiac deformity (Table 111.2). Gynecological consultation should be requested so that problems such as pelvic deformity or a genital anomaly can be considered. An obstetri-

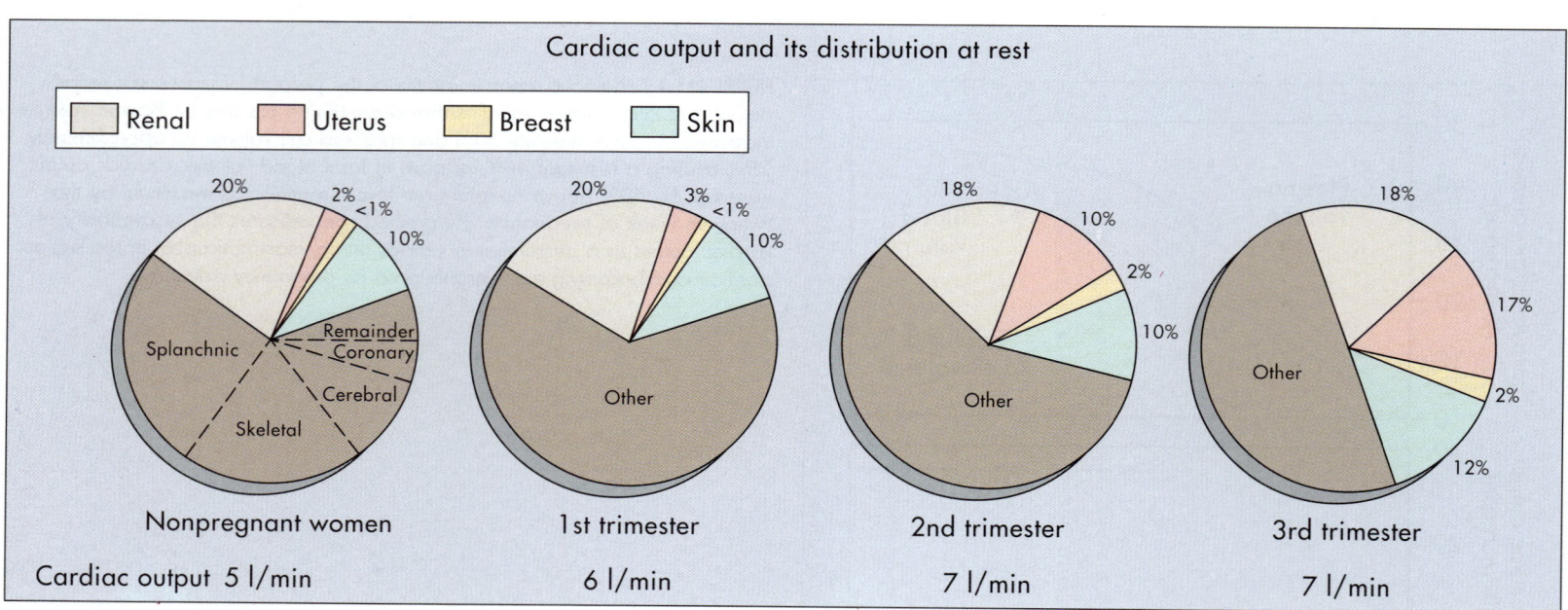

FIGURE 111.2 The increase in cardiac output during pregnancy is associated with a redistribution of blood flow. This results in an 11-fold increase in uterine blood flow and a 1.5- to 2-fold increase in renal blood flow. There is little available information on the distribution of flow to the "other" systems of the body during pregnancy.

cal colleague who deals well with complicated pregnancies should be identified and should share in advice regarding family planning. When the patient has a lesion that is recognized as jeopardizing fetal health and development, careful attention to monitoring fetal growth and fetal well-being should be planned and discussed early in pregnancy to minimize anxiety later.

When cardiac output is limited by maternal heart disease, measures that diminish the total cardiac burden should be outlined early in pregnancy and introduced as pregnancy advances. These include prescription of regular periods of rest, limitation of activity, and avoidance of anemia and infections. Prospective discussion minimizes anxiety, itself a burden on the heart. Attention to general health habits can increase the chance of successful pregnancy. This is especially important in women with heart disease. The woman should be advised to stop or avoid all unnecessary medications. Cigarette smoking is demonstrably dangerous to maternal health and fetal development and should be stopped before, during, and after pregnancy.[12-16] The same is true for alcohol[17] (we advise a limitation of alcohol to one drink per day) and "street drugs." Although there is not a great deal of information available about these latter, there is some evidence of danger to the fetus[18,19] and the uncertainty about the content of many of these drugs supports this recommendation. Vaccination, particularly against rubella, should be completed before pregnancy. Activity during pregnancy should be regularly reviewed and limited in patients who have any symptoms or when there is evidence of fetal distress.

DIAGNOSTIC STUDIES DURING PREGNANCY

Because of their inherent risks and expense, and because misinterpretation of findings in a pregnant woman is possible, it is essential that cardiac diagnostic studies be ordered and interpreted by individuals familiar with their use and with the altered findings that occur during pregnancy. Some are obviously safe. The electrocardiogram can be helpful by revealing findings for specific cardiac abnormalities. Caution with some interpretations is necessary, however, since changes can occur in a normal pregnancy. A leftward shift in the axis is common, presumably the result of cardiac displacement by the distended abdomen; left axis deviation of minus 30 degrees or less is not a normal pregnancy variant.[20] The ST-T wave changes that have occasionally been attributed to pregnancy may simply be normal electrocardiographic variations of the young.

Because of its safety and diagnostic power, the echocardiogram is especially attractive for use during pregnancy. However, it is expensive and misinterpretation is common. Normal pregnancy alters left ventricular size and dynamics and this must be taken into account when interpreting a study.[9,10]

Exposure to ionizing radiation should be avoided when possible, especially during early pregnancy. It poses a number of potential risks. There is some controversy about whether radiation exposure results in subsequent malignancies in the offspring[21-23] but there is no doubt that the incidence of congenital abnormalities is increased by exposure. The highest incidence results from exposure during weeks 3 through 10 of gestation.[24] Additionally, the risk of a congenital abnormality increases with the dose of radiation. There is no conclusive evidence of an increase in the incidence of congenital abnormalities with exposures of less than 10 rad.[25,26] Thus, a woman who has received less than this, particularly when it is not focused on the uterus and when it occurs far removed from the time of greatest vulnerability, is unlikely to have an increased risk of a deformed child. A chest x-ray film (approximately 0.15 rad) performed inadvertently, even early in pregnancy, is not a reason to consider interruption of the pregnancy. Still, the problems with radiation lead to a number of recommendations. Every woman of child-bearing age should be questioned about the possibility of pregnancy before diagnostic x-ray procedures. If an x-ray study is required, shielding of the abdomen is advised. The procedure that gives the least amount of radiation should be performed and, whenever possible, the radiation exposure should be delayed until at least the completion of the first trimester.

TABLE 111.1 INDICATORS OF HEART DISEASE DURING PREGNANCY

Symptoms
- Severe or progressive dyspnea
- Progressive orthopnea
- Paroxysmal nocturnal dyspnea
- Hemoptysis
- Syncope with exertion
- Chest pain related to effort or emotion

Signs
- Cyanosis
- Clubbing
- Persistent neck vein distention
- A systolic murmur greater than grade III or VI in intensity
- Diastolic murmur
- Cardiomegaly, general or localized
- A documented sustained arrhythmia
- A split second sound, persisting unchanged during expiration
- Criteria for pulmonary hypertension
    - Left parasternal lift
    - Loud P_2

TABLE 111.2 RISK OF CONGENITAL HEART DISEASE IN OFFSPRING IF ONE PARENT IS AFFECTED*†

Type of Heart Defect	Risk
Intracardiac Shunts	
Atrial septal defect	3%–11%
Ventricular septal defect	4%–22%
Patent ductus arteriosus	4%–11%
Obstruction to Flow	
Left-sided obstruction‡	3%–26%
Right-sided obstruction	3%–22%
Complex Abnormalities	
Tetralogy of Fallot	4%–15%
Ebstein's anomaly	Uncertain
Transposition of the great arteries	Uncertain

* The higher number in each range comes from one large series.[51] The incidence in congenital heart disease in the offspring tends to be closer to the lower numbers for most other reported series.[85,91]

† The risk of congenital heart disease in the offspring of women with obstructive lesions is decreased by corrective surgery prior to pregnancy.[51]

‡ Includes coarctation, aortic stenosis, discrete subaortic stenosis, supravalvular stenosis. It does not include idiopathic hypertrophic subaortic stenosis; with this the child has a 50% chance of having idiopathic hypertrophic subaortic stenosis.

Radionuclides are another source of ionizing radiation. Until more is known about the distribution of these substances, whenever possible radionuclide procedures should be avoided during pregnancy.[27]

SPECIFIC COMPLICATIONS OF CARDIOVASCULAR DISEASE

The major complications of cardiac disease will be discussed, reviewing the approach to management as well as the use of selected drugs in pregnancy. Table 111.3 reviews important features of groups of cardiac drugs as they relate to pregnancy.

PULMONARY ARTERY HYPERTENSION

Irreversible pulmonary hypertension is a contraindication to pregnancy. Primary pulmonary hypertension and Eisenmenger's syndrome are associated with a maternal mortality rate of 50%. The mechanism is often obscure but death is frequently sudden and the woman is at particular risk during labor and in the postpartum period.[28-31] Even if the woman survives pregnancy, there is a high incidence of spontaneous abortions[29] and congenital cardiac malformations.[28]

When pregnancy occurs in a patient with recognized pulmonary hypertension, prompt pregnancy interruption is advised. With interruption, careful hemodynamic monitoring and attempts to avoid hypotension and venous pooling are essential. If interruption as an option is refused or not feasible, careful in-hospital monitoring with bed rest is recommended. Particular attention to avoidance of hypovolemia is essential. Central venous and pulmonary capillary wedge pressure measurements with serial evaluation of cardiac output are recommended at the time of labor and delivery, during the first postpartum week, and when treatment of right-sided heart failure and chest pain is considered necessary. Adequate analgesia and anesthesia are important during labor. A combination narcotic with a local anesthesia epidermal technique can achieve this without causing major hemodynamic alterations.

PULMONARY VASCULAR CONGESTION

The standard approach to management of congestive heart failure—limitation of activity and sodium intake, correction of precipitating factors such as arrhythmias or structural abnormalities, and use of medication—is as important during pregnancy as at any other time. The emphasis on each measure, however, should be different. While limitation of activity or strict dietary restriction may not be acceptable long-term options, they are a small sacrifice for the duration of pregnancy and, when feasible, are preferable to use of medications or to surgical correction of structural abnormalities. However, if pulmonary vascular congestion cannot be controlled despite close attention to

TABLE 111.3 CARDIOVASCULAR DRUGS DURING PREGNANCY

Drug Group	Use During Pregnancy	Adverse Effects
Diuretics[116,117]	Use as in nonpregnant women. Should not be used prophylactically or to treat pedal edema unless there is associated pulmonary vascular congestion.	May exacerbate preeclampsia by reducing uterine blood flow
Inotropic agents[32,118-120]	Pregnancy does not alter the indications for digitalis therapy. An increased dose may be required to achieve acceptable serum levels. Digitalis crosses the placenta and is excreted in breast milk but fetal or infant toxicity is unusual.	Labor potentially earlier and shorter in women on digitalis
	Beta-stimulating or dopaminergic agents should be reserved for life-threatening situations.	May decrease uterine blood flow
Vasodilator agents[119,121,122]	Afterload-reducing agents: adverse fetal effects not reported with hydralazine. There is little experience during pregnancy with captopril, enalapril, clonidine, diazoxide.	Hypotension may jeopardize uterine blood flow
	Preload-reducing agents; nitrates indicated as in nonpregnant state. Nitroprusside justified in life-threatening situations. There is little experience with prazosin.	Concern about but no documentation of cyanide toxicity with nitroprusside
Antiarrhythmic agents[119,120,123]	Indications for use as in nonpregnant state. Greatest experience with quinidine but procainamide and disopyramide not clearly inferior. Lidocaine crosses placenta but no teratogenic effects reported. No information is available on tocainide, mexiletine, flecainide, or encainide.	Potential fetal dysrhythmias Phenytoin can cause fetal abnormalities and should be avoided
Beta-blocking agents[119,123,124]	May be used to treat hypertension, angina, and supraventricular tachyarrhythmias when there are no reasonable alternatives. Close fetal and newborn monitoring required. Selective beta$_1$ blockers may result in fewer adverse fetal effects.	May depress intrauterine growth Newborn bradycardia, hypotension, hypoglycemia, and respiratory depression
Calcium channel blockers[119,123-125]	Verapamil use as in nonpregnant state. There is little information on nifedipine and diltiazem.	
Anticoagulants[75,76,126]	Coumadin is *contraindicated* at time of conception and during pregnancy because of teratogenic effects and placental and fetal bleeding.	Teratogenic effect—10%–20% in first trimester
	When anticoagulation is required, heparin via subcutaneous administration at home is preferred. It does not cross the placenta.	Maternal, placental bleeding
	Acetylsalicylic acid may be used but there is some increased risk of bleeding.	Maternal plus fetal bleeding. Potential premature closure of ductus arteriosus by prostaglandin inhibition
	There is no reported experience with dipyridamole or sulfinpyrazone.	

activity and sodium limitation, standard medications should be used (Table 111.3).

Digitalis preparations are as effective during pregnancy as at other times although increased doses may be required to achieve acceptable serum levels.[32] These preparations do cross the placenta and are excreted in breast milk but have not resulted in recognized fetal or infant abnormalities. Although diuretics should not be used on a prophylactic basis or simply to treat pedal edema, they can be used for uncontrolled pulmonary vascular congestion. There is less experience with the use of vasodilator therapy during pregnancy but standard agents can be employed and have not been shown to jeopardize the fetus.

Correction of an underlying structural cardiac defect with surgery is rarely required during pregnancy. It should be reserved for life-threatening situations.

ARRHYTHMIAS

Pregnancy should not alter the indications for, or the approach to, arrhythmia management. It is preferable to avoid pharmacologic therapy but drugs should be used if a patient is particularly symptomatic or health is jeopardized. Arrhythmias cannot be attributed to pregnancy itself and their presence is an indication to consider underlying causes, some of which may be correctable.

The incidence of tachycardias is not clearly increased by pregnancy. The sinus rate increases progressively throughout pregnancy but it is unusual for a pregnant woman to have a rate at rest exceeding 100 beats per minute, and rates this fast indicate the need to look for a potentially correctable cause.

Atrial and ventricular tachyarrhythmias can be treated in a standard fashion (see drug profiles in Table 111.3). Direct-current cardioversion can be used without adverse fetal effects although fetal monitoring is advised at the time of the procedure.[33]

Management of bradycardias should not be influenced by the pregnancy. Unless they cause symptoms, treatment is generally not indicated. Women with congenital complete heart block can accomplish an uneventful and successful pregnancy.[34,35] If required, a temporary or permanent pacemaker can be inserted during pregnancy with no apparent increased risk to the fetus other than the exposure to radiation during fluoroscopy.[36]

Increased antepartum and intrapartum fetal monitoring has demonstrated a higher than expected incidence of *fetal arrhythmias*.[37–39] It is not clear that this occurs more commonly in women with heart disease. Tachyarrhythmias in the fetus can occasionally be treated by administration of drugs to the mother with placental transfer to the fetus.[40,41] Even transplacental electrical cardioversion for fetal dysrhythmias has been successful.[42] Fetal arrhythmia treatment should be considered when there is development of fetal ascites and edema, which is best detected by serial fetal ultrasonography, or when there is evidence of retardation of normal fetal growth. Fetal bradyarrhythmias are more likely than the tachyarrhythmias to be associated with congenital heart disease.[43–45] The likelihood of congenital heart block in the fetus or the newborn is increased if the mother has a collagen vascular disease.[46,47]

SUDDEN DECREASES IN CARDIAC OUTPUT

Because of the risks to both the mother and the fetus from this complication it is important to anticipate and prevent a sudden fall in cardiac output. It is a common and lethal complication in women with elevated pulmonary vascular resistance. During pregnancy, careful attention to venous return and to hydration is necessary, particularly at the time of labor, delivery, and in the puerperium. Fluid or blood loss should be replaced immediately when recognized.

INFECTIVE ENDOCARDITIS

The approach to the prevention and management of endocarditis should not be influenced by pregnancy. Antibiotic prophylaxis for the purpose of preventing bacterial endocarditis is indicated for the usual reasons.[48] Although the value of routine antibiotic prophylaxis at the time of labor and delivery is uncertain,[49,50] the high mortality associated with the infection and the relative safety of antibiotic prophylaxis lead us and others[51] to recommend its use beginning with labor and continuing for 24 hours following delivery. If endocarditis occurs, aggressive antibiotic therapy is warranted, and the usual indications for cardiac surgery apply, even during pregnancy (see below).

STRUCTURAL LESIONS REQUIRING URGENT CARDIAC SURGERY

Since the vast majority of structural abnormalities can be tolerated during pregnancy, cardiac surgery should be reserved for extreme cases.[52,53] Open heart surgery is associated with an increased fetal and maternal loss but it can be performed successfully if both the mother and the fetus are monitored closely.[54,55] Induced hypothermia appears to be safe during pregnancy.[54] Although there are no established rules, it seems appropriate to recommend an increase in extracorporeal pump flow during cardiac surgery at a somewhat higher level then usual, preferably to the range of 3 liters/min/m^2 without hypothermia and 2 liters/min/m^2 with adequate hypothermia.[56] Fetal monitoring for bradycardia should be instituted during the surgery.[57,58]

SPECIFIC CARDIAC ABNORMALITIES
VALVE DISEASE

A number of issues should be addressed each time a patient with valve disease is seen. These include attention to the hemodynamic status with measures for correction if it is not optimal, attention to the need for antibiotic prophylaxis at the time of dental or surgical procedures, attention to the need for antibiotic prophylaxis against rheumatic fever, a consideration of the need for anticoagulation, and the need to relate a patient's symptoms to her known heart disease. Finally, it is important to decide if diagnostic or therapeutic plans should be changed because the individual is pregnant or planning pregnancy. The woman of child-bearing age is unique and it may be necessary to change otherwise routine management because of this.

MITRAL STENOSIS

Although the incidence of rheumatic heart disease and the incidence of mitral stenosis are decreasing in the United States, they continue to be the leading cause of death from heart disease in young women throughout the world.[59,60] Women with mitral stenosis who are asymptomatic prior to pregnancy usually tolerate pregnancy well. Those with pulmonary congestion have an increased incidence of pulmonary edema and a higher mortality with pregnancy.[30] The risk of death is greatest during labor and in the postpartum period.[61] In addition to the risk of pulmonary edema, women with mitral stenosis are also in danger of sudden decreases in venous return with a resultant fall in cardiac output; hypovolemia should be avoided. If significant mitral stenosis is recognized prior to pregnancy, surgery is recommended, utilizing a mitral commissurotomy when possible.[62,63] If a prosthesis is required in a woman of child-bearing age, a tissue valve is preferable so that coumadin anticoagulation can be avoided despite the concerns of subsequent deterioration of the tissue valve.[64] If symptomatic pulmonary congestion occurs in a woman with mitral stenosis during pregnancy, standard medical therapy is appropriate with particular emphasis on limitation of physical activity including strict bed rest if necessary. If congestive heart failure is refractory to treatment, valve surgery can be performed during pregnancy.

MITRAL REGURGITATION

Most women with mitral regurgitation remain asymptomatic through the child-bearing years. If symptoms develop, limitation of sodium intake and activity is appropriate and, if necessary, standard medical treatment can be used. In our experience, surgical correction has never been required. Mitral regurgitation due to acute uncontrollable endocarditis or to an acute myocardial infarction may dictate the need for surgery.

AORTIC STENOSIS

Aortic valve stenosis is uncommon in women of child-bearing age and there is little experience with its effect on pregnancy. While well tolerated in some pregnant women,[30,65] a summary of the reports in the English literature[66] revealed a maternal mortality rate of 18%, with 40% of the deaths occurring at the time of therapeutic abortions. In addition, the spontaneous abortion rate was high. In one series of women with obstruction to left ventricular outflow, some of whom had aortic valve stenosis, there was no maternal mortality.[51] There was a high incidence of congenital heart disease in the live offspring of women with uncorrected obstruction to left ventricular outflow (37%) which declined to 16% when surgery was performed prior to pregnancy.[51] If a pregnant woman has the signs of aortic stenosis, an echo-Doppler study can support the diagnosis and help determine the severity. Even if the stenosis is considered severe, surgery during pregnancy is not appropriate in the asymptomatic woman. If symptoms develop and cannot be controlled with reduction of activity and medications, valve surgery or valvuloplasty is indicated.

AORTIC REGURGITATION

Like aortic stenosis, isolated aortic regurgitation (or mixed aortic regurgitation and stenosis) is uncommon in young women during pregnancy.[30,67] As with other regurgitant lesions, it is generally well tolerated during pregnancy. If arrhythmia or congestive heart failure develops it should be managed in the standard fashion. If aortic regurgitation develops suddenly as the result of bacterial endocarditis or aortic root dissection, emergency angiography and surgery must be performed even during pregnancy.[68-70]

PULMONIC VALVE DISEASE

Stenosis of the pulmonic valve is almost exclusively a congenital abnormality. With the increased recognition of pulmonic stenosis in childhood, the number of women reaching child-bearing age with this abnormality is increasingly fewer and much of the experience in relation to pregnancy comes from the older literature.[30,65,67,71] Even in these older series, no maternal deaths were reported during pregnancy, labor, or delivery.

If a patient with severe pulmonic stenosis develops severe right-sided heart failure or recurrent syncope, surgery or balloon valvuloplasty may be necessary.

There are variable reports about the incidence of congenital heart disease in the offspring of women with pulmonic stenosis. As many as 20% of infants born to women with obstructive lesions of the right ventricle may have congenital heart disease.[51] This incidence may be reduced if correction of the obstruction is achieved before pregnancy.[51]

Primary pulmonic insufficiency is so uncommon that there is no reported experience with pregnancy. In women who have undergone surgical correction of tetralogy of Fallot (as noted below), pregnancy can be well tolerated. Although all of these women have some pulmonic insufficiency, it appears not to cause problems for the mother or the child.

TRICUSPID VALVE DISEASE

Tricuspid stenosis is rare in the United States. It does occur occasionally in women with severe rheumatic heart disease involving also the aortic and mitral valves.[72] Experience during pregnancy is limited.[30]

Tricuspid regurgitation is also uncommon but the incidence is increasing due to the increasing abuse of intravenous drugs with resultant endocarditis of the tricuspid valve.[73] Doppler studies may reveal regurgitation not detected by physical examination.[74] There is no evidence that tricuspid regurgitation increases the risk during pregnancy and the lesion should be managed as in the nonpregnant woman.

PROSTHETIC HEART VALVE DISEASE

The woman who is pregnant or who is contemplating pregnancy is affected by and emphasizes a number of the features of prosthetic heart valve disease. Being young, a woman of child-bearing age should best receive a valve with proven longevity. The use of a mechanical prosthesis would seem optimal. However, all available mechanical prostheses require the use of warfarin anticoagulants. These drugs are contraindicated during pregnancy and at the time of conception because they cross the placenta and can cause congenital abnormalities.[75,76] Thus, when considering a prosthesis in a patient of this age group it is preferable to use a tissue valve with its lower association with thromboemboli even though it may not be as durable as a mechanical prosthesis.[77-80] Surgical repair of a patient's own valve is always preferable to replacement when this is possible.

There is some experience with prosthetic valve disease in pregnancy. Of interest, in three series[81,82] warfarin derivatives were used in women with mechanical prostheses. Although there was a high fetal loss in these series (up to 60%) the warfarin embryopathy syndrome was not seen in any live-born infants. This is not typical of others' experience.[83] Administration of the warfarin derivatives is associated with a 10% to 20% incidence of the warfarin embryopathy syndrome when the drugs are used in the first trimester.[75,76] The concern for this is greatest when coumadin is used in weeks 6 through 12 of the pregnancy.[83] Women with tissue prostheses have a lower incidence of fetal loss and have not required exposure to coumadin but they do have a significantly increased requirement for valve re-replacement in the two years after pregnancy.[80]

Management of women with prosthetic valves should include the use of antibiotic prophylaxis with dental and surgical procedures. Antibiotics are recommended with the onset of labor and should be continued for 48 hours after delivery. It is important to avoid coumadin use, particularly in the first trimester but preferably throughout pregnancy. Self-administered twice daily deep subcutaneous heparin administration is recommended throughout pregnancy. Some have advocated coumadin use in the middle trimester.[84]

CONGENITAL HEART DISEASE

It is increasingly common for infants with congenital heart disease to survive into the reproductive years. Many will have had corrective or palliative surgery and many will be able to have children. This, along with the decline in rheumatic fever, is making congenital heart disease increasingly important as the major form of heart disease in women considering pregnancy.

Some generalizations about management are appropriate. First, genetic counseling is essential. While congenital heart disease occurs in 0.8%[85] of children born in the United States, 4% to 20% of the offspring will be affected if either parent has congenital heart disease[51,85]; it is frequently the same cardiac abnormality as in the parent (see Table 111.2). Second, when congenital heart disease requiring correction is recognized, surgery should be performed prior to pregnancy. In addition to making pregnancy safer for the mother, it is likely to improve the environment for the fetus by optimizing uterine blood flow and oxygenation; this may decrease the chance that the child will be born with congenital heart disease.[51] Third, in this population fetal growth and development should be monitored carefully, particularly in women with cyanosis.

LESIONS IMPEDING BLOOD FLOW IN THE HEART OR GREAT VESSELS

The two most common abnormalities resulting in impedance of *left-sided* heart flow are aortic valve stenosis (previously discussed) and coarctation of the aorta.[30,86,87]

Maternal mortality associated with coarctation of the aorta ranges from 3% to 8%.[30,86,87] Death is most commonly due to dissection or rupture of the aorta.[88] On occasion it may be caused by complications from associated abnormalities, including an aneurysm of the circle of Willis in 10% (which may rupture),[89] aortic valve stenosis in 10%, a patent ductus arteriosus, ventricular septal defect, or a mitral valve deformity.

The majority of deaths occur prior to labor and delivery. The collateral vessels that develop as a result of a coarctation may make cesarean section particularly hazardous. (Cheitlin M: personal communication). Death from uncontrolled hemorrhage in a woman with an unrecognized coarctation has occurred. Pregnancy is less hazardous for women whose coarctation has been surgically corrected in childhood. When recognized in an adult, correction prior to pregnancy is preferable.[90] Fetal mortality with maternal coarctation approaches 20%. The incidence of subsequent congenital heart disease in the offspring of patients with obstruction of left ventricular outflow may exceed 20%; this can be diminished by one half with surgical correction prior to pregnancy.[51]

Obstruction to *right* ventricular outflow is uncommon as an isolated abnormality in women of child-bearing age. It can be the result of pulmonic valve stenosis (previously discussed) or rarely to isolated subpulmonic valve obstruction. When obstruction causes ventricular hypertrophy or symptoms, correction prior to pregnancy is recommended.

SHUNTS BETWEEN THE HEART CHAMBERS OR GREAT VESSELS

Women with an uncomplicated *left-to-right* shunt do well during pregnancy unless ventricular failure or arrhythmias complicate the lesion. *Right-to-left* shunts put the woman at substantial risk; when due to Eisenmenger's syndrome, maternal mortality can exceed 50%. The incidence of cardiac abnormalities in the offspring of women with a left-to-right shunt can approach 15%[51] and it is higher still in surviving infants of mothers with right-to-left shunts.

An *atrial septal defect* is a common site of shunting in women of child-bearing age and is well tolerated when uncomplicated by pulmonary hypertension or heart failure. Since the resistances of the pulmonary and peripheral vascular circuits decrease equally during pregnancy, there is no significant change in the degree of shunting during pregnancy. Unless severe pulmonary hypertension is suspected, an atrial septal defect recognized during pregnancy requires no further evaluation until after the postpartum period. Women who have had surgical correction of an atrial septal defect also tolerate pregnancy well but their children continue to have approximately a 4% to 5% chance of congenital heart disease.[51,91]

A ventricular septal defect is also well tolerated during pregnancy.[30,51] No treatment is required during pregnancy unless the lesion is complicated by pulmonary hypertension, heart failure, or arrhythmias. The incidence of congenital heart disease in offspring can exceed 15%, with approximately half of these being ventricular septal defects.[52]

Patency of the *ductus arteriosus*, when uncomplicated, is unlikely to influence a pregnancy. If the lesion is recognized prior to pregnancy, surgical closure is recommended.

COMBINED LESIONS: SHUNTS PLUS OBSTRUCTIVE LESIONS

This combination of abnormalities is generally associated with cyanosis. Women with uncorrected lesions can become pregnant but the pregnancy is associated with a high maternal morbidity and mortality and with a high rate of fetal loss. Whenever possible, surgical repair before pregnancy is recommended.

If a woman is first recognized to have complex congenital heart disease during pregnancy and is cyanotic, accurate evaluation is essential; pulmonary hypertension, if present, requires interruption of the pregnancy for maternal safety. Even in the absence of pulmonary hypertension, cyanosis that results in a maternal hematocrit exceeding 60% increases maternal risks and is virtually incompatible with fetal survival. Interruption of the pregnancy is advisable. If this is not acceptable, women with cyanotic congenital heart disease involving both shunts and obstruction should be followed closely; activity should be restricted below that causing symptoms, chronic oxygen administration at 3 to 4 liters/min by nasal prongs is recommended, and venous pooling and major changes in vascular resistance should be avoided.

TETRALOGY OF FALLOT

This is the most common of the cyanotic congenital heart diseases compatible with survival into adulthood and with pregnancy. Women can survive pregnancy with an uncorrected tetralogy of Fallot but maternal morbidity and fetal loss are high, especially if the hematocrit is above 60 and right ventricular pressure exceeds 120 mm Hg.[30,71,92–94] Because of this, pregnancy should be discouraged until after surgery. Surgical correction of tetralogy of Fallot, either in childhood or in the adult, increases the safety of pregnancy.[23,30,93,94] In one series of 18 women, there was no maternal mortality with 40 pregnancies. There were 5 therapeutic and 5 spontaneous abortions in this group but only one of the live-born offspring had congenital heart disease.[91]

If a patient with tetralogy of Fallot becomes pregnant, interruption is advised for maternal safety. If this is not accepted or if the pregnancy has progressed beyond 12 weeks, surgical correction of the maternal cardiac lesion may be preferable. It is not clear that this type of heart surgery carries greater risk for the woman who is pregnant and fetal loss is high even without surgery.

EBSTEIN'S ANOMALY

This congenital abnormality may also be associated with significant obstruction and shunting; in the mild form with little obstruction and shunting it may go unrecognized both before and during pregnancy. When severe, it increases the risk associated with pregnancy, but successful pregnancies have been reported.[95] When pregnancy does occur in a patient with uncorrected Ebstein's anomaly it is important to maintain adequate venous return in order to sustain pulmonary blood flow.

TRANSPOSITION OF THE GREAT ARTERIES

Even this complex abnormality can be associated with a successful pregnancy.[96] There is very little experience with pregnancy in women with this abnormality but surgical correction is recommended prior to the woman becoming pregnant. In the nonoperated patient, severe cyanosis or symptoms are a reason to consider interruption of the pregnancy.

DEVELOPMENTAL ABNORMALITIES

Some cardiac lesions have a genetic component but are not apparent in childhood. Because they are either common or possibly could cause difficulty during pregnancy, it is appropriate to discuss them. These include the prolapsing mitral valve syndrome, idiopathic hypertrophic subaortic stenosis, and Marfan's syndrome.

Mitral valve prolapse is common in young women and therefore is frequently associated with pregnancy. The changes in volume and hemodynamics may change the physical examination findings. There is no evidence that any of the uncommon complications of prolapse (arrhythmias, endocarditis, or emboli) is more likely to occur during pregnancy.[97,98] Management during pregnancy should not differ from that in the nonpregnant state.

Idiopathic hypertrophic subaortic stenosis (IHSS) is transmitted as an autosomal dominant trait; thus, 50% of the offspring will be affected. It is appropriate to be concerned that the normal hemodynamic changes of pregnancy could adversely affect the woman with IHSS. Although the increased blood volume might be considered beneficial, the fall in arterial blood pressure and the tendency to sudden decreases in venous return are potential dangers. Additionally, changing circulating catecholamine levels, especially at the time of labor and delivery, could be detrimental. Although symptoms may increase, pregnancy in women with IHSS is generally well tolerated.[99] Management of IHSS during pregnancy should not differ from that at other times although it is particularly important to avoid sudden hypovolemia. Beta blockers may be used for persistent symptoms but routine use should be avoided because of possible depression of fetal growth; use of selective beta$_1$-blocking agents is less likely to affect the fetus adversely. In a symptomatic woman, nifedipine or verapamil may reduce left ventricular compliance and favorably affect symptoms.

Pregnancy with *Marfan's syndrome* is complicated. First, because Marfan's syndrome is transmitted as an autosomal dominant trait, half of the offspring will inherit the syndrome. Second, the life span of the mother will be shortened, with 50% of affected women dying before age 40.[100] Most importantly, pregnancy is a particularly high-risk event for these women, with death from aortic root dissection or rupture being common. While some have shown a low incidence of maternal mortality,[101] there are a large number of reports of maternal death with pregnancy. Because of this we advise women with Marfan's syndrome to avoid pregnancy, and should they become pregnant, we discuss pregnancy interruption. The risk of maternal death may increase when the aortic root diameter exceeds 40 mm as measured by echocardiography.[101] When a woman with Marfan's syndrome accepts the risks of pregnancy, physical activity restriction and beta-blocking agents are used on theoretical grounds.

DISEASES OF THE MYOCARDIUM

The classification of myocardial diseases is difficult even unrelated to pregnancy. Myocardial disease occurring as the result of pregnancy makes classification even more difficult. Whether associated with, or caused by, the pregnancy, myocardial dysfunction is associated with significant maternal risk.

MYOCARDITIS

The pregnant woman has no clear increase in susceptibility to myocarditis but it can occur during gestation and in the postpartum period. In one series of 34 patients with myocarditis, 12 patients were women and in five of these the myocarditis was associated with pregnancy.[102] When the myocarditis causes heart failure or arrhythmias, treatment should be carried out in the standard fashion. As in the nonpregnant state, it is not clear that further intervention will be of benefit to the woman with myocarditis. On occasion anti-inflammatory agents have been used in this group.[102,103]

DILATED CARDIOMYOPATHY

Women of child-bearing age can develop a dilated cardiomyopathy. In the woman symptomatic with heart failure who has a persistently enlarged heart, the risks to the mother are sufficient to advise avoidance of pregnancy. If the cardiomyopathy is first recognized during pregnancy, endomyocardial biopsy should be considered to search for a potentially reversible cause, a myocarditis; the value of treatment of inflammation, however, is as yet unproven.[102-104]

When a dilated cardiomyopathy is first recognized late in pregnancy or in the postpartum period, it is considered a "peripartum cardiomyopathy." Because of the tendency to develop late in pregnancy, it appears that this is a distinct entity from other dilated cardiomyopathies and is presumably the result of the pregnancy.[105,106] The etiology is unclear but endomyocardial biopsy results in a very few patients have suggested that myocarditis is the cause in some.[102,103] The syndrome occurs often but not exclusively in lower socioeconomic groups, in black women, and in older multiparous women.[106-108] Treatment should be directed toward the complications of a cardiomyopathy. If a woman continues to have cardiomegaly with symptoms following pregnancy, further pregnancies should be discouraged.

CORONARY ARTERY DISEASE

Chest pain is a common symptom during pregnancy and is most commonly due to rib cage dynamics, a hiatal hernia, or esophagitis. Still, coronary artery disease can occur in pregnancy. It can on occasion be due to atherosclerosis[109] and the risk of this may be increased by the use of oral contraceptives, particularly in women who smoke.[15,110-112] Other mechanisms include coronary emboli, coronary spasm, or coronary artery dissection.[113,114] If a myocardial infarction occurs, the patient should be treated in the coronary care unit in the usual manner. If the woman is asymptomatic following the infarction, further evaluation is not appropriate until the conclusion of the pregnancy. Angina should be treated with standard medical therapy and only if this fails to relieve symptoms should diagnostic procedures be undertaken. If angina cannot be controlled during pregnancy, angioplasty or coronary bypass surgery can be performed.[115]

REFERENCES

1. Ueland K, Novy MJ, Peterson EN, Metcalfe J: Maternal cardiovascular dynamics: IV. The influence of gestational age on the maternal cardiovascular response to posture and exercise. Am J Obstet Gynecol 104:856, 1969
2. Lees MM, Taylor SH, Scott DB, Kerr MG: A study of cardiac output at rest throughout pregnancy. J Obstet Gynaecol Br Commonw 74:319, 1967
3. Ueland K, Gills RE, Hansen J: Maternal cardiovascular dynamics: I. Cesarean section under subarachnoid block anesthesia. Am J Obstet Gynecol 100:42, 1968
4. Lindheimer MD, Katz AI: Sodium and diuretics in pregnancy. N Engl J Med 288:891, 1973
5. Wood JE: The cardiovascular effects of oral contraceptives. Mod Concepts Cardiovasc Dis 41:37, 1972
6. Keates JD, FitzGerald DE: Limb volume and blood flow changes during the menstrual cycle: I. Limb volume changes during the menstrual cycle. Angiology 20:618, 1969
7. Burg JR, Dodek A, Kloster FE, Metcalfe J: Alterations of systolic time intervals during pregnancy. Circulation 49:560, 1974
8. Liebson PR, Mann LI, Evans MI et al: Cardiac performance during pregnancy: Serial evaluation using external systolic time intervals. Am J Obstet Gynecol 122:1, 1975
9. Katz R, Karliner JS, Resnik R: Effects of a natural volume overload state (pregnancy) on left ventricular performance in normal human subjects. Circulation 58:434, 1978
10. Rubler S, Damani PM, Pinto ER: Cardiac size and performance during pregnancy estimated with echocardiography. Am J Cardiol 40:534, 1977
11. Hart MV, Hosenpud JD, Hohimer AR, Morton MJ: Hemodynamics during pregnancy and sex steroid administration in the guinea pig. Am J Physiol, *in press*
12. Abel EL: Smoking during pregnancy: A review of effects on growth and development of offspring. Hum Biol 52:593, 1980
13. Elliot J: Maternal smoking and the fetus: One fear buried but others arise. JAMA 241:867, 1979
14. Baird DD, Wilcox AJ: Cigarette smoking associated with delayed conception. JAMA 253:2979, 1985
15. Slone D, Shapiro S, Rosenberg L et al: Risk of myocardial infarction in relation to current and discontinued use of oral contraceptives. N Engl J Med 305:420, 1981
16. Nieberg P, Marks JS, McLaren NM, Remington PL: The fetal tobacco syndrome. JAMA 253:2998, 1985
17. Loser H, Majewski F: Type and frequency of cardiac defects in embryofetal alcohol syndrome: Report of 16 cases. Br Heart J 39:1374, 1977
18. Amarose AP: Chromosome aberrations in the mother and the newborn from drug-addiction pregnancies. J Reprod Med 20:323, 1978
19. Robinson DS: Evaluation of drugs used in pregnancy and pediatric age groups. Ann Intern Med 82:841, 1975
20. Schwartz DB, Schamroth L: The effect of pregnancy on the frontal plane QRS axis. Journal of Electrocardiography 12:279, 1979
21. Capizzi RL: Hematologic neoplasms during pregnancy. In Brodsky I, Kahn SB, Moyer JH (eds): Cancer Chemotherapy II: The 22nd Hahnemann Symposium, pp 131–146. New York, Grune & Stratton, 1972
22. Sternberg J: Irradiation and radiocontamination during pregnancy. Am J Obstet Gynecol 108:590, 1970
23. Sweet DL Jr, Kinzie J: Consequences of radiotherapy and antineoplastic therapy for the fetus. J Reprod Med 17:241, 1976
24. Dekaban A: Abnormalities in children exposed to x-radiation during various stages of gestation: Tentative timetable of radiation injury to the human fetus: Part I. J Nucl Med 9:471, 1968
25. Mossman KL, Hill LT: Radiation risks in pregnancy. Obstet Gynecol 60:237, 1982
26. Barron WM: The pregnant surgical patients: Medical evaluation and management. Ann Intern Med 101:683, 1984
27. Mitchell MS, Capizzi RL: Neoplastic diseases. In Burrow GN, Ferris TF (eds): Medical Complications During Pregnancy, 2nd ed, pp 510–537. Philadelphia, WB Saunders, 1972
28. Elkayam U, Gleicher N: Primary pulmonary hypertension and pregnancy. In Elkayam U, Gleicher N (eds): Cardiac Problems in Pregnancy, pp 153–160. New York, Alan R Liss, 1982
29. McCaffrey RN, Dunn LJ: Primary pulmonary hypertension in pregnancy.

30. Szekely P, Snaith L: Heart Disease and Pregnancy. Edinburgh, Churchill Livingston, 1974
31. Nielsen NC, Fabricius J: Primary pulmonary hypertension with special reference to prognosis. Acta Med Scand 170:731, 1961
32. Rogers MC, Willerson JT, Goldblatt A, Smith TW: Serum digoxin concentrations in the human fetus, neonate, and infant. N Engl J Med 287:1010, 1972
33. Schroeder JS, Harrison DC: Repeated cardioversion during pregnancy: Treatment of refractory paroxysmal atrial tachycardia during 3 successive pregnancies. Am J Cardiol 27:445, 1971
34. Kenmure ACB, Cameron AJV: Congenital complete heart block in pregnancy. Br Heart J 29:910, 1967
35. Esscher EB: Congenital complete heart block in adolescence and adult life: A follow-up study. Eur Heart J 2:281, 1981
36. Ginns HM, Hollinrake K: Complete heart block in pregnancy treated with an internal cardiac pacemaker. J Obstet Gynaecol Br Commonw 77:710, 1970
37. Schreiner RL, Hurwitz RA, Rosenfeld CR, Miller W: Atrial tachyarrhythmias associated with massive edema in the newborn. J Perinat Med 6:274, 1978
38. Klapholz H, Schifrin BS, Rivo E: Paroxysmal supraventricular tachycardia in the fetus. Obstet Gynecol 43:718, 1974
39. Klein AM, Holzman IR, Austin EM: Fetal tachycardia prior to the development of hydrops—attempted pharmacologic cardioversion: Case report. Am J Obstet Gynecol 134:347, 1979
40. Teuscher A, Bossi E, Imhof P et al: Effect of propranolol on fetal tachycardia in diabetic pregnancy. Am J Cardiol 42:304, 1978
41. Kerenyi TD, Gleicher N, Meller J et al: Transplacental cardioversion of intrauterine supraventricular tachycardia with digitalis. Lancet 2:393, 1980
42. Meitus ML: Fetal electrocardiography and cardioversion with direct current countershock: Report of a case. Dis Chest 48:324, 1965
43. Schneider H, Weinstein HM, Young BK: Fetal trigeminal rhythm. Obstet Gynecol (Suppl) 50:58, 1977
44. Gochberg SH: Congenital heart block. Am J Obstet Gynecol 88:238, 1964
45. Teteris NJ, Chisholm JW, Ullery JC: Antenatal diagnosis of congenital heart block: Report of a case. Obstet Gynecol 32:851, 1968
46. McCue CM, Mantakas ME, Tingelstad JB, Ruddy S: Congenital heart block in newborns of mothers with connective tissue disease. Circulation 56:82, 1977
47. Chameides L, Truex RC, Vetter V et al: Association of maternal systemic lupus erythematosus with congenital complete heart block. N Engl J Med 297:1204, 1977
48. Kaplan EL, Anthony BF, Bisno A et al: Prevention of bacterial endocarditis. Circulation 56:139A, 1977
49. Fleming HA: Antibiotic prophylaxis against infective endocarditis after delivery. Lancet 1:144, 1977
50. Sugrue D, Blake S, Troy P, MacDonald D: Antibiotic prophylaxis against infective endocarditis after normal delivery—is it necessary? Br Heart J 44:499, 1980
51. Whittemore R, Hobbins JC, Engle MA: Pregnancy and its outcome in women with and without surgical treatment of congenital heart disease. Am J Cardiol 50:641, 1982
52. Whittemore R: Congenital heart disease: Its impact on pregnancy. Hosp Pract 18:65, 1983
53. Collins HA, Daniel RA Jr, Scott HW Jr: Cardiac surgery during pregnancy. Ann Thorac Surg 5:300, 1968
54. Matsuki A, Oyama T: Operation under hypothermia in a pregnant woman with an intracranial arteriovenous malformation. Can Anaesth Soc J 19:184, 1972
55. Levy DL, Warriner RA III, Burgess GE III: Fetal response to cardiopulmonary bypass. Obstet Gynecol 56:112, 1980
56. Estafanous FG, Buckley S: Management of anesthesia for open heart surgery during pregnancy. Cleve Clin Q 43:121, 1976
57. Koh KS, Friesen RM, Livingstone RA, Peddle LJ: Fetal monitoring during maternal cardiac surgery with cardiopulmonary bypass. Can Med Assoc J 112:1102, 1975
58. Trimakas AP, Maxwell KD, Berkay S et al: Fetal monitoring during cardiopulmonary bypass for removal of a left atrial myxoma during pregnancy. Johns Hopkins Med J 144:156, 1979
59. Padmavati S: Rheumatic fever and rheumatic heart disease in developing countries. Bull WHO 56:543, 1978
60. Stollerman GH: Connective tissue disease of the cardiovascular system. In Braunwald E (ed): Heart Disease, 4th ed, pp 1723–1770. Philadelphia, WB Saunders, 1988
61. Jones M: Heart disease in pregnancy. Proc R Soc Med 52:767, 1959
62. Schenker JG, Polishuk WZ: Pregnancy following mitral valvotomy: A survey of 182 patients. Obstet Gynecol 32:214, 1968
63. Wallace WA, Harken DE, Ellis LB: Pregnancy following closed mitral valvuloplasty. A long-term study with remarks concerning the necessity for careful cardiac management. JAMA 217:297, 1971
64. Limet R, Grondin CM: Cardiac valve prostheses, anticoagulation, and pregnancy. Ann Thorac Surg 23:337, 1977
65. Howitt G: Heart disease and pregnancy. Practitioner 206:765, 1971
66. Arias F, Pineda J: Aortic stenosis and pregnancy. J Reprod Med 20:229, 1978
67. Metcalf J, McAnulty JH, Veland K: Burwell and Metcalf's Heart Disease and Pregnancy: Physiology and Management, 2nd ed, pp 203–206. Boston, Little, Brown & Co, 1986
68. Wheat MW Jr: Acute dissecting aneurysm of the aorta: Diagnosis and treatment—1979. Am Heart J 99:373, 1980
69. Wilson WR, Danielson GK, Giuliani ER et al: Valve replacement in patients with active infective endocarditis. Circulation 58:585, 1978
70. Richardson JV, Karp RB, Kirklin JW, Dismukes WE: Treatment of infective endocarditis: A 10-year comparative analysis. Circulation 58:589, 1978
71. Mendelson CL: Cardiac Disease in Pregnancy: Medical Care, Cardiovascular Surgery, and Obstetrical Management as Related to Maternal and Fetal Welfare, p 135. Philadelphia, FA Davis, 1960
72. Morgan JR, Forker AD, Coates JR, Myers WS: Isolated tricuspid stenosis. Circulation 44:729, 1971
73. Dreyer NP, Fields BN: Heroin-associated infective endocarditis. A report of 28 cases. Ann Intern Med 78:699, 1973
74. Limacher MC, Ware JA, O'Meara ME et al: Tricuspid regurgitation due to pregnancy: Two-dimensional and pulsed Doppler echocardiographic observations. Am J Cardiol 55:1059, 1985
75. Hall JG, Pauli RM, Wilson KM: Maternal and fetal sequelae of anticoagulation during pregnancy. Am J Med 91:808, 1977
76. Stevenson RE, Burton OM, Ferlauto GJ, Taylor HA: Hazards of oral anticoagulants during pregnancy. JAMA 243:1549, 1980
77. Kutshe LM, Oyer P, Shumway N, Baum D: An important complication of Hancock mitral valve replacement in children. Circulation 60(Suppl 1):198, 1979
78. Geha AS, Laks H, Stansel HC Jr et al: Late failure of porcine heterografts in children. J Thorac Cardiovasc Surg 78:351, 1979
79. Sanders SP, Freed MD, Norwood WI et al: Early failure of porcine valves implanted in children. Am J Cardiol 45:499, 1980
80. McAnulty JH, Blair N, Walance C, Ueland K: Prosthetic heart valves and pregnancy: Maternal and infant outcome (abstr). J Am Coll Cardiol 7:171A, 1986
81. Ibarra-Perez C, Arevalo-Toledo N, Alvarez-De la Cadena O, Noriega-Guerra L: The course of pregnancy in patients with artificial heart valves. Am J Med 61:504, 1976
82. Lutz DJ, Noller KL, Spittell JA Jr et al: Pregnancy and its complications following cardiac valve prostheses. Am J Obstet Gynecol 131:460, 1978
83. Iturbe-Alessio I, Fonesco MC, Mutchinik O et al: Risk of anticoagulant therapy in pregnant women with artificial heart valves. N Engl J Med 315:1390, 1986
84. Lee P-K, Wang RYC, Chow JSF et al: Combined use of warfarin and adjusted subcutaneous heparin during pregnancy in patients with an artificial heart valve. J Am Coll Cardiol 8:221, 1986
85. Nora JJ, Nora AH: The evolution of specific genetic and environmental counseling in congenital heart disease. Circulation 57:205, 1978
86. Deal K, Wooley CF: Coarctation of the aorta and pregnancy. Ann Intern Med 78:706, 1973
87. Barash PG, Hobbins JC, Hook R et al: Management of coarctation of the aorta during pregnancy. J Thorac Cardiovasc Surg 69:781, 1975
88. Goodwin JF: Pregnancy and coarctation of the aorta. Clin Obstet Gynecol 4:645, 1961
89. Maron BJ, Humphries JO, Rowe RD, Mellits ED: Prognosis of surgically corrected coarctation of the aorta: A twenty-year postoperative appraisal. Circulation 47:119, 1973
90. Mortensen JD, Ellsworth HS: Coarctation of the aorta and pregnancy. Obstetric and cardiovascular complications before and after surgical correction. JAMA 191:596, 1965
91. Morris C, Menashe VD: Recurrence of congenital heart disease in offspring of parents with surgical correction (abstr). Clin Res 33:68A, 1985
92. Higgins CB, Mulder DG: Tetralogy of Fallot in the adult. Am J Cardiol 29:837, 1972
93. Batson GA: Cyanotic congenital heart disease and pregnancy. J Obstet Gynaecol Br Commonw 81:549, 1974
94. Loh TF, Tan NC: Fallot's tetralogy and pregnancy: A report of a successful pregnancy after complete correction. Med J Aust 2:141, 1971
95. Kahler RL: Cardiac disease. In Burrow GN, Ferris TF (eds): Medical Complications During Pregnancy, pp 105–149. Philadelphia, WB Saunders, 1975
96. Neilson G, Galea EG, Blunt A: Congenital heart disease and pregnancy. Med J Aust 1:1086, 1970
97. Haas JM: The effect of pregnancy on the midsystolic click and murmurs of the prolapsing posterior leaflet of the mitral valve. Am Heart J 92:407, 1976
98. Devereux RB, Perloff JK, Reichek N, Josephson MD: Mitral valve prolapse. Circulation 54:3, 1976
99. Kolibash AJ, Ruiz DE, Lewis RP: Idiopathic hypertrophic subaortic stenosis in pregnancy. Ann Intern Med 82:791, 1975
100. Pyeritz RE, McKusick VA: The Marfan syndrome: Diagnosis and management. N Engl J Med 300:772, 1979
101. Pyeritz RE: Maternal and fetal complications of pregnancy in the Marfan syndrome. Am J Med 71:784, 1981
102. Fenoglio JJ, Ursell PC, Kellogg CF et al: Diagnosis and classification of myocarditis by endomyocardial biopsy. N Engl J Med 308:12, 1983
103. Melvin KR, Richardson PJ, Olsen EGJ et al: Peripartum cardiomyopathy due to myocarditis. N Engl J Med 307:731, 1982
104. Hosenpud JD, McAnulty JH, Niles NR: Lack of objective improvement in systolic function in patients with myocarditis treated with azathioprine and prednisone. J Am Coll Cardiol 6:797, 1985
105. Homans DC: Peripartum cardiomyopathy. N Engl J Med 312:1432, 1985

106. O'Connell JB, Costanzo-Nordin MR, Subtamanian R et al: Peripartum cardiomyopathy: Clinical, hemodynamic, histologic and prognostic characteristics. J Am Coll Cardiol 8:52, 1986
107. Walsh JJ, Burch GE, Black WC et al: Idiopathic myocardiopathy of the puerperium (postpartal heart disease). Circulation 32:19, 1965
108. Demakis JG, Rahimtoola SH: Peripartum cardiomyopathy. Circulation 44:964, 1971
109. Ginz B: Myocardial infarction in pregnancy. J Obstet Gynaecol Br Commonw 77:610, 1970
110. Slone D, Shapiro S, Rosenberg L et al: Relation of cigarette smoking to myocardial infarction in young women. N Engl J Med 298:1273, 1978
111. Maleki M, Lange RL: Coronary thrombosis in young women on oral contraceptives: Report of two cases and review of the literature. Am Heart J 85:749, 1973
112. Rosenberg L, Kaufman DW, Helmrich SP et al: Myocardial infarction and cigarette smoking in women younger than 50 years of age. JAMA 253:2965, 1985
113. Jewett JF: Two dissecting coronary-artery aneurysms postpartum. N Engl J Med 298:1255, 1978
114. Beary JF, Summer WR, Bulkley BH: Postpartum acute myocardial infarction: A rare occurrence of uncertain etiology. Am J Cardiol 43:158, 1979
115. Majdan JF, Walinsky P, Cowchock SF et al: Coronary artery bypass surgery during pregnancy. Am J Cardiol 52:1145, 1983
116. Gant NF, Madden JD, Siiteri PK, MacDonald PC: The metabolic clearance rate of dehydroisoandrosterone sulfate. IV. Acute effects of induced hypertension, hypotension, and anuresis in normal and hypertensive pregnancies. Am J Obstet Gynecol 124:143, 1976
117. Maclean AB, Doig JR, Aickin DR: Hypovolemia, pre-eclampsia and diuretics. Br J Obstet Gynaecol 85:597, 1978
118. Chan V, Tse TF, Wang V: Transfer of digoxin across the placenta and into breast milk. Br J Obstet Gynaecol 85:605, 1978
119. Tamari I, Eldar M, Rabinowitz B, Neufeld HN: Medical treatment of cardiovascular disorders during pregnancy. Am Heart J 104:1357, 1982
120. Brinkman CR 3rd, Woods JR Jr: Effects of cardiovascular drugs during pregnancy. Cardiovasc Med 1:231, 1976
121. Ferris TF: Toxemia and hypertension. In Burrow GN, Ferris TF (eds): Medical Complications During Pregnancy, 2nd ed, pp 1–35. Philadelphia, WB Saunders, 1982
122. Drayer JIM, Weber MA: The use of antihypertensive drugs. In Elkayam U, Gleicher N (eds): Cardiac Problems in Pregnancy, pp 245–260. New York, Alan R Liss, 1982
123. Rotmensch HH, Elkayam U, Frishman W: Antiarrhythmic drug therapy during pregnancy. Ann Intern Med 98:487, 1983
124. Rubin DC: Beta-blockers in pregnancy. N Engl J Med 305:1323, 1981
125. Ueland K, McAnulty JH, Ueland FR, Metcalfe J: Special considerations in the use of cardiovascular drugs. In Ueland K, Beck WW (eds): Clinical Obstetrics and Gynecology, pp 809–823. New York, Harper & Row, 1981
126. Stuart MJ, Gross SJ, Elrad H, Graeber SE: Effects of acetylsalicylic-acid ingestion on maternal and neonatal hemostasis. N Engl J Med 307:909, 1982

THE ELDERLY PATIENT WITH CARDIOVASCULAR DISEASE

Nanette Kass Wenger

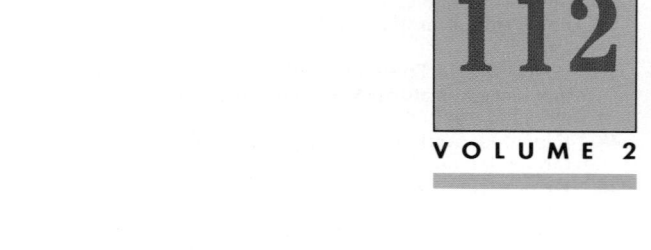

CHAPTER 112
VOLUME 2

The presentation of cardiovascular disease in elderly patients reflects both its superimposition on the physiologic processes and structural changes of aging that occur in the cardiovascular system and its typical association with multiple disorders affecting other organ systems, which also may have functional compromise related to aging.

The changes in cardiac function that occur with aging may potentiate the disease-related impairment of cardiovascular performance. There is an increase in vascular stiffness, increasing the impedance to left ventricular ejection, prolongation of the cardiac contraction and relaxation times, decreased sympathetic (catecholamine) responsiveness, and decreased myocardial compliance. No age-related changes occur in resting cardiac output, end-diastolic or end-systolic volumes, or ejection fraction. Even with vigorous exercise, cardiac output is not altered with age. However, there is an age-related increase in end-diastolic volume and stroke volume, emphasizing the dependence of the increase in stroke volume on diastolic filling. There is an age-related decrease in exercise heart rate and exercise ejection fraction.[1] This decrease in intrinsic heart rate with aging is independent of habitual physical activity. However, the maximal oxygen uptake of elderly sedentary individuals is from 10% to 20% less than that of their physically active counterparts.

These changes of aging, as well as the decrease in maximal oxygen uptake, decrease the functional reserve capacity of the heart and result in a diminished capacity for work and a lessened ability to tolerate a variety of stresses. The resting filling pressures of the heart are not significantly altered with aging, but there is an accentuated pressure rise with exercise as an adjustment to decreased myocardial wall distensibility; this, combined with the increase in left ventricular mass with aging, places the aged heart at a mechanical disadvantage. The increased filling pressure with exercise compensates for the decrease in myocardial compliance and enables the ventricles to increase their stroke volume.[1] Nevertheless, the ejection fraction may decrease with exercise in elderly subjects, even in the absence of heart disease. The rate of early diastolic left ventricular filling may decrease by as much as 50% with aging, reflecting decreased ventricular compliance; the increased late diastolic left ventricular filling mediated by atrial contraction helps preserve overall diastolic volume.

The number of disorders affecting the heart also increases progressively with age[2]; there may be associated protein–calorie malnutrition, and an increased likelihood of adverse drug reactions is encountered. These variables reinforce the observation that chronologic age among the elderly poorly predicts physiologic age and functional ability.

Despite the prominent decrease in cardiovascular mortality in the United States in recent years, the impact has been less in the elderly population because of the increasing number of individuals in this population group; 11% of the US population is currently age 65 or older, and about half of these 25 million people have cardiovascular disease. Cardiovascular disease remains a major cause of death in the elderly; in addition, as a major contributor to the disability of elderly individuals, it exerts an enormous impact on the need for hospital, ambulatory, and custodial care.[3,4] Atherosclerotic coronary heart disease is the most prevalent cardiac problem, followed by hypertensive cardiovascular disease. Other important etiologies include valvular heart disease and pulmonary heart disease.

The more common cardiovascular problems encountered in elderly patients are discussed in this chapter; despite their frequency and significant contribution both to morbidity and to health care costs, cerebrovascular disease and peripheral vascular disease are not addressed.

DIAGNOSIS AND FUNCTIONAL ASSESSMENT

APPROACH TO DIAGNOSIS

When blood pressure is measured in the elderly, it is essential to document the effect of postural change because of the frequent occurrence of orthostatic hypotension.[5,6] Disease and medications, rather than aging, account for the preponderance of postural hypotension—a relatively uncommon finding in healthy elderly persons.[7] The increased vascular stiffness renders peripheral arterial pulsations characteristically, and at times factitiously, brisk; this includes the carotid arterial pulsation. The increased ventricular filling pressure with aging, reflecting a decrease in ventricular compliance, is responsible for the S_4; neither the increased filling pressure nor the S_4 are evidence of heart failure. The presence of an S_3 suggests heart failure. S_2 is often single in the elderly patient, or there is less prominent inspiratory splitting. The apical impulse, even in patients with left ventricular hypertrophy, may not be readily palpated owing to a combination of chest wall alterations and emphysema. Soft, spindle-shaped, early peaking, basal systolic murmurs may reflect dilatation of the ascending aorta and/or decreased aortic compliance[8] or may be due to aortic vascular sclerosis.

Elderly patients are at increased risk for complications of most diagnostic procedures. However, because co-morbidity and the physiologic and mental consequences of aging, illness, and drug therapy limit the information available from the history and physical examination, diagnostic tests assume greater importance.

As in younger cardiac patients, noninvasive diagnostic methods should be initially selected, with echocardiography and particularly echo-Doppler studies often of value. Treadmill exercise testing, particularly with a low-level or intermittent protocol, may be feasible for selected elderly patients; alternatively, arm ergometry may be considered for patients in whom musculoskeletal problems, instability, or claudication limit treadmill exercise testing. Exercise thallium scintigraphy may be helpful when electrocardiographic conduction abnormalities or repolarization changes related to left ventricular hypertrophy or digitalis use limit the interpretation of the exercise electrocardiogram; the presence and extent of exercise-induced thallium-201 scan abnormalities are described to effectively stratify elderly patients into different risk groups.[9] Myocardial perfusion scintigraphy after intravenous administration of dipyridamole (Persantine) is well tolerated by aged patients and may help identify myocardial ischemia in elderly patients unable to exercise.[10] Nevertheless, it is important to appreciate that cardiovascular catheterization and coronary arteriography are well tolerated in the elderly and may be an important procedure both because cardiovascular surgery can be selected if appropriate and because a precise diagnosis may enable more successful therapy.

FUNCTIONAL ASSESSMENT

The combination of the increased life expectancy and the progressively increased proportion of aged persons in the population, many of whom have reasonably well-maintained levels of function, mandates an approach to assess their capacity for suitable vocational and recreational or leisure activities. Remunerative work continuing into the eighth decade may soon be usual and, since deconditioning due to inactivity occurs more rapidly in the elderly, encouraging recreational and leisure activities is also important.

Both the physiologic characteristics of aging and the superimposed limitations due to cardiovascular dysfunction must be considered in formulating recommendations for activity for elderly patients. Inappropriate prolonged activity restriction imposed for a variety of medical problems accelerates the progressive limitation of cardiovascular functional capacity with aging and often threatens the independent life-style of elderly individuals. The institution of a suitable physical activity regimen, even in previously sedentary elderly patients, can often improve their endurance and functional capacity.[11]

ATHEROSCLEROTIC CORONARY HEART DISEASE

Atherosclerotic coronary heart disease is the most prevalent cardiac disease in the aged and responsible for more than two thirds of all cardiac deaths in the elderly population. Although coronary atherosclerosis is almost uniformly present at autopsy examination of elderly patients, many of these persons have never had clinical manifestations of myocardial ischemia. The male predominance in the occurrence of myocardial infarction and in mortality from atherosclerotic coronary heart disease decreases with age; there is an essentially equal sex incidence of myocardial infarction beyond age 70.[12] More than half of all US patients hospitalized for acute myocardial infarction are older than age 65. Furthermore, elderly patients tend to have a significantly different presentation, clinical course, and prognosis of myocardial infarction than their younger counterparts.[12,13]

ANGINA PECTORIS

A decrease in the habitual level of activity of aged persons may lessen their frequency of angina or render the presentation of angina pectoris deceptive, in that it is less likely to be effort-induced; arthritis, claudication, or musculoskeletal problems limit the activity of many older patients before anginal pain occurs. Dyspnea and fatigue may be the prominent manifestations of myocardial ischemia. Occasionally angina may be precipitated by eating. Additionally, patients with memory lapses or memory loss may not remember the transitory anginal pain, and patients with a variety of chronic brain syndromes may not adequately appreciate, describe, and/or express the occurrence of chest discomfort. In patients with previously asymptomatic coronary atherosclerosis, angina is often precipitated by associated medical problems such as infection, blood loss, hypertension or hypotension, and arrhythmia; and angina may be misinterpreted as presenting an unstable pain pattern because it occurs at rest in patients who are generally inactive.

Therapy is comparable to that for younger patients. Most elderly patients with stable angina who have a good symptomatic response to drug therapy and have no evidence of early ischemic abnormality at exercise testing are best suited for medical management.

MYOCARDIAL INFARCTION

Chest pain as the presenting manifestation of myocardial infarction is less frequent in elderly patients. The elderly have an increased prevalence of problems commonly associated with painless myocardial infarction (e.g., diabetes mellitus, systemic arterial hypertension); in addition, there may be a lesser or altered sensitivity to pain with aging. This is despite the fact that acute myocardial infarction is one of the most common causes for hospital admission in the elderly, as well as one of the most common causes of in-hospital death. The Goteborg Study identified that 60% of patients with electrocardiographic evidence of myocardial infarction gave no history of an acute episode,[14] suggesting that painless infarction or infarction with atypical pain is not unusual, even among elderly patients without impairment of mental function.

In addition to painless myocardial infarction, the elderly patient often has an atypical, although not asymptomatic, presentation[15]; pulmonary edema is frequent at onset, and myocardial infarction may also be manifest initially as cerebrovascular accident or peripheral arterial embolism. It may present in a more subtle manner as profound weakness or fatigue, dyspnea, acute confusion or agitation, exacerbation of chronic congestive heart failure, giddiness or vertigo, or nausea and vomiting. Less commonly, renal failure, decompensation of diabetes mellitus, unexplained hypotension, or general "ill health" may herald myocardial infarction. Unrecognized myocardial infarctions have as serious a prognosis as do identified episodes of infarction. Additionally, the onset of symptoms of myocardial infarction in elderly patients is more likely to occur at rest or during sleep, possibly reflecting the more sedentary life-style of elderly persons.[16] Myocardial infarction is also more likely to complicate surgery characterized by hypotension or major blood loss or occur subsequent to other serious medical problems such as stroke, serious infection, and transient ischemic attacks. In addition to the atypical presentation, the diagnosis may be further obscured by the fact that elevated CK-MB isoenzymes tend to occur in the setting of a normal total creatine kinase (CK) level; this occurs twice as frequently in patients older than 70 years of age.[17] Preexisting abnormalities on the electrocardiogram, such as those of left ventricular hypertrophy, conduction abnormalities, or prior myocardial infarction, may also limit the diagnostic information to be gained from this examination, adding to the challenge of recognizing myocardial infarction in the elderly.

Age typically adversely affects survival after myocardial infarction.[18] Of the approximately 500,000 Americans estimated to die annually of myocardial infarction, the majority will be elderly.[19] Myocardial infarction in the elderly tends to be more severe because, in general, infarctions are larger and are characterized by more and typically severe complications than encountered in a younger population. Common complications of infarction include congestive heart failure, cardiogenic shock, arrhythmias, and cardiac rupture; although these are the same complications as in younger individuals, they occur with increased frequency in the elderly. Cardiac rupture during the first week following myocardial infarction is more frequent in elderly patients; the classic presentation is of recurrent chest pain, hypotension, and, preterminally, electromechanical dissociation, in that cardiac electrical activity transiently persists in the absence of ventricular pumping function. The data from Williams and associates[16] delineate a 74%, 25%, and 22% respective occurrence of pulmonary edema, cardiogenic shock, and congestive heart failure in elderly patients; this can be compared with 52%, 15%, and 8%, respectively, for individuals younger than 70 years of age. An increased frequency of conduction defects, heart block, and arrhythmias is also described. Indeed, some reports identify a hospital mortality for patients older than age 70 of 30% to 40%, approximately twice that encountered in younger patients. It is not surprising, therefore, that elderly patients often have a more protracted hospital stay for an episode of myocardial infarction. The increased severity of infarction, often superimposed on prior infarction, accounts for the increased residual invalidism, as well as the increase in late deaths, among elderly patients.

The management of the acute episode of myocardial infarction is as for younger patients, except that elderly individuals are more prone to lidocaine toxicity, as well as to adverse effects from narcotic analgesic medications; initial therapy with one half of the dose usual for younger individuals is recommended. Prophylactic administration of lidocaine, even in coronary care units where this is routine for younger patients, is probably unwise for an elderly population; elderly individuals appear less likely to develop ventricular tachycardia or fibrillation, whereas their likelihood of adverse responses to lidocaine is increased. There is, at best, limited information about approaches designed to limit infarct size in the elderly population, since patients older than 65 to 70 years have typically been excluded from studies of these interventions. Although not studied in a randomly assigned fashion, favorable results of intracoronary thrombolysis have been described in selected elderly patients. However, in the large randomized Italian trial of intravenous streptokinase, short-term survival from myocardial infarction was not improved in patients older than age 65.[20] Increased bleeding complications, including increased hemorrhagic stroke, are described as more frequent in the elderly. More recent studies of thrombolytic therapy, however, have document survival benefit in the elderly.

In patients with cardiogenic shock due to surgically remediable lesions resulting from myocardial infarction, favorable responses to surgical intervention have been described.[21]

In the early years of acute coronary care, elderly patients were arbitrarily excluded from coronary or intensive care facilities on the basis of age alone. However, elderly patients are now known to benefit equally well from intensive coronary care,[22] electrocardiographic monitoring, and arrhythmia prevention and reversion; in particular, they have an equally favorable response to defibrillation as do younger persons. The increased occurrence of congestive heart failure in the elderly,[23] as well as other complications of infarction and frequent complicating illnesses warrant meticulous surveillance. Elderly patients with congestive heart failure more often require measurement of cardiac output and intracardiac pressures through a pulmonary artery catheter to guide therapy. Other problems encountered more frequently in the elderly patient with myocardial infarction include difficulty with urination, particularly in the male with prostatic enlargement who receives diuretic therapy; constipation and a variety of nonspecific gastrointestinal symptoms; and the precipitation of glaucoma, urinary retention, or confusion when atropine is used to reverse sinus bradycardia. The early mortality of elderly patients following myocardial infarction has been reduced from an estimated 43% to 79% to as low as 25% to 27% with coronary care unit management.

When there is no age limitation for coronary care unit admission, more than one fifth of all patients are over the age of 70 years. Comparison of the prior medical history in younger and older patients admitted to coronary care units reveals a similar occurrence of antecedent angina pectoris, myocardial infarction, hypertension, and diabetes mellitus.[16] However, elderly patients have a far greater delay in seeking medical care for coronary episodes than do younger patients.[24] The reasons suggested include that elderly patients were often unable to recognize their symptoms as life-threatening or suggestive of myocardial infarction and that they were not able to differentiate between their prior angina and the more severe pain of infarction. It is not known whether the patient's decision time currently varies as much with age as was the case some years ago.

It deserves emphasis that a substantial number of elderly patients have an essentially uncomplicated myocardial infarction; in these individuals, the prognosis is excellent for recovery and rehabilitation. Elderly patients with uncomplicated myocardial infarction are ideal candidates for early ambulation, since older persons are particularly susceptible to the deleterious effects of prolonged immobilization; the latter results in an excess of pulmonary atelectasis and thromboembolic complications. Activity as low-level as sitting in a chair for several hours each day may limit the orthostatic intolerance associated with protracted bed rest; the exposure to gravitational stress, rather than the intensity of the activity, seems to be the major determinant limiting orthostatic intolerance.[25] Reassurance is also offered to the patient by the demonstration that physical activity does not produce cardiac symptoms. Education and counseling are important components of care for the elderly. Elderly patients in the coronary care unit have added needs for concise and repeated explanations about equipment and procedures. The combination of the more severe disease and the frequent adverse or excessive reactions to medications is associated with a greater likelihood of disorientation and confusion; reinforcement of time and place orientation is important for these individuals. Elderly patients also tend to be excessively concerned about the potential failure of life-sustaining equipment, such as cardiac pacemakers. At discharge, they require a careful review of all medications; written instructions are essential, and the help of family members may have to be enlisted in giving medications. Specific recommendations and explanations should be given for diet, activity, and smoking cessation; and patients with significant impairment of physical activity should be taught energy-conserving techniques in self-care and household management. When feasible, a return to prior social and recreational activities should be encouraged, as should the return to the pre-illness patterns of sexual activity.[26] Predischarge exercise testing appears safe for selected elderly patients and offers prognostic data comparable to that reported for younger patients.

Preliminary information suggests that, in view of the continued progression of atherosclerotic lesions even in old age, a variety of coronary risk interventions may arrest the progression or produce regression of atherosclerosis even into the 60s and 70s. Because data are less firm than for younger patients, preventive efforts should entail few if any risks, involve few adverse effects, and have limited costs. These preventive approaches include control of hypertension, weight reduction or control, dietary sodium and fat restriction, and emphasis on the avoidance of cigarette smoking. Recommendations for the recognition and management of hyperlipidemia are as for younger persons.[27] Reasonable modest-intensity physical activity appears beneficial, and continued socialization is important in reinforcing recommendations for care and potentially in delaying the need for institutional care. The maintenance of an appropriate level of physical activity may require encouragement from both the physician and the family.

The drug therapy for angina pectoris following myocardial infarction does not differ substantially from that in younger patients, but adverse responses to drug therapy are more likely to occur. Nitrate drugs are the cornerstone of management, but attention must be paid to orthostatic hypotension; in particular, elderly patients must be cautioned to sit when taking sublingual nitroglycerin for relief of angina. β-Blockade carries the risk of inducing congestive cardiac failure and the development or exacerbation of atrioventricular conduction defects but is the only drug category shown to improve survival and reduce reinfarction following a myocardial infarction; this protective effect is evident both in younger and in elderly patients.[28] Calcium antagonist drugs may be of value if there is monitoring for potential complications including postural hypotension, constipation, ankle edema, depression of myocardial function, and/or exacerbation of atrioventricular conduction defects. In one study, elderly patients recovered from myocardial infarction were more often prescribed diuretic drugs at discharge from the hospital, whereas younger patients more often were directed to take β-blocking drugs and calcium channel blocking drugs; the increase in diuretic use and the decrease in β-blocking drug prescription is not unexpected, given the more frequent left ventricular dysfunction in the elderly.[13] Comparable recommendations for reduced dosage to those cited previously are warranted for antiarrhythmic drugs used on a more chronic basis.

REHABILITATIVE EXERCISE TRAINING

The rehabilitative approach to care of the elderly coronary patient is designed to preserve physical function, mental function, and alertness; to limit anxiety and depression; and to encourage readjustment to the prior life-style. Exercise testing is recommended before embarking on physical activity in excess of slow walking as a basis for prescribing the appropriate intensity of activity to be undertaken; a target exercise heart rate range between 60% and 75% of the highest rate safely achieved at exercise testing is recommended. The lowered heart rate with aging compensates in part for the increase in systemic vascular resistance, effecting a maintenance of cardiac work; therefore, in recommending a target heart rate range for exercise, because the heart rate does not directly reflect cardiac work, a lower heart rate range than that suggested for younger individuals is preferred.

Warm-up exercises are particularly important in permitting training to occur; and elderly patients require an increased duration of warm-up and of cool-down activities as well, the latter because of the more gradual return to normal of their exercise heart rate; this necessitates longer rest periods or periods of low-level activity between the components of exercise training.[29] Elderly persons also typically take longer to attain a training effect because of the appropriately low intensity of the recommended training stimulus; the desired decrease in the heart rate and blood pressure responses to submaximal work occurs only after a more prolonged period of exercise training. Because the energy expenditure of walking often entails a significant proportion of their aerobic capacity, walking, even as slowly as 3½ miles an hour, is an excellent physical conditioning stimulus for elderly patients. An ideal activity regimen after discharge from the hospital is a walking program, with a gradual increase in the pace and distance of walking; advantages of a walking program are that it requires no specific skills, equipment, or facilities. Running and jumping activities are inappropriate, since they are associated with an increase in orthopedic complications. There is also a reduced effectiveness of thermal regulation with aging owing to inadequate sweating; this requires that even moderate physical activity be limited in hot, and particularly in humid, environments.

Exercise training of elderly persons is associated with maintenance of physical work capacity and with a general increase in well-being. The major physiologic effect is a decrease in the heart rate response to submaximal work. However, elderly individuals who can exercise at a greater intensity may have improvement in their maximal oxygen uptake, as well as stroke volume and cardiac output. One should expect comparable benefits, and exercise should entail no greater risks in elderly than in younger coronary patients.[30] Additional benefits of exercise training include an improvement in neuromuscular coordination, in joint mobility, and in coordination and flexibility and the potential of limiting of bone demineralization; weight control may be facilitated, and patients may be encouraged to continue a more active life-style.

MYOCARDIAL REVASCULARIZATION

There is a greater occurrence of multivessel and left main coronary stenoses in older than in younger patients with myocardial infarction. Elderly patients with severe or unstable angina pectoris or with life-threatening obstructive coronary lesions at arteriography are candidates for myocardial revascularization. When the severity of the anginal pain, or the side effects of medications used to control angina, significantly interfere with the prior and desired life-style, consideration should also be given to myocardial revascularization. An additional option when the coronary anatomy is suitable is percutaneous transluminal coronary angioplasty (PTCA); favorable results with this procedure in the elderly population have been reported in several series.

Substantial improvements in surgical technique, anesthesia, and myocardial preservation, with a resultant decrease in operative mortality, have made coronary bypass surgery a reasonable alternative for selected elderly patients.[31] This is the case despite their increased perioperative morbidity, in great part related to cerebrovascular and peripheral vascular atherosclerotic disease complications. Additional common complications include psychosis, supraventricular tachyarrhythmias, complete heart block requiring permanent pacing, pulmonary embolism, and the need for intra-aortic balloon pump support.[32] In the Coronary Artery Surgery Study,[33] elderly patients who had functional class III or IV disease and those with unstable angina had a higher morbidity and mortality than encountered in comparable younger patients; and all elderly patients were more liable to perioperative neuropsychiatric complications. Thus the duration of hospital stay is increased, with more time spent in an intensive care unit.

Nevertheless, elderly patients appear to have equally favorable results as do younger persons from coronary bypass surgery,[34] often with complete symptomatic relief and characteristically with marked improvement of their chest pain. Graft patency also compares favorably. A resultant improvement is described in quality of life and in restoration of activity status, but detailed prospectively acquired data about cost-effectiveness are not available. In the Coronary Artery Surgery Study, 81% of elderly patients were free of recurrent angina, myocardial infarction, the requirement for repeat coronary bypass surgery, or death at 1 year; and 40% were free of such events at 5 years; these results were comparable to those in patients younger than age 65.[35]

High-risk patients older than age 65 in the Coronary Artery Surgery Study had a greater improvement in survival and freedom from chest pain with surgical than with medical management.[36] Nevertheless, careful selection of patients is requisite, particularly because a major favorable effect on longevity is doubtful in the general elderly population. Early ambulation and gradually progressive physical activity are recommended after coronary bypass surgery to limit complications and improve the functional status at the time of discharge from the hospital.

SYSTEMIC ARTERIAL HYPERTENSION AND ITS CONSEQUENCES

The pulse pressure tends to widen in old age owing to a continued rise in systolic blood pressure with a decrease in diastolic blood pressure.[37–39] In most populations, systolic blood pressure consistently continues to increase into the seventh and eighth decades, whereas diastolic blood pressure levels off in the 50s and 60s. The widened pulse pressure probably reflects diminished arterial elasticity.[40] It remains uncertain whether the age-related increase in systemic arterial pressure is a phenomenon related to aging or whether it can be prevented. Also there is a greater variability among individuals in the level of systolic blood pressure with age. The World Health Organization definition of hypertension is a blood pressure in excess of 160/95 mm Hg. Either isolated systolic hypertension or combined systolic and diastolic hypertension occurs in 63% of US whites and over 75% of blacks older than age 65[41]; major elevation of the diastolic blood pressure, in excess of 110 mm Hg, is three times as common in elderly blacks as in elderly whites.[42]

Much of the cardiovascular morbidity in the elderly is related to hypertension, either isolated systolic hypertension or combined elevation of the systolic and diastolic blood pressures. In addition to accelerating the occurrence of myocardial infarction and congestive heart failure, hypertension also adversely effects renal function and cerebral blood flow, increases the incidence of aortic dissection and aortic aneurysm rupture, and increases the occurrence of cerebrovascular bleeding and stroke.[43,44] In the Veterans Administration Cooperative Study on Antihypertensive Agents, although only 20% of patients were older than 60 years of age, they sustained half of all the morbidity, heart failure, and stroke.[45] Hypertension remains a powerful predictor of cardiovascular mortality at all ages; even borderline systolic or diastolic hypertension doubles the risk of cardiovascular events in the elderly. However, systolic hypertension occurs more commonly with aging (owing, at least in part, to decreased arterial compliance) than does diastolic hypertension and may be more prominently related to the occurrence of congestive heart failure.[46] As in younger populations, hypertension is associated with overweight and with diabetes mellitus.

Because control of hypertension may decrease cardiovascular morbidity and mortality, antihypertensive medications are designed to prevent the consequences of this disease; however, the clinical trials that provided recommendations for pharmacotherapy have rarely included patients with isolated systolic hypertension nor patients over 70 years of age. Thus, although isolated systolic hypertension in the elderly increases cardiovascular morbidity and mortality, there are only limited and conflicting data as to whether control of this problem in asymptomatic elderly individuals will effect clinical improvement[40]; and the extent of adverse consequences of excessive lowering of the blood pressure is not known. In the pilot phase of the Systolic Hypertension in the Elderly Program, adverse effects were comparable in the drug intervention and placebo groups.[47] In the Hypertension Detection and Follow-Up Program, more intensive hypertension control produced a modest benefit for patients between ages 50 and 69[48]; a 60% reduction in fatal myocardial infarctions was documented in the European Working Party trial.[49] Much of the treatment of hypertension in the elderly continues to be based on extrapolation from data acquired in younger patients.[50]

In elderly patients with orthostatic hypotension, most antihypertensive medications are likely to accentuate this problem. Hygienic measures such as reduction of sodium intake, weight reduction, moderation in alcohol consumption, and low-level exercise should thus be tried initially to control modest elevations of blood pressure,[51] since they do not entail the risk, expense, and inconvenience of pharmacotherapy. Weight reduction can decrease blood pressure even without dietary sodium restriction. Elderly patients should be cautioned that their frequent use of nonsteroidal anti-inflammatory drugs decreases the efficacy of virtually all antihypertensive drugs.

It seems prudent to initiate pharmacologic therapy for all elderly hypertensive patients with a diastolic pressure in excess of 104 mm Hg to 110 mm Hg, even if symptomless, as well as for elderly patients with complications of hypertension.[52] The goal of drug therapy is to reduce the diastolic pressure below 90 mm Hg; a target blood pressure of 140 mm Hg to 160 mm Hg is recommended if isolated systolic hypertension is treated.[41,53] Complications of antihypertensive therapy occur more frequently in the aged patient and must be anticipated[54,55]; once antihypertensive therapy is instituted, blood pressure should be checked both in the sitting and standing positions. Thiazide diuretics are a reasonable first-step drug, or β-adrenergic blocking drugs may be given to elderly patients without contraindications to their use. Elderly hypertensive patients treated with β-blockade should be carefully monitored for development of congestive heart failure or conduction system disease; β-blocking drugs have the advantage of lowering the blood pressure of elderly persons without associated orthostatic hypotension. However, in patients with aortic regurgitation in addition to hypertension, β-blockade may be contraindicated, because the longer diastolic interval associated with the slower heart rate allows for an increase in regurgitant flow. Patients receiving even the milder thiazide diuretics should be observed to ensure that hypovolemia and its orthostatic complications and electrolyte disturbances, particularly hypokalemia, do not occur; hypokalemia may predispose to serious ventricular arrhythmias. Furthermore, hyperglycemia resulting from thiazide therapy may aggravate preexisting glucose intolerance. Often, starting with one half of the usual adult antihypertensive dose will provide satisfactory control of the blood pressure without adverse reactions; drug dosage may be gradually increased if needed. If satisfactory blood pressure control is not achieved, one of the above drugs can be combined with another, or vasodilator therapy may be added; patients often complain of headaches and palpitations as complications of vasodilator therapy. Orthostatic falls may complicate both vasodilator and diuretic therapy because of diminished baroreceptor sensitivity, limited compensatory cardiovascular responses, and decreased central blood flow autoregulation as homeostatic mechanisms. Of the antiadrenergic drugs, methyldopa is often satisfactory; reserpine may be effective but may potentiate depression. Calcium antagonist drugs, when used to control blood pressure, require careful surveillance to avoid hypovolemia and hypotension[56] but effectively control hypertension in the elderly. Dizziness and syncope may be averted if patients are instructed to assume the upright posture gradually. Angiotensin converting enzyme inhibitors may be particularly valuable in that they favorably affect both preload and afterload, and are generally well tolerated; excessive hypotension appears more likely in patients taking diuretics. Hypotension may be delayed in onset and protracted in duration following administration of enalapril.[57] The goal of antihypertensive therapy in the elderly should be not only the reduction of cardiovascular morbidity and mortality but the accomplishment of this without adverse impact on the patients' well-being.[58]

Data from the pilot study of the Systolic Hypertension in the Elderly Program showed high levels of compliance with antihypertensive medications in elderly patients, including those older than age 80.[59]

Of interest is that methyldopa, angiotensin converting enzyme inhibitors, and β-blocking drugs seem to limit or reverse left ventricular hypertrophy, whereas this is not the case with arteriolar vasodilators that effect a comparable control of blood pressure; since left ventricular hypertrophy adversely affects prognosis, consideration must be given to this aspect.

In the rare elderly patient with secondary hypertension, medical therapy should be tried initially; an exception may be the patient with renovascular hypertension, both those whose lesions are amenable to renal angioplasty and those who require surgery.[60]

VALVULAR HEART DISEASE, CONGENITAL HEART DISEASE, AND INFECTIVE ENDOCARDITIS

VALVULAR HEART DISEASE

Degeneration of collagen and secondary calcification occur commonly in the heart valves with increasing age; about one third of patients over age 70 have evidence of calcium deposition in either the mitral or the aortic valve.[61,62] This calcific degeneration is primarily responsible for the aortic valvular disease, both aortic stenosis and aortic regurgitation, in elderly patients. Mitral annular calcification also increases in frequency with age. Echocardiography, supplemented by Doppler studies as needed, is often recommended as the initial diagnostic procedure.

AORTIC STENOSIS

There seems to be frequent underdiagnosis of hemodynamically important aortic stenosis; this is of concern since aortic valve replacement in the elderly entails an acceptably low risk and significantly improves the outlook. Aortic stenosis is often confused with the far more frequent aortic sclerosis of the elderly; one third to one half of elderly patients have a short, early peaking, basal systolic murmur without hemodynamic consequences, associated with a normal carotid pulse.

Aortic stenosis of hemodynamic significance in the elderly is typically calcific, but the underlying disease may be rheumatic, a congenitally bicuspid aortic valve, or a number of nonrheumatic valvular disorders[63]; in the elderly patient with calcific aortic stenosis, in excess of 90% of aortic valves are tricuspid. Features in the clinical history suggesting hemodynamically significant aortic valvular obstruction include the occurrence of angina pectoris, congestive heart failure, or effort syncope; however, these symptoms are not specific, commonly are present as manifestations of coronary atherosclerotic heart disease, and may occur with other cardiovascular problems as well. Furthermore, because of the relatively sedentary life-style of many elderly patients, reliance on activity-precipitated symptoms is less appropriate. At times the initial presentation is of congestive heart failure as a result of the onset of atrial fibrillation, because of the importance of atrial contraction in filling a poorly compliant ventricle. Aortic stenosis of hemodynamic significance is one of the most common anatomical causes of syncope in elderly patients.

Physical findings of significant aortic valvular obstruction include a slow rise and small volume of the carotid pulse, occasionally with a thrill; a late-peaking harsh basal systolic murmur, often with a thrill, that radiates into the neck; a diminished aortic component of S_2 and rarely reversed splitting of S_2; an S_4; evidence on physical examination and on the electrocardiogram of left ventricular hypertrophy; and a narrow pulse pressure. In contrast to findings in younger patients, severe elevation of systolic blood pressure may be present with severe aortic valve obstruction in the elderly. The high-frequency components of the basal systolic murmur are often heard along the lower left sternal border throughout most of systole and may be transmitted toward the cardiac apex; thus, a misdiagnosis of mitral regurgitation may be made. In some instances, there may be an associated murmur of aortic regurgitation. Unfortunately, sclerosis and decreased elasticity of the carotid vessels may mask the classic slowly rising carotid pulse and, with advanced disease, an increased anteroposterior chest diameter, and a markedly restricted cardiac output, the cardiac basal systolic murmur may be soft as well.

Aortic valvular calcification is often evident on the chest film and can be confirmed by echocardiography; it is virtually universal in patients with hemodynamically significant aortic valve obstruction, and its absence is powerful evidence against severe aortic valvular stenosis. Echocardiography and, in particular, echocardiography with Doppler studies may noninvasively assess the severity of aortic stenosis and help select patients for whom cardiac catheterization is indicated. Exercise testing is hazardous if critical aortic stenosis is suspected, since sudden death has been precipitated; indeed, the use of exercise testing to define the etiology of chest pain must be reevaluated in any elderly patient with a basal systolic murmur if there are findings suggesting hemodynamically important outflow obstruction. Cardiac catheterization appears indicated for most symptomatic elderly patients in that many noninvasive tests cannot reliably assess the severity of the aortic stenosis, particularly when dense valvular calcification is present; limited experience with Doppler echocardiography[64] shows reasonable correlation with aortic valve area as measured by cardiac catheterization in elderly persons. Additionally, coronary arteriography is mandatory if aortic valve replacement is considered.

Aortic valve replacement for critical aortic stenosis is indicated at virtually all ages in independent otherwise functional elderly patients,[65] because of their excessive mortality after the onset of heart failure, angina pectoris, or syncope. Only a minority of patients with hemodynamically significant calcific aortic stenosis survive more than 3 years after the onset of heart failure, angina, or syncope; and sudden death is common. Calcific aortic stenosis is the most prevalent valvular lesion requiring surgery in elderly patients. Even in old age, aortic valve replacement significantly increases survival and substantially improves the quality of life.[66] Valve replacement can be performed with a 5% to 10% mortality, even in cardiac patients with class III and class IV disease, because left ventricular function is often well preserved, even after the onset of heart failure. A favorable 10-year postoperative survival, with maintenance of improved functional status, is described.[67] Concurrent coronary bypass surgery may be indicated for selected patients[68] and has been safely and successfully accomplished.

Balloon valvuloplasty may offer palliation for selected patients and can be accomplished in the aged patient with low morbidity and mortality. The long-term benefits are at present uncertain, but appear limited. Balloon valvuloplasty may be best used to improve the status of the elderly patient with severe aortic stenosis and congestive heart failure, increasing the likelihood of subsequent successful valve replacement.

AORTIC REGURGITATION

Aortic regurgitation, the most common cause of a diastolic murmur in old age, is typically managed medically, with combinations of dietary sodium restriction, diuretics, vasodilator drugs, and digitalis to control the cardiac failure. The causes vary widely and include hypertension, infective endocarditis, aortic dissection, and rheumatoid processes. A rheumatic etiology is likely when there is associated mitral valvular disease, although this characteristic may not persist with the decreasing prevalence of rheumatic heart disease. Luetic aortic regurgitation has a less favorable outlook because of its typically increased hemodynamic significance and the frequently associated luetic aortic aneurysm.

Acute aortic regurgitation, as may occur with infective endocarditis or trauma, is often overlooked because of lack of the characteristic wide pulse pressure and the brief and at times inaudible murmur due to overwhelming cardiac failure. These patients typically present with acute pulmonary edema and may be misdiagnosed as having myocardial infarction. Valve replacement is typically needed.

MITRAL VALVULAR DISEASE

Mitral valvular disease in the elderly patient is more commonly mitral regurgitation than stenosis and may be due to rheumatic heart disease, papillary muscle dysfunction resulting from coronary artery disease, myxomatous degeneration of the mitral valve cusps, or calcification of the mitral annulus. The latter is more frequent in women than in men and can often be diagnosed either by its characteristic roentgenographic configuration (C-shaped calcification) or at echocardiography. Myxomatous degeneration of the mitral valve may cause mitral valve prolapse, which at times is associated with chest pain atypical for myocardial ischemia and disturbances of cardiac rhythm. Despite the frequency of mitral valve prolapse in younger individuals, its prevalence in an elderly population is not known. Many elderly patients with mitral valvular disease are essentially asymptomatic, particularly when there is maintenance of sinus rhythm; the onset of atrial fibrillation often heralds hemodynamic deterioration. There is, however, an age-related increase in left ventricular end-diastolic pressure, probably due to an increase in myocardial stiffness.[69] Mitral stenosis is rarely diagnosed *de novo* in the elderly, save for the occasional patient with mitral stenosis of mild or moderate hemodynamic significance who suddenly develops atrial fibrillation and/or a peripheral arterial embolism; rarely, modest mitral stenosis occurs with progressive mitral annular calcification.

Usually medical therapy is appropriate unless there is associated significant mitral stenosis or the mitral regurgitation is of major hemodynamic importance. The latter may be due to chordal rupture or the development of a flail mitral leaflet, as occurs with infective endocarditis; papillary muscle rupture in the setting of myocardial ischemia is another cause. Emergency valve replacement is required; and the hemodynamic instability may mandate intra-aortic balloon counterpulsation support to enable cardiac catheterization to be performed.

The results of mitral valve replacement are less satisfactory than those of aortic valve replacement,[66,70] and the surgical mortality approximates 10% to 14%; this may, in part, be due to the frequently associated left ventricular dysfunction. The risks and benefits are comparable with those of younger patients. The common need for long-term anticoagulant therapy imposes a greater risk of bleeding than in a younger population.

In patients with atrial fibrillation, long-term anticoagulant therapy is often indicated. Detailed education of these elderly patients may minimize the bleeding complications of ambulatory anticoagulation.

With all valvular diseases, the need for antibiotic prophylaxis against infective endocarditis is occasioned by the invasive procedures frequently performed in hospitalized elderly patients and the attendant bacteremia. The revised recommendations for prophylaxis against infective endocarditis apply to both older and younger patients.[71]

CONGENITAL HEART DISEASE

Atrial septal defect is the most frequent congenital cardiac lesion encountered in elderly patients; these patients are characteristically asymptomatic in the absence of complicating pulmonary hypertension or supraventricular tachyarrhythmias. In elderly patients with atrial septal defects who develop dyspnea and fatigue and whose pulmonary vascular resistance is not elevated, closure of the shunt improves these symptoms. The occasional elderly patient with a small calcified persistent ductus arteriosus does not require surgical correction; this entails an unacceptable surgical risk, without defined benefit.

INFECTIVE ENDOCARDITIS

The clinical presentation of infective endocarditis is also often atypical in the elderly, so that the diagnosis is less commonly made or recognition is delayed, although one third of all cases of infective endocarditis occur in elderly persons.[72] Invasive vascular procedures are the most common source of infection in the elderly; almost one fourth of all episodes are nosocomially acquired. Coagulase-negative staphylococci were also more common organisms in the elderly and were typically traceable to invasive vascular or skin sources.[73] Aortic valve endocarditis is most common, with mitral regurgitation the second most frequent predisposing valvular lesion. The increased occurrence of *Streptococcus bovis* appears to be due to gastrointestinal problems and that of enterococcus to genitourinary procedures in elderly men.[73] Elderly patients report fewer symptoms. At times a cardiac murmur may not be prominent, and the patients may not manifest a febrile response; the major features may include anemia, renal failure, otherwise unexplained coma, hemiplegia, and so forth. Infective endocarditis may result from surgical or diagnostic procedures if prophylactic antibiotics are not given. Because the prognosis of endocarditis tends to be less favorable in the elderly, a high index of suspicion should be maintained in elderly patients with otherwise unexplained fever, weight loss, embolic episodes, and confusion.

The management is as for younger patients, initially with appropriate antibiotics, with consideration given to valve replacement for significant hemodynamic abnormalities.

CARDIOMYOPATHY
HYPERTROPHIC CARDIOMYOPATHY

Hypertrophic cardiomyopathy occurs relatively frequently in the elderly population and is often either not suspected or confused with valvular aortic stenosis or the papillary muscle dysfunction of atherosclerotic coronary heart disease.[74,75] About one third of individuals with hypertrophic cardiomyopathy are believed to be older than age 60; despite this, little is known about the natural history of hypertrophic cardiomyopathy in the elderly save that, in this subset of patients, it appears compatible with a long life. This may represent the survival of a low-risk population, or the lessened physical activity with aging may limit risk. Differentiation from valvular aortic stenosis is important in that nitroglycerin, diuretic drugs, and digitalis may exacerbate the outflow obstruction, and β-blocking drugs may effect a remission of symptoms.[76] Hypovolemia of any cause increases risk and should be avoided. The identification of hypertrophic cardiomyopathy at physical examination may not be easy in that brisk carotid pulsations are erroneously ascribed to decreased vascular elasticity and an S_4 and nonspecific systolic murmurs are common in an elderly population. However, a bisferiens character to the carotid pulse or a double cardiac apex impulse may provide the clue to perform appropriate maneuvers; the systolic murmur of hypertrophic cardiomyopathy increases with a Valsalva maneuver and decreases on squatting.

The presentation may be of dizziness, palpitations, syncope, chest pain, or dyspnea; dyspnea may be the prominent complaint. There is disagreement as to whether these symptoms differ from those of younger patients. However, women predominate among elderly patients with hypertrophic cardiomyopathy.

The electrocardiogram is consistent with left ventricular hypertrophy; the Q waves, reflecting septal hypertrophy, may mimic myocardial infarction. Echocardiography, with or without provocative maneuvers can confirm the diagnosis. Free wall myocardial hypertrophy may often equal that of the ventricular septum. β-Blocking agents are generally indicated for symptomatic patients. Verapamil may improve left ventricular compliance and thus be helpful in patients with dyspnea due to decreased ventricular compliance. On occasion, surgical intervention may be warranted for severely symptomatic elderly patients.[77] Prophylaxis against infective endocarditis is needed for these patients.

DILATED AND RESTRICTIVE CARDIOMYOPATHIES

The dilated (congestive) cardiomyopathies are uncommon in an elderly population, probably related to the shortened survival of patients with this problem, save for the dilated cardiomyopathy that results from amyloidosis. The treatment is that of heart failure due to ventricular systolic dysfunction. Less commonly, amyloidosis may be confused with hypertrophic cardiomyopathy or may present as a restrictive cardiomyopathy; the latter may also occur with hemochromatosis, which is another, although uncommon, cause of heart failure in the elderly. The electrocardiographic voltage is characteristically low in the patient with cardiac amyloidosis, and a "sparkling" appearance to the myocardium may be seen on two-dimensional echocardiography.

The development of the pathophysiologic and clinical picture of restrictive cardiomyopathy is increasingly encountered as a consequence of coronary bypass surgery and postoperative pericarditis.

CARDIAC DISEASE SECONDARY TO PULMONARY DISEASE: COR PULMONALE
CHRONIC COR PULMONALE

Right-sided heart failure resulting from pulmonary hypertension in elderly patients is most often due to chronic bronchitis and emphysema; recurrent pulmonary embolism is another important etiology, especially in the setting of prolonged immobilization at bed rest. Although very severe pulmonary heart disease is uncommon in old age, possibly because of the shortened life expectancy in patients with this problem, pulmonary heart disease frequently coexists with atherosclerotic coronary heart disease and hypertensive cardiovascular disease. Because maximal breathing capacity, vital capacity, and forced expiratory volume (FEV) decrease with aging, with an associated increase in residual volume, pulmonary dysfunction is typically accentuated by the superimposition of specific disorders. Both ventilatory function and pulmonary diffusing capacity decline progressively with age.

The clinical findings of pulmonary hypertension and right ventricular decompensation include an accentuated pulmonic component of S_2, often with wide splitting; jugular venous distention with prominent a and v waves; a right-sided S_3; a parasternal impulse; hepatomegaly; peripheral edema; and often the holosystolic murmur of tricuspid regurgitation that is accentuated with inspiration. The electrocardiogram may show a rightward deviation of the QRS axis or evidence of right ventricular hypertrophy; P wave abnormalities may be present. Radioisotope angiography has been described as useful in differentiating left-sided heart disease, pulmonary hypertension, and subsequent right-sided heart failure from pulmonary hypertension due to pulmonary vascular obstruction with right-sided heart failure.

Cigarette smoking and, occasionally, environmental pollutants are chronic contributors to the increased severity of the cardiac decompensation, and respiratory infections often cause an exacerbation on an intermittent basis.

Cardinal features of therapy include discontinuation of cigarette smoking, avoidance of environmental pollutants, appropriate antibiotic treatment of respiratory infections, bronchodilator drugs, liquefaction of sputum, and, less frequently, corticosteroid hormones. Chronic oxygen therapy is helpful in patients with chronic hypoxemia if respiratory depression does not occur with oxygen administration. Sodium restriction should be advised, and diuretic therapy may lessen the heart failure. The use of digitalis is controversial, except to control the ventricular response to rapid supraventricular tachyarrhythmias; digitalis toxicity occurs commonly in elderly patients with chronic lung disease receiving digitalis. Verapamil, given intravenously, often is effective in terminating supraventricular tachycardia and at times may revert multiform atrial tachycardia; however, verapamil may concomitantly depress myocardial contractility. There is no evidence that any of the pulmonary vasodilator drugs have a beneficial effect on a long-term basis, despite the demonstration of acute hemodynamic improvement. Similarly, phlebotomy to reduce blood viscosity in patients with moderate erythrocytosis remains a controversial therapy in that the oxygen-carrying capacity of the blood is reduced and little hemodynamic benefit is attained.

β-Agonist drugs and theophylline used to treat chronic obstructive pulmonary disease may induce arrhythmias or ventricular dysfunction in elderly coronary patients; nonselective β-blocking drugs used to treat coronary disease or hypertension may worsen coexisting chronic lung disease.

ACUTE COR PULMONALE: PULMONARY EMBOLISM

Pulmonary embolism occurs more frequently in the elderly, in part related to their increased immobilization and in part to the multiple concomitant serious illnesses; it is often misdiagnosed as pneumonia or congestive cardiac failure.

The clinical presentation varies from an acute cardiovascular emergency characterized by dyspnea, orthopnea, chest discomfort, syncope, and/or shock to increased cough, mild chest discomfort, transient dyspnea, or often an exacerbation of congestive heart failure. Sudden unexplained dyspnea should be considered as due to pulmonary embolism until proved otherwise; isotopic perfusion lung scanning abnormalities, however, may occur in the absence of embolism, rendering this test of lesser value than in a younger population. The clinical findings include tachypnea, tachycardia, often a low-grade fever, an accentuated pulmonic component of S_2 with wide splitting, a prominent parasternal impulse, an accentuated a wave in the jugular venous pulse, and at times evidence of right ventricular decompensation; deep vein thrombosis of the leg may also be evident.

The treatment of choice is anticoagulation, initially with heparin and subsequently with coumadin. Thrombolytic therapy may be indicated for massive pulmonary embolism with hemodynamic instability; both with thrombolysis and with conventional anticoagulation, the risk of bleeding is increased in the elderly. In patients for whom anticoagulation is contraindicated, vena caval obstruction, usually with a transvenously inserted filter device, is the preferable management.

MANIFESTATIONS OF CARDIAC DISEASE
CONGESTIVE HEART FAILURE

There is probably an equal frequency of underdiagnosis and overdiagnosis of congestive heart failure in elderly patients. Elderly patients often fail to report progressive dyspnea and ankle edema, deeming them a consequence of aging; or early evidence of heart failure may not be apparent because of maintenance of a cardiac output adequate for the habitually limited activity levels. On the other hand, shortness of breath, basal lung crackles and rales, and relatively larger heart volumes, which are normal in an older population, may often be misinterpreted and managed as heart failure. Also, ankle edema is more often due to venous stasis and decreased tissue turgor than to heart failure. Changes in the lungs associated with aging may decrease the tolerance to exercise, even in the absence of congestive heart failure. Concomitant pulmonary disease may also cause breathlessness. Fewer than half of the elderly individuals receiving digitalis in one survey had evidence of cardiovascular disease.[14] Many elderly patients with heart failure may have disordered mental function and behavior as a reflection of diminished cerebral blood flow; because of their limited activity, at times the only complaint encountered in elderly persons may be profound fatigue, rather than effort dyspnea. However, comparable fatigue and exhaustion are often described with excessive diuresis. At times, only anorexia may be reported as the presentation of heart failure or patients may describe insomnia and a nocturnal cough.

The incidence and prevalence of congestive heart failure increase with increasing age. There was an almost eightfold increase in congestive heart failure in men in the seventh as compared with the fifth decade in the Framingham population.[78] As expected, elderly patients are more likely to be receiving digitalis, diuretic drugs, and nitrate or other vasodilator preparations. Intercurrent infections and fever more frequently precipitate or exacerbate heart failure in elderly than in younger patients, as do fluid overload, acute blood loss, pulmonary embolism, anemia, thyrotoxicosis, major dietary indiscretions, acute lower urinary tract obstruction in the male, drugs causing myocardial depression, and/or poor compliance with the medical regimen. The limited cardiac reserve of elderly persons renders them increasingly liable to cardiac failure, and remediable factors should be carefully sought and corrected as complications of the underlying cardiovascular disease.

Heart failure in elderly patients is most commonly due to hypertensive cardiovascular disease or atherosclerotic coronary heart disease as the underlying problem; exacerbations also may result from tachyarrhythmias or bradyarrhythmias. Left ventricular systolic dysfunction or overt congestive cardiac failure is an important contributor to the excessive mortality among elderly patients in the early months following myocardial infarction. Calcific aortic stenosis of hemodynamic significance is another common cause of heart failure. Thyrotoxic heart disease may cause high-output cardiac failure in the elderly patient, and this etiology is often unrecognized because the hypermetabolic aspects of thyrotoxicosis are subtle or inapparent.[79] The decrease in renal function, common with aging, may be accentuated by congestive heart failure and then may further exacerbate the heart failure. Echocardiography is often useful in defining an otherwise inapparent etiology of the congestive heart failure and in differentiating systolic and diastolic dysfunction. The characteristics of the heart valves can be assessed, as can the size and function of the cardiac chambers, the presence of pericardial effusion, and localized wall motion abnormalities.

In elderly patients with preserved systolic function, pulmonary congestion and other clinical manifestations of heart failure are often due to diastolic dysfunction. Differentiation is important in that therapy differs; diuretic and venodilator drugs alone may reduce ventricular filling volume and potentiate diastolic dysfunction. Clues to decreased ventricular complicance (diastolic dysfunction) as the mechanism for heart failure include a normal or near-normal heart size and a cause for left ventricular hypertrophy such as hypertension or hypertrophic cardiomyopathy.[80]

Common physical findings with predominantly left-sided decompensation, in addition to tachycardia, include cardiac enlargement, gallop sounds, lung rales, and, with severe congestive heart failure, acute pulmonary edema; the patient with predominant right-sided heart failure has dependent edema, hepatomegaly, ascites, and jugular venous distention. The elderly patient is often restless and agitated, in part related to increased sympathetic activity, when congestive heart failure occurs; control of the cardiac problem more effectively limits these symptoms than does sedation. Weight gain may be evident, and pulsus alternans is evidence of profound cardiac decompensation. The skin, particularly of the extremities, may be cool as a result of peripheral vasoconstriction.

As in younger patients, the major components of therapy for heart failure due to systolic dysfunction include restriction of dietary sodium, activity limitation, digitalis, and diuretic drugs, supplemented, if needed, by vasodilator therapy. This regimen improves cardiac function by decreasing the cardiac workload, limiting sodium and water retention, and improving myocardial contractility. Sodium restriction, as previously discussed, is an important feature both in encouraging the diuresis and in limiting the resultant hypokalemia; however, major dietary alterations are often difficult to accomplish in an elderly population. Difficulties with the purchasing and preparation of food, lack of interest in meals when eating alone, dental problems that may impair the chewing of food, and financial constraints often hamper dietary alterations. A sizeable component of the diet of elderly individuals is frequently the preprocessed "convenience foods" that have an excessive sodium content. Although some limitation of physical activity is advisable, protracted immobilization is unwise in that it predisposes to deep vein thrombosis and resultant pulmonary embolism; sitting in a bedside chair, preferably with the legs elevated, or sitting upright in bed are reasonable compromises that may also favorably affect the loading conditions of the heart. When the level of activity is increased after initial control of the heart failure, the patient should be carefully observed for fatigue, breathlessness, edema, and weight gain, as evidence of recurrent decompensation. Patients with severe congestive cardiac failure, particularly when it is associated with atrial fibrillation, are candidates for anticoagulant therapy.

Digitalis remains the cornerstone of management, with the proviso that smaller doses should be prescribed to elderly patients. Digitalis improves myocardial contractility and may limit the ventricular response to supraventricular tachyarrhythmias. Often 0.125 mg of digoxin given daily is a satisfactory dose; the dosage should be further reduced if quinidine is given concomitantly or if renal function is compromised. Because of the decrease in lean body mass,[81] the volume in which digitalis is distributed is lessened, causing an increase in plasma concentration; also, digoxin excretion is decreased because of the reduction in glomerular filtration. Digitalis overdosage should be suspected if any of a variety of nonspecific findings occur, including confusion, bizarre behavior, altered mental status, fatigue, and anorexia, in addition to the usual nausea and vomiting. Digitalis, given for heart failure precipitated by an acute problem that has resolved, can often be safely discontinued.

Common complications of excessive diuretic therapy include dehydration and electrolyte abnormalities (often manifest as altered mental status), an increased likelihood of digitalis toxicity, and orthostatic hypotension with resultant orthopedic complications. The expected reflex tachycardia in response to hypotension and hypovolemia is delayed and limited in the elderly because of attenuated baroreceptor reflexes; therefore, patients are increasingly susceptible to adverse effects of excessive diuresis, as may occur with potent loop diuretics, as well as to overzealous antihypertensive therapy.

The newer vasodilator drugs (nitrates in sizeable doses, prazosin, hydralazine, and the converting enzyme inhibitors) used judiciously with gradual increases in dosage appear to improve cardiac status in patients with ventricular systolic dysfunction by favorably altering the loading conditions of the heart. Data derived from a younger population suggest an improvement in survival when vasodilator therapy is added to digitalis and diuretics.[82] The role of the newer inotropic agents (*e.g.*, milrinone) is not known for patients in this age-group.

Because of the significant morbidity and mortality associated with congestive cardiac failure, elderly patients with this problem require frequent and meticulous surveillance and caution is warranted about the prognosis, since the development of heart failure adversely influences the outlook for most cardiovascular diseases.

ARRHYTHMIAS AND CONDUCTION ABNORMALITIES

Both arrhythmias and other electrocardiographic abnormalities increase in incidence with increasing age.[83] Any tachyarrhythmia or bradyarrhythmia may compromise cardiac function because of the resultant decrease in cardiac output. Although arrhythmias may present as syncope or an alteration of consciousness, many aged patients have significant disturbances of cardiac rhythm without symptoms of palpitations. Electrocardiographic abnormalities (*e.g.*, left axis deviation of the QRS, incomplete right bundle branch block, first-degree atrioventricular block) have little prognostic significance in themselves, since their adverse consequences relate to the underlying disease rather than to the electrocardiographic abnormality.

The number of pacemaker cells in the sinoatrial node, as well as the number of fibers in the bundle branches, decrease with age, but the loss of sinoatrial node pacemaker cells is far more pronounced. Baroreceptor responsiveness also decreases with aging, at least in part due to loss of distensibility of the vascular wall; myocardial catecholamine responsiveness also decreases. There is a diminution both in the number and in the function of β-adrenergic receptors with increasing age.

The combination of atrial fibrosis and atrial dilatation may underlie the increased prevalence of atrial arrhythmias in an elderly population.

It is not surprising, therefore, that both cardiac arrhythmias[84,85] and conduction defects are common in an elderly population; there is an increased occurrence of atrioventricular block progressing to complete heart block, of intraventricular conduction delays and bundle branch blocks, as well as of the sick sinus syndrome with advancing age.[86] These findings may be accentuated by drugs used to treat hypertension and coronary disease, such as β-blockers and calcium antagonist drugs. A 24-hour electrocardiographic recording is the most appropriate diagnostic procedure to correlate symptoms with spontaneous arrhythmias. This test is indicated to evaluate for and identify cardiac rhythm disturbances when elderly patients have otherwise unexplained lightheadedness, dizziness, giddiness, falls, or frank syncope or when they describe uncomfortable palpitations. Identification of a specific dysrhythmia is needed before the institution of drug therapy or pacemaker implantation because comparable symptoms often result from orthostatic hypotension of varied cause and from hemodynamically significant aortic stenosis; additionally, there is a poor correlation of symptoms even with documented arrhythmias in elderly patients. How much of this reflects inadequate reporting by the patient is not known. Symptoms of low cardiac output, in the absence of documented arrhythmias, rarely respond favorably to pacemaker implantation. Carotid sinus hypersensitivity should also be considered when evaluating the etiology of syncope in elderly patients, particularly elderly men.

The pharmacologic management of both supraventricular and ventricular arrhythmias is as in younger patients, except that lower doses of medication are usually indicated. There is concern when antiarrhythmic drugs used to treat ventricular tachyarrhythmias prolong the QT interval, since this may induce additional ventricular tachyarrhythmias; ambulatory electrocardiography or electrophysiologic study is indicated to gauge the efficacy of therapy.[87] The prognostic significance of ventricular ectopy in the absence of significant ventricular dysfunction or myocardial ischemia is not known. Ventricular arrhythmias are pervasive in elderly persons, including multiform ventricular ectopic complexes and nonsustained ventricular tachycardia, even in the absence of cardiac disease. Asymptomatic ventricular arrhythmias rarely require therapy in the absence of myocardial ischemia or significant ventricular dysfunction. In excess of 1,000 ventricular premature beats in 24 hours, however, was unusual in very old healthy persons; it generally occurred in association with coronary heart disease, where it heralded a poor prognosis.[88] Antiarrhythmic drugs are more likely to potentiate conduction abnormalities and ventricular dysfunction in an elderly population, and problems with drug elimination or drug interactions increase the likelihood of other toxic manifestations as well.

In elderly patients with refractory symptomatic life-threatening ventricular arrhythmias, electrophysiologic testing was well tolerated and identified patients requiring drug therapy or surgical intervention that included coronary artery bypass grafting, endocardial resection, aneurysmectomy, and/or implantation of an automatic defibrillator.[89]

Sick sinus syndrome is a frequent problem in elderly persons but does not generally require treatment in the absence of symptoms. Pacemaker implantation may be necessary to permit the pharmacologic management of the tachyarrhythmias. Atrial fibrillation is also more common, often as a consequence of hypertensive cardiovascular disease or atherosclerotic coronary heart disease. Chronic atrial fibrillation, in the absence of valvular disease, is associated with an increased incidence of stroke that increases steadily with age; antiplatelet agents have not been effective in preventing stroke. Evaluation of the relative risks and benefits of warfarin anticoagulation appears warranted.[90]

Pacemaker implantation is appropriate at all ages, since pacemakers can improve both the quantity and quality of life. Prior to permanent pacing, more than half of all patients with complete heart block died within 2 years. Although ventricular demand pacemakers are currently the most common units in use, dual-chambered pacemakers have the advantages that atrial contraction may contribute importantly to ventricular function when ventricular compliance is abnormal, and the cardiac rate is proportional to the activity need. Disadvantages of these complex pacemakers are their higher cost and lesser life expectancy, as well as the increased skill of the physician needed for implantation and surveillance. Sinus bradycardia is a common rhythm in elderly patients; when asymptomatic, it is not an indication for pacemaker implantation or other intervention. Similarly, asymptomatic complete atrioventricular block does not warrant pacing. A consensus guideline for indications for pacemaker implantation prepared by the American College of Cardiology is equally appropriate for younger and older patients.[91] In elderly patients with limited mobility, transtelephonic pacemaker surveillance may be helpful.

DRUG THERAPY

There is an increased frequency of drug administration to the elderly, who comprise approximately 10% of the US population but account for 25% of the drug use. The multiple vague somatic complaints offered by elderly patients are more often palliatively managed with drugs rather than with reassurance and counseling; and many elderly cardiac patients are often overmedicated to relieve vague discomfort and ensure rest. Any drug therapy is more likely to be associated with unwanted effects in an elderly population,[92] despite the fact that many elderly patients are willing and able to adhere to medical care regimens.

This increase in adverse drug reactions relates both to the age-related pharmacokinetic and the pharmacodynamic changes.[93] The former involve a lesser volume of distribution of water-soluble drugs and an increased volume of distribution of lipid-soluble drugs, owing to changes in body composition. Diminished hepatic blood flow reduces the metabolism and excretion of drugs by the liver, and decreased renal blood flow limits elimination of drugs by the kidney. A normal serum creatinine level cannot be equated with normal renal function since the reduced creatine production secondary to a lessened lean body mass can be adequately handled even with the lower glomerular filtration rate. There is also an increase in drug bioavailability that reflects a reduction in first-pass metabolism. Additionally, a number of pharmacodynamic changes reflect alterations at the site of action of drugs. β-Receptor effect appears diminished in the elderly,[94] and older persons also seem more sensitive to the effect of warfarin.[95,96]

A study of adverse drug reactions showed that 30% of persons age 65 and over had an unwanted drug effect, in contrast to 15% with these episodes in the general population. The adverse reactions were due to cardiovascular drugs in about one third of instances,[97] with major adverse drug effects related to the use of digitalis, diuretics, antihypertensive drugs, antiarrhythmic agents, and anticoagulant drugs.

The purpose of and schedule for medications should be clearly and simply explained to elderly patients, but often the help of a family member is needed for medication administration. Hearing and vision impairment may further limit the medication-taking ability of elderly patients, and medication costs may be a major consideration. Memory impairment may pose an added problem in that elderly patients may either forget to take their medication or may inappropriately repeatedly take the same drug. Emphasis should be to devise a simple regimen, using the smallest number of drugs in the lowest effective dosage,[98] realizing that multidrug treatment is often given for concomitant multisystem chronic diseases.

Drug therapy may also lead to psychologic complications; sedatives and tranquilizers may produce confusion; *Rauwolfia* preparations and methyldopa may induce or potentiate depression, as may β-adrenergic blockade; and electrolyte disturbances and dehydration may also produce confusion and an altered mental status that often mimics dementia.

PSYCHOSOCIAL CONCERNS, PREVENTION, AND REHABILITATION

PSYCHOSOCIAL CONCERNS

The diagnosis of cardiovascular disease in an elderly patient typically initiates anxiety and concern that even a modest further deterioration of function can threaten the ability to continue independent living. The restoration of normal physical activity and prior life-style patterns are major deterrents to both anxiety and depression. They may avert the use of psychotropic drugs, which often have adverse effects on heart rate, blood pressure, and cardiac rhythm; if these drugs must be used, benzodiazepine compounds appear to have the fewest unwanted responses.

On the other hand, many elderly persons do not report cardiovascular or other symptoms because their general expectation of health in old age is low. At times, they may have been discouraged by attitudes suggesting that valuable health care resources should not be expended on elderly patients; alternatively, they may have failed to understand the explanations and recommendations of physicians and other health care personnel.

Both anxiety and depression may limit the return of elderly patients to their prior life-style, possibly accounting for the frequent persistence of psychosocial impairment identified in the early months after myocardial infarction.[99] Social and environmental changes more profoundly affect the elderly cardiac patient. Mortality is greater in widows and widowers than in the married elderly, and is also greater in socially isolated individuals.[100]

PREVENTION

Risk attributes continue to predict cardiovascular disease at an advanced age,[40] and most alterable risk characteristics are highly prevalent in the aged. Although hypertension remains the dominant cardiovascular risk factor in the elderly population (even through the seventh decade), hyperlipidemia and cigarette smoking still impart risk, although less than in middle age.[101] The association between hyperlipidemia and coronary risk appears less in old age, although elevated lipid levels remain good predictors of stroke and of noncoronary death[102]; lowered levels of high-density lipoprotein cholesterol remain a significant predictor of atherosclerosis in elderly men into their 60s. Cigarette smoking continues to be associated with an increase in sudden cardiac death and in fatal reinfarction.[103] Diabetes mellitus or glucose intolerance is an independent predictor of cardiovascular risk. A concern in assuming that older persons have a lesser susceptibility to coronary risk factors is that the individuals at highest risk may have already died. Furthermore, the absolute impact of preventive interventions may be greater in the elderly, despite their lesser relative impact.

Control of blood pressure helps both to limit cerebrovascular complications and to facilitate the management of angina pectoris and congestive heart failure; restriction of dietary sodium is an important component of blood pressure control. Control of obesity, in addition to decreasing cardiac work and cardiovascular risk, also favorably affects glucose tolerance, serum lipid levels, and blood pressure.

REHABILITATION

Many physicians characteristically underestimate the habitual activity level of their older patients with cardiovascular disease and inappropriately recommend that these patients restrict their activity.[104] Excessive immobilization may be associated with detrimental physical and psychologic consequences; however, only limited information is available about the appropriate levels of physical activity for aged individuals.

On the other hand, many elderly individuals may have also decreased their activity levels because any submaximal task is perceived as requiring increased work; this is because of its increase in relative energy cost owing to the lessened aerobic capacity of aging. Even with the usual daily activities, there is a greater increase in heart rate in the elderly population.[105] Additionally, combinations of musculoskeletal instability, emotional problems (particularly depression), and often inappropriate admonitions from family members and friends further decrease activity levels.

Both appropriate physical activity and correct nutrition, including weight control, contribute importantly to the maintenance of cardiovascular function in the elderly.

NONCARDIOVASCULAR SURGERY IN ELDERLY PATIENTS WITH CARDIOVASCULAR DISEASE

Noncardiovascular surgery in elderly cardiac patients is often complicated, in addition to the cardiovascular disease, by cerebrovascular and peripheral vascular disease; atherosclerosis of the aorta and great vessels; impaired renal function and/or prostatic obstruction; pulmonary disease; and problems of general debility and malnutrition.[106,107] Overall recovery is more protracted with an increased need for nursing care and more time spent in an intensive care setting.

As with younger patients, the highest risk for noncardiac surgery is within 6 months of acute myocardial infarction; in this setting, only emergency surgery should be considered. Other features associated with an adverse prognosis for noncardiac surgery are unstable angina pectoris, uncontrolled hypertension, and decompensated congestive cardiac failure.

Careful preoperative assessment should be directed toward metabolic status and mental status, in addition to general physical health. Meticulous intraoperative and postoperative surveillance should be directed toward ensuring adequate oxygenation, electrolyte balance, and control of congestive cardiac failure and arrhythmias. "Prophylactic" digitalis administration is not indicated, and pulmonary artery catheter monitoring is warranted only for specific indications. Similarly, prophylactic pacemaker insertion is not routinely indicated. In patients with potential or established atherosclerotic coronary heart disease with unknown anatomy, preoperative exercise testing may define the risk status and suggest whether further investigation is necessary before scheduling semielective or elective noncardiac surgery. Continuous electrocardiographic monitoring is recommended intraoperatively for most patients with known or suspected cardiovascular disease; evaluation for an acute event by means of cardiac enzymes, electrocardiograms, and chest films daily for at least 3 days following surgery shows that the highest occurrence of acute coronary events is on the second or third postoperative day.

Early mobilization helps prevent thromboembolic complications.

SOCIAL IMPACT/COST CONTAINMENT

In 1978 in the United States almost one third of all hospitalized elderly patients were hospitalized for cardiovascular diseases, predominantly atherosclerotic coronary heart disease.[108]

The elderly are intensive users of emergency medical services[109] and of medical services in general. However, since most elderly cardiovascular patients entering hospitals are discharged, the majority of elderly patients appear to benefit from active treatment rather than using the hospital for custodial care. The aim of ongoing care should be to return elderly patients to independent living in their own home setting for as long as is reasonable.

The increasing proportion of elderly patients will unquestionably increase their demands for health care and related services.[110] This approximately 10% of the population now over age 65 currently uses up to 30% of the health resources, and the population over age 65 is estimated to increase by about 1600 people each day. A significant proportion of the health care expense is incurred in the treatment of cardiovascular disease.

The admission diagnosis of elderly patients tends to vary with age, although there is a general progressive increase in hospitalization with increasing age; younger elderly patients are more likely to have myocardial infarction, whereas heart failure and arrhythmias are preeminent in the oldest age-groups. Multiple concomitant medical problems will increase the need for emergency services and office and hospital care; and progressive incapacity will increase the requirements for residential or custodial care. Systems designed to maintain dependent elderly individuals in the community, although requiring considerable organization, appear a reasonable approach to cost containment. One US survey[111] showed that home nursing services for individuals older than age 85 were ten times the average for all ages.

The use of health services by the elderly only partially indicates their need, since much of the statistical data is determined by the patients' access to and the general availability of health care, rather than by the patients' needs.[112] Thus health service use appears more dependent on the provision, availability, and accessibility of these services than on the morbidity of the population or their need for care; thus statistics cannot be considered to adequately reflect the prevalence of disease and disability.

CONCLUSIONS

In planning for health care in the 21st century, the increased proportion of elderly patients, who often will have cardiovascular disease and often will require high technology diagnostic and therapeutic interventions, must be addressed. The use of health care resources will increase not only with increasing age but with the improved expectations of older persons about their health status.

At the same time, it will be necessary to avoid overzealous and redundant diagnostic and therapeutic interventions. Preventive aspects will increasingly become important components of care for elderly cardiac patients,[113,114] although it remains uncertain how much extension of years of health and decrease in disability can be anticipated in later life. The decline in cardiovascular mortality in recent decades appears an important component in the longevity of the elderly population; however, it is not certain whether these preventive efforts, by limiting or delaying cardiovascular disease, will ultimately decrease overall health care costs.

REFERENCES

1. Rodeheffer RJ, Gerstenblith G, Becker LC et al: Exercise cardiac output is maintained with advancing age in healthy human subjects: Cardiac dilatation and increased stroke volume compensate for a diminished heart rate. Circulation 69:203, 1984
2. Pomerance A: Pathology of the heart with and without cardiac failure in the aged. Br Heart J 27:697, 1965
3. Lopez AD, Hanada K: Mortality patterns and trends among the elderly in developed countries. World Health Stat Q 35:203, 1982
4. Manton KG: Changing concepts of morbidity and mortality in the elderly population. Milbank Mem Fund Q 60:183, 1982
5. Caird FI, Andrews GR, Kennedy RD: Effect of posture on blood pressure in the elderly. Br Heart J 35:527, 1973
6. Kirkendall WM, Hammond JJ: Hypertension in the elderly. Arch Intern Med 140:1155, 1980
7. Mader SL, Josephson KR, Rubenstein LZ: Low prevalence of postural hypotension among community-dwelling elderly. JAMA 258:1511, 1987
8. Kotler MN, Mintz GS, Parry WR et al: Bedside diagnosis of organic murmurs in the elderly. Geriatrics 36:107, 1981
9. Iskandrian AS, Heo J, Decoskey D et al: Use of exercise thallium-201 imaging for risk stratification of elderly patients with coronary artery disease. Am J Cardiol 61:269, 1988
10. Gerson MC, Moore EN, Ellis K: Systemic effects and safety of intravenous dipyridamole in elderly patients with suspected coronary artery disease. Am J Cardiol 60:1399, 1987
11. Hodgson JL, Buskirk ER: Physical fitness and age, with emphasis on cardiovascular function in the elderly. J Am Geriatr Soc 25:385, 1977
12. Latting CA, Silverman ME: Acute myocardial infarction in hospitalized patients over age 70. Am Heart J 100:311, 1980
13. Hill RD, Glazer MD, Wenger NK: Myocardial infarction in the elderly. In Hurst JW (ed): Clinical Essays on the Heart, vol 5, p 293. New York, McGraw-Hill, 1985
14. Svanborg A, Bergstrom G, Mellstrom D: Epidemiological studies on social and medical conditions of the elderly. European Reports and Studies 62, Copenhagen, WHO Regional Office for Europe, 1982
15. Pathy MS: Clinical features of ischemic heart disease. In Caird FI, Dall JLC, Kennedy RD (eds): Cardiology in Old Age, p 193. New York, Plenum Press, 1976
16. Williams BO, Begg TB, Semple T et al: The elderly in a coronary unit. Br Med J 2:451, 1976
17. Heller GV, Blaustein AS, Wei JY: Implications of increased myocardial isoenzyme level in the presence of normal serum creatine kinase activity. Am J Cardiol 51:24, 1983
18. Marchionni N, Pini R, Vannucci A et al: Intensive care for the elderly with acute myocardial infarction. J Clin Exp Gerontol 3:46, 1981
19. American Heart Association: Heart Facts. Dallas, Texas, 1984
20. GISSI: Study of streptokinase in acute myocardial infarction. Lancet 1:397, 1986
21. Weintraub RM, Wei JY, Thurer RL: Surgical repair of remediable post-infarction cardiogenic shock in the elderly: Early and long-term results. J Am Geriatr Soc 34:389, 1986
22. Berman ND: The elderly patient in the coronary care unit: I. Acute myocardial infarction. J Am Geriatr Soc 27:145, 1979
23. Akman D: Treatment of acute myocardial infarction in the elderly. Geriatrics 38:46, 1983
24. Moss AJ, Wynar B, Goldstein S: Delay in hospitalization during the acute coronary period. Am J Cardiol 24:659, 1969
25. Convertino V, Hung J, Goldwater D et al: Cardiovascular responses to exercise in middle-aged men after 10 days of bed rest. Circulation 65:134, 1982
26. Peach H, Pathy J: Disability in elderly after myocardial infarction. J R Coll Physicians Lond 13:154, 1979
27. Report of the National Cholesterol Education Program Expert Panel on Detection, Evaluation and Treatment of High Blood Cholesterol in Adults. Arch Intern Med 148:36, 1988
28. Gundersen T, Abrahamsen AM, Kjekshus J et al: Timolol-related reduction in mortality and reinfarction in patients ages 65–75 years surviving acute myocardial infarction. Circulation 66:1179, 1982
29. Montoye HJ, Willis PW, Cunningham DA: Heart rate response to submaximal exercise: Relation to age and sex. J Gerontol 23:127, 1968
30. Williams MA, Maresh CM, Esterbrooks DJ et al: Early exercise training in patients older than age 65 years compared with that in younger patients after acute myocardial infarction or coronary artery bypass grafting. Am J Cardiol 55:263, 1985
31. Elayda MA, Hall RJ, Gray AG et al: Coronary revascularization in the elderly patient. J Am Coll Cardiol 3:1398, 1984
32. Knapp WS, Douglas JS Jr, Craver JM et al: Efficacy of coronary artery bypass grafting in elderly patients with coronary artery disease. Am J Cardiol 47:923, 1981
33. Gersh BJ, Kronmal RA, Frye RL et al: Coronary arteriography and coronary artery bypass surgery: Morbidity and mortality in patients ages 65 years or older. Circulation 67:483, 1982
34. Cron JP, Adolph WL, Barthes PX et al: Indications and results of coronary surgery in patients age 70 or more. Presse Med 13:2303, 1984
35. Gersh BJ, Schaff HV, Kronmal RA et al: Five-year survival after coronary artery bypass surgery in 1,096 elderly patients. Circulation 66(suppl II):II-220, 1982
36. Gersh BJ, Kronmal RA, Schaff HV et al: Comparison of coronary artery surgery and medical therapy in patients 65 years of age or older: A nonrandomized study from CASS registry. N Engl J Med 313:217, 1985
37. Messerli FH, Ventura HO, Glade LB et al: Essential hypertension in the elderly: Haemodynamics, intravascular volume, plasma renin activity, and circulating catecholamine levels. Lancet 2:983, 1983
38. Amery A, Hansson L, Andren L et al: Hypertension in the elderly: Hypertension seminars at Ostra Hospital, Goteborg, Sweden. Acta Med Scand 210:221, 1981
39. Finnerty FA: Hypertension in the elderly: Special considerations in treatment. Postgrad Med 65:119, 1979
40. Kannel W, Gordon T: Evaluation of cardiovascular risk in the elderly: The Framingham Study. Bull NY Acad Med 54:573, 1978
41. The Working Group on Hypertension in the Elderly: Statement on hypertension in the elderly. JAMA 256:70, 1986
42. Moser M: Hypertension in the elderly. In Rossman I (ed): Clinical Geriatrics, p 606. Philadelphia, JB Lippincott, 1979
43. Ostfeld AM: Elderly hypertensive patients: Epidemiologic review. NY State J Med 78:1125, 1978

44. Forette F, de la Fuente X, Golmard JL et al: The prognostic significance of isolated systolic hypertension in the elderly: Results of ten year longitudinal study. Clin Exp Hyper (Theory and Practice) A4:117, 1982
45. Veterans Administration Cooperative Study Group on Antihypertensive Agents: Effects of treatment on morbidity in hypertension. III. Influence of age, diastolic pressure, and previous cardiovascular disease: Further analysis of side effects. Circulation 45:991, 1972
46. Rowe JW: Systolic hypertension in the elderly. N Engl J Med 309:1246, 1983
47. Hulley SB, Furberg CD, Gurland B et al: The Systolic Hypertension in the Elderly Program (SHEP): Antihypertensive effect of chlorthalidone. Am J Cardiol 56:913, 1985
48. Hypertension Detection and Follow-Up Program Cooperative Group: Five-Year Findings of the Hypertension Detection and Follow-Up Program: II. Mortality by race, sex, and age. JAMA 242:2572, 1979
49. Amery A, Birkenhäger W, Brixko P et al: Mortality and morbidity results from the European Working Party on High Blood Pressure in the Elderly trial. Lancet 1:1349, 1985
50. Larochelle P, Bass MJ, Birkett NJ et al: Recommendations from the Consensus Conference on Hypertension in the Elderly. Can Med Assoc J 135:741, 1986
51. Amery A, Bulpitt C, Fagard R et al: Does diet matter in hypertension? Eur Heart J 1:299, 1980
52. Amery A, Beard K, Birkenhager W et al: Antihypertensive therapy in patients above age 60 years. Eighth Interim Report of the European Working Party on High Blood Pressure in the Elderly (EWPHE). Curr Med Res Opin 8(suppl 1):5, 1982
53. National High Blood Pressure Education Program Coordinating Committee: Statement on hypertension in the elderly. Bethesda, MD, National Institutes of Health, 1979
54. O'Malley K, O'Brien E: Management of hypertension in the elderly. N Engl J Med 302:1397, 1980
55. Wood AJJ, Feely J: Management of hypertension in the elderly. South Med J 74:1503, 1981
56. Buhler RF: Age and cardiovascular response adaptation: Determinants of antihypertension treatment concept based primarily on beta blockers and calcium entry blockers. Hypertension 5(suppl II):II-94, 1983
57. Reid JL: Angiotensin converting enzyme inhibitors in the elderly. Br Med J 295:943, 1987
58. Emerian JP, Decamps A, Manciet G et al: Hypertension in the elderly. Am J Med 84(suppl 3B):92, 1988
59. Black DM, Brand RJ, Greenlich M et al: Compliance to treatment for hypertension in elderly patients: The SHEP Pilot Study. J Gerontol 42:552, 1987
60. Delin K, Aurell M, Granerus G et al: Surgical treatment of renovascular hypertension in the elderly patient. Acta Med Scand 211:169, 1982
61. Sugiura M, Matsushita S, Ueda K et al: A clinicopathological study of valvular diseases in 3,000 consecutive autopsies of the aged. Jpn Circ J 46:337, 1982
62. Jamieson WRE, Dooner J, Munro I et al: Cardiac valve replacement in the elderly: A review of 320 consecutive cases. Circulation 64(suppl II):II-177, 1981
63. Pomerance A: Pathogenesis of aortic stenosis and its relationship to age. Br Heart J 34:569, 1972
64. Come PC, Riley MF, McKay RG et al: Echocardiographic assessment of aortic valve area in elderly patients with aortic stenosis and of changes in valve area after percutaneous balloon valvuloplasty. J Am Coll Cardiol 10:115, 1987
65. Logeais Y, Leguerrier A, Rioux C et al: Surgery of calcified aortic stenosis in patients age 70 and over: Immediate results: Apropos of the series of 229 cases. Ann Cardiol Angeiol 33:385, 1984
66. Stephenson LW, Mac Vaugh H III, Edmunds LH Jr: Surgery using cardiopulmonary bypass in the elderly. Circulation 58:250, 1978
67. Murphy ES, Lawson RM, Starr A et al: Severe aortic stenosis in patients 60 years of age and older: Left ventricular function and 10-year survival after valve replacement. Circulation 64(suppl II):II-184, 1981
68. Smith JM, Lindsay WG, Lillehei RC et al: Cardiac surgery in geriatric patients. Surgery 80:443, 1976
69. Clancy KF, Iskandrian AS, Hakki A-H et al: Age-related changes in cardiovascular performance in mitral regurgitation: Analysis of 61 patients. Am Heart J 109:442, 1985
70. Hochberg MS, Derkac WM, Conkle DM et al: Mitral valve replacement in elderly patients: Encouraging postoperative clinical and hemodynamic results. J Thorac Cardiovasc Surg 77:422, 1979
71. Committee on Rheumatic Fever and Infective Endocarditis of the Council on Cardiovascular Disease in the Young: Prevention of Bacterial Endocarditis. Circulation 70:1123A, 1984
72. Thell R, Martin FH, Edwards JE: Bacterial endocarditis in subjects 60 years of age and older. Circulation 51:174, 1975
73. Terpenning MS, Buggy BP, Kauffman CA: Infective endocarditis: Clinical features in young and elderly patients. Am J Med 83:626, 1987
74. Whiting RB, Powell WJ Jr, Dinsmore RE et al: Idiopathic hypertrophic subaortic stenosis in the elderly. N Engl J Med 285:196, 1971
75. Krasnow N, Stein RA: Hypertrophic cardiomyopathy in the aged. Am Heart J 96:326, 1978
76. Hamby RI, Aintablian A: Hypertrophic subaortic stenosis is not rare in the eighth decade. Geriatrics 31:71, 1976
77. Koch J-P, Maron BJ, Epstein SE et al: Results of operation for obstructive hypertrophic cardiomyopathy in the elderly: Septal myotomy and myectomy in 20 patients 65 years of age or older. Am J Cardiol 46:963, 1980
78. McKee PA, Castelli WP, McNamara PM et al: The natural history of congestive heart failure: The Framingham Study. N Engl J Med 285:1441, 1971
79. Kennedy RD: Drug therapy for cardiovascular disease in the aged. J Am Geriatr Soc 23:113, 1975
80. Topol EJ, Traill TA, Fortuin NJ: Hypertensive hypertrophic cardiomyopathy of the elderly. N Engl J Med 312:277, 1985
81. Fentem PH, Jones PRM, MacDonald IC et al: Changes in the body composition of elderly men following retirement from the steel industry. J Physiol 258:29P, 1976
82. Cohn JN, Archibald DG, Ziesches S et al: Effect of vasodilator therapy on mortality in chronic congestive heart failure: Results of a Veterans Administration cooperative study. N Engl J Med 314:1547, 1986
83. Martin A, Bembo LJ, Butrous GS et al: Five-year follow-up of 101 elderly subjects by means of long-term ambulatory cardiac monitoring. Eur Heart J 5:592, 1984
84. Fleg JL, Kennedy HL: Cardiac arrhythmias in a healthy elderly population: Detection by 24-hour ambulatory electrocardiography. Chest 81:302, 1982
85. Kantelip JP, Sage E, Duchene-Marulla ZP: Findings on ambulatory electrocardiographic monitoring in subjects older than 80 years. Am J Cardiol 57:398, 1986
86. Nejat M, Greif E: The aging heart: A clinical review. Med Clin North Am 60:1059, 1976
87. Dunbar DN: Ventricular arrhythmias in elderly patients. Evaluation and management. Postgrad Med 81:281, 1987
88. Ingerslev J, Bjerregaard P: Prevalence and prognostic significance of cardiac arrhythmias detected by ambulatory electrocardiography in subjects 85 years of age. Eur Heart J 7:570, 1986
89. Tresch DD, Platia EV, Guarnieri T et al: Refractory symptomatic ventricular tachycardia and ventricular fibrillation in elderly patients. Am J Med 83:399, 1987
90. Wolf PA, Abbott RD, Kannel WB: Atrial fibrillation: A major contributor to stroke in the elderly. The Framingham Study. Arch Intern Med 147:1561, 1987
91. Report of the Joint American College of Cardiology/American Heart Association Task Force on Assessment of Cardiovascular Procedures (Subcommittee on Pacemaker Implantation): Guidelines for Permanent Cardiac Pacemaker Implantation, May 1984. J Am Coll Cardiol 4:434, 1984
92. Greenblatt DJ, Sellers EM, Shader RI: Drug disposition in old age. N Engl J Med 306:1081, 1982
93. Ouslander JG: Drug therapy in the elderly. Ann Intern Med 95:711, 1981
94. Vestal RE, Wood AJJ, Shand DG: Reduced β-adrenoceptor sensitivity in the elderly. Clin Pharmacol Ther 26:181, 1979
95. Wintzen AR, Tijssen JGP, de Vries WA et al: Risk of long-term oral anticoagulant therapy in elderly patients after myocardial infarction: Second report of the sixty plus Reinfarction Study Research Group. Lancet 1:64, 1982
96. O'Malley K, Stevenson IH, Ward CA et al: Determinants of anticoagulant control and patients receiving warfarin. Br J Clin Pharmacol 4:309, 1977
97. Lavarenne J, Dumas R, Cayrol C: Effects indesirable des médicaments chez les persones agées: Bilan des observation recueilliés pendant un an par l'Association Francaise des Centres de Pharmacovigilance. Therapie 36:485, 1983
98. Lowenthal DT, Affrime MB: Cardiovascular drugs for the geriatric patient. Cardiology 36:65, 1981
99. Pathy MS, Peach H: Disability among the elderly after myocardial infarction: A 3-year follow-up. J R Coll Physicians Lond 14:221, 1980
100. Strasser T (ed): Cardiovascular Care of the Elderly. Geneva, World Health Organization, 1987
101. Mellstrom D, Rundgren A, Jagenburg R et al: Tobacco smoking, ageing and health among the elderly: A longitudinal population study of 70-year-old men and an age cohort comparison. Age Ageing 11:45, 1982
102. Gordon T, Kannel WB, Castelli WP et al: Lipoproteins, cardiovascular disease, and death: The Framingham Study. Arch Intern Med 141:1128, 1981
103. Jajich CL, Ostfeld AM, Freeman DH Jr: Smoking and coronary heart disease mortality in the elderly. JAMA 252:2831, 1984
104. Wenger NK: The elderly coronary patient. In Wenger NK, Hellerstein HK (eds): Rehabilitation of the Coronary Patient, 2nd ed, p 397. New York, John Wiley & Sons, 1984
105. Kostis JB, Moreyra AE, Amendo MT et al: The effect of age on heart rate in subjects free of heart disease: Studies by ambulatory electrocardiography and maximal exercise stress test. Circulation 65:141, 1982
106. Goldman L: Cardiac risks and complications of noncardiac surgery. Ann Intern Med 98:504, 1983
107. Wells PH, Kaplan JA: Optimal management of patients with ischemic heart disease for noncardiac surgery by complementary anesthesiologist and cardiologist interaction. Am Heart J 102:1029, 1981
108. Haupt BJ: Utilization of shortstay hospitals: Annual summary for the United States, 1978. In Vital and Health Statistics, Series 13, No. 46, DHEW Publication No. (PHS) 80-1797. Hyattsville, MD, Office of Health Research, Statis-

109. Gerson LW, Skvarch L: Emergency medical service utilization by the elderly. Ann Emerg Med 11:610, 1982
110. Haynes SG, Feinleib M (eds): Epidemiology of Aging. Proceedings of the Second Conference, March 28–29, 1977, NIH publication No. 80-969. Bethesda, MD, US Department of Health and Human Services, National Institutes of Health, National Institute on Aging, National Heart, Lung, and Blood Institute, July 1980
111. Feller BA: Americans needing help to function at home, publication No. 92. Washington, DC, US Department of Health and Human Services, National Center for Health Statistics, September 14, 1983
112. Heller TA, Larson EB, LoGerfo JP: Quality of ambulatory care of the elderly: An analysis of five conditions. J Am Geriatr Soc 32:782, 1984
113. Epstein FH: Is there an age limit to the prevention of coronary heart disease? G Arteriosclerosi 1983, suppl 1, p 30
114. Blankenhorn DH, Brooks SH, Selzer RH et al: The rate of atherosclerosis change during treatment of hyperlipoproteinemia. Circulation 57:355, 1978

GENERAL REFERENCES

Caird FI, Dall JLC, Kennedy RD (eds): Cardiology in Old Age. New York, Plenum Press, 1976
Coodley EL (ed): Geriatric Heart Disease. Littleton, MA, PSG Publishing Co, 1985
Messerli FH: Cardiovascular Disease in the Elderly, 2nd ed. Boston, Martinus Nijhoff, 1988
Noble RJ, Rothbaum DA (eds): Geriatric Cardiology. Philadelphia, FA Davis, 1982
Weisfeldt ML (ed): The Aging Heart: Its Function and Response to Stress. New York, Raven Press, 1980

ASSESSMENT AND MANAGEMENT OF THE CARDIAC PATIENT BEFORE, DURING, AND AFTER NONCARDIAC SURGERY

Lee Goldman

Anesthesia and surgery may represent major stresses to the patient with compromised cardiac function. It is vital that cardiac disease be assessed adequately before surgery to aid in risk assessment and in the planning of any preoperative, intraoperative, or postoperative interventions that may reduce risk. In this process, the physician must be prepared to assess the patient with known or suspected cardiac disease, understand the physiologic stresses and potential consequences of the anesthesia and surgery, and appreciate how general principles of cardiologic care should be applied to the perioperative patient.

PREOPERATIVE EVALUATION, RISK ASSESSMENT, AND MANAGEMENT STRATEGIES

The preoperative evaluation must begin with a careful medical history and physical examination. In patients with known heart disease, this evaluation will often focus on an assessment of the severity of the condition and the determination of whether the current therapy is optimal. In many situations, however, one may evaluate a patient in whom cardiac disease is newly suspected and for whom further evaluation might precede elective surgery.

ROUTINE PREOPERATIVE EVALUATION

For the patient with known heart disease, the careful history and physical examination should be supplemented by an electrocardiogram (ECG) and a chest radiograph. The history must emphasize the determination of the stability of symptoms, the adequacy of current therapy, and the functional status of the patient.

Even if an adult has no prior evidence of heart disease, the history and physical examination should commonly be supplemented by routine ECG in men over 40 years of age and women over 55 years of age.[1]

An ECG is also indicated in patients with systemic diseases or other conditions that may be associated with unrecognized but clinically important cardiac conditions. Thus, an ECG normally would be recommended in patients with hypertension, peripheral vascular disease, diabetes mellitus, and collagen vascular diseases. An ECG is also generally recommended in patients taking medications that may have cardiac side effects or in patients who are at major risk for electrolyte abnormalities[1].

The value of a routine preoperative chest radiograph is less clear. Such radiographs appear to be indicated in patients with clinical evidence of cardiopulmonary disease by history or physical examination. In other patients, the yield of the preoperative chest radiograph, like the yield of any routine screening chest radiograph, is very low,[2] and the procedure is difficult to justify in terms of cost-effectiveness except in patients undergoing chest procedures. Other tests, such as serum electrolytes, creatinine, and glucose, should be ordered selectively in persons in whom underlying diseases or medications increase the likelihood of an abnormal result[3,4].

CORONARY ARTERY DISEASE (KNOWN OR SUSPECTED)

The risk of a perioperative myocardial infarction during or after major noncardiac surgery in adults over 40 years of age without known ischemic heart disease is less than about 1%. In patients with known ischemic heart disease, however, the risk is higher, averaging closer to 2% to 4%.[5,6]

The available literature has considered three groups of patients with coronary artery disease: patients with a known prior myocardial infarction, patients with symptomatic angina, and patients at high risk for having asymptomatic coronary artery disease. Although a patient may sometimes be in more than one group, it is helpful to consider the groups sequentially.

PATIENTS WITH A PRIOR MYOCARDIAL INFARCTION

While patients whose prior myocardial infarction occurred 6 or more months before surgery have about a 2%–5% risk of a major cardiac complication with noncardiac surgery, the risks are higher in patients whose operation occurs within 6 months of the infarction.[7-12] In data pooled from some of the larger studies[7,10,11] from the 1960s and 1970s, recurrent myocardial infarction or cardiac death developed in about 30% of patients who underwent operation within 3 months after a preoperative myocardial infarction and in about 15% of patients who underwent operation between 3 to 6 months after a myocardial infarction. Of note was that these percentages seemed to have changed little, if at all, during the 2 decades up to the mid-1970s. However, more recent data suggest that the risks of operation in patients having surgery less than 6 months after a myocardial infarction may be substantially lower now than was reported a decade or more ago, principally because of the application of modern cardiovascular anesthetic techniques to cardiac patients undergoing major non-cardiac surgical procedures.[6,13] In the most notable series, Rao and colleagues[6] reported a reinfarction rate of 6% in patients who underwent surgery less than 3 months after a preoperative myocardial infarction and a rate of only 2% in patients who underwent surgery between 3 and 6 months after a myocardial infarction during a consecutive series gathered between 1977 and 1982. Similarly, Wells and Kaplan[13] recently reported no reinfarctions in 48 patients who had surgical procedures within 3 months of a preoperative myocardial infarction. In both series,[6,13] rigorous protocols were followed to optimize hemodynamic management: pulmonary artery catheters were placed if the surgery was expected to last for more than 30 minutes, monitored pressures were maintained within 20% of their preanesthesia values, and blood gases, electrolytes, and the hematocrit were followed closely, with any abnormalities treated aggressively.

In addition to the improved outcome in recent series, there are several general clinical guidelines that may be used to select patients in whom the likely risk of cardiac complications is acceptable despite the presence of a recent preoperative myocardial infarction, just as the recent literature has allowed for improved prognostic stratification of the survivors of a myocardial infarction.[14-17] These studies have emphasized that exercise tolerance, the left ventricular ejection fraction, and the presence of congestive heart failure are important and easily obtainable predictors of prognosis. These data suggest that estimating cardiac risk by relying exclusively on the presence or absence of a recent preoperative myocardial infarction may be far too simplistic.

Based on these considerations, several recommendations can be made for risk assessment in the patient with a history of myocardial infarction. First, if more than 6 months has elapsed since the infarction, there is no appreciable benefit from further delay, unless such delay will help improve the management of manifest cardiac problems. Second, if surgery is truly elective, with no strong reasons why it must be performed immediately, it would be ideal to wait a full 6 months before such surgery. If surgery is not purely elective but should not be delayed for a full 6 months, such as the potential complete resection of a carcinoma, one would normally try to delay for 4 to 6 weeks after the infarction so that full healing and scar formation may occur and the early post–myocardial infarction rehabilitation may progress. Submaximal exercise testing, performed either in the hospital or after discharge,[16-19] may aid in the overall assessment by demonstrating whether the patient is able to exercise to levels that equal or exceed the stress that may be associated with the planned surgery. Of course, if urgent or emergent surgery is necessary, such that the surgical risk of delay outweighs the cardiac risk of surgery, one must try to maximize preoperative management but not delay the surgery. In patients with a recent preoperative myocardial infarction, consideration of other factors (multifactorial cardiac risk assessment) will play a major role in determining which patients may be more likely to survive surgery without major complications.

PATIENTS WITH ANGINA

Patients with a history of stable angina have risks similar to those in patients who have survived for 6 or more months after a myocardial infarction, and the preoperative evaluation of such patients therefore should be similar. The clinical assessment of the patient with angina should address several key issues. First, is the angina stable or unstable? Second, what is the degree of functional limitation, and can the patient perform activities that equal or exceed the myocardial stress that is expected with the planned surgical procedure? Third, is the medical regimen optimal, or could it be improved prior to surgery? This includes an assessment for conditions such as poorly controlled hypertension or congestive heart failure that may contribute to the severity of the angina. Fourth, are any diagnostic tests indicated to improve the assessment of the severity of the anginal syndrome because the history or physical examination is inadequate for risk assessment? Fifth, is there an indication for coronary angiography to assess risk and/or as a prelude to coronary artery bypass surgery or percutaneous transluminal coronary angioplasty?

The differentiation between stable and unstable angina is usually a clinical distinction, based on a careful medical history. In some cases, however, the stability of the angina, as well as the patient's functional status, may be difficult to assess because the patient's progressive noncardiac disease, such as a severe orthopaedic or peripheral vascular problem, may mask the severity of the angina.

While the New York Heart Association Functional Classification System[20,21] has long been the standard for assessing functional status, recent data suggest that it is neither sufficiently reproducible nor well correlated with objective exercise capacity by treadmill testing to be particularly useful.[22,23] The Canadian Cardiovascular Society Scale[24] is more reproducible but only slightly more valid.[22] The author has shown that functional classification based on specific questions about what the patient can and cannot do, which has been termed the Specific Activity Scale,[22,23] is the most reproducible and valid of the available easily administered systems for the assessment of functional status. Patients who are class I on the Specific Activity Scale questionnaire are able to perform activities such as carrying 80-pound objects, jogging, or doing heavy recreational or outdoor work, activities that are more stressful than what would be expected with routine surgical procedures. Most class II patients, who can be expected to exercise for more than 3 minutes but less than 6 minutes of a standard Bruce protocol,[22] also perform activities, such as carrying objects up a flight of stairs, that exceed the expected stress associated with most surgical procedures, except in some cases for complicated procedures such as abdominal aortic aneurysm repair. Conversely, patients who are a cardiac functional class III or IV by the Specific Activity Scale or the Canadian Cardiovascular Society criteria commonly may be unable to perform activities that correspond to the stresses that are usually associated with surgical procedures.

If patients do not have a functional class that implies an exercise capacity greater than the stress to be expected with surgery, one must ask whether the medical regimen can be improved. In general, the approach to the control of angina in the preoperative patient is analogous to what one would use in other circumstances. Of course, if the surgery is urgent, intravenous medication such as nitroglycerin may be required for urgent therapy.

There is currently much controversy about the role of diagnostic tests to assess the severity of coronary artery disease preoperatively. Treadmill exercise tolerance tests have a limited sensitivity and specificity as screening tests for the presence or absence of coronary artery disease,[25] but are very helpful in assessing the degree of functional disability in patients with known angina. Since one is worried principally about functional status, not coronary anatomy, in assessing a patient's suitability for surgical stress, the principal role of preoperative exercise testing is in patients in whom the history is unreliable, and therefore exercise testing is required for an objective assessment of functional status. In such situations, the inability to exercise for 3 minutes in the standard Bruce protocol implies a functional class III or IV status,[22] and if this is due to coronary artery disease, one should improve the medical regimen or, if this is impossible or unsuccessful, strongly consider angiography and possible surgical treatment of the coronary disease.

The preoperative cardiac assessment of patients with angina pectoris should begin with a good medical history. If the patient is clearly class I or early class II by history, further diagnostic tests are not usually necessary. If the history is not reliable, formal exercise testing is advised to quantify exercise capacity. In patients over 65 years of age undergoing elective abdominal or non-cardiac thoracic surgery, the inability to raise the heart rate to 100 beats per minute with supine bicycle exercise correlates with a significant increase in the risk of cardiac and pulmonary complications.[26,27] Although some data suggest that patients with depressed left ventricular ejection fractions by radionuclide angiography are at markedly increased risk,[28] other authors have not confirmed these results.[26]

The incremental risk attributable to stable class I or class II angina pectoris for major noncardiac surgery is probably no more than a 1% to 2% risk of a perioperative myocardial infarction,[11] which then carries a mortality rate of about 50%.[5] Cardiac catheterization and elective coronary artery bypass grafting carry about a 1% to 2% risk of death, with about a 5% to 10% risk of a Q-wave myocardial infarction among the survivors.[40] Thus, the risks of catheterization and bypass grafting for patients with stable class I or class II angina pectoris are probably reasonably similar to the potential benefits, even assuming that successful coronary artery bypass grafting would eliminate nearly all of the incremental risk associated with the coronary artery disease. Although patients who have had coronary artery bypass surgery commonly do well with subsequent noncardiac surgery if their functional status is good,[29-33] no randomized trials have been conducted to determine the precise circumstances in which such surgery does more good than harm. Thus, it is vital that the potential risks and benefits be carefully weighed before recommending prophylactic coronary artery bypass surgery prior to or concomitant with noncardiac surgery.

Further information relevant to this issue is provided by the Coronary Artery Surgery Study (CASS).[34] Among patients who had mild angina or who were asymptomatic after a myocardial infarction and were followed as part of the CASS registry, the mortality for subsequent noncardiac surgery was 2.4% among patients whose coronary disease was managed medically and 0.9% among patients whose coronary disease was managed with bypass grafting. Although this difference is appealing, the mortality from elective coronary bypass grafting in the CASS was 1.4%. Thus, the combined mortality from both the coronary artery bypass grafting and the subsequent noncardiac surgery was essentially identical to the mortality from the noncardiac surgery alone in patients whose coronary disease was managed medically. Coronary bypass surgery did not reduce the risk of subsequent cardiac death, and the risk of perioperative myocardial infarction with the noncardiac surgery was also not affected by prior coronary bypass grafting. These results emphasize the rather low absolute risk of major perioperative coronary events with noncardiac surgery in patients with stable and relatively mild coronary disease, and argue against routine prophylactic coronary revascularization prior to noncardiac surgery.

Nevertheless, there certainly are subgroups of patients in whom preoperative cardiac catheterization may be indicated. If patients have unstable angina despite medical intervention or have more than class II angina despite optimal medical management, then one should strongly consider cardiac catheterization prior to major noncardiac surgery. These are patients in whom the expected stress of anesthesia and the following surgical procedure may be substantially greater than the stresses that usually precipitate myocardial ischemia, stresses that the patient therefore either avoids or is prohibited from performing on a voluntary basis. Thus, anesthesia and surgery may represent an unusual stress that may greatly change the patient's expected natural history by precipitating severe myocardial ischemia or infarction.

In patients in whom noncardiac conditions such as orthopaedic or peripheral vascular disease may mask the severity of angina and in whom these same conditions may also prohibit treadmill exercise testing, several diagnostic options have been suggested. One approach is cardiac catheterization with right atrial pacing.[35] If typical anginal pain is precipitated at paced heart rates that are no higher than to be expected by the surgical procedure, especially rates below 100 or 120 beats per minute, and if the pain is associated with hemodynamic changes, such as a rise in the left ventricular end-diastolic pressure, then any observed coronary stenoses are presumably of physiologic importance, and coronary artery bypass grafting may be of benefit. The second option is thallium scanning during pacing[35] to assess transient myocardial ischemia, but it may be no better to use the size of the thallium defect instead of the left ventricular hemodynamics to estimate the severity of the ischemia.

A promising noninvasive approach is dipyridamole thallium imaging.[37-41] Since normal coronary vessels will be dilated by dipyridamole but stenosed arteries will not be dilated, a thallium defect may be precipitated in regions of myocardium supplied by stenosed coronary arteries. In one recent study,[38] the absence of a defect by dipyridamole thallium scanning correlated with a benign cardiac course in patients undergoing major vascular surgery. By comparison, eight ischemic events were noted among 16 patients with transient dipyridamole thallium abnormalities. However, only one of the 16 patients died, and that was a patient who had chest pain during the dipyridamole thallium imaging and who underwent an intra-abdominal vascular procedure. Subsequent studies have suggested that patients who do not have electrocardiographic Q waves, a history of ventricular ectopic activity, diabetes, or a history of angina, and who are not over 70 years of age, are at such low risk that dipyridamole thallium imaging is not needed, while patients with three or more of these factors are at such high risk that one might proceed directly to cardiac catheterization without dipyridamole thallium imaging. In patients with one or two factors, the presence of a thallium redistribution abnormality was associated with about a 30% risk of a coronary ischemic event, while a normal thallium redistribution scan was associated with only a 3% risk.[38] Six (20%) of the 30 ischemic events were fatal. More recently, however, the limitations of dipyridamole thallium scintigraphy in this setting have been emphasized.[40] This technique represents a potentially powerful investigative method in patients whose exercise capacity cannot be determined reliably by the history or even by exercise testing.

In another recent study in patients undergoing peripheral vascular surgery, ambulatory ischemia found on preoperative monitoring was associated with a 38% risk of major postoperative ischemic events, while the rate was only 1% in patients without ischemia on monitor.[42] Ambulatory ischemia remained a statistically significant correlate even after controlling for all other clinical data. Low-risk patients, defined as those who had no history of angina, myocardial infarction, or diabetes and who were class I on the cardiac risk index[11] appeared not to require ambulatory ischemia monitoring. Because it is less expensive, this monitoring may be preferable to dipyridamole thallium imaging in patients whose electrocardiograms do not preclude its use.

In addition to issues regarding the potential for catheterization and surgery, the patient with coronary artery disease often is taking a variety of medications. In general, nitrates cause peripheral vasodilatation, especially in the venous system, but do not pose any major problem for surgical patients. Nitrates have the advantage of being available for intravenous, topical, sublingual, or oral administration, thus making them an ideal class of drugs for the perioperative patient.

Calcium channel antagonists have direct myocardial depressant activity, which may be a theoretic problem in patients whose myocardial contractility may also be reduced by general anesthetic agents. However, at the present time, there are insufficient data about the clinical implications of these theoretic problems, and no firm recommendation can be made regarding the discontinuation of calcium channel antagonists in patients undergoing surgery. In general, the safest option is to continue such medications up to and including the morning of surgery, because at the present time their beneficial effects for anginal control in patients who rely upon them would seem to outweigh any theoretic hemodynamic disadvantages.

While it was initially felt that β-adrenergic antagonists might cause hemodynamic problems during major surgery,[43] it is clear that such medications can be used safely up to and including the morning of surgery.[44,45] In fact, pretreatment with β-adrenergic blocking agents reduces the incidence of arrhythmias, hypertension, and ECG ischemia during laryngoscopy and intubation in hypertensive patients.[46] In patients who are taking less than about 480 mg/day of propranolol, a normal response to atropine and neostigmine is usually preserved.[47] However, the response to β-adrenergic agents such as isoproterenol may be blunted, and it has been suggested that to achieve a 20-beat/min increase in heart rate in a patient taking 120 mg of propranolol per day, a 10-μg bolus of isoproterenol is required; a 30-μg bolus may be required if the daily dose of propranolol is 240 mg, and an 80-μg bolus if the daily dose is 480 mg.[47]

While the potential acute adverse hemodynamic effects of propranolol can be easily reversed by pharmacologic maneuvers, the adverse effects of discontinuing propranolol are less predictable. Among patients who rely on β-adrenergic blockade for the control of ischemic heart disease, a marked exacerbation upon discontinuation of the drugs is not infrequent,[48,49] and in some situations an actual propranolol withdrawal rebound phenomenon may occur.[49]

The signs of inadequate β-blockade include tachycardia, hypertension, and ECG evidence of ischemia, even though sedated patients may not complain of chest pain.[48] The physician must be sure that tachycardia and hypertension do not represent other conditions, such as fluid overload, and must be prepared to reinstitute β-blockade immediately. Since the half-life of propranolol in tissue is approximately 24 hours, such problems will not usually occur until about one day after the last dose. Even with longer-acting β-adrenergic antagonist preparations, the first signs of withdrawal will commonly appear within 48 hours.

Several different regimens have been recommended for patients who cannot take β-adrenergic antagonists orally but who should be given medication post-operatively.[48] Propranolol can be administered through a nasogastric tube, and in many instances, sufficient drug will be absorbed within 30 minutes to prevent or reverse signs of insufficient drug levels. Alternatively, propranolol can be given in 1-mg intravenous boluses up to a total loading dose of 10 mg, followed by 1 mg intravenously every 20 to 60 minutes. A second option is a loading dose of 5 mg to 10 mg over 60 minutes followed by an infusion of 0.01 mg to 0.05 mg/min[50] or about 3 mg/hour.[51] Alternatively, either metoprolol or esmolol can be used. In general, if a patient's angina has been more severe than stable class II *prior* to the institution of medical treatment, expectant therapy with propranolol is commonly indicated. In patients whose angina has always been milder, propranolol may be reserved for the treatment of observed problems. Although one might argue for the more aggressive use of intravenous propranolol in less symptomatic patients, such a policy would require a large number of low-risk patients to remain in an intensive care setting solely for the administration of intravenous propranolol during the several days that may be required to resume full gastrointestinal tract function after an abdominal operation. In some situations, increased doses of nitrates or calcium channel antagonists may substitute for intravenous propranolol, but since nifedipine and nitrates may cause tachycardia, they may actually exacerbate angina in patients who have been dependent on β-adrenergic blocking agents.[52]

PATIENTS AT HIGH RISK OF ASYMPTOMATIC CORONARY ARTERY DISEASE

Elderly patients and patients with diabetes or peripheral vascular disease are at increased risk of asymptomatic coronary artery disease. Unfortunately, exercise tolerance testing is neither perfectly sensitive nor perfectly specific, and a positive test in a symptomatic patient will frequently be a false positive. Even if the test is a true positive and does indicate the presence of coronary artery disease, the key issue for preoperative risk assessment is the patient's functional class, which commonly should be estimated reasonably accurately even without exercise testing. Thus, the key role for preoperative evaluation of the asymptomatic patient for suspected coronary artery disease is in patients who are at high risk and in whom exercise capacity cannot be adequately assessed by the history; this usually implies that the patient cannot exercise sufficiently, because of orthopaedic or vascular problems, for a reliable exercise tolerance test to be performed. In these patients, dipyridamole thallium imaging[37-41] or ambulatory ischemia monitoring[42] can be employed, but such testing would seem to be appropriate and cost-effective in asymptomatic patients only in high-risk circumstances.

HYPERTENSION

There are three types of hypertensive patients who may raise questions during the preoperative evaluation. First are patients with untreated hypertension, second are those with inadequately treated hypertension, and finally those with well-controlled hypertension. Despite recent advances in the diagnosis and control of the hypertensive patient, a substantial proportion of hypertensive patients are undiagnosed or inadequately treated. On admission to the hospital, a patient's blood pressure may be elevated as a result of the acute stress of the situation. A careful preoperative examination may be the first documentation that hypertension exists and that chronic therapy should be instituted. Later, however, the bed rest associated with hospitalization may actually lead to lower blood pressures than would be observed during ambient blood pressure monitoring. In patients in whom hypertension appears to be treated inadequately, observation in the hospital, with the associated mandatory compliance with medications, may distinguish unresponsive hypertension from poor compliance.

Hypertensive patients are more likely to have coronary artery disease and congestive heart failure, both of which may increase the risk of perioperative cardiac complications. Nevertheless, after controlling for other evidence of cardiac disease, such as ischemia, congestive heart failure, and arrhythmias, hypertension itself is not a major independent risk factor for noncardiac surgery,[53] even though it is a univariate correlate.

Hypertensive patients do, however, appear to be more subject to major blood pressure variations during anesthesia and surgery. Prys-Roberts and colleagues demonstrated more perioperative blood pressure lability in patients with higher preoperative blood pressures.[54,55] Patients with a preoperative history of hypertension are also more likely to develop marked postoperative hypertension.[53] However, it is not clear whether the degree of preoperative blood pressure control is a major determinant of perioperative blood pressure lability. Prys-Roberts and colleagues reported conflicting results in two studies, one of which showed markedly lower intraoperative blood pressure values among untreated hypertensive patients but the latter of which showed no significant difference.[54,55] In my experience,[53] the mean intraoperative systolic blood pressure nadir, the need for a fluid challenge or adrenergic agents to maintain intraoperative blood pressure, and the development of marked postoperative hypertension were not significantly different based on whether the hypertension was untreated, inadequately treated, or well controlled. There are several caveats, however. Available data apply only to patients with stable, asymptomatic hypertension and with diastolic blood pressures no higher than about 110 mm Hg; also, all reported data are in major medical centers with expert anesthesiologic care.

Thus, the preoperative evaluation should determine whether the blood pressure is stable and whether there are any symptoms related to it. The physicians involved in the patient's care must recognize the potential that all hypertensive patients have for perioperative blood pressure lability. In general, surgery need not be postponed until tight antihypertensive control has been established if the preceding conditions are met.

The risk of perioperative hypertension is strongly related to the type of operative procedure. Hypertensive events may occur in 50% to 60% of patients undergoing abdominal aortic aneurysm repair; in about 30% of patients having peripheral vascular procedures, including carotid endarterectomies; in about 8% of patients having other major intraperitoneal or intrathoracic procedures; and in fewer than 5% of patients having other noncardiac, nonneurologic surgery.[53]

One of the principal concerns regarding hypertensive patients is the management of their chronic antihypertensive therapy. Guidelines for propranolol are similar to those outlined above for patients with coronary artery disease, with the exception that intravenous postoperative propranolol will be required less commonly because of the availability of medications such as methyldopa or nitroprusside for the control of postoperative hypertension in patients who cannot take oral medications.

Although early authors were concerned about the risk of antihypertensive medications in patients who were about to have surgery,[56] numerous subsequent investigators have shown that it is not only safe but also preferable[54,55,57,58] to continue medications up to, and often including, the morning of surgery. Clonidine especially should be continued up to and including the morning of surgery because of the risk of postoperative hypertension.[59,60] Guanethidine and reserpine cause depletion of norepinephrine at adrenergic sites, so that the perioperative use of indirect adrenergic agents such as ephedrine may not be efficacious, while the use of direct adrenergic agents such as norepinephrine, methoxamine, or phenylephrine may cause a marked hypertensive response because of the principle of denervation-hypersensitivity.

Patients receiving chronic thiazide diuretic therapy will often have some chronic reduction in their blood volumes, but these reductions are less than those that are associated with acute thiazide therapy.[61,62] Patients who take diuretics chronically do not appear to have a markedly increased risk of developing intraoperative hypotension.[53]

ARRHYTHMIAS AND ELECTROCARDIOGRAPHIC ABNORMALITIES

In addition to the risk associated with the ECG finding of a possible recent myocardial infarction, certain arrhythmias and other ECG changes may be associated with increased risk. If the patient has a Q wave consistent with a myocardial infarction of uncertain age, every attempt must be made to obtain prior ECGs. In general, if one cannot date the likely time of the infarction, and assuming that there are no symptoms, enzyme changes, or ECG evolution suggesting that the event is acute, one must usually assume that the infarction may have occurred as recently as 7 to 10 days previously. The safest course of action is to consider such patients as having had a recent myocardial infarction, to assess their risks in such a way, and to follow the management strategies that are suggested for patients with a recent myocardial infarction.

Electrocardiographic ST and T wave changes of ischemia or strain raise the possibility of coronary artery disease, valvular heart disease, hypertensive heart disease, or cardiomyopathy. In the absence of symptoms, such ECG changes probably do not represent a major risk factor for noncardiac surgery.[5,11] Nevertheless, such findings on the ECG should prompt a redoubled effort to be sure that the patient does not have symptoms that may be consistent with unstable or advanced angina, which certainly would change risk assessment and perioperative management.

The presence of atrial or ventricular arrhythmias is often a marker of the severity of any underlying coronary artery disease or ventricular dysfunction[63,64] and is thus associated with an increased risk during major noncardiac surgery. Rhythms other than normal sinus or the presence of frequent ventricular premature contractions in patients with heart disease clearly confers increased risk.[5,11,27] Interestingly, in my experience,[5,11] patients with known heart disease and preoperative atrial or ventricular arrhythmias have had an increased risk of perioperative ischemia and congestive heart failure, as well as of the worsening of perioperative arrhythmias. It is unlikely that patients with arrhythmias but without evident heart disease have an increased risk of perioperative complications, just as such patients do not have a diminished life expectancy.[65,66]

Since arrhythmias are principally a marker of the severity of underlying heart disease and not a predictor of specific arrhythmic complications, preoperative interventions designed specifically to treat asymptomatic arrhythmias *per se* are not routinely indicated. Intravenous prophylactic lidocaine is recommended, however, in patients with a history of *symptomatic* ventricular arrhythmias or a history of an arrest from ventricular arrhythmias. In patients with chronic, asymptomatic ventricular ectopy, lidocaine commonly may be reserved for patients who develop symptoms or a worsening of their ventricular arrhythmias, or for patients who have arrhythmias with concomitant evidence of myocardial ischemia. It must be remembered that the reduction in myocardial performance and hepatic function caused by many general anesthetic agents may greatly lengthen the half-life of lidocaine, and anesthesia may mask the usual early signs of lidocaine's neurologic toxicity. All antiarrhythmic medications should be restarted as soon as possible postoperatively, with the understanding that quinidine can be given intramuscularly and procainamide can be given intravenously.

The patients who are most at risk for postoperative atrial arrhythmias are elderly patients with rales either from a cardiac or pulmonary standpoint who undergo major abdominal or thoracic procedures[67]; elderly patients undergoing lung resections are at especially high risk. Data suggest that digitalis may reduce the ventricular response rate to new postoperative atrial fibrillation[67,68] and may therefore be helpful in elderly patients undergoing pulmonary surgery, in patients with subcritical valvular heart disease who may tolerate such an arrhythmia poorly, or in patients who are not currently receiving medication but who have a history of symptomatic supraventricular tachycardias. Patients with asymptomatic premature atrial contractions do not have a sufficiently high risk of postoperative supraventricular tachycardias for routine prophylactic preoperative digitalis to be indicated.[67] The availability of verapamil hydrochloride has greatly aided the acute therapy of postoperative supraventricular tachyarrhythmias and thus reduced the indications for prophylactic preoperative digitalis; verapamil is a successful drug for slowing the ventricular response rate even in multifocal atrial tachycardia.[69]

Patients with conduction system abnormalities, such as atrioventricular block, fascicular block, or bundle branch block have an increased prevalence of underlying heart disease. If the patient with first-degree or more advanced atrioventricular block has had a history of intermittent complete heart block, vagal stimulation associated with surgery may precipitate complete heart block again. In general, prophylactic preoperative pacemakers for bradyarrhythmias such as sick sinus syndrome or atrioventricular block should be reserved for patients who warrant chronic pacing. If the operative procedure is likely to produce a transient bacteremia, a temporary pacemaker should be inserted and then replaced with a permanent pacemaker after the risk of bacteremia has passed.

Patients with bundle branch blocks, even if they have bifascicular block with a prolonged PR interval, do not have an appreciable risk of developing complete heart block during the perioperative period,[5,70] even though they may have an increased risk of developing complete heart block during long-term follow-up.[71,72] The presence of a bundle branch block is not an independent predictor of major postoperative cardiac complications after controlling for other evidence of more serious heart disease.[5,11]

CONGESTIVE HEART FAILURE

Many general anesthetic agents cause direct myocardial depression, which may make it difficult for the patient to handle the large amounts of fluid that are often given intraoperatively and postoperatively. Thus, it is not surprising that preoperative congestive heart failure increases the risk of noncardiac surgery.[11,27,73,74] The risk of perioperative cardiogenic pulmonary edema in patients over age 40 undergoing major noncardiac surgery ranges from about 2% in patients with no history of congestive heart failure, to about 6% in patients with a history of heart failure that is no longer evident on the preoperative physical examination or chest radiograph, to about 16% in patients in whom left-sided heart failure persists as diagnosed by the preoperative physical examination or chest radiograph.[5] The risk of complications increases as the preoperative functional class of heart failure worsens,[5,73] and over 20% of patients with a history of pulmonary edema may redevelop pulmonary edema in the perioperative period.[5] The most specific predictors of the risk of postoperative pulmonary edema are the presence of an S_3 gallop or jugular venous distention with coexistent signs of left-sided heart failure on the preoperative examination: either of these findings carries up to a 30% risk of postoperative pulmonary edema,[5] which is not surprising since these physical findings are also the most specific predictors of congestive heart failure at catheterization.[75] When congestive heart failure develops perioperatively in a patient with no history of congestive heart failure, it is usually in elderly patients who have preexisting ECG abnormalities or other evidence of heart disease and who have undergone major abdominal or thoracic surgery.[5]

It is imperative that preoperative congestive heart failure be as well controlled as possible before surgery but that one be careful not to dehydrate the patient in the process. Both general and spinal anesthetics commonly cause marked peripheral vasodilatation, which may result in severe intraoperative hypotension in the volume-depleted patient. A good general rule of thumb is to be sure the patient does not have a postural reduction of blood pressure or increase in pulse rate before surgery. In the patient with severe heart failure, there may be some advantage to spinal anesthesia or to general anesthetic techniques that do not cause a decrease in cardiac performance. Hemodynamic monitoring is indicated when patients with severe heart failure undergo major surgical procedures in which marked fluid shifts will be anticipated.

VALVULAR HEART DISEASE

Patients with late class II or more severe valvular heart disease are at increased risk of congestive heart failure, hypovolemia or hypervolemia, and arrhythmias in the perioperative period. Since congestive heart failure is a common accompaniment of valvular heart disease, it is vital that congestive failure be controlled preoperatively in such patients. Nevertheless, as many as 20% of patients with late class II or more severe valvular heart disease will develop new or worsening heart failure during major surgery.[5] Patients with aortic stenosis appear to be at especially high risk[11] because they tolerate hypovolemia and hypervolemia so poorly. Patients with mitral valve disease, especially mitral stenosis, have an increased risk of developing atrial arrhythmias, which may be tolerated especially poorly.

It is crucial that a patient who is suspected of having important valvular heart disease be evaluated preoperatively. In the presence of a murmur suggestive of aortic stenosis, echocardiography, perhaps combined with Doppler studies, may help assess the severity of any suspected aortic stenosis. If the patient has symptoms of congestive heart failure, syncope, or angina and if aortic stenosis cannot be excluded by the noninvasive evaluation, cardiac catheterization will be required. In general, if the patient is asymptomatic, prophylactic aortic valve replacement is not required before elective surgery even if important valvular aortic stenosis is documented by catheterization.[76] The exception is patients in whom regularly performed activities do not meet or exceed the expected stress of the planned noncardiac surgery. In patients with severe peripheral vascular disease or orthopaedic or other conditions that limit activity to a bed-to-chair existence, aggressive preoperative evaluation to exclude the possibility of severe aortic stenosis is recommended even in the absence of cardiac symptoms.

Aortic valvuloplasty is a reasonable alternative to valve replacement in high-risk patients.[77]

In patients with mitral stenosis, the development of marked sinus tachycardia, atrial fibrillation with a rapid ventricular response, or an excessive increase in intravascular volume raises the risk of pulmonary edema. These issues must be considered when deciding whether a patient with mitral stenosis can tolerate planned surgery. In patients with aortic or mitral regurgitation, the increased afterload that is caused by hypertension may greatly reduce cardiac output; thus, hypertension should be controlled preoperatively and treated aggressively if it develops during or after surgery. Decreased intracardiac volume and enhanced contractility worsen left ventricular outflow obstruction in patients with hypertrophic cardiomyopathy; pharmacologic and nonpharmacologic interventions that decrease ventricular volume and increase contractility should be avoided.

Patients with valvular heart disease are at risk of developing bacterial endocarditis if the operative procedure may be associated with a transient bacteremia. This risk is especially high in patients with prosthetic valves. Recent recommendations[78,79] have outlined the approach to antibiotic prophylaxis in patients with valvular heart disease who are undergoing major noncardiac procedures.

If a patient with valvular heart disease has been receiving anticoagulant therapy, one must decide whether to discontinue the anticoagulation before surgery. In general, if the patient is anticoagulated because of native valvular heart disease or atrial fibrillation, the risk of a major embolus during the perioperative period in the absence of anticoagulation is very low, and discontinuation of anticoagulants for a week or two is safe. In patients with non–tissue prosthetic heart valves, discontinuation of anticoagulants for up to 3 days is usually safe,[80-82] except in the occasional patient with a caged-disk valve, in whom anecdotal evidence suggests that even several days without anticoagulation carries a major risk of thromboembolic complications.

Several alternative strategies have been suggested for anticoagulation management in patients with prosthetic valves. Warfarin can be discontinued about 2 days preoperatively and then resumed 1 to 3 days after surgery.[81] Alternatively, warfarin can be discontinued 3 to 5 days preoperatively, the patient can be treated with full-dose heparin until about 6 hours before surgery, heparin can be reinstituted about 12 to 24 hours after surgery, and warfarin can be restarted when the patient can take oral medication.[82] Both of these regimens are associated with hemorrhagic complication rates of 10% to 15%, of which very few of the episodes are life-threatening.[81,82] Despite these risks, one must remember that bleeding complications can usually be controlled, whereas a cerebral embolus may cause irreversible damage.

AGE, URGENCY, AND GENERAL MEDICAL STATUS

Even after controlling for the degree of evident cardiac disease, the general status of the patient will be an important correlate of cardiac complications because of its contribution to the expected cardiac stress. One way to estimate the patient's general status is by the American Society of Anesthesiologists' Classification System, in which a class I patient is a healthy patient having a limited operation, class II represents a patient with a mild to moderate systemic disturbance, class III represents a patient with a severe systemic disturbance, and class IV is a patient with a life-threatening disturbance.[83,84] Although this system is somewhat vague and subjective and hence is poorly reproducible,[85] it does correlate with postoperative cardiac complications.[11,86]

One can also use more objective data for estimating the contribution of the patient's general medical status to the risk of major cardiac complications. For example, the elderly are at increased risk of cardiac complications even after controlling for evident cardiac disease[11,27,74]; the risk is especially high in patients over the age of 70. Risk is also increased in patients who have electrolyte abnormalities, renal insufficiency, hypoxia or hypercarbia, or abnormal liver status, and in those who are chronically bed-ridden for any reason.[11,73,74] In part because of the severity of the surgical condition and in part because of the occasional inability to correct the preceding abnormalities, patients undergoing emergency surgery have a fourfold to fivefold increased risk of perioperative myocardial infarction or of dying of cardiac causes.[5,11]

Although truly emergent surgery should always proceed without unnecessary delay, attention to possible reversible medical problems will likely reduce the risk of postoperative complications. In many situations, the medical consultant's role is not to recommend the cancellation of surgery, but rather to advise as to the optimum timing from a medical standpoint.

UNDERSTANDING THE ANESTHETIC AND SURGICAL STRESS

Although no attempt is made here to be totally comprehensive, it is important to understand the stresses of anesthesia and surgery in order to appreciate how to make recommendations for the perioperative management of the cardiac patient. Anesthesia begins with induction. Intravenous sodium thiopental is generally an excellent agent, although it is often associated with myocardial depression and vasodilatation. Agents such as sodium thiopental may cause a 20% to 30% decrease in blood pressure in healthy patients and even larger decreases in hypertensive patients.[87] Alternatively, ketamine hydrochloride usually results in mild sympathetic stimulation, thus making it a good agent for patients who are hypotensive but creating potential problems in patients who are hypertensive.

During laryngoscopy and intubation, normotensive patients usually have about a 20-mm to 30-mm Hg increase in their arterial blood pressures, but much more impressive increases may occur in the hypertensive patient,[87] often associated with ECG evidence of myocardial ischemia.[54,55,64] This hypertensive response can be reduced by intubation without laryngoscopy or by pretreating patients with β-adrenergic blockade.[88]

During the phase when anesthesia is maintained, both general and spinal forms of anesthesia cause similar reductions in systolic blood pressures,[5] but sometimes even larger decreases occur with epidural anesthesia.[89] It is not uncommon for systolic blood pressure to fall to the 95-mm to 100-mm Hg range and then to be raised by a lightening of anesthesia or, in about 20% to 30% of patients, by a fluid challenge or the use of an intravenous adrenergic agent.[53]

Halothane and enflurane are myocardial depressants, while isoflurane probably produces less dose-dependent depression.[90] Nitrous oxide also can result in a modest decrease in cardiac performance,[91] but it is usually associated with a reflex vasoconstriction such that blood pressure is better maintained than with halothane, with which the reflex vasoconstriction is commonly inhibited. Thus, several studies[53,54] found that halothane tended to be associated with larger reductions in systolic blood pressure and might therefore increase the risk of intraoperative hypotension. Droperidol and fentanyl produce less depression in cardiac performance,[92] and intravenous narcotics also are usually well tolerated in cardiac patients.

Despite these theoretic issues, the medical physician must recognize that the literature has shown essentially no difference in the outcome in cardiac patients based on the type of general anesthesia that was used.[5-10] Furthermore, from a cardiac standpoint, there appears to be little if any difference in the outcome in patients having general anesthesia compared with those having spinal or regional anesthesia.[93,94] Perhaps the one exception is that spinal anesthesia does not cause myocardial depression and may be preferable to general anesthetic agents that are associated with myocardial depression in patients with severe heart failure. However, even in that situation, one now can choose from among various general anesthetic techniques that do not cause myocardial depression. The best rule of thumb is for the medical physician to avoid entering into the discussion about the anesthetic technique and to leave that decision in the hands of a well-trained anesthesiologist. The medical physician must remember that the principal goal of anesthesia is to maintain acceptable hemodynamics and to provide complete anesthesia; inappropriate recommendations suggesting techniques that may provide inadequate anesthesia will only tend to increase the likelihood that pain will produce myocardial ischemia and that the medical physician will lose credibility in the eyes of more experienced colleagues from other specialties.

Intraoperative hypotension is usually managed by lightening the anesthesia, by a fluid challenge, or by the use of intravenous adrenergic agents. However, intraoperative hypotension, especially if it causes the systolic blood pressure to be reduced by 50% or more or to be reduced by 33% for 10 minutes or longer,[5,6,95,96] or reduces mean arterial pressure by 20 mm Hg or more[97] is associated with marked increases in cardiac complications.

In my experience, intraoperative hypotension led anesthesiologists to administer a fluid challenge or adrenergic agents to maintain blood pressure in about 40% of patients undergoing abdominal aneurysm resections; in about 25% of patients having major intraperitoneal, intrathoracic, or peripheral vascular procedures; but in only about 15% of patients having other major noncardiac procedures.[53] However, since anesthesiologists are well aware of the causes, risks, and treatment of intraoperative hypotension, the medical consultant should avoid making trite recommendations such as "avoid intraoperative hypotension."

The type of surgery is clearly related to cardiovascular risk. Major intra-abdominal or intrathoracic procedures carry substantially higher cardiac risks than do peripheral procedures, and abdominal aortic aneurysm repairs carry an even higher risk.[5,11,73,74,98,99] This risk, however, is not related to the length of anesthesia and surgery, since the length of surgery does not correlate with cardiac complications after controlling for the type of surgery.[5,9] It is likely, therefore, that the higher complication rates associated with intra-abdominal, intrathoracic, and aortic procedures are a function of the greater fluid shifts, the greater difficulty in postoperative oxygenation, and the longer and more difficult recuperative processes that are involved in such types of surgery. Patients who undergo peripheral vascular surgery often have advanced diabetes or atherosclerosis and may have advanced coronary artery disease as well. Such patients may have an increased cardiac risk not because of the location of surgery but because their inability to exercise preoperatively may lead one to underestimate the true severity of their underlying cardiac disease.

At the conclusion of positive pressure ventilation, left ventricular filling pressures will commonly increase because of increased venous return. At the same time, the awakening patient may be frightened, be in pain, but still be sufficiently sedated to have suboptimal ventilation. These phenomena often lead to hypertension in the early postoperative period, and they also increase the risk of pulmonary congestion, arrhythmias, and myocardial ischemia.

A second risk period for postoperative hypertension and congestive heart failure is about 1 to 2 days after surgery, when fluid that was "third-spaced" during the surgical procedure is mobilized into the intravascular space. However, the peak risk of myocardial infarction is somewhat later, perhaps because of changes in the clotting system or because the combination of aggressive ambulation and less careful hemodynamic monitoring usually occurs about 3 to 5 days after surgery.

MULTIFACTORIAL CARDIAC RISK ASSESSMENT

Although a number of individual cardiac conditions are associated with an increased risk of perioperative cardiac complications, it is desirable to have a more global assessment of risk to identify patients in whom surgery may be more risky than nonsurgical alternatives or in whom special interventions may reduce risks. The classification system of the American Society of Anesthesiologists[83-86,100] performs such a role for the prediction of anesthetic and surgical complications but may not be as good in predicting specific cardiac complications.[11,33]

In a series of 1001 patients over 40 years of age who underwent major noncardiac and nonneurologic surgery,[11] nine findings from the history, physical examination, ECG, laboratory, and the operation were independent correlates of the development of major cardiac complications and retrospectively grouped patients into four categories of varying risk (Table 113.1). In prospective testing at several institutions, this index has been accurate in identifying high-risk patients,[33,74,98,101,102] and it was found to be superior to the index of the American Society of Anesthesiologists in assessing risk among patients who had general surgery after prior coronary artery bypass grafting.[33] In elderly patients, Gerson and colleagues showed that the index's factors identified high-risk operations.[26,27,33] In the most complete prospective evaluation of the cardiac risk index, Zeldin[102] reported complication rates that were remarkably similar to the predicted rates (Table 113.2).

The principal difference between the original results[11] and the validation series of Zeldin[102] was that class IV patients fared better in the later series, which is consistent with other data suggesting that high-risk patients may fare better now than in the mid-1970s because they are recognized preoperatively and monitored aggressively.[6,13,103] In addition, more detailed investigation of certain situations has identified areas in which the cardiac risk index should be modified for particular patient subgroups. For example, increased experience with patients undergoing abdominal aortic aneurysm resections indicates that the risks of major cardiac complications in classes I, II, and III are about 7%, 11%, and 38% respectively.[99] and are at higher risk than patients who have other types of abdominal and thoracic surgery.[73] Also, patients who have peripheral vascular disease and in whom exercise capacity cannot be adequately evaluated may benefit from noninvasive dipyridamole thallium scanning or ambulatory ischemic monitoring to aid in the identification of groups at high risk.[37–42,104] More recently, Detsky and associates[74,98] proposed a revised multifactorial risk index. It included factors for a myocardial infarction within 6 months, a myocardial infarction more than 6 months ago, class III angina, class IV angina, unstable angina within 6 months, and a history of pulmonary edema. When used by Detsky and colleagues on their own patients, its performance was about equivalent to that of the original multifactorial risk index.[37–42,104]

TABLE 113.1 COMPUTATION OF CARDIAC RISK INDEX

Risk Factor	Points
On preoperative physical examination, presence of (1) an S_3 gallop, or (2) jugular venous distention and evidence of left-sided heart failure	11
A myocardial infarction (Q wave or non–Q wave) in the preceding 6 months	10
More than 5 premature ventricular contractions per minute noted routinely (not including Holter monitoring) at any time	7
Rhythm other than sinus or presence of premature atrial contractions on last preoperative ECG	7
Age ≥ 70 years	5
Emergency operation	4
Intrathoracic, intraperitoneal, or aortic operation	3
Evidence of important valvular aortic stenosis on physical examination, noninvasive testing, or catheterization	3
Poor general medical condition, including potassium < 3.0 mEq/liter; $HCO_3 < 20$ mEq/liter; blood urea nitrogen > 50 mg/dl; creatinine > 3.0 mg/dl; $Po_2 < 60$ mm Hg; $Pco_2 > 50$ mm Hg; elevated aspartate transaminase levels or physical examination signs of chronic liver disease, or any condition that has caused the patient to be chronically bed-ridden	3

(Adapted from Goldman L, Caldera DL, Nussbaum SR et al: Multifactorial index of cardiac risk in noncardiac surgical procedures. N Engl J Med 297:845, 1977. Reprinted by permission)

TABLE 113.2 PERFORMANCE OF CARDIAC RISK INDEX AT TWO HOSPITALS

				No. of Patients With					
		No. of Patients		No or Minor Cardiac Complications (%)		Life-Threatening Complications		Cardiac Death	
Class	Points	Boston	Toronto	Boston	Toronto	Boston	Toronto	Boston	Toronto
I	0–5	537	590	532 (99)	586 (99)	4 (0.7)	3 (0.5)	1 (0.2)	1 (0.2)
II	6–12	316	453	295 (93)	440 (97)	16 (5)	9 (2)	5 (2)	4 (1)
III	13–25	130	74	112 (86)	63 (85)	15 (12)	8 (11)	3 (2)	3 (4)
IV	≥ 26	18	23	4 (22)	16 (70)	4 (22)	1 (4)	10 (56)	6 (26)
Total		1001	1140	943 (94)	1105 (97)	39 (4)	21 (2)	19 (2)	14 (1)

(Data from Goldman L, Calders DL, Nussbaum SR et al: Multifactorial index of cardiac risk in noncardiac surgical procedures. N Engl J Med 297:845, 1977; Zelden RA: Assessing cardiac risk in patients who undergo noncardiac surgical procedures. Can J Surg 27:402, 1984)

There are insufficient data regarding surgical risk in patients with unstable angina or hypertrophic obstructive cardiomyopathy to derive risk predictors in such patients. However, in patients with unstable angina, risks are likely to be very high, and these patients commonly warrant special attention and therapeutic interventions to control their angina, often including coronary artery bypass grafting prior to all but truly emergent surgery.

INTRAOPERATIVE AND POSTOPERATIVE MONITORING AND COMPLICATIONS

Modern hemodynamic monitoring with arterial catheters and pulmonary artery catheters[6,13] probably reduces complication rates in high-risk patients. Although precise guidelines are controversial, such monitoring is suggested in patients with severe heart failure or a recent myocardial infarction, patients who are class IV on the cardiac risk index, some patients who are class III, and in patients undergoing abdominal aortic aneurysm surgery. Some authors have recommended such hemodynamic monitoring in all patients who are over age 65 and are having major surgery,[105,106] but risk commonly can be assessed without these interventions,[107] and I reserve them for defined high-risk subjects.

About 80% of perioperative hypertensive events will occur within 30 minutes after the end of anesthesia, and virtually all will occur in the first 60 minutes.[108] Unless hypertension remains severe for 3 or more hours, perioperative hypertension is usually not associated with other cardiac complications.[53,108]

Perioperative hypertension is commonly precipitated by a reaction to or discomfort with the endotracheal tube, poor oxygenation, pain, excitement, temperature abnormalities, and fluid overload.[108] In view of the usual precipitants of perioperative hypertension, the preferred therapy should be clear: oxygen, sedation, and adequate analgesia are cornerstones of therapy. Morphine is especially helpful for relieving pain and decreasing venous return, and it can be given into the epidural space to decrease hypertension postoperatively.[109]

The exact degree of hypertension requiring treatment with medications is controversial. Some anesthesiologists do not allow the diastolic blood pressure to remain over 100 mm Hg for a prolonged period, while others will treat only if the diastolic blood pressure is above 120 mm Hg or the systolic is above 200 mm Hg.

One excellent medication for the treatment of severe hypertension in the early postoperative period probably is nitroprusside, prepared as 50 mg/500 ml in 5% glucose in water. It will have its onset of action in less than 1 minute and maximum action within 2 minutes; its duration is no more than about 5 minutes. An alternative is intravenous labetalol.[110]

In less severe cases, hydralazine is often administered. As an intramuscular preparation, absorption is potentially erratic and such use should be avoided. If hydralazine is to be used intravenously, it is most safely begun as about a 2.5-mg test dose followed by 5-mg to 10-mg intravenous doses every 5 to 10 minutes. If therapy is begun with 10 mg intravenously, the dose may precipitate supraventricular tachycardia or ischemia.[67] Intravenous propranolol, metroprolol, or esmol can also be used to keep the heart rate below 100 beats/min in a patient who is receiving hydralazine. Intravenous beta blockers should be avoided in patients with congestive heart failure or postoperative fluid overload.

In addition to any specific antihypertensive therapy, morphine is usually administered in increments of 2 mg or 2.5 mg intravenously. Intravenous furosemide is usually given as a 20-mg or 40-mg bolus, which causes immediate peripheral vasodilatation that will be followed by a brisk diuresis. Intravenous methyldopa will not have its onset of action for about 2 to 3 hours, and its peak action will not occur until 3 to 5 hours after it is given. However, intravenous methyldopa is very effective for maintaining an antihypertensive effect several hours later when one wishes to discontinue other intravenous therapies. Clonidine can be given intramuscularly in doses about one half as large as those used in chronic daily therapy[60] in a patient who has evidence of potential clonidine withdrawal hypertension.

Hypertension that develops 24 to 48 hours after surgery, when the patient is mobilizing fluid that was given in the perioperative period, will usually respond to mild diuretics or simply to the restriction of oral intake. As soon as the patient is able to resume oral medications, the chronic antihypertensive regimen should be resumed as tolerated.

The risk of postoperative heart failure peaks at the same times as does postoperative hypertension. Postoperative heart failure may sometimes be caused by myocardial ischemia or infarction, but over half of the cases can be attributed directly to excess fluid administration.[111] Diuretics are the cornerstone of management, and most patients will not require chronic treatment of congestive heart failure if the heart failure was precipitated by excess fluid administration during the perioperative period.

Postoperative supraventricular tachycardias are caused directly by specific cardiac problems in only about 30% of cases[67]; they are more commonly precipitated by electrolyte abnormalities, hypoxia, infection, or new medications. The cornerstone of therapy is therefore the identification and management of these noncardiac problems. Medical interventions with verapamil, digoxin, quinidine, and other drugs may be helpful but should not interfere with the investigation and treatment of these noncardiac problems. Electrical cardioversion will rarely be required, since most arrhythmias will subside with treatment of the underlying condition. In fact, electroconversion may not be very successful if these other conditions have not first been corrected. The mortality rate in patients with new postoperative supraventricular tachycardias is high[67] because of mortality from the underlying noncardiac causes; patients will rarely die as a result of complications from the postoperative supraventricular tachycardia per se. If a patient has had one episode of supraventricular tachycardia during the early postoperative period but has not had further problems later on during the hospital course, any new medications that were started to control the tachycardia may often be discontinued before discharge, with the patient then observed for a day or so in the hospital without the medication.

Postoperative ventricular arrhythmias tend to be produced by the same precipitants that are commonly responsible for postoperative hypertension or supraventricular arrhythmias. In patients who have no clinical evidence of underlying heart disease, treatment is rarely indicated. However, if the ventricular arrhythmia is associated with evidence of ischemia or of hemodynamic compromise, intravenous lidocaine is the drug of choice.

Intraoperative hemodynamic abnormalities[5,6,95-97] are associated with postoperative ischemic complications, but the precise cause and effect is uncertain. In coronary artery bypass surgery, intraoperative ischemia correlates with postoperative myocardial infarction.[112] Asymptomatic postoperative ischemia, as detected by continuous electrocardiographic monitoring, usually precedes postoperative clinical ischemic events.[113] There may be two different syndromes of postoperative myocardial infarction. Non-Q-wave infarctions, which are commonly diagnosed by transient ST-T changes and enzyme elevations,[114,115] tend to occur within 24 to 48 hours after surgery. By comparison, Q-wave infarctions tend to have their peak incidence about 3 to 5 days after surgery.[7,11]

Postoperative ischemic complications are often precipitated by postoperative noncardiac surgical complications. Postoperative recuperation, especially if complicated by surgical problems, is more likely to cause myocardial ischemia than is closely monitored general anesthesia. In high-risk ischemic heart disease patients, it may be wise to moderate the usual aggressive postoperative recuperative process in order to minimize ischemic risk. Such patients may be maintained on prophylactic anticoagulation,[116] since their risk of thromboembolic disease may be higher if the mobilization process is delayed.

About 50% of postoperative myocardial infarctions will be painless,[5] presumably because the patient either has more severe pain at the operative site or is still sufficiently sedated so that the pain is not appreciated. Thus, one must be alert for other signs, such as hypertension, hypotension, arrhythmias, or altered mental status, that may signify postoperative ischemia. Routine daily postoperative ECGs may be indicated only in high-risk patients,[114] although a single postoperative ECG on days 3 to 5 is reasonable for patients with a history of angina or infarction. Routine postoperative myocardial enzymes are not generally indicated in patients who have no signs or symptoms of ischemia.

If a patient has signs or symptoms suggestive of infarction, serum enzyme studies will usually be helpful. The aspartate transaminase (AST) and lactic acid dehydrogenase (LDH) levels will commonly be elevated in patients who have had biliary surgery, and AST and creatine kinase (CK) levels will be elevated after abdominal or orthopaedic procedures.[117-119] CK isoenzyme determination will usually be required.[115,120] Abnormal CK MB isoenzyme fractions commonly are not seen in patients who have had muscle trauma only, and even when they are seen they should not have the same serial evolution that would be seen in patients with myocardial infarctions. LDH isoenzyme determination may be helpful in patients in whom the creatine kinase levels are thought to be unreliable, but hemolytic anemia or renal procedures may cause elevation of the cardiac LDH isoenzyme and make this test unreliable.[121] Technetium pyrophosphate scans often are not helpful in evaluating the postoperative patient.[122,123]

If hemodynamic monitoring has been instituted because of the risk of severe heart failure, it can usually be discontinued by 48 hours after surgery, since by that time the risk of worsening heart failure will have largely subsided. If, however, such monitoring was instituted in a patient with a recent myocardial infarction or potentially unstable ischemic heart disease, one must often continue monitoring for 3 to 5 days after the surgical procedure.[21]

REFERENCES

1. Goldberger AL, O'Konski M: Utility of the routine electrocardiogram before surgery and on general hospital admission. Critical review and new guidelines. Ann Intern Med 105:552,1986
2. Tape TG, Mushlin AL: The utility of routine chest radiographs. Ann Intern Med 104:663, 1986
3. Charpak Y, Blery C, Chastang CL et al: Usefulness of selectively ordered preoperative tests. Med Care 26:95, 1988
4. Turnbull JM, Buck C: The value of preoperative screening investigations in otherwise healthy individuals. Arch Intern Med 147:1101, 1987
5. Goldman L, Caldera DL, Southwick FS et al: Cardiac risk factors and complications in non-cardiac surgery. Medicine 57:357, 1978
6. Rao TLK, Jacobs KH, El-Etr AA: Reinfarction following anesthesia in patients with myocardial infarction. Anesthesiology 59:499, 1983
7. Tarhan S, Moffitt EA, Taylor WF et al: Myocardial infarction after general anesthesia. JAMA 220:1451, 1972
8. Arkins R, Smessaert AA, Hicks RG: Mortality and morbidity in surgical patients with coronary artery disease. JAMA 190:485, 1964
9. Topkins MJ, Artusio JF: Myocardial infarction and surgery: A five year study. Anesth Analg 43:716, 1964
10. Steen PA, Tinker JH, Tarhan S: Myocardial reinfarction after anesthesia and surgery. JAMA 239:2566, 1978
11. Goldman L, Caldera DL, Nussbaum SR et al: Multifactorial index of cardiac risk in noncardiac surgical procedures. N Engl J Med 297:845, 1977
12. Fraser JG, Ramachandran PR, Davis HS: Anesthesia and recent myocardial infarction. JAMA 199:318, 1967
13. Wells PH, Kaplan JA: Optimal management of patients with ischemic heart disease for noncardiac surgery by complementary anesthesiologist and cardiologist interaction. Am Heart J 102:1029, 1981
14. Sanz G, Castaner A, Betriu A et al: Determinants of prognosis in survivors of myocardial infarction. N Engl J Med 306:1065, 1982
15. The Multicenter Postinfarction Research Group: Risk stratification and survival after myocardial infarction. N Engl J Med 309:331, 1983
16. DeBusk RF, Blomqvist CG, Kouchoukos NT et al: Identification and treatment of low-risk patients after acute myocardial infarction and coronary-artery bypass graft surgery. N Engl J Med 314:161, 1986
17. Beller GA, Gibson RS: Risk stratification after myocardial infarction. Mod Concepts Cardiovasc Dis 55:5, 1986
18. DeBusk RF, Kraemer HC, Nash E et al: Stepwise risk stratification soon after acute myocardial infarction. Am J Cardiol 52:1161, 1983
19. De Feyter PJ, van Eenige MJ, Dighton DH et al: Prognostic value of exercise testing, coronary angiography and left ventriculography 6–8 weeks after myocardial infarction. Circulation 66:527, 1982
20. The Criteria Committee of the New York Heart Association, Inc.: Diseases of the Heart and Blood Vessels; Nomenclature and Criteria for Diagnosis, 6th ed. Boston, Little, Brown & Co, 1964
21. Harvey RM, Doyle EF, Ellis K et al: Major changes made by the Criteria Committee of the New York Heart Association. Circulation 49:390, 1974
22. Goldman L, Hashimoto B, Cook EF et al: Comparative reproducibility and validity of systems for assessing cardiovascular functional class: Advantages of a new Specific Activity Scale. Circulation 64:1227, 1981
23. Goldman L, Cook EF, Mitchell N et al: Pitfalls in the serial assessment of cardiac functional status. J Chronic Dis 35:763, 1982
24. Campeau L: Grading of angina pectoris. Circulation 54:522, 1975
25. Rifkin RD, Hood WB Jr: Bayesian analysis of electrocardiographic exercise stress testing. N Engl J Med 297:681, 1977
26. Gerson MC, Hurst JM, Hertzberg VS et al: Cardiac prognosis in noncardiac geriatric surgery. Ann Intern Med 103:832, 1985
27. Gerson MC, Hurst JM, Hertzberg VS et al: Prediction of cardiac and pulmonary complications related to elective abdominal and noncardiac thoracic surgery in geriatric patients. Am J Med 88:101, 1990
28. Pasternack PF, Imparato AM, Bear G et al: The value of radionuclide angiography as a predictor of perioperative myocardial infarction in patients undergoing abdominal aortic aneurysm resection. J Vasc Surg 1:320, 1984
29. Hertzer NR, Young JR, Kramer JR et al: Routine coronary angiography prior to elective aortic reconstruction: Results of selective myocardial revascularization in patients with peripheral vascular disease. Arch Surg 114:1336, 1979
30. Bernhard VM, Johnson WD, Peterson JJ: Carotid artery stenosis; Association with surgery for coronary artery disease. Arch Surg 105:837, 1972
31. Mahar LJ, Steen PA, Tinker JH et al: Perioperative myocardial infarction in patients with coronary artery disease with and without aorto-coronary bypass grafts. J Thorac Cardiovasc Surg 76:533, 1978
32. Crawford ES, Morris GC, Howell JF et al: Operative risk in patients with previous coronary artery bypass. Ann Thorac Surg 26:215, 1978
33. Kaplan JA, Dunbar RW: Anesthesia for noncardiac surgery in patients with cardiac disease. In Kaplan JA (ed): Cardiac Anesthesia, pp 377–389. New York, Grune & Stratton, 1979
34. Foster ED, Davis KB, Carpenter JA, Abele S, Fray D: Risk of noncardiac operation in patients with defined coronary disease: The Coronary Artery Surgery Study (CASS) registry experience. Ann Thorac Surg 41:42, 1986
35. Heller GV, Aroesty JM, Parker JA et al: The pacing stress test: Thallium-201 myocardial imaging after atrial pacing: Diagnostic value in detecting coronary artery disease compared with exercise testing. J Am Coll Cardiol 3:1197, 1984
36. Leppo JA, Boucher CA, Okada RD et al: Serial thallium-201 myocardial imaging after dipyridamole infusion: Diagnostic utility in detecting coronary stenoses and relationship to regional wall motion. Circulation 66:649, 1982
37. Boucher CA, Brewster DC, Darling RC et al: Determination of cardiac risk by dipyridamole-thallium imaging before peripheral vascular surgery. N Engl J Med 312:389, 1985
38. Eagle KA, Coley CM, Newell JB et al: Combining clinical and thallium data optimizes preoperative assessment of cardiac risk before major vascular surgery. Ann Intern Med 110:859, 1989
39. Leppo J, Plaja J, Gionet M, Tumolo J, Paraskos JA, Cutler BS: Noninvasive evaluation of cardiac risk before elective vascular surgery. J Am Coll Cardiol 9:269, 1987
40. Chin WL, Go R, Lenehan S, Underwood DA. Failure of dipyridamole-thallium myocardial imaging to detect severe coronary disease. Cleveland Clinic J Med 56:587, 1989
41. Lette J, Waters D, Lapointe J et al: Usefulness of the severity and extent of reversible perfusion defects during thallium-dipyridamole imaging for cardiac risk assessment before noncardiac surgery. Am J Cardiol 64:276, 1989
42. Raby KE, Goldman L, Creager MA et al: Correlation between preoperative ischemia and major cardiac events after peripheral vascular surgery. N Engl J Med 321:1296, 1989
43. Viljoen JF, Estafanous FG, Kellner GA: Propranolol and cardiac surgery. J Thorac Cardiovasc Surg 64:826, 1972
44. Moran JM, Mulet J, Caralps JM et al: Coronary revascularization in patients receiving propranolol. Circulation 50(Suppl 2):116, 1974
45. Kopriva CJ, Brown ACD, Pappas G: Hemodynamics during general anesthesia in patients receiving propranolol. Anesthesiology 48:28, 1978
46. Prys-Roberts C, Foex P, Roberts JG: Studies of anaesthesia in relation to hypertension. Br J Anaesthesiol 45:671, 1973
47. Prys-Roberts C: Hemodynamic effects of anesthesia and surgery in renal hypertensive patients receiving large doses of beta-receptor antagonists. Anesthesiology 51(suppl):122, 1979
48. Goldman L: Noncardiac surgery in patients on propranolol: Case reports and a recommended approach. Arch Intern Med 141:193, 1981
49. Nattel S, Rangno RE, Van Loon G: Mechanism of propranolol withdrawal phenomena. Circulation 59:1158, 1979
50. Woolsey RL, Shand DG: Pharmacokinetics of antiarrhythmic drugs. Am J Cardiol 41:986, 1978
51. Smulyan H, Weinberg SE, Howanitz PJ: Continuous propranolol infusion

following abdominal surgery. JAMA 247:2539, 1982
52. Boden WE, Korr KS, Bough EW: Nifedipine-induced hypotension and myocardial ischemia in refractory angina pectoris. JAMA 253:1131, 1985
53. Goldman L, Caldera DL: Risks of general anesthesia and elective operative in the hypertensive patient. Anesthesiology 50:285, 1979
54. Prys-Roberts C, Meloche R, Foex P: Studies of anesthesia in relation to hypertension: I. Cardiovascular responses of treated and untreated patients. Br J Anaesthesiol 43:122, 1971
55. Prys-Roberts C, Foex P, Greene LT et al: Studies of anaesthesia in relation to hypertension: IV. The effects of artificial ventilation on the circulation and pulmonary gas exchanges. Br J Anaesthesiol 44:335, 1972
56. Ziegler CH, Lovette JB: Operative complications after therapy with reserpine and reserpine compounds. JAMA 176:916, 1961
57. Katz RL, Weintraub HD, Papper EM: Anesthesia, surgery and rauwolfia. Anesthesiology 25:142, 1964
58. Foex P, Prys-Roberts C: Anaesthesia and the hypertensive patient. Br J Anaesthesiol 46:575, 1974
59. Hansson L, Hunyor SN, Julius S et al: Blood pressure crisis following withdrawal of clonidine (Catapres, Catapresan), with special reference to arterial and urinary catecholamine levels, and suggestions for acute management. Am Heart J 85:605, 1973
60. Bruce DL, Croley TF, Lee JS: Perioperative clonidine withdrawal syndrome. Anesthesiology 51:90, 1979
61. Leth A: Changes in plasma and extracellular fluid volumes in patients with essential hypertension during long-term treatment with hydrochlorothiazide. Circulation 42:479, 1970
62. Tarazi RC, Dustan HP, Frohlich ED: Long-term thiazide therapy in essential hypertension. Evidence for persistent alteration in plasma volume and renin activity. Circulation 41:709, 1970
63. Schulze RA Jr, Rouleau J, Rigo P et al: Ventricular arrhythmias in the late hospital phase of acute myocardial infarction: Relation to left ventricular function detected by gated cardiac blood pool scanning. Circulation 52:1006, 1975
64. Schulze RA Jr, Strauss HW, Pitt B: Sudden death in the year following myocardial infarction: Relation to ventricular premature contractions in the late hospital phase and left ventricular ejection fraction. Am J Med 62:192, 1977
65. Fisher FD, Tyroler HA: Relationship between ventricular premature contractions on routine electrocardiography and subsequent death from coronary heart disease. Circulation 47:712, 1973
66. Kennedy HL, Whitlock JA, Sprague MK et al: Long-term follow-up of asymptomatic healthy subjects with frequent and complex ventricular ectopy. N Engl J Med 312:193, 1985
67. Goldman L: Supraventricular tachyarrhythmias in hospitalized adults after surgery: Clinical correlates in patients over 40 years of age after major noncardiac surgery. Chest 73:450, 1978
68. Selzer A, Walter RM: Adequacy of preoperative digitalis therapy in controlling ventricular rate in postoperative atrial fibrillation. Circulation 34:119, 1966
69. Levine JH, Michael JR, Guarnieri T: Treatment of multifocal atrial tachycardia with verapamil. N Engl J Med 312:21, 1985
70. Pastore JO, Yurchak PM, Janis KM et al: The risk of advanced heart block in surgical patients with right bundle branch block and left axis deviation. Circulation 57:677, 1978
71. Rotman M, Triebwasser JH: A clinical and follow-up study of right and left bundle branch block. Circulation 51:477, 1975
72. Scanlon PJ, Pryor R, Blount SG Jr: Right bundle branch block associated with left superior or inferior intraventricular block: Clinical setting, prognosis and relation to complete heart block. Circulation 42:1123, 1970
73. Larsen SF, Olesen KH, Jacobsen E et al: Prediction of cardiac risk in noncardiac surgery. Eur Heart J 8:179, 1987
74. Detsky AS, Abrams HB, McLaughlin JR et al: Predicting cardiac complications in patients undergoing non-cardiac surgery. J Gen Intern Med 1:211, 1986
75. Harlan WR, Oberman A, Grimm R et al: Chronic congestive heart failure in coronary artery disease: Clinical criteria. Ann Intern Med 86:133, 1977
76. O'Keefe JH Jr, Shub C, Rettke SR: Risk of noncardiac surgical procedures in patients with aortic stenosis. Mayo Clin Proc 64:400, 1989
77. Hayes SN, Holmes DR, Nishimura RA, Reeder GS: Palliative percutaneous aortic balloon valvuloplasty before noncardiac operations and invasive diagnostic procedures. Mayo Clin Proc 64:753, 1989
78. Recommendations from the Endocarditis Working Party of the British Society for Antimicrobial Chemotherapy. Antibiotic prophylaxis of infective endocarditis. Lancet 335:88, 1990.
79. Shuman ST, Amren DP, Bisno AL et al: Prevention of bacterial endocarditis: A statement for health professionals by the Committee on Rheumatic Fever and Infective Endocarditis of the Council on Cardiovascular Disease in the Young. Circulation 70:1123A, 1984
80. Katholi RE, Nolan SP, McGuire LB: Living with prosthetic heart valves: Subsequent noncardiac operations and the risk of thromboembolism and hemorrhage. Am Heart J 92:162, 1976
81. Tinker JH, Tarhan S: Discontinuing anticoagulant therapy in surgical patients with cardiac valve prostheses: Observations in 180 operations. JAMA 239:738, 1978
82. Katholi RE, Nolan SP, McGuire LB: The management of anticoagulation during noncardiac operations in patients with prosthetic heart valves: A prospective study. Am Heart J 96:163, 1978
83. Dripps RD, Lamont A, Eckenhoff JE: The role of anesthesia in surgical mortality. JAMA 178:261, 1961
84. New classification of physical status. Anesthesiology 24:111, 1963
85. Owens WD, Felts JA, Spitznagel EL Jr: ASA Physical Status Classifications: A study of consistency of ratings. Anesthesiology 49:239, 1978
86. Lewin I, Lerner AG, Green SH et al: Physical class and physiological status in the prediction of operative mortality in the aged sick. Ann Surg 174:217, 1971
87. Prys-Roberts C, Meloche R: Management of anesthesia in patients with hypertension or ischemic heart disease. Int Anesthesiol Clin 18:181, 1980
88. Prys-Roberts C, Greene LT, Meloche R et al: Studies of anaesthesia in relation to hypertension: II. Haemodynamic consequences of induction and endotracheal intubation. Br J Anaesth 43:531, 1971
89. Defalque RJ: Compared effects of spinal and extradural anesthesia upon the blood pressure. Anesthesiology 23:627, 1962
90. Merin RG, Basch S: Are the myocardial functional and metabolic effects of isoflurane really different from those of halothane and enflurane? Anesthesiology 55:398, 1981
91. Eisele JH, Reitan JA, Massumi RA et al: Myocardial performance and N_2O analgesia in coronary-artery disease. Anesthesiology 44:16, 1976
92. Bille-Brahe NE, Sorensen MB, Mondorf T et al: Central haemodynamics during induction of neurolept anaesthesia in patients with arteriosclerotic heart disease. Acta Anaesth Scand Suppl 67:47, 1978
93. Yeager MP: Pro: Regional anesthesia is preferable to general anesthesia for the patient with heart disease. J Cardiothorac Anesth 3:793, 1989
94. Beattie C: Con: Regional anesthesia is not preferable to general anesthesia for the patient with heart disease. J Cardiothorac Anesth 3:797, 1989
95. Mauney FM, Ebert PA, Sabiston DC Jr: Postoperative myocardial infarction: A study of predisposing factors, diagnosis and mortality in a high risk group of surgical patients. Ann Surg 172:497, 1970
96. Von Knorring J: Postoperative myocardial infarction: A prospective study in a risk group of surgical patients. Surgery 90:55, 1981
97. Charlson ME, MacKenzie CR, Gold JP et al: The preoperative and intraoperative hemodynamic predictors of postoperative myocardial infarction or ischemia in patients undergoing noncardiac surgery. Ann Surg 210:637, 1989
98. Detsky AS, Abrams HB, Forbath N, Scott JG, Hilliard JR: Cardiac assessment for patients undergoing noncardiac surgery. Arch Intern Med 146:2131, 1986
99. Jeffrey CC, Kunsman J, Cullen DJ et al: A prospective evaluation of cardiac risk index. Anesthesiology 58:462, 1983
100. Vacanti CJ, vanHouten RJ, Hill RC: A statistical analysis of the relationship of physical status to postoperative mortality in 68,388 cases. Anesth Analg 49:564, 1970
101. Weathers LW, Paine R: The risk of surgery in cardiac patients. Intern Med 2:57, 1981
102. Zeldin RA: Assessing cardiac risk in patients who undergo noncardiac surgical procedures. Can J Surg 27:402, 1984
103. Shah K, Kleinman B, Rao T, Mestan K, Schaafsma M: Reduction in mortality from cardiac causes in Goldman Class IV patients. J Cardiothorac Anesth 2:789, 1988
104. Eagle KA, Boucher CA: Cardiac risk of noncardiac surgery. (Editorial) N Engl J Med 321:1330, 1989
105. Del Guercio LRM, Cohn JD: Monitoring operative risk in the elderly. JAMA 243:1350, 1980
106. Babu SC, Sharma PVP, Raciti A et al: Monitor-guided responses: Operability with safety is increased in patients with peripheral vascular diseases. Arch Surg 115:1384, 1980
107. Bille-Brahe NE, Eickhoff JH: Measurement of central haemodynamic parameters during preoperative exercise testing in patients suspected of arteriosclerotic heart disease: Value in predicting postoperative cardiac complications. Acta Chir Scand 502:38, 1980
108. Gal TJ, Cooperman LH: Hypertension in the immediate postoperative period. Br J Anaesth 47:70, 1975
109. Breslow MJ, Jordan DA, Christopherson R et al: Epidural morphine decreases postoperative hypertension by attenuating sympathetic nervous system hyperactivity. JAMA 261:3577, 1989
110. Orlowski JP, Vidt DG, Walker S, Haluska JF: The hemodynamic effects of intravenous labetalol for postoperative hypertension. Cleveland Clin J Med 56:29, 1989
111. Cooperman LH, Price HL: Pulmonary edema in the operative and postoperative period: A review of 40 cases. Ann Surg 172:883, 1970
112. Slogoff S, Keats AS: Does perioperative myocardial ischemia lead to postoperative myocardial infarction? Anesthesiology 62:107, 1985
113. Ouyang P, Gerstenblith G, Furman WR, Golueke PJ, Gottlieb SO: Frequency and significance of early postoperative silent myocardial ischemia in patients having peripheral vascular surgery. Am J Cardiol 64:1113, 1989
114. Charlson ME, MacKenzie CR, Ales K, Gold JP, Fairclough G Jr, Shires GT: Surveillance for postoperative myocardial infarction after noncardiac operations. Surg Gyn & Obstet 167:407, 1988
115. Lee TH, Gold man L: Serum enzyme essays in the diagnosis of acute myocardial infarction. Recommendations based on a quantitative analysis. Ann Intern Med 105:221, 1986
116. Oster G, Tuden RL, Colditz GA: Prevention of venous thromboembolism

117. Person DA, Judge RD: Effect of operation on serum transaminase levels. Arch Surg 77:892, 1958
118. Aryes PR, Williard TB: Serum glutamic oxaloacetic transaminase levels in 266 surgical patients. Ann Intern Med 52:1279, 1960
119. Kelley JL, Campbell DA, Brandt RL: The recognition of myocardial infarction in the early postoperative period. Arch Surg 94:673, 1966
120. Charlson ME, MacKenzie CR, Ales KL, Gold JP, Fairclough GF Jr, Shires GT. The post-operative electrocardiogram and creatine kinase: Implications for diagnosis of myocardial infarction after non-cardiac surgery. J Clin Epidemiol 42:25, 1989
121. Vasudevan G, Mercer DW, Varat MA: Lactic dehydrogenase isoenzyme determination in the diagnosis of acute myocardial infarction. Circulation 57:1055, 1978
122. Massie BM, Botvinick EH, Werner JA et al: Myocardial scintigraphy with technetium-99m stannous pyrophosphate: An insensitive test for non-transmural myocardial infarction. Am J Cardiol 43:186, 1979
123. Goldman L, Feinstein AR, Batsford WP et al: Ordering patterns and clinical impact of cardiovascular nuclear medicine procedures. Circulation 62:680, 1980

CHAPTER 114

RESPIRATORY AND HEMODYNAMIC MANAGEMENT AFTER CARDIAC SURGERY

Michael A. Matthay • Kanu Chatterjee

The purpose of this chapter is to consider guidelines for the respiratory and hemodynamic management of patients following cardiac surgery. There will be particular emphasis on management of patients with preoperative evidence of impaired cardiac and/or pulmonary function. In addition, the importance of heart and lung interactions will be discussed.

RESPIRATORY MANAGEMENT

Management of the respiratory system after cardiac surgery depends on multiple factors, including preoperative cardiac and pulmonary function, intraoperative events, and postoperative hemodynamic status. This section will consider the effects of anesthesia, thoracic surgery, and cardiopulmonary bypass on pulmonary function. Then, respiratory management of patients following cardiac surgery will be discussed.

EFFECTS OF ANESTHESIA, THORACIC SURGERY, AND CARDIOPULMONARY BYPASS ON PULMONARY FUNCTION

A number of studies have documented that an increased alveolar-arterial oxygen gradient is common in patients both during anesthesia and following major surgical procedures.[1] In addition, it has been appreciated for many years that some degree of respiratory functional impairment occurs after thoracic surgery.[2] More recently, it has been demonstrated that following cardiac surgery, patients develop a significant worsening of oxygenation that requires higher inspiratory concentrations of oxygen (FIO_2) in order to achieve a reasonable oxygen tension.[3,4] The physiologic basis for the widened alveolar-arterial oxygen gradient after cardiac surgery is primary right-to-left intrapulmonary shunting due to the lack of ventilation to some air spaces that still receive pulmonary blood flow.[5,6] If there is no ventilation to an alveolus (either because it is collapsed or filled with edema fluid), then it is called a shunt unit, because the blood flowing by the alveolus cannot be oxygenated (Fig. 114.1). If the air space receives some ventilation, though less than normal, oxygenation of pulmonary blood flowing to the underventilated alveoli can be improved with supplemental oxygen, which increases the FIO_2 in the alveolar gas. Following cardiac surgery, a number of investigators have found that right-to-left intrapulmonary shunting constitutes the major cause for the widened alveolar-arterial oxygen gradient; others found ventilation–perfusion mismatch is a secondary cause for the oxygenation defect.[3,6] The relationship of inspired oxygen concentration, arterial PaO_2, and shunt fraction assuming a normal hemoglobin concentration, a normal arterial carbon dioxide concentration, and a normal cardiac output is shown in Figure 114.2.

The explanation for right-to-left intrapulmonary shunting and ventilation–perfusion mismatch in patients following cardiac surgery may be multifactorial. Most patients have no evidence for intracardiac or intrapulmonary shunting during preoperative catheterization. Postoperatively, some have suggested that the oxygenation defect may result from noncardiogenic pulmonary edema that develops after cardiopulmonary bypass.[7] However, the increase in lung water that usually occurs causes only mild interstitial pulmonary edema, which is not adequate to explain the widened alveolar-arterial oxygen gradient. It is more likely that the ventilation–perfusion mismatch and the intrapulmonary shunting after cardiac surgery develops from scattered regions of atelectasis from airway closure secondary to retained secretions and to alveolar collapse, perhaps from alterations in surface active material (Fig. 114.3).[1,3,6,8] In fact, experimental studies have shown that mild increases in interstitial lung water do not result in major gas exchange abnormalities unless there is alveolar edema as well.[9,10] Another mechanism that may worsen the alveolar-arterial oxygen gradient is administration of anesthetic agents that decrease hypoxic pulmonary vasoconstriction.[11,12] In addition, use of vasodilating agents, such as nitroprusside, in the postoperative period will inhibit hypoxic pulmonary vasoconstriction.[13]

Postoperative respiratory function will also be influenced by alterations in the mechanics of breathing that may be produced by inhalational anesthetics and the use of muscle paralyzing agents.[14] There has been some controversy over the effect of inhaled anesthetics on respiratory compliance, although a number of investigators have found a reduced respiratory compliance during general anesthesia and muscle paralysis.[1,15–17] Anesthesia seems to affect the chest wall and diaphragm first, perhaps from central nervous system effects, and later secondary changes in lung function occur with a reduction in functional residual capacity.[18]

Some studies have demonstrated that carbon dioxide elimination is impaired during anesthesia with a significant increase in the dead space fraction.[19,20] Osborne and co-workers[8] reported a rise in alveolar dead space in patients following cardiac surgery, perhaps because of abnormalities in perfusion to the lung following cardiopulmonary bypass. Inadequate alveolar ventilation following cardiac surgery may also be related to decreased ventilatory drive because of the effects of general anesthesia or narcotics, as well as inadequate tidal volume because of neuromuscular weakness.

In addition, cardiopulmonary bypass has been shown to alter pulmonary function. Although most patients tolerate cardiopulmonary bypass well, a number of studies have established that cardiopulmonary bypass may result in a systemic and pulmonary capillary leak syndrome associated with fever, leukocytosis, renal dysfunction, transient neurologic dysfunction, and a bleeding diathesis.[21] These multisystem effects have been called the "postpump syndrome." The mechanisms for this syndrome may be related to exposure of the blood to nonendothelial surfaces with subsequent complement activation, platelet aggregation, and effects on the fibrinolytic system.[21,22] In addition, pulmonary sequestration of neutrophils may occur from complement activation and from shear stress generated during cardiopulmonary bypass by blood pumps, air bubbles, tissue debris, and platelet aggregates. Thus, pulmonary and systemic microembolization may occur

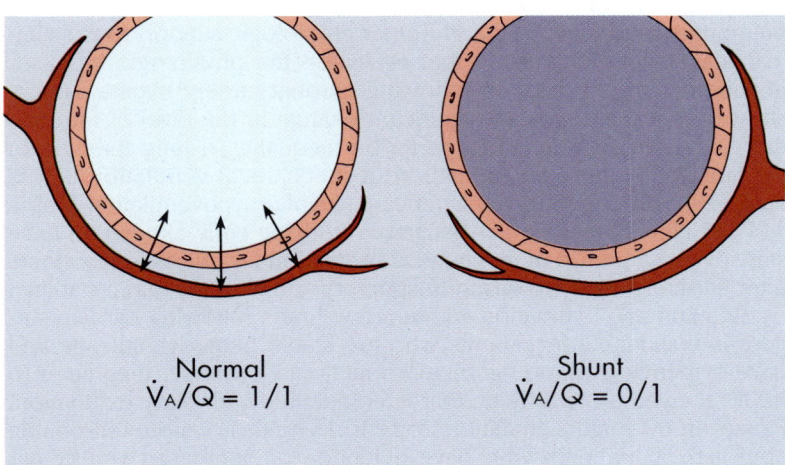

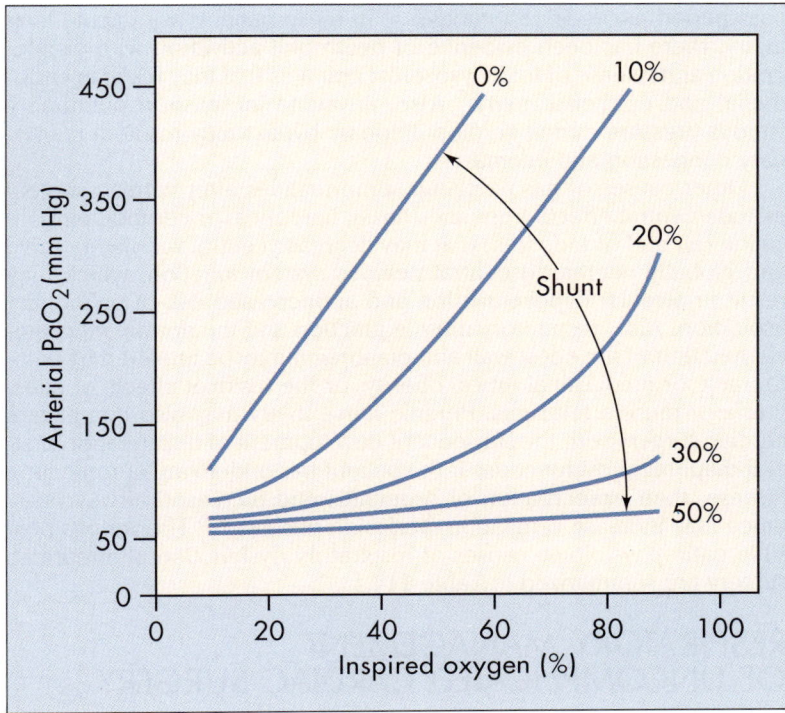

FIGURE 114.1 Left. Schematic diagram of an alveolus with normal perfusion and ventilation with a ventilation–perfusion ratio ($\dot{V}_A/\dot{Q}$) of 1:1. **Right.** Diagram of an alveolus filled with fluid, so it cannot participate in gas exchange. Thus, the ventilation to perfusion ($\dot{V}_A/\dot{Q}$) ratio is 0:1. The same physiologic effect occurs if the alveoli are atelectatic (see Figure 114.3 for a clinical example of a widened alveolar-arterial oxygen gradient and right-to-left intrapulmonary shunting in a patient following cardiac surgery). (Modified from Wiener-Kronish J, Matthay MA: Diagnosis and treatment of acute respiratory failure. In Scheinman M (ed): Cardiac Emergencies, pp 366–383. Philadelphia, WB Saunders, 1984)

FIGURE 114.2 The relationship among the inspired oxygen concentration, the arterial PaO_2, and the shunt fraction is shown. The patient is assumed to have a normal hemoglobin concentration, a normal $PaCO_2$, and a normal cardiac output. (Modified from Flenley DC: Blood gas and acid–base interpretations. Basics of Respiration Disease, ATS News, Fall 1981)

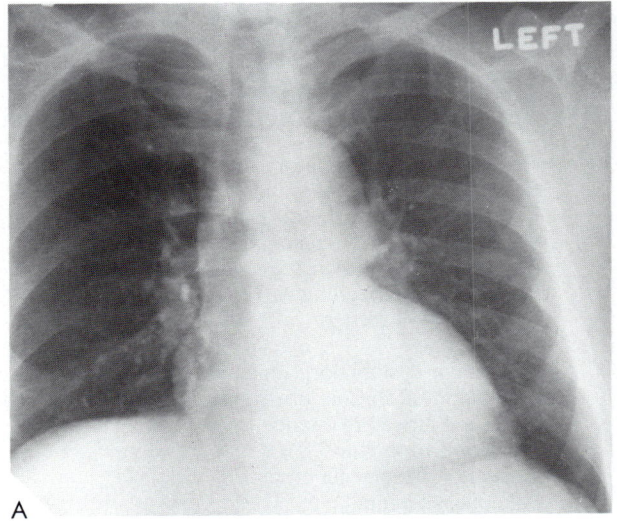
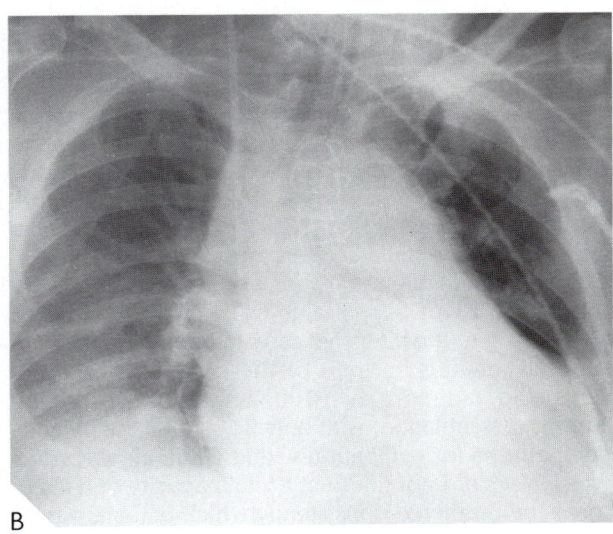

FIGURE 114.3 A. Posteroanterior chest roentgenogram of a 68-year-old man 2 days prior to coronary artery bypass surgery. Lung fields are clear. **B.** Anteroposterior chest film taken 1 day after coronary artery bypass surgery. An endotrachial tube is in place. There is evidence of both right and left lower lobe atelectasis with blurring of the right and left hemidiaphragms. There may also be small pleural effusions. The PaO_2 was 65 mm Hg with an FIO_2 of 0.7 on mechanical ventilation with a tidal volume of 1000 ml plus 5 cm H_2O positive end-expiratory pressure.

during cardiopulmonary bypass. It is controversial whether the nonpulsatile blood flow usually used during cardiopulmonary bypass causes additional damage when compared with pulsatile blood flow.[21]

It has been well established that the duration of cardiopulmonary bypass has some relationship to postoperative respiratory problems.[21,23,24] For example, the severity of interstitial pulmonary edema after cardiopulmonary bypass is directly proportional to the duration of cardiopulmonary bypass.[7] Morphologic studies have shown sequestered neutrophils in the lung after cardiopulmonary bypass.[7] However, it has also been demonstrated in experimental studies that neutrophils may migrate across the lung endothelium and epithelium without causing lung injury; in order to injure the lung, neutrophils need to be activated.[25] Nevertheless, there are some patients who do sustain acute lung injury following cardiopulmonary bypass, especially when the bypass period exceeds 150 minutes.[21] In these patients with acute lung injury, there has been evidence of neutrophil activation with disintegration and release of toxic lysosomal granules that may result in endothelial and epithelial injury.[7] Also, an acute increase in pulmonary venous pressure during cardiopulmonary bypass may result in pulmonary congestion and edema.

Other causes of gas exchange abnormalities after cardiac surgery include central effects from anesthesia, narcotics, or cerebral embolization (air and blood clots) that may decrease central ventilatory drive and globally decreased central nervous system function, which may result in alveolar hypoventilation and an increased risk of pulmonary aspiration. Also, respiratory muscle function and the normal mechanical function of the chest wall and diaphragm may be impaired by pain, thoracic or mediastinal tubes, obesity, or the residual effects of anesthesia or muscle relaxants. Phrenic nerve injury may also complicate cardiac surgery with the subsequent development of unilateral or bilateral diaphragm dysfunction. If the patient has underlying chronic lung disease, then exacerbation of bronchitis and increased airway resistance may increase ventilation–perfusion mismatch.[6] The various possible pathophysiologic causes of respiratory dysfunction after cardiac surgery are summarized in Table 114.1.

RESPIRATORY MANAGEMENT OF UNCOMPLICATED CARDIAC SURGERY

In general, most patients are ventilated for 6 to 18 hours following open heart surgery in order to establish a period of hemodynamic stability and to reduce the immediate postoperative work of breathing. There have been numerous investigators that have considered the routine use of mechanical ventilation for postoperative care of cardiac surgical patients. In addition, some investigators have tested various guidelines for determining the optimal timing for extubation and withdrawal of mechanical ventilation. Most of the early literature from the 1950s through the early 1970s supports the value of mechanical ventilation for respiratory support following cardiac surgery.[26-29]

Subsequently, however, some investigators have offered criteria that would guide extubation within a few hours of surgery. For example, Bendixen and colleagues noted that following cardiac surgery, the average patient could be weaned successfully from mechanical ventilation if the vital capacity was greater than 10 ml/kg.[30] Other investigators have used assessment of mental alertness, muscle strength, hemodynamic stability, and adequate pulmonary gas exchange as a basis for extubation. In one study, 18 of 22 patients (82%) were extubated within 10 hours of returning to the intensive care unit if the total bypass time was less than 100 minutes.[31] None of these patients required reintubation. Patients who had more than 100 minutes of bypass time required longer periods of ventilation, with only 9 (41%) of the patients in this group meeting criteria for extubation within 10 hours of cardiac surgery. These investigators did not find that a vital capacity or a maximum inspiratory pressure predicted consistently which patients would tolerate extubation and spontaneous ventilation. Other studies have indicated that the majority of patients can be extubated safely within a few hours following cardiac surgery. For example, one group of investigators reported that 90% of patients were successfully extubated following coronary artery bypass surgery without any increase in pulmonary morbidity.[32] In another study, 63% of patients were successfully extubated within 5 hours of arrival in the intensive care unit.[33]

More recently, from our own institution, a prospective trial of early versus late extubation following coronary artery bypass surgery was undertaken. Thirty-eight patients were randomly assigned to either early extubation (2 hours post bypass) or late extubation (18 hours post bypass). Anesthesia technique consisted of inhalation agents followed by reversal of muscle relaxants in the patients who were extubated early. There were no significant differences between the two groups in subsequent respiratory or hemodynamic stability. The investigators concluded that early endotracheal extubation following uncomplicated coronary artery bypass procedures with halothane anesthesia is safe and does not increase postoperative cardiac or pulmonary morbidity.[34] To add further physiologic support to this clinical trial, results of a study that evaluated the physiologic basis for impairment of oxygenation following coronary artery bypass surgery showed that there was no significant change in the level of intrapulmonary shunt or ventilation–perfusion inequality in lung function in patients following discontinuation of mechanical ventilation unless analgesia or sedation led to significant alveolar hypoventilation (Table 114.2).[6] Nevertheless, all investigators studying early extubation have still advised a period of mechanical ventilation for at least a few hours after cardiac surgery to ensure respiratory and hemodynamic stability.

In summary, extubation within a few hours following cardiac surgery is reasonable in patients who are stable hemodynamically and have evidence of good ventricular function. Of course, they need to have received an anesthetic that is compatible with early extubation. However, overnight ventilation for 12 to 18 hours is a more reasonable approach in patients who have evidence of decreased ventricular function or who have moderate-to-severe chronic obstructive lung disease. In addition, patients who have had hemodynamic instability intraoperatively or in the immediate postoperative period should be mechanically ventilated until their hemodynamic abnormalities are stabilized. Overall, the risk of continuing mechanical ventilation for 12 to 18 hours postoperatively is minimal, especially when weighed against the possible complications of premature extubation in patients with postoperative arrhythmias, a low cardiac output, a decreased or an agitated mental status, or exacerbated chronic obstructive lung disease or pulmonary edema.[35]

In order to wean patients from mechanical ventilation, it is reasonable to use either a T-piece or CPAP trial to assess their work of breathing in terms of minute ventilation, tidal volume, and respiratory

---

TABLE 114.1 CAUSES OF RESPIRATORY DYSFUNCTION AFTER CARDIAC SURGERY

Decreased central respiratory drive
   General anesthesia, narcotics
   Primary neurologic injury (ischemia from emboli)
Decreased respiratory muscle function
   Residual effect of muscle relaxants
   Pain, chest drainage tubes
   Poor cardiac function
   Obesity, age
   Diaphragm dysfunction (unilateral or bilateral)
Exacerbation of chronic obstructive pulmonary disease
   Increased airway resistance
   Worsened bronchitis
Disorders of alveolar function
   Pulmonary edema
      Cardiogenic
      Noncardiogenic (adult respiratory distress syndrome)
   Atelectasis
   Pneumonia

rate, as well as the effect of spontaneous ventilation on arterial blood gases and vital signs. If the patients are stable for 1 to 2 hours on T-piece or CPAP ventilation, then extubation is ordinarily well tolerated.

RESPIRATORY MANAGEMENT OF PULMONARY EDEMA AFTER CARDIAC SURGERY

The most common cause of pulmonary edema following cardiac surgery is high pressure in the pulmonary microcirculation from elevated pressure in the left side of the heart. The usual cause is related to poor ventricular function, although there may be a specific valvular defect as well (Fig. 114.4). Some patients develop a low cardiac output in association with elevated left ventricular end-diastolic pressure in the absence of any clear evidence of myocardial ischemia. These patients frequently require vasodilator and/or inotropic therapy; the pulmonary edema will gradually clear as the patient's ventricular function improves. Mechanical ventilation is required to support the patients during this time period, both to preserve adequate oxygenation as well as to decrease myocardial oxygen demand by having the mechanical ventilator assume the work of breathing. Other patients require prolonged ventilatory support because of biventricular heart failure in the presence of valvular disease.

Patients who develop the adult respiratory distress syndrome (ARDS) after cardiopulmonary bypass may have severe respiratory failure that requires a longer period of mechanical ventilatory support.[21] The adult respiratory distress syndrome may become the patient's primary clinical problem. Figure 114.5 shows an electron micrograph from a patient with pulmonary endothelial and epithelial injury after cardiopulmonary bypass.

TABLE 114.2 GAS EXCHANGE IN PATIENTS AFTER CARDIAC SURGERY DURING MECHANICAL VENTILATION (MV) AND SPONTANEOUS BREATHING (SB)

Patient	Arterial P_{O_2} (mm Hg)		Arterial P_{CO_2} (mm Hg)		Arterial pH		Minute Ventilation (liters/min)		Dead Space (%)		Shunt (%)	
	MV	SB	MV	SB	MV	SB	MV	SB	MV	SB	MV	SB
1	90	91	35	46	7.49	7.38	14.3	6.0	31.9	38.2	17.9	21.4
2	83	81	35	46	7.49	7.38	12.6	6.6	33.0	38.0	26.1	22.8
3	153	138	38	52	7.48	7.36	12.1	5.0	34.2	25.6	19.1	23.0
4	81	78	41	43	7.44	7.43	5.6	3.7	37.2	39.9	19.3	21.9
5	113	89	34	44	7.48	7.38	10.3	5.6	43.7	31.1	11.9	17.5
6	141	90	38	47	7.51	7.42	10.1	6.3	30.0	29.7	13.6	21.3
7	88	85	35	43	7.48	7.41	10.9	7.6	40.8	46.3	13.8	20.5
8	80	92	53	53	7.36	7.35	7.1	7.5	42.2	35.0	27.7	18.7
9	84	79	43	56	7.37	7.29	10.7	7.5	45.0	48.3	16.4	21.0
Mean	101	91	39	48	7.46	7.38	10.4	6.2	37.6	36.9	17.9	19.9
Standard deviation	28	18	6	5	0.5	0.5	2.8	1.3	5.5	7.5	6.3	2.4
P value (MV vs SB)	NS		0.1		0.001		0.02		NS		NS	

(Adapted from Dantzker DR et al: Gas exchange alterations associated with weaning from mechanical ventilation following coronary artery bypass grafting. Chest 82:674, 1982)

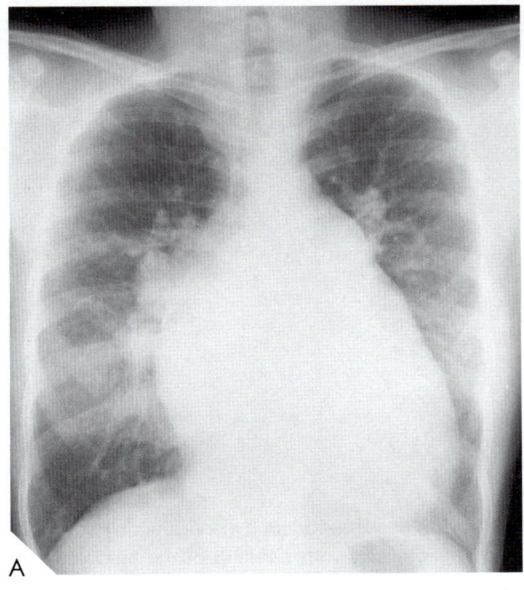 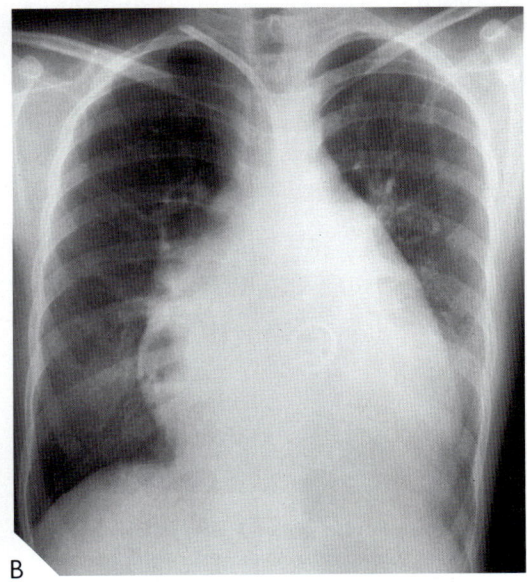

FIGURE 114.4 A. Anteroposterior chest film of a 45-year-old woman with cardiomegaly and pulmonary edema from aortic and mitral regurgitation. **B.** Anteroposterior film shows clearing of pulmonary edema 2 weeks after aortic and mitral valve replacement.

The possibility of sepsis must be considered and ruled out in patients who develop acute lung injury following cardiopulmonary bypass. In most cases, however, the source of the acute lung injury can be related to the duration of cardiopulmonary bypass, a blood transfusion reaction, or a protamine reaction.[36,37] The natural history of ARDS following cardiopulmonary bypass has not been carefully studied. However, our own experience indicates that many patients with ARDS following cardiac surgery have a more limited form of acute lung injury which appears to be restricted primarily to pulmonary endothelial injury. The prognosis for recovery from ARDS following cardiopulmonary bypass may be better than recovery from ARDS associated with sepsis or gastric aspiration.[38] More studies along the lines of recently proposed guidelines for expanding the definition of acute lung injury are needed to evaluate the prognosis of patients with ARDS following cardiopulmonary bypass.[39]

The goals of managing patients with ARDS following cardiac surgery are the same as in all patients with ARDS. Respiratory support depends primarily on the use of positive end expiratory pressure (PEEP) to maintain adequate oxygenation. PEEP significantly improves oxygenation in patients with ARDS by increasing the functional residual capacity, thereby allowing ventilation with a lower fraction inspired oxygen.[40] By lowering the fraction of inspired oxygen, PEEP may reduce further lung injury from oxygen toxicity. In normal lungs, lung impairment from oxygen toxicity can develop after 40 hours of breathing 100% oxygen.[41] Diseased lungs may be more susceptible to injury from oxygen toxicity based on experimental work.[42] However, the safe level of oxygen delivery in ARDS is certainly not established. In one experimental study, dogs were exposed either to air or to fraction inspired oxygen of 0.5 continuously for 8 days after mild lung injury caused by oleic acid.[43] There were no differences in the clinical course, in the lung water content, or in the lung histology for the dogs breathing air or for those breathing oxygen. In this model of moderate lung injury, a fraction of inspired oxygen of 0.5 appeared to be safe. It is certainly possible that higher levels of oxygen concentration may also be safe, though this has not been systematically studied experimentally or clinically.

Other possible benefits of PEEP have not been clearly demonstrated. When given prophylactically, PEEP does not protect against the development of lung injury.[44] Therefore, PEEP does not treat the lung injury, but may be useful in protecting the lung from further injury by allowing a decrease in the fraction of oxygen to safer levels. In patients following cardiac surgery, it is important that cardiac function not be impaired by the use of PEEP. PEEP reduces cardiac output by decreasing ventricular preload. Ordinarily, this will not be a major problem in patients who are treated with levels of PEEP in the range of 5 cm to 10 cm H_2O. However, with higher levels of PEEP, a decrease in cardiac output may result from a decrease in venous return.[45]

It should not be forgotten that oxygenation may be improved by other measures. Increasing the mixed venous oxygen saturation by increasing the cardiac output will improve oxygenation in many patients.[46] Also, paralysis or sedation of agitated patients can decrease oxygen utilization especially when the patient is shivering, because paralysis improves the efficiency of ventilation by relaxing the diaphragm and chest wall.[47] If the pulmonary disease appears assymetric on the chest radiograph then repositioning the patient so that the better lung is dependent may decrease right-to-left shunting and improve oxygenation.[48]

Careful management of hemodynamics is of course important for cardiac stability and minimizing the quantity of edema fluid that collects in the lung. The pulmonary arterial wedge pressure should be maintained as low as possible without compromising stroke volume. An elevated pulmonary arterial wedge pressure will amplify the amount of edema fluid that collects in the lung if there is an increase in lung vascular permeability.[45]

Currently, all treatment is supportive. In particular, corticosteroids are not beneficial in ARDS.[49] A number of review articles provide more information regarding the outlook for advances in treatment of ARDS.[50-52]

MANAGEMENT OF PATIENTS WITH CHRONIC LUNG DISEASE AFTER CARDIAC SURGERY

Preoperative assessment of pulmonary function may indicate restrictive disease with a reduction in lung compliance secondary to pulmonary venous congestion, pleural effusions, or simply a large, dilated heart that compresses the lungs (Fig. 114.6).[24] Occasionally, of course, patients with interstitial lung disease from sarcoidosis, collagen vascular diseases, pneumoconiosis, or idiopathic pulmonary fibrosis will require cardiac surgery.

The most common cause, however, of preoperative pulmonary

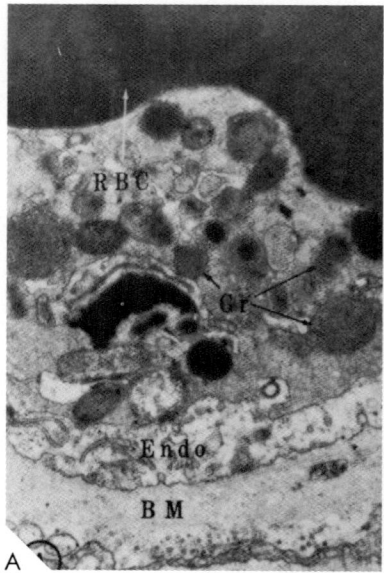
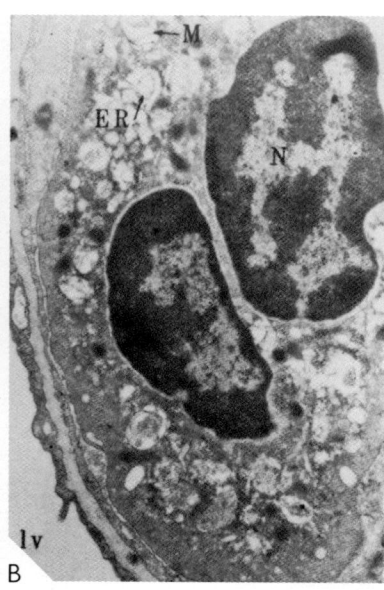
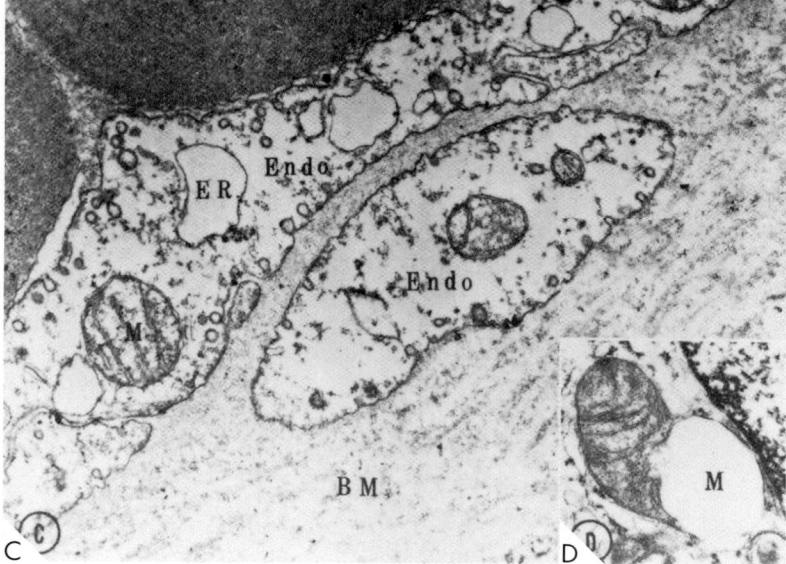

FIGURE 114.5 Electron micrographs taken from a patient's lung following cardiopulmonary bypass. **A.** Granules (Gr) from a neutrophil are floating freely along with red blood cells (RBC) within the lumen of a pulmonary capillary. There is also some cytoplasmic swelling of the endothelial cell (Endo). (BM, basement membrane) **B.** An abnormal neutrophil (N) is within the lumen of a capillary; note the absence of granules and marked swelling of the endoplasmic reticulum (ER) and mitochondria (M). (Alv, alveoli) **C.** Marked endothelial injury with swelling of the cytoplasm, endoplasmic reticulum, and mitochondria. **D.** An example of marked mitochondrial swelling. (Modified from Ratliff ND, Young WG Jr, Hachel DB et al: Pulmonary injury secondary to extracorporeal circulation. J Thorac Cardiovasc Surg 65:425, 1973)

dysfunction in patients undergoing cardiac surgery is chronic obstructive pulmonary disease. A number of patients have mild chronic obstructive pulmonary disease that has no significant influence on their postoperative management. In general, if the forced expiratory volume in 1 second (FEV_1) is greater than 65% of the vital capacity, then the possibility that the patient will have severe pulmonary difficulties postoperatively is low. However, patients who undergo cardiac surgery with moderate-to-severe obstructive lung disease (forced expiratory FEV_1 < 65% of vital capacity, or an FEV_1 < 1.5 liters) do have an increased risk of postoperative respiratory failure. In particular, oxygenation and carbon dioxide excretion may be markedly worse than in patients with normal lung function preoperatively. One classic study of risk factors for patients undergoing elective surgery indicated that identification of high-risk patients with chronic obstructive pulmonary disease is useful, since a preoperative regimen combining antibiotics, bronchodilators, and cessation of smoking did help prevent significant respiratory failure from postoperative atelectasis and pneumonia.[53]

In general, postoperative management of patients with chronic obstructive pulmonary disease should be treated first with inhaled, β_2 bronchodilators.[54] The β_2 agonists (terbutaline, metaproterenol) have a rapid onset of action, are potent bronchodilators, have minimal cardiovascular effects, and have a more prolonged duration of action than aerosols such as isoproterenol.[55–60] Terbutaline (0.25 mg every eight hours) subcutaneously may be given with the goal of dilating small airways that aerosols cannot reach, although with parenteral administration these agents lose much of their β_2 selectivity. There is some evidence that subcutaneous terbutaline can improve right and left ventricular ejection fraction and decrease pulmonary and systemic vascular resistance.[60] Also, β_2 agonists may augment mucociliary transport and thus help patients clear secretions.[55]

In general, the second level of pharmacologic treatment for patients with significant obstructive lung disease following cardiac surgery is intravenous theophylline. Much has been learned about the therapeutic and toxic range for theophylline. A number of studies have demonstrated that theophylline is metabolized more quickly by smokers than by nonsmokers, but patients with liver disease, congestive heart failure, severe hypoxia, or cor pulmonale require smaller doses.[55,57] Generally, a maintenance dose of 0.4 mg/kg/hr should be used in patients with severe chronic obstructive pulmonary disease and moderate-to-severe heart disease. It is important to monitor plasma levels of theophylline to maintain a range of 10 μg to 20 μg/ml. Theophylline toxicity can be heralded by agitation, central nervous system symptoms, supraventricular tachycardia, and gastrointestinal side effects. Grand mal seizures are the dreaded complication of theophylline toxicity and have a high mortality rate.[55]

Theophylline therapy has at least four mechanisms of action that may be beneficial to patients with chronic obstructive pulmonary disease and respiratory failure. First, theophylline produces bronchodilation by relaxing airway smooth muscle. This effect may be mediated by an inhibition of phosphodiesterase (and thereby an increase in cyclic adenosine monophosphate), or it may even act as a prostaglandin antagonist.[57] Second, theophylline stimulates the central nervous system, which may increase ventilatory drive in some patients after cardiac surgery. Third, theophylline can improve right ventricular ejection fraction and decrease pulmonary artery pressure in patients with severe chronic obstructive pulmonary disease and cor pulmonale.[58] Some of these patients, in fact, will show improved left-sided heart function as well.[58] Finally, there are some preliminary data that theophylline may improve respiratory muscle function.[59] However, one recent prospective study in medical patients with an acute exacerbation of COPD demonstrated no benefit of theophylline when added to a standard treatment regimen.[60] The side effects of combined theophylline and β_2-agonist therapy may be more of a problem in cardiac surgical patients because of the propensity of these therapies to cause tachycardia or arrythmias. No general rule can be established indicating exactly what the effects might be in a given patient, but close monitoring of these patients is especially warranted in patients with a history in cardiac disease.

In patients with severe obstructive pulmonary disease following cardiac surgery or severe bronchoconstriction from asthma, it may be necessary to treat the patient with parenteral corticosteroids. It has been shown that corticosteroids are useful in decreasing airway obstruction in patients with acute asthma, and it has also been shown that in patients with acute respiratory failure from chronic obstructive pulmonary disease that corticosteroids result in a more rapid clinical recovery from acute respiratory failure.[61] Corticosteroids may increase the sensitivity of the airway to bronchodilatation with β agonists. In general, a brief course of corticosteroids for 1 to 2 weeks will not result in serious susceptibility to the longer term side effects of corticosteroid administration. The use of corticosteroids may also allow the use of lower doses of β_2 agonists or theophylline as well.

Weaning patients from mechanical ventilation following cardiac surgery is usually not difficult. However, in the case of patients with severe obstructive pulmonary disease preoperatively, it may be necessary to wean the patient very slowly. In addition, it is important to ventilate patients by keeping the arterial carbon dioxide tension similar to the patient's preoperative level. For example, if a patient has baseline hypercapnia with a compensated respiratory acidosis, then it is important to wean the patient from mechanical ventilation starting at this higher level of arterial carbon dioxide tension. Patients can be gradually weaned from mechanical ventilation once their acute cardiopulmonary problems are clearing. This involves an assessment of their hemodynamic stability, airway resistance, mental alertness, and overall nutritional status. Then they can be weaned from mechanical ventila-

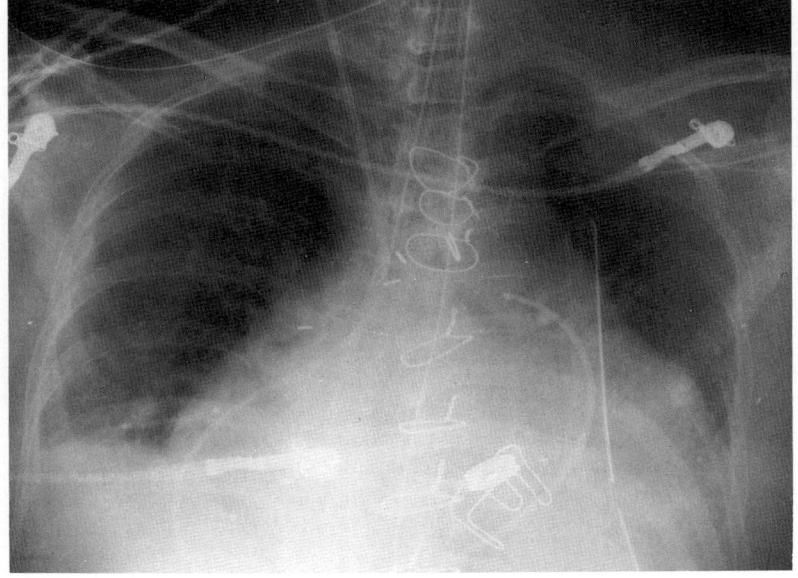

FIGURE 114.6 Anteroposterior chest film of a 58-year-old woman with a history of severe rheumatic heart disease and pulmonary hypertension. Note the massive cardiomegaly due to an enlarged right ventricle after mitral and aortic valve replacement. There is interstitial pulmonary edema and small bilateral pleural effusions. Preoperative pulmonary function tests showed moderate restrictive disease.

tion with a gradual decrease in their ventilatory support.[62] When a patient can maintain spontaneous ventilation for a few hours with adequate arterial blood gases and a minute ventilation of less than 10 to 12 liters for a few hours, then most patients will be ready for extubation.[63] More information on weaning patients from mechanical ventilation, including guidelines for nutritional supplement, is available in a recent review article.[63]

MANAGEMENT OF PATIENTS WITH DIAPHRAGM DYSFUNCTION AFTER CARDIAC SURGERY

A very small percentage of patients (<1%) will develop unilateral (or rarely bilateral) diaphragm paralysis from phrenic nerve injury following cardiac surgery. This may complicate weaning from mechanical ventilation, especially in patients with underlying pulmonary disease. Recovery of diaphragm function generally occurs within 6 weeks, provided that the phrenic nerve has only been injured and not ligated. The diagnosis of diaphragm dysfunction should be suspected when a patient's failure to wean from mechanical ventilation is associated with a vital capacity less than 500 ml. The diagnosis can be confirmed with fluoroscopy or ultrasound to demonstrate paradoxic movement of the diaphragm. Plication of the diaphragm has resulted in respiratory improvement when the paralysis was unilateral.[64]

HEMODYNAMIC MONITORING

Heart rate and rhythm, arterial pressure, and right and left ventricular filling pressures are usually monitored in adult patients who have undergone cardiac surgery, especially if they have preoperative evidence of a decrease in left ventricular function. Although direct left atrial cannulation is still used to determine left atrial pressure in some institutions, flow-directed, balloon-tipped pulmonary artery catheters are now almost universally employed for hemodynamic monitoring. Determination of cardiac output is necessary, not only for confirmation of the diagnosis of postoperative "low output syndrome," but also for evaluation of prognosis. In adults, a cardiac index between 1.6 and 2 liters/min/m^2 during the immediate postoperative period has been noted to be adequate in the majority of patients.[65] The probability of cardiac death increases considerably when the cardiac index is less than 1.6 liters/min/m^2 (Fig. 114.7).[66] Although systemic arteriovenous oxygen difference reflects tissue perfusion and overall oxygen extraction, repeated and direct measurements of cardiac output are frequently required, particularly during assessment of response to therapy of low output syndrome. The thermodilution technique has virtually replaced other methods of determination of cardiac output, including the use of indocyanine green. Arterial pressure is monitored by direct cannulation of a superficial artery, most frequently the radial artery. Arterial cannulation is also necessary for repeated determination of arterial blood gases.

Pulmonary capillary wedge pressure and pulmonary artery end-diastolic pressure are frequently used to approximate left ventricular filling pressure. One study indicated that in the first few hours after coronary artery bypass graft surgery, the correlation between changes in pulmonary capillary wedge pressure and left ventricular end-diastolic volumes determined by radioisotope angiograms was poor.[67] Thus, in some patients, pulmonary capillary wedge pressure may not reflect left ventricular preload. The mechanisms for the lack of correlation between pulmonary capillary wedge pressure and left ventricular diastolic volumes following coronary artery bypass graft surgery remain unclear; open pericardium and alteration in left ventricular compliance might be contributory. Nevertheless, these observations suggest that in some patients, monitoring of pulmonary capillary wedge pressure may not be sufficient to detect changes in left ventricular preload, and other investigations, such as echocardiography or radioisotope angiography, may be required. Monitoring of pulmonary capillary wedge pressure, however, is still useful because it is the major determinant of cardiogenic pulmonary edema.

POSTOPERATIVE HYPERTENSION

Systemic hypertension is common following cardiopulmonary bypass, occurring in 33% to 58% of patients undergoing cardiac surgery. Arterial hypertension results from increased systemic vascular resistance. The mechanisms for peripheral vasoconstriction during the immediate postoperative period are not entirely clear; activation of the renin–angiotensin system, increased catecholamines and serotonin, and abnormalities of prostaglandins have been thought to be contributory.[68–70] Abnormal vasomotor responses associated with altered cardiac and aortic baroreceptor function and nonpulsatile perfusion during cardio-

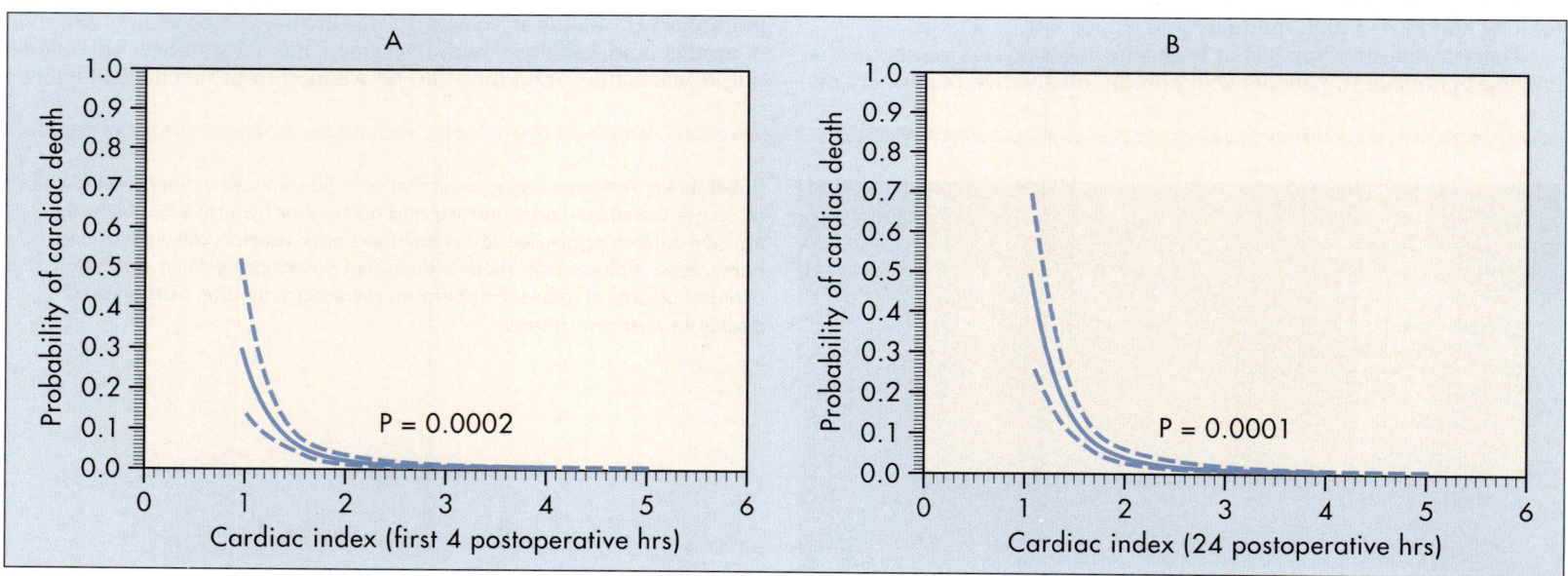

FIGURE 114.7 Relation between the probability of cardiac death and cardiac index during first 4 postoperative hours. **A.** Four hours after surgery. **B.** Twenty-four hours after surgery. (The solid line in both **A** and **B** is the point estimate and the dotted lines are the 70% confidence limits.) (Modified from Kirklin JW, Barrat-Boyes BG: Postoperative care. In Kirklin JW, Barrat-Boyes BG (eds): Cardiac Surgery: Morphology, Diagnostic Criteria, Natural History, Techniques, Results and Indications, p 139. New York, Wiley Medical Publications, 1986)

pulmonary bypass may also influence peripheral vascular tone and cause postoperative hypertension.

Postoperative hypertension tends to occur more frequently in patients who are known to be hypertensive preoperatively. Arterial pressure greater than 160/90 mm Hg, detected the day prior to surgery, also predisposes to postoperative hypertension. Patients with left main coronary artery stenosis greater than 50% have been found more prone to develop postoperative hypertension.[71]

Uncontrolled hypertension during the immediate postoperative period may produce adverse effects on cardiac performance and, therefore, require prompt treatment. Increased arterial pressure may stress suture lines and increase bleeding. Hypertension is also associated with increased tension in the aortic wall with enhanced risk for disruption of the aortic repair. Thus, controlled hypotension is preferable after certain surgical procedures. Hypertension increases left ventricular systemic wall tension, and, hence, myocardial oxygen requirements, which may be contributory to myocardial ischemia, dysrhythmias, and even infarction. Postoperative hypertension has also been associated with an increased incidence of cerebrovascular accidents.[72,73] Increased arterial pressure and systemic vascular resistance also increase resistance to left ventricular ejection, which then decreases forward stroke volume and causes further depression of cardiac function.[74]

Antihypertensive drugs should not be discontinued preoperatively in patients with a history of hypertension. Abrupt withdrawal of certain antihypertensive agents, such as clonidine, may be associated with a profound rebound hypertension. Adequate sedation and an analgesic, usually morphine sulfate, should be the first treatment of postoperative hypertension. Hypoxia and hypercapnia must be corrected. If hypertension persists, then treatment with intravenous vasodilators with a short duration of action are preferable, and their dosage should be titrated to achieve a desirable level of arterial pressure. Intravenous infusion of sodium nitroprusside to 8 $\mu g/kg/min$ is usually very effective for control of hypertension. Infusion should always be started with a small dose, and the infusion rate should be gradually increased every 10 to 15 minutes to lower the arterial pressure to an adequate range. The infusion rate is then adjusted to maintain arterial pressure in the same range. In the absence of heart failure, reflex tachycardia may result during nitroprusside infusion. Concomitant administration of intravenous fluids to maintain adequate preload or β-blocking agents (such as propranolol or metoprolol) may be required to prevent excessive tachycardia. Prolonged administration of large doses of sodium nitroprusside (exceeding 8 $\mu g/kg/min$) may be associated with adverse effects, such as sudden hypotension, thiocyanate and cyanide toxicity, and methemoglobinemia.

Intravenous nitroglycerin has also been found to be effective in controlling postoperative hypertension in most patients. Antihypertensive effects of sodium nitroprusside and intravenous nitroglycerin have been compared in patients following coronary artery bypass surgery.[75,76] Both drugs were found to decrease blood pressure and central venous pressure and to increase heart rate. In 18% of patients, adequate control of blood pressure was not achieved with large doses of nitroglycerin, but nitroprusside was effective. Arterial dilatation with nitroprusside is more pronounced than with nitroglycerin, which is predominantly a venodilator. Nitroglycerin, however, may be more effective in relieving myocardial ischemia, not only due to reduced myocardial oxygen demand, but also due to decreased epicardial coronary arterial tone. Thus, when myocardial ischemia is suspected, nitroglycerin is the preferred drug for control of postoperative hypertension.

Intravenous hydralazine (5 mg to 10 mg every 3 to 4 hours) and intravenous α-methyldopa are occasionally used to control postoperative hypertension, but these agents are less effective than sodium nitroprusside or nitroglycerin and their doses cannot be easily titrated for smooth control of blood pressure. Adenosine and adenosine triphosphate, physiologic vasodilators with little or no acute toxicity and that also do not produce reflex tachycardia, have been used for treatment of postoperative hypertension.[77] More clinical experience will be required, however, to establish the superiority of these agents compared with other vasodilators in use.

HYPOTENSION AND LOW OUTPUT SYNDROME

During the immediate postoperative period, hypotension usually results from inadequate cardiac output and rarely from inappropriately low systemic vascular resistance. The latter mechanism is the principal hemodynamic cause of hypotension in postoperative sepsis. Transient hypotension is not infrequently encountered during vasodilator therapy of postoperative hypertension, particularly when patients start "warming up" 6 to 8 hours after surgery. In these circumstances, hypotension can usually be corrected by discontinuation of vasodilator therapy. Low cardiac output can be caused or aggravated by a number of postoperative complications (Table 114.3), and the correct diagnosis of the underlying mechanism is essential for appropriate management. Low cardiac output decreases oxygen delivery to the various end organs, resulting in tissue hypoxia. Associated hypotension further compromises organ perfusion. Lower hemoglobin concentration impairs oxygen delivery if cardiac output is also reduced. Thus, adequate hemoglobin level (10 g to 12 g/dl) must be maintained in patients with low cardiac output by blood transfusion.

The clinical manifestations of low cardiac output in postoperative patients are often difficult to recognize. Cold extremities may result from hypothermia or peripheral vasoconstriction. Neurologic function cannot be assessed because of the effects of anesthesia and sedation. Decreased urine output, mottled skin, and persistently cold extremities, along with hypotension, should raise suspicion of low cardiac output. With declining cardiac output, tissue oxygen extraction increases, which is reflected in lower mixed venous oxygen tension (P-VO_2). Metabolic acidosis and oliguria also indicates inadequate tissue perfusion. Thus, the mixed venous oxygen tension and the parameters for metabolic acidosis can be monitored to determine the adequacy of cardiac output and tissue perfusion. A mixed venous oxygen tension of less than 30 mm Hg and an arterial–mixed venous oxygen content difference of greater than 6 vol% should be considered evidence for inadequate cardiac output.[78] A mixed venous oxygen tension of 23 mm Hg or less indicates severe inadequacy of cardiac output and is associated with a high probability of acute cardiac death.[79] It needs to be emphasized that mixed venous oxygen tension and arteriovenous oxygen difference (oxygen extraction) parallel the metabolic demand. Thus, even when the cardiac output appears adequate and is in the normal range, a low P-VO_2 suggests increased metabolic demand and a further increase in cardiac output may be desirable. Furthermore, P-VO_2 may be higher than anticipated, despite a low cardiac output. A marked reduction in cardiac output may be associated with reduced perfusion of some peripheral tissues, resulting in reduced oxygen consumption. Hypothermia may also decrease metabolic demand, and P-VO_2 may be higher than expected for cardiac output. A proper interpretation of P-VO_2, therefore, requires consideration of metabolic demand and oxygen consumption, which may vary according to the body temperature as well as alterations in the circulatory and metabolic status in the postoperative period. Thus, concomitant measurements of cardiac output and mixed venous oxygen tension plus calculation of oxygen extraction are preferable to assess adequacy of cardiac performance in postoperative patients.

HYPOVOLEMIA

A decrease in circulating intravascular volume may occur despite increased body water and total extracellular fluid volume following cardiopulmonary bypass.[80] Both inadequate volume replacement after cardiopulmonary bypass and increased capillary permeability causing "third space" fluid loss contribute to intravascular hypovolemia. A positive fluid balance in these circumstances does not exclude a decreased circulating blood volume. Thus, body weight changes cannot be used to determine the intravascular volume status.

During the immediate postoperative period, peripheral venous tone is increased, probably related to hypothermia and increased sympathetic activity. During rewarming, vasodilation is associated with increased vascular capacitance, decreased venous return, decreased intracardiac volumes, and further reduction in cardiac output. These circulatory adjustments should be anticipated, and appropriate volume expansion should be provided to avoid low cardiac output and hypotension.

Hypovolemia is usually diagnosed by demonstrating that both right atrial (central venous) and pulmonary capillary wedge pressures are less than normal. Decreased right atrial pressure alone may not be a sufficient indicator of hypovolemia, since it can be normal or even relatively low in the presence of elevated pulmonary capillary wedge pressure, either because of isolated left ventricular failure or decreased left ventricular compliance. Furthermore, in postcoronary bypass surgery patients, changes in pulmonary capillary wedge pressure may not always reflect changes in left ventricular preload.[67] In these circumstances, an estimate of ventricular volumes by echocardiography or radioisotopic angiography may be necessary to determine the adequacy of ventricular preloads.

Therapy for hypovolemia is intravenous administration of fluids to maintain adequate right atrial and pulmonary capillary wedge pressures. The type of fluid is guided by the hemoglobin concentration. If it is low, whole blood transfusions are desirable. As in patients with acute myocardial infarction, the increase in cardiac output usually reaches a plateau when pulmonary capillary wedge pressure increases to between 15 mm Hg and 18 mm Hg, except in patients who have a marked decrease in ventricular compliance.[81,82] During volume expansion, if there is an inadequate increase in cardiac output, other causes of low cardiac output should be suspected.

CARDIAC TAMPONADE

Cardiac tamponade results from decreased diastolic filling of the heart secondary to increased intrapericardial pressure, which is usually due to intrapericardial bleeding in the early postoperative phase. The diagnosis of cardiac tamponade during the early postoperative period is often difficult because the expected physical findings may not be present. Decreased heart sounds and a quiet precordium are not usually present because the anterior pericardium may be open. Pulsus paradoxus may result from artificial ventilation; partial or total electrical alternans are rare in the postoperative patient. Cardiac tamponade can occur despite an open pericardium and the use of large-caliber mediastinal drainage. Demonstration of a pericardial collection of blood by echocardiography or by radioisotope angiography does not necessarily indicate cardiac tamponade. Routine echocardiography performed during the early postoperative period demonstrates intrapericardial fluid in the vast majority of patients following cardiac surgery.[83] In approximately 83% of patients, pericardial effusion was detected postoperatively, and in the majority of patients (70%), it was already present, as expected, on the second postoperative day. The pericardial effusion reached maximum size by the tenth postoperative day. Although echocardiographically demonstrable pericardial effusion was very common, the incidence of cardiac tamponade was only 1%.

In postcardiac surgical patients, tamponade can occur, not only from the nonloculated pericardial effusions surrounding both ventricles, but also from the presence of a loculated effusion, usually located posteriorly.[84] Loculated pericardial effusion or localized pericardial hematomas can cause compression of any intracardiac chamber and may be associated with clinical and hemodynamic abnormalities of cardiac tamponade. Two-dimensional echocardiography has been found useful for diagnosing both nonloculated and loculated pericardial effusion.[84] Computed tomography is also useful for detecting localized hematomas.[85] Wide mediastinum is also a frequent radiologic finding after cardiac surgery. Determination of the hemodynamic abnormalities, which include increasing right atrial and pulmonary capillary wedge pressure and frequently equalization of right and left ventricular filling pressures along with hypotension and low cardiac output, helps in the diagnosis of tamponade.[86] However, diagnosis primarily depends on the clinical suspicion and the detection of the clinical correlates of hemodynamic abnormalities, such as elevated systemic venous pressure, tachycardia, and falling arterial pressure. Cardiac tamponade may occur several days or several weeks after cardiac surgery (delayed cardiac tamponade), usually in patients who are on long-term anticoagulation therapy. If unrecognized, delayed tamponade may cause serious morbidity and mortality.[87,88] Weakness, lethargy, dyspnea on exertion, increased jugular venous pressure, peripheral edema, and occasionally ascites and prerenal azotemia may

TABLE 114.3 POTENTIAL CAUSES OF LOW CARDIAC OUTPUT IN THE POSTOPERATIVE PERIOD

Hypovolemia:
  Blood loss
  Third space loss
Mechanical:
  Tamponade
  Pneumothorax
  Pulmonary embolism
Increased left ventricular afterload:
  Postoperative hypertension
Increased right ventricular afterload:
  Increased pulmonary artery pressure
  Increased pulmonary vascular resistance
Decreased left ventricular contractility:
  Poor myocardial preservation
  Perioperative myocardial infarction
  Incomplete revascularization
  Coronary artery spasm
  Coronary artery or graft embolism
    (air or particulates)
  Preoperative left ventricular dysfunction
Decreased right ventricular contractility:
  Right ventricular infarction
	Dysrhythmias:
	  Inadequate heart rate: atrioventricular block,
	    junctional rhythm
	  Ventricular and supraventricular tachyarrhythmias
	Acid–base imbalance
	Hypoxemia, hypercarbia, and hypocarbia
	Electrolyte abnormalities: hypocalcemia, hyperkalemia
	Drug toxicity: procainamide, verapamil, amiodarone
	Anaphylactic reactions
	Inadequate surgical correction of mechanical lesions
	    or mechanical
	    complications of surgical corrections:
	  Residual ventricular or atrial septal defect
	  Paraprosthetic leak, patient–prosthetic valve mismatch

be mistaken clinically as evidence for severe congestive heart failure. Pulsus paradoxus, widening of the cardiac silhouette on the chest film, and absence of atrial and ventricular gallops, as well as lack of physical findings of pulmonary arterial hypertension, should raise suspicion of cardiac tamponade. Diagnosis can be confirmed by echocardiography, which demonstrates intrapericardial fluid, normal ventricular systolic function, and compression of the right atrium and right ventricle. It is rarely necessary to perform hemodynamic studies in these patients. If right-sided heart catheterization is done, hemodynamics demonstrate equalization of right atrial, right ventricular end-diastolic, pulmonary artery end-diastolic, and pulmonary capillary wedge pressures.

Early postoperative cardiac tamponade requires emergency sternotomy for decompression, and this can be done at the bedside in the intensive care unit. Pericardial decompression in delayed cardiac tamponade is accomplished either by pericardiocentesis or surgical drainage. It needs to be emphasized that if cardiac tamponade is suspected in a hypotensive patient, decompression should not be delayed to determine the hemodynamics or to assess response to pharmacotherapy.

LEFT VENTRICULAR FAILURE

Introduction of cold cardioplegic solution to induce cardiac arrest intraoperatively has decreased the incidence of severe myocardial injury during cardiopulmonary bypass significantly.[89] Despite the improved techniques for myocardial preservation, varying degrees of myocardial dysfunction occur postoperatively, particularly in patients with severe valvular heart disease, coronary artery disease with preoperative depressed left ventricular function, and severe left ventricular hypertrophy. Perioperative myocardial infarction, residual surgically uncorrected abnormalities, inadequate myocardial revascularization, and poor myocardial preservation during cardiopulmonary bypass may also precipitate a low output state postoperatively.

Left ventricular failure should be suspected when low cardiac output is associated with elevated pulmonary capillary wedge pressure. Since these hemodynamic abnormalities may also occur due to decreased left ventricular compliance, assessment of left ventricular size and systolic function by echocardiography or radioisotope angiography should be considered to confirm the diagnosis. Left ventricular failure is associated with increased left ventricular size and decreased systolic wall motion.

Once left ventricular failure is diagnosed, a search should be made for the etiology. New Q waves along with ST segment elevation, particularly in the anterior precordial electrocardiographic leads, almost always suggest recent perioperative myocardial infarction.[90] Myocardial necrosis can occur in the absence of electrocardiographic signs of myocardial infarction; the electrocardiograms may reveal only nonspecific ST-T wave changes, which are common postoperatively. In patients undergoing myocardial revascularization, total creatine kinase (CK) is always abnormally elevated and CK-MB is also detectable in the absence of clinically relevant perioperative myocardial infarction. Technetium-99m myocardial scintigraphy is more useful in the diagnosis of perioperative myocardial infarction.[90] Perioperative myocardial infarction does not always result from closure of the aortocoronary artery bypass grafts. In many patients, infarcted myocardial segments are perfused by patent bypass grafts, as demonstrated by contrast computerized tomography.[91]

Coronary artery spasm can occur during the early postoperative phase, but is a rare cause of postoperative myocardial necrosis and left ventricular failure. The incidence has been estimated to be approximately 0.8%.[92] Spasm has also been demonstrated in the aortocoronary saphenous vein grafts.[93] Coronary artery spasm should be suspected if there is acute ST segment elevation on the electrocardiogram, particularly in the area of the coronary artery without a critical stenosis.[94] Therapy is directed to relieve the spasm using intravenous nitroglycerin, intravenous verapamil, or sublingual nifedipine. If hypotension occurs as a result of large doses of intravenous nitroglycerin, concomitant infusion of phenylephrine or norepinephrine may be required to maintain arterial pressure.[95] Intracoronary nitroglycerin in boluses of 0.1 mg to 1 mg has been required to relieve postoperative coronary artery spasm associated with hemodynamic compromise in occasional patients who failed to respond to conventional therapy.[92] It has been suggested that abrupt withdrawal of nifedipine may predispose to postoperative coronary artery spasms[96]; when such a cause is suspected, reinstitution of nifedipine therapy should be considered, and it can be administered either sublingually or via a nasogastric tube.

Air embolization of the coronary arteries can occur up to 24 hours after cardiac surgery involving the ascending aorta or left heart chambers. Most frequently, the right coronary artery is involved in the supine position—the ostium of the right coronary artery is in its most anterior position (at the highest elevation of the aortic root). Air embolization of a coronary artery is often temporally related to the physical repositioning of the patient.[97] The electrocardiographic changes and the consequences of coronary artery embolism are similar to those of coronary artery spasm. Administration of catecholamines to increase coronary artery perfusion pressure and intravenous nitroglycerin to increase the caliber of the epicardial coronary arteries have been suggested as the appropriate therapeutic approach.[98]

MANAGEMENT

In most patients, the cause of left ventricular failure is not apparent and frequently therapy is directed to improve left ventricular function and to correct the hemodynamic abnormalities rather than to reverse the etiologic mechanism. The acid-base status should be normalized to avoid cardiac depression from acidosis and vasoconstriction from alkalosis. If the hematocrit is low, blood transfusion is required to increase the hematocrit, which is associated with increased oxygen-carrying capacity and improved oxygen delivery. A hematocrit of 33% has been suggested as the optimal for maximum oxygen delivery and minimal viscosity.[99] Adequate sedation and ventilation should be maintained to prevent an undue increase in ventilatory work and oxygen consumption.

The goals of therapy in patients with left ventricular failure and a low cardiac output are to increase cardiac output, to optimize right and left ventricular filling pressure, and to correct hypotension if it is present. It is preferable to achieve these goals without causing an excessive increase in myocardial oxygen consumption, which may enhance myocardial ischemia. During management of postoperative pump failure, one should always consider that the patient's clinical and hemodynamic status and cardiac performance can change spontaneously over time. Thus, the hemodynamic parameters that may be appropriate early postoperatively may be inappropriate several hours after or during the second or third postoperative day. Impaired myocardial function and low cardiac output immediately following cardiopulmonary bypass tend to return toward normal after 24 hours.[100] In critically ill patients, repeated hemodynamic measurements are also necessary to evaluate response to therapy and for titration of drugs to optimize the hemodynamic response without producing adverse effects. Prompt change of therapy should be considered if response to one type of therapy is inadequate or associated with undesirable side effects.

For correction of hypotension accompanying low cardiac output, the use of catecholamines is usually necessary. The pharmacologic and systemic hemodynamic effects and relative advantages and disadvantages of commonly used catecholamines (epinephrine, norepinephrine, dopamine, dobutamine, and isoproterenol) have been fully described elsewhere in this volume.

In patients with moderate hypotension, dopamine is frequently adequate to increase arterial pressure. Cardiac output may also increase significantly. When the increase in cardiac output is not adequate but the blood pressure rises, either addition of dobutamine or a vasodilator may increase cardiac output considerably. Vasodilator therapy may be particularly effective when systemic vascular resistance is very high. In patients following cardiac surgery, dobutamine (7.5 µg/kg/min) increased cardiac index without any increase in heart rate, mean arterial and pulmonary capillary wedge pressure, or pulmonary vascular resistance. Dopamine, with a similar dose, produced no increase in cardiac index, but increased mean arterial pressure, pulmonary capillary wedge pressure, and pulmonary vascular resistance.[101] With a dose of 5 µg/kg/min or less, both drugs improved hemodynamics.[102] Thus, when a significant increase in arterial pressure is desired and the use of larger doses of dopamine are necessary, cardiac output may not increase and the addition of dobutamine or other cardiotonic agents is frequently required. Low-dose dopamine (1 µg to 2 µg/kg/min) is frequently used to enhance renal perfusion. For treatment of oliguria, intermittent intravenous administration of a diuretic (e.g., furosemide) is often required. Initially, a low dose, such as 10 mg to 20 mg of furosemide, should be administered, since even a low dose may produce prompt diuresis in the postcardiac surgical patient. Intravenous furosemide may also cause a significant reduction in pulmonary capillary wedge pressure.

In some intensive care units, epinephrine is preferred as the catecholamine of choice for treatment of hypotension and low cardiac output due to left ventricular failure. Epinephrine, in doses of 1 µg to 3 µg/min, primarily stimulates β-receptors; with doses between 3 µg to 10 µg/min, both β- and α-receptor agonist effects are evident; with doses greater than 10 µg/min, primarily α-stimulation causes marked vasoconstriction and increased arterial pressure. Intrarenal vasoconstriction may also occur with decreased renal perfusion. Increased left ventricular outflow resistance resulting from peripheral vasoconstriction can be attenuated with concomitant administration of sodium nitroprusside.[103] Calcium chloride is sometimes combined with epinephrine to increase contractility in patients with severe left ventricular dysfunction who fail to respond to other inotropic agents.

Norepinephrine is seldom used except in patients with severe hypotension who remain unresponsive to dopamine or epinephrine. Norepinephrine increases arterial blood pressure, but cardiac output usually does not change, or even decreases owing to a reflex decrease in heart rate and marked increase in systemic vascular resistance (increased afterload). Norepinephrine is usually ineffective in the treatment of low output state due to left ventricular dysfunction, unless it is used in combination with vasodilators that reduce its intense vasoconstriction. The hemodynamic effects of combined norepinephrine-phentolamine in a fixed ratio (1:2.5) have been compared with those of dobutamine and dopamine in patients with low cardiac output after cardiac surgery. With the norepinephrine-phentolamine combination, cardiac output increased even with a significantly increased arterial pressure and systemic vascular resistance.[104] Tachycardia and dysrhythmias were less common compared with dobutamine or dopamine. Nevertheless, this combination does not appear to be superior to the combination of dopamine and nitroprusside, the doses of which can be more easily titrated to achieve the desired hemodynamic responses. Furthermore, phentolamine is a very expensive drug.

Isoproterenol is a potent positive inotropic agent, and its hemodynamic effects are characterized by a significant increase in cardiac output and systolic arterial pressure, but lower diastolic and mean arterial pressure. Pulmonary artery pressure and pulmonary vascular resistance also decrease. Its propensity to induce arrhythmias, to increase myocardial oxygen consumption, and to reduce coronary artery perfusion pressure limit its clinical use. Isoproterenol is useful in patients without coronary artery disease (postvalve replacement) particularly when low cardiac output is associated with bradyarrhythmias or high pulmonary and systemic vascular resistance.

Amrinone, a phosphodiesterase inhibitor, possesses positive inotropic and vasodilatory effects, increases cardiac output, and decreases pulmonary capillary wedge and right atrial pressure without causing any significant change in heart rate or arterial pressure. With larger doses, however, hypotension may occur due to a marked reduction in systemic vascular resistance. Amrinone can be added to other inotropic agents to further increase cardiac output. Clinical experience with amrinone for the treatment of low cardiac output in patients after cardiac surgery is limited; nevertheless, it has the potential to be very effective in some patients. It should not be used in patients with significant hypotension.

In patients with low cardiac output, elevated pulmonary capillary wedge pressure, and adequate arterial pressure, vasodilator therapy may be effective in increasing cardiac output. In the intensive care unit, the most commonly used vasodilators are sodium nitroprusside, nitroglycerin, hydralazine, and phentolamine.[105-107] The pharmacokinetics, hemodynamic effects, and relative advantages and disadvantages of these vasodilators, along with their clinical uses, are described elsewhere in this volume.

Sodium nitroprusside is most effective when systemic vascular resistance is significantly elevated. The initial starting dose should be low, 10 µg to 15 µg/min, and the dose should be increased gradually by 5 µg to 10 µg/min every 10 to 15 minutes, monitoring changes in arterial pressure, cardiac output, pulmonary capillary wedge pressure, and systemic vascular resistance. The minimum dose that increases cardiac output adequately without producing significant hypotension should be used for maintenance therapy.

The addition of dobutamine or dopamine to nitroprusside frequently enhances cardiac output. The hemodynamic effects of sodium nitroprusside have been compared with those of chlorpromazine, nitroglycerin, and trimethaphan in patients immediately after cardiac surgery.[107] The magnitude of increase in cardiac output with nitroprusside is considerably greater than that with nitroglycerin. Nitroglycerin tends to decrease pulmonary capillary wedge pressure by a greater magnitude than with nitroprusside. Thus, nitroglycerin is preferable in those patients with only slightly reduced cardiac output but markedly elevated pulmonary capillary wedge pressure. Nitroglycerin is also the vasodilator of choice when coexistent myocardial ischemia is suspected. Nitroglycerin may decrease myocardial ischemia, not only by decreasing myocardial oxygen demands, but also by improving myocardial perfusion by decreasing epicardial coronary arterial tone and increasing collateral blood flow to the ischemic myocardium. The relative changes in intrapulmonary shunt (decreased arterial oxygen tension) following sodium nitroprusside and nitroglycerin remain controversial; in some studies, worsened intrapulmonary shunting with nitroprusside and improvement with nitroglycerin have been observed.[76] In other studies no differences between nitroglycerin and nitroprusside were found.[108]

The hemodynamic effects of phentolamine, an α-blocking agent, are similar to those of nitroprusside, and for practical purposes it does not provide any advantage over sodium nitroprusside. It may be more useful in the treatment of right ventricular dysfunction because it decreases pulmonary vascular resistance. It is, however, much more expensive to use as a continuous intravenous infusion than sodium nitroprusside.

Hydralazine is a potent direct-acting arteriolar dilator, and its hemodynamic effects include a significant increase in cardiac output along with decreased systemic vascular resistance. Pulmonary capillary wedge pressure usually does not decrease significantly, and arterial pressure and heart rate may not decrease appreciably in patients with heart failure.[105] In postoperative patients, tachycardia and hypotension may develop, particularly after intravenous administration of hydralazine. Hydralazine is usually recommended during weaning from intravenous nitroprusside therapy in those patients who are likely to require long-term vasodilator therapy for pump failure. In patients with severe pump failure, combined vasodilator and inotropic therapy increases cardiac output considerably and also maintains arterial pressure.

When the hemodynamic response is inadequate, particularly if the arterial diastolic pressure remains low, intra-aortic balloon counterpulsation should be considered. Intra-aortic balloon counterpulsation increases diastolic arterial pressure (diastolic augmentation) and decreases peak systolic pressure and left ventricular developed pressure (systolic unloading). Cardiac output increases, and left ventricular end-diastolic pressure and volume and pulmonary capillary wedge pressure decrease. Diastolic augmentation increases coronary artery perfusion pressure, which may increase coronary blood flow in the presence of myocardial ischemia. Transmyocardial pressure gradient also increases owing to concomitant reduction in left ventricular diastolic pressure and can cause improved subendocardial perfusion. The overall myocardial oxygen requirements, however, decrease owing to decreased arterial pressure and decreased left ventricular developed pressure and diastolic volume. With a marked reduction in myocardial oxygen requirements, total coronary blood flow may actually decrease. In some patients, intra-aortic balloon counterpulsation alone is not effective in producing hemodynamic improvement and the addition of vasodilators and/or inotropic agents is required. Nevertheless, intra-aortic balloon counterpulsation seems effective for correcting low cardiac output and it potentially can decrease myocardial necrosis by decreasing left ventricular afterload and increasing coronary blood flow.[109-111] Thus, it has been recommended when substantial impairment of cardiac function occurs during or soon after cardiac surgery (Fig. 114.8).[112]

RIGHT VENTRICULAR FAILURE

Right ventricular failure may result from postoperative right ventricular infarction or ischemia or due to persistently elevated pulmonary artery pressure and pulmonary vascular resistance (e.g., in patients with mitral valve disease with preoperative severe pulmonary arterial hypertension). The hemodynamic abnormalities in predominant right ventricular failure are a disproportionate elevation of right atrial pressure compared with pulmonary capillary wedge pressure and, not infrequently, equalization of right atrial and pulmonary capillary wedge pressure. It is apparent that severe right ventricular failure cannot be differentiated from cardiac tamponade based on the hemodynamic abnormalities. Assessment of right ventricular function by either echocardiography or by radioisotope angiography is required, and such evaluation demonstrates a dilated, poorly contracting right ventricle in right ventricular failure. In cardiac tamponade, however, right ventricular volume is decreased and its systolic function is normal. The mechanism for decreased systemic output in predominant right ventricular failure is decreased left ventricular preload, resulting primarily from a decreased right ventricular stroke output.[113] The principal therapeutic goal is to promote left ventricular filling by increasing right ventricular stroke volume. Enhanced contractility or decreased outflow resistance are associated with an increased right ventricular stroke volume. Dobutamine increases right ventricular contractility and also has the potential to decrease pulmonary artery pressure and pulmonary vascular resistance (right ventricular afterload). Dobutamine is effective in increasing cardiac output in patients with mild-to-moderate right ventricular dysfunction. In patients with severe right ventricular failure, isoproterenol may be more effective, particularly in patients with severe pulmonary hypertension (post mitral valve replacement) and without associated coronary artery disease. Pulmonary vasodilators, such as nitroglycerin or nitroprusside, can be used to decrease right ventricular outflow resistance, provided arterial pressure is adequate and right atrial and pulmonary capillary wedge pressures are not low. Concomitant administration of fluids intravenously is necessary to maintain adequate ventricular preload when vasodilators are used. Phentolamine, also a pulmonary vasodilator, may be effective occasionally. Phentolamine may also decrease systemic vascular resistance and arterial pressure. These adverse effects of phentolamine may be attenuated by the simultaneous administration of norepinephrine via a left atrial line. Administration of norepinephrine directly into the left atrium avoids an increase in pulmonary vascular resistance and first-pass metabolism of norepinephrine in the lung.[114,115] In refractory cases, pulmonary artery counterpulsation and right ventricular assist with the use of a pneumatic pump have been used with some success.[116]

It is apparent that hemodynamic monitoring is extremely useful in the diagnosis of the causes of low output and hypotension in postoperative patients. It is also necessary to determine the changes in hemodynamics to assess responses to therapy. The diagnosis of the causes of low output state is summarized in Table 114.4. The suggested stepwise therapeutic approach for treatment of hypotension, see Figure 39.6 (Volume 1).

PULMONARY EMBOLISM

Massive pulmonary embolism is a rare, but usually catastrophic, complication that may precipitate low cardiac output and sudden, unexpected death in patients after cardiac surgery. Unexplained episodes of dyspnea and deterioration in arterial blood gases should raise the suspicion of pulmonary embolism.[117] Signs of deep venous thrombosis may or may not be evident. If deep vein thrombosis or minor, submassive pulmonary embolism exists, intravenous heparin therapy should be started without delay. Thrombolytic therapy with streptokinase is contraindicated in the immediate postoperative period. An echocardiogram should be performed to detect right atrial or right ventricular thrombus, and when a large mobile thrombus is visualized, surgical removal is recommended since the majority of patients die suddenly of

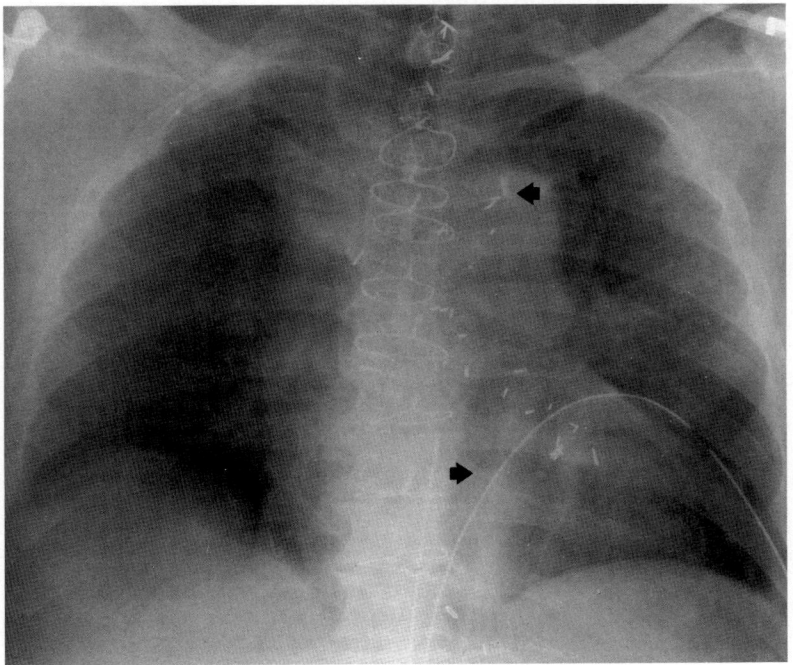

FIGURE 114.8 Anteroposterior chest film of a 60-year-old patient who underwent three-vessel coronary artery bypass grafting that was complicated by severe hypotension when coming off cardiopulmonary bypass. An intra-aortic balloon was inserted via the femoral artery to improve cardiac output and myocardial blood flow. The top arrow indicates the position of the balloon tip in the superior portion of the descending aorta. The lower arrow shows the radiolucent shadow of the balloon inflated in the descending aorta. The patient also has a left chest tube, mediastinal tube, endotracheal tube, sternal sutures, and temporary pacer wires. A pulmonary artery line was subsequently inserted for monitoring of pulmonary and systemic hemodynamics.

massive pulmonary embolism, despite anticoagulation therapy. Should massive pulmonary embolism occur and accurate diagnosis is made, treatment is urgent pulmonary embolectomy.[118]

PNEUMOTHORAX

Clinically insignificant pneumothorax occurs in approximately 5% of patients after cardiopulmonary bypass.[98] Serial chest films are required to diagnose enlargement of the pneumothorax. With positive-pressure ventilation, any pneumothorax can rapidly increase to tension pneumothorax with cardiovascular collapse. Rapid decompression therapy should be immediately undertaken.

DYSRRHYTHMIAS

Postoperative tachyarrhythmias or bradyarrhythmias may precipitate a low output state, and their prompt recognition is required for appropriate management. In many institutions, atrial and ventricular pacing wires are routinely placed at surgery. These temporary atrial and ventricular electrodes are useful, not only for the treatment of arrhythmias but also for correct diagnosis.

Premature ventricular contractions are common during the early postoperative period. Several potential causes have been identified: hypoxia, hypokalemia, hypocalcemia, hypomagnesemia, acidosis, myocardial ischemia or myocardial injury, hypercapnia, increased sympathetic activity, and insertion of a balloon-flotation catheter. There appears to be a correlation between the incidence of premature ventricular contractions and hypokalemia, which is common after cardiac surgery.[119] Potassium replacement is required to keep the potassium level at 3.9 mEq to 4.2 mEq/liter. A higher serum potassium level greater than 4.5 mEq/liter is desirable in patients on digitalis therapy. The other potential causes that may precipitate premature ventricular contractions should also be corrected. The initial treatment for unifocal or multifocal premature ventricular contractions (>5/min) is intravenous administration of lidocaine, initially as a bolus, 50 mg to 100 mg (or 1 mg/kg), followed by a maintenance infusion of 1 mg to 4 mg/kg/min. Nonsustained ventricular tachycardia is also initially treated by lidocaine. In the absence of hemodynamic compromise, and when the ventricular rate is relatively slow (e.g., <150 beats per minute), the initial treatment of sustained ventricular tachycardia is also intravenous lidocaine. If, however, a favorable response is not observed, electroversion should be employed. Sustained ventricular tachycardia associated with hemodynamic deterioration (e.g., hypotension) requires immediate electroversion. Overdrive or underdrive ventricular pacing is occasionally effective for termination of relatively slow ventricular tachycardia. Ventricular fibrillation should be treated with immediate cardioversion.

If lidocaine is ineffective to control ventricular arrhythmias, intravenous procainamide is the next drug of choice. The loading dose is about 10 mg/kg, but it should be infused slowly (50 mg/min) to avoid hypotension, and a maintenance infusion rate of 2 mg to 4 mg/min should be started after the loading dose. Recurrent ventricular tachycardia refractory to lidocaine and/or procainamide is treated with bretylium tosylate. An intravenous loading dose (5 mg to 10 mg/kg) is given, followed by a maintenance infusion of 1 mg to 2 mg/min. Bretylium may cause tachycardia and hypertension initially, followed by prolonged hypotension and bradycardia.[120]

After initial control of ventricular tachyarrhythmias, oral procainamide therapy (500 mg to 1000 mg four times daily) is usually continued for 6 to 8 weeks after the patient is discharged from the hospital. Quinidine, 200 mg to 400 mg, four times daily, or disopyramide, 100 mg to 300 mg, three to four times daily can also be used instead of procainamide. In patients with depressed left ventricular function, disopyramide should be avoided because of its potent negative inotropic effect. The adverse effects of these antiarrhythmic agents, and the patient's tolerance to the drug, should be considered when an antiarrhythmic agent is chosen for maintenance therapy.

Premature atrial contractions are frequent in the immediate postoperative period and usually precede the onset of atrial fibrillation. The incidence of atrial fibrillation or atrial flutter is quite high, approximately 30% in patients undergoing coronary artery surgery; the incidence is much higher, close to 70%, following valve surgery. In the absence of hemodynamic compromise, atrial fibrillation or flutter is initially treated with digoxin. Digoxin, 0.5 mg to 1 mg, is administered intravenously, slowly in 10 to 15 minutes, and 0.125 to 0.25 mg is then repeated every 3 to 4 hours until the ventricular response has decreased (less than 100 beats per minute), or a total of 1.5 mg to 2 mg has been administered. After cardiac surgery digoxin alone is frequently ineffective to control the ventricular response. Propranolol may be given intravenously in doses of 0.5 mg every 2 minutes to a maximum dose of 1 mg/kg; alternatively, verapamil may be infused slowly in a dose of 5 to 10 mg. Both propranolol and verapamil should be avoided in patients with overt heart failure due to left ventricular dysfunction. In these patients, severe hypotension may be precipitated.

TABLE 114.4 DIAGNOSIS OF CAUSES OF POSTOPERATIVE LOW OUTPUT SYNDROME

		Echocardiographic or Radioisotope Angiographic Findings
Hypovolemia	Decreased right atrial and pulmonary capillary wedge pressures	Normal or decreased right and left ventricular size; normal or slightly depressed right and left ventricular systolic function
Cardiac tamponade	Equalization of right atrial, pulmonary artery diastolic, and pulmonary capillary wedge pressures	Decreased right and left ventricular size; normal right and left ventricular systolic function; diastolic compression of right atrium and right ventricle
Predominant right ventricular failure	Disproportionate elevation of right atrial pressure compared with pulmonary capillary wedge pressure. Right atrial/pulmonary capillary wedge pressure ratio greater than 0.7; equalization of right atrial and pulmonary capillary wedge pressure; normal or increased pulmonary artery pressure and pulmonary vascular resistance, depending on the etiology of right-sided heart failure	Dilated, poorly contracting right ventricle
Predominant left ventricular failure	Pulmonary capillary wedge pressure is higher than right atrial pressure; right atrial/pulmonary capillary wedge pressure ratio less than 0.7	Dilated, poorly contracting left ventricle

Paroxysmal atrial tachycardia can sometimes be terminated by carotid artery massage. However, in the majority of patients, intravenous verapamil therapy is required and is extremely effective for the termination of supraventricular tachycardia. Frequent premature atrial contractions, atrial fibrillation or flutter, and supraventricular tachycardia can be occasionally suppressed by atrial pacing. When hemodynamic deterioration occurs with supraventricular tachyarrhythmias, synchronized cardioversion should be attempted. After the initial control of atrial arrhythmias, maintenance therapy with type I antiarrhythmic drugs (quinidine, procainamide, or disopyramide) is instituted and continued for 6 to 8 weeks. Electrical cardioversion should be considered prior to maintenance antiarrhythmic drug therapy in patients who remain in atrial fibrillation or flutter for 7 days or more after surgery.

The most effective treatment for atrioventricular block is ventricular or atrioventricular sequential pacing with the use of pacing wires placed at the time of surgery. In some patients, ventricular pacing alone may prove to be inadequate to improve cardiac output and correct hypotension. Timed atrial contribution to ventricular filling with atrioventricular sequential pacing may be more effective in increasing cardiac output. In patients with right ventricular infarction and predominant right ventricular failure, atrioventricular sequential pacing is always preferable to ventricular pacing.[121] The chronotropic catecholamines (isoproterenol, dopamine) are used only when pacemaker therapy is not available and before the transvenous pacemaker electrode catheters are placed.

CONCLUSIONS

In a modern intensive care unit, with the capability of monitoring respiratory and hemodynamics status, most of the postoperative complications can be identified. Due to advances in the therapeutic modalities, these complications can be treated. However, the awareness of potential postoperative complications and their consequences is essential for effective management of the patient after cardiac surgery. Monitoring of respiratory function and systemic hemodynamics provides useful guidelines in the management of these complications. However, the primary therapeutic goal is to avoid complications, rather than to treat their consequences.

REFERENCES

1. Rehder K, Sessler AD, Marsh HM: General anesthesia and the lung. Am Rev Respir Dis 112:541, 1975
2. Maier HS, Cournand A: Studies of arterial oxygen saturation in the postoperative period after pulmonary resection. Surgery 13:199, 1943
3. Hedley-White J, Corning H, Laver MB et al: Pulmonary ventilation–perfusion relations after valve replacement or repair in man. J Clin Invest 44:406, 1965
4. Geha AS, Sessler AD, Kirklin JW: Alveolar-arterial oxygen gradients after open intracardiac surgery. J Thorac Cardiovasc Surg 51:609, 1966
5. McClenahan JB, Young WE, Sykes MK: Respiratory changes after open heart surgery. Thorax 20:545, 1965
6. Dantzkar DR, Cowenhaven WM, Willoughby WJ et al: Gas exchange alternations associated with weaning from mechanical ventilation following coronary artery bypass surgery. Chest 82:674, 1982
7. Ratliff NB, Young WG Jr, Hachel DB et al: Pulmonary injury secondary to extracorporeal circulation. J Thorac Cardiovasc Surg 65:425, 1973
8. Osborne JJ, Proper RM, Kerth WJ et al: Respiratory insufficiency following open heart surgery. Ann Surg 1565:638, 1962
9. Bongard FS, Matthay MA, Machersie RC et al: Morphologic and physiologic correlates of increased extravascular lung water. Surgery 96:395, 1984
10. Matthay MA: Pathophysiology of pulmonary edema. Clin Chest Med 6:301, 1985
11. Benumof JL, Wahrenbrock EA: Local effects of anesthetics on regional hypoxic pulmonary vasoconstriction. Anesthesiology 43:525, 1975
12. Marshall BE, Marshall C: Anesthesia and the pulmonary circulation. In Corino BG et al (eds): Effects of Anesthesia, p 121. Bethesda, MD, American Physiologic Society, 1985
13. Prewitt RM, McCarthy J, Wood LDH: Treatment of acute low pressure pulmonary edema in dogs. J Clin Invest 67:409, 1981
14. Nims RG, Connjer EH, Comroe JH: The compliance of the human thorax in anesthetized patients. J Clin Invest 34:744, 1955
15. Westbrook PR, Stubbs SE, Sessler AD et al: Effects of anesthesia and muscle paralysis on respiratory mechanics in normal man. J Appl Physiol 34:81, 1973
16. Gold MI, Helrich M: Pulmonary compliance during anesthesia. Anesthesiology 26:281, 1965
17. Foster CA, Heaf PJD, Semple SJG: Compliance of the lung in anesthetized paralyzed subjects. J Appl Physiol 11:383, 1957
18. Rehder K: Anesthesia and the mechanics of respiration. In Covino BG et al (eds): Effects of Anesthesia, p 91. Bethesda, MD, American Physiologic Society, 1985
19. Severinghaus JW, Stupfel M: Respiratory dead space increases following atropine in man and atropine, vagal or ganglionic blockade and hypothermia in dogs. J Appl Physiol 8:81, 1957
20. Camplebell EJM, Nunn JF, Peckett BW: A comparison of artificial ventilation and spontaneous respiration with particular reference to ventilation–blood flow relationships. Br J Anaesth 30:106, 1958
21. Kirklin JW, Blackstone EH, Kirklin JK: General principles of cardiac surgery. In Braunwald EG (ed): Cardiovascular Disease, p 1797. Philadelphia, WB Saunders, 1984
22. Chenowith PE, Cooper SW, Hugh TE et al: Complement activation during cardiopulmonary bypass-evidence for generation of C_{3a} and C_{5a} anaphylotoxins. N Engl J Med 304:497, 1981
23. Edmunds LH Jr, Alexander JA: Effect of cardiopulmonary bypass on the lungs. In Fishman AP (ed): Pulmonary Disease and Disorders, p 1728. New York, McGraw-Hill, 1980
24. Litwak RS, Jurado RA: Cardiac Surgical Patient. Norwalk, CT, Appleton-Century-Crofts, 1982
25. Matthay MA, Berthiaume Y, Staub NC: Long-term clearance of liquid and protein from the lungs of unanesthetized sheep. J Appl Physiol 59:928, 1985
26. Spencer FC, Benson DW, Liu WC et al: Use of a mechanical respirator in the management of respiratory insufficiency following trauma or operation for cardiac or pulmonary disease. J Thorac Cardiovasc Surg 38:758, 1959
27. Bjork VO, Engstrom CG: The treatment of ventilatory insufficiency by tracheostomy and artificial ventilation. J Thorac Surg 34:228, 1957
28. Pontoppidan H, Laver MB, Geffin B: Acute respiratory failure in the surgical patients. Adv Surg 4:163, 1970
29. Lowenstein E, Bland JHL: Anesthesia in cardiac surgery. In Norman JC (ed): Cardiac Surgery, 2nd ed, p 75. New York, Appleton-Century-Crofts, 1972
30. Bendixen HH, Hedley-White J, Laver MB: Impaired oxygenation in surgical patients during general anesthesia with controlled ventilation: A concept of atelectasis. N Engl J Med 269:991, 1963
31. Michael L, McMichan JC, Marsh HM et al: Measurement of ventilatory reserve as an indication for early extubation after cardiac operation. J Thorac Cardiovasc Surg 78:761, 1979
32. Prakash O, Jonson B, Meji S et al: Criteria for early extubation after intracardiac surgery in adults. Anesth Analg 56:703, 1977
33. Klineberg PL, Geer RT, Hirsh RA et al: Early extubation after coronary artery bypass graft surgery. Crit Care Med 5:272, 1977
34. Quasha AC, Loeber N, Feeley TW et al: Postoperative respiratory care: A controlled trial of early and late extubation following coronary artery bypass grafting. Anesthesiology 52:135, 1980
35. Matthay MA, Wiener-Kronish JP: Respiratory management after cardiac surgery. Chest 95:424, 1989
36. Swerdlow BN, Mihm FG, Goetzl EJ, Matthay MA: Leukotrienes in pulmonary edema fluid after cardiopulmonary bypass. Anesth Analg 65:306, 1986
37. Maggart M, Stewart S: The mechanisms and management of noncardiogenic pulmonary edema following cardiopulmonary bypass. Ann Thorac Surg 43:231, 1987
38. Wiener-Kronish JP, Matthay MA: Sequential measurements of pulmonary edema protein concentration provide a reliable index of alveolar epithelial function and prognosis in patients with the adult respiratory distress syndrome. Clin Res 37:112, 1989
39. Murray JF, Matthay MA, Luce JM, Flick MR: An expanded definition of the adult respiratory distress syndrome. Am Rev Resp Dis 138:720, 1988
40. Lowenstin E, Ashbough DG, Bigelow DD et al: Continuous positive-pressure ventilation in acute respiratory failure: effects on hemodynamics and lung function. N Engl J Med 283:1430, 1970
41. Barber RE, Lee J, Hamilton WK: Oxygen toxicity in man: A prospective study in patients with irreversible brain damage. N Engl J Med 283:1478, 1970
42. Clark JM, Lamberston CJ: Pulmonary oxygen toxicity: A review. Pharm Rev 23:37, 1971
43. Cheney FW, Huang TW, Gronka R: The effects of 50% oxygen on the resolution of pulmonary injury. Am Rev Respir Dis 122:373, 1980
44. Pepe PE, Hudson LD, Carrico CJ: Early application of positive end-expiratory pressure in patients at risk for the adult respiratory distress syndrome. N Engl J Med 311:281, 1984
45. Broaddus C, Berthiaume Y, Biondi J, Matthay MA: Hemodynamic management of the adult respiratory distress syndrome. J Intensive Care Med 2:190, 1987
46. Dantzker DR. Gas exchange in acute lung injury. In Wiedemann HP, Matthay MA, Matthay RA (eds): Critical care clinics: Acute lung injury. Philadelphia:

WB Saunders, 527, 1986
47. Coggeshall JW, Marini JJ, Newman JH: Improved oxygenation after muscle relaxation in adult respiratory distress syndrome. Arch Intern Med 145:1718, 1985
48. Zack MB, Pontoppidan H, Kazemi H: The effect of lateral position on gas exchange in pulmonary disease: a prospective evaluation. Am Rev Respir Dis 110:49, 1974
49. Luce JW, Montgomery AB, Marks JD et al: Ineffectiveness of high dose methylprednisolone in preventing parenchymal lung injury and improving mortality in patients with septic shock. Am Rev Respir Dis 138:62, 1988
50. Matthay MA: The adult respiratory distress syndrome: New insights into diagnosis, pathophysiology, and treatment. West J Med 150:187, 1989
51. Rinaldo JE, Rogers RM: Adult respiratory distress syndrome: changing concepts of lung injury and repair. N Engl J Med 306:900, 1982
52. Wiedeman H, Matthay MA, Matthay RA (eds): Acute lung injury. Critical Care Clinics. Philadelphia, WB Saunders, 1986
53. Stein M, Cassara EL: Preoperative pulmonary evaluation and therapy for surgery patients. JAMA 211:787, 1970
54. Plummer AL: Bronchodilator drugs and the cardiac patients. In Kaplan JA (ed): Cardiac Anesthesia, vol 2, p 581. New York, Grune & Stratton, 1983
55. Weinberger M, Hendeles L, Ahrens R: Pharmacologic management of reversible obstructive airways disease: Symposium on chronic lung obstructive airways disease. Med Clin North Am 65:579, 1980
56. Brent BN, Mahler PA, Burger HJ et al: Augmentation of right ventricular performance by terbutaline: A combined radionuclide and hemodynamic study. Am J Cardiol 50:313, 1982
57. Patterson JW, Woolcock AJ, Shenfield GM: Bronchodilator drugs. Am Rev Respir Dis 120:1149, 1979
58. Matthay RA: Effects of theophylline on cardiovascular performance in chronic obstructive pulmonary disease. Chest 88:1125, 1985
59. Aubier M, Roussos S: Effect of theophylline on respiratory muscle function. Chest 88:915, 1985
60. Rice KL, Leatherman JW, Duane PG et al: Aminophylline for acute exacerbations of chronic obstructive disease. Ann Intern Med 92:753, 1980
61. Albert RK, Martin TR, Lewis SW: Controlled clinical trial of methylprednisolone in patients with chronic bronchitis and acute respiratory insufficiency. Ann Intern Med 92:753, 1980
62. Morgenroth ML, Morgenroth JL, Nett LM et al: Criteria for weaning from prolonged mechanical ventilation. Arch Intern Med 144:1012, 1984
63. Pierson DJ: Weaning from mechanical ventilation in acute respiratory failure. Resp Care 28:646, 1983
64. Wright CD, Williams JG, Ogilvie CM et al: Results of diaphragmatic plication for unilateral diaphragmatic paralysis. J Thorac Cardiovasc Surg 90:195, 1985
65. Dietzman RH, Ersek RA, Lillehei CW et al: Low output syndrome: Recognition and treatment. J Thorac Cardiovasc Surg 57:138, 1969
66. Kirklin JW, Barrat-Boyes BG: Postoperative care. In Kirklin JW, Barrat-Boyes BG (eds): Cardiac Surgery: Morphology, Diagnostic Criteria, Natural History, Techniques, Results and Indications, p 139. New York, Wiley Medical Publications, 1986
67. Hansen R, Viquerat C, Matthay MA et al: Poor correlation between pulmonary artery wedge pressure and left ventricular end-diastolic volume after coronary artery bypass surgery. Anesthesiology 64:764, 1986
68. Salerno TA, Henderson M, Keith FM et al: Hypertension after coronary operation. J Thorac Cardiovasc Surg 81:396, 1981
69. Fee HJ, Viljoen JF, Cukingnam RA et al: Right stellate ganglion block for treatment of hypertension after cardiopulmonary bypass. Ann Thorac Surg 27:5192, 1979
70. Estafanous FG, Tarazi RC, Viljoen JF et al: Systemic hypertension following myocardial revascularization. Am Heart J 74:732, 1973
71. Roberts AJ, Niarchos AP, Subramanian VA et al: Systemic hypertension associated with coronary artery bypass surgery. J Thorac Cardiovasc Surg 74:846, 1977
72. Viljoen JF, Estafanous FG, Tarazi RC: Acute hypertension immediately after coronary artery surgery. J Thorac Cardiovasc Surg 71:548, 1976
73. Kaplan JA: Nitroglycerin for the treatment of hypertension during coronary artery surgery. In Robinson BF, Kaplan JA (eds): International Symposium on the Clinical Use of Tridil, Intravenous Nitroglycerin, p 26. Oxford, England, Oxford Medicine Publishing Foundation, 1982
74. Chatterjee K, Parmley WW: The role of vasodilator therapy in heart failure. Prog Cardiovasc Dis 19:301, 1977
75. Kaplan JA, Finlayson DC, Woodward S: Vasodilator therapy after cardiac surgery: A review of the efficacy and toxicity of nitroglycerin and nitroprusside. Can Anaesth Soc J 27:254, 1980
76. Flaherty JT, Magee PA, Gardner TL et al: Comparison of intravenous nitroglycerin and sodium nitroprusside for treatment of acute hypertension developing after coronary artery bypass surgery. Circulation 65:1072, 1982
77. Fukunaga AF, Flacke WE, Bloor BC: Hypertensive effects of adenosine and adenosine triphosphate compared with sodium nitroprusside. Anesth Analg 61:273, 1982
78. Shapiro BA, Harrison RA, Walton JR: Clinical application of blood gases. In Year Book of Medicine, 2nd ed. Chicago, Year Book Medical Publishers, 1977
79. Parr GVS, Blackstone EH, Kirklin JW: Cardiac performance and mortality early after intracardiac surgery in infants and young children. Circulation 51:867, 1975
80. Beattie HW, Evars G, Garnett ES et al: Sustained hypovolemia and extracellular fluid volume expansion following cardiopulmonary bypass. Surgery 71:891, 1972
81. Kouchoukos NT, Karp RB: Management of the postoperative surgical patient. Am Heart J 92:513, 1976
82. Crexells C, Chatterjee K, Forrester JS et al: Optimal level of filling pressure in the left side of the heart in acute myocardial infarction. N Engl J Med 289:1263, 1973
83. Weitzman LB, Tinker PW, Kronzon I et al: The incidence and natural history of pericardial effusion after cardiac surgery. Circulation 69:506, 1984
84. D'Cruz IA, Kensey K, Campbell C et al: Two-dimensional echocardiography in cardiac tamponade occurring after cardiac surgery. J Am Coll Cardiol 5:1250, 1985
85. Fyke III FE, Tancredi RG, Shub C et al: Detection of intrapericardial hematoma after open heart surgery: The roles of echocardiography and computed tomography. J Am Coll Cardiol 5:1496, 1985
86. Weeks KR, Chatterjee K, Block S et al: Bedside hemodynamic monitoring—its value in the diagnosis of tamponade complication cardiac surgery. J Thorac Cardiovasc Surg 71:250, 1976
87. Hockberg MS, Merrill WH, Bruber H et al: Delayed cardiac tamponade associated with prophylactic anticoagulants. J Thorac Cardiovasc Surg 75:777, 1978
88. Merrill W, Donahoo JS, Brawley RK et al: Late cardiac tamponade: A potentially lethal complication of open heart surgery. J Thorac Cardiovasc Surg 72:919, 1976
89. Guyton RD: Method and magic in myocardial preservation. In Hurst JW (ed): Clinical Essays on the Heart. New York, McGraw-Hill, 1982
90. Klausner SC, Botvinick EH, Shames D et al: The application of radionuclide infarct scintigraphy to diagnose perioperative myocardial infarction following revascularization. Circulation 56:173, 1977
91. McKay CR, Brundage BH, Ullyot DJ et al: Evaluation of early postoperative coronary artery bypass graft patency by contrast-enhanced computed tomography. J Am Coll Cardiol 2:312, 1983
92. Buxton AE, Goldberg S, Harken A et al: Coronary artery spasm immediately after myocardial revascularization. N Engl J Med 304:1249, 1981
93. Heupler FA Jr: Aortocoronary vein graft spasm. Chest 80:4123, 1981
94. Zeff RH, Iannone LA, Kongtahworn C et al: Coronary artery spasm following coronary artery revascularization. Ann Thorac Surg 34:196, 1982
95. Curling PE, Eapal JA: Indications and uses of intravenous nitroglycerin during cardiac surgery. Angiology 33:302, 1982
96. Kay R, Blake I, Rubin D: Possible coronary spasm rebound to abrupt nifedipine withdrawal. Am Heart J 103:308, 1982
97. Goldfarb D, Bahnson HT: Early and late effects on the heart of small amounts of air in the coronary circulation. J Thorac Cardiovasc Surg 46:368, 1963
98. Curling PE, Duke PG, Levy JH et al: Management of the postoperative cardiac patient. In Hurst JW (ed): Clinical Essays on the Heart, vol 1, p 257. New York, McGraw-Hill, 1982
99. Messmer K, Kessler M, Sunder-Plassman L: Hemorrhagic effects of intentional hemodilution. In Tavares B (ed): Current Topics in Critical Care Medicine (Third International Symposium, Rio de Janeiro), p 130, Basel, S Karger, 1974
100. Berger RL, Weisel RD, Vito L et al: Cardiac output measurement by thermodilution during cardiac operation. Ann Thorac Surg 21:43, 1976
101. Salomon NW, Plachetka JR, Copeland JG: Comparison of dopamine and dobutamine following coronary artery bypass grafting. Ann Thorac Surg 33:48, 1982
102. Makabali C, Weil MH, Henning RJ: Dobutamine and other sympathomimetic drugs for the treatment of low cardiac output failure. Semin Anesth 1:63, 1982
103. Strum JT, Fuhrman TM, Lgo SR et al: Efficacy of nitroprusside therapy in postcardiotomy low output syndrome necessitating intra-aortic balloon counterpulsation. J Thorac Cardiovasc Surg 78:254, 1979
104. Gray R, Shah PK, Singh B et al: Low cardiac output states after open heart surgery. Chest 80:16, 1981
105. Parmley WW, Chatterjee K: Vasodilator therapy for chronic heart failure. Cardiovasc Med 1:17, 1976
106. Lappas DC, Lowenstein E, Waller J et al: Hemodynamic effects of nitroprusside infusion during coronary artery operation in man. Circulation 54(suppl 3):4, 1976
107. Stinson EB, Holloway EL, Derby G et al: Comparative hemodynamic responses to chlorpromazine, nitroprusside, nitroglycerin and trimethaphan immediately after open heart operations. Circulation 51-52(suppl 1):26, 1974-75
108. Brooks JL, Kaplan JA, Finlayson DC et al: Vasodilators and pulmonary venous admixture after myocardial revascularization. Anesth Analg 59:532, 1980
109. Gill CC, Wechsler AS, Newman GE et al: Augmentation and redistribution of myocardial blood flow during acute ischemia by intra-aortic balloon pumping. Ann Thorac Surg 16:445, 1973
110. Scanlon PJ, O'Connell J, Johnson SA et al: Balloon counterpulsation following surgery for ischemic heart disease. Circulation 54(suppl 3):III-90, 1976

111. Chatterjee S, Rosenweig J: Evaluation of intra-aortic balloon counterpulsation. J Thorac Cardiovasc Surg 61:405, 1971
112. Kirklin JW, Conti VR, Blackstone EH: Prevention of myocardial damage during cardiac operations. N Engl J Med 301:135, 1979
113. Goldstein JA, Vlahakes GJ, Verrier ED et al: The role of right ventricular systolic function and evaluated intrapericardial pressure in the genesis of low output in experimental right ventricular infarction. Circulation 65:513, 1982
114. McEnany MT, Morgan RJ, Mundth ED et al: Circumvention of detrimental pulmonary vasoactivity of exogenous catecholamines in cardiac resuscitation. Surg Forum 26:98, 1975
115. Block ER, Stalcup SA: Metabolic functions of the lung. Chest 81:215, 1982
116. Miller DC, Moreno-Cabral RJ, Stinson EB et al: Pulmonary artery balloon counterpulsation for acute right ventricular failure. J Thorac Cardiovasc Surg 80:760, 1980
117. Broaddus C, Matthay MA: Pulmonary embolism and deep venous thrombosis. Postgrad Med 79:333, 1986
118. Hoaglund PM: Massive pulmonary embolism. In Goldhaber SZ (ed): Pulmonary Embolism and Deep Venous Thrombosis, p 179. Philadelphia, WB Saunders, 1985
119. Rao G, Ford WB, Zikria EA et al: Prevention of arrhythmias after direct myocardial revascularization surgery. Vasc Surg 8:82, 1974
120. Chatterjee K, Mandel WJ, Vyden JK et al: Cardiovascular effects of bretylium tosylate in acute myocardial infarction. JAMA 223:757, 1973
121. Topol EJ, Goldschlager N, Ports TA et al: Hemodynamic benefit of atrial pacing in right ventricular infarction. Ann Intern Med 96:594, 1982

THE RELATIONSHIP OF EMOTIONS AND CARDIOPATHOLOGY

Robert S. Eliot • Hugo M. Morales-Ballejo

There are many anecdotes of persons who died suddenly after an emotional shock. In the last two decades, scientific studies have confirmed the links between emotions and illness or death. This chapter describes the pathologic results of emotions and stress as seen in laboratory animals and in clinical tests; discusses the mechanisms believed to mediate these results; and then relates these mechanisms to the pathogenesis of hypertension, atherosclerosis, ischemia, and sudden death. Some implications for management are also offered.

ANIMAL STUDIES

Although animal models are less complex than their human counterparts, they leave little doubt that emotional stress can induce changes in cardiovascular physiology and promote pathophysiologic mechanisms.

For example, Henry and Ely[1] have demonstrated that socially deprived mice, when introduced into a colony with an established hierarchy, develop a significant incidence of hypertension, myocardial hypertrophy, progressive arteriosclerosis, myocardial fibrosis, and renal failure.

A study by Lapin and Cherkovich[2] utilized hamadryas baboons, which mate for life and form very strong attachments to their mates. After the original male was removed from the cage and placed in another cage in full view of his original habitat, a new male of the same age was moved into the original cage with the original female. Although neither the diet nor any other component of the experiment was changed, the original males were reported to have developed hypertension, coronary insufficiency, or myocardial infarction within 6 months to a year.

McGuire and Raleigh[3] found a correlation between status and serotonin levels in vervet monkeys. The dominant male had whole blood serotonin levels of about 1000 ng/ml, whereas subordinate males had levels of about 650 ng/ml. If a dominant male was removed from the group, the subordinate with the greatest responsivity to serotonin stimulation was most likely to become dominant. The serotonin level of the new dominant would gradually rise over a period of 3 to 7 days to the average level for dominants. The status changes also affected cortisol levels: after a dominant male was removed, the basal cortisol levels of the subordinates doubled, and the probable dominant replacement could be identified by determining which male had the highest basal cortisol concentration during the first 10 days. Cortisol levels in all the animals remained elevated for several weeks, even after the serotonin levels had stabilized.

In Von Holst's[4] experiments with tree shrews, a subordinate male was introduced into a cage with a dominant one. In every such pair, the dominant animal immediately attacked, and the subordinate one submitted. Each subordinate was removed before it was injured. If the subordinate was placed so that it could not see the other shrew, it recovered rapidly; but if it was placed so that it could see and hear the dominant male, it lay still, watching the dominant animal's every move 90% of the time. Such subordinate animals rapidly lost weight and died in 2 to 20 days of renal failure, despite adequate food and water. On the other hand, if two males were placed in a strange cage, an initial fight established the hierarchy. In some instances, the subordinate males showed active avoidance behavior; their weight stabilized after a few days, and they were able to survive even while remaining in the dominant's cage, unlike those animals who responded with the more submissive behavior. Heartbeat rates and hormone levels were reportedly unchanged in dominant males, except for a tendency to increased testosterone levels. Cortisol was markedly elevated in very submissive males. Active subordinate males had normal cortisol levels, elevated norepinephrine, and more rapid heartbeats.

Henry[5] has observed that, in general, animal responses can be divided into three types: aggressive–dominant, defensive–subordinate, and hopeless–submissive. In the first two groups, there is active coping, characterized by stimulation of the sympathetic nervous system with the release of catecholamines (epinephrine and norepinephrine). In successful coping, when the animal feels in control, there is a decrease in adrenocorticotropic hormone (ACTH) and an increase in gonadotropins. In submissive animals, the pituitary adrenocortical system is aroused, resulting in the release of ACTH and cortisol and a reduction in testosterone. Von Holst's experiments with tree shrews afford a good example of these reactions.

The first two responses may correspond with the so-called fight or flight or defense pattern, first developed by Cannon, and the third is the vigilance or playing dead pattern. The defense pattern has been elicited by such stressors as shock avoidance and sudden threats that arouse fear or require active coping. The vigilance pattern has been elicited by stressors of a more chronic type such as placement in an overcrowded or otherwise unpleasant environment or perceiving a threat to status without a possibility of doing anything about it.

The resulting effects of the defense reaction—increase in blood flow to the muscles; decrease in blood flow to the gastrointestinal tract, kidneys, and skin; faster heartbeat; and increase in alertness—all serve the animal to react more effectively to a threat requiring muscular activity.[6] The increased stickiness of platelets that follows the release of catecholamines adds the advantage of limiting bleeding from wounds. Vasopressin and cholesterol, which also tend to increase during stress, act synergistically with epinephrine to increase the sensitivity of the platelets.[7]

The submissive "playing dead" reaction also can be lifesaving in certain situations, such as when hiding from a predator. In intraspecies confrontations, it may be a mechanism for survival of the fittest. The lower levels of testosterone in submissive males would favor procreation by the dominants even when subordinate animals survive.

HUMAN STUDIES

Both epidemiologic studies and controlled laboratory tests have indicated that emotions and stress can have profound effects on the cardiovascular system.

EPIDEMIOLOGIC STUDIES

Harburg and colleagues[8] have shown that blacks living in areas of Detroit with low ecologic stress had less hypertension than their counterparts living in high-stress areas. Gampel and associates[9] noted a lower incidence of hypertension among Zulus in rural areas than among those who moved to the cities; the urban Zulus who were hypertensive tended to be those who clung to traditional cultural practices and seemed unable to adapt to the demands of urban living.

In the Alameda County study[10] a poverty area was compared with a more affluent area. Incidence of hypertension was 50% higher in the poverty area regardless of considerations of social interaction, medical care, smoking, and other accepted risk factors. However, among a group of more affluent people living in the area, the pattern of hypertension reflected that of the poverty area as a whole rather than that of the similar income group in the affluent area. Interviews with the individuals revealed fears of robbery and violence. It was then noted that the distribution of hypertension within the community correlated with the concentration of police and fire department calls.

Several studies of widowers indicate bereavement increases susceptibility to illness and death.[11,12]

REACTIVITY STUDIES

Measurements of cardiovascular responses to psychological stressors have demonstrated that blood pressure and heart rate can be as greatly affected by such stimuli as by physical exertion.

One method with which to relate emotions and blood pressure is to use ambulatory monitoring of blood pressure. Such studies have shown interesting patterns. In the course of daily activities, a given individual will have marked variability in blood pressure, with frequent spikes, particularly during work hours.[13] In addition, there is a diurnal rhythm, the lowest pressures being manifested during sleep and the highest pressure being noted during worktime.[14] Devereux and co-workers[15] found that left ventricular hypertrophy in hypertensives correlated with their average workday blood pressures but not with their nonworkday pressures, suggesting that the recurrent stress of working plays a part in this development. Public speaking is apparently a particularly stressful activity, but even friendly conversations with peers or superiors are usually accompanied by hypertensive surges.[16] Conversely, conversations with a pet or a subordinate tend to lower the blood pressure.[17]

Laboratory tests using various types of stressors show that reactions differ according to the degree of active participation, the perception of the stressor, the novelty of the situation, and the degree of control allowed to the participant.

Frankenhaeuser,[18] for instance, finds three categories that roughly parallel those of Henry. She describes them as responses to effort without distress, effort with distress, and distress without effort. In experiments with healthy subjects performing a choice-reaction task with a high degree of control or a vigilance task with no control, subjects reported they were pleasantly challenged by the high-control task and felt some distress from the low-control task. Frankenhaeuser[18] noted increased epinephrine and decreased cortisol in high-control circumstances and increased levels of both epinephrine and cortisol in low-control situations. In a review of the literature, Glass[19] concluded that active coping in response to a threat to status but without fear markedly increased plasma norepinephrine, while epinephrine stayed the same or even decreased. Cortisol levels were related to fear in a study by Ursin and associates[20] of trainees at a parachute school. Cortisol levels in plasma samples obtained immediately after the jumps decreased from day to day, then increased again when criteria for jumps changed. The levels correlated with the men's self-ratings of fear of failure.

Williams[21] noted that mental arithmetic elicited increases in forearm blood flow, prolactin, norepinephrine, epinephrine, and cortisol, accompanied by decreases in forearm vascular resistance and no change in testosterone. During reaction time tests, the same subjects showed no change in forearm vascular resistance and significant increases only in norepinephrine and testosterone. Type A subjects who also had a family history of hypertension showed the largest cortisol and diastolic blood pressure responses to the reaction-time task.

In a more natural and realistic situation, urinary excretion of epinephrine, norepinephrine, and 11-hydroxycorticosteroids were measured during varied working conditions.[22] Levels of all three hormones increased on days when the workers were paid by the piece compared to fixed-salary periods, even with the same oxygen expenditure. Similarly, working on the assembly line induced greater excretion of these compounds than work off the assembly line. Familiarity with the procedures did not reduce the effects, which were essentially the same when the testing was repeated 6 months later.

Cholesterol also can be grossly elevated by chronic work stress. As early as the 1950s, Friedman, Rosenman, and Carroll[23] demonstrated that certified public accountants who were followed from January 1 to April 15 had as much as a 100 mg/dl rise in serum cholesterol without a change in diet. Francis[24] has shown that high-density (HDL) and low-density lipoprotein (LDL) ratios are consistently altered 10 days after stress. He found that cortisol levels in students peaked shortly after taking examinations and that soon afterward LDL rose, while HDL fell. The flip side of the cholesterol picture may also be related to psychological factors. Nerem and co-workers[25] showed that rabbits that were fondled and petted while on a high-cholesterol diet had a markedly lower rate of atheromatous plaque formation than a matched group that was not fondled or petted.

In reviewing the literature relating plasma lipid levels and emotion, Dimsdale and Herd[26] noted that free fatty acids often were elevated in anticipation of a stress and could continue to rise for hours after a stressful task. Active tasks such as race car driving produced larger elevations in free fatty acids than more passive stressors such as watching violent films. Changes in cholesterol were not usually significant in studies of short-term stressors but were observed in comparisons of stress periods versus nonstress periods such as medical student's exam periods versus vacation; accountants at tax time versus least stressful time; workers during unemployment versus during reemployment, and so on. Triglyceride changes were inconsistent, increasing markedly in some cases and decreasing in others. Variable cholesterol responses to short-term stressors suggested that some individuals are more labile in this respect than others.

ROLE OF ENDOCRINES AND THE AUTONOMIC NERVOUS SYSTEM

Raab[27] and Selye,[28] among others, identified the importance of the endocrines and the autonomic nervous system in the stress response, and later work has confirmed and expanded their observations. The defense reaction can be inititated experimentally by stimulation of the hypothalamic area, which controls the autonomic responses.[29]

CATECHOLAMINES

Although both epinephrine and norepinephrine increase during acute stress, plasma norepinephrine is mainly supplied by the sympathetic nerve terminals in activated skeletal muscles, while the adrenal medulla is the principal source of the circulating epinephrine. The two hormones evidently serve different functions. Robertson and associates[30] found that different stimuli induced differing proportions of each. For instance, sodium restriction increased plasma norepinephrine but not epinephrine. Caffeine had a greater effect on epinephrine levels than the treadmill test, but the treadmill exercise was more effective in raising norepinephrine levels. Orthostasis was also a potent stimulus for sympathetic nervous function but not for adrenomedullary discharge.

ORGANIZATION OF RESPONSE

As described by Bohus,[31] the stress response involves four levels of physiologic reactions. The first level is the limbic–midbrain system in conjunction with cerebral cortical areas. Here sensory information from the environment and internal hormonal signals are integrated and then appropriate activating or inhibitory signals are sent out by neural transmission.

At the second level is the hypothalamus, which translates the neural messages into hormonal messages by the synthesis or release of appropriate stimulating or inhibitory factors. The hypothalamus synthesizes neurosecretory peptides that are sent to the posterior pituitary. By means of nerves through the spinal cord, it also activates the release of catecholamines from the adrenal medulla.

The pituitary gland, which constitutes the third level, responds to the hormones both from the hypothalamus and in the circulation. The substances released seem to vary with the different stimuli, but vasopressin, prolactin, growth hormone, and the endorphins have all been related to stress, as well as ACTH. As Skinner[29] has emphasized, the reaction is not determined by the stressor itself but by the individual's interpretation regarding the stressfulness and importance of the event.

The final level of organization includes target organs in the various physiologic systems—heart, blood vessels, liver, kidney, and others. Indeed, the brain itself is affected by the stress-induced hormones, thus completing and closing the circuit of brain–neuroendocrine interactions.

CONTROL OF CARDIOVASCULAR SYSTEM

One of the major targets in this process is the cardiovascular system. Nerves of both the sympathetic and parasympathetic types supply the heart. The sympathetic nervous system acts through the effects of epinephrine, secreted by the adrenal medulla, and of norepinephrine, mainly released at the sympathetic nerve endings. Receptors for these hormones are found not only in the heart but also on smooth muscle throughout the body and are divided into α_1, α_2, β_1, and β_2. The vasodepressive α_1-receptors are the predominant type on innervated postjunctional sites of cardiovascular tissues. The heart contains predominantly β_1-receptors. Norepinephrine acts on the α-receptors and the β_1-receptors. Epinephrine can act on all four and is preferentially accepted by all but the α_1-receptors. The β-adrenergic receptors in the heart activate adenylate cyclase, thus increasing intracellular cyclic AMP.[32]

Overall, sympathetic activity tends to enhance smooth muscle contractility, thus increasing the total systemic resistance (TSR) and also increasing heart rate and force.

While the sympathetic system acts in response to environmental changes, the parasympathetic system reacts to internal clues to maintain homeostasis. The parasympathetic system achieves its effects by means of acetylcholine from stimulation of the vagus nerve. Its receptors are found in the heart and in prejunctional areas of sympathetic nerve endings where their stimulation can prevent the release of norepinephrine from the associated nerve ending. The acetylcholine from parasympathetic activity can also interfere with β-adrenergic effects by antagonizing the cyclic AMP within the cell. Atrial and ventricular portions of the heart do not respond to parasympathetic activity in the same way. In the ventricles, the predominant effect is inhibition of the β-adrenergic agonists. In the atrial tissues, an additional effect is an increase in the outward flow of potassium ions. The result is a decrease in the contractility of the heart and slowing of the heartbeat.[32]

Cholinergic factors stimulate the release of ACTH, which in turn increases the formation of cortisol and aldosterone.

CORTISOL AND ALDOSTERONE

The effects of cortisol and other glucocorticoids include increased plasma cholesterol; increased sensitivity of arterioles to catecholamines; increased angiotensin; increased gluconeogenesis in the liver; enhanced lipid mobilization; and depletion of myocardial potassium and magnesium. The increased angiotensin and aldosterone raise the blood pressure by the retention of sodium and water in the kidney and the pressor activity of angiotensin II on vascular tissues. In sum, the overall effect is increased cardiac output and vascular resistance.

Thus, the sympathetic and the parasympathetic nervous systems and various hormones interact to modulate the cardiovascular responses to environmental stimuli.

CORONARY HEART DISEASE AND ATHEROSCLEROSIS

Current theories regarding the development of atherosclerosis postulate several phases, starting with injury to the intima, followed by platelet aggregation and fibrosis at the site, infiltration of monocytes, proliferation of vascular smooth muscle, and adherence or incorporation of lipids and thrombi.[33]

Many of the observed responses to stress can possibly facilitate this process. For instance, injury to intima is more apt to occur when blood flow increases in velocity due to hypertension, surges in blood pressure, or turbulence, as at sites of bifurcating or originating vessel branches. Platelet stickiness, increased by the presence of catecholamines, enhances the possibilities of platelet aggregation and thrombus formation. Then growth factor released by the platelets fosters endothelial growth. Furthermore, the increased availability of free fatty acids and cholesterol associated with stress certainly aids the atherosclerotic build-up.[33]

HYPERTENSION

Blood pressure is determined by the interrelationships among cardiac output, arterial blood pressure, total peripheral resistance, blood volume, and extracellular fluid volume. The feedback control governing these elements involves neurogenic mechanisms, renal excretion, cardiac function, and circulatory function. As has been discussed, stress effects resulting from the release of cortisol and catecholamines tend to increase total peripheral resistance, blood volume, cardiac output, and arterial blood pressure.

Frequent elevations in blood pressure in response to stress may contribute to essential hypertension. Overreactivity has been found to be predictive for persons already at risk because of borderline hypertension or family history of hypertension. As a group, such persons respond to mental stress with greater increments in blood pressure and heart rates than normotensives with negative family history.[34-36] In a study of high-risk borderline hypertensives followed for 5 years, 54 of 80 progressed to sustained hypertension. These had a strong family history of essential hypertension and a high cardiovascular response to mental stress (subtraction problems), as compared with both low-risk controls and the high-risk group who maintained borderline levels of blood pressure.[36]

Folkow and co-workers[37] have postulated that in time the adaptation of the cardiovascular tissues to repeated hypertensive episodes may lead to permanent changes. In experiments with spontaneously hypertensive rats, they found evidence that the vascular musculature thickened in response to the raised pressure, thus increasing peripheral resistance. If normal rats were made hypertensive artificially, as by clipping the renal artery, they too showed vascular hypertrophy but to a lesser extent.

An alternative explanation proposed by Obrist and colleagues[38] is that autoregulation of the vasculature adapts to the β-adrenergic–mediated increase in cardiac output by increasing vascular tone to normalize the flow. They point out that retention of sodium outside metabolic needs by β-adrenergic stimulation of the kidney can expand plasma volume and start the chain of events leading to essential hypertension. Since not everyone develops hypertension despite daily fluctuations in blood pressure, they suggest that genetic susceptibility as well as physiologic overreactivity is requisite for essential hypertension. Indeed, Light and her co-workers[39] observed that high-risk young men (borderline hypertensives or positive family history) who had high heart rates in response to mental stress also had significantly greater decreases in sodium and fluid excretion than low-risk groups with either high or low heart rate reaction or than a high-risk group with low heart rates. In comparing the hemodynamic responses to stress after salt loading, Falkner and associates[36] noted little change in the findings for normotensive adolescents with a negative family history but significant increases in both diastolic and systolic blood pressures and reductions in heart rate in normotensive adolescents with a positive family history. This suggests that renal abnormalities may mediate and amplify the pathogenetic effects of stress.

ISCHEMIA, INFARCTION, AND SUDDEN DEATH

Marked increases in myocardial oxygen demand such as by increased physical or mental activity or some reduction in the available blood supply or oxygen such as by atherosclerosis sets the stage for ischemia, angina, or myocardial infarction. The precipitating event is likely to be blockage by a thrombus or spasm, particularly in a vulnerable area. Such a thrombus can be precipitated by increased platelet stickiness induced by sympathetic overstimulation from psychological stress. Vasospasm also has been induced by emotional stress[40] and may be related to the release of potent substances by platelets. Ambulatory monitoring has shown that ischemic events are often related to psychological arousal in patients with angina, both typical and atypical types.

Increased sympathetic arousal has been demonstrated to lower the threshold for ventricular fibrillation[41] and is also capable of creating myocardial damage. Both are predisposing factors for sudden death. Myocardial damage has usually occurred on a long-term basis before the final event. However, studies by Reich and colleagues[42] indicate that approximately 20% of resuscitated victims of sudden death have no structural heart disease. In these cases, lethal arrhythmias may be precipitated exclusively by psychological stress. In many instances, depression has been documented as preceding sudden death, and this suggests the deleterious effects of cortisol and perhaps the depletion of protective substances such as endorphins.

In a series of 208 witnessed sudden cardiac deaths, Baroldi and co-workers[43] reported coagulation necrosis in only 17% while coagulative myocytolysis (contraction-band necrosis) was present in 86% and was the unique lesion detected in 72%. Contraction-band lesions have been described in clinical cases of pheochromocytoma[44] and in animals subjected to experimental stress.[45] We also observed these changes in dogs given boluses of catecholamines.[46] In these animal studies, the coagulative myocytolysis appeared in a matter of minutes. Interestingly, we have found that β-blockers such as propranolol[46] and calcium blockers,[47] particularly diltiazem, provide some degree of protection against such norepinephrine-induced lesions in dogs.

In a discussion of the electrocardiographic responses to behavioral stimuli, deSilva[48] cited numerous demonstrations that stressful states can evoke dysrhythmias, including tachycardia, ventricular premature beats, and ventricular fibrillation, both in patients with and without heart disease. Furthermore, animal studies showed that the incidence of arrhythmias increased in aversive environments as compared with tranquil ones. The role of stress and sympathetic arousal is also indicated by studies with animals or susceptible patients demonstrating the protective effects of tranquilizers, β-adrenergic blockade, α-adrenergic blockade, serotonin, or vagal stimulation to counteract the effects of catecholamines.[49]

Although rarely effective alone, emotional stress can lead to sudden death either as the "softening up" process that increases vulnerability or as the final blow in a system already compromised by the presence of myocardial damage, electrical instability, or coronary artery disease. In addition, it can be a factor in facilitating the occurrence of the compromising conditions.

IDENTIFYING THOSE AT RISK

To elucidate the relationship of mental stress and physiologic reactivity, we have developed an objective system of testing that measures the physiologic responses to standardized low-challenge mental tasks, selected because of their similarity to mild routine daily stresses.[50] Using impedance cardiography, various hemodynamic factors are monitored while a subject does mental arithmetic under time pressure, plays a competitive video game, and performs the cold pressor test. (These are three of 14 challenges given in our overall program of evaluation.) With the aid of computerized calculations, we obtain data on 17 hemodynamic variables. We designed a coordinate system graph to display the hemodynamic changes during the standardized stress test.[51]

About one in five apparently healthy individuals responds with abnormal increases in cardiovascular reactivity. Among the changes observed are elevations in total systemic resistance or in cardiac output. The latter changes are as great as might be seen with maximum physical effort. Such physiologic overreactivity, which we call *hot reacting*, has been correlated with hyperlipidemia,[52] family history of hypertension,[52] and susceptibility to illness.[53] However, it does not correlate with the type A behavior pattern.[54] Also, the mean blood pressure obtained in 15 minutes of such testing correlates with the mean systolic blood pressure of a day of ambulatory monitoring[55] and has better test–retest reliability.[56] In addition, it correlates with blood pressure in the workplace and with average 24-hour blood pressure as obtained by ambulatory monitoring.[57] Hypertensives and hot reactors can be treated according to the mechanism by which the blood pressure is elevated. Figures 115.1 and 115.2 show the blood pressure and hemodynamic changes in a double-blind study of mild hypertensives using a calcium channel blocker.[58]

IMPLICATIONS FOR TREATMENT

Obviously, control of emotions and stress can be important for prevention and delay of cardiovascular diseases both in the primary and secondary sense. This requires behavioral modification. The first step in getting people to change their behavior is to determine what their values and beliefs are with regard to life and health. By this we mean clarifying what they expect out of life and how they wish to be remembered. Indeed, helping patients to sort out their values is not only the first step but is probably the most fundamental to their evaluation and subsequent management.

Later, one can review their belief systems to enable them to see the origin of their feelings and attitudes. This is accomplished very quickly, using rational cognitive approaches. By bringing their beliefs to their conscious minds, they can become aware of self-destructive habits and substitute healthy ones in their place. Often people are not really conscious of their belief systems because they have practiced them so often they have become automatic. We try to bring these subconscious products of the limbic portion of the brain back to conscious levels by a variety of methods.

Physiologic stress responses are determined by a person's interpretation of an event, not by the event itself. Therefore, if a person's beliefs are irrational, his or her stress responses may be totally inappropriate. By enabling individuals to examine their own thinking patterns, we can help them to substitute rational for irrational beliefs. For example, clues to irrational perfectionist patterns include words such as "should" and "must." These indicate inflexible rules, portend frequent "failures," and lead to many self-inflicted guilt trips. "What if" may indicate catastrophizing, and "everybody," "never," "always," and other similar words indicate globalization. Projection, or the blaming of others when things go wrong, and constant measuring of oneself by others' opinions are additional signs of faulty thinking. Substituting rational for irrational thinking leads to a more healthful performance and reduction in physiologic overreactivity.

When patients adopt more rational modes of thinking, they realize they have more control in many aspects of their lives and are more open to new options. Eliminating irrational approaches unloads their "circuits" by reducing the "tail chasing" of pursuing irrational goals. This not only is a way of reducing stress, but also facilitates other changes in behavior such as smoking cessation, improving the diet, increasing exercise, and learning other stress-management techniques. Success breeds success.

For selected hypertensives and "hot reactors," self-hypnosis and relaxation techniques can reduce blood pressure to the extent that medications may not be necessary or can be used in lower dosages. Side effects diminish, quality of life increases, and adherence can be expected.

It is necessary to teach patients how to do these things. Besides the clinical counseling, tapes of progressive relaxation, demonstration of abdominal breathing, and supervised training in self-hypnosis by qualified personnel are possible teaching modes. It is better to have the patient practice these techniques for a few days before relating them to blood pressure readings. This will ensure improvement when the blood pressure determination is finally made and will engender enthusiasm for continued practice and improvement. Again, success is a great motivator.

Practice of progressive relaxation twice a day for 4 to 6 weeks, with weekly supervised sessions is the recommended regimen for training. Additional biofeedback methods are not needed by most patients but can enhance motivation in those who respond mainly to concrete evidence rather than intellectual concepts.

Engel and associates[59] achieved reductions in blood pressure with

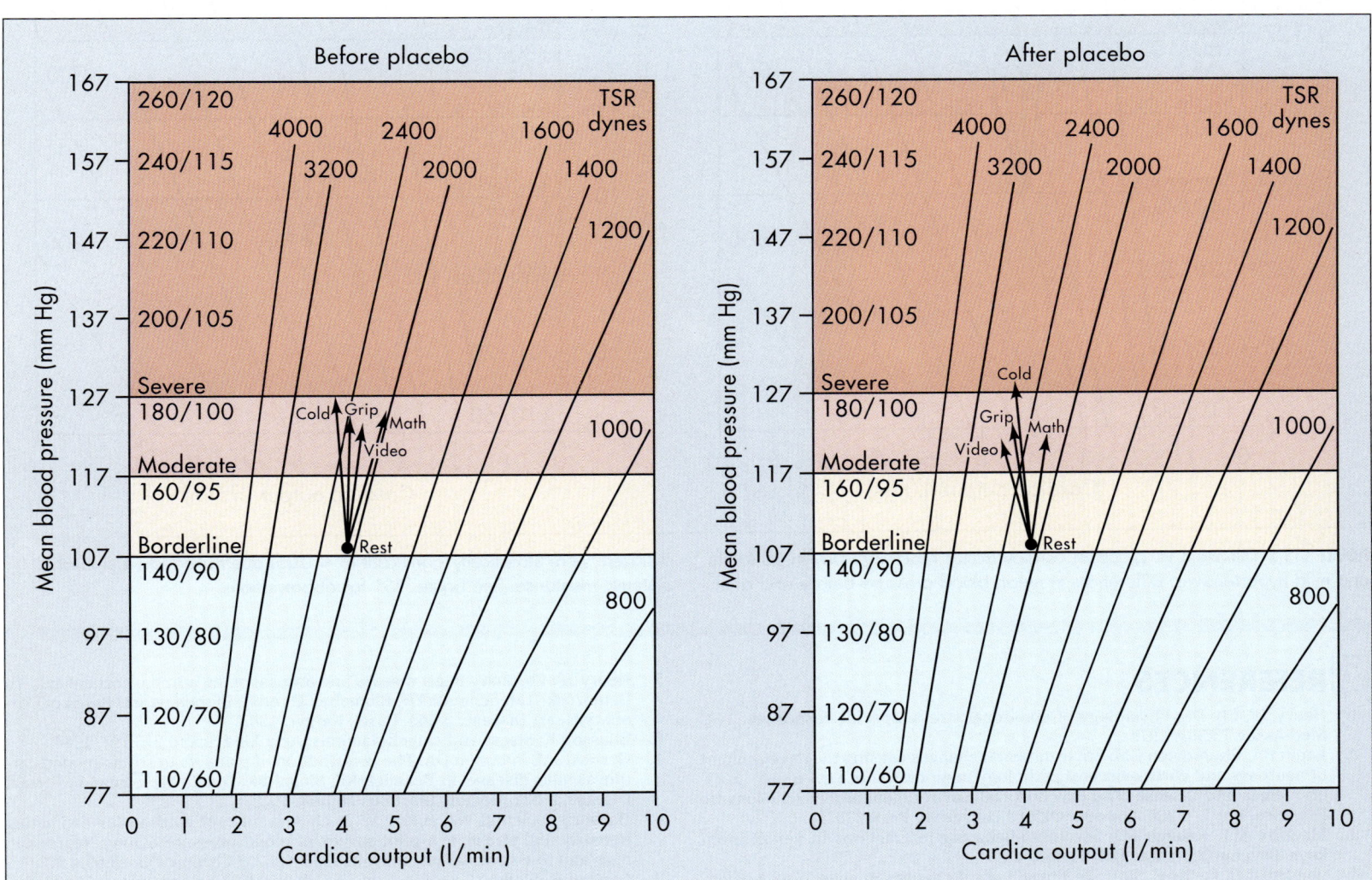

FIGURE 115.1 Diltiazem vs. placebo: cardiovascular reactivity study in 20 labile and mild hypertensives. Differences in mean blood pressure before and after placebo were not statistically significant. (*Cold*, cold pressor test; *Grip*, hand grip test; *Math*, mental arithmetic test; *Video*, competitive video game test).

either relaxation or biofeedback training, and even better results with patients given both types of training. The benefits were maintained at the 6-month follow-up.

Other behavioral methods have been effective in achieving improvements in blood pressure, response to emotional stress, incidence of cardiac arrhythmias, and cholesterol level. These methods have included non-cultist meditation, dietary changes, moderate daily exercise, anger management, assertiveness training, and cognitive restructuring.[60-63] Each of these methods has helped some individuals, although the results tend to be variable. While individual physiologic differences may account for some of the variability, it has also been noted that a strategy is more apt to work if the patient believes it will be effective, is motivated to make a behavioral change, and believes the consequences of the change will be important to overall health or quality of life.

We have tried a comprehensive approach, incorporating relaxation therapy, cognitive restructuring, stress management, diet changes, group instruction, and individual counseling that includes finding key attitudes, behaviors, and situations. In a pilot study of "hot reactors," this comprehensive approach has resulted in reductions in physiologic overreactivity to emotional stress, reductions in both resting and stress-induced blood pressure, reductions in cholesterol levels, and subjective improvements in their quality of life that included increases in income from 40% to 200%.

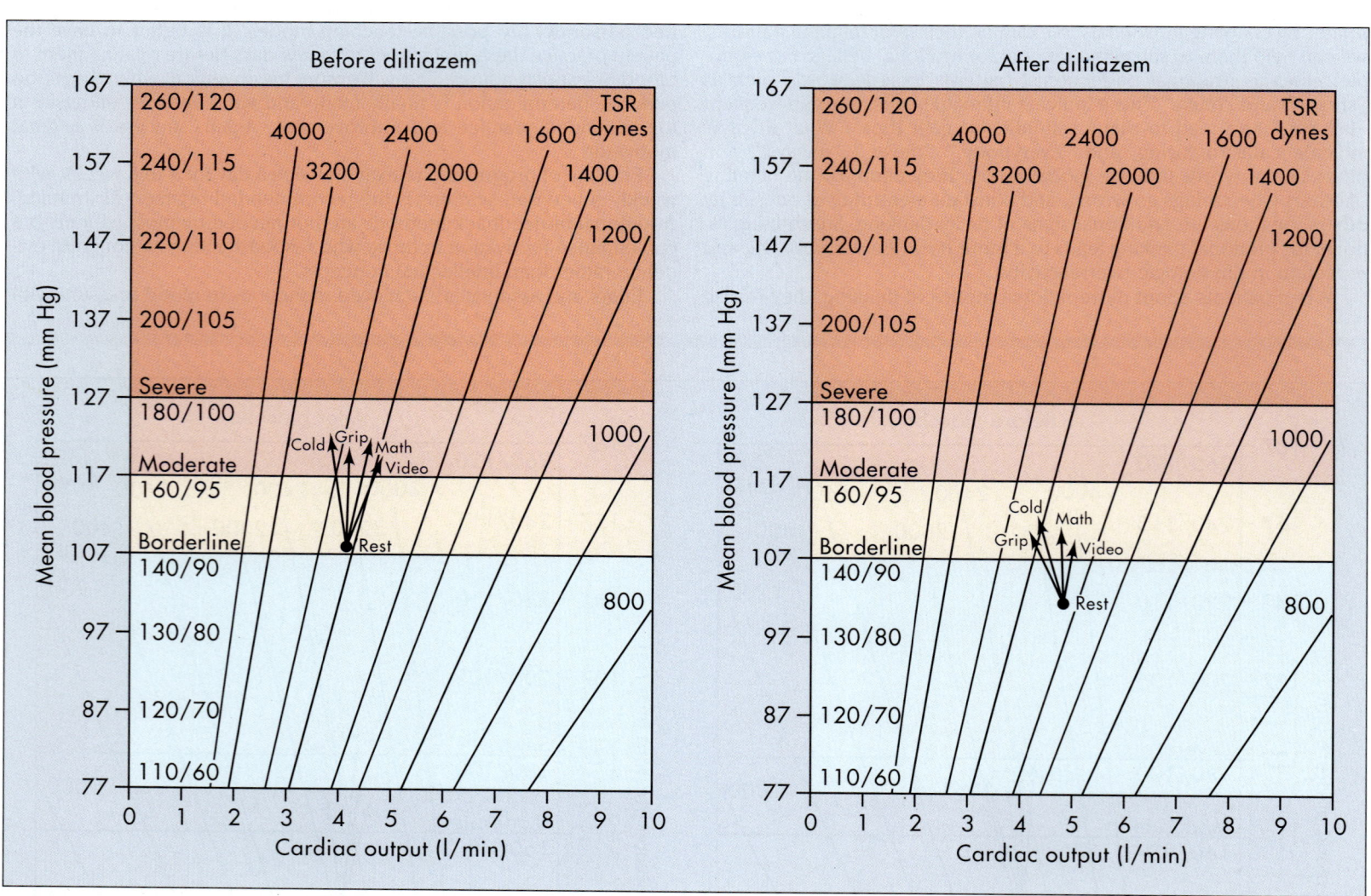

FIGURE 115.2 Diltiazem vs. placebo: cardiovascular reactivity study in 20 labile and mild hypertensives. Differences in mean blood pressure before and after diltiazem were statistically significant (P < 0.05) due to reduction in total systemic resistance. See Figure 115.1 for abbreviations.

REFERENCES

1. Henry JP, Ely DL: Physiology of emotional stress. Specific responses. J SC Med Assoc 75:501, 1979
2. Lapin BA, Cherkovich GM: Environmental changes causing the development of neuroses and corticovisceral pathology in monkeys. In Levi L (ed): Society, Stress and Disease: The Psychosocial Environment and Psychosomatic Diseases, Vol 1, p 266. London, Oxford University Press, 1971
3. McGuire MT, Raleigh MJ: Serotonin-behavior interactions in vervet monkeys. Psychopharmacol Bull 21:458, 1985
4. von Holst D, Fuchs E, Stohr W: Physiological changes in male Tupaia belangeri under different types of social stress. In Dembroski TM, Schmidt TH, Blumchen G: Biobehavioral Bases of Coronary Heart Disease, p 382. Basel, Karger, 1983
5. Henry JP: Coronary heart disease and arousal of the adrenal cortical axis. In Dembroski TM, Schmidt TH, Blumchen G (eds): Biobehavioral Bases of Coronary Heart Disease, p 365. Basel, Karger, 1983
6. Eliasson K: Stress and catecholamines. Acta Med Scand 215:197, 1984
7. Gerrard JM, Peterson DA: The contribution of platelets to stress-related cardiovascular disease. In Beamish RE, Singal PK, Dhalla SN: Stress and Heart Disease, p 331. Boston, Martinus Nijhoff, 1985
8. Harburg E, Schull WJ, Erfurt JC et al: A family set method for estimating heredity and stress. I. A pilot survey of blood pressure among Negroes in high and low stress areas, Detroit, 1966–1967. J Chronic Dis 23:69, 1970
9. Gampel B, Slome C, Scotch N et al: Urbanization and hypertension among Zulu adults. J Chronic Dis 15:67, 1962
10. Berkman LF, Syme SL: Social networks, host resistance, and mortality: A nine-year follow-up study of Alameda County residents. Am J Epidemiol

109:186, 1979
11. Parkes CM, Benjamin B, Fitzgerald RG: Broken hearts: A statistical study of increased mortality among widowers. Br Med J 1:740, 1969
12. Ward AM: Mortality of bereavement. Br Med J 1:700, 1976
13. Surwit RS: Pharmacologic and behavioral modulators of cardiovascular reactivity: An overview. In Matthews KA, Weiss SM, Detre T et al (eds): Handbook of Stress, Reactivity, and Cardiovascular Disease, p 385. New York, John Wiley & Sons, 1986
14. Harshfield GA, Pickering TG, Kleinert HD et al: Situational variations of blood pressure in ambulatory hypertensive patients. Psychosom Med 44:237, 1982
15. Devereux RB, Pickering TG, Harshfield GA et al: Left ventricular hypertrophy in patients with hypertension: Importance of blood pressure response to regularly recurring stress. Circulation 68:470, 1983
16. Lynch JJ: The Language of the Heart. New York, Basic Books, 1985
17. Kangilaski J: Dialogue: A link to psychosomatic illness. JAMA 247:2760, 1982
18. Frankenhaeuser M: The sympathetic-adrenal and pituitary-adrenal response to challenge: Comparison between the sexes. In Dembroski TM, Schmidt TH, Blumchen G (eds): Biobehavioral Bases of Coronary Heart Disease, p 91. Basel, Karger, 1983
19. Glass DC: Behavior Patterns, Stress and Coronary Disease. Hillsdale, NJ, Lawrence Erlbaum Associates, 1977
20. Ursin H, Baade E, Levine S (eds): Psychobiology of Stress. A Study of Coping Men. New York, Academic Press, 1978
21. Williams RB Jr: Patterns of reactivity and stress. In Matthews KA, Weiss SM, Detre T et al (eds): Handbook of Stress, Reactivity, and Cardiovascular Disease, p 109. New York, John Wiley & Sons, 1986
22. Timio M, Gentili S, Pede S: Free adrenaline and noradrenaline excretion related to occupational stress. Br Heart J 42:471, 1979
23. Friedman M, Rosenman RH, Carroll V: Changes in the serum cholesterol and blood clotting time in men subjected to cyclic variation of occupational stress. Circulation 17:852, 1958
24. Francis KT: Psychologic correlates of serum indicators of stress in man: A longitudinal study. Psychosom Med 41:617, 1979
25. Nerem RM, Levesque MJ, Cornhill JF: Social environment as a factor in diet-induced aortic atherosclerosis in rabbits. Science 208:1475, 1980
26. Dimsdale JE, Herd JA: Variability of plasma lipids in response to emotional arousal. Psychosom Med 44:413, 1982
27. Raab W: Emotional and sensory stress factors in myocardial pathology. Am Heart J 72:538, 1966
28. Selye H: Stress in Health and Disease. Boston, Butterworth, 1976
29. Skinner JE: Psychosocial stress and sudden cardiac death: Brain mechanisms. In Beamish RE, Singal PK, Dhalla NS (eds): Stress and Heart Disease, p 44. Boston, Martinus Nijhoff, 1985
30. Robertson D, Johnson GA, Robertson RM et al: Comparative assessment of stimuli that release neuronal and adrenomedullary catecholamines in man. Circulation 59:637, 1979
31. Bohus B: Neuroendocrine interactions with brain and behavior: A model for psychoneuroimmunology? In Breakdown in Human Adaptation to "Stress," p 638. Boston, Martinus Nijhoff, 1984
32. Watanabe SN, Lindemann JP: Mechanisms of adrenergic and cholinergic regulation of myocardial contractibility. In Sperelakis N (ed): Physiology of the Heart, p 377. Boston, Martinus Nijhoff, 1984
33. Ross R, Faggiotto A, Bowen-Pope D, Raines E: The role of endothelial injury and platelet and macrophage interactions in atherosclerosis. Circulation (Suppl) 70:III–77, 1984
34. Falkner B, Onesti G, Angelakos ET et al: Cardiovascular response to mental stress in normal adolescents with hypertensive parents. Hypertension 1:23, 1979
35. Falkner B, Onesti G, Hamstra B: Stress response characteristics of adolescents with high genetic risk for essential hypertension: A five-year follow-up. Clin Exp Hypertens 3:583, 1981
36. Falkner B, Onesti G, Angelakos E: Effect of salt loading on the cardiovascular response to stress in adolescents. Hypertension (Suppl) 3:II–195, 1981
37. Folkow BUB, Hallback MIL, Lundgren Y et al: Importance of adaptive changes in vascular design for establishment of primary hypertension, studies in man and in spontaneously hypertensive rat. Circ Res (Suppl) 32/33:I–2, 1973
38. Obrist PA, Langer AW, Light KC, Koepke JP: A cardiac-behavioral approach in the study of hypertension. In Dembroski TM, Schmidt TH, Blumchen G (eds): Biobehavioral Bases of Coronary Heart Disease, p 290. Basel, Karger, 1983
39. Light KC, Koepke JP, Obrist PA, Willis PW IV: Psychological stress induces sodium and fluid retention in men at high risk for hypertension. Science 220:429, 1983
40. Schiffer F, Hartley LH, Schulman CL, Anelmann WH: Evidence for emotionally-induced coronary arterial spasm in patients with angina pectoris. Br Heart J 44:62, 1980
41. Skinner JE, Lie JT, Entman ML: Modification of ventricular fibrillation latency following coronary artery occlusion in the conscious pig: The effects of psychological stress and beta-adrenergic blockade. Circulation 51:656, 1975
42. Reich P, DeSilva RA, Lown B, Murawski BJ: Acute psychological disturbance preceding life-threatening ventricular arrhythmias. JAMA 246:233, 1981
43. Baroldi G, Falzi G, Mariani F: Sudden coronary death: A postmortem study in 208 selected cases compared to 97 "control" subjects. Am Heart J 98:20, 1979
44. Szakacs JE, Cannon A: L-norepinephrine myocarditis. Am J Clin Pathol 30:425, 1958
45. Raab W, Chaplin JP, Bajusz E: Myocardial necrosis produced in domesticated rats and in wild rats by sensory and emotional stresses. Proc Soc Exp Biol 116:665, 1964
46. Eliot RS, Todd GL, Clayton FC, Pieper GM: Experimental catecholamine-induced acute myocardial necrosis. Adv Cardiol 25:107, 1978
47. Todd GL, Sterns DA, Plambeck MS et al: Protective effects of slow channel calcium antagonists on noradrenaline-induced myocardial necrosis. Cardiovasc Res 20:645, 1986
48. deSilva RA: Electrocardiographic responses to behavioral stimuli. In United States Department of Health and Human Services: Applicability of New Technology to Biobehavioral Research, p 121. NIH publication No. 84-1654, 1984
49. Lown B, DeSilva RA, Reich P, Murawski BJ: Psychophysiologic factors in sudden cardiac death. Am J Psychiatry 137:11, 1980
50. Eliot RS, Buell JC: Utilization of a new objective, non-physical stress test. In Beamish RE, Singal PK, Dhalla NS (eds): Stress and Heart Disease, p 116. Boston, Martinus Nijhoff, 1985
51. Eliot RS, Morales-Ballejo HM: Stress and the heart: Measuring and evaluating reactivity. Illustrated Medicine 2(3):2, 1987
52. McKinney ME, McIlain HE, Hofschire PJ et al: Cardiovascular changes during mental stress: Correlations with presence of coronary risk factors and cardiovascular disease in physicians and dentists. Unpublished paper, 1986
53. Dembroski TM, MacDougall JM, Slaats S et al: Challenge-induced cardiovascular response as a predictor of minor illnesses. J Human Stress 7:2, 1981
54. Ruddel H, Langewitz JW, McKinney ME et al: Hemodynamic responses during the type A interview: A comparison with mental challenge and a clinical interview. J Auton Nerv Syst (Suppl) 15:685, 1986
55. Ruddel H, McKinney ME, Dembroski T et al: Reliability of ambulatory blood pressure monitoring and blood pressure response to mental challenge in the laboratory. J Auton Nerv Syst (Suppl) 15:247, 1986
56. McKinney ME, Miner MH, Ruddel H et al: The standardized mental stress test protocol: Test-retest reliability and comparison with ambulatory blood pressure monitoring. Psychophysiology 22:453, 1985
57. Morales-Ballejo HM, Eliot RS, Boone JL, Hughes JS: Psychophysiological stress testing as a predictor of mean daily blood pressure. Am Heart J 116:673, 1988
58. Morales-Ballejo HM, Eliot RS, Boone JL: Influence of diltiazem and placebo on the hemodynamic changes caused by mental and physical stress. Institute of Stress Medicine (in press).
59. Engel BT, Glasgow MS, Gaarder KR: Behavioral treatment of high blood pressure. III. Follow-up results and treatment recommendations. Psychosom Med 45:23, 1983
60. Patel C: A new dimension in the prevention of coronary heart disease. In Dembroski TM, Schmidt TH, Blumchen G (eds): Biobehavioral Bases of Coronary Heart Disease, p 416. Basel, Karger, 1983
61. Chesney MA, Ward MM: Biobehavioral treatment approaches for cardiovascular disorders. J Cardiopulmonary Rehabil 5:226, 1985
62. Barnard RJ, Zifferblatt SM, Rosenberg JM, Pritikin N: Effects of a high-complex-carbohydrate diet and daily walking on blood pressure and medication status of hypertensive patients. J Cardiac Rehabil 3:839, 1983
63. Nonpharmacological approaches to the control of high blood pressure: Final report of the Subcommittee on Nonpharmacological therapy of the 1984 Joint National Committee on Detection, Evaluation, and Treatment of High Blood Pressure. Hypertension 8:444, 1986

The International Stress Foundation and the Monsour Medical Foundation provided grants for editorial assistance with this paper.

CARDIAC COMPLICATIONS OF SUBSTANCE ABUSE

Michael Callaham • Kanu Chatterjee

CHAPTER 116
VOLUME 2

Use and abuse of various mood-altering substances is rife in modern society and ranges from oral intake of ethanol to the intravenous administration of cocaine, heroin, and other illegal substances. Many of these substances produce cardiac complications, particularly if taken in large enough quantities or over a long enough period of time. Certain cardiac complications, such as those produced by ethanol abuse (which is not discussed in this chapter), are fairly common. Also relatively common are infectious complications (such as endocarditis) due to intravenous drug use or cardiac complications such as arrhythmias or shock seen in the setting of frank drug overdose.

However, neither of the above categories is discussed in this chapter, which instead focuses on the noninfectious cardiac complications of substance abuse. This distinction is a bit arbitrary, as substance abuse often merges almost indistinguishably into frank overdose, but it is a useful one because the clinical scenarios of substance abuse and frank overdose are usually very different. In overdose, the patient often presents with a history of ingestion or overdose and usually has an altered mental status (and is frequently comatose). In this setting the cardiac symptoms and signs are usually promptly connected in the clinician's mind with the offending substance and appropriate diagnosis and treatment follows. However, the situation is quite different in the type of substance abuse discussed in this chapter. In this clinical setting, patients often present with cardiac symptoms or signs in a normal mental state after the intoxication has passed. The possibility of substance abuse is often not thought of at all by the physician and is typically minimized or denied by the patient. Furthermore, overdose is an acute event that can be treated and reversed satisfactorily whereas the cardiac complications of substance abuse are more often the result of long-standing behavior patterns and substance usage, and the physician has the additional task of convincing the patient of the danger of the practice.

Although the problem of cardiac complications of substance abuse is a significant one, there are really few reports in the literature about such complications, considering the frequent use of many of the offending substances. In addition, the state of medical knowledge regarding these complications is remarkably rudimentary, and, in most cases, pathophysiology is poorly understood.

■ SYMPATHOMIMETICS
COCAINE

Cocaine is the single most common drug of abuse with significant cardiac effects, owing to its incredible surge in popularity in the past decade. Between 1976 and 1985 the number of emergency department visits related to cocaine increased ninefold, and the number of cocaine-related deaths increased almost 12-fold.[1] An estimated 30 million Americans have used cocaine, and an estimated 5 million use it regularly.[2] In 1987, the National Institute of Drug Abuse reported that 5,000 persons per day became new cocaine users, and 200,000 to 1 million persons are compulsive users.[3] During the past 2 decades a 300% increase in emergency department visits for cocaine-related complications has been reported.[4] The incidence of cocaine-related deaths has also increased, and most of these deaths could be attributed to the cardiovascular complications.

Until recently, cocaine was believed to be a relatively benign and nonaddicting drug, but new evidence suggests that it may be more harmful than heroin.[2] Our level of scientific ignorance of this drug is illustrated by the fact that as recently as 1978 it was an accepted "fact" that oral cocaine was pharmacologically inactive, despite the fact that Peruvian Indians had been chewing cocoa leaves for 2,000 years (presumably for some good reason).[5] The truth is that the oral and nasal forms of cocaine are just as potent as the intravenous form and that many of the major cardiac complications occur with nasal use. The cardiac complications of cocaine use were only first reported in 1982, although a series of cases since then demonstrate that cardiac complications are not rare.[6-14]

PHARMACOLOGY

Cocaine is an alkaloid derived from the leaves of the erythroxylon coca plant. Cocaine hydrochloride, which is available for medicinal use, is prepared by dissolving the alkaloid in hydrochloric acid to form a water-soluble salt. The cocaine alkaloid ("free base") is soluble in alcohol, acetone, oils, and ether. Cocaine free base is absorbed from all sites, including mucous membranes of nasal passages, gastrointestinal tract, and vagina. Absorption through mucous membranes is slow, which results in a delayed onset and longer duration of action. It is metabolized by plasma and liver cholinesterases to water-soluble metabolites, benzoylecgonine and ecgonine methyl ester, which are then excreted in the urine.[15] When cholinesterase activity is low or deficient, as in fetuses, infants, elderly men, pregnant women, or patients with liver disease or congenital cholinesterase deficiency, an exaggerated response to small doses of cocaine might occur. Cocaine may be detected in the urine for 24 to 36 hours, depending on the route of administration and cholinesterase activity.

The local anesthetic effect of cocaine, which was recognized as early as 1884,[2] results from the prevention of the rapid increase in the nerve cell membrane permeability to sodium ions during depolarization, which blocks the initiation and conduction of electrical impulses within the nerve cells.[16] Its systemic effects on the nervous system, however, are probably mediated by alterations in synaptic transmission (Fig. 116.1). Cocaine inhibits the presynaptic reuptake of the neurotransmitters norepinephrine and dopamine, producing an excess of the neurotransmitters at the postsynaptic receptor sites.[16] Activation of the postsynaptic vascular α-adrenergic receptors results in vasoconstriction and acute rise in arterial pressure, and that of myocardial β-adrenergic receptors causes tachycardia and enhanced contractility. Sympathetic activation may also cause mydriasis, hyperglycemia, and hyperthermia.[2]

Dopaminergic effects of cocaine have been regarded as contributory in producing addiction. Short-term use of cocaine appears to stimulate dopaminergic neurotransmission by blocking the reuptake of dopamine and causing euphoria. However, with long-term use of cocaine, the nerve terminals may become depleted of dopamine, and it has been suggested that dopamine depletion may be a potential mechanism for the dysphoria and subsequent craving for the drug that develops during withdrawal.[17] Dopamine depletion may also be contributory to the pathogenesis of the adverse cardiovascular effects of chronic cocaine abuse.[18]

CARDIOVASCULAR COMPLICATIONS

In volunteers, intravenous cocaine has been shown to cause a dose-dependent increase in systolic and diastolic blood pressures.[19] These effects of cocaine were virtually identical to those produced by dextroamphetamine and were blocked by the calcium channel blocker nitrendipine in rats.[20] Plasma cocaine levels are not, however, linearly related to central nervous system effects, and the subjective "high" sought by the user dissipates at a time when plasma levels are still significantly elevated. Thus, the practice of repeating cocaine administration to maintain a "high" over hours can lead to progressively more elevated plasma levels (with corresponding cardiac toxicity) without the similarly improved mood sought by the use.[5]

A number of cardiovascular adverse effects associated with cocaine abuse have been recognized and are listed in Table 116.1. Sinus tachycardia, ventricular fibrillation, and asystole have been reported in patients indulging in cocaine abuse. A reported case of asystole and ventricular fibrillation is typical of many anecdotes in the literature, in that a drug abuser was found unresponsive and by the time medical care arrived was in a terminal arrhythmia.[10] Whether this was due to a direct drug effect, seizures, hypoxia, or other causes could not be determined, and thus cocaine was not convincingly shown to have directly caused the final arrhythmia. However, it is known that cocaine use during anesthesia is associated with a greater incidence of arrhythmias, particularly premature ventricular beats,[21] and a case of self-resolving accelerated ventricular rhythm after intravenous cocaine abuse has been reported.[22] Accelerated idioventricular rhythm with hypotension was seen in a case of frank cocaine poisoning.[23]

The mechanisms of the arrhythmogenic effects of cocaine have not been clearly elucidated. Arrhythmias may result from its direct effects on the myocardium or from the effects of catecholamines. Due to inhibition of presynaptic norepinephrine uptake, surplus neurotransmitters are available for activation of postsynaptic adrenergic receptors. Thus, excessive stimulation of myocardial β-receptors may result that may promote arrhythmias. Arrhythmias may also occur due to

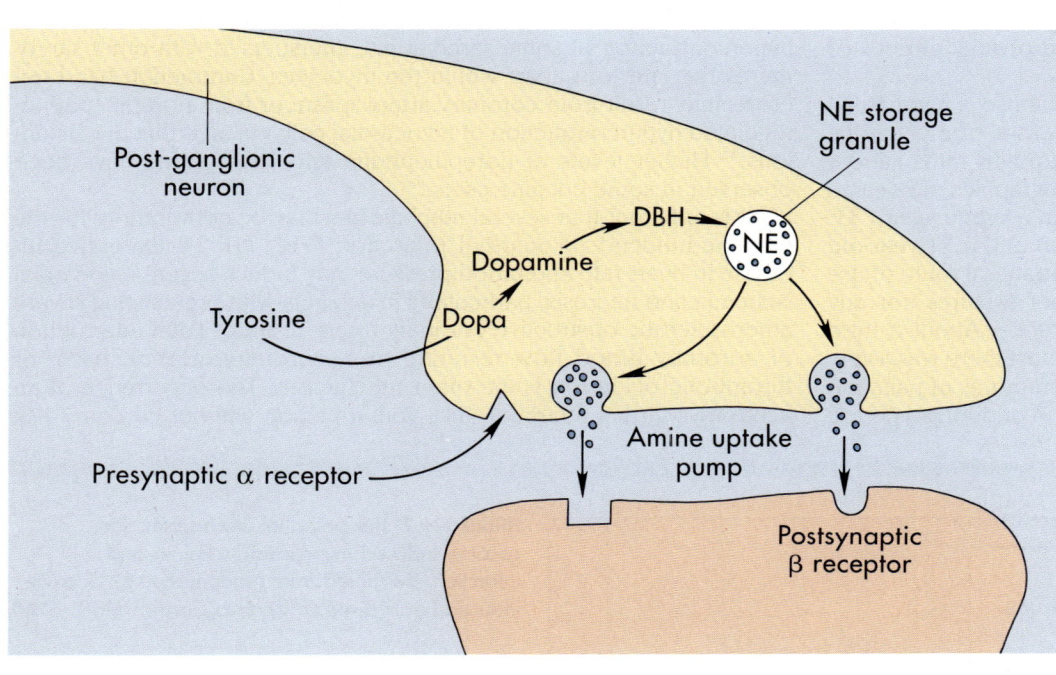

FIGURE 116.1 Effects of cocaine on the presynaptic reuptake of the neurotransmitter norepinephrine (*NE*). Decreased reuptake of NE results in surplus of NE, which then enhances activation of adrenergic receptors. (Modified from Nademanee K: Cocaine-induced heart disease. Choices Cardiol 3:180, 1989)

TABLE 116.1 CARDIOVASCULAR COMPLICATIONS OF COCAINE ABUSE

Dysrhythmias
Sinus tachycardia
Ventricular premature contractions
Ventricular tachycardia
Ventricular fibrillation
Asystole
Atrioventricular block and intraventricular conduction disturbance

Myocardial Ischemic Syndromes
Acute myocardial infarction
Angina
Spontaneous silent myocardial ischemia
Sudden death

Myocarditis and Cardiomyopathy

Miscellaneous
Hypertension
Rupture of the ascending aorta
Dissecting thoracic aortic aneurysm
Noncardiogenic pulmonary edema
Pneumopericardium and pneumomediastinum
Interaction with ganglion blocking drugs

cocaine-induced myocardial ischemia or infarction. In addition, cocaine can produce hyperpyrexia, which can lead to seizures and possibly cardiac arrhythmias.

Electrophysiologic studies in animals have attempted to elucidate the potential mechanism of cocaine-related arrhythmias. Cocaine overdose has been shown to cause significant prolongation of QRS complex duration and induce bundle branch block.[24] In conscious dogs, intravenous cocaine infusion produced sinus bradycardia progressing to asystole and ventricular tachycardia and fibrillation, and these arrhythmias were delayed several hours after cocaine infusion.[25] High-dose cocaine infusion in anesthetized dogs may also cause acute prolongation of atrial refractoriness and ventricular repolarization along with ventricular tachycardia, low-grade sinoatrial block, and atrioventricular nodal block.[26] These electrophysiologic abnormalities, however, have not been consistently detected in all studies, during either acute or chronic cocaine administration.[27,28]

Bradyarrhythmias require standard treatment, including atropine and transvenous pacing. For the treatment of ventricular arrhythmias, propranolol and amitriptyline have been recommended.[23,29–31] Calcium channel blocking agents such as nitrendipine have also been found to be effective antagonists to the cardiotoxic effects of cocaine.[20]

The most significant cardiac effect of cocaine abuse is myocardial ischemia and infarction. There have been many cases of myocardial infarction reported since the first in 1982, with a mortality rate of about 13%.[6,8,11,13,14] As might be expected from the demographics of cocaine use, the patients were predominantly male, with an average age of 31. However, cases also include a 28-year-old woman and a 21-year-old man, both with normal coronary arteries.[8,9] The intranasal route of use predominated. Most of these patients had neither seizures nor any other major manifestation of frank cocaine overdose. About a third had no risk factors for coronary artery disease. In most there was a very clear temporal relationship to cocaine use, with symptoms of pain and nausea starting either immediately on using cocaine or during a period of prolonged and heavy use involving many doses within a period of hours or days. In several cases there have been recurrent episodes of ischemia and infarction associated with cocaine use in the same person, and cessation of use has resulted in complete absence of further ischemic symptoms.[11,14] There thus seems to be little doubt about a causal relationship.

Autopsy studies in the victims of cocaine-related sudden death have reported the presence of severe atherosclerotic coronary artery disease in many patients.[32] Healed myocardial infarction, acute myocardial infarction, and complete thrombotic occlusion of the coronary arteries have also been reported. Thus, in many patients, atherosclerotic obstructive coronary artery disease appears to be the pathologic basis for myocardial ischemia and infarction. However, the coronary arteriograms of patients with acute myocardial infarction who abuse cocaine reveal frequently normal or near-normal coronary arteries that are free of atherosclerosis.[6,33] Coronary artery spasm and other mechanisms have been proposed as the pathogenetic process for myocardial infarction. The incidence of contraction band necrosis in the myocardium of patients who died of complications of cocaine abuse varies between 25% and 93%.[32,34] Contraction band necrosis is defined as the hypercontraction of some sarcomeres, interspersed with other sarcomeres that are torn apart within the myocytes. Contraction band necrosis may result from coronary artery spasm or from norepinephrine-mediated hypercontraction of myocardial cells via an influx of calcium ions.[35] Higher levels of norepinephrine and epinephrine have been observed in some cocaine users.[35]

It is apparent that several mechanisms may be contributory for the cocaine-induced myocardial infarction (Fig. 116.2). Excessive increase in heart rate and blood pressure may induce severe myocardial ischemia and necrosis, particularly in subjects with pre-existing severe atherosclerotic obstructive coronary artery disease. Total interruption of coronary blood flow resulting from coronary arterial spasm or thrombotic occlusion is the other mechanism. The occurrence of an acute myocardial infarction in a young person without coronary risk

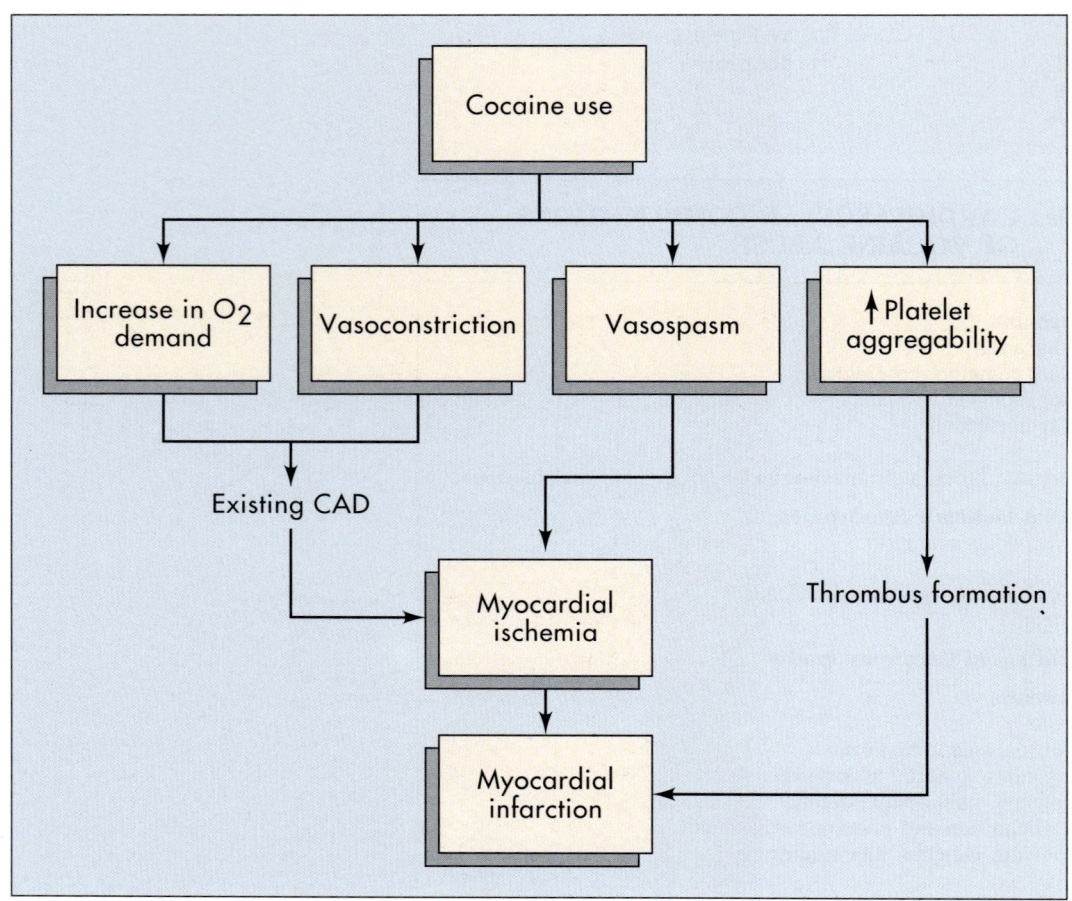

FIGURE 116.2 The potential mechanisms for cocaine-induced myocardial ischemia and infarction. (Modified from Nademanee K: Cocaine-induced heart disease. Choices Cardiol 3:180, 1989)

factors should raise the suspicion of coronary artery spasm related to recreational use of cocaine.[2] Even in the presence of anatomically normal coronary arteries, thrombosis may cause acute myocardial infarction.[36,37] Whether cocaine can precipitate coronary artery thrombosis without inducing coronary spasm is not known. The procoagulant effects of cocaine such as combined protein C and antithrombin III deficiency may promote in situ thrombosis, which remains another possible mechanism for myocardial infarction related to cocaine abuse.[38] Catecholamine-mediated direct myocardial injury is another potential mechanism of myocardial infarction related to abuse of cocaine.

Angina and silent myocardial ischemia may occur in subjects indulging in cocaine use. Electrocardiographic ST segment elevations or T wave abnormalities accompany ischemic episodes.[18,39] The incidence of episodes of silent ischemia may be as high as 87% in these patients[18] and may be observed during the first weeks of withdrawal.

There are a number of different mechanisms that might account for the myocardial ischemic effect of cocaine. Cocaine increases both heart rate and blood pressure, increasing cardiac work, but this is not necessarily different than during exercise and most of the patients were in fact able to exercise vigorously without evidence of ischemia. Of course, details of just how high the blood pressure and pulse rate might have increased at the peak of intoxication are unknown. Many of the patients reported in the literature have had coronary angiography, and about half had significant stenoses that might have caused ischemia during extreme stress. However, most of these patients were able to tolerate exercise alone without any symptoms and remained free of symptoms when abstaining from cocaine, suggesting that the coronary lesions alone were not sufficient to explain their ischemia. Thus, increased myocardial oxygen demand, resulting from increased heart rate and blood pressure, is unlikely to induce myocardial ischemia, particularly in patients without atherosclerotic obstructive coronary artery disease.

Animal studies of the effect of cocaine on coronary blood flow are contradictory, with one showing increasing coronary blood flow and another increased coronary resistance.[40,41] The latter study found that at cocaine blood levels frequently found in humans, coronary blood flow in anesthetized dogs decreased about 40% with almost 30% decrease in cardiac output but no significant change in peripheral vascular resistance. Studies of animals administered exogenous norepinephrine found that cocaine administration dramatically decreased the coronary extraction of norepinephrine (from about 80% to about 25%) but that there was no increased overflow of norepinephrine in coronary sinus blood (as there is with sympathetic nerve stimulation of the heart), possibly because the increased perineuronal norepinephrine concentrations caused by cocaine stimulate presynaptic α_2-adrenergic receptors and thus inhibit norepinephrine release.[40] This fact is important because one potential explanation for cocaine-induced ischemia is the direct cardiac injury known to be produced by elevated catecholamine levels[42] or the intravascular platelet aggregation seen with prolonged norepinephrine infusion.[43]

In intact dogs, intravenous cocaine may cause dose-dependent reduction of the epicardial coronary artery diameters, resulting in progressive reduction in coronary blood flow.[44] The cocaine metabolite norcocaine has also been reported to produce constriction of ring segments of rabbit aorta.[45] In patients with or without atherosclerotic coronary artery disease, intranasal administration of cocaine (10% cocaine hydrochloride, 2 mg/kg, the commonly used local anesthetic dose) caused significant reduction of the diameters of the epicardial coronary arteries.[46] The overall coronary vascular resistance increased with a substantial reduction of coronary blood flow despite an increase in heart rate–blood pressure product. These findings suggest that the primary reduction of coronary blood flow, due either to coronary artery spasm or to global increase in coronary vascular resistance, induces myocardial ischemia, even though myocardial oxygen requirements may increase concomitantly. Focal spasm of the epicardial coronary artery segments have been demonstrated during angiographic studies in patients who developed cocaine-related acute myocardial infarction.[33,47] The mechanism for cocaine-induced vasoconstriction has not yet been clearly elucidated. Although in some studies, α-adrenergic blockade prevented cocaine-induced increase in coronary vascular resistance and constriction of epicardial coronary arteries,[46] other studies have indicated that cocaine-induced vasoconstriction occurs in the presence of intact or disrupted endothelium in in vitro experiments.[48] However, vasoconstriction of rabbit aortic rings could be prevented in experimental studies with pretreatment with the calcium channel blocking agent diltiazem.[48] These observations suggest that the vasoconstrictor effect of cocaine on vascular smooth muscle is independent of endothelium and adrenergic stimulation and may be dependent on calcium flux. Platelet aggregation and release of platelet-derived vasoactive substances may also be contributory to cocaine-induced vasoconstriction.[49]

Cocaine has been found to lower the threshold level for platelet aggregation.[50] In a case in which a 21-year-old man died of infarction within 2 hours after cocaine abuse and was examined at autopsy within 6 hours, acute coronary obstruction was found due solely to platelet thrombi.[51] This is of particular significance because other causes of thrombosis were ruled out in this case and because platelet thrombi are fragile, do not persist long, and are seldom seen unless autopsy occurs within a short time, making their occurrence usually very difficult to document. Other potential causes of the ischemia seen with cocaine is that cocaine is usually mixed and administered with other drugs, including procaine, phencyclidine, and amphetamines, which also have cardiac effects. However, infarction has occurred with cocaine alone and has not been reported with any of these other drugs, so this is an unlikely explanation.[2] It is apparent that the mechanisms for myocardial ischemia associated with cocaine abuse are multifactorial.

Dilated cardiomyopathy after long-term use of cocaine has been reported.[7] A 42-year-old man with normal coronary arteries had recurrent myocardial infarction progressing to severe global systolic dysfunction, and a 28-year-old woman without risk factors had other causes of cardiomyopathy ruled out. Long-term follow-up could not be obtained. It is possible that myocardial damage may occur comparable to that seen in long-term catecholamine excess, such as exogenous catechol administration or pheochromocytoma, but this possibility remains unstudied and unsupported by evidence at this time.[42,52] Several studies have reported the presence of lymphocytic and eosinophilic myocarditis in patients with detectable cocaine or its metabolites in body fluids.[6,32,35] In experimental animal studies, cocaine can cause direct impairment of myocardial and cardiac function, independent of any changes in coronary blood flow.[53,54]

Sudden cardiac deaths have been reported to occur in cocaine addicts.[3] Ventricular or supraventricular tachyarrhythmias and asystole are likely mechanisms in some patients. However, intracranial hemorrhage, seizure, respiratory arrest, hyperpyrexia, or rupture of aneurysm may also cause sudden death.[3] In cocaine abuse patients who died suddenly, autopsy studies have demonstrated smooth muscle cell–rich fibrous plaques in the coronary arteries with medial inflammation and thrombosis without underlying plaque hemorrhage. A significant increase in mural mast cells was also found.[55] The significance of such pathologic findings, however, remains to be elucidated.

Acute rupture of the ascending aorta has been reported in cocaine addicts. Rupture of the aorta was most likely caused by a large increase in systemic arterial pressure due to the extremely high levels of cocaine.[56] Systemic hypertension results from its effects on catecholamines. Inhaling or smoking free-base cocaine may cause lung damage and noncardiac pulmonary edema.[57] Spontaneous pneumomediastinum and pneumopericardium have been reported after "free-basing" smoking, which probably results as a consequence of alveolar rupture due to a sudden rise in intra-alveolar pressure.[2] Increased risk for endocarditis has been reported in association with cocaine use compared with use of other intravenous drugs.[58] Stress predisposes to endocarditis. Cocaine use and addiction produce physiologic stress, which has been suggested to explain the increased risk for endocarditis.[58]

Treatment of cocaine-induced ischemia has generally been the same as for other forms of myocardial ischemia and infarction. A calcium channel blocker has been effective in blocking direct cocaine cardiotoxicity in a briefly described study in rats but has not been studied in humans.[20] Another very brief and unconvincing report claimed that amitriptyline administration conveyed significant protection against sudden cardiac death after cocaine poisoning in rats, even up to 10 days later.[59] The actual mechanism of death was not studied and electrocardiographic monitoring was not done. Unfortunately this "treatment" has become very popular among chronic cocaine users as supposed protection against the cardiac effects of cocaine. Their adoption of this therapy is unfortunate because tricyclic antidepressants inhibit the α_2-adrenergic receptors at synapses and thus increase neuronal norepinephrine release after long-term administration.[29] Tricyclic antidepressants and cocaine also have the same effect of blocking neuronal reuptake of norepinephrine, so patients on tricyclic antidepressants experience synergistic effects with cocaine use and can have toxic effects or frank overdose at levels of cocaine use that are not normally toxic.

In summary, the major cardiac risk of cocaine use is ischemia and infarction, and cocaine use should be considered a significant risk factor that should be actively sought in taking any patient's history. The mechanism of injury is not really known, and there does not appear to be any particular "safe" route or dose of cocaine. Treatment of ischemia and infarction once it does occur is conventional, as would be treatment of hypertension contributing to ischemia.

OTHER STIMULANTS: AMPHETAMINES, PHENYLPROPANOLAMINE, PHENCYCLIDINE

Amphetamines possess cardiac stimulant properties virtually identical to those of cocaine.[19] Intravenous and oral use have caused acute cardiomyopathy and myocardial injury.[60] Four patients have been reported with left ventricular dysfunction and congestive cardiomyopathy after chronic intravenous abuse of propylhexedrine, an amphetamine analogue[61]; the one patient who later abstained from the drug clinically improved. In a series of 15 deaths due to intravenous propylhexedrine abuse, there was a finding of right ventricular hypertrophy and pulmonary hypertension in most of these patients. This is a common finding in those persons chronically using illicit intravenous substances that cause inflammation and scarring of pulmonary arteries. However, in Europe, aminorex fumarate, an oral α-sympathomimetic anorectic agent similar to propylhexedrine, caused a 20-fold increase in primary pulmonary hypertension. Animal studies showed the drug elevated pulmonary artery pressures and that these elevations were prolonged.[62,63] Such pulmonary hypertensive effects may also occur with propylhexedrine, although they have not been documented. A number of propylhexedrine deaths also occurred after abuse followed by sudden exertion or stress; these patients had atrioventricular dissociation or idioventricular rhythm on presentation, leading to speculation that the drug may predispose to arrhythmias.[62]

Phenylpropanolamine is another common drug of abuse, particularly among adolescents, with the expected range of sympathetic stimulant effects. Cardiac arrest has been reported in a 16-year-old girl who had a series of hypertensive episodes and seizures and who was evaluated thoroughly over a period of 3 months for suspected pheochromocytoma.[64] It was not until the third series of toxicologic tests that phenylpropanolamine was detected, and even then not at excessive levels. Sympathomimetic abuse should be part of the differential diagnosis of paroxysmal hypertension and should be sought vigilantly, because it is probably more common than pheochromocytoma. Toxicologic tests should be obtained, preferably on urine, and should probably be repeated several times if not initially positive.

Phencyclidine is an anesthetic and analgesic agent developed 25 years ago for humans but limited to veterinary use after widespread reports of serious psychomimetic and pressor side effects.[65] It became a very popular drug of abuse during the 1970s and has many of the stimulant properties of amphetamines.[66] Emergency department visits related to this drug peaked in 1979 and have remained level since; deaths peaked in 1983 and declined to 190 in 1985.[1] Nineteen deaths were reported due to this drug in two counties in California in a 6-year period, but in none of them could a cardiac cause be considered primary.[65] One case has been reported of hypertensive crisis (with a blood pressure of 220/130 mm Hg) and death during apparent recovery 48 hours after phencyclidine overdose, but this seems more likely to have been due to increased intracranial pressure than to the drug itself.[67] Careful review of 1000 cases found self-limited systolic and diastolic hypertension in 75%; in 2.1% systolic pressure exceeded 200 mm Hg, and diastolic exceeded 110 mm Hg in 3.3%.[68] However, hypertension abated spontaneously and no drug treatment was needed in any of these cases. There were two cases of delayed onset of hypertension, but these were possibly due to other causes rather than a direct action of phencyclidine. There were no cases of the delayed "dopaminergic storm," with malignant hypertension claimed by one author to occur 72 to 96 hours after ingestion.[69] In all, phencyclidine does not seem to have prominent or major cardiovascular toxicity even in most overdoses, and certainly not in ordinary phencyclidine abuse. In recent years there has been little literature on this drug of abuse and its usage seems to be on the wane.

INHALANTS

The ability of humans to find substances to abuse seems virtually unlimited, and during the past few decades inhalation of various volatile agents has been common. Such substances include toluene, glue vapors, gasoline, freon, and other halogenated hydrocarbon propellants of various commercial products, and their use is most frequent among adolescents and lower socioeconomic groups. No doubt new agents of inhalation abuse will continue to be discovered. The common theme of their popularity seems to be ready availability at a low price and chemical vapors that alter mental status. Unfortunately for the users, many of these agents are well known to be toxic and have significant cardiac effects.

MISUSE OF ISOPROTERENOL

Probably the earliest concerns about cardiotoxic effects of inhalants arose over the use of isoproterenol inhalers in asthmatics.[70] A number of cases of cardiac toxicity in humans after isoproterenol drip and inhalation have been reported, involving two cases of acute myocardial infarction and about five cases of ischemia after inhaler use.[71,72] Isoproterenol inhaler use in asthmatics increased dramatically in the early 1960s, and so did the case–fatality rate from asthma.[70] In many cases death seemed to have been sudden and unexpected; in 39% of these cases the physician had thought the terminal episode "not severe," and in 80% the physician did not expect a fatal outcome.[70] The vast majority of victims had been using isoproterenol by inhalation, sometimes consuming as much as two inhalers a day. All of this suggested sudden death by arrhythmia possibly due to the β-adrenergic stimulation of isoproterenol superimposed on a hypoxic heart. Another mechanism of death is suggested by the fact that prolonged infusion of norepinephrine causes intravascular platelet aggregation[43] and myofibrillar degeneration.[42] Similar changes have been found after isoproterenol administration.[73] As a result of this implied association with sudden death and their other less dramatic but unpleasant adrenergic side effects, isoproterenol inhalers have fallen out of favor. With the switch to more β_2-adrenergic specific bronchodilator drugs, no further reports of serious cardiac toxicity have occurred.

GLUE SNIFFING

Although the toxic effects of isoproterenol were ascribed to its sympathomimetic effects, studies in mice showed that isoproterenol inhaled under anoxic conditions in fact caused rapid heart block and sinus bradycardia.[74] About the same time there appeared a report of 110 "sudden sniffing deaths" in American youths who were inhaling solvents such as glue (toluene, benzene), gasoline, aerosol household products with fluorocarbon propellants, trichlorethane, spray paints, and cleaning fluids to become intoxicated.[75] These deaths occurred without anoxia and often during physical activity. A dramatic and typical example was a 17-year-old boy sniffing airplane glue who suddenly shouted "I think my heart is stopping," became wild, collapsed in the back seat of the car, and was dead on arrival at the hospital.[75] Many of the substances inhaled were fluorocarbons very similar to anesthetic agents that had already been shown to trigger arrhythmias.[76] Studies in dogs revealed that inhaling these agents sensitized the heart to epinephrine, producing ectopy, ventricular beats, and ventricular fibrillation.[77] It was shown in mice and dogs that glue sniffing could cause rapid onset of sinus bradycardia and then complete heart block followed by asystole; this effect was potentiated by hypoxia but could occur with normal oxygenation. It was not prevented or reversed by atropine, and its progression was not stopped by reversing the hypoxia.[78,79] Similar bradycardia has been documented in a patient with toluene abuse.[80]

Probably as a result of the publicity arising from these cases the abuse of such substances has declined; a contributing factor has been the replacement of fluorocarbon propellants in commercial aerosol products by other gases. Certain socioeconomic groups still indulge in these practices; toluene sniffing continues to be reported and produces multifocal premature ventricular beats and supraventricular tachycardia, usually in association with acidosis, hypophosphatemia, hyperchloremia, hypobicarbonemia, and hypokalemia.[81] Although current case reports are few, the problem still exists. Paint sniffers made up 7.5% of patients admitted for drug or inhalant abuse at Denver General Hospital in 1979,[81] and fatal cases of inhalant abuse continue to be reported in significant numbers.[82] There has been one case reported of fatal dilated cardiomyopathy after chronic abuse of shoe cleaning fluid containing trichloroethylene, an anesthetic agent.[83]

In addition, abusers continually find new substances to inhale; in recent years intoxication with typewriter correction fluid, which also contains chlorinated hydrocarbons, has resulted in sudden death during exercise, presumably due to arrhythmia.[84,85] In Australia, adolescents have inhaled the contents of fire extinguishers, which contain bromochlorotrifluoroethane, with similar results suggesting sudden arrhythmias.[86] Similar results were seen in a student who abused chloroform, with resultant unconsciousness and ventricular tachycardia.[87]

There is no specific treatment for the arrhythmias caused by inhalants; in most cases they occur long before the patient is seen by a physician. When present they should be treated by oxygenation, correction of acid–base and electrolyte abnormalities, and conventional pharmacologic treatment. The cause of such arrhythmias can often be suspected from patient age and appearance, history, the characteristic odors of the inhaled agents, or telltale traces of paint or white typewriter correction fluid on the hands, nose, or mouth. Probably the most useful service the physician can perform is to warn such patients and their families of the very significant risks of death with such abuse and urge them to seek counseling and discontinue this practice.

IPECAC AND WEIGHT-LOSS REGIMENS

In recent years there has been a growing epidemic among Americans of pathologic concern about weight, particularly among young women, leading to the widespread use of various techniques of induced vomiting, abuse of furosemide and other diuretics, and purging with laxatives.[88] Physicians often fail to think of these practices or believe that they could be present in their patients. Abusing patients perceive themselves as being overweight even though usually underweight and must be questioned aggressively about their ability to control their appetite. They often express fears of losing control if they should eat three regular meals a day. Eating disorders must always be considered in the workup of persistent unexplained hypokalemia. Patients may present with bradycardia, ST and T wave changes on electrocardiogram, low voltage, a prolonged QT interval, and U waves due to hypokalemia. Prolonged QT interval due to anorexia nervosa has led to ventricular arrhythmias and death.[89]

Cardiomyopathy has been seen as well.[90] Patients who abuse ipecac are at particular risk, because they may ingest very large quantities of this over-the-counter medication over long periods of time, accumulating a large tissue burden of the cardiotoxic ingredient emetine.[91] A fatal overdose can be taken in a few days, particularly by underweight women.[92] In reported cases, patients have presented and died with fulminant biventricular failure.[91,93] There is no specific treatment, and ipecac abuse should be aggressively sought in patients with unexplained hypokalemia or cardiac failure.

MISCELLANEOUS
ANABOLIC STEROIDS

Synthetic anabolic-androgenic steroids are widely used by professional athletes in many sports, but particularly among weight lifters and body builders. There are over 24 such compounds available through the black market, an estimated 1 million Americans use them, and their annual market value is over $100 million.[94] Calls have been issued to make them controlled substances. They have major effects on muscle mass, libido, performance, and aggression, but of major concern here is their effects on the cardiovascular system. Their use is a major risk factor for coronary artery disease. These drugs are some of the most potent atherogenic agents known, at least partly due to their significant depression of high-density lipoprotein levels.[94–98] In addition, they cause fluid retention, hypertension, and clotting abnormalities. Scientific research on them outside the Soviet Union is almost nonexistent. Physicians seeing coronary artery disease or thrombosis in patients without other risk factors should actively pursue the possibility of anabolic steroid use and should discuss the risk of such use with any patients engaged in athletics.

ASTEMIZOLE

There is a brief report of torsade de pointes occurring after ingestion of astemizole (a new long-acting H_1 antihistamine) in an awake 16-year-old girl.[99] There are no similar reports for other antihistamines. The dose ingested was 200 mg, not much greater than doses used daily for the treatment of mastocytosis.

CONCLUSIONS

Substance abuse is endemic in modern society but seldom is considered or vigorously pursued in the evaluation of patients with cardiac complaints. A detailed history of such usage should be sought in all such patients, with particular inquiries about the use of cocaine, amphetamines, phenylpropanolamine, or phencyclidine; sniffing of glue or other volatile solvents; laxative or ipecac use; or use of anabolic steroids. Certain patients are at particularly high risk for certain kinds of abuse, such as glue sniffing in adolescent rural ethnic minorities, use of anabolic steroids in competitive body builders, and ipecac use in thin young female college students. However, abuse of these agents is probably much more widespread than suspected, and stereotypes of users should not prevent the taking of a complete history whenever appropriate.

All of these agents can cause long-term and irreversible damage to the heart, and the inhalants can cause fatal arrhythmias at the time of intoxication. In general, the treatment of the side effects of these agents is the same as when these effects are induced by nondrug causes. However, it is very important for the physician to identify the use of these agents and to convince the patient of the seriousness of the complications. Probably the most useful service the physician can perform is to urge such patients and their families to seek counseling and discontinue their substance abuse.

REFERENCES

1. Services USDoHaH: Trends in drug abuse–related hospital emergency room episodes and medical examiner cases for selected drugs. National Institute for Drug and Alcohol Statistics Series H, Vol 3, pp 24–156, 1987
2. Creagler L, Mark H: Special report: Medical complications of cocaine abuse. N Engl J Med 315:1495, 1986
3. Gawin FH, Ellinwood EH Jr: Cocaine and other stimulants: Actions, abuse and treatment. N Engl J Med 318:1173, 1988
4. Kozel NJ, Adams EH: Epidemiology of drug abuse: An overview. Science 234:970, 1986
5. Van Dyke C, Jatlow P, Ungerer J: Oral cocaine: Plasma concentrations and central effects. Science 200:211, 1978
6. Isner J, Estes N, Thompson P: Acute cardiac events temporally related to cocaine abuse. N Engl J Med 315:1438, 1986
7. Weiner R, Lockhart J, Schwartz R: Dilated cardiomyopathy and cocaine abuse. Am J Med 81:699, 1986
8. Smith H, Liberman H, Brody S et al: Acute myocardial infarction temporally related to cocaine abuse. Ann Intern Med 107:13, 1987
9. Howard R, Hueter D, Davis G: Acute myocardial infarction following cocaine abuse in a young woman with normal coronary arteries. JAMA 254:95, 1985
10. Nanji A, Filipenko J: Asystole and ventricular fibrillation associated with cocaine intoxication. Chest 85:132, 1984
11. Weiss R: Recurrent myocardial infarction caused by cocaine abuse. Am Heart J 111:793, 1986
12. Boag F, Havard C: Cardiac arrhythmia and myocardial ischemia related to cocaine and alcohol consumption. Postgrad Med J 61:997, 1985
13. Kossowsky W, Lyon A: Cocaine and myocardial infarction: A probable connection. Chest 86:729, 1984
14. Coleman D, Ross T, Naughton J: Myocardial ischemia and infarction related to recreational cocaine use. West J Med 136:444, 1982
15. Stewart DJ, Inaba T, Lucassen M et al: Cocaine metabolism: Cocaine and norcocaine hydrolysis by liver and serum esterases. Clin Pharmacol Ther 25:464, 1979
16. Ritchie J, Greene N: Local anesthetics. In Gilman A, Goodman L, Rall T, Murad F (eds): The Pharmacological Basis of Therapeutics, 7th ed, pp 309–310. New York, Macmillan, 1985
17. Dackis CA, Gold MS: New concepts in cocaine addictions: The doputamine depletion hypothesis. Neurosci Biobehav Rev 9:469, 1985
18. Nademanee K, Gonelick DA, Josephson MA et al: Myocardial ischemia during cocaine withdrawal. Ann Intern Med 111:876, 1989
19. Fischman M, Schuster C, Resnekow L, Shick J: Cardiovascular and subjective effects of intravenous cocaine administration in humans. Arch Gen Psychiatry 33:983, 1976
20. Nahas G, Trouve R, Demus J: Letter: A calcium channel blocker as antidote to the cardiac effects of cocaine intoxication. N Engl J Med 313:519, 1985
21. Koehntop D, Liao J, Van Bergen F: Effects of pharmacologic alterations of adrenergic mechanisms by cocaine, tropolone, aminophylline, and ketamine on epinephrine-induced arrhythmias during halothane–nitrous oxide anesthesia. J Anesthesiol 46:83, 1977
22. Benchimol A, Bartall H, Desser K: Accelerated ventricular rhythm and cocaine abuse. Ann Intern Med 75:519, 1978
23. Jonsson S, O'Meara M, Young J: Acute cocaine poisoning: Importance of treating seizures and acidosis. Am J Med 75:1061, 1983
24. Crumb WJ Jr, Clarkson CW, Xu Y et al: Electrocardiographic evidence for cocaine cardiotoxicity in cats (abstr). Circulation (Suppl II)80:II-132, 1989
25. Temesy-Armus PM, Fraker TD Jr, Wilkerson RD: Cocaine causes delayed cardiac arrhythmias in conscious dogs (abstr). Circulation (Suppl II)80:II-132, 1989
26. Kanter RJ, DeVane CL, Epstein MJ: Electrophysiologic effects of high-dose intravenous cocaine in dogs (abstr). J Am Coll Cardiol 11:60A, 1988
27. Bedotto JB, Lee RW, Lancaster LD et al: Cocaine and cardiovascular function in dogs: Effects on heart and peripheral circulation. J Am Coll Cardiol 11:1337, 1988
28. Coptrad-Jackle A, Jackle SE, Kates RE et al: Electrophysiological and biochemical effect of chronic cocaine administration. Circulation (Suppl II)80:II-15, 1989
29. Garcia-Sevilla J, Zis A, Zelnik T, Smith C: Tricyclic antidepressant drug treatment decreases alpha-2 adrenoreceptors on human platelet membranes. Eur J Pharmacol 69:121, 1981
30. Wesson DR, Smith DE: Cocaine: Treatment perspectives. Natl Inst Drug Abuse Res Monogr Serv 61:193, 1985
31. Gay GR: Clinical management of acute and chronic cocaine poisoning. Ann Emerg Med 11:562, 1982
32. Mittleman RE, Wetli CV: Cocaine and sudden "natural" death. J Forensic Sci Soc 32:11, 1987
33. Zimmerman FH, Gustafson GM, Kemp HG: Recurrent myocardial infarction associated with cocaine abuse in a young man with normal coronary arteries: Evidence for coronary artery spasm culminating in thrombosis. J Am Coll Cardiol 9:964, 1987
34. Tazelaar H, Karch SB, Billingham ME et al: Cocaine cardiotoxicity. Hum Pathol 18:195, 1987
35. Karch SB, Billingham ME: The pathology and etiology of cocaine induced heart disease. Arch Pathol Lab Med 112:225, 1988
36. Fernandez MS, Pichard AD, Marchyant E et al: Acute myocardial infarction with normal coronary arteries: In vivo demonstration of coronary thrombosis during the acute episode. Clin Cardiol 6:553, 1983
37. Vincent GM, Anderson JL, Marshall HW: Coronary spasm producing coronary thrombosis and myocardial infarction. N Engl J Med 309:220, 1983
38. Chokshi SK, Miller G, Rongione A et al: Cocaine and cardiovascular disease: The leading edge. Cardiology 3:1, 1989
39. Mazid PA, Patel B, Kim H-S et al: Cocaine-induced chest pain: Angiographic and histologic study (abstr). Circulation (Suppl II)80:II-352, 1989
40. Levy M, Blattberg B: The influence of cocaine and desipramine on the cardiac responses to exogenous and endogenous norepinephrine. Eur J Pharmacol 48:37, 1978
41. Pierre A, Kossowsky W, Chou S, Abadir A: Coronary and systemic hemodynamics after intravenous injection of cocaine. Anesthesiology 63(3A):A28, 1985
42. Reichenbach D, Benditt E: Catecholamines and cardiomyopathy: The pathogenesis and potential importance of myofibrillar degeneration. Hum Pathol 1:125, 1970
43. Haft J, Kranz P, Albert F, Fani K: Intravascular platelet aggregation in the heart induced by norepinephrine. Circulation 46:698, 1972
44. Hayes SM, Moyer TP, Bove AA: Intravenous cocaine causes epicardial coronary vasoconstriction in the intact dog (abstr). J Am Coll Cardiol 11:49A, 1988
45. Chokshi SK, Gal D, Isner JM: Vasospasm caused by cocaine metabolite: A possible explanation for delayed onset of cocaine-related cardiovascular toxicity (abstr). Circulation (Suppl II)80:II-35, 1989
46. Lange RA, Cigarroa RG, Yaney CW et al: Cocaine-induced coronary artery vasoconstriction. N Engl J Med 321:1557, 1989
47. Ascher EK, Stauffer JC, Gaasch WH: Coronary artery spasm, cardiac arrest, transient electrocardiographic Q-waves and stunned myocardium in cocaine-associated acute myocardial infarction. Am J Cardiol 61:939, 1988
48. Isher JM, Chokshi SK: Cocaine and vasospasm. N Engl J Med 321:1604, 1989
49. Robinowitz M, Virmani R: Cocaine-associated cardiovascular disease. Cardiol Board Rev 6:71, 1989
50. Togna G, Tempesta E, Togna A, Dolci N: Platelet responsiveness and biosynthesis of thromboxane and prostacyclin in response to in vitro cocaine treatment. Haemostasis 15:100, 1985
51. Simpson R, Edwards W: Pathogenesis of cocaine-induced ischemic heart disease. Arch Pathol Lab Med 110:479, 1986
52. Stenstrom G, Holmber S: Cardiomyopathy in pheochromocytoma: Report of a case with a 16-year follow-up after surgery and review of the literature. Eur Heart J 6:539, 1985
53. Morcos NC, Fairhurst AS, Henry WL: Direct but reversible effects of cocaine on the myocardium (abstr). J Am Coll Cardiol 11:71A, 1988
54. Johnson MN, Karas SP, Hursey TL et al: Cocaining "binging" produces progressive left ventricular dysfunction. Circulation (Suppl II)80:II-15, 1989
55. Virmani R, Kolodgie FK, Robinowitz M et al: Cocaine associated coronary thrombosis coexists with atherosclerosis and increased adventitial mast cells. Circulation (Suppl II)80:II-647, 1989
56. Barth C, Bray M, Roberts W: Rupture of the ascending aorta during cocaine intoxication. Am J Cardiol 57:496, 1986
57. Itkonen J, Schnoll S, Glassroth J: Pulmonary dysfunction in "free base" cocaine users. Arch Intern Med 144:2195, 1984
58. Chanbers JF, Morris L, Tauber MG et al: Cocaine use and the risk for endocarditis in intravenous drug users. Ann Intern Med 106:833, 1987
59. Antelman S, Kocan D, Rowland N: Amitriptylline provides long-lasting immunization against sudden cardiac death from cocaine. Eur J Pharmacol 1981:119, 1981
60. Call T, Hartneck J, Dickinson W et al: Acute cardiomyopathy secondary to intravenous amphetamine abuse. Ann Intern Med 97:559, 1982
61. Croft C, Frith B, Hillis L: Propylhexedrine-induced left ventricular dysfunction. Ann Intern Med 97:560, 1982
62. Anderson R, Garza H, Garriott J, Dimaio V: Intravenous propylhexedrine (Benzedrex) abuse and sudden death. Am J Med 67:15, 1979

63. Brunner H, Stepanek J: Effects of aminorex on the pulmonary circulation of the dog. Proc Eur Soc Study Drug Tox 12:123, 1971
64. Hyams J, Leichtner A, Breiner R et al: Pseudopheochromocytoma and cardiac arrest associated with phenylpropanolamine. JAMA 253:1609, 1985
65. Burns R, Lerner S: Phencyclidine deaths. JACEP 7:135, 1978
66. Benowitz N, Rosenberg J, Becker C: Cardiopulmonary catastrophes in drug-overdosed patients. Med Clin North Am 63:267, 1979
67. Eastman J, Cohen S: Hypertensive crisis and death associated with phencyclidine poisoning. JAMA 231:1270, 1975
68. McCarron M, Schulze B, Thompson G et al: Acute phencyclidine intoxication: Incidence of clinical findings in 1000 cases. Ann Emerg Med 10:237, 1981
69. Rappolt R, Gay G, Farris R: Emergency management of acute phencyclidine intoxication. JACEP 8:68, 1979
70. Speizer F, Doll R, Half P, Strang L: Investigation into use of drugs preceding death from asthma. Brit Med J 1:339, 1968
71. Winsor T, Wright R, Berger H: Isoproterenol toxicity. Am Heart J 89:814, 1975
72. Jacobs R, Koppes G: Myocardial necrosis associated with isoproterenol abuse: A ten year follow-up. Texas Med 78:58, 1982
73. Rona G, Chappel C, Balazs T, Goudry R: An infarct-like myocardial lesion and other manifestations produced by isoproterenol in the rat. Arch Pathol 67:443, 1959
74. Azar A, Zapp J, Reinhardt C, Stopps G: Cardiac toxicity of aerosol propellants. JAMA 215:1501, 1971
75. Bass M: Sudden sniffing death. JAMA 212:2075, 1970
76. Baerg R, Kinberg D: Centrilobular hepatic necrosis and acute renal failure in "solvent sniffers." Ann Intern Med 73:713, 1970
77. Reinhardt C, Azar A, Maxfield M et al: Cardiac arrhythmias and aerosol "sniffing." Arch Environ Health 22:265, 1971
78. Taylor G, Harris W: Glue sniffing causes heart block in mice. Science 170:866, 1970
79. Flower N, Horan L: Nonanoxic aerosol arrhythmias. JAMA 219:33, 1972
80. Zee-Cheng C, Mueller C, Gibbs H: Letter: Toluene sniffing and severe sinus bradycardia. Arch Intern Med 103:482, 1985
81. Streicher H, Gabow P, Moss A et al: Syndromes of toluene sniffing in adults. Ann Intern Med 94:758, 1981
82. Garriott J, Petty C: Death from inhalant abuse: Toxicological and pathological evaluation of 34 cases. Clin Toxicol 16:305, 1980
83. Mee S, Wright P: Congested (dilated) cardiomyopathy in association with solvent abuse. J R Soc Med 73:671, 1980
84. King G, Smialek J, Troutman W: Sudden death in adolescents resulting from the inhalation of typewriter correction fluid. JAMA 253:1604, 1985
85. Greer J: Adolescent abuse of typewriter correction fluid. South Med J 77:297, 1984
86. Steadman C, Dorrington L, Kay P, Stephens H: Abuse of a fire-extinguishing agent and sudden death in adolescents. Med J Aus 141:115, 1984
87. Hutchens K, Kung M: "Experimentation" with chloroform. Am J Med 78:715, 1985
88. Herzog D, Copeland P: Eating disorders. N Engl J Med 313:295, 1985
89. Isner J, Roberts W, Heymsfield S: Anorexia nervosa and sudden death. Ann Intern Med 102:49, 1985
90. Manno B, Manno J: Toxicology of ipecac: A review. Clin Toxicol 10:221, 1977
91. Adler A, Walinsky P, Drall R, Cho S: Death resulting from ipecac syrup poisoning. JAMA 243:1927, 1980
92. Romig R: The potential toxicity of ipecac. Am J Psychiatry 141:1639, 1984
93. Dawson J, Yager J: A case of the abuse of syrup of ipecac resulting in death. J Am Coll Health 34:280, 1986
94. Taylor W: Synthetic anabolic-androgenic steroids: A plea for controlled substance status. Phys Sports Med 150:140, 1987
95. Kantor M, Bianchini A, Bernier D: Androgens reduce HDL2-cholesterol and increase hepatic triglyceride lipase activity. Med Sci Sports Exer 17:462, 1985
96. Webb O, Laskarzwski P, Glueck C: Severe depression of high density lipoprotein cholesterol levels in weight lifters and body builders by self-administered exogenous testosterone and anabolic-androgenic steroids. Metabolism 33:971, 1974
97. Services DoHaH: Anabolic steroid abuse. FDA Drug Bull 17(3):27, 1987
98. Alen M, Rahkila P: Reduced high density lipoprotein-cholesterol in power athletes: Use of male sex hormone derivates, an atherogenic factor. Int J Sports Med 5:341, 1984
99. Craft T: Torsade de pointes after astemizole overdose. Br Med J 292:660, 1986

Endocrine Diseases and the Cardiovascular System

Leon Resnekov

Only in the past few decades has the availability of techniques to measure concentrations of circulating hormones provided insight into the effects of the endocrine system on the heart. This knowledge has been slow in coming: it has been well over 150 years since Robert James Graves described the cardiac effects of thyrotoxicosis, and nearly as long since Thomas Addison recorded the circulatory effects of the disease bearing his name.[1,2]

This chapter summarizes current views on the effects of diseases of the endocrine system on the heart and circulation.

DIABETES MELLITUS

Whereas ketoacidosis was the major cause of death in diabetics prior to the availability of insulin, associated cardiovascular disease has now emerged as the major cause of fatality in such patients.

In the United States it has been estimated that some 10 million individuals have diabetes, and the associated cardiac and renal morbidity is extremely high (Table 117.1). It should be noted that diabetic females are more prone to cardiovascular disease, including coronary artery disease, than nondiabetic females. In the cardiovascular system, pathologic changes include nonspecific effects such as arteriosclerosis or a specific proliferative endothelial change affecting the arterioles as a microangiopathy (Fig. 117.1). This specific microangiopathy causes thickening of the capillary basement membranes and affects many organs, including the myocardium, the retina and other eye tissues, the kidneys, the brain, and the pancreas. At times a more severe proliferative effect follows, causing occlusion of the small arterioles.

ARTERIOSCLEROSIS

Arteriosclerosis tends to be more severe in diabetics than in nondiabetics. There is a distressingly high incidence of associated cerebral, coronary, and renal arterial disease, as well as disease of the peripheral vasculature.[3] Myocardial infarction and the effects on the myocardium of coronary arteriosclerosis are three times more common in diabetics than in nondiabetics. It is the duration of diabetes rather than its severity that results in the high incidence of coronary arteriosclerosis.

Arteriosclerosis in diabetics occurs prematurely and more severely than in nondiabetics. Its pathogenesis in diabetics has recently been reviewed by Stolar[4] and is illustrated in Figure 117.2. Hyperinsulinemia stimulates the subintimal smooth muscle cells and fibroblasts, increasing both the uptake and local synthesis of lipids by these cells. It is injury to the endothelial lining of arteries that begins the formation of arteriosclerotic plaque. The actual injury can be caused by a variety of factors that include hyperlipidemia, hypertension, smoking tobacco, hyperglycemia, and various immune processes. Later in life, direct injury to the endothelial lining of coronary arteries becomes important. This may result from aging, coronary artery bypass graft surgery, or percutaneous transluminal coronary angioplasty.

The common pathway of all these processes is a loss of endothelial structure. A variety of biochemical substances that promote platelet and white cell aggregation are released. Thromboxane-B_2 from agglutinating platelets and some of the leucotrienes from the white cells precipitate vasoconstriction. In addition, platelet adhesion to the endothelial lining is enhanced by other elements, including various growth factors and von Willebrand factor, which is known to be elevated in diabetics, especially those with non-insulin-dependent diabetes (type II).[5] Plasminogen activation in diabetics is depressed. Vague and colleagues[6] have suggested that increased amounts of circulating insulin may reduce fibrinolytic activity because of the presence of increased amounts of plasminogen activator.

Platelet-derived growth factor in combination with circulating plasma insulin stimulates smooth muscle cell growth and proliferation of macrophages, especially in diabetics.[7] Furthermore, it is found in high concentration in persons with poorly controlled diabetes and reduced in well controlled diabetes. Insulin also stimulates smooth muscle proliferation[8] and can enhance the synthesis of lipids in cells of diabetic animals.[9]

These abnormal changes combine with the circulating atherogenic lipoproteins commonly found in diabetics. Lipid is deposited into the arterial wall and eventually an atherosclerotic plaque forms. It is important to consider that although each of the steps outlined above may eventually result in development of an atherosclerotic plaque, all are potentially reversible, particularly in diabetics.[4]

HYPERLIPIDEMIA

Many lipoprotein abnormalities accompany insulin-dependent and non-insulin-dependent diabetes.

Specific dyslipoproteinemias include the following: over-production of very-low-density lipoprotein (VLDL), inappropriate lipolysis of the VLDL triglycerides, inadequate low-density lipoprotein (LDL) receptor activity, and even, on occasion, type III hyperlipidemia.[10–12]

It is easier to understand why VLDL metabolism is abnormal in diabetics than to comprehend why high-density lipoprotein (HDL) is lowered.[13] However, since there is an inverse relationship between plasma triglyceride and HDL concentration, it is likely that the causes are interrelated and associated with resistance to insulin stimulated glucose uptake.[14] In contrast to type I diabetics, those with non-insulin-dependent diabetes have elevated levels of plasma glucose but are normoinsulinemic in absolute terms. With relative deficiencies of insulin, lipoprotein lipase activity is reduced, and LDL levels are therefore high. Carbohydrate intolerance occurs in approximately 30% of individuals with familial hyperlipoproteinemia.[15,16]

TABLE 117.1 CARDIOVASCULAR RISK OF DIABETES MELLITUS AMONG THE ESTIMATED 10 MILLION DIABETICS IN THE U.S.

Risk	Incidence per 10,000	
	Diabetics	Nondiabetics
Coronary artery disease	225	144
Acute myocardial infarction	100	64
Sudden death	26	18

There continues to be a great deal of interest in the role of HDL in diabetics. Calvert and colleagues found a correlation between HDL cholesterol and concentrations of glycosylated hemoglobin.[17] As the concentration of glycosylated hemoglobin was lowered, HDL concentration rose.

Currently, diabetic dyslipidemia is managed mainly by lifestyle modification—diet, exercise, and smoking cessation. The usual drugs of choice for treatment of hypercholesterolemia, such as bile acid sequestrants and nicotinic acid, are best avoided because they may have adverse effects in patients with diabetes.[12] Bile acid sequestrants accentuate hypertriglyceridemia; nicotinic acid worsens glucose intolerance.

It is fortunate that recent reports document the ability of HMG-CoA reductase inhibitors to reduce levels of VLDL and LDL cholesterol in those with non-insulin-dependent diabetes.[18,19] As yet, the effects of long-term management of diabetic dyslipoproteinemia with such drugs are unknown.

EFFECT ON THE HEART

Myocardial infarction occurs more commonly in diabetics (see Table 117.1). Complications emerge more frequently and include acute heart failure, cardiogenic shock, and cardiac rhythm disturbances. Because of the associated stimulation of the sympathetic nervous system following myocardial infarction, the diabetic state is frequently worsened. High concentrations of circulating free fatty acids occur and lead, in turn, to the emergence of ventricular rhythm disturbances.[20]

In addition there appears to be an autonomic neuropathy that re-

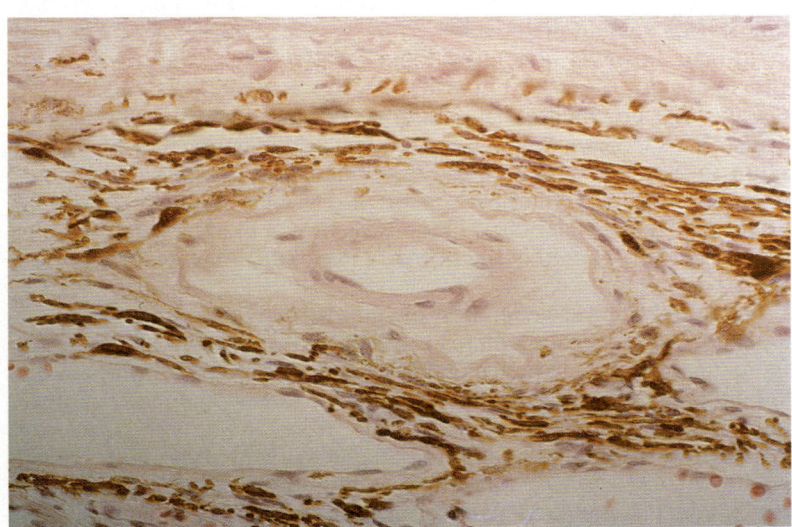

FIGURE 117.1 Diabetic microangiopathy, a specific proliferative endothelial lesion of arterioles.

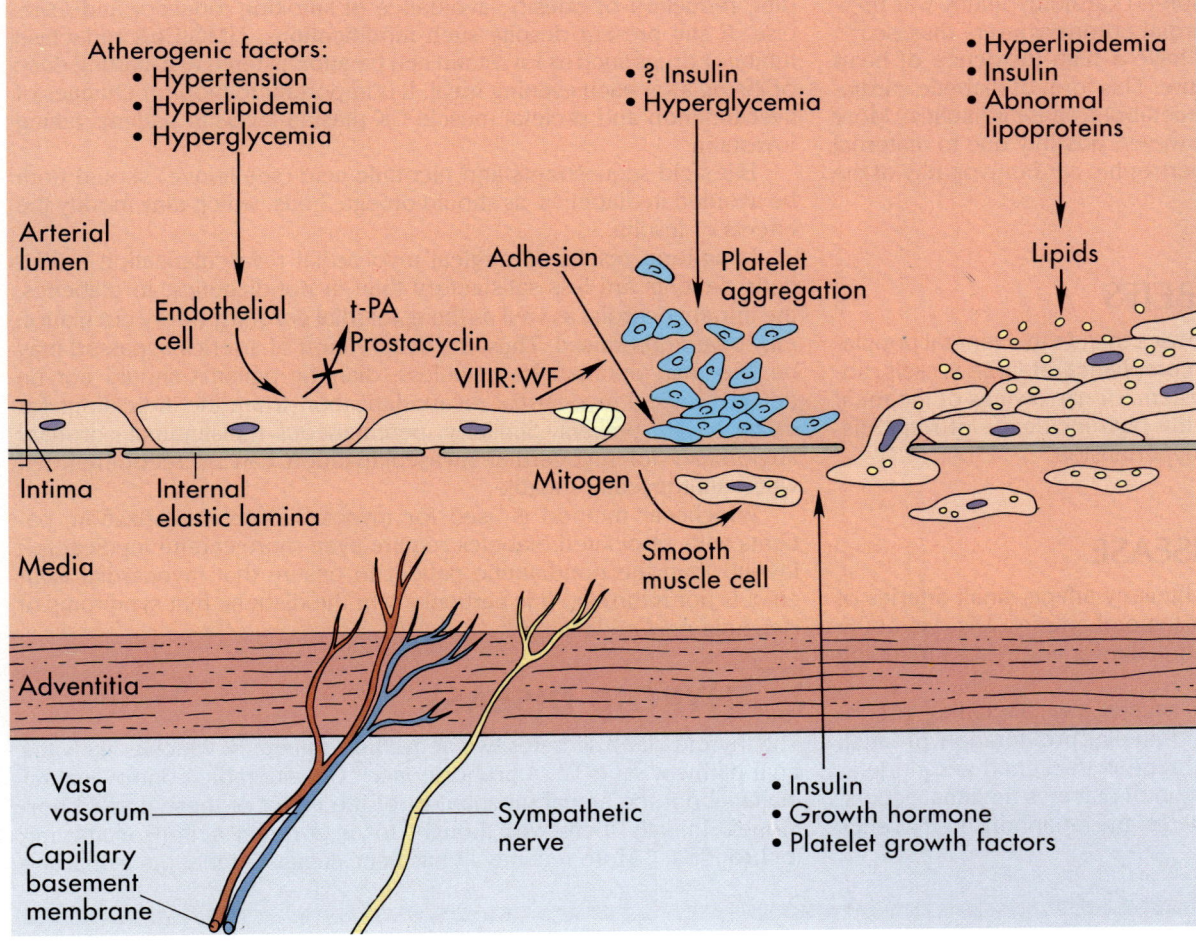

FIGURE 117.2 Pathogenesis of atherosclerosis in diabetes. (t-PA, tissue-type plasminogen activator; VIIIR:WF, von Willebrand factor, component of clotting factor VIII) (Modified from Stolar MW: Atherosclerosis in diabetes: The role of hyperinsulinemia. Metabolism 37(suppl 1):2; Colwell JA, Halushik PV, Sarji KE et al: Vascular disease in diabetes: Pathophysiological mechanisms and therapy. Arch Intern Med 139:228, 1979)

sults in cardiac denervation. In diabetics, myocardial infarction without pain has been noted frequently over the years,[21] possibly due to the loss of nerve fibers in the ischemic area. Not only does myocardial infarction occur without symptoms but chronic silent ischemia is not uncommon in diabetics,[22] particularly those with peripheral autonomic nervous system abnormalities.[23]

Since silent myocardial ischemia is common in diabetics, these patients should have periodic objective measurements of ischemia. Coronary risk factors should be determined and modified as needed. Exercise stress testing with myocardial scintigraphy and ambulatory ECG monitoring may reveal the occurrence of silent myocardial ischemia and can be used to observe the progress of the disease as well as the effects of therapeutic interventions.[24,25]

Many additional factors combine to result in a higher incidence of heart disease in the diabetic. These include hypertension, hyperlipidemia (see above), obesity, and hyperglycemia. In addition, there may be coagulation changes such as increased platelet adhesiveness[26] and changes in blood viscosity.[27]

Diabetic neuropathy involving both the sympathetic and parasympathetic nervous systems may have profound effects on the heart, resulting in persistent tachycardias that respond little to physiologic stimuli and may, in turn, lead to more serious dysrhythmias.

CONGESTIVE HEART FAILURE

Heart failure is common among diabetics.[28] Its increased incidence is probably caused by a microangiopathy that is common and specific to diabetes, although metabolically induced myocardial cellular dysfunction may also be responsible. A specific histologic pattern described in diabetic cardiomyopathy includes accumulation of periodic acid–Schiff (PAS)-positive material between muscle fibers and collections of collagen and glycoprotein extending into T tubules.[29] It should be noted that small vessel disease is rare in nondiabetic patients with cardiomyopathy. Regan and colleagues studied diabetic patients who had no evidence of clinical heart failure but in whom left ventricular end-diastolic pressure was raised.[29] Hamby and colleagues showed by hemodynamic challenges that a widespread cardiomyopathy was present, despite the absence of any epicardial coronary artery disease.[30]

Infants born to diabetic mothers have a high incidence of heart enlargement and congestive heart failure. This form of diabetic cardiomyopathy is at times transient when a metabolic cause is likeliest. More prolonged heart failure may occur, however, possibly due to maternal hormonal influences resulting in a hypertrophic cardiomyopathy of the infant.[31]

HYPERTENSION AND DIABETES

Hypertension is more common in diabetics than in the general population.[32] This may result from impaired compliance of large vessels, abnormalities of the renin-angiotensin system, or narrowings of the renal arteries.[33] In juvenile-onset diabetes, the high incidence of renal disease contributes greatly to emerging hypertension.

PERIPHERAL VASCULAR DISEASE

This often occurs in diabetics and particularly affects small arteries of the feet rather than the iliacs, aorta, or femoral arteries. Disease of the arteries of the brain is also common in diabetics and results in a high incidence of cerebral infarction.

The kidney circulation is affected in several ways, including arteriosclerosis of the larger vessels and endothelial proliferation of small arteries. The capillary basement membrane is thickened and nodular glomerulosclerosis, a characteristic lesion of diabetes mellitus, occurs. Because of these various pathologic states, pyelonephritis in diabetics is common and renal failure frequent.

TREATMENT OF DIABETES AND PREVENTION OF CARDIOVASCULAR COMPLICATIONS

In the diabetic state, therapy must be directed to control of excess fatty acid mobilization, to oxidation, and to protein catabolism. Most recommend controlling the blood glucose level to within physiologic ranges, to prevent the emergence of cardiovascular complications.

In type I diabetics, the combination of diet and insulin remains the mainstay of treatment. Treating non-insulin-dependent diabetes with exogenous insulin, however, causes hyperinsulinemia. Furthermore, insulin-binding antibodies may develop following insulin injections, thereby increasing daily requirements, and antibody-bound insulin may be released into the circulation.

Controversy has arisen concerning the efficacy of oral hypoglycemic agents in non-insulin-dependent diabetics.[34] It has been suggested, for example, that the sulfonylureas may increase still further the reduced diastolic compliance of the ventricle because of an accumulation of PAS-staining material.[35]

In man, however, it is not yet known how long tissues need exposure to insulin each 24 hours before the emergence of metabolic changes that precipitate macrovascular disease. Note that the plasma levels of insulin are normally exceedingly low during the night and return to usual levels during the day, stimulated by the glucose challenge of eating. Such diurnal variation may be important in maintaining a normal cellular metabolic homeostasis. It would appear reasonable, therefore, to try to mimic the normal physiologic changes when therapy is needed.

Thus, the second generation of sulfonylurea compounds (such as glipizide and gliclazide) that do not cause hyperinsulinemia, as do first-generation oral hypoglycemics (such as tolbutamide, propamide, and giburide), can be recommended for the management of non-insulin-dependent diabetes mellitus.[4]

The hyperosmolar diabetic state requires urgent correction, since it has been shown to cause reduced ventricular systolic contraction.[36] Insulin injections reverse hyperosomolarity very successfully.

The dyslipoproteinemia in association with diabetes responds to diet, reduction of obesity, avoidance of smoking tobacco, and exercise. If still present despite such modifications, HMG-CoA reductase inhibitor drugs such as lovastatin can be administered at a starting dose of 20 mg after each evening meal. It is important to monitor changes of liver function and skeletal muscle CK plasma levels in patients taking lovastatin.

Bile acid sequestrants and nicotinic acid (see above) should both be avoided in diabetics, as should omega-3 oils, which may modify the effects of insulin.

Long-term results of surgical myocardial revascularization in diabetic patients are less satisfactory than in nondiabetics. In diabetics, the intramyocardial as well as the epicardial coronary artery circulation may be compromised. Thus, the distal runoff of arteries bypassed may be less than optimal. Nevertheless, diabetic patients should not be denied surgical myocardial revascularization when the indications for doing so are present. Similarly, percutaneous transluminal coronary angioplasty for myocardial revascularization can be recommended when anatomically suitable.

Whichever method is used for myocardial revascularization, patients with associated diabetes require even more careful medical follow-up than the nondiabetic patient to ensure that myocardial ischemia is not returning. It is particularly in the diabetic that symptoms of ischemia may be lacking.[22]

THYROID DISEASE

The thyroid gland secretes two active hormones: T3, which is likely the final pathway, and T4, a prohormone.[37] Considerable controversy remains about the actual mechanism of the effect of these thyroid hormones. Initially there was thought to be a direct action on the mitochondria.[38] More recently, it has been suggested that the actual site of action is the nucleus of the cell itself.[39] Thyroid hormone also increases the activity of sodium-potassium ATPase,[40] and this may enhance cellular respiration.

HYPERTHYROIDISM

For many years it has been recognized that among the most striking features of thyrotoxicosis are its effects on the heart and circulation. These include a hyperdynamic circulation; heart murmurs, particularly ejection systolic, suggesting rapid flow; a widened pulse pressure; rapid filling during diastole; and even engorgement of neck veins and peripheral edema in the absence of true congestive heart failure.

Atrial fibrillation may occur: Premature beats, ventricular and atrial, are frequent and, in addition, the electrocardiogram may record changes indicative of myocardial infarction even when the epicardial coronary arteries are documented as normal.[41,42] It should be recognized that myocardial ischemia may emerge more easily when thyrotoxicosis is present. Consequently, symptoms of coronary arteriosclerosis are often more frequent and more severe in hyperthyroidism.

Conduction disturbances are common, including first-degree heart block (up to 30% of thyrotoxicosis patients).[43] Higher degrees of heart block are also common and include fascicular blocks, complete heart block, and even ventricular asystole.[44,45] The likely cause of the conduction disturbances is a histiocytic infiltration of the myocardium that comes about in thyrotoxicosis. There may also be an acute direct effect of T3 on the myocardium.

Congestive heart failure is common and often worsened by hyperthyroidism. Of 460 patients with hyperthyroidism, 150 were found to have evidence of myocardial dysfunction and atrial fibrillation.[46] More than 40% of these patients, however, were young and had no other evidence of heart disease.

In the presence of thyrotoxicosis there is a greatly increased myocardial oxygen demand. At times such hearts produce lactate during induced stress even when epicardial coronary arteries are normal.[47]

Among the many controversies regarding the effects of thyrotoxicosis on the heart has been the role of catecholamines. Early investigators reported an increased sensitivity to circulating catecholamines[48] but recently, with more specific techniques to assess β-receptor activity, alternative explanations have been suggested. It is very likely that there is a direct effect of T3 on the β-receptors rather than an effect mediated through circulating catecholamine.[49–51]

Thyroid hormone directly effects the myocardium by enhancing contractility.[52] Thyroid hormone changes cardiac myosin to be more contractile[53] and in addition there is enhancement of the synthesis of myosin isoenzyme with ATPase activity.[54] Finally it has been shown that in the presence of thyrotoxicosis calcium exchange is increased, potentiating myocardial contraction and enhancing relaxation.[55]

TREATMENT

Therapeutic options for hyperthyroidism include irradiation using radioactive iodine, surgical removal of the hyperthyroid gland, and medical therapy.

MEDICAL TREATMENT.

1. *β-Adrenergic blocking drugs*. These agents are often successful in reducing cardiac manifestations that include tachycardia and premature beats as well as the more general symptoms of tremor, heat intolerance, and muscular weakness. It is likely that benefit occurs by β-adrenergic-blocking drugs inhibiting the conversion of thyroxine to T3 in the peripheral tissues. The effect of propranolol appears within 1 or 2 hours of oral administration; the dose required varies but is usually in the range of 10 to 40 mg each 6 hours. Even in the presence of thyroid storm, propranolol can be very beneficial in improving hyperpyrexia and acute rhythm disturbances. It is important, however, that specific antithyroid treatment also be used in the management of thyroid storm or when congestive heart failure and hyperthyroidism occur.[56]

2. *Digitalis preparations*. Cardiac glycosides are less effective in hyperthyroidism[57,58] and serum levels are lower because of the increased volume of distribution. In addition, digitalis toxicity occurs not infrequently in hyperthyroid patients.[58]

3. *Propylthiouracil and the thionamides*. These drugs, which reduce the production of thyroid hormone, should always be used with β-adrenergic blocking drugs. An initial dose is 300 to 800 mg. Careful monitoring for side effects is essential; these include suppression of bone marrow activity, gastrointestinal upsets, and even vasculitis.

4. *Saturated potassium* iodine acts rapidly by inhibiting release of thyroid hormone from the gland. It will therefore greatly benefit a patient with hyperthyroidism and cardiac manifestations. It should not be used long-term, however, since its benefit is usually short-lived, with the return of thyrotoxic manifestations in some 2 to 4 weeks.

5. *Conversion of atrial fibrillation to sinus rhythm*. Only about one-half of thyrotoxic patients made euthyroid by treatment convert spontaneously to sinus rhythm.[59] The remainder remain at risk of systemic embolism. An incidence of just under 10% has been reported.[60] In consequence, once a euthyroid state has been achieved, sinus rhythm should be reestablished by synchronized DC shock unless there are definite contraindications.

HYPOTHYROIDISM

Hypothyroidism comes about due to a lack of adequate secretion of both T3 and T4. Often this follows an inflammatory disease of the thyroid gland, but it may result from diseases of the hypothalamus or pituitary gland that reduce secretion or availability of thyrotropin.

Cardiovascular symptoms and signs are common. Patients present with breathlessness, edema, enlargement of the heart and pericardial effusions. Systemic effects of hypothyroidism include constipation, intolerance to cold, physical weakness, impairment of memory, skin dryness, and menstrual abnormalities frequently occur. There may also be slowness of speech and partial deafness. The skin is often somewhat yellowish because of difficulty converting carotene into vitamin A.

Histologic examination of the heart reveals considerable dilation of all chambers and there is interstitial fibrosis, loss of striations and swelling of myofibrils.[61]

Electrocardiographic changes are very common. These include bradycardia, diffuse reduction of voltage, QRS widening, and generalized flat or inverted T waves. Conduction disturbances are common particularly prolongation of the PR interval.[62] In general, conduction disturbances are rapidly normalized by treatment of the hypothyroid state. At times more serious conduction disturbances may emerge, including abnormalities beneath the bundle of His and complete heart block.[61]

Rhythm disturbances are also common and include ventricular tachycardia even in the absence of any other associated cardiac abnormality.[63]

Pericardial effusions are particularly common.[64,65] There is little correlation between initial values of levels of thyroid hormone and the presence or absence of the effusion that occurs in about 30% of hypothyroid patients.[65] Treatment with thyroid hormone is followed by a gradual absorption of the fluid.

Very rarely in hypothyroidism the pericardial fluid accumulates rapidly and to an extent that can cause tamponade.[66] When examined, the pericardial fluid has predominance of lymphocytes, some bleeding into the fluid may be found and cholesterol crystals are common.

The cardiac output in myxedema is low, and overall myocardial function is greatly reduced.[64] It is likely that the reduction in overall myocardial function relates to reduced metabolic requirements in hypothyroidism, since exercise causes appropriate increases in cardiac output.

Congestive heart failure commonly occurs and at times is severe. It is more frequent when other forms of heart disease are present.

HYPOTHYROIDISM AND ARTERIOSCLEROSIS

Although there is an association with hyperlipidemia that includes elevations of both serum cholesterol and triglycerides, the relationship has not been clearly elucidated. There is an impairment in the mobilization of free fatty acid and coronary arteriosclerosis occurs twice as commonly in patients with myxedema compared to age- and sex-matched euthyroid individuals.[67] Both the hypercholesterolemia and hypertriglyceridemia decline following treatment with thyroid hormone. In animal studies, it has been shown that the extent of the experimentally created myocardial infarction is larger in hypothyroid animals.[68] On the other hand, clinical studies have reported a relatively low incidence of angina pectoris and myocardial infarction in hypothyroid individuals.[68]

TREATMENT

The elderly hypothyroid patient should be treated cautiously with thyroid hormone replacement. Any underlying coronary artery disease may exacerbate symptoms, or cause symptoms to appear for the first time, as treatment with thyroxine begins. Levo-thyroxine doses of 25 to 50 μg should be given daily to such patients, with gradual increments each two to four weeks as tolerated. Any worsening or precipitation of angina pectoris requires reduction of the dose.

Although in the past myxedema was considered a contraindication to cardiovascular surgery, several series have now been reported in which patients have undergone successful myocardial revascularization surgery with no heightened risk of increased complications.[69]

ACROMEGALY

The effects on the heart of acromegaly are still ill understood and controversial. Fatal cases of acromegaly have considerable and at times massive enlargement of the heart, but it is the actual cause of the enlargement that is still elusive.

Growth hormone, one of the seven polypeptide hormones secreted by the anterior pituitary gland, has anabolic effects influencing many metabolic processes. For example, it increases the synthesis of transfer and messenger RNA, and augments the substrate for protein synthesis; in addition, it brings about changes in fat and carbohydrate metabolism to increase lipogenesis.[70-72] Growth hormone increases gluconeogenesis, peripheral resistance to insulin, and plasma glucose levels. The heart, as do many other organs, then uses free fatty acids and ketones as changed energy substrates.

The usual cause of acromegaly is a growth hormone-secreting eosinophilic or chromophobic adenoma of the pituitary gland. Typical changes of the exaggerated effects of growth hormone on bone and muscle follow; organomegaly is common, and abnormalities of carbohydrate metabolism occur. Hyperlipidemia is usually found only in persons with both acromegaly and diabetes mellitus.

CARDIAC EFFECTS

There is considerable enlargement of the heart, a result of many contributing factors.[73] Although hypertension is present in 30% of cases, the cardiac hypertrophy is also a result of the direct effect of growth hormone on myocardial protein synthesis. Histologically, there is a diffuse increase in collagen and fibrous connective tissue that may result in poor contractility.[74]

It is interesting to note that the cardiac output is usually well-preserved, suggesting that an associated cause for cardiac hypertrophy may be an increased work demand due to the associated visceromegaly.

The cause of the hypertension so common in acromegaly remains uncertain. It is likely to be associated with changes in circulating plasma volume resulting from alterations in renin, angiotensin and aldosterone.[75,76] It is usual to find among acromegalics reduced plasma renin and aldosterone responses.[77] Others have suggested that sodium retention may occur as a primary effect of the growth hormone independent of aldosterone.[78]

Heart failure and rhythm disturbances are common. Both improve once growth hormone levels are normalized by treatment.[79] Of the known clinical parameters of acromegalic heart disease (namely ECG abnormalities, rhythm disturbances, cardiac hypertrophy, and heart failure), the only one that statistically correlates with the level of growth hormone is hypertension.[79]

There is generalized enlargement of the heart, and at times asymmetric hypertrophy, but the clinical syndrome of hypertrophic cardiomyopathy with ventricular outflow obstruction is rare.[80]

Except for ventricular premature beats and tachycardia, conduction disturbances are common. These include abnormalities of sinus node function, AV nodal conduction disturbances, fascicular blocks, and even complete heart block.[81]

Premature atherosclerosis occurs, but its frequency is uncertain in acromegalics. Epicardial coronary artery disease is estimated as occurring in 10% of acromegaly patients.[82]

DIAGNOSIS AND TREATMENT

The diagnosis is established by demonstrating that serum growth hormone levels cannot be suppressed after glucose loading. Treatment is by surgery and by irradiation, using proton beam rather than conventional irradiation techniques.[83]

The cardiovascular abnormalities associated with acromegaly do respond to usual treatments for hypertension, heart failure, and rhythm disturbances. Hypertension, as could be predicted from its possible cause in acromegaly, reportedly responds well to diuretic therapy.

PHEOCHROMOCYTOMA

The pheochromocytomata are tumors arising from sympathetic nervous tissue and are particularly common in the adrenal medulla. All paraganglionic or embryologic rest tissue of the sympathetic nervous system, however, may develop such tumors. Although often sporadic, there is a familial occurrence in association with diseases of the neuroectoderm. These include von Recklinghausen's disease, von Hippel-Lindau disease, and type III multiple endocrine neoplasia syndrome often associated with bilateral pheochromocytomata of the adrenal glands, medullary carcinoma of the thyroid, and adenoma or hyperplasia of the parathyroid glands. The type III syndrome is an autosomal dominant.

Pheochromocytomata secrete norepinephrine, epinephrine, and occasionally dopamine. Therefore, apart from effects on the cardiovascular system, more generalized effects are increased production of glucose from glycogen, stimulation of lipolysis, mobilization of free fatty acids, and inhibition of insulin secretion.

The pheochromocytomata that do not arise from the adrenal chromaffin cells are called paragangliomas. Both types are very vascular. The majority are solitary, with 10% being bilateral and 20% being away from the adrenal glands. Fewer than 1% are malignant. Only about 0.1% of hypertension is due to pheochromocytoma.

CARDIAC EFFECTS

The particular features suggesting pheochromocytoma in a patient with elevated blood pressure include excess sweating, a hypermetabolic state, orthostasis, exaggerated elevation of the blood pressure in response to stress or trauma, and excessive headaches. It is the paroxysmal nature of these symptoms that should lead the physician to suspect pheochromocytoma.

Cardiovascular features result from the effects of catecholamines on the peripheral vasculature, myocardial contractility, and cardiac conduction tissues. In addition, pheochromocytoma occasionally causes a myocarditis that may induce severe cardiac dysfunction.[84]

Elevation of blood pressure is common and frequently sustained; at times there may be wide variations. In certain patients, elevation of the blood pressure can be shown to relate to sudden increased release of catecholamine from the tumor or nerve endings. All symptoms are likely to be caused by dysfunction of the autonomic nervous system, a result of the excess circulating catecholamines.[85] Cardiac chest discomfort may occur even when the epicardial coronary arteries are normal and probably relates to increased work of the heart.[86] In the presence of the associated rare myocarditis, severe congestive heart failure may ensue.[87]

Electrocardiographic changes are common, including patterns of left ventricular hypertrophy and strain, sinus tachycardia, diffuse nonspecific T-wave changes, and ventricular rhythm disturbances (either isolated ectopic beats or paroxysmal ventricular tachycardia). At times during a paroxysm of hypertension, severe bradycardia and junctional escape rhythms may be recorded.[88] The mechanism is interesting, since in the presence of excess circulation of catecholamines the exaggerated vagal response to sudden elevations of blood pressure would have to be postulated.

In animals a direct toxic action of catecholamines on the heart has been documented.[89] The hearts of patients dying with pheochromocytoma often reveal widespread focal myocardial lesions, including endocardial fibrosis.[84] Tumors that predominantly secrete epinephrine may be associated with such myocardial changes even in the absence of hypertension. It is possible that excess catecholamine secretion so greatly increases oxygen demand by the myocardium that it leads to ischemic damage.[90]

DIAGNOSIS AND TREATMENT

The diagnosis is suggested by the typical history of paroxysmal attacks in a patient with hypertension. It is confirmed by demonstrating increased levels of catecholamines and their metabolites in urine, blood and platelets. The commonly employed tests are measurement of total catecholamine, metanephrine, and vanillylmandelic acid. Although clonidine administration has been shown in normals to reduce catecholamine levels via its central α-adrenergic effect, and to have no effect on the level of catecholamines in individuals with pheochromocytoma, the test can provoke profound and prolonged hypotension and is not recommended as a routine confirmatory investigation.[91]

Medical treatment is begun with phenoxybenzamine hydrochloride, a usual starting dose being 10 mg each 12 hours, increasing each 2–3 days to normalize the blood pressure. It is important to ensure an adequate sodium intake to prevent severe postural hypotension, a result of associated vasodilation, and consequent hypovolemia. It is essential that the blood pressure be brought under proper control before surgery or intravascular diagnostic studies. Similarly, using β-adrenergic blocking drugs without first administering α-blocking drugs can be hazardous. The resulting hypertension, because of the unopposed α-stimulating effect of circulating catecholamines, could be extremely severe and precipitate dire consequences.

The definitive treatment is surgery. The tumor or tumors are first localized, either by computerized axial tomographic scanning techniques or by demonstrating their presence following an injection of guanethidine labeled with iodine-131.[92]

The more unusual malignant form of pheochromocytoma has been treated with α-methylthyrosine that inhibits biosynthesis of the catecholamine.[93]

▎DISEASES OF THE ADRENAL CORTEX

In 1849 Addison described the clinical syndrome of adrenal insufficiency,[2] and in 1932 Cushing described a syndrome resulting from excess production of glucocorticoids and androgens.[94]

The adrenal cortex secretes three types of steroids: the glucocorticoids, the mineralocorticoids, and the androgens. Cortisol, a glucocorticoid, forms a complex with a receptor (its specific acceptor site being nuclear chromatin tissue) to increase RNA production and protein synthesis. The glucocorticoids, being catabolic and anti-insulin, promote gluconeogenesis. They also help vascular tissue maintain a normal response to circulating norepinephrine, thus influencing the distribution and excretion of water. In addition, they alter calcium absorption from the gastrointestinal tract.

Aldosterone, the most important mineralocorticoid, causes sodium retention, regulates extracellular fluid volume, and controls potassium metabolism.

The adrenal cortex can therefore influence the cardiovascular system by bringing about changes to blood pressure and volume homeostasis.

CUSHING'S DISEASE

Cardiovascular complications are the cause of death in about 40% of patients with Cushing's disease. The manifestations are cardiac failure in association with myocardial infarction or renal dysfunction. The full clinical picture includes hypertension, osteoporosis, diabetic glucose tolerance curves, striae of the skin, menstrual disturbances in females, and impotence in males. The predominant cause of heart involvement in Cushing's disease is associated hypertension. It is unclear whether cortisol has a direct effect on the heart muscle. The cause of the associated glucocorticoid hypertension may be increased production of renin substrate, as occurs with the use of oral contraceptives.[95] In addition, cortisol enhances the vascular response to circulating catecholamines and other pressor agents.

On occasion, skin lentigines occur in patients with Cushing's disease; there are also myxomas of the heart and breast tissue. The total clinical entity is familial and inherited as an autosomal dominant.[96]

DIAGNOSIS AND TREATMENT

The diagnosis is established by demonstrating that dexamethasone does not suppress cortisol secretion.

Treatment depends on the specific cause. Those with adenoma or carcinoma of the adrenal gland are treated surgically. If surgery cannot be performed, chemotherapy is used. When the cause is bilateral hyperplasia of the gland, appropriate treatment is still uncertain. At times bilateral adrenalectomy has been recommended; alternatively, surgery or irradiation of the pituitary gland has been recommended.[97]

Hypertension and hypokalemia should be treated but potassium-depleting diuretics should be avoided, if at all possible, since patients with Cushing's disease are prone to hypokalemia. The β-adrenergic blocking drugs or converting enzyme inhibitors are particularly useful alternatives for treating the hypertension. In addition, they block both the production and action of renin.

HYPERALDOSTERONISM

When excess production of aldosterone occurs, there is elevation of the blood pressure, excess excretion of potassium, and retention of sodium and water.[98] The condition is termed hyperaldosteronism when elevated levels of aldosterone occur with suppression of the renin-angiotensin system. Conn's syndrome results from a single adenoma of the adrenal gland, bilateral hyperplasia or, less frequently, carcinoma of the adrenal cortex.[99] Such patients present with elevation of the blood pressure that may rapidly increase in severity, leading to accelerated coronary atherosclerosis and congestive heart failure. Congestive heart failure is associated with increased levels of aldosterone as well as retention of both sodium and water.

The diagnosis is made by demonstrating increased secretion of aldosterone that is not suppressed as it should be during volume expansion. Moreover, there is inadequate secretion of renin, hypokalemia, and increased potassium loss in the urine during salt loading.

It is important to recognize that about 20% of patients with essential hypertension have low renin levels in the absence of any demonstrable excess secretion of mineralicorticoids.

Primary aldosteronism is treated by surgical removal of the adenoma. If this is not possible, spironolactone (which blocks the effects of aldosterone) has been given long-term. Unfortunately, it causes impotence in males as well as considerable gynecomastia, limiting its use.

When hyperaldosteronism is due to bilateral hyperplasia, the best treatment is a combination of spironolactone and antihypertensive therapy.

ADRENAL INSUFFICIENCY

Addison's disease[2] occurs in both sexes and at any age. The usual cause is bilateral atrophy of the adrenal glands, a result of an autoimmune process, although, less commonly, infection may be responsible. There is increased skin pigmentation, physical weakness, nausea, vomiting, and hypotension. The serum levels of sodium chloride and bicarbonate are lessened, serum potassium is increased, a result of lessened aldosterone, and impaired glomerular filtration rates.

CARDIOVASCULAR MANIFESTATIONS

Hypotension occurs in 90% of cases,[100] and circulatory collapse may be a terminal event. The causes of cardiac failure in adrenal insufficiency are many and include reduced blood volume, decreased myocardial contractility, and impaired vascular tone.[101,102]

ECG changes that are frequently recorded include increased T-wave amplitude, flattened P waves, and abnormalities of QRS complexes, probably resulting from hyperkalemia; sinus bradycardia and prolongation of the QT time are also common.

DIAGNOSIS AND TREATMENT

The diagnosis is confirmed by demonstrating decreased response of the adrenal cortex to an injection of ACTH.

Treatment is to administer hydrocortisone in a dose of 20 to 30 mg each day. If there is any associated aldosterone deficiency, 9-α-fluorohydrocortisone (0.05 to 0.10 mg daily) should be given.

PARATHYROID DISEASE

Changes in levels of calcium and phosphorus occur and are responsible for the major cardiac effects of parathyroid disease, namely hypertension and the precipitation of cardiac rhythm disturbances. Aside from changes in calcium metabolism, parathyroid hormone may also have a direct effect on the heart.

Parathyroid hormone mobilizes calcium from various tissues. The increase in serum calcium concentration, in turn, reduces the release of parathyroid hormone. Hyperparathyroidism usually results from a single adenoma of the parathyroid glands. Clinical manifestations may at first be slight, and the diagnosis is not infrequently established by a routine chemical screen. Hypercalcemia produces renal dysfunction and polyuria; renal stones and calcification of the kidneys, leading to renal failure, are common. Bone pain and, at times, spontaneous fractures may occur.

CARDIOVASCULAR MANIFESTATIONS

Parathyroid hormone can have a direct effect on the heart, causing an increased contractility and tachycardia.[103] In contrast, hypoparathyroidism may present as a dilated cardiomyopathy due to hypocalcemia, hypomagnesemia, and reduced concentrations of circulating parathyroid hormone.[104]

In hyperparathyroidism, serum calcium values rarely exceed 14 mg/dl, but any additional dehydration or immobilization may lead to much higher levels. When hyperparathyroidism is due to malignancy of the parathyroid glands, levels of serum calcium increase, owing to parathyroid hormone-like substances produced by the malignant cells. Chronic hypercalcemia may lead to depositions of calcium in the mitral valve annulus, tricuspid valve, and aortic and pulmonary valve tissues.[105]

DIAGNOSIS AND TREATMENT

The demonstration of hypercalcemia with an elevated or even normal level of parathyroid hormone establishes the diagnosis. In many patients, hypercalcemia emerges as thiazide treatment is given for high blood pressure. If the serum calcium level is elevated, it should be retested within a few months; if elevation of serum calcium continues after thiazides are stopped, hyperparathyroidism should be suspected.

HYPOPARATHYROIDISM

This condition occurs without obvious cause, may appear following inadvertent surgical removal of the parathyroid glands, or can be associated with chronic renal failure and vitamin D deficiency. When the serum calcium level is 6 mg/dl or less, the electrocardiogram records reduced QRS voltages and prolongations of the QT time. The effects of digitalis may be diminished by the presence of hypocalcemia but, once the serum calcium has returned to normal, digitalis toxicity may emerge.

Hyperparathyroidism results in a urinary loss of phosphate. Hypophosphatemia may deplete myocardial ATP stores and thereby reduce contractility[106]; thus, part of the cardiac effects of hyperparathyroidism may result from hypophosphatemia.

ROLE OF SEX HORMONES

Coronary artery disease and myocardial infarction are rare in women under 45 years of age but common in men. Consequently, a hypothesis developed that estrogens protected against cardiovascular arteriosclerotic disease. Confirmation seemed possible, since women having oophorectomy before the menopause, or experiencing premature spontaneous menopause, had an increased incidence of coronary artery disease at a younger age.[107,108]

However, when such women were treated with estrogens, no protection against the development of myocardial infarction occurred.[109] On the other hand, men treated with diethylstilbestrol because of carcinoma of the prostate gland had an increased mortality from coronary artery disease, suggesting that estrogens might adversely influence the development of atherosclerosis in a certain age group.[110,111]

These observations led to a study of the effects of oral contraceptives on the emergence of coronary artery disease and myocardial infarction in younger women. A significantly greater incidence of infarction was found among women using oral contraceptive drugs.[112] However, cigarette smoking, hypertension, obesity, diabetes, and toxemia of pregnancy were also more common in these women. It is particularly in women over 40 years that the risk of oral contraceptives precipitating myocardial infarction occurs.[113-115] The effect of oral contraceptives, most of which contain estrogen, is to increase total cholesterol and the LDL fraction while decreasing HDL.

Oral contraceptives may increase the frequency of hypertension, diabetes mellitus and thromboembolism.

Estrogen administration causes hypertension by raising concentrations of renin substrate and angiotensin II.[116] It is possible, however, that the disease emerges only in those females predisposed to hypertension, since it does not develop in all women using oral contraceptives.

In regard to thromboembolism, estrogen-containing oral contraceptives increase platelet adhesion leading to aggregation, increase blood viscosity, and enhance the biosynthesis of clotting factors from the liver.[117]

Although further studies are needed regarding oral contraceptives as a risk factor for cardiovascular disease, it has been recommended that oral contraceptives be avoided by specific groups: women over the age of 40, those known to have other risk factors (namely hypertension, hyperlipidemia, diabetes mellitus, or smoking), and those in whom there is a strong family history of premature and severe coronary atherosclerosis. Whether there is a risk in women below 30 years old remains uncertain, although thromboembolism has been reported with an increased frequency in younger women on oral contraceptives.[118]

More recently, the issue of accelerated atherogenesis in postmenopausal women has been challenged. Investigators have shown that in females, the incidence of myocardial infarction from the early adult years into the menopause and beyond does not increase at the time of menopause.[119] In men, the rate of increase may decline at about age 50. This suggests that some males may have a higher propensity for coronary artery disease at a younger age, but subsequently the incidence is similar to that of women in the same age group.

NUTRITION AND THE CARDIOVASCULAR SYSTEM
OBESITY

Obesity may be present during early childhood and continue throughout life or may commence in the adult age group; the latter is much more common, a result of an imbalance between the amount of calories consumed and the degree of physical activity.

It seems that in persons who are obese from early childhood and throughout their lives, there is an increase in both the number and size of adipose cells; in persons with later-onset obesity, an increase in the size rather than the number of cells is found.[120]

There are data to suggest that obesity may have a genetic determination.[121] When the weights of children adopted in early life were compared with the weights of their natural and adoptive parents, it was the natural rather than the adoptive parents to whom the weights of the children most closely related—both for obese children and for those of normal weight. No doubt this genetic determination can be modified and modulated by environmental factors.

The metabolic consequences of obesity of all types include increased sensitivity to insulin, non-insulin-dependent diabetes mellitus, dyslipoproteinemias (including hypercholesterolemia and hypertriglyceridemia), and changes in amino acids.

CARDIOVASCULAR EFFECTS

Hypertension, hyperlipidemia, and premature death are all more common in those who are overweight.

The associated circulatory dysfunction has been studied extensively since pioneer investigations were undertaken by Smith and Willeus in the early 1930s.[122] Obese persons have an increased circulating blood volume and a high cardiac output. Since there is usually no associated tachycardia, the high cardiac output is caused by an increase in stroke volume. On exercise, filling pressures of the ventricles rise quickly and to abnormal levels, presumably in association with reduced diastolic compliance. In addition, any tendency to systemic hypertension worsens during exercise, when hypertensive levels in the obese are frequently recorded.

More detailed investigations of ventricular function have demonstrated that even in the young obese individual without any evidence of overt heart disease, maximum velocity of myocardial fiber shortening and other indices of ventricular performance are abnormal.[123]

Pathologic studies of the heart of the obese demonstrate hypertrophy and dilatation of both ventricles and atria. The hypertrophy of the heart in the obese tends to be eccentric rather than concentric.[124] Long-term ECG monitoring documents that episodic ventricular dysrhythmias are common in the obese, particularly in association with eccentric ventricular hypertrophy.[125]

Eventually, cardiac failure supervenes as increasing pulmonary and systemic congestion manifest.

It has been demonstrated that in those who are obese and exhibit the cardiovascular changes documented above, dieting improves not only exercise capacity and tolerance but brings about a significant reduction in left ventricular mass and an important improvement in overall ventricular performance.[126,127]

Once cardiac failure supervenes, treatment includes dieting to reduce body weight, sodium restriction, control of any associated hypertension, appropriate use of diuretics, and digitalization.

MALNUTRITION

Malnourishment with reduced protein and calorie intake can be associated with myocardial atrophy and the precipitation of congestive heart failure.[128] In addition, dangerous ventricular rhythm disturbances may emerge, followed by sudden cardiac death.

A hyponutritional state in patients going forward for major cardiac surgery can have disastrous consequences resulting from severely reduced postoperative ventricular performance. Associated abnormalities of liver function are common and serious. In addition, there is an increased predilection to postoperative infections.[129] Every effort should therefore be made, in the preoperative state, to ensure adequate nutrition before such surgery is undertaken.

REFERENCES

1. Graves RJ: Clinical lectures. Med Surg J 7:516, 1835
2. Addison T: On the constitutional and local effects of diseases of the suprarenal capsules. London, Highley, 1855
3. Rimoin DL: Inheritance in diabetes mellitus. Med Clin North Am 55:807, 1971
4. Stolar MW: Atherosclerosis in diabetics: The role of hyperinsulinemia. Metabolism 37(suppl 1):1, 1988
5. Rak K, Beck P, Udvardy M et al: Plasma levels of beta thromboglobulin and factor VIII-related antigen in diabetic children and adults. Thromb Res 29:155, 1983
6. Vague P, Juhan-Vague I, Ailland MF et al: Correlation between blood fibrinolytic activity, plasminogen activator inhibitor level, plasma insulin level, and relative body weight in normal and obese subjects. Metabolism 35:250, 1986
7. Koschinsky T, Bunting CE, Rutter R et al: Vascular growth factors and the development of macrovascular disease in diabetes mellitus. Hum Metab Res 17(suppl):23, 1985
8. Stout RW, Bierman FL, Ross R: Effect of insulin on the proliferation of cultured primate arterial smooth muscle cells. Circ Res 36:319, 1975
9. Stout RW: The effect of insulin and glucose on sterol synthesis in cultured rate arterial smooth muscle cells. Atherosclerosis 27:271, 1977
10. Albrink MJ: Dietary and drug treatment of hyperlipidemia in diabetes. Diabetes 23:913, 1974
11. Bagdade JD, Porte D Jr, Bierman EL: Diabetic lipemia: Form of acquired fat induced lipemia. N Engl J Med 276:427, 1967
12. Grundy SM: HMG-CoA reductase inhibitors for treatment of hypercholesterolemia. N Engl J Med 319:24, 1988
13. Reaven GM: Non-insulin-dependent diabetes mellitus, abnormal lipoprotein metabolism, and atherosclerosis. Metabolism 36(suppl):1, 1987
14. Reaven GM: Insulin resistance in non-insulin dependent diabetes mellitus: Does it exist, and can it be measured? Am J Med 74:3, 1983
15. Santen RJ, Willis PW, Fajans SS: Atherosclerosis in diabetes mellitus: Correlation with serum lipid levels, adiposity, and serum insulin levels. Arch Int Med 130:833, 1972
16. Bradley R: Cardiovascular disease. In Marble A, White R, Bradley R, Kroll L (eds): Joslin's Diabetes Mellitus, ch. 15. Philadelphia, Lea & Febinger 1971
17. Calvert GD, Mannick R, Graham JJ, Wise PH, Yeates RA: Effects of therapy on plasma high density lipoprotein cholesterol concentration in diabetes mellitus. Lancet 1:66, 1978
18. Yoshino G, Kazumi T, Kasama T et al: Effects of CS-514, an inhibitor on 3-hydroxy-3-methylglutaryl coenzyme A reductase, on lipoprotein and apolipoprotein in plasma of hypercholesterolemic diabetics. Diab Res Clin Pract 2:179, 1986
19. Garg A, Grundy SM: Lovastatin for lowering cholesterol levels in non-insulin-dependent diabetes mellitus. N Engl J Med 318-81, 1988
20. Oliver MF: Metabolic response during impending myocardial infarction. II. Clinical implications. Circulation 42:981, 1970
21. Bennett T, Hosking DJ, Hampton JR: Cardiovascular control in diabetes mellitus. Brit Med J 2:585, 1975
22. Resnekov L: Silent myocardial ischemia: Therapeutic implications. Am J Med 79(3A):30, 1985
23. Ewing DJ, Campbell IW, Clarke BF: Assessment of cardiovascular effects in diabetic autonomic neuropathy and prognostic implications. Ann Int Med 92:308, 1980
24. Phillips R, Kett KG, Perper E, Hill T, Nesto RW: Is silent exertional ischemia really more common in diabetics than non-diabetics. Circulation 76(suppl

IV):IV, 1987
25. Chipkin SR, Frid D, Alpert JS et al: Frequency of painless myocardial ischemia during exercise tolerance testing in patients with and without diabetes mellitus. Am J Cardiol 59:61, 1987
26. Bern M: Platelet function in diabetes mellitus. Diabetes 27:342, 1977
27. Peterson C, Jones R, Koenig RJ, Melvin ET, Lehrman ML: Reversible hematologic sequelae of diabetes mellitus. Ann Int Med 86:425, 1977
28. Kannel W, Hjortland M, Castelli W: Role of diabetes in congestive heart failure. The Framingham Study. Am J Cardiol 34:29, 1974
29. Regan FJ, Lyons MM, Ahmed SS et al: Evidence of cardiomyopathy in familial diabetes mellitus. J Clin Invest 60:885, 1977
30. Hamby RI, Zoneraich S, Sherman L: Diabetic cardiomyopathy. JAMA 229:1749, 1974
31. Wolfe RR, Way GL: Cardiomyopathies in infants of diabetic mothers. Johns Hopkins Med J 140:177, 1977
32. Pell S, D'Alonzo A: Some aspects of hypertension in diabetes mellitus. JAMA 202:104, 1967
33. Rubler S: Cardiac manifestations of diabetes mellitus. Cardiovasc Med 2:823, 1977
34. University Group Diabetes Program: A study of the effects of hypoglycemic agents on vascular complications in patients with adult-onset diabetes. V. Evaluation of phenformin therapy. Diabetes 24(suppl):65, 1975
35. Wu CF, Haideo B, Ahmed SS et al: The effects of tolbutamide on the myocardium in experimental diabetes. Circulation 55:200, 1977
36. Bielefeld OR, Pace CS, Boshen BR: Hyperosmolarity and cardiac function in chronic diabetic rat heart. Am J Physiol 245:E568, 1983
37. Schimmel M, Utiger RD: Thyroidal and peripheral production of thyroid hormones. Review of recent findings and their clinical implications. Ann Intern Med 87:760, 1977
38. Lardy HA, Feldott HG: Metabolic effects of thyroxine in vitro. Ann NY Acad Sci 54:636, 1951
39. Stocker WW, Samaha FJ, Degroot LJ: Coupled oxidative phosphorylation in muscle of thyrotoxic patients. Am J Med 44:900, 1968
40. Edelman IS, Ismail-Beigi F: Thyroid thermogenesis and active sodium transport. Recent Progr Horm Res 30:235, 1974
41. Proskey MD, Saksina T, Towne WD: Myocardial infarction associated with thyrotoxicosis. Chest 72:109, 1977
42. Symmes JC, Lenkei SCM, Berman ND: Myocardial infarction, hyperthyroidism and normal coronary arteries: Report of two cases. Calif Med Assoc J 117:489, 1977
43. Stern MP, Jacobs RL, Duncan GW: Complete heart block complicating hyperthyroidism. JAMA 212:2117, 1970
44. Campus S, Rappelli A, Malavasi A, Satta A: Heart block and hyperthyroidism. Arch Int Med 135:1091, 1975
45. Davis AC, Smith JL: Complete heart block in hyperthyroidism following acute infections: A report of six cases with necropsy findings in one case. Am Heart J 9:81, 1933
46. Sandler G, Wilson GM: The nature and prognosis of heart disease in thyrotoxicosis: A review of 150 patients treated with [131]I. Quart J Med 28:347, 1959
47. Resnekov L, Falicov R: Thyrotoxicosis and lactate-producing angina pectoris with normal coronary arteries. Brit Heart J 39:1051, 1977
48. Brester WR, Isaacs JR, Osgood PF: The hemodynamic and metabolic interrelationships in the activity of epinephrine, norepinephrine, and the thyroid hormones. Circulation 13:1, 1956
49. Wildenthal K: Studies of isolated fetal mouse hearts in organ culture: Evidence for a direct effect of triiodothyronine in enhancing cardiac responsiveness to norepinephrine. J Clin Invest 51:2702, 1972
50. Wildenthal K: Studies on fetal mouse hearts in organ culture: Influence of prolonged exposure to triiodothyronine on cardiac responsiveness to isoproterenol, glucagon, theophylline, acetylcholine, and dibutyryl cyclic 3',5'-adenosine monophosphate. J Pharmacol Exp Ther 109:272, 1974
51. Williams LT, Lefkowitz RJ, Watanabe AM, Hathaway DR, Besch HR: Thyroid hormone regulation of beta-adrenergic receptor number. J Biol Chem 272:2787, 1977
52. Rutherford JP, Vatner SF, Braunwald E: Adrenergic control of myocardial contractility in conscious hypertrophied dogs. Am J Physiol 237:590, 1980
53. Hoh GFY, McGrath PA, Hale PT: Electrophoretic analysis of multiple forms of cardiac myosin: Effect of hypophysectomy and thyroxine replacement. J Mol Cell Cardiol 10:1053, 1978
54. Litten RZ, Martin BJ, Howe ER, Alpert NR, Solaro RJ: Phosphorylation and adenosine triphosphate activity of myofibrils from thyrotoxic rabbit hearts. Circ Res 48:498, 1981
55. Suko J: The calcium pump of cardiac sarcoplasmic reticulum. Functional alterations at different levels of thyroid state in rabbits. J Physiol (Lond) 228:563, 1973
56. Eriksson M, Rubenfield S, Garber A, Kohler P: Propranolol does not prevent thyroid storm. NEJM 296:263, 1977
57. Doherty JE, Perkins WH: Digoxin metabolism in hypo- and hyperthyroidism. Studies with tritiated digoxin in thyroid disease. Ann Intern Med 64:489, 1966
58. Morrow DH, Gaffney TE, Braunwald E: Studies on digitalis VIII. Effect of autonomic innervation and of myocardial catecholamine stores upon the cardiac action of ouabain. J Pharmacol Exp Ther 140:236, 1963
59. Nakazawa HK, Sakurai K, Hamada N, Momotani N, Ito K: Management of atrial fibrillation in the post-thyrotoxic state. Am J Med 72:903, 1982
60. Staffurth JS, Gibberd MC, Fui ST: Arterial embolism in thyrotoxicosis with atrial fibrillation. Br Med J 2:688, 1977
61. Singh JB, Starobin OE, Guerrant R, Manders E: Reversible atrio-ventricular block in myxedema. Chest 63:582, 1973
62. Gavrilescu S, Luca C, Streian C, Lungo G, Deutsch G: Monophasic action potentials of right atrium and electrophysiological properties of AV conducting system in patients with hypothyroidism. Brit Heart J 38:1350, 1976
63. Keating FR, Parkin TW: Treatment of heart disease associated with myxedema. Prog Cardiovasc Dis 3:364, 1960
64. Crowley WF, Ridgeway EC, Bough E et al: Noninvasive evaluation of cardiac function in hypothyroidism. NEJM 296:1, 1977
65. Kerber RE, Sherman B: Echocardiographic evaluation of pericardial effusion in myxedema. Circulation 52:823, 1975
66. Smolar EN, Rubin JE, Avramides A, Carter A: Cardiac tamponade in primary myxedema and review of the literature. Am J Med Sci 272:345, 1976
67. Steinberg AD: Myxedema and coronary artery disease—a comparative study. Ann Int Med 68:338, 1968
68. Littman DS, Jeffers WA, Rose E: The infrequency of myocardial infarction in patients with thyrotoxicosis. Am J Med Sci 233:10, 1957
69. Paine TD, Rogers WJ: Coronary arterial surgery in patients with incapacitating angina pectoris and myxedema. Am J Cardiol 40:226, 1977
70. Sonenberg M, Cohen H: Growth hormone. Ann NY Acad Sci 148:291, 1968
71. Daughaday W: The adenohypophysis. In Williams RH (ed): Textbook of Endocrinology, p 31. Philadelphia, WB Saunders, 1974
72. Mautalen CA, Mellinger RC, Smith RW Jr: Lipolytic effect of growth hormone in acromegaly. J Cin Endocrinol 28:1031, 1968
73. Joplin GF, Lewis P: A case of acromegalic heart disease. Brit Med J 1:718, 1973
74. Pepine CJ, Aloia J: Heart muscle disease in acromegaly. Am J Med 48:530, 1970
75. Falkheden T, Sjogren B: Extracellular fluid volume and renal function in pituitary insufficiency and acromegaly. Acta Endoc 46:80, 1964
76. Hirsch EZ, Sloman JB, Martin FIR: Cardiac function in acromegaly. Am J Med Sci 257:1, 1969
77. Cain JP, Williams GH, Dluhy RG: Plasma renin activity and aldosterone secretion in patients with acromegaly. J Clin Endoc 34:73, 1972
78. Ikkos D, Luft R, Gemzell CA: The effect of human growth hormone in man. Acta Endoc 34:341, 1959
79. McGuffin WL, Sherman BM, Roth J et al: Acromegaly and cardiovascular disorders: A prospective study. Ann Int Med 81:11, 1974
80. O'Keefe J, Grant S, Wiseman J: Acromegaly and the heart echocardiographic and nuclear imaging studies. Austral & NZJ Med 12:603, 1982
81. Rossi Y, Thiene G, Caregaro J: Dysrhythmias and sudden death in acromegalic heart disease: A clinicopathologic study. Chest 72:495, 1977
82. Lie JT, Grossman SJ: Pathology of the heart in acromegaly: Anatomic findings in 27 autopsied patients. Am Heart J 100:41, 1980
83. Kjellberg RM: Proton-beam therapy in acromegaly. N Engl J Med 278:689, 1968
84. Van Vliet P, Burchell HB, Titus JL: Focal myocarditis associated with pheochromocytoma. NEJM 274:1102, 1966
85. Engleman K: Catecholamines: Pheochromocytoma. Clin Endoc Metab 6(3):769, 1977
86. Cheng TO, Bashour TT: Striking electrocardiographic changes associated with pheochromocytoma. Chest 70:397, 1976
87. Baker G, Zeller NH, Weitzner S, Leach JK: Pheochromocytoma with hypertension presenting as cardiomyopathy. Am Heart J 83:688, 1972
88. Forde TP, Yormak SS, Killip T: Reflex bradycardia and nodal escape rhythm in pheochromocytoma. Am Heart J 76:388, 1968
89. Szakacs JE, Mehlman B: Pathologic changes induced by 1-norepinephrine: Quantitative aspects. Am J Cardiol 5:619, 1960
90. James TN: Pathology of small coronary arteries. Am J Cardiol 20:679, 1967
91. Bravo EL, Tarazi RC, Fouad FM, Vidt DG, Gifford Jr RW: Clonidine-suppression test: A useful aid in the diagnosis of pheochromocytoma. NEJM 305:623, 1981
92. Sisson JC, Frager MS, Valk TW et al: Scintigraphic localization of pheochromocytoma. NEJM 305:12, 1981
93. Hengstmann JH, Gugler R, Dengler HJ: Malignant pheochromocytoma. Effect of oral a-methyl-p-tyrosine upon catecholamine metabolism. Klin Wochenschr 57:351, 1979
94. Rose LI, Underwood RH, Newmark SR, Kisch ES, Williams GH: Pathophysiology of spironolactone-induced gynecomastia. Ann Intern Med 87:398, 1977
95. Krakoff L, Nicolis G, Amsel B: Pathogenesis of hypertension in Cushing's syndrome. Am J Med 58:216, 1975
96. Carney JA, Hruska LA, Beauchamp GD, Gordon H: Dominant inheritance of the complex of myxomas, spotty pigmentation and endocrine overactivity. Mayo Clin Proc 61:165, 1986
97. Tyrrel JB, Brooks RM, Fitzgerald PA, Cofoid PB, Forsham PH, Wilson CB: Cushing's disease: Selective transphenoidal resection of pituitary microadenomas. NEJM 298:753, 1978
98. Brown JJ, Fraser R, Lever AF, Robertson JIS: Diseases of the adrenal cortex: Aldosterone: Physiological and pathophysiological variations in man. Clin Endoc Metab 1:397, 1972
99. Salti IS: Non-tumorous "primary" aldosteronism I. type relieved by glucocorticoid. Canad Med Assoc J 101:1, 1969

100. Nerup J: Addison's disease—clinical studies: A report of 108 cases. Acta Endoc 76:127, 1974
101. Lefer AM, Sutfin DC: Cardiovascular effects of catecholamines in experimental adrenal insufficiency. Am J Physiol 206:1151, 1964
102. Webb WR, Degerli IU, Hardy JD, Unal M: Cardiovascular responses in adrenal insufficiency. Surgery 58:273, 1965
103. Katoh Y, Klein KL, Kaplan RA, Sanborn WG, Kurokawa K: Parathyroid hormone has a positive inotropic action in the rat. Endocrinology 109:2252, 1981
104. Giles TD, Iteld BJ, Rires KL: The cardiomyopathy of hypoparathyroidism. Chest 79:225, 1981
105. Roberts T, Waller B: Chronic hypercalcemia on the heart: An analysis of 18 necropsy patients. Am J Med 71:371, 1981
106. O'Connor LR, Wheeler WS, Bethune JE: Effect of hypophosphatemia on myocardial performance in man. NEJM 297:901, 1977
107. Higano N, Robinson RW, Cohen WD: Increased incidence of cardiovascular disease in castrated women. NEJM 268:1123, 1963
108. Sznajderman M, Oliver MF: Spontaneous premature menopause, ischemic heart disease, and serum lipids. Lancet 1:962, 1963
109. Rosenberg F, Armstrong B, Jick H: Myocardial infarction and estrogen therapy in postmenopausal women. NEJM 294 23:1256, 1976
110. Byar DP: The Veterans Administration Cooperative Urological Research Group's studies of cancer of the prostate. Cancer 32 5:1126, 1973
111. Blackard CE, Doe RP, Mellinger GT, Byer DP: Incidence of cardiovascular disease and death in patients receiving diethylstilbestrol for carcinoma of the prostate. Cancer 26 2:249, 1970
112. Mann JI, Vessey MP, Thorogood M, Doll R: Myocardial infarction in young women with special reference to oral contraceptive practice. Brit Med J 2:241, 1975
113. Vessey M, Doll R, Peto R: A longterm followup study of women using different methods of contraception—an interim report. J Biosoc Sci 8:373, 1976
114. Beral V: Cardiovascular disease mortality trends and oral contraceptive use in young women. Lancet 2:1047, 1976
115. Jick H, Dinan B: Myocardial infarction and other vascular diseases in young women: role of estrogens and other factors. JAMA 240:2548, 1978
116. Hollenberg NK, Williams GH, Burger B, Chenitz W, Hooshmand I, Adams DF: Renal blood flow and its response to A II: An interaction between oral contraceptive agents, sodium intake and the renin-angiotensin system in healthy young women. Circ Res 38:35, 1976
117. Wood JE: The cardiovascular effects of oral contraceptives. Mod. Concepts Cardiovasc Dis 41:37, 1972
118. Sartwell PE, Masi AT, Arthes FG: Thromboembolism and oral contraceptives: An epidemiologic case-control study. Am J Epidemiol 90:365, 1969
119. Furman RH: Are gonadal hormones (estrogens and androgens) of significance in the development of ischemic heart disease? Ann NY Acad Sci 149:822, 1968
120. Hirsch J, Knittle JL: Cellularity of obese and non-obese human adipose tissue. Fed Proc. 29:1516, 1970
121. Stunkard AJ, Sorensen TIA, Hanis C et al: An adoption study of human obesity. N Engl J Med 314:193, 1988
122. Smith HL, Willius RA: Adiposity of the heart. A clinical and pathological study of one hundred and thirty-six obese patients. Ann Intern Med 52:911, 1933
123. De Diritiis O, Fazio S, Petitto M et al: Obesity and cardiac function. Circulation 64:477, 1981
124. Ventura HO, Messerli FH, Dunn FG et al: Left ventricular hypertrophy in obesity: Discrepancy between echo and electrocardiogram. J Am Coll Cardiol 1:682, 1983
125. Messerli FH, Ventura HO, Elizardi DJ et al: Hypertension and sudden death: Increased ventricular ectopic activity in left ventricular hypertrophy. Am J Med 77:18, 1984
126. Reisin E, Frohlich ED, Messerli FH et al: Cardiovascular changes after weight reduction in obesity hypertension. Ann Intern Med 98:315, 1983
127. MacMahon SW, Wicken DEL, MacDonald GJ: The effect of weight reduction on left ventricular mass: A randomized controlled trial in young, overweight hypertensive patients. N Engl J Med 314:334, 1986
128. Abel RM, Fischeer JE, Buckley MJ et al: Malnutrition in cardiac surgical patients. Arch Surg 111:45, 1976
129. Blackburn GL, Gibbons GW, Bothe A et al: Nutritional support in cardiac cachexia. J Thorc Cardiovasc Surg 43:489, 1977

Cardiac and Cardiopulmonary Transplantation

Mark E. Thompson • J. Stephen Dummer
Bartley P. Griffith

CARDIAC TRANSPLANTATION
HISTORY

In 1960 at Stanford University, Lower and Shumway established the experimental basis for cardiac transplantation as it is now practiced.[1] By 1965, extended survival of experimental animals undergoing cardiac transplantation was attained using steroids, azathioprine, or mercaptopurine as immunosuppressive agents.[1,2] The excitement and enthusiasm generated by the first successful cardiac transplantation performed by Dr. Christiaan Barnard was reflected in the 103 transplant operations performed in 17 countries over the next 12 months.[3] Following this initial burst of exuberance, however, the difficulties associated with human cardiac transplantation began to surface, foremost among them being control of rejection and concomitant serious infection in the immunocompromised host. Enthusiasm waned as the reality of a 20% one-year survival rate was recognized throughout the medical community. It remained for Stanford University, the Medical College of Virginia, and Groote Schuur Hospital to continue pioneering efforts in cardiac transplantation for another decade, until widespread acceptance of this procedure was reestablished.

SELECTION OF CANDIDATES

Candidates for cardiac transplantation are severely disabled (New York Heart Association Classification IV) as the result of end-stage cardiac disease, usually related to idiopathic cardiomyopathy (50%), ischemic cardiomyopathy (40%), end-stage valvular heart disease (5%), and other miscellaneous causes (5%).[4] In all instances, candidates for cardiac transplantation should undergo thorough cardiac evaluation, including complete cardiac catheterization, in order to identify those who may benefit from alternative treatment modalities and promising experimental therapy.

An extensive screening process has been established to select those candidates most likely to benefit from cardiac transplantation. A thorough review of the medical history and a complete physical examination are essential. Routine laboratory studies, including complete blood cell count, urinalysis, electrocardiography, chest roentgenography, pulmonary function, blood urea nitrogen, creatinine, electrolytes, bilirubin, alkaline phosphatase, serum glutamic oxaloacetic transaminase, serum glutamic pyruvic transaminase, lactic dehydrogenase, 2-hour postprandial blood sugar, 24-hour urine for creatinine clearance, ABO blood typing, human leukocyte antigen (HLA) typing, and percent reactive antibodies, are obtained as part of the preoperative evaluation. Restoration of good oral hygiene is indicated, to avoid dental sources of postoperative infection. Patients are also evaluated for previous exposure to Epstein-Barr virus, *Toxoplasma gondii*, cytomegalovirus, *Mycobacterium tuberculosis,* and fungi. These studies are of particular value postoperatively, when there may be reactivation of latent infections or transmission of Epstein-Barr virus, cytomegalovirus or *Toxoplasma* from donor to recipient.[5] A complete history of drug allergy, especially to antibiotics, is essential so that adverse reactions to drugs may be avoided. A careful inquiry into sites of recurrent infection, such as the bronchial tree or urinary tract, is useful, as is a description of foreign travel or unusual environmental exposures caused by activities such as spelunking. Stool specimens should be examined for ova and parasites in individuals endemically exposed to intestinal parasites such as *Strongyloides* (Table 118.1).

The purpose of this extensive pretransplantation screening is to identify underlying systemic illnesses that may hamper recuperation and rehabilitation following cardiac transplantation. It must also be determined that there has been no irreversible damage to the central nervous system, liver, or kidneys that would preclude recovery. Additionally, it is important to assess the patient's economic situation and psychosocial support system.[6] The cost of cardiac transplantation has been estimated to be between $22,000 (Veterans Administration Medical Center, Richmond, Virginia) and $100,000 (Stanford University)[7]; this cost may be covered by insurance in many instances. The patient must have a demonstrated ability to cooperate with and fully understand the medical treatment programs, be willing to accept the risks of cardiac transplantation as a prerequisite for eventual recovery and rehabilitation, and be committed to a long-term follow-up program. A strong supportive family unit is of immeasurable value in tiding the patient over the rigors of the postoperative period. In addition, there must be sufficient financial resources to pay expenses not covered by

TABLE 118.1 INFECTION SURVEILLANCE PROTOCOL

Pre-Transplantation	Post-Transplantation
Cytomegalovirus IgG antibody	Viral surveillance cultures
Epstein-Barr IgG antibody	Repeat pretransplant titers if infection with these agents is suspected
Varicella-zoster IgG antibody	
Toxoplasma IgG antibody	
Legionella antibody	
Tubercular skin test	
Hepatitis B screening	
Stool for ova/parasites*	

* For residents of tropical and subtropical regions.

(Adapted from Dummer JS, Montero CG, Griffith BP et al: Infections in heart–lung transplant recipients. Transplantation 41:725, 1986)

Adapted from Thompson ME: Selection of candidates for cardiac transplantation. J Heart Transplant 3(1):65, 1983; from Thompson ME, Dummer JS, Griffith BP et al: Cardiac transplantation 1985: Hope—promise—reality. In Yu PN, Goodwin JF (eds): Progress in Cardiology, vol 14, chap 7. Philadelphia, Lea & Febiger, 1986; and from Thompson ME, Dummer JS, Paradis I et al: Heart–lung transplantation. In Yu PN, Goodwin JF (eds): Progress in Cardiology, vol 16, chap 3. Philadelphia, Lea & Febiger, 1988.

insurance such as travel and lodging before and after transplantation. Social service support in these areas is invaluable.

This highly select group of patients, once chosen for cardiac transplantation, has a median survival of 30 days without transplantation and a life expectancy of less than 6 to 9 months overall.[4] In the initial experience at Stanford University, approximately 10% of patients referred for cardiac transplantation were selected as candidates and approximately half of these eventually underwent the procedure. These percentages may vary from center to center, but they do serve to emphasize the highly selective indications for cardiac transplantation and the relatively circumscribed situations under which it is actually accomplished. It is estimated that 1,000 to 8,000 individuals per year are suitable candidates for cardiac transplantation but only about 2,000 hearts are available.[8,9] These figures highlight the importance of choosing the best available candidates and indicate that a large percentage of patients die before transplantation because of the limitations imposed by available facilities. Similarly, the importance of early identification and evaluation of possible candidates for cardiac transplantation is stressed, so that one is not faced with the problem of trying, in a relatively short time, to evaluate and to transplant a desperately ill patient requiring maximal cardiovascular support.

The primary criteria for recipient selection include the following[4,9,10]:

1. Terminal heart disease with an estimated life expectancy of less than 6 to 12 months
2. Age younger than 50 to 55 years (ideally)
3. Normal or reversible renal and hepatic function
4. Absence of active infection
5. Absence of pulmonary infarction in the preceding 8 weeks
6. Absence of insulin-dependent diabetes mellitus or hyperglycemia requiring treatment with insulin or oral hypoglycemic agents
7. Psychosocial stability and a supportive social milieu

There are also absolute contraindications to cardiac transplantation[4,9]:

1. A pulmonary vascular resistance in excess of 6 Wood units (orthotopic transplantation)
2. Crossmatch incompatibility between recipient and donor
3. Significant peripheral vascular or cerebrovascular disease
4. Active peptic ulcer disease
5. Drug addiction
6. Alcoholic cardiomyopathy and continued alcohol abuse
7. Coexisting systemic illness that may limit life expectancy or compromise recovery from cardiac transplantation
8. Preexisting malignancy
9. Chronic bronchitis and chronic obstructive pulmonary disease

The screening criteria for selection of ideal patients for cardiac transplantation are based on identification of those characteristics that provide the patient with the greatest opportunity for survival and rehabilitation following cardiac transplantation. A lower age for cardiac transplantation requires a young individual who is fully cognizant of the ramifications of the proposed procedure and who is fully prepared to cooperate completely during the extended postoperative recovery phase and lifelong follow-up. Under unusual circumstances the upper age limit for cardiac transplantation may be extended. Likewise, clinical judgment must be employed when faced with a decision regarding patients requiring insulin for control of diabetes or those with modest impairment of renal and hepatic function. The normal right ventricle of a transplanted heart cannot acutely adapt to a fixed pulmonary vascular resistance in excess of 6 Wood units, defined as one that does not respond to interventions such as improvement in arterial oxygen saturation, vasodilator therapy, or inotropic therapy.[4] Additionally, the absolute pressure gradient across the pulmonary vascular bed has been shown to be of prognostic significance postoperatively.[11] Peptic ulcer disease is also exacerbated by postoperative stress and high corticosteroid doses. Drug addiction and continued excessive alcohol consumption are psychological factors that may adversely affect outcome. Finally, preexisting malignancy and chronic bronchitis and emphysema (with their predisposition to infection) are two common examples of coexisting illness that may limit life expectancy or compromise recovery from cardiac transplantation.[4,9] The introduction of cyclosporine as an alternative immunosuppressive agent has raised the hopes of many that the selection of candidates for transplantation may be liberalized. However, experience to date with cyclosporine has not indicated that such changes can be made.

All institutions with an active cardiac transplantation program are faced with seriously ill patients having life expectancy numbered in days as a result of severe congestive failure unless extraordinary measures for circulatory support are used. Not infrequently, these patients require parenteral administration of inotropic drugs and, in some instances, the use of an intra-aortic balloon assist device to maintain adequate blood pressure and renal perfusion prior to cardiac transplantation. Experience has shown that the survival statistics following cardiac transplantation in this group are similar to those in patients who are not so ill, provided irreversible cerebral, gastrointestinal (including hepatic), or renal failure has not supervened.[12-14]

USE OF THE MECHANICAL HEART AS A BRIDGE TO TRANSPLANTATION

Present experience indicates that mechanical assist devices (total artificial heart, left ventricular assist or biventricular assist) may be used for interim support of critically ill patients. Successful staged cardiac transplantation has been reported in patients in whom mechanical assistance has been used as a "bridge to transplant."[13,15,16] However, hemorrhage, infection, embolization, and multiorgan failure are potential complications of mechanical circulatory assistance that may ultimately preclude transplantation in this group of patients. Even though mechanical assistance prior to cardiac transplantation is still limited in its availability, the temporary use of these devices provides additional experience that may result in their future improvement. The overall problem of limited donor availability is not ameliorated, however, by the use of mechanical devices.

SELECTION CRITERIA FOR RETRANSPLANTATION

Selection of patients for a second or third cardiac transplantation procedure may be required under certain circumstances.[17] In some instances, acute severe irreversible rejection has necessitated a second procedure shortly after the first. In other instances, chronic rejection or the development of accelerated atherosclerosis has resulted in graft failure and the need for a second transplant. The guidelines for selection of persons for repetitive transplantations are the same as for the initial procedure. The survival statistics for second and third transplants indicate that approximately 30% of these patients survive an additional 2 years. Until further progress is made, the number of sequential cardiac transplantation procedures will be limited.

HETEROTOPIC CARDIAC TRANSPLANTATION

Up to this point, the discussion has been directed to the selection of recipients for orthotopic cardiac transplantation. Alternatively, heterotopic transplantation has been developed and championed by Dr. Christiaan Barnard and his associates in Cape Town.[19] The major advantage of heterotopic transplantation is that under some circumstances the recipient's own heart may be sufficiently functional to tide him over a period of graft failure as a result of an arrhythmia or rejection that would otherwise have proven fatal. In addition, it may be possible to consider heterotopic transplantation in persons with elevated pulmonary resistance, since the recipient's right ventricle remains functional and has previously adapted to the pressure overload. With time, the transplanted right ventricle may also undergo significant hypertrophy so that it, too, may contribute to forward pulmonary flow.

The disadvantage of the heterotopic procedure lies in the fact that the dilated diseased hypofunctional native heart may be the source of systemic emboli or the site of a mural thrombus that may become infected. The native heart must not be compromised by right-sided heart failure or tricuspid insufficiency. Likewise, the recipient heart should have no prosthetic valvular device that may provide a nidus for infection, thus posing an extremely difficult management problem, complicated by the necessity for continued immunosuppression. Nevertheless, one published review of heterotopic cardiac transplantation indicates that this procedure compares favorably with orthotopic transplantation, while less favorable results are reported by others.[19,20]

CADAVERIC ORGAN PROCUREMENT
IDENTIFICATION OF DONORS

A procurement organization is crucial to the success of a program for cardiac transplantation. These professionals identify potential donors locally, obtain permission for donation, manage the donor until organ removal, account for expenses incurred, and reimburse the hospital in which the donation took place. When a donor is identified in a distant area, they arrange necessary transportation by ground and/or air.

SELECTION OF DONORS

The criteria for certification of brain death are determined by the staff of the hospital in which the heart-beating cadaver is located.[21] Coronary artery disease of the donor heart is minimized by selecting males under age 35 and females under age 40. The relative lack of donors has prompted liberalization of donor age to 50 years in some centers.[22,23] When the potential donor exceeds the age limit, coronary arteriography may be done to exclude or identify disease in a specific donor. The absence of a history of cardiac disease, a normal cardiac examination, a normal cardiac silhouette on the chest roentgenogram, and a normal electrocardiogram are the primary criteria to ensure that the heart is satisfactory for transplantation. A donor heart too small for the recipient may be avoided by using hearts from donors whose weight is not more than 10 kg less than that of the recipient. A somewhat larger donor heart in proportion to the recipient's is preferred to one that is smaller, especially in the presence of an elevated pulmonary vascular resistance (4-6 Wood units).

In spite of adequate volume replacement, most donors require inotropic support, presumably necessitated by an absence of vasomotor regulation. Donor hearts requiring in excess of 10 $\mu g/kg/min$ of dopamine or its equivalent does not exclude selection of the heart, provided that the usual clinical indices of adequate cardiac output are satisfactory on low-dose (5 $\mu g/ml/min$) inotropic drugs following stabilization. Hypoxia resulting from neurogenic pulmonary edema does not preclude use of the heart, nor does pneumonia or other infections in the absence of septicemia.

MULTIPLE CADAVERIC ORGAN PROCUREMENT

The cardinal principle of multiple organ procurement is the *in situ* cooling of different organs in the same donor.[24] Using this approach, it is possible to obtain the liver and kidneys in addition to the heart, from a single donor for transplantation into multiple recipients.

CARDIECTOMY

The donor heart is arrested by infusion of a cold cardioplegic solution. The excised donor heart is immersed in a cold crystalloid solution (4°C), placed in a sterile plastic container, and covered with three plastic bags to maintain sterility. It is then packed in an ice chest and transported for reimplantation. It is preferable to limit the total ischemic time to 3 hours, but this has been extended to 5 to 6 hours (including the 45 minutes allotted to implantation) without undue impairment of cardiac function in some instances.

ANESTHESIA

The general approach to anesthetic management of the cardiac transplantation candidate is similar to that used in other patients undergoing routine cardiovascular surgical procedures.[25,26]

OPERATIVE PROCEDURE FOR ORTHOTOPIC CARDIAC TRANSPLANTATION

The operative technique for orthotopic cardiac transplantation was described by Lower and Shumway.[1] This technique employs biatrial anastomosis of the recipient and donor, avoiding difficult and time-consuming caval and pulmonary venous anastomoses. The right atrium of the donor heart is opened posterolaterally from the inferior caval-atrial junction. This avoids injury to the sinus node, which is solely responsible for the maintenance of sinus rhythm in the transplanted heart. Reperfusion of the transplanted heart can be accomplished following completion of the aortic anastomosis prior to completing the pulmonary artery anastomosis. Reimplantation is usually accomplished in 45 to 60 minutes.

Most recipients require small doses of isoproterenol, dobutamine or dopamine for up to 48 hours postoperatively to improve chronotropic and inotropic function of the graft. Adequate filling pressures are maintained to maximize cardiac output, which is dependent on the Frank-Starling principle. Temporary pacemaker wires are frequently used to maintain an adequate heart rate during the immediate post-transplant period.

REJECTION

The rejection response to a transplanted organ proceeds along multiple pathways that involve both cellular and humoral components.[27-29] The cell-mediated immune response depends on lymphocytes of thymic derivation (T-lymphocytes). Each subset of T-lymphocytes assumes a specialized role in the rejection of transplanted tissue. The T-helper and T-cytotoxic lymphocytes actively support and carry out the rejection response, while the T-suppressor lymphocytes inhibit this reaction.[30] Two additional types of lymphocytes (neither T- nor B-lymphocytes) play less well defined roles in response to transplanted tissue. One of these is the killer (K) lymphocyte, which is involved in an antibody-dependent cellular cytotoxic response; the other is the natural killer (NK) lymphocyte.

The humoral response to transplanted tissue is dependent on antibody production by B-lymphocytes. Immature B-lymphocytes originate from lymphoid stem cells within the bone marrow and evolve into mature B-lymphocytes and antibody-producing plasma cells. The humoral rejection response results in tissue lysis, inflammation, and possible binding and activation of the complement system by antigen antibody reaction, which takes place on the cell surface of transplanted tissue. Complement activation results in the production of chemotactic factors, which promote the influx of inflammatory cells. The migration of inflammatory cells occurs in association with altered vascular permeability, which is also brought about by complement activation. Phagocytosis of the damaged tissue occurs in conjunction with the influx of macrophages and phagocytes at the site of the rejection reaction.[30,31]

Rejection is characterized by a cellular infiltration of the transplanted organ. The mode of sensitization of the host by the transplanted organ, the number of donor leukocytes (often more immunogenic than the organ itself) transferred along with the transplanted organ, the manner of vascularization of the transplanted organ, the lymphatic drainage of the organ, and the specific organ transplanted are all factors that influence the severity of the rejection reaction.[28] The basic immunologic rules for organ transplantation are derived from experience gained in renal allograft procedures. One universal principle in organ transplantation is that ABO blood group compatibility between donor and recipient be honored.[32] The human leukocyte antigen (HLA) system also plays an important part in organ transplantation. Retrospective studies have shown no correlation between HLA matching and survival in heart transplantation patients.[33]

Each potential candidate for cardiac transplantation is tested for the presence of preformed antibodies by reacting the patient's serum with a panel of T-lymphocytes representing the major HLA antigens. Patients reacting to more than 15% of the panel of lymphocytes should undergo a direct crossmatch of recipient serum and donor lymphocytes prior to transplantation. The direct crossmatch is usually not done prospectively because of logistical reasons for patients with less than 15% reactive antibodies. The presence of preformed antibodies in patients prior to cardiac transplantation may identify a group of individuals who are hyperresponders and who may have more difficulty with rejection postoperatively, even in the presence of a negative crossmatch. Likewise, patients with preformed antibodies who have experienced prior rejection may have a predisposition to recurrent rejection if retransplantation is accomplished.[34] While the presence of a positive crossmatch between recipient serum and donor T-lymphocytes may lead to acute rejection, a more likely outcome is the presence of difficult-to-control rejection that smoulders during the ensuing postoperative course.[26] Hyperacute rejection has been attributed to antibodies directed against an antigenic system present on the vascular endothelial cells.[35]

IMMUNOSUPPRESSION

Immunosuppressive protocols for cardiac transplantation have evolved from experience gained with renal transplantation.[36] The most significant advances in immunosuppressive therapy occurred in the 1970s with the introduction of the endomyocardial biopsy and the addition of antithymocyte globulin to the immunosuppressive regimen of azathioprine and prednisone. Using this approach, a 1-year survival rate of 65% and a 5-year survival rate of 40% were achieved by the end of the decade.[4]

The complexion of immunosuppression for cardiac transplantation has changed since the introduction of cyclosporine. This cyclic polypeptide, a metabolite of the fungal species *Tolypocladium inflatum* Gams, was found to be immunosuppressive by Borel.[37] Early experience in renal transplantation showed superior results, and cyclosporine was quickly adopted into trials of cardiac transplantation. The initial experiences at Stanford University and the University of Pittsburgh indicated that cyclosporine is a superior but imperfect drug for immunosuppression. Chronic unresolved rejection of the allograft occurred in 30% of Pittsburgh patients when cyclosporine was combined with corticosteroids alone. However, this could be reversed when rabbit antithymocyte globulin was added for severe or persisting rejection as a "rescue" agent.[38] At Stanford, rabbit antithymocyte globulin was used prophylactically and rejection was rare, but there was an unacceptably high incidence of lymphoma.[39]

Because cyclosporine is associated with serious nephrotoxicity and hypertension, recent trends have been toward the use of lower doses of this drug than initially thought necessary to prevent rejection. Many centers have incorporated the old and new drugs into current protocols for treatment because experimental and clinical evidence in renal transplantation have suggested that the combination of low-dose cyclosporine and azathioprine provides adequate immunosuppression with less toxicity.[40] It appears that the nephrotoxicity and hypertension can be lessened, but not eliminated, in patients who develop the complications of cyclosporine administration over a period of some months. The cardiac transplant recipient appears to be uniquely at risk for acute renal failure when cyclosporine is used in the traditional perioperative doses. The combination of low cardiac output, cardiopulmonary bypass, and unstable cardiovascular status preoperatively and postoperatively is most likely responsible for this complication. Avoidance of cyclosporine until the recipient is hemodynamically stable has virtually eliminated acute renal failure.[41]

While most centers exhibit individuality to some degree in their postoperative immunosuppressive protocols, most are avoiding cyclosporine during the perioperative period of cardiovascular instability, using much lower chronic doses—between 2.5 and 5 mg/kg/day (less than 200 ng/ml plasma and less than 700 ng/ml whole blood radioimmunoassay). Azathioprine has generally been used during the early postoperative period (1–3 days), when cyclosporine has been avoided because of its nephrotoxicity. Recently, rabbit antithymocyte globulin or OKT3 has been used prophylactically in the immediate perioperative period, in an effort to suppress the initial rejection response.[42] Trials are in progress to test the advisability of continuing azathioprine with low doses of cyclosporine and maintenance doses of prednisone in doses of 10 to 20 mg/day. This three-drug regimen is believed to have fewer side effects and a lower incidence of infection than previously used immunosuppressive strategies.[44] In some instances, the use of prophylactic OKT3 has allowed discontinuation of maintenance corticosteroids in approximately half of the cardiac transplant recipients.[42]

Recalcitrant rejection is treated by pulse intravenous doses of corticosteroids or by temporarily increasing the oral dose of prednisone. Recalcitrant or severe rejection requires treatment with rabbit antithymocyte globulin or OKT3. If significant nephrotoxicity (creatinine value greater than 2.5 mg/dl) develops postoperatively, azathioprine is again substituted for cyclosporine. In the late postoperative period, a combination of low-dose cyclosporine (2.5 mg/kg/day) and azathioprine has been used in patients with nephrotoxicity in an effort to slow the progressive deterioration in renal function.

The use of rabbit antithymocyte globulin or OKT3 has been associated with allergic responses and liberation of lymphokines and other substances associated with the destruction of T cells. In order to reduce the severity of the systemic response to these agents, pretreatment with corticosteroids, antihistamines, and an antipyretic agent is recommended. The response to these agents is characterized by the development of hives, fever, chills, hypotension, local erythema, induration, pain, and other characteristics of an anaphylactoid reaction. Some patients develop serum sickness–like symptoms later in the course of the administration of these agents. In addition, OKT3 is associated with a decrease in myocardial function, hypoxia, pulmonary edema, bronchospasm, and aseptic meningitis in some instances. OKT3 is best avoided in patients with excess intravascular volume or a poorly functioning transplanted heart.[42]

POSTOPERATIVE SURVEILLANCE

The frequency of acute rejection decreases over the first year following cardiac transplantation. The incidence of acute rejection for patients receiving azathioprine has been calculated to be one episode per 23 patient-days during the first 3 months, and one episode per 325 patient-days 2 to 5 years following transplantation.[4,45] Continued efforts to find more acceptable immunosuppressive agents have led to the experimental use of FK506.[43] No precise statistics are available for patients receiving cyclosporine, but it is estimated that acute rejection occurs with approximately the same incidence.[46]

CLINICAL MANIFESTATIONS

Rejection classified as mild to moderate is unassociated with symptoms or significantly abnormal physical findings. Not until severe rejection occurs are the clues to cardiac dysfunction present. Patients often relate a history of lethargy, easy fatigability, weakness, and return of breathlessness. In our experience with cyclosporine-treated patients, the abrupt development of hypotension (often over a 12-hour period within the first 2 postoperative weeks) has been associated with moderately severe to severe rejection, frequently requiring the supportive use of inotropic agents, and the addition of rabbit antithymocyte globulin or OKT3 to the immunosuppressive regimen until the rejection crisis has resolved. Moderately severe rejection may be manifested by the presence of a third or fourth heart sound. Other concomitants of congestive heart failure such as an increase in venous pressure, hepatic congestion, development of peripheral edema, and weight gain usually occur later in the course of rejection.[4]

ENDOMYOCARDIAL BIOPSY DIAGNOSIS OF REJECTION

Ideally, a diagnosis of acute rejection of the transplanted heart is established by the technique of transvenous endomyocardial biopsy introduced by Caves in 1972.[47] This advance contributed greatly to the prolonged survival of transplant recipients by allowing earlier initiation of augmented immunosuppressive therapy. With the use of local anesthesia, a biopsy forceps is percutaneously inserted into the internal jugular vein and fluoroscopically guided into the body of the right ventricle, where a number of endomyocardial biopsy specimens can be obtained. This is done weekly for the first 6 weeks following transplantation, with decreasing frequency thereafter, unless clinical circumstances suggest otherwise. Episodes of rejection beyond 6 months are infrequent.[4,45]

Experience in interpretation of these biopsy specimens has been reported by Billingham.[48] Mild acute rejection is manifested by a sparse perivascular lymphocytic infiltrate and a minor degree of subendocardial lymphocytic accumulation. Activated lymphocytes may be identified by the pyroninophilic reaction. Moderate acute rejection is identified by a more prominent infiltration of lymphocytes in a pattern similar to that shown in mild rejection reaction, with the addition of an increased interstitial mononuclear infiltration and focal myocytolysis. Severe acute rejection is characterized by more intense mononuclear infiltration, infiltration of neutrophils, eosinophils, interstitial hemorrhage, intravascular microthrombi, and more prominent myocyte necrosis. Resolving and resolved rejection show a decreased or absent cellular infiltration, active fibrosis and scar formation, inactive mononuclear cells (absence of pyroninophilic reaction), and residual lipochrome pigment. The rejection reaction seen in patients treated with cyclosporine is similar to that for patients receiving azathioprine, with the following exceptions: (1) widely dispersed interstitial mononuclear cells are not necessarily associated with rejection; (2) moderate rejection is associated with more extensive myocyte necrosis and hemorrhage; (3) acute rejection reactions resolve less quickly and have more prolonged evidence of myocyte damage; and (4) a fine diffuse interstitial fibrotic reaction has been observed, which is believed to result from cyclosporine administration alone and to be independent of prior rejection episodes.

DETECTION OF REJECTION USING NONINVASIVE TECHNIQUES

Methods to monitor cardiac rejection following transplantation have been diligently sought. Since the introduction of cyclosporine as an immunosuppressive agent, serial monitoring of electrographic voltage has not been useful in detecting rejection. Likewise, serial M-mode and two-dimensional echocardiography and radionuclide scanning procedures have been of little use in the diagnosis of rejection. Thus, despite the time, expense, and inconvenience of myocardial biopsy, it remains the standard for detection of myocardial rejection.

PHYSIOLOGY OF THE TRANSPLANTED HEART

Following cardiac transplantation, an opportunity exists to study cardiovascular physiology of the denervated heart in the presence of a normally innervated peripheral vascular system. Permanent cardiac denervation in the transplanted heart has been established by observing the lack of heart rate response to baroreceptor stimulation using carotid massage, Valsalva maneuver, and amyl nitrite inhalation, phenylephrine infusion, and tilting.[49,50]

CARDIAC OUTPUT IMMEDIATELY AFTER TRANSPLANTATION

In the immediate postoperative period, the cardiac output of the donor heart is severely depressed. An increase in heart rate results in an increase in cardiac output because the stroke volume remains fixed for the first 4 to 5 days. During this period, the normal inverse relationship between heart rate and stroke volume is not observed. Administration of inotropic agents augments cardiac output during the immediate postoperative period, and cardiac output gradually returns toward normal during the first postoperative week.[51] Later, the normal inverse relationship between heart rate and stroke volume again becomes operative.

RESPONSE OF THE DENERVATED HEART TO DYNAMIC EXERCISE

Dynamic exercise creates a response in a denervated heart that differs from that of the innervated heart. In the normal circumstance, the onset of exercise is associated with an increased heart rate, primarily as a result of withdrawal of vagal tone at moderate levels of exercise. At increased exercise levels, heart rate increases as a result of the direct chronotropic effect of sympathetic stimulation.[52] In the transplanted heart, the initial increase in heart rate is more gradual, probably reflecting an increase in circulating catecholamines. Additional increases in exercise-induced heart rate occur in direct proportion to an increase in circulating catecholamines and can be attenuated by β-adrenergic blocking agents.[53] The peak heart response is less than that of normal controls. When exercise is stopped, the heart rate and cardiac output only gradually return to normal as the catecholamine level falls.[54] With submaximal exercise, the initial response of the cardiac output in the denervated heart is dependent on the Frank-Starling principle: An increase in venous return results in an increase in left ventricular filling, followed in turn by an increase in stroke volume. As the exercise period is extended, a rise in circulating catecholamines results in an increased heart rate and an increased velocity of circumferential fiber shortening, that is, a positive inotropic and chronotropic effect.[50,52]

Peak heart rate and cardiac output response to exercise is blunted following cardiac transplantation.[55] The cardiac transplantation patient relies on an increased oxygen extraction and experiences greater lactate production at the time of maximal exercise, thus indicating a greater degree of anaerobic metabolism.[55]

RESPONSE OF THE DENERVATED HEART TO DYNAMIC EXERCISE AND HAND GRIP

The interplay between the denervated heart and the innervated peripheral vascular system has been studied by observing the response to isometric exercise in the form of hand grip. In normal persons and transplant recipients, the major response to isometric exercise is an increase in blood pressure and peripheral vascular resistance, with little change in cardiac output and only a slight increase in heart rate in subjects with normally innervated hearts.[56]

PHYSIOLOGY OF HETEROTOPIC CARDIAC TRANSPLANTATION

The physiology of the patient with heterotopic cardiac transplantation is more complex.[57] The parallel arrangement between the native and donor hearts dictates that the relative compliance of the native and donor ventricles will determine the relative contribution of each heart to the cardiac output. In patients with high pulmonary vascular resistance, the native right ventricle will support pulmonary flow to a greater extent, while the more compliant donor left ventricle will support the systemic circulation. The interplay between the cardiac output of the native and donor hearts may alter with time, since there is a gradual fall in the pulmonary vascular resistance as the function of the native heart continues to deteriorate or as the function of the donor heart is altered by the onset of rejection.[57] Alterations in preload and afterload occur on a beat-to-beat basis and have marked influence on the cardiac function at any given moment.

ELECTROPHYSIOLOGY OF THE TRANSPLANTED HEART

The denervated transplanted heart offers an ideal opportunity to study the intrinsic electrical activity of the heart in the absence of the autonomic influences.[58] Because the suture line between the donor and recipient atria effectively blocks electrical interchange at the atrial level, no relationship exists between donor and recipient atrial activity, both of which can be recorded separately. In fact, independent atrial arrhythmias such as sinus rhythm in the recipient atrium and atrial flutter in the donor atrium (and vice versa) have been observed. The sinus node and the adrenergic receptors of the cardiac conduction system function normally, in the absence of autonomic innervation. Sinus node dysfunction has been demonstrated in approximately 50% of the patients studied in the early postoperative period and may portend a poor prognosis.[59] Sinus node dysfunction in long-term survivors of cardiac transplantation is associated with abnormal sinus node automaticity and prolongation of the PR interval while in sinus rhythm. A comparison of the electrophysiologic characteristics of the denervated atrioventricular node and the innervated atrioventricular node indicates that the autonomic nervous system has little influence on atrioventricular conduction under resting conditions.[60]

Extensive studies of the electrophysiology of the ventricles have not been conducted. However, permanent perioperative right bundle branch block is a frequent concomitant of cardiac transplantation.

PHARMACOLOGY

A thorough understanding of the effects of drugs on the transplanted heart is important when one wishes to intervene therapeutically. The direct cardiac effect of physiologic and pharmacologic manipulation may be dissociated from the autonomically mediated effects of these interventions by observing the divergent response of the innervated recipient atrium and the denervated donor atrium. The effect of a drug on the peripheral vascular system is characterized by changes induced in the venous capacitance and arterial resistance. The following general rules apply[57]:

1. The transplanted heart is not affected by drugs that act via the autonomic nervous system.
2. The cardiac receptors may be more responsive to β-agonists.
3. Drugs with intrinsically negative inotropic or chronotropic effects may not be well tolerated, since these effects cannot be offset by autonomically mediated increases in sympathetic tone.

Similarly, drugs that cause peripheral vasodilation and a reduction in venous return may compromise left ventricular function, which is dependent mainly on the Frank-Starling principle for maintenance of cardiac output.

DRUGS ACTING VIA THE AUTONOMIC NERVOUS SYSTEM

DIGOXIN. The predominant mechanism of the electrophysiologic effect of digoxin in the normally innervated heart results from its interaction with the autonomic nervous system. In the transplanted denervated heart, however, there is minimal prolongation of the atrioventricular node conduction time when digoxin is administered acutely.[61] Chronic administration may have more of an effect on atrioventricular conduction; however, tachycardia is required for this effect to be manifest. From a therapeutic standpoint, digoxin is of little value in the treatment of supraventricular arrhythmias in the transplanted heart. Digitalis does exert a direct inotropic effect on the denervated heart and a vasoconstrictive effect on the peripheral vascular tree.

ATROPINE AND EDROPHONIUM. Since the effect is mediated vagally, these drugs have no effect on the transplanted heart.

ANTIARRHYTHMIC AGENTS

QUINIDINE SULFATE. The administration of quinidine sulfate has two consequences: a direct electrophysiologic effect and a peripheral vasodilatory effect. In the denervated heart, quinidine significantly increases sinus cycle length, the atrial refractory period, and the HV interval. It also results in significant vasodilation resulting in a decrease in venous return, cardiac output, and arterial pressure. These effects are not offset by an increase in sympathetic tone, as would occur in the normally innervated cardiovascular system. Cardiac contractility *per se* is unchanged.[62] From a therapeutic standpoint, the direct electrophysiologic effect of quinidine sulfate makes it useful in controlling atrial and ventricular arrhythmias. Most patients tolerate quinidine without difficulty, despite the peripheral hemodynamic effects of quinidine sulfate.

PROCAINAMIDE. No study of the electrophysiologic and hemodynamic consequences of procainamide administration has been reported. One would expect its effects to be similar to other type 1 antiarrhythmics. This drug is well tolerated in our experience and has been therapeutically useful for the control of atrial and ventricular arrhythmias.

DISOPYRAMIDE PHOSPHATE. The acute administration of disopyramide phosphate causes a significant prolongation of donor atrial cycle length and all conduction intervals in the transplanted heart. The marked negative inotropic effect of disopyramide phosphate, combined with the depression of electrical activity, suggests that caution should be exercised in the therapeutic application of this drug.[63]

CATECHOLAMINES

The adrenergic receptors of the denervated heart remain functional in the absence of autonomic influences,[49] but catecholamine depletion of the denervated heart increases its sensitivity to catecholamine infusion.[57] Norepinephrine and isoproterenol infusion decrease the sinus cycle length and shorten the AH interval. In circumstances in which direct inotropic and chronotropic support of the transplanted heart is required, catecholamine infusion is of benefit. Dobutamine is especially helpful in supporting patients during a rejection crisis, which is often associated with a decreased cardiac output and systemic arterial pressure.

β-ADRENERGIC BLOCKADE

The chronotropic response of the transplanted heart to stress is mediated by circulating catecholamines.[53] Stroke volume is augmented in part by an increase in venous return using the Frank-Starling principle and in part by the inotropic effect of circulating catecholamines. The administration of β-blocking drugs impairs the functional response of the transplanted heart.[53] β-Blockade also competitively inhibits the cardiac response to catecholamine infusion. Nevertheless, β-blocking drugs have been well tolerated when used for treatment of the hypertension that develops following cyclosporine administration.[26] Usually, the addition of β-blocking agents has not resulted in significant lowering of the resting heart rate, thus indicating that the intrinsic rate of the transplanted heart is influenced little by the sympathetic nervous system.

CALCIUM ANTAGONISTS

VERAPAMIL. The intravenous administration of verapamil results in an immediate increase in the sinus node cycle length, indicating suppression of sinus node automaticity. Verapamil prolongs the AH interval and increases the antegrade refractory period of the atrioventricular node.[64] There has been little experience with verapamil in patients following cardiac transplantation. It may be useful in situations in which an increase in atrioventricular node refractory period is desirable, such as in the treatment of supraventricular tachycardia. The direct depressant effect on myocardial contractility and the conduction system, combined with its lesser peripheral vascular effects, may be associated with unwanted side effects, however.

NIFEDIPINE. Nifedipine has no direct electrophysiologic effect on the heart. It does, however, result in systemic hypotension as a result of its vasodilatory effect.[54] Therapeutically, nifedipine has been used in the treatment of postoperative hypertension developing in transplant patients receiving cyclosporine and has been well tolerated. Whether this drug will have any role in the management of coronary vasospasm—rarely reported in the denervated heart—remains to be seen.

CARDIZEM. Cardizem has been used to treat hypertension following cardiac transplantation. One of the main and most important side effects of this drug is an interaction with cyclosporine which causes an elevation of the cyclosporine level. This interaction must be taken into account when Cardizem and cyclosporine are to be used simultaneously.

VASODILATOR THERAPY

Hydralazine and minoxidil have been used to control the hypertension associated with cyclosporine administration.[65] The reflex tachycardia usually associated with these agents has not been a problem clinically in our heart transplantation patients, probably because the transplanted heart is denervated. Further controlled observation of this phenomena is necessary.

ARRHYTHMIAS

Cardiac arrhythmias are common following cardiac transplantation. Atrial arrhythmias have been reported in as many as 70% of post-transplant patients.[66] In the early postoperative period, sinus bradycardia, junctional rhythm, and junctional escape rhythms are not uncommon, perhaps as a result of reversible operative injury to the sinoatrial node. Permanent pacemakers have been used to treat patients with symptomatic bradyarrhythmias resulting from sinus node dysfunction.

The development of atrial premature beats, atrial flutter, and atrial fibrillation frequently coincides with the occurrence of a rejection reaction.[66] These atrial arrhythmias may be successfully treated with overdrive atrial pacing, synchronized direct-current cardioversion, or the use of type 1 antiarrhythmic agents.[66] Late in the post-transplant period, atrial arrhythmias continue to be common, with atrial premature contractions, paroxysmal atrial tachycardia, and sinus arrest being manifest.[66]

In the early post-transplant period, ventricular premature beats occur in more than 50% of patients.[56] Ventricular arrhythmias are less frequently reported with acute rejection reactions than atrial arrhythmias, but two patients experienced ventricular fibrillation at the height of a rejection crisis.[66] As the time following cardiac transplantation lengthens, nearly 100% of patients ultimately develop premature ventricular activity.[66] Complex ventricular ectopy is a precursor of sudden death in many patients following transplantation and is associated with extensive accelerated atherosclerosis in a majority of instances.[66,67] These complex arrhythmias may be identified using ambulatory electrocardiographic monitoring and are useful in identifying patients with extensive left ventricular damage as a result of myocardial fibrosis for whom cardiac retransplantation may be considered.

INFECTIONS

In the first decade of cardiac transplantation, infections accounted for a large portion of all postoperative deaths.[68] Although mortality from infection was highest in the first 3 months, 40% of all deaths within 2 years of transplantation were still attributed to infection. At Stanford University, 61% of all infections were caused by bacteria, 22% by viruses (predominantly members of the herpes group), and 13% by fungi. Protozoa and nocardia made up the remaining 10% of significant pathogens.[9] The organisms most frequently associated with a fatal outcome were gram negative bacteria and aspergillus.[9] The lungs were the most frequently involved site (47% of all episodes), followed by the bloodstream (10%), urinary tract (6%), and a host of sites of lesser importance.[69] Data acquired in the 1980s suggest that both infection rates and the death rate from infection have declined.[136,137] It is not clear to what extent this is due to the superiority of cyclosporine-containing immunosuppressive regimens, and to what extent it is due to general advances in medical and surgical care. In Dr. Dummer's recent review of infectious complications of transplantation, 56 of 119 patients (47%) died during the followup period. In this group, 30 of the 56 patients who died had infection. However, in only 15 of 56 patients (13%) was infection thought to be primarily responsible for death. Similarly, in recent published data from Stanford, approximately 8% of the first year postoperative deaths were attributed to infection, but only 6% of deaths *after* one year.[85] The lungs still remain the major site of infection, even in patients treated with cyclosporine. Infectious complications in cardiac allograft recipients on cyclosporine are certainly no more severe, and probably somewhat milder, than those in patients on conventional azathioprine regimens.[26]

Individual variations in immunosuppression related to rejection treatment are also important determinants of infectious morbidity. For example, patients with significant rejection episodes requiring augmented immunosuppression with pulse doses of corticosteroids and antithymocyte globulin demonstrate a 2.5- to 12-fold increase in infectious rates during the 3 months following treatment of a rejection episode.

SITES OF INFECTION

LUNGS. A wide range of pathogens can involve the lungs in the transplant patient, and infections with multiple organisms are sometimes seen. Therefore, empiric treatment is rarely possible or justified. Expectorated sputum is often adequate to make a presumptive diagnosis, particularly when the gram stain is inspected by a trained observer and the clinical course suggests acute bacterial pneumonia. In situations where the patient cannot produce a sputum sample, various invasive techniques can be used to obtain material for culture: transtracheal aspiration, bronchoscopy, bronchoalveolar lavage, and open lung biopsy. Percutaneous lung aspiration is also useful in the diagnosis of peripheral lung nodules. Bronchoalveolar lavage is especially useful when *Pneumocystic carinii* is suspected.[19]

MEDIASTINUM AND STERNUM. Mediastinitis and sternal infections are unusual following transplantation but may occur as late as 4 weeks after surgery and present with relatively subtle clinical signs. Treatment consists of surgical drainage and long courses of intravenously administered antibiotics. Cure is possible with combined surgical and medical therapy.[19]

CENTRAL NERVOUS SYSTEM. Central nervous system infections occur in about 5% of cardiac transplant patients and involve a wide range of pathogens, including *Aspergillus, Toxoplasma, Cryptococcus, Listeria,* varicella zoster virus, *Nocardia,* and routine bacterial pathogens.[70] The onset of central nervous system infection may be indolent and the presentation subtle, particularly in cryptococcal meningitis. A high index of suspicion must be maintained if an early diagnosis of treatable central nervous system disease is to be made.

SKIN. Minor skin infections occur frequently after transplantation. Most common are folliculitis, herpetic eruptions, warts, and dermatophyte infections. These are a significant nuisance and often require persistent or intermittent topical care. The skin may be involved in disseminated infections, and attention should be given to unusual skin lesions. Skin biopsy has helped diagnose disseminated cryptococcal and nocardial infections.

TYPES OF INFECTION

HERPES SIMPLEX VIRUS. About half of all transplant patients shed herpes simplex virus postoperatively, and about half of these patients have clinical stomatitis, esophagitis, or genital lesions.[26] In general, we treat all cases of documented esophagitis, and most cases of genital herpes are also severe enough to require intravenous antiviral therapy. Oral herpes is treated if pain is present and impairs eating. Most cases occur in the first 2 to 3 weeks, but some occur later. On rare occasions, herpes simplex virus may cause visceral disease such as hepatitis or pneumonia in transplant patients.[68,71] Although these infections are uncommon, one must be alert to their potential occurrence because antiviral therapy may be lifesaving.

CYTOMEGALOVIRUS. Cytomegalovirus (CMV) is a significant cause of morbidity and mortality after heart transplantation. Eighty to 90% of individuals have evidence of infection by positive viral cultures.[72,138] Many of these infections are asymptomatic, but 15% to 40% of infected patients may have symptoms varying from a self-limited febrile illness to severe pneumonitis. In the azathioprine era, 10% to 20% of patients were reported to have pneumonitis due to CMV, but rates of 6% or less have been reported recently.[72,136,137] Antibody titers from CMV should be measured on all candidates before transplantation. Since the donor heart may transmit CMV infection to the recipient, many centers also measure donor CMV antibody titers. Surveillance cultures for CMV should be performed every 2 to 3 weeks for the first 2 to 3 months after transplantation to assess the presence of active infection. In recent years there have been a number of promising new approaches to the treatment or prophylaxis of CMV infection in transplant recipients. These include the prophylactic use of I.V. hyperimmune globulin or high-dose oral acyclovir and the therapeutic use of ganciclovir.[150-152] Although these approaches have not been specifically validated or approved for heart or heart-lung transplant recipients, each is promising in its own right, and further investigation of their uses in heart and heart-lung transplantation can be expected.

HERPES ZOSTER. Herpes zoster (shingles) occurs in about 10% of transplant patients.[73] Most cases are uncomplicated; routine antiviral therapy should be employed if there is any evidence of cutaneous or visceral dissemination. Patients who develop varicella (chickenpox) after cardiac transplantation may have a severe or fatal course, and antiviral therapy is probably indicated in all patients as soon as the diagnosis is made. Patients known to be susceptible to varicella are candidates for prophylaxis with varicella-zoster immune globulin after household or other close exposure to chickenpox.[74]

TOXOPLASMA. Evidence of toxoplasmosis at autopsy has been shown in the heart, lungs, pericardium, and brain of patients with primary infection.[75] Diagnosis is difficult in the absence of tissue evidence of disease, but pre- and post-transplant serologic testing may help provide evidence of infection. Because this infection is usually derived from the donor heart, serum should be obtained from heart donors to test for toxoplasma antibody titers. If a serum-negative recipient receives a heart from a serum-positive donor, he should be carefully followed for toxoplasma infection. Some centers recommend the institution of prophylaxis (Pyrimethamine) in such patients, but the risks and benefits of such treatments have not yet been clearly defined.[153]

NOCARDIA. *Nocardia* represents approximately 5% of all clinical infectious episodes encountered at Stanford University during the post-transplant period.[68] *Nocardia* is restricted to the lungs in about 80% of cases but may disseminate to the skin or brain. The discovery of a lung nodule or abscess on the chest roentgenogram may lead to the diagnosis, and the response to antimicrobial therapy (sulfamethoxazole) is good.

PNEUMOCYSTIS CARINII. *Pneumocystis carinii* pneumonia occurs in up to 3% to 10% of all cardiac transplant recipients, usually presenting between the 2nd and 12th months.[69,136] The onset may be acute or subacute. Breathlessness and fever are the most common symptoms; cough, when present, is nonproductive. The classic radiographic pattern is diffuse interstitial and alveolar infiltrates, but focal patterns may be seen and occasionally chest roentgenograms are initially clear. About 75% of patients respond to either pentamidine isethionate or sulfamethoxazole-trimethoprim.[76] The latter drug is usually used because of lower toxicity. Prophylaxis with orally administered sulfamethoxazole-trimethoprim effectively prevents the disease and should be considered when the incidence of the disease is high.[77]

PERIOPERATIVE MANAGEMENT

At the time of transplant surgery, patients should receive prophylactic antibiotics highly active against staphylococci. The choice of antibiotic depends on local factors such as the presence of methicillin-resistant staphylococci in the hospital flora. During the initial post-transplant hospitalization, patients are kept in private rooms, masks are worn, and strict handwashing is implemented. Nystatin is administered orally three to four times a day to suppress fungal colonization and prevent thrush. Surveillance cultures for bacteria and fungi are not performed.

MALIGNANT TUMORS

Administration of cytotoxic agents is associated with an increased incidence of malignant neoplasms, regardless of indication for use, that is, for immunosuppressive or chemotherapeutic purposes. The incidence of malignancy following transplantation is estimated to be 4% (1–6%), or 100 times greater than in the general population.[78]

The experience of the Groote Schuur Hospital suggests that patients undergoing cardiac transplantation have a threefold increase in incidence of neoplasm when compared with the renal transplant recipients.[79] It has been proposed that the observed increase in neoplastic disease in cardiac transplant patients may be related to their more intensive immunosuppressive therapy.[39] Whether the use of rabbit antithymocyte globulin in conjunction with cyclosporine increases the risk of neoplasm remains to be determined. The tumors most frequently seen are squamous cell carcinoma, acute leukemia, adenocarcinoma (lung and gastrointestinal), Kaposi's sarcoma, and lymphomas (often involving the central nervous system).[9,45]

LYMPHOPROLIFERATIVE DISEASE

Transplant patients have an increased risk of developing neoplasms of the lymphoid system.[79] Many of these lymphoproliferative lesions contain the genome of Epstein-Barr virus (EBV) and their occurrence is frequently associated with serologic evidence of EBV infection.[80,81] The observation that some of these tumors regress following reduction of immunosuppression places them in a unique category of immune-responsive tumors.[82] The underlying biology of these lesions is being investigated at a number of centers, and many factors are still unclear. Hanto and co-workers suggest that two separate clinical groups may be represented: (1) a younger population with infectious mononucleosis–like symptoms and polyclonal proliferation of virally infected cells and (2) an older group presenting with localized tumor masses composed of a monoclonal population of B-cells. The older patients presented later after transplantation; 91% had a malignant course and fatal outcome.[80] In cyclosporine-treated patients, the tumors present earlier (often within the first 8 months), and no association between the behavior of the tumor and the patient's age or clonality of the lesion is seen.[81,82] A strong association with serologic evidence of EBV infection and EBV markers was found in 82% of all tumors. Patients with primary EBV infection were at particularly high risk of developing these syndromes.[81]

The management of the tumors is controversial. Currently, a substantial reduction in the dose of cyclosporine, and frequent cardiac biopsies to monitor rejection, are recommended. Acyclovir has been promoted as a possible treatment because of its known *in vitro* effect against EBV replication.[80,82,83] Localized tumors may respond to resection or radiation.[80,84]

PATHOLOGIC FINDINGS FOLLOWING CARDIAC TRANSPLANTATION

Pathologic findings in transplant recipients can be placed in three categories—acute rejection, infection, and chronic rejection—depending on the duration of elapsed time since transplantation. In the absence of other complications, initial interest in the post-transplant period (fewer than 90 days) is directed toward identification of the acute rejection response so that necessary modifications of the immunosuppressive therapy may be made.

Graft failure accounts for approximately half of the initial 10% mortality that occurs within the first 30 days following cardiac transplantation.[114] In some instances graft failure is attributed to hyperacute rejection caused by complement-fixing antibodies directed against DR antigens on the vascular endothelium.[29,35] Postmortem examination of patients who die within 90 days of cardiac transplantation usually demonstrate one of three findings: 1) graft failure (of undetermined cause), 2) acute cardiac rejection (as previously described), or 3) evidence of overwhelming infection. In one series of postmortem examinations reported by Uys and Rose, 14 of 29 patients died within 3 months of cardiac transplantation.[86] Acute rejection accounted for 2 deaths and was complicated by infection in a third, 2 patients died of acute right heart failure as a result of pulmonary hypertension, infections (pulmonary in 3 cases) resulted in the deaths of 4 patients, and miscellaneous causes accounted for the deaths of the remaining patients. This experience is in keeping with the cause of death within 30 days reported by the Registry of the International Heart Transplantation Society.[114]

MYOCARDIAL FIBROSIS AND ACCELERATED CORONARY ARTERY ATHEROSCLEROSIS AS A MANIFESTATION OF CHRONIC REJECTION

Myocardial fibrosis has two etiologies. The first is the result of previous rejection episodes resulting in scar formation. The second is the result of myocardial ischemia leading to myocardial necrosis and scar formation, undoubtedly the result of accelerated atherosclerosis, which impairs myocardial blood supply.

While the etiology of atherosclerosis of the transplanted heart has not been fully evaluated, it is postulated that it develops in response to the rejection reaction that takes place at the endothelial surface of the graft vasculature, representing the interface between graft and host. In experimental animals, the transplanted heart has been used as a model to study coronary atherosclerosis in an attempt to modify its development using interventional therapy.[87]

Accelerated atherosclerosis is one of the limiting factors in the long-term survival of transplant recipients and may become clinically important as early as 12 months postoperatively. In the experience at Stanford University, 40% of patients develop angiographic coronary vascular disease within 5 years of transplantation.[88] The vascular disease associated with transplantation represents a mixture of proximal lesions simulating typical atherosclerotic plaques and diffuse obliterative coronary disease with an immunologic component. Numerous studies have been done in an effort to identify factors such as hyperlipidemia, immunologic markers, and a number of rejection episodes that correlate with the development of accelerated coronary atherosclerosis.[89,90] To date, no widely demonstrable correlates have been identified. The use of interventional therapy such as anticoagulants or antiplatelet therapy has been inadequate to prevent the rapid development of atherosclerosis in the transplanted heart.[89] Thus, new approaches for the control of the immunologic and hyperlipidemic contributions to accelerated atherosclerosis are required.

OTHER LATE COMPLICATIONS ASSOCIATED WITH CARDIAC TRANSPLANTATION

In long-term survivors of cardiac transplantation, death has been associated with chronic rejection, cerebral embolus, bacterial and viral infections, and malignancy, including carcinoma of the lung and gastrointestinal tract, as well as melanoma and lymphoproliferative disease.[85] The importance of chronic rejection as a cause of death in the long-term survivors of cardiac transplantation is emphasized.[86] Old and recent myocardial infarction and chronic severe vascular disease contribute to graft failure. Evidence of acute rejection was also found in association with chronic rejection in some of the long-term survivors.

COMPLICATIONS OF IMMUNOSUPPRESSIVE AGENTS
CYCLOSPORINE

Since its introduction into clinical practice in 1978, cyclosporine has received widespread acceptance as the immunosuppressive agent of choice in renal, liver, and cardiac transplantation procedures.[91-94] As further experience with this agent has been gained, however, two notable and unexpected side effects have been observed: the almost universal development of systemic hypertension and progressive nephrotoxicity.[36,91-94] These side effects may ultimately limit the long-term usefulness of this drug as an immunosuppressive agent.

HYPERTENSION. Hypertension is a frequent concomitant of cyclosporine administration, occurring in 60% to 95% of patients undergoing cardiac transplantation; in 13% of renal transplantation patients; and in 27% of liver transplant patients. The etiology of the hypertension (which develops between 6 days and 6 months) has not been fully elucidated but has been associated with an increase in intravascular volume as a result of salt and water retention, normalization of the cardiac output, maintenance of an abnormally elevated peripheral vascular resistance, distorted autonomic innervation, and modest renal dysfunction.[41,65] Carruthers and co-workers have also suggested that vascular α-receptor hypersensitivity may contribute to the development of accelerated systemic hypertension following transplantation.[95] As the renal failure becomes more severe, marked elevation of peripheral renin activity suggests a renovascular component to the *de novo* hypertension. When the cyclosporine dose is lowered to 2 mg/kg/day in combination with azathioprine, there is a modest fall in blood pressure.[26]

Twenty-four-hour blood pressure monitoring in patients who have undergone cardiac transplantation demonstrates failure of the systolic and diastolic pressures to fall during sleep, in sharp contrast with the response of patients having essential hypertension in whom there is a night-time fall of the systolic and diastolic blood pressures of 10% to 15%. The sleeping heart rate also falls to a lesser extent in patients who undergo cardiac transplantation compared with those having essential hypertension. Both of these observations are believed to be related to the denervated state of the heart following transplantation via an associated imbalance between the increase in central circulating volume occurring during sleep, a persistently increased systemic vascular resistance in the innervated peripheral vascular system, and absence of neural autoregulation of the transplanted heart.[26]

The hypertension associated with cyclosporine administration is relatively resistant to treatment. Management of this hypertension is empiric and involves the stepwise use of a diuretic in an effort to reduce intravascular volume, use of a vasodilator to reduce the peripheral vascular resistance, and the use of β-blockade. Angiotensin-converting enzyme inhibitor has been useful in the treatment of hypertension, especially in patients who demonstrate an elevation of the peripheral renin activity a year or more following transplantation. In patients with more resistant hypertension, the use of minoxidil has become increasingly necessary.[26,96]

NEPHROTOXICITY. Nephrotoxicity of cyclosporine represents the most serious side effect and has acute and chronic components. The acute renal failure at the time of cardiac transplantation is characterized by oliguria and an increased sodium avidity.[97] Impairment of renal function in the immediate postoperative period occurs in approximately 60% of patients receiving cyclosporine and may require dialysis in approximately 10% of patients.[97] This immediate postoperative complication may be avoided by delaying cyclosporine administration until an adequate postoperative urinary output has been established. This experience is in contrast to the finding of only modest postoperative impairment of renal function in transplant patients receiving azathioprine.

Chronic impairment of renal function after long-term administration of cyclosporine is also a frequent finding in patients undergoing cardiac transplantation,[97] as well as in those undergoing renal transplantation[98,99] and liver transplantation.[94] The rise in the serum creatinine value has been gradual over time, with the prevalence of renal impairment increasing in the same group of patients as well. The mean serum creatinine level and the prevalence of renal impairment at 6, 12, and 36 months is 1.7 mg/dl and 38%, 2.3 mg/dl and 78%, and 2.5 mg/dl and 100%, respectively.[26] The nephrotoxicity of cyclosporine has reversible and irreversible components. The reversible component of renal dysfunction has been demonstrated in a group of 20 patients with a mean serum creatinine value of 3.6 ± 0.85 mg/dl, in whom this value fell to 2.2 ± 0.5 mg/dl when the patients were switched to a combination of low-dose cyclosporine and azathioprine.[19] Even with the low dose of cyclosporine, the renal function remained impaired. The irreversible component of renal failure may be related to the tubular atrophy and interstitial parenchymal fibrosis seen in renal biopsies obtained in this group of patients. As the nephrotoxicity progresses, there is glomerular loss and arteriolar hyalinization.[100]

MODIFICATION OF DOSAGE. These observations on the combination of systemic hypertension and progressive renal failure have prompted an alteration in the immunosuppressive protocols in which cyclosporine is used. These modifications have been described in the section on immunosuppression.

MISCELLANEOUS SIDE EFFECTS. Other less serious complications of cyclosporine administration have been reported. Hepatotoxicity is characterized by a rise in the serum bilirubin level and the alkaline phosphatase activity; serum transaminase activity is elevated to a lesser extent, and the overall picture is one of cholestasis.[99,101] Gingival hyperplasia and hirsutism have also been noted.[102] Gastrointestinal symptoms characterized by nausea, vomiting, and disorders of motility are seen in association with higher doses of cyclosporine. Acute pancreatitis has also been reported. Seizures have been seen in persons receiving cyclosporine and may be related in part to the development of hypertension.[93,103] Pericardial effusion is a not infrequent postoperative finding in patients receiving cyclosporine and may require pericardiocentesis and/or subxiphoid drainage in some instances because of the development of postoperative cardiac tamponade.

Intravenous administration of cyclosporine may be associated with significant systemic side effects, including shortness of breath, hypotension, nausea, vomiting, and, under extreme circumstances, anaphylaxis.[104] Important drug interactions that must be considered when cyclosporine is administered are summarized in Table 118.2.[105] The ethanol used in preparation of oral and intravenous forms of cyclosporine may react adversely in patients receiving disulfiram, cefamandole, cefaperazone, moxalactam, chlorpropamide, and metronidazole. Hyperkalemia may be associated with concomitant administration of potassium-sparing drugs, angiotensin-converting enzyme inhibitors, or excess potassium supplementation because of cyclosporine-induced hypoaldosteronism.[106]

SIDE EFFECTS OF OTHER IMMUNOSUPPRESSIVE AGENTS

The side effects of the conventionally used immunosuppressive agents —corticosteroids, azathioprine, antithymocyte globulin, and OKT3— have been described.[43,107]

PSYCHIATRIC ADJUSTMENT TO CARDIAC TRANSPLANTATION

Study of the psychiatric aspects of cardiac transplantation has led to the identification of seven transitional psychological stages.[108-110]

The *first stage* begins when transplantation is proposed. The patient frequently expresses fear and disbelief that his physical condition demands such drastic intervention.

The *second stage* is the evaluation period, characterized by hope for future improvement, often in association with a large element of denial of the potential hazards of the procedure. A great deal of anxiety and distress is experienced by the patient and the family until a final decision is made regarding acceptance into the program.

The *third stage*, the waiting period following acceptance into the program, is often characterized by relief and by fear that a donor will not become available in time. Frequently, the patient simply wants to have the operation completed, regardless of the outcome, just to be able to escape this time of uncertainty.

The immediate post-transplant period (*fourth stage*) is characterized by relief and often euphoria in patients who make a rapid recovery. Patients must also resolve the psychological issue of having a "new" heart. The symbiotic nature of this relationship is best described by the question, "Is the new heart keeping me alive, or am I keeping the new heart alive?"

The first rejection episode (*fifth stage*) represents the fifth stressful period in the recipient's life. The patient must now come to understand that long-term treatment is still required, in spite of the significant improvement in physical well-being that is being experienced. The recovery period is characterized by gradual improvement, punctuated by minor setbacks as a result of rejection or infection. Often, depression and withdrawal are noted in association with these complications.

The time of hospital discharge—the *sixth stage*—again raises anxiety associated with separation from the hospital and staff, while at the same time bringing to fruition the hope of recovery. Reestablishment of a normal life-style must be emphasized. The emotional and physical "rebirth" of the patient cannot be denied and contributes substantially to the perceived attitude of the patient and the family.

The final stage, the *seventh*, is the long-term follow-up period. During this time, the importance of long-term compliance with therapy must be emphasized. In the Cape Town center experience, 25% of late deaths were attributed (directly or indirectly) to noncompliance.[111] Emotional problems frequently arise as a result of role reversal following transplantation and the inability to accept a state of dependency.[108]

LONG-TERM FOLLOW-UP

The initial period of hospitalization is 4 to 6 weeks. The majority of recipients return to their homes, and arrangements are made for intermittent evaluation for possible rejection, infection, and the side effects of renal toxicity and hypertension due to cyclosporine administration.

TABLE 118.2 DRUG INTERACTIONS AFFECTING CYCLOSPORINE

Increased Blood Levels	Increased Nephrotoxicity	Decreased Blood Levels
Corticosteroids	Melphalan	Phenytoin
Ketoconazole	Aminoglycosides	Phenobarbital
Cimetidine	Amphotericin B	Rifampin
Erythromycin	Cephalosporins	Carbamazepine
Diltiazem	Trimethoprim-sulfamethoxazole	Primidone
		Glutethimide
		Sulfatrimethoprim I.V.

(Hansten PD: Cyclosporin Interactions. Adapted from the Drug Interactions Newsletter 4/8, August 1984, published by Applied Therapeutics, Inc., P.O. Box 1903, Spokane, WA 99210)

During the first 6 months, the endomyocardial biopsy, whole blood cyclosporine trough level, and renal and hepatic functions are monitored at 2- to 4-week intervals; after 6 months, the frequency of these evaluations depends primarily on the presence or absence of rejection and renal toxicity.

Coronary arteriography, endomyocardial biopsy, and an assessment of hemodynamic status are performed annually. Noninvasive evaluation of cardiovascular function may be conducted in addition to the routine annual catheterization, which is done primarily to detect the development of accelerated graft atherosclerosis. Thallium treadmill testing may be used to document exercise-induced myocardial ischemia.[112] Ambulatory electrocardiographic monitoring is useful to document the presence of complex ventricular ectopy, which is associated with extensive graft atherosclerosis.[57] These long-term observations are used to identify patients in whom retransplantation may be considered.

During long-term followup of transplant recipients, complications requiring general surgical intervention occur in approximately 30% of patients. These problems require close cooperation with the general surgical consultant and prompt, aggressive intervention if a favorable outcome is to be achieved.[113]

SURVIVAL STATISTICS

Through the cooperation of 118 transplantation centers worldwide, the International Heart Transplantation Society Registry has been compiled.[114] At the present time, data accumulated from 1968 through 1988 are available; during that time, 9,139 patients undergoing orthotopic cardiac transplantation were entered into the Registry. The mean age was 43.8 years (range newborn to 48 years). The earlier exponential increase in the number of patients undergoing cardiac transplantation has slowed, with a plateau of 1500 to 1600 transplantation procedures per year performed in the United States. This is in accord with the estimated number of 2,000 donor hearts that are available each year within the U.S.

Long-term followup data on patients through 1989 is now available: the 1-year actuarial survival rate for orthotopic cardiac transplantation is 73.9%. For patients receiving cyclosporine, the 5-year actuarial survival rate is 78%. For those patients receiving triple immunosuppressive therapy, the actuarial survival rate for 5 years is 81.9%. Recent information shows that the indication for cardiac transplantation and the age of the recipient have no influence on the actuarial survival rate.

The overall improvement in survival rate from the initial 20% 1-year survival (1968) to the present 70% to 80% 5-year actuarial survival rate is a truly remarkable achievement in less than 2 decades. Likewise, the 73% 10-year actuarial survival rate is a testimony to the therapeutic benefit of the procedure.

QUALITY OF LIFE ASSOCIATED WITH CARDIAC TRANSPLANTATION

Renal and cardiac transplantation patients adapt well to their situations when compared with the general population.[115] The functional rehabilitation of patients under age 30 is especially encouraging.[116] These patients can walk 1 mile or more and experience only moderate limitations during daily living. Perhaps the most compelling testimony to the contribution made by transplantation to the well-being of these patients and their families is embodied in the Transplantation Recipients International Organization (TRIO), a volunteer group established to provide transplant patients with support based on the experience of previous transplant recipients.*

---

* TRIO, P.O. Box 19791, Pittsburgh, PA 15213

THE FUTURE OF CARDIAC TRANSPLANTATION

Great strides have been made in the field of cardiac transplantation over the past 18 years. Yet no more than 6,500 people have had the opportunity to benefit from this procedure, the majority having done so within the past 5 years. Currently, limited donor availability is the major constraint on the number of transplant procedures that can be performed. Based on the present indications for cardiac transplantation and the number of available donors, it appears that it is now appropriate to have one transplantation program for every 15 million persons.[117] Further progress in the field of cardiac transplantation will require continued dedication to find solutions to problems now being encountered.

Finally, one possible alternative to cardiac transplantation lies in the development of a mechanical heart.[15,16] This device may provide a viable alternative to cardiac transplantation as it is now being practiced. Nevertheless, many of the same considerations discussed in this paper remain applicable, regardless of the procedure used.

CARDIOPULMONARY TRANSPLANTATION

Long-term survival following cardiopulmonary transplantation was first achieved at Stanford University by Dr. Bruce Reitz in 1981.[118] The experimental basis for cardiopulmonary transplantation was established in primates by Reitz using cyclosporine as the immunosuppressive agent.[119] The limited number of suitable donors for cardiopulmonary transplantation results in extended and often unrewarding waiting periods and accounts for the relatively few procedures that have been accomplished in the past 8 years. Early postoperative mortality and an increased incidence of postoperative complications, including the long-term development of obliterative bronchiolitis, make the results of cardiopulmonary transplantation less satisfactory than that of cardiac transplantation alone,[120] and these limitations must be fully understood by all who become involved with this procedure.

SELECTION OF CANDIDATES

Candidates for cardiopulmonary transplantation have severe pulmonary vascular disease as a result of primary pulmonary hypertension or pulmonary hypertension secondary to congenital heart disease complicated by Eisenmenger's syndrome.[118,120–122] Cardiopulmonary transplantation may also be considered for primary pulmonary disorders such as emphysema, idiopathic pulmonary fibrosis, recurrent pulmonary emboli, eosinophilic granuloma, cystic fibrosis, pulmonary veno-occlusive disease, sarcoidosis, angiomyomatosis, or α_1-antitrypsin deficiency.[120] Some of these conditions may be treated by single or bilateral lung transplantation alone, as opposed to combined cardiopulmonary transplantation.[120] Patients with preexisting infection in the tracheobronchial tree that cannot be eradicated, those with chest wall deformities, and those with systemic enzymatic deficiencies are not ideal candidates for cardiopulmonary transplantation. Candidates should not have had prior extensive intrathoracic operative procedures because these persons often experience difficult-to-control hemorrhage postoperatively. Even prior lung biopsy or prior pulmonary emboli may have associated pleural adhesions that result in postoperative hemorrhage. Extensive bronchial collateral circulation to the lungs is another source of bleeding, which may be fatal.

Candidates for cardiopulmonary transplantation should be symptomatic at rest. They often have P_{O_2} values of less than 50 mm Hg on room air and may require supplemental oxygen at rest. The primary criteria for selecting candidates are similar to those for cardiac transplantation[120]:

1. Terminal pulmonary vascular disease with a life expectancy of 6 to 12 months, recognizing that it is difficult to project life expectancy, especially in patients with Eisenmenger's syndrome

2. Age preferably younger than 50 years. Currently, the youngest surviving cardiopulmonary recipient is 3 years old.
3. Normal renal and hepatic function (bilirubin < 3.5 mg/dl)[106]
4. Absence of active infection
5. Absence of insulin-dependent diabetes mellitus and hyperglycemia
6. Absence of steroid dependence and a short duration of disability is ideal
7. Psychosocial stability and a supportive social milieu

Significant cachexia or tricuspid insufficiency with resultant hepatic dysfunction have been emphasized as contraindications to cardiopulmonary transplantation because of the hepatotoxicity and nephrotoxicity of cyclosporine.[118] A relatively close size match between recipient and donor lung volumes is also important.

The immunologic considerations for cardiopulmonary transplantation are similar to those for cardiac transplantation; the major difference in the criteria between cardiac and cardiopulmonary transplantation is that one can consider patients for cardiopulmonary transplantation regardless of the extent of pulmonary vascular disease.

SELECTION OF DONORS

It is estimated that the donor pool for cardiopulmonary transplantation is only 10% to 20% the size of the cardiac pool, which currently is estimated to be 2,000 hearts per year.[111,112] The heart and lung donor should be younger than 35 years, there should be no thoracic injury, preexisting cardiopulmonary disease, pulmonary infiltrate on the chest roentgenogram, or sepsis. The electrocardiogram should be normal. Extensive inotropic support of the cardiovascular system should not be required.[118,125] Every effort should be made to ensure sterility in the tracheobronchial tree since postoperative infection is a frequent complication even under optimal circumstances. Screening bronchoscopy may be done in some instances. Arterial oxygen tension in the donor should exceed 100 mm Hg on 40% oxygen and 300 mm Hg on 100% inspired oxygen. Lung compliance should be normal, with a peak inspiratory pressure of less than 30 mm Hg and a normal tidal volume. The donor and recipient should be closely matched with respect to weight and thoracic circumference. Other criteria are similar to those for cardiac alone.

OPERATIVE PROCEDURE

The technique for the cardiopulmonary donor and recipient procedure has evolved in stepwise fashion and has been described in detail in several publications.[120,126-128] Basically, the donor operation involves procurement of a heart-lung bloc using a median sternotomy and bilateral thoracotomy. Flush perfusion of the heart-lung preparation with a Euro-Collins solution has allowed distant transport of the organs.[129] This method of preservation and transport is generally acceptable and satisfactory and may be augmented by the addition of prostaglandins to the perfusate.[126]

The recipient operation involves the removal of the native heart and lungs through a median sternotomy.[118,120-122] The most important part of this operation is meticulous attention to establishment of hemostasis, especially in the posterior mediastinum, as well as preservation of the left and right phrenic nerves. Phrenic nerve function is essential for maintenance of adequate postoperative diaphragmatic innervation. During implantation of the donor organs, the tracheal anastomosis is performed one or two rings above the carina. Incorporation of adventitial tissue from the peritracheal region and the use of an omental wrap at the completion of the operation may supplement the bronchial collateral circulation and improve healing at the site of anastomosis. Circumferential anastomosis at the right atrium of the donor and recipient hearts and that of the ascending donor aorta with the recipient aorta reestablishes the circulation.

IMMUNOSUPPRESSION

Immunosuppression consists of azathioprine, 4 mg/kg intravenously, and methylprednisolone, 500 mg, intraoperatively. Postoperatively, cyclosporine is given in a dose that achieves a target whole blood level of approximately 700 ng/ml; the dose is then modified according to renal function.[63] After the initial bolus, corticosteroids are not administered during the first 14 days in order to facilitate healing of the tracheal anastomosis. A combination of azathioprine and cyclosporine supplemented by rabbit antithymocyte globulin constitutes the immunosuppressive protocol during the immediate postoperative period. Prednisone is added to the regimen beginning 2 to 3 weeks postoperatively, at a dose of 20 mg/day. Bolus corticosteroids are used for the treatment of cardiac or pulmonary parenchymal rejection after the first 2 weeks.[118,124,129]

EARLY POSTOPERATIVE CARE

Positive end-expiratory pressure of 5 to 15 cm H_2O is maintained in order to reduce the incidence of postoperative pulmonary edema. Inotropic support is usually required for the first 24 to 72 hours. Isoproterenol (Isuprel) is a useful inotropic agent following cardiopulmonary transplantation because of its bronchodilator effect. Other inotropic agents such as dopamine, dobutamine, and, in some cases, epinephrine are also useful. Denervation of the carina and tracheobronchial tree results in an absence of the cough reflex below the site of tracheal anastomosis. Blunted ciliary action and impaired clearing of pulmonary secretions make frequent endotracheal suction necessary.[120]

Postoperative bronchoscopic examination is useful to observe the suture line and to remove inspissated secretions. Reimplantation pulmonary edema occurs within the first 2 days, and a tendency to develop interstitial edema persists for the first 7 to 10 days.

COMPLICATIONS OF CARDIOPULMONARY TRANSPLANTATION

SURVEILLANCE FOR REJECTION

The ability to detect and treat acute and chronic pulmonary rejection following lung transplantation is essential for the long-term success of the procedure. Because there is no convenient and readily available diagnostic test to confirm this diagnosis, it must be made on clinical grounds.[130]

ACUTE LUNG REJECTION

Acute lung rejection is manifested clinically by the rapid development of diffuse roentgenographic infiltrates in the absence of infection after the ninth postoperative day. Clearing of these infiltrates following augmentation of the immunosuppressive regimen confirms the clinical judgment. Acute lung rejection occurs more frequently than cardiac rejection, and isolated pulmonary rejection is much more common than synchronous rejection of the heart and lungs. The differential diagnosis of radiographic infiltrates during the first 6 weeks may be facilitated by the use of bronchoalveolar lavage. Analysis of the lavage fluid may be useful in identifying infection but currently is not of great value in identifying characteristics of rejection.[120]

CHRONIC LUNG REJECTION

The most significant long-term complication of cardiopulmonary or pulmonary transplantation is the development of chronic rejection, characterized by recurrent respiratory tract infections and a combined obstructive and restrictive defect identified by pulmonary function testing.[120] Histologically, chronic rejection is characterized by obliterative bronchiolitis, with or without associated severe bronchitis and/or bronchiectasis.[131] It has been postulated that pneumocystis infection or "graft vs. host" disease may contribute to the development of obliterative bronchiolitis.[132] Chronic lung rejection occurs in approximately one third of long-term survivors of cardiopulmonary transplantation.[85]

More recent experience suggests that intensification of the immunosuppressive regimen may be of some benefit in retarding the development of this syndrome.

INFECTION

Infection is the most common cause of morbidity and mortality in cardiopulmonary recipients.[133,134] Infectious complications in these patients occur twice as frequently as in recipients of cardiac transplants alone, and the infections that occur are judged to be severe in 80% of these patients. Of long-term survivors, infection is a contributing factor to death in the majority of patients, whereas death in long-term survivors of cardiac transplantation alone is associated with infection in fewer than half.[135,136]

The lungs, mediastinum, and pleural spaces are the sites of infection in 60% to 90% of cardiopulmonary recipients.[134,137] Disseminated viral or fungal infections constitute the majority of the remaining infections. Invasive fungal infection occurring in approximately 25% of patients is usually fatal. Invasive *Candida* infections occur most often in conjunction with antibiotic-resistant bacterial infections and complicate the terminal illnesses in these patients.

Characteristic patterns of infection have been identified, depending on the length of time elapsed since the transplant procedure. The peak incidence of infection occurs within the first 3 to 6 months and usually involves serious viral infections (cytomegalovirus) and serious fungal infections (*Candida* and *Aspergillus*).[138] *Pneumocystis* infections do not occur until 3 months following transplant but then are prevalent throughout the subsequent follow-up period. Bacterial infections occur with equal frequency throughout the entire post-transplant period.

As might be expected, a number of unusual infections have been identified following cardiopulmonary transplantation. These include mediastinitis due to *Mycoplasma hominis*, toxoplasmosis, and documented lymphoproliferative syndromes related to primary EBV infection.[137]

The incidence of cytomegalovirus infection may be reduced by the use of cytomegalovirus-seronegative blood products following transplantation.[133,134,139] For cardiopulmonary recipients surviving for 6 months or longer, a syndrome characterized by chronic colonization of the tracheobronchial tree with *Pseudomonas aeruginosa* has been identified.[134] This infection is the source of significant morbidity and mortality.

INFECTIOUS SURVEILLANCE PROTOCOL

In addition to the monitoring recommended for heart transplant recipients, lung transplant recipients can be followed with routine surveillance gram stains and cultures of the sputum every few days while they are intubated in the intensive care unit. This practice is generally most helpful if a trained observer routinely assesses the gram stain for dramatic changes in white cells or bacterial populations that may signal an episode of pneumonia. It may also provide warning of antibiotic sensitivity patterns of colonizing bacteria. Colonization or subclinical infection of the donor lung is frequent, and monitoring of donor respiratory secretions by gram stain, and, if possible, culture is recommended before harvest.[154] A donor tracheal gram stain and culture should be performed at the time of implantation.

PATHOLOGIC FINDINGS FOLLOWING CARDIOPULMONARY TRANSPLANTATION

In animals, the acute rejection response as modified by cyclosporine immunosuppression is characterized by moderate perivascular and interstitial round cell infiltration.[140] Monocytes, desquamated pneumocytes, macrophages, and fibrous debris fill alveolar spaces, which are surrounded by hypoplastic alveolar lining cells. The interstitium of the lung is edematous, with fibrin deposits and fibrocytes. Predominating focal edema and round cell infiltrates are seen in the peribronchial and perivascular tissues.

CHRONIC PULMONARY REJECTION MODIFIED BY IMMUNOSUPPRESSIVE THERAPY

In humans, the gross pathology of the transplanted lung shows abnormalities of the visceral pleura.[85,131] Dense adhesions involve the chest wall and are associated with diffuse pleural fibrosis. The development of pleural thickening and the associated pleural adhesions make cardiopulmonary retransplantation more difficult, if not impossible, because of inability to control intrathoracic bleeding at the time of reoperation.

The pulmonary parenchyma shows cylindrical dilation of the bronchial tree with associated fibrous destruction of the bronchus and mucus plugging.[131] Histologically, bronchiolitis obliterans has been identified. Bronchial mucosal abnormalities include submucosal scarring, loss of ciliary epithelial cells, disruption of the elastic lamina, and loss of smooth muscle in the bronchial walls.[141] Concentric proliferative fibroelastosis in the elastic and muscular pulmonary arteries is associated with severe proliferative intimal thickening in the coronary arteries of the transplanted heart. Accelerated phlebosclerosis is also present in the pulmonary veins.

PHYSIOLOGIC ASSESSMENT

HEMODYNAMIC OBSERVATIONS

Postoperatively, the circulatory response to exercise is the major limiting factor. The heart rate and maximal oxygen consumption is blunted.[142] These observations are similar to those following cardiac transplantation.[143] Exercise is nevertheless well tolerated in patients without obliterative bronchiolitis.[142] Compared with the preoperative state, the cardiac output increases, the oxygen extraction decreases, and the tissue oxygen delivery improves in these patients postoperatively.[144]

PULMONARY FUNCTION TESTING

A mild restrictive defect is identified by pulmonary function testing 12 to 18 months postoperatively. Approximately 2 years postoperatively, a decrease in airway function is demonstrated by reduction in the $FEF_{25-75\%}$. The restrictive defect identified after the first year also becomes more prominent during the third year.[145] These changes in pulmonary function parallel those changes in recipients with chronic lung rejection and symptomatic bronchiolitis obliterans. These abnormalities in pulmonary function may be the physiologic manifestations of chronic rejection.[146]

LONG-TERM FOLLOW-UP

Follow-up of the cardiopulmonary recipient is similar to that of the cardiac recipient. Because *Pneumocystis carinii* infection frequently occurs in this group, all patients receive prophylactic trimethoprim-sulfamethoxazole. The transplanted lung is monitored by chest roentgenography, pulmonary function testing, and bronchial alveolar lavage every 3 months for the first year and once or twice a year thereafter. Complete pulmonary function tests are performed at 6 and 12 months.[120]

The relative lack of cardiopulmonary donors severely limits the number of retransplantation procedures. The major reason for considering retransplantation of the heart and lungs is the development of accelerated atherosclerosis of the donor heart and/or the development of obliterative bronchiolitis. Retransplantation for bronchiectasis and chronic pulmonary infection is relatively unsatisfactory because of the inability to sterilize the tracheobronchial tree prior to the procedure.

ALTERNATIVES TO CARDIOPULMONARY TRANSPLANTATION

SINGLE AND/OR DOUBLE LUNG TRANSPLANTATION

Under selected circumstances, single or double lung transplantation may be considered for some patients in whom combined cardiopulmonary transplantation is not required.[147-149] Patients with pulmonary fibrosis or alpha-1 antitrypsin deficiency and well-maintained cardiac function are ideal candidates for unilateral lung transplantation. Favorable results have been reported by the Toronto Lung Transplantation Group for patients undergoing unilateral lung transplantation.[147] Bilateral lung transplantation has been undertaken in selected patients having either primary pulmonary hypertension or cystic fibrosis. In these patients, cardiac function must be satisfactory at the time of the procedure. Additional experience must be gained before the role of these alternatives to cardiopulmonary transplantation can be assessed.

SURVIVAL STATISTICS[102]

The registry of cardiopulmonary transplantation now has data on approximately 501 procedures, half of which were performed in the United States.[114] Over the past several years, the number of cardiopulmonary transplants performed in this country has plateaued at approximately 70 per year, again reflecting the limited number of donors. The average age of the cardiopulmonary recipient is 29.4 years, with 59% being female. The actuarial survival rate for patients operated on between 1981 and 1986 is 55.7%, whereas for patients operated on in 1987, the one-year actuarial survival rate is 61%. Thus, there has been some improvement in the outlook for patients undergoing cardiopulmonary transplantation. It remains to be seen, however, whether favorable long-term survival can be achieved. In a cohort of 16 patients, the five-year actuarial survival rate is 55.4%.

THE FUTURE OF CARDIOPULMONARY TRANSPLANTATION

Cardiopulmonary transplantation has been practiced clinically only for the past 8 years. The operation should be limited primarily to those candidates with Eisenmenger's syndrome and primary pulmonary hypertension until better results are obtained. The prevention, diagnosis, and management of postoperative infections remain important goals. At present, there is a critical need to develop a reliable technique for the diagnosis of pulmonary rejection, which is as clinically applicable as is the endomyocardial biopsy technique for the identification of cardiac rejection. Refinement of the immunosuppressive protocols may lead to a reduction in both acute and chronic lung rejection and the concomitant development of obliterative bronchiolitis. With time and additional experience, it is anticipated that progress in cardiopulmonary transplantation will parallel that of cardiac transplantation.

REFERENCES

1. Lower RR, Shumway NE: Studies on the orthotopic homotransplantation of the canine heart. Surg Forum 11:18, 1960
2. Lower RR, Dong E, Shumway NE: Suppression of rejection crisis in the cardiac homograft. Ann Thorac Surg 1:645, 1965
3. Barnard CN: The operation: A human heart transplantation: An interim report of the successful operation performed at Groote Shuur Hospital, Cape Town, South Africa. S Afr Med J 41:1271, 1967
4. Baumgartner WA, Reitz BA, Oyer PE et al: Cardiac homotransplantation. Curr Probl Surg 16:1, 1979
5. Hakim M, Wreghitt T, Cory-Pearce R et al: Significance of donor-transmitted disease in cardiac transplantation. Heart Transplant 4:120, 1985
6. Thomas FT, Lower RR: Heart transplantation—1978. Surg Clin North Am 58:335, 1978
7. Evans RW: Economic and social costs of heart transplantation. Heart Transplant 1:243, 1982
8. Evans RW, Manninen DL, Garrison LP et al: Donor availability as the primary determinant of the future of heart transplantation. JAMA 255:1892, 1986
9. Pennock JL, Oyer PE, Reitz BA et al: Cardiac transplantation in perspective for the future: Survival, complications, rehabilitation, and cost. J Thorac Cardiovasc Surg 83:168, 1982
10. Medicare Program: Criteria for Medicare coverage of heart transplants. Fed Register 46:10935, 1987
11. Kormos RL, Thompson M, Hardesty RL et al: Utility of preoperative right heart catheterization data as a predictor of survival after heart transplantation. J Heart Transplant 5:391, 1986
12. Hardesty RL, Griffith BP, Trento A et al: Mortally ill patients and excellent survival following cardiac transplantation. Ann Thorac Surg 41:126, 1986
13. Kormos RL, Borovetz HS, Gasior T et al: Experience with univentricular support in mortally ill cardiac transplant candidates. Ann Thorn Surg 49:1, 1990
14. Pae WE, Miller CA, Pierce WS: Combined registry for the clinical use of mechanical ventricular assist pumps and the total artificial heart: Third official report—1988. J Heart Transplant 8:276, 1989
15. Kolff WJ: For the clinical application of the artificial heart. Heart Transplant 1:159, 1982
16. Pennock JL, Wisman CB, Pierce WS: Mechanical support of the circulation prior to cardiac transplantation. Heart Transplant 1:299, 1982
17. Watson DC, Reitz BA, Oyer PE et al: Sequential orthotopic heart transplantation in man. Transplantation 30:401, 1980
18. Gao SZ, Schroeder JS, Hunt S et al: Retransplantation for severe accelerated coronary artery disease in heart transplant recipients. Am J Cardiol 62:876, 1988
19. Barnard CN, Barnard MS, Cooper DKC et al: Present status of heterotopic cardiac transplantation. J Thorac Cardiovasc Surg 81:433, 1981
20. Kawaguchi A, Gandjbakhch I, Pavie A et al: Cardiac transplant recipients with preoperative pulmonary hypertension: Evolution of pulmonary hemodynamics and surgical options. Circulation (suppl 80/5):III–90, 1989
21. Griepp RB, Stinson EB, Clark DA et al: The cardiac donor. Surg Gynecol Obstet 133:792, 1971
22. Mulvagh SL, Thornton B, Frazier H et al: The older cardiac transplant donor: Relation to graft function and recipient survival longer than 6 years. Circulation (suppl 80/5):III–126, 1989
23. Schuler S, Warnecke H, Loebe M et al: Extended donor age in cardiac transplantation. Circulation (suppl 80/5):III–133, 1989
24. Starzl TE, Hakala TR, Shaw BW et al: A flexible procedure for multiple cadaveric organ procurement. Surg Gynecol Obstet 158:223, 1984
25. Schertz CW: Anesthesia for organ transplantation. In Flye MW (ed): Principles of Organ Transplantation. Philadelphia, WB Saunders, 1985
26. Thompson ME, Dummer JS, Griffith BP et al: Cardiac transplantation 1985: Hope—promise—reality. In Yu PN, Goodwin JF (eds): Progress in Cardiology, vol 14, ch 7. Philadelphia, Lea & Febiger, 1986
27. Bieber C, Stinson E, Shumway N: Immunology of cardiac transplantation. In Zabriskie JB, Engle MA, Villareal H (eds): Clinical Immunology of the Heart. Philadelphia, John Wiley & Sons, 1981
28. Carpenter CB, Strom TB: Transplantation immunology. In Parker CW (ed): Clinical Immunology. Philadelphia, WB Saunders, 1980
29. Duquesnoy R, Cramer DV: Immunologic mechanisms of cardiac transplant rejection. In Thompson ME (ed): Cardiac Transplantation, p. 87. Brest AN (ed-in-chief): Cardiovascular Clinics: 20/2. Philadelphia, FA Davis, 1990
30. Rabin BS: Immunologic aspects of human cardiac transplantation. Heart Transplant 2:188, 1983
31. Hall BM, Dorsch S, Roser B: The cellular basis of allograft rejection *in vivo*. J Exp Med 148:878, 1978
32. Dausset J, Rapaport FT: The role of blood group antigens in human histocompatibility. Ann NY Acad Sci 129:408, 1966
33. Stinson EB, Griepp RB, Payne R, Dong E Jr: Correlation of histocompatibility matching with graft rejection and survival after cardiac transplantation in man. J Thorac Cardiovasc Surg 63:344, 1982
34. Lanza RP, Campbell EM, Cooper DKC et al: The problem of the presensitized heart transplant recipient. Heart Transplant 2:151, 1983
35. Trento A, Hardesty R, Griffith B et al: Role of the antibody to vascular endothelial cells in hyperacute rejection of patients undergoing cardiac transplantation. J Thor Cardiovasc Surg 95:37, 1988
36. Kahan BD: Cyclosporine. N Engl J Med 321:1725, 1989
37. Borel JF: Cyclosporine: Historical perspectives. In Kahan DB (ed): Cyclosporine: Biological Activity and Clinical Applications, p 3. New York, Grune & Stratton, 1984
38. Griffith BP, Hardesty RL, Bahnson HT: Powerful but limited immunosuppression for cardiac transplantation with cyclosporine and low-dose steroid. J Thorac Cardiovasc Surg 87:35, 1984
39. Brumbaugh J, Baldwin J, Stinson EB et al: Quantitative analysis of immunosuppression in cyclosporine-treated cardiac transplant patients with lymphoma. Heart Transplant 4:121, 1985
40. Copeland JG: Cardiac transplantation. Curr Prob Cardiol 13, 1988
41. Greenberg A, Thompson ME: Cyclosporine-related hypertension and renal

failure after cardiac allografting. In Gallucci V, Bortolotti U, Faggian G et al (eds): Heart and Heart–Lung Transplantation Update. Padua, Italy, USES Edizioni Scientifiche Firenze, 1988

42. Bristow MR, Gilbert EM, Renlund DG et al: Use of OKT3 monoclonal antibody in heart transplantation: Review of the initial experience. J Heart Transplant 7:1, 1988
43. Starzl TE, Fung J, Venkataramman R et al: FK506 for liver, kidney, and pancreas transplantation. Lancet II:1000, 1989
44. Andreone PA, Olivari MT, Elick B et al: Reduction of infectious complications following heart transplantation with triple-drug immunotherapy. J Heart Transplant 5:13, 1986
45. Hunt SA, Stinson EB: Cardiac transplantation. Ann Rev Med 32:213, 1981
46. Cooper DKC, Novitzky D: Diagnosis and management of acute rejection. In Cooper DKC, Lanza RP (eds): Heart Transplantation. Boston, MTP Press, 1984
47. Caves PK, Stinson EB, Billingham ME et al: Serial transvenous biopsy of the transplanted human heart: Improved management of acute rejection episodes. Lancet 1:821, 1974
48. Billingham ME: Diagnosis of cardiac rejection by endomyocardial biopsy. Heart Transplant 1:25, 1980
49. Mason JW, Stinson EB, Harrison DC: Autonomic nervous system and arrhythmias: Studies in the transplanted denervated human heart. Cardiology 61:75, 1976
50. Stinson EB, Griepp RB, Schroeder JS et al: Hemodynamic observations one and two years after cardiac transplantation in man. Circulation 45:1183, 1972
51. Ingels NB Jr, Ricci DR, Daughters GT II et al: Effects of heart rate augmentation on left ventricular volumes and cardiac output of the transplanted human heart. Circulation 56(suppl 2):11, 1967
52. Hammond HK, Froelicher VF: Normal and abnormal heart rate response to exercise. Prog Cardiovasc Dis 27:271, 1985
53. Bexton RS, Hellestrand KJ, Cory-Pearce R et al: Effect of beta-blockade on the exercise response following cardiac transplantation. J Am Coll Cardiol 1:722, 1983
54. Pope SE, Stinson EB, Daughters GT II et al: Exercise response of the denervated heart in long-term cardiac transplant recipients. Am J Cardiol 46:213, 1980
55. Savin WM, Gordon E, Green S et al: Comparison of exercise training effects in cardiac denervated and innervated humans. J Am Coll Cardiol 1:722, 1968
56. Haskell WL, Savin WM, Schroeder JS et al: Cardiovascular responses to hand grip isometric exercise in patients following cardiac transplantation. Circ Res 48(suppl 1):156, 1981
57. Horak AR: Physiology and pharmacology of the transplanted heart. In Cooper DKC, Lanza RP (eds): Heart Transplantation. Boston, MTP Press, 1984
58. Bexton RS, Nathan AW, Hellestrand KJ et al: Sinoatrial function after cardiac transplantation. J Am Coll Cardiol 3:712, 1984
59. Mackintosh AF, Carmichael DJ, Wren C et al: Sinus node function in the first three weeks after cardiac transplantation. Br Heart J 48:485, 1982
60. Bexton RS, Nathan AW, Hellestrand KJ et al: The electrophysiologic characteristics of the transplanted human heart. Am Heart J 107:1, 1984
61. Goodman DJ, Rossen RM, Cannom DS et al: Effect of digoxin on atrioventricular conduction: Studies in patients with and without cardiac autonomic innervation. Circulation 51:251, 1975
62. Mason JW, Winkle RA, Rider AK et al: The electrophysiologic effects of quinidine in the transplanted human heart. J Clin Invest 59:481, 1977
63. Bexton RS, Hellestrand KJ, Cory-Pearce R et al: The direct electrophysiological effects of disopyramide phosphate in the transplanted heart. Circulation 3:97, 1984
64. Bexton RS, Nathan AW, Cory-Pearce R et al: Electrophysiologic effects of disopyramide phosphate in the transplanted heart. Circulation 67:38, 1983
65. Thompson ME, Shapiro AP, Johnsen AM et al: New onset of hypertension following cardiac transplantation: A preliminary report and analysis. Transplant Proc 15:2573, 1983
66. Berke DK, Graham AF, Schroeder JS et al: Arrhythmias in the denervated transplanted human heart. Circulation 48(suppl 2):112, 1973
67. Pomhilt DW, Doyle M, Sagar KB et al: Prevalence and significance of arrhythmias in long-term survivors of cardiac transplantation. Circulation 66(suppl 1):219, 1982
68. Baumgartner WA: Infection in cardiac transplantation. Heart Transplant 3:75, 1983
69. Copeland JG, Stinson EB: Human heart transplantation. Curr Probl Cardiol 3:4, 1980
70. Hooper DC, Pruitt AA, Rubin RH: Central nervous system infection in the chronically immunosuppressed. Medicine 61:166, 1982
71. Taylor RJ, Saul SH, Dowling JH et al: Primary disseminated herpes simplex infection with fulminant hepatitis following renal transplantation. Arch Intern Med 141:1519, 1981
72. Pollard RB, Rand KH, Arvin AM et al: Cell-mediated immunity to cytomegalovirus infection in normal subjects and cardiac transplant patients. J Infect Dis 137:541, 1978
73. Ho M, Wajszczuk CP, Hardy A et al: Infections in kidney, heart and liver transplant recipients on cyclosporine. Transplant Proc 15:2768, 1983
74. Weller TH: Varicella and herpes zoster: Changing concepts of the natural history, control and importance of a not-so-benign virus. N Engl J Med 309:1362, 1983
75. Luft BJ, Naot Y, Araujo FG et al: Primary and reactivated *Toxoplasma* infection in patients with cardiac transplants. Ann Intern Med 99:27, 1983
76. Young LS: Trimethoprim-sulfamethoxazole in the treatment of adults with pneumonia due to *Pneumocystis carinii.* Rev Infect Dis 4:608, 1982
77. Hughes WT, Kuhn S, Chaudhary S et al: Successful chemoprophylaxis for *Pneumocystis carinii* pneumonitis. N Engl J Med 297:1419, 1977
78. Penn I: Tumor incidence in human allograft recipients. Transplant Proc 11:1047, 1979
79. Lanza RP, Hingham MA: Malignant neoplasm in the immunocompromised patient. In Cooper DKC, Lanza RP (eds): Heart Transplantation. Boston, MTP Press, 1984
80. Hanto DW, Cajl-Peczalska KJ, Frizzera G et al: Epstein-Barr virus (EBV)–induced polyclonal and monoclonal B-cell lymphoproliferative diseases occurring after renal transplantation: Clinical, pathologic, and virologic findings and implications for therapy. Ann Surg 198:356, 1983
81. Ho M, Miller G, Atchison RW et al: Epstein-Barr virus infections and DNA hybridization studies in post-transplantation lymphoma and lymphoproliferative lesions: Role of primary infection. J Infect Dis 152:876, 1985
82. Starzl TE, Nalesnik MA, Porter KA et al: Reversibility of lymphomas and lymphoproliferative lesions developing under cyclosporine-steroid therapy. Lancet 1:583, 1984
83. Hanto DW, Frizzera G, Gajl-Peczalska KJ et al: Epstein-Barr virus–induced B-cell lymphoma after renal transplantation: Acyclovir therapy and transition from polyclonal to monoclonal B-cell proliferation. N Engl J Med 306:913, 1982
84. Thiru S, Caine RY, Hagington J: Lymphoma in renal allograft patients treated with cyclosporin-A as one of the immunosuppressive agents. Transplant Proc 18:359, 1981
85. Billingham ME: The pathology of combined heart-lung transplantation. In Thompson ME (ed): Cardiac Transplantation, ch. 4. Brest AN, (ed-in-chief): Cardiovascular Clinics 20/2. Philadelphia, FA Davis, 1990
86. Uys CJ, Rose AG: Pathologic findings in long-term cardiac transplants. Arch Pathol Lab Med 108:112, 1984
87. Lurie KG, Billingham ME, Jamieson SW et al: Pathogenesis and prevention of graft arteriosclerosis in an experimental heart transplant model. Transplantation 31:41, 1981
88. Gao SZ, Alderman EL, Schroeder JS et al: Accelerated coronary vascular disease in the heart transplant patient: Coronary arteriographic findings. J Am Coll Cardiol 12:334, 1988
89. Hess ML, Hastillo A, Mohanakumar T et al: Accelerated atherosclerosis in cardiac transplantation: Role of cytotoxic B-cell antibodies and hyperlipidemia. Circulation 68(suppl II):94, 1983
90. Eich DM, Johnson DE, Hastillo A et al: Accelerated coronary atherosclerosis in cardiac transplantation. In Thompson ME (ed): Cardiac Transplantation, ch. 13. Brest AN, (ed-in-chief): Cardiovascular Clinics 20/2. Philadelphia, FA Davis, 1990
91. Bennett WM, Pulliam JP: Letter: Cyclosporine nephrotoxicity. Ann Intern Med 99:851, 1983
92. Calne RY, Rolles K, White DJ et al: Cyclosporin-A initially as the only immunosuppressant in 34 recipients of cadaveric organs: 32 kidneys, 2 pancreas, 2 livers. Lancet 2:1033, 1979
93. Griffith BP, Hardesty RL, Deeb GM et al: Cardiac transplantation with cyclosporin-A and prednisone. Ann Surg 196:324, 1982
94. Klintmalm GBG, Iwatsuki S, Starzl TE: Nephrotoxicity of cyclosporine in liver and kidney transplant patients. Lancet 1:470, 1981
95. Carruthers SG, Webster EC, Kostuk WJ et al: Accelerated systemic hypertension after cardiac transplantation—possible vascular alpha-receptor hypersensitivity. Am J Cardiol 53:334, 1984
96. Shapiro AP, Rutan G, Thompson ME et al: Hypertension following orthotopic cardiac transplantation. In Brest AN (ed): Cardiovascular Clinics. Philadelphia, FA Davis, 1988
97. Greenberg A, Egel JW, Thompson ME et al: Early and late forms of cyclosporine nephrotoxicity: Studies in cardiac transplant recipients. Am J Kidney Dis 9:12, 1986
98. Canadian Multicentre Transplant Study Group: A randomized clinical trial of cyclosporine in cadaveric renal transplantation. N Engl J Med 309:809, 1983
99. European Multicentre Trial Group: Cyclosporine in cadaveric renal transplantation: One-year follow-up of a multicentre trial. Lancet 2:986, 1983
100. Myers BD, Ross J, Newton L et al: Cyclosporine-associated chronic nephropathy. N Engl J Med 311:699, 1984
101. Schade RR, Guglielmi A, VanThiel DH et al: Cholestasis in heart transplant recipients treated with cyclosporine. Transplant Proc 15:2757, 1983
102. Cohen DJ, Loertscher R, Rubin MF et al: Cyclosporine—a new immunosuppressive agent for organ transplantation. Ann Intern Med 101:667, 1984
103. Joss DV, Barrett AJ, Kendra JR et al: Hypertension and convulsions in children receiving cyclosporin-A. Lancet 1:906, 1982
104. Chapuis B, Helg C, Jeannet M et al: Letter: Anaphylactic reactions to I.V. cyclosporine-A. N Engl J Med 312:1259, 1985
105. Hansten PD: Cyclosporin Interactions. Adapted from the Drug Interactions Newsletter 4/8, August 1984, published by Applied Therapeutics, Inc., P.O.

Box 1903, Spokane, WA 99210

106. Bantle JP, Nath KA, Sutherland DE et al: Effects of cyclosporine in the renin-angiotensin-aldosterone system and potassium excretion in renal transplant recipients. Arch Intern Med 145:505, 1985
107. Lanza RP: Other complications of transplantation and immunosuppression. In Cooper DKC, Lanza RP (eds): Heart Transplantation. Boston, MTP Press, 1984
108. Allender J, Shisslak C, Kaszniak A et al: Stages of psychological adjustment associated with heart transplantation. Heart Transplant 2:228, 1983
109. Lunde DT: Psychiatric complications of heart transplants. Am J Psychiatry 126:369, 1969
110. Watts D, Freeman AM III, McGiffin DG et al: Psychiatric aspects of cardiac transplantation. Heart Transplant 3:243, 1984
111. Cooper DKC, Lanza RP, Barnard CN: Noncompliance in heart transplant recipients: The Cape Town experience. Heart Transplant 3:248, 1984
112. Hess ML, Hastillo A, Wolfgang TC et al: The noninvasive diagnosis of acute and chronic cardiac allograft rejection. Heart Transplant 1:31, 1984
113. Steed DL, Brown B, Reilly JJ et al: The general surgical complications in heart and heart/lung transplantation. Surgery 98:739, 1985
114. Heck CF, Shumway SJ, Kaye MP: The registry of the International Society for Heart Transplantation: Sixth official report—1989. J Heart Transplant 8:271, 1989
115. Evans RW, Manninen DL, Maier A et al: The quality of life of kidney and heart transplant recipients. Transplant Proc 17:1579, 1985
116. Samuelsson RG, Hunt SA, Schroeder JS: Functional and social rehabilitation of heart transplant recipients under age thirty. Scand J Thorac Cardiovasc Surg 18:97, 1984
117. Copeland JG: Facts to be considered prior to undertaking a heart transplantation program. Heart Transplant 3:275, 1984
118. Reitz BA, Wallwork JL, Hunt SA et al: Heart-lung transplantation: Successful therapy for patients with pulmonary vascular disease. N Engl J Med 306:557, 1982
119. Reitz BA, Bieber CP, Raney AA et al: Orthotopic heart and combined heart and lung transplantation with cyclosporin-A immune suppression. Transplant Proc 13:393, 1981
120. Thompson ME, Dummer JS, Paradis I et al: Heart-lung transplantation. In Yu PN, Goodwin JF (eds): Progress in Cardiology, vol 16, chap 3. Philadelphia: Lea & Febiger, 1988
121. Lower RR: Heart-lung transplantation. Ann Thorac Surg 38:551, 1984
122. Starnes VA, Jamieson SW: Current status of heart and lung transplantation. World J Surg 10:442, 1986
123. Evans RW, Manninen D, Gersh BJ et al: The need for and supply of donor hearts for transplantation. Heart Transplant 4:57, 1984
124. Jamieson SW, Baldwin J, Stinson EB et al: Clinical heart-lung transplantation. Transplantation 37:81, 1984
125. Jamieson SW, Stinson EB, Oyer PE et al: Heart-lung transplantation for irreversible pulmonary hypertension. Ann Thorac Surg 38:554, 1984
126. Baldwin JC: Technique of heart-lung graft procurement and preservation. In Gallucci V, Bortolotti U, Faggian G et al (eds): Heart and Heart-Lung Transplantation Update. Padua, Italy, USES Edizioni Scientifiche Firenze, 1988
127. Hardesty RL, Griffith BP: Procurement for combined heart-lung transplantation: Bilateral thoracotomy with sternal transection, cardiopulmonary bypass, and profound hypothermia. J Thorac Cardiovasc Surg 89:795, 1985
128. Ladowski JS, Hardesty RL, Griffith BP: Protection of the heart-lung allograft during procurement. Heart Transplant 3:351, 1984
129. Griffith BP, Hardesty RL, Trento A et al: Heart-lung transplantation: Lessons learned and future hopes. Ann Thorac Surg 43:6, 1987
130. Chiles C, Guthaner DF, Jamieson SW et al: Heart-lung transplantation: The postoperative chest radiograph. Radiology 154:299, 1985
131. Yousem SA, Burke CM, Billingham ME: Pathologic pulmonary alterations in long-term human heart-lung transplantation. Hum Pathol 16:911, 1985
132. Epler GR: Bronchiolotis obliterans and airways obstruction associated with graft-versus-host disease. Clin Chest Med 9:551, 1988
133. Brooks RG, Hofflin JM, Jamieson SW et al: Infectious complications in heart-lung transplant recipients. Am J Med 79:412, 1985
134. Dummer JS: Infectious complications in heart and heart-lung transplant recipients: Incidence and management. Proceedings of the First European Congress on Transplantation, Venice, Italy, March 1987
135. Dummer JS, Bahnson HT, Griffith BP et al: Infection in patients on cyclosporine and prednisone following cardiac transplantation. Transplant Proc 15:2779, 1983
136. Hofflin JM, Potasman I, Baldwin JC et al: Infectious complications in heart transplant recipients receiving cyclosporine and corticosteroids. Ann Intern Med 106:209, 1987
137. Dummer JS: Infectious complications of transplantation. In Thompson ME (ed): Cardiac Transplantation, ch. 10. Brest AN, (ed-in-chief): Cardiovascular Clinics 20/2 Philadelphia, FA Davis, 1990
138. Dummer JS, White LT, Ho M et al: Morbidity of cytomegalovirus infection in recipients of heart or heart-lung transplantation who received cyclosporine. J Infect Dis 152:1182, 1985
139. Dummer JS, Montero CG, Griffith BP et al: Infections in heart-lung transplant recipients. Transplantation 41:725, 1986
140. Griffith BP, Hardesty RL, Trento A et al: Asynchronous rejection of heart and lungs following cardiopulmonary transplantation. Ann Thorac Surg 40:488, 1985
141. McDowell E, Barrett L, Harris C et al: Abnormal cilia in human bronchial epithelium. Arch Pathol Lab Med 100:429, 1976
142. Theodore J, Burke CM, Dawkins K et al: Circulatory versus respiratory limitations to exercise before and after human heart-lung transplantation. J Am Coll Cardiol 3:509, 1984
143. Savin WM, Haskell WL, Schroeer JS et al: Cardiorespiratory responses of cardiac transplant patients to graded, symptom-limited exercise. Circulation 62:55, 1980
144. Theodore J, Robin ED, Burke CM et al: Impact of profound reductions of PaO_2 on O_2 transport and utilization in congenital heart disease. Chest 87:293, 1985
145. Burke CM, Theodore J, Dawkins K et al: Post-transplant obliterative bronchiolitis and other late lung sequelae in human heart-lung transplantation. Chest 86:824, 1984
146. Theodore J, Jamieson SW, Burke CM et al: Physiologic aspects of human heart-lung transplantation: Pulmonary function status of the post-transplanted lung. Chest 86:349, 1984
147. Toronto Lung Transplant Group: Unilateral lung transplantation for pulmonary fibrosis. N Engl J Med 314:1140, 1986
148. Copeland JG: Editorial: Heart-lung transplantation: Current status. Ann Thorac Surg 43:2, 1987
149. Montefusco CM, Veith FJ: Lung transplantation. Surg Clin North Am 66:503, 1986
150. Snydman DR, Werner BG, Heinze-Lacey B et al: Use of cytmegalovirus immune globulin to prevent CMV disease in renal transplant recipients. N Engl J Med 317:1049, 1987
151. Balfour HH, Chase BA, Stapleton JT et al: A randomized, placebo-controlled trial of oral acyclovir for the prevention of cytomegalovirus disease in recipients of renal allografts. N Engl J Med 320:1381, 1989
152. Keay S, Bisset J, Merigan TC: Ganciclovir treatment of cytomegalovirus infections in iatrogenically immunocompromised patients. J Infect Dis 156:1016, 1987
153. Wreghitt TG, Hakim M, Gray JJ et al: Toxoplasmosis in heart and heart and lung transplant recipients. J Clin Pathol 42:194, 1989
154. Zenati M, Dowling RD, Dummer JS et al: Influence of the donor lung on the development of early infections in heart-lung transplant recipients. J Heart Transplant 8:95, 1989

INDEX

Numbers followed by *f* refer to figures; those followed by *t* refer to tables.

A

Abdominal examination, 3.14
Abscess, myocardial, color-flow Doppler of, 4.87, 28.126f
Absorption
  of drugs, 2.5
    and bioavailability, 2.5, 2.6, 12.7f
  of salt and water in renal tubules, 2.19–2.20, 13.1f–13.2f
Acebutolol, 8.22, 77.7t
  pharmacology of, 2.96, 2.97, 16.2t, 16.3t
Acetazolamide, 2.27, 13.1t
Acetylcholine
  effects on cellular electrophysiology, 6.6
  receptors for. See Muscarinic cholinergic receptors
Acetylsalicylic acid. See Aspirin
Acidosis
  effects of verapamil in, 1.69, 4.1f
  intracellular, in myocardial infarction, 7.121
Acrocyanosis, 12.41, 12.43
Acromegaly, 13.86
  hypertension in, 8.42
Acrosclerosis, cardiovascular disorders in, 3.12
ACTH production by pheochromocytomas, 8.37, 78.6f
Actin, 1.20–1.21, 1.22, 2.1f–2.2f
Action potential, cardiac, 1.24, 1.25, 2.6f, 6.2
  characteristics in different regions of heart, 6.4–6.5, 40.4f
  cycle-length dependency in steady state, 6.75–6.76, 45.10f–45.11f
  duration of
    antiarrhythmic drugs affecting, 6.77–6.78, 45.15f
    electrical restitution curve in, 6.74, 45.9f
    heart rate and rhythm affecting, 6.74–6.77
    and refractoriness, 6.5, 6.78, 45.16f
  and electrocardiography, 4.14, 4.15, 27.1f
  fast-response, 6.4
  ionic basis for, 6.3–6.5
  monophasic, recordings of. See MAP recording
  phases of, 6.3–6.4, 40.3f
  premature, 6.74
  rate adaptation in, 6.76, 6.77, 45.12f–45.13f
  relation to surface electrocardiography, 6.3, 40.2f
  slow-response, 6.4
  supernormal, 6.74
Addison's disease, 13.88
  electrocardiography in, 4.31
Adenosine
  and coronary resistance, 1.105–1.106
  intravenous, hemodynamic effects of, 2.66
Adenosine diphosphate (ADP) release from platelets, 2.143–2.144
Adhesions, pericardial, 10.40, 10.41, 92.3t
Adson maneuver in peripheral arterial disease, 12.36, 108.9f
Adrenal glands
  cortical diseases, 13.87–13.88
  disorders with hypertension, 8.36–8.41
  pheochromocytoma in, 13.86
  response to angiotensin II, 8.5–8.14, 76.4f–76.13f
α-Adrenergic blocking drugs, 2.91–2.94, 16.1f
  and activity of β-adrenergic blockers, 2.91, 2.97
  adverse effects of, 2.94
  in angina pectoris, 2.93
  in arrhythmias, 2.93
  in arterioconstriction, 2.94
  in bronchospasm, 2.94
  in heart failure, 2.93
  in hypertension, 2.92–2.93
  pharmacology of, 2.91
  in pheochromocytoma, 2.93–2.94
    preoperative, 8.83–8.39
  in prostatic obstruction, benign, 2.94
  in pulmonary hypertension, 2.94
  in shock, 2.94
β-Adrenergic blocking drugs, 2.94–2.103, 6.25–6.26, 6.39, 16.2f
  adverse effects of, 2.101–2.103
  in angina pectoris, 2.98–2.99, 7.71–7.72, 62.3t–62.4t
  compared to other antianginal drugs, 2.116, 17.6t
  in unstable angina, 7.78, 7.81–7.83, 63.3t–63.4t, 63.5f–63.7f
  in arrhythmias, 2.99–2.100, 6.15
  in cardiomyopathies, 2.100
    dilated, 10.16
    hypertrophic, 10.34
  characteristics of, 8.22–8.23, 77.7t
  choice of, factors in, 2.103, 16.5t
  concomitant activity of
    α-adrenergic blockage, 2.91, 2.97
    calcium channel blockage, 2.97
  in digitalis toxicity, 2.49
  in dissecting aneurysms, 2.101
  effects on transplanted heart, 13.97
  in epinephrine-induced hypokalemia, 2.101
  equivalent dosage of, 7.72, 62.4t
  in essential tremor, 2.101
  in hypertension, 2.98, 8.22–8.23, 77.7t–77.8t
  in elderly patients, 13.32
  in hyperthyroidism, 13.85
  interactions with other drugs, 2.102, 2.103, 2.177–2.178, 16.4t, 21.4t
    antiarrhythmic drugs, 2.175, 21.2t
    calcium entry blockers, 2.179, 21.5t
    nonsteroidal anti-inflammatory drugs, 2.181, 21.7t
    sympathomimetic drugs, 2.184, 21.8t
  in left ventricular hypertrophy, 2.101
  membrane stabilizing activity of, 2.96
  in migraine prophylaxis, 2.101
  in mitral valve prolapse, 2.100–2.101
  in myocardial infarction, 7.155–7.156
  in open angle glaucoma, 2.101
  partial agonist activity of, 2.96–2.97
  pharmacodynamic properties of, 2.96, 16.2t
  pharmacokinetic properties of, 2.97–2.98, 16.3t
  pharmacology of, 2.94
  in postinfarction prophylaxis, 7.233–7.234, 72.8t–72.9t
  potency of, 2.95
  in pregnancy, 13.22, 111.3t
  preoperative, in noncardiac surgery, 13.43–13.44
  in QT interval prolongation syndrome, 2.101
  selectivity of, 2.96
  in silent myocardial ischemia, 2.100, 7.98
  in supraventricular tachycardia, 6.138
  in survivors of acute myocardial infarction, 2.100
  sympathomimetic activity of, intrinsic, 2.96–2.97
  in tetralogy of Fallot, 2.101
  in thyrotoxicosis, 2.101
  withdrawal of, 2.101–2.102
Adrenergic nervous system, effects on cellular electrophysiology, 6.6
Adrenoreceptors, 1.47–1.59, 3.7f
  agonists and antagonists of, 1.49, 3.3t. See also α-Adrenergic blocking drugs; β-Adrenergic blocking drugs
  and blood flow to limbs, 1.117–1.118, 7.4f
  G proteins of, 1.45–1.47, 3.1t, 3.5f–3.6f
  in Raynaud's disease, 1.125
  responses mediated by, 1.48, 3.2t
β-Adrenoreceptors, 1.48, 1.56–1.59, 2.51–2.52, 3.2t, 8.23
  in cardiovascular disease, 1.59
  in pathologic conditions, 1.56
  pharmacology of, 1.56–1.57
  radioligand binding studies, 1.57
  receptor-effector coupling, 1.57–1.58, 3.10f
  regulation of, 1.58–1.59
  structure of, 1.57

I.1

β-Adrenoreceptors, 1.49–1.56, 2.51–2.52
 agonists of, 2.58
  partial, 2.57–2.58
 in cardiovascular disease, 1.55–1.56
 desensitization of, 1.51, 1.52–1.53, 3.9f
 distribution of, 1.50, 3.4t
 in pathologic conditions, 1.54–1.55, 3.5t
 radioligand binding studies, 1.49–1.50
 receptor-effector coupling, 1.50–1.52, 3.8f
 regulation of, 1.52
  down-regulation, 1.52
  up-regulation, 1.52–1.54
 structure of, 1.50
 supersensitivity of, 1.53–1.54
Aerospace medicine, G-force tolerance in, 1.172
After depolarizations, 6.7–6.9
 and arrhythmias, 6.16–6.17
 delayed, 6.8–6.9, 6.16–6.17, 40.8f
 early, 6.7–6.8, 6.17, 40.7f
 in long QT syndrome, 6.81–6.82
 MAP recordings of, 6.73
Afterload
 affecting ejection fraction, 5.8, 5.9, 34.8f
 and left ventricular performance, 1.85–1.86
 mismatch with preload reserve, 1.98, 5.21f
 reduction of, and colloid osmotic pressure, 1.150, 9.9f
Afterload agents, 9.6, 81.2t
Age
 and β-adrenoreceptor changes, 1.54, 1.55, 3.5t
 affecting drug disposition, 2.15
 and amyloid deposits in heart, 10.113
 and electrocardiography, 4.18
 and intracellular calcium levels, 1.71
 and rheumatic fever incidence, 10.98
Aging. See Elderly patients
AIDS, echocardiography in, 4.89
Alcohol interaction with anticoagulants, 2.153, 20.2t
Alcoholic heart disease, 12.1–12.11
 arrhythmias in, 12.9, 12.10, 12.11, 106.11f–106.12f
 cardiomyopathy in, 10.3, 12.2–12.5, 106.1f–106.6f
 chest pain in, 12.8–12.9
 course of, 12.9
 diagnosis of, 12.9–12.11
 heart failure in, 12.5–12.6, 12.7, 106.7f–106.9f
 hypertension in, 7.20, 7.21, 12.6–12.8, 59.10t, 106.10f
 management of, 12.11
 and negative inotropic action of ethanol, 12.11, 106.13f
Aldosterone, in renin-angiotensin-aldosterone system, 8.3–8.5, 76.1f–76.3f
Aldosteronism, 13.87–13.88
 clinical features of, 8.39
 computed tomography in, 8.39, 8.40, 78.7f
 hypertension in, 8.39–8.40
 laboratory studies in, 8.39–8.40
 pathophysiology of, 8.39
Aliasing, in pulsed-wave Doppler echocardiography, 4.36, 4.71, 28.93f
Alinidine in unstable angina. 7.86
Alkalosis, digitalis toxicity in, 2.46
Allen test in peripheral arterial disease, 12.36, 108.6f
Allergic angiitis and granulomatosis, 13.11
Allopurinol
 interaction with anticoagulants, 2.153, 2.187, 20.2t, 21.10t
 interaction with theophylline, 2.186, 21.9t
Alprenolol in postinfarction prophylaxis, 7.233, 72.9t
Alveolar hypoxia, 10.72
Amebiasis
 myocarditis in, 10.95
 pericarditis in, 10.59
Amiloride, 2.27, 13.1t
Amiodarone, 6.24–6.25, 6.48–6.49
 antiarrhythmic spectrum of, 6.48
 in dilated cardiomyopathy, 10.15
 dosage of, 6.49
 effects on heart and circulation, 6.25
 effects on transmembrane potential, 6.24–6.25
 electrophysiologic properties of, 6.48
 interactions with other drugs, 2.175, 2.176–2.177, 21.2t–21.3t
  β-adrenergic blocking drugs, 2.177, 21.4t
  anticoagulants, 2.153, 2.187, 20.2t, 21.10t
  digoxin, 2.47, 2.172, 21.1t
 oral therapy with, 6.48
 pharmacokinetics of, 6.48
 side effects of, 6.48–6.49
 in supraventricular tachycardia, 6.138
 in unstable angina, 7.80, 7.86–7.87, 63.3t
Amoxicillin in endocarditis prevention, 11.60
cAMP
 and cardiac contraction, 1.21, 1.23
 in platelets, drugs increasing, 2.148–2.149
Amphetamines
 abuse, 13.78
 interactions with antihypertensive drugs, 2.184, 21.8t
Amplatz catheters, 5.29, 35.23f
Amrinone, 2.61–2.62, 14.10f
 adverse effects of, 2.66, 14.7t
 in dilated cardiomyopathy, 10.15
 hemodynamic effects of, 2.66, 14.7t
Amyl nitrite inhalation
 in mitral valve prolapse, 9.32
 murmurs in, 3.40, 3.50, 23.11t
Amyloid heart disease, 10.112–10.114
 biopsy in, S.71, 5.72, 38.6f
 clinical features of, 10.113
 diagnosis of, 10.113–10.114, 97.7f
 in rheumatoid arthritis, 13.4
Anaerobic threshold in exercise, 1.129–1.130
Anatomy of heart, 1.2–1.3
 anterior view, 1.2f, 1.4
 aortic valve, 1.8f, 1.9, 1.10, 1.11f, 1.11–1.12
 conduction system, 1.12–1.13, 1.12f–1.15f
 coronary arteries, 1.9, 1.9f, 1.13–1.15, 1.16f–1.17f
 external configuration, 1.2f, 1.3–1.5
 internal structure, 1.5–1.12
 intramural vessels, 1.15–1.16, 1.18f
 left atrium, 1.8f–1.10f, 1.9–1.10
 left ventricle, 1.6f, 1.7, 1.10, 1.11, 1.11f
 lymphatics, 1.16
 mitral valve, 1.9–1.10, 1.10f–1.11f
 nerve supply, 1.17–1.18, 1.19f
 pericardium, 10.38, 10.39, 92.1f
 posterior view, 1.2f, 1.4
 pulmonary arteries, 1.2f, 1.4, 1.8–1.9, 1.14, 1.16f
 pulmonic valve, 1.8, 1.8f–1.9f, 1.9
 right atrium, 1.3f–1.5f, 1.5–1.7
 right ventricle, 1.5f, 1.6, 1.8
 tricuspid valve, 1.6f–1.7f, 1.7–1.8
 venous system, 1.16f–1.17f, 1.14, 1.15, 1.16
Androgenic steroids, toxic effects of, 13.79
Anemia
 cardiac output increase in, 1.157
 coronary blood flow in, 1.112
Anesthesia
 interaction of agents with sympathomimetic drugs, 2.184, 21.8t
 physiologic effects of, 13.47
 in cardiac surgery, 13.52–13.53, 114.1f–114.3f
Aneurysms
 aortic, 12.27–12.33 See also Aorta, aneurysms of
 of aortic sinus, 3.66–3.67
 coronary artery, congenital, 11.23–11.24, 11.25, 99.14f–99.15f
 mycotic
  of aorta, 12.34–12.35
  arterial, in endocarditis, 9.79
  peripheral arterial, 12.40–12.41, 108.13f–108.15f
 ventricular
  chronic, antithrombotic therapy in, 2.164
  length-tension relations in, 1.156, 10.1f
  in myocardial infarction, 7.126–7.127, 7.198, 7.199, 70.8f
  surgery in, 7.272–7.273
  postinfarction, echocardiography of, 4.48, 4.49, 4.50, 28.26f–28.38f, 28.42f–28.43f
  traumatic, 12.17
  in viral myocarditis, 10.88
Angina pectoris, 7.48–7.50, 7.62–7.73
 α-adrenergic blocking drugs in, 2.93

β-adrenergic blocking drugs in,
2.98–2.99, 7.71–7.72,
62.3t–62.4t
in aortic valvular stenosis, 9.109
calcium channel blockers in,
2.113–2.115, 7.72–7.73, 17.5t,
62.5t
β-adrenergic blocking drugs with,
2.99
characteristics of, 7.49, 61.1t
clinical features of, 7.64–7.65
coronary angiography in, 7.68
after coronary angioplasty, 7.243
coronary vasomotion in, 7.63–7.64
differential diagnosis of, 7.65–7.66
in elderly patients, 13.29
evaluation of, 3.4–3.6
exercise in, 7.69
exercise tolerance test in, 7.67–7.68
glycosides in, 2.43
grading by Canadian Cardiovascular
Society, 7.69, 62.1t
natural history of, 7.68–7.69
nitrates in, 2.80–2.81, 7.70–7.71, 62.2t
β-adrenergic blocking drugs with,
2.99
mechanisms of efficacy in, 2.80, 15.3t
selection of patients in, 2.81, 15.4t
nocturnal, 3.5
noncardiac surgery in, 13.42–13.44
pathology of, 7.62
physiologic considerations in, 7.62–7.64
placebo effect in, 7.70
postinfarction, 3.5
bypass surgery in, 7.265–7.266
at rest, 7.48–7.49, 7.65
in rheumatoid arthritis, 13.5
sexual activity in, 7.69–7.70
and silent ischemia, 7.94–7.95,
64.4f–64.5f
smoking affecting, 7.69
stable, 7.62–7.73
antithrombotic therapy in, 2.162
bypass surgery in, 7.249–7.250
calcium channel blockers in,
2.114–2.115
clinical features of, 7.107, 65.3t
nitrates in, 2.80–2.81
thallium–201 scintigraphy in, 7.68
treatment of, 7.69–7.73
unstable, 7.49, 7.75–7.88
β-adrenergic blockers in, 7.80,
7.81–7.83, 63.3t–63.4t,
63.5f–63.7f
aggravating factors in, 7.78, 63.2t
alinidine in, 7.86
amiodarone in, 7.80, 7.86–7.87, 63.3t
anticoagulants in, 7.80, 7.85, 63.3t
antiplatelet agents in, 7.80, 7.85–7.86,
63.3t
antithrombotic therapy in, 2.159–2.161
bypass surgery in, 7.250, 7.252–7.253
calcium channel blockers in,
2.113–2.114, 7.80, 7.83–7.85,
63.3t, 63.5f–63.6f

clinical features of, 7.107, 65.3t
coronary artery spasm in, 7.76, 7.77,
63.1f
coronary vascular factors in, 7.75–7.78,
63.1t
electrocardiography in, 7.76, 7.80, 63.1f
intra-aortic balloon pumping in, 7.87
natural history of, 7.78–7.80,
63.3f–63.4f
nitrates in, 2.81
pathophysiology of, 7.75–7.78
percutaneous transluminal coronary
angioplasty in, 7.86, 7.87, 63.8f
pharmacologic agents in, 7.80–7.87,
63.3t
silent ischemia in, 7.96
surgical therapy in, 7.87–7.88, 63.9f
thrombolytic agents in, 2.160–2.161,
7.80, 7.85, 63.3t
thrombosis in, 2.158
tissue plasminogen activator in, 7.80,
7.85
treatment of, 7.80–7.88, 63.6t
variant or Prinzmetal, 3.5, 7.49,
7.76–7.77, 7.100–7.111
arrhythmias in, 7.108
calcium channel blockers in, 2.113,
2.114, 7.83, 7.108–7.110, 17.7f,
65.7f–65.9f
clinical features of, 7.100, 7.107, 65.3t
and coronary artery spasm,
7.100–7.101, 7.119
diagnosis of, 7.101–7.107
differential diagnosis of, 7.107, 65.3t
electrocardiography in, 7.101–7.103,
65.1f–65.4f
medical therapy in, 7.107–7.110,
65.7f–65.9f
pathophysiology of, 7.110–7.101
physical examination in, 7.101
prognosis of, 7.110–7.111
provocative testing in
cold pressor test in, 7.106–7.107
ergonovine in, 7.104–7.106,
65.1t–65.2t, 65.5f–65.6f
histamine in, 7.107
hyperventilation in, 7.106
methacholine in, 7.106
surgery in, 7.110
treatment of, 7.107–7.110
vasodilator reserve reduction in, 7.64
"walk-through," 3.5
Angiocardiography
in aortic insufficiency, chronic,
9.23–9.24
in atrial septal defect, 11.48
in cyanotic congenital heart disease,
11.29, 11.30, 11.32, 11.33 11.37,
100.4f–100.5f, 100.7f–100.9f
digital, 5.43–5.52
contrast enhancement in, 5.43–5.45,
36.2f
gray scale alterations in, 5.43
image subtraction methods in,
5.43–5.44, 36.2f

spatial filtering in, 5.44–5.45
coronary analysis in, 5.47–5.51,
36.4f–36.7f
image quality in, 5.45
myocardial perfusion imaging in,
5.51–5.52, 36.8f
quantitative measurements of
myocardial function in,
5.45–5.47, 36.3f
technical considerations in, 5.43, 5.44,
36.1f
in ductus arteriosus patency,
11.57–11.58
in Eisenmenger syndrome, 11.58–11.59,
11.82
in endocarditis, 9.83–9.85, 86.8f
in left atrial myxomas, 12.49
in mitral insufficiency, chronic, 9.15
in mitral valve prolapse, 9.16
radionuclide
in atrial septal defect, 11.47–11.48
in ischemic heart disease, 7.56–7.57
in myocardial contusion, 12.19
in tricuspid regurgitation, 9.99–9.100,
87.14f
in ventricular septal defect, 11.57–11.58,
102.7f
Angioplasty
coronary, percutaneous transluminal,
7.237–7.245
abrupt reclosure in, 7.243
management of, 7.243, 73.8f
risk factors for, 7.238, 73.2t
antithrombotic therapy in, 2.163
balloon dilatation systems in,
7.241–7.242, 73.6f
bypass surgery after, in myocardial
infarction, 7.265
compared to bypass surgery, 7.241
complications of, 7.243–7.244
in elderly patients, 13.31
history of, 7.237–7.238, 73.1f
indications for, 7.239–7.241, 73.1t
mechanisms of, 7.238, 73.2f–73.4f
in myocardial infarction, 7.170–7.173
restenosis in, 2.158, 2.163, 7.244–7.245,
73.9f
risk factors for, 7.244, 73.3t
in silent ischemia, 7.97
technique of, 7.241–7.243, 73.7f
in unstable angina, 7.86, 7.87, 63.8f
in vein graft dilatation, 7.240–7.241,
73.5f
laser, 7.246, 73.12f
percutaneous balloon, in peripheral
arterial occlusive disease,
12.40
renal, percutaneous transluminal, in
renovascular hypertension,
8.35
Angiosarcoma, cardiac, 12.52, 109.9f
Angiotensin
converting enzyme inhibitors
captopril, 2.129–2.130
enalapril, 2.130

I.3

in heart failure, 2.129–2.131
hemodynamic effects of, 2.129–2.131, 18.9f–18.11f
hydralazine with, 2.131
in hypertension, 8.24
in myocardial infarction, 7.158
and nonmodulation of responses in hypertension, 8.11–8.13, 76.13f–76.16f
in renovascular hypertension, 8.31, 8.35
and norepinephrine release, 1.118, 7.4f
renin-angiotensin-aldosterone system, 8.3–8.5, 76.1f–76.3f
responsiveness to, in hypertension, 8.5–8.14, 76.4f–76.7f
Ankylosing spondylitis, 13.6
Annuloplasty, tricuspid, 9.103
Annulus of mitral valve, calcification of, 9.17
Antabuse in alcoholic heart disease, 12.11
Antacids
interaction with antiarrhythmic drugs, 2.175, 21.2t
interaction with digoxin, 2.172, 21.1t
Antecubital fossae, anatomy of, 5.31, 35.27f
Anthracycline cardiotoxicity
biopsy in, 5.72–5.75, 38.11f–38.12f
morphologic grading system in, 5.74, 38.2t
Antiarrhythmic drugs
β-adrenergic blockers, 6.25–6.26, 6.39
in atrial fibrillation, 6.131
in atrial flutter, 6.132
in atrioventricular nodal tachycardia, 6.133–6.134
bioavailability of, 6.31
in bundle branch block, 6.123
calcium channel blocking drugs, 6.39
clearance of, 6.31
complications of, 6.34–6.35, 6.36, 42.1f–42.3f
depressing fast inward current
and acceleration of repolarization, 6.21–6.23
with no effect on repolarization, 6.23–6.24
and prolongation of repolarization, 6.20–6.21
in digitalis toxicity, 2.48
antiarrhythmic drugs
in dilated cardiomyopathy, 10.15
dosing history of, 6.32
effects on action potential duration, 6.77–6.78, 45.15f
effects on transplanted heart, 13.97
in elderly patients, 13.37
factors affecting actions of, 6.17–6.19
guarded receptor hypothesis of actions, 6.19, 41.7f
half-life of, 6.31–6.32
interactions with other drugs, 2.174–2.177, 6.32–6.34, 21.2t–21.3t, 42.1t

with major effect on repolarization, 6.24–6.25
mechanisms of action, 6.20–6.26
metabolites of, 6.32
modifying slow inward current, 6.25
molecular weight affecting actions of, 6.19, 41.6f
newer agents, 6.44–6.51
pharmacokinetics of, 6.31–6.32
plasma concentrations of, 6.32
in pregnancy, 13.22, 111.3t
protein binding of, 6.32
in reentry suppression, 6.14–6.16
sodium channel blocking drugs, 6.35–6.39
in supraventricular tachycardia, 6.138
volume of distribution of, 6.31
Antibiotic therapy
in endocarditis, 9.85–9.86, 86.6t
allergy to penicillin in, 9.86
prophylactic, 9.87, 11.60, 86.8t–86.10t
in rheumatic fever prevention, 10.105–10.106
Antibodies
to digoxin, 2.49–2.50
to myosin, in viral myocarditis, 10.88
to streptococci, tests for, 10.102
Anticoagulants, oral, 2.152–2.154
in atrial fibrillation, 6.131
contraindications to, 2.152
guidelines for therapy with, 2.153
interactions with other drugs, 2.153, 2.186–2.188, 20.2t, 21.10t–21.11t
mechanism of action, 2.152
in myocardial infarction, 7.152–7.153, 68.2t–68.3t
in pregnancy, 13.22, 111.3t
with prosthetic heart valves, 9.47–9.48
in pulmonary embolism, 10.81
side effects of, 2.153–2.154
in unstable angina, 7.80, 7.85, 63.3t
in viral myocarditis, 10.90
Antidepressants, tricyclic, interactions with other drugs
antihypertensive drugs, 2.184, 21.8t
monoamine oxidase inhibitors, 2.184, 21.8t
sympathomimetic drugs, 2.184, 21.8t
Antihypertensive agents, 8.20–8.25
classification of, 8.20–8.21, 77.5t
in elderly patients, 13.32
hemodynamic effects of, 8.21
interactions with other drugs, 2.183–2.185, 21.8t
in renovascular hypertension, 8.34–8.35
and reversal of left ventricular hypertrophy, 8.44–8.52
and cardiac performance, 8.47–8.49, 79.2f–79.5f
clinical correlates of, 8.45–8.46
and coronary blood flow, 8.49–8.51, 79.3f–79.4f
factors affecting, 8.45, 79.1t
inotrophic responses in, 8.48–8.49, 79.4f–79.5f

relation to vascular hypertrophy, 8.49
type of therapy affecting, 8.46–8.47, 79.2t
ventricular pump function in, 8.47–8.48, 79.2f–79.3f
Anti-inflammatory drugs, nonsteroidal, interactions with other drugs, 2.181–2.183, 21.2f, 21.7t
diuretics, 2.180, 21.6t
warfarin, 2.187, 21.10t
Antiplatelet agents
in myocardial infarction, 7.153
in unstable angina, 7.85–7.86
in vein graft patency, 7.255–7.256
Antithrombin III
deficiency of, and venous thrombosis, 10.78
and thrombosis inhibition, 2.146
Antithrombotic therapy, 2.143–2.166
in angina
stable, 2.162
unstable, 2.159–2.161
in atrial fibrillation, 2.163
in coronary angioplasty, 2.162
in coronary artery disease, 2.159–2.163, 20.4t
in dilated cardiomyopathy, 2.164
heparin in, 2.149–2.152
in left ventricular aneurysm, 2.164
in myocardial infarction, 2.164
in noncardiac surgery, 2.165
oral anticoagulants in, 2.152–2.154
in organic heart disease, 2.160, 2.163–2.164, 20.4t
platelet inhibitors in, 2.147–2.149
postinfarction use of, 2.162
in pregnancy, 2.165–2.166
in prevention of atherosclerosis progression, 2.162–2.163
in prosthetic valve use, 2.160, 2.164–2.165, 20.4t
thrombolytic agents in, 2.154–2.156
in vein graft disease after bypass surgery, 2.163
Antithymocyte globulin, rabbit, immunosuppressive effects of, 13.95, 13.103
Anxiety
chest discomfort in, 3.6, 7.65
in myocardial infarction, 7.143–7.144
palpitations in, 3.8
Aorta
aneurysms of, 12.27–12.33
abdominal, 12.28–12.30, 108.2f
chest film in, 4.8, 4.12, 4.13, 26.15f, 26.23f–26.24f
chest pain in, 3.6
dissecting, 12.30–12.33. *See also* Aorta, dissection
etiology of, 12.27–12.28
mycotic, 12.34–12.35
thoracic, 12.28
anomalous origin of coronary arteries from, 11.19–11.20
atherosclerosis of, 12.27

balloon pumping. *See* Balloon pump, intra-aortic
baroreceptors, 1.168–1.169, 11.7f
  and blood flow to limb muscles, 1.122–1.123
  interactions with cardiopulmonary receptors, 1.170, 1.171, 11.8f–11.9f
chemoreceptors in, and blood flow to limb muscles, 1.123
coarctation of, 3.63, 3.64, 11.73–11.75, 25.8f–25.9f, 103.10f
  in aortic valvular stenosis, 9.109
  cardiac catheterization in, 5.18
  chest film in, 4.13
  in pregnancy, 13.24–13.25
  surgery in, 11.74–11.75, 103.11f
    long-term outcome of, 11.6–11.7
dissection, 12.30–12.33
  β-adrenergic blocking drugs in, 2.101
  in aortic valvular stenosis, 9.109
  aortography in, 12.32, 108.4f
  chest films in, 12.32, 108.1t
  chest pain in, 7.66
  classification of, 12.31, 108.3f
  medical management of, 12.31–12.33, 108.2t
  pericarditis in, 10.61
in giant cell arteritis, 12.33
in rheumatic disease, 12.35
rupture
  in cocaine abuse, 13.77
  traumatic, 12.11–12.24, 12.28, 12.29, 107.6f–107.7f, 108.1f
sclerosis of, murmur in, 3.40
stenosis
  arterial pulse in, 3.21–3.22, 23.3t, 23.5f
  subvalvular, 3.63
    congenital, 11.68–11.69, 103.5f
    echocardiography in, 11.92, 105.7f
  supravavular, congenital, 11.71–11.73, 103.9f
  valvular. *See* Aortic valve, stenosis of
in Takayasu's disease, 12.33–12.34, 108.5f
transposition of. *See* Transposition of great vessels
trauma of, 12.22–12.24, 12.28, 12.29, 107.6f–107.7f, 108.1f
Aortic sinus
  aneurysm of, 3.66–3.67
  anomalous origin of coronary arteries from, 11.15–11.19, 99.1f–99.9f
Aortic valve
  anatomy of, 1.8f, 1.9, 1.10, 1.11f, 1.11–1.12
  balloon valvuloplasty, 9.59–9.67, 9.113
    cardiac catheterization in, 5.13, 5.15, 34.18f
    complications of, 9.65–9.67, 85.7t
    history of, 9.60–9.62
    mechanism of dilatation in, 9.63
    patient selection in, 9.62
    procedure in, 9.62–9.63, 9.64, 85.7f–85.9f
    results of, 9.63–9.65, 9.66, 85.6t
    simultaneous procedures with, 9.67
  bicuspid, 11.69, 103.6f
    echocardiography of, 4.40, 4.77, 28.28f, 10.104f
  echocardiography of, 4.75–4.81, 28.100f
    in endocarditis, 4.80, 4.81, 28.111f
    in Marfan syndrome, 4.81, 28.112f
  normal area of, 9.55, 85.2t
  prosthetic replacement, 9.25–9.27, 9.113
    coronary bypass surgery with, 7.257–7.258
    in elderly patients, 13.33
    hypertension after, 8.43
    indications for, 9.25, 82.3t
    in regurgitation, 9.41
    results of, 9.25–9.27, 82.15f–82.18f
    in stenosis, 9.40–9.41
    technique of, 9.42, 9.43, 84.1f
  regurgitation or insufficiency
    acute
      causes of, 9.3, 81.1t
      pathophysiology of, 9.2
      vasodilators in, 9.5
    in aortic valvular stenosis, 9.109
    cardiac catheterization in, 5.16
    chronic, 9.10, 9.18–9.27
      auscultation in, 9.20–9.21
      blood pressure in, 9.20
      diagnosis of, 9.24
      differential diagnosis of, 9.24
      echocardiography in, 9.20, 9.21–9.23, 9.24, 82.9f, 82.11f–82.14f
      electrocardiography in, 9.21
      etiology of, 9.18–9.19
      hemodynamic effects of, 9.23–9.24
      inspection in, 9.20
      medical treatment of, 9.24–9.25
      natural history and prognosis of, 9.20
      noninvasive tests in, 9.21–9.23
      palpation in, 9.20, 82.9f
      pathophysiology of, 9.19, 82.8f
      physical examination in, 9.20–9.21
      physical working capacity in, 9.23
      pulmonary function in, 9.23
      radioisotope studies in, 9.23
      radiology in, 9.21, 82.10f
      surgery in, 9.25–9.27, 82.3t, 82.15f–82.18f
      symptoms of, 9.20
      systolic time intervals in, 9.23
      vasodilators in, 9.9
    color-flow Doppler of, 4.88, 28.128f–28.129f
    coronary blood flow in, 1.112
    echocardiography of, 4.77–4.80, 28.105f–28.110f
    in elderly patients, 13.33
    lesions simulating, 3.66–3.67
    murmurs in, 3.45, 3.47
    pregnancy, 13.24
    prosthetic replacement in, 9.41
    pulsus bisferiens in, 9.110
    traumatic, 12.21
    vasodilators in, 2.133, 9.9
  stenosis of, 3.62–3.63, 9.106–9.114, 25.7f
    acquired, 9.106
    in bicuspid valve, 9.106, 9.107, 88.1f
    cardiac catheterization in, 5.13–5.16, 9.112, 34.19f, 88.6f
    chest films in, 9.110, 9.111, 88.4f
    in children and infants, management of, 9.113
    complications of, 9.109
    congenital, 9.106, 11.69–11.71, 103.7f
      balloon valvuloplasty in, 11.71, 103.7f
    coronary blood flow in, 1.112
    debridement valvulotomy in, 9.60, 9.61, 85.4f
    echocardiography in, 4.76–4.77, 9.110–9.111, 11.90–11.92, 28.103f, 88.5f, 105.6f
    in elderly patients, 13.33
    electrocardiography in, 9.110
    etiology of, 9.59, 9.106–9.107
    long-term outcome of surgery in, 11.6
    management of, 9.113–9.114
    Mönckeberg, 9.106–9.107, 88.3f
    murmur in, 3.39
    natural history and prognosis of, 9.59–9.60, 9.112–9.113
    noncardiac surgery in, 13.46
    pathophysiology of, 9.107–9.108
    phonocardiography and pulse recordings in, 9.112
    physical findings in, 9.109–9.110
    in pregnancy, 13.24
    prosthetic replacement in, 9.40–9.41
    rheumatic, 9.106, 9.107, 88.2f
    surgical experience in, 9.60
    symptoms of, 9.108–9.109
    vegetations in, echocardiography of, 4.75, 28.102f
Aortitis, 12.33–12.35
  in rheumatic disease, 12.35
  syphilitic, 12.34
Aortography, 5.8
  in aortic dissection, 12.32, 108.4f
Aortopulmonary collaterals with tetralogy of Fallot and pulmonary atresia, 3.59, 3.60, 25.2f
Apolipoproteins, 7.39, 60.3f
  C-II deficiency, familial, 7.42, 7.45, 60.4t
Apex cardiograms, 3.23–3.25, 23.6f–23.7f
  in mitral insufficiency, chronic, 9.15
Apex impulse
  in aortic stenosis, 9.110
  in mitral stenosis, 9.119
Apical diastolic rumble in mitral stenosis, 9.120
Apical hypertrophic cardiomyopathy, 10.31
Aprindine, 6.23
  effects on heart and circulation, 6.23
  effects on transmembrane potential, 6.23
Arachidonic acid metabolism, inhibitors of, 2.147–2.148

Arrhythmias
  α-adrenergic blocking drugs in, 2.93
  β-adrenergic blocking drugs in,
      2.99–2.100
  in after depolarizations, 6.16–6.17
  in alcoholic heart disease, 12.9, 12.10,
      12.11, 106.11f–106.12f
  antiarrhythmic drugs in. See
      antiarrhythmic drugs
  automaticity in, 6.16
  calcium channel blockers in,
      2.116–2.118, 17.7t
  cardiac biopsy in, 5.78
  from cardiac catheterization, 5.39–5.40
  cocaine-induced, 13.75–13.76
  in digitalis toxicity, 2.45, 14.4t
  in dilated cardiomyopathy, 10.12
  in elderly patients, 13.36
  exacerbation by antiarrhythmic drugs,
      6.34–6.35
  glycosides in, 2.44
  heart failure in, 1.157
  Holter monitoring in, 6.95, 6.96, 6.97,
      46.6f–46.8f
  in hyperthyroidism, 13.85
  in hypertrophic cardiomyopathy,
      10.30–10.31
    management of, 10.34, 10.36
  in hypothyroidism, 13.85
  impulse conduction abnormalities in,
      6.14–6.16
  impulse initiation abnormalities in,
      6.16–6.17
  in mitral valve prolapse, 9.36
    treatment of, 9.38
  in myocardial contusion, 12.18, 107.1t
  lt in myocardial infarction, 7.148–7.151
    continuous monitoring for, 7.143, 7.145,
      68.2f
  noncardiac surgery in, 13.45
  in normal population, 6.94–6.95
  postinfarction, 7.226–7.229
    bypass surgery in, 7.266
    in exercise testing, 7.221–7.222
    relation to left ventricular ejection
      fraction, 7.227 7.228, 72.4f
  postoperative
    in cardiac surgery, 13.64–13.65
    in noncardiac surgery, 13.49
    in transplantation of heart, 13.98
  in pregnancy, 13.23
  reentrant, 6.9–6.11, 6.14–6.16
  in variant angina, 7.108
  in viral myocarditis, 10.86, 10.88
    treatment of, 10.90
Arterial injury from cardiac
    catheterization, 5.39
Arteriography
  coronary, 5.20–5.42
    Amplatz catheters in, 5.29, 35.23f
    in angina pectoris, 7.68
      unstable, 7.76–7.77, 63.1f–63.2f
      variant, 7.104
    anomalous origin of arteries in, 5.40,
      5.42, 35.39f–35.40f
    brachial approach in, 5.30–5.33
      bypass graft cannulation in, 5.32
      catheters used in, 5.32, 35.29f
      closure techniques in, 5.32, 35.30f
      cutdown technique in, 5.30, 5.31,
        35.28f
      internal mammary artery cannulation
        in, 5.32
      left coronary artery cannulation in,
        5.32
      percutaneous, 5.33
      right coronary artery cannulation in,
        5.32
    catheter-induced coronary spasm in,
      5.41–5.42
    complications of, 5.38–5.40, 35.2t
    coronary artery spasm evaluation in,
      5.33, 5.34, 35.31f
    correlation with postinfarction
      exercise tests, 7.222
    in dilated cardiomyopathy, 10.9–10.10
    in estimates of stenosis severity, 1.108,
      1.109–1.110, 6.8f
    femoral approach in, percutaneous,
      5.27–5.30
      Amplatz catheters in, 5.29, 35.23f
      bypass graft cannulation in, 5.30,
        35.25f
      guidewires in, 5.28, 35.20f
      inguinal area anatomy in, 5.27–5.28,
        35.19f
      internal mammary artery cannulation
        in, 5.30, 35.26f
      Judkins catheters in, 5.28–5.30,
        35.21f–35.22f,
        35.24f–35.26f
      left artery cannulation in, 5.28–5.29
      right artery cannulation in,
        5.29–5.30
    inadequate x-ray penetration in, 5.41
    incomplete study in, 5.40–5.41
    interpretation of, 5.35–5.37
      errors in, 5.40–5.42
    in ischemic heart disease, 7.58–7.60
    myocardial bridging in, 5.41, 5.42,
      35.41f
    normal anatomy in, 5.20–5.25
    poor contrast injection in, 5.41
    in postinfarction prognosis, 7.224
    quantitative, 1.109, 5.38
    selective injections in, 5.40, 5.41,
      35.38f
    techniques in, 5.25–5.33
    total occlusion of artery in, 5.41, 5.42,
      35.42f
    transaxillary approach, percutaneous,
      5.33
  in ergotism, 12.39, 108.12f
  pulmonary, in pulmonary embolism,
      10.80, 94.6f
  renal, in renovascular hypertension,
      8.32, 8.33, 8.34, 78.1f–78.3f
  in scleroderma, 13.12
Arteriolar vasodilators, 2.124–2.125
Arteriosclerosis. See Atherosclerosis

Arteriovenous fistula. See Fistula,
    arteriovenous
Arteritis
  allergic angiitis and granulomatosis,
      13.11
  giant cell, 12.33, 13.11
  in Kawasaki disease, 13.10–13.11
  periarteritis nodosa, 13.9–13.10
  in rheumatic disease, 12.35
  syphilitic, 12.34
  Takayasu, 12.33–12.34, 13.11, 108.5f
  in Wegener's granulomatosis, 13.11
Arthritis
  in rheumatic fever, 10.100–10.101
  rheumatoid. See Rheumatoid arthritis
Artifacts in cardiac biopsy, 5.69, 5.70,
    5.71, 38.2f–38.4f
Artificial heart, 13.93
Aschoff nodules in rheumatic fever, 10.99
Ascites, diuretics in, 2.28
Ashman's phenomenon, 6.5
Aspartate aminotransferase levels in
    myocardial infarction, 7.146
Aspergillosis, myocarditis in, 10.93
Aspirin
  chemical structure of, 2.148, 20.4f
  as inhibitor of platelet cyclo-oxygenase,
      2.147
  interaction with anticoagulants, 2.153,
      20.2t
  in myocardial infarction, 7.153
    streptokinase with, 7.153, 7.166
  postinfarction use of, 2.162, 7.234–7.235,
      72.10t
  in pregnancy, 13.22, 111.3t
  in prevention of myocardial infarction,
      2.162, 7.115–7.116
  in prevention of restenosis after
      coronary angioplasty, 2.163
  in rheumatic fever, 10.104
  in unstable angina, 2.159–2.160, 7.80,
      7.86, 63.3t
  and vein graft patency, 2.163,
      7.255–7.256
Astemizole, toxic effects of, 13.79
Asthma
  cardiac, 3.54
  exercise-induced, calcium channel
      blockers in, 2.120
Atenolol, 8.22, 77.7t
  pharmacology of, 2.96, 2.97, 7.71. 16.2t,
      16.3t, 62.3t
  in unstable angina, 7.81–7.83, 63.4t
Atherectomy, percutaneous, 7.245, 73.10f
Atherosclerosis
  aorta in, 12.27
  calcium channel blockers affecting,
      2.116
  in diabetes mellitus, 13.82, 13.83, 117.2f
  in elderly patients, 13.29–13.32
  and hypothyroidism, 13.86
  International Atherosclerosis Project
      (IAP), 7.16
  lipoprotein role in, 7.40–7.42
  in lupus erythematosus, 13.9

multi-system, coronary bypass surgery in, 7.258–7.259, 74.1f, 74.2t
obliterans, limb blood vessels in, 1.126–1.127, 7.10f
plaque formation in, and myocardial infarction, 7.113–7.114
prevention of progression of, 2.162–2.163
renal artery, hypertension in, 8.31–8.36, 78.3f
in rheumatoid arthritis, 13.5
stress affecting, 13.69
of transplanted heart, 13.100
vascular injury in, 2.156, 2.157–2.158
Athletes. *See also* Exercise, training programs
electrocardiography in, 4.18
ATP
plasma levels in myocardial infarction, 7.121
synthesis in myocardium, 1.78–1.79, 4.13f–4.14f
substrates for, 1.79–1.80
Atrial septal defect, 3.63–3.65, 11.43–11.50
catheterization and angiography in, 5.17–5.18, 11.48
chest films in, 11.46, 11.47, 101.2f–101.5f
computed tomography in, 11.48
coronary sinus, 3.64
course and natural history of, 11.49
diagnosis of, 11.48
differential diagnosis of, 10.13, 10.14, 11.48–11.49, 90.5f
echocardiography in, 4.62–4.63, 11.47, 11.88–11.89, 28.74f–28.76f, 101.6f–101.7f, 105.1f–105.3f
in elderly patients, 13.34
electrocardiography in, 11.46–11.47
indications for surgery in, 11.49–11.50
left-to-right shunt in, 11.43–11.45
long-term outcome of surgery in, 11.4–11.5
magnetic resonance imaging in, 11.48
mitral stenosis with, 11.43
murmur in, 3.47, 23.15f
ostium primum, 3.63–3.64, 3.65, 11.43, 11.44, 25.10f, 101.1f
pulmonary vascular disease with, 11.85–11.86
clinical features of, 11.85–11.86
management of, 11.86
ostium secundum, 3.63, 3.65, 11.43, 11.44, 101.1f
pulmonary vascular disease in, 11.83–11.85
clinical features of, 11.84
management of, 11.85
pathophysiology of, 11.43–11.45
physical examination in, 11.45–11.46
postoperative history in, 11.50
in pregnancy, 13.25
pulmonary vascular disease with, 11.83–11.86
in primum defect, 11.85–11.86
in secundum defect, 11.83–11.85

radioisotope shunt studies in, 11.47–11.48
right-to-left shunt in, 11.45
sinus venosus, 3.64, 11.43, 11.44, 101.1f
traumatic, 12.20
Atrial systole, 5.65
Atriogenic reflux, 9.17
Atrioventricular block, 6.113
clinical implications of, 6.123
in elderly patients, 13.37
first-degree, 6.115, 6.117, 48.1t
in rheumatoid arthritis, 13.5
infranodal, 6.119, 48.2t
in myocardial infarction, 6.123
nodal, 6.113, 6.118–6.119
and noncardiac surgery, 13.45
paroxysmal, 6.115
pathologic findings in, 6.113
second-degree, 6.115–6.116, 6.117, 48.1t, 48.4f
third-degree, 6.116, 6.117, 6.118, 48.1t, 48.6f
2:1 or greater, 6.116, 6.117, 48.1t, 48.5f
vagotonic, 6.116, 6.117, 6.118, 48.1t, 48.7f
Atrioventricular canal defect, partial. *See* Atrial septal defect, ostium primum
Atrioventricular junctional tachycardias, 6.132–6.135, 49.2f–49.5f
treatment of, 6.138
Atrioventricular node, 1.12, 1.13, 1.14f, 6.111–6.112, 48.1f
action potential in, 6.4, 6.5, 40.4f
block in, 6.113, 6.118–6.119
calcification in aortic valvular stenosis, 9.109
conduction delay from β-adrenergic blocking drugs, 2.101
electrophysiologic studies of conduction in, 6.55–6.58, 6.59, 44.2f–44.3f, 44.5f–44.6f
physiology of, 6.113–6.114
Atrium
common, 11.35
management of, 11.39
cor triatriatum, 3.62, 11.66–11.67
left, 1.8f–1.10f, 1.9–1.10
chest films of, 4.5, 4.6–4.7, 26.9f–26.12f
echocardiography of, 4.64–4.65, 4.66, 28.80f–28.84f
in tumors, 4.96–4.97, 28.145f–28.146f
enlargement of, electrocardiography in, 4.19, 4.20, 27.8f
myxomas of, 12.46–12.49
pressure pulse in mitral stenosis, 9.117, 89.1f
right
anatomy of, 1.3f–1.5f, 1.5–1.7
chest films of, 4.3–4.4, 4.5, 26.5f
echocardiography of, 4.65
in tumors, 4.97–4.98, 28.147f
enlargement of, electrocardiography in, 4.19, 4.20, 27.7f
myxomas of, 12.49–12.50
tricuspid valve in, 9.96

oxygen step-up in, 11.48, 101.1t
pressure pulse in tricuspid stenosis, 9.101, 87.18f
thrombosis of, 12.50, 109.7f
echocardiography in, 4.97–4.98, 28.147f
septal defect. *See* Atrial septal defect
structure-function relationships, 1.19
Atropine
in digitalis toxicity, 2.48
in sinus node function tests, 6.102, 6.103, 47.2t
Auscultation
of heart sounds and murmurs, 3.25–3.50. *See also* Heart sounds; Murmurs
of lung sounds, 3.56–3.57, 24.1t–24.2t
of voice sounds, 3.57
Austin Flint murmur, 3.47
in aortic insufficiency, 9.21
differential diagnosis of, 9.120
in pulmonic insufficiency, chronic, 9.27
Automaticity in cardiac cells, 6.6–6.7, 40.6f
abnormal, 6.7
and abnormal conduction, 6.11–6.12
antiarrhythmic drugs affecting, 6.34
and arrhythmias, 6.16
Autonomic nervous system
blockade of, and sinus node recovery time, 6.105–6.106, 47.4f–47.5f
cardiac glycosides affecting, 2.39
and cardiac performance, 1.98–1.99
dysfunction in mitral valve prolapse, 1.173–1.174, 11.10f
effects on cellular electrophysiology, 6.6
failure of, 1.174–1.175, 11.3t
in reentry of cardiac impulses, 6.15
stress affecting, 13.69
Autoregulation
of blood flow in limbs, 1.116
coronary vascular, 7.63
Autoregulatory resistance in coronary blood flow, 1.102, 1.103–1.104, 6.2f, 6.4f
adenosine affecting, 1.105–1.106
control of, 1.105–1.106
myogenic factors in, 1.106
neurohumaral factors in, 1.106
transmural variations in, 1.102, 1.104, 6.2f
Axillary artery in coronary arteriography, 5.33
Axon reflex, local sympathetic, and blood flow to limbs, 1.118–1.119
Azathioprine in transplantation of heart, 13.95, 13.103

B

Bachmann bundle, 1.12
Balloon catheters, interventional procedures with, 9.54, 9.55, 85.1t

in coronary angioplasty, 7.241–7.242, 73.6f
in pulmonary artery stenosis, 9.58–9.59
in valvuloplasty, 9.54–9.72. *See also* Valvuloplasty, balloon
Balloon pump, intra-aortic, 7.194, 70.6f
  in mitral regurgitation, acute, 9.4
  in postinfarction shock, 7.194, 7.266, 70.11t
  in postoperative hypotension and low cardiac output, 13.63, 114.8f
  in unstable angina, 7.87
Barbiturates, interaction with anticoagulants, 2.153, 2.187, 20.2t, 21.11t
Barlow syndrome. *See* Mitral valve, prolapse
Baroreceptors
  aging affecting, 8.56
  cardiopulmonary, 1.169–1.170
  carotid and aortic, 1.168–1.169, 11.7f
    and blood flow to limb muscles, 1.122–1.123
    interactions with cardiopulmonary receptors, 1.170, 1.171, 11.8f–11.9f
Bay K 8644, inotropic effects of, 2.66
Bed rest
  effects of gravity in, 7.209
  in myocardial infarction, 7.145–7.146
  prolonged
    orthostatic intolerance in, 1.173
    responses to, 1.140–1.142, 8.9f
  in rheumatic fever, 10.103
Bedside evaluation of patients
  analysis of symptoms in, 3.4–3.9
  in angina, 3.4–3.6
  in cardiomyopathy, 3.50, 23.14t
  in chest pain or discomfort, 3.4
  in congenital heart disease presenting initially in adults, 3.58–3.67
  in coughing and hemoptysis, 3.9
  in cyanosis, 3.7
  in dyspnea, 3.6–3.7
  in edema, 3.9
  ejection systolic murmurs in, 3.41, 23.12t–23.13t
  history-taking in, 3.2–3.9
  lung examination in, 3.54–3.57
  in mitral valve prolapse, 9.32
  in palpitation, 3.7–3.8
  physical examination in, 3.11–3.51
  in syncope, 3.8–3.9
Behçet's disease, 13.6
Benzocaine, antiarrhythmic effects of, factors affecting, 6.18, 41.5f
Bepridil, 2.106, 2.107, 6.49–6.50, 17.1t
  antiarrhythmic spectrum of, 6.50 dosage of, 6.50
  electrophysiologic properties of, 6.49
  interactions with other drugs, 6.50
  pharmacokinetics of, 6.49–6.50
  side effects of, 6.50
Berberine, 2.66
Bernheim phenomenon, 9.108

reversed, 9.108
Bernoulli equation for Doppler echocardiography, 4.63
Betaxolol
  in glaucoma, 2.101
  pharmacology of, 2.96, 2.97, 16.2t, 16.3t
Bethanidine, interactions with other drugs, 2.184, 2.185, 21.8t
Bevantolol, pharmacology of, 2.96, 2.97, 16.2t, 16.3t
Bile acid binding resins, 2.137–2.138
Bioavailability of drugs, 2.5, 2.6, 12.7f
Bioprosthetic heart valves, 9.46–9.47, 84.3f
  aortic, 9.113
  degeneration of, 9.48–9.49
  durability of, 9.51
  evaluation of, 9.83
Biopsy, cardiac, 5.67–5.78
  in amyloidosis, 5.71, 5.72, 38.6f
  in anthracycline cardiotoxicity, 5.72–5.75, 38.11f–38.12f
  in arrhythmias, 5.78
  artifacts in, 5.69, 5.70, 5.71, 38.2f–38.4f
  bioptomes in, 5.67
  in dilated cardiomyopathy, 5.75–5.76, 10.4, 10.11, 38.13f–38.15f
  in hypertrophic cardiomyopathy, 5.76
  indications for, 5.71–5.78, 38.1t
  in infants and children, 5.69
  interpretation of, 5.70
  in myocarditis, 5.76, 5.77, 5.78, 10.85, 38.3t, 38.5f, 38.16f–38.18f
  in rejection of transplanted heart, 13.96
  in restrictive cardiomyopathy, 5.78, 10.109–10.110, 97.4f
  in right ventricular dysplasia, 5.78, 39.19f
  right versus left ventricular, 5.69
  safety and complications of, 5.68–5.69
  sampling error in, 5.69
  in sarcoidosis, 5.71, 38.5f
  size of specimens in, 5.68, 38.1f
  in specific heart muscle diseases, 5.78, 38.6t
  technique of, 5.68
  tissue handling and processing in, 5.69–5.70
  in transplanted heart, 5.71–5.72, 5.73, 38.7f–38.10f
Biot's respiration, 3.55
Bisoprolol, pharmacodynamic properties of, 2.96, 16.2t
Bjork-Shiley valves, 9.45, 84.2f
  orifice areas in, 9.44, 84.1t
Blalock-Taussig operation in cyanotic heart disease, 11.27, 11.40
Bleeding from oral anticoagulants, 2.153–2.154
Blood chemistries in hypertension, 8.18–8.19, 77.2t
Blood count in hypertension, 8.18, 77.2t
Blood flow
  aortic, as index of contractile state, 1.89, 5.4f

cerebral, in orthostatic hypotension, 1.164–1.165
coronary
  in anemia, 1.112
  in aortic insufficiency, 1.112
  in aortic stenosis, 1.112
  autoregulation of, 7.63
  calcium channel blockers affecting, 2.111
  cocaine affecting, 13.77
  collateral vessels in, 1.110
  driving pressure in, 1.102, 1.103, 6.2f
  exercise affecting, 1.135, 7.48, 7.204–7.205
  in hypertrophy of heart, 1.76–1.77, 1.112
  impedance in, 1.102, 1.103, 5.2f
  in left ventricular hypertrophy reversal with antihypertensive drugs, 8.49–8.51, 79.3t–79.4t
  measurements of, 1.112–1.113
  nitrates affecting, 2.79–2.80, 15.2t, 15.5f
  physiologic factors in, 1.102–1.105
  in polycythemia, 1.112
  relation to coronary arterial pressure, 1.105, 6.5f
  and reperfusion in myocardial infarction, 7.163–7.176
  reserve in, measurements of, 1.110–1.111, 6.10f
  resistance in, 1.102, 1.103–1.105, 6.2f
    autoregulatory, 1.102, 1.103–1.104, 6.2f, 6.4f
    basal viscous, 1.102, 1.103, 6.2f
    calculation of, 1.104–1.105
    compressive, 1.102, 1.103, 1.104, 6.2f, 6.3f
  in scleroderma, 13.12
  in silent ischemia, 7.92
  in stenotic lesions, 1.106–1.110, 6.6f–6.9f
  in tachycardia, 1.105, 1.112, 6.5f, 6.128
  vasomotor regulation of, 1.106
in limbs, 1.114–1.127. *See also* Limb circulation
pulmonary
  in cyanotic congenital heart disease
    deficient flow in, 11.28–11.30, 11.35–11.37, 11.39–11.41, 100.3f–100.6f
    excessive flow in, 11.28, 11.38–11.39, 100.1f–100.2f
  increased, 10.71
  obstruction to, 3.58–3.62
in skin, 1.119–1.121, 7.5f
  in cold exposure, 1.121
  cooling affecting, 1.120
  and reactive hyperemia, 1.121
  and reflexes involving blood vessels, 1.121
  triple response in, 1.121
  warming affecting, 1.120–1.121

systemic
  in exercise, 7.204–7.205
  in limb, 1.114–1.127
  obstruction in congenital heart disease, 3.62–3.63
  in peripheral arterial disease. *See* Peripheral arterial disease
Blood gases
  postoperative exchange in mechanical ventilation and spontaneous breathing, 13.54, 13.55, 114.2t
  in pulmonary embolism, 10.79
Blood pressure. *See also* Hypertension; Hypotension
  in aortic insufficiency, 9.20
  control with nitrates during surgery, 2.84
  and coronary heart disease risk, 7.7–7.10
  diastolic, 3.18
    relation to systolic pressure, 8.54, 80.1f–80.2f
  in exercise, 7.204, 7.205, 71.1f
    in peripheral arterial disease, 12.35, 12.37, 108.5t
  measurements of, 3.18–3.19
    in elderly persons, 8.56, 13.29
  and progress in control efforts, 7.28
  regulation of
    neurohumoral, 1.168–1.170, 11.6f–11.7f
    renin-angiotensin-aldosterone system in, 8.3–8.5, 76.1f–76.3f
  stress affecting, 13.68, 13.69–13.70
  systolic, 3.18
    relation to diastolic pressure, 8.54, 80.1f–80.2f
Blood viscosity, and pulmonary hypertension, 10.71
Blood volume
  hypovolemia in myocardial infarction, 7.189, 7.199, 80.7t
    hypotension in, 7.154
  in orthostatic hypotension, 1.166–1.167, 1.173–1.174, 11.4f
  postoperative hypovolemia, 13.59–13.60
Body build affecting electrocardiography, 4.18
Body surface mapping, 4.19
Borg scale, for perceived level of exertion, 7.207, 71.4t
Brachial artery
  in cardiac catheterization, 5.2
  in coronary arteriography, 5.30–5.33
Bradycardia
  sinus, in myocardial infarction, 7.152
  bradytachycardia syndrome, 6.100, 6.101, 47.1f
Braking phenomenon in renal response to diuretics, 2.25–2.26, 2.28, 2.30, 13.9f
Bretylium, 6.24, 6.40
  contraindications in digitalis toxicity, 2.49
  dosage and pharmacokinetic properties of, 6.37, 42.2t
  effects on heart and circulation, 6.24
  effects on transmembrane potential, 6.24
  interaction with other drugs, 6.33, 42.1t
Broadbent's sign, 3.22
Brockenbrough sign, 5.17
Bromocriptine, inotropic effects of, 2.59
Bronchoconstriction from β-adrenergic blocking drugs, 2.102
Bronchophony, 3.57
Bronchospasm, α-adrenergic blocking drugs in, 2.94
Buerger's disease, 12.39, 108.8t
Bumetanide, 2.27, 13.1t
Bundle branch block
  antiarrhythmic drugs in, 6.123
  chronic, 6.119–6.123
  clinical implications of, 6.123
  deceleration-dependent, 6.11–6.12
  in elderly patients, 13.37
  epidemiologic studies, 6.119, 6.120, 48.3t–48.4t
  exercise testing in, 6.122–6.123, 48.10f
  invasive electrophysiologic studies in, 6.119–6.121, 48.5t, 48.8f
  left
    electrocardiography in, 4.22–4.23, 27.9f
    ventricular activation in, 6.115
  in myocardial infarction, 6.123–6.125, 48.6t–48.8t
  and noncardiac surgery, 13.45
  pathology of, 6.113
  phase 3, 6.115, 6.116, 48.2f
  phase 4, 6.115, 6.116, 48.3f
  prophylactic pacemakers in, 6.121–6.122, 48.9f
  in rheumatoid arthritis, 13.5
  right
    electrocardiography in, 4.22
    incomplete, 11.46
    ventricular activation in, 6.114–6.115
  surgery in, 6.123
Butopamine, 2.58
Bypass surgery
  coronary, 7.249–7.259
    affecting left ventricular performance, 7.253
    in angina
      stable, 7.249–7.250
      unstable, 7.250, 7.252–7.253
    and angioplasty for dilatation of vein graft, 7.240–7.241, 73.5f
    and catheters for visualization of grafts, 5.30, 35.25f
    compared to angioplasty, 7.241
    critical appraisals of, 7.254
    in elderly patients, 13.31–13.32
    as emergency procedure, 7.173–7.174, 7.253–7.254, 7.263–7.264
    follow-up randomized studies of, 7.249–7.250
    heart failure after, 10.3
    hypertension after, 8.43
    internal mammary artery in, 7.256–7.257
    in multi-system atherosclerosis, 7.258–7.259, 74.1f, 74.2t
    in myocardial infarction, 7.173–7.174, 7.262–7.273. *See also* Infarction, myocardial, bypass surgery in
    occlusion of graft in, 7.254–7.255
      antiplatelet agents affecting, 7.255–7.256
      lipid-lowering regimens and smoking affecting, 7.256
    perioperative myocardial infarction in, 7.257
    and reoperations, 7.253
    and return to work and other activities, 7.259
    saphenous vein in, 7.249–7.256
    in silent ischemia, 7.97
    and size of recurrent infarctions, 7.253
    survival rate in, 7.251–7.252
      age affecting, 7.253
      compared to medical therapy, 7.251, 74.1t
      in left main equivalent disease, 7.252
      and sudden death reduction, 7.253
      in unstable angina, 7.252–7.253
    timing of, 7.253
      in myocardial infarction, 7.263, 7.267–7.268, 75.2f
    valve replacement procedures with, 7.257–7.258
    vein graft disease after
      antithrombotic therapy in, 2.163
      thrombosis in, 2.158
    visualization with brachial approach, 6.32
  renal, in renovascular hypertension, 8.35–8.36

C

Calcifications
  of aortic valve, 9.59, 9.106–9.107, 88.3f
  in elderly patients, 13.33
  cardiovascular, chest films of, 4.7, 4.9, 4.11–4.12, 26.10f–26.12f, 26.16f, 26.21f–26.22f
  of mitral annulus, 9.17
    echocardiography of, 4.69–4.70, 28.91f
Calcium
  cardiac concentrations of, 6.2, 40.1t
  channel blockers, 1.68, 2.105–2.121, 6.4, 6.25, 6.39, 17.1f
    and activity of β-adrenergic blocking drugs, 2.97
    in angina pectoris, 2.113–2.115, 7.72–7.73, 17.5t, 62.5t
    β-adrenergic blocking drugs with, 2.99
    compared to other antianginal drugs, 2.116, 17.6t
    in unstable angina, 7.80, 7.83–7.85, 63.3t, 63.5f–63.6f

in variant angina, 7.108–7.110,
    65.7f–65.9f
in arrhythmias, 2.116–2.118, 17.7t
as arteriolar vasodilators, 2.125, 2.126,
    18.4f
in cerebrovasoconstriction, 2.120
choice of, 2.121
classification of, 2.106–2.107, 17.1t
with complex pharmacologic profile,
    2.106, 2.107, 17.1t
dihydropyridine subgroup of, 2.106,
    2.107, 17.1t
effects in atherosclerosis, 2.116
effects on coronary circulation, 2.111
effects at rest in in exercise, 2.115,
    17.8f
effects on transplanted heart,
    13.97–13.98
electrophysiologic effects of,
    2.107–2.109, 17.2t, 17.2f–17.3f
in exercise-induced asthma, 2.120
in gastrointestinal disorders, 2.120
in heart failure, 2.120
in hypertension, 2.118–2.119, 8.25
  in elderly patients, 13.32
in hypertrophic cardiomyopathy,
    2.119
interactions with other drugs, 2.112,
    2.178–2.180, 21.5t
  β-adrenergic blocking drugs, 2.177,
    21.4t
  antiarrhythmic drugs, 2.176, 21.3t
in ischemic myocardial syndromes,
    2.112–2.113
with myocardial effects *in vivo*,
    2.106–2.107, 17.1t
in myocardial infarction, 7.156–7.157
pharmacokinetics of, 2.111–2.112,
    17.3t
pharmacology of, 2.105–2.106
piperazine derivatives, 2.106, 2.107,
    17.1t
in pregnancy, 13.22, 111.3t
protective effects of, 1.69, 1.70, 1.71,
    2.115–2.116, 4.1f, 4.4f
in pulmonary hypertension,
    2.119–2.120, 11.80
in Raynaud phenomenon, 2.120
selective vascular effects, 2.106, 2.107,
    17.1t
serum levels after bolus injection,
    2.117, 2.118, 17.9f
side effects of, 2.120–2.121, 17.8t
in silent ischemia, 7.98
systemic hemodynamic effects of,
    2.109–2.111, 17.4f–17.6f
therapeutic applications of,
    2.112–2.121, 17.4t
vascular effects *in vivo*, 2.106, 2.107,
    17.1t
and electrical excitation of myocardial
    fibers, 1.24
exchange with sodium, 1.68–1.70, 4.3f
flux in depolarization, 1.68, 1.69, 4.2f
intracellular

in aging, 1.71
in hypertension and hypertrophy,
    1.70–1.71
overload of, 1.70
regulation of, 1.68–1.70
  abnormalities in, 1.70–1.71
metabolism in myocardial infarction,
    7.121
sarcolemma channels, 1.68, 6.2, 6.3, 40.1f
sarcoplasmic reticulum channels, 1.68
serum levels
  affecting electrocardiogram, 4.30
  and digitalis toxicity, 2.46
Calmodulin and cardiac contractility, 1.21
Canadian Cardiovascular Society
    Functional Classification, 3.3,
    22.1t
Cannon waves, 9.97
Captopril, 9.6, 9.7, 81.2t
in dilated cardiomyopathy, 10.15
hemodynamic effects of, 2.129–2.130,
    2.131, 18.9f–18.11f
hydralazine with, 2.131
in hypertension, 8.24
interactions with other drugs, 2.184,
    2.185, 21.8t
  nonsteroidal anti-inflammatory drugs,
    2.181, 21.7t
in myocardial infarction, 7.158
in renal hypertension, 8.31
in reversal of left ventricular
    hypertrophy, 8.46–8.47, 79.2t
Carbamazepine
  interactions with theophylline, 2.186,
    21.9t
  interactions with warfarin, 2.187, 21.11t
Carbenicillin, interactions with warfarin,
    2.187, 21.10t
Carcinoid heart disease, 10.117
  echocardiography in, 4.83, 28.117f
Carcinoid syndrome
  hypertension in, 8.42
  tricuspid valve in, 9.95, 87.9f
Carcinoma metastasis to heart,
    12.52–12.53, 109.10f–109.11f
Cardiac output
  determinations of
    angiographic method, 5.5
    Fick method, 5.3–5.4
    indicator dilution method, 5.4–5.5,
      34.2f–34.3f
    thermodilution method, 5.5
  increased, causes of, 1.156, 1.157, 10.4t
  postoperative low output in cardiac
    surgery, 13.59, 13.60, 114.3t
    diagnosis of causes of, 13.64, 114.4t
    management of, 13.61–13.63, 114.8f
  post-transplantation, 13.96
Cardiofacial syndrome, cardiovascular
    disorders in, 3.13, 23.1t
Cardiomegaly
  in rheumatic fever, 10.101
  in viral myocarditis, 10.88
Cardiomyopathy
  in alcoholism, 10.3, 12.2–12.11

dilated, 10.2–10.16
  β-adrenergic blocking drugs in, 2.100
  in alcoholism, 10.3
  antithrombotic therapy in, 2.164
  arrhythmias in, 10.12
  assessment of functional status in,
    10.11–10.12
  bedside diagnosis of, 3.50, 23.14t
  biopsy in, 5.75–5.76, 10.4, 10.11,
    38.13f–38.15f
  cardiac catheterization in, 5.17,
    10.9–10.11
  catecholamine levels in, 10.12
  chest films in, 10.7, 90.2f
  clinical course of, 10.12–10.13
  clinical findings in, 10.6–10.7
  cocaine-induced, 13.77
  definition and classification of, 10.2
  in diabetes mellitus, 10.3
  diagnosis of, 10.13
  differential diagnosis of, 10.13–10.14,
    10.89, 90.5f–90.6f
  echocardiography in, 4.51–4.53,
    10.8–10.9, 28.29f–28.46f,
    90.3f–90.4f
  in elderly patients, 13.34–13.35
  electrocardiography in, 10.8
  etiology of, 10.2–10.3
  familial, 10.3
  functional abnormalities in, 10.4–10.5,
    90.1t
  heart failure in, 10.2
  hemodynamic effects of, 10.10
  in hypertension, 10.3
  initial presentation in, 10.5–10.6
  laboratory studies in, 10.9
  and myocarditis, 10.2, 10.89, 10.91
  in obesity, 10.3
  pathology of, 10.3–10.4, 90.1f
  peripartum, 10.3
  in pregnancy, 13.26
  prognosis of, 10.12
  radionuclide studies in, 10.9
  right ventricular pressure in, 10.10
  symptoms of, 10.5–10.6
  toxic, 10.3
  treatment of, 10.14–10.16
  ventricular function in, 10.12
  in virus infections, 10.2–10.3
echocardiography in, 4.39, 4.51–4.55,
    4.61, 28.15f, 28.46f–28.57f
Holter monitoring in, 6.94
hypertrophic, 10.18–10.36
  β-adrenergic blocking drugs in, 2.100
  apical, 10.31
  arrhythmias in, 10.30–10.31
    management of, 10.34, 10.36
  atrial fibrillation in, 6.130, 10.31, 10.36
  bedside diagnosis of, 3.50, 23.14t
  biopsy in, 5.76
  calcium channel blockers in, 2.119
  cardiac catheterization in, 5.17
  clinical course of, 10.36
  complications of, 10.36
  diastolic filling in, 10.26–10.29, 10.31, 91.5t

diastolic relaxation in, 10.28, 10.29–10.30, 91.6t
echocardiography in, 4.53–4.55, 10.20, 10.21, 28.52f–28.57f, 91.4f
  in elderly patients, 13.34
electrocardiography in, 10.30
endocarditis in, 10.36
extent of hypertrophy in, 10.28–10.29, 10.30, 91.11f
genetic factors in, 10.19
heart failure in, 10.36
hemodynamic classification of, 10.20–10.21, 91.2t–91.3t
  subgroups in, 10.32, 91.7t
intraventricular pressure differences in, 10.25, 91.4t
latent obstruction in, 10.32, 91.7t
  treatment of, 10.33, 10.34, 91.8t
left ventricular filling in, 5.61
midventricular obstruction in, 10.31
murmur in, 3.39, 3.40, 23.11t
myocardial fiber disarray in, 10.19–10.20, 91.3f
nonobstructive, 10.24–10.26, 10.32, 91.7t
  treatment of, 10.33, 10.34, 91.8t
outflow tract obstruction and mitral regurgitation in, 10.21–10.24, 91.5f–91.7f
pathology of, 10.18, 10.19–10.20, 91.1f–91.3f
in pregnancy, 13.25–13.26
resting obstruction in, 10.32, 91.7t
  treatment of, 10.33–10.34, 10.35, 91.8t, 91.12f
right ventricular involvement in, 10.31
  septal perforator artery compression in, 10.30
sudden death in, 10.36
treatment of, 10.32–10.36
types of, 10.18, 91.1t
ventricular tachycardia in, 10.30–10.31, 10.36
peripartum, 10.3
and viral myocarditis, 10.91
restrictive, 10.107–10.117
  in amyloid heart disease, 10.112–10.114
  bedside diagnosis of, 3.50, 23.14t
  biopsy in, 10.109–10.110, 97.4f
  in carcinoid heart disease, 10.117
  cardiac catheterization in, 5.17, 10.109, 97.3f
  in carnitine deficiency, 10.115–10.116
  clinical features of, 10.109
  compared to constrictive pericarditis, 10.109, 10.110, 97.2t
  diastolic function in, 10.108
  echocardiography in, 4.55
  in elderly patients, 13.35
  in endocardial fibroelastosis, 10.115

  in endomyocardial fibrosis, 10.111–10.112
  in Fabry's disease, 10.115
  in Gaucher's disease, 10.115
  hemodynamic effects of, 10.109, 97.3f
  in hemosiderosis and hemochromatosis, 10.114–10.115, 97.8f
  incidence and prevalence of, 10.108
  in neoplastic disease, 10.116
  pathology of, 10.108–10.109, 97.2f
  in pseudoxanthoma elasticum, 10.116
  radiation-induced, 10.117
  in sarcoidosis, 10.116–10.117
  in scleroderma, 10.116
  treatment of, 10.110–10.111
  in rheumatoid arthritis, 13.4
  in scleroderma, 10.116, 13.13
Cardioprotection, calcium channel blocking drugs in, 1.69, 1.70, 1.71, 2.115–2.116, 4.1f, 4.4f
Cardiopulmonary bypass
  and digitalis toxicity, 2.47
  physiologic effects of, 13.52–13.54
Cardiopulmonary receptors, 1.169–1.170
Cardioversion, direct-current
  in atrial fibrillation, 6.131
  in atrial flutter, 6.132
  contraindications in digitalis toxicity, 2.49
Carditis in rheumatic fever, 10.101
  differential diagnosis of, 10.89
Cardizem, effects on transplanted heart, 13.98
Carey-Coombs murmur, 3.47
Carnitine deficiency, restrictive cardiomyopathy in, 10.115–10.116
Carotid baroreceptors, 1.168–1.169, 11.7f
  and blood flow to limb muscles, 1.122–1.123
Carotid chemoreceptors, and blood flow to limb muscles, 1.123
Carotid pulse
  in aortic stenosis, 3.21–3.22, 23.3t, 23.5f
  configurational changes in, 3.20, 23.4f
Carotid sinus
  massage contraindications in digitalis toxicity, 2.49
  stimulation in sinus node evaluation, 6.102, 6.103, 47.2t
Carpentier-Edwards bioprosthetic valve, 9.46, 84.3f
  orifice areas in, 9.44, 84.1t
Carteolol, pharmacology of, 2.97, 9.96, 16.2t, 16.3t
Carvallo's sign, 3.46
Carvedilol, pharmacodynamic properties of, 2.96, 16.2t
Catalase, in myocardial infarction, 7.157
Catecholamines
  receptors for, 2.91, 7.191, 70.9t
  serum levels

    in dilated cardiomyopathy, 10.12
    in exercise, 1.137, 8.4t
    in myocardial infarction, 7.122
    in pheochromocytoma, 8.38
  therapy with, 2.50–2.59. *See also* Sympathomimetic drugs
    clinical applications of, 2.52–2.59, 2.66–2.68
    interactions with antihypertensive drugs, 2.184, 21.8t
    myocarditis from, 10.95
    in postinfarction shock, 7.191–7.192, 7.193, 70.10t
    vasodilators with, 7.194
Catheter(s)
  in ablation therapy of supraventricular tachycardia, 6.138
  balloon flotation, for right heart pressures, 5.80–5.81
  in brachial cutdown approach in angiography, 5.32, 35.29f
  coronary artery
    Amplatz, 5.29, 35.23f
    Judkins, 5.28–5.30, 35.21f–35.22f, 35.24f–35.26f
    for coronary bypass graft visualization, 5.30, 35.25f
    internal mammary artery, 5.30, 35.26f
  for MAP recording, 6.68, 6.70, 45.3f
  placement for intracardiac electrograms, 6.54, 6.55, 44.1f–44.2f
  pulmonary artery, knotting of, 5.92–5.93
Catheterization
  cardiac, 5.2–5.18
    in aortic valvular stenosis, 9.112, 88.6f
    in aortic valvuloplasty, 5.13, 5.15, 34.18f
    aortography in, 5.8
    in atrial septal defect, 11.48
      ostium primum with pulmonary vascular disease, 11.86
      ostium secundum with pulmonary vascular disease, 11.84
    brachial approach in, 5.2
    cardiac function evaluation in, 5.8–5.12
      contractile function indices in, 5.8–5.11
      pump function indices in, 5.11–5.12
      cardiac output calculations in, 5.3–5.5
    complications of, 5.38–5.40, 35.2t
    conduction defects from, 6.123
    in congenital heart disease in adults, 5.17–5.18
    in cyanotic congenital heart disease, 11.29, 11.31, 11.32, 11.33, 100.4f, 100.7f–100.8f
    in dilated cardiomyopathy, 10.9–10.11
    in ductus arteriosus patency, 11.57–11.58
      with pulmonary vascular disease, 11.83
    in Eisenmenger syndrome, 11.58–11.59, 11.82
    in endocarditis, 9.83–9.85
    femoral approach in, 5.3

indications for, 5.13–5.18, 7.59, 61.4f
and interventional procedures with balloon catheters, 9.54, 9.55, 85.1t
in left atrial myxoma, 12.48–12.49
left heart, 5.3
in mitral valvuloplasty, 5.12–5.23, 5.14, 34.17f
in myocardial and pericardial disease, 5.17
newer uses for, 5.13, 34.1t
patient preparation in, 5.2
in pulmonary heart disease, 10.74–10.75, 94.3f
in restrictive cardiomyopathy, 10.109, 97.3f
right heart, 5.3
risks and contraindications in, 5.18
simultaneous recording of left ventricular and pulmonary capillary wedge pressure in, 5.3, 5.4, 34.1f
systemic and pulmonary resistance calculations in, 5.5–5.6
transseptal approach in, 5.3
in valvular disease, 5.13–5.17
in ventricular septal defect, 11.57–11.58
ventriculography in, 5.6–5.8
pulmonary artery, 5.80–5.81
Caves-Stanford bioptome, 5.67
Cefamandole, interactions with warfarin, 2.187, 21.10t
Cefoperazone, interactions with warfarin, 2.187, 21.10t
Celiprolol, pharmacology of, 2.96, 2.97, 16.2t, 16.3t
Cellular electrophysiology, communication in, 6.5–6.6
Central venous pressure, 5.82
and plethora of inferior vena cava, 4.92–4.93
Cerebral blood flow in orthostatic hypotension, 1.164–1.165
Cerebrovascular disease
and anticoagulation after embolic strokes, 2.165
and complications of cardiac catheterization, 5.38–5.39
and coronary bypass surgery, 7.258–7.259, 74.1f, 74.2t
embolism from left atrial myxomas, 12.46
vasoconstriction in, calcium channel blockers in, 2.120
Cervical disk disease, chest pain in, 7.67
Chagas disease
echocardiography in, 4.52, 4.53, 28.50f–28.51f
myocarditis in, 10.94–10.95
Chemoreceptors, carotid and aortic, and blood flow to limb muscles, 1.123
Chemotaxis in myocardial ischemia, 7.118
Chest examination, 3.14, 3.54–3.57
inspection in, 3.55

palpation in, 3.55–3.56
percussion in, 3.56
Chest films, 4.2–4.13
in adult respiratory distress syndrome, 1.151, 9.10f
in aortic aneurysm, 4.8, 4.12, 4.13, 26.15f, 26.23f–26.24f
in aortic dissection, 12.32, 108.1t
in aortic insufficiency, chronic, 9.21, 82.10f
in aortic valvular stenosis, 9.110, 9.111, 88.4f
in atrial septal defect, 11.46, 11.47, 101.2f–101.5f
ostium primum with pulmonary vascular disease, 11.86
ostium secundun with pulmonary vascular disease, 11.84
borders of cardiac silhouette in, 4.3, 4.4, 26.1f–26.2f
calcifications in, 4.7, 4.9, 4.11–4.12, 26.10f–26.12f, 26.16f, 26.21f–26.22f
chamber size estimation in, 4.3
in constrictive pericarditis, 10.51
in cyanotic congenital heart disease, 11.28–11.30, 11.32, 100.1f–100.4f, 100.6f
in dilated cardiomyopathy, 10.7, 90.2f
in ductus arteriosus patency, 11.55, 11.56, 102.4f
with pulmonary vascular disease, 11.83
in Eisenmenger syndrome, 11.55, 11.82
in endocarditis, 9.82
epicardial fat stripe sign in, 4.3, 4.4, 26.4f
evaluation of cardiac size in, 4.3
examination of, 4.2–4.3
in great vessel abnormalities, 4.5, 4.12–4.13, 26.6f, 26.23f–26.25f
in hypertension, 8.19
in ischemic heart disease, 7.50–7.51
Kerley A lines in, 4.9
Kerley B lines in, 4.9, 4.10, 26.17f–26.18f
left atrium in, 4.5, 4.6–4.7, 26.9f–26.10f
enlargement of, 4.5, 4.7, 26.11f–26.12f
in myxoma, 12.47, 109.2f
left ventricle in, 4.5
enlargement of, 4.5, 4.7–4.8, 26.13f–26.14f
in mitral insufficiency, chronic, 9.13–9.14, 82.3f
in mitral valve prolapse, 9.34
in mitral valve stenosis, 9.120, 9.121, 89.2f
in myocardial infarction, 7.148
in myocarditis, viral, 10.87
in myocardial effusion, 4.3, 4.4, 10.41, 10.42, 26.3f–26.4f, 92.2f–92.3f
in positional abnormalities of heart, 4.10, 4.11, 26.19f–26.20f
in pulmonary edema, 1.148–1.149, 9.1t
in pulmonary embolism, 10.79
in pulmonary heart disease, 10.73, 94.1f
in pulmonary vascular disease, 11.80
pulmonary vasculature in, 4.8–4.9

enlargement of, 4.6, 4.9, 26.8f, 26.16f
in heart failure, 4.9–4.11, 26.17f–26.18f
right atrium in, 4.3–4.4
enlargement of, 4.4, 4.5, 26.5f
right ventricle in, 4.4–4.5, 26.5f–26.6f
enlargement of, 4.5, 4.6, 26.7f–26.8f
superior part of cardiac border in, 4.8
in tricuspid regurgitation, 9.98
in tricuspid stenosis, 9.101
unusual bulge of left cardiac border in, 4.13
in ventricular septal defect, 11.55
Chest pain or discomfort
in alcoholism, 12.8–12.9
in angina pectoris. See Angina pectoris
in anxiety and hyperventilation, 7.65
in aortic dissection, 7.66
atypical, 7.65–7.66
in Barlow's syndrome, 7.65
differential diagnosis of, 7.64–7.65
evaluation of, 3.4
in gastrointestinal disease, 7.67
in mediastinal emphysema, 7.66
in myocarditis, viral, 10.86
in neurovascular and neuromuscular disorders, 7.67
in pericarditis, 7.66
in pneumonia, 7.66
in pneumothorax, 7.66
in pulmonary arterial hypertension, 7.66
in pulmonary infarction, 7.66
Chest wall pain, 7.66
Cheyne-Stokes respiration, 3.6, 3.55
Chiari network, echocardiography of, 4.82, 4.98, 28.115f
Children and infants
aortic valvular stenosis in, management of, 9.113
biopsy of heart in, 5.69
cardiac failure in, differential diagnosis of, 10.89
cyanotic congenital heart disease in, 11.27–11.41
life-style of, and coronary heart disease risk, 7.23
viral myocarditis in neonates, 10.87
Chloral hydrate, interaction with anticoagulants, 2.153, 2.187, 20.2t, 21.10t
Chloramphenicol, interaction with anticoagulants, 2.153, 20.2t
Chloride
cardiac concentrations of, 6.2, 40.1t
channels across sarcolemma, 6.2
Chloroquine, myocarditis from, 10.95
Chlorpromazine, interactions with antihypertensive drugs, 2.184, 21.8t
Chlorthalidone, 2.27, 13.1t
Cholecystitis, chest pain in, 7.67
Cholesterol
content in foods, 7.4, 59.1t
crystals in pericarditis, 10.63

dietary, and coronary heart disease, 7.3, 7.14, 7.21
hypercholesterolema
  familial, 2.141, 7.41–7.43, 60.4t
  polygenic, 7.42, 7.43, 60.4t
  serum levels
    and coronary heart disease risk, 7.4–7.7, 7.36–7.38, 59.2t–59.3t, 60.1f–60.2f
    declines in American population, 7.26, 7.28
    diagnosis of abnormalities in, 7.46
    heritable disorders in, 7.42–7.43, 60.4t
    hypolipidemic agents, 2.137–2.141
    normal levels, 7.38, 60.1t
    stress affecting, 13.68
    and vein graft patency, 7.256
Cholestyramine, 2.137–2.138
  interaction with anticoagulants, 2.153, 2.187, 20.2t, 21.11t
  interaction with digoxin, 2.172, 21.1t
Cholinergic nerves, and blood flow to limbs, 1.119
Cholinergic receptors. See Muscarinic cholinergic receptors
Chorea in rheumatic fever, 10.101–10.102
  management of, 10.105
Chylomicrons, 7.40, 60.3t
  in lipoprotein metabolism, 7.39
Chylopericardium, 10.63
Cibenzoline, 6.47–6.48
  antiarrhythmic spectrum of, 6.47
  dosage of, 6.48
  electrophysiologic properties of, 6.47
  pharmacokinetics of, 6.47
  side effects of, 6.47–6.48
Cimetidine, interaction with other drugs
  β-adrenergic blocking drugs, 2.177, 21.4t
  antiarrhythmic drugs, 2.175, 21.2t
  anticoagulants, 2.153, 2.187, 20.2t, 21.10t
  theophylline, 2.186, 21.9t
Cinnarizine, 2.106, 2.107, 17.1t
Ciprostene, as platelet inhibitor, 2.149
Cicardian rhythm of silent ischemia, 7.94, 7.95, 64.3f
Circulation. See Blood flow
Cirrhosis, diuretics in, 2.28
C1–914, inotropic effects of, 2.65
Claudication, intermittent
  in atherosclerosis of limb vessels, 1.126–1.127
  misinterpretation of, 12.39, 108.10f, 108.12f
  in occlusive peripheral arterial disease, 12.37
Clicks, systolic
  ejection, 3.35
  non-ejection, 3.35–3.36
Clofibrate, 2.139
  interaction with anticoagulants, 2.153, 2.187, 20.2t, 21.10t
Clonidine
  interactions with other drugs, 2.184, 2.185, 21.8t

in orthostatic hypotension, 1.175–1.176, 11.11f
Clotting factors. See Coagulation factors
Clubbing of fingers and toes, 3.14
Coagulation, mechanisms in, 2.145, 20.2f
Coagulation factors
  deficiency of, and venous thrombosis, 10.78
  interactions of, 2.145
  oral anticoagulants affecting, 2.152
Coanda effect in supravalvular aortic stenosis, 11.72
Coarctation of aorta, 3.63, 3.64, 11.73–11.75, 25.8f–25.9f, 103.10f. See also Aorta, coarctation of
Cocaine, 13.74–13.78
  arrhythmias from, 13.75–13.76
  cardiovascular complications of, 13.75–13.78, 116.1t
  myocardial infarction from, 13.76–13.77, 116.2f
  treatment of, 13.78
  pharmacology of, 13.74–13.75, 116.1f
Coccidioidomycosis, pericarditis in, 10.59
Coeur en sabot, 3.59
Cold exposure
  and Raynaud's disease, 1.124–1.126, 7.8f
  vasodilation in, 1.121
Cold pressor testing in variant angina, 7.106
Colestipol, 2.137–2.138
  interactions with warfarin, 2.187, 21.11t
Collagen
  diseases of, 13.2–13.16, 110.1t
    rheumatoid arthropathy, 13.2–13.6
    sclerosing syndrome, 13.12–13.16
    vasculitis syndrome, 13.6–13.11
  and platelet adhesion and aggregation, 2.143–2.144
Collateral vessels
aortopulmonary, with tetralogy of Fallot and pulmonary atresia, 3.59, 3.60, 25.2f
  coronary, 1.110, 5.25, 5.26–5.27, 35.13f–35.18f
  in ischemic heart disease, 7.64
Colloid osmotic pressure, in plasma, 1.145
  compared to endobronchial fluid, 1.151, 1.152, 9.11f
  and effects of afterload reduction, 1.150, 9.9f
  posture affecting, 1.148, 9.8f
  in pulmonary edema, 1.145–1.147, 9.4f
Commissurotomy, mitral
  closed, 9.123
  open, 9.123
Compliance
  arterial, 8.55–8.56, 80.3f
  ventricular, 5.62
    vasodilators affecting, 2.131, 2.132, 18.12f
Compressive resistance in coronary flow, 1.102, 1.103, 1.104, 6.2f, 6.3f
Computed tomography

in aldosteronism, 8.40, 78.7f
  in aortic dissection, 12.32
  in atrial myxomas, 12.48
  in atrial septal defect, 11.48
  in measurements of infarct size, 7.135–7.137, 67.6f
  in myocardial contusion, 12.19
  in pericardial effusion, 10.43, 92.6f
  in pheochromocytoma, 8.38
Computer use
  in digital angiography, 5.43–5.52
  in quantitative coronary angiography, 5.38
Conduction
  abnormalities in, 6.9–6.12
    catheter-induced, 6.123
    in elderly patients, 13.36–13.37
    electrocardiography in, 4.22–4.24, 27.9f–27.11f
    noncardiac surgery in, 13.45
    in rheumatoid arthritis, 13.5
  anatomy of system, 1.12–1.13, 1.12f–1.15f
    in lower system, 6.111–6.112, 48.1f
  antiarrhythmic drugs affecting, 6.34
  delayed
    generalized depolarization in, 6.9, 6.10, 40.10f
    premature stimulation in, 6.9, 6.10, 40.9f
  sinoatrial conduction time, 6.104–6.105
  ventricular physiology of, 6.113–6.115
Congenital heart disease
  aortic valvular stenosis, 9.106, 11.6
  atrial septal defect, 11.43–11.50
  bedside diagnosis in adults, 3.58–3.67
  blood flow obstruction in
    pulmonary, 3.58–3.62
    systemic, 3.62–3.63
  cardiac catheterization in, 5.17–5.18
  coronary artery anomalies, 11.14–11.25
  cyanotic, 11.27–11.41
  differential diagnosis of, 10.13, 10.14, 90.5f–90.6f
  ductus arteriosus patency, 11.51–11.60
  echocardiography in, 11.88–11.96
  in elderly patients, 13.34
  identification of lesions in, 11.2
  isolated obstructive lesions, 11.61–11.76
  left-to-right shunt lesions, 3.63–3.66
  lesions simulating valvar aortic regurgitation, 3.66–3.67
  long-term outcome of surgically corrected lesions, 11.3–11.11
    in atrial septal defect, 11.4–11.5
    in coarctation of aorta, 11.6–11.7
    in conduit replacements, 11.11, 98.5f–98.6f
    in Ebstein's anomaly, 11.10–11.11
    in patent ductus arteriosus, 11.3–11.4, 98.1f
    in pulmonary valve stenosis, 11.6
    in tetralogy of Fallot, 11.7–11.8, 92.2f
    in transposition of great vessels, 11.8–11.10, 98.3f–98.4f
    in tricuspid atresia, 11.10

in ventricular septal defect, 11.5–11.6
mitral insufficiency in, 9.17
pericardial, 10.64
in postoperative adult patients, 3.67
in pregnancy, 13.24–13.25
pulmonary vascular disease in, 3.58, 11.77–11.86
right ventricular obstruction
  inflow, 11.61–11.62
  outflow, 11.62–11.64, 103.1f
risk in offspring of parents with heart disease, 13.21, 111.2t
tetralogy of Fallot, 3.59
transposition of great arteries, congenitally corrected, 3.67, 3.68, 25.13f–25.14f
tricuspid valve abnormalities, 9.96–9.97
unoperated lesions in adult, 11.2–11.3
ventricular septal defect, 11.51–11.60
Conn syndrome, 13.87–13.88
Connective tissue disease, mixed, 13.15–13.16
Conotruncal anomalies, complex, with pulmonary stenosis, 3.62
Constrictive pericarditis, 10.48–10.52
Contraceptives, oral
  cardiovascular effects of, 13.88
  and coronary heart disease risk, 7.22
  interaction with anticoagulants, 2.153, 2.187, 20.2t, 21.11t
  interaction with theophylline, 2.186, 21.9t
Contractile function indices, 5.8–5.11
  ejection fraction, 5.8
    corrected for afterload, 5.8–5.9, 34.8f
  end-systolic relationships, 5.9–5.11, 34.9f–34.12f
  mean velocity of circumferential fiber shortening, 5.8
Contractile proteins, 1.20–1.21, 1.22, 1.23, 2.2f–2.4f
Contraction band necrosis in cocaine abuse, 13.76
Contraction of cardiac muscle, 1.19–1.40
  antiarrhythmic drugs affecting, 6.34
  aortic flow trace in, 1.89, 5.4f
  energy metabolism in, 1.79, 1.80, 4.15f
  excitation-contraction coupling in, 1.24–1.26, 2.6f–2.8f
  force-velocity relations in, 1.86–1.87, 1.88, 5.2f–5.3f
  heart rate affecting, 1.31, 2.16f–2.17f
  hypoxia affecting, 1.81, 4.17f
  isometric, 1.30–1.31, 2.12f–2.15f
    relation to isotonic contractions, 1.35–1.36, 2.25f–2.26f
  isotonic, 1.32–1.34, 2.18f–2.22f
    relation to isometric contractions, 1.35–1.36, 2.25f–2.26f
  and left ventricular performance, 1.86–1.89
  in myocardial infarction, 7.180–7.181, 70.2f
  length-tension relations in, 1.27–1.28, 2.9f–2.10f

loading conditions affecting, 1.36, 1.37, 2.27f–2.28f
maximum rate of pressure development in, 1.88–1.89
mechanics of, 1.27–1.38
mitochondria in, 1.23–1.24
modulators of membrane function in, 1.21–1.23
myocardial cells in, 1.19–1.24
and relaxation, 1.26, 1.36–1.40, 2.8f, 2.29f–2.32f
sarcomere apparatus in, 1.20–1.21, 1.22, 1.23, 2.1f–2.4f
sarcoplasmic reticulum in, 1.23, 1.24, 2.5f
superficial membrane system in, 1.21, 1.24, 2.5f
velocity of fiber shortening in, 1.87–1.88
velocity-length relations in, 1.34–1.35, 2.23f–2.24f
Contusions, myocardial, 12.16–12.20
  clinical features of, 12.17
  diagnosis of, 12.17
  laboratory data in, 12.18–12.19
  management of, 12.19
Cor pulmonale, 10.70–10.77
  cardiac catheterization in, 10.74–10.75, 94.3f
  causes of pulmonary hypertension in, 10.71–10.72, 94.1t
  chest films in, 10.73, 94.1f
  diagnosis of, 10.73–10.75
  differential diagnosis of, 10.14
  digitalis in, 10.76–10.77
  diuretics in, 10.76
  echocardiography in, 4.63, 4.64, 10.74, 28.79f
  in elderly patients, 13.35
  electrocardiography in, 4.28, 10.73–10.74, 94.2f
  heart-lung transplantation in, 10.76
  management of, 10.75–10.77
  pathophysiology of, 10.70
  physical examination in, 10.73
  in pulmonary embolism, 10.77–10.82
  in scleroderma, 13.14
  vasodilators in, 10.76, 94.2t
Cor triatriatum, 3.62, 11.66–11.67
Cordis bioptome, 5.67–5.68
Cornelia de Lange syndrome, cardiovascular disorders in, 3.13, 23.1t
Coronary arteries
  absent arteries, 11.15, 11.20, 99.2f, 99.10f
  anatomy of, 1.9, 1.9f, 1.13–1.15, 1.16f–1.17f, 5.20–5.25
  aneurysms, 11.23–11.24, 11.25, 99.14f–99.15f
  angioplasty. See Angioplasty, coronary, percutaneous transluminal
  anomalies of, 11.14–11.25
    classification of, 11.14, 99.1t
    secondary to primary cardiac defects, 11.24
  arteriography, 5.25–5.42
  arteritis, 13.9–13.11, 110.3f

collateral supply, 5.25, 5.26–5.27, 35.13f–35.18f
dominant systems, 5.24–5.25, 35.12f
ectopic origin
  from aorta, 11.19–11.20
  from aortic sinus, 11.15–11.19, 99.1f–99.9f
  from pulmonary artery, 11.20–11.22, 99.11f
fistulas, 11.22–11.23, 99.12f–99.13f
hypoplasia or atresia, 11.23
left, 1.13–1.14, 5.20, 5.22–5.24, 35.1f, 35.8f–35.11f
anterior descending, stenosis of, Dock's murmur in, 3.45, 3.46, 23.14f
normal, myocardial infarction with, 7.113
radiographic projections of, 5.33–5.38, 35.1t
restenosis after percutaneous coronary angioplasty, 2.158
right, 1.14–1.15, 5.20, 5.22, 35.1f–35.7f
spasm
  catheter-induced, 5.41–5.42
  and myocardial infarction, 7.119–7.120
  nitrates in, 2.81–2.82
  provocative testing in
    ergonovine in, 5.33, 5.34, 7.104–7.106, 35.31f, 65.1t–65.2t, 65.5f–65.6f
    histamine in, 7.107
    methacholine in, 7.106
  unstable angina in, 7.76, 7.77, 63.1f
  in variant Prinzmetal angina, 7.100–7.101, 7.119
stenosis
  assessment by angiography, 1.108, 1.109–1.110, 5.37–5.38, 6.8f
  coronary circulation in, 1.106–1.110, 6.6f–6.9f
  thrombosis and embolism in, 2.156–2.158
  and myocardial infarction, 7.112, 7.114–7.115
  in trauma, 12.22
trauma of, 12.22
in unstable angina, 7.75–7.78, 63.1t
vasomotion of, 7.63–7.64
Coronary arteriovenous fistula, 3.67
Coronary care units, 7.143
  admission orders in, 7.144–7.145, 68.1f
  mobile, 7.142
  step-down or intermediate, 7.143
Coronary circulation. See Blood flow, coronary
Coronary heart disease
  α-adrenergic receptors in, 1.56–1.57
  β-adrenergic receptors in, 1.54–1.55, 3.5
  angina pectoris in, 7.48–7.50, 7.62–7.73, 61.1f
  angioplasty in, percutaneous transluminal, 7.237–7.245
  antithrombotic therapy in, 2.159–2.163, 20.4t
  association with mitral regurgitation, 7.268, 7.269, 75.2t

asymptomatic, 7.91–7.92
  surgery in, 7.97
behavioral-psychosocial factors in, 7.22
blood pressure in, 7.7–7.10
  diastolic, 7.7–7.8, 59.4t
  and progress in control efforts, 7.28
  systolic, 7.8, 7.9, 59.1f, 59.5t
bypass surgery in, 7.249–7.259
chest films in, 7.50–7.51
childhood life-style as factor in, 7.23
cholesterol levels in, 7.4–7.7, 7.36–7.38, 59.2t–59.3t, 60.1f–60.2f
  reduction of, effects of, 7.37
collateral circulation in, 7.64
coronary arteriography in, 7.58–7.60
decline in mortality and incidence, 7.28–7.32, 59.9f–59.10f, 59.14t–59.15t
in diabetes mellitus, 7.11–7.12, 59.6t–59.7t
dietary factors in, 7.3–7.4, 7.14–7.21, 59.2f
  autopsy studies, 7.15–7.16, 59.2f
  and guidelines for Americans, 7.24, 59.5f
  interpopulation research in, 7.14–7.19
  intrapopulation research in, 7.19–7.22, 59.10t
  living population studies, 7.16–7.19, 59.3f–59.4f
  migration affecting, 7.15, 7.17, 7.36
  and recent changes by Americans, 7.25–7.27, 59.6f, 59.12t–59.13t
differential diagnosis of, 10.13
echocardiography in, 4.48, 7.57–7.58, 61.3f
and effects of reperfusion, 1.82
in elderly patients, 13.29–13.32
electrocardiography in, 4.24, 4.25, 7.51–7.54, 27.11f
  ambulatory, 7.58
  exercise testing in, 7.52–7.54, 61.1f, 61.2f–61.3t
epidemiology of, 7.3
exercise in, cardiac changes from, 7.214
heart failure in, 1.156, 10.2t
indications for cardiac catheterization in, 7.59, 61.4f
infarction in. *See* Infarction, myocardial
left ventricular dysfunction in, 7.63
left ventricular filling in, 5.61
left ventriculography in, 7.60–7.61, 61.5f
in lupus erythematosus, 13.9
MAP recordings in, 6.82–6.84, 45.22f–45.24f
metabolic alterations in, 7.63
Multiple Risk Factor Intervention Trial (MRFIT), 7.5–7.10
myocardial metabolism in, 1.81
nitrates in, 2.79–2.80
noncardiac surgery in, 13.41–13.44
and obesity, 7.21–7.22
and oral contraceptive use, 7.22
physical examination in, 7.50
platelets in, 7.115

Pooling Project Research studies, 7.13, 59.8t
in pregnancy, 13.26
primary prevention of, 7.2
  recommendations for, 7.23–7.25, 59.5f, 59.11t
  and risk factor concept, 7.2–7.3
radionuclide angiocardiography in, 7.56–7.57
regional myocardial function in, 1.81, 1.82, 4.18f
in rheumatoid arthritis, 13.5
risk factors in, 7.38, 60.2t
  combinations of, 7.12–7.14, 59.7t–59.8t
sedentary life-style as risk, 7.22
Seven Countries Study, 7.10, 7.16, 7.17, 7.36, 59.1f, 59.3f
silent ischemia in, 7.65, 7.91–7.98
  β-adrenergic blocking drugs in, 2.100
  and angina pectoris, 7.94–7.95, 64.4f–64.5f
  circadian rhythm of, 7.94, 7.95, 64.3f
  definition and classification of, 7.91
  diagnosis of, 7.92–7.93, 64.1t
  electrocardiography in, 7.92
  hemodynamics in, 7.92
  medical therapy in, 7.97–7.98
  mechanisms for absence of discomfort in, 7.93–7.94, 64.2f
  metabolism in, 7.93
  postinfarction, 7.96
  prognosis of, 7.96–7.97, 64.6f
  surgery in, 7.97
  thallium–201 scintigraphy in, 7.92
  in unstable angina, 7.96
smoking status in, 7.6, 7.10, 59.3t
  and recent changes by Americans, 7.28, 59.8f
stress related to, 13.60, 13.69
subclinical, signs of, 7.22
thallium–201 myocardial imaging in, 7.54–7.57, 61.2f
time course of necrosis in, 1.81–1.82, 1.83, 4.19f–4.20f
Western Electric Company Study, 7.20–7.21, 59.10t
Coronary sinus, 1.4f, 1.6, 1.16
  septal defect, 3.64
  thebesian valve of, 1.4f, 1.6
Corrigan's pulse, in aortic insufficiency, 9.20
Corticosteroid therapy
  β-adrenergic receptors in, 1.54, 1.55, 3.5t
  in lupus erythematosus, 13.7
  in myocardial infarction, 7.157
  in myocarditis, 10.90, 10.92
  in rheumatic fever, 10.104
  in transplantation of heart, 13.95, 13.103
Cortisol levels, stress affecting, 13.68
Costochondral separation, palpation in, 3.55
Costochondritis, chest pain in, 3.6

Costoclavicular maneuver in peripheral arterial disease, 12.36, 108.7f
Coughing, evaluation of, 3.9
Coumarin drugs, 2.152–2.154. *See also* Warfarin
Coxsackievirus infections, myocarditis in, 10.90
Crackles, 3.56, 24.1t
  inspiratory, 3.56–3.57, 24.2t
  post-tussive, 3.57
C–reactive protein in rheumatic fever, 10.102
Creatine kinase
  in estimation of infarct size, 7.134–7.135
  in myocardial contusion, 12.18
  in myocardial infarction, 7.147
Crista terminalis, 1.6
Critically ill patients, hemodynamic monitoring in, 5.90–5.91, 39.7f
Cryptococcosis, myocarditis in, 10.93
Cultures, throat, in rheumatic fever, 10.102
Curare, interaction with antiarrhythmic drugs, 2.176, 21.3t
Cushing's disease, 13.87
Cushing's syndrome, hypertension in, 8.40–8.41
Cyanosis
  central, 3.7
  clubbing with, 3.14
  evaluation of, 3.7
  peripheral, 3.7
  in pregnancy, 13.25
Cyanotic congenital heart disease, 11.27–11.41
  chest films in, 11.28–11.30, 11.32, 100.1f–100.4f, 100.6f
  determination of cardiac and visceral situs in, 11.31
  diagnosis of, 11.30–11.37
  differential diagnosis of, 11.33–11.37, 100.1t
  in neonates, 11.41
  electrocardiography in, 11.31
  invasive studies in, 11.29, 11.31, 11.32, 11.33, 100.4f, 100.7f–100.8f
  management of, 11.37–11.41
    with deficient pulmonary blood flow, 11.39–11.41
    with excessive pulmonary blood flow, 11.38–11.39
  noninvasive studies in, 11.31
  pulmonary blood flow in
    deficient, 11.28–11.30, 11.35–11.37, 100.3f–100.6f
      management of, 11.39–11.41
    excessive, 11.28, 11.33–11.35, 100.1f–100.2f
      management of, 11.38–11.39
Cyclo-oxygenase, platelet, inhibitors of, 2.147
Cyclophosphamide, myocarditis from, 10.95–10.96
Cyclosporine
  complications of, 13.100–13.101

interactions with other drugs, 13.101, 118.2f
in transplantation of heart, 13.95, 13.103
Cyst, pericardial
  congenital, 10.64
  inflammatory, 10.64
Cysticercosis, myocarditis in, 10.94
Cytomegalovirus infections, after transplantation of heart, 13.98–13.99

D

D13625, inotropic effects of, 2.66
Death, sudden
  after bypass surgery, 7.253
  in cocaine abuse, 13.77
  in emotional stress, 13.70
  in hypertrophic cardiomyopathy, 10.36
  in mitral valve prolapse, 9.36
    prevention of, 9.37–9.38
  in viral myocarditis, 10.86, 10.88
Debrisoquin, interactions with other drugs, 2.184, 2.185, 21.8t
Denervation, sympathetic, and blood flow to limbs, 1.119
Densitometry, video, 5.38, 5.45–5.47
Depolarization, 1.24, 6.3, 6.4, 40.43f
  after depolarizations, 6.7–6.9, 40.7f–40.8f
  calcium flux in, 1.68, 1.69, 4.2f
  electrocardiography in, 4.14, 4.16, 27.3f
  ionic basis for, 6.6
Dermatomyositis, 13.15
Desensitization of β-adrenergic receptors, 1.51, 1.52–1.53, 3.9f
Deslanoside, 2.37
  pharmacokinetics of, 2.37, 14.2t
Dextran, as platelet inhibitor, 2.149
Dextrocardia, mirror image, electrocardiography in, 4.18
Diabetes mellitus, 13.82–13.84
  atherosclerosis in, 13.82, 13.83, 117.2f
  cardiovascular risk in, 13.82, 117.1t
  coronary heart disease in, 7.11–7.12, 59.6t–59.7t
  dilated cardiomyopathy in, 10.3
  electrocardiography in, 4.31
  heart failure in, 13.84
  hyperlipidemia in, 13.82–13.83
  hypertension in, 8.42, 13.84
  microangiopathy in, 13.83, 117.1f
  myocardial infarction in, 13.83–13.84
  peripheral vascular disease in, 13.84
  treatment of, 13.84
Diagnostic procedures
  in bedside evaluation, 3.2. See also Bedside evaluation of patients of patients
  in elderly patients, 13.29
  invasive tests in. See Invasive tests
  noninvasive tests in, 4.2–4.98
Dialysis
  in digitalis toxicity, 2.49
  and endocarditis, 9.81
  and pericarditis, 10.62

Diaphragm dysfunction, postoperative, management of, 13.58
Diastole
  apical, rumble in, in mitral stenosis, 9.120
  MAP recording in, 6.70
  mitral regurgitation in, 9.17
  murmurs in, 3.45–3.48
Diastolic function of ventricles, 5.55–5.65, 10.107–10.108, 97.1f
  aortic valvular stenosis affecting, 9.108
  and atrial systole, 5.65
  hypertrophic cardiomyopathy affecting, 10.26–10.29, 10.31, 91.5t
  isovolumic relaxation in, 5.55–5.59, 10.26–10.28, 91.9f
    duration of, 5.55–5.57, 37.1f–37.2f
    pressure changes in, 5.57–5.58, 37.3f
    regional wall motion in, 5.58, 37.4f
    significance of abnormalities in, 5.58–5.59, 37.5f
  myocardial infarction affecting, 7.123–7.125, 7.181–7.184, 70.3f–70.5f
  passive ventricular filling in, 5.62–5.65, 37.7f
    abnormalities of, 5.65
    pressure-volume relations in, 5.63–5.64
    stiffness affecting, 5.62–5.63
    stress-strain relations in, 5.64–5.65
  phases in, 5.55
  rapid ventricular filling in, 5.59–5.62
    abnormal, 5.61
    mechanisms in, 5.61–5.62
    normal, 5.59–5.60, 37.6f
    and pulmonary artery wedge pressure, 5.84
Dibutyryl-cAMP, inotropic effects of, 2.60
Diet. See Nutrition
Diflunisal, interactions with other drugs, 2.181, 21.7t
  warfarin, 2.187, 21.10t
Digital angiography, cardiac, 5.43–5.52
Digitalis glycosides. 2.34–2.36, 6.40. See also Glycosides, cardiac
  digitoxin, 2.36
  digoxin, 2.34–2.36
  in dilated cardiomyopathy, 10.15
  in heart failure, in elderly patients, 13.36
  in hyperthyroidism, 13.85
  interaction with calcium entry blockers, 2.179, 21.5t
  interaction with diuretics, 2.180, 21.6t
  pharmacology of, 2.34
  in postinfarction shock, 7.191
  in pregnancy, 13.22, 111.3t
  prophylactic use of, 2.44
  in pulmonary heart disease, 10.76–10.77
  in supraventricular tachycardia, 6.138
  toxicity of, 2.44–2.50, 14.3t–14.4t
    arrhythmias in, 2.45–2.46, 14.4t
    diagnosis of, 2.47–2.48
    extracardiac manifestations of, 2.44–2.45, 24.3t

    management of, 2.48–2.50, 2.51, 14.5t
    predisposing factors for, 2.46–2.47
Digitoxin, 2.36
  pharmacokinetics of, 2.37, 14.2t
Digoxin, 2.34–2.36
  antibodies to, 2.49–2.50
  effects on transplanted heart, 13.97
  Fab fragment infusions in digitalis toxicity, 2.49–2.50
  interactions with other drugs, 2.172–2.174, 21.1f, 21.1t
    antiarrhythmic drugs, 2.176, 21.3t
    calcium entry blockers, 2.179, 21.5t
    monoamine oxidase inhibitors, 2.184, 21.8t
  pharmacokinetics of, 2.37, 14.2t
  structure of, 2.34, 2.35, 14.1f
Dilevalol, pharmacology of, 2.96, 2.97, 16.2t, 16.3f
Diltiazem, 2.106–2.107, 17.1t
  adverse effects of, 2.121, 17.8t
  as arteriolar vasodilator, 2.125
  characteristics of, 7.72, 62.5t
  interactions with other drugs, 2.179, 21.5t
    digoxin, 2.172, 21.1t
  in myocardial infarction, 7.157
  pharmacokinetics of, 2.111, 2.112, 17.3t
  in pulmonary hypertension, 11.80
  systemic hemodynamic effects of, 2.109–2.110, 17.5f
  in unstable angina, 7.83, 7.84
  in variant angina, 7.108–7.110, 65.7f, 65.9f
Diphtheria, myocarditis in, 10.92–10.93
Dipyridamole
  chemical structure of, 2.148, 20.4f
  as platelet inhibitor, 2.148
  warfarin with, in thrombosis prevention with prosthetic valves, 2.165
Dipyridamole-thallium scintigraphy, preoperative, 13.43
Disopyramide, 6.21, 6.35–6.37
  contraindications in digitalis toxicity, 2.49
  dosage and pharmacokinetic properties of, 6.37, 42.2t
  effects on heart and circulation, 6.21
  effects on transmembrane potential, 6.21
  effects on transplanted heart, 13.97
  in hypertrophic cardiomyopathy, 10.33–10.34
  interaction with other drugs, 6.33, 42.1t
  in pregnancy, 13.22, 111.3t
  in supraventricular tachycardia, 6.138
Dissection, aortic, 12.30–12.33
Disulfiram
  in alcoholic heart disease, 12.11
  interaction with anticoagulants, 2.153, 2.187, 20.2t, 21.10t
Diuretics, 2.19–2.31
  actions of, 3.21–2.24, 13.3f
    cellular mechanisms of, 2.21–2.22, 2.23, 13.4f–13.5f
    on nephron segments, 2.22–2.24, 13.6f
  in ascites, 2.28

in cirrhosis, 2.28
clinical uses of, 2.26–2.30, 13.1t
complications of, 2.30–2.31, 13.2t
in dilated cardiomyopathy, 10.14
in heart failure, 1.161, 2.26–2.28,
    13.10f–13.12f
  in elderly patnets, 13.36
in hypertension, 2.29–2.30, 8.21–8.22,
    77.6t
  in elderly patients, 13.32
in idiopathic edema, 2.29
interactions with other drugs,
    2.180–2.181, 21.6t
  antihypertensive drugs, 2.184, 21.8t
  digoxin, 2.172, 21.1t
  nonsteroidal anti-inflammatory drugs,
    2.181, 21.7t
in nephrotic syndrome, 2.28–2.29
in pregnancy, 13.22, 111.3t
in pulmonary heart disease, 10.76
renal handling of, 2.24–2.25, 13.7f–13.8f
  braking phenomenon in, 2.25–2.26,
    2.28, 2.30, 13.9f
in renal hypertension, 8.30–8.31
Diving reflex, 1.123
Dizziness in dilated cardiomyopathy,
  10.6
DNA, recombinant, in receptor studies,
  1.44–1.45
Dock's murmur, 3.45, 3.46, 23.14f
Dobutamine, 2.55–2.57, 14.8f, 9.7–9.8
  effects on transplanted heart, 13.97
  hemodynamic effects of, 2.53,
    14.6t
  in postinfarction shock, 7.191–7.192,
    7.193, 70.10t
  receptors for, 7.191, 70.9t
L-Dopa, 2.58–2.59
  hemodynamic effects of, 2.53, 14.6t
Dopamine, 2.54–2.55, 9.7–9.8, 14.7f
  hemodynamic effects of, 2.53, 14.6t
  interactions with other drugs, 2.184,
    21.8t
  in postinfarction shock, 7.191, 7.193,
    70.10
  receptors for, 7.191, 70.9t
Dopexamine, 2.59
  hemodynamic effects of, 2.53, 14.6t
Doppler echocardiography, 4.43–4.36,
  28.3f–28.5f
  aliasing in, 4.36, 4.71, 28.93f
  in aortic insufficiency, chronic, 9.22,
    9.23, 9.24, 82.11f–82.14f
  in aortic stenosis, 4.76–4.77, 28.103f
  in atrial septal defect, 11.88–11.89, 105.2f
  color-flow, 4.86–4.89, 28.125f–28.131f
    in aortic abscess, 4.87, 28.126f
    in aortic regurgitation, 4.88,
      28.128f–28.129f
    in mitral regurgitation, 4.86, 4.88,
      28.125f, 28.127f
    in mitral stenosis, 4.88, 28.130f
    in tricuspid regurgitation, 4.86, 4.89,
      9.98–9.99, 28.125f, 28.131f,
      87.12f–87.13f
  in ventricular septal defect,
    4.59, 28.68f
  continuous-wave, 4.36
  in dilated cardiomyopathy, 10.8, 10.9,
    90.4f
  exercise testing in, 4.55–4.56, 28.58f
  for left ventricular stroke volume, 4.44,
    28.24f
  in mitral regurgitation, 4.71, 9.14–9.15,
    28.93f–28.94f, 82.4f–82.6f
  in mitral stenosis, 4.69, 9.121, 28.90f,
    89.3f
  in mitral valve prolapse, 9.35
  normal ventricular flow patterns in, 4.68,
    28.86f
  Nyquist limit in, 4.36, 4.71, 4.86, 28.93f
  peak velocity ranges in, 4.36, 28.1t
  in pulmonary heart disease, 10.74
  pulsed-wave, 4.34, 4.36
Dose-response relationships in
    pharmacology, 2.2–2.4,
    12.1f–12.3f
  dose-response relationships in
    pharmacology
  receptor systems in, 2.2–2.4, 12.4f
  and structure-activity relationships,
    2.4, 12.5f
Down's syndrome, cardiovascular
    disorders with, 3.11, 3.13,
    23.1t
Doxazosin, 2.91
Doxorubicin (adriamycin) toxicity
  cardiac biopsy in, 5.72–5.75,
    38.11f–38.12f
  myocarditis in, 10.95
Dozazosin, pharmacokinetics of, 2.92,
  16.1t
Dressler's syndrome, 7.201–7.202
  pericarditis in, 10.61
Driving pressure in coronary flow, 1.102,
  1.103, 6.2f
Drug abuse, 13.74–13.80
  amphetamines, 13.78
  anabolic steroids, 13.79
  astemizole, 13.79
  cocaine, 13.74–13.78
  endocarditis in, 9.80–9.81
  glue sniffing, 13.79
  inhalants, 13.78–13.79
  isoproterenol inhalers, 13.78
  phencyclidine, 13.78
  phenylpropanolamine, 13.78
Drug-induced conditions
  anthracycline cardiotoxicity, 5.72–5.75,
    38.11f–38.12f
  digitalis toxicity, 2.44–2.50,
    14.3t–14.4t
  in elderly patients, 13.37
  electrocardiographic changes, 4.30–4.31
  hypertension, 8.42
  myocarditis, 5.77, 38.4t, 10.95–10.96
    hypersensitivity in, 10.96, 95.5t
  pericardial effusions, 10.63
  pulmonary hypertension, 10.72
  sinus node disorders, 6.100

Drug interactions, 2.172–2.188
  with β-adrenergic blocking drugs, 2.102,
    2.103, 2.177–2.178, 16.4t, 21.4t
  pharmacodynamic interactions, 2.178
  pharmacokinetic interactions,
    2.177–2.178
  with antiarrhythmic drugs, 2.174–2.177,
    6.32–6.34, 42.1t
  with antihypertensive drugs,
    2.183–2.185, 21.8t
  with calcium channel blockers, 2.112,
    2.178–2.180, 21.5t
  pharmacodynamic interactions,
    2.179–2.180
  pharmacokinetic interactions,
    2.178–2.179
  with cardiac glycosides, 2.172–2.174,
    21.1t
  bioavailability in, 2.172–2.173
  distribution in, 2.173
  elimination in, 2.173–2.174
  pharmacologic interactions in, 2.174
  with cyclosporine, 13.101, 118.2t
  and digitalis toxicity, 2.47
  with diuretics, 2.180–2.181, 21.6t
  with monoamine oxidase inhibitors,
    2.183, 2.184, 21.8t
  with oral anticoagulants, 2.153, 20.2t
  with sympathomimetic drugs, 2.183,
    2.184, 21.8t
Ductus arteriosus patency, 3.66,
  11.51–11.60
  catheterization and angiocardiography
    in, 5.18, 11.57–11.58
  chest films in, 11.55, 11.56, 102.4f
  clinical features of, 11.54
  echocardiography in, 11.55–11.57, 102.5f
  in elderly patients, 13.34
  electrocardiography in, 11.55
  long-term outcome of surgery in,
    11.3–11.4, 98.1f
  management of, 11.59–11.60, 11.83
  pathologic anatomy in, 11.51–11.53
  pathophysiology of, 11.53–11.54
  in pregnancy, 13.25
  pulmonary vascular disease in,
    11.82–11.83
    clinical features of, 11.82–11.83
Duroziez's sign in aortic insufficiency,
  9.20
Dyspnea, 3.54
  in aortic valvular stenosis, 9.108
  conditions with, 7.63
  in dilated cardiomyopathy, 10.6
  episodic, 3.7, 22.3t
  evaluation of, 3.6–3.7
  exertional, 3.6
  in heart failure, 1.154
  in mitral stenosis, 9.117
  in myocardial ischemia, 7.49
  paroxysmal nocturnal, 3.6
    in pulmonary edema, 1.148
  in pulmonary vascular disease, 11.80
  in viral myocarditis, 10.86
Dysrhythmias. *See* Arrhythmias

E

E-point separation, mitral-septal, echocardiography of, 4.40, 4.78, 28.16f–28.17f, 28.106f
Eating disorders, drug abuse in, 13.79
Ebstein's anomaly of tricuspid valve, 3.60–3.61, 9.96, 11.36, 25.4f–25.5f
  differential diagnosis of, 10.13, 10.14, 90.6f
  echocardiography of, 4.83–4.84, 28.118f–28.120f
  long-term outcome of surgery in, 11.10–11.11
  management of, 11.41
  in pregnancy, 13.25
Echocardiography, 4.33–4.98
  in AIDS, 4.89
  in amyloid heart disease, 10.113–10.114, 97.7f
  in aortic stenosis, subvalvular, 11.92, 105.7f
  aortic valve and root in, 4.75–4.81, 28.100f
    in bicuspid valve, 4.40, 4.77, 28.28f, 28.104f
    in cardiomyopathy, 4.40, 4.75, 28.19f, 28.101f
    diastolic vibrations in, 4.75, 28.102f
    in endocarditis, 4.80, 4.81, 28.111f
    flow velocity in, 4.44, 4.76, 28.24f
    in left ventricular outflow obstruction, 4.76–4.77
    in Marfan syndrome, 4.81, 28.112f
    motion of aortic root in, 4.40–4.41, 4.46, 4.75, 28.18f–28.20f, 28.30f, 28.100f–28.101f
    in regurgitation, 4.77–4.80, 25.105f–28.110f
    in stenosis, 4.76–4.77, 9.110–9.111, 11.90–11.91, 28.103f, 88.5f, 105.6f
  in atrial septal defect, 11.47, 11.88–11.89, 101.6f–101.7f, 105.1f–105.3f
    ostium primum with pulmonary vascular disease, 11.86
    ostium secundum with pulmonary vascular disease, 11.84
  in atrial tumors, 4.96–4.97, 28.145f–28.146f
  cardiac valves in, 4.65–4.86
  in cardiomyopathy, 4.39, 28.15f
    dilated, 10.8–10.9, 90.3f–90.4f
    hypertrophic, 10.20, 10.21, 91.4f
  Chiari network in, 4.82, 4.98, 28.115f
  in congenital heart disease, 11.88–11.96
  Doppler, 4.34–4.36, 28.3f–28.5f. *See also* Doppler echocardiography
    in ductus arteriosus patency, 11.55–11.57, 102.5f
      with pulmonary vascular disease, 11.83
    in Ebstein's anomaly, 9.96
    in Eisenmenger syndrome, 11.82
    in endocarditis, 9.82
  in endomyocardial fibrosis, 10.66–10.67, 10.112, 97.6f
  exercise testing in, 4.55–4.56
  four-chamber views in, 4.39, 28.12f–28.14f
  in ischemic heart disease, 7.57–7.58, 61.3f
  left atrium in, 4.64–4.65, 4.66, 28.80f–28.84f
    in myxoma, 12.47–12.48, 109.3f–109.5f
  left ventricle in, 4.37–4.56, 28.6f–28.11f
    algorithms for volume calculations in, 4.41, 4.42–4.43, 28.21f–28.23f, 28.2t
    in cardiomyopathies, 4.51–4.55, 28.46f–28.57f
    in coronary artery disease, 4.48
    diastolic function studies, 4.45–4.46, 4.47, 28.30f–28.32f
    E-point septal separation in, 4.40, 4.78, 28.16f–28.17f, 28.106f
    in endomyocardial fibrosis, 4.48, 4.55, 28.35f
    mass measurements in, 4.44–4.45, 4.46, 28.4t, 28.26f–28.29f
    in myocardial infarction, 4.48, 4.49, 28.39f–28.41f
    in postinfarction aneurysms, 4.48, 4.49, 4.50, 28.36f–28.38f, 28.42f–28.43f
    shape changes in, 4.44
    size measurements in, 4.41, 4.44
    systolic function assessment in, 4.37–4.41, 28.16f–28.20f
    in thrombi, 4.46–4.47, 4.48, 4.49, 4.97, 28.33f–28.34f, 28.37f
    in tumors, 4.48
    wall thickness in, 4.44, 4.45, 26.25f–28.26f
  M-mode, 4.33, 4.34–4.35, 28.1f–28.2f
    in mitral valve prolapse, 9.34
  mitral valve in, 4.35, 4.38, 4.39, 4.40, 4.51, 4.52, 4.66–4.74, 28.2f, 28.11f, 28.13f, 28.16f, 28.46f–28.47f, 28.49f, 28.85f, 28.95f
    in annular calcification, 4.69–4.70, 28.91f
    in endocarditis, 4.74, 28.99f
    in inflow obstruction, 4.67–4.70, 28.87f–28.91f
    in insufficiency, chronic, 9.14
    in prolapse, 4.71–4.74, 9.16, 9.34–9.35, 28.95f–28.98f
    in stenosis, 4.67–4.69, 28.87f–28.90f
    systolic vibrations in, 4.74, 28.99f
  in myocardial contusion, 12.19
  in myocardial infarction, 7.148
  pericardium in, 4.89–4.96, 28.132f
    in absence of pericardium, 4.63, 4.96
    in constriction, 4.94–4.95, 10.50–10.51, 28.143f, 92.6t
    in cysts, 4.96
    in effusion, 4.35, 4.89–4.94, 10.41–10.43, 28.2f, 28.133f–28.136f, 92.4t, 92.4f–92.5f
    tamponade with, 4.90–4.94, 28.137f–28.141f
    in thickening, 4.94, 28.142f
    in tumors, 4.95–4.96
  in pleural effusion, 4.96, 28.144f
  in postoperative cardiac evaluation, 11.92–11.96
    in Fontan procedure, 11.94
    in Mustard or Senning procedure, 11.92–11.94, 105.8f–105.9f
    in tetralogy of Fallot, 11.94–11.95, 105.10f–105.11f
    transesophageal images in, 11.95, 105.12f
  in pulmonary heart disease, 10.74
  pulmonary valve and artery in, 4.84–4.86, 28.121f–28.124f
    in insufficiency, 4.85, 9.27, 28.122f
    in stenosis, 4.85, 28.121f
  in pulmonary vascular disease, 11.80
  right atrium in, 4.65
    in masses and tumors, 4.97–4.98, 12.50, 28.147f, 109.6f
  right ventricle in, 4.59–4.64
    in atrial septal defect, 4.62–4.63, 28.74f–28.76f
    in cardiomyopathy, 4.61
    in conditions associated with dilation, 4.61–4.64
    contractile function assessment in, 4.60
    in cor pulmonale, 4.63, 4.64, 28.79f
    in endomyocardial fibrosis, 4.61, 28.73f
    in infarction, 4.50, 4.60–4.61, 28.44f, 28.72f
    peak pulmonary systolic pressure estimation in, 4.63, 4.83, 28.78f
    in pulmonary hypertension, 4.64
    segmental abnormalities, 4.60–4.61
    in thrombi, 4.61
    in tricuspid insufficiency, 4.63, 28.77f
    in tumors, 4.61
    in volume overload, 4.59–4.60, 28.69f–28.71f
    wall thickness evaluation in, 4.60
  in scleroderma, 13.13
  in shunt lesions, 11.88–11.92
  in tamponade, cardiac, 10.47, 92.11f–92.12f
  transesophageal, 4.56–4.59, 28.59f–28.68f
    in congenital heart disease, 11.95–11.96, 105.12f–105.13f
    in endocarditis, 9.83, 9.84, 86.7f
  tricuspid valve in, 4.81–4.84, 28.113f–28.115f
    in carcinoid heart disease, 4.83, 28.117f
    in Ebstein's anomaly, 4.83–4.84, 28.118f–28.120f
    in insufficiency, 4.60, 4.63, 4.81–4.84, 9.98, 28.71f, 28.77f, 28.116f–28.120f
    in stenosis, 4.83, 4.84, 9.101, 9.103, 28.117f
  two-dimensional, 4.33, 4.34, 28.1f
    in dilated cardiomyopathy, 10.8–10.9
    in mitral valve prolapse, 9.34

in ventricular septal defects, 11.57, 11.89–11.90, 102.6f, 105.4f–105.5f
in viral myocarditis, 10.88
Ectopic beats
   atrial tachycardia, 6.129
   atrioventricular junctional tachycardia, 6.134–6.135, 49.4f-49.5f
   and postectopic potentiation in mitral valve prolapse, 9.32
   supraventricular, β-adrenergic blocking drugs in, 2.99
   ventricular, variability of, Holter monitoring of, 6.96
Edema
   disorders with, 3.11, 3.14
   evaluation of, 3.9
   idiopathic, diuretics in, 2.29
   pulmonary, 1.144–1.153
      cardiogenic, 1.144, 1.147–1.151
      clinical features of, 1.147
      colloid-hydrostatic pressure relationships in, 1.145–1.147, 9.4f
      dyspnea in, paroxysmal nocturnal, 1.148
      etiology of, 1.149
      heart failure in, 1.148
      hemodynamic, 1.144, 1.147–1.151
      management of, 1.149–1.151
      in myocardial infarction, 7.187–7.188, 70.6t
         shock syndrome with, 7.188–7.199
      noncardiogenic, 1.144, 1.151–1.153
      pathophysiology of, 1.144–1.147
      permeability, 1.144–1.145, 1.151–1.153. See also Respiratory distress syndrome, adult
   postoperative, 13.55, 114.4f–114.5f
   radiographic features of, 1.148–1.149, 9.1t
Education programs in mitral valve prolapse, 9.37
Effusions
   pericardial. See Pericardium, effusions in
   pleural, echocardiography in, 4.96, 28.144f
Egophony, 3.57
Ehler-Danlos syndrome, cardiovascular disorders in, 3.13, 23.1t
Eicosanoids, affecting coronary vessels, 1.106
Einthoven's triangle, 4.16, 27.5f
Eisenmenger reaction, 11.77
   causes of, 11.81, 104.3t
   hemodynamic effects of, 11.80
   management of, 11.81
Eisenmenger syndrome, 11.30, 11.36–11.37, 11.51, 11.52, 11.77, 11.81–11.82, 100.6f
   catheterization and angiocardiography in, 11.58–11.59
   chest films in, 11.55

clinical features of, 11.54–11.55, 11.81–11.82
electrocardiography in, 11.55
heart-lung transplantation in, 13.102
management of, 11.41, 11.59–11.60, 11.82
pathophysiology of, 11.53
in pregnancy, 13.25
Ejection fraction, left ventricular, 1.91–1.92, 5.10f
   as index of contractile function, 5.8
      corrected for afterload, 5.8–5.9, 34.8f
   postinfarction, 7.225–7.226, 72.5t
      relation to ventricular arrhythmias, 7.227–7.228, 72.4f
Ejection sounds
   aortic, 3.35
   pulmonary, 3.35
   systolic murmurs, 3.39–3.41
   vascular, 3.35
Elderly patients, 13.28–13.39
   arrhythmias and conduction abnormalities in, 13.36–13.37
   baroreceptor reflexes in, 8.56
   blood pressure measurements in, 8.56, 13.29
   cardiac function in, 13.28
   cardiomyopathy in, 13.34–13.35
   congenital heart disease in, 13.34
   cor pulmonale in, 13.35
   coronary bypass surgery in, 7.253, 13.31–13.32
   coronary heart disease in, 13.29–13.32
   diagnostic procedures in, 13.29
   drug therapy in, 13.37
   endocarditis in, 13.34
   exercise training in, 13.31
   functional assessment of, 13.29
   health care services for, 13.38–13.39
   heart failure in, 13.35–13.36
   hypertension in, 8.53–8.57, 13.32–13.33
   orthostatic hypotension in, 1.170, 1.172, 13.32
   preventive measures in, 13.38
   psychosocial concerns in, 13.38
   rehabilitation in, 13.31, 13.38
   surgery in, noncardiovascular, 13.38
   valvular heart disease in, 13.33–13.34
Electrical alternans in cardiac tamponade, 10.47, 10.56, 92.13f
Electrical excitation of myocardial fibers, 1.24
Electrical properties of cardiac cells, 6.2–6.12
   action potential in. See Action potential, cardiac
   afterdepolarizations and triggered activity in, 6.7–6.9, 40.7f–40.8f
   automatic mechanisms in, 6.6–6.7, 40.6f
      abnormal, 6.7
   electrotonic interactions in, 6.6, 6.7
Electrocardiography, 4.14–4.31
   abnormalities in absence of heart disease, 4.31
   age affecting, 4.18

ambulatory (Holter), 6.87–6.98
   analysis systems in, 6.89–6.90, 6.91–6.92, 46.1f–46.4f
      comparison of, 6.90, 46.2t
   in aortic valve disease, 6.94
   in cardiomyopathy, 6.94
   in chronic obstructive pulmonary disease, 6.94
   in diagnostic procedures, 6.94
   duration of recording cycle in, 6.96–6.97
   in hemodialysis, 6.94
   in high-risk patients with ventricular arrhythmias, 6.95, 6.97, 46.8f
   indications for, 6.93
   in ischemic heart disease, 7.58
   in mitral valve prolapse, 6.94, 9.35
   in normal population, 6.94–6.95
   in pacemaker evaluation, 6.98
   in palpitations, 6.93–6.94
   in prolonged QT interval syndrome, 6.94
   recording modes in, 6.88–6.89
   in sick sinus syndrome, 6.102–6.103
   in silent ischemia, 7.92
   in ST segment change evaluation, 6.97–6.98
   in supraventricular arrhythmias, 6.95, 6.96, 46.6f–47.7f
   symptom evaluations in, 6.93–6.94
   types of recorders in, 6.87–6.88, 46.1t
   in variability of ventricular ectopy, 6.96
   in variant angina, 7.102–7.103, 65.2f–65.3f
   in Wolff-Parkinson-White syndrome, 6.94
in aortic dissection, 12.32
in aortic insufficiency, chronic, 9.21
in aortic valvular stenosis, 9.110
in atrial fibrillation, 6.131
in atrial flutter, 6.131–6.132
in atrial septal defect, 11.46–11.47
   ostium primum with pulmonary vascular disease, 11.86
   ostium secundum with pulmonary vascular disease, 11.84
in atrioventricular nodal tachycardia, 6.132
basis of, 4.14–4.16
body build affecting, 4.18
and body surface mapping, 4.19
calcium levels affecting, 4.30
in cardiac chamber enlargements, 4.19–4.22, 27.7f–27.8f
in cardiomyopathy
   dilated, 10.8
   hypertrophic, 10.30
in conduction disturbances, 4.22–4.24, 27.9f–27.22f
in cor pulmonale, 4.28
in cyanotic congenital heart disease, 11.31
disease-specific patterns in, 4.31
drugs affecting, 4.30–4.31
in ductus arteriosus patency, 11.55

with pulmonary vascular disease, 11.83
in Ebstein's anomaly, 9.96
Einthoven's triangle in, 4.16, 27.5f
in Eisenmenger syndrome, 11.55, 11.82
electric field created by dipole in, 4.14–4.15, 4.16, 27.4f
electrical position of heart in, 4.18–4.19
in endocrine disorders, 4.31
exercise testing in. *See* Exercise tests
in hypertension, 8.19–8.20
in hypothyroidism, 13.85
in ischemia, 4.24, 4.25, 7.51–7.54, 27.11f
leads in, 4.16–4.17, 27.5f–27.6f
in metabolic disorders, 4.31
in mirror image dextrocardia, 4.18
in mitral valve disorders
   insufficiency, chronic, 9.13, 82.2f
   prolapse, 9.33–9.34
   stenosis, 9.120
monitoring in exercise programs, 7.213, 71.9t
in myocardial contusion, 12.18
in myocardial infarction, 4.24–4.28, 27.12f–27.14f
   in subendocardial infarction, 4.25
normal patterns in, 4.17–4.19
P wave in, 4.17
   abnormalities in, 4.19, 4.20, 27.7f–27.8f
in pericarditis, 4.28
   acute, 10.54–10.56, 92.18f–92.20f
   constrictive, 10.51, 92.16f
in pheochromocytoma, 13.87
potassium levels affecting, 4.30
PR interval in, 4.18
preexcitation pattern in, 4.24, 27.10f
in pulmonary embolism, 4.28, 10.79
in pulmonary heart disease, 10.73–10.74, 94.2f
in pulmonary vascular disease, 11.80
in pulmonary insufficiency, chronic, 9.27
QRS complex in, 4.18
QRS precordial mapping in estimation of infarct size, 7.137–7.138
QTc lengthening in, 4.30, 27.2t–27.3t
relation to action potential, 6.3, 40.2f
sex of patient affecting, 4.18
signal-averaged, postinfarction, 7.230–7.231, 72.5f, 72.6t
in silent ischemia, 7.92
in sinus node disorders, 6.100–6.110
ST segment in, 4.18
in supraventricular tachycardia, 6.128, 6.129, 49.1f
T wave in, 4.18
   abnormalities in, 4.28–4.29, 27.1t
in tamponade, cardiac, 10.47, 92.13f
temperature affecting, 4.19
training affecting, 4.18
transtelephonic transmission in variant angina, 7.103, 65.4f
in tricuspid regurgitation, 9.98
in tricuspid stenosis, 9.101
U wave in, 4.18
   abnormalities in, 4.29–4.30
in unstable angina, 7.76, 7.80, 63.1f

in variant angina, 7.101–7.103, 65.1f–65.4f
vectorcardiography, 4.19
in ventricular septal defect, 11.55, 102.3f
in viral myocarditis, 10.86, 10.88
in Wolff-Parkinson-White syndrome, 6.136, 49.1t
Electrograms, intracardiac, 6.54–6.66
  in atrioventricular conduction studies, 6.55–6.58, 6.59, 44.2f–44.3f, 44.5f–44.6f
  in atrioventricular nodal tachycardia, 6.113, 6.134, 49.3f
  in bundle branch block, 6.119–6.121, 48.5t, 48.8f
  catheter placement in, 6.54, 6.55, 4.41f, 44.2f
  complications of, 6.64
  diagnostic use of, 6.57–6.62
  filtering frequencies in, 6.56, 44.3f
  problems in, 6.64, 6.65–6.66, 44.15f–44.17f
  sinus node recordings in, 6.57, 6.106–6.107, 44.4f, 47.6f–47.8f
  in supraventricular tachycardia, 6.58–6.60
  therapeutic use of, 6.62–6.64
  in wide QRS tachycardia, 6.58–6.62, 44.7f–44.10f
Electrolyte replacement therapy in digitalis toxicity, 2.49
Electrophysiologic studies
  in control of inducible tachycardia, 6.62–6.65, 44.13f–44.15f
  in dilated cardiomyopathy, 10.8
  in drug effects
    from calcium channel blockers, 2.107–2.109, 17.2t, 17.2f–17.3f
    from cardiac glycosides, 2.38
  His bundle electrograms in, 6.57–6.58, 6.71, 44.5f. 45.5f. *See also* Electrograms, intracardiac
  invasive studies in, 6.54–6.66
  postinfarction, 7.229–7.230
  in recordings of monophasic action potentials, 6.68–6.84
  in sinus node dysfunction, 6.102, 6.103–6.109, 47.2t, 47.3f–47.8f
    indications for, 6.107–6.109, 47.9f–47.10f
  in transplantation of heart, 13.96–13.97
  in unexplained syncope, 6.61–6.62
  in ventricular tachycardia, 6.60–6.61, 6.63, 44.11f–44.12f
  in Wolff-Parkinson-White syndrome, 6.137–6.138
Ellis van Creveld syndrome, cardiovascular disorders in, 3.13, 23.1t
Embolectomy, pulmonary, 10.82
Embolism
  pathogenesis of, 2.156–2.159
  pulmonary, 10.77–10.82
    anticoagulants in, 10.81
    chest pain in, 3.6

clinical features of, 10.77, 94.3t
diagnosis of, 10.78–10.80
dyspnea in, 3.7
electrocardiography in, 4.28
in elderly patients, 13.35
in endocarditis, 9.79
fibrinolytic therapy in, 10.81–10.82
heart failure in, 1.158
pathophysiology of, 10.77–10.78
and pericarditis, 10.61
physical examination in, 10.77
possible sources of, 10.78, 94.4t
postoperative, in cardiac surgery, 13.63–13.64
and prevention of venous thrombosis, 10.80–10.81
treatment of, 10.81–10.82
venous interruption in, 10.81
in viral myocarditis, 10.86
systemic
  in atrial fibrillation, 6.131
  in endocarditis, 9.79
  in left atrial myxomas, 12.46
  in mitral valve prolapse, 9.37
    prevention of, 9.38
  in viral myocarditis, 10.86
Embryopathy, coumarin-induced, 2.154
Emetine, myocarditis from, 10.96
Emergencies
  bypass surgery in, 7.253–7.254, 7.263–7.264
  hypertensive, treatment of, 8.26–8.27, 77.10t
Emotional stress, 13.67–13.72
  animal studies of, 13.67–13.68
  autonomic responses in, 13.69
  blood pressure in, 13.68, 13.69–13.70
  management of, 13.70–13.72
  physiologic changes in, 13.70, 13.71, 13.72, 115.1f–115.2f
  reactivity studies in, 13.68
Emphysema
  mediastinal
    auscultation in, 3.57
    chest pain in, 7.66
  pulmonary, genetic factors in, 10.72
Employment. *See* Work
Enalapril, 9.6, 9.7, 81.2t
  in hypertension, 8.24
  in reversal of left ventricular hypertrophy, 8.46–8.47, 79.2t
  vasodilating effects of, 2.130
Encainide, 6.23, 6.45–6.46
  antiarrhythmic spectrum of, 6.45–6.46
  dosage of, 6.46
  effects on heart and circulation, 6.23
  effects on transmembrane potential, 6.23
  electrophysiologic properties of, 6.45
  interactions with other drugs, 6.46
  pharmacokinetics of, 6.45
  side effects of, 6.46
  in supraventricular tachycardia, 6.138
Endocarditis
  infective, 9.73–9.89
    angiocardiography in, 9.83–9.85

antibiotics in, 9.85–9.86, 86.6t
  allergy to penicillin in, 9.86
  prophylactic, 9.87, 86.8t–86.10t
aortic valvular
  echocardiography in, 4.80, 4.81, 28.111f
  in stenosis, 9.109
blood cultures in, 9.81–9.82
clinical features of, 9.77–9.78, 86.4t
clinical implications of, 9.87–9.89
complications of, 9.78–9.80
  extravalvular, 9.78–9.79, 86.3f–86.4f
culture-negative, 9.86
cutaneous manifestations of, 9.78
in ductus arteriosus patency, 11.59
echocardiography in, 9.82
  transesophageal, 9.83, 9.84, 86.7f
in elderly patients, 13.34
embolism in, 9.79
enterococcal, 9.86
fungal, 9.86
heart failure in, 9.78
hematologic disorders in, 9.80
in hemodialysis patients, 9.81
in hypertrophic cardiomyopathy, 10.36
incidence of, 9.73
laboratory studies in, 9.81–9.82
in lupus erythematosus, 13.7, 13.8, 110.2f
microorganisms found in, 9.74–9.75, 86.2t
of mitral valve
  echocardiography in, 4.74, 28.99f
  in prolapse, 9.36–9.37, 9.38, 9.81
mycotic aneurysms in, 9.79
in narcotic drug abusers, 9.80–9.81
neurologic disorders in, 9.79–9.80, 86.5t
nosocomial, 9.81
ocular manifestations of, 9.78
pathogenesis of, 9.75–9.77
pathology in, 9.76–9.77, 86.1f–86.2f
  cardiac, 9.76
physical findings in, 9.77
predisposing factors in, 9.73–9.74, 86.1t
in pregnancy, 13.23
prevention of, 9.87, 11.60, 86.8t–86.10t
of prosthetic valves, 9.47, 9.50, 9.81
  treatment of, 2.165, 9.86
radionuclide studies in, 9.82
renal involvement in, 9.80, 86.5f
in rheumatic fever, 10.99
roentgenography in, 9.82
source of infection in, 9.75–9.76, 86.3t
staphylococcal, 9.86
streptococcal, 9.86
surgery in, 9.86–9.87, 86.7t
symptoms of, 9.77
treatment of, 9.85–9.87
tricuspid valve in, 9.93–9.94
vegetations in, 9.76–9.77, 86.1f–86.2f
  identification of, 9.82–9.83, 86.3f
in ventricular septal defect, 11.59
noninfective
  Libman-Sacks, 13.7, 13.8, 110.2f

  Löffler's, 10.67–10.69, 10.107, 10.111, 97.5f
  thrombotic, 10.65–10.66, 93.1f
Endocardium
  fibroelastosis of, 10.115
  in rheumatoid arthritis, 13.4–13.5
Endocrine disorders, 13.82–13.89
  acromegaly, 13.86
  adrenal cortex diseases, 13.87–13.88
  diabetes mellitus, 13.82–13.84
  and effects of sex hormones, 13.88–13.89
  hypertension in, 8.36–8.42
  parathyroid disease, 13.88
  pheoehromocytoma, 13.86–13.87
  thyroid disease, 13.84–13.86
Endomyocardial disease
  eosinophilic, 10.67–10.69, 10.107, 10.111, 93.2f, 93.2t, 97.5f
    treatment of, 10.68–10.69
  fibrosis, 10.66–10.67, 10.107, 10.111–10.112, 93.1t, 97.5f–97.6f
    treatment of, 10.67
  tropical, 10.111–10.112
Endothelin affecting coronary vessels, 1.106
Endothelium
  action on vascular smooth muscle, 1.125, 1.127, 7.9f
  functions of, 1.115–1.116
  injury of, and thrombosis, 2.156, 2.159
  interaction with platelets, 7.116–7.118
Endothelium-derived relaxing factor, 1.115–1.116, 7.1f–7.2f
  affecting coronary vessels, 1.106
End-systolic indices of ventricular function, 5.9–5.11, 34.9f–34.12f
Energy metabolism, myocardial, 1.78–1.80
  in contraction-relaxation cycle, 1.79, 1.80, 4.15f
  ischemia affecting, 1.81
  nucleotide utilization in, 1.80–1.81, 4.16f
Energy requirements for muscular work, 1.129–1.130
Enlargement of heart. See Hypertrophy, myocardial
Enoximone, 2.53–2.65, 14.13f–14.14f
  adverse effects of, 2.66, 14.7t
  hemodynamic effects of, 2.66, 14.7t
Enterococcal endocarditis, 9.86
Enzymes
  in estimation of infarct size, 7.134–7.135
  in myocardial contusion, 12.18
  in myocardial infarction, 7.146–7.148, 68.3f
Eosinophilic endomyocardial disease, 10.67–10.69, 10.107, 10.111, 93.2f, 93.2t, 97.5f
Ephedrine, 2.57
Epicardial fat stripe sign in chest films, 4.3, 4.4, 26.4f
Epidemiology, and risk factor concept, 7.2–7.3
Epinephrine
  clinical applications of, 2.52–2.53
  hemodynamic effects of, 2.53, 14.6t

  hypokalemia from, β-adrenergic blocking drugs in, 2.101
  interactions with other drugs, 2.184, 21.8t
    β-adrenergic blocking drugs, 2.177, 21.4t
  receptors for, 7.191, 70.9t
  serum levels
    in exercise, 1.137, 8.4t
    in pheochromocytoma, 13.86–13.87
    stress affecting, 13.68, 13.69
Epstein-Barr virus infection, and tumors after transplantation of heart, 13.99
Ergonovine test
  in coronary artery spasm evaluation, 5.33, 5.34, 35.31f
  in variant angina, 7.104–7.106, 65.1t–65.2t, 65.5f–65.6f
Ergotism, arteriography in, 12.39, 108.12f
Erythema marginatum, in rheumatic fever, 10.101
Erythrocyte sedimentation rate in rheumatic fever, 10.102
Erythromycin, interaction with other drugs
  digoxin, 2.172, 21.1t
  theophylline, 2.186, 21.9t
  warfarin, 2.187, 21.10t
Esmolol, pharmacology of, 2.96, 2.97, 16.2t, 16.3t
Esophageal echo studies, 4.56–4.59, 28.59f–28.68f
  in congenital heart disease, 11.95–11.96, 105.12f–105.13f
  in endocarditis, 9.83, 9.84, 86.7f
Esophagitis, reflux, chest pain in, 7.67
Esophagus
  rupture of, chest pain in, 7.67
  spasm of
    nitrates in, 2.84
    provocative testing in, 7.106
Estrogens, cardiovascular effects of, 13.88
Ethacrynic acid, 2.27, 13.1t
Ethmozin, 6.23
  effects on heart and circulation, 6.23
  effects on transmembrane potential, 6.23
Eustachian valve, 1.4f, 1.6
Examination procedures. See Bedside evaluation of patients; Chest examination; Diagnostic procedures; Physical examination
Excitability of cardiac cells, 6.5, 6.6, 40.5f
  spread of, 4.14, 4.15, 27.2f
Excitation-contraction coupling, 1.24–1.26, 2.6f–2.8f
Exercise
  activity scale in, 7.205, 7.206, 71.2t
  anaerobic threshold in, 1.129–1.130
  angina in, 7.48, 7.69
  arm work compared to leg exercise, 1.132–1.133
  basic physiology of, 7.204
  blood flow in, 7.204–7.205

to limb muscles, 1.123
blood pressure in, 7.204, 7.205, 71.1f
cardiac changes from, 7.206, 7.207, 71.3t
 in coronary heart disease patients, 7.214
cardiac output and oxygen uptake in, 1.131–1.132, 8.1t–8.2t, 8.2f
in cardiac rehabilitation, 7.204–7.216
cardiovascular and pulmonary function in, 1.130–1.131, 8.1t
and coronary heart disease, 7.22
and determinants of performance capacity, 1.129–1.131
dynamic, 7.204
 responses to, 1.131–1.133
and effects of physical training, 1.138–1.140, 8.8f
and functional classifications, 3.3, 22.1t, 22.2t
heart rate in, 7.204, 7.205, 71.1f
and hyperemia in muscles, 1.121
isometric, 7.204
 responses to, 1.133–1.135, 8.3t, 8.5f
left ventricular performance in, 1.97–1.98, 1.132, 1.133, 5.20f, 8.3f
maximum oxygen uptake in, 1.129
 genetic factors affecting, 1.137–1.138, 8.7f
in myocardial infarction, 7.145–7.146, 68.1t
myocardial perfusion and performance in, 1.135, 7.214–7.215, 71.12f
normal postexercise hemodynamic data, 1.172, 11.2t
and orthostatic tolerance, 1.172
oxygen consumption in, 7.205–7.206, 71.1t
perceived level of exertion in, 7.207, 71.4t
and physical working capacity in
 aortic insufficiency, 9.23
 in mitral insufficiency, 9.15
physiologic responses to, 1.130, 8.1f
prescription of, 7.206–7.207
pump function in, 5.12, 5.13, 34.16f
reflex mechanisms in, 1.135–1.136, 8.6f
regulatory mechanisms in, 1.135–1.137
response of denervated heart to, 13.96
training programs
 adaptations to, 7.206, 7.207, 71.3t
 affecting electrocardiogram, 4.18
 assessment of patient in, 7.211–7.212, 71.8t
 contraindications to, 7.212
 duration of, 7.213
 for elderly persons, 13.31
 monitoring in, 7.213, 71.9t
 mortality from, 7.214, 71.11t
 and responses to exercise, 1.138–1.140, 8.8f
 safety of, 7.213
vasoregulatory mechanisms in, 1.136–1.137
Exercise tests
in angina pectoris, 7.67–7.68
in bundle branch block, 6.122–6.123, 48.10f
in dilated cardiomyopathy, 10.11–10.12
and double product index of left ventricular oxygen demand, 1.102
in echocardiography, 4.55–4.56
in ischemic heart disease, 7.52–7.54, 61.1f, 61.2t–61.3t
in mitral valve prolapse, 9.35
in peripheral arterial disease, systolic pressure in, 12.35, 12.37, 108.5t
postinfarction, 7.217–7.225
 advantages of, 7.217
 angiographic correlations with, 7.222
 before hospital discharge, 7.210, 7.211, 7.217, 71.7t
 blood pressure abnormalities in, 7.222
 candidates for, 7.217–7.218, 72.1t
 heart-rate-limited, 7.218
 normal test in, 7.221
 predictive value of, 7.224
 prognostic value of, 7.221–7.222
 radionuclide ventriculography in, 7.224–7.225, 72.4t
 reproducibility of results in, 7.222–7.223, 72.3f
 sign-limited, 7.218–7.219, 7.220, 71.1f–71.2f
 ST segment in, 7.218–7.219, 7.220, 7.221, 71.1f–71.2f
 symptom-limited, 7.219–7.220
 termination of, indications for, 7.218, 72.2t
 thallium–201 scintigraphy with, 7.223–7.224
 ventricular arrhythmias in, 7.221–7.222
 workload-limited, 7.218
in sinus node evaluation, 6.102, 6.103, 47.2t
in variant angina, 7.103
in Wolff-Parkinson-White syndrome, 6.137
Extrasystole. See Premature beats
Extremities, examination of, 3.14
Extubation procedures, postoperative, 13.54–13.55
Eyes
in endocarditis, 9.78
examination of, 3.12

F

Fabry's disease, restrictive cardiomyopathy in, 10.115
Factor V, interaction with factor X, 2.145
Factor VIII, interaction with factor IX, 2.145
Factor IX, interaction with factor VIII, 2.145
Factor X, interaction with factor V, 2.145
Fallot tetralogy. See Tetralogy of Fallot
Familial conditions. See Genetic factors
Fascicular block, left, electrocardiography in, 4.23
Fat
 content in foods, 7.4, 59.1t
 in take of, and coronary heart disease, 7.3, 7.14–7.21
Fat necrosis, pericardial, 10.64
Fatigue in dilated cardiomyopathy, 10.6
Fatty acids, omega–3, as platelet inhibitor, 2.147
Felodipine, 2.106, 2.107, 17.1t
Femoral artery
 in cardiac catheterization, 5.3
 in coronary arteriography, 5.27–5.30
Fenoldopam, 2.59
 hemodynamic effects of, 2.53, 14.6t
Fiber, dietary, affecting lipid levels, 7.46
Fibers, myocardial, 1.19, 1.20, 2.1f
 disarray in hypertrophic cardiomyopathy, 10.19–10.20, 91.3f
Fibric acid derivatives as hypolipidemic agents, 2.139
Fibrillation
 atrial, 6.129–6.131
  β-adrenergic blocking drugs in, 2.99–2.100
  in alcoholic heart disease, 12.9, 12.10, 106.11f
  antithrombotic therapy in, 2.163–2.164
  in aortic valvular stenosis, 9.109
  calcium channel blockers in, 2.117, 2.118, 17.10f
  clinical patterns and precipitating illnesses in, 6.130–6.131
  complications of, 6.131
  in elderly patients, 13.37
  electrocardiography in, 6.131
  glycosides in, 2.44
  in hyperthyroidism, 13.85
  in hypertrophic cardiomyopathy, 10.31, 10.34
  mechanisms in, 6.130
  in mitral stenosis, 9.118–9.119
  in myocardial infarction, 7.152
  pathologic features of, 6.130
  physical findings in, 6.131
  prevalance of, 6.130
  sick sinus rhythm with, 6.100, 6.101, 47.2f
  treatment of, 6.131, 6.138
 ventricular
  MAP recordings in, 6.76–6.77, 45.14f
  in myocardial infarction, 7.148, 7.149
  prevention with β-adrenergic blocking drugs, 2.100
Fibrin and thrombogenesis, 2.149, 2.156
Fibrinolysis and thrombosis inhibition, 2.146–2.147
Fibrinolytic therapy in pulmonary embolism, 10.81–10.82
Fibroelastoma, papillary, 12.52
Fibroelastosis, endocardial, 10.115
Fibromas, cardiac, 12.51–12.52, 109.8f
Fibrosis

endomyocardial, 10.66–10.67, 10.107, 10.111–10.112, 93.1t, 97.5f–97.6f
   echocardiography in, 4.48, 4.55, 4.61, 28.35f, 28.73f
   tropical, 10.111–10.112
  myocardial
   in scleroderma, 13.12–13.13
   in transplanted heart, 13.100
  pericardial, 10.40, 10.41, 92.3t
Fibrous renal artery lesions, hypertension in, 8.31–8.32, 78.1f–78.2f, 78.2t
Fick equation, 1.132
Fick method for cardiac output determination, 5.3–5.4
Fish
  consumption affecting lipid levels, 7.46
  oils as platelet inhibitors, 2.147
Fistula
  arteriocameral, coronary, 3.67
  arteriovenous
   cardiac output increase in, 1.157
   coronary, 3.67
   pulmonary, 11.36
    management of, 11.41
  coronary artery, congenital, 11.22–11.23, 99.12f–99.13f
  intracardiac, traumatic, 12.21–12.22
Fitness, and orthostatic tolerance, 1.172
Flail mitral valve syndrome, 9.36
Flecainide, 6.23–6.24, 6.46
  antiarrhythmic spectrum of, 6.46
  dosage of, 6.46
  effects on heart and circulation, 6.24
  effects on transmembrane potential, 6.23–6.24
  electrophysiologic properties of, 6.46
  hemodynamic effects of, 6.46
  molecular weight affecting actions of, 6.19
  pharmacokinetics of, 6.46
  side effects of, 6.46
  in supraventricular tachycardia, 6.138
Floppy mitral valve. *See* Mitral valve, prolapse
Flunarizine, 2.106, 2.107, 17.1t
Fluoroscopy, in silent ischemia, 7.93
Flutter, atrial, 6.131–6.132
  β-adrenergic blocking drugs in, 2.99
  calcium channel blockers in, 2.117
  electrocardiography in, 6.131–6.132
  in myocardial infarction, 7.151–7.152
  sick sinus rhythm with, 6.100, 6.101, 47.2f
  treatment of, 6.132
Fontan operation in cyanotic heart disease, 11.39, 11.41
  and postoperative echocardiography, 11.94
Foramen ovale, 1.4f, 1.5, 1.6
  blown-open, 11.43
  patency of, pulmonic valve stenosis with, 11.29, 100.4f

Force-velocity relations, and left ventricular performance, 1.86–1.87, 1.88, 5.2f–5.3f
Foreign bodies in heart, 12.24, 107.8f–107.9f
Forskolin, inotropic effects of, 2.59–2.60
Fossa ovalis, 1.5
  limbus of, 1.4f, 1.5, 1.6
Frank-Starling mechanism, ultrastructural basis of, 1.28
Free radicals, oxygen-derived, in myocardial infarction, 7.118–7.119, 7.122, 7.157, 7.174
Fremitus, vocal, 3.55–3.56
Friction rub
  pericardial, 3.48–3.49, 10.54, 92.17f
  pleural, 3.57
Friedreich's ataxia, cardiovascular disorders in, 3.11, 3.13, 23.1t
Fromm graft catheter, 5.30, 35.25f
Fungus infections
  endocarditis in, 9.86
  myocarditis in, 10.93
  pericarditis in, 10.58
Furosemide, 2.27. 13.1t
  interactions with digoxin, 2.172, 21.1t
  interactions with nonsteroidal anti-inflammatory drugs, 2.181, 21.7t

G

G-force levels in aerospace medicine, 1.172
G proteins in cardiovascular tissues, 1.45–1.47, 3.1t, 3.5f–3.6f
Gait, abnormalities in, 3.11
Gallavardin phenomenon, 3.39
Gallium–67 citrate scans
  in endocarditis, 9.82
  in viral myocarditis, 10.88
Gallop sounds, 3.34–3.35
  left ventricular origin of, 3.34
  right ventricular origin of, 3.34–3.35
Gallopamil, 2.106–2.107, 17.1t
Gap junctions of cardiac cells, 6.5
Gases in arterial blood
  postoperative exchange in mechanical ventilation and spontaneous breathing, 13.54, 13.55, 114.2t
  in pulmonary embolism, 10.79
Gastrointestinal disorders
  in aortic valvular stenosis, 9.109
  calcium channel blockers in, 2.120
  chest pain in, 7.67
Gaucher's disease, restrictive cardiomyopathy in, 10.115
Gemfibrozil, 2.139
Genetic factors in familial cardiomyopathy, 10.3
  in familial myocarditis, 10.91
  in hypertrophic cardiomyopathy, 10.19

in lung disease, 10.72
in nonmodulation of responses to angiotensin in hypertension, 8.13–8.14
in rheumatic fever, 10.98
Giant cell arteritis, 12.33, 13.11
Giant cell myocarditis, 10.96
Gibson's murmurs, 3.48
Glaucoma, open-angle, β-adrenergic blocking drugs in, 2.101
Glenn anastomosis in cyanotic heart disease, 11.40
Glucagon, inotropic effects of, 2.59
Glucose-insulin-potassium infusions in myocardial infarction, 7.157
Glucose tolerance test in hypertension, 8.18
Glue sniffing, toxic effects of, 13.79
Glutamic oxaloacetic transaminase in myocardial contusion, 12.18
Glutethimide, interaction with anticoagulants, 2.153, 2.187, 20.2t, 21.11t
Glycolysis, pathway for, 1.78, 4.11f
Glycoproteins, and platelet adhesions, 2.143
Glycosides, cardiac
  in angina pectoris, 2.43
  in arrhythmias, 2.44
  in chronic obstructive pulmonary disease, 2.43–2.44
  clinical applications of, 2.39–2.40
  deslanoside, 2.37
  digitalis, 2.34–2.36. *See also* Digitalis glycosides
  electrophysiologic effects of, 2.38
  in heart failure, 2.41–2.43, 14.5f–14.6f
  interactions with autonomic nervous system, 2.39
  interactions with other drugs, 2.172–2.174, 21.1f, 21.1t
  mechanisms of action, 2.37–2.38, 14.2f
  in myocardial infarction, 2.40–2.41, 14.3f–14.4f
  ouabain, 2.36, 2.37
  pharmacokinetics of, 2.37, 14.2t
  prophylactic digitalization, 2.44
  toxicity of digitalis, 2.44–2.50, 14.3t–14.4t
Gold paint pericarditis, 10.63
Gorlin formula in valve area calculation, 9.122–9.123, 89.4f
  for aortic valve area, 5.15
Graham Steell murmur, 3.45
  in pulmonic insufficiency, 9.27
Granulomas
  myocardial, in rheumatoid arthritis, 13.4
  nodular, in rheumatoid arthritis, 13.3, 110.1f
Granulomatosis
  in allergic angiitis, 13.11
  Wegener's, 13.11
Griseofulvin, interaction with angicoagulants, 2.153, 2.187, 20.2t, 21.11t

I.23

Growth hormone secretion in acromegaly, 13.86
Guanethidine, interactions with other drugs, 2.184, 2.185, 21.8t

H

Halo sign in constrictive pericarditis, 4.95, 28.143f
Hamman's crunch, 3.57
Hancock bioprosthetic valve, 9.46, 84.3f
  orifice areas in, 9.44, 84.1t
Hand grip, and differential diagnosis of murmurs, 3.40, 3.49, 23.11t
Hangout time, aortic and pulmonary, 3.31, 3.32, 23.10f
Head-down tilt, responses to, 1.41, 1.165, 1.173, 11.2f
Heart block
  atrioventricular. *See* Atrioventricular block
  bundle branch. *See* Bundle branch block
  in elderly patients, 13.37
  fascicular, left, electrocardiography in, 4.23
  in hyperthyroidism, 13.85
  and noncardiac surgery, 13.45
  peri-infarction, 4.28
  in rheumatoid arthritis, 13.5
Heart failure, congestive, 1.154–1.162
  in acromegaly, 13.86
  acute
    inotropic agents in, 2.66–2.67, 14.8t
    nitrates in, 2.83
  α-adrenergic blocking drugs, in, 2.93
  from β-adrenergic blocking durgs, 2.101
  in alcoholism, 12.5–12.6, 12.7, 106.7f–106.9f
  in aortic valvular stenosis, 9.109
  approach to patient with, 1.161–1.162, 106.9t
  autonomic dysfunction in, 1.137
  biochemical changes in, 1.77
  calcium channel blockers in, 2.120
  in cardiomyopathy
    dilated, 10.2
    hypertrophic, 10.36
  causes of, 1.156–1.158, 10.3t–10.5t
  chest films in, 4.9–4.11, 26.17f–26.18f
  chronic
    glycosides in, 2.41–2.43, 14.5f–14.6f
    inotropic drugs in, 2.67–2.68
    nitrates in, 2.83
  clinical features of, 1.154–1.155
  combination therapy in, 1.161, 10.3f
  compensatory mechanisms in, 1.159–1.160, 10.7t
  in diabetes mellitus, 13.84
  diuretics in, 2.26–2.28, 13.20f–13.12f
  efficacy of therapeutic agents in, 1.161–1.162, 10.10t
  in elderly patients, 13.35–13.36
  in endocarditis, 9.78
  hormonal vasoconstrictor mechanisms in, 1.159, 10.2f
  in hyperthyroidism, 13.85
  in hypothyroidism, 13.85
  in infancy, differential diagnosis of, 10.89
  left ventricular
    hemodynamic monitoring in, 5.84–5.85, 39.2t
    postoperative, 13.61–13.63
  limb blood vessels in, 1.124
  in mitral valve prolapse, 9.35–9.36
    treatment of, 9.38
  in mitral stenosis, 9.119
  in myocardial infarction, 7.180–7.184, 70.1f
    bypass surgery in, 7.266
    categories of, 7.186, 70.5t
    clinical syndromes of, 7.184–7.200
  myocardium in, 1.158–1.159, 10.6t
  nitrates in, 2.82–2.83
  noncardiac surgery in, 13.45–13.46
  pathophysiology of, 1.155–1.156, 10.1t–10.2t
  postoperative
    after coronary artery bypass, 10.3
    left ventricular, 13.61–13.63
    right ventricular, 13.63
  in pregnancy, 13.22–13.33
  in pulmonary edema, 1.148
  response to exercise in, 1.133, 1.137, 8.4t
  in rheumatic fever, 10.101
    control of, 10.104
  right ventricular
    hemodynamic monitoring in, 5.85–5.86, 39.2f, 39.2t
    postoperative, 13.63
  therapeutic principles in, 1.160, 10.8t
  vasodilator drugs in, 2.123–2.135
  in viral myocarditis, 10.86, 10.88
    treatment of, 10.90
Heart-lung transplantation, 13.102–13.105
Heart rate
  and action potential duration, 6.74–6.77
  autonomic blockade affecting, 6.105–6.106, 47.4f–47.5f
  and contractility of cardiac muscle, 1.31, 2.16f–2.17f
  drug-induced changes in, antiarrythmic effects of, 6.14. 6.16, 41.3f
  in exercise, 7.204, 7.205, 71.1f
  and left ventricular performance, 1.86
  in pericarditis, 10.56
  in viral myocarditis, 10.86
Heart sounds, 3.25–3.50
  in aortic insufficiency, chronic, 9.20–9.21
  in aortic valvular stenosis, 9.110
  in atrial myxoma, 12.47, 109.2f
  in atrial septal defect, 11.45
  in constricitive pericarditis, 10.50
  differential diagnosis of, maneuvers in, 3.49–3.50
  in dilated cardiomyopathy, 10.6
  in ductus arteriosus patency, 11.54
  in Ebstein's anomaly, 9.96
  ejection sounds, 3.35
  first
    abnormalities in, 3.29, 23.4t
    intensity of, 3.26–3.27
    interval to midsystolic click, 3.35–3.36, 23.8t
    splitting of, 3.27–3.28, 23.9f
      differential diagnosis of, 3.29, 23.5t
  fourth, 3.33–3.34
    gallop sounds, 3.34–3.35
  high-frequency, in early diastole, 3.36–3.37, 23.9t
  in hypertension, 8.17–8.18
  in mitral valve prolapse, 9.32
  in mitral valve stenosis, 9.119–9.120
  murmurs in. *See* Murmurs
  non-ejection systolic clicks, 3.35–3.36
  pericardial friction rub, 3.48–3.49
  pericardial knock, 3.35
  with prosthetic and tissue valves, 3.37–3.38, 23.10t
  in pulmonic insufficiency, 9.27
  scratchy, 3.49
  second
    abnormalities in, 3.34, 23.7t
    aortic component of, 3.28
    hangout time in, 3.31, 3.32, 23.10f
    intensity of, 3.28–3.31
    pulmonic component of, 3.28, 3.30
    single, 3.33, 3.34, 23.7t
    splitting of, 3.31–3.32
      fixed, 3.33, 3.34, 23.7t
      reversed (paradoxic), 3.33, 3.34, 23.7t
      wide, 3.32–3.33, 3.34, 23.7t
  third, 3.33–3.34
    gallop sounds, 3.34–3.35
  in tricuspid stenosis, 9.101, 87.18f
Helminthic infections, myocarditis in, 10.94
Hemochromatosis, 10.114–10.155, 97.8f
Hemodialysis
  and endocarditis, 9.81
  Holter monitoring in, 6.94
  and pericarditis, 10.62
Hemodynamic monitoring, 5.80–5.93
  in adult respiratory distress syndrome, 5.85, 5.88, 39.2t
  arterial pressure in, 5.80
  catheter design and placement for right heart pressures, 5.80–5.82, 39.1f
  central venous pressure in, 5.82
  clinical applications of, 5.85, 39.2t
  complications of, 5.92–5.93
  in critically ill patients, 5.90–5.91, 39.7f
  equal right atrial and pulmonary artery wedge pressures in, 5.86, 39.3f
  heart rate and rhythm in, 5.80
  in hypovolemic shock, 5.84, 5.85, 39.2t
  intraoperative, in noncardiac surgery, 13.49
  in intravenous vasodilator therapy, 5.89, 39.4t
  in left ventricular failure, 5.84–5.85, 39.2t
  in mitral regurgitation, 5.85, 5.87, 39.2t, 39.4f

in response to therapy, 5.89, 5.90, 39.6f
in myocardial infarction, 5.88, 39.3t
  during therapeutic interventions, 5.88–5.91, 39.4t, 39.6f–39.7f
normal values in, 5.80, 39.1t
postoperative, in cardiac surgery, 13.58–13.61, 114.7f
prognostic indices in, 5.91
pulmonary artery end-diastolic pressure in, 5.83
pulmonary artery wedge pressure in, 5.82–5.83
in pulmonary congestion with normal cardiac output, 5.85
in right ventricular failure, 5.85–5.86, 39.2f, 39.2t
in septic shock, 5.85, 5.88, 39.2t
in ventricular septal defect, 5.85, 5.87–5.88, 39.2t, 39.5f
in response to therapy, 5.89–5.90
Hemoptysis
  evaluation of, 3.9
  in mitral stenosis, 9.119
Hemorrhage from oral anticoagulants, 2.153–2.154
Hemosiderosis, 10.114–10.115
Heparin, 2.149–2.152
  chemical structure of, 2.148, 20.4f
  dosage of, 2.150, 20.1t
  in embolic strokes, 2.165
  intravenous administration of, 2.150–2.151, 20.1t, 20.5f
    continuous, 2.150, 2.151, 20.5f
    intermittent, 2.151, 20.5f
  mechanisms of action, 2.149–2.150
  in myocardial infarction, 2.161–2.162, 2.164, 7.152–7.153, 68.2t–68.3t
  neutralization with protamine, 2.152
  overlapping of coumarin with, 2.152
  in pregnancy, 2.166, 13.22, 111.3t
  in prevention of vein graft disease after bypass surgery, 2.163
  side effects of, 2.151–2.152
  subcutaneous injection of, 2.150, 2.151, 20.1t, 20.5f
  in unstable angina, 2.160, 7.85
  in venous thromboembolism, 10.81
Hepatitis, viral, myocarditis in, 10.91
Herpes simplex infection after transplantation of heart, 13.98
Herpes zoster infection after transplantation of heart, 13.99
Heterophyiasis, myocarditis in, 10.94
Hirudin as thrombin inhibitor, 2.149
His bundle, 1.12, 1.13, 1.15f, 6.112, 48.1f
  branches, 6.112, 48.1f
    block in. See Bundle branch block
    left, 1.12–1.13
    right, 1.12
  electrogram recordings, 6.57–6.58, 6.71, 44.5f, 45.5f
  physiology of, 6.114
Histamine
  inotropic effects of, 2.59

and norepinephrine release, 1.118, 7.4f
provocative testing with, in variant angina, 7.107
Histoplasmosis, pericarditis in, 10.59
History-taking in bedside evaluation, 3.2–3.9
HMG-CoA reductase inhibitors as hypolipidemic agents, 2.140–2.141
Holiday heart syndrome, 12.9
Holt-Oram syndrome, cardiovascular disorders in, 3.13, 23.1t
Holter monitoring, 6.87–6.98. See also Electrocardiography, ambulatory (Holter)
Homocystinuria, cardiovascular disorders in, 3.13, 23.1t
Hospital-acquired infections, endocarditis, 9.81
Hum, venous, 3.48
Hurler's syndrome, cardiovascular disorders in, 3.13, 23.1t
Hyaluronidase, in myocardial infarction, 7.157
Hydatid disease, myocarditis in, 10.94
Hydralazine, 2.124, 9.6, 18.2f, 81.2t
  in aortic regurgitation, acute, 9.5
  captopril with, 2.131
  in dilated cardiomyopathy, 10.15
  interaction with β-adrenergic blocking drugs, 2.177, 21.4t
  interaction with digoxin, 2.172, 21.1t
  in mitral regurgitation, acute, 9.4
  nitrates with, in heart failure, 2.127, 18.6f
  in pregnancy, 13.22, 111.3t
  in sinus node dysfunction, 6.109
11-β-Hydroxylase deficiency, hypertension in, 8.41
17-α-Hydroxylase deficiency, hypertension in, 8.41
5-Hydroxytryptamine. See Serotonin
Hyperabduction maneuver in peripheral arterial disease, 12.36, 108.8f
Hypercholesterolemia
  familial, 7.41–7.43, 60.4t
  polygenic, 7.42, 7.43, 60.4t
Hypercoagulability and venous thrombosis, 10.78
Hyperemia
  exercise, in muscles, 1.121
  reactive, 1.121–1.122
Hyperlipidemia
  in diabetes mellitus, 13.82–13.83
  familial combined, 7.42, 7.43, 7.44, 60.4t
  secondary, 7.45–7.46
Hyperlipoproteinemia
  type I, 7.42, 7.45, 60.4t
  type III, 7.40–7.41, 7.42, 7.45, 60.4t
  type V, familial, 7.42, 7.44–7.45, 60.4t
Hyperparathyroidism, 13.88
  hypertension in, 8.41–8.42
Hypersensitivity, and myocarditis, 10.96, 95.5t
Hypertension, 8.1–8.57
  in acromegaly, 8.42, 13.86

in adrenal disorders, 8.36–8.41
α-adrenergic blocking drugs in, 2.92–2.93
β-adrenergic blocking drugs in, 2.98, 8.22–8.23, 77.7t–77.8t
in alcoholism, 7.20–7.21, 12.6–12.8, 59.10t, 106.10f
in aldosteronism, 8.39–8.40
angiotensin converting enzyme inhibitors in, 8.24
antihypertensive agents in, 8.20–8.25
blood chemistries in, 8.18–8.19, 77.2t
blood count in, 8.18, 77.2t
calcium channel blockers in, 2.118–2.119, 8.25
calcium levels in, intracellular, 1.70–1.71
in carcinoid syndrome, 8.42
centrally acting adrenergic inhibiting drugs in, 8.23
chest films in, 8.19
clinical features of, 8.17
and coronary heart disease risk, 7.7–7.10
and progress in control efforts, 7.28
in Cushing's syndrome, 8.40–8.41, 13.87
in diabetes mellitus, 8.42, 13.84
dilated cardiomyopathy in, 10.3
diuretics in, 2.29–2.30, 8.21–8.22, 77.6t
drug-induced, 8.42
  from cyclosporine, 13.100
in elderly persons, 8.53–8.57, 13.32–13.33
  arterial compliance in, 8.55–8.56, 80.3f
  baroreceptor function in, 8.56
  blood pressure recordings in, 8.56
  evaluation of patients in, 8.56
  hemodynamic effects of, 8.54–8.55, 80.1t
  morbidity in, 8.57, 80.2t
  systolic hypertension in, 8.53–8.54
  therapy in, 8.56–8.57
electrocardiography in, 8.19–8.20
emergencies in, treatment of, 8.26–8.27, 77.10t
in endocrine disorders, 8.36–8.42
evaluation of patients in, 8.17–8.20, 77.4t
heart disease in
  atrial fibrillation in, 6.130
  classification of, 8.18, 77.1t
  differential diagnosis of, 10.14
in 11-β-hydroxylase deficiency, 8.41
in 17-α-hydroxylase deficiency, 8.41
in hyperparathyroidism, 8.41–8.42
in hyperthyroidism, 8.41
in hypothyroidism, 8.41
laboratory studies in, 8.18–8.19, 77.2t
in Liddle's syndrome, 8.41
mild, management of, 8.25
moderate-to-severe, management of, 8.25–8.26
in myocardial infarction, 7.154
in neurologic diseases, 8.42
nitrates in, 2.83–2.84
noncardiac surgery in, 13.44–13.45, 13.49
pathogenesis of, 8.2–8.3, 76.1t
peripheral pulses in, 8.17
in pheochromocytoma, 8.36–8.39, 13.86–13.87

postoperative, 8.43
  in cardiac surgery, 13.58–13.59
pulmonary
  α-adrenergic blocking drugs in, 2.94
  bedside diagnosis of, 3.30, 23.6t
  calcium channel blockers in,
      2.119–2.120
  chest pain in, 7.66
  drug-induced, 10.72
  echocardiography in, 4.64
  in elderly patients, 13.35
  heart-lung transplantation in, 13.102
  management of, 10.75–10.76
  mechanisms and causes of,
      10.71–10.72, 94.1t
  in mitral stenosis, 9.117
  nitrates in, 2.83
  in pregnancy, 13.22
  primary, 10.72–10.73, 11.79
    clinical features of, 11.79
    etiology of, 11.79
    treatment of, 11.80
  vasodilators in, 10.76, 94.2t
in renal disease, 8.29–8.31
  in bilateral disease, 8.29–8.30
  clinical features of, 8.29
  laboratory studies in, 8.30
  pathophysiology of, 8.29–8.30
  treatment of, 8.30–8.31
  in unilateral disease, 8.30
renovascular, 8.31–8.36
  in atherosclerotic renal artery disease,
      8.31–8.36, 78.3f
  clinical features of, 8.31–8.32
  in fibrous renal artery lesions,
      8.31–8.32, 78.1f–78.2f, 78.2t
  laboratory studies in, 8.33–8.34, 78.4f
  pathophysiology of, 8.32–8.33
  renin-angiotensin system in, 8.32–8.33,
      8.34
  revascularization procedures in,
      8.35–8.36
  in thromboembolic diseases, 8.36
  treatment of, 8.34–8.36
responsiveness to angiotensin II in,
    8.5–8.14
  nonmodulation in, 8.6–8.14
    characteristics of, 8.7, 76.2t
    classification of, 8.7
    heritability of, 8.13–8.14
    potential mechanisms in, 8.11–8.13,
        76.13f–76.16f
    and production of hypertension,
        8.7–8.11, 76.3t, 76.8f–76.12f
    as subgroup of patients, 8.13, 76.17f
secondary, 8.28–8.43
  causes of, 8.28–8.29, 78.1t
severe, management of, 8.26–8.27
sodium-sensitive, 8.3
  causes of, 8.11, 76.3t
stepped-care approach in, 8.25, 77.9t
stress factors in, 13.68, 13.69–13.70
survey data in, 8.16–8.17
urine studies in, 8.18, 8.19, 77.2t
vasodilators in, 8.23–8.24

Hyperthyroidism, 13.85
  β-adrenergic receptors in, 1.54, 1.55, 3.5t
  cardiac output increase in, 1.157
  hypertension in, 8.41
  treatment of, 13.85
Hypertriglyceridemia, familial, 7.42, 7.44,
    60.4t
Hypertrophic cardiomyopathy,
    10.18–10.36
Hypertrophic subaortic stenosis,
    idiopathic. See
    Cardiomyopathy,
    hypertrophic
Hypertrophy, myocardial, 1.72–1.75
  in athletes, 1.139
  calcium levels in, intracellular, 1.70–1.71
  cell size and volume in, 1.72, 1.73,
      4.6f–4.7f
  coronary blood flow in, 1.76–1.77, 1.112
  diastolic volume overload in, 1.76
  early stages of, 1.72–1.73, 1.74, 4.8f
  induction of, 1.74–1.75
  pathologic, 1.76
  patterns of, 1.76, 1.77, 4.10f
  physiologic, 1.76
  progression of, 1.75
  regression of, 1.77
  RNA synthesis in, 1.73, 1.74, 4.9f
  systolic pressure overload in, 1.76
Hyperventilation
  chest pain in, 7.65
  as test in variant angina, 7.106
Hypoglycemic agents, oral
  in diabetes, 13.84
  interaction with β-adrenergic blocking
      drugs, 2.177, 21.4t
  interaction with calcium entry blockers,
      2.179, 21.5t
Hypokalemia
  in aldosteronism, 8.39
  causes of, 8.19, 77.3t
  in Cushing's disease, 13.87
  epinephrine-induced, β-adrenergic
      blocking drugs in, 2.101
  postoperative, in cardiac surgery, 13.64
  in weight-loss regimens, 13.75
Hypolipidemic agents, 2.137–2.141
  bile acid binding resins, 2.137–2.138
  clofibrate, 2.139
  combinations of, 2.141
  in familial hypercholesterolemia,
      homozygous, 2.141
  gemfibrozil, 2.139
  HMG-CoA reductase inhibitors,
      2.140–2.141
  neomycin, 2.139
  nicotinic acid (niacin), 2.138–2.139
  probucol, 2.139
  d-thyroxine, 2.140
Hypoparathyroidism, 13.88
Hypopituitarism, electrocardiography in,
    4.31
Hypoplastic left heart syndrome, 11.35
  management of, 11.39
Hypotension

hypovolemic, in myocardial infarction,
    7.154
orthostatic, 1.163–1.177
  in autonomic failure, 1.174–1.175
  blood volume changes in, 1.166–1.167,
      11.4f
  causes of, 1.163
  cerebral perfusion in, 1.164–1.165
  diastolic pressure-volume
      characteristics in,
      1.167–1.168, 11.5f
  and effects of fitness and exercise,
      1.172
  in elderly patients, 1.70, 1.72, 13.32
  hypovolemic hyperreactive,
      1.173–1.174
    treatment of, 1.175–1.176
  neurogenic causes of, 1.174–1.175
  normovolemic hyporeactive,
      1.174–1.175
    treatment of, 1.176
  pathophysiology of, 1.163–1.168
  treatment of, 1.75–1.76
    drugs used in, 1.177t
  vascular pressure-volume relationships
      in, 1.163–1.164, 11.1f
in postinfarction exercise testing, 7.222
postoperative, in cardiac surgery, 13.59
  diagnosis of causes in, 13.64, 114.4t
  management of, 13.61–13.63, 114.8f
and shock in myocardial infarction,
    7.188
Hypothyroidism, 13.85–13.86
  β-adrenergic receptors in, 1.54, 1.55, 3.5t
  and atherosclerosis, 13.86
  digitalis toxicity in, 2.47
  hypertension in, 8.41
  and myxedematous pericardial disease,
      10.62–10.63
  treatment of, 13.86
Hypoventilation, alveolar hypoxia in,
    10.72
Hypovolemia
  in myocardial infarction, 7.189, 7.199,
      70.7t
  hypotension in, 7.154
  and orthostatic hypotension,
      1.166–1.167, 1.173–1.174, 11.4f
  postoperative, in cardiac surgery,
      13.59–13.60
Hypoxemia in myocardial infarction,
    7.153–7.154
Hypoxia
  β-adrenergic receptors in, 1.54, 1.55, 3.5t
  alveolar, 10.72
  contraction mechanics in, 1.81, 4.17f

I

Ibopamine, 2.59
  hemodynamic effects of, 2.53, 14.6t
Iloprost, as platelet inhibitor, 2.149
Immune mechanisms in rheumatic fever,
    10.100
Immunosuppressive therapy

in chronic active myocarditis, 10.91–10.92
complications of, 13.100–13.101
in transplantation of heart, 13.95
  in heart-lung transplants, 13.103
in viral myocarditis, 10.90
Impedance in coronary flow, 1.102, 1.103, 6.2f
Impedance plethsymography, in venous thrombosis detection, 10.78–10.79, 94.4f
Impotence in dilated cardiomyopathy, 10.6
Indapamide, 2.27, 13.1t
Indicator dilution method for cardiac output determination, 5.4–5.5, 34.2f–34.3f
Indomethacin, interactions with other drugs, 2.181, 21.7t
  β-adrenergic blocking drugs, 2.177, 21.4t
  antihypertensive drugs, 2.184, 21.8t
  diuretics, 2.180, 21.6t
Indoramin, 2.91
  pharmacokinetics of, 2.92, 16.1t
Infants. See Children and infants
Infarction, myocardial, 7.112–7.127
  accelerated idioventricular rhythm in, 7.150
  β-adrenergic blockade in, 7.155–7.156
    for survivors, 2.100
  β-adrenergic receptors in, 1.54–1.55, 3.5t
  anticoagulant therapy in, 7.152–7.153, 68.2t–68.3t
  antiplatelet therapy in, 7.153
  antithrombotic therapy in, 2.161–2.162, 2.164
  anxiety in, 7.143–7.144
  aspirin in prevention of, 7.115–7.116
  atherosclerotic plaques in, 7.113–7.114
  atrioventricular block in, 6.123
  bed rest and physical activity in, 7.145–7.146, 68.1t
  bradyarrhythmias in, 7.152
  bundle branch block in, 6.123–6.125, 48.6t–48.8t
  bypass surgery in, 7.262–7.273
    after angioplasty, 7.265
    with correction of mechanical complications, 7.268–7.273
    evolution of, 7.262–7.263
    as primary therapy, 7.263–7.264
    in recurrent ventricular arrhythmias, 7.266
    results of, 7.266–7.267
    after thrombolytic therapy, 7.264–7.265
    timing of, 7.263, 7.267–7.268, 75.2f
    in uncomplicated infarction, 7.267–7.268, 75.2f
  calcium channel blockers in, 7.156–7.157
  in cardiac catheterization, 5.38
  causes of, 7.112–7.113
  chest films in, 7.148
  clinical subsets in, 7.184–7.185, 70.2t
  cocaine-induced, 13.76–13.77, 116.2f
    treatment of, 13.78
  complicated, criteria for, 7.208, 71.5t
  complications of, 7.148–7.155, 7.179–7.101, 70.1t
  coronary artery spasm in, 7.119–7.120
  coronary artery thrombosis in, 7.112, 7.114–7.115
  coronary care units for, 7.143
    admission orders in, 7.144–7.145, 68.1f
    mobile, 7.142
  in diabetes mellitus, 13.83–13.84
  diagnosis of, 7.146–7.148
  diastolic alterations in, 7.123–7.125
  diet in, 7.144–7.145
  differentiation from acute myocarditis, 10.86–10.87, 95.3t
  and Dressler's syndrome, 7.201–7.202
    pericarditis in, 10.61
  drug disposition in, 2.14–2.15, 12.4t
  early ambulation in, 7.209–7.210
  echocardiography in, 4.48, 4.49, 7.148, 28.39f–28.41f
    in postinfarction complications, 4.48–4.51, 28.36f–28.38f, 28.42f–28.45f
  in elderly patients, 13.29–13.32
    management of, 13.30–13.31
  electrocardiography in, 4.24–4.28, 27.12f–27.14f
  in emotional stress, 13.70
  enzyme changes in, 7.146–7.148, 68.3f
  expansion of, 7.126
    postinfarction, 7.201
  free wall rupture in, ventricular, 7.198
    surgery in, 7.272
  functional effects of, 7.122–7.127
    site affecting, 7.125
    size affecting, 7.125
    time course of, 7.125–7.126
  glycosides in, 2.40–2.41, 14.3f–14.4f
  hemodynamic complications of, 7.154–7.155
  hemodynamic monitoring in, 5.88, 39.3t
  hemodynamic subsets in, 7.185, 70.2t
  historical aspects of, 7.112
  hypertension in, 7.154
  hypotension in, hypovolemic, 7.154
  hypovolemia in, 7.189, 7.199, 70.7t
  hypoxemia in, 7.153–7.154
  invasive monitoring in, 7.185–7.186, 70.3t
  and later noncardiac surgery, 13.42
  left ventricular dysfunction prevention in, 7.157–7.158
  in lupus erythematosus, 13.9
  management of, 7.142–7.159
    optimal strategy in, 7.175, 7.176, 69.7f
    postinfarction, 7.217–7.235
    mechanical complications of, 7.195–7.199, 7.262, 75.1t
    surgery in, 7.268–7.273
  metabolic effects of, 7.120–7.122
  mitral regurgitation with, 7.189, 7.195–7.197, 70.7f, 70.7t
    in papillary muscle dysfunction, 7.195–7.196, 7.268–7.269
    in papillary muscle rupture, 7.196–7.197, 70.13t
  surgery in, 7.268–7.271, 73.3f–75.6f
  monitoring for arrhythmias in, 7.143, 7.145, 68.2f
  and mural thrombi in left ventricle, 7.127
  neutrophils in, 7.118–7.119
  nitrates in, 2.81, 2.82, 15.5t
  nitroglycerin in, 7.156
  noninvasive assessment of, 7.186, 70.4t
  oxygen-derived free radicals in, 7.118–7.119, 7.122, 7.157, 7.174
  oxygen therapy in, 7.154
  pain relief in, 7.143–7.144
  pathophysiology of, 7.179–7.180
  percutaneous transluminal coronary angioplasty in, 7.170–7.173
  pericarditis in, 7.201, 10.60–10.61
    and peri-infarction block, 4.28
  perioperative
    in bypass surgery, 7.257
    in noncardiac surgery, 13.49–13.50
  platelets in, 7.115–7.116
  postinfarction management in, 7.217–7.235
    analysis of risk in, 7.231–7.233, 72.6f, 72.7t
    aspirin therapy in, 7.234–7.235, 72.10t
    bypass surgery in, 7.265–7.266
    electrophysiologic studies in, 7.229–7.230
    exercise testing in, 7.210, 7.211, 7.217–7.225, 71.7t
    left ventricular ejection fraction assessment in, 7.225–7.226, 72.5t
    prophylactic β-adrenergic blocking agents in, 7.233–7.234, 72.8t–72.9t
    rehabilitation in, 7.204–7.216
    right atrial pacing in, 7.225
    signal-averaged electrocardiography in, 7.230–7.231, 72.5f, 72.6t
    in ventricular arrhythmias, 7.226–7.229
  in pregnancy, 13.26
  prehospital care in, 7.142
  pseudoaneurysm in, 7.198–7.199, 70.8f
  pulmonary congestion in, 7.185–7.187
  pulmonary edema in, acute, 7.187–7.188, 70.6t
  pump failure in, 7.180–7.184, 70.1f
    bypass surgery in, 7.266
    categories of, 7.186, 70.5t
    clinical syndromes of, 7.184–7.200
  radionuclide studies in, 7.148
  and recurrent ischemia, 7.200–7.201
  rehabilitation and prognosis in, 7.158–7.159, 7.204–7.216
  reperfusion in, 7.163–7.176
    detrimental effects of, 7.174
    emergency surgical revascularization in, 7.173–7.174
    late, 7.174
    percutaneous transluminal coronary angioplasty in, 7.170–7.173

thrombolytic therapy in, 7.163–7.170, 69.1t–69.2t
and time course of functional changes, 7.125–7.126
right ventricular, 7.154–7.155, 7.189, 7.199–7.200, 70.7t, 70.9f
echocardiography of, 4.50, 4.60–4.61, 28.44f, 28.72f
tricuspid regurgitation in, 9.93
salvage measures in, 7.155–7.158
shock syndrome in, 7.188–7.200, 70.7t
catecholamines in, 7.191–7.192, 7.193, 70.10t
vasodilators with, 7.194
digitalis in, 7.191
dobutamine in, 7.191–7.192, 7.193, 70.10t
dopamine in, 7.191, 7.193, 70.10
intra-aortic balloon pumping in, 7.194, 70.6f, 70.11t
from mechanical complications, 7.195–7.199
nitroglycerin in, intravenous, 7.192–7.193, 70.10t
nitroprusside sodium in, 7.192, 7.193, 70.10t
norepinephrine in, 7.192, 7.193, 70.10t
phentolamine in, 7.193–7.194, 70.10t
with pulmonary congestion or edema, 7.188–7.199
without pulmonary congestion or edema, 7.199–7.200
surgery in, 70.12t, 7.28, 7.195
treatment of, 7.189, 7.190–7.195, 70.7t
beneficial and adverse effects of, 7.190, 70.8t
vasodilators in, 7.192–7.194, 70.10t
catecholamines with, 7.194
ventriculopenic, 7.188–7.195, 70.7t
silent, 7.96
silent ischemia after, 7.96
site of, affecting functional alterations, 7.125
size of, 7.134–7.140
affecting functional alterations, 7.125
bypass surgery affecting, 7.253
computed tomography of, 7.135–7.137, 67.6f
and death with cardiogenic shock, 7.134, 67.1f
enzymatic estimates of, 7.134–7.135
magnetic resonance imaging of, 7.136–7.138, 67.7f
metabolic perfusion imaging of, 7.138, 7.139, 67.9f
pyrophosphate scintigrams of, 7.135, 7.136–7.137, 67.2f–67.5f
QRS precordial mapping of, 7.137–7.138
radionuclide ventriculography of, 7.138–7.140, 67.10f
reduction of, 7.157
thallium-201 scintigraphy of, 7.138, 67.8f

and ventricular end-diastolic volume, 7.183–7.184, 70.4f
streptokinase in, 7.153, 7.164–7.167, 69.2f, 69.2t
administration of, 7.164–7.165
anologues in, 7.166–7.167
aspirin with, 7.153, 7.166
efficacy of, 7.165, 69.1t
intracoronary, 7.165–7.166
intravenous, 7.166
percutaneous transluminal coronary angioplasty with, 7.170–7.171
subendocardial, 4.25
supraventricular tachyarrhythmias in, 7.151–7.152
systolic alterations in, 7.122–7.123
thromboembolic complications from, 2.158, 7.152, 7.153, 7.202
thrombolytic therapy in, 2.161, 7.117, 7.163–7.170, 69.1t–69.2t
bypass surgery after, 7.174, 7.264–7.265
combination therapy in, 7.169–7.170, 69.4f
cost-effectiveness of, 7.175–7.176
fibrin-specific, 7.175
new approaches in, 7.170
percutaneous transluminal coronary angioplasty with, 7.170–7.173, 69.3t
tissue-type plasminogen activator in, 7.167, 7.168–7.169, 69.2t
percutaneous transluminal coronary angioplasty with, 7.171–7.173, 69.3t
triage procedures in, 7.264, 75.1f
urokinase and prourokinase in, 7.167–7.168, 69.2t
intracoronary, 7.168
intravenous, 7.168
ventricular aneurysm in, 7.126–7.127, 7.198, 7.199, 70.8f
surgery in, 7.272–7.273
ventricular septal defect in, 7.189, 7.197–7.198, 70.7t, 70.13t
surgery in, 7.269–7.272
ventricular tachyarrhythmias in, 7.148–7.151
Infections
aortic, 12.34–12.35
endocarditis. See Endocarditis, infective
myocarditis, 10.84–10.96
pericarditis, 10.57–10.58
postoperative, in transplantation of heart, 13.98–13.99
in heart-lung transplantation, 13.104
rheumatic fever, 10.98–10.106
Inguinal area, anatomy of, 5.27–5.28, 35.19f
Inosine, intravenous, hemodynamic effects of, 2.66
Inotropic drugs
catecholamines, 2.50–2.59
classification of, 2.35, 14.1t
clinical use of, 2.66–2.68
deslanoside, 2.37

dibutyryl-cAMP, 2.60
digitalis glycosides, 2.34–2.50
forskolin, 2.59–2.60
glucagon, 2.59
in heart failure, 2.66–2.67, 14.8t
histamine, 2.59
nitrates, 2.75–2.89
ouabain, 2.36–2.37
phosphodiesterase inhibitors, 2.60–2.65, 14.9f
piroximone, 2.65
posicor (ro 13-6438), 2.65
in pregnancy, 13.22, 111.3t
sulmazole (ARL 115BS), 2.65
Inspection
in aortic insufficiency, chronic, 9.20
of chest, 3.55
diagnostic clues in, 3.11–3.14
Insulin therapy in diabetes, 13.84
Intercalated disks, 1.21, 6.5
in alcoholic heart disease, 12.9, 12.11, 106.12f
International Atherosclerosis Project (IAP), 7.16
Invasive tests
in bedside hemodynamic monitoring, 5.80–5.93
biopsy, cardiac, 5.67–5.78
in bundle branch block, 6.119–6.121
cardiac catheterization, 5.2–5.18
coronary arteriography, 5.20–5.42
digital angiography, cardiac, 5.43–5.52
electrophysiologic studies, 6.54–6.66
in myocardial infarction, 7.185, 7.186, 70.3t
in ventricular diastolic function assessment, 5.55–5.65
Ionescu-Shiley bioprosthetic valve, 9.46, 84.3f
orifice areas in, 9.44, 94.1t
Ipecac abuse, toxic effects of, 13.79
Iron deposits in heart, 10.114–10.115
Ischemia, myocardial, 1.77–1.83. See also Coronary heart disease
Isometric exercise, 7.204
responses to, 1.133–1.135, 8.3t, 8.5f
Isometric contraction of muscle, 1.30–1.31, 2.12f–2.15f
Isoproterenol, 2.53–2.54
effects on transplanted heart, 13.97
hemodynamic effects of, 2.53, 14.6t
inhalation of, cardiac toxicity of, 13.78
receptors for, 7.191, 70.9t
in sinus node function tests, 6.102, 6.103, 47.2t
Isosorbide dinitrate, 9.6, 9.7
in angina pectoris, 7.70–7.71, 62.2t
unstable, 7.80, 63.3t
variant, 7.107, 65.8f
in dilated cardiomyopathy, 10.15
metabolism of, 2.84, 15.6t
as venodilator, 2.125–2.127, 18.5f
Isotonic contraction of muscle, 1.32–1.34, 2.18f–2.22f
Isozymes, myosin, 1.75–1.76

I.28

J

James fibers, 1.13
Janeway lesions in endocarditis, 3.14, 9.78
Jatene procedure in cyanotic heart disease, 11.38
Jaundice, disorders with, 3.12
Joints, rheumatic fever affecting, 10.99
Jones criteria for rheumatic fever diagnosis, 10.103, 95.1t
Judkins coronary catheters
　left, 5.28–5.29, 35.21f-35.22f
　right, 5.29, 5.30, 35.24f-35.26f
Jugular venous pulse
　a wave in, 3.15, 23.1f
　　abnormalities in, 3.16, 3.17, 23.2t
　in aortic valvular stenosis, 9.109
　compared to arterial pulse, 3.15
　in dilated cardiomyopathy, 10.6
　examination of, 3.14–3.18, 23.1f
　normal, 9.97, 87.10f
　in systemic venous pressure elevation, 3.16
　in tricuspid regurgitation, 9.97, 87.10f
　in tricuspid stenosis, 9.100, 9.101, 87.16f-87.17f
　v wave in, 3.15, 23.1f
　　abnormalities in, 3.17
　x descent in, 3.15, 23.1f
　　abnormalities in, 3.18, 23.3f
　y descent in, 3.15, 23.1f
　　abnormalities in, 3.17–3.18, 23.3f

K

Kawasaki disease, 13.10–13.11
Kent bundles, 1.13
Kerley A and B lines, 4.9, 4.10, 26.17f–26.18f
Kidney
　clearance of drugs, 2.7
　compensatory responses to diuretics, braking phenomenon in, 2.25–2.26, 2.28, 2.30, 13.9f
　cyclosporine nephrotoxicity, 13.100–13.101
　diseases of
　　drug disposition in, 2.14
　　hypertension in, 8.29–8.31
　diuretics affecting, 2.22–2.24, 13.6f
　　in collecting system, 2.23, 2.24, 13.5f
　　in distal convoluted tubules, 2.23, 2.24, 13.5f
　　in glomerulus, 2.22
　　in loop of Henle, 2.23, 2.24, 13.4f
　　in proximal tubule, 2.22
　in endocarditis, 9.80, 86.5f
　failure of, digitalis toxicity in, 2.46
　function tests in hypertension, 8.19
　handling of diuretic drugs, 2.24–2.25, 13.7f–13.8f
　nephrotic syndrome, diuretics in, 2.28–2.29
　renin-angiotensin-aldosterone system, 8.3–8.5, 76.1f–76.3f
　renovascular hypertension, 8.31–8.36
　salt and water handling in, 2.19–2.21, 13.1f–13.2f
　thromboembolism in, and hypertension, 8.36
　uremic pericarditis, 10.62
　vasculature affected by nitrates, 2.79
Klinefelter's syndrome, cardiovascular disorders in, 3.11, 3.13, 23.1t
Klippel-Feil syndrome, cardiovascular disorders in, 3.13, 23.1t
Knock, pericardial, 3.35, 10.50
Knotting of pulmonary artery catheter, 5.92–5.93
Konno-Sakakibara bioptome, 5.67
Korotkoff sounds, 3.18
Krebs cycle, 1.78, 4.12f
Kussmaul respiration, 3.55

L

Labetalol, 2.91, 2.97, 8.22, 77.7t
　pharmacology of, 2.96, 2.97, 16.2t, 16.3t
Lacerations
　of aorta, 12.22
　of heart, 12.16, 12.17, 107.1f–107.4f
　pericardial, 12.16
Lactate dehydrogenase
　in myocardial contusion, 12.18
　in myocardial infarction, 7.146–7.147
Lactic acid metabolism
　in myocardial infarction, 7.121
　in silent ischemia, 7.93
Laplace law, 1.114
　in end-systolic wall stress, 5.9
Laser angioplasty, 7.246, 73.12f
Lebobunolol in glaucoma, 2.101
Leg-raising, and differentiation of murmurs, 3.40, 23.11t
Length-tension relations, in contraction of cardiac muscle, 1.27–1.28, 2.9f–2.10f
Leptospirosis, myocarditis in, 10.93
Leukocytes, accumulation in myocardial infarction, 7.118
Leukotrienes, affecting coronary vessels, 1.106
Libman-Sacks endocarditis, 13.7, 13.8, 110.2f
Liddle's syndrome, hypertension in, 8.41
Lidocaine, 6.21–6.22, 6.37–6.38
　antiarrhythmic effects of, 6.14
　　factors affecting, 6.18, 41.5f
　in digitalis toxicity, 2.48–2.49
　dosage and pharmacokinetic properties of, 6.37, 42.2t
　effects on heart and circulation, 6.22
　effects on transmembrane potential, 6.21–6.22
　interactions with other drugs, 2.174–2.175, 6.33, 21.2t, 42.1t
　　β-adrenergic blocking drugs, 2.177, 21.4t
　molecular weight affecting actions of, 6.19
　in pregnancy, 13.22, 111.3t
　toxicity in elderly patients, 13.30
Lidoflazine, 2.106, 2.107, 17.1t
Life-style
　in childhood, and coronary heart disease risk, 7.23
　recent changes in Americans, 7.25–7.28
　sedentary, and coronary heart disease risk, 7.22
Limb circulation, 1.114–1.127
　adrenergic nerves affecting, 1.117–1.119, 7.3f–7.4f
　in atherosclerosis obliterans, 1.126–1.127, 7.10f
　autoregulation of, 1.116
　cholinergic nerves affecting, 1.119
　critical closing pressure in, 1.116
　cutaneous, 1.119–1.121
　dynamics of, 1.114–1.116
　in heart failure, 1.124
　metabolic regulation of, 1.117
　nitrates affecting, 2.78, 15.4f
　in Raynaud's disease, 1.124–1.126, 7.8f
　in skeletal muscle, 1.121–1.123, 7.6f
　sympathetic denervation affecting, 1.119
　veins in, 1.123–1.124, 7.7f
Lipid
　dietary, and coronary heart disease, 7.3, 7.14–7.21, 59.9t
　hyperlipidemia
　　dietary treatment of, 7.46
　　familial combined, 7.42, 7.43, 7.44, 60.4t
　　secondary, 7.45–7.46
　hypolipidemic agents, 2.137–2.141
　serum levels
　　in diabetes mellitus, 13.82–13.83
　　diagnosis of abnormalities in, 7.46
　　recommended levels, 7.38, 60.1t
　　and vein graft patency, 7.256
Lipoprotein
　apolipoproteins of, 7.39, 60.3f
　classification and characterization of, 7.39–7.40, 60.3t
　in diabetes mellitus, 13.82–13.83
　high-density, 7.40, 60.3t
　hyperlipoproteinemia
　　type I, 7.42, 7.45, 60.4t
　　type III, 7.40–7.41, 7.42, 7.45, 60.4t
　　type V, familial, 7.42, 7.44–7.45, 60.4t
　intermediate-density, 7.40, 60.3t
　low-density, 7.40, 60.3t
　metabolism of, 7.39–7.40, 60.4f–60.5f
　　heritable disorders of, 7.42–7.45, 60.4t
　serum levels
　　and atherosclerosis, 7.40–7.42
　　and coronary heart disease risk, 7.4–7.7
　　recommended levels, 7.38, 60.1t
　very-low-density, 7.40, 60.3t
Lipoprotein lipase deficiency, familial, 7.42, 7.45, 60.4t
Lisinopril, in hypertension, 8.24
Lithium

interaction with diuretics, 2.180, 21.6t
myocarditis from, 10.96
Livedo reticularis, 3.12, 12.41, 12.43
  classification of, 12.43, 108.18
  management of, 12.43
Liver
  cirrhosis of, diuretics in, 2.28
  clearance of drugs, 2.6
  diseases affecting drug disposition, 2.13
  enzyme induction or inhibition by drugs, 2.6–2.7
Löffler's endocarditis, 10.67–10.69, 10.107, 10.111, 97.5f
Lorcainide, 6.50–6.51
  antiarrhythmic spectrum of, 6.51
  dosage of, 6.51
  electrophysiologic properties of, 6.50
  pharmacokinetics of, 6.51
  side effects of, 6.51
Lovastatin, 2.140–2.141
Lungs
  cardiopulmonary transplantation, 13.102–13.105
  chronic obstructive disease
    glycosides in, 2.43–2.44
    Holter monitoring in, 6.94
    hypoventilation in, 10.72
    and management of pulmonary hypertension, 10.75–10.76
    postoperative management in, 13.56-13.58
    theophylline in, 13.57
  colloid-hydrostatic pressure relationships in, 1.145–1.147, 9.3f
    in hypoproteinemia, 1.146, 9.5f
    measurements of, 1.147
    in pulmonary edema, 1.145–1.147, 9.4f
  congestion in myocardial infarction, 7.185–7.187
    shock with, 7.188–7.199
  edema in, 1.144–1.153
  embolism, pulmonary, 10.77–10.82
  examination of, 3.54–3.57
  function studies
    in aortic insufficiency, 9.23
    in mitral insufficiency, 9.15
  infections after transplantation of heart, 13.98
  perfusion scans in pulmonary embolism, 10.79-10.80, 94.5f
  pulmonary heart disease, 10.70–10.77. See also Cor pulmonale
  respiratory management after cardiac surgery, 13.52–13.58
  in rheumatic fever, 10.99
  sounds in
    classification of, 3.56, 24.1t
    inspiratory crackles in, 3.56, 24.2t
  structure and function of, 1.145
  surfactant in, 1.145
  transplantation of, 13.105
  vasculature of. See Pulmonary vessels
Lupus erythematosus, 13.6–13.9
  coronary artery disease in, 13.9
  electrophysiologic disorders in, 13.9

endocarditis in, 13.7, 13.8, 110.2f
myocarditis in, 13.8
pericarditis in, 10.60, 13.7–13.8
Lutembacher syndrome, 11.43
  murmur in, 3.48
Lymphatics, cardiac, 1.16
Lymphoproliferative disease after transplantation of heart, 13.99

M

Magnesium
  replacement therapy in digitalis toxicity, 2.49
  serum levels and digitalis toxicity, 2.46
Magnesium sulfate, 6.40–6.41
  dosage and pharmacokinetic properties of, 6.37, 42.2t
  interaction with other drugs, 6.33, 42.1t
Magnetic resonance imaging
  in atrial myxomas, 12.48
  in atrial septal defect, 11.48
  in measurement of infarct size, 7.136–7.138, 67.7f
  in myocardial contusion, 12.19
  in pericardial effusion, 10.43, 92.7f
Mahaim fibers, 1.13, 6.138–6.139
Malaria, myocarditis in, 10.95
Malnutrition, 13.89
Mammary artery, internal cannulation
  brachial approach in, 5.32
  percutaneous femoral approach, 5.30, 35.26f
  in coronary bypass surgery, 7.256–7.257
Mammary souffle, 3.48
Mannitol, 2.27, 13.1t
MAP (monophasic action potential) recordings, 6.68–6.84
  accuracy of, 6.72, 45.7f
  afterdepolarizations in, 6.73
  analysis of amplitude and duration in, 6.73, 45.8f
  of antiarrhythmic drug effects, 6.77–6.82, 45.15f–45.21f
  clinical applications of, 6.73–6.84, 45.1t
  duration of action potential in, rate and rhythm affecting, 6.74–6.77
  early techniques in, 6.68, 6.69, 45.1f–45.2f
  electronic recording equipment in, 6.68
  endocardial, 6.69, 6.71, 45.4f–45.5f
    recording catheters in, 6.68, 6.70, 45.3f
  epicardial, 6.70, 6.71, 45.4f
    recording probes in, 6.68, 6.70, 45.3f
  genesis of MAP in, 6.70–6.72, 45.6f
  in myocardial ischemia, 6.82–6.84, 45.22f–45.24f
  Purkinje fiber activity in, 6.73
  resting potential changes in, 6.73
  upstroke velocity in, 6.72
  ventricular fiber activity in, 6.73
  in ventricular tachycardia or fibrillation, 6.76–6.77, 45.14f
Mapping

of body surface, 4.19
precordial, in estimation of infarct size, 7.137–7.138
Marfan syndrome
  aortic dissection in, 12.30
  aortic rupture in, 12.28
  cardiovascular disorders in, 3.11, 3.13, 23.1t
  in pregnancy, 13.26
Means-Lerman scratch, 3.49
Mechanical devices, as bridge to cardiac transplantation, 13.93
Mediastinal emphysema
  auscultation in, 3.57
  chest pain in, 7.66
  postoperative, in transplantation of heart, 13.98
Medtronic-Hall valves, 9.45, 84.2f
  orifice areas in, 9.44, 84.1t
Mefenamic acid, interactions with warfarin, 2.187, 21.10t
Meningococcal infection, myocarditis in, 10.93
Meperidine, interactions with monoamine oxidase inhibitors, 2.184, 21.8t
Mephentermine, 2.57
Mercurial diuretics, 2.27, 13.1t
Meromyosin, 1.21
Mesenteric circulation, nitrates affecting, 2.78
Mesotheliomas, cardiac, 12.52
Metabolism
  of drugs, 2.6–2.7, 12.1t
  energy. See Energy metabolism, myocardial
  in ischemic heart disease, 7.63
  lipoprotein, 7.39–7.40, 60.4f–60.5f
  in myocardial infarction, 7.120–7.122
  in silent ischemia, 7.93
Metaraminol, 2.57
  hemodynamic effects of, 2.53, 14.6t
Metastases to heart, 12.52–12.53, 109.10f–109.11f
Methacholine, provocative testing with, in variant angina, 7.106
Methemoglobinemia, skin color in, 3.7
Methoxamine
  in differentiation of murmurs, 3.50
  hemodynamic effects of, 2.53, 14.6t
Methyldopa, interaction with other drugs, 2.184, 2.185, 21.8t
  anticoagulants, 2.153, 20.2t
Metolazone, 2.27, 13.1t
  interaction with diuretics, 2.180, 21.6t
Metoprolol, 8.22, 77.7t
  in dilated cardiomyopathy, 10.16
  interaction with other drugs, 2.177, 21.4t
  in myocardial infarction, 7.155
  pharmacology of, 2.96, 2.97, 7.71, 16.2t, 16.3t, 62.3t
  in postinfarction prophylaxis, 7.233, 72.9t
  in unstable angina, 7.82

Metronidazole, interaction with anticoagulants, 2.153, 2.187, 20.2t, 21.10t
Mexiletine, 6.22, 6.44–6.45
  antiarrhythmic spectrum of, 6.44–6.45
  dosage of, 6.45
  effects on heart and circulation, 6.22
  effects on transmembrane potential, 6.22
  electrophysiologic properties of, 6.44
  interactions with other drugs, 2.175, 2.177, 21.2t
  molecular weight affecting actions of, 6.19
  pharmacokinetics of, 6.44
  side effects of, 6.45
Microangiopathy in diabetes mellitus, 13.83, 117.1f
Migraine prophylaxis with, β-adrenergic blocking drugs, 2.101
Milrinone, 2.62–2.63, 14.11f–14.12f
  adverse effects of, 2.66, 14.7t
  in dilated cardiomyopathy, 10.15
  hemodynamic effects of, 2.66, 14.7t
Minoxidil, 2.124–2.125, 18.3f
Mirsky formula for wall stress, 5.10
Mitochondria, myocardial, 1.23–1.24
Mitral-septal E-point separation, echocardiography of, 4.40, 4.78, 28.16f–28.17f, 28.106f
Mitral valve
  anatomy of, 1.9–1.10, 1.10f–1.11f
  in aortic insufficiency, echocardiography of, 4.78–4.79, 28.105f–28.107f
  balloon valvuloplasty, 9.67–9.72, 9.124
    cardiac catheterization in, 5.12–5.13, 5.14, 34.17f
    complications of, 9.71–9.72, 85.9t
    double-balloon technique in, 9.67–9.68, 85.10f
    history of, 9.67–9.69
    mechanism of dilatation in, 9.70
    procedure in, 9.69–9.70, 85.10f–85.11f
    results of, 9.70–9.71, 85.8t
  calcification of annulus, 9.17
    in aortic valvular stenosis, 9.109
    echocardiography of, 4.69–4.70, 28.91f
  commissurotomy
    closed, 9.123
    open, 9.123
  echocardiography of, 4.35, 4.38, 4.39, 4.40, 4.51, 4.52, 4.66–4.74, 28.2f, 28.11f, 28.13f, 28.16f, 28.46f–28.47f, 28.49f, 28.85f, 28.95f
  normal area of, 9.55, 85.2t
  prolapse, 9.16, 9.30–9.38
    β-adrenergic blocking drugs in, 2.100–2.101
    amyl nitrite inhalation in, 9.32
    arrhythmias in, 9.36
      treatment of, 9.38
    associated diseases with, 9.31
    auscultation in, 9.32
    absence of signs in, 9.33
    autonomic nervous system dysfunction in, 1.173–1.174, 11.10f
    bedside maneuvers in, 9.32
    chest films in, 9.34
    chest pain in, 3.6, 7.65
    clinical features of, 9.31–9.33
    complications of, 9.35–9.38
      prevention of, 9.37–9.38
      treatment of, 9.38
    definitions of, 9.30–9.31
    echocardiography in, 4.71–4.74, 9.16, 9.34–9.35, 28.95f–28.98f
    effects of posture in, 9.32
    electrocardiography in, 9.33–9.34
      ambulatory, 6.94, 9.35
    embolism in, systemic, 9.37
      prevention of, 9.38
    endocarditis in, 9.36–9.37, 9.81
      prevention of, 9.37
      treatment of, 9.38
    etiology and prevalence of, 9.31
    exercise testing in, 9.35
    flail valve syndrome in, 9.36
    hemodynamic effects of, 9.16
    management of, 9.37–9.38
    midsystolic click in, 3.35–3.36, 23.8t
    murmur in, 3.44
    natural history of, 9.16, 9.37
    orthostatic intolerance in, 1.173–1.174
    pathogenesis of, 9.33
    pathology of, 9.16, 9.31
    patient education and reassurance in, 9.37
    physical examination in, 9.16
    physical signs of, 9.32
      intermittency of, 9.33
    postectopic potentiation in, 9.32
    in pregnancy, 13.25
    progressive regurgitation and heart failure in, 9.35–9.36
      treatment of, 9.38
    sudden death in, 9.36
      prevention of, 9.37–9.38
    symptoms of, 9.31–9.32
    thallium stress test in, 9.35
    Valsalva maneuver in, 9.32
  prosthetic replacement, 9.17, 9.41, 9.123
    coronary bypass surgery with, 7.257
    in elderly patients, 13.34
    technique in, 9.41–9.42
  reconstruction of, 9.17–9.18, 82.2t–82.7f
  regurgitation or insufficiency, 9.11–9.18
    acute
      causes of, 9.3, 81.1t
      intra-aortic balloon pump in, 9.4
      pathophysiology of, 9.3
      vasodilators in, 9.3–9.4, 81.1f
    apexcardiogram in, 9.15
    association with ischemic heart disease, 7.268–7.269, 75.2t
    atrial fibrillation in, 6.130
    in calcification of annulus, 9.17
    cardiac catheterization in, 5.17
    chest films in, 9.13–9.14, 82.3f
    chronic, 9.10
    color-flow Doppler of, 4.86, 4.88, 28.125f, 28.127f
    in congenital heart disease, 9.17
    diagnosis of, 9.16
    diastolic, 9.17
    differential diagnosis, 9.16, 10.89
    Doppler echocardiography in, 9.14–9.15, 82.4f–82.6f
    in elderly patients, 13.34
    electrocardiography in, 9.13, 82.2f
    etiology of, 4.70, 9.11, 28.5t, 82.1t
    hemodynamic effects of, 9.15
    hemodynamic monitoring in, 5.85, 5.87, 39.2t, 39.4f
      in response to therapy, 5.89, 5.90, 39.6f
    in hypertrophic cardiomyopathy, 10.21–10.22
    in left ventricular cavity enlargement, 9.17
    medical treatment of, 9.17
    murmur in, 3.40, 3.41–3.43, 23.11t, 23.13f
    nitrates in, 2.84
    noninvasive tests in, 9.13–9.15
    in papillary muscle dysfunction, 9.16–9.17
    pathophysiology of, 9.11, 9.12, 82.1f
    physical examination in, 9.13
    postinfarction, 7.189, 7.195–7.197, 70.7f, 70.7t
      echocardiography of, 4.50, 28.45f
      surgery in, 7.268–7.271, 75.3f–75.6f
    in pregnancy, 13.23
    prognosis and natural history of, 9.12
    in prolapse, 9.16
      progressive increase and heart failure in, 9.35, 9.38
    prosthetic replacement in, 9.17, 9.41
    pulmonary function in, 9.15
    radioisotope studies in, 9.15
    rheumatic, 9.11, 9.16
      echocardiography in, 4.70–4.71, 28.92f–28.94f
    surgery in, 9.17–9.18
      indications for, 9.18, 82.2t
      results of, 9.17–9.18, 82.7f
    symptoms of, 9.13
    traumatic, 12.21
    vasodilators in, 2.131–2.133, 9.9, 18.13f–18.14f
    in viral myocarditis, 10.86
  stenosis, 9.116–9.124
    arterial pressure in, 9.119
    atrial fibrillation in, 9.118–9.119
    with atrial septal defect, 11.43
    cardiac catheterization in, 5.16–5.17, 34.20f
    chest films in, 9.120, 9.121, 89.2f
    color-flow Doppler of, 4.88, 28.130f
    congenital, 11.67–11.68
    diagnosis of, 9.122–9.123
    diastolic pressure gradient in, 9.117, 89.1f

differential diagnosis of, 11.49, 12.49, 109.3t
Doppler recordings in, 9.121, 89.3f
echocardiography of, 4.67–4.69, 9.121–9.122, 28.87f–28.90f
electrocardiography in, 9.120
heart failure in, 9.119
hemoptysis in, 9.119
left ventricular filling in, 5.61
murmurs in, 3.46, 3.47
noncardiac surgery in, 13.46
opening snap in, 3.36–3.37
pathology of, 9.116
peripheral pulse in, 9.119
physical and laboratory examinations in, 9.119–9.122
precordial examination in, 9.119–9.120
in pregnancy, 13.23
pulmonary artery wedge pressure in, 9.123, 89.5f
pulmonary capillary hypertension in, 9.117
pulmonary vascular disease in, 9.117–9.118
signs and symptoms of, 9.116–9.119
surgery in, 9.123–9.124
valve area calculation in, 9.122–9.123, 89.4f
supravalve mitral ring, 11.67
systolic anterior motion of leaflets, 10.21–10.22
vegetations, echocardiography of, 4.74, 28.99f
Mönckeberg's aortic valvular stenosis, 9.106–9.107, 88.3f
Monitoring
of drug plasma concentrations, 2.15
hemodynamic, 5.80–5.93
Monoamine oxidase inhibitors, interactions with other drugs, 2.183, 2.184, 21.8t
Mononucleosis, infectious, myocarditis in, 10.90
Moricizine, 6.51
antiarrhythmic spectrum of, 6.51
dosage of, 6.51
electrophysiologic properties of, 6.51
pharmacokinetics of, 6.51
side effects of, 6.51
Morphine
in myocardial infarction, 7.14–7.143
in pulmonary edema, 1.150
Morquio's syndrome, cardiovascular disorders in, 3.13, 23.1t
Mortality
in bypass surgery, 7.251
in postinfarction exercise programs, 7.214, 71.11t
Moxalactam, interactions with warfarin, 2.187, 21.10t
Mulibrey nanism, cardiovascular disorders in, 3.13, 23.1t
Müller's sign, in aortic insufficiency, 9.20

Multiple Risk Factor Intervention Trial (MRFIT), in coronary heart disease, 7.5–7.10
Murmurs, 3.38–3.50
in aortic insufficiency, 9.21
in aortic valvular stenosis, 9.109, 9.110
Austin Flint, 3.47. See also Austin Flint murmur
Carey-Coombs, 3.47
continuous, 3.48
diastolic, 3.38–3.39, 3.45–3.48, 23.11f
early, 3.45–3.46
late (presystolic), 3.47–3.48
mid-diastolic, 3.46–3.47
Dock's, 3.45, 3.46, 23.14f
Gibson's, 3.48
Graham Steell, 3.45
in pulmonic insufficiency, 9.27
innocent, 11.48
maneuvers in differential diagnosis of, 3.49–3.50
in mitral insufficiency, chronic, 9.13
in mitral valve prolapse, 9.32
in mitral valve stenosis, 9.120
in pulmonic insufficiency, chronic, 9.27
in rheumatic fever, 10.101
Still's, 3.41
systolic, 3.38, 3.39–3.45, 23.11f
early, 3.44
ejection, 3.39–3.41
bedside diagnosis of, 3.41, 23.12t–23.13t
holosystolic, 3.40, 3.41–3.44, 23.11t
differential diagnosis of, 3.42, 23.12f
late, 3.44–3.45
in tricuspid regurgitation, 9.97–9.98, 9.100, 87.11f, 87.15f
in tricuspid stenosis, 9.101, 9.102, 87.19f
in ventricular septal defect, 11.54
Muscarinic cholinergic receptors, 1.48, 1.59–1.64, 3.7f
agonists and antagonists of, 1.60, 3.7t
in cardiovascular disease, 1.64
G proteins of, 1.45–1.47, 3.1t, 3.5f–3.6f
and norepinephrine release, 1.118, 7.4f
pharmacology of, 1.59–1.60
radioligand binding studies, 1.60
receptor-effector coupling, 1.61–1.63, 3.11f–3.12f
regulation of, 1.63–1.64
responses mediated by, 1.59, 3.6t
structure of, 1.60–1.61
Muscle, skeletal
blood flow in, 1.121–1.123, 7.6f
reflex control of, 1.122–1.123
characteristics of, 1.130
compared to cardiac muscle, 1.28–1.29, 2.2t, 2.11f
dystrophy of
facioscapulohumeral, cardiovascular disorders in, 3.13, 23.1t
pseudohypertrophic, cardiovascular disorders in, 3.13, 23.1t
exercise hyperemia in, 1.121
reactive hyperemia in, 1.121–1.122

training affecting, 1.138, 1.139, 8.8f
Musculoskeletal disorders, chest pain in, 7.67
Musset's sign, in aortic insufficiency, 9.20
Mustard procedure in cyanotic heart disease, 11.38
echocardiography after, 11.92–11.94, 105.8f
and postoperative venous obstruction, 11.61
surgical revision of, 11.66
Mycoplasma pneumoniae infection, myocarditis in, 10.91
Mycotic aneurysm
aortic, 12.34–12.35
in endocarditis, 9.79
Myocarditis, 10.84–10.96
bacterial, 10.92–10.93
biopsy in, 5.76, 5.77, 5.78, 38.3t, 38.5t, 38.16f–38.18f
from bites and stings, 10.95
in candidiasis, 10.93
chronic active, 10.91–10.92
and dilated cardiomyopathy, 10.2
drug-induced, 5.77, 10.95–10.96, 38.4t
hypersensitivity in, 10.96, 95.5t
fungal, 10.93
giant cell, 10.96
helminthic, 10.94
hypersensitivity, 10.96, 95.5t
in lupus erythematosus, 13.8
nonviral, 10.92–10.96
in pregnancy, 13.26
protozoal, 10.94–10.95
in rheumatic fever, 10.99
in rheumatoid arthritis, 13.4
rickettsial, 10.93–10.94
spirochetal, 10.93
viral, 10.84–10.92
arrhythmias in, 10.86, 10.88
treatment of, 10.90
biopsies in, 10.85
causative agents in, 10.84, 95.1t
chest films in, 10.87
chronic active, 10.91–10.92
clinical features of, 10.85–10.86, 95.2t
in coxsackievirus infections, 10.90
death from, 10.86, 10.88
diagnosis of viral disease in, 10.87
differential diagnosis, 10.89
differentiation from infarction, 10.86–10.87, 95.3t
and dilated cardiomyopathy, 10.89, 10.91
echocardiography in, 10.88
electrocardiography in, 10.86, 10.88
heart failure in, 10.86, 10.88
treatment of, 10.90
in hepatitis, 10.91
laboratory data in, 10.87
management of, 10.89–10.90
in mononucleosis, 10.90
in *Mycoplasma pneumoniae* infection, 10.91
neonatal, 10.87
nuclear imaging in, 10.88

pathology of, 10.84–10.85
pericardial effusion in, 10.89
  treatment of, 10.90
and peripartum cardiomyopathy, 10.91
in psittacosis, 10.91
valvular heart disease in, 10.91
Myocardium
  cardiomyopathy. See Cardiomyopathy
  cells in, 1.19–1.24
  contusions of, 12.16–12.20
  energy metabolism in, 1.78–1.80
  fiber disarray in hypertrophic cardiomyopathy, 10.19–10.20, 91.3f
  in heart failure, 1.158–1.159, 10.6t
  ischemia of. See Coronary heart disease
  oxygen demand in, determinants of, 7.62
  oxygen supply of
    in acute infarction, 7.112–7.113
    determinants of, 7.63
  perfusion imaging with thallium-201, 7.54–7.56, 61.2f
  in rheumatoid arthritis, 13.4
  in scleroderma, 13.13
Myofibrils, 1.19
Myopericarditis, 10.52
  recurrent, 10.89
  viral, 10.7
Myosin, 1.20–1.21, 1.22, 1.23, 2.1f, 2.3f–2.4f
  antibody to, in viral myocarditis, 10.88
  isozymes in atria and ventricles, 1.75
Myositis, chest pain in, 3.6
Myotonia dystrophilia, cardiovascular disorders in, 3.13, 23.1t
Myxedema, 13.85–13.86
  pericarditis in, 10.62–10.63
Myxomas, cardiac, 12.45–12.51
  early diastolic sounds in, 3.37
  left atrial, 12.46–12.49
    chest films in, 12.47, 109.2f
    clinical features of, 12.46, 109.2t
    differential diagnosis of, 12.49, 109.3t
    echocardiography in, 4.96, 12.47–12.48, 28.145f, 109.3f–109.5f
    invasive testing in, 12.48–12.49
    noninvasive testing in, 12.47–12.48
    tumor plop in, 12.46, 12.47t, 109.1f
  murmurs in, 3.46–3.47, 3.48
  right atrial, 12.49–12.50
    clinical features of, 12.50
    differential diagnosis of, 12.50
    echocardiography of, 4.97, 4.98, 28.147t
  surgery in, 12.51
  tricuspid valve in, 9.96

N

Nadolol, 8.22, 77.7t
  pharmacology of, 2.96, 2.97, 7.71, 16.2t, 16.3t, 62.3t
Neck pulsations, disorders with, 3.12
Neck veins, examination of, 3.14
Necrosis
  contraction band, in cocaine abuse, 13.76
  of epicardial fat, 10.64
  of ischemic myocardium, time course of, 1.81–1.82, 1.83, 4.19f–4.20f
  of skin, coumarin-induced, 2.154
Neomycin, as hypolipidemic agent, 2.139
Neoplastic disorders. See Tumors of heart
Nephrotic syndrome, diuretics in, 2.28–2.29
Nerve supply of heart, 1.17–1.18, 1.19f
Neurohumoral regulation of blood pressure, 1.168–1.170, 11.6f–11.7f
Neurologic disorders
  from cardiac catheterization, 5.39
  hypertension in, 8.42
  infections after transplantation of heart, 13.98
  in rheumatic fever, 10.99
Neuromuscular blocking agents, interaction with anti-arrhythmic drugs, 2.176, 21.3t
Neurovascular disorders, chest pain in, 7.67
Neutrophils, in myocardial infarction, 7.118–7.119
New York Heart Association Functional Classification, 3.3, 22.1t
Nicardipine, 2.106, 2.107, 17.1t
  systemic hemodynamic effects of, 2.110, 2.111, 17.6f
Nicotinic acid, as hypolipidemic agent, 2.138–2.139
Nifedipine, 2.106, 2.107, 9.6, 9.7, 17.1t, 81.2t
  adverse effects of, 2.121, 17.8t
  in aortic regurgitation, acute, 9.5
  as arteriolar vasodilator, 2.125, 2.126, 18.4f
  characteristics of, 7.72, 62.5t
  effects on transplanted heart, 13.97
  in hypertension, 8.25
  in myocardial infarction, 7.157
  pharmacokinetics of, 2.111, 2.112, 17.3t
  in pulmonary hypertension, 11.80
  systemic hemodynamic effects of, 2.110–2.111
  in unstable angina, 7.82, 7.84, 63.7f
  in variant angina, 7.107, 7.108–7.110, 65.9f
Niludipine, 2.106, 2.107, 17.1t
Nimodipine, 2.106, 2.107, 17.1t
Nisoldipine, 2.106, 2.107, 17.1t
Nitrates, 2.75–2.89
  adverse effects of, 2.88, 15.11f
  in angina pectoris, 2.80–2.81
    β-adrenergic blocking drugs with, 2.99
    compared to other antianginal drugs, 2.116, 17.6t
    mechanisms of efficacy, 2.80, 15.3t
    selection of patients in, 2.81, 15.4t
    stable angina, 2.80–2.81
    unstable angina, 2.81
  in blood pressure control during surgery, 2.84
  buccal or transmucosal, 2.86, 15.7t
    dosage of, 2.86, 15.7t
  in coronary vasospasm, 2.81–2.82
  delivery systems for, 2.86–2.88
  dosage of, 2.86, 15.7t
    affecting activity, 2.78
  in esophageal spasm, 2.84
  guidelines for therapy with, 2.89, 15.8t
  in heart failure, 2.82–2.83
    acute, 2.83
    chronic, 2.83
    hydralazine with, 2.127, 18.6f
  hemodynamic effects of, 2.75–2.80, 15.2t, 15.2f–15.5f
  in hypertension, 2.83–2.84
  indications for, 2.80–2.84
  in interventional cardiology, 2.84
  intravenous, 2.87–2.88
  in ischemic heart disease, 2.79–2.80
  and left ventricular diameter reduction, 2.77, 15.3f
  long-acting, 2.86–2.87, 15.7t
    dosage of, 2.86, 15.7t
  mechanism of action, 2.75, 2.76, 15.1f
  metabolism of, 2.84, 15.6t
  in mitral regurgitation, 2.84
  modulators of action, 2.77–2.78, 15.1t
  in myocardial infarction, 2.81, 2.82, 15.5t
    improved mortality with, 2.81, 2.82, 15.6f
  ointment, 2.87
    dosage of, 2.86, 15.7t
  oral, 2.86–2.87, 15.7t
  pharmacology of, 2.84–2.85
  plasma concentrations of, 2.85, 15.8f–15.9f
  in pregnancy, 13.22, 111.3t
  in pulmonary hypertension, 2.83
  rapid-onset formulations, 2.86
    dosage of, 2.86, 15.7t
  regional circulatory responses to, 2.78–2.79
    coronary, 2.79–2.80, 15.2t, 15.5f
    limb, 2.78, 15.4f
    pulmonary, 2.79
    renal, 2.79
    splanchnic and mesenteric, 2.78
  in silent ischemia, 7.98
  sublingual, 2.86, 15.7t
    dosage of, 2.86, 15.7t
  systemic responses to, 2.78
  tolerance to, 2.75, 2.76, 2.78, 2.88–2.89, 15.1f
  transdermal, 2.87, 15.10f
  venodilation from, 2.76–2.77, 2.125–2.127, 15.2f
Nitrendipine, 2.106, 2.107, 17.1t
Nitroglycerin, 9.6, 9.7, 81.2t
  in angina pectoris, 7.70–7.71, 62.2t
    unstable, 7.80–7.81, 63.3t
    variant, 7.107
  in differentiation of murmurs, 3.40, 23.11t

metabolism of, 2.84, 15.6t
in myocardial infarction, 7.156
in postinfarction shock, 7.192–7.193, 70.10t
in postoperative hypertension, 13.59
transdermal, dosage of, 2.86, 15.7
Nitroprusside sodium, 9.5–9.6, 81.2t
in aortic regurgitation, acute, 9.5
interaction with digoxin, 2.172, 21.1t
in mitral regurgitation, 2.131–2.133, 9.4, 18.13f–18.14f
in postinfarction shock, 7.192, 7.193, 70.10t
in pregnancy, 13.22, 111.3t
vasodilating effects of, 2.128, 2.129, 18.8f
Nocardiosis, after transplantation of heart, 13.99
Node of Tawara, 1.12
Nodules
 Aschoff, in rheumatic fever, 10.99
 subcutaneous, in rheumatic fever, 10.99, 10.101
Noninvasive tests
 in aortic insufficiency, 9.21–9.23
 chest films in, 4.2–4.13
 in cyanotic congenital heart disease, 11.31
 echocardiography in, 4.33–4.98
 electrocardiography in, 4.14–4.31
 in mitral insufficiency, 9.13–9.15
 in sinus node evaluation, 6.102–6.109, 47.2t
Noonan's syndrome, cardiovascular disorders in, 1.13, 23.1t
Norepinephrine
 and cardiac contractility, 1.23
 clinical applications of, 2.52
 effects on transplanted heart, 13.97
 hemodynamic effects of, 2.53, 14.6t
 interactions with other drugs, 2.184, 21.8t
 modulation of release from sympathetic nerve endings, 1.118, 7.4f
 in postinfarction shock, 7.192, 7.193, 70.10t
 receptors for, 7.191, 70.9t
 serum levels
  in exercise, 1.137, 8.4t
  in pheochromocytoma, 13.86–13.87
  stress affecting, 13.68, 13.69
  and sympathetic activity, 1.117
Nosocomial endocarditis, 9.81
Nuclear studies. See Radionuclide studies
Nucleotide utilization, pathways for, 1.80–1.81, 4.16f
Nutrition
 dietary factors in coronary heart disease, 7.3–7.4, 7.14–7.21, 59.2f
 and guidelines for Americans, 7.24, 59.5f
 dietary treatment of hyperlipidemia, 7.46

and drug abuse in eating disorders, 13.79
fat and cholesterol content of foods, 7.4, 59.1t
malnutrition, 13.89
in myocardial infarction, 7.144–7.145
recent changes by Americans, 7.25–7.27, 59.6f, 59.12t–59.13t
Nyquist limit, in pulsed-wave Doppler echocardiography, 4.36, 4.71, 4.86, 28.93f

O

Oat bran intake, affecting lipid levels, 7.46
Obesity, 13.89
 and coronary heart disease, 7.21–7.22
 dilated cardiomyopathy in, 10.3
Ochronosis, cardiovascular disorders in, 3.12
Occlusive peripheral arterial disease, 12.37–12.40
Ohm's law 5.5
OKT3, immunosuppressive effects of, 13.95
Oliver-Cardarelli's sign, in aortic insufficiency, 9.20
Omega-3 fatty acids, as platelet inhibitors, 2.147
Omniscience valves, 9.45, 84.2f
 orifice areas in, 9.44, 84.1t
OPC-8212, inotropic effects of, 2.65
Ornithosis, myocarditis in, 10.91
Orthopnea, 3.6, 3.54
Orthostatic hypotension, 1.163–1.177
Orthostatic intolerance, 1.163
 after bed rest, 1.141
Osler's nodes, in endocarditis, 9.78
Osteogenesis imperfecta, cardiovascular disorders in, 3.13, 23.1t
Ostium primum atrial septal defect, 3.63–3.64, 3.65, 25.10f
Ostium secundum atrial septal defect, 3.63, 3.65
Ouabain, 2.36–2.37
 pharmacokinetics of, 2.37, 14.2t
Oxprenolol pharmacology of, 2.96, 2.97, 16.2t, 16.3t
 in postinfarction prophylaxis, 7.233, 72.9t
Oxygen
 hypoxia
  β-adrenergic receptors in, 1.54, 1.55, 3.5t
  alveolar, 10.72
  contraction mechanics in, 1.81, 4.17f
 maximal uptake of, 1.129
  genetic factors affecting, 1.137–1.138, 8.7f
 myocardial consumption of, 1.78
  in exercise, 7.205–7.206, 71.1t
  in right and left ventricles, 1.101–1.102
 myocardial demand and supply, 1.101–1.102, 6.1f
  in acute infarction, 7.112–7.113

determinants of, 7.62–7.63
 in exercise, 1.135
 variations in left ventricle, 1.102
step-up in right atrium, 11.48, 101.1t
therapy with
 in myocardial infarction, 7.153–7.154
 in pulmonary edema, 1.149
 in pulmonary hypertension, 10.75–10.76
 in viral myocarditis, 10.90
Oxygen-derived free radicals in myocardial infarction, 7.118–7.119, 7.122, 7.157, 7.174
Oxyphenbutazone, interactions with warfarin, 2.187, 21.10t

P

P wave in electrocardiography, 4.17
 abnormalities in, 4.19, 4.20, 27.7f–27.8f
Pacemaker activity
 automaticity in, 6.6–6.7
 currents in, 6.6, 6.16
 ectopic, 6.11, 6.16
Pacing studies, endocardial, in ventricular tachycardia, 6.60–6.61, 6.63, 44.11f–44.12f
Pacing therapy
 in atrial flutter, 6.132
 in atrioventricular nodal tachycardia, 6.134
 in elderly patients, 13.37
 evaluation with Holter monitoring, 6.98
 postoperative, in cardiac surgery, 13.64
 prophylactic, in bundle branch block, 6.121–6.122, 48.9f
 right atrial, postinfarction, 7.225
 in sick sinus syndrome, 6.110
 in tachycardias, 6.63
 transvenous ventricular endocardial, in digitalis toxicity, 2.48
Pain
 in chest. See Chest pain in chest wall, 7.66
 relief of, in myocardial infarction, 7.143–7.144
Pallor in elevation of extremities, grading of, 12.35, 108.3t
Palpation
 in aortic insufficiency, 9.20, 82.9f
 of chest, 3.55–3.56
 in mitral insufficiency, 9.13
 of precordium, 3.23–3.25
Palpitation, evaluation of, 3.7–3.8
 Holter monitoring in, 6.93–6.94
Pancreatitis, chest pain in, 7.67
Papillary muscle
 dysfunction of
  mitral insufficiency in, 9.16–9.17
  in myocardial infarction, 7.195–7.196, 7.268–7.269
 rupture in myocardial infarction, 7.196–7.197, 70.13t
Paracentesis in cardiac tamponade, 10.48
Paragangliomas, 13.86
Parasitic diseases

myocarditis in, 10.94
pericarditis in, 10.59
Parasympathetic nervous system, and cardiac performance, 1.98–1.99
Parasystole, 6.11
Parathyroid disease, 13.88
  electrocardiography in, 4.31
Parchment ventricle, 4.64
Patent ductus arteriosus. See Ductus arteriosus patency
Pectoriloquy, whispered, 3.57
Pectus excavatum, murmurs in, 11.49
Penbutolol, pharmacology of, 2.96, 2.97, 16.2t, 16.3t
Penicillin
  allergy to, and treatment of endocarditis, 9.86
  in rheumatic fever prophylaxis, 10.105–1.106
Percussion of chest, 3.56
Perhexiline, 2.106, 2.107, 17.1t
Periarteritis nodosa, 13.9–13.10
Pericardial fluid, 10.40
Pericardial friction rub, 3.48–3.49
Pericardial knock, 3.35, 10.50
Pericardial reflections, 1.1f, 1.2, 1.3
Pericarditis
  acute, 10.52, 10.63
    cholesterol, 10.63
  in connective tissue disorders, 10.59–10.60
  in dialysis patients, 10.62
  in dissecting aortic hematoma, 10.61
  effusions in, 10.56
  electrocardiography in, 10.54–10.56, 92.10f–92.18f
  in esophageal diseases, 10.61
  etiology of, 10.52, 10.53, 92.7t
  friction rub in, 10.54, 92.17f
  in fungus diseases, 10.59
  in immunopathies and hypersensitivity states, 10.60
  laboratory studies in, 10.54
  in metabolism disorders, 10.62–10.63
  in myocardial infarction, 10.60–10.61
  in myxedema, 10.62–10.63
  noneffusive, 10.53–10.54
  in parasitic diseases, 10.59
  postinfarction, 10.61
  in postpericardiotomy syndrome, 10.61–10.62
  in pulmonary embolism, 10.61
  radiation-induced, 10.62
  rate and rhythm abnormalities in, 10.56
  in renal failure, 10.62
  suppurative, 10.58
  symptoms and signs of, 10.53–10.54
  traumatic, 10.62, 12.16
  treatment of, 10.57
  tuberculous, 10.58–10.59
  viral, 10.57–10.58
  chest pain in, 3.5–3.6, 7.66
  constrictive, 10.48–10.52
    cardiac catheterization in, 5.17
    chest films in, 10.51
    compared to restrictive cardiomyopathy, 10.109, 10.110, 97.2t
    diagnosis of, 10.52
    differential diagnosis of, 10.13–10.14
    echocardiography in, 10.50–10.51, 92.6t
    effusive, 10.51
    elastic, 10.51
    electrocardiography in, 10.51, 92.16f
    latent (occult), 10.52
    management of, 10.52
    pathogenesis of, 10.48
    pathophysiology of, 10.48–10.50, 92.14f–92.15f
    physical examination in, 10.50
    physiology of constriction in, 10.50
    precordial pulsations in, 3.25, 3.26, 23.8f
    symptoms of, 10.50
  in viral myocarditis, 10.89
  echocardiography in, 4.94, 28.142f
  electrocardiography in, 4.28
  in lupus erythematosus, 13.7–13.8
  postinfarction, 7.201
  in rheumatic fever, 10.59–10.60. 10.99, 10.101
  in rheumatoid arthritis, 13.3–13.4
  in scleroderma, 13.13
Pericardium
  absence of, 4.63, 4.96
  acute pericarditis, 10.52–10.63
  adhesions and fibrosis of, 10.40, 10.41, 92.3t
  anatomy of, 1.2–1.3, 10.38, 10.39, 92.1f
  chylopericardium, 10.63
  congenital defects of, 10.64
  constrictive disease, 10.48–10.52. See also Pericarditis, constrictive
  cysts of
    congenital, 10.64
    echocardiography of, 4.96
    inflammatory, 10.64
  diseases of, 10.41, 92.2t
  drug-associated disease, 10.63
  echocardiography of, 4.89–4.96, 28.132f–28.144f
  effusions in, 10.40–10.44
    chest films in, 4.3, 4.4, 10.41, 10.42, 26.3f–26.4f, 92.2f–92.3f
    chronic, 10.63–10.64
    clinical features of, 10.41
    computed tomography in, 10.43, 92.6f
    decompensated, and cardiac tamponade, 10.44–10.48, 92.8f
    differential diagnosis of, 10.13, 10.89
    echocardiography of, 4.35, 4.89–4.94, 10.41–10.43, 28.2f, 28.133f–28.136f, 92.4t, 92.4f–92.5f
    in hypothyroidism, 13.85
    magnetic resonance imaging in, 10.43, 92.7f
    management of, 10.44
  pathophysiology of, 10.40–10.41
  in viral myocarditis, 10.89
    treatment of, 10.90
  fat necrosis, 10.64
  inflammation of, 10.40
  lacerations of, 12.16
  normal physiology of, 10.38–10.40, 92.1t
  tumors of, 10.63
    echocardiography in, 4.95–4.96
Peripheral arterial disease, 12.35–12.43
  Allen test in, 12.36, 108.6f
  aneurysmal, 12.40–12.41, 108.13f–108.15f
  color return after elevation in, 12.35, 108.4t
  and coronary bypass surgery, 7.258–7.259, 74.1f, 74.2t
  costoclavicular maneuver in, 12.36, 108.7f
  in diabetes mellitus, 13.84
  diagnosis of, 12.35–12.37
  grading of elevation pallor in, 12.35, 108.3t
  hyperabduction maneuver in, 12.36, 108.8f
  occlusive, 12.37–12.40
    balloon angioplasty in, 12.40
    differential diagnosis of, 12.41, 108.13t
    etiology of, 12.38, 108.6t
    intermittent claudication in, 12.37
    ischemic ulceration in, 12.37, 12.39, 108.11f
    management of, 12.40, 108.10t–108.11t
    occupational, 12.37, 12.39, 108.9t
    uncommon types of, 12.38, 108.7t
  scalene or Adson maneuver in, 12.36, 108.9f
  systolic pressure after exercise in, 12.35, 12.37, 108.5t
  thoracic outlet maneuvers in, 12.36, 108.7f–108.9f
  thromboangiitis obliterans, 12.39, 108.8t
  vasospastic, 12.41–12.43, 108.12t. See also Vasospastic disorders
Pernio, 12.41, 12.43, 108.17f, 108.19t
Pharmacokinetics, 2.8–2.11
  of cardiac glycosides, 2.37, 14.2t
  concept of compartments in, 2.8–2.10, 12.9f–12.12f
  loading dose in, 2.10–2.11, 2.12, 12.15f
  multiple doses in, 2.10, 2.11, 2.13f
  nitrate, factors affecting, 2.85, 15.8f
  steady state in, 2.10, 2.11, 12.2t, 12.14f
Pharmacology
  absorption in, 2.5
  active metabolites of drugs, 2.11–2.13, 12.16f–12.17f
  adrenergic blocking drugs, 2.91–2.103
  age affecting drug disposition, 2.15
  antithrombotic therapy, 2.143–2.166
  calcium channel blockers, 2.105–2.121, 17.1f
  cardiac glycosides, 2.34–2.50
  cardiovascular drug interactions, 2.172–2.188. See also Drug interactions

I.35

catecholamines, 2.50–2.59
diseases affecting drug disposition, 2.13–2.15
   acute myocardial infarction, 2.14–2.15, 12.4t
   cardiac failure, 2.13–2.14, 12.18f
   liver disease, 2.13
   renal disease, 2.14
distribution in, 2.5–2.6
   volume of, 2.5–2.6
diuretics, 2.19–2.31
dose-response relationships in, 2.2–2.4, 12.1f–12.3f
effects of drugs on transplanted heart, 13.97–13.98
hypolipidemic agents, 2.137–2.141
mathematical relationships in, 2.16–2.17
metabolism and elimination in, 2.6–2.7, 12.1t
   hepatic clearance in, 2.6–2.7
   renal clearance in, 2.7
monitoring of plasma concentrations of drugs, 2.15, 2.16, 12.19f
nitrates, 2.75–2.89
protein binding by drugs, 2.7–2.8
   concentration-dependent, 2.8, 12.8f
   structure-activity relationships in, 2.4, 12.5f
therapeutic window in, 2.4, 2.5, 12.6f
vasodilator drugs in heart failure, 2.123–2.135
Phencyclidine abuse, 13.78
Phenobarbital, interaction with other drugs
   β-adrenergic blocking drugs, 2.177, 21.4t
   antiarrhythmic drugs, 2.175, 21.2t
   theophylline, 2.186, 21.9t
Phenothiazines, myocarditis from, 10.96
Phenoxybenzamine, 2.94
   in pheochromocytoma, 13.87
Phentolamine, 2.94, 9.6, 9.7, 81.2t
   in postinfarction shock, 7.193–7.194, 70.10t
   vasodilating effects of, 2.128
Phenylbutazone, interactions with other drugs, 2.181, 21.7t
   anticoagulants, 2.153, 2.187, 20.2t, 21.10t
Phenylephrine, 2.57
   in differentiation of murmurs, 3.40, 3.50, 23.11t
   hemodynamic effects of, 2.53, 14.6t
   interactions with other drugs, 2.184, 21.8t
Phenylpropanolamine
   abuse of, 13.78
   interactions with other drugs, 2.184, 21.8t
Phenytoin, 6.22–6.23, 6.38
   antiarrhythmic effects of, 6.14, 6.15
   in digitalis-induced arrhythmias, 2.48
   dosage and pharmacokinetic properties of, 6.37, 42.2t
   effects on heart and circulation, 6.22–6.23
   effects on transmembrane potential, 6.22

interaction with other drugs, 6.33, 42.1t
   β-adrenergic blocking drugs, 2.177, 21.4t
   antiarrhythmic drugs, 2.175, 21.2t
   anticoagulants, 2.153, 2.187, 20.2t, 21.11t
   theophylline, 2.186, 21.9t
Pheochromocytoma, 8.36–8.39, 13.86–13.87
   ACTH production in, 8.37, 78.6f
   α-adrenergic blocking drugs in, 2.93–2.94
   clinical features of, 8.36–8.37, 78.3t
   diagnosis of, 13.87
   differential diagnosis of, 8.37, 78.4t
   hypertension in, 8.36–8.39
   laboratory studies in, 8.38
   pathophysiology of, 8.37–8.38
   treatment of, 8.38–8.39, 13.87
Phlebotomy, in hemochromatosis, 10.15, 97.8f
Phonocardiography
   in aortic valvular stenosis, 9.112
   in atrial myxoma, 12.46, 109.1f
   in tricuspid regurgitation, 9.100, 87.15f
Phosphodiesterase inhibitors
   adverse effects of, 2.66, 14.7t
   amrinone, 2.61–2.62, 14.10f
   enoximone, 2.63–2.65, 14.13f–14.14f
   hemodynamic effects of, 2.66, 14.7t
   inotropic effects of, 2.60–2.65, 14.9f
   milrinone, 2.62–2.63, 14.11f–14.12f
Phospholipids, platelet membrane, inhibitors of, 2.147
Phosphorylation, oxidative, myocardial, 1.78–1.79
Phthalazinol in Prinzmetal angina, 7.86
Physical activity. See Exercise
Physical examination, 3.11–3.51
   in aortic insufficiency, 9.20–9.21
   arterial pressure and pulse in, 3.18–3.22
   in atrial septal defect, 11.45–11.46
      ostium primum, with pulmonary vascular disease, 11.86
      ostium secundum, with pulmonary vascular disease, 11.84
   auscultation in, 3.25–3.50
   in ductus arteriosus patency with pulmonary vascular disease, 11.83
   in Eisenmenger syndrome, 11.81–11.82
   in hypertension, 8.17–8.20
   inspection in, 3.11–3.14
   in ischemic heart disease, 7.50
   jugular venous pulse in, 3.14–3.16, 23.1f
   in mitral insufficiency, 9.13
   in mitral prolapse, 9.16
   in mitral stenosis, 9.119–9.120
   precordial pulsations in, 3.22–3.25
   in pulmonary embolism, 10.77
   in pulmonary heart disease, 10.73
   in pulmonic insufficiency, 9.27
   in variant angina, 7.101
Physiology of cardiac muscle contraction, 1.19–1.40
   principles of, 1.19, 2.1t

Pierre Robin syndrome, cardiovascular disorders in, 3.13, 23.1t
Pimobendan, 2.66
Pindolol, 8.22, 77.7t
   interaction with other drugs, 2.177, 21.4t
   pharmacology of, 7.71, 62.3t
   in postinfarction prophylaxis, 7.233, 72.9t
Pirbuterol, 2.57
   hemodynamic effects of, 2.53, 14.6t
Pirmenol, 6.50
   antiarrhythmic spectrum of, 6.50
   dosage of, 6.50
   electrophysiologic properties of, 6.50
   pharmacokinetics of, 6.50
   side effects of, 6.50
Piroximone, 2.65
   adverse effects of, 2.66, 14.7t
   hemodynamic effects of, 2.66, 14.7t
Pituitary adenomas, growth hormone secretion in, 13.86
Plasminogen activators
   inhibition of, 2.146–2.147
   single-chain urokinase, 7.167–7.168
   tissue-type (tPA)
      in myocardial infarction, 7.118, 7.167, 7.168–7.169, 69.2t
         percutaneous transluminal coronary angioplasty with, 7.171–7.173, 69.3t
      in pulmonary embolism, 10.81–10.82
      recombinant, 2.155
      in unstable angina, 7.80, 7.85, 63.3t
Plasminogen-streptokinase-activator complex
   acylated, 2.155–2.156
   anisoylated, in myocardial infarction, 7.166–7.167, 69.2t
Platelets
   activation of, and thrombogenesis, 2.143–2.147, 20.1f–20.3f
   aggregation of, and thrombus formation, 2.156
   cAMP levels in, drugs increasing, 2.148–2.149
   cyclo-oxygenase inhibitors, 2.147
   inhibitors of, 2.147–2.149
      anticoagulants with, in thrombosis prevention with prosthetic valves, 2.165
      aspirin, 2.147
      dextran, 2.149
      dipyridamole, 2.148
      in myocardial infarction, 2.161
      postinfarction use of, 2.162
      in prevention of vein graft disease after bypass surgery, 2.163
      prostacyclin, 2.148–2.149
      prostaglandin E_1, 2.148–2.149
      sulfinpyrazone, 2.149
      ticlopidine, 2.149
      in unstable angina, 2.160
   interactions with vascular endothelium, 7.116–7.118

membrane phospholipid inhibitors, 2.147
in myocardial infarction, 7.115–7.116
thrombin inhibitors, 2.149
thromboxane synthetase inhibitors, 2.148
Plethora of inferior vena cava, 4.92–4.93
Plethysmography, impedance, in venous thrombosis detection, 10.78-10.79, 94.4f
Pleural effusion, echocardiography in, 4.96, 28.144f
Pleural friction rub, 3.57
Pneumocystic carinii pneumonia, after transplantation of heart, 13.99
Pneumocytes, 1.145
Pneumonia
  chest pain in, 7.66
  postoperative, in transplantation of heart, 13.98
Pneumothorax
  chest pain in, 7.66
  postoperative, in cardiac surgery, 13.64
Poiseuille's law, 1.114, 10.71
Polycythemia
  coronary blood flow in, 1.112
  venesection in, 11.59
Polymerase chain reaction in DNA sequencing, 1.45
Polymyositis, 13.15
Posicor, 2.65
  adverse effects of, 2.66, 14.7
  hemodynamic effects of, 2.66, 14.7t
Positional abnormalities of heart, chest films in, 4.1, 4.11, 26.19f–26.20f
Positron emission tomography in silent ischemia, 7.92, 7.93, 64.1f
Postectopic beat, and differentiation of murmurs, 3.40, 3.49–3.50, 23.11t
Posture
  cardiovascular adjustment to changes in, 1.164, 1.165, 11.1t
  and colloid osmotic pressure changes, 1.148, 9.8f
  and normal responses to orthostatic stress, 1.165–1.166, 11.3f
  and orthostatic hypotension, 1.163–1.177
  and orthostatic intolerance, 1.163
  after bed rest, 1.141
  and physical signs in mitral prolapse, 9.32
Potassium
  cardiac concentrations of, 6.2, 40.1t
  channels across sarcolemma, 6.2
  and electrical excitation of myocardial fibers, 1.24
  excretion in hypertension, 8.19
  hypokalemia
    in aldosteronism, 8.39
    causes of, 8.19, 77.3t
    in Cushing's disease, 13.87
    epinephrine-induced, β-adrenergic blocking drugs in, 2.101

postoperative, in cardiac surgery, 13.64
in weight-loss regimens, 13.75
Na/K pump, 6.2
replacement therapy in digitalis toxicity, 2.49
serum levels
  affecting electrocardiogram, 4.30
  and digitalis toxicity, 2.46
supplements of
  interactions with antihypertensive drugs, 2.184, 21.8t
  interactions with nonsteroidal anti-inflammatory drugs, 2.181, 21.7t
Potts anastomosis in cyanotic heart disease, 11.40
PR interval in electrocardiography, 4.18
Practolol, in postinfarction prophylaxis, 7.233, 72.9t
Prazosin, 2.91, 9.6–9.7, 81.2t
  adverse effects of, 2.94
  in aortic regurgitation, 9.5
  in mitral regurgitation, 9.4
  pharmacokinetics of, 2.92, 16.1t
  vasodilating effects of, 2.127–2.128, 18.7f
Precordium
  mapping of, in estimation of infarct size, 7.137–7.138
  palpation of, 3.23–3.25
    left ventricular impulse in, 3.23–3.25, 23.6f–23.7f
    right ventricular impulse in, 3.25
  pulsations in, 3.22–3.25
    apex beat in, 3.23–3.25
    systolic retraction in, 3.25
Preexcitation syndromes
  electrocardiography in, 4.24, 27.10f
  Holter monitoring in, 6.94
  Wolff-Parkinson-White syndrome, 6.135–6.136
Pregnancy
  antithrombotic therapy in, 2.165–2.166
  aortic dissection in, 12.30
  in cardiac patients, 13.19–13.26
    arrhythmias in, 13.23
    cardiac output decrease in, 13.23
    in congenital heart disease, 13.24–13.25
    in developmental abnormalities, 13.25–13.26
    diagnostic studies in, 13.21–13.22
    drugs used in, 13.22, 111.3t
    endocarditis in, 13.23
    indicators of heart disease in, 13.20, 13.21, 111.1t
    management of, 13.20–13.21
    pulmonary hypertension in, 13.22
    pulmonary vascular congestion in, 13.22–13.33
    and risk of congenital heart disease in offspring, 13.21, 111.2t
    structural lesions in, 13.23
    valvular disease in, 13.23–13.24
    cardiovascular changes in, 13.19–13.20, 111.1f–111.2f
    coronary artery disease in, 13.26

myocardial diseases in, 13.26
and peripartum cardiomyopathy, 10.3
and viral myocarditis, 10.91
Preload
  and left ventricular performance, 1.85
  reducing agents, 9.6, 81.2t
  reserve mismatch with afterload, 1.98, 5.21f
Premature beats
  atrial
    in myocardial infarction, 7.151
    postoperative, in cardiac surgery, 13.64–13.65
    post-transplant, 13.98
    and murmur during postectopic potentiation, 3.40, 3.49–3.50, 23.11t
  ventricular, 6.41
    in myocardial infarction, 7.150–7.151
    postoperative, in cardiac surgery, 13.64
    post-transplant, 13.98
Prenalterol, 2.57–2.58
  hemodynamic effects of, 2.53, 14.6t
Pressure-volume relations
  left ventricular, 1.92–1.95, 5.11f–5.15f
  passive, 1.95–1.97, 5.17f–5.19f
  and performance, 1.85, 1.86, 5.1f
  in orthostatic hypotension, 1.167–1.168, 11.5f
Prinzmetal angina. See Angina pectoris, variant or Prinzmetal
Probucol, as hypolipidemic agent, 2.139–2.140
Procainamide, 6.20–6.21, 6.38
  antiarrhythmic effects of, 6.14
  contraindications in digitalis toxicity, 2.49
  dosage and pharmacokinetic properties of, 6.37, 42.2t
  effects on heart and circulation, 6.21
  effects on transmembrane potential, 6.20–6.21
  effects on transplanted heart, 13.97
  interactions with other drugs, 2.175, 2.176, 6.33, 21.2t–21.3t, 42.1t
  in pregnancy, 13.22, 111.3t
  in supraventricular tachycardia, 6.138
Progeria, cardiovascular disorders in, 3.13, 23.1t
Prolapse
  of mitral valve, 9.16, 9.30–9.38
  of tricuspid valve, 9.94–9.95, 87.7f–87.8f
Propafenone, 6.46–6.47
  antiarrhythmic spectrum of, 6.47
  dosage of, 6.47
  electrophysiologic effects of, 6.46–6.47
  pharmacokinetics of, 6.47
  side effects of, 6.47
Propranolol, 6.25–6.26, 8.22, 77.7t
  in cyanotic heart disease, 11.40
  effects on heart and circulation, 6.26
  effects on transmembrane potential, 6.25–6.26
  interaction with other drugs, 2.177, 21.4t

antiarrhythmic drugs, 2.175, 2.176, 21.2t–21.3t
sympathomimetic agents, 2.184, 21.8t
in myocardial infarction, 7.155
pharmacology of, 2.96, 2.97, 7.71, 16.2t, 16.3t, 62.3t
in postinfarction prophylaxis, 7.233, 72.9t
and sinus node recovery time, 6.105–6.106
in unstable angina, 7.81–7.83, 63.5f–63.6f
withdrawal syndrome, 1.54
Propylbutyl dopamine, 2.59
hemodynamic effects of, 2.53, 14.6t
Propylthiouracil, in hyperthyroidism, 13.85
Prostacyclin
affecting coronary vessels, 1.106
formation in endothelial cells, 1.115, 7.1f
interaction with thromboxane A_2, 7.116
as platelet inhibitor, 2.148–2.149
therapy with
in pulmonary hypertension, 11.80
in unstable angina, 7.85–7.86
and thrombosis inhibition, 2.146
Prostaglandin E_1, as platelet inhibitor, 2.148–2.149
Prostatic obstruction, benign, α-adrenergic blocking drugs in, 2.94
Prosthetic heart valves, 9.40–9.51
antithrombotic therapy with, 2.164–2.165
aortic, 9.113
indications for, 9.40–9.41
operative technique, 9.42, 9.43, 84.1f
ball, 9.45, 84.2f
bileaflet, 9.45, 9.46, 84.2f
bioprosthetic, 9.46–9.47, 84.3f
aortic, 9.113
degeneration of, 9.48–9.49
durability of, 9.51
evaluation of, 9.83
complications of, 9.47–9.49
endocarditis of, 9.47, 9.50, 9.81
treatment of, 9.86
failure of, 9.50–9.51, 84.5f
heart sounds with, 3.37–3.38, 23.10t
history of, 9.40
indications for, 9.40–9.41
mitral, 9.123
indications for, 9.41
operative technique, 9.41–9.42
and noncardiac surgery, 13.46
operative technique in, 9.41–9.43
orifice areas in, 9.44, 84.1t
postoperative care in, 9.42–9.44
in pregnancy, 13.24
reoperations in, 9.51
results with, 9.49–9.51
survival of, 9.49–9.50, 84.2t
thromboembolism from, 2.159, 9.47–9.48, 9.50
tilting disc, 9.45–9.46, 84.2f
tricuspid, 9.103

indications for, 9.41
Protamine, for heparin neutralization, 2.152
Protein C, and thrombosis inhibition, 2.146
Proteins
contractile, 1.20–1.21, 1.22, 1.23, 2.2f–2.4f
plasma, binding by drugs, 2.7–2.8, 12.8f
concentration-dependent, 2.8, 12.8f
Proteinuria, in hypertension, 8.19
Prothrombin time, 2.153
Protodiastole, 5.55
Protozoal infections, myocarditis in, 10.94–10.95
Pseudoaneurysm, ventricular
echocardiography of, 4.50, 28.43f
in myocardial infarction, 7.198–7.199, 70.8f
traumatic, 12.16–12.17, 107.1f–107.4f
Pseudotruncus arteriosus, management of, 11.40
Pseudoxanthoma elasticum, restrictive cardiomyopathy in, 10.116
Psittacosis, myocarditis in, 10.91
Psychologic aspects
of cardiac transplantation, 13.101
of emotional stress, 13.67–13.72
Psychosocial factors
in coronary heart disease, 7.22
in elderly patients, 13.38
Pulmonary artery
abnormalities of, chest films in, 4.5, 4.12–4.13, 26.6f
anomalous origin of coronary arteries from, 11.20–11.22, 99.11f
atresia with tetralogy of Fallot and aortopulmonary collaterals, 3.59, 3.60, 25.2f
banding in cyanotic heart disease, 11.38
catheterization of, 5.80–5.81
knotting of catheter in, 5.92–5.93
echocardiography of, 4.84–4.86, 28.123f–28.124f
end-diastolic pressure, 5.83
pressure in, 10.70
stenosis of branches, 11.64
balloon dilatation in, 9.58–9.59
transposition of. See Transposition of great vessels
wedge pressure, 5.82–5.83
equal to right atrial pressure, 5.86, 39.3f
and left ventricular filling pressure, 5.84
in mitral stenosis, 9.123, 89.5f
Pulmonary conditions. See Lungs
Pulmonary heart disease, 10.70–10.77. See also Cor pulmonale
Pulmonary valve
anatomy of, 1.8, 1.8f–1.9f, 1.9
atresia with tetralogy of Fallot and aortopulmonary collaterals, 3.59, 3.60, 25.2f
balloon valvuloplasty, 9.54–9.59, 11.64, 103.2f

complications of, 9.57
history of, 9.54
mechanism of dilatation in, 9.57–9.58
patient selection in, 9.56
physiologic and anatomical effects of, 9.54–9.56
procedure in, 9.56–9.57, 9.58, 85.3f
reported series of, 9.54, 9.55, 85.3t
results of, 9.58
echocardiography of, 4.84–4.86, 28.121f–28.124f
normal area of, 9.55, 85.2t
regurgitation or insufficiency
acute, vasodilators in, 9.5
chronic, 9.27–9.28
echocardiography in, 4.85, 28.122f
murmur in, 3.45–3.46
traumatic, 12.21
stenosis of, 9.54
complex conotruncal anomalies with, 3.62
congenital, 3.58–3.59, 3.60, 11.29, 11.36, 11.63–11.64, 25.1f
management of, 11.41
echocardiography in, 4.85, 28.121f
long-term outcome of surgery in, 11.6
mild, differential diagnosis of, 11.48
in pregnancy, 13.24
Pulmonary vascular disease
in atrial septal defect
ostium primum, 11.85–11.86
clinical features of, 11.85–11.86
management of, 11.86
ostium secundum, 11.83–11.85
clinical features of, 11.84
management of, 11.85
clinical features of, 11.80–11.81
in congenital heart disease, 11.77–11.86
in ductus arteriosus patency, 11.82–11.83
clinical features of, 11.82–11.83
management of, 11.83
histologic classification of, 11.78, 104.1t
management of, 11.81
in mitral stenosis, 9.117–9.118
natural history of, 11.80–11.81
obstructive disease, congenital, 3.58
pathology and pathophysiology of, 11.77–11.79, 104.2t
in ventricular septal defect, 11.81–11.82
clinical features of, 11.81–11.82
management of, 11.82
Pulmonary vessels
arteries, 1.2f, 1.4, 1.8–1.9, 1.14, 1.16f. See also Pulmonary artery
arteriovenous fistula, 11.36
management of, 11.41
blood flow in. See Blood flow, pulmonary
capillary wedge pressure
reduction of, in postinfarction acute pulmonary edema, 7.188
in silent ischemia, 7.92
chest films of, 4.6, 4.8–4.9, 26.8f, 26.26f
in heart failure, 4.9–4.11, 26.17f–26.18f

decreased radius of arterial bed, 10.71–10.72
diseases of. *See* Pulmonary vascular disease
hypertension in. *See* Hypertension, pulmonary
nitrates affecting, 2.79
resistance in, 10.70–10.71
  calculation of, 5.5–5.6
venous congestion, normal cardiac output with, 5.85
venous obstruction, 11.64–11.66, 103.3f–103.4f
  in cor triatriatum, 11.66–11.67
venous return
  partial anomalous, 3.65, 25.11f
  total anomalous, 11.35
    chest film in, 4.13
    differential diagnosis of, 11.49
    management of, 11.38, 11.39
Pulsations
  in neck, 3.12
  precordial, examination of, 3.22–3.25
Pulse
  arterial, 3.18–3.22
    in aortic valvular stenosis, 9.109
    in mitral stenosis, 9.119
  carotid
    in aortic stenosis, 3.21–3.22, 23.3t, 23.5f
    configurational changes in, 3.20, 23.4f
  dicrotic, 3.21
  in hypertension, 8.17
  jugular venous, 3.14–3.18
  parvus et tardus, in aortic valvular stenosis, 9.109
Pulseless disease, 12.33
Pulsus
  alternans, 3.19
    in aortic valvular stenosis, 9.109
  bisferiens, 3.20–3.21
    in aortic regurgitation, 9.110
  paradoxus, 3.19–3.20
    in cardiac tamponade, 10.45–10.46, 92.9f–92.10f
    absence of, 10.46
  reversed, 3.20
Pump function indices, 5.11–5.12
  in exercise, 5.12, 5.13, 34.16f
  plotting of ventricular function curves in, 5.11–5.12, 34.14f–34.15f
  stroke work index, 5.11, 34.13f
Purkinje fibers, 1.13, 6.112
  activity in MAP recordings, 6.73
Pyelography, intravenous, in renal artery disease, 8.33
Pyrophosphate scanning. *See* Technetium-99m pyrophosphate scans

Q

Q fever, myocarditis in, 10.94
Q waves in electrocardiography
  abnormalities of, 4.27
  in myocardial infarction, 4.25
Quality of life after cardiac transplantation, 13.102
QRS complex in electrocardiography, 4.18
  abnormalities in, 4.27–4.28
  in estimation of infarct size, 7.137–7.138
  narrow QRS tachycardia, 6.58–6.60, 6.62, 44.10f
  wide QRS tachycardia, 6.58–6.62, 44.7f–44.10f
QT interval prolongation syndrome, 6.81–6.82
  β-adrenergic blocking drugs in 2.101
  Holter monitoring in, 6.94
Quinidine, 6.20, 6.38–6.39
  antiarrhythmic effects of, 6.14
  contraindications in digitalis toxicity, 2.49
  dosage and pharmacokinetic properties of, 6.37, 42.2t
  effects on heart and circulation, 6.20
  effects on transmembrane potential, 6.20
  effects on transplanted heart, 13.97
  interactions with other drugs, 2.175–2.176, 6.33, 21.2t–21.3t, 42.1t
    anticoagulants, 2.153, 2.187, 20.2t, 21.10t
    calcium entry blockers, 2.179, 21.5t
    digoxin, 2.47, 2.172, 21.1f, 21.1t
  in pregnancy, 13.22, 111.3t
  in supraventricular tachycardia, 6.138
QX-314, antiarrhythmic effects of, factors affecting, 6.18, 41.5f

R

R waves in electrocardiography, abnormalities in, 4.27
Radiation
  heart disease from, 10.117
  pericarditis from, 10.62
Radioisotope studies in aortic insufficiency, 9.23
Radioligand receptor binding assays, 1.41–1.44, 3.1f–3.4f
Radiology
  chest films in, 4.2–4.13. *See also* Chest films
  projections of coronary arteries in, 5.33–5.38, 5.35, 35.1t
    identification of vessels in, 5.35–5.37, 35.33f–35.37f
    stenosis evaluation in, 5.37–5.38
    terminology for, 5.34, 35.32f
Radionuclide studies
  angiocardiography
    in atrial septal defect, 11.47–11.48
    in ischemic heart disease, 7.56–7.57
    in myocardial contusion, 12.19
  scintigraphy in. *See* Scintigraphy
  ventriculography
    in estimation of infarct size, 7.138–7.140, 67.10f
  in postinfarction exercise testing, 7.224–7.225, 72.4t
Rales, 3.56
Rashkind procedure in cyanotic heart disease, 11.38
Rastelli procedure in cyanotic heart disease, 11.39, 11.40
Raynaud disease, 1.124–1.126, 7.8f, 12.41
  management of, 12.43
Raynaud phenomenon, 1.124, 12.41
  α-adrenergic blocking drugs in, 2.94
  from β-adrenergic blocking drugs, 2.102
  calcium channel blockers in, 2.120
  differential diagnosis of, 12.42, 108.15t
  evaluation of, 12.42, 108.16t
  management of, 12.42, 12.43, 108.17t
  in scleroderma, 13.12
  secondary, causes of, 12.42, 108.14t
Receptors
  cardiopulmonary, 1.169–1.170
  cardiovascular, 1.41–1.64
    adrenergic, 1.47–1.59, 3.7f
    G proteins of, 1.45–1.47, 3.1t, 3.5f–3.6f
    muscarinic cholinergic, 1.59–1.64
    radioligand binding assays of, 1.41–1.44, 3.1f–3.4f
    studies with recombinant DNA and immunological techniques, 1.44–1.45
  carotid and aortic baroreceptors, 1.168–1.169, 11.7f
  and responses to drugs, 2.2–2.4, 12.4f
Reentry of cardiac impulses
  arrhythmias in, 6.9–6.11, 6.14–6.16
  and atrioventricular nodal tachycardia, 6.132–6.134
  circuits in, 6.9, 6.10, 40.11f
  leading circle mechanism in, 6.11, 6.12, 40.13f
  reflection mechanism in, 6.9, 6.11, 40.12f
  suppression by drugs, 6.14–6.16
Reflection and reentry of cardiac impulses, 6.9, 6.11, 40.12f
Reflex sympathetic dystrophy, 12.41
Reflexes
  and blood flow to limb muscles, 1.122–1.123
  and blood flow to skin, 1.121
  in exercise, 1.135–1.136, 8.6f
Reflux, atriogenic, 9.17
Refractoriness
  of cardiac cells, 6.5
  relation to action potential duration, 6.78, 45.16f
  sinus node, assessment of, 6.107
Refsum's disease, cardiovascular disorders in, 3.13, 23.1t
Rehabilitation, cardiac, 7.204–7.216
  eight levels of activity in, 7.209–7.210, 71.6t
  in elderly patients, 13.31, 13.38
  exercise in. *See* Exercise
  in-hospital, postinfarction, 7.208–7.211
    exercise testing in, 7.210, 7.211, 71.7t

maintenance of behavior modification in, 7.213–7.214
in myocardial infarction, 7.158
out-of-hospital, postinfarction, 7.211–7.213
return to work in, 7.210–7.211
sexual activity in, 7.210–7.211
survey of procedures in, 7.213–7.214, 71.10t
Reiter's disease, 13.6
Rejection of transplanted heart, 13.94–13.96, 13.100
in heart-lung transplantation, 13.103–13.104
Relapsing fever, myocarditis in, 10.93
Relaxation of cardiac muscle, 1.26, 1.36–1.40, 2.8f, 2.29f–2.32f
diastolic, 10.26–10.28, 91.9f
abnormal, measures of, 10.29–10.30, 91.6t
in hypertrophic cardiomyopathy, 10.28, 91.10f
isovolumic, 5.55–5.59
left ventricular, 1.97
Renal artery disease, hypertension in, 8.31–8.35
Renin activity in plasma
in aldosteronism, 8.39
in renovascular hypertension, 8.34
Renin-angiotensin-aldosterone system, 8.3–8.5, 76.1f–76.3f
in renovascular hypertension, 8.32–8.33, 8.34
Reperfusion of myocardium, effects of, 1.82
Repolarization, 1.24, 6.3, 6.4, 40.3f
acceleration by antiarrhythmic drugs, 6.21–6.23
antiarrhythmic drugs affecting, 6.20–6.21, 6.24–6.25
electrocardiography in, 4.14, 4.16, 27.3f
time course of. See Action potential, duration of
Resins, bile acid binding, 2.137–2.138
Resistance
in coronary flow, 1.102, 1.103–1.105, 6.2f
autoregulatory, 1.102, 1.103–1.104, 6.2f, 6.4f
control of, 1.105–1.106
transmural variations in, 1.102, 1.104, 6.2f
calculation of, 1.104–1.105
compressive, 1.102, 1.103, 1.104, 6.2f, 6.3f
pulmonary vascular, 10.70–10.71
calculation of, 5.5–5.6
Respiration, observation of, 3.55
Respiratory distress syndrome, adult, 1.144–1.145, 1.147, 1.151–1.153, 9.7f
after cardiopulmonary bypass, 13.55–13.56
clinical features of, 1.151–1.152, 9.2t
etiology of, 1.151
hemodynamic monitoring in, 5.85, 5.88, 39.2t

management of, 1.152–1.153
mechanisms and pathology in, 1.151
pathologic changes in, 1.146–1.147, 9.6f
roentgenography in, 1.151, 9.10f
Rest
in bed. See Bed rest
in viral myocarditis, 10.89–10.90
Restrictive cardiomyopathy, 10.107–10.117
Revascularization procedures. See Bypass surgery, coronary
Rhabdomyoma, cardiac, 12.51
Rheumatic fever, 10.98–10.106
age and sex factors in, 10.98
arteritis in, 12.35
Aschoff nodules in, 10.99
carditis in, differential diagnosis of, 10.89
chorea in, 10.101–10.102
management of, 10.105
clinical features of, 10.100–10.102
diagnosis of, 10.103
endocarditis in, 10.99
etiology and pathogenesis of, 10.99–10.100
extracardiac lesions in, 10.99
genetic factors and ethnicity in, 10.98
heart failure in, 10.101
control of, 10.104
immune mechanisms in, 10.100
incidence of, 10.98
Jones criteria for diagnosis of, 10.103, 96.1t
laboratory data in, 10.102
myocarditis in, 10.99
pathology of, 10.98–10.99
pericarditis in, 10.99, 10.101
post-therapeutic rebounds in, 10.104
prevention of, 10.105–10.106
and residual heart disease, 10.105. See also Rheumatic heart disease
seasonal variations in, 10.98
socioeconomic factors in, 10.98
in streptococcal infections, 10.98, 10.99–10.100
tests for antibodies in, 10.102
treatment of, 10.103
treatment of, 10.103–10.105
vasculitis in, 10.99
Rheumatic heart disease
aortic valvular stenosis in, 9.59, 9.106, 9.107, 88.2f
differential diagnosis of, 10.13
mitral regurgitation in, 9.11, 9.16
echocardiography of, 4.70–4.71, 28.92f–28.94f
mitral stenosis in, 9.116
pericarditis in, 10.59–10.60, 10.99, 10.101
tricuspid valve in, 9.93, 87.5f
Rheumatoid arthritis, 13.2–13.5
arteritis in, 12.35
cardiovascular disorders in, 3.14
conduction system disorders in, 13.5
coronary artery disease in, 13.5

endocardial and valvular involvement in, 13.4–13.5
myocardial involvement in, 13.4
nodular granuloma in, 13.3, 110.1f
pericarditis in, 10.60, 13.3–13.4
Rhonchus, 3.56, 3.57, 24.1t
Rickettsial infections, myocarditis in, 10.93–10.94
Rifampin, interactions with other drugs
β-adrenergic blocking drugs, 2.177, 21.4t
antiarrhythmic drugs, 2.175, 21.2t
anticoagulants, 2.153, 20.2t
digoxin, 2.172, 21.1t
theophylline, 2.186, 21.9t
warfarin, 2.187, 21.11t
Risk factors for coronary heart disease, 7.3–7.23, 7.38, 60.2t
RNA synthesis in myocardial hypertrophy, 1.73, 1.74, 4.9f
Rocky Mountain spotted fever, myocarditis in, 10.94
Roth spots in endocarditis, 3.12, 9.78
Rub
pericardial, 3.48–3.49
pleural, 3.57
Rubella syndrome, cardiovascular disorders in, 3.13, 23.1t
Rubidium-82 PET studies, in silent ischemia, 7.92, 7.93, 64.1f
Rubinstein-Taybi syndrome, cardiovascular disorders in, 3.13, 23.1t
Rumble, apical diastolic, in mitral stenosis, 9.120

S

St. Jude valves, 9.45, 84.2f
orifice areas in, 9.44, 84.1t
Salbutamol, 2.57
hemodynamic effects of, 2.53, 14.6t
Salicylates, interactions with warfarin, 2.187, 21.10t
Salmonellosis, myocarditis in, 10.93
Saphenous vein
bypass catheters, 5.30, 35.25f
grafts in coronary bypass surgery, 7.249–7.256
visualization with brachial approach, 5.32
Saralasin, and renal function, 8.4
Sarcoid heart disease, 10.116–10.117
biopsy in, 5.71, 38.5f
Sarcolemma of cardiac cells, 1.21, 6.2
calcium channels in, 1.68
Sarcoma, cardiac, 12.52
Sarcomeres, 1.20, 2.1f
Sarcoplasmic reticulum, 1.23, 1.24, 2.5f
calcium channels in, 1.68
Scalene maneuver in peripheral arterial disease, 12.36, 108.9f
Schistosomiasis, myocarditis in, 10.94
Scimitar syndrome, 3.65, 25.11f
Scintigraphy

gallium-67 citrate scans
    in endocarditis, 9.82
    in viral myocarditis, 10.88
gated techniques
    in atrial myxomas, 12.48
    in dilated cardiomyopathy, 10.9
    in myocardial contusion, 12.19
    in pulmonary embolism, 10.79–10.80, 94.5f
    in pulmonary heart disease, 10.74
technetium-99m pyrophosphate scans
    in measurement of infarct size, 7.135, 7.136–7.137, 67.2f–67.5f
    in myocardial contusion, 12.19
    in viral myocarditis, 10.88
thallium-201 scans
    in angina pectoris, 7.68
    in estimation of infarct size, 7.138, 67.8f
    in ischemic heart disease, 7.54–7.56, 61.2f
    in postinfarction prognosis, 7.224
    preoperative, 13.43
    in scleroderma, 13.13, 13.14, 110.4f
    in silent ischemia, 7.92
    stress imaging
        in coronary artery disease, 7.55, 61.2f
        in mitral valve prolapse, 9.35
        postinfarction, 7.223–7.224
Scleroderma, 10.116, 13.12–13.15
    cor pulmonale, 13.14
    coronary perfusion disorders in, 13.13–13.14, 110.4f
    hypertensive-renal crisis of, 8.31
    management of, 13.14
    myocardial disease in, 13.13
    pericarditis in, 10.60, 13.13
Sclerosing syndrome, 13.12–13.16
    mixed connective tissue disease, 13.15–13.16
    polymyositis-dermatomyositis complex, 13.15
    scleroderma, 13.12–13.15
Scratchy heart sounds, 3.49
Scrub typhus, myocarditis in, 10.94
Sedimentation rate, erythrocyte, in rheumatic fever, 10.102
Senning operation in cyanotic heart disease, 11.38
    and postoperative echocardiography, 11.92–11.94, 105.9f
    venous obstruction after, 11.61
Septal defects. See Atrial septal defect; Ventricular septal defect
Septal perforator artery compression in hypertrophic cardiomyopathy, 10.30
Serotonin
    and norepinephrine release, 1.118, 7.4f
    receptor activation in Raynaud's disease, 1.125
    receptor antagonists in myocardial infarction, 7.117, 7.118
    release from platelets, 2.143–2.144
Sexual activity
    in angina pectoris, 7.69–7.70

after bypass surgery, 7.259
postinfarction, 7.210–7.211
Shock
    α-adrenergic blocking drugs in, 2.94
    hypovolemic, hemodynamic monitoring in, 5.84, 5.85, 39.2t
    in myocardial infarction, 7.188–7.200, 70.7t
        with pulmonary congestion or edema, 7.188–7.199
        without pulmonary congestion or edema, 7.199–7.200
    septic
        hemodynamic monitoring in, 5.85, 5.88, 39.2t
        inotropic drugs in, 2.67
Shingles after transplantation of heart, 13.99
Shunt lesions
    echocardiography in, 11.88–11.92
    left-to-right, 3.63–3.66
        in atrial septal defect, 3.63–3.65, 11.43–11.45
        in ductus arteriosus patency, 3.66
        in partial anomalous pulmonary venous connection, 3.65
        in pregnancy, 13.25
        in ventricular septal defect, 3.66, 25.12f
    right-to-left
        in atrial septal defect, 11.45
        in Eisenmenger syndrome, 11.81
        in pregnancy, 13.25
Shy-Drager syndrome, 3.11
Sick sinus syndrome, 6.100–6.110
    atrial fibrillation or flutter in, 6.100, 6.101, 47.2f
    bradytachy syndrome with, 6.100, 6.101, 47.1f
    etiology of, 6.100, 6.101, 47.1t
    in elderly patients, 13.37
    noninvasive tests in, 6.102–6.109
    pathophysiology of, 6.101–6.102
    therapy in, 6.109–6.110
Simpson's rule to calculate ventricular volume, 4.41, 4.43, 28.2t, 28.21f–28.23f
Sinoatrial node, 1.12, 1.13, 1.13f
    action potential in, 6.4, 6.5, 40.4f
    antiarrhythmic drugs affecting, 6.34, 6.35, 42.1f
    conduction time in, 6.104–6.105
    disorders of, 6.100–6.110. See also Sick sinus syndrome
    from β-adrenergic blocking drugs, 2.101
    electrogam recordings, 6.106–6.107, 47.6f–47.8f
    function tests, 6.102–6.109, 47.2t
        carotid sinus stimulation in, 6.102, 6.103, 47.2t
        electrophysiologic studies in, 6.57, 6.106, 6.103–6.109, 44.4f, 47.2t, 47.3f–47.10f
        exercise testing in, 6.102, 6.103, 47.2t
        Holter monitoring in, 6.102–6.103, 47.2t

pharmacologic agents in, 6.102, 6.103, 47.2t
recovery time assessment, 6.104, 47.3f
    after autonomic blockade, 6.105–6.106, 47.4f–47.5f
refractoriness assessment, 6.107
Sinus node. See Sinoatrial node
Sinus tachycardia, 6.128–6.129
Sinus venarum cavarum, 1.6
Sinus venosus defects, 3.64, 11.43, 11.44, 101.1f
Size of heart, evaluation in chest films, 4.3
Skeletal muscle, compared to cardiac muscle, 1.28–1.29, 2.2t, 2.11f
Skin
    anatomy of, 1.119
    blood flow in, 1.119–1.121, 7.5f
    in endocarditis, 9.78
    infections after transplantation of heart, 13.98
    necrosis of, coumarin-induced, 2.154
    pigmentation
        in cyanosis, 3.7, 3.12
        disorders with, 3.12
    thermoregulation, 1.119–1.121
Sleep disorders in dilated cardiomyopathy, 10.6
Smoking
    and angina pectoris, 7.69
    and coronary heart disease risk, 7.6, 7.10t, 59.3t
    recent changes by Americans, 7.28, 59.8f
    and vein graft patency, 7.256
Snakebite, myocarditis from, 10.95
Socioeconomic factors in rheumatic fever incidence, 10.98
Sodium
    cardiac concentrations of, 6.2, 40.1t
    channels across sarcolemma, 6.2, 6.3, 6.17, 40.1f, 41.4f
        blocking drugs, 6.3, 6.4, 6.35–6.39
        heart rate affecting action of, 6.79
    and electrical excitation of myocardial fibers, 1.24
    exchange with calcium, 1.68–1.70, 4.3f
    excretion of
        in aldosteronism, 8.39
        in hypertension, 8.19
    intake of
        and hypertension pathogenesis, 8.3
        and responses to angiotensin II, 8.4–8.7, 76.4f–76.7f
    restriction in heart failure, 1.161
    Na/K pump, 6.2
    renal handling of, 2.19–2.21, 13.1f–13.2f
Sones catheter, in brachial cutdown approach in angiography, 5.32, 35.29f
Sonography. See Echocardiography
Sotalol, 6.49
    antiarrhythmic spectrum of, 6.49
    dosage of, 6.49
    electrophysiologic effects of, 6.49
    pharmacokinetics of, 6.49
    pharmacology of, 2.96, 2.97, 16.2t, 16.3t

in postinfarction prophylaxis, 7.233, 72.9t
  side effects of, 6.49
Souffle, mammary, 3.48
Space flight, responses to, 1.140–1.141
Spasm
  coronary artery. See Coronary arteries, spasm
  esophageal
    nitrates in, 2.84
    provocative testing in, 7.106
  vasospastic disorders. See Vasospastic disorders
Spirochetal infections, myocarditis in, 10.93
Spironolactone, 2.27, 13.1t
  interaction with digoxin, 2.172, 21.1t
Splanchnic circulation, nitrates affecting, 2.78
Spondylitis, ankylosing, 13.6
Spondyloarthropathy, seronegative, 13.5–13.6
Squatting, heart sounds and murmurs in, 3.40, 3.49, 23.11t
ST segment in electrocardiography, 4.18
  changes in, evaluation with Holter monitoring, 6.97–6.98
  in ischemic heart disease, 7.51
  in postinfarction exercise testing, 7.218–7.219, 7.220, 7.221, 71.1f–71.2f
Standing, abrupt, heart sounds and murmurs in, 3.40, 3.49, 23.11t
Staphylococcal endocarditis, 9.86
Starling equation, 1.144, 9.1f
  relation to pulmonary edema, 1.144, 9.2f
Starr-Edwards valves, 9.45, 84.2f
  orifice areas in, 9.44, 84.1t
Stenosis
  aortic. See Aorta, stenosis
  idiopathic hypertrophic subaortic. See Cardiomyopathy, hypertrophic
  valvular. See specific valves
Stenting of arterial lesions, 7.245–7.246, 73.11f
Sternal infections, postoperative, in transplantation of heart, 13.98
Steroids, anabolic
  interaction with anticoagulants, 2.153, 2.187, 20.2t, 21.10t
  toxic effects of, 13.79
Stiffness, ventricular, 5.62
Still's murmur, 3.41
Stings from scorpions, wasps and spiders, myocarditis from, 10.95
Stokes-Adams syndrome, syncope in, 3.8
Streptococcal infections
  endocarditis in, 9.86
  myocarditis in, 10.93
  rheumatic fever in, 10.98, 10.99–10.100
  tests for antibodies in, 10.102
  vaccines in, 10.106
Streptokinase, 2.154–2.155
  actions of, 2.154–2.155, 7.164, 69.1f
  complications from, 2.155

intracoronary administration of, 2.155
in myocardial infarction, 7.153, 7.164–7.167, 69.2f, 69.2t
  aspirin with, 7.153, 7.166
  bypass surgery after, 7.264–7.265
  percutaneous transluminal coronary angioplasty with, 7.170–7.171
in unstable angina, 7.80, 7.85, 63.3t
Stress, emotional, 13.67–13.72
Stress-strain relations, left ventricular, 5.64–5.65
Stroke work index, 5.11, 34.13f
Substance abuse. See Drug abuse
Succinylcholine, interaction with antiarrhythmic drugs, 2.176, 21.3t
Sulfinpyrazone
  interaction with anticoagulants, 2.153, 20.2t
  interaction with theophylline, 2.186, 21.9t
  as platelet inhibitor, 2.149
  warfarin with, in thrombosis prevention with prosthetic valves, 2.165
Sulfonamides, interaction with anticoagulants, 2.153, 2.187, 20.2t, 21.10t
Sulfonylurea compounds in diabetes, 13.84
Sulmazole, 2.65
Superoxide dismutase therapy in myocardial infarction, 7.157, 7.174
Supersensitivity, denervation, 1.53–1.54
Surfactant, pulmonary, 1.145
Surgery
  cardiac
    in aortic insufficiency, chronic, 9.25–9.27
    in aortic valvular stenosis, 9.113
    arrhythmias after, 13.64–13.65
    in atrial septal defect
      indications for, 11.49–11.50
      with pulmonary vascular disease, 11.84
    in bundle branch block, 6.123
    causes of respiratory dysfunction in, 13.54, 114.1t
    in cyanotic congenital heart disease, 11.37–11.41
    effects of anesthesia in, 13.52–13.53, 114.1f–114.3f
    in endocarditis, 9.86–9.87, 87.7t
    hemodynamic monitoring in, 13.58–13.61, 114.7f
    hypertension after, 8.43, 13.58–13.59
    in hypertrophic cardiomyopathy, 10.33, 10.34, 91.8f
    hypotension and low output syndrome after, 13.59, 13.60, 114.3t
      diagnosis of causes, 13.64, 114.4t
      management of, 13.61–13.63, 114.8f
    long-term outcome of, 11.3–11.11

in mitral insufficiency, chronic, 9.17–9.18
in mitral stenosis, 9.123–9.124
in myxomas, 12.51
pericarditis after, 10.61–10.62
pneumothorax after, 13.64
prosthetic valve replacement, 9.40–9.51
pulmonary embolism after, 13.63–13.64
respiratory management after, 13.52–13.58
  in chronic lung disease, 13.56–13.58, 114.6f
  in diaphragm dysfunction, 13.58
  extubation procedures in, 13.54–13.55
  and postoperative gas exchange in mechanical ventilation and spontaneous breathing, 13.54, 13.55, 114.2t
  in pulmonary edema, 13.55–13.56
  in uncomplicated surgery, 13.54–13.55
in tamponade, 10.48
tamponade after, 13.60–13.61
in tricuspid valve disease, 9.103
in ventricular septal defect, 11.59
noncardiac, 13.41–13.50
  in angina, 13.42–13.44
  antithrombotic therapy in, 2.165
  in arrhythmias, 13.45
  complications from, 13.49–13.50
  in coronary artery disease, 13.41–13.44
  in elderly patients, 13.38
  in heart failure, 13.45–13.46
  in hypertension, 13.44–13.45, 13.49
  intraoperative monitoring in, 13.49
  postinfarction, 13.42
  preoperative evaluation in, 13.41
  risk assessment in, 13.47–13.49, 113.1t–113.2t
  and stress from anesthesia and surgery, 13.47
  in valvular heart disease, 13.46
vascular
  angioplasty, percutaneous transluminal, 7.237–7.245
  in aortic dissection, 12.33
  in asymptomatic coronary artery disease, 7.97
  atherectomy, percutaneous, 7.245, 73.10f
  in coarctation of aorta, 11.74–11.75, 103.11f
  coronary bypass procedures, 7.249–7.259. See also Bypass surgery, coronary
  embolectomy, pulmonary, 10.82
  laser angioplasty, 7.246, 73.12f
  in postinfarction shock, 7.195, 7.268, 70.12t
  stenting of arterial lesions, 7.245–7.246, 73.11f
  in unstable angina, 7.87–7.88, 63.9f
  in variant angina, 7.110
Sutter valves, 9.45, 84.2f
  orifice areas in, 9.44, 84.1t
Suzman's sign, 3.48

Sympathetic dystrophy, reflex, 12.41, 12.43
Sympathetic nervous system
  and cardiac performance, 1.98
  in exercise, 1.136
  in modulation of nitrate activity, 2.77
Sympathomimetic drugs
  abuse of, 13.74–13.78
  bromocriptine, 2.59
  butopamine, 2.58
  clinical applications of, 2.52–2.59, 2.66–2.68
  L-dopa, 2.58–2.59
  dobutamine, 2.55–2.57, 14.8f
  dopamine, 2.54–2.55, 14.7f
  dopexamine, 2.59
  ephedrine, 2.57
  epinephrine, 2.52–2.53
  fenoldopam, 2.59
  hemodynamic effects of, 2.53, 14.6t
  ibopamine, 2.59
  interactions with other drugs, 2.183, 2.184, 21.8t
    antihypertensive drugs, 2.184, 21.8t
  isoproterenol 2.53–2.54
  mephentermine, 2.57
  metaraminol, 2.57
  norepinephrine, 2.52
  phenylephrine, 2.57
  pirbuterol, 2.57
  prenalterol, 2.57–2.58
  propylbutyl dopamine, 2.59
  salbutamol, 2.57
  TA—064, 2.58
  xamoterol, 2.58
Syncope
  in aortic valvular stenosis, 9.109
  in dilated cardiomyopathy, 10.6
  evaluation of, 3.8–3.9
  in orthostatic hypotension, 1.163
Syphilis, cardiovascular, 3.11
  aortitis in, 12.34
  myocarditis in, 10.93
Systole
  anterior motion of mitral leaflets in, 10.21–10.22
  atrial, 5.65
  dysfunction in aortic valvular stenosis, 9.108
  hypertension in elderly persons, 8.53–8.54
  MAP recording in, 6.70
  murmurs in, 3.38, 3.39–3.45, 23.11f
  myocardial infarction affecting, 7.122–7.123
  time intervals in aortic insufficiency, chronic, 9.23
  ventricular function disturbances in myocardial infarction, 7.180–7.181, 70.2f

T

T system in cardiac contraction, 1.21, 1.24, 2.5f
T wave in electrocardiography, 4.18
  abnormalities in, 4.28–4.29, 27.1t
  in ischemic heart disease, 7.51
TA-064, 2.58
  hemodynamic effects of, 2.53, 14.6t
Tachycardia
  atrial
    ectopic, 6.129
    multifocal, 6.129
      calcium channel blockers in, 2.117
  atrioventricular junctional, 6.132–6.135, 49.2f–49.5f
    ectopic, 6.134–6.135, 49.4f–49.5f
    electrocardiography in, 6.132
    electrophysiologic findings in, 6.133, 6.134, 49.3f
    mechanisms in, 6.132, 6.133, 49.2f
    nonparoxysmal, 6.134
    paroxysmal, 6.133–6.134
    reciprocating, permanent form of, 6.139
    treatment of, 6.133–6.134
  coronary blood flow in, 1.105, 1.112, 6.5f
  sinus, 6.128–6.129
    β-adrenergic blocking drugs in, 2.99
    in myocardial infarction, 7.151
  supraventricular, 6.128–6.137
    ablative therapy in, 6.63–6.64
    clinical features of, 6.128
    coronary blood flow in, 6.128
    electrocardiography in, 6.128, 6.129, 49.1f
    electrophysiologic studies in, 6.58–6.60, 6.62, 44.10f
    hemodynamic effects of, 6.128
    in myocardial infarction, 7.151
    pacing therapy in, 6.63
    paroxysmal
      β-adrenergic blocking drugs in, 2.99
      calcium channel blockers in, 2.117
    treatment of, 6.138
  in tachy-brady syndrome, 6.100, 6.101, 47.1f
  ventricular
    ablative therapy in, 6.63–6.64
    β-adrenergic blocking drugs in, 2.100
    calcium channel blockers in, 2.117–2.118
    drug-induced, 6.35, 6.36, 42.2f–42.3f
    in elderly patients, 13.37
    electrophysiologic studies in, 6.60–6.61, 6.63, 44.11f, 44.12f
    in hypertrophic cardiomyopathy, 10.30–10.31, 10.36
    MAP recordings in, 6.76–6.77, 45.14f
    in myocardial infarction, 7.148, 7.149–7.150
    pacing therapy in, 6.63
    polymorphous, 6.81–6.82, 45.21f
    wide QRS complex in, 6.58–6.62, 44.7f–44.10f
Takayasu's disease, 12.33–12.34, 13.11, 108.5f
Tamponade, cardiac, 10.44–10.48, 92.8f
  atypical, 10.45
  chamber collapse in, 10.47, 10.48, 92.11f
  compensatory responses in, 10.44, 10.45, 92.8f
  diagnosis of, 10.46–10.48
  echocardiography in, 4.90–4.94, 10.47, 28.137f–28.141f, 92.11f, 92.12f
  electrical alternans in, 10.47, 10.56, 92.13f
  electrocardiography in, 10.47, 92.13f
  etiology of, 92.5t
  low-pressure, 10.45
  management of, 10.48
  pathophysiology of, 10.44–10.45, 92.8f
  in penetrating cardiac injury, 12.15
  postoperative, in cardiac surgery, 13.60–13.61
  pulsus paradoxus in, 10.45–10.46, 92.9f–92.10f
    absence of, 10.46
  right-sided, 10.45
Taussig-Bing anomaly, 11.34
  management of, 11.39
Tawara node. 1.12
Technetium-99m pyrophosphate scans
  in measurement of infarct size, 7.135, 7.136–7.137, 67.2f–67.5f
  in myocardial contusion, 12.19
  in viral myocarditis, 10.88
Telephone transmission of ECG in variant angina, 7.103, 65.4f
Temperature
  affecting electrocardiography, 4.19
  and blood flow to skin, 1.120–1.121
Tendon of Todara, 1.7
Terazosin, 2.91
  adverse effects of, 2.94
  pharmacokinetics of, 2.92, 16.1t
Tetracycline, interaction with digoxin, 2.172, 21.1t
Tetralogy of Fallot, 3.59, 11.29, 11.36, 11.37, 100.3f, 100.9f
  β-adrenergic blocking drugs in, 2.101
  long-term outcome of surgery in, 11.7–11.8, 98.2f
  management of, 11.40
  postoperative echocardiography in, 11.93–11.95, 105.10f–105.11f
  in pregnancy, 13.25
  with pulmonary atresia and aortopulmonary collaterals, 3.59, 3.60, 25.2f
Tetralogy-like lesions
  diagnosis of, 11.34, 100.1t
  management of, 11.41
Tetrodotoxin, blocking sodium channels, 6.3, 6.4
Thallium-201 scans. *See* Scintigraphy, thallium-201 scans
Thebesian valve, 1.4f, 1.6
Thebesian veins, 1.15
Theophylline
  in chronic obstructive pulmonary disease, 13.57
  interactions with other drugs, 2.185–2.186, 21.9t

I.43

diuretics, 2.180, 21.6t
  intravenous, in sinus node dysfunction, 6.109
Therapeutic window for drugs, 2.4, 2.5, 12.6f
Thermodilution method in cardiac output determination, 5.5
Thermography, liquid crystal color, in venous thrombosis, detection, 10.79
Thermoregulation, and blood flow in skin, 1.119–1.121
Thiazide diuretics, 2.27, 13.1t
  in hypertension, in elderly patients, 13.32
  interaction with loop diuretics, 2.180, 21.6t
Thoracic outlet
  maneuvers in peripheral arterial disease, 12.36, 108.7f–108.9f
  syndrome of, chest pain in, 7.67
Throat cultures in rheumatic fever, 10.102
Thrombin
  inhibitors of, 2.149
  and platelet aggregation, 2.143–2.144
Thromboangiitis obliterans, 12.39, 108.8t
Thromboembolism
  in myocardial infarction, prevention of, 7.152–7.153
  from prosthetic heart valves, 9.47–9.48, 9.50
  renal, hypertension in, 8.36
Thrombolytic therapy, 2.154–2.156
  acylated plasminogen-streptokinase-activator complex in, 2.155–2.156
  in elderly patients, 13.30
  in myocardial infarction, 2.161, 7.118, 7.163–7.170, 69.1t–69.2t. See also Infarction, myocardial, thrombolytic therapy in
  and rethrombosis, 2.161
  streptokinase in, 2.154–2.155. See also Streptokinase
  tissue plasminogen activator in, 2.155. See also Plasminogen activators, tissue type (tPA)
  in unstable angina, 2.160–2.161, 7.80, 7.85, 63.3t
  urokinase, 2.156
Thromboplastin, commercial, variations in, 2.153, 20.3t
Thrombosis
  in acute coronary syndromes, 2.158
  antithrombotic therapy in, 2.143–2.166
  in cardiac chambers, 2.159
  in coronary arteries, 2.156–2.158
    and myocardial infarction, 7.112, 7.114–7.115
  in injuries, 12.22
  endogenous inhibitors of, 2.146–2.147, 20.3f
  left ventricular
    echocardiography of, 4.46–4.47, 4.48, 4.49, 4.97, 28.33f–28.34f, 28.37f
  mural, in myocardial infarction, 7.127, 7.202
  noninfective thrombotic endocarditis, 10.65–10.66, 93.1f
  pathogenesis of, 2.156–2.159
  platelet activation and fibrin formation in, 2.143–2.147, 20.1f–20.3f
  and postangioplasty restenosis, 2.158
  in prosthetic heart valves, 2.159
  right atrial, 12.50, 109.7f
    echocardiography of, 4.97–4.98, 28.147f
  right ventricular, echocardiography of, 4.61
  vascular injury in, 2.156–2.158
  in vein graft disease, 2.158, 2.163
  venous
    detection of, 10.78–10.80
    in myocardial infarction, 7.202
    predisposing factors in, 10.77–10.78, 94.5t
    prevention of, 10.80–10.81
Thromboxane A_2
  affecting coronary vessels, 1.106
  interaction with prostacyclin, 7.116
  release from platelets, 2.143–2.144
Thromboxane synthetase, inhibitors of, 2.148
Thyroid disease, 13.84–13.86
  electrocardiography in, 4.31
  hypertension in, 8.41
  hyperthyroidism, 13.85. See also Hyperthyroidism
  hypothyroidism, 13.85–13.86. See also Hypothyroidism
  myxedematous pericardial disease, 10.62–10.63
Thyroid hormones, interaction with warfarin, 2.187, 21.10t
d-Thyroxine
  as hypolipidemia agent, 2.140
  interaction with anticoagulants, 2.153, 20.2t
Thyrotoxicosis, 13.85. See also Hyperthyroidism
Tiapamil, 2.106–2.107, 17.1t
Ticlopidine
  as platelet inhibitor, 2.149
  in unstable angina, 2.160
Tietze syndrome, 7.66
  chest pain in, 3.6
Timolol, 8.22, 77.7t
  pharmacology of, 2.96, 2.97, 7.71, 16.2t, 16.3t, 62.3t
  in postinfarction prophylaxis, 7.233, 72.9t
Tissue plasminogen activators. See Plasminogen activators, tissue-type (tPA)
Tocainide, 6.22, 6.45
  antiarrhythmic spectrum of, 6.45
  dosage of, 6.45
  effects on heart and circulation, 6.22
  effects on transmembrane potential, 6.22
  electrophysiologic properties of, 6.45
  interaction with other drugs, 2.177
  pharmacokinetics of, 6.45
  side effects of, 6.45
Todara tendon, 1.7
Toluene sniffing, toxic effects of, 13.79
Torsade de pointes, 6.35, 6.36, 6.81–6.82, 42.2f, 45.21f
Toxocariasis, myocarditis in, 10.94
Toxoplasmosis
  myocarditis in, 10.95
  pericarditis in, 10.59
  after transplantation of heart, 13.99
Training programs. See Exercise, training programs
Transplantation of heart, 13.92–13.105
  arrhythmias after, 13.98
  and atherosclerosis development, 13.100
  cardiac biopsy in, 5.71–5.72, 5.73, 38.7f–39.10f
  contraindications to, 13.93
  criteria for retransplantation in, 13.93
  donor selection in, 13.94
  and effects of drugs on transplanted heart, 13.97–13.98
  heart-lung, 13.102–13.105
    alternatives to, 13.105
    complications of, 13.103–13.104
    donor selection in, 13.103
    early postoperative care in, 13.103
    in Eisenmenger syndrome, 11.41
    immunosuppressive therapy in, 13.103
    long-term follow-up in, 13.104
    operative procedure in, 13.103
    pathologic findings after, 13.104
    physiologic assessment in, 13.104
    in pulmonary heart disease, 10.76
    rejection of, 13.103–13.104
    selection of recipients in, 13.102–13.103
    survival statistics, 3.105
  heterotopic, 13.93–13.94
    physiology of, 13.96
  history of, 13.92
  hypertension after, 8.43
  immunosuppressive therapy in, 13.95
    complications of, 13.100–13.101
  infections after, 13.98–13.99
  long-term follow-up in 13.101–13.102
  lymphoproliferative disease after, 13.99
  mechanical heart as bridge to, 13.93
  myocardial fibrosis in, 13.100
  operative procedure in, 13.94
  pathologic findings after, 13.99–13.100
  physiology of transplanted heart, 13.96
  psychiatric adjustment to, 13.101
  quality of life after, 13.102
  rejection of, 13.94–13.96, 13.100
    biopsy diagnosis of, 13.96
    clinical features of, 13.95
  selection of recipients, 13.92–13.94
    infection surveillance protocol in, 13.92, 118.1t
  survival statistics in, 13.102
  tumors after, 13.99
Transposition of great vessels, 11.28, 11.32, 11.33–11.34, l00.1f–100.2f, 100.7f

congenitally corrected, 3.67, 3.68, 11.34, 25.13f–25.14f
  management of, 11.38
long-term outcome of surgery in, 11.8–11.10, 98.3f–98.4f
management of, 11.38
in pregnancy, 13.25
Trauma, cardiovascular, 12.13–12.25
  in acutely injured patients, 12.14–12.15
  aortic, 12.22–12.24, 12.28, 12.29, 107.6f–107.7f, 108.1f
  aortic valve insufficiency in, 12.21
  arrhythmias in, 12.18, 107.1t
  atrial septal defect from, 12.20
  from cardiac catheterization, 5.39
  contusions of myocardium, 12.16, 12.20
  coronary artery, 12.22
  and foreign body retention, 12.24, 107.8f–107.9f
  iatrogenic, 12.24–12.25, 107.10f–107.11f
  intracardiac, 12.20–12.22
    fistulas in, 12.21–12.22
  lacerations, 12.16, 12.17, 107.1f–107.4f
  mitral valve insufficiency in, 12.21
  and occupational occlusive arterial disease, 12.37, 12.39, 108.9t
  pathologic classification of, 12.14
  penetrating, and pericardial tamponade, 12.15
  pericarditis from, 10.62, 12.16
  physical causes of, 12.13–12.14
  pulmonic valvular insufficiency in, 12.21
  respiratory distress from, 1.151, 9.10f
  and thrombus formation, 2.156–2.158
  of tricuspid valve, 9.94, 22.21, 87.6f
  valvular, 12.20–12.21
  ventricular septal defect from, 12.20
Tremors, essential, β-adrenergic blocking drugs in, 2.101
Triacetyloleandomycin, interactions with theophylline, 2.186, 21.9t
Triage procedures in myocardial infarction, 7.264, 75.1f
Triamterene, 2.27, 13.1t
Trichinosis, myocarditis in, 10.94
Tricuspid valve, 9.91–9.103
  acquired disease, 9.92–9.96
  anatomy of, 1.6f–1.7f, 1.7–1.8, 9.91, 9.92, 87.1f–87.3f
  annuloplasty of, 9.103
  atresia, 11.30, 11.36, 100.5f
    long-term outcome of surgery in, 11.10
    management of, 11.41
  in atrial myxomas, 9.96
  balloon valvuloplasty, 9.59
  in carcinoid syndrome, 9.96, 87.9f
  congenital abnormalities, 9.96–9.97
  Ebstein's anomaly, 3.60–3.61, 9.96, 11.36, 25.4f–25.5f
  echocardiography of, 4.81–4.84, 28.113f–28.115f
  endocarditis of, 9.93–9.94
  normal area of, 9.55, 85.2t
  normal physiology of, 9.91–9.92, 9.93, 87.4f
  prolapse of, 9.94–9.95, 87.7f–87.8f
    midsystolic click in, 3.36
  prosthetic replacement of, 9.41, 9.103
  regurgitation and insufficiency, 9.97–9.100
    acute, vasodilators in, 9.5
    angiography in, 9.99–9.100, 87.14f
    cardiac catheterization in, 5.17
    chest films in, 9.98
    clinical findings in, 9.97–9.98
    color-flow Doppler of, 4.86, 4.89, 28.125f, 28.131f
    Doppler flow studies in, 9.98–9.99, 87.12f–87.13f
    echocardiography in, 4.60, 4.63, 4.81–4.84, 9.98, 28.71f, 28.77f, 28.116f–28.120f
    electrocardiography in, 9.98
    functional, 9.92–9.93
    hemodynamic effects of, 9.99
    jugular venous pulse in, 9.97, 87.10f
    management of, 9.103
    murmurs in, 3.43, 9.97–9.98, 9.100, 87.11f, 87.15f
    phonocardiography in, intracardiac, 9.100, 87.15f
    in pregnancy, 13.24
    traumatic, 12.21
    in viral myocarditis, 10.86
  in rheumatic disease, 9.93, 87.5f
    differential diagnosis of, 12.50
  in right ventricular infarction, 9.93
  stenosis of, 9.100–9.103
    chest films in, 9.101
    clinical findings in, 9.100–9.101
    echocardiography of, 4.83, 4.84, 9.101, 28.117f
    electrocardiography in, 9.101
    hemodynamic effects of, 9.103
    jugular venous pulse in, 9.100, 9.101, 87.16f–87.17f
    management of, 9.103
    murmurs in, 3.46, 3.47, 9.101, 9.102, 87.19f
    opening snap in, 3.37
    in pregnancy, 13.24
    right atrial pressure pulse in, 9.101, 87.18f
    right ventricular inflow obstruction in, 11.61–11.62
  trauma of, 9.94, 87.6f
Tricyclic antidepressants, interactions with other drugs
  antihypertensive drugs, 2.184, 21.8t
  monoamine oxidase inhibitors, 2.184, 21.8t
  sympathomimetic drugs, 2.184, 21.8t
Triggered activity
  and afterdepolarizations, 6.7–6.9
  and arrhythmias, 6.16–6.17
Triglycerides
  hypertriglyceridemia, familial, 7.42, 7.44, 60.4t
  serum levels
    diagnosis of abnormalities in, 7.46
    heritable disorders in, 7.42, 7.43–7.45, 60.4t
    normal levels, 7.38–7.39
Trimazosin, 2.91
  pharmacokinetics of, 2.92, 16.1t
  vasodilating effects of, 2.128
Trimethoprim-sulfamethoxazole, interactions with warfarin, 2.187, 21.10t
Triple response, cutaneous, 1.121
Trisomy 13-15, cardiovascular disorders in, 3.13, 23.1t
Trisomy 18, cardiovascular disorders in, 3.13, 23.1t
Trisomy 21, cardiovascular disorders with, 3.11, 3.13, 23.1t
Tropomyosin, 1.21, 1.22, 2.2f
Troponin, 1.21, 1.22, 2.2f
Truncus arteriosus, 11.33, 11.35, 100.8f
  management of, 11.38, 11.39
Trypanosomiasis
  echocardiography in, 4.52, 4.53, 28.50f–28.51f
  myocarditis in, 10.94–10.95
Tuberculosis
  myocarditis in, 10.93
  pericarditis in, 10.58–10.59
Tubular system, transverse, 1.21, 1.24, 2.5f
Tumors
  adrenal, and Cushing's disease, 13.87
  of heart, 12.45–12.53, 109.1t
    angiosarcoma, 12.52, 109.9f
    benign, 12.45–12.52
    fibroelastomas, papillary, 12.52
    fibromas, 12.51–12.52, 109.8f
    left atrial, echocardiography of, 4.96–4.97, 28.145f–28.146f
    left ventricular, 4.48
    malignant, 12.51–12.53
    mesotheliomas, 12.52
    metastatic, 12.51–12.53, 109.10f–109.11f
    myxomas, 12.45–12.51
      left atrial, 4.96, 12.46–12.49, 28.145f
      right atrial, 12.49–12.50
      ventricular, 12.50
  pericardial, 10.63
    echocardiography in, 4.95–4.96
    restrictive cardiomyopathy in, 10.116
  rhabdomyoma, 12.51
  right atrial, 12.49–12.50
    echocardiography in, 4.97–4.98, 28.147f
  right ventricular, echocardiography of, 4.61
  pheochromocytoma, 13.86–13.87
  pituitary, growth hormone-secreting, 13.86
  after transplantation of heart, 13.99
Turner's syndrome, cardiovascular disorders in, 3.12
Typhus, scrub, myocarditis in, 10.94
Tyramine, interactions with monoamine oxidase inhibitors, 2.184, 21.8t

U

U wave in electrocardiography, 4.18
 abnormalities in, 4.29–4.30
UD-CG 115, inotropic effects of, 2.66
UD-CG 212, inotropic effects of, 2.65
Uhl's disease, 4.64
Ulcers
 ischemic, in occlusive peripheral arterial disease, 12.37, 12.39, 108.11f
 peptic, chest pain in, 7.67
Ultrasound. See Echocardiography
Urapadil, 2.91
Uremia, pericarditis in, 10.62
Uric acid levels in hypertension, 8.19
Urine studies in hypertension, 8.18, 8.19, 77.2t
Urokinase, 2.156
 in myocardial infarction, 7.167–7.168, 69.2t
 proenzyme of, 7.167–7.168
 single-chain plasminogen activator, 7.167–7.168

V

Vagus nerve, effects on cellular electrophysiology, 6.6
Valsalva maneuver
 heart sounds and murmurs in, 3.40, 3.49, 23.11t
 in mitral valve prolapse, 9.32
Valsalva sinus. See Aortic sinus
Valvular heart disease
 balloon valvuloplasty in, 9.54–9.72. See also Valvuloplasty, balloon
 cardiac catheterization in, 5.13–5.17
 echocardiography in, 4.65–4.86. See also Echocardiography in elderly patients, 13.33–13.34
 endocarditis
  infective, 9.73–9.89
  noninfective thrombotic, 10.65–10.66, 93.1f
 noncardiac surgery in, 13.46
 in pregnancy, 13.23–13.24
 prosthetic valve replacement in, 9.40–9.51. See also Prosthetic heart valves
 regurgitation or insufficiency
  acute, 9.2–9.8
   causes of, 9.3, 81.1t
   management of, 9.8
   pathophysiology of, 9.2–9.3
   vasodilators in, 9.3–9.8
  aortic, 9.18–9.27
  chronic, 9.8–9.28
  mitral, 9.11–9.18
  pathophysiology of, 9.8–9.9
  pulmonary, 9.27–9.28
  tricuspid, 9.97–9.100
 stenosis
  aortic, 3.62–3.63, 9.106–9.114, 25.7f
  mitral, 9.116–9.124
  pulmonary, 9.54
  tricuspid, 9.100–9.103
 in rheumatoid arthritis, 13.4–13.5
 traumatic, 12.20–12.21
 valve areas in, 9.55, 85.2t
 vegetations in. See Vegetations, valvular
 in viral myocarditis, 10.91
Valvuloplasty, balloon, 9.54–9.72
 aortic, 9.59–9.67, 9.113, 11.71, 103.7f
  cardiac catheterization in, 5.13, 5.15, 34.18f
 dilatation catheters in, 9.56–9.57, 9.62, 85.2f, 85.4t, 85.5f
 dual-balloon area equivalents in, 9.62, 9.65, 85.5t
 mitral, 9.67–9.72, 9.124
 pulmonary, 9.54–9.59, 11.41, 11.64, 103.2f
 sheaths used in, 9.62, 9.63, 85.6f
 tricuspid, 9.59
Valvulotomy
 debridement, aortic, 9.60, 9.61, 85.4f
 mitral commissurotomy, 9.123
Vasculature
 cerebral. See Cerebrovascular disease
 constriction of
  β-adrenergic blocking drugs in, 2.94
  cerebral, calcium channel blockers in, 2.120
  cocaine-induced, 13.77
 coronary. See Coronary arteries
 dilation of
  in cold exposure, 1.121
  nitrate-induced, 2.76, 2.77, 15.2f
 endothelium of. See Endothelium
 injury of, and thrombus formation, 2.156–2.158
 peripheral arterial disease, 12.35-12.43
 pulmonary. See Pulmonary vessels
 regulatory mechanisms in exercise, 1.136–1.137
 renovascular hypertension, 8.31–8.36
 resistance in
  coronary, 1.102, 1.103–1.105, 6.2f
  pulmonary, 10.70–10.71
   calculation of, 5.5–5.6
  systemic, calculation of, 5.5–5.6
Vasculitis syndromes, 13.6–13.11, 110.3f
 coronary arteritis, 13.9–13.11
 in lupus erythematosus, 13.6–13.9
 in rheumatic fever, 10.99
Vasodilator reserve, reduced, in ischemic heart disease, 7.64
Vasodilator therapy, 9.6–9.8
 adverse effects of, 2.133
 in aortic regurgitation, 2.133
  acute, 9.5
  chronic, 9.9
 arteriolar agents, 2.124–2.125
  calcium channel blockers, 2.125, 2.126, 18.4f
  hydralazine, 2.124, 18.2f
  minoxidil, 2.124–2.125, 18.3f
 in dilated cardiomyopathy, 10.15
 effects on left ventricular compliance, 2.131
 effects on transplanted heart, 13.98
 in heart failure, 2.123–2.135
  in elderly patients, 13.36
  pathophysiologic basis of, 2.123–2.124, 18.1f
  selection of agents in, 2.134, 18.15f
 in hypertension, 8.23–8.24
 intravenous, hemodynamic monitoring in, 5.89, 39.4t
 in mitral regurgitation, 2.131–2.133, 18.13f–18.14f
  acute, 9.3–9.4, 81.1f
  chronic, 9.9
 with mixed effects on arteries and veins, 2.127–2.128
  nitroprusside, 2.128, 2.129, 18.8f
  phentolamine, 2.128
  prazosin, 2.127–2.128, 18.7f
  trimazosin, 2.128
 in myocardial infarction, 7.156
 in pulmonary hypertension, 10.76, 94.2t
 in postinfarction shock, 7.192–7.194, 70.10t
  catecholamines with, 7.194
 in pregnancy, 13.22, 111.3t
 in pulmonary edema, 1.150
 in pulmonic regurgitation, acute, 9.5
 in tricuspid regurgitation, acute, 9.5
 in valvular regurgitation, acute, 9.3–9.8
 venodilators, 2.125–2.127
 in ventricular septal rupture, 2.133
Vasospastic disorders, 12.41-12.43, 108.12t
 coronary. See Coronary arteries, spasm
 differential diagnosis of, 12.42, 108.13t
 Raynaud's disease, 1.124–1.126, 7.8f
 in scleroderma, 13.12
Vectorcardiography, 4.19
Vegetations, valvular
 aortic, echocardiography of, 4.75, 28.102f
 in endocarditis, 9.76–9.77, 86.1f–86.2f
  identification of, 9.82–9.83, 86.6f
 mitral, echocardiography of, 4.74, 28.99f
 in noninfective thrombotic endocarditis, 10.65, 93.1f
Vein graft disease after bypass surgery
 antithrombotic therapy in, 2.163
 thrombosis in, 2.158
Velocity-length relations in contraction of cardiac muscle, 1.34–1.35, 2.23f–2.24f
Vena cava, inferior, 1.6
 eustachian valve of, 1.4f, 1.6
 interruption of, in venous thrombosis, 10.81
 plethora of, 4.92–4.93
Venesection in polycythemia, 11.59
Venodilators, 2.125–2.127
 nitrates, 2.76–2.77, 2.125–2.127, 15.2f
Venous drainage
 pulmonary. See Pulmonary vessels, venous return

systemic
  anomalous, 11.36
    management of, 11.41
  postoperative obstruction to, 11.61
Venous hum, 3.48
Venous pressure
  central, 5.82
    and plethora of inferior vena cava,
      4.92–4.93
  pulmonary, increased, 10.72
Venous pulse, jugular, normal, 9.97, 87.10.
    See also Jugular venous pulse
Venous system
  coronary, 1.14, 1.15, 1.16, 1.16f–1.17f
  in limbs, 1.123–1.124, 7.7f
Ventilation, mechanical
  in adult respiratory distress syndrome,
    1.152
  and extubation procedures after
    surgery, 13.54–13.55
  postoperative gas exchange in, 13.54,
    13.55, 114.2t
  in pulmonary edema, 1.149
Ventricles
  activation of, 6.114
    in conduction defects, 6.114–6.115
  biventricular hypertrophy,
    electrocardiography in, 4.22
  diastolic function, 10.107–10.108, 97.1f
    assessment of, 5.55–5.65
  free wall rupture in myocardial
    infarction, 7.198
  surgery in, 7.272
  left, 1.6f, 1.7, 1.10, 1.11, 1.11f
    aneurysms of. See Aneurysms,
      ventricular
    in aortic valvular stenosis, 9.107–9.108
    apex impulse palpation, 3.23–3.25
    bypass surgery affecting, 7.253
    chest films of, 4.5, 4.7–4.8, 26.13f–26.14f
    compliance affected by vasodilators,
      2.131, 2.132, 18.12f
    contractile dysfunction in myocardial
      infarction, 7.180–7.181, 70.2f
    diameter reduction from nitrates, 2.77,
      15.3f
    diastolic dysfunction in myocardial
      infarction, 7.181–7.184,
      70.3f–70.5f
    diastolic filling in hypertrophic
      cardiomyopathy, 10.26–10.29,
      10.31, 91.5t
    in dilated cardiomyopathy, 10.12
    double-outlet, 11.34
      management of, 11.39
    dysfunction in ischemic heart disease,
      7.63
    dysfunction in myocardial infarction,
      prevention of, 7.157–7.158
    echocardiography of, 4.37–4.56,
      28.6f–28.11f
    ejection fraction, 1.91–1.92, 5.10f
      postinfarction, 7.225–7.226, 72.5t
    failure of. See Heart failure, left
      ventricular

  function curves, 1.89–1.91, 5.5f–5.9f
  function status as modulator of nitrate
    activity, 2.77–2.78
  gallop sounds, 3.34
  in hypertrophic cardiomyopathy,
    10.18–10.36
  hypertrophy
    β-adrenergic blocking drugs in, 2.101
    electrocardiography in, 4.20–4.21,
      27.8f
    mitral insufficiency in, 9.17
    reversal by antihypertensive agents,
      8.44–8.52
  indices of muscle performance,
    1.86–1.89
  indices of pump performance,
    1.89–1.98
  inflow tract pressure concept, 10.25-
    10.26, 91.8f
  mural thrombi in myocardial
    infarction, 7.127, 7.202
  myxomas of, 12.50
  outflow obstruction in aortic stenosis,
    11.68–11.73
    in coarctation of aorta, 11.73–11.75
    echocardiography in, 4.76–4.77
    in hypertrophic cardiomyopathy,
      10.21–10.24, 91.5f–91.7f
    murmur in, 3.39, 3.40. 23.11t
  oxygen consumption in, 1.101–1.102
    double product index of, 1.102
  passive filling of, 5.62–5.65, 37.7f
  performance determinants of, 1.85–1.86
  pressure-volume relations in, 1.85, 1.86,
    1.92–1.95, 5.1f, 5.11f–5.15f
    passive, 1.95–1.97, 5.17f–5.19f
  regional wall motion in, 1.95, 1.96, 5.16f
  relaxation rate in, 1.97
    in diastole, 10.26–10.28, 91.9f
  response to exercise, 1.132, 1.133, 8.3f
  stress affecting, 1.97–1.98, 5.20f
  stress-strain relations, 5.64–5.65
  thrombi of, echocardiography of, 4.97
  ventriculography of, 5.7, 34.7f
  myxomas of, 12.50
  postoperative function abnormalities,
    11.3
  pressures between, 11.53, 102.2f
  pump failure in myocardial infarction,
    7.180–7.184, 70.1f. See also
    Heart failure
  pump function after reversal of left
    ventricular hypertrophy,
    8.47–8.48, 79.2f–79.3f
  regional functional alterations in
    myocardial infarction,
    7.122–7.127
  right
    anatomy of, 1.5f, 1.6, 1.8
    anomalous muscle bundle in, 3.59
    chest films of, 4.4–4.5, 4.6, 26.5f–26.8f
    double-chambered, 3.59–3.60, 25.3f
    double-outlet, 11.34
      management of, 11.39
    dysplasia of, biopsy in, 5.78, 38.19f

    echocardiography of, 4.59–4.64
    failure of. See Heart failure, right
      ventricular
    gallop sounds, 3.34–3.35
    in hypertrophic cardiomyopathy, 10.31
    hypertrophy
      absence of pericardium with, 4.63,
        4.96
      electrocardiography in, 4.20,
        4.21–4.22, 27.7f
      infarction of, 7.154, 7.155, 7.189,
        7.199–7.200, 70.7t, 70.9f
      echocardiography of, 4.50, 4.60–4.61,
        28.44f, 28.72f
    inflow obstruction, 11.61–11.62
    infundibular stenosis, 11.62–11.63
    myxomas of, 12.50
    outflow obstruction, 11.62–11.64,
      103.1f
      in infundibular stenosis, 11.62–11.63
      muscle bundle in, 11.62
      in pulmonary artery branch stenosis,
        11.64
      in pulmonic valve stenosis,
        11.63–11.64
    oxygen consumption in, 1.101–1.102
    pressure studies in dilated
      cardiomyopathy, 10.10
    in pulmonary heart disease, 10.70
    systolic impulse palpation, 3.25
    volume changes affecting left
      ventricular diastolic function,
      5.63–5.64
  single, 3.62, 11.33, 11.35, 25.6f, 100.8f
    management of, 11.38, 11.39
  structure-function relationships, 1.19
Ventricular septal defect, 3.66, 11.51–11.60
  associated anomalies with, 11.53
  catheterization and angiocardiography
    in, 5.18, 11.57–11.58, 102.7f
  chest films in, 11.55
  clinical features of, 11.54–11.55
  color-flow Doppler of, 4.59, 28.68f
  congenital, 11.28, l00.1f
  echocardiography in, 11.57, 11.89–11.90,
    102.6f, 105.4f–105.5f
  electrocardiography in, 11.55, 102.3f
  hemodynamic monitoring in, 5.85,
    5.87–5.88, 39.2t, 39.5f
  in response to therapy, 5.89–5.90
  long-term outcome of surgery in,
    11.5–11.6
  management of, 11.59–11.60
  murmur in, 3.43–3.44
  pathological anatomy in, 11.51–11.53,
    102.1f
  pathophysiology of, 11.53–11.54,
    102.2f
  postinfarction, 7.189, 7.197–7.198, 70.7t,
    70.13t
    echocardiography of, 4.50, 28.44f
  surgery in, 7.269–7.272
  in pregnancy, 13.25
  pulmonary vascular disease in,
    11.81–11.82

I.47

clinical features of, 11.81–11.82
  management of, 11.82
subsets of, 3.59
traumatic, 12.20
vasodilators in, 2.133
Ventriculography, 5.6–5.8, 34.4f–34.6f
  augmentation, 5.7–5.8
  cardiac output determination in, 5.5
  digital, 5.45–5.47
  left ventricular, 5.7, 34.7f
    in ischemic heart disease, 7.60–7.61, 61.5f
  radionuclide
    in estimation of infarct size, 7.138–7.140, 67.10f
    in postinfarction exercise testing, 7.224–7.225, 72.4t
Ventriculomyectomy, in hypertrophic cardiomyopathy, 10.34
Ventriculopenic shock, in myocardial infarction, 7.188–7.195, 70.7t
Venturi effect, and systolic anterior motion of mitral leaflets, 10.21–10.22
Verapamil, 2.106–2.107, 6.25, 6.39, 17.1t
  adverse effects of, 2.121, 17.8t
  antiarrhythmic effects of, 6.14
  as arteriolar vasodilator, 2.125
  characteristics of, 7.72, 62.5t
  contraindications in digitalis toxicity, 2.49
  effects on heart and circulation, 6.25
  effects on transmembrane potential, 6.25
  effects on transplanted heart, 13.97
  in hypertension, 8.25
  interactions with other drugs, 2.179, 21.5t
    β-adrenergic blocking drugs, 2.177, 21.4t
    antiarrhythmic drugs, 2.176, 21.3t
    digoxin, 2.47, 2.172, 21.1t
  in myocardial infarction, 7.157
  pharmacokinetics of, 2.112, 17.3t
  in pregnancy, 13.22, 111.3t

protective effects of, 1.69, 1.70, 1.71, 4.1f, 4.4f
  in supraventricular tachycardia, 6.138
  systemic hemodynamic effects of, 2.109, 2.110, 17.4f
  in unstable angina, 7.84
  in variant angina, 2.113–2.114, 7.108–7.110, 17.7f
Video densitometry, 5.38, 5.45–5.47
Virus infections
  dilated cardiomyopathy in, 10.2–10.3
  myocarditis in, 10.84–10.92
  pericarditis in, 10.57–10.58
Viscosity of blood, and rate of flow, 1.114–1.115
Viscous resistance in coronary flow, 1.102, 1.103, 6.2f
Vitamin K, interaction with anticoagulants, 2.153, 2.187, 20.2t, 21.11t
Vitiligo, disorders with, 3.12
Voice sounds, auscultation of, 3.57
Von Willebrand factor, and platelet adhesions, 2.143

W

Wall-motion studies in silent ischemia, 7.92
Warfarin, 2.152–2.154
  chemical structure of, 2.148, 20.4f
  interactions with other drugs, 2.186–2.188, 21.10t–21.11t
    antiarrhythmic drugs, 2.176, 21.3t
    nonsteroidal anti-inflammatory drugs, 2.181, 21.7t
  in myocardial infarction, 2.164
  overlapping with heparin, 2.152
  postinfarction use of, 2.162
  in pregnancy, 2.166, 13.22, 111.3t
  in prevention of vein graft disease after bypass surgery, 2.163
  in prosthetic valve replacement, 9.47–9.48
  in thrombosis prevention with prosthetic valves, 2.164–2.165
  in venous thromboembolism, 10.81

Water, renal handling of, 2.19–2.21, 13.1f–13.2f
Waterston shunt, in cyanotic heart disease, 11.40
Wegener's granulomatosis, 13.11
Weight gain. *See* Obesity
Weight-loss regimens, drug abuse in, 13.79
Weightlessness, responses to, 1.140–1.141
Werner's syndrome, cardiovascular disorders in, 3.13, 23.1t
Wheezes, 3.56, 3.57, 24.1t
Williams syndrome, 11.64, 11.72, 103.8f
Wolff-Parkinson-White syndrome, 6.135–6.137
  arrhythmias with, 6.136–6.137, 49.7f–49.8f
  electrocardiography in, 4.24, 6.136, 27.10f, 49.1t
  electrophysiologic studies in, 6.137–6.138
  Holter monitoring in, 6.94
  noninvasive evaluation of, 6.137
  pathology of, 6.135–6.136, 49.6f
  treatment of, 6.138
  wide QRS tachycardia in, 6.58, 6.59, 6.62, 44.7f, 44.10f
Work
  and occupational occlusive arterial disease, 12.37, 12.39, 108.9t
  return to
    after bypass surgery, 7.259
    postinfarction, 7.210–7.211

X

Xamoterol, 2.58
  in dilated cardiomyopathy, 10.15–10.16
Xanthomas, disorders with, 3.14

Y

YM 151, 2.97
  pharmacodynamic properties of, 2.96, 16.2t
Yohimbine, 2.91
  adverse effects of, 2.94